Pharmacology & Physiology in Anesthetic Practice

FOURTH EDITION

ROBERT K. STOELTING, M.D.
Emeritus Professor and Chair, Department of Anesthesia
Indiana University School of Medicine
Indianapolis, Indiana

SIMON C. HILLIER, M.B., Ch.B., FRCA
Associate Professor
Department of Anesthesia
Indiana University School of Medicine
Indianapolis, Indiana

LIPPINCOTT WILLIAMS & WILKINS
A **Wolters Kluwer** Company
Philadelphia • Baltimore • New York • London
Buenos Aires • Hong Kong • Sydney • Tokyo

Acquisitions Editor: Brian Brown
Developmental Editor: Fran Murphy
Project Manager: Dave Murphy
Manufacturing Manager: Ben Rivera
Marketing Manager: Angela Panetta
Compositor: TechBooks
Printer: Courier

530 Walnut Street
Philadelphia, PA 19106 USA
LWW.com

Printed in the USA

Library of Congress Cataloging-in-Publication Data

Pharmacology & physiology in anesthetic practice / edited by Robert K. Stoelting, Simon Hillier. — 4th ed.
p. ; cm.
Rev. ed. of: Pharmacology and physiology in anesthetic practice / Robert K. Stoelting. 3rd ed. c1999.
Includes bibliographical references and indexes.
ISBN 0-7817-5469-0 (case)
1. Anesthesiology—Physiological effect—Handbooks, manuals, etc.
I. Stoelting, Robert K. II. Hillier, Simon. III. Stoelting, Robert K. Pharmacology and physiology in anesthetic practice. IV. Title: Pharmacology and physiology in anesthetic practice.
[DNLM: 1. Anesthetics—pharmacology. 2. Physiology. QV 81 P5362 2006]
RD82.2.S688 2006
615'.781—dc22

2005020012

Care has been taken to confirm the accuracy of the information presented and to describe generally accepted practices. However, the authors, editors, and publisher are not responsible for errors or omissions or for any consequences from application of the information in this book and make no warranty, expressed or implied, with respect to the currency, completeness, or accuracy of the contents of the publication. Application of this information in a particular situation remains the professional responsibility of the practitioner.

The authors, editors, and publisher have exerted every effort to ensure that drug selection and dosage set forth in this text are in accordance with current recommendations and practice at the time of publication. However, in view of ongoing research, changes in government regulations, and the constant flow of information relating to drug therapy and drug reactions, the reader is urged to check the package insert for each drug for any change in indications and dosage and for added warnings and precautions. This is particularly important when the recommended agent is a new or infrequently employed drug.

Some drugs and medical devices presented in this publication have Food and Drug Administration (FDA) clearance for limited use in restricted research settings. It is the responsibility of the health care provider to ascertain the FDA status of each drug or device planned for use in their clinical practice.

10 9 8 7 6 5 4 3 2 1

To purchase additional copies of this book, call our customer service department at (800) 638-3030 or fax orders to (301) 824-7390. International customers should call (301) 714-2324.

Visit Lippincott Williams & Wilkins on the Internet: http://www.LWW.com. Lippincott Williams & Wilkins customer service representatives are available from 8:30 am to 6:00 pm, EST.

Contents

Preface

This fourth edition of *Pharmacology and Physiology in Anesthetic Practice* is intended to meet the same goals as the first three editions—to provide students as well as practicing anesthesiologists with an in-depth but concise presentation of those aspects of pharmacology and physiology that are relevant either directly or indirectly to the perioperative anesthetic management of patients. For this fourth edition, Simon C. Hillier, M.B., Ch.B., FRCA, joins as a coauthor with special input in the physiology section as reflected by new chapters on thermoregulation and physiology of the newborn and elderly.

During the brief period since the last edition, the number of drugs available to anesthesiologists has continued to proliferate. The pharmacologic features of these drugs, as well as improved understanding of the uses and side effects of drugs available for many years, necessitates frequent revisions of a pharmacology textbook. Dr. Hillier has devoted his efforts to expanding and updating the physiology section.

It is the authors' goal to fill the voids created by new information and to update the information on drug behavior and organ function that has become available since the third edition. Although the discussions of drug classes and organ systems remain similar to the first three editions, the content of each chapter, as well as the figures, tables, and references, reflects the most recent information available.

Robert K. Stoelting, M.D.
Simon C. Hillier, M.B., Ch.B., FRCA

Acknowledgments

The authors wish to acknowledge the understanding and support of their wives and families during the long periods of time required for the preparation of this fourth edition of *Pharmacology and Physiology in Anesthetic Practice*. The preparation of several new computer-generated illustrations reflects the efforts of Dr. Hillier's son, Christopher. Our colleagues in the Department of Anesthesia, Indiana University School of Medicine were generous with their patience and encouragement, which helped facilitate the completion of the final product in a timely manner. Secretarial support for this and all the previous editions was provided by Deanna Walker. A special thank you and recognition from the authors is sincerely extended to the professionals at Lippincott, Williams & Wilkins, particularly Brian Brown, Senior Acquisitions Editor, and Fran Murphy, Development Editor, for making this edition both possible and a pleasant experience.

Robert K. Stoelting, M.D.
Indianapolis, Indiana

Simon C. Hillier, M.B., Ch.B., FRCA
Indianapolis, Indiana

Pharmacology

I

Pharmacokinetics and Pharmacodynamics of Injected and Inhaled Drugs

1

Pharmacokinetics is the quantitative study of the absorption, distribution, metabolism, and excretion of injected and inhaled drugs and their metabolites. Thus, pharmacokinetics may be viewed as what the body does to a drug. Combined with the dose of drug administered, pharmacokinetics determines the concentration of drug at its sites of action (receptors) and thus the intensity of the drug's effects with time. Pharmacokinetics may also determine variability in drug responses between patients, reflecting individual differences in absorption, distribution, and elimination (Wood, 1989). Selection and adjustment of drug dosage schedules and interpretation of measured plasma concentrations of drugs are facilitated by an understanding of pharmacokinetic principles.

Pharmacodynamics is the study of the intrinsic sensitivity or responsiveness of receptors to a drug and the mechanisms by which these effects occur. Thus, pharmacodynamics may be viewed as what the drug does to the body. Structure-activity relationships link the actions of drugs to their chemical structure and facilitate the design of drugs with more desirable pharmacologic properties. The intrinsic sensitivity of receptors is determined by measuring plasma concentrations of a drug required to evoke specific pharmacologic responses. The intrinsic sensitivity of receptors varies among patients. As a result, at similar plasma concentrations of a drug, some patients show a therapeutic response, others show no response, and in others, toxicity develops.

STEREOCHEMISTRY

Stereochemistry is the study of how molecules are structured in three dimensions (Egan, 1996; Nau and Strichartz, 2002). *Chirality* is a unique subset of stereochemistry, and the term *chiral* is used to designate a molecule that has a center (or centers) of three-dimensional asymmetry. This kind of molecular configuration is almost always a function of the unique, tetrahedral bonding characteristics of the carbon atom.

Chirality is the structural basis of *enantiomerism*. Enantiomers (substances of opposite shape) are a pair of molecules existing in two forms that are mirror images of one another (right- and left-hand) but cannot be superimposed. In every other aspect, enantiomers are chemically identical. A pair of enantiomers is distinguished by the direction in which, when dissolved in solution, they rotate polarized light, either clockwise (dextrorotatory, d [+]) or counterclockwise (levorotatory, l [−]). These observed signs of rotation, d(+) and l(−), are often confused with the designations D and L used in protein and carbohydrate chemistry. The characteristic of rotation of polarized light is the origin of the term *optical isomers*. When the two enantiomers are present in equal proportions (50:50), they are referred to as a *racemic mixture*. A racemic mixture does not rotate polarized light because the optical activity of each enantiomer is canceled by the other. The most applicable and unambiguous convention for designating isomers is the *sinister (S)* and *rectus (R)* classification that specifies the absolute configuration in the name of the compound (Nau and Strichartz, 2002). Molecular interactions that are the mechanistic foundation of pharmacokinetics and pharmacodynamics are stereoselective (relative difference between enantiomers) or stereospecific (absolute difference between enantiomers) (Fig. 1-1) (Nau and Strichartz, 2002). The "lock and key" hypothesis of enzyme-substrate activity emphasizes that biologic systems are inherently stereospecific. The pharmacologic extension

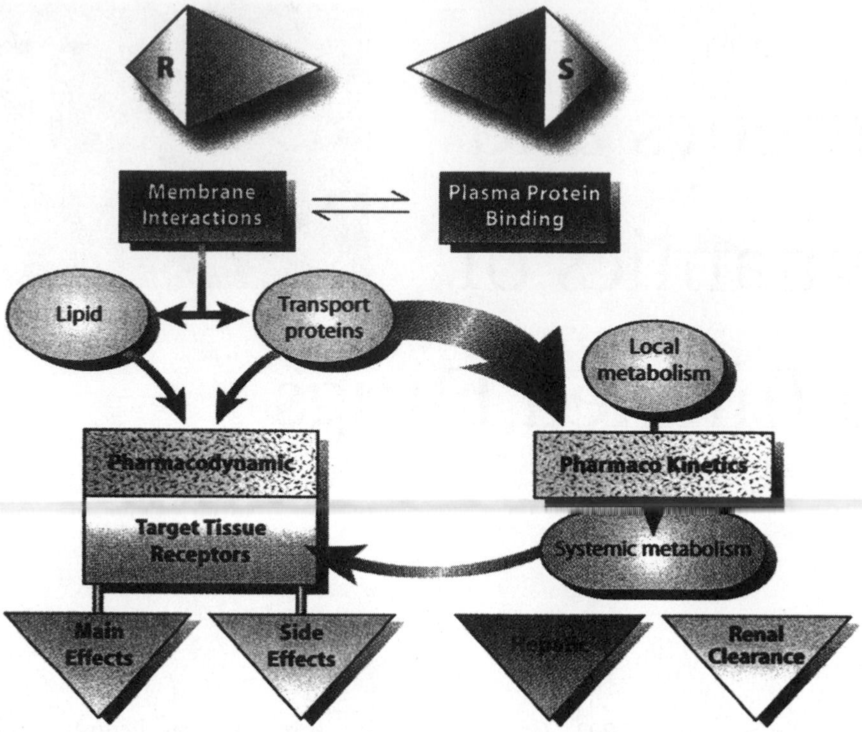

Figure 1-1. Potential sources for chiral contributions to anesthetic drug actions. Differences caused by pharmacokinetic and pharmacodynamic interactions may influence the disposition of drugs throughout the body and their actions at target tissues or receptors. (From Nau C, Strichartz GR. Drug chirality in anesthesia. *Anesthesiology* 2002;97:497–502; with permission.)

of this concept is that drugs can be expected to interact with other biologic components in a geometrically specific way (Egan, 1996). Pharmacologically, not all enantiomers are created equal. Drug-specific, drug-enzyme, and drug-protein binding interactions are virtually always three-dimensionally exacting. Enantiomers can exhibit differences in absorption, distribution, clearance, potency, and toxicity (drug interactions). Enantiomers can even antagonize the effects of one another.

The administration of a racemic drug mixture may in fact represent pharmacologically two different drugs with distinct pharmacokinetic and pharmacodynamic properties. The two enantiomers of the racemic mixture may have different rates of absorption, metabolism, and excretion as well as different affinities for receptor-binding sites. Although only one enantiomer is therapeutically active, it is possible that the other enantiomer contributes to side effects. The therapeutically inactive isomer in a racemic mixture should be regarded as an impurity (Ariens, 1984). A cogent theoretical argument is that studies on racemic mixtures may be scientifically flawed if the enantiomers have different pharmacokinetics or pharmacodynamics (Egan, 1996). An estimated one-third of drugs in clinical use are administered as racemic mixtures, but this practice is likely to decrease in the future although the clinical advantages of single enantiomers must be balanced against the increased costs of drugs (Nau and Strichartz, 2002). Enantiomer-specific drug studies are likely to become more common in the future. Regulatory agencies and pharmaceutical companies are increasingly aware of the importance of enantiomers in pharmacology and are likely to avoid the scientific ambiguities associated with the development of racemic drugs (Egan, 1996; Nation, 1994). Progress in chemical technology has greatly simplified the separation and the preparation of individual enantiomers.

Clinical Aspects of Chirality

More than one-third of all synthetic drugs are chiral although most of them are utilized clinically as racemic mixtures (Burke and Henderson, 2002; Nau and Strichartz, 2002) In addition to thiopental, methohexital and ketamine are administered as racemic mixtures. The majority of inhaled anesthetics are chiral with the notable exception of sevoflurane. Most evidence suggests that enantiomer-selective effects for volatile anesthetics are relatively weak in contrast to much stronger evidence for specific drug-receptor interactions for intravenous (IV) anesthetics (Burke and Henderson, 2002). Local anesthetics, including mepivacaine, prilocaine, and bupivacaine, have a center of molecular asymmetry. The S (+) enantiomer of ketamine is more potent than the R (−) form and is also less likely to produce emergence delirium. Similarly, in addition to pharmacokinetic differences, the cardiac toxicity of bupivacaine is thought to be predominantly due to the *R*-bupivacaine isomer. Ropivacaine is the S-enantiomer of a bupivacaine homolog which has decreased cardiac toxicity. Likewise, the S-enantiomer of bupivacaine, levobupivacaine is associated with less cardiac toxicity than bupivacaine. Cisatracurium is an isomer of atracurium that lacks histamine-releasing potential. Drugs used in anesthesia that occur naturally reflect the importance of stereochemistry, with morphine (actually *l*-morphine) and *d*-tubocurarine being examples. Because these drugs are synthesized by nature's stereospecific enzymatic machinery, they exist in a single form before they are extracted and purified (Egan, 1996).

DESCRIPTION OF DRUG RESPONSE

Hyperreactive is the term used for people in whom an unusually low dose of drug produces its expected pharmacologic effects. *Hypersensitive* is the term usually reserved for individuals who are allergic (sensitized) to a drug. *Hyporeactive* describes persons who require exceptionally large doses of drug to evoke expected pharmacologic effects. Hyporeactivity acquired from chronic exposure to a drug is better termed *tolerance*. Cross-tolerance develops between drugs of different classes that produce similar pharmacologic effects (alcohol and inhaled anesthetics). Tolerance that develops acutely within only a few doses of a drug, such as thiopental, is termed *tachyphylaxis*. The most important factor in the development of tolerance to drugs such as opioids, barbiturates, and alcohol is neuronal adaptation, referred to as *cellular tolerance*. Other mechanisms of tolerance may include enzyme induction and depletion of neurotransmitters caused by sustained stimulation. Immunity is present when hyporeactivity is due to formation of antibodies. Idiosyncrasy is present when an unusual effect of a drug occurs in a small percentage of individuals regardless of the dose of drug administered. More appropriately, unusual effects of drugs should be described precisely in terms of their documented or likely mechanisms, such as allergy or genetic differences.

An *additive effect* means that a second drug acting with the first drug will produce an effect equal to an algebraic summation. For example, the anesthetic effects of two different inhaled anesthetics are additive (see the section on Minimal Alveolar Concentration). *Synergistic effect* means that two drugs interact to produce an effect greater than an algebraic summation. Antagonism means that two drugs interact to produce an effect less than an algebraic summation.

A drug that activates a receptor by binding to that receptor is called an *agonist*. An *antagonist* is a drug that binds to the receptor without activating the receptor and at the same time prevents an agonist from stimulating the receptor. *Competitive antagonism* is present when increasing concentrations of the antagonist progressively inhibit the response to an unchanging concentration of agonist. *Noncompetitive antagonism* is present when, after administration of an antagonist, even high concentrations of agonist cannot completely overcome the antagonism.

PHARMACOLOGY OF INJECTED DRUGS

The pharmacokinetics of injected drugs usually is defined initially in healthy adults with a low fat-to-lean body ratio. Conversely, drugs are most likely to be administered to patients with chronic diseases (renal failure, cirrhosis of the liver, cardiac failure) at various extremes of age, hydration, and nutrition. General anesthesia and surgery may alter the pharmacokinetics of injected drugs relative to the awake state because of alterations in renal blood flow, hepatic blood flow, and hepatic enzyme activity. Drug-induced changes in peripheral blood flow may further alter perioperative distribution of injected anesthetics.

An understanding of the pharmacokinetics of injected drugs is the basis for choosing rational dosing intervals or continuous IV infusion rates of these drugs during anesthesia. As with all drugs, the pharmacologic response depends on the receptor concentration achieved and the sensitivity of these receptors to the drug. Measured or calculated pharmacokinetic parameters of injected drugs include bioavailability, clearance, and volume of distribution (Vd), elimination half-time, context-sensitive half-time, effect-site equilibration time, and recovery time (Hughes et al., 1992; Shafer and Stanski, 1992). Context-sensitive half-time and effect-site equilibration time are more useful than elimination half-time in characterizing the clinical responses to drugs (Fisher, 1996).

Compartmental Models

The pharmacokinetics of injected drugs has been simplified by considering the body to be composed of a number of compartments representing theoretical spaces with calculated volumes. A two-compartment model can be used to illustrate basic concepts of pharmacokinetics that also apply to more complex models (Fig. 1-2) (Stanski and Watkins, 1982). In the two-compartment model, the drug is introduced by IV injection directly into the central compartment. The drug subsequently distributes to the peripheral compartment only to return eventually to the central compartment, where clearance from the body occurs.

The central compartment includes intravascular fluid and highly perfused tissues (lungs, heart, brain, kidneys,

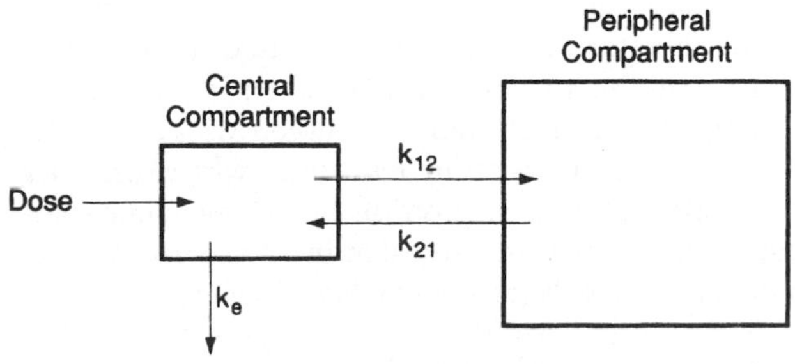

Figure 1-2. A two-compartment pharmacokinetic model as derived from a biexponential plasma decay curve (see Fig. 1-3). The rate constants that characterize intercompartmental transfer of drugs are k_{12} and k_{21}, and k_e is the rate constant for overall drug elimination from the body. (From Stanski DR, Watkins WD. *Drug disposition in anesthesia*. New York: Grune & Stratton, 1982; with permission.)

liver) into which uptake of the drug is rapid. In adults, these highly perfused tissues receive almost 75% of the cardiac output but represent about 10% of the body mass. This central compartment is defined only in terms of its apparent volume, which is calculated and does not necessarily correspond to actual anatomic volumes (see the section on Volume of Distribution). Likewise, the peripheral compartment (which consists of multiple compartments) is defined in terms of its calculated volume. A large calculated volume for the peripheral compartment suggests extensive uptake of drug by those tissues that constitute the peripheral compartment. The rate of drug transfer (rate constant, K) between compartments (intercompartmental clearance) may decrease with aging, resulting in higher plasma concentrations of drugs such as thiopental in elderly patients, despite identical injected doses and similar Vd in young adults and elderly patients (see Fig. 4-5) (Avram et al, 1990; Stanski and Maitre, 1990). Any residual drug present in the peripheral compartment at the time of repeat IV injection will diminish the effect of distributive processes on the reduction of the plasma concentration and lead to exaggerated (cumulative) effects of the repeat dose. The degree of cumulative drug effect can be calculated knowing the drug's dosing interval and elimination half-time.

Alternative Concepts in the Interpretation of Compartment Modeling

The strict application of traditional compartment modeling may be limited or even flawed, especially when applied to rapid IV injection of drugs that attain a maximum effect in <2 minutes (Fisher, 1996; Kisor et al., 1996). For example, the traditional application of compartmental models to pharmacokinetics assumes that a drug is eliminated only from the central compartment. Nevertheless, elimination of drugs by nonorgan clearance mechanisms will result in clearance from both central and peripheral compartments (Fisher, 1996). For instance, atracurium and cisatracurium are eliminated by pathways (Hoffman elimination, ester hydrolysis) that do not depend on the usual organs of clearance as depicted by the central compartment. Therefore, application of the traditional compartmental model to the pharmacokinetics of drugs that undergo nonorgan clearance is flawed (Kisor et al., 1996). Furthermore, elimination half-time, which provides a description of drug disposition in a single compartment model, may be of limited value in describing multicompartmental models (Shafer and Varvel, 1991).

Plasma Concentration Curves

A graphic plot of the logarithm of the decrease in the plasma concentration of a drug versus time after a rapid (bolus) IV injection characterizes the distribution (alpha) and elimination (beta) phase of that drug (Fig. 1-3) (Stanski and Watkins, 1982). Logarithms provide a convenient means for plotting the large range in plasma concentrations present after IV injection of a drug. In addition, logarithms are appropriate for depiction of the first-order kinetics characteristic of the distribution and elimination of most drugs.

The distribution phase of the plasma concentration curve begins immediately after IV injection of a drug and reflects that drug's distribution from the circulation (central compartment) to peripheral tissues (peripheral compartments) (see Figs. 1-2 and 1-3) (Stanski and Watkins, 1982). The elimination phase of the plasma concentration curve follows the initial distribution phase and is characterized by a more gradual decline in the drug's plasma concentration (see Fig. 1-3) (Stanski and Watkins, 1982). This gradual decline reflects the drug's elimination from the circulation (central compartment) by renal and hepatic clearance mechanisms.

Alternative Concepts in Interpretation of Plasma Drug Concentration

The traditional concept that a drug's pharmacologic effect parallels its plasma (presumably receptor) concentration is not always valid. For example, 1 minute after the bolus administration of cisatracurium, the plasma concentration is already decreasing, whereas the pharmacologic effect is increasing (Boyd et al., 1995). For this reason, it has been proposed that a drug's pharmacologic effect should not be related to its plasma concentration but rather to its concentration in a hypothetical peripheral compartment (an effect compartment) that is linked to plasma by a rate constant (Fisher, 1996). Effect compartment modeling provides insights into the time course of onset and offset of many drugs.

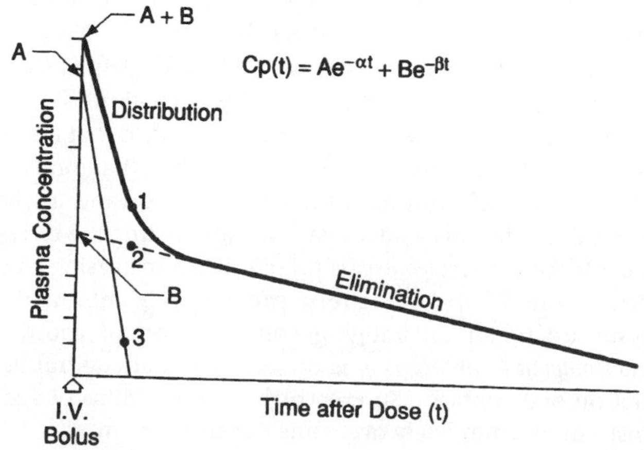

Figure 1-3. Schematic depiction of the decrease in plasma concentration of a drug with time after rapid intravenous injection into the central compartment (see Fig. 1-2). Two distinct phases (biexponential) that characterize this curve are designated the distribution (alpha) and elimination (beta) phases. (From Stanski DR, Watkins WD. *Drug disposition in anesthesia*. New York: Grune & Stratton, 1982; with permission.)

Elimination Half-Time

The rate of drug elimination is defined by the slope of the line representing the log plasma concentration of drug plotted against the time during the elimination phase. *Elimination half-time* is the time necessary for the plasma concentration of a drug to decrease to 50% during the elimination phase. Elimination half-time of a drug is directly proportional to its Vd and inversely proportional to its clearance. For this reason, renal or hepatic disease that alters Vd and/or clearance will alter the elimination half-time. Conversely, elimination half-time is independent of the dose of drug administered.

Elimination half-life, in contrast to elimination half-time, defines the time necessary to eliminate 50% of the drug from the body after its rapid IV injection. Elimination half-time and elimination half-life are not equal when the decrease in the drug's plasma concentration does not parallel its elimination from the body. The amount of drug remaining in the body is related to the number of elimination half-times that have elapsed (Table 1-1). For example, if 50% of a drug is eliminated in 10 minutes, another 10 minutes will be needed for elimination of one-half of the remaining drug. About five elimination half-times are required for nearly total (96.9%) elimination of drug from the body. For this reason, drug accumulation is predictable if dosing intervals are less than this period of time. Drug accumulation continues until the rate of its elimination equals the rate of its administration. As with drug elimination, the time necessary for a drug to achieve a steady-state plasma concentration (Cp_{ss}) with intermittent dosing is about five elimination half-times.

Alternative Concepts in Interpretation of the Elimination Half-Time

Elimination half-time is the descriptor used most often to characterize a drug's pharmacokinetic behavior. In a strictly mathematical construct, however, half-time is useful in the computation of central compartment drug concentration only in the one-compartment model (Hughes et al., 1992). Elimination half-time may be of little value in describing drug pharmacokinetics in multicompartmental models. Furthermore, of more importance to the clinician is how long it will take the plasma concentration to decrease to a level that allows the patient to awaken, rather than the slope of the plasma drug concentration–time curve (Fisher, 1996). It has been suggested that clinical conclusions based on elimination half-times of anesthetic drugs administered IV should be replaced by recovery times using computer simulations of specific clinical scenarios (Shafer and Stanski, 1992). Elimination half-times alone provide virtually no insight into the rate of decrease in the plasma concentration after discontinuation of a continuous IV drug infusion. Instead of focusing on elimination half-time, clinicians should consider the value of the concept of context-sensitive half-time (Hughes et al., 1992).

TABLE 1-1.
RELATIONSHIP OF HALF-TIMES TO AMOUNT OF DRUG ELIMINATED

Number of Half-Times	Fraction of Initial Amount Remaining	Percent of Initial Amount Eliminated
0	1	0
1	1/2	50
2	1/4	75
3	1/8	87.5
4	1/16	93.8
5	1/32	96.9
6	1/64	98.4

Context-Sensitive Half-Time

The concept of context-sensitive half-time was introduced to circumvent the limitations of the elimination half-time in describing postinfusion central compartment drug pharmacokinetics (Hughes et al., 1992). The effect of distribution on plasma drug concentrations varies in magnitude and direction over time and depends on the drug concentration gradients between various compartments. The context-sensitive half-time describes the time necessary for the plasma drug concentration to decrease by 50% (or any other percentage) after discontinuing a continuous infusion of a specific duration (*context* refers to infusion duration). Computer simulation of multicompartmental pharmacokinetic models of drug disposition has been used to calculate context-sensitive half-times for drugs administered as continuous infusions during anesthesia (Fig. 1-4) (Hughes et al., 1992).

Context-sensitive half-time, in contrast to elimination half-time, considers the combined effects of distribution

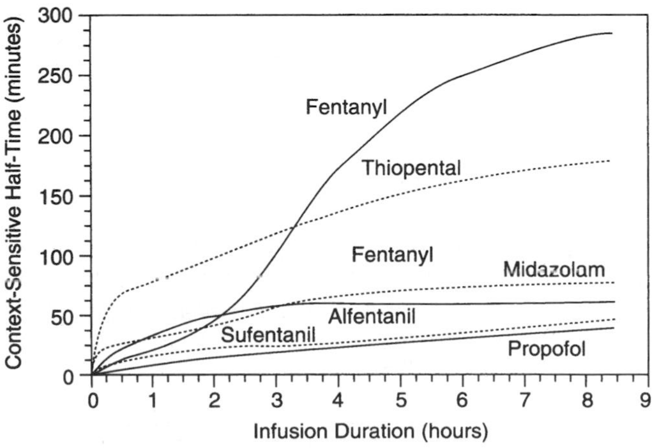

Figure 1-4. Context-sensitive half-times as a function of the duration of intravenous drug infusion for each of the computer-simulated pharmacokinetic models. (From Hughes MA, Glass PSA, Jacobs JR. Context-sensitive half-time in multicompartment pharmacokinetic models for intravenous anesthetic drugs. *Anesthesiology* 1992; 76:334–341; with permission.)

and metabolism as well as duration of continuous IV administration on drug pharmacokinetics. For example, depending largely on the lipid solubility of the drug and the efficiency of its clearance mechanisms, the context-sensitive half-time increases in parallel with the duration of continuous IV administration (see Fig. 1-4) (Hughes et al., 1992). The context-sensitive half-time bears no constant relationship to the drug's elimination half-time.

Time to Recovery

The time to recovery depends on how far the plasma concentration of drug must decrease to reach levels compatible with awakening (Fig. 1-5). For example, if the concentration of drug maintained by continuous infusion is only just above that required for awakening, the time to recovery will be more rapid than that after a continuous infusion that maintains the plasma drug concentration at a level much higher than associated with awakening (see Fig. 1-5). Thus, the difference between the plasma concentration at the time the continuous infusion of drug is discontinued and the plasma concentration below which awakening can be expected is an important factor in determining time to recovery. In this regard, the context-sensitive half-time does not directly describe how long it will take a patient to awaken. Furthermore, elimination half-time does not allow prediction of recovery after drug administration as this parameter only sets an upper limit on how much time will be required for a 50% decrease in plasma drug concentration (Shafer and Stanski, 1992).

Effect-Site Equilibration

The delay between the IV administration of a drug and the onset of its clinical effect reflects the time necessary for the circulation to deliver the drug to its site of action (tissues such as the brain). This delay reflects the fact that the plasma is not usually the site of drug action but rather the circulation is merely the route by which the drug reaches its effect site (biophase). If some parameter of drug effect can be measured (time to produce a specific effect on the electroencephalogram), the half-time of equilibration between drug concentration in the plasma and the drug effect can be measured. This time is characterized as the effect-site equilibration time.

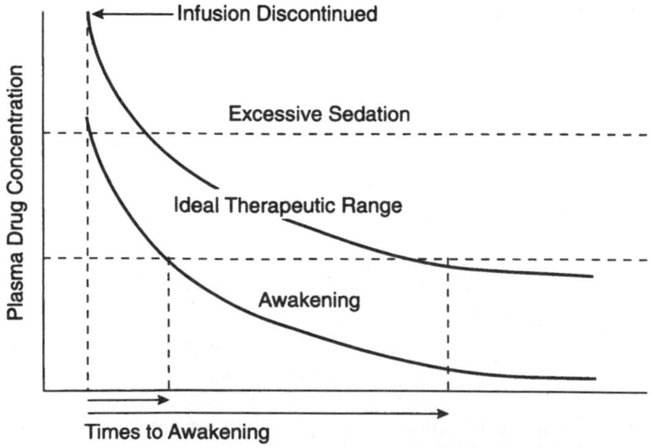

Figure 1-5. The time necessary for the plasma concentration of drug to decrease to a level associated with awakening depends on the plasma concentration present when the infusion of drug is discontinued.

Effect-site equilibration time is a particularly relevant concept in the logical timing of IV drug administration. Drugs with a short effect-site equilibration time (remifentanil, alfentanil, thiopental, propofol) will produce a more rapid onset of pharmacologic effect compared with drugs that have a longer effect-site equilibration time (fentanyl, sufentanil, midazolam). Knowledge of effect-site equilibration time is important in determining dosing intervals, especially when titrating IV drugs to a given clinical effect. For example, doses of midazolam should be spaced at sufficient intervals to permit the peak pharmacologic effect to be apparent clinically before further drug administration. Failure to appreciate the importance of effect-site equilibration time could result in unnecessary administration of drug. In addition to effect-site equilibration time, dosing intervals will also be influenced by redistribution to inactive tissue sites. This redistribution depends on tissue blood flow, which may be altered by cardiac output.

Route of Administration and Systemic Absorption of Drugs

The choice of route of administration for a drug should be determined by factors that influence the systemic absorption of drugs. The systemic absorption rate of a drug determines its intensity and duration of action. Changes in the systemic absorption rate may necessitate an adjustment in the dose or time interval between repeated drug doses.

Systemic absorption, regardless of the route of drug administration, depends on the drug's solubility. Local conditions at the site of absorption alter solubility, particularly in the gastrointestinal tract. Blood flow to the site of absorption is also important in the rapidity of absorption. For example, increased blood flow evoked by rubbing or applying heat at the injection site enhances systemic absorption, whereas decreased blood flow due to vasoconstriction impedes drug absorption. Finally, the area of the absorbing surface available for drug absorption is an important determinant of drug entry into the circulation.

Oral Administration

Oral administration of a drug is the most convenient and economic route of administration. Disadvantages of the oral route include (a) emesis caused by irritation of the gastrointestinal mucosa by the drug, (b) destruction of the drug by digestive enzymes or acidic gastric fluid, and (c) irregularities in absorption in the presence of food or other drugs. Furthermore, drugs may be metabolized by enzymes or bacteria in the gastrointestinal tract before systemic absorption can occur.

With oral administration, the onset of drug effect is largely determined by the rate and extent of absorption from the gastrointestinal tract. The principal site of drug absorption after oral administration is the small intestine due to the large surface area of this portion of the gastrointestinal tract. Changes in the pH of gastrointestinal fluid that favor the presence of a drug in its nonionized (lipid-soluble) fraction thus favor systemic absorption. Drugs that exist as weak acids (such as aspirin) become highly ionized in the alkaline environment of the small intestine, but absorption is still great because of the large surface area. Furthermore, absorption also occurs in the stomach, where the fluid is acidic.

First-Pass Hepatic Effect

Drugs absorbed from the gastrointestinal tract enter the portal venous blood and thus pass through the liver before entering the systemic circulation for delivery to tissue receptors (Fig. 1-6). This is known as the *first-pass hepatic effect*, and for drugs that undergo extensive hepatic extraction and metabolism (propranolol, lidocaine), it is the reason for large differences in the pharmacologic effect between oral and IV doses.

Oral Transmucosal Administration

The sublingual or buccal route of administration permits a rapid onset of drug effect because it bypasses the liver and thus prevents the first-pass hepatic effect on the initial plasma concentration of drug. For example, venous drainage from the sublingual area is into the superior vena cava. Evidence of the value of bypassing the first-pass hepatic effect is the efficacy of sublingual nitroglycerin. Conversely, oral administration of nitroglycerin is ineffective because extensive first-pass hepatic metabolism prevents establishment of a therapeutic plasma concentration. Buccal administration is an alternative to sublingual placement of a drug; it is better tolerated and less likely to stimulate salivation. The nasal mucosa also provides an effective absorption surface for certain drugs.

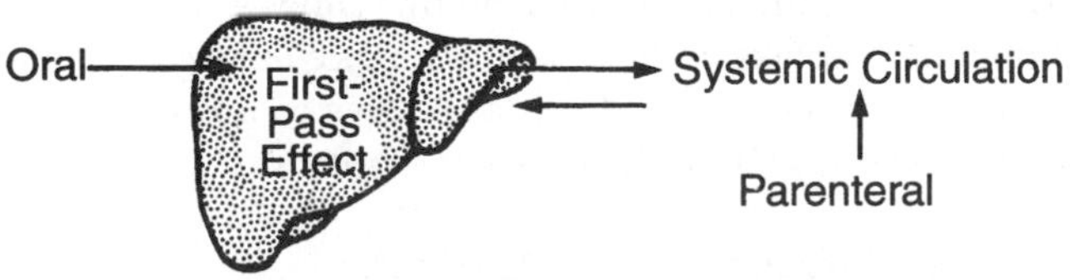

Figure 1-6. Drugs administered orally are absorbed from the gastrointestinal tract into the portal venous blood and pass through the liver (first-pass hepatic effect) before entering the systemic circulation for distribution to receptors. Conversely, intravenous administration of drugs allows rapid access to the systemic circulation without an initial impact of metabolism in the liver.

Transdermal Administration

Transdermal administration of drugs provides sustained therapeutic plasma concentrations of the drug and decreases the likelihood of loss of therapeutic efficacy due to peaks and valleys associated with conventional intermittent drug injections. This route of administration is devoid of the complexity of continuous infusion techniques, and the low incidence of side effects (because of the small doses used) contributes to high patient compliance. Characteristics of drugs that favor predictable transdermal absorption include (a) combined water and lipid solubility, (b) molecular weight of <1,000, (c) pH 5 to 9 in a saturated aqueous solution, (d) absence of histamine-releasing effects, and (e) daily dose requirements of <10 mg. Scopolamine, fentanyl, clonidine, and nitroglycerin are drugs available in transdermal delivery systems (see Chapters 3, 10, 15, and 16). Unfortunately, sustained plasma concentrations provided by transdermal absorption of scopolamine and nitroglycerin may result in tolerance and loss of therapeutic effect.

It is likely that transdermal absorption of drugs initially occurs along sweat ducts and hair follicles that function as diffusion shunts. The rate-limiting step in transdermal absorption of drugs is diffusion across the stratum corneum of the epidermis. Differences in the thickness and chemistry of the stratum corneum are reflected in the skin's permeability. For example, skin may be 10 to 20 μm thick on the back and abdomen compared with 400 to 600 μm on the palmar surfaces of the hands. Likewise, skin permeation studies have shown substantial regional differences for systemic absorption of scopolamine. The postauricular zone, because of its thin epidermal layer and somewhat higher temperature, is the only area that is sufficiently permeable for predictable and sustained absorption of scopolamine. The stratum corneum sloughs and regenerates at a rate that makes 7 days of adhesion the duration limit for one application of a transdermal system. Contact dermatitis at the site of transdermal patch applications occurs in a significant number of patients.

Rectal Administration

Drugs administered into the proximal rectum are absorbed into the superior hemorrhoidal veins and subsequently transported via the portal venous system to the liver (first-pass hepatic effect), where they are exposed to metabolism before entering the systemic circulation. On the other hand, drugs absorbed from a low rectal administration site reach the systemic circulation without first passing through the liver. These factors, in large part, explain the unpredictable responses that follow rectal administration of drugs. Furthermore, drugs may cause irritation of the rectal mucosa.

Parenteral Administration

Parenteral administration may be required to ensure absorption of the active form of the drug and is the only acceptable route of administration in an unconscious or otherwise uncooperative patient. Systemic absorption after subcutaneous or intramuscular injection is usually more rapid and predictable than after oral administration. Rate of systemic absorption is limited by the surface area of the absorbing capillary membranes and by solubility of the drug in interstitial fluid. Large aqueous channels in vascular endothelium account for the unimpeded diffusion of drug molecules, regardless of their lipid solubility.

The desired concentration of drug in the blood can be achieved more rapidly and precisely by the IV route of administration, which circumvents those factors that limit systemic absorption by other routes. Irritant drugs are administered more comfortably by the IV route because blood vessel walls are relatively insensitive and the injected drug is rapidly diluted, especially if the drug is injected into a large forearm vein.

TABLE 1-3.
RATE AND CAPACITY OF TISSUE UPTAKE OF DRUGS

Determinants of tissue uptake of drug
Blood flow
Concentration gradient
Blood-brain barrier
Physicochemical properties of drug
Ionization
Lipid solubility
Protein binding
Determinants of capacity of tissue to store drug
Solubility
Tissue mass
Binding to macromolecules
pH

Distribution of Drugs after Systemic Absorption

After systemic absorption of a drug, the highly perfused tissues (heart, brain, kidneys, liver) receive a disproportionately large amount of the total dose (see page 7, Table 1-2). As the plasma concentration of drug decreases below that in highly perfused tissues, drug leaves these tissues to be redistributed to less well-perfused sites, such as skeletal muscles and fat (see Table 1-2). For example, awakening after a single dose of thiopental principally reflects redistribution of drug from the brain to less well-perfused tissue sites such as skeletal muscles and fat, where thiopental is considered to be pharmacologically inactive.

Uptake of a drug by tissues is principally determined by tissue blood flow if the drug in question can penetrate membranes rapidly. The concentration gradient for the diffusible fraction of drug (nonionized, lipid soluble, and unbound to protein) determines both the rate and direction of net transfer between plasma and the tissue. Initially, after administration of a drug, the concentration gradient favors drug passage from plasma into tissues. With continuing elimination of drug, the plasma concentration declines below that in tissues, and drug leaves tissues to reenter the circulation. Therefore, a tissue that accumulates drug preferentially may act as a reservoir to maintain the plasma concentration and thus prolong its duration of action. Similarly, repeated or large doses of drug may saturate inactive tissue sites, thus negating the role of these tissues in providing an inactive tissue site for redistribution. When this occurs, the duration of action of drugs such as thiopental and fentanyl is likely to be prolonged as waning of drug effect now depends on metabolism rather than redistribution.

The capacity of tissues to accept a drug depends largely on the drug's solubility in the tissue and the mass of the tissue (Table 1-3). For example, a drug could exhibit limited solubility in skeletal muscles, but the large mass of this tissue (about 50% of the body weight) would exert a dominant role in tissue distribution of the drug.

TABLE 1-2.
BODY TISSUE COMPOSITION

	Body Mass (% of 70-kg Adult)	Blood Flow (% of Cardiac Output)
Vessel-rich group	10	75
Muscle group	50	19
Fat group	20	6
Vessel-poor group	20	<1

Uptake into the Lungs

The lungs have important functions in pharmacokinetics as reflected by uptake of injected drugs, especially basic lipophilic amines (pK 8). For example, first-pass pulmonary uptake of the initial dose of lidocaine, propranolol, meperidine, fentanyl, sufentanil, and alfentanil exceeds 65% of the dose (Boer et al., 1994). Spontaneous versus controlled ventilation versus apnea does not influence the magnitude of the first-pass pulmonary effect observed for alfentanil or sufentanil (Boer et al., 1994). Pulmonary uptake of drugs may influence the peak arterial concentration of these drugs and serve as a reservoir to release drug back into the systemic circulation.

Central Nervous System Distribution

Distribution of ionized water-soluble drugs to the central nervous system (CNS) from the circulation is restricted because of the limited permeability characteristics of brain capillaries, known as the *blood-brain barrier*. Conversely, cerebral blood flow is the only limitation to permeation of the CNS by nonionized lipid-soluble drugs. It is important to recognize that the blood-brain barrier is subject to change and can be overcome by administration of large doses of the drug. Furthermore, acute head injury and arterial hypoxemia may be associated with disruption of the blood-brain barrier.

Volume of Distribution

Vd of a drug is a mathematical expression of the sum of the apparent volumes of the compartments that constitute the compartmental model (see Fig. 1-2) (Stanski and Watkins, 1982). As such, this value depicts the distribution characteristics of a drug in the body. Volume of distribution is calculated as the dose of drug administered IV divided by the resulting plasma concentration of drug before elimination begins (initial Vd, or Vd_i) or when steady-state conditions have been achieved (Vd_{ss}). As such, Vd is influenced by physicochemical characteristics of the drug, including: (a) lipid solubility, (b) binding to plasma proteins, and (c) molecular size. Binding to plasma proteins and poor lipid solubility limit passage of drug to tissues, thus maintaining a high concentration in the plasma and a small calculated Vd. Examples of poorly lipid-soluble drugs with a Vd similar to extracellular fluid volume are the nondepolarizing neuromuscular blocking drugs. A lipid-soluble drug that is highly concentrated in tissues with a resulting low plasma concentration will have a calculated Vd that exceeds total body water. Examples of lipid-soluble drugs with a Vd that exceeds total body water are thiopental and diazepam. Traditional pharmacokinetic models that do not account for nonorgan drug clearance (Hofmann elimination, ester hydrolysis) underestimate Vd_{ss} (Fisher, 1996).

Ionization

Most drugs are weak acids or bases that are present in solutions as both ionized and nonionized molecules. Solubility characteristics of the ionized and nonionized molecules determine the ease with which drugs may diffuse through lipid components of cell membranes. This diffusion is particularly important because drugs are often too large to pass through membrane channels.

Characteristics of Ionized and Nonionized Molecules

The nonionized molecule is usually lipid soluble and can diffuse across cell membranes that constitute the blood-brain barrier, renal tubular epithelium, gastrointestinal epithelium, and hepatocytes (Table 1-4). As a result, this fraction of drug is pharmacologically active, undergoes reabsorption across renal tubules, is absorbed from the gastrointestinal tract, and is susceptible to hepatic metabolism. Conversely, the ionized fraction is poorly lipid soluble and cannot penetrate lipid cell membranes easily (see Table 1-4). Ionization causes the drug to be repelled from portions of cells with similar charges. A high degree of ionization thus impairs absorption of drug from the gastrointestinal tract, limits access to drug-metabolizing enzymes in the hepatocytes, and facilitates excretion of unchanged drug, as reabsorption across the renal tubular epithelium is unlikely.

TABLE 1-4.
CHARACTERISTICS OF NONIONIZED AND IONIZED DRUG MOLECULES

	Nonionized	Ionized
Pharmacologic effect	Active	Inactive
Solubility	Lipids	Water
Cross lipid barriers (gastrointestinal tract, blood-brain barrier, placenta)	Yes	No
Renal excretion	No	Yes
Hepatic metabolism	Yes	No

Determinants of Degree of Ionization

The degree of drug ionization is a function of its dissociation constant (pK) and the pH of the surrounding fluid. When the pK and the pH are identical, 50% of the drug exists in both the ionized and nonionized form. Small changes in pH can result in large changes in the extent of ionization, especially if the pH and pK values are similar. Acidic drugs, such as barbiturates, tend to be highly ionized at an alkaline pH, whereas basic drugs, such as opioids and local anesthetics, are highly ionized at an acid pH.

Ion Trapping

A concentration difference of total drug can develop on two sides of a membrane that separates fluids with different pHs (Fig. 1-7) (Hug, 1978). As a result of this pH difference, the degree of ionization of a drug is also different on each side of the membrane. The nonionized lipid-soluble fraction of drug equilibrates across cell membranes, but the total concentration of drug is very different on each side of the membrane because of the impact of pH on the fraction of drug that exists in the ionized form. This is an important consideration because one fraction of the drug may be more pharmacologically active than the other fraction.

Systemic administration of a weak base, such as an opioid, can result in accumulation of ionized drug (*ion trapping*) in the acid environment of the stomach. A similar phenomenon occurs in the transfer of basic drugs, such as local anesthetics, across the placenta from mother to fetus because the fetal pH is lower than maternal pH. The lipid-soluble nonionized fraction of local anesthetic crosses the placenta and is converted to the poorly lipid-soluble ionized fraction in the more acidic environment of the fetus.

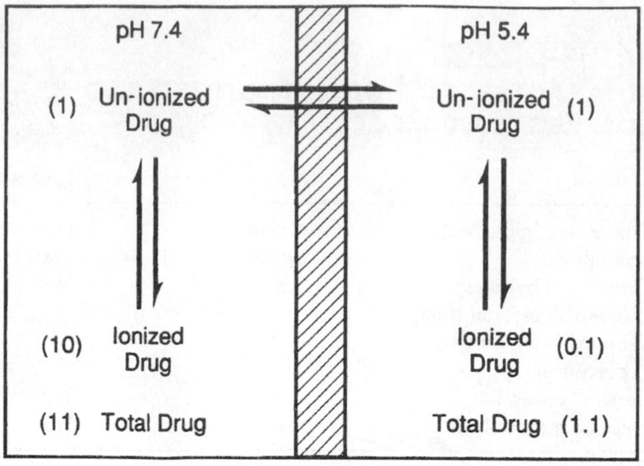

Figure 1-7. A concentration difference of total drug can develop on two sides of a membrane that separates fluids with different pHs. At steady state, the nonionized (un-ionized) drug concentration on both sides of the membrane is similar, but the concentration of ionized drug differs. (From Hug CC. Pharmacokinetics of drugs administered intravenously. *Anesth Analg* 1978;57:704–723; with permission.)

The ionized fraction in the fetus cannot easily cross the placenta to the maternal circulation and thus is effectively trapped in the fetus. At the same time, conversion of the nonionized to ionized fraction maintains a gradient for continued passage of local anesthetic into the fetus. The resulting accumulation of local anesthetic in the fetus is accentuated by the acidosis that accompanies fetal distress.

Protein Binding

A variable amount of most drugs is bound to plasma proteins that include albumin, alpha$_1$-acid glycoprotein, and lipoproteins (Wood, 1986). Most acidic drugs bind to albumin, whereas basic drugs select alpha$_1$-acid glycoprotein. Protein binding has an important effect on distribution of drugs because only the free or unbound fraction is readily available to cross cell membranes. Furthermore, Vd of a drug is inversely related to protein binding. For example, high protein binding limits passage of drug into tissues, thus resulting in high drug plasma concentrations and a small calculated Vd. Clearance of a drug is also influenced by protein binding because it is the unbound fraction in the plasma that has ready access to hepatic drug-metabolizing enzymes, and it is also this unbound fraction of drug that undergoes glomerular filtration.

The drug-protein complex is maintained by a weak bond (ionic, hydrogen, van der Waals bond) and can dissociate when the plasma concentration of drug declines as a result of hepatic or renal clearance of the unbound drug fraction. In this regard, protein binding of drugs may actually facilitate elimination by acting as a transport mechanism to deliver drugs to sites of clearance.

Alterations in protein binding are usually important only for drugs that are highly protein bound, such as warfarin, propranolol, phenytoin, and diazepam. For example, for a drug that is 98% protein bound, a decrease in binding to 96% will double the plasma fraction of unbound drug, with potential associated increases in pharmacologic effects. Conversely, a decrease in protein binding from 70% to 68% results in only a 7% increase in the free fraction of drug in plasma.

Determinants of Protein Binding

The extent of protein binding parallels lipid solubility of the drug. For example, pentobarbital is less highly bound to protein than is its more lipid-soluble thioanalogue, thiopental. In addition to lipid solubility, the fraction of total drug in plasma that is protein bound is determined by the drug's plasma concentration and the number of available binding sites. Low plasma concentrations of drugs are likely to be more highly protein bound than are higher plasma concentrations of the same drug. Statements about the percentage of protein binding of a drug are not meaningful unless the plasma concentration of drug and availability of binding sites (plasma concentration of albumin) are also known.

Binding of drugs to plasma albumin is often nonselective; thus, many drugs with similar physicochemical characteristics can compete with each other and with endogenous substances for the same protein-binding sites. For example, sulfonamides can displace unconjugated bilirubin from binding sites on albumin, leading to the risk of bilirubin encephalopathy in the neonate. It is important to consider protein binding when comparing maternal to fetal ratios for drugs. For example, total body concentrations of drugs may be different, but the pharmacologic effects are similar because the free concentrations of drugs are similar.

Renal failure may decrease the fraction of a drug bound to protein even in the absence of changes in plasma concentrations of albumin or other proteins. For example, the free fraction of phenytoin is increased in patients with renal failure such that toxic plasma concentrations are likely to occur if the total dose of a drug is not decreased. This occurrence in the presence of normal plasma concentrations of albumin suggests that an alteration in protein structure or displacement of phenytoin from its protein-binding sites by a metabolic factor that is normally excreted by the kidneys has occurred. Albumin concentrations tend to be lower in elderly patients, but the impact of this change is small compared with the effect of disease states that result in renal or hepatic dysfunction.

Increases in the plasma concentration of alpha$_1$-acid glycoprotein occur in response to surgery, chronic pain, and acute myocardial infarction (Wood, 1986). An increase of this protein fraction in patients with rheumatoid arthritis leads to increased protein binding of lidocaine and propranolol. The plasma concentrations of alpha$_1$-acid glycoprotein are decreased in neonates, resulting in decreased protein binding of several drugs, including diazepam, propranolol, sufentanil, and lidocaine (Wood and Wood, 1981).

Clearance of Drugs from the Systemic Circulation

Clearance is the volume of plasma cleared of drug by renal excretion and/or metabolism in the liver or other organs. Examples of nonorgan clearance of drugs are Hofmann elimination and ester hydrolysis that are responsible for the elimination of succinylcholine, atracurium, cisatracurium, and mivacurium. Almost all drugs administered in the therapeutic dose ranges are cleared from the circulation at a rate proportional to the amount of drug present in the plasma (*first-order kinetics*). More drug is cleared from the plasma per unit time at the beginning when plasma concentrations are the highest (elimination rate is proportional to the concentration). Even at therapeutic doses, however, a few drugs will exceed the metabolic or excretory capacity of the body to clear drugs by first-order kinetics. In this situation, a constant amount of drug is cleared per unit of time (*zero-order kinetics*).

Clearance is one of the most important pharmacokinetic variables to consider when defining a constant drug infusion regimen. To maintain an unchanging plasma concentration of drug (steady state), the infusion rate must be equal to the rate of drug clearance by hepatic and renal clearance mechanisms. Knowledge of the elimination half-time for a drug is important for achieving a constant plasma concentration of drug. Nevertheless, individual variations in Vd and clearance may alter the elimination half-time of a drug in an individual patient compared with values calculated from normal patients.

Hepatic Clearance

Hepatic clearance of a drug is the product of hepatic blood flow and the hepatic extraction ratio. If the hepatic extraction ratio is high (>0.7), the clearance of drug will depend on hepatic blood flow, whereas changes in enzyme activity will have minimal influence (Fig. 1-8) (Wilkinson and Shand, 1975). Thus, a high hepatic extraction ratio results in *perfusion-dependent elimination*. If the hepatic extraction ratio is <0.3, only a small fraction of the drug delivered to the liver is removed per unit of time. As a result, an excess of drug is available for hepatic-elimination mechanisms, and changes in hepatic blood flow will not greatly influence hepatic clearance. A decrease in protein binding or an increase in enzyme activity, as associated with enzyme induction, will greatly increase hepatic clearance of a drug with a low hepatic extraction ratio. This type of hepatic elimination is termed *capacity-dependent elimination*.

Biliary Excretion

Most of the metabolites of drugs produced in the liver are excreted in bile into the gastrointestinal tract. Often, these metabolites are reabsorbed from the gastrointestinal tract into the circulation for ultimate elimination in the urine. Organic anions, such as glucuronides, are transported actively into bile by carrier systems similar to those that transport these anions into renal tubules.

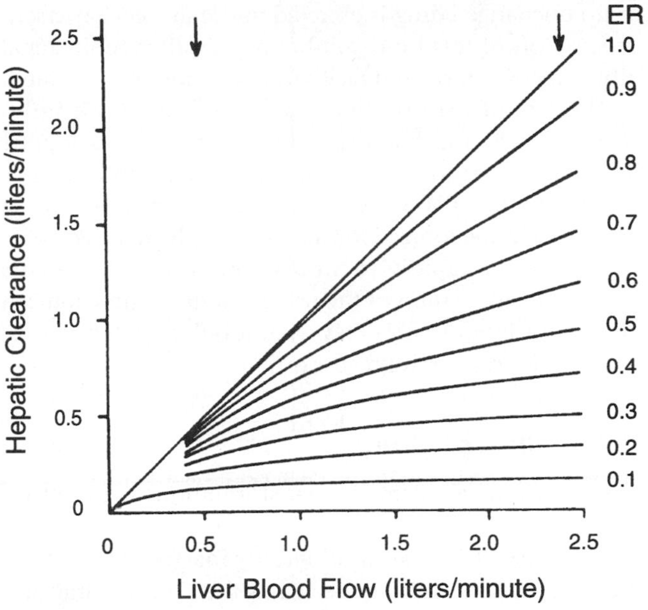

Figure 1-8. An increase in hepatic blood flow within the physiologic range denoted by the arrows produces minimal changes in hepatic clearance of drugs with a low extraction ratio (ER). Conversely, for drugs with a high ER, an increase in hepatic blood flow produces a nearly proportional increase in hepatic clearance. (From Wilkinson GR, Shand DG. A physiologic approach to hepatic drug clearance. *Clin Pharmacol Ther* 1975;18:377–390; with permission.)

Renal Clearance

The kidneys are the most important organs for the elimination of unchanged drugs or their metabolites. Water-soluble compounds are excreted more efficiently by the kidneys than are compounds with high lipid solubility. This emphasizes the important role of metabolism in converting lipid-soluble drugs to water-soluble metabolites. Drug elimination by the kidneys is correlated with endogenous creatinine clearance or serum creatinine concentration. The magnitude of increase of these indices provides an estimate of the necessary downward adjustment in drug dosage.

Renal excretion of drugs involves (a) glomerular filtration, (b) active tubular secretion, and (c) passive tubular reabsorption. The amount of drug that enters the renal tubular lumen depends on the fraction of drug bound to protein and the glomerular filtration rate. Renal tubular secretion involves active transport processes, which may be selective for certain drugs and metabolites, including protein-bound compounds. Reabsorption from renal tubules removes drug that has entered tubules by glomerular filtration and tubular secretion. This reabsorption is most prominent for lipid-soluble drugs that can easily cross cell membranes of renal tubular epithelial cells to enter pericapillary fluid. Indeed, a highly lipid-soluble drug, such as thiopental, is almost completely reabsorbed such that little or no unchanged drug is excreted in the urine. Conversely, production of less lipid-soluble metabolites limits renal tubule reabsorption and facilitates excretion in the urine.

The rate of reabsorption from renal tubules is influenced by factors such as pH and rate of renal tubular urine flow. Passive reabsorption of weak bases and acids is altered by urine pH, which influences the fraction of drug that exists in the ionized form. For example, weak acids are excreted more rapidly in an alkaline urine. This occurs because alkalinization of the urine results in more ionized drug that cannot easily cross renal tubular epithelial cells, resulting in less passive reabsorption.

Metabolism of Drugs

The role of metabolism (biotransformation) is to convert pharmacologically active, lipid-soluble drugs into water-soluble and often pharmacologically inactive metabolites. Increased water solubility decreases the Vd for a drug and enhances its renal excretion and occasionally gastrointestinal elimination. A lipid-soluble parent drug is not likely to undergo extensive renal excretion because of the ease of reabsorption from the lumens of renal tubules into pericapillary fluid. In the absence of metabolism, a lipid-soluble drug, such as thiopental, would continue to undergo reabsorption from renal tubules and have an elimination half-time of about 100 years. Metabolism to water-soluble metabolites, however, decreases its reabsorption from renal tubules and thus facilitates elimination in the urine.

It is important to recognize that metabolism does not always lead to production of pharmacologically inactive metabolites. For example, diazepam and propranolol may be metabolized to active compounds. In some instances, an inactive parent compound (prodrug) is administered and subsequently undergoes metabolism to active metabolites allowing a route of administration that would be precluded by solubility characteristics of the active molecule. These examples emphasize that metabolism is not always synonymous with inactivation or even detoxification.

Rate of Metabolism

The rate of metabolism of most drugs is determined by the concentration of drug at the site of metabolism and by the intrinsic rate of the metabolism process. Hepatic blood flow often determines delivery and thus concentration of drug at the site of metabolism. The intrinsic rate of metabolism reflects factors that influence enzyme activity, such as genetics and enzyme induction.

First-Order Kinetics

Most drug metabolism follows linear or first-order kinetics such that a constant fraction of available drug is metabolized in a given time period. First-order kinetics depends on the plasma concentration of drug in the sense that the absolute amount of drug eliminated per unit of time is greatest when its plasma concentration is greatest. However, the fraction of total drug that is eliminated during first-order kinetics is independent of the plasma concentration of drug.

Zero-Order Kinetics

Zero-order kinetics occurs when the plasma concentration of drug exceeds the capacity of metabolizing enzymes. This reflects saturation of available enzymes and results in metabolism of a constant amount of drug per unit of time. This contrasts with the constant fraction of drug metabolized during first-order kinetics. As a result, the absolute amount of drug eliminated per unit of time during zero-order kinetics is the same, regardless of the drug's plasma concentration. The intrinsic activity of enzymes determines the constant amount of drug metabolized per unit of time. Alcohol, aspirin, and phenytoin are drugs that exhibit zero-order kinetics at even therapeutic concentrations.

Pathways of Metabolism

The four basic pathways of metabolism are (a) oxidation, (b) reduction, (c) hydrolysis, and (d) conjugation. Traditionally, metabolism has been categorized as phase I and phase II reactions. Phase I reactions include oxidation, reduction, and hydrolysis which increase the drug's polarity and prepare it for phase II reactions. Phase II reactions are conjugation reactions that covalently link the drug or metabolites with a highly polar molecule (carbohydrate or an amino acid) that renders the conjugate more water soluble for subsequent excretion. Hepatic microsomal enzymes are responsible for the metabolism of most drugs. Other sites of drug metabolism include the plasma (Hofmann elimination, ester hydrolysis), lungs, kidneys, and gastrointestinal tract. The evolutionary development of drug-metabolizing enzymes is most likely related to ingestion of toxic alkaloids in plants. In this regard, drug metabolism has evolved as a means of protection against environmental toxins.

Hepatic microsomal enzymes, which participate in the metabolism of many drugs, are located principally in hepatic smooth endoplasmic reticulum. These microsomal enzymes are also present in the kidneys, gastrointestinal tract, and adrenal cortex. The term *microsomal enzyme* is derived from the fact that centrifugation of homogenized cells (usually hepatocytes) concentrates fragments of the disrupted smooth endoplasmic reticulum in what is designated as the microsomal fraction.

Although the gastrointestinal tract is traditionally considered an organ of absorption, it is recognized that the small intestine has considerable drug metabolizing activity involving both phase I and phase II reactions. Cytochrome P-450 enzymes are located throughout the gastrointestinal system but the majority of these enzymes are located in the small intestine. The kidneys are also capable of oxidizing and conjugating drugs and endogenous substrates utilizing cytochrome P-450 enzymes and phase II enzymes.

Phase I Enzymes

Enzymes responsible for phase I reactions include cytochrome P-450 enzymes, noncytochrome P-450 enzymes, and flavin-containing monooxygenase enzymes.

Cytochrome P-450 Enzymes

The cytochrome P-450 enzyme (CYP) system is a superfamily of membrane-bound heme proteins that catalyze the metabolism of endogenous compounds. P-450 enzymes are predominantly hepatic microsomal enzymes although there are also mitochondrial P-450 enzymes. The designation *cytochrome P-450* emphasizes this substance's absorption peak at 450 nm when it combines with carbon monoxide. The cytochrome P-450 system is also known as the *mixed function oxidase system* or *monooxygenases* because it involves both oxidation and reduction steps. Cytochrome P-450 functions as the terminal oxidase in the electron transport scheme.

Individual cytochrome P-450 enzymes (more than 50 CYP genes have been identified) have evolved from a common protein (Nelson, 1999). Cytochrome P-450 enzymes that share more than 40% sequence homology are grouped in a family designated by a number (CYP2), those that share more than 55% homology are grouped in a subfamily designated by a letter (CYP2A), and individual CYP enzymes are identified by a third number (CYP2A6). Ten isoforms of cytochrome P-450 are responsible for the oxidative metabolism of most drugs. The preponderance of CYP activity is generated by CYP2D6 and CYP3A4/5 isozymes. P-450 3A4 is the most abundantly expressed P-450 isoform, comprising 20% to 60% of total P-450 activity. P-450 3A4/5 is considered to be responsible for metabolizing more than one-half of all currently available drugs, including opioids (alfentanil, sufentanil, fentanyl), benzodiazepines, local anesthetics (lidocaine, ropivacaine), immunosuppressants (cyclosporine), and antihistamines (terfenadine). Systemic clearance of several drugs that serve as substrates for P-450 3A4/5 is gender dependent, with clearance being 20% to 40% higher in women than in men. This reflects stimulation of P-450 3A4/5 activity by steroid hormones, which may vary during the menstrual cycle. Nevertheless, alfentanil clearance has not been shown to vary on different days in the menstrual cycle (Kharasch et al., 1997a). CYP2D6 is responsible for phase I reactions involving nearly 25% of all drugs including analgesics, antidysrhythmics, amide local anesthetics, ketamine, propofol, antiemetics, and beta-blockers.

Microsomal enzymes catalyze most of the oxidation, reduction, and conjugation reactions that lead to metabolism of drugs. Lipid solubility of a drug favors passage across cell membranes and thus facilitates access by drugs to microsomal enzymes in hepatocytes and other cells. Hepatic microsomal enzyme activity is low in neonates, especially premature infants. Individual differences in microsomal enzyme activity are determined genetically. Indeed, rate of drug metabolism may vary sixfold or more among individuals as a reflection of differences in microsomal enzyme activity.

Enzyme Induction

A unique feature of hepatic microsomal enzymes is the ability of drugs or chemicals to stimulate activity of these enzymes. Increased enzyme activity produced by drugs or chemicals is known as *enzyme induction*. Enzyme induction also occurs to a limited extent in the lungs, kidneys, and gastrointestinal tract. Phenobarbital and polycyclic hydrocarbons are examples of substances that induce microsomal enzymes. The resulting increase in microsomal enzyme activity produced by phenobarbital is attributed to increased synthesis of cytochrome P-450 and cytochrome P-450 reductase.

Noncytochrome P-450 Enzymes (Esters)

Noncytochrome P-450 enzymes (nonmicrosomal enzymes) catalyze reactions responsible for metabolism of drugs by conjugation, by hydrolysis, and, to a lesser extent, by oxidation and reduction. These noncytochrome P-450 enzymes are present principally in the liver but are also found in plasma and the gastrointestinal tract. All conjugation reactions except for conjugation of glucuronic acid are catalyzed by noncytochrome P-450 enzymes. Nonspecific esterases in the liver, plasma, and gastrointestinal tract are examples of noncytochrome P-450 enzymes responsible for hydrolysis of drugs that contain ester bonds (succinylcholine, atracurium, mivacurium, esmolol, ester local anesthetics). Noncytochrome P-450 enzymes such as plasma cholinesterase and acetylating enzymes do not, however, undergo enzyme induction. The activity of these enzymes is determined genetically, as emphasized by patients with atypical cholinesterase enzyme and individuals who are classified as being rapid or slow acetylators. It is estimated that 1 of 2500 individuals are homozygous for "atypical cholinesterase" which reflects a genetic mutation (glycine is substituted for an aspartate in the anionic binding site of the protein) resulting in loss of electrostatic interactions necessary for drug-substrate binding. As a result, duration of action of drugs such as succinylcholine and mivacurium is dramatically prolonged.

Flavin-Containing Monooxygenase Enzymes

Flavin-containing monooxygenase (FMO) enzymes are nicotinamide adenine dinucleotide (NAD)-dependent microsomal enzymes that oxidize (phase I reactions) nitrogen, sulfur and phosphorus-containing compounds. FMO3 catalyzes oxygenation of tricyclic antidepressants and H_2-receptor antagonists.

Phase II Enzymes

Phase II enzymes include glucuronosyltrasferases, glutathione-*S*-transferases, *N*-acetyl-transferases, and sulfotransferases.

Glucuronosyltransferase

The uridine diphosphate glucuronosyltransferase enzymes are a family of hepatic microsomal enzymes that catalyze the covalent addition of glucuronic acid to a variety of endogenous and exogenous compounds rendering them more water soluble. The intestine contains beta-glucuronidase which hydrolyzes glucuronides back to their parent compounds which can be reabsorbed from the intestine and transported to the liver to undergo reconjugation (enterohepatic recirculation). Glucuronides may be more or less pharmacologically active than their parent drugs.

Glucuronidation is an important metabolic pathway for several drugs used during anesthesia. Propofol undergoes glucuronidation in the liver and kidneys. Opioids undergo glucuronidation as reflected by morphine-3-glucuronide and morphine-6-glucuronide. The glucuronide metabolite, 1-hydroxymidazolam is pharmacologically active and may contribute to prolonged midazolam effects in patients with renal insufficiency.

Glutathione-S-Transferase

Glutathione-*S*-transferase (GST) enzymes are primarily a defensive system for detoxification and protection against oxidative stress. The two superfamilies of GST enzymes are the large number of hepatic cytosolic enzymes and a smaller number of membrane-bound microsomal GST enzymes. Compound A nephrotoxicity in rats is attributed to GST-dependent activation whereas absence of similar toxicity in humans most likely reflects a species difference in GST enzyme activity.

N-Acetyl-Transferase

N-acetylation catalyzed by *N-acetyl-transferase* (NAT) is a common phase II reaction for heterocyclic aromatic amines and arylamine hydrazine. *N*-acetylation reactions are responsible for inactivation of isoniazid and genetic polymorphisms of this enzyme result in fast- and slow-acetylators. Slow acetylators have a greater therapeutic response to drugs that are inactivated by NAT enzymes and these individuals may be at greater risk for drug-induced side effects (isoniazid hepatotoxicity, hydralazine or procainamide lupus-like syndrome).

Oxidative Metabolism

Hepatic microsomal enzymes, including cytochrome P-450 enzymes, are crucial for the oxidation and resulting metabolism of many drugs. These enzymes require an electron donor in the form of reduced nicotinamide adenine dinucleotide (NAD) and molecular oxygen for their activity. The molecule of oxygen is split, with one atom of oxygen oxidizing each molecule of drug and the other oxygen atom being incorporated into a molecule of water. A loss of electrons results in oxidation, whereas a gain of electrons results in reduction.

Examples of oxidative metabolism of drugs catalyzed by cytochrome P-450 enzymes include hydroxylation, deamination, desulfuration, dealkylation, and dehalogenation. Demethylation of morphine to normorphine is an example of oxidative dealkylation. Dehalogenation involves oxidation of a carbon-hydrogen bond to form an intermediate metabolite that is unstable and spontaneously loses a halogen atom. Halogenated volatile anesthetics are susceptible to dehalogenation, often leading to release of bromide, chloride, and fluoride ions. Aliphatic oxidation is oxidation of a side chain. For example, oxidation of the side chain of thiopental converts the highly lipid-soluble parent drug to the more water-soluble carboxylic acid derivative. Thiopental also undergoes desulfuration to pentobarbital by an oxidative step.

Epoxide intermediates in the oxidative metabolism of drugs are capable of covalent binding with macromolecules and may be responsible for drug-induced organ toxicity, such as hepatic dysfunction. Normally, these highly reactive intermediates have such a transient existence that they exert no biologic action. When enzyme induction occurs, however, large amounts of reactive intermediates may be produced, leading to organ damage. This is especially likely to occur if the antioxidant glutathione, which is in limited supply in the liver, is depleted by the reactive intermediates.

Reductive Metabolism

Reductive pathways of metabolism, like oxidative pathways, involve cytochrome P-450 enzymes. Under conditions of low oxygen partial pressures, cytochrome P-450 enzymes transfer electrons directly to a substrate such as halothane rather than to oxygen. This electron gain imparted to the substrate occurs only when insufficient amounts of oxygen are present to compete for electrons.

Hydrolysis

Enzymes responsible for hydrolysis of drugs (often an ester bond) do not involve the cytochrome P-450 enzyme system (see the section on Nonmicrosomal Enzymes). Hydrolysis of glucuronide conjugates secreted into the bile occurs in the gastrointestinal tract and is necessary for release of a drug to become available for enterohepatic recirculation.

Conjugation

Conjugation with glucuronic acid involves cytochrome P-450 enzymes. Glucuronic acid is readily available from glucose. When conjugated to a lipid-soluble drug or metabolite, hydrophilic glucuronic acid renders the substance pharmacologically inactive and more water soluble. The resulting water-soluble glucuronide conjugates are unlikely to be reabsorbed into the systemic circulation and are thus preferentially excreted in bile and urine.

Reduced microsomal enzyme activity interferes with conjugation, leading to hyperbilirubinemia of the neonate and the risk of bilirubin encephalopathy. This decreased microsomal enzyme activity is responsible for increased toxicity in the neonate of drugs that are normally inactivated by conjugation with glucuronic acid. Conjugation with glucuronic acid is also decreased during pregnancy, presumably because of increased blood levels of progesterone.

Dose-Response Curves

Dose-response curves depict the relationship between the dose of drug administered and the resulting pharmacologic effect (Fig. 1-9). Logarithmic transformation of dosage is frequently used, because it permits display of a wide range of doses. Dose-response curves are characterized by differences in (a) potency, (b) slope, (c) efficacy, and (d) individual responses.

Potency

The potency of a drug is depicted by its location along the dose axis of the dose-response curve. Factors that influence the potency of a drug include (a) absorption, (b) distribution, (c) metabolism, (d) excretion, and (e) affinity for the receptor. For clinical purposes, the potency of a drug makes little difference as long as the effective dose of the drug can be administered conveniently. The dose required to produce a specified effect is designated as the effective dose (ED) necessary to produce that effect in a given percentage of patients (ED_{50}, ED_{90}). Increased affinity of a drug for its receptor moves the dose-response curve to the left.

Slope

The slope of the dose-response curve is influenced by the number of receptors that must be occupied before a drug effect occurs. For example, if a drug must occupy a majority of receptors before an effect occurs, the slope of the dose-response curve will be steep. A steep dose-response curve is characteristic of neuromuscular blocking drugs and inhaled anesthetics (minimal alveolar concentration [MAC]); it means that small increases in dosage evoke intense increases in drug effect. For example, a 1 MAC concentration of volatile anesthetic prevents skeletal muscle movement in response to a surgical skin incision in 50% of patients, whereas a modest increase to about 1.3 MAC prevents movement in at least 95% of patients. Furthermore, when the dose-response curve is steep, the difference between a therapeutic and toxic concentration may be small. This is true for volatile anesthetics that are characterized by small differences between the doses that produce desirable degrees of central nervous system (CNS) depression and undesirable degrees of cardiac depression (see Chapter 2).

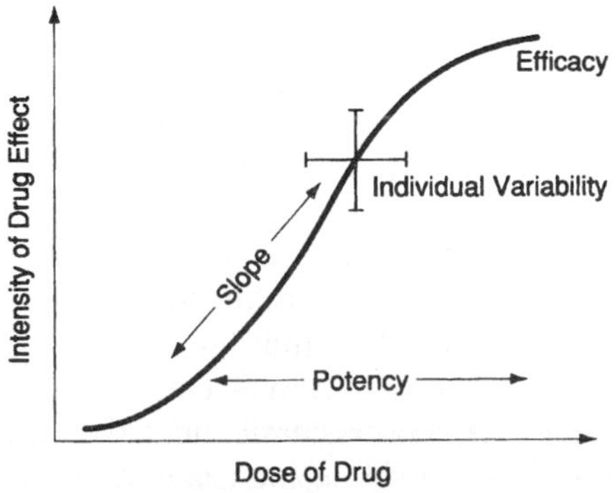

Figure 1-9. Dose-response curves are characterized by differences in potency, slope, efficacy, and individual responses.

Efficacy

The maximal effect of a drug reflects its intrinsic activity or efficacy. This efficacy is depicted by the plateau in dose-response curves. It must be recognized that undesirable effects (side effects) of a drug may limit dosage to below the concentration associated with its maximal desirable effect. Differences in efficacy are emphasized by the pharmacologic effects of opioids versus aspirin in relieving pain. Opioids relieve pain of high intensity, whereas maximal doses of aspirin are effective only against mild discomfort. The efficacy and potency of a drug are not necessarily related.

The *therapeutic index*, or margin of safety, is the difference between the dose of drug that produces a desired effect and the dose that produces undesirable effects. In laboratory studies, the therapeutic index is often defined as the ratio between the median lethal dose and the median effective dose (LD_{50}/ED_{50}). Drugs have multiple therapeutic indices, depending on the therapeutic response being considered and the dose of drug necessary to evoke that response. For example, the therapeutic index for aspirin to relieve headache is greatly different from the therapeutic index to relieve pain of rheumatoid arthritis.

Individual Variability

The response to many drugs varies greatly among patients (Caraco, 2004). After administration of identical doses, some patients may have clinically significant adverse effects whereas others may exhibit no therapeutic response. Some of this diversity of response can be ascribed to differences in the rate of drug metabolism, particularly by the cytochrome P-450 superfamily of enzymes. The incorporation of pharmacogenetics into clinical medicine may become useful in predicting patient responses to drugs.

Variability of individual responses to a drug often reflects differences in pharmacokinetics and/or pharmacodynamics among patients (Table 1-5) (Wood, 1989). This may account even for differences in pharmacologic effects of drugs in the same patient at different times. Accurate dosing is difficult to acheive in the presence of interindividual variability and it is not unusual to find at least a twofold variation in plasma concentrations achieved in different individuals using the same dosing scheme. This is true for

TABLE 1-5.
EVENTS RESPONSIBLE FOR VARIATIONS IN DRUG RESPONSES BETWEEN INDIVIDUALS

Pharmacokinetics
Bioavailability
Renal function
Hepatic function
Cardiac function
Patient age
Pharmacodynamics
Enzyme activity
Genetic differences
Drug Interactions

inhaled as well as injected drugs. Furthermore, there may be a fivefold range in the plasma concentrations of a drug required to achieve the same pharmacologic effect in different individuals and this range may be even greater if tolerance has developed in some of these individuals.

The relative importance of the numerous factors that contribute to variations in individual responses to drugs depends, in part, on the drug itself and its usual route of excretion. Drugs excreted primarily unchanged by the kidneys tend to exhibit smaller differences in pharmacokinetics than do drugs that are metabolized. The most important determinant of metabolic rate is genetic. Changes in metabolic rate have little impact on drugs with a high-extraction ratio as the efficiency of extraction is so great that hepatic blood flow is a more rate-limiting factor than metabolism. Conversely, the systemic clearance of low-extraction drugs is highly susceptible to small changes in the rate of metabolism. For example, the systemic clearance of alfentanil is exquisitely sensitive to CYP induction and inhibition, whereas clearance of high-extraction opioids such as fentanyl and sufentanil is minimally influenced (Kharasch et al., 1997b). Interindividual variability in the response to the prodrug codeine is determined by activity of CYP2D6-mediated *O*-demethylation to morphine and morphine-6-glucuronide. CYP2D6-deficient individuals have diminished or absent morphine formation following administraiton of codeine, whereas individuals with CYP2D6 gene amplification experience exaggerated opioid effects following administraiton of codeine ("codeine intoxication) (Gasche et al., 2004). Quinidine inhibits CYP2D6 and markedly diminishes codeine bioactivation and morphine formation. The dynamic state of receptor concentrations, as influenced by diseases and other drugs, also influences the variation in drug responses observed among patients (see the section on Concentration of Receptors). Finally, inhaled anesthetics, by altering circulatory, hepatic, and renal function, may influence the pharmacokinetics of injected drugs.

In clinical practice, the impact of interpatient variability may be masked by the administration of high doses of a drug. For example, the administration of 2-3 × ED_{95} of a nondepolarizing neuromusuclar blocking drug is common practice to achieving a desired effect (skeletal muscle paralysis) in all patients. Interpatient variability, however, is manifest if the level of neuromuscular blockade and duration of action is monitored. Furthermore, it is common practice in anesthesia to administer drugs in proportion to body weight although pharmacokinetic and pharmacodynamic principles may not support this practice. In attempts to minimize interindividual variability, computerized infusion systems (target-controlled infusion systems) have been developed to deliver intravenous drugs (alfentanil, remifentanil, etomidate, propofol) to achieve a desired (target) concentration (White and Kenny, 1990).

Elderly Patients

In elderly patients, variations in drug response most likely reflect (a) decreased cardiac output, (b) enlarged fat content, (c) decreased protein binding, and (d) decreased renal function. Decreased cardiac output decreases hepatic blood flow and thus delivery of drug to the liver for metabolism. This decreased delivery, combined with the possibility of decreased hepatic enzyme activity, may prolong the duration of action of drugs such as lidocaine and fentanyl (Bentley et al., 1982). An enlarged fat compartment may increase the Vd and lead to the accumulation of lipid-soluble drugs such as diazepam and thiopental (Jung et al., 1982). Increased total body fat content and decreased plasma protein binding of drugs accounts for the increased Vd that accompanies aging. A parallel decrease in total body water accompanies increased fat stores. The net effect of these changes is an increased vulnerability of elderly patients to cumulative drug effects. Aging does not seem to be accompanied by changes in receptor responsiveness.

Enzyme Activity

Alterations in enzyme activity as reflected by enzyme induction may be responsible for variations in drug responses among individuals. For example, cigarette smoke contains polycyclic hydrocarbons that induce mixed-function hepatic oxidases, leading to increased dose requirements for drugs such as theophylline and tricylic antidepressants. Acute alcohol ingestion can inhibit metabolism of drugs. Conversely, chronic alcohol use (>200 g/day) induces microsomal enzymes that metabolize drugs. Because of enzyme induction, this accelerated metabolism may manifest as tolerance to drugs such as barbiturates.

Genetic Disorders

Variations in drug responses among individuals are due, in part, to genetic differences that may also affect receptor sensitivity. Genetic variations in metabolic pathways (rapid versus slow acetylators) may have important clinical implications for drugs such as isoniazid and hydralazine. *Pharmacogenetics* describes genetically determined disease states that are initially revealed by altered responses to specific drugs. Examples of diseases that are unmasked by drugs include (a) atypical cholinesterase enzyme revealed by prolonged neuromuscular blockade after administration of succinylcholine or mivacurium, (b) malignant hyperthermia triggered by succinylcholine or volatile anesthetics, (c) glucose-6-phosphate dehydrogenase deficiency, in which certain drugs cause hemolysis, and (d) intermittent porphyria, in which barbiturates may evoke an acute attack.

Drug Interactions

A drug interaction occurs when a drug alters the intensity of pharmacologic effects of another drug given concurrently. Drug interactions may reflect alterations in pharmacokinetics (increased metabolism of neuromuscular blocking drugs in patients receiving anticonvulsants chronically) or pharmacodynamics (decrease in volatile anesthetic requirements produced by opioids). The net result of a drug interaction may be enhanced or diminished effects of one or both drugs, leading to desired or undesired effects. A physicochemical drug interaction occurs when two incompatible drugs are mixed in the same solution (precipitate of the conjugate salt of a weak acid and weak base when pancuronium and thiopental are mixed together in the same intravenous tubing). The potential for drug interactions in the perioperative period is great considering the large number of drugs from different chemical classes that are likely to be part of anesthesia management. For example, a typical "balanced anesthetic" may include benzodiazepines, sedative-hypnotics, barbiturates, opioids, neuromuscular blocking drugs, anticholinergics, anticholinesterases, sympathomimetics, sympathetic nervous system blocking drugs, and antibiotics.

An example of a beneficial drug interaction is the concurrent administration of propranolol with hydralazine to prevent compensatory increases in heart rate that would offset the blood pressure–lowering effects of hydralazine. Interactions between drugs are frequently used to counter the effects of agonist drugs, as reflected by the use of naloxone to antagonize opioids. Adverse drug interactions typically manifest as impaired therapeutic efficacy and/or enhanced toxicity. In this regard, one drug may interact with another to (a) impair absorption, (b) compete with the same plasma protein-binding sites, (c) alter metabolism by enzyme induction or inhibition, or (d) change the rate of renal excretion.

PHARMACODYNAMICS OF INJECTED DRUGS

The most important mechanism by which drugs exert pharmacologic effects is by the interaction of the drug with a specific protein molecule in the lipid bilayer of cell membranes (Fig. 1-10) (Schwinn, 1993). This transmembrane protein macromolecule is referred to as a *receptor*. Receptors

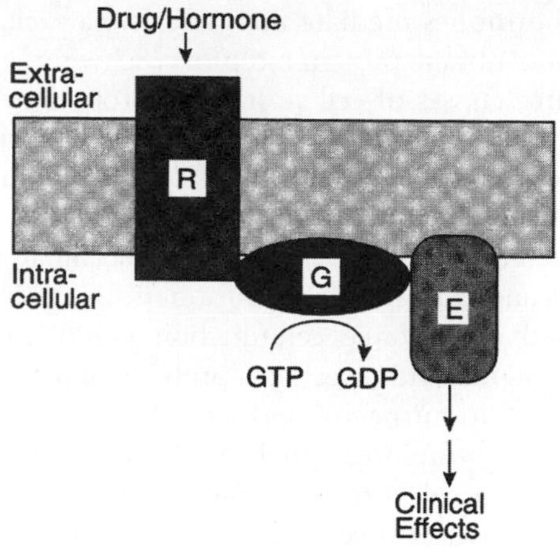

Figure 1-10. Transmembrane receptors (R) are located in the cell membrane and bind drugs or hormones on the extracellular surface. Agonist-bound receptors then interact with guanine nucleotide proteins (G proteins). With the energy provided by the hydrolysis of guanine triphosphate (GTP) to guanine diphosphate (GDP), activated G proteins are able to interact with effector systems (E), leading to clinically recognized responses. (From Schwinn DA. Adrenoceptors as models for G protein–coupled receptors: structure, function, and regulation. *Br J Anaesth* 1993;71:77–85; with permission.)

are classified as surface receptors or intracellular receptors depending on their cellular location. Similar receptors exist for endogenous regulatory substances such as hormones and neurotransmitters. A drug administered as an exogenous substance is an incidental "passenger" for these receptors. A drug-receptor interaction alters the function or conformation of a specific cellular component that initiates or prevents a series of changes that characterize the pharmacologic effects of the drug.

In addition to excitable transmembrane protein receptors, drugs could evoke cellular changes (pharmacologic effects) via cytoplasmic (intracellular) receptors (present in the nucleus or cytosol) and stimulation or inhibition of enzyme systems (Schwinn, 1993). Cytoplasmic receptors may be represented by steroid hormone receptors. Because steroids are lipophilic, they cross the lipid bilayer of the cell membrane and interact with steroid receptors in the cytoplasm. The steroid hormone-receptor complex acts as a ligand regulated transcription factor to modulate gene expression by binding to regulatory DNA sequences in target genes that alter their transcription and thus target cell function. In addition to cytoplasmic receptors, various enzyme systems are also located in the cytoplasm. Inhibition or stimulation of these enzymes may be important in the pharmacologic effects of certain drugs, such as amrinone and milrinone, which inhibit a specific type of phosphodiesterase enzyme. Other mechanisms of action for drugs include formation of strong bonds with metallic cations (chelating drugs) and direct neutralization of gastric acid (antacids). Despite examples of drugs exerting pharmacologic effects via cytoplasmic receptors or enzymes, the vast majority of clinically useful drugs and endogenously secreted hormones mediate their effects via excitable surface transmembrane protein receptors (Schwinn, 1993).

The three classes of cell surface receptors as defined by their signal transduction mechanisms are categorized at G protein-coupled receptors, ligand-gated ion channels, and receptor-linked enzymes. These surface receptor proteins act as signal transudcers by binding extracellular signaling molecules and converting this information into intracellular signals that alter target cell function. G protein-coupled receptors interact with specific G proteins in plasma membranes which in turn activates or inhibits enzymes or ion channels. G protein-coupled receptors constitute the largest family of cell surface receptors and they mediate the cellular responses to diverse extracellular signals including hormones, neurotransmitters and local mediators. A hallmark of signal transduction by G protein-coupled receptors is their ability to amplify extracellular signals. Enzyme-linked cell surface receptors are a heterogeneous group of receptors that are associated with intracellular enzymes (tyrosine kinases, guanylate cyclases) and receptor binding activates intrinsic catalytic activity.

Excitable Transmembrane Proteins

Excitable transmembrane proteins are represented by (a) voltage-sensitive ion channels, (b) ligand-gated ion channels (ionotropic receptors), and (c) transmembrane receptors (Schwinn, 1993).

Voltage-Sensitive Ion Channels

Voltage-sensitive ion channels open and close in response to changes in voltage across cell membranes and are represented by classic ion channels, such as sodium, chloride, potassium, and calcium channels. Voltage-gated ion channels are present in neurons, skeletal muscles, and endocrine cells. At normal resting membrane potentials (usually −60 to −80 mV) these channels remain closed. When cell membranes are depolarized (become less negative) these ion channels undergo conformational changes such that the ion channel pore opens and ions pass through (10^4 to 10^5 ions flow per millisecond and thousands of channels may open during a single action potential). Voltage-gated ion channels are protein complexes formed by the association of several individual subunits. The largest subunit of each voltage-gated ion channel is termed the alpha subunit.

Ligand-Gated Ion Channels

Ligand-gated ion channels include acetylcholine receptors (nAChRs), serotonin receptors ($5HT_3$), gamma-aminobutyric acid receptors ($GABA_A$), and glycine receptors. These receptors function as receptor-ion channel complexes in which the ion channel is an integral part of a larger and more complex transmembrane protein. Each of these receptors is a pentamer, composed of five homologous subunits, each with four transmembrane segments and an extracellular terminus that contains residues that form the neurotransmitter binding sites. Two ligand-gated ion channels are cation-selective and excitatory (nAChRs, $5HT_3$) and two are anion-selective and inhibitory ($GABA_A$, glycine). A second family of ligand-gated ion channels is activated by glutamate, the principal excitatory neurotransmitter in the CNS. Different combinations of subunits form ligand-gated ion channels that are activated by the selective ligands *N*-methyl-D-aspartate (NMDA), alpha-amino-3-hydroxy-5-methylisoxazole-4-propionic acid (AMPA) and kainate. Ligand-gated ion channels open and close in response to changes in the presence of extracellular ligands (neurotransmitters) and are involved primarily in fast synaptic transmission between excitable cells. Specific neurotransmitters bind to these receptors and transiently open or close the associated ion channels in the absence of second messengers to alter ion permeability of the plasma membrtanes and thus membrane potentials. The common structural pattern for ligand-gated ion channels is a pentamer of subunits surrounding a central ion pore (Yost, 1993). Activation of ion channels is dependent on continued occupation of the receptors by ligand and is rapidly reversible on ligand dissociation allowing these channels to mediate rapid onset and rapidly reversible cell signalling. NMDA receptors possess unique properties among ligand-gated ion channels that includes voltage sensitivity in addition to glutamate sensitivity, the requirement for glycine as a co-agonist, and blockade by magnesium ions. Baseline potassium ion channels are not voltage-gated but are always open and thus are likely to function to maintain negative transmembrane potentials.

Ligand-gated ion channels are important targets for drugs administered during anesthesia (Dingledine et al., 1999). Examples include actions of neuromuscular blocking drugs on nAChRs, barbiturates and benzodiazepines on $GABA_A$ receptors and ketamine on NMDA receptors. Excitatory neurotransmitters (acetylcholine, glutamate) open sodium ion channels which results in depolarization of cell membranes. Inhibitory neurotransmitters (GABA, glycine) open chloride ion channels and hyperpolarize cell membranes thus preventing depolarization. A subclass of ligand-gated ion channels includes receptors for intracellular messengers that control calcium ion channels and regulation of intracellular calcium concentrations (ryanodine receptors, IP_3 receptors).

There is compelling evidence for the role of the $GABA_A$ receptor-chloride ion complex in the neuronal mechanism of anesthesia (Tanelian et al., 1993). For example, anesthetics at clinically relevant concentrations enhance GABA-mediated inhibition by two primary actions (a) an increase in agonist affinity for $GABA_A$ receptors, and (b) a prolongation or augmentation of the chloride conductance that is gated by these receptors. Either of these actions results in CNS depression. Anesthetics comprising several chemically distinct classes of drugs can enhance GABA-mediated inhibition without an apparent structural requirement for the molecule involved. A lack of structural requirement has long been recognized among anesthetics and has been attributed to a lack of a specific anesthetic receptor. This view may now be modified as the existence of multiple receptor subtypes may explain the apparent lack of structural requirement for anesthetic molecules (Tanelian et al., 1993).

Transmembrane Receptors

The third type of excitable transmembrane proteins is transmembrane receptors that interact selectively with extracellular compounds (drugs, hormones, neurotransmitters) to initiate a cascade of biochemical changes that lead to the ultimate pharmacologic or physiologic response. Because transmembrane receptors are located in the lipid cell membrane, they are able to bind hydrophilic ligands located in the extracellular space. Thus, many water-soluble drugs do not have to cross lipid bilayers to interact with cells. This process, however, necessitates a mechanism by which transmembrane receptors notify the cell of receptor occupancy by a ligand such as an exogenous drug. This process is frequently referred to as *signal transduction*, which often involves guanine nucleotide proteins (G proteins) (see Fig. 1-10) (Schwinn, 1993).

Receptor Families

Receptors are grouped and categorized as members of membrane receptor families.

Gamma-Aminobutyric Acid Receptors

Activation of the $GABA_A$-chloride channel (receptor) results in cell hyperpolarization or an increase in ion conductance that prevents depolarization, thereby inhibiting neuronal activity. Such activation by benzodiazepines, barbiturates, and propofol enhances endogenous $GABA_A$-mediated inhibition in the CNS, providing a neurobiologic basis for the hypnotic and sedative effects of these drugs (Fig. 1-11) (Lynch and Pancrazio, 1994; Tanelian et al., 1993). Volatile anesthetics have a similar action with regard to activation of the $GABA_A$-chloride channel (see Fig. 1-11) (Lynch and Pancrazio, 1994). GABA is the major inhibitory neurotransmitter of the mammalian brain and is responsible for most fast synaptic inhibition of neurons. Approximately one-third of all synapses in the CNS are responsive to GABA. GABA is not pharmacologically active when administered systemically because it cannot cross the blood-brain barrier.

A complete anesthetic adequate for surgery cannot be provided by the $GABA_A$-agonist activity of drugs such as benzodiazepines, barbiturates, propofol, or etomidate. Likewise, even large doses of opioids and $alpha_2$ agonists induce an incomplete anesthetic state that usually requires the addition of a hypnotic drug. Many of the opioids and $alpha_2$ agonists act by inhibiting presynaptic calcium ion

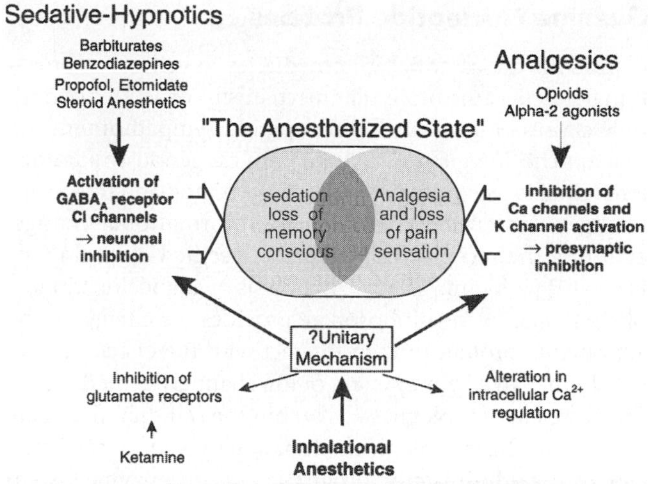

Figure 1-11. The major pathways for sedative-hypnotics and analgesics in generating the anesthetized state considered to be characteristic of volatile anesthetics. (From Lynch C, Pancrazio JJ. Snails, spiders, and stereospecificity—is there a role for calcium channels in anesthetic mechanisms? *Anesthesiology* 1994;81:1–5; with permission.)

channels responsible for activating transmitter release (see Fig. 1-11) (Lynch and Pancrazio, 1994). Activation of $GABA_A$ channels and decreased calcium influx produced independently by hypnotic drugs and opioids, respectively, may be a singular response produced by volatile anesthetics.

Glycine Receptors

Glycine receptors are closely related to $GABA_A$ receptors. They are inhibitory receptors that are selectively permeable to anions and mediate rapid inhibitory synaptic transmission, primarily in the spinal cord. Unlike $GABA_A$ receptors which form functional receptors only as heteromers, glycine receptors are homonomers of alpha subunits, of which several subtypes exist. Like $GABA_A$ receptors, the activity of glycine receptors is enhanced by volatile anesthetics (Mihic et al., 1997).

5-Hydroxytryptamine (5-HT) Receptors

Many subtypes of 5-HT receptors exist but with the execption of the $5HT_3$ subtype, all are metabotropic (G-protein coupled). Ionotropic 5-HT receptors are excitatory, selectively permeable to cations and exert a variety of effects in the CNS including anxiolysis, analgesia, and emetic.

Glutamate Receptors

Glutamate is an excitatory neurotransmitter and receptors are widely expressed in various types of glial cells. Because glutamic acid does not cross the blood-brain barrier, it must originate from local metabolism. Glutamate acts via metabotropic and ionotropic receptors. Ionotropic glutamate receptors include AMPA, NMDA, and kainate receptors. AMPA receptors mediate fast excitatory transmission at most synapses in the CNS.

Guanine Nucleotide Proteins

G proteins are essential intermediaries in cell communication that reflect the molecular mechanisms of actions of multiple classes of drugs including opioids, sympathomimetics, and anticholinergics (Yost, 1993). An exogenously administered drug is recognized by a specific receptor, and this receptor-ligand interaction induces a conformational change, enabling the receptor to activate a specific G protein (see Fig. 1-10) (Schwinn, 1993). Hydrolysis of guanosine triphosphate to guanosine diphosphate provides the energy for the activated G protein to then interact with the effector molecule (either an enzyme system or ion channel) to mediate the final cascade of biologic steps within the cell that ultimately lead to the pharmacologic or physiologic response characteristic of the administered drug. The effector enzyme system may be activated or inhibited, whereas the ion channel may open or close in response to the G protein activation.

Many different transmembrane receptors are part of the large superfamily of G protein–coupled receptors. Examples of clinically important protein-coupled receptor systems include adrenergic, opioid, muscarinic cholinergic, dopamine, and histamine receptors. Multiple subtypes of receptors ($alpha_1$ and $alpha_2$, $beta_1$ and $beta_2$, mu_1 and mu_2, H_1 and H_2) exist, and for adrenergic receptors these distinct subtypes have been cloned (Schwinn, 1993). For example, there are differences in the ligand-binding properties for acetylcholine at cholinergic nicotinic receptors present in ganglia of the autonomic nervous system compared with those at the neuromuscular junction. This difference is emphasized by nondepolarizing neuromuscular-blocking drugs that act at nicotinic receptors at the neuromuscular junction but exert minimal or no effect at nicotinic receptors in autonomic ganglia.

Concentration of Receptors

The concentration of receptors in the lipid portion of cell membranes is dynamic, either increasing (up-regulation) or decreasing (down-regulation) in response to specific stimuli. For example, an excess of endogenous ligand, as in a patient with a pheochromocytoma, results in a decrease in the concentration of beta-adrenergic receptors in cell membranes in an attempt to decrease the intensity of stimulation. Likewise, prolonged treatment of asthma with a beta agonist may result in tachyphylaxis associated with a decrease in the concentration of receptors. Conversely, chronic interference with the activity of receptors as produced by a beta antagonist may result in increased numbers of receptors in cell membranes such that an exaggerated response (hypersensitivity) occurs if the blockade is abruptly reversed, as by the sudden discontinuation of propranolol in the perioperative period. Disease states may reflect the inappropriate regulation of the concentration of receptors in cell membranes. For example, antibodies against beta-adrenergic receptors may occur in patients with asthma, leading to a predominance of bronchoconstrictor activity. Patients with myasthenia gravis often manifest antibodies to receptors that respond to acetylcholine.

Changing concentrations of receptors in cell membranes emphasize that receptors determine that pharmacologic responses to drugs are not static but rather dynamic. This dynamic state is modulated by a variety of exogenous and endogenous factors that may influence the pharmacologic responses to drugs in different people or the same individual at different times. If this concept is kept in mind, variable pharmacologic responses often evoked by drugs become more predictable.

Characteristics of Drug-Receptor Interaction

A drug or endogenous substance (ligand) is an agonist if the drug-receptor interaction elicits a pharmacologic effect by an alteration in the functional properties of receptors. A drug is an antagonist when it interacts with receptors but does not alter their functional properties and, at the same time, prevents their response to an agonist. If inhibition can be overcome by increasing the concentration of agonist, the antagonist drug is said to produce *competitive blockade*. This type of antagonism is produced by neuromuscular-blocking drugs and beta-adrenergic antagonists that act reversibly at receptors. An agonist drug that binds only weakly to receptors may produce minimal pharmacologic effects even though a maximal concentration is present. Such a drug is known as a *partial agonist*. Examples of partial agonists are the opioid agonist-antagonist drugs.

Receptor Occupancy Theory

Traditionally, it is assumed that the intensity of effect produced by binding of drugs to receptors is proportional to the fraction of receptors occupied by the drug. Conceptually, maximal drug effects occur when all the receptors are occupied. This *receptor occupancy theory*, however, does not explain differences in intrinsic activity between drugs that occupy the same number of receptors and produce responses ranging from full stimulation to antagonism.

State of Receptor Activation

A modification of the receptor occupancy theory that is consistent with differences in intrinsic activity of drugs is the concept of activated and nonactivated states for receptors. In this theory, when an agonist binds to receptors, it converts the receptors from a nonactivated to an activated state. Full agonists are able to convert most of the receptors they occupy to the activated state; partial agonists convert only a fraction of the receptors they occupy to the activated state; and antagonists do not activate any of the receptors they occupy to the activated state. Increasing doses of a partial agonist in the presence of a maximal effect produced by an agonist results in competitive antagonism of the effect of the agonist. Conversely, addition of a partial agonist in the presence of less than a maximal effect produced by the agonist will result in additional drug action to the maximal effect of the partial agonist. It is likely that opioid agonist-antagonists act in this way when administered in the presence of opioid agonists (see Chapter 3).

Drug-Receptor Bond

The action of drugs on receptors requires binding between drugs and receptors by a physicochemical force. It is likely that multiple types of bonds between drugs and receptors occur involving reactive groups on drugs and complementary regions of receptors. A covalent bond is formed by sharing a pair of electrons between atoms, thus forming a strong bond that plays little role in reversible binding of drugs to receptors. *Covalent* bonding is involved in the inactivation of cholinesterase enzyme by organophosphates (insecticides) and alpha-adrenergic blockade as produced by pheoxybenzamine. *Ionic* bonds arise from electrostatic forces existing between groups of opposite charge. Acidic or basic drugs that are ionized at plasma pH can combine readily with charged groups on proteins. *Hydrogen* bonds occur between hydroxyl or amino groups and an electronegative carboxyl oxygen group. *Van der Waals forces* are weak bonds between two atoms or groups of atoms of different molecules. When the configuration between drug and receptor is sterically similar, these bonds can form readily.

Plasma Drug Concentrations

Plasma drug concentrations are a reliable monitor of therapy only when interpreted in parallel with the clinical course of the patient. Furthermore, serial measurements of plasma drug concentrations at selected intervals are more informative than isolated determinations. It is misleading to measure the plasma concentrations of drugs during the rapidly changing distribution phase. For example, after the rapid IV administration of a nondepolarizing muscle relaxant, the plasma concentration is decreasing before the peak pharmacologic effect of the drug is manifest. At a later time, when the gradient is reversed, drug concentrations at receptors are probably higher than that existing in plasma. In this regard, individual pharmacokinetic characteristics of each drug must be considered to determine an optimal time during the elimination phase for measurement of a steady-state plasma concentration of drug.

It is important to know whether the analytical technique used to determined the plasma concentration of drug measures both free and protein-bound drug. Most often, the technique for determining the plasma concentration of drug measures the total concentration of drug and does not discriminate between protein-bound or free drug. Nevertheless, pharmacologic effects usually reflect only the free fraction of drug in the plasma. Indeed, drug toxicity from phenytoin or diazepam is more frequent in patients with associated hypoalbuminemia, suggesting that measurement of the free fraction of these drugs would permit better prediction of drug toxicity.

Relationship of Plasma and Receptor Drug Concentration

In patients, the plasma concentration of a drug is the most practical measurement for monitoring the receptor concentration. The plasma concentration should be representative of the receptor concentration of drug during Vd_{ss}. Typically, there is a direct relationship between the (a) dose of drug administered, (b) resulting plasma concentration, and (c) intensity of drug effect. Likewise, the onset and duration of drug effect are related to the increase and decrease of the drug concentration at responsive receptors as reflected by corresponding changes in the plasma concentration.

Initial and Maintenance Doses

An initial loading dose is necessary to establish a therapeutic concentration of drug promptly. This initial dose will be larger than the subsequent maintenance dose. Changes in Vd will influence the size of the initial dose. For example, in the presence of an increased Vd, the drug is diluted in a large volume, and thus a larger initial dose is required to produce the same plasma concentration of drug that would be obtained with a smaller dose and a normal Vd. The maintenance dose of a drug must be adjusted downward in the presence of renal or hepatic dysfunction to prevent drug accumulation due to a prolonged elimination half-time. This adjustment can be achieved by decreasing the maintenance dose or increasing the time interval between doses.

Intermittent doses result in abrupt increases followed by decreases in the plasma concentration of drug such that a therapeutic plasma level is not sustained. A continuous variable-rate infusion of drug is more likely to maintain the plasma concentration in a therapeutic range without the wide oscillations characteristic of intermittent injections.

PHARMACOKINETICS OF INHALED ANESTHETICS

The pharmacokinetics of inhaled anesthetics describes their (a) absorption (uptake) from alveoli into pulmonary capillary blood, (b) distribution in the body, (c) metabolism, and (d) elimination, principally via the lungs. The pharmacokinetics of volatile anesthetics may be influenced by aging reflecting decreases in lean body mass and increases in body fat (Strum et al., 1991). These factors should increase the apparent Vd of these drugs in the elderly, especially for those anesthetics most soluble in fat. In addition, decreased hepatic function, together with decreased pulmonary gas exchange (secondary to lower metabolic rate) may decrease anesthetic clearance with age. Furthermore, decreased cardiac output in the elderly decreases tissue perfusion, increases time constants, and

$$P_A \rightleftharpoons Pa \rightleftharpoons Pbr$$

Figure 1-12. The alveolar partial pressure (PA) of an inhaled anesthetic is in equilibrium with the arterial blood (Pa) and brain (Pbr). As a result, the PA is an indirect measurement of anesthetic partial pressure at the brain.

may be associated with an altered regional distribution of anesthetics. Opposite effects on the pharmacokinetics of inhaled anesthetics might be expected in the very young.

A series of partial pressure gradients beginning at the anesthetic machine serve to propel the inhaled anesthetic across various barriers (alveoli, capillaries, cell membranes) to their sites of action in the CNS. The principal objective of inhalation anesthesia is to achieve a constant and optimal brain partial pressure of the inhaled anesthetic.

The brain and all other tissues equilibrate with the partial pressures of inhaled anesthetics delivered to them by arterial blood (Pa) (Fig. 1-12). Likewise, arterial blood equilibrates with the alveolar partial pressures (PA) of anesthetics. This emphasizes that the PA of inhaled anesthetics mirrors the brain partial pressure (Pbr). This is the reason that PA is used as an index of (a) depth of anesthesia, (b) recovery from anesthesia, and (c) anesthetic equal potency (MAC). It is important to recognize that equilibration between the two phases means the same partial pressure exists in both phases. Equilibration does not mean equality of concentrations in two biophases. Understanding those factors that determine the PA and thus the Pbr permits control of the doses of inhaled anesthetics delivered to the brain so as to maintain a constant and optimal depth of anesthesia.

Determinants of Alveolar Partial Pressure

The PA and ultimately the Pbr of inhaled anesthetics are determined by input (delivery) into alveoli minus uptake (loss) of the drug from alveoli into arterial blood (Table 1-6). Input of anesthetics into alveoli depends on the (a) inhaled partial pressure (PI), (b) alveolar ventilation, and (c) characteristics of the anesthetic breathing (delivery) system. In addition, the patient's functional residual capacity (FRC) influences the PA that is achieved. Uptake of inhaled anesthetics from alveoli into the pulmonary capillary blood depends on (a) solubility of the anesthetic in body tissues, (b) cardiac output, and (c) alveolar to venous partial pressure differences (A-vD).

Inhaled Partial Pressure

A high PI delivered from the anesthetic machine is required during initial administration of the anesthetic. A high initial input offsets the impact of uptake, accelerating induction of anesthesia as reflected by the rate of rise in the PA and thus the Pbr. With time, as uptake into the blood decreases, the PI should be decreased to match the decreased anesthetic uptake and therefore maintain a constant and optimal Pbr. If the PI is maintained constant with time, the PA and Pbr will increase progressively as uptake diminishes.

TABLE 1-6.
FACTORS DETERMINING PARTIAL PRESSURE GRADIENTS NECESSARY FOR ESTABLISHMENT OF ANESTHESIA

Transfer of inhaled anesthetic from anesthetic machine to alveoli (anesthetic input)
Inspired partial pressure
Alveolar ventilation
Characteristics of anesthetic breathing system
Functional residual capacity
Transfer of inhaled anesthetic from alveoli to arterial blood (anesthetic loss)
Blood:gas partition coefficient
Cardiac output
Alveolar-to-venous partial pressure difference
Transfer of inhaled anesthetic from arterial blood to brain (anesthetic loss)
Brain:blood partition coefficient
Cerebral blood flow
Arterial-to-venous partial pressure difference

Concentration Effect

The impact of PI on the rate of rise of the PA of an inhaled anesthetic is known as the *concentration effect* (Fig. 1-13) (Eger, 1963). The concentration effect states that the higher

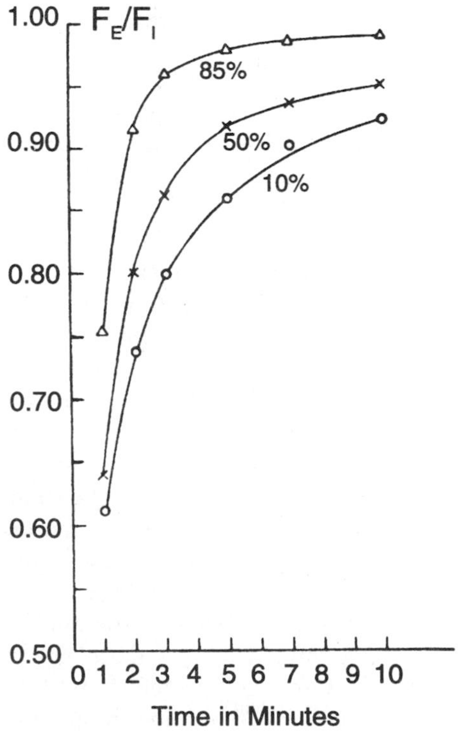

Figure 1-13. The impact of the inhaled concentration of an anesthetic on the rate at which the alveolar concentration increases toward the inspired (F_E/F_I) is known as the *concentration effect*. (From Eger EI. Effect of inspired anesthetic concentration on the rate of rise of alveolar concentration. *Anesthesiology* 1963;24: 153–157; with permission.)

the PI, the more rapidly the PA approaches the PI. The higher PI provides anesthetic molecule input to offset uptake and thus speeds the rate at which the PA increases.

The concentration effect results from (a) a concentrating effect, and (b) an augmentation of tracheal inflow (Stoelting and Eger, 1969a). The concentrating effect reflects concentration of the inhaled anesthetic in a smaller lung volume due to uptake of all gases in the lung. At the same time, anesthetic input via tracheal inflow is increased to fill the space (void) produced by uptake of gases.

Second-Gas Effect

The second-gas effect reflects the ability of high-volume uptake of one gas (first gas) to accelerate the rate of increase of the PA of a concurrently administered "companion" gas (second gas) (Fig. 1-14) (Epstein et al., 1964). For example, the initial large-volume uptake of nitrous oxide accelerates the uptake of companion (second) gases such as oxygen and volatile anesthetics. This increased uptake of the second gas reflects increased tracheal inflow of all the inhaled gases (first and second gases) and concentration of the second gas or gases in a smaller lung volume (concentrating effect) due to the high-volume uptake of the first gas (Fig. 1-15) (Stoelting and Eger, 1969a). Conceptually, the loss of lung volume may be compensated for by decreased expired ventilation or reduction in lung volume as well as increased inspired ventilation (increased tracheal inflow). The implication that extra gas is routinely drawn into the lungs to compensate for loss of lung volume, is misleading if compensatory changes are based on decreased expired ventilation and/or a decrease in lung volume (Korman and Mapleson, 1997).

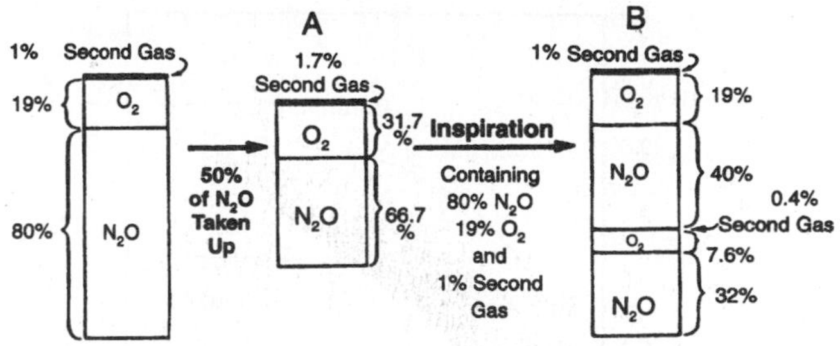

Figure 1-15. The second-gas effect results from a concentrating effect (**A**) and an augmentation of tracheal inflow (**B**). (From Stoelting RK, Eger EI. An additional explanation for the second gas effect: a concentrating effect. *Anesthesiology* 1969; 30:273–277; with permission.)

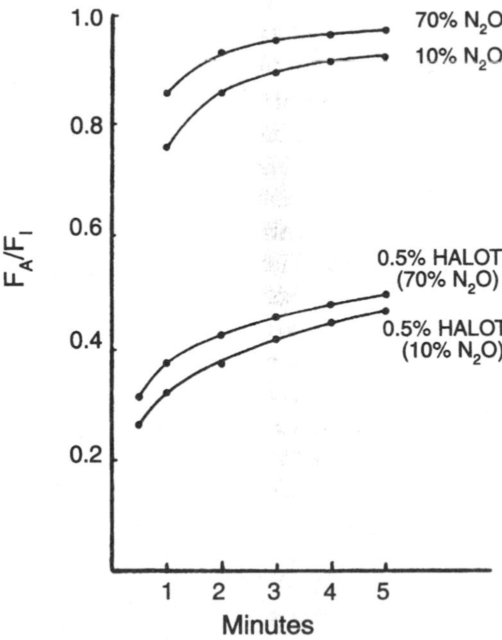

Figure 1-14. The second-gas effect is the accelerated increase in the alveolar concentration of a second gas, halothane (HALOTH), toward the inspired (F_A/F_I) in the presence of a high inhaled concentration of the first gas (N_2O). (From Epstein RM, Rackow H, Salanitre E, et al. Influence of the concentration effect on the uptake of anesthetic mixtures: the second gas effect. *Anesthesiology* 1964; 25:364–371; with permission.)

Alveolar Ventilation

Increased alveolar ventilation, like PI, promotes input of anesthetics to offset uptake. The net effect is a more rapid rate of increase in the PA toward the PI and thus induction of anesthesia. In addition to the increased input, the decreased $Pa{CO_2}$ produced by hyperventilation of the lungs decreases cerebral blood flow. Conceivably, the impact of increased input on the rate of rise of the PA would be offset by decreased delivery of anesthetic to the brain. Decreased alveolar ventilation decreases input and thus slows the establishment of a PA and a Pbr necessary for the induction of anesthesia. The greater the alveolar ventilation to FRC ratio, the more rapid is the rate of increase in the PA. In neonates, this ratio is approximately 5:1 compared with only 1.5:1 in adults, reflecting the greater metabolic rate in neonates compared with adults. As a result, the rate of increase of PA toward the PI and thus the induction of anesthesia is more rapid in neonates than in adults (Fig. 1-16) (Salanitre and Rackow, 1969).

Spontaneous versus Mechanical Ventilation

Inhaled anesthetics influence their own uptake by virtue of dose-dependent depressant effects on alveolar ventilation. This, in effect, is a negative-feedback protective mechanism that prevents establishment of an excessive depth of anesthesia (delivery of anesthesia is decreased when ventilation is decreased) when a high PI is administered during spontaneous breathing (Fig. 1-17) (Gibbons et al., 1977). As anesthetic input decreases in parallel with decreased ventilation, anesthetic present in tissues is redistributed from tissues in which it is present in high concentrations (brain) to other tissues in which it is present in low concentrations (skeletal muscles). When the concentration (partial pressure) in the brain decreases to a certain threshold, ventilation increases

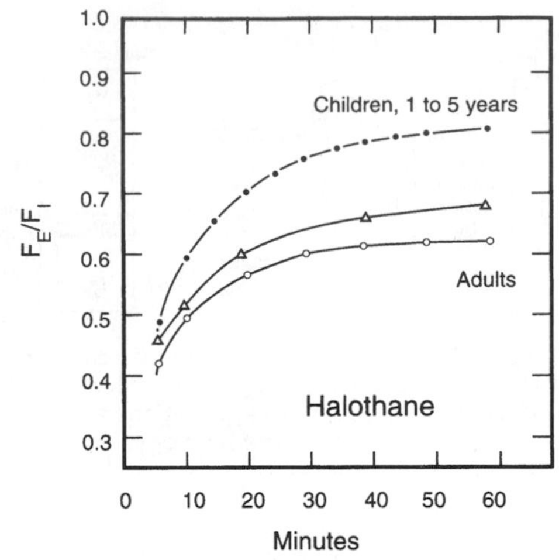

Figure 1-16. The rate at which the alveolar concentration (F_E) increases toward the inspired (F_I) for halothane (HALO 0.5%) in children 1 to 5 years of age is more rapid than in adults. (From Salanitre E, Rackow H. The pulmonary exchange of nitrous oxide and halothane in infants and children. *Anesthesiology* 1969; 30:388–392; with permission.)

and delivery of the anesthetic to the lungs increases. This protective mechanism against development of an excessive depth of anesthesia (anesthetic overdose) is lost when mechanical ventilation of the lungs replaces spontaneous breathing.

Impact of Solubility

The impact of changes in alveolar ventilation on the rate of increase in the PA toward the PI depends on the solubility of the anesthetic in blood. For example, changes in alveolar ventilation influence the rate of increase of the PA of a soluble anesthetic (halothane, isoflurane) more than a poorly soluble anesthetic (nitrous oxide, desflurane, sevoflurane). Indeed, the rate of increase in the PA of nitrous oxide is rapid regardless of the alveolar ventilation. This occurs because uptake of nitrous oxide is limited because of its poor solubility in blood. Conversely, uptake of a more blood-soluble anesthetic is larger, and increasing alveolar ventilation will accelerate the rate at which the PA of the soluble anesthetic approaches the PI. This emphasizes that changing from spontaneous breathing to mechanical (controlled) ventilation of the lungs, which also is likely to be associated with increased alveolar ventilation, will probably increase the depth of anesthesia (PA) produced by a more blood-soluble anesthetic.

Anesthetic Breathing System

Characteristics of the anesthetic breathing system that influence the rate of increase of the PA are the (a) volume of the external breathing system, (b) solubility of the inhaled anesthetics in the rubber or plastic components of the breathing system, and (c) gas inflow from the anesthetic machine. The volume of the anesthetic breathing system acts as a buffer to slow achievement of the PA. High gas inflow rates (5 to 10 liters/minute) from the anesthetic machine negate this buffer effect. Solubility of inhaled anesthetics in the components of the anesthetic breathing system initially slows the rate at which the PA increases. At the conclusion of the administration of an anesthetic,

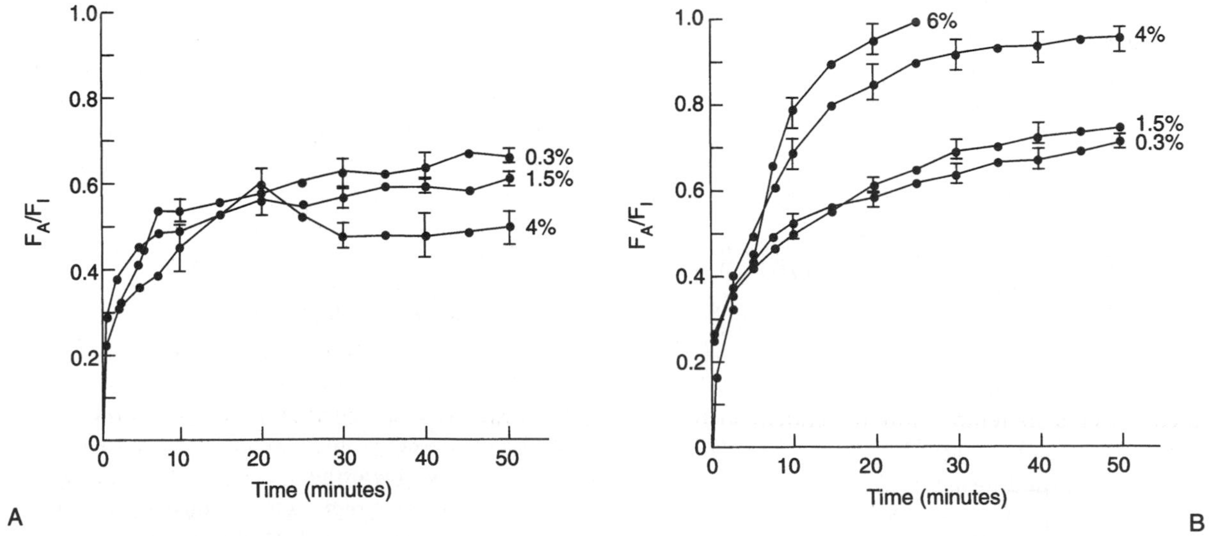

Figure 1-17. Effect of the mode of ventilation on the rate of increase of the alveolar concentration (F_A) of halothane toward the inspired concentration (F_I) as determined in an animal model. Negative feedback inhibition of spontaneous ventilation (**A**) limits the F_A/F_I to 0.6 for all the inspired concentrations of halothane. The positive feedback effect of controlled ventilation (**B**) results in ratios of the F_A/F_I that approach 1.0 and excessive depressant effects of halothane on the cardiovascular system at the higher inspired concentrations of the anesthetic. (Data are mean ± SD.) (From Gibbons RT, Steffey EP, Eger EI. The effect of spontaneous versus controlled ventilation on the rate of rise in the alveolar halothane concentration in dogs. *Anesth Analg* 1977;56:32–37; with permission.)

TABLE 1-7.
COMPARATIVE SOLUBILITIES OF INHALED ANESTHETICS

	Blood:Gas Partition Coefficient	Brain:Blood Partition Coefficient	Muscle:Blood Partition Coefficient	Fat:Blood Partition Coefficient	Oil:Gas Partition Coefficient
Soluble					
Methoxyflurane	12	2	1.3	48.8	970
Intermediately soluble					
Halothane	2.54	1.9	3.4	51.1	224
Enflurane	1.90	1.5	1.7	36.2	98
Isoflurane	1.46	1.6	2.9	44.9	98
Poorly soluble					
Nitrous oxide	0.46	1.1	1.2	2.3	1.4
Desflurane	0.42	1.3	2.0	27.2	18.7
Sevoflurane	0.69	1.7	3.1	47.5	55
Xexon	0.115				

Source: Data from Eger EI. *Desflurane (Suprane): a compendium and reference.* Nutley, NJ: Anaquest, 1993:1–119; and Yasuda N, Targ AC, Eger EI. Solubility of I-653, sevoflurane, isoflurane, and halothane in human tissues. *Anesth Analg* 1989;69:370–373.

however, reversal of the partial pressure gradient in the anesthetic breathing system results in elution of the anesthetic, which slows the rate at which the PA decreases.

Solubility

The solubility of the inhaled anesthetics in blood and tissues is denoted by the partition coefficient (Table 1-7) (Eger, 1993; Yasuda et al., 1989). A partition coefficient is a distribution ratio describing how the inhaled anesthetic distributes itself between two phases at equilibrium (partial pressures equal in both phases). For example, a blood:gas partition coefficient of 0.5 means that the concentration of inhaled anesthetic in the blood is half that present in the alveolar gases when the partial pressures of the anesthetic in these two phases is identical. Similarly a brain:blood partition coefficient of 2 indicates a concentration of anesthetic in the brain is twice that in the blood when the partial pressures of anesthetic are identical at both sites.

Partition coefficients may be thought of as reflecting the relative capacity of each phase to accept anesthetic. Partition coefficients are temperature dependent such that the solubility of a gas in a liquid is decreased when the temperature of the liquid increases.

Blood:Gas Partition Coefficients

The rate of increase of the PA toward the PI (maintained constant by mechanical ventilation of the lungs) is inversely related to the solubility of the anesthetic in blood (Fig. 1-18) (Yasuda et al., 1991). Based on their blood:gas partition coefficients, inhaled anesthetics are categorized traditionally as soluble, intermediately soluble, and poorly soluble (see Table 1-7) (Eger, 1993; Yasuda et al., 1989). Blood can be considered a pharmacologically inactive reservoir, the size of which is determined by the solubility of the anesthetic in blood. When the blood:gas partition coefficient is high, a large amount of anesthetic must be dissolved in the blood before the Pa equilibrates with the PA. For example, the high blood solubility of methoxyflurane slows the rate at which the PA and Pa increase relative to the PI, and the induction of anesthesia is slow. The impact of high blood solubility on the rate of increase of the PA can be offset to some extent by increasing the PI above that required for maintenance of anesthesia. This is termed the *overpressure* technique and may be used to speed the induction of anesthesia, recognizing that sustained delivery of a high PI will result in an anesthetic overdose.

When blood solubility is low, minimal amounts of inhaled anesthetic must be dissolved before equilibration is achieved; therefore, the rate of increase of PA and Pa, and thus onset-of-drug effects such as the induction of anesthesia, are rapid. For example, the inhalation of a constant PI of nitrous oxide, desflurane, or sevoflurane for about 10 minutes results in a PA that is ≥80% of the PI (see Fig. 1-18) (Yasuda et al., 1991). Use of an overpressure technique with sevoflurane is more readily accepted by patients because this anesthetic is less pungent than desflurane. Indeed, one or more vital capacity breaths of high concentrations of sevoflurane (7% with 66% nitrous oxide) may result in loss of the eyelash reflex (Meretoja et al., 1996).

Associated with the rapid increase in the Pa of nitrous oxide is the absorption of several liters (up to 10 liters during the first 10 to 15 minutes) of this gas, reflecting its common administration at inhaled concentrations of 60% to 70%. This high-volume absorption of nitrous oxide is

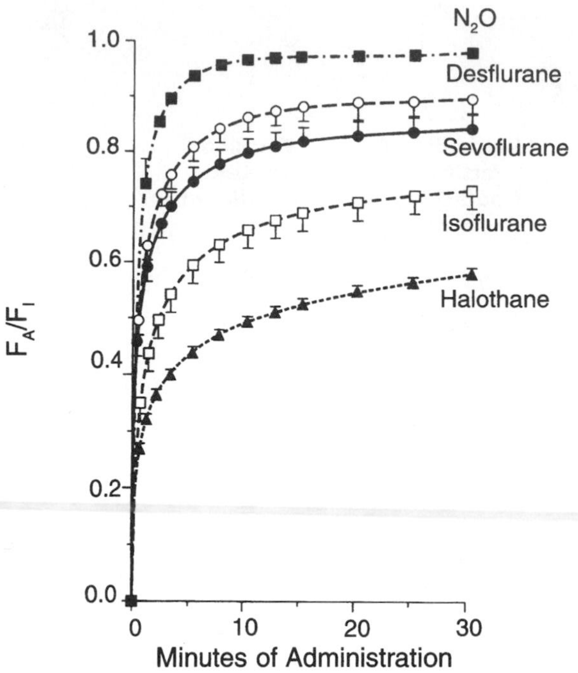

Figure 1-18. The pharmacokinetics of inhaled anesthetics during the induction of anesthesia is defined as the ratio of the end-tidal anesthetic concentration (F_A) to the inspired anesthetic concentration (F_I). Consistent with their relative blood:gas partition coefficients, the F_A/F_I of poorly soluble anesthetics (nitrous oxide, desflurane, sevoflurane) increases more rapidly than that of anesthetics with greater solubility in blood. A decrease in the rate of change in the F_A/F_I after 5 to 15 minutes (three time constants) reflects decreased tissue uptake of the anesthetic as the vessel-rich group tissues become saturated. (Data are mean ± SD.) (From Yasuda N, Lockhart SH, Eger EI, et al. Comparison of kinetics of sevoflurane and isoflurane in humans. *Anesth Analg* 1991;72:316–324; with permission.)

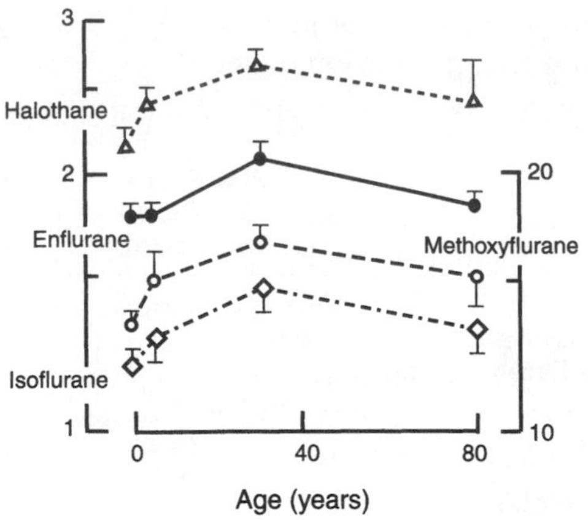

Figure 1-19. Blood:gas partition coefficients are 18% less in neonates compared with adults. (Mean ± SD.) (From Lerman J, Gregory GA, Willis MM, Eger EI II. Age and solubility of volatile anesthetics in blood. *Anesthesiology* 1984;61:139–143; with permission.)

responsible for several unique effects of nitrous oxide when it is administered in the presence of volatile anesthetics or air-containing cavities (see the sections on Concentration Effect, Second-Gas Effect, and Nitrous Oxide Transfer to Closed Gas Spaces).

Percutaneous loss of inhaled anesthetics occurs but is too small to influence the rate of increase in the PA (Stoelting and Eger, 1969b). With the possible exception of methoxyflurane, the magnitude of metabolism of inhaled anesthetics is too small to influence the rate of increase of the PA. This lack of effect reflects the large excess of anesthetic molecules administered and the saturation, by anesthetic concentrations of inhaled drugs, of enzymes responsible for anesthetic metabolism (Sawyer et al., 1971).

Blood:gas partition coefficients are altered by individual variations in water, lipid, and protein content and by the hematocrit of whole blood (Laasberg and Hedley-White, 1970; Ellis and Stoelting, 1975). For example, blood:gas partition coefficients are about 20% less in blood with a hematocrit of 21% compared with blood with a hematocrit of 43%. Presumably, this decreased solubility reflects the decrease in lipid-dissolving sites normally provided by erythrocytes. Conceivably, decreased solubility of volatile anesthetics in anemic blood would manifest as an increased rate of increase in the PA and a more rapid induction of anesthesia. Ingestion of a fatty meal alters the composition of blood, resulting in an approximately 20% increase in the solubility of volatile anesthetics in blood (Munson et al., 1978).

The solubility of inhaled anesthetics in blood varies with age (Fig. 1-19) (Lerman et al., 1984). The blood solubilities of halothane, enflurane, methoxyflurane, and isoflurane are about 18% less in neonates and the elderly compared to young adults. In contrast, the solubility of the less soluble anesthetic sevoflurane (presumably also true for desflurane) is not different in neonates and adults (Malviya and Lerman, 1990).

Tissue:Blood Partition Coefficients

Tissue:blood partition coefficients determine uptake of anesthetic into tissues and the time necessary for equilibration of tissues with the Pa. This time for equilibration can be estimated by calculating a time constant (amount of inhaled anesthetic that can be dissolved in the tissue divided by tissue blood flow) for each tissue. One time constant on an exponential curve represents 63% equilibration. Three time constants are equivalent to 95% equilibration. For volatile anesthetics, equilibration between the Pa and Pbr depends on the anesthetic's blood solubility and requires 5 to 15 minutes (three time constants). Fat has an enormous capacity to hold anesthetic, and this characteristic, combined with low blood flow to this tissue, prolongs the time required to narrow anesthetic partial pressure differences between arterial blood and fat. For example, equilibration of fat with isoflurane (three time constants) based on this drug's fat:blood partition coefficient and an assumed fat blood flow of 2–3/100 g/minute is estimated to be 25 to 46 hours. Fasting before elective operations results in transport of fat to the liver, which could increase anesthetic uptake by this organ and modestly slow the rate of increase in the PA of a volatile anesthetic during induction of anesthesia (Fassoulaki and Eger, 1986).

Oil:Gas Partition Coefficients

Oil:gas partition coefficients parallel anesthetic requirements. For example, an estimated MAC can be calculated as 150 divided by the oil:gas partition coefficient. The constant, 150, is the average value of the product of oil:gas solubility and MAC for several inhaled anesthetics with widely divergent lipid solubilities. Using this constant, the calculated MAC for a theoretical anesthetic with an oil:gas partition coefficient of 100 would be 1.5%.

Nitrous Oxide Transfer to Closed Gas Spaces

The blood:gas partition coefficient of nitrous oxide (0.46) is about 34 times greater than that of nitrogen (0.014). This differential solubility means that nitrous oxide can leave the blood to enter an air-filled cavity 34 times more rapidly than nitrogen can leave the cavity to enter blood. As a result of this preferential transfer of nitrous oxide, the volume or pressure of an air-filled cavity increases. Passage of nitrous oxide into an air-filled cavity surrounded by a compliant wall (intestinal gas, pneumothorax, pulmonary blebs, air bubbles) causes the gas space to expand. Conversely, passage of nitrous oxide into an air-filled cavity surrounded by a noncompliant wall (middle ear, cerebral ventricles, supratentorial space) causes an increase in intracavitary pressure.

The magnitude of volume or pressure increase is influenced by (a) partial pressure of nitrous oxide, (b) blood flow to the air-filled cavity, and (c) duration of nitrous oxide administration. In an animal model, the inhalation of 75% nitrous oxide doubles the volume of a pneumothorax in 10 minutes (Fig. 1-20) (Eger and Saidman, 1965). The finding emphasizes the high blood flow to this area.

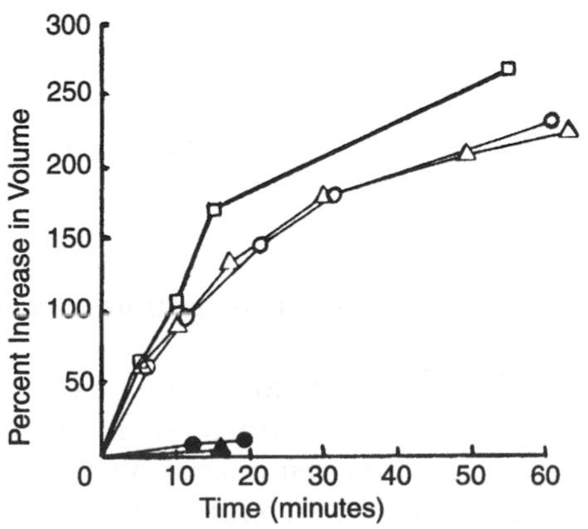

Figure 1-20. Inhalation of 75% nitrous oxide rapidly increases the volume of a pneumothorax (*open symbols*). Inhalation of oxygen (*solid symbols*) does not alter the volume of the pneumothorax. (From Eger EI, Saidman LJ. Hazards of nitrous oxide anesthesia in bowel obstruction and pneumothorax. *Anesthesiology* 1965;26: 61–66; with permission.)

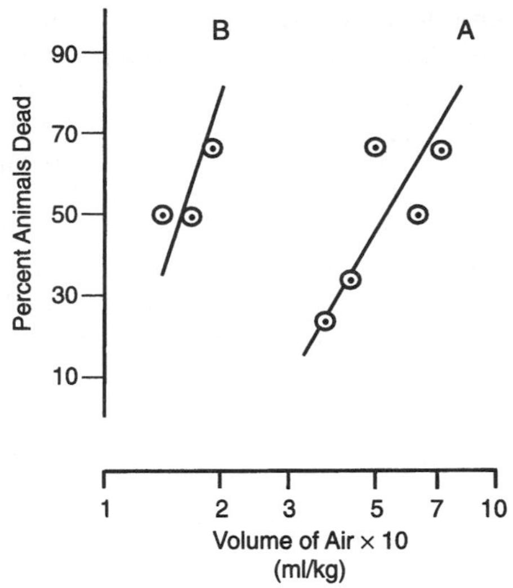

Figure 1-21. Nitrous oxide rapidly expands air bubbles as reflected by the volume of injected air necessary to produce 50% mortality in animals breathing nitrous oxide (0.16 mL/kg) (**A**) compared with animals breathing oxygen (0.55 mL/kg) (**B**). (From Munson ES, Merrick HC. Effect of nitrous oxide on venous air embolism. *Anesthesiology* 1966;27:783–787; with permission.)

Likewise, air bubbles (emboli) expand rapidly when exposed to nitrous oxide (Fig. 1-21) (Munson and Merrick, 1966). Nevertheless, in neurosurgical patients operated on in the sitting position, 50% nitrous oxide has no measurable effect on the incidence or severity of venous air embolism if its administration is discontinued immediately upon Doppler detection of venous air embolism (LoSasso et al., 1992). In contrast to the rapid expansion of a pneumothorax, the increase in bowel gas volume produced by nitrous oxide is slow and of questionable clinical significance in the absence of bowel obstruction.

The middle ear is an air-filled cavity that vents passively via the eustachian tube when pressure reaches 20 to 30 cm H_2O. Nitrous oxide diffuses into the middle ear more rapidly than nitrogen leaves, and middle ear pressures may increase if eustachian tube patency is compromised by inflammation or edema. Indeed, tympanic membrane rupture has been attributed to this mechanism after administration of nitrous oxide. Negative middle ear pressures may develop after discontinuation of nitrous oxide, leading to serous otitis. Nausea and vomiting that may follow general anesthesia may be due to multiple mechanisms, but the role of altered middle ear pressures as a result of nitrous oxide is a consideration.

Intraocular gas bubbles as used for internal retinal tamponade (retinal detachment, macular hole repair, complicated vitrectomy) may persist in the eye for up to 10 weeks following ocular surgery. Administration of nitrous oxide for periods as brief as 1 hour during this time period may result in rapid increases in the volume of intraocular gas within the rigid closed eye that is sufficient to compress the retinal artery with resulting visual loss (Vote et al., 2002).

Cardiopulmonary Bypass

Cardiopulmonary bypass produces changes in blood-gas solubility that depend on the constituents of the priming solution and temperature (Gedney and Ghosh, 1995). Nevertheless, the overall effect of hypothermic cardiopulmonary bypass and a crystalloid prime on blood-gas solubility is only 2%. Volatile anesthetics initiated during cardiopulmonary bypass take longer to equilibrate, whereas the same drugs already present when cardiopulmonary bypass is initiated are diluted, potentially changing the depth of anesthesia.

Cardiac Output

Cardiac output (pulmonary blood flow) influences uptake and therefore PA by carrying away either more or less anesthetic from the alveoli. An increased cardiac output results in more rapid uptake, so the rate of increase in the PA and thus the induction of anesthesia is slowed. A decreased cardiac output speeds the rate of increase of the PA, because there is less uptake to oppose input.

The effect of cardiac output on the rate of increase in the PA may seem paradoxical. For example, the uptake of more drug by an increased cardiac output should speed the rate of increase of partial pressures in tissues and thus narrow the A-vD for anesthetics. Indeed, an increase in cardiac output does hasten equilibration of tissue anesthetic partial pressures with the Pa. Nevertheless, the Pa is lower than it would be if cardiac output were normal. Conceptually, a change in cardiac output is analogous to the effect of a change in solubility. For example, doubling cardiac output increases the capacity of blood to hold anesthetic, just as solubility increases the capacity of the same volume of blood.

As with alveolar ventilation, changes in cardiac output most influence the rate of increase of the PA of a soluble anesthetic. Conversely, the rate of increase of the PA of a poorly soluble anesthetic, such as nitrous oxide, is rapid regardless of physiologic deviations of the cardiac output around its normal value. As a result, changes in cardiac output exert little influence on the rate of increase of the PA of nitrous oxide. In contrast, doubling the cardiac output will greatly increase the uptake of soluble anesthetic from alveoli, slowing the rate of increase of the PA. Conversely, a low cardiac output, as with shock, could produce an unexpectedly high PA of a soluble anesthetic.

Volatile anesthetics that depress cardiac output can exert a positive feedback response that contrasts with the negative (protective) feedback response on spontaneous breathing exerted by these drugs. For example, decreases in cardiac output due to an excessive dose of volatile anesthetic results in an increase in the PA, which further increases anesthetic depth and thus cardiac depression. The administration of a volatile anesthetic that depresses cardiac output, plus controlled ventilation of the lungs, results in a situation characterized by unopposed input of anesthetic via alveolar ventilation combined with decreased uptake because of decreased cardiac output. The net effect of this combination of events can be an unexpected, abrupt increase in the PA and an excessive depth of anesthesia.

Distribution of cardiac output will influence the rate of increase of the PA of an anesthetic. For example, increases in cardiac output are not necessarily accompanied by proportional increases in blood flow to all tissues. Preferential perfusion of vessel-rich group tissues when the cardiac output increases results in a more rapid increase in the PA of anesthetic than would occur if the increased cardiac output was distributed equally to all tissues. Indeed, infants have a relatively greater perfusion of vessel-rich group tissues than do adults and, consequently, show a faster rate of increase of the PA toward the PI (see Fig. 1-16) (Salanitre and Rackow, 1969).

Impact of a Shunt

In the absence of an intracardiac or intrapulmonary right-to-left shunt, it is valid to assume that the PA and Pa of inhaled anesthetics are essentially identical. When a right-to-left shunt is present, the diluting effect of the shunted blood on the partial pressure of anesthetic in blood coming from ventilated alveoli results in a decrease in the Pa and a slowing in the induction of anesthesia. Monitoring the end-tidal concentration of anesthetic or carbon dioxide reveals a gradient between the PA and Pa in which the PA underestimates the Pa. A similar mechanism is responsible for the decrease in Pa_{O_2} and the gradient between the PA and Pa in the presence of a right-to-left shunt.

The relative impact of a right-to-left shunt on the rate of increase in the Pa depends on the solubility of the anesthetic. For example, a right-to-left shunt slows the rate of increase of the Pa of a poorly soluble anesthetic more than that of a soluble anesthetic (Stoelting and Longnecker, 1972). This occurs because uptake of a soluble anesthetic offsets dilutional effects of shunted blood on the Pa. Uptake of a poorly soluble drug is minimal, and dilutional effects on the Pa are relatively unopposed. This impact of solubility in the presence of a right-to-left shunt is opposite to that observed with changes in cardiac output and alveolar ventilation. All factors considered, it seems unlikely that a right-to-left shunt alone will alter the speed of induction of anesthesia significantly.

Left-to-right tissue shunts (arteriovenous fistulas, volatile anesthetic–induced increases in cutaneous blood flow) result in delivery to the lungs of blood containing a higher partial pressure of anesthetic than that present in blood that has passed through tissues. As a result, left-to-right shunts offset the dilutional effects of a right-to-left shunt on the Pa. Indeed, the effect of a left-to-right shunt on the rate of increase in the Pa is detectable only if there is a concomitant presence of a right-to-left shunt. Likewise, the effect of a right-to-left shunt on the rate of increase in the PA is maximal in the absence of a left-to-right shunt.

Alveolar-to-Venous Partial Pressure Differences

The A-vD reflects tissue uptake of the inhaled anesthetic. Tissue uptake affects uptake at the lung by controlling the rate of increase of the mixed venous partial pressure of anesthetic. Factors that determine the fraction of anesthetic removed from blood traversing a tissue parallel those factors that determine uptake at the lungs (tissue solubility, tissue blood flow, and arterial-to-tissue partial pressure differences).

Highly perfused tissues (brain, heart, kidneys) in the adult account for <10% of body mass but receive 75% of the cardiac output (see Table 1-2). As a result of the small mass and high blood flow, these tissues, known as vessel-rich group tissues, equilibrate rapidly with the Pa. Indeed, after about three time constants, approximately 75% of the returning venous blood is at the same partial pressure as the PA. For this reason, uptake of a volatile anesthetic is decreased greatly after three time constants (5 to 15 minutes depending on the blood solubility of the inhaled anesthetic), as reflected by a narrowing of the inspired-to-alveolar partial pressure difference. Continued uptake of anesthetic after saturation of vessel-rich group tissues reflects principally the entrance of anesthetic into skeletal muscles and fat. Skeletal muscles and fat represent about 70% of the body mass but receive only about 25% of the cardiac output (see Table 1-2). As a result of the large tissue mass, sustained tissue uptake of the inhaled anesthetic continues and the effluent venous blood is at a lower partial pressure than the PA. For this reason, the A-vD difference for anesthetic is maintained and uptake from the lungs continues, even after several hours of continuous administration of inhaled anesthetics.

The time for equilibration of vessel-rich group tissues is more rapid for neonates and infants than for adults. This difference reflects the greater cardiac output to vessel-rich group tissues in the very young as well as decreased solubility of anesthetics in the tissues of neonates. Furthermore, skeletal muscle bulk comprises a small fraction of body weight in neonates and infants.

Recovery from Anesthesia

Recovery from anesthesia is depicted by the rate of decrease in the Pbr as reflected by the PA (Fig. 1-22) (Yasuda et al., 1991). The rate of washout of anesthetic from the brain should be rapid because inhaled anesthetics are not highly soluble in brain and the brain receives a large fraction of the cardiac output. Although similarities exist between the rate of induction and recovery, as reflected by changes in the PA of the inhaled anesthetic, there are important differences between the two events. In contrast to induction of anesthesia, which may be accelerated by the concentration effect, it is not possible to speed the decrease in PA by this mechanism (you cannot administer less than zero).

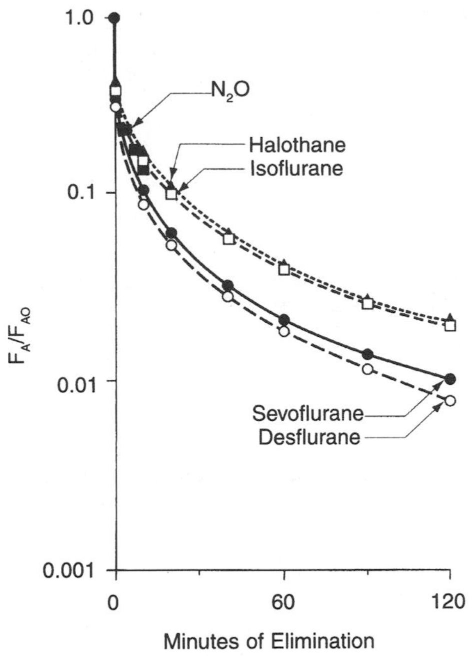

Figure 1-22. Elimination of inhaled anesthetics is defined as the ratio of the end-tidal anesthetic concentration (F_A) to the F_A immediately before the beginning of elimination (F_{AO}). The rate of decrease (awakening from anesthesia) in the F_A/F_{AO} is most rapid with the anesthetics that are least soluble in blood (nitrous oxide, desflurane, sevoflurane). (From Yasuda N, Lockhart SH, Eger EI, et al. Comparison of kinetics of sevoflurane and isoflurane in humans. *Anesth Analg* 1991;72:316–324; with permission.)

Furthermore, at the conclusion of every anesthetic, the concentration of the inhaled anesthetic in tissues depends highly on the solubility of the inhaled drug and the duration of its administration. This contrasts with tissue concentrations of zero at the initiation of induction of anesthesia. The failure of certain tissues to reach equilibrium with the PA of the inhaled anesthetic during maintenance of anesthesia means that the rate of decrease of the PA during recovery from anesthesia will be more rapid than the rate of increase of the PA during induction of anesthesia (see Figs. 1–18 and 1–22) (Yasuda et al., 1991). Indeed, even after a prolonged anesthetic, skeletal muscles probably, and fat almost certainly, will not have equilibrated with the PA of the inhaled anesthetic. Thus, when the PI of an anesthetic is abruptly decreased to zero at the conclusion of an anesthetic, these tissues initially cannot contribute to the transfer of drug back to blood for delivery to the liver for metabolism or to the lungs for exhalation. As long as gradients exist between the Pa and tissues, the tissues will continue to take up anesthetic. Thus, during recovery from anesthesia, the continued passage of anesthetic from blood to tissues, such as fat, acts to speed the rate of decrease in the PA of that anesthetic. Continued tissue uptake of anesthetic will depend on the solubility of the inhaled anesthetic and the duration of anesthesia, with the impact being most important with soluble anesthetics (Stoelting and Eger, 1969c). For example, time to recovery

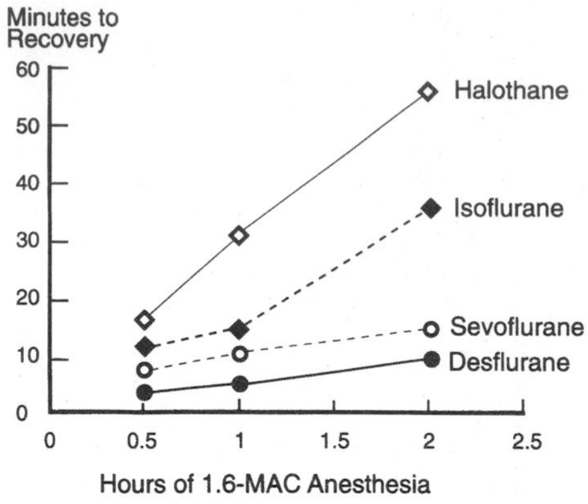

Figure 1-23. An increase in the duration of anesthesia during a constant dose of anesthetic (1.6 MAC) is associated with increases in the time to recovery (motor coordination in an animal model), with the greatest increases occurring with the most blood-soluble anesthetics. [From Eger EI. *Desflurane (Suprane): a compendium and reference*. Nutley, NJ: Anaquest, 1993:1–119; with permission.]

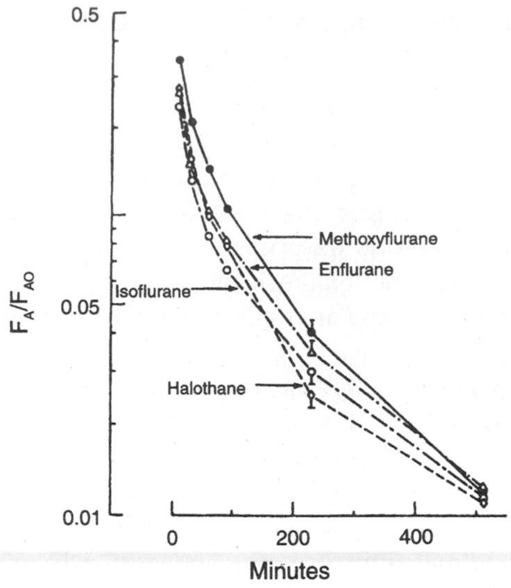

Figure 1-24. The decrease in the alveolar concentration is expressed as the ratio of the alveolar partial pressure at a given time (F_A) to the alveolar concentration present immediately before discontinuation of the administration of the anesthetic (F_{AO}). Unlike induction of anesthesia, the rate of decrease in anesthetic concentrations during recovery from anesthesia does not precisely follow predictions based on blood:gas partition coefficients of halothane and methoxyflurane due to the influence of metabolism of these drugs. (From Carpenter RL, Eger EI, Johnson BH, et al. Pharmacokinetics of inhaled anesthetics in humans: measurements during and after the simultaneous administration of enflurane, halothane, isoflurane, methoxyflurane, and nitrous oxide. *Anesth Analg* 1986;65:575–582; with permission.)

is prolonged in proportion to the duration of anesthesia for soluble anesthetics (halothane and isoflurane), whereas the impact of duration of administration on time to recovery is minimal with poorly soluble anesthetics (sevoflurane and desflurane) (Fig. 1-23) (Eger, 1993).

Anesthetic that has been absorbed into the components of the anesthetic breathing system will pass from the components back into the gases of the breathing circuit at the conclusion of anesthesia and retard the rate of decrease in the PA of the anesthetic. Likewise, exhaled gases of the patient contain anesthetic that will be rebreathed unless fresh gas flow rates are increased (at least 5 liters/minute of oxygen) at the conclusion of anesthesia.

In contrast to the rate of increase of the PA during induction of anesthesia, the rate of decrease in the PA during recovery from anesthesia is not entirely consistent with what might be predicted from the inhaled anesthetic's blood:gas partition coefficient (Fig. 1-24) (Carpenter et al., 1986). For example, the PA for halothane decreases more rapidly than that for isoflurane and enflurane despite the greater blood solubility of halothane. Similarly, the PA of methoxyflurane decreases below that of enflurane even though methoxyflurane is about six times more soluble in blood than is enflurane. The more rapid decrease in the PA for halothane and methoxyflurane is, in large part, due to the metabolism of these drugs in the liver (Carpenter et al., 1986) (see Chapter 2). This suggests that metabolism can significantly influence the rate of recovery from halothane and methoxyflurane anesthesia. In contrast, the rate of induction of anesthesia is not influenced by the magnitude of metabolism even for drugs such as halothane and methoxyflurane.

Context-Sensitive Half-Time

The pharmacokinetics of the elimination of inhaled anesthetics depends on the length of administration and the blood-gas solubility of the inhaled anesthetic. As with injected anesthetics, it is possible to use computer simulations to determine context-sensitive half-times for volatile anesthetics. In this regard, the time needed for a 50% decrease in anesthetic concentration of enflurane, isoflurane, desflurane, and sevoflurane is <5 minutes and does not increase significantly with increasing duration of anesthesia (Bailey, 1997). Presumably, this is a reflection of the initial phase of elimination, which is primarily a function of alveolar ventilation. Determination of other decrement times (80% and 90%) reveals differences between various inhaled anesthetics. For example, the 80% decrement times of desflurane and sevoflurane are <8 minutes and do not increase significantly with the duration of anesthesia, whereas 80% decrement times for enflurane and isoflurane increase significantly after about 60 minutes, reaching plateaus of approximately 30 to 35 minutes. The 90% decrement time of desflurane increases slightly from 5 minutes after 30 minutes of anesthesia to 14 minutes after 6 hours of anesthesia, which is significantly less than sevoflurane (65 minutes), isoflurane (86 minutes), and enflurane (100 minutes) after 6 hours of administration. Based on the simulated context-sensitive half-times and assuming that MAC-awake is 0.5 MAC, there would be little difference in recovery time among these volatile anesthetics when a pure inhalation anesthetic technique is used. The major differences in the rates at which desflurane, sevoflurane, isoflurane, and enflurane are eliminated occur in the final 20% of the elimination process.

Diffusion Hypoxia

Diffusion hypoxia occurs when inhalation of nitrous oxide is discontinued abruptly, leading to a reversal of partial pressure gradients such that nitrous oxide leaves the blood to enter alveoli (Fink, 1955). This initial high-volume outpouring of nitrous oxide from the blood into the alveoli can so dilute the P_{AO_2} that the Pa_{O_2} decreases. In addition to dilution of the P_{AO_2} by nitrous oxide, there is also dilution of the P_{ACO_2}, which decreases the stimulus to breathe (Sheffer et al., 1972). This decreased stimulus to breathe exaggerates the impact on Pa_{O_2} of the outpouring of nitrous oxide into the alveoli. Outpouring of nitrous oxide into alveoli is greatest during the first 1 to 5 minutes after its discontinuation at the conclusion of anesthesia. Thus, it is common practice to fill the lungs with oxygen at the end of anesthesia to ensure that arterial hypoxemia will not occur as a result of dilution of the P_{AO_2} by nitrous oxide.

PHARMACODYNAMICS OF INHALED ANESTHETICS

Minimal Alveolar Concentration

Minimal alveolar concentration (MAC) of an inhaled anesthetic is defined as that concentration at 1 atm that prevents skeletal muscle movement in response to a supramaximal painful stimulus (surgical skin incision) in 50% of patients (Merkel and Eger, 1963). MAC is an anesthetic 50% effective dose (ED_{50}). Immobility produced by inhaled anesthetics as measured by MAC is mediated principally by effects of these drugs on the spinal cord and only a minor component of immobility results from cerebral effects (Sonner et al., 2003). For example, in animals, MAC for isoflurane is 1.2% when delivered to the intact animal but delivery of inhaled anesthetic only to the brain results in isoflurane MAC increasing to nearly 3% (Antognini et al. 1993). Further evidence that MAC reflects effects of the inhaled anesthetics at the spinal cord is the observation that decerebration does not change MAC (Fig. 1-25) (Rampil et al., 1993; Rampil 1994).

MAC is among the most useful concepts in anesthetic pharmacology as it establishes a common measure of potency (partial pressure at steady state) for inhaled anesthetics. This concept is used to provide uniformity in dosages of inhaled anesthetics, to establish relative amounts of inhaled anesthetics to reach specific endpoints (MAC_{awake}; MACBAR), and to guide the search for mechanisms responsible for mechanisms of anesthetic action (Sani and Shafer, 2002). A unique feature of MAC is its consistency varying only 10% to 15% among individuals.

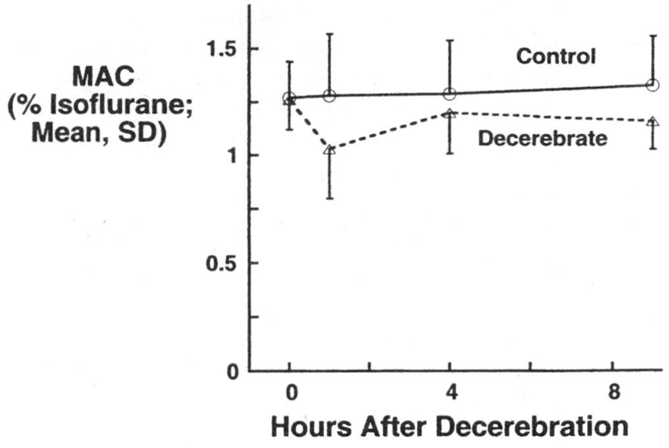

Figure 1-25. Decerebration does not change the minimum alveolar anesthetic concentration of isoflurane in rats confirming that the effects of volatile anesthetics on the spinal cord determine MAC. (From Rampil IJ, Mason P, Singh H. Anesthetic potency (MAC) is independent of forebrain structures in the rat. *Anesthesiology* 1993;78:707–712; with permission.)

This small degree of pharmacodynamic variability for inhaled anesthetics is unique in pharmacology. The use of equally potent doses (comparable MAC concentrations) of inhaled anesthetics is mandatory for comparing effects of these drugs not only at the spinal cord but at all other organs (Table 1-8). For example, similar MAC concentrations of inhaled anesthetics produce equivalent depression of the spinal cord whereas effects on cardiopulmonary parameters may be different for each drug (see Chapter 2). This emphasizes that MAC represents only one point on the dose-response curve of effects produced by inhaled anesthetics and that these dose-response curves are not parallel.

Factors that Alter MAC

Inhalation anesthetic requirements are remarkably uniform in humans, mainly being affected by age and body

TABLE 1-8.
COMPARATIVE MINIMUM ALVEOLAR CONCENTRATION (MAC) OF INHALED ANESTHETICS

	MAC (%, 30 to 55 Years Old at 37°C, PB 760 mm Hg)
Nitrous oxide*	104
Halothane	0.75
Enflurane	1.63
Isoflurane	1.17
Desflurane	6.6
Sevoflurane	1.80
Xenon	63–71

*Determined in a hyperbaric chamber in males 21 to 55 years old.

temperature. MAC allows a quantitative analysis of the effect, if any, of various physiologic and pharmacologic factors on anesthetic requirements (Table 1-9) (Hall and Sullivan, 1990; Quasha et al., 1980). For example, increasing age results in a progressive decrease in MAC of about 6% per decade that is similar for all inhaled anesthetics (Figs. 1-26 and Fig. 1-27) (Eger, 2001; Mapleson, 1996). MAC is decreased nearly 30% in the early postpartum period, returning to normal values in 12 to 72 hours (Chan and Gin, 1995; Zhou et al., 1995). Nevertheless, gender does not influence MAC (Fig. 1-28) (Eger et al., 2003; Wadhwa et al., 2003). MAC is increased in women with natural red hair presumably reflecting mutations of the melanocortin-1 receptor gene and increased pheomelanin concentrations (Fig. 1-29) (Liem et al. 2004). Although most reports describe MAC as independent of the duration of anesthesia, there is evidence that MAC for isoflurane decreases during the administration of anesthesia and the performance of surgery (Fig. 1-30) (Petersen-Felix et al., 1993). The effect of cardiopulmonary bypass on MAC is uncertain, with some studies showing a decrease, whereas others fail to demonstrate any change (Gedney and Ghosh, 1995). Despite prolongation of sleeping times in animals, cyclosporine increases rather than decreases isoflurane MAC (Niemann et al., 2002). MAC values may vary with the type of stimulus; tetanic stimulation and trapezius squeeze are considered noninvasive stimulation patterns that are equivalent to surgical skin incision, though in contrast to skin incision, these events can be repeated (Fig. 1-31) (Zbinden et al., 1994). Tracheal intubation requires the highest MAC to prevent skeletal muscle responses (see Fig. 1-31) (Zbinden et al., 1994).

MAC values for inhaled anesthetics are additive. For example, 0.5 MAC of nitrous oxide plus 0.5 MAC isoflurane has the same effect at the brain as does a 1 MAC concentration of either anesthetic alone. The fact that 1 MAC for nitrous oxide is >100% means that this anesthetic cannot be used alone at 1 atm and still provide an acceptable inhaled concentration of oxygen. Opioids significantly decrease anesthetic requirements for volatile anesthetics. For example, 25 minutes after the administration of fentanyl, 3 μg/kg or 6 μg/kg IV, MAC for desflurane is decreased 48% and 68%, respectively (Sebel et al., 1992).

TABLE 1-9.
IMPACT OF PHYSIOLOGIC AND PHARMACOLOGIC FACTORS ON MINIMUM ALVEOLAR CONCENTRATION (MAC)

Increases in MAC
Hyperthermia
Excess pheomelanin production (red hair)
Drug-induced increases in central nervous system catecholamine levels
Cyclosporine
Hypernatremia
Decreases in MAC
Hypothermia
Increasing age
Preoperative medication
Drug-induced decreases in central nervous system catecholamine levels
Alpha-2 agonists
Acute alcohol ingestion
Pregnancy
Postpartum (returns to normal in 24 to 72 hours)
Lithium
Lidocaine
Neuraxial opioids (?)
Ketanserin
Pa_{O_2} <38 mm Hg
Blood pressure <40 mm Hg
Cardiopulmonary bypass
Hyponatremia
No change in MAC
Anesthetic metabolism
Chronic alcohol abuse
Gender
Duration of anesthesia (?)
Pa_{CO_2} 15 to 95 mm Hg
Pa_{O_2} >38 mm Hg
Blood pressure >40 mm Hg
Hyperkalemia or hypokalemia
Thyroid gland dysfunction

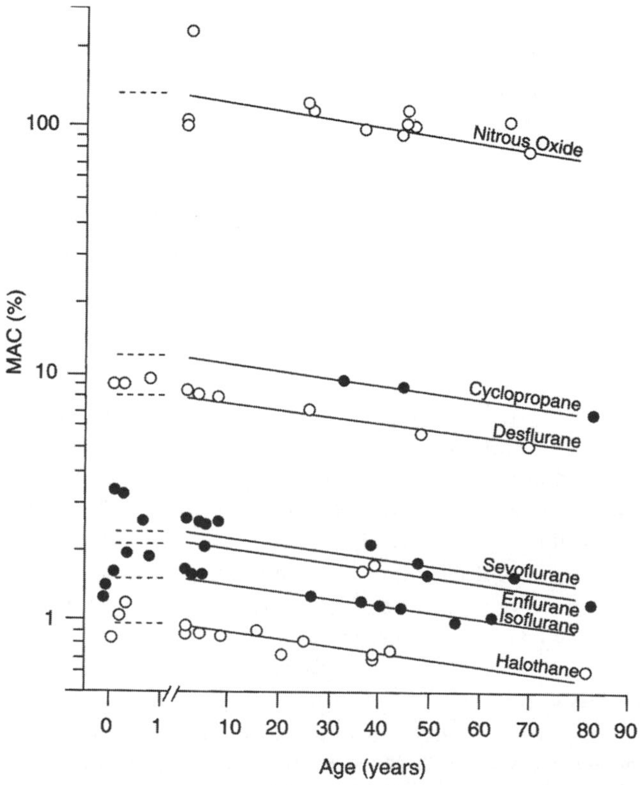

Figure 1-26. Effect of age on minimum alveolar concentration (MAC). (From Mapleson WW. Effect of age on MAC in humans: a meta-analysis. *Br J Anaesth* 1996;76:179–185; with permission.)

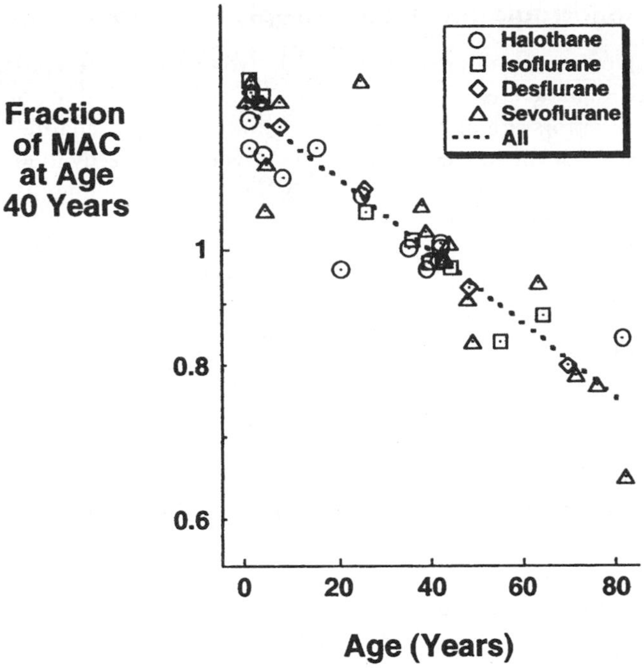

Figure 1-27. Minimum alveolar anesthetic concentration (MAC) (as a fraction of MAC at 40 years of age) with increasing age. (From Eger EI. Age, minimum alveolar anesthetic concentration, and minimum alveolar anesthetic concentration-awake. *Anesth Analg* 2001;93:947–953; with permission.)

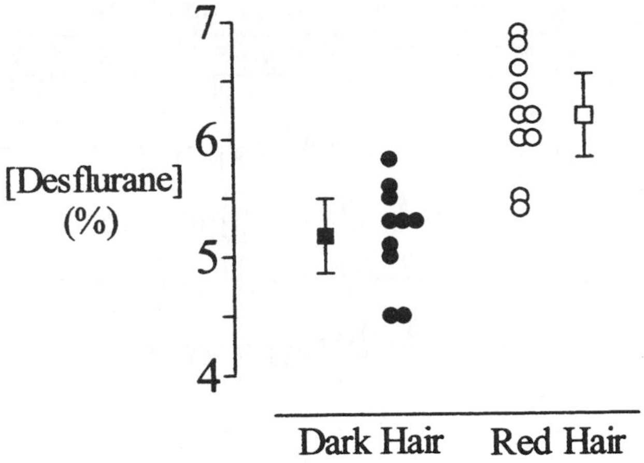

Figure 1-29. Anesthetic requirements for individual participants (circles) with group means (squares). The desflurane requirement in redheads (6.2%) was significantly greater than in dark-haired women (5.2%) (From Liem ER, Lin C-M, Suleman M-I, et al. Anesthetic requirement is increased in redheads. *Anesthesiology* 2004;101:279–83, with permission.)

Similar decreases in isoflurane MAC are also produced by these doses of fentanyl.

Dose-response curves for inhaled anesthetics, although not parallel, are all steep. This is emphasized by the fact that a 1 MAC dose prevents skeletal muscle movement in response to a painful stimulus in 50% of patients, whereas a modest increase to about 1.3 MAC prevents movement in at least 95% of patients.

Mechanism of Immobility

MAC is based on the characteristic ability of inhaled drugs to produce immobility by virtue of actions of these drugs principally on the spinal cord rather than on higher centers (Sonner et al., 2003). The observation that immobility during noxious stimulation does not correlate with electroencephalographic activity reflects the fact that cortical electrical activity does not control motor responses to noxious stimulation. Effects of inhaled anesthetics on the spinal cord leading to immobility are diverse and likely reflect

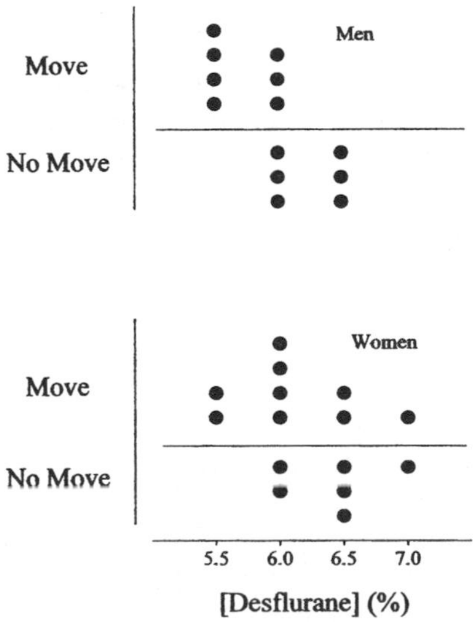

Figure 1-28. End-tidal concentrations of desflurane were tested for "Move" or "No Move" in men and women. MAC for desflurane in men was 6.0 ≠ 0.3% and in women it was 6.2 ≠ 0.4%. P = 0.31 (mean ≠ SD). (From Wadhwa A, Durrani J, Sengupta P, et al. Women have the same desflurane minimum alveolar concentration as men: A prospective study. *Anesthesiology* 2003;99:1062–1065; with permission.)

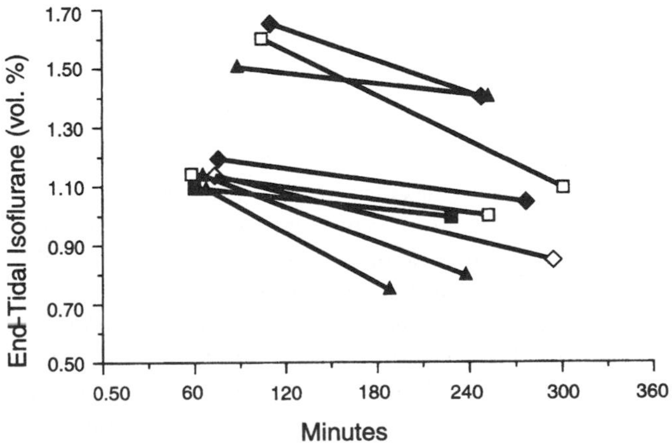

Figure 1-30. Preoperative (60 minutes) and postoperative (180 to 300 minutes) individual minimum alveolar concentration (MAC) determinations using continuous electrical stimulation (MAC tetanus). Each line represents an individual patient. (From Petersen-Felix S, Zbinden AM, Fischer M, et al. Isoflurane minimum alveolar concentration decreases during anesthesia and surgery. *Anesthesiology* 1993;79:959–965; with permission.)

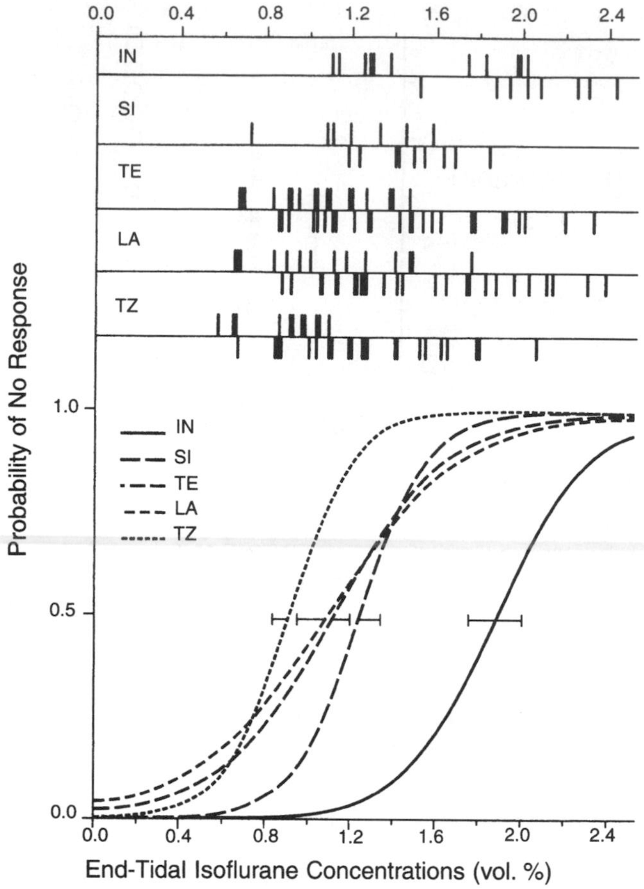

Figure 1-31. Responses (movement [*horizontal line above*]) or no movement (*horizontal line below*) to preoperative stimulation represented by tracheal intubation (IN), skin incision (SI), response to a continuous (tetanus) electrical stimulation (TE), direct laryngoscopy (LA), and trapezius muscle squeeze (TZ). The probability of response versus end-tidal isoflurane concentration is plotted. (From Zbinden AM, Maggiorini M, Peterson-Felix S, et al. Anesthetic depth defined using multiple noxious stimuli during isoflurane/oxygen anesthesia. I. Motor reactions. *Anesthesiology* 1994;80:253–260; with permission.)

drug-induced depression of excitation as well as enhancement of inhibition. In this regard, inhaled anesthetics depress excitatory alpha-amino-3- AMPA and NMDA receptor-mediated currents by actions independent of inhibitory $GABA_A$ and glycine receptor-mediated currents. Actions on sodium ion channels but not potassium channels may also be important in producing immobility. Conversely, cholinergic receptors do not seem to exert a significant role in anesthetic-induced immobility at the spinal cord level (Eger et al., 2002). Likewise, although opioids and stimulation of $alpha_2$ adrenergic receptors (clonidine) decrease MAC, it is unlikely that immobility produced by inhaled anesthetics is due to activation of these receptors (Eger et al., 2003a). Inhaled anesthetics do not act via opioid receptors. Overall, no inhaled anesthetic action on a single group of receptors can explain immobility, and immobility as a result of concurrent actions on many receptors is unlikely (Eger et al., 2001b; Sonner et al., 2003).

Ionotropic and Metabotropic Receptors

Neurotransmitters signal through two families of receptors designated as ionotropic and metabotropic. Ionotropic receptors are also known as ligand-gated ion channels because the neurotransmitter (GABA) binds directly to ion channel proteins and this interaction causes opening (gating) of the ion channels allowing transmission of specific ions (chloride ions) with resulting changes in membrane potentials. Ionotropic receptors are composed of several subunits (pentameric receptors) and each subunit consists of four transmembrane segments. In contrast, metabotropic receptors are monomeric receptors consisting of seven transmembrane segments. Binding of neurotransmitters (acetylcholine) to metabotropic receptors causes activation of guanosine triphosphate binding proteins (G-proteins) associated with the receptors, and these G-proteins act as second messengers to activate other signaling molecules such as protein kinases, or potassium or calcium channels (Sonner et al., 2003).

Inhaled anesthetics do not seem to stimulate the release of endogenous opioids and do not suppress autonomic or ventilatory responses to surgical stimulation at concentrations that suppress movement. The fact that small doses of opioids decrease MAC reflects their ability to provide an effect (analgesia) that is not present with inhaled anesthetics alone. Evidence that $alpha_2$ receptors participate in the immobility produced by inhaled anesthetics is provided by decreases in MAC produced by clonidine although $alpha_2$ adrenergic receptors are not considered to mediate the capacity of inhaled anesthetics to produce immobility (Eger et al., 2003). A small portion of the ability of inhaled anesthetics to produce immobility may be mediated by 5-HT receptors.

Inhibitory Ligand-Gated and Voltage Gated Channels (Glycine and $GABA_A$ Receptors)

Glycine receptors are major mediators of inhibitory neurotransmission in the spinal cord and mediate part of the immobility produced by inhaled anesthetics (Zhang et al., 2003). Their spinal localization and potentiation by volatile anesthetics is consistent with immobility as defined by MAC. Intravenous and intrathecal administration of strychnine, a glycine receptor antagonist increases MAC. Although $GABA_A$ receptors mediate immobility produced by injected anesthetics (propofol, etomidate) there is evidence that $GABA_A$ receptors do not mediate immobility produced by inhaled anesthetics (Zhang et al., 2004). In this regard, the enhancing effects of inhaled anesthetics on $GABA_A$ receptors minimally influences MAC.

Glutamate (NMDA, AMPA, and Kainate Receptors)

Glutamate is the principal excitatory neurotransmitter in the mammalian central nervous system. Glutamate receptors include G-protein coupled receptors and the ligand-gated receptors (NMDA, AMPA and kainate). NMDA receptors likely are important mediators of the immobilizing effects of inhaled anesthetics. AMPA receptors mediate the initial (fast) component of excitatory postsynaptic transmission and are likely targets for volatile anesthetic-induced immobility. Kainate receptors are a subtype of ionotropic glutamate receptors although the importance of these receptors on MAC is unclear (Sonner et al., 2003).

Sodium Channels

Despite the historical notion that inhaled anesthetics do not block axonal conduction and thus voltage-dependent sodium channels, there is evidence that these drugs can inhibit presynaptic terminal release of neurotransmitters, particularly glutamate. Indeed, intravenous administration of lidocaine decreases MAC.

Mechanism of Anesthesia-Induced Unconsciousness

A comprehensive explanation of the mechanism by which anesthetics cause loss of consciousness (suppression of awareness) has not yet been developed (John and Prichep, 2005). Subtle differences in the clinical effects of inhaled anesthetics may be attributed to distinct actions on a number of critical molecular targets. There is evidence that loss of consciousness (hypnosis and amnesia) and the response to skin incision (immobility as reflected by MAC) are not a single continuum of increasing anesthetic depth but rather two separate phenomena (Glass, 1998; Mashour, 2004). Combining these two observations it has been proposed that general anesthesia is a process requiring a state of unconsciousness of the brain (produced by volatile or injected anesthetics) plus immobility in response to a noxious stimulus (surgical skin incision) that is mediated by the action of volatile anesthetics on the spinal cord administered at concentrations equivalent to MAC for that drug. Immobility may also be produced by the action of opioids at opioid receptors in the spinal cord or the action of local anesthetics on peripheral nerves.

The mechanism by which inhaled anesthetics produce progressive, and occasionally selective, depression of the CNS is not known although the relationship between anesthetic activity of gases and molecular structure indicates that inhaled anesthetics must act through specific interactions with target molecules (presumably proteins) in the CNS (Campagna and Miller, 2003; Pocock and Richards, 1991). A single theory to explain the mechanism of anesthesia is no longer viewed as tenable as there are now multiple recognized potential targets of anesthetic action and this vast array of targets varies among different classes of anesthetics (Harrison, 2000). This constrasts with the fact that only a single family of receptors ($GABA_A$) is likely to be responsible for mediating the effects of propofol and etomidate. It is likely the two universal effects of inhaled anesthetics (immobility in response to noxious stimuli and unconsciousness) result from actions at separate molecular and anatomic sites and that they are produced by different mechanisms. There is strong evidence that a variety of inhaled anesthetics can hyperpolarize cortical and spinal neurons and there is a correlation between the ability to hyperpolarize neurons and anesthetic potency (MacIver and Kendig, 1991). There is widespread agreement that volatile anesthetics enhance inhibitory synaptic transmission especially at synapses where GABA is the major inhibitory neurotransmitter in the brain (Franks and Lieb, 1994). This inhibition of synaptic transmission through multineuronal polysynaptic pathways is especially prominent in the reticular activating system. Glycine is another important inhibitory neurotransmitter particularly in the spinal cord and brainstem and inhaled anesthetics potentiate glycine-activated currents. It is likely that the actions of halogenated volatile anesthetics on inhibitory neurotransmission via $GABA_A$ and glycine receptors is important in producing some components of anesthesia (Greenblatt and Meng, 2001). Inhibition of neurotransmitter release may explain how certain inhaled anesthetics can inhibit synaptic transmission. Inhibition of neurotransmitter release by inhaled anesthetics appears to be mediated by inhibition of neurosecretion rather than by inhibition of transmitter synthesis or storage. The mechanism by which anesthetics act to inhibit neurotransmitter release might reflect actions at presynaptic sodium ion channels or voltage-gated calcium ion channels. In contrast, nitrous oxide and xenon are virtually devoid of any effect on inhibitory $GABA_A$ receptors suggesting a distinct group of inhaled anesthetics with a completely different mechanism of action (Mennerick et al., 1998).

Inhaled anesthetics could theoretically have effects on excitatory neurotransmission in the CNS. The major excitatory neurotrasmitter in the CNS is glutamate and the three categories of postsynaptic glutamate receptors are AMPA, kainate, and NMDA receptors. Evidence indicates that all three types of glutamate receptors are insensitive to clinical concentrations of inhaled anesthetics. It is generally thought that peripheral nerves conduct normally during general anesthesia. Inhaled anesthetics do not appear to have significant effects on the generation or propagation of action potentials.

Molecular and Cellular Mechanisms

There is increasing evidence that general anesthetics may act by binding to only a small number of targets in the CNS. At the molecular level, anesthetics almost certainly act by binding directly to proteins rather than by perturbing lipid bilayers (Franks and Lieb, 1994). Stereoselective effects of volatile anesthetics on ion channel function suggest the existence of specific binding sites on membrane proteins. For example, the R(+) isomer of isoflurane is more potent than the S(−) isomer with respect to the loss of righting reflex in animals (Dickinson et al., 2000). There is accumulating evidence that $GABA_A$ and glycine receptors provide the molecular binding sites for inhaled anesthetics. Nevertheless, inhaled anesthetics are a heterogenous group of drugs and do not all interact with the same molecular target. $GABA_A$ and glycine receptors are members of a superfamily of ligand-gated ion channels, which also includes nAChR and 5-HT receptors. $GABA_A$ and glycine receptors are members of a subfamily of these channel proteins that are selective for chloride ions.

Voltage-Gated Ion Channels

Although it is conceivable that small changes in voltage-gated ion channels could change patterns of neuronal activity, it seems unlikely that voltage-gated sodium, potassium, or calcium ion channels play a substantial role in the production of the anesthetic state (Franks and Lieb, 1994).

Ligand-Gated Ion Channels

Ligand-gated ion channels (glutamate, glycine) may be important sites of anesthetic action. It is estimated that about one-third of all synapses in the CNS are responsive to GABA, with resulting activation leading to increased chloride permeability of neurons. GABA is not effective when administered systemically because it cannot easily cross the blood-brain barrier. The $GABA_A$ chloride ion channel (receptor) is a prime anesthetic target, and most anesthetics are effective in potentiating responses to GABA (enhance currents induced by this inhibitory neurotransmitter), either by enhancing the affinity of GABA for its receptor or augmenting the chloride conductance that is gated by this receptor, both of which result in CNS depression (Fig. 1-32) (Franks and Lieb, 1994; Tanelian et al., 1993). With the exception of ketamine, almost all injected and inhaled anesthetics enhance current flow induced by low concentrations of GABA by >50%. This potentiation of postsynaptic currents is presumed to translate into enhancement of synaptic inhibition. Anesthetic potentiation of inhibitory synaptic $GABA_A$ receptors best matches the pharmacologic profile of a wide variety of drugs that produce anesthesia in mammals. Consistent with the suggestion that $GABA_A$ receptors are relevant to the production of anesthetic-induced immobility is the fact that maximum enhancement of GABA and $GABA_A$ receptors occurs at anesthetic partial pressures required to produce immobility in vivo. This also makes the $GABA_A$ receptor a less likely target for the amnesia component of anesthesia because the partial pressures of anesthetics that cause amnesia in vivo have only a slight effect on $GABA_A$ receptors (Eger et al., 1997a). There is little evidence that second messenger systems are involved in general anesthesia.

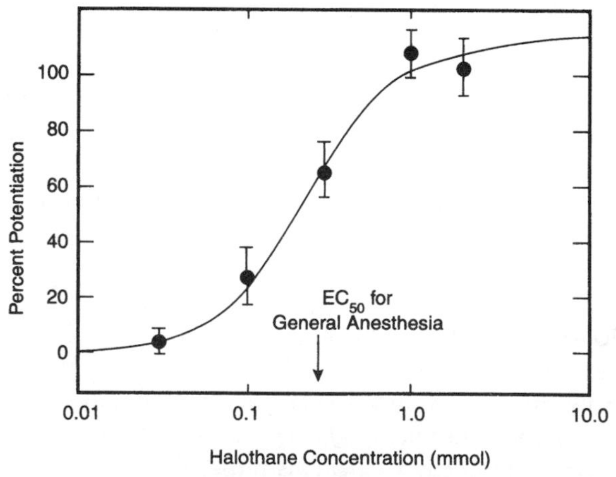

Figure 1-32. Clinically relevant concentrations of halothane (0.23 mmol is near the EC_{50} for anesthesia) potentiate responses to low levels of gamma-aminobutyric acid in dissociated rat brain neurons. (From Franks NP, Lieb WR. Molecular and cellular mechanisms of general anesthesia. *Nature* 1994;367:607–614; with permission.)

Stereoselectivity

The most definitive evidence that general anesthetics act by binding directly to proteins and not a lipid bilayer comes from observations of stereoselectivity (Lynch and Pancrazio, 1994). Inhalation anesthetics exist as isomers, and isoflurane has been shown to act stereoselectively on neuronal channels, with the levoisomer being more potent than the dextroisomer in enhancing potassium conductance in neurons (Franks and Lieb, 1991). This finding suggests the possibility of a specific protein receptor interaction as the basis for anesthesia. The dextroisomer, but not the levoisomer, of medetomidine, an $alpha_2$ agonist, produces dose-dependent decreases in MAC in animals (Doze et al., 1989; Segal et al., 1988). The stereospecificity of the MAC-decreasing effects of dexmedetomidine suggests that this hypnotic-anesthetic effect is mediated through a homogenous receptor population. It is speculated that $alpha_2$ agonists act on postsynaptic $alpha_2$ receptors in the CNS so as to activate an inhibitory G protein and to increase potassium ion conductance. The inhibitory G protein and hyperpolarization produced by increased potassium conductance results in depression of neuronal excitability characteristic of general anesthesia. Indeed, pertussis toxin (a specific inactivator of inhibitory G proteins) and 4-aminopyridine (a blocker of potassium channels) produce dose-dependent decreases in the hypnotic-anesthetic effects of dexmedetomidine (Doze et al., 1990).

The relevance to anesthetic mechanisms of the differing effects of enantiomers of volatile anesthetics on in vitro nerve conduction would be supported by parallel changes in MAC in the intact animal. Indeed, in rats, MAC for the levoisomer of isoflurane was 60% more potent than the dextroisomer (Lysko et al., 1994). In contrast, others have not found a significant difference in the effects of the enantiomers of isoflurane and desflurane on anesthetic effects in animals (Eger et al., 1997b). The steep slope of the dose-response curve (MAC) for inhaled anesthetics is possible evidence of a protein receptor in the CNS as a site and mechanism of action of inhaled anesthetics. Indeed, a crucial degree of receptor occupancy is characteristic of a steep dose-response curve. Receptor specificity is also suggested by conversion of an anesthetic to a nonanesthetic by increasing the molecular weight, despite corresponding increases in lipid solubility. Nevertheless, there is evidence that molecular shape (bulkiness) and size provide limited insight into the structure of the anesthetic site of action (Fang et al., 1996).

Meyer-Overton Theory (Critical Volume Hypothesis)

Correlation between the lipid solubility of inhaled anesthetics (oil:gas partition coefficient) and anesthetic potency has historically been presumed to be evidence that inhaled anesthetics act by disrupting the structure or dynamic properties of the lipid portions of nerve membranes. For example, when a sufficient number of molecules dissolve (critical concentration) in crucial hydrophobic sites such as lipid cell membranes, there is distortion of channels necessary for ion flux and the subsequent development of action potentials needed for synaptic transmission. Likewise, changes in the lipid matrix produced by dissolved anesthetic molecules could alter the function of proteins in cell membranes, thus decreasing sodium conductance. Evidence supporting distortion of sodium channels by dissolved anesthetic molecules is the observation that high pressures (40 to 100 atm) partially antagonize the action of inhaled anesthetics (pressure reversal), presumably by returning (compressing) lipid membranes and their sodium channels to their "awake" contour (Halsey and Smith, 1975).

The most compelling evidence against the Meyer-Overton theory of anesthesia is the fact that effects on lipid bilayers of inhaled anesthetics are implausibly small and can generally be mimicked by temperature changes of 1°C (Franks and Lieb, 1994). Furthermore, not all lipid-soluble drugs are anesthetics, and, in fact, some are convulsants. For example, the observation that, among *n*-alcohols, dodecanol is anesthetic and decol is not (for *n*-alkanes the cutoff is after octane) suggests that anesthetic binding to protein pockets or clefts and not lipid membranes is important in the mechanism of anesthesia. Based on these negative observations, lipid theories have been refined to postulate that specialized domains in membranes (boundary membranes surrounding proteins) are not only particularly sensitive to anesthetics but also are critical to membrane function. Indeed, both binding to proteins and dissolving in lipids can account for the Meyer-Overton correlation.

PHARMACOECONOMICS

Pharmacoeconomics is the application of economics to drug selection and usage relative to the expenditure of financial resources that could be used for other purposes (Fisher and Macario, 1997). It is recognized that additional financial resources spent for small improvements in drug profiles may not be practical. Physicians recognize that cost-effectiveness should be considered when evaluating different treatment options. Recognized obstacles to cost-effective care are society's unwillingness to accept the reality of limited resources and patients who have unrealistic expectations regarding the role of medical care in their lives. Anesthesia-related medications account for 8% to 12% of a hospital's total drug expenditures (Watcha and White, 1997, White and White, 1994). The economic cost of limiting or preventing postoperative nausea and vomiting and surgical pain are examples of applying pharmacoeconomics to common side effects of anesthesia (Macario and Vasanawala, 2001).

REFERENCES

Antognini JF, Schwartz K. Exaggerated anesthetic requirements n the preferentially anesthetized brain. *Anesthesiology* 1993;79:1244–1299.

Ariens EJ. Stereochemistry, a basis for sophisticated nonsense in pharmacokinetics and clinical pharmacology. *Eur J Clin Pharmacol* 1984;26:663–668.

Avram MJ, Krejcie TC, Henthorn TK. The relationship of age to the pharmacokinetics of early drug distribution: the concurrent disposition of thiopental and indocyanine green. *Anesthesiology* 1990;72:403–411.

Bailey JM. Context-sensitive half-times and other decrement times of inhaled anesthetics. *Anesth Analg* 1997;85:681–686.

Bentley JB, Borel JD, Nad RE, et al. Age and fentanyl pharmacokinetics. *Anesth Analg* 1982;61:968–971.

Boer F, Bovill JG, Burm AGL, et al. Effect of ventilation on first-pass pulmonary retention of alfentanil and sufentanil in patients undergoing coronary artery surgery. *Br J Anaesth* 1994;73: 458–463.

Boyd AH, Eastwood NB, Parker CJ, et al. Pharmacodynamics of the 1R cis1'R cis isomer of atracurium (51W89) in health and chronic renal failure. *Br J Anaesth* 1995;74:400–404.

Campagna JA, Miller KW, Forman SA. Mechanisms of actions of inhaled anesthetics. *N Engl J Med* 2003;352:2110–2124.

Caraco Y. Genes and the response to drugs. *N Engl J Med* 2004;351: 2867–2869.

Carpenter RL, Eger EI, Johnson BH, et al. Pharmacokinetics of inhaled anesthetics in humans: measurements during and after the simultaneous administration of enflurane, halothane, isoflurane, methoxyflurane, and nitrous oxide. *Anesth Analg* 1986;65: 575–582.

Chan MTV, Gin T. Postpartum changes in the minimum alveolar concentration of isoflurane. *Anesthesiology* 1995;82:1360–1363.

Dickinson R, White I, Lieb WR, et al. Stereoselective loss of righting reflex in rats by isoflurane. *Anesthesiology* 2000;93:837–845.

Dingledine R, Borgas K, Bowie D, et al. The glutamate receptor ion channels. *Pharmacol Rev* 1999;51:7–61.

Doze VA, Chen BX, Maze M. Dexmedetomidine produces a hypnotic-anesthetic action in rats via activation of central alpha-2 adrenoceptors. *Anesthesiology* 1989;71:75–79.

Doze VA, Chen BX, Tinklenberg JA, et al. Pertussis toxin and 4-aminopyridine differently affect the hypnotic-anesthetic action of dexmedetomidine and pentobarbital. *Anesthesiology* 1990;73: 304–307.

Egan TD. Stereochemistry and anesthetic pharmacology: joining hands with the medicinal chemists. *Anesth Analg* 1996;83: 447–450.

Eger EI, Fisher DM, Dilger JP, et al. Relevant concentrations of inhaled anesthetics for in vitro studies of anesthetic mechanisms. *Anesthesiology* 2001a;94:915–921.

Eger EI, Koblin DD, Harris RA, et al. Hypothesis: inhaled anesthetics produce immobility and amnesia by different mechanisms at different sites. *Anesth Analg* 1997a;84:915–918.

Eger EI, Koblin DD, Laster MJ, et al. Minimum alveolar anesthetic concentration values for the enantiomers of isoflurane differ minimally. *Anesth Analg* 1997b;85:188–192.

Eger EI, Laster MJ, Gregory GA, et al. Women appear to have the same alveolar concentration as men: A retrospective study. *Anesthesiology* 2003;99:1059–1061.

Eger EI, Saidman LJ. Hazards of nitrous oxide anesthesia in bowel obstruction and pneumothorax. *Anesthesiology* 1965;26:61–66.

Eger EI, Zhang Y, Laster M, et al. Acetylcholine receptors doe not mediate the immobilization produced by inhaled anesthetics. *Anesth Analg* 2002;94:1500–1504.

Eger EI. Age, minimum alveolar anesthetic concentration, and minimum alveolar anesthetic concentration-awake. *Anesth Analg* 2001b;93:947–953.

Eger EI. *Desflurane (Suprane): a compendium and reference.* Nutley, NJ: Anaquest, 1993:1–119.

Eger EI. Effect of inspired anesthetic concentration on the rate of rise of alveolar concentration. *Anesthesiology* 1963;24:153–157.

Ellis DE, Stoelting RK. Individual variations in fluroxene, halothane and methoxyflurane blood-gas partition coefficients, and the effect of anemia. *Anesthesiology* 1975;42:748–750.

Epstein RM, Rackow H, Salanitre E, et al. Influence of the concentration effect on the uptake of anesthetic mixtures: the second gas effect. *Anesthesiology* 1964;25:364–371.

Fang Z, Sonner J, Laster MJ, et al. Anesthetic and convulsant properties of aromatic compounds and cycloalkanes: implications for mechanisms of narcosis. *Anesth Analg* 1996;83:1097–1104.

Fassoulaki A, Eger EI. Starvation increases the solubility of volatile anesthetics in rat liver. *Br J Anaesth* 1986;58:327–329.

Fink BR. Diffusion anoxia. *Anesthesiology* 1955;16:511–519.

Fisher D, Macario A. Economics of anesthesia practice: a call to arms. *Anesthesiology* 1997;86:1018–1019.

Fisher DM. (Almost) everything you learned about pharmacokinetics was (somewhat) wrong! *Anesth Analg* 1996;83:901–903.

Franks NP, Lieb WR. Molecular and cellular mechanisms of general anaesthesia. *Nature* 1994;367:607–614.

Franks NP, Lieb WR. Stereospecific effects of inhalational general anesthetic optical isomers on nerve ion channels. *Science* 1991;254:427–430.

Gasche Y, Daali Y, Fathi M, et al. Codeine intoxication associated with ultrarapid CYP2D6 metabolism. *N Engl J Med* 2004;351: 2827–2831.

Gedney JA, Ghosh S. Pharmacokinetics of analgesics, sedatives and anaesthetic agents during cardiopulmonary bypass. *Br J Anaesth* 1995;75: 344–351.

Gibbons RT, Steffey EP, Eger EI. The effect of spontaneous versus controlled ventilation on the rate of rise in the alveolar halothane concentration in dogs. *Anesth Analg* 1977;56:32–37.

Glass PSA. Anesthetic drug interactions: an insight into general anesthesia—its mechanisms and dosing strategies. *Anesthesiology* 1998; 88:5–6.

Greenblatt EP, Meng X. Divergence of volatile anesthetic effects in inhibitory neurotransmitter receptors. *Anesthesiology* 2001;94: 1026–1033.

Hall RI, Sullivan JA. Does cardiopulmonary bypass alter enflurane requirements for anesthesia? *Anesthesiology* 1990;73:249–255.

Halsey MJ, Smith B. Pressure reversal of narcosis produced by anesthetics, narcotics and tranquilizers. *Nature* 1975;257:811–813.

Harrison NL. Ion channels take center stage. Twin spotlights on two anesthetic targets. *Anesthesiology* 2000;92:936–938.

Hug CC. Pharmacokinetics of drugs administered intravenously. *Anesth Analg* 1978;57:704–723.

Hughes MA, Glass PSA, Jacobs JR. Context-sensitive half-time in multicompartment pharmacokinetic models for intravenous anesthetic drugs. *Anesthesiology* 1992;76:334–341.

John ER, Prichep LS. The anesthetic cascade. A theory of how anesthesia suppresses consciousness. *Anesthesiology* 2005;102:447–471.

Jung D, Mayersohn M, Perrie D, et al. Thiopental disposition as a function of age in female patients undergoing surgery. *Anesthesiology* 1982; 56:263–268.

Kharasch E, Russell M, Garton K, et al. Assessment of cytochrome P450 3A4 activity during the menstrual cycle using alfentanil as a noninvasive probe. *Anesthesiology* 1997a;87:26–35.

Kharasch ED, Russell M, Mautz D, et al. The role of cytochrome P450 3A4 in alfentanil clearance: implications for interindividual variability in disposition and perioperative drug interactions. *Anesthesiology* 1997b;87:36–50.

Kisor DF, Schmith VD, Wargin WA, et al. Importance of the organ-independent elimination of cisatracurium. *Anesth Analg* 1996;83:1065–1071.

Korman B, Mapleson WW. Concentration and second gas effects: can the accepted explanation be improved? *Br J Anaesth* 1997; 78:618–625.

Laasberg HL, Hedley-White J. Halothane solubility in blood and solutions of plasma proteins: effects of temperature, protein composition and hemoglobin concentration. *Anesthesiology* 1970;32: 351–356.

Lerman J, Gregory GA, Willis MM, Eger EI II. Age and solubility of volatile anesthetics in blood. *Anesthesiology* 1984;61:139–143.

Liem EB, Lin C-M, Suleman M-I, et al. Anesthetic requirement is increased in redheads. *Anesthesiology* 2004;101:279–283.

LoSasso TJ, Muzzi DA, Dietz NM, et al. Fifty percent nitrous oxide does not increase the risk of venous air embolism in neurosurgical patients operated upon in the sitting position. *Anesthesiology* 1992;77:21–30.

Lynch C, Pancrazio JJ. Snails, spiders, and stereospecificity—is there a role for calcium channels in anesthetic mechanisms? *Anesthesiology* 1994;81:1–5.

Lysko GS, Robinson JL, Casto R, et al. The stereospecific effects of isoflurane isomers in vivo. *Eur J Pharmacol* 1994;263:25–29.

Macario A, Vasanawala A. Improving quality of anesthesia care: opportunities for the new decade. *Can J Anesth* 2001;48:6–11.

Malviya S, Lerman J. The blood/gas solubilities of sevoflurane, isoflurane, halothane, and serum constituent concentrations in neonates and adults. *Anesthesiology* 1990;72:79–83.

Mapleson WW. Effect of age on MAC in humans: a meta-analysis. *Br J Anaesth* 1996;76:179–185.

Mashour GA. Consciousness unbound. Toward a paradigm of general anesthesia. *Anesthesiology* 2004;100:428–433.

Mennerick S, Jevtovic-Todorovic V, Todorovic SM, et al. Effects of nitrous oxide on excitatory and inhibitory synaptic transmission in hippocampal cultures. *J Neurosci* 1998;18:971–976.

Meretoja OA, Taivainen T, Raiha L, et al. Sevoflurane-nitrous oxide or halothane-nitrous oxide for pediatric bronchoscopy and gastroscopy. *Br J Anaesth* 1996;76:767–770.

Merkel G, Eger EI. A comparative study of halothane and halopropane anesthesia: including method for determining equipotency. *Anesthesiology* 1963;24:346–357.

Mihic SJ, Ye Q, Wick MJ, et al. Sites of alcohol and volatile anaesthetic action on GABA(A) and glycine receptors. *Nature* 1997;389: 385–389.

Munson ES, Eger EI, Tham MK, et al. Increase in anesthetic uptake, excretion and blood solubility in man after eating. *Anesth Analg* 1978;57: 224–231.

Munson ES, Merrick HC. Effect of nitrous oxide on venous air embolism. *Anesthesiology* 1966;27:783–787.

Nation RL. Chirality in new drug development-clinical pharmacokinetic considerations. *Clin Pharmacokinet* 1994;27:249–255.

Nelson DR. Cytochrome P450 and the individuality of species. *Arch Biochem Biophys* 1999;369:1–10.

Niemann CU, Stabernack C, Serkova, et al. Cyclosporine can increase isoflurane MAC. *Anesth Analg* 2002;95:930–934.

Petersen-Felix S, Zbinden AM, Fischer M, et al. Isoflurane minimum alveolar concentration decreases during anesthesia and surgery. *Anesthesiology* 1993;79:959–965.

Pocock G, Richards CD. Cellular mechanisms in general anaesthesia. *Br J Anaesth* 1991;66:116–128.

Quasha AL, Eger EI, Tinker JH. Determination and application of MAC. *Anesthesiology* 1980;53:315–334.

Rampil IJ, Mason P, Singh H. Anesthetic potency (MAC) is independent of forebrain structures in the rat. *Anesthesiology* 1993;78: 707–712.

Rampil IJ. Anesthetic potency is not altered after hypothermic spinal cord transection in rats. *Anesthesiology* 1994;80:606–610.

Salanitre E, Rackow H. The pulmonary exchange of nitrous oxide and halothane in infants and children. *Anesthesiology* 1969;30:388–394.

Sani O, Shafer SL. MAC attack? *Anesthesiology* 2003;99:1249–1250.

Sawyer DC, Eger EI, Bahlman SH, et al. Concentration dependence of hepatic halothane metabolism. *Anesthesiology* 1971;34:230–234.

Schwinn DA. Adrenoceptors as models for G protein–coupled receptors: structure, function, and regulation. *Br J Anaesth* 1993; 71:77–85.

Sebel PS, Glass PSA, Fletcher JE, et al. Reduction of the MAC of desflurane with fentanyl. *Anesthesiology* 1992;76:52–59.

Segal IS, Vickery RG, Walton JK, et al. Dexmedetomidine diminishes halothane anesthetic requirements in rats through a postsynaptic alpha-2 adrenergic receptor. *Anesthesiology* 1988;69:818–823.

Shafer SL, Stanski DR. Improving the clinical utility of anesthetic drug pharmacokinetics. *Anesthesiology* 1992;76:327–330.

Shafer SL, Varvel JR. Pharmacokinetics, pharmacodynamics, and rational opioid selection. *Anesthesiology* 1991;74:53–63.

Sheffer L, Steffenson JL, Birch AA. Nitrous oxide-induced diffusion hypoxia in patients breathing spontaneously. *Anesthesiology* 1972;37: 436–439.

Sonner JM, Antognini JF, Dutton RC, et al. Inhaled anesthetics and immobility: Mechanisms, mysteries, and minimum alveolar anesthetic concentration. *Anesth Analg* 2003;97:718–740.

Stanski DR, Maitre PO. Population pharmacokinetics and pharmacodynamics of thiopental: the effect of age revisited. *Anesthesiology* 1990; 72:412–422.

Stanski DR, Watkins WD. *Drug disposition in anesthesia.* New York: Grune & Stratton, 1982.

Stoelting RK, Eger EI. An additional explanation for the second gas effect: a concentrating effect. *Anesthesiology* 1969a;30:273–277.

Stoelting RK, Eger EI. Percutaneous loss of nitrous oxide, cyclopropane, ether and halothane in man. *Anesthesiology* 1969b; 30:278–283.

Stoelting RK, Eger EI. The effects of ventilation and anesthetic solubility on recovery from anesthesia: an in vivo and analog analysis before and after equilibration. *Anesthesiology* 1969c;30:290–296.

Stoelting RK, Longnecker DE. Effect of right-to-left shunt on rate of increase in arterial anesthetic concentration. *Anesthesiology* 1972;36:352–356.

Strum DP, Eger EI, Unadkat JD, et al. Age affects the pharmacokinetics of inhaled anesthetics in humans. *Anesth Analg* 1991;73:310–318.

Tanelian DL, Kosek P, Mody I, et al. The role of the $GABA_A$ receptor/chloride channel complex in anesthesia. *Anesthesiology* 1993;78:757–776.

Vote BJ, Hart RH, Worsley DR, et al. Visual loss after use of nitrous oxide gas with general anesthetic in patients with intraocular gas still persistent up to 30 days after vitrectomy. *Anesthesiology* 2002;97:1305–1308.

Wadhwa A, Durrani J, Sengupta P, et al. Women have the same desflurane minimum alveolar concentration as men: a prospective study. *Anesthesiology* 2003;99:1062–1065.

Watcha MF, White PF. Economics of anesthesia practice. *Anesthesiology* 1997;86:1170–1196.

White M, Kenny GN. Intravenous propofol anaesthesia using a computerized infusion system. *Anaesthesia* 1990;45:204–209.

White PF, White LD. Cost containment in the operating room: who is responsible? *J Clin Anesth* 1994;6:351-356.

Wilkinson GR, Shand DG. A physiologic approach to hepatic drug clearance. *Clin Pharmacol Ther* 1975;18:377–390.

Wood M, Wood AJJ. Changes in plasma drug binding and $alpha_1$ acid glycoprotein in mother and newborn infant. *Clin Pharmacol Ther* 1981; 29:522–526.

Wood M. Plasma drug binding: implications for anesthesiologists. *Anesth Analg* 1986;65:786–804.

Wood M. Variability of human drug response. *Anesthesiology* 1989;71: 631–633.

Yasuda N, Lockhart SH, Eger EI, et al. Comparison of kinetics of sevoflurane and isoflurane in humans. *Anesth Analg* 1991; 72:316–324.

Yasuda N, Targ AC, Eger EI. Solubility of I-653, sevoflurane, isoflurane, and halothane in human tissues. *Anesth Analg* 1989;69:370–373.

Yost CS. G proteins: basic characteristics and clinical potential for the practice of anesthesia. *Anesth Analg* 1993;77:822–834.

Zbinden AM, Maggiorini M, Peterson-Felix S, et al. Anesthetic depth defined using multiple noxious stimuli during isoflurane/oxygen anesthesia. I. Motor reactions. *Anesthesiology* 1994;80:253–260.

Zhang Y, Laster MJ, Hara K, et al. Glycine receptors mediate part of the immobility produced by inhaled anesthetics. *Anesth Analg* 2003;96:97–101.

Zhang Y, Sonner JM, Eger EI, et al. Gamma-aminobutyric $acid_A$ receptors do not mediate the immobility produced by isoflurane. *Anesth Analg* 2004;95:85–90.

Zhou HH, Norman P, DeLima LGR, et al. The minimum alveolar concentration of isoflurane in patients undergoing bilateral tubal ligation in the postpartum period. *Anesthesiology* 1995;82: 1364–1368.

Inhaled Anesthetics

2

HISTORY

The discovery of the anesthetic properties of nitrous oxide, diethyl ether, and chloroform in the 1840s was followed by a hiatus of about 80 years before other inhaled anesthetics were introduced (Figure 2-1) (Eger, 1993). In 1950, all inhaled anesthetics, with the exception of nitrous oxide, were flammable or potentially toxic to the liver. Recognition that combining carbon with fluorine decreased flammability led to the introduction, in 1951, of the first halogenated hydrocarbon anesthetic, fluroxene. Fluroxene was used clinically for several years before its voluntary withdrawal from the market due to its potential flammability and increasing evidence that this drug could cause organ toxicity (Johnston et al., 1973).

Halothane was synthesized in 1951 and introduced for clinical use in 1956. However, the tendency for alkane derivatives such as halothane to enhance the dysrhythmogenic effects of epinephrine, led to the search for new inhaled anesthetics derived from ethers. Methoxyflurane, a methyl ethyl ether, was the first such derivative, being introduced for clinical use in 1960. Although this drug does not enhance the dysrhythmogenic effects of epinephrine, its high solubility in blood and lipids results in a prolonged induction and slow recovery from anesthesia. More important, its extensive hepatic metabolism results in increased plasma concentrations of fluoride that could produce nephrotoxicity, especially with prolonged exposures to the anesthetic. Enflurane, the next methyl ethyl ether derivative, was introduced for clinical use in 1973. This anesthetic, in contrast to halothane, does not enhance the dysrhythmogenic effects of epinephrine, and hepatotoxicity seems less likely. Nevertheless, side effects were present, including metabolism to inorganic fluoride and stimulation of the central nervous system (CNS) as evidenced by spike and wave activity on the electroencephalogram (EEG) at high concentrations. In search of a drug with fewer side effects, isoflurane, the isomer of enflurane, was introduced in 1981. This drug was resistant to metabolism, making organ toxicity an unlikely occurrence after its administration.

Inhaled Anesthetics for the Present and Future

The search for even more pharmacologically "perfect" inhaled anesthetics did not end with the introduction and widespread use of isoflurane. The exclusion of all halogens except fluorine results in nonflammable liquids that are poorly lipid soluble and extremely resistant to metabolism. Desflurane, a totally fluorinated methyl ethyl ether, was introduced in 1992 and was followed in 1994 by the totally fluorinated methyl isopropyl ether, sevoflurane (Eger, 1994; Smith et al., 1996). The low solubility in blood of these newest anesthetics was desirable because it would facilitate the rapid induction of anesthesia, permit precise control of anesthetic concentrations during maintenance of anesthesia, and favor prompt recovery at the end of anesthesia independent of the duration of administration. Indeed, the development, introduction, and clinical acceptance of desflurane and sevoflurane reflects in large part the impact of market forces (ambulatory surgery and the desire for rapid awakening possible with poorly soluble but potent anesthetics) more than an improved pharmacologic profile on various organ systems as compared with isoflurane. The challenge to the anesthesiologist is to exploit the pharmacokinetic advantages of these drugs while minimizing the risks (airway irritation, sympathetic nervous system stimulation, carbon monoxide production, complex vaporizer technology, and compound A production) and increased expense associated with the manufacture and increased cost of administration of these new drugs.

Cost Considerations

Cost is an increasingly important consideration in the adoption of new drugs, including inhaled anesthetics, into clinical practice. Factors that may influence the cost of a new inhaled anesthetic include (a) its price (cost per mL of liquid) as determined by the manufacturer; (b) inherent characteristics of the anesthetic, such as its vapor pressure (mL of vapor available per mL of liquid), potency, and solubility; and (c) flow rate selected for delivery of the anesthetic (Weiskopf and Eger, 1993). The costs of new inhaled anesthetics can be decreased somewhat by using low flow

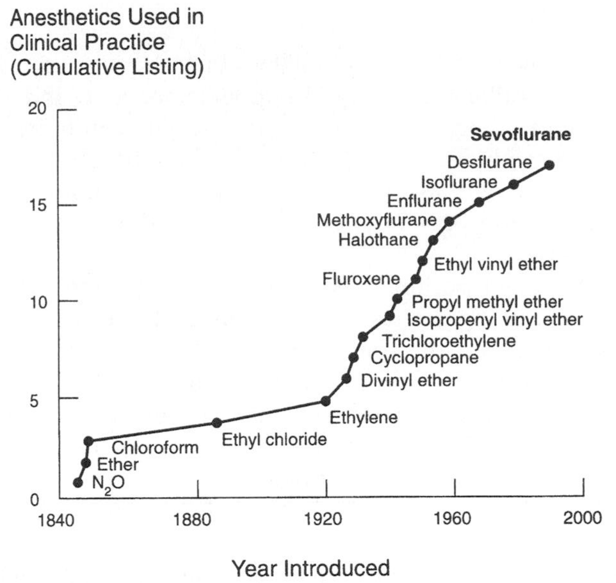

Figure 2-1. Inhaled anesthetics introduced into clinical practice beginning with the successful use of nitrous oxide in 1844 for dental anesthesia followed by recognition of the anesthetic properties of ether in 1846 and of chloroform in 1847. Modern anesthetics, beginning with halothane, differ from prior anesthetics in being fluorinated and nonflammable. [Modified from Eger EI. *Desflurane (Suprane): a compendium and reference*. Nutley, NJ: Anaquest, 1993:1–119; with permission.]

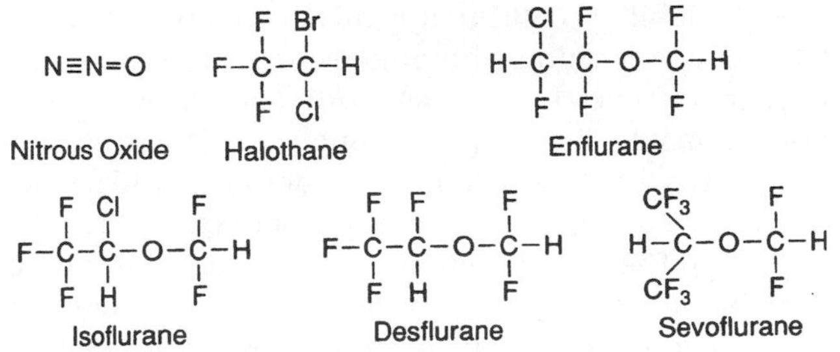

Figure 2-2. Inhaled anesthetics.

rates. Less soluble anesthetics are more suitable for use with low gas flow rates because their poor solubility permits better control of the delivered concentration. Furthermore, there is less depletion of these anesthetics from the inspired gases so that fewer molecules need to be added to the returning rebreathed gases. This conservation offsets the decreased potency of a drug such as desflurane compared with isoflurane. For example, desflurane is one-fifth as potent as isoflurane, yet the amount of desflurane that must be delivered to sustain minimal alveolar concentration (MAC) is only slightly more than threefold the amount of isoflurane. Similarly, although MAC of sevoflurane is 74% greater than isoflurane, the amount of sevoflurane that must be delivered to sustain MAC is only 30% greater.

CLINICALLY USEFUL INHALED ANESTHETICS

Commonly administered inhaled anesthetics include the inorganic gas nitrous oxide and the volatile liquids isoflurane, desflurane, and sevoflurane (Table 2-1) (Fig. 2-2) (Eger, 1994; Smith et al., 1996). Halothane and enflurane are administered infrequently but are included in the discussion of the comparative pharmacology of volatile anesthetics since halothane in particular has been studied extensively (Table 2-1) (Fig. 2-2) (Eger, 1994; Smith et al., 1996).

Volatile liquids are administered as vapors after their evaporation in devices known as *vaporizers*. Available but rarely administered inhaled anesthetics include the volatile liquids methoxyflurane and diethyl ether and the cyclic hydrocarbon gas cyclopropane. Xenon is an inert gas with anesthetic properties, but its clinical use is hindered by its high cost (Goto et al., 2003).

Nitrous Oxide

Nitrous oxide is a low-molecular-weight, odorless to sweet-smelling nonflammable gas of low potency and poor

TABLE 2-1.
PHYSICAL AND CHEMICAL PROPERTIES OF INHALED ANESTHETICS

	Nitrous Oxide	Halothane	Enflurane	Isoflurane	Desflurane	Sevoflurane
Molecular weight	44	197	184	184	168	200
Boiling point (°C)		50.2	56.5	48.5	22.8	58.5
Vapor pressure (mmHg; 20°C)	Gas	244	172	240	669	170
Odor	Sweet	Organic	Ethereal	Ethereal	Ethereal	Ethereal
Preservative necessary	No	Yes	No	No	No	No
Stability in soda lime (40°C)	Yes	No	Yes	Yes	Yes	No
Blood:gas partition coefficient	0.46	2.54	1.90	1.46	0.42	0.69
MAC (37°C, 30 to 55 years old, P_B 760 mmHg) (%)	104	0.75	1.63	1.17	6.6	1.80

blood solubility (0.46) that is most commonly administered in combination with opioids or volatile anesthetics to produce general anesthesia. Although nitrous oxide is nonflammable, it will support combustion (Neuman et al., 1993). Its poor blood solubility permits rapid achievement of an alveolar and brain partial pressure of the drug (see Fig. 1-18). The analgesic effects of nitrous oxide are prominent, but it causes minimal skeletal muscle relaxation. The speculated role of nitrous oxide in postoperative nausea and vomiting is unsettled, although meta-analysis of published studies suggest this inhaled anesthetic does increase the incidence of nausea and vomiting (Divatia et al., 1996; Fisher, 1996; Hartung, 1996). Nitrous oxide has no effect on polarographic Po_2 measurements but does cause a small increase in the P_{50} (about 1.6 mm Hg) (Kambam and Holiday, 1987). The routine use of nitrous oxide must be balanced against its possible adverse effects related to the high-volume absorption of nitrous oxide (see Chapter 1), and appreciation of potential toxic effects on organ function and ability to inactivate vitamin B_{12}.

Halothane

Halothane is a halogenated alkane derivative that exists as a clear, nonflammable liquid at room temperature. The vapor of this liquid has a sweet, nonpungent odor. An intermediate solubility in blood, combined with a high potency, permits rapid onset and recovery from anesthesia using halothane alone or in combination with nitrous oxide or injected drugs such as opioids.

Halothane was developed on the basis of predictions that its halogenated structure would provide nonflammability, intermediate blood solubility, anesthetic potency, and molecular stability. Specifically, carbon-fluorine decreases flammability, and the trifluorocarbon contributes to molecular stability. The presence of a carbon-chlorine and carbon-bromine bond plus the retention of a hydrogen atom ensures anesthetic potency. Despite its chemical stability, halothane is susceptible to decomposition to hydrochloric acid, hydrobromic acid, chloride, bromide, and phosgene. For this reason, halothane is stored in amber-colored bottles, and thymol is added as a preservative to prevent spontaneous oxidative decomposition. Thymol that remains in vaporizers after vaporization of halothane can cause vaporizer turnstiles or temperature-compensating devices to malfunction.

Enflurane

Enflurane is a halogenated methyl ethyl ether that exists as a clear, nonflammable volatile liquid at room temperature and has a pungent, ethereal odor. Its intermediate solubility in blood combined with a high potency permits rapid onset and recovery from anesthesia, using enflurane alone or in combination with nitrous oxide or injected drugs such as opioids.

Isoflurane

Isoflurane is a halogenated methyl ethyl ether that exists as a clear, nonflammable liquid at room temperature and has a pungent, ethereal odor. Its intermediate solubility in blood combined with a high potency permits rapid onset and recovery from anesthesia using isoflurane alone or in combination with nitrous oxide or injected drugs such as opioids.

Although isoflurane is an isomer of enflurane, their manufacturing processes are not similar. The compounds used at the start of manufacturing are different, with 2,2,2-trifluoroethanol the starting compound for isoflurane and chlorotrifluoroethylene for enflurane. The subsequent purification of isoflurane by distillation is complex and expensive. Isoflurane is characterized by extreme physical stability, undergoing no detectable deterioration during 5 years of storage or on exposure to carbon dioxide absorbents or sunlight. The stability of isoflurane prevents the need to add preservatives such as thymol to the commercial preparation.

Desflurane

Desflurane is a fluorinated methyl ethyl ether that differs from isoflurane only by substitution of a fluorine atom for the chlorine atom found on the alpha-ethyl component of isoflurane. Fluorination rather than chlorination increases vapor pressure (decreases intermolecular attraction), enhances molecular stability, and decreases potency. Indeed, the vapor pressure of desflurane exceeds that of isoflurane by a factor of three such that desflurane would boil at normal operating room temperatures. A new vaporizer technology addresses this property, producing a regulated concentration by converting desflurane to a gas (heated and pressurized vaporizer that requires electrical power), which is then blended with diluent fresh gas flow. The only evidence of metabolism of desflurane is the presence of measurable concentrations of serum and urinary trifluoroacetate that are one-fifth to one-tenth those produced by the metabolism of isoflurane. The potency of desflurane as reflected by MAC is about fivefold less than isoflurane.

Unlike halothane and sevoflurane, desflurane is pungent, making it unlikely that inhalation induction of anesthesia will be feasible or pleasant for the patient. Indeed, the pungency of desflurane produces airway irritation and an appreciable incidence of salivation, breath-holding, coughing, or laryngospasm when >6% inspired desflurane is administered to an awake patient (Eger, 1994). Carbon monoxide results from degradation of desflurane by the strong base present in desiccated carbon dioxide absorbents. Desflurane produces the highest carbon monoxide concentrations, followed by enflurane and isoflurane, whereas amounts produced from halothane and sevoflurane are trivial.

Solubility characteristics (blood:gas partition coefficient 0.45) and potency (MAC 6%) permit rapid achievement of an alveolar partial pressure necessary for anesthesia followed by prompt awakening when desflurane is discontinued. It is this lower blood-gas solubility and more precise control over the delivery of anesthesia and more rapid recovery from anesthesia that distinguish desflurane (and sevoflurane) from earlier volatile anesthetics.

Sevoflurane

Sevoflurane is a fluorinated methyl isopropyl ether. The vapor pressure of sevoflurane resembles that of halothane and isoflurane, permitting delivery of this anesthetic via a conventional unheated vaporizer. The blood:gas partition coefficient of sevoflurane (0.69) resembles that of desflurane, ensuring prompt induction of anesthesia and recovery after discontinuation of the anesthetic. Compared with isoflurane, recovery from sevoflurane anesthesia is 3 to 4 minutes faster and the difference is magnified in longer duration surgical procedures (>3 hours) (Fig. 2-3) (Ebert et al., 1998). Sevoflurane is nonpungent, has minimal odor, produces bronchodilation similar in degree to isoflurane, and causes the least degree of airway irritation among the currently available volatile anesthetics. For these reasons, sevoflurane, like halothane, is acceptable for inhalation induction of anesthesia.

Sevoflurane may be 100-fold more vulnerable to metabolism than desflurane, with an estimated 3% to 5% of the dose undergoing biodegradation. The resulting metabolites include inorganic fluoride (plasma concentrations exceed those that occur after enflurane) and hexafluoroisopropanol. The chemical structure of sevoflurane is such that it cannot undergo metabolism to an acyl halide. Sevoflurane metabolism does not result in the formation of trifluoroacetylated liver proteins and therefore cannot stimulate the formation of antitrifluoroacetylated protein antibodies. In this regard, sevoflurane differs from halothane, enflurane, isoflurane, and desflurane, all of which are metabolized to reactive acyl halide intermediates with the potential to produce hepatotoxicity as well as cross-sensitivity between drugs (Kharasch, 1995). Sevoflurane is the least likely volatile anesthetic to form carbon monoxide on exposure to carbon dioxide absorbents. In contrast to other volatile anesthetics, sevoflurane breaks down in the presence of the strong bases present in carbon dioxide absorbents to form compounds that are toxic in animals (Fig. 2-4) (Smith et al., 1996). The principal degradation product is fluoromethyl-2,2-difluoro-1-(trifluoromethyl) vinyl-ether (compound A). Compound A is a dose-dependent nephrotoxin in rats, causing renal proximal tubular injury. Although this finding is a concern, the levels of these compounds (principally compound A) that occur during administration of sevoflurane to patients are far

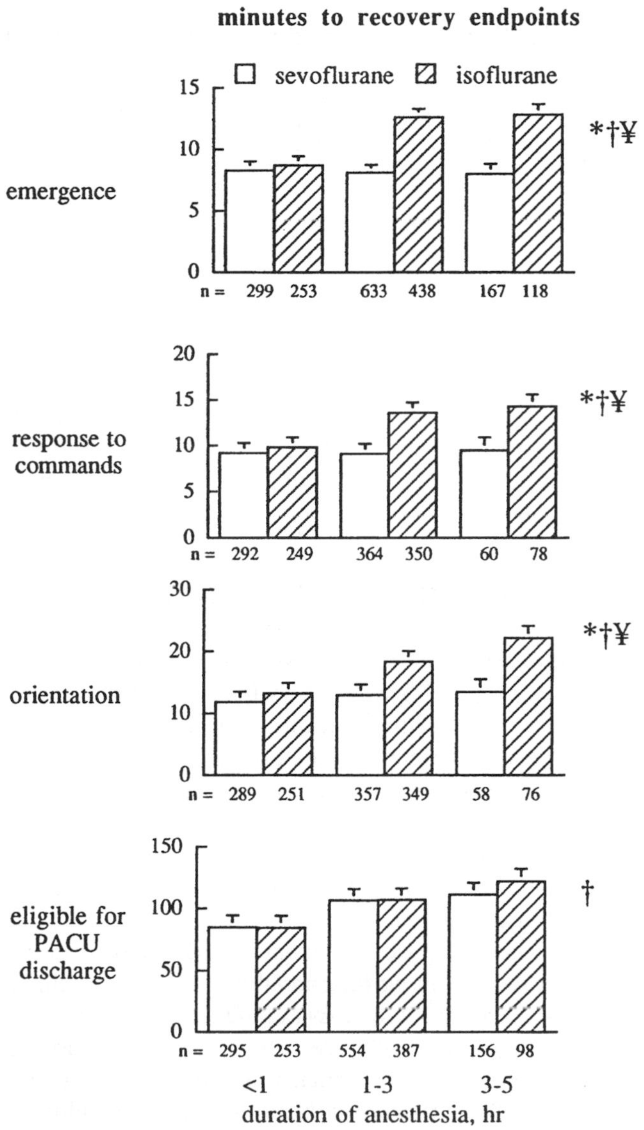

Figure 2-3. Analysis of variance results showing times to emergence, responses to commands, orientation, and discharge from the postanesthesia care unit (PACU) with differing durations of anesthesia. Mean ≠ SEM. (From Ebert TJ, Robinson BJ, Uhrich TD, et al. Recovery from sevoflurane anesthesia: A comparison to isoflurane and propofol anesthesia. *Anesthesiology* 1998;89:1524–1531; with permission.)

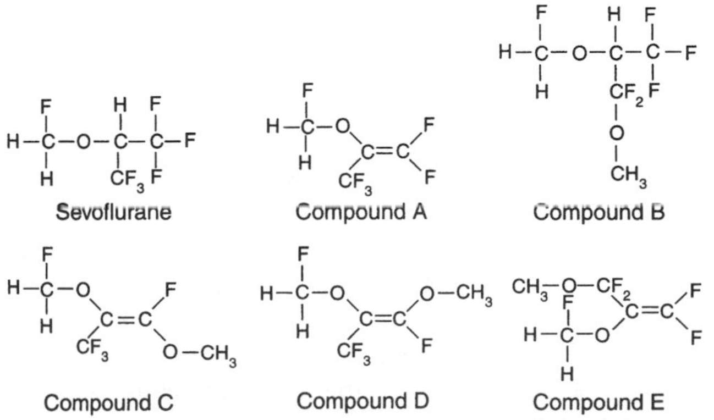

Figure 2-4. Degradation products of sevoflurane on exposure to soda lime. The formation of these degradation products is increased under experimental conditions in which the soda lime is heated to ≥65°C.

below speculated toxic levels, even when total gas flows are 1 liter per minute (Bito et al., 1997; Kharasch et al., 1997).

Xenon

Xenon is an inert gas with many of the characteristics considered important for an ideal inhaled anesthetic (Goto et al., 2003). MAC is 63% to 71% in humans, suggesting that this gas is more potent than nitrous oxide (MAC, 104%) (Nakata et al., 2001). MAC-awake for xenon is 33% (Goto et al., 2000). Unlike MAC for other volatile anesthetics, there is evidence that xenon MAC is gender-dependent, being less in females (Goto et al., 2002). Xenon is nonexplosive, nonpungent and odorless, and chemically inert as reflected by absence of metabolism and low toxicity. Unlike other inhaled anesthetics, it is not harmful to the environment because it is prepared by fractional distillation of the atmospheric air. To date, its high cost has hindered its acceptance in anesthesia practice. This disadvantage may be offset to some degree by using low fresh gas flow rates and development of a xenon-recycling system. Nevertheless, even if cost considerations can be negated, acceptance of xenon as a replacement for current inhaled anesthetics (that also share many of the same advantages of xenon) will be based more on evidence that morbidity and mortality is less when this drug is administered during anesthesia (Goto et al., 2003).

Xenon has a blood:gas partition coefficient of 0.115 which is lower than that of other clinically useful anesthetics and even lower than that of nitrous oxide (0.46), sevoflurane (0.69), and desflurane (0.42). Like nitrous oxide, xenon anesthesia results in gas exchange conditions that favor air bubble expansion which could worsen neurologic injury from venous air embolism (Maria and Eckmann, 2003). Diffusion of xenon into highly compliant bowel occurs but is less compared with nitrous oxide (Fig. 2-5) (Reinelt, et al., 2001). It is possible this minimal effect on bowel may be different when xenon diffuses into less compliant cavities as represented by pneumothorax, pneumoperitoneum and pneumopericardium. Xenon does not trigger malignant hyperthermia in susceptible swine (Froeba et al., 1999). Emergence from xenon anesthesia, regardless of the duration of anesthesia, is two to three times faster than that from equal-MAC nitrous oxide plus isoflurane or sevoflurane (Rossaint et al., 2003). Xenon is a potent hypnotic and analgesic, resulting in suppression of hemodynamic and catecholamine responses to surgical stimulation. Unlike other inhaled and injected anesthetics, xenon does not produce hemodynamic depression in healthy adults. Neuromuscular blocking effects of rocuronium are not different when given during propofol versus xenon anesthesia (Kunitz et al., 2004). A risk of recall would seem to be present but has not been observed in small numbers of patients. Like ketamine, xenon exerts antagonist effects at *N*-methyl-D-aspartate (NMDA) subtypes of glutamate receptors which have been shown to have both neuroprotective and neurotoxic properties. Xenon is unique among known NMDA antagonists in exhibiting neuroprotection without coexisting psychotomimetic behavioral changes (Ma et al. 2002). The reason why ketamine and nitrous oxide, but not xenon, produce neurotoxicity may reflect actions on dopaminergic pathways that does not occur in the presence of xenon.

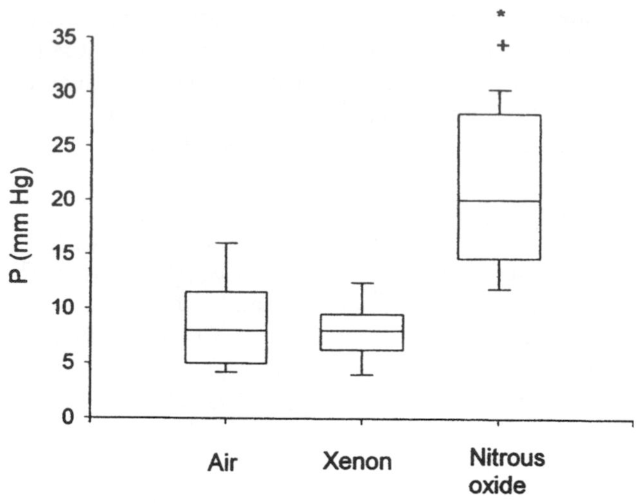

Figure 2-5. Pressures in obstructed bowel segments after 4 hours of air or anesthesia administration. After 4 hours of anesthesia, intraluminal pressures were significantly higher in the presence of nitrous oxide. (From Reinelt H, Schirmer U, Marx T, et al. Diffusion of xenon and nitrous oxide into the blood. *Anesthesiology* 2001;94:475-7; with permission.)

COMPARATIVE PHARMACOLOGY

Inhaled anesthetics often evoke differing pharmacologic effects at comparable MAC concentrations, emphasizing that dose-response curves for these drugs are not necessarily parallel. Measurements obtained from normothermic volunteers exposed to equal potent concentrations of inhaled anesthetics during controlled ventilation of the lungs to maintain normocapnia have provided the basis of comparison for pharmacologic effects of these drugs on various organ systems (Eger, 1985a). In this regard, it is important to recognize that surgically stimulated patients who have other confounding variables may respond differently than healthy volunteers (Table 2-2).

Desflurane and sevoflurane provide one specific advantage over other currently available potent inhaled anesthetics (Eger, 1994). Their lower blood and tissue solubilities permit more precise control over the induction of anesthesia and a more rapid recovery when the drug is discontinued. Most of the other properties of these new volatile anesthetics resemble their predecessors, especially at concentrations of ≤1 MAC.

TABLE 2-2.
VARIABLES THAT INFLUENCE PHARMACOLOGIC EFFECTS OF INHALED ANESTHETICS

Anesthetic concentration
Rate of increase in anesthetic concentration
Spontaneous versus controlled ventilation
Variations from normocapnia
Surgical stimulation
Patient age
Coexisting disease
Concomitant drug therapy
Intravascular fluid volume
Preoperative medication
Injected drugs to induce and/or maintain anesthesia or skeletal muscle relaxation
Alterations in body temperature

CENTRAL NERVOUS SYSTEM EFFECTS

Mental impairment is not detectable in volunteers breathing 1,600 ppm (0.16%) nitrous oxide or 16 ppm (0.0016%) halothane (Frankhuizen et al., 1978). It is therefore unlikely that impairment of mental function in the personnel who work in the operating room can result from inhaling trace concentrations of anesthetics. Reaction times do not increase significantly until 10% to 20% nitrous oxide is inhaled (Garfield et al., 1975).

Volatile anesthetics do not cause retrograde amnesia or prolonged impairment of intellectual function. Cerebral metabolic oxygen requirements are decreased in parallel with drug-induced decreases in cerebral activity. Drug-induced increases in cerebral blood flow may increase intracranial pressure (ICP) in patients with space-occupying lesions. The effects of desflurane and sevoflurane on the CNS do not differentiate these inhaled anesthetics from the other commonly used inhaled drugs.

Electroencephalogram

Volatile anesthetics in concentrations of <0.4 MAC similarly increase the frequency and voltage on the EEG. At about 0.4 MAC, there is an abrupt shift of high-voltage activity from posterior to anterior portions of the brain (Tinker et al., 1977). Cerebral metabolic oxygen requirements also begin to decrease abruptly at about 0.4 MAC. It is likely that these changes reflect a transition from wakefulness to unconsciousness. Furthermore, amnesia probably occurs at this dose of volatile anesthetic. As the dose of volatile anesthetic approaches 1 MAC, the frequency on the EEG decreases and maximum voltage occurs. During administration of isoflurane, burst suppression appears on the EEG at about 1.5 MAC, and at 2 MAC electrical silence predominates (Eger et al., 1971). Electrical silence does not occur with enflurane, and only unacceptably high concentrations of halothane (>3.5 MAC) produce this effect. The effects of nitrous oxide on the EEG are similar to those produced by volatile anesthetics. Slower frequency and higher voltage develop on the EEG as the dose of nitrous oxide is increased or when nitrous oxide is added to a volatile anesthetic to provide a greater total MAC concentration.

Desflurane and sevoflurane cause dose-related changes in the EEG similar to those that occur with isoflurane (Eger, 1994). With desflurane, the EEG progresses from an initial increase in frequency and lowering of voltage at nonanesthetic MAC concentrations to increased voltage at anesthetizing concentrations. Higher concentrations of desflurane produce decreasing voltage and increasing periods of electrical silence with an isoelectric EEG at 1.5 to 2.0 MAC. The addition of nitrous oxide to a given level of anesthesia with desflurane causes little or no change in the EEG.

Seizure Activity

Enflurane can produce fast frequency and high voltage on the EEG that often progresses to spike wave activity that is indistinguishable from changes that accompany a seizure. This EEG activity may be accompanied by tonic-clonic twitching of skeletal muscles in the face and extremities. The likelihood of enflurane-induced seizure activity is increased when the concentration of enflurane is >2 MAC or when hyperventilation of the lungs decreases the Pa_{CO_2} to <30 mm Hg. Repetitive auditory stimuli can also initiate seizure activity during the administration of enflurane. There is no evidence of anaerobic metabolism in the brain during seizure activity produced by enflurane. Furthermore, in an animal model, enflurane does not enhance preexisting seizure foci, with the possible exception being certain types of myoclonic epilepsy and photosensitive epilepsy (Oshima et al., 1985).

Isoflurane does not evoke seizure activity on the EEG, even in the presence of deep levels of anesthesia, hypocapnia, or repetitive auditory stimulation. Indeed, isoflurane suppresses convulsant properties; it is able to suppress seizure activity produced by flurothyl (Koblin et al., 1980). An undocumented speculation is that the greater MAC value for enflurane compared with its isomer, isoflurane, reflects the need for a higher concentration to suppress the stimulating effects of enflurane in the CNS.

Desflurane and sevoflurane, like isoflurane, do not produce evidence of convulsive activity on the EEG either at deep levels of anesthesia or in the presence of hypocapnia or auditory stimulation. Nevertheless, there are reports of pediatric patients with epilepsy and otherwise healthy adults who developed EEG evidence of seizure activity during sevoflurane anesthesia (Kaisti et al., 1999; Komatsu et al., 1994). Sevoflurane can suppress convulsive activity induced with lidocaine.

The administration of nitrous oxide may increase motor activity with clonus and opisthotonus even in clinically used concentrations (Henderson et al., 1990). When nitrous oxide is administered in high concentrations in a hyperbaric chamber, abdominal muscle rigidity, catatonic movements of extremities, and periods of skeletal muscle activity may alternate with periods of skeletal muscle relaxation, clonus, and opisthotonus (Russell et al., 1990). Although very rare, tonic-clonic seizure activity has been described after administration of nitrous oxide to an otherwise healthy child (Lannes et al., 1997). Animals suspended by their tails may experience seizures in the first 15 to 90 minutes after discontinuation of nitrous oxide but not of volatile anesthetics (Smith et al., 1979). It is possible that these withdrawal seizures reflect acute nitrous oxide dependence. In patients, delirium or excitement during recovery from anesthesia that included nitrous oxide could reflect this phenomenon.

Evoked Potentials

Volatile anesthetics cause dose-related decreases in the amplitude and increases in the latency of the cortical component of median nerve somatosensory evoked potentials, visual evoked potentials, and auditory evoked potentials (Boisseau et al., 2002; Iohom et al. 2001). Decreases in amplitude are more marked than increases in latencies. In the presence of 60% nitrous oxide, waveforms adequate for monitoring cortical somatosensory evoked potentials are present during administration of 0.50 to 0.75 MAC halothane and 0.5 to 1.0 MAC enflurane and isoflurane (Pathak et al., 1987). Increasing concentrations of desflurane (0.5 to 1.5 MAC) increasingly depress somatosensory evoked potentials in patients (Eger, 1994). Even nitrous oxide alone may decrease the amplitude of cortical somatosensory evoked potentials.

Mental Function and Awareness

Inhaled anesthetics cause loss of response to verbal command at MAC-awake concentrations. Subtle effects on mental function (learning) may occur at lower anesthetic concentrations (trace concentrations to 0.2 MAC) (Ghoneim and Block, 1997). Volatile anesthetics may not be equally effective in preventing awareness. For example, 0.4 MAC isoflurane prevents recall and responses to commands whereas nitrous oxide requires greater than 0.5 to 0.6 MAC to produce similar effects. Surgical stimulation may increase the anesthetic requirement to prevent awareness.

Cerebral Blood Flow

Volatile anesthetics produce dose-dependent increases in cerebral blood flow (CBF). The magnitude of this increase is dependent on the balance between the drug's intrinsic vasodilatory actions and vasoconstriction secondary to flow-metabolism uncoupling. Volatile anesthetics administered during normocapnia in concentrations of >0.6 MAC produce cerebral vasodilation, decreased cerebral vascular resistance, and resulting dose-dependent increases in CBF (Fig. 2-6) (Eger, 1985a). This drug-induced increase in CBF occurs despite concomitant decreases in cerebral metabolic requirements. Sevoflurane has an intrinsic dose-dependent cerebral vasodilatory effect but this effect is less than that of isoflurane (Matta et al., 1999). Desflurane and isoflurane are similar in terms of increases in CBF and the preservation of reactivity to carbon dioxide (Fig. 2-7) (Ornstein et al., 1993). Nitrous oxide also increases CBF, but its restriction to concentrations of <1 MAC limits the magnitude of this change. In fact, nitrous oxide may be a more potent cerebral vasodilator than an equipotent dose of isoflurane alone in humans (Lam et al., 1994).

Anesthetic-induced increases in CBF occur within minutes of initiating administration of the inhaled drug and whether blood pressure is unchanged or decreased, emphasizing the cerebral vasodilating effects of these drugs. Animals exposed to halothane demonstrate a time-dependent decrease in the previously increased CBF begin-

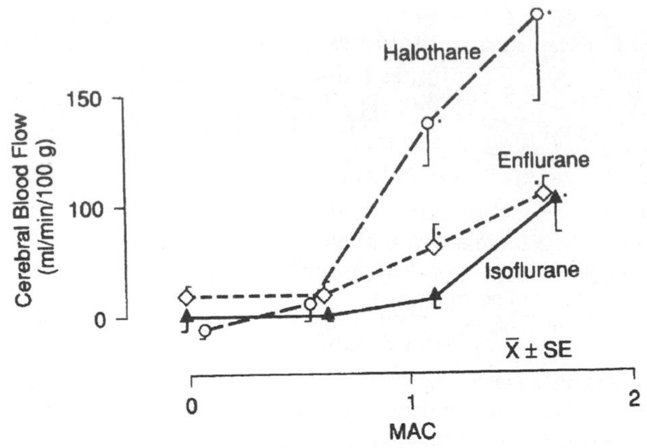

Figure 2-6. Cerebral blood flow measured in the presence of normocapnia and in the absence of surgical stimulation. ($P < .05$.) [From Eger EI. *Isoflurane (Forane): a compendium and reference,* 2nd ed. Madison, WI: Ohio Medical Products, 1985:1–110; with permission.] (From Eger EI. Pharmacology of isoflurane. *Br J Anaesth* 1984;56:71S–99S; with permission.)

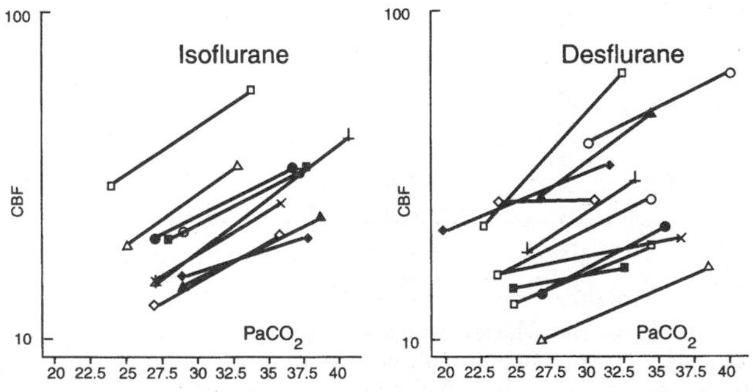

Figure 2-7. Individual cerebral blood flow (CBF) measurements (mL/100 g/min) plotted against $PaCO_2$ (mm Hg) in patients receiving 1.25 MAC isoflurane or desflurane. (From Ornstein E, Young WL, Fleischer LH, et al. Desflurane and isoflurane have similar effects on cerebral blood flow in patients with intracranial mass lesions. *Anesthesiology* 1993;79:498–502; with permission.)

ning after about 30 minutes and reaching predrug levels after about 150 minutes (Albrecht et al., 1983). This normalization of CBF reflects a concomitant increase in cerebral vascular resistance that is not altered by alpha- or beta-adrenergic blockade and is not the result of changes in the pH of the cerebrospinal fluid (Warner et al., 1985).

Unlike the decay in CBF with time observed in animals, CBF remains increased relative to cerebral metabolic oxygen requirements for as long as 4 hours during administration of halothane, isoflurane, or sevoflurane to patients during surgery (see Fig. 2-6) (Kuroda et al., 1996). Furthermore, in these patients, isoflurane possesses greater capability to maintain global CBF relative to cerebral metabolic oxygen requirements than does halothane or sevoflurane (Fig. 2-8) (Kuroda et al., 1996). An unchanging EEG during this period suggests that CBF is increased over time without a decay rather than a parallel change in CBF and cerebral metabolic oxygen requirements.

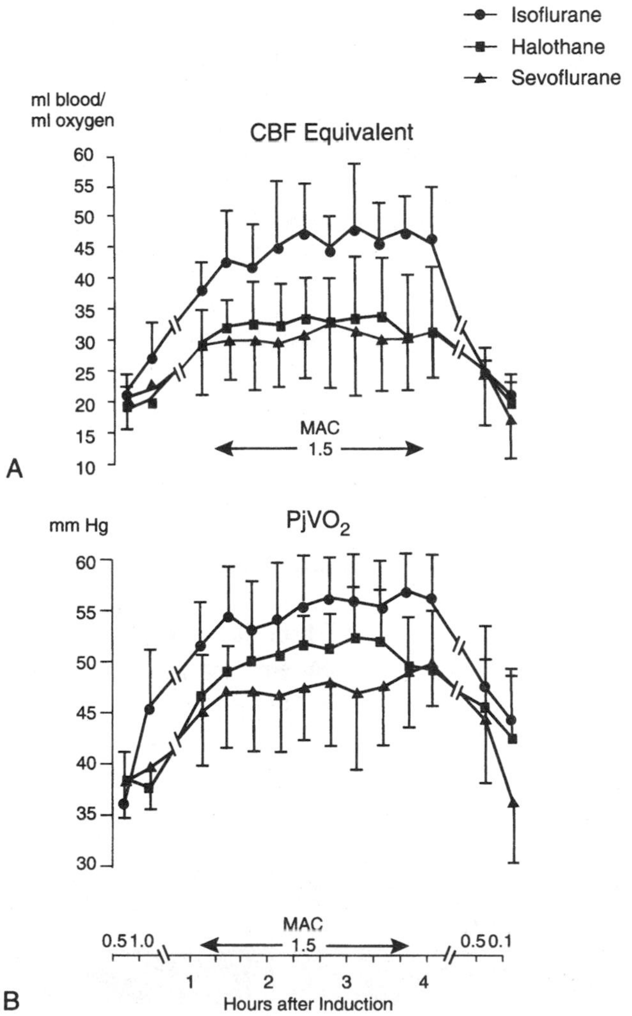

Figure 2-8. **A:** When compared at 1.5 MAC, the average increase in cerebral blood flow (CBF) in the patients receiving isoflurane is greater than in those receiving halothane and isoflurane. **B:** Likewise, the average value of the internal jugular venous oxygen tension ($PjVO_2$) is higher in patients receiving isoflurane. The increased CBF present at 1.5 MAC was sustained over time. (From Kuroda Y, Murakami M, Tsuruta J, et al. Preservation of the ratio of cerebral blood flow/metabolic rate for oxygen during prolonged anesthesia with isoflurane, sevoflurane, and halothane in humans. *Anesthesiology* 1996;84:555–561; with permission.)

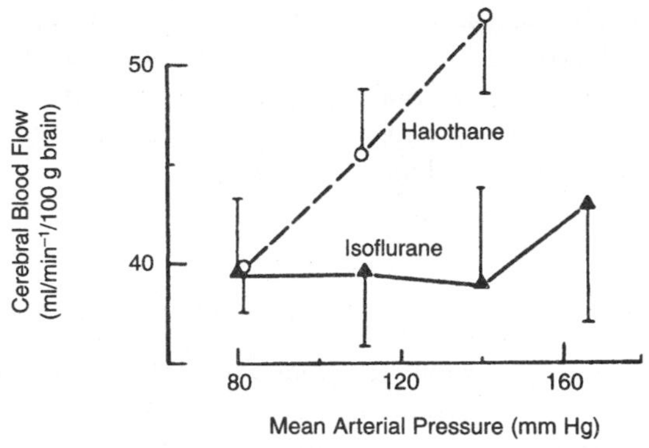

Figure 2-9. Autoregulation of cerebral blood flow (mean ≠ SE) as measured in animals. (From Eger EI. Pharmacology of isoflurane. *Br J Anaesth* 1984;56:71S-99S; with permission.)

In animals, autoregulation of CBF in response to changes in systemic blood pressure is retained during administration of 1 MAC isoflurane but not halothane (Fig. 2-9) (Drummond et al., 1982; Eger, 1985a). Indeed, increases in systemic blood pressure produce smaller increases in brain protrusion during administration of isoflurane and enflurane compared with halothane (Drummond et al., 1982). It is speculated that loss of autoregulation during administration of halothane is responsible for the greater brain swelling seen in animals anesthetized with this drug. Inhaled anesthetics including desflurane and sevoflurane do not alter autoregulation of CBF as reflected by the responsiveness of the cerebral circulation to changes in $Pa{CO_2}$ (Cho et al., 1996; Kitaguchi et al., 1993; Ornstein et al., 1993). For example, cerebrovascular carbon dioxide reactivity is described as intact during administration of 1 MAC desflurane (Mielck et al., 1998). Nevertheless, others describe impairment of autoregulation by desflurane with 1.5 MAC nearly abolishing autoregulation (Bedforth et al., 2001).

Cerebral Metabolic Oxygen Requirements

Inhaled anesthetics produce dose-dependent decreases in cerebral metabolic oxygen requirements that are greater during the administration of isoflurane than with an equivalent MAC concentration of halothane (Todd and Drummond, 1984). When the EEG becomes isoelectric, an additional increase in the concentration of the volatile anesthetics does not produce further decreases in cerebral metabolic oxygen requirements. The greater decrease in cerebral metabolic oxygen requirements produced by isoflurane may explain why CBF is not predictably increased by this anesthetic at concentrations lower than 1 MAC. For example, decreased cerebral metabolism means less carbon dioxide is produced, which thus opposes any increase in CBF. It is conceivable that isoflurane could evoke unexpected increases in CBF if administered to a patient in whom cerebral metabolic oxygen requirements were already decreased by drugs. Desflurane and sevoflurane decrease cerebral metabolic oxygen requirements similar to isoflurane.

Cerebral Protection

In animals experiencing temporary focal ischemia, there is no difference in neurologic outcome when cerebral function is suppressed by isoflurane or thiopental if systemic blood pressure is maintained (Milde et al., 1988). In humans undergoing carotid endarterectomy, the CBF at which ischemic changes appear on the EEG is lower during administration of isoflurane than during enflurane or halothane (Fig. 2-10) (Michenfelder et al., 1987). Although neurologic outcome is not different based on the volatile anesthetic administered, these data suggest that relative to enflurane and halothane, isoflurane may offer a degree of cerebral protection (blunts necrotic processes resulting from cerebral ischemia) from transient incomplete regional cerebral ischemia during carotid endarterectomy (Warner, 2000). Unchanged CBF and decreased cerebral metabolic oxygen requirements during isoflurane-induced controlled hypotension for clipping of cerebral aneurysms indicates that global cerebral oxygen supply-demand balance is favorably altered in patients anesthetized with this anesthetic (Newman et al., 1986).

Intracranial Pressure

Inhaled anesthetics produce increases in ICP that parallel increases in CBF produced by these drugs. Patients with space-occupying intracranial lesions are most vulnerable to these drug-induced increases in ICP. In hypocapnic humans with intracranial masses, desflurane concentrations of <0.8 MAC do not increase ICP whereas 1.1 MAC increases ICP by 7 mm Hg (Muzzi et al., 1992). Hyperventilation of the lungs to decrease the $Pa{CO_2}$ to about 30 mm Hg opposes the tendency for inhaled anesthetics to increase ICP (Adams et al., 1981). In this regard, isoflurane differs from halothane in that hyperventilation of the lungs can be instituted at the time the anesthetic is administered rather than before its introduction. With enflurane, it must be remembered that hyperventilation of the lungs increases the risk of seizure activity, which could lead to increased cerebral metabolic oxygen requirements and carbon dioxide production. These enflurane-induced changes will tend to increase CBF, which could further increase ICP. The ability of nitrous oxide to increase ICP is probably less than that of volatile anesthetics, reflecting the restriction of the dose of this drug to <1 MAC.

Cerebrospinal Fluid Production

Enflurane increases both the rate of production and the resistance to reabsorption of cerebrospinal fluid (CSF), which may contribute to sustained increases in ICP associated with administration of this drug (Artru, 1984a). Conversely, isoflurane does not alter production of CSF

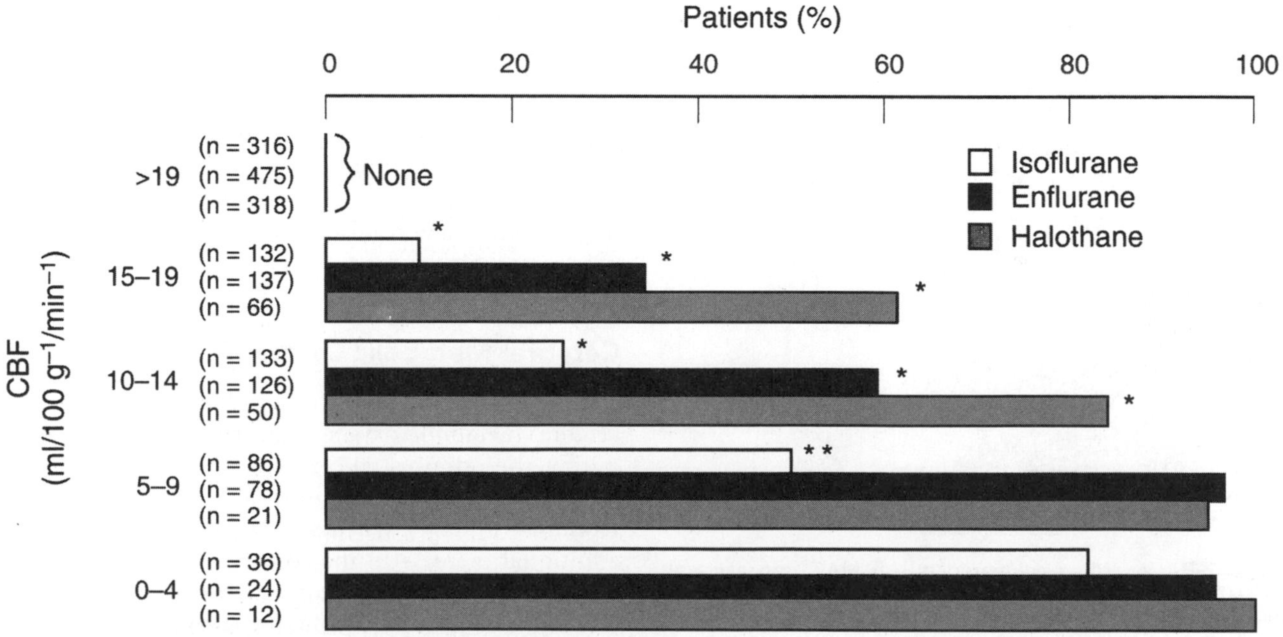

Figure 2-10. The number of patients (%) manifesting signs of cerebral ischemia on the electroencephalogram during administration of different volatile anesthetics and various ranges of cerebral blood flow (CBF). (*Significantly different from each other; **significantly different from the other two.) (From Michenfelder JD, Sundt TM, Fode N, et al. Isoflurane when compared to enflurane and halothane decreases the frequency of cerebral ischemia during carotid endarterectomy. *Anesthesiology* 1987;67:336–340; with permission.)

and, at the same time, decreases resistance to reabsorption (Artru, 1984b). These observations are consistent with minimal increases in ICP observed during the administration of isoflurane. Increases in ICP associated with administration of nitrous oxide presumably reflect increases in CBF, because enhanced production of CSF does not occur in the presence of this inhaled anesthetic (Artru, 1982).

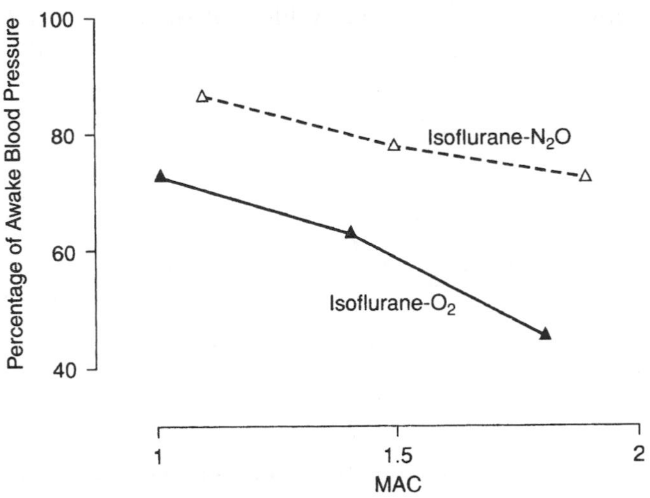

Figure 2-12. The substitution of nitrous oxide for a portion of isoflurane produces less decrease in blood pressure than the same dose of volatile anesthetic alone. [From Eger EI. *Isoflurane (Forane): a compendium and reference*, 2nd. ed. Madison, WI: Ohio Medical Products, 1985:1–110; with permission.]

CIRCULATORY EFFECTS

Inhaled anesthetics produce dose-dependent and drug-specific circulatory effects. The circulatory effects of desflurane and sevoflurane parallel many of the characteristics of older inhaled anesthetics with desflurane most closely resembling isoflurane, whereas sevoflurane has characteristics of both isoflurane and halothane (Eger, 1994; Malan et al., 1995).

Drug-induced circulatory effects manifest as changes in systemic blood pressure, heart rate, cardiac output, stroke volume, right atrial pressure, systemic vascular resistance, cardiac rhythm, and coronary blood flow. Circulatory effects of inhaled anesthetics may be different in the presence of: (a) controlled ventilation of the lungs compared with spontaneous breathing, (b) preexisting cardiac disease, or (c) drugs that act directly or indirectly on the heart. The mechanisms of circulatory effects are diverse but often reflect the effects of inhaled anesthetics on (a) myocardial contractility, (b) peripheral vascular smooth muscle tone, and (c) autonomic nervous system activity (see the section on Mechanisms of Circulatory Effects).

Mean Arterial Pressure

Halothane, isoflurane, desflurane, and sevoflurane produce similar and dose-dependent decreases in mean arterial pressure when administered to healthy human volunteers (Fig. 2-11) (Cahalan, 1996). The magnitude of decrease in mean arterial pressure in volunteers is greater than that which occurs in the presence of surgical stimulation. Likewise, artificially increased preoperative levels of systemic blood pressure, as may accompany apprehension, may be followed by decreases in blood pressure that exceed the true pharmacologic effect of the volatile anesthetic. In contrast with volatile anesthetics, nitrous oxide produces either no change or modest increases in systemic blood pressure (Eger, 1985a; Hornbein et al., 1982). Substitution of nitrous oxide for a portion of the volatile anesthetic decreases the magnitude of blood pressure decrease produced by the same MAC concentration of the volatile anesthetic alone (Fig. 2-12) (Eger, 1985a). The decrease in blood pressure produced by halothane is, in part or in whole, a consequence of decreases in myocardial contractility and cardiac output, whereas with isoflurane, desflurane, and sevoflurane, the decrease in systemic blood pressure results principally from a decrease in systemic vascular resistance (see the section on Mechanisms of Anesthesia).

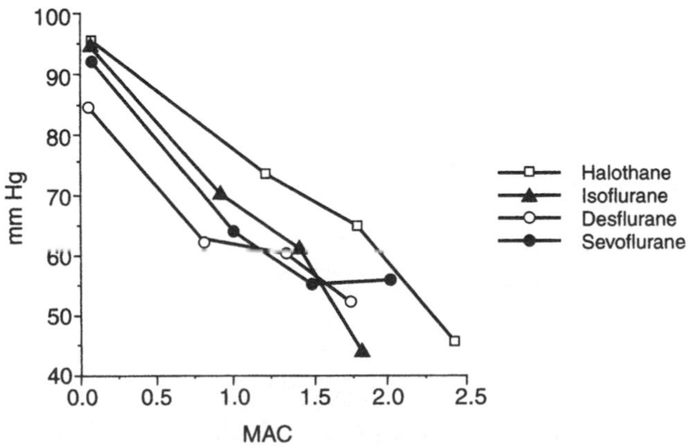

Figure 2-11. The effects of increasing concentrations (MAC) of halothane, isoflurane, desflurane, and sevoflurane on mean arterial pressure (mm Hg) when administered to healthy volunteers. [From Cahalan MK. Hemodynamic effects of inhaled anesthetics (review courses). Cleveland: International Anesthesia Research Society, 1996:14–18; with permission.]

Heart Rate

Isoflurane, desflurane, and sevoflurane, but not halothane, increase heart rate when administered to healthy human volunteers (Fig. 2-13) (Cahalan, 1996). Sevoflurane increases heart rate only at concentrations of >1.5 MAC, whereas isoflurane and desflurane tend to increase heart rate at lower concentrations. Heart rate effects seen in patients undergoing surgery may be quite different than those documented in volunteers because so many confounding variables influence heart rate. For example, a small dose of opioid (morphine in the preoperative medication or fentanyl intravenously immediately before induction of anesthesia) can prevent the heart rate increase associated with

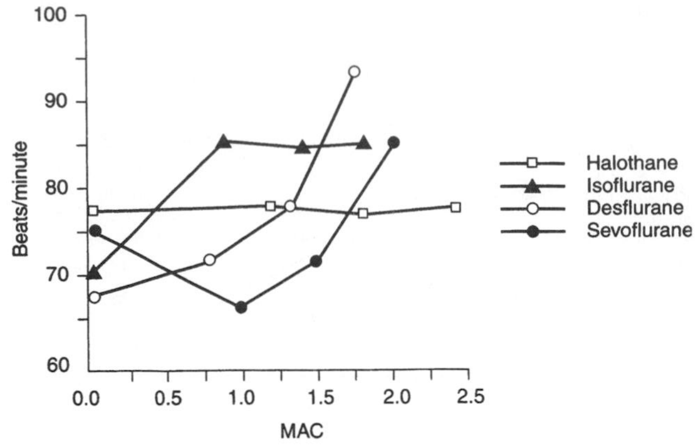

Figure 2-13. The effects of increasing concentrations (MAC) of halothane, isoflurane, desflurane, and sevoflurane on heart rate (beats/minute) when administered to healthy volunteers. [From Cahalan MK. Hemodynamic effects of inhaled anesthetics (review courses). Cleveland: International Anesthesia Research Society, 1996:14–18; with permission.]

isoflurane and presumably the other volatile anesthetics (Fig. 2-14) (Cahalan et al., 1987). Increased sympathetic nervous system activity, as accompanies apprehension, may artificially increase heart rate and the magnitude of the true pharmacologic effect of the volatile anesthetic. Similarly, excessive parasympathetic nervous system activity may result in unexpected increases in heart rate when anesthesia is established.

The common observation of an unchanged heart rate despite a decrease in blood pressure during the administration of halothane may reflect depression of the carotid sinus (baroreceptor-reflex response) by halothane, as well as drug-induced decreases in the rate of sinus node depolarization. Junctional rhythm and associated decreases in systemic blood pressure most likely reflect suppression of sinus node activity by halothane. Halothane also decreases the speed of conduction of cardiac impulses through the atrioventricular node and His-Purkinje system. At 0.5 MAC anesthesia, desflurane produces decreases in systemic blood pressure similar to those caused by isoflurane but does not evoke an increased heart rate as does isoflurane. This difference is not explained by disparate effects of these anesthetics on the baroreceptor-reflex response (Muzi and Ebert, 1995). In neonates, administration of isoflurane is associated with attenuation of the carotid sinus reflex response, as reflected by drug-induced decreases in blood pressure that are not accompanied by increases in heart rate (Murat et al., 1989). Heart rate responses during administration of isoflurane also seem to be blunted in elderly patients, whereas isoflurane-induced increases in heart rate are more likely to occur in younger patients and may be accentuated by the presence of other drugs (atropine, pancuronium) that exert vagolytic effects. Nitrous oxide also depresses the carotid sinus, but quantitating this effect is difficult because of its limited potency and its frequent simultaneous administration with other injected or inhaled drugs.

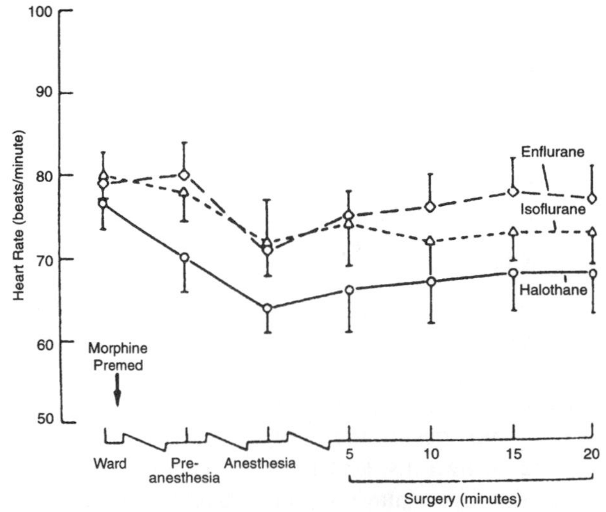

Figure 2-14. Morphine premedication is not associated with increases in heart rate (mean ± SE) during administration of volatile anesthetics with or without surgical stimulation. (From Cahalan MK, Lurz FW, Eger EI, et al. Narcotics decrease heart rate during inhalational anesthesia. *Anesth Analg* 1987;66:166–170; with permission.)

Cardiac Output and Stroke Volume

Halothane, but not isoflurane, desflurane, and sevoflurane, produces dose-dependent decreases in cardiac output when administered to healthy human volunteers (Fig. 2-15) (Cahalan, 1996). Sevoflurane did decrease cardiac output at 1 and 1.5 MAC, but at 2 MAC cardiac output had recovered to nearly awake values. Sevoflurane causes a smaller decrease in cardiac output than does halothane when administered to infants (Wodey et al., 1997). Due to different effects on heart rate (halothane causes no change and heart rate increases in the presence of the other volatile anesthetics), the calculated left ventricular stroke volume

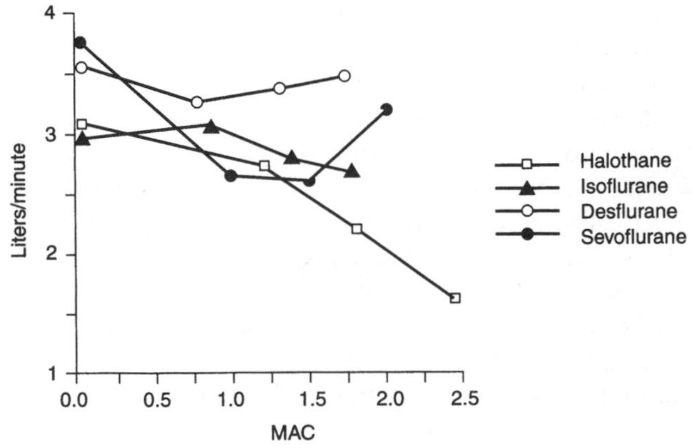

Figure 2-15. The effects of increasing concentrations (MAC) of halothane, isoflurane, desflurane, and sevoflurane on cardiac index (liters/minute) when administered to healthy volunteers. [From Cahalan MK. Hemodynamic effects of inhaled anesthetics (review courses). Cleveland: International Anesthesia Research Society, 1996:14–18; with permission.]

was similarly decreased 15% to 30% for all the volatile anesthetics. In patients, the increase in heart rate may tend to offset drug-induced decreases in cardiac output. Cardiac output is modestly increased by nitrous oxide, possibly reflecting the mild sympathomimetic effects of this drug.

In addition to better maintenance of heart rate, isoflurane's minimal depressant effects on cardiac output could reflect activation of homeostatic mechanisms that obscure direct cardiac depressant effects. Indeed, volatile anesthetics, including isoflurane, produce similar dose-dependent depression of myocardial contractility when studied in vitro using isolated papillary muscle preparations. The vasodilating effects of the ether-derivative volatile anesthetics make the direct myocardial depression produced by these drugs less apparent than that of halothane. Indeed, excessive concentrations of these drugs administered to patients can produce cardiovascular collapse. In vitro depression of myocardial contractility produced by nitrous oxide is about one-half that produced by comparable concentrations of volatile anesthetics. Direct myocardial depressant effects in vivo are most likely offset by mild sympathomimetic effects of nitrous oxide.

Another possible explanation for the lesser impact of isoflurane on myocardial contractility may be its greater anesthetic potency relative to that of halothane (Eger, 1985a). For example, the multiple of MAC times the oil:gas partition coefficient for halothane is 168 and 105 for isoflurane. The implication is that isoflurane may more readily depress the brain and thus, at a given MAC value, appear to spare the heart. Indeed, in animals, the lesser myocardial depression associated with the administration of isoflurane manifests as a greater margin of safety between the dose that produces anesthesia and that which produces cardiovascular collapse (Wolfson et al., 1978).

Right Atrial Pressure

Halothane, isoflurane, and desflurane, but not sevoflurane, increase right atrial pressure (central venous pressure) when administered to healthy human volunteers (Fig. 2-16) (Cahalan, 1996). These differences are not predictable based on the many other similarities between sevoflurane, desflurane, and isoflurane. The peripheral vasodilating effects of volatile anesthetics would tend to minimize the effects of direct myocardial depression on right atrial pressure produced by these drugs. Increased right atrial pressure during administration of nitrous oxide most likely reflects increased pulmonary vascular resistance due to the sympathomimetic effects of this drug (Smith et al., 1970).

Systemic Vascular Resistance

Isoflurane, desflurane, and sevoflurane, but not halothane, decrease systemic vascular resistance when administered to healthy human volunteers (Fig. 2-17) (Cahalan, 1996).

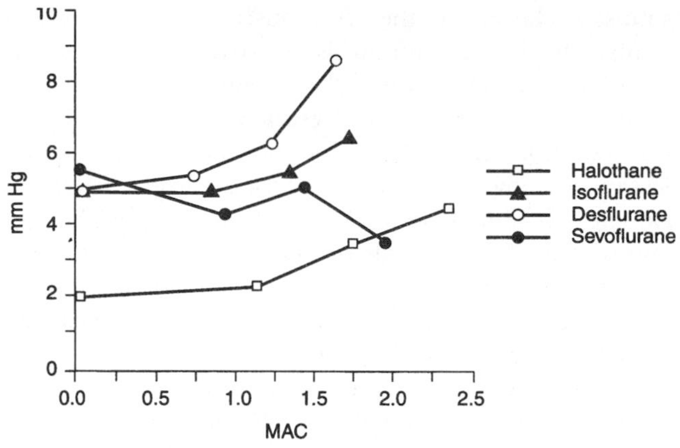

Figure 2-16. The effects of increasing concentrations (MAC) of halothane, isoflurane, desflurane, and sevoflurane on central venous pressure (mm Hg) when administered to healthy volunteers. [From Cahalan MK. Hemodynamic effects of inhaled anesthetics (review courses). Cleveland: International Anesthesia Research Society, 1996:14–18; with permission.]

Thus, although these four volatile anesthetics decrease systemic blood pressure comparably, only halothane does so principally by decreasing cardiac output. For example, the absence of changes in systemic vascular resistance during administration of halothane emphasizes that decreases in systemic blood pressure produced by this drug parallel decreases in myocardial contractility. The other volatile anesthetics decrease blood pressure principally by decreasing systemic vascular resistance. Nitrous oxide does not change systemic vascular resistance.

Decreases in systemic vascular resistance during administration of isoflurane principally reflect substantial (up to fourfold) increases in skeletal muscle blood flow (Stevens et al., 1971). Cutaneous blood flow is also increased by isoflurane. The implications of these alterations in blood flow may include (a) excess (wasted) perfusion relative to oxygen needs, (b) loss of body heat due to increased cutaneous blood flow, and (c) enhanced delivery of drugs, such

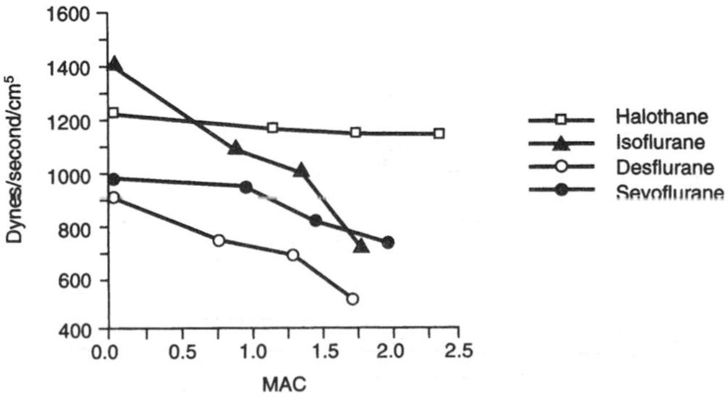

Figure 2-17. The effects of increasing concentrations (MAC) of halothane, isoflurane, desflurane, and sevoflurane on systemic vascular resistance (dynes/second/cm^5) when administered to healthy volunteers. [From Cahalan MK. Hemodynamic effects of inhaled anesthetics (review courses). Cleveland: International Anesthesia Research Society, 1996:14–18; with permission.]

as muscle relaxants, to the neuromuscular junction. A beta agonist effect of isoflurane is consistent with vascular smooth muscle relaxation in skeletal muscles.

Failure of systemic vascular resistance to decrease during administration of halothane does not mean that this drug lacks vasodilating effects on some organs. Clearly, halothane is a potent cerebral vasodilator, and cutaneous vasodilation is prominent. These vasodilating effects of halothane, however, are offset by absent changes or vasoconstriction in other vascular beds such that the overall effect is unchanged calculated systemic vascular resistance.

The increase in cutaneous blood flow produced by all volatile anesthetics arterializes peripheral venous blood, providing an alternative to sampling arterial blood for evaluation of pH and $PaCO_2$ (Fig. 2-18) (Williamson and Munson, 1982). These drug-induced increases in cutaneous blood flow most likely reflect a central inhibitory action of these anesthetics on temperature-regulating mechanisms. In contrast to volatile anesthetics, nitrous oxide may produce constriction of cutaneous blood vessels (Smith et al., 1978).

Pulmonary Vascular Resistance

Volatile anesthetics appear to exert little or no predictable effect on pulmonary vascular smooth muscle. Conversely, nitrous oxide may produce increases in pulmonary vascular resistance that are exaggerated in patients with preexisting pulmonary hypertension (Hilgenberg et al., 1980; Schulte-Sasse et al., 1982). The neonate with or without preexisting pulmonary hypertension may also be uniquely vulnerable to the pulmonary vascular vasoconstricting effects of nitrous oxide (Eisele et al., 1986). In patients with congenital heart disease, these increases in pulmonary vascular resistance may increase the magnitude of right-to-left intracardiac shunting of blood and further jeopardize arterial oxygenation.

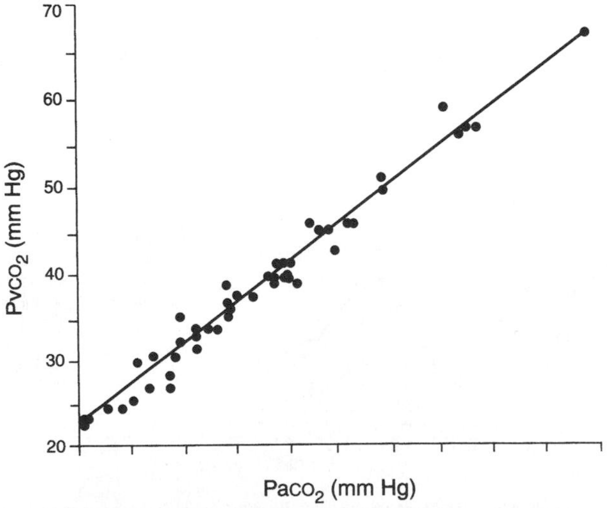

Figure 2-18. There is a linear relationship between $PvCO_2$ measured in "arterialized" peripheral venous blood and the $PaCO_2$. (From Williamson DC, Munson ES. Correlation of peripheral venous and arterial blood gas values during general anesthesia. *Anesth Analg* 1982;61:950–952; with permission.)

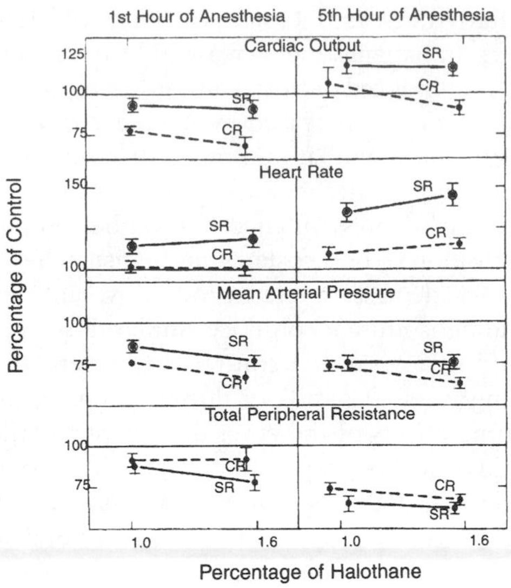

Figure 2-19. Comparison of circulatory effects of halothane during spontaneous breathing (SR) and controlled ventilation of the lungs (CR) after 1 and 5 hours of administration of halothane. (From Bahlman SH, Eger EI, Halsey MJ, et al. The cardiovascular effects of halothane in man during spontaneous ventilation. *Anesthesiology* 1972;36:494–502; with permission.)

Duration of Administration

Administration of a volatile anesthetic for 5 hours or longer is accompanied by recovery from the depressant effects of these drugs. For example, compared with measurements at 1 hour, the same MAC concentration after 5 hours is associated with a return of cardiac output toward predrug levels (Figs. 2-19 and 2-20) (Bahlman et al., 1972; Calverley et al., 1978b). After 5 hours, heart rate is also increased, but systemic blood pressure is unchanged, as the increase in cardiac output is offset by decreases in systemic vascular resistance. Evidence of recovery with time is most apparent during administration of halothane and is minimal during inhalation of isoflurane. Minimal evidence of recovery during administration of isoflurane (and presumably desflurane and sevoflurane) is predictable, because this drug does not substantially alter cardiac output even at 1 hour.

The return of cardiac output toward predrug levels with time, in association with increases in heart rate and peripheral vasodilation, resembles a beta-adrenergic agonist response. Indeed, pretreatment with propranolol prevents evidence of recovery with time from the circulatory effects of volatile anesthetics (Price et al., 1970).

Cardiac Dysrhythmias

The ability of volatile anesthetics to decrease the dose of epinephrine necessary to evoke ventricular cardiac dysrhythmias is greatest with the alkane derivative halothane and

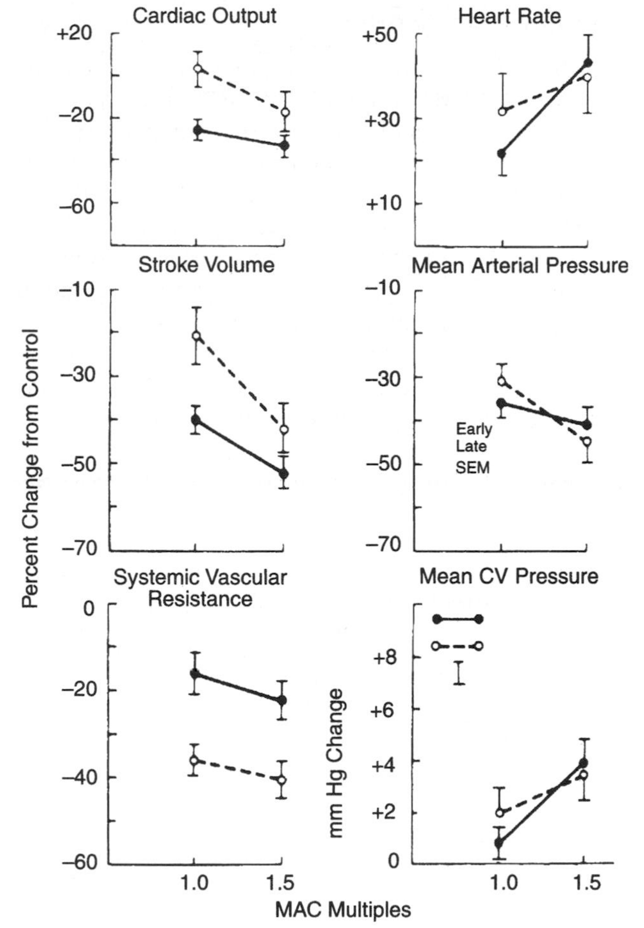

Figure 2-20. Comparison of circulatory effects of enflurane after 1 hour (*solid line*) and 6 hours (*broken line*) of administration during controlled ventilation of the lungs to maintain normocapnia. (CV, cardiovascular.) (From Calverley RK, Smith NT, Prys-Roberts C, et al. Cardiovascular effects of enflurane anesthesia during controlled ventilation in man. *Anesth Analg* 1978;57:619–628; with permission.)

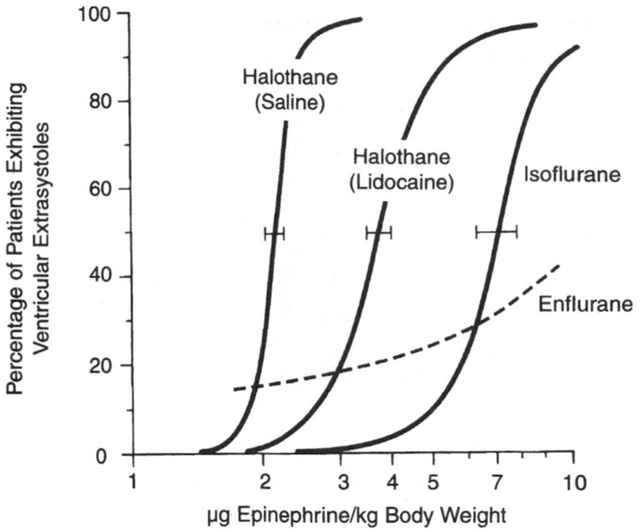

Figure 2-21. Percentage of patients developing ventricular cardiac dysrhythmias [three or more premature ventricular contractions (PVCs)] with increasing doses of submucosal epinephrine injected during administration of 1.25 MAC of halothane, isoflurane, or enflurane. (From Johnston PR, Eger EI, Wilson C. A comparative interaction of epinephrine with enflurane, isoflurane, and halothane in man. *Anesth Analg* 1976;55:709–712; with permission.)

minimal to nonexistent with the ether derivatives isoflurane, desflurane, and sevoflurane (Figs. 2-21, 2-22, and 2-23) (Johnston et al., 1976; Moore et al., 1993; Navarro et al., 1994). In contrast to adults, children tolerate larger doses of subcutaneous epinephrine (7.8 to 10.0 μg/kg) injected with or without lidocaine during halothane anesthesia (Karl et al., 1983; Ueda et al., 1983). Mechanical stimulation associated with injection of epinephrine for repair of cleft palate has been associated with cardiac dysrhythmias (Ueda et al., 1983).

Inclusion of lidocaine 0.5% in the epinephrine solution that is injected submucosally nearly doubles the dose of epinephrine necessary to provoke ventricular cardiac dysrhythmias (see Fig. 2-21) (Johnston et al., 1976). A similar response occurs when lidocaine is combined with epinephrine injected submucosally during administration of enflurane (Horrigan et al., 1978). Despite the apparent protective effect of lidocaine, the systemic concentrations of the local anesthetic are <1 μg/mL after its subcutaneous injection with epinephrine (Stoelting, 1978).

In animals, enhancement of the dysrhythmogenic potential of epinephrine is independent of the dose of halothane between alveolar concentrations of 0.5% and 2% (Metz and Maze, 1985). If true in patients, it is likely that cardiac dysrhythmias due to epinephrine will persist until the halothane concentration decreases to <0.5%. For this reason, therapeutic interventions other than decreasing the inhaled concentration of halothane may be required to treat cardiac dysrhythmias promptly due to epinephrine.

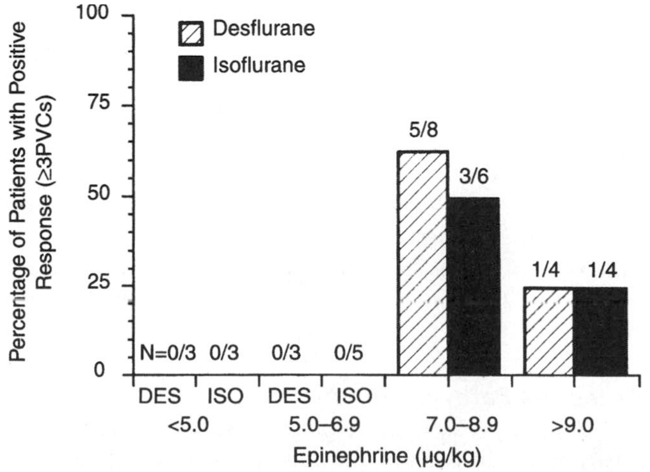

Figure 2-22. Responses to submucosally injected epinephrine in patients receiving desflurane (DES) or isoflurane (ISO) anesthesia. (PVCs, premature ventricular contractions.) (From Moore MA, Weiskopf RB, Eger EI, et al. Arrhythmogenic doses of epinephrine are similar during desflurane or isoflurane anesthesia in humans. *Anesthesiology* 1993;79:943–947; with permission.)

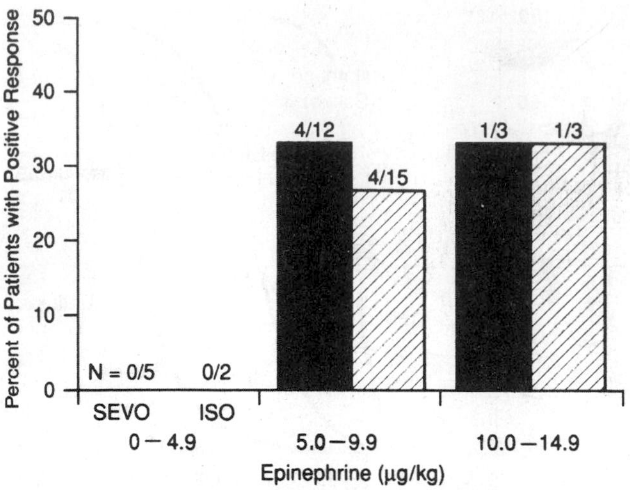

Figure 2-23. Responses to submucosally injected epinephrine in patients receiving sevoflurane (SEVO) or isoflurane (ISO) anesthesia. (From Navarro R, Weiskopf RB, Moore MA, et al. Humans anesthetized with sevoflurane or isoflurane have similar arrhythmic response to epinephrine. *Anesthesiology* 1994;80:545–549; with permission.)

The explanation for the difference between volatile anesthetics and the dysrhythmogenic potential of epinephrine may reflect the effects of these drugs on the transmission rate of cardiac impulses through the heart's conduction system. Nevertheless, halothane and isoflurane both slow the rate of sinoatrial node discharge and prolong His-Purkinje and ventricular conduction times (Atlee and Bosnjak, 1990) (see Chapter 48).

QTc Interval

Halothane, enflurane, and isoflurane prolong the QTc interval on the ECG in healthy patients (Schmeling et al., 1991). Nevertheless, similar changes may not occur in patients with idiopathic long QTc interval syndrome suggesting that generalizations from healthy patients to patients with long QTc interval syndrome may not be valid. Likewise, thiopental prolongs the QTc interval in healthy patients but has no effect in patients with long QTc syndrome. Conversely, there is a report of a patient with long QTc syndrome of prolongation of the QT interval in response to the administration of sevoflurane (Gallagher et al., 1998). Furthermore, in healthy patients, administration of sevoflurane, but not propofol, results in prolongation of the QTc interval on the ECG (Kleinsasser et al., 2000).

Accessory Pathway Conduction

Isoflurane increases the refractoriness of accessory pathways and the atrioventricular conduction system thus interfering with interpretation of postablative studies used to determine successful ablation. In contrast, sevoflurane has no effect on the atrioventricular or accessory pathways and is considered an acceptable anesthetic drug for patients undergoing ablative procedures (Sharpe et al., 1999).

Spontaneous Breathing

Circulatory effects produced by volatile anesthetics during spontaneous breathing are different from those observed during normocapnia and controlled ventilation of the lungs. This difference reflects the impact of sympathetic nervous system stimulation due to accumulation of carbon dioxide (respiratory acidosis) and improved venous return during spontaneous breathing. In addition, carbon dioxide may have direct relaxing effects on peripheral vascular smooth muscle. Indeed, systemic blood pressure, and heart rate are increased and systemic vascular resistance is decreased compared with measurements during administration of volatile anesthetics in the presence of controlled ventilation of the lungs to maintain normocapnia (see Figs. 2-19 and 2-20) (Bahlman et al., 1972; Calverley et al., 1978a; Cromwell et al., 1971).

Coronary Blood Flow

Volatile anesthetics induce coronary vasodilation by preferentially acting on vessels with diameters from 20 µm to 50 µm, whereas adenosine, in addition, has a pronounced impact on the small precapillary arterioles (Conzen et al., 1992). It has been suggested that isoflurane as well as other coronary vasodilators (adenosine, dipyridamole, nitroprusside) that preferentially dilate the small coronary resistance coronary vessels would be capable of redistributing blood from ischemic to nonischemic areas, producing the phenomenon known as *coronary steal syndrome*. Nevertheless, this phenomenon is not clinically significant and volatile anesthetics, including isoflurane, are cardioprotective (see the section on Cardiac Protection [Anesthetic Preconditioning]).

Neurocirculatory Responses

The solubility characteristics of desflurane make this volatile anesthetic a good choice to treat abrupt increases in systemic blood pressure and/or heart rate as may occur in response to sudden changes in the intensity of surgical stimulation. Nevertheless, abrupt increases in the alveolar concentrations of isoflurane and desflurane from 0.55 MAC (0.71% isoflurane and 4% desflurane) to 1.66 MAC (2.12% isoflurane and 12% desflurane) increase sympathetic nervous system and renin-angiotensin activity and cause transient increases in mean arterial pressure and heart rate (Figs. 2-24, 2-25, and 2-26) (Weiskopf et al., 1994b). Desflurane causes significantly greater increases than isoflurane. The magnitude of the response to a rapid increase from 4% to 8% desflurane was similar to that produced by a rapid increase from 4% to 12%, suggesting that the stimulus provided by 8% desflurane produced a maximum response. Small (1%) increases in the desflurane concentration also transiently increase systemic blood pressure and heart rate, but the magnitude is less than those same changes that

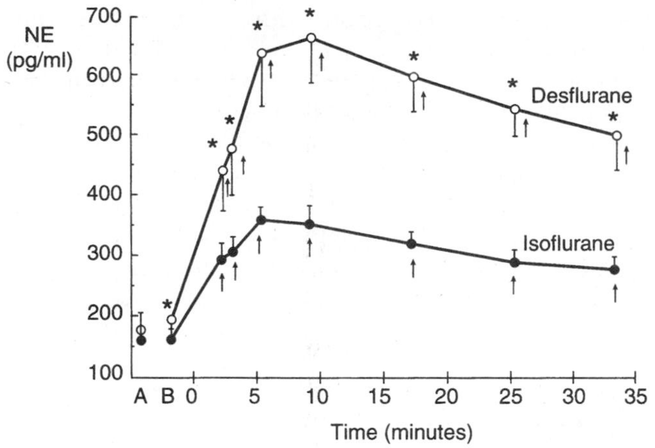

Figure 2-24. Plasma norepinephrine (NE) concentrations increased from awake levels (A) and those present during administration of 0.55 MAC desflurane or isoflurane (B) when the anesthetic concentrations were abruptly increased to 1.66 MAC (0). The increase was greater in the presence of desflurane than isoflurane (*$P < .05$). Data are mean ± SE. (From Weiskopf RB, Moore MA, Eger EI, et al. Rapid increase in desflurane concentration is associated with greater transient cardiovascular stimulation than with rapid increases in isoflurane concentration in humans. *Anesthesiology* 1994;80:1035–1045; with permission.)

occur with an increase from 4% to 12% (Moore et al., 1994). Sites mediating sympathetic nervous system activation in response to desflurane are present in the upper airway (larynx and above) and in the lungs (Muzi et al., 1996). These sites may respond to direct irritation. The increase in

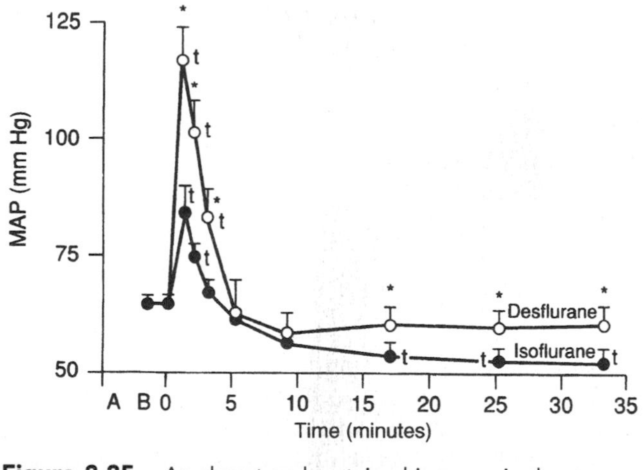

Figure 2-25. An abrupt and sustained increase in the concentration of desflurane from 0.55 MAC to 1.66 MAC (0) resulted in a substantial but transient increase in mean arterial pressure (MAP). A similar increase in isoflurane MAC produced an increase in MAP that was substantially less than that observed in patients receiving desflurane. Within 5 minutes after increasing the anesthetic concentration, the MAP had decreased below awake (A) and 0.55 MAC values (B) reflecting the greater depth of anesthesia present at this time. (t, $P < .05$ compared with the value at 0.55 MAC of the same anesthetic; *$P < .05$ compared with isoflurane at the same time point.) (From Weiskopf RB, Moore MA, Eger EI, et al. Rapid increase in desflurane concentration is associated with greater transient cardiovascular stimulation than with rapid increases in isoflurane concentration in humans. *Anesthesiology* 1994;80:1035–1045; with permission.)

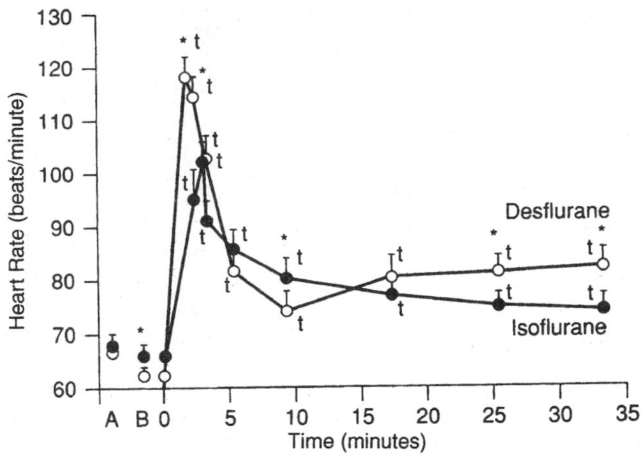

Figure 2-26. An abrupt and sustained increase in the concentration of desflurane from 0.55 MAC to 1.66 MAC (0) resulted in a substantial but transient increase in heart rate. A similar increase in isoflurane MAC produced an increase in heart rate that was substantially less than that observed in patients receiving desflurane. Within 5 minutes after increasing the anesthetic concentration, the heart rate remained above awake (A) and baseline values at 0.55 MAC (B), reflecting the greater depth of anesthesia present at this time. (t, $P < .05$ compared with the value at 0.55 MAC of the same anesthetic; *$P < .05$ compared with isoflurane at the same time point.) (From Weiskopf RB, Moore MA, Eger EI, et al. Rapid increase in desflurane concentration is associated with greater transient cardiovascular stimulation than with rapid increases in isoflurane concentration in humans. *Anesthesiology* 1994;80:1035–1045; with permission.)

basal levels of sympathetic nervous system activity that accompany increasing inhaled concentrations of desflurane does not reflect the effects of drug-induced hypotension or alterations in baroreceptor activity.

In contrast to desflurane and isoflurane, neurocirculatory responses do not accompany abrupt increases in the delivered concentration of sevoflurane (Fig. 2-27) (Ebert et al., 1995).

Fentanyl (1.5 to 4.5 μg/kg IV administered 5 minutes before the abrupt increase in desflurane concentration), esmolol (0.75 mg/kg IV 1.5 minutes before), and clonidine (4.3 μg/kg orally 90 minutes before) blunt the transient cardiovascular responses to rapid increases in desflurane concentration (Weiskopf et al., 1994a). Fentanyl may be the most clinically useful of these drugs because it blunts the increase in heart rate and blood pressure, has minimal cardiovascular depressant effects, and imposes little postanesthetic sedation. Alfentanil, 10 μg/kg IV, in conjunction with the induction of anesthesia, also blunts the hemodynamic responses to an abrupt increase in the delivered concentration of desflurane (Yonker-Sell et al., 1996). The increase in plasma norepinephrine concentrations that accompany the abrupt increase in desflurane concentration are not predictably prevented by the prior administration of opioids.

Preexisting Diseases and Drug Therapy

Preexisting cardiac disease may influence the significance of circulatory effects produced by inhaled anesthetics. For example, volatile anesthetics decrease myocardial

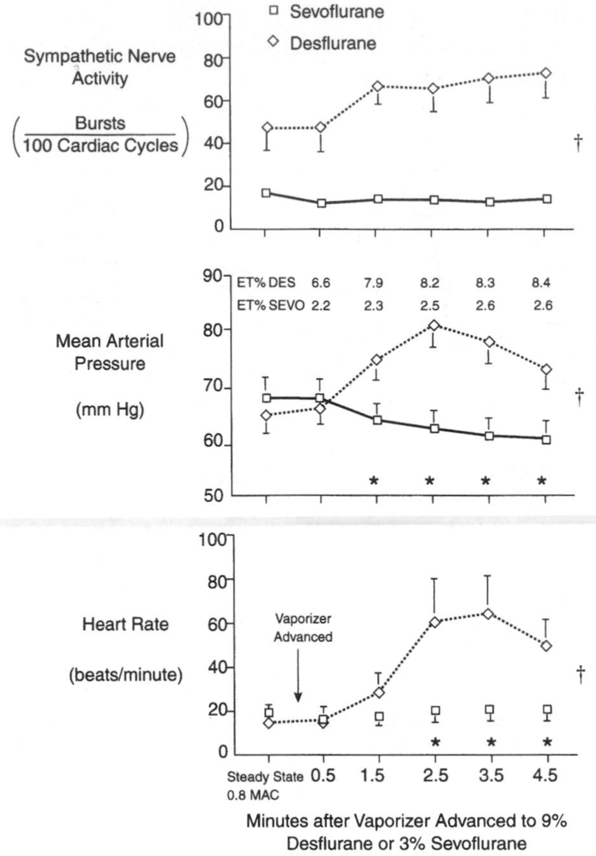

Figure 2-27. A rapid increase in the inspired concentration of sevoflurane (SEVO) from 0.8 MAC to 3% did not alter sympathetic nerve activity, mean arterial pressure, or heart rate. Conversely, a rapid increase in the inspired concentration of desflurane (DES) from 0.8 MAC to 9% significantly increased sympathetic nerve activity, mean arterial pressure, and heart rate. (Mean ± SE; $^*P < .05$; ET, end-tidal.) (From Ebert TJ, Muzi M, Lopatka CW. Neurocirculatory responses to sevoflurane in humans: a comparison to desflurane. *Anesthesiology* 1995;83:88–95; with permission.)

contractility of normal and failing cardiac muscle by similar amounts, but the significance is greater in diseased cardiac muscle because contractility is decreased even before administration of depressant anesthetics. Neurocirculatory responses evoked by abrupt increases in the concentration of desflurane may be undesirable in patients with coronary artery disease. In patients with coronary artery disease, administration of 40% nitrous oxide produces evidence of myocardial depression that does not occur in patients without heart disease (Eisele and Smith, 1972). Valvular heart disease may influence the significance of anesthetic-induced circulatory effects. For example, peripheral vasodilation produced by isoflurane (presumably also desflurane and sevoflurane) is undesirable in patients with aortic stenosis but may be beneficial in those with mitral or aortic regurgitation. Arterial hypoxemia may enhance the cardiac depressant effects of volatile anesthetics. Conversely, anemia does not alter anesthetic-induced circulatory effects compared with measurements from normal animals.

Prior drug therapy that alters sympathetic nervous system activity (antihypertensives, beta-adrenergic antagonists) may influence the magnitude of circulatory effects produced by volatile anesthetics. Calcium entry blockers decrease myocardial contractility and thus render the heart more vulnerable to direct depressant effects of inhaled anesthetics. In animals, the depressant effects of verapamil on cardiac output are greater during administration of enflurane than of isoflurane (see Chapter 18).

Mechanisms of Circulatory Effects

There is no single mechanism that explains the depressant effects of volatile anesthetics in all situations. Proposed mechanisms include (a) direct myocardial depression, (b) inhibition of CNS sympathetic outflow, (c) peripheral autonomic ganglion blockade, (d) attenuated carotid sinus reflex activity, (e) decreased formation of cyclic adenosine monophosphate, (f) decreased release of catecholamines, and (g) decreased influx of calcium ions through slow channels. Indeed, negative inotropic, vasodilating, and depressant effects on the sinoatrial node produced by volatile anesthetics are similar to the effects produced by calcium entry blockers (Lynch et al., 1981). Plasma catecholamine concentrations typically do not increase during administration of volatile anesthetics, which is evidence that these drugs do not activate and may even decrease activity of the central and peripheral sympathetic nervous systems.

Isoflurane may be unique among the volatile anesthetics in possessing mild beta-adrenergic agonist properties. This effect is consistent with the maintenance of cardiac output, increased heart rate, and decreased systemic vascular resistance that may accompany administration of isoflurane (Stevens et al., 1971). A beta agonist effect of isoflurane, however, is not supported by animal data that fail to demonstrate a difference between volatile anesthetics with or without beta-adrenergic blockade (Philbin and Lowenstein, 1976).

Nitrous oxide administered alone or added to unchanging concentrations of volatile anesthetics produces signs of mild sympathomimetic stimulation characterized by (a) increases in the plasma concentrations of catecholamines, (b) mydriasis, (c) increases in body temperature, (d) diaphoresis, (e) increases in right atrial pressure, and (f) evidence of vasoconstriction in the systemic and pulmonary circulations. Evidence of the sympathomimetic effect is more prominent when nitrous oxide is administered in the presence of halothane than of enflurane or isoflurane. It is presumed that this mild sympathomimetic effect masks any direct depressant effects of nitrous oxide on the heart. Nitrous oxide–induced increases in sympathetic nervous system activity may reflect activation of brain nuclei that regulate beta-adrenergic outflow from the

CNS (Fukunaga and Epstein, 1973). Sympathetic nervous system stimulation may also result because nitrous oxide can inhibit uptake of norepinephrine by the lungs, making more neurotransmitter available to receptors (Naito and Gillis, 1973).

In contrast to sympathomimetic effects observed with the administration of nitrous oxide alone or added to volatile anesthetics, the inhalation of nitrous oxide in the presence of opioids results in evidence of profound circulatory depression, characterized by decreases in systemic blood pressure and cardiac output and increases in left ventricular end-diastolic pressure and systemic vascular resistance (Lappas et al., 1975; Stoelting and Gibbs, 1973). It is possible that opioids inhibit the centrally mediated sympathomimetic effects of nitrous oxide, thus unmasking its direct depressant effects on the heart.

Cardiac Protection (Anesthetic Preconditioning)

Brief episodes of myocardial ischemia occurring before a subsequent longer period of myocardial ischemia providing protection against myocardial dysfunction and necrosis is termed ischemic preconditioning (IPC) (Lynch, 1999). The preconditioning protection seems to be mediated by release of adenosine which binds to adenosine receptors and increases protein kinase C activity. The resulting phosphorylation of adenosine triphosphate (ATP) sensitive mitochondrial potassium channels (K_{ATP}) results in these channels being less sensitive to inhibition by ATP. These channels are important in regulating vascular smooth muscle tone by causing hyperpolarization and relaxation when oxygen delivery results in decreased ATP production. When K_{ATP} channel activity is increased there is a decrease in the voltage gradient and decrease in calcium ion accumulation, the cardiac action potential shortens, accompanied by a mild negative inotropic action and remarkable protection against subsequent sustained ischemic or hypoxic insult. Opening of K_{ATP} channels is critical for the beneficial cardioprotective effects of IPC. Brief exposure to a volatile anesthetic (isoflurane, sevoflurane, desflurane) can activate K_{ATP} channels resulting in cardioprotection (anesthetic preconditioning) against subsequent prolonged ischemia and myocardial reperfusion injury that is identical to IPC (Hanouz et al., 2002; Tanaka et al., 2004: Warltier et al., 2002; Yvon et al., 2003; Zaugg et al., 2002). Concentrations of isoflurane as low as 0.25 MAC are sufficient to precondition myocardium against ischemic injury although higher doses may provide even greater cardiac protection (Kehl et al., 2002). Combined administration of isoflurane and morphine enhances protection against myocardial infarction to a greater extent than either drug alone (Ludwig et al., 2003).

Reperfusion injury is defined as cellular injury that is caused by reperfusion itself and not the preceding ischemia. Manifestations of reversible reperfusion injury include cardiac dysrhythmias, contractile dysfunction ("stunning"), and microvascular injury (Ross and Foex, 1999). In addition to myocardium, a similar effect induced by volatile anesthetics on vascular endothelium may result in protection from ischemia in other tissues. Conversely, certain intravenous anesthetics may have deleterious effects on IPC and protection against reperfusion injury as produced by opening of K_{ATP} channels. If anesthetic preconditioning is to be of clinical value, it will most likely be because it affords additional time before occurrence of dysfunction and/or infarction that will allow either spontaneous reperfusion or application of therapies such as angioplasty to relieve a coronary occlusion (Kevin et al., 2003). The preconditioning effects of volatile anesthetics may be beneficial in patients who are susceptible to myocardial infarction during and following surgery. Indeed, patients receiving sevoflurane for cardiac surgery (off-bypass or cardiopulmonary bypass) had less myocardial injury (lower release of troponin I) during the first 24 postoperative hours than patients receiving propofol (Figs. 2-28 and 2-29) (Conzen et al., 2003; DeHert et al., 2002). In patients undergoing coronary artery surgery with cardiopulmonary bypass, the cardioprotective effects of sevoflurane were clinically more apparent when this volatile anesthetic was administered throughout the operation compared with administration during only a part of the anesthetic (Fig. 2-29) (DeHert, et al., 2004). Cardiac output was improved in patients receiving sevoflurane but

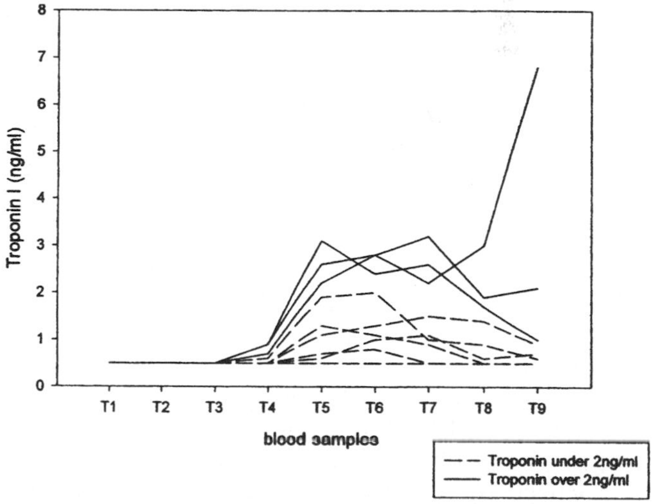

Figure 2-28. Cardiac troponin I concentrations in sevoflurane-anesthetized patients during and after anesthesia. Samples were obtained before induction of anesthesia (T1), before ischemia (T2), 15 minutes after reperfusion (T3), at arrival in the postanesthesia care unit (T4), and 3 (T5), 6 (T6), 12 (T7), 18 (T8), and 24 hours (T9) after arrival. (From Conzen PF, Fischer S, Detter C, et al. Sevoflurane provides greater protection of the myocardium than propofol in patients undergoing off-pump coronary artery bypass surgery. *Anesthesiology* 2003;99:826-833; with permission.)

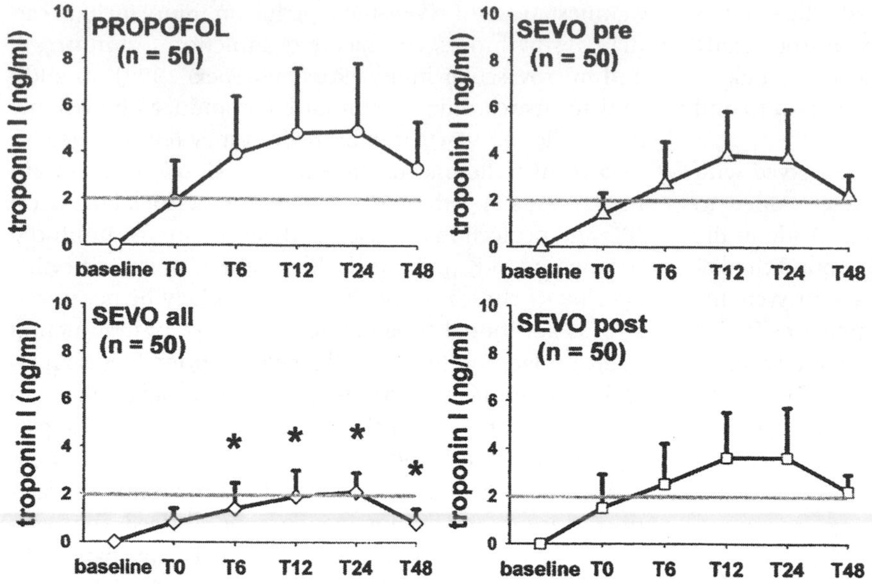

Figure 2-29. Cardiac troponin I concentrations in four patient groups before surgery (baseline), at arrival in the intensive care unit (T0), and after 6 (T6), 12 (T12), 24 (T24), and 48 (T48) hours. Mean ≠ SD. A transient increase in troponin I concentrations was observed in all groups. The increase in the SEVO (sevoflurane) group was significantly less than in the propofol group. (From DeHert, Van der Linden PJ, Cromheecke S, et al. Cardioprotective properties of sevoflurane in patients undergoing coronary surgery with cardiopulmonary bypass are related to its modalities of its administration. *Anesthesiology* 2004;101: 299-310, with permission.)

not propofol suggesting better maintenance of myocardial function.

IPC is a fundamental endogenous protective mechanism against tissue injury (best characterized in the heart but also present in other tissues) ubiquitous to all species in which it has been studied. An early phase of IPC persists for 1 to 2 hours before disappearing and then reoccurring 24 hours. This second or late window of preconditioning may last for as long as 3 days.

VENTILATION EFFECTS

Inhaled anesthetics produce dose-dependent and drug-specific effects on the (a) pattern of breathing, (b) ventilatory response to carbon dioxide, (c) ventilatory response to arterial hypoxemia, and (d) airway resistance. The $Pa{O_2}$ predictably declines during administration of inhaled anesthetics in the absence of supplemental oxygen. Drug-induced inhibition of hypoxic pulmonary vasoconstriction as a mechanism for this decrease in oxygenation has not been confirmed during one-lung ventilation in patients breathing halothane or isoflurane (see Fig. 46-4). Changes in intraoperative $Pa{O_2}$ and the incidence of postoperative pulmonary complications are not different in patients anesthetized with halothane, enflurane, or isoflurane (Gold et al., 1983).

Pattern of Breathing

Inhaled anesthetics, except for isoflurane, produce dose-dependent increases in the frequency of breathing (Eger, 1985b). Isoflurane increases the frequency of breathing similarly to other inhaled anesthetics up to a dose of 1 MAC. At a concentration of >1 MAC, however, isoflurane does not produce a further increase in the frequency of breathing. Nitrous oxide increases the frequency of breathing more than other inhaled anesthetics at concentrations of >1 MAC. The effect of inhaled anesthetics on the frequency of breathing presumably reflects CNS stimulation. Activation of pulmonary stretch receptors by inhaled anesthetics has not been demonstrated. The exception may be nitrous oxide, which at anesthetic concentrations of >1 MAC, may also stimulate pulmonary stretch receptors.

Tidal volume is decreased in association with anesthetic-induced increases in the frequency of breathing. The net effect of these changes is a rapid and shallow pattern of breathing during general anesthesia. The increase in frequency of breathing is insufficient to offset decreases in tidal volume, leading to decreases in minute ventilation and increases in $Pa{CO_2}$. There is evidence in patients that isoflurane produces a greater decrease in minute ventilation than does halothane (Fig. 2-30) (Canet et al., 1994). The pattern of breathing during general anesthesia is also characterized as regular and rhythmic in contrast to the awake pattern of intermittent deep breaths separated by varying intervals.

Ventilatory Response to Carbon Dioxide

Volatile anesthetics produce dose-dependent depression of ventilation characterized by decreases in the ventilatory response to carbon dioxide and increases in the $Pa{CO_2}$ (Fig. 2-31) (Eger, 1993). Desflurane and sevoflurane depress ventilation, producing profound decreases in ventilation leading to apnea between 1.5 and 2.0 MAC. Both of these volatile anesthetics increase $Pa{CO_2}$ and decrease the ventilatory response to carbon dioxide. Depression of ventilation

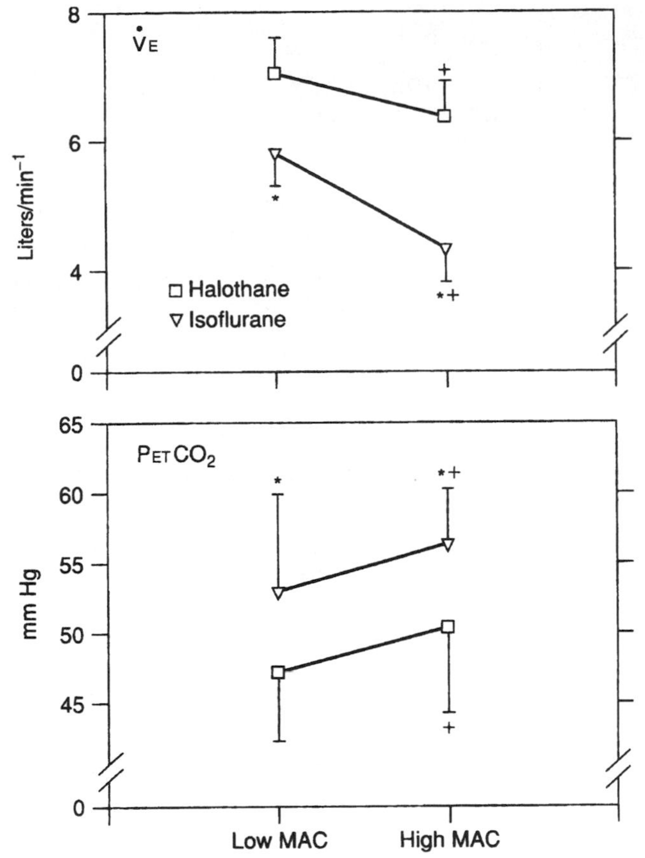

Figure 2-30. Minute ventilation (V̇E) and end-tidal carbon dioxide concentration (PETCO$_2$), as measured in volunteers breathing halothane or isoflurane in oxygen spontaneously at 1.2 (low) and 2.0 (high) MAC. (**P* <.05 compared with halothane; +, *P* <.05 compared with low MAC.) (From Canet J, Sanchis J, Zegri A, et al. Effects of halothane and isoflurane on ventilation and occlusion pressure. *Anesthesiology* 1994;81:563–571; with permission.)

produced by anesthetic concentrations up to 1.24 MAC desflurane are similar to the depression produced by isoflurane (Lockhart et al., 1991).

The presence of chronic obstructive pulmonary disease may accentuate the magnitude of increase in PaCO_2 produced by volatile anesthetics (Pietak et al., 1975). Nitrous oxide does not increase the PaCO_2, suggesting that substitution of this anesthetic for a portion of the volatile anesthetic would result in less depression of ventilation. Indeed, nitrous oxide combined with a volatile anesthetic produces less depression of ventilation and increase in PaCO_2 than does the same MAC concentration of the volatile drug alone (Lam et al., 1982). This ventilatory depressant-sparing effect of nitrous oxide is detectable with all volatile anesthetics (see Fig. 2-29) (Eger, 1993).

Despite the apparent benign effect of nitrous oxide on ventilation, the slope of the carbon dioxide response curve is decreased similarly and shifted to the right by anesthetic concentrations of all inhaled anesthetics (Fig. 2-32) (Eger, 1993). Subanesthetic concentrations (0.1 MAC) of inhaled anesthetics, however, do not alter the ventilatory response

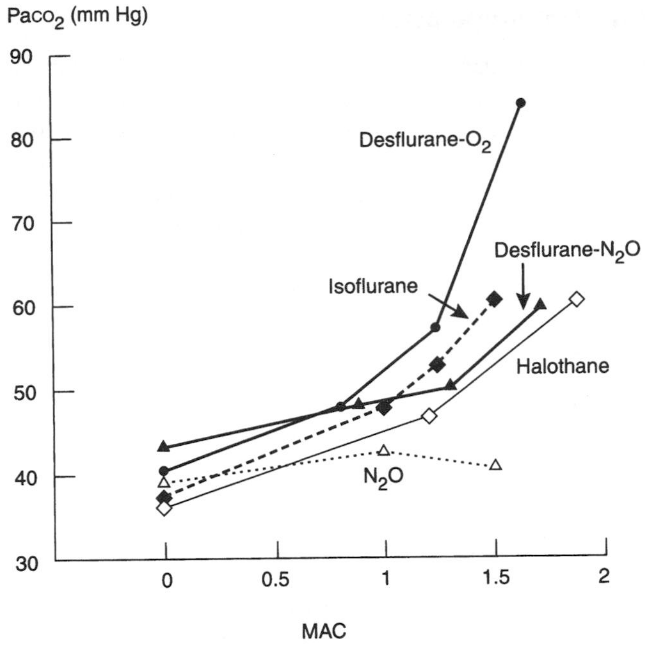

Figure 2-31. Inhaled anesthetics produce drug-specific and dose-dependent increases in PaCO_2. [From Eger EI. *Desflurane (Suprane): a compendium and reference.* Nutley, NJ: Anaquest, 1993:1–119; with permission.]

to carbon dioxide. In addition to nitrous oxide, painful stimulation (surgical skin incision) and duration of drug administration influence the magnitude of increase in PaCO_2 produced by volatile anesthetics.

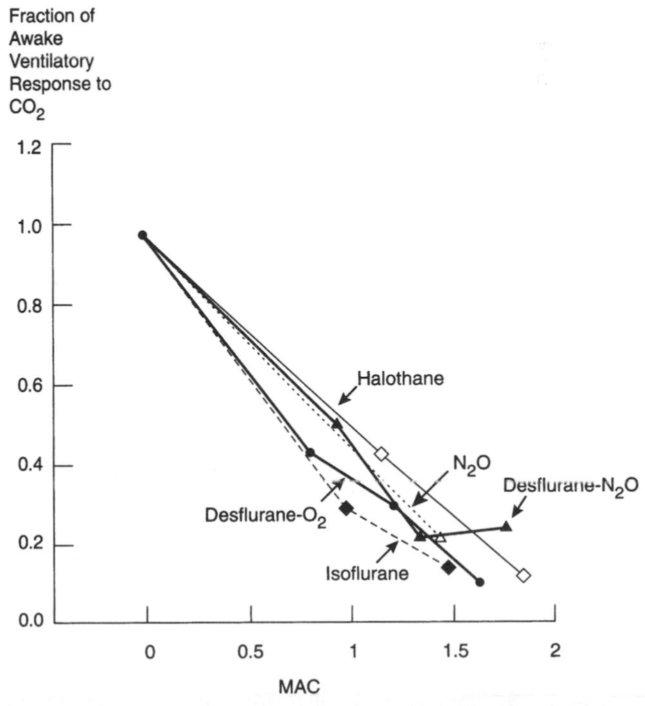

Figure 2-32. All inhaled anesthetics produce similar dose-dependent decreases in the ventilatory response to carbon dioxide. [From Eger EI. *Desflurane (Suprane): a compendium and reference.* Nutley, NJ: Anaquest, 1993:1–119; with permission.]

Surgical Stimulation

Surgical stimulation increases minute ventilation by about 40% because of increases in tidal volume and frequency of breathing. The Pa_{CO_2}, however, decreases only about 10% (4 to 6 mm Hg) despite the larger increase in minute ventilation (Fig. 2-33) (Eger, 1985a). The reason for this discrepancy is speculated to be an increased production of carbon dioxide resulting from activation of the sympathetic nervous system in response to painful surgical stimulation. Increased production of carbon dioxide is presumed to offset the impact of increased minute ventilation on Pa_{CO_2}.

Duration of Administration

After about 5 hours of administration, the increase in Pa_{CO_2} produced by a volatile anesthetic is less than that present during administration of the same concentration for 1 hour (Table 2-3) (Calverley et al., 1978a). Likewise, the slope and position of the carbon dioxide response curve returns toward normal after about 5 hours of administration of the volatile anesthetics (Lam et al., 1982). The reason for this apparent recovery from the ventilatory depressant effects of volatile anesthetics with time is not known.

Mechanism of Depression

Anesthetic-induced depression of ventilation as reflected by increases in the Pa_{CO_2} most likely reflects the direct depressant effects of these drugs on the medullary ventilatory center. An additional mechanism may be the ability of halothane and possibly other inhaled anesthetics to selectively interfere with intercostal muscle function, contributing to loss of chest wall stabilization during spontaneous breathing (Tusiewicz et al., 1977). This loss of chest wall stabilization could interfere with expansion of the chest in response to chemical stimulation of ventilation as normally produced by increases in the Pa_{CO_2} or arterial hypoxemia. Furthermore, this loss of chest wall stabilization means the descent of the diaphragm tends to cause the chest to collapse inward during inspiration, contributing to decreases in lung volumes, particularly the functional residual capacity. It is thus likely that halothane-induced depression of ventilation reflects both central and peripheral effects of the drug. The ventilatory depression associated with sevoflurane may result from a combination of central depression of medullary inspiratory neurons and depression of diaphragmatic function and contractility (Ide et al., 1992).

TABLE 2-3.
EVIDENCE FOR RECOVERY FROM THE VENTILATORY DEPRESSANT EFFECTS OF VOLATILE ANESTHETICS

	Arterial P_{CO_2}	
	1 Hour of Administration	**5 Hours of Administration**
Enflurane	(mm Hg)	(mm Hg)
1 MAC	61	46
2 MAC	Apnea	67

Source: Data from Calverley RK, Smith NT, Jones CW, et al. Ventilatory and cardiovascular effects of enflurane anesthesia during controlled ventilation in man. *Anesth Analg* 1978;57:610–618.

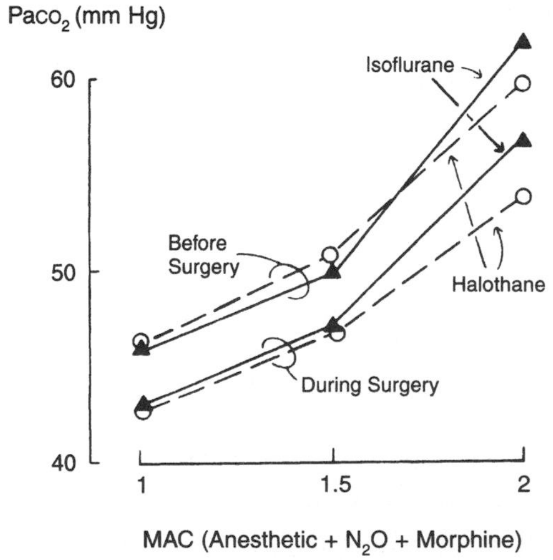

Figure 2-33. Impact of surgical stimulation on the resting Pa_{CO_2} (mm Hg) during administration of isoflurane or halothane. [From Eger EI. *Isoflurane (Forane): a compendium and reference*, 2nd ed. Madison, WI: Ohio Medical Products, 1985:1–110; with permission.]

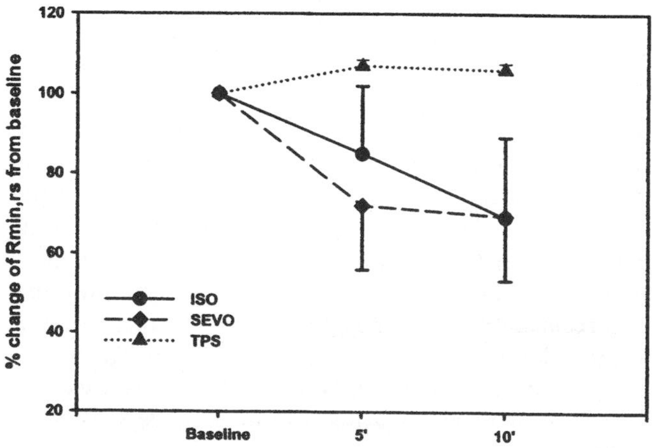

Figure 2-34. The percentage change (mean ≠ SD) in respiratory system resistance (Rmin, rs) after 5 and 10 minutes of maintenance of anesthesia with thiopental (TPS), 1.1 MAC isoflurane (ISO) or 1.1 MAC sevoflurane (SEVO) administered to patients with chronic obstructive pulmonary disease. (From Volta CA, Alvisi V, Petrini S, et al. The effect of volatile anesthetics on respiratory system resistance in patients with chronic obstructive pulmonary disease. *Anesth Analg* 2005;100:348-353; with permission.)

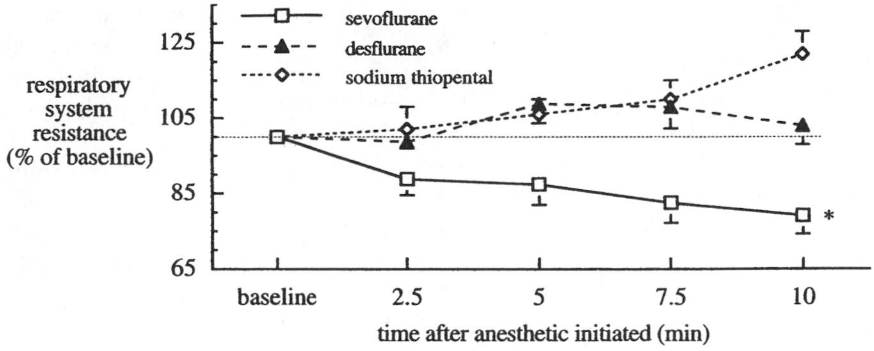

Figure 2-35. Changes in respiratory system resistance as a percentage of the thiopental baseline recorded after tracheal intubation but before the addition of sevoflurane or desflurane to the inhaled gases or beginning the infusion of thiopental. Airway resistance responses to sevoflurane were significantly different from desflurane and thiopental. *P<0.05 (From Goff MJ, Arain SR, Ficke DJ, et al. Absence of bronchodilation during desflurane anesthesia. *Anesthesiology* 2000;93:404-408; with permission.)

Management of Ventilatory Depression

The predictable ventilatory depressant effects of volatile anesthetics are most often managed by institution of mechanical (controlled) ventilation of the patient's lungs. In this regard, the inherent ventilatory depressant effects of volatile anesthetics facilitate the initiation of controlled ventilation. Assisted ventilation of the lungs is a questionably effective method for offsetting the ventilatory depressant effects of volatile anesthetics. For example, the apneic threshold (maximal Pa_{CO_2} that does not initiate spontaneous breathing) is only 3 to 5 mm Hg lower than the Pa_{CO_2} present during spontaneous breathing (Ravin and Olsen, 1972). As a result, a Pa_{CO_2} increase to 50 mm Hg due to ventilatory depressant effects of a volatile anesthetic could only be lowered to 45 to 46 mm Hg by assisted ventilation of the lungs before apnea occurs.

Ventilatory Response to Hypoxemia

All inhaled anesthetics, including nitrous oxide, profoundly depress the ventilatory response to hypoxemia that is normally mediated by the carotid bodies. For example, 0.1 MAC produces 50% to 70% depression, and 1.1 MAC produces 100% depression of this response (Knill and Clement, 1982; Nagyova et al., 1997). This contrasts with the absence of significant depression of the ventilatory response to carbon dioxide during administration of 0.1 MAC of volatile anesthetics. Inhaled anesthetics also attenuate the usual synergistic effect of arterial hypoxemia and hypercapnia on stimulation of ventilation. Sevoflurane-induced decreases in hypoxic responses are not different in men and women which contrasts with morphine which produces greater depression of the ventilatory response to hypoxia in women (Sarton et al., 1999). Sevoflurane is useful during thoracic surgery as it is a potent bronchodilator, its low blood-gas solubility permits rapid adjustment of the depth of anesthesia, and effects on hypoxic pulmonary vasoconstriction are small (Beck et al., 2001).

Airway Resistance and Irritability

Risk factors for developing bronchospasm during anesthesia include young age (<10 years), perioperative respiratory infection, endotracheal intubation and the presence of chronic obstructive pulmonary disease (COPD) (Olsson, 1987). Nevertheless, isoflurane and sevoflurane produce bronchodilation in patients with COPD (Fig. 2-34) (Volta et al., 2005). Sevoflurane causes moderate bronchodilation that is not observed in patients receiving desflurane or thiopental (Fig. 2-35) (Goff et al., 2000). Bronchoconstriction produced by desflurane is most likely to occur in patients who smoke (Fig. 2-36) (Goff et al.,

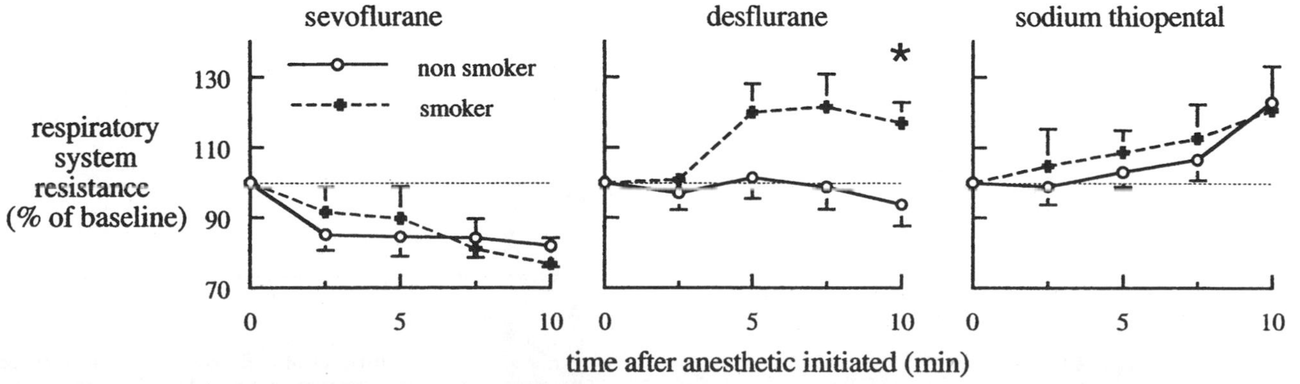

Figure 2-36. Respiratory system resistance during the 10 minutes after thiopental (baseline) based on current smoking status. Administration of desflurane to patients who were smokers was associated with significant bronchoconstriction compared with nonsmokers receiving desflurane. *P<0.05 (From Goff MJ, Arain SR, Ficke DJ, et al. Absence of bronchodilation during desflurane anesthesia. *Anesthesiology* 2000;93:404-408; with permission.)

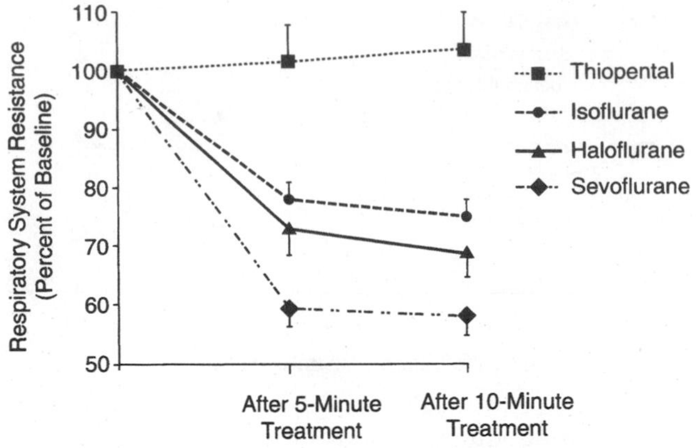

Figure 2-37. Respiratory system resistance decreased in the presence of 1.1 MAC isoflurane, halothane, or sevoflurane, whereas no change occurred in patients receiving thiopental 0.25 mg/kg/minute plus 50% nitrous oxide. (From Rooke GA, Choi JH, Bishop MJ. The effect of isoflurane, halothane, sevoflurane, and thiopental/nitrous oxide on respiratory system resistance after tracheal intubation. *Anesthesiology* 1997;86:1294–1299; with permission.)

2000). Administration of fentanyl 1 μg/kg IV or morphine 100 μg/kg IV prior to inhalation induction with desflurane and nitrous oxide significantly decreases airway irritability associated with desflurane (Kong et al., 1999). After tracheal intubation in patients without asthma, sevoflurane decreases airway resistance as much or more than isoflurane (Fig. 2-37) (Rooke et al., 1997). Sevoflurane and desflurane have been administered without evidence of bronchospasm to patients with bronchial asthma (Eger, 1994).

The assessment of the cough response to tracheal stimulation by endotracheal tube cuff inflation is a reliable and clinically meaningful measure of upper airway reactivity. At 1 MAC, sevoflurane is superior to desflurane for suppressing moderate and severe responses to this stimulus (Fig. 2-38) (Klock et al., 2001).

Despite the typical lack of irritant effects of sevoflurane on the airways there is evidence that exposure of sevoflurane to desiccated carbon dioxide absorbents, especially those containing potassium hydroxide, may result in production of toxic gases and subsequent inhalation of these products causing airway irritation and impaired gas exchange (Funk et al., 1998; Holak et al., 2003). This airway irritation may be caused by formaldehyde which is generated in isomolar concentrations with methanol. Compound A is not an airway irritant.

In the absence of bronchoconstriction, the bronchodilating effects of volatile anesthetics are difficult to demonstrate, because normal bronchomotor tone is low and only minimal additional relaxation is possible. Inhaled anesthetics are not irritating to airways; thus, increased secretions or increases in airway resistance by this mechanism are unlikely. Administration of desflurane, 1.8% to 5.4%, does not produce secretions, coughing, or breath-holding in human volunteers (Eger, 1993). Like other inhaled anesthetics, nitrous oxide decreases functional residual capacity; this may be exaggerated by nitrous oxide–induced skeletal muscle rigidity.

HEPATIC EFFECTS

Hepatic Blood Flow

In patients receiving 1.5% end-tidal isoflurane, total hepatic blood flow and hepatic artery blood flow was maintained while portal vein blood flow was increased confirming that isoflurane was a vasodilator of the hepatic

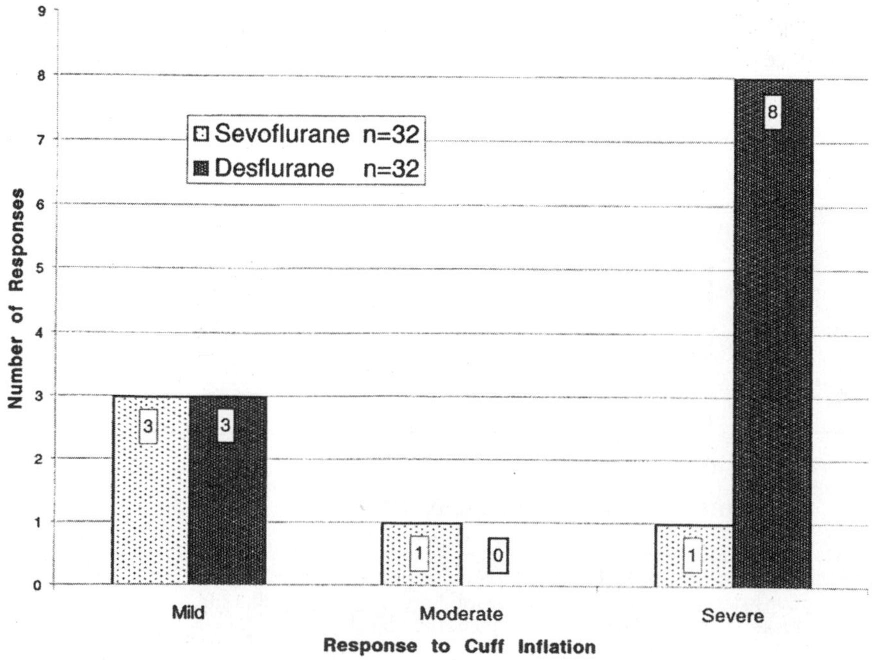

Figure 2-38. Responses to tracheal tube cuff inflation during 1MAC anesthesia with sevoflurane or desflurane. (From Klock PA, Czeslick EG, Klafta JM, et al. The effect of sevoflurane and desflurane on upper airway reactivity. *Anesthesiology* 2001;94:963-967; with permission.)

circulation providing beneficial effects on hepatic oxygen delivery (Gatecel et al., 2003). In contrast, halothane acts as a vascoconstrictor on the hepatic circulation. In another report, patients receiving 1 MAC isoflurane plus nitrous oxide demonstrated increases in hepatic blood flow and increased hepatic venous oxygen saturation, whereas hepatic blood flow did not change in patients receiving 1 MAC halothane plus nitrous oxide (Goldfarb et al., 1990). Selective hepatic artery vasoconstriction has been reported in otherwise healthy patients during the administration of halothane (Benumof et al., 1976). Hepatic blood flow during administration of desflurane and sevoflurane is maintained similar to isoflurane (Fig. 2-39) (Eger, 1994; Frink et al., 1992a). Maintenance of hepatic oxygen delivery relative to demand during exposure to anesthetics is uniquely important in view of the evidence that hepatocyte hypoxia is a significant mechanism in the multifactorial etiology of postoperative hepatic dysfunction.

Drug Clearance

Volatile anesthetics may interfere with clearance of drugs from the plasma as a result of decreases in hepatic blood flow or inhibition of drug-metabolizing enzymes. Intrinsic clearance by hepatic metabolism of drugs such as propranolol is decreased by 54% to 68% by inhaled anesthetics (Whelan et al., 1989). In the overall hepatic clearance of drugs, decreases in hepatic blood flow seem less important than anesthetic-induced inhibition of hepatic drug-metabolizing enzymes (Reilly et al., 1985).

Liver Function Tests

Transient increases in the plasma alanine aminotransferase activity follow administration of enflurane and desflurane, but not isoflurane administration, to human volunteers (Fig. 2-40) (Eger, 1993; Weiskopf et al., 1992). Transient increases in plasma concentrations of alpha glutathione transferase (sensitive indicator of hepatocellular injury) follow administration of isoflurane or desflurane for surgical anesthesia (Tiainen et al., 1998). In the presence of surgical stimulation, bromsulphalein retention and increases in liver enzymes follow transiently the administration of even isoflurane, suggesting that changes in hepatic blood flow evoked by painful stimulation can adversely alter hepatic function independent of the volatile anesthetic.

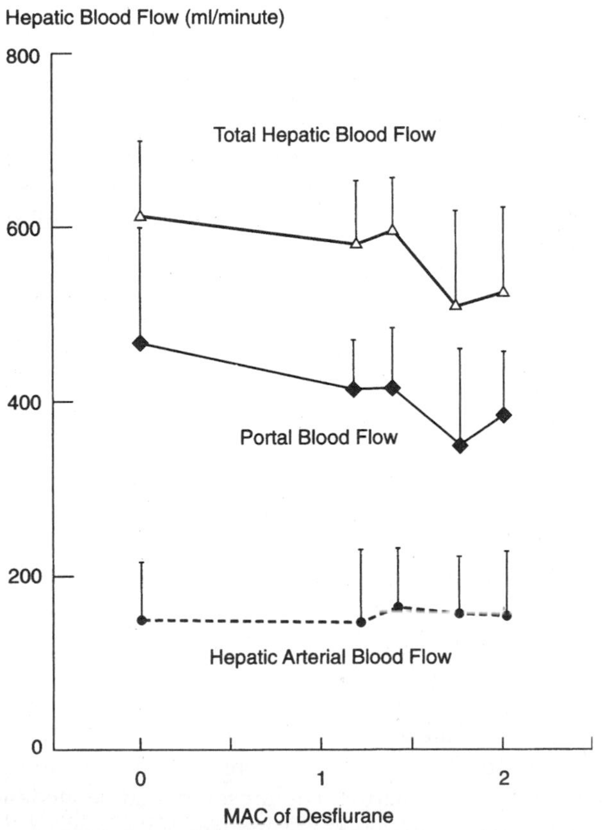

Figure 2-39. Administration of desflurane to dogs does not significantly alter hepatic perfusion. (Mean ± SD.) [Modified from Eger EI. *Desflurane (Suprane): a compendium and reference.* Nutley, NJ: Anaquest, 1993:1–119; with permission.]

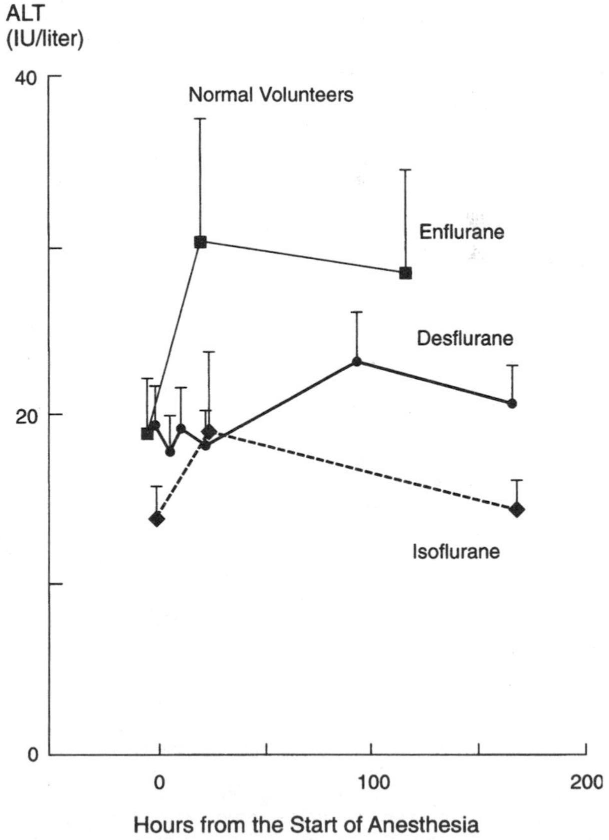

Figure 2-40. Plasma alanine aminotransferase (ALT) levels do not change significantly when enflurane, desflurane, or isoflurane are administered to healthy volunteers. (Mean ± SE.) [Modified from Eger EI. *Desflurane (Suprane): a compendium and reference.* Nutley, NJ: Anaquest, 1993:1–119; with permission.]

Hepatotoxicity

Postoperative liver dysfunction has been associated with most volatile anesthetics, with halothane receiving the most attention (Elliott and Strunin, 1993). Injected and inhaled anesthetics studied in the hypoxic rat model that includes enzyme induction may produce centrilobular necrosis, but the incidence is greatest with halothane (Fig. 2-41) (Shingu et al., 1983). It is likely that inadequate hepatocyte oxygenation (oxygen supply relative to oxygen demand) is the principal mechanism responsible for hepatic dysfunction that follows anesthesia and surgery. Any anesthetic that decreases alveolar ventilation and/or decreases hepatic blood flow could interfere with adequate hepatocyte oxygenation. Enzyme induction increases oxygen demand and could make patients vulnerable to decreased hepatic oxygen supply due to anesthetic-induced ventilatory or circulatory events that decrease hepatic oxygen delivery. Preexisting liver disease, such as hepatic cirrhosis, may be associated with marginal hepatocyte oxygenation, which would be further jeopardized by the depressant effects of anesthetics on hepatic blood flow and/or arterial oxygenation. Indeed, liver transaminase enzymes are increased more in cirrhotic than noncirrhotic animals exposed to halothane (Fig. 2-42) (Baden et al., 1987). Hypothermia, which decreases hepatic oxygen demand, may protect the liver from drug-induced events that decrease hepatic oxygen delivery.

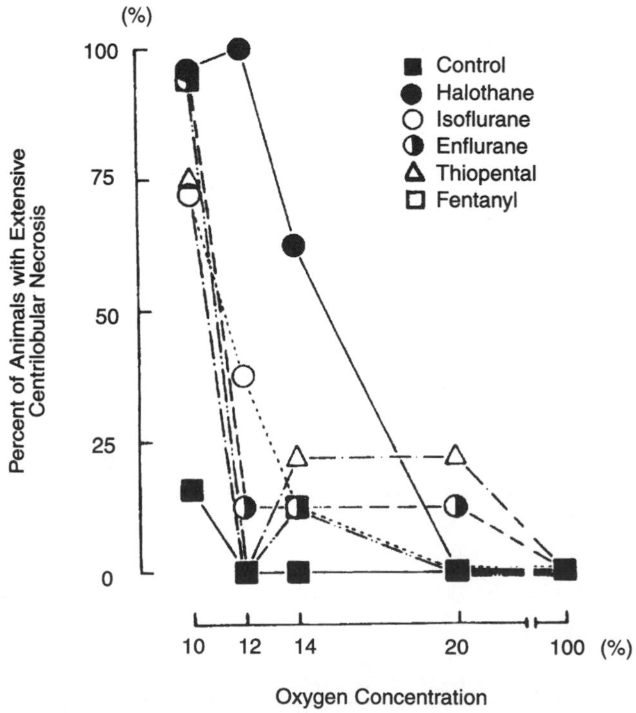

Figure 2-41. Hepatic damage may occur in the rat model after administration of inhaled or injected drugs when the inhaled oxygen concentration is 10%. Conversely, hepatic damage occurs after administration of halothane, but not enflurane or isoflurane, when the inhaled concentration of oxygen is 12% or 14%. (From Shingu K, Eger EI, Johnson BH, et al. Effect of oxygen concentration, hyperthermia, and choice of vendor on anesthetic-induced hepatic injury in rats. *Anesth Analg* 1983;62:146–150; with permission.)

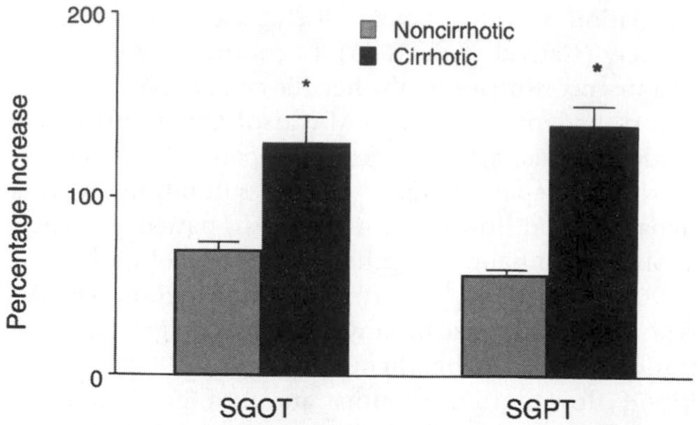

Figure 2-42. Increases (mean ± SE) in liver transaminase enzymes after administration of 1.05% halothane for 3 hours to noncirrhotic or cirrhotic rats. (From Baden JM, Serra M, Fujinaga ME, et al. Halothane metabolism in cirrhotic rats. *Anesthesiology* 1987;67:660–664; with permission.)

Halothane

Halothane produces two types of hepatotoxicity in susceptible patients. An estimated 20% of adult patients receiving halothane develop a mild, self-limited postoperative hepatotoxicity that is characterized by nausea, lethargy, fever, and minor increases in plasma concentrations of liver transaminase enzymes (Wright et al., 1975). The other and rarer type of hepatotoxicity (halothane hepatitis) is estimated to occur in 1 in 10,000 to 1 in 30,000 adult patients receiving halothane and may lead to massive hepatic necrosis and death (Moult and Sherlock, 1975). Children seem to be less susceptible to this type of hepatotoxicity than adults (Kenna et al., 1987; Warner et al., 1984). It is likely that the more common self-limited form of hepatic dysfunction following halothane is a nonspecific drug effect due to changes in hepatic blood flow that impair hepatic oxygenation. Conversely, the rarer, life-threatening form of hepatic dysfunction characterized as halothane hepatitis is most likely an immune-mediated hepatotoxicity (Elliott and Strunin, 1993).

Halothane Hepatitis

Clinical manifestations of halothane hepatitis that suggest an immune-mediated response include eosinophilia, fever, rash, arthralgia, and prior exposure to halothane. Risk factors commonly associated with halothane hepatitis include female gender, middle age, obesity, and multiple exposures to halothane. The predominant histologic feature is acute hepatitis. The most compelling evidence for an immune-mediated mechanism is the presence of circulatory immunoglobulin G antibodies in at least 70% of those patients with the diagnosis of halothane hepatitis (Elliott and Strunin, 1993). These antibodies are directed

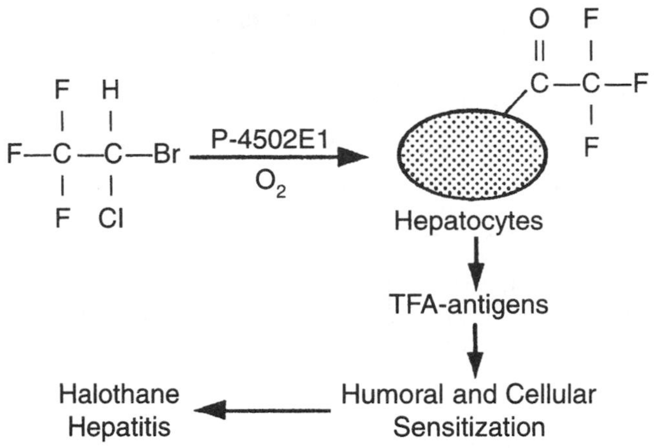

Figure 2-43. Halothane is metabolized to a trifluoroacetylated (TFA) adduct that binds to liver proteins. In susceptible patients, this adduct (altered protein) is seen as nonself (neoantigen), generating an immune response (production of antibodies). Subsequent exposure to halothane may result in hepatotoxicity. A similar process may occur in genetically susceptible individuals after anesthetic exposure to other fluorinated volatile anesthetics (enflurane, isoflurane, desflurane) that also generate a TFA adduct. (From Njoku D, Laster MJ, Gong DH, et al. Biotransformation of halothane, enflurane, isoflurane, and desflurane to trifluoroacetylated liver proteins: association between protein acylation and hepatic injury. *Anesth Analg* 1997;84:173–178; with permission.)

against liver microsomal proteins on the surface of hepatocytes that have been covalently modified by the reactive oxidative trifluoroacetyl halide metabolite of halothane to form neoantigens (Fig. 2-43) (Njoku et al., 1997). This acetylation of liver proteins in effect changes these proteins from self to nonself (neoantigens), resulting in the formation of antibodies against this new protein. It is presumed that the subsequent antigen-antibody interaction is responsible for the liver injury characterized as halothane hepatitis. The possibility of a genetic susceptibility factor is suggested by case reports of halothane hepatitis in closely related relatives (Farrell et al., 1985; Gourlay et al., 1981). Indeed, metabolism of halothane appears to be under genetic influence in humans (Cascorbi et al., 1970).

Several observations suggest that reductive metabolism is not the primary mechanism in the development of halothane hepatitis. For example, neither enflurane nor isoflurane undergoes reductive metabolism, yet these drugs both produce centrilobular necrosis in the hypoxic rat model. Furthermore, metabolites produced by reductive metabolism of halothane do not themselves produce hepatotoxicity. Finally, fasting does not alter metabolism but enhances hepatotoxicity by volatile anesthetics.

Enflurane, Isoflurane, and Desflurane

The mild, self-limited postoperative hepatic dysfunction that is associated with all the volatile anesthetics most likely reflects anesthetic-induced alterations in hepatic oxygen delivery relative to demand that results in inadequate hepatocyte oxygenation. More disturbing, however, is the realization that enflurane, isoflurane, and desflurane are oxidatively metabolized by liver cytochrome P-450 enzymes to form acetylated liver protein adducts by mechanisms similar to that of halothane (Fig. 2-44) (Christ et al., 1988; Martin et al., 1995; Njoku et al., 1997). As a result, acetylated liver proteins capable of evoking an antibody response could occur after exposure to halothane, enflurane, isoflurane, or desflurane. Indeed, trifluoroacetyl-modified proteins have been described in a patient with hepatitis associated with isoflurane (Njoku et al., 2002a). This raises the possibility that enflurane, isoflurane, and desflurane could produce hepatotoxicity by a mechanism similar to that of halothane but at a lower incidence because the degree of anesthetic metabolism appears to be directly related to the potential for hepatic injury. Considering the magnitude of metabolism of these volatile anesthetics, it is predictable that the incidence of anesthetic-induced hepatitis would be greatest with halothane, intermediate with enflurane, and rare with isoflurane (Brunt et al., 1991; Eger et al., 1986; Stoelting et al., 1987). Desflurane is metabolized even less than isoflurane, and from the standpoint of immune-mediated hepatotoxicity, desflurane should be very safe because it would have the lowest level of adduct formation. Nevertheless, even very small amounts of adduct may be able to precipitate massive hepatotoxicity, particularly if the patient was previously sensitized against trifluoroacetyl proteins. Indeed, hepatotoxicity after desflurane anesthesia has been described in a patient who may have been previously sensitized by exposure to halothane 18 years and 12 years previously (Martin et al., 1995). Fulminant hepatic failure accompanied by high plasma concentrations of CYP2A6 autoantibodies has been observed in a patient 22 years following exposure to enflurane (Martin et al., 2001). Similarly, halothane may be able to sensitize patients against protein adducts formed by other fluorinated volatile anesthetics (Christ et al., 1988; Sigurdsson et al., 1985).

Development of an enzyme-linked immunosorbent assay for detection of antibodies evoked by acetylation may help detect those rare patients who have become sensitized due to a prior exposure to halothane and who are thus at presumed increased risk for subsequent exposure to other fluorinated volatile anesthetics. The risk of fulminant hepatic failure after exposure to enflurane, isoflurane, or desflurane after previous exposure to halothane is probably less than the overall risk associated with anesthesia (Elliott and Strunin, 1993).

Environmental exposure of operating room personnel to trace concentrations of volatile anesthetics could stimulate antibody production. Indeed, measurement of plasma autoantibody concentrations demonstrated increased levels in pediatric anesthesiologists (especially females) compared with general anesthesiologists and controls (Fig 2-45) (Njoku et al., 2002b). It is presumed that pediatric anesthesiologists experience greater occupational exposure to trace concentrations of volatile anesthetics due to the

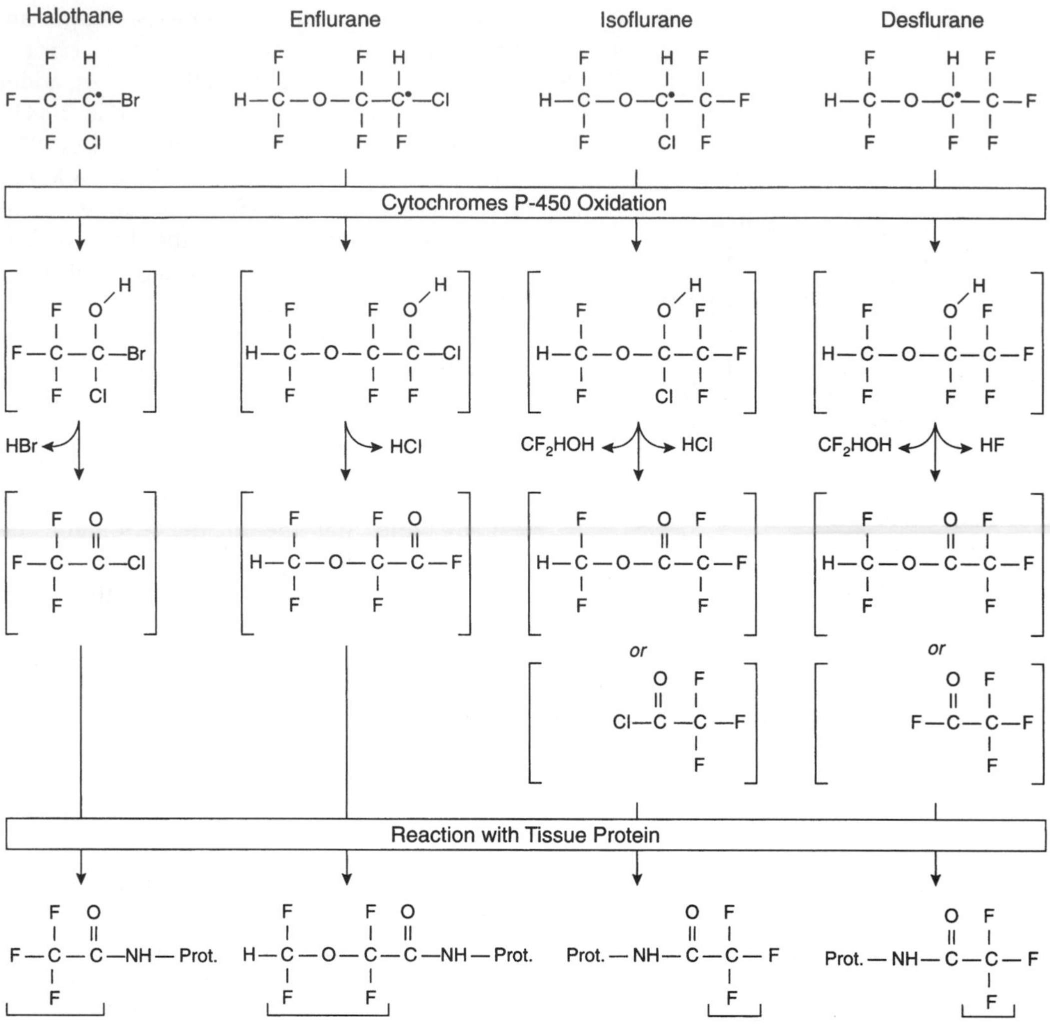

Figure 2-44. Pathways for the oxidative metabolism of fluorinated volatile anesthetics by cytochrome P-450 enzymes to form acetylated protein adducts. In genetically susceptible individuals, the resulting trifluoroacetylates are thought to produce an immune response manifesting clinically as drug-induced hepatitis. (From Martin JL, Plevak DJ, Flannery KD, et al. Hepatotoxicity after desflurane anesthesia. *Anesthesiology* 1995;83:1125–1129; with permission.)

frequent use of nonrebreathing anesthesia delivery systems and use of uncuffed endotracheal tubes. Despite these higher antibody levels, pediatric anesthesiologists did not have increased liver transaminase enzymes compared with general anesthesiologists suggesting these antibodies may be insufficient to cause appreciable damage to normal hepatic cells (Eger, 2002).

Sevoflurane

The chemical structure of sevoflurane, unlike that of other fluorinated volatile anesthetics, dictates that it cannot undergo metabolism to an acetyl halide (Fig. 2-46) (Kharasch, 1995). Sevoflurane metabolism does not result in the formation of trifluoroacetylated liver proteins and therefore cannot stimulate the formation of antitrifluoroacetylated protein antibodies. In this regard, sevoflurane differs from halothane, enflurane, and desflurane, all of which are metabolized to reactive acetyl halide metabolites. Therefore, unlike all the other fluorinated volatile anesthetics, sevoflurane would not be expected to produce immune-mediated hepatotoxicity or to cause cross-sensitivity in patients previously exposed to halothane. Rare reported cases of sevoflurane hepatotoxicity are without explanation or proven cause and effect (Eger, 1994; Reich et al., 2004).

Compound A is hepatotoxic in animals, but the concentration present in the anesthesia breathing circuit are far below the toxic level in animals. Nevertheless, small increases in the plasma alanine aminotransferase have been observed in volunteers receiving sevoflurane for prolonged periods of time during which the compound A concentration averaged 41 ppm. Similar changes in the plasma transaminase concentrations did not occur in volunteers receiving desflurane, suggesting that mild transient hepatic injury was limited to the sevoflurane-treated individuals (Eger et al., 1997a). Conversely, others have not observed differences in liver function enzyme changes in patients

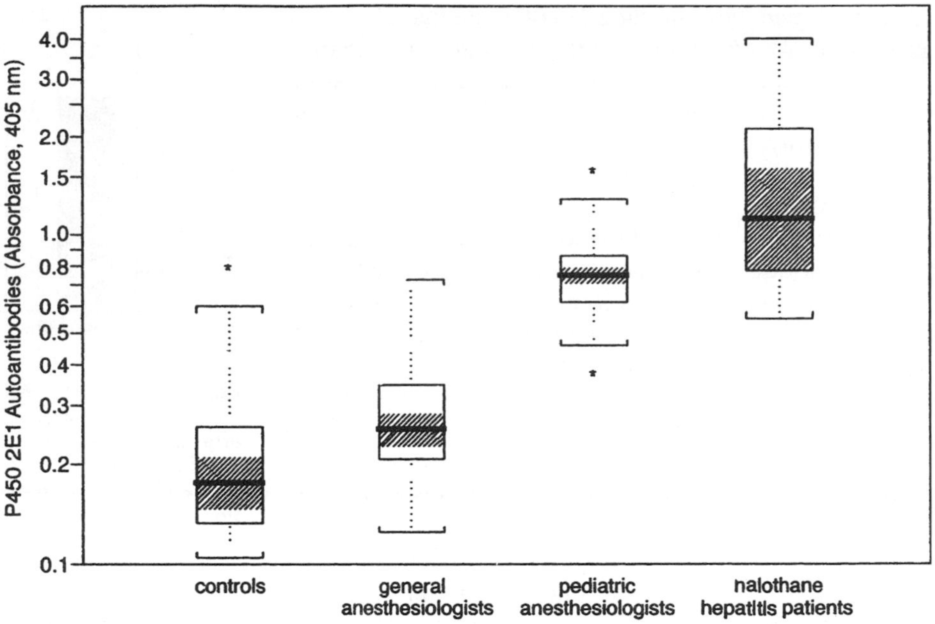

Figure 2-45. Plots of cytochrome P-450 2E1 autoantibody levels in four groups. The median of the P-450 2E1 autoantibodies plasma levels for control patients are significantly lower than for the median levels of the other groups. There was a highly significant increasing trend for the median levels of general anesthesiologists, pediatric anesthesiologists, and halothane hepatitis patients. (From Njoku DB, Greenberg RS, Bourdi M, et al. Autoantibodies associated with volatile anesthetic hepatitis found in the sera of a large cohort of pediatric anesthesiologists. *Anesth Analg* 2002b; 94:243-249; with permission.)

receiving sevoflurane compared with isoflurane (Kharasch et al., 1997).

RENAL EFFECTS

Volatile anesthetics produce similar dose-related decreases in renal blood flow, glomerular filtration rate, and urine output. These changes are not a result of the release of arginine vasopressin hormone but rather most likely reflect the effects of volatile anesthetics on systemic blood pressure and cardiac output. Preoperative hydration attenuates or abolishes many of the changes in renal function associated with volatile anesthetics. Renal function after

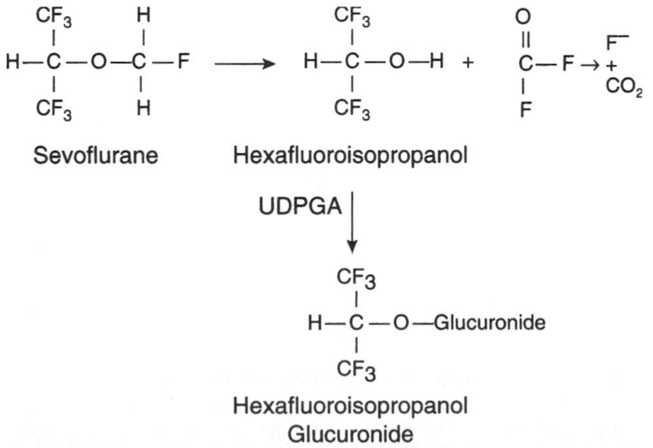

Figure 2-46. Proposed pathway for oxidative metabolism of sevoflurane. (UDPGA, uridine diphosphate glucuronic acid.) (From Frink EJ, Ghantous H, Malan TP, et al. Plasma inorganic fluoride with sevoflurane anesthesia: correlation with indices of hepatic and renal function. *Anesth Analg* 1992;74:231–235; with permission.)

kidney transplantation is not uniquely influenced by the volatile anesthetic administered (Cronnelly et al., 1984).

Fluoride-Induced Nephrotoxicity

Fluoride-induced nephrotoxicity (polyuria, hypernatremia, hyperosmolarity, increased plasma creatinine, inability to concentrate urine) was first recognized in patients after the administration of methoxyflurane, which undergoes extensive metabolism (70% of the absorbed dose) to inorganic fluoride, which acts as a renal toxin. In these patients, no renal effects were observed when peak plasma fluoride was <40 μm/liter; subclinical toxicity was accompanied by peak plasma fluoride concentrations of 50 to 80 μm/liter; and clinical toxicity occurred when peak plasma fluoride concentrations were >80 μm/liter. The methoxyflurane nephrotoxicity theory has been extended to other fluorinated volatile anesthetics despite the absence of data to support this extrapolation. Furthermore, a plasma fluoride concentration of 50 μm/liter has been adopted as an indicator that renal toxicity may occur from other volatile anesthetics. Nevertheless, all volatile anesthetics introduced since methoxyflurane undergo significantly less metabolism, and their decreased solubility compared with methoxyflurane means that substantial amounts of the anesthetic are exhaled and thus not available for hepatic metabolism to fluoride. The absence of renal toxicity despite peak plasma fluoride concentrations exceeding 50 μm/liter after administration of enflurane or sevoflurane suggests that this peak value alone cannot be accepted as an indicator for fluoride-induced nephrotoxicity after administration of these volatile anesthetics. Reversible depression of urine concentrating ability observed in healthy volunteers following prolonged enflurane administration (8 hours) may reflect alkaline degradation products of enflurane that are conjugated to thiol compounds, forming S-conjugates (Orhan et al., 2001). Enzyme induction, obesity, and preexisting renal dysfunction appear to be risk factors for enflurane nephrotoxicity.

Sevoflurane

Sevoflurane is metabolized to inorganic fluoride, and peak plasma fluoride concentrations consistently exceed those peak levels that occur after a comparable dose of enflurane (Fig. 2-47) (Conzen et al., 1995; Frink et al., 1992b; Frink et al., 1994; Munday et al., 1995). Despite higher peak plasma fluoride concentrations compared with enflurane, prolonged sevoflurane anesthesia does not impair renal concentrating function as evaluated with desmopressin testing 1 and 5 days postanesthesia in healthy volunteers (Fig. 2-48) (Conzen et al., 1995; Frink et al., 1994). In the same report, two patients receiving enflurane developed transient impairment of renal concentrating ability despite lower peak plasma fluoride concentrations than the patients receiving sevoflurane (Frink et al., 1994). In another report, there were no significant differences between urine concentrating abilities after enflurane (6 MAC hours) or sevoflurane (9 MAC hours) (Munday et al., 1995).

Despite reports failing to show renal impairment after the administration of sevoflurane, there are observations of transient impairment of renal concentrating ability and increased urinary excretion of beta-*N*-acetylglucosaminidase (NAG) in patients exposed to sevoflurane and developing peak plasma inorganic fluoride concentrations >50 μm/liter (Figs. 2-49 and 2-50) (Higuchi et al., 1995). Urinary excretion of NAG is considered an indicator of acute proximal renal tubular injury. Despite these changes, the blood urea nitrogen and plasma creatinine did not change, and the authors concluded that clinically significant renal damage did not accompany administration of sevoflurane to patients with no preexisting renal disease. Concern that administration of sevoflurane to patients with preexisting renal disease could accentuate renal dysfunction was not confirmed when this volatile anesthetic was administered to patients with chronic renal disease as reflected by increased plasma creatinine concentrations (Conzen et al., 1995; Mazze and Jamison, 1995). Likewise, administration of desflurane or isoflurane did not aggravate renal impairment in patients with preexisting chronic renal insufficiency (Fig. 2-51) (Litz et al., 2002).

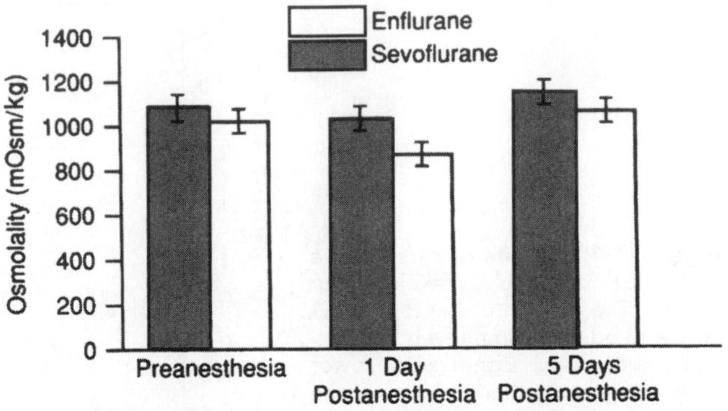

Figure 2-48. Maximal urinary osmolalities (mean ± SE) in adult male volunteers after administration of desmopressin before and after prolonged administration (>9 MAC hours) of enflurane or sevoflurane. (From Frink EJ, Malan TP, Isner RJ, et al. Renal concentrating function with prolonged sevoflurane or enflurane anesthesia in volunteers. *Anesthesiology* 1994;80:1019–1025; with permission.)

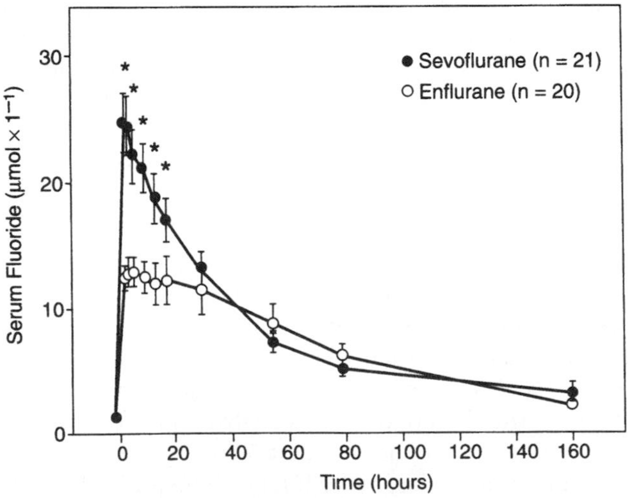

Figure 2-47. Plasma fluoride concentrations during and after sevoflurane or enflurane anesthesia. (Mean ± SE.) (From Conzen PF, Nuscheler M, Melotte A, et al. Renal function and serum fluoride concentrations in patients with stable renal insufficiency after anesthesia with sevoflurane or enflurane. *Anesth Analg* 1995;81:569–575; with permission.)

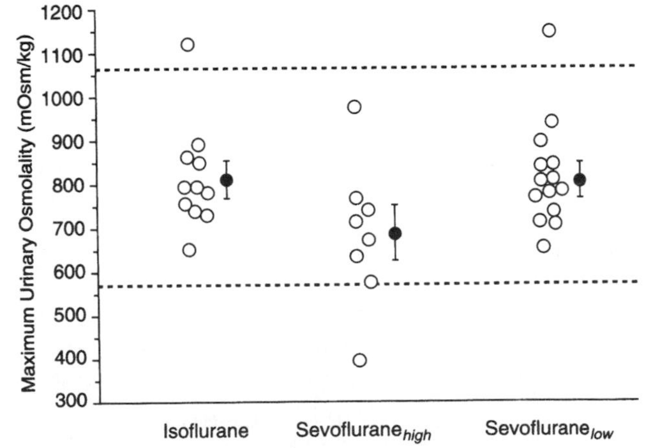

Figure 2-49. Maximum urinary osmolality in response to vasopressin 16.5 hours after cessation of anesthesia was not significantly different between the three anesthesia groups. Sevoflurane$_{high}$ included only patients with a peak plasma inorganic fluoride concentration >50 μm/liter. Solid circles and bars represent mean ± SE. (From Higuchi H, Sumikura H, Sumita S, et al. Renal function in patients with high serum fluoride concentrations after prolonged sevoflurane anesthesia. *Anesthesiology* 1995;83:449–458; with permission.)

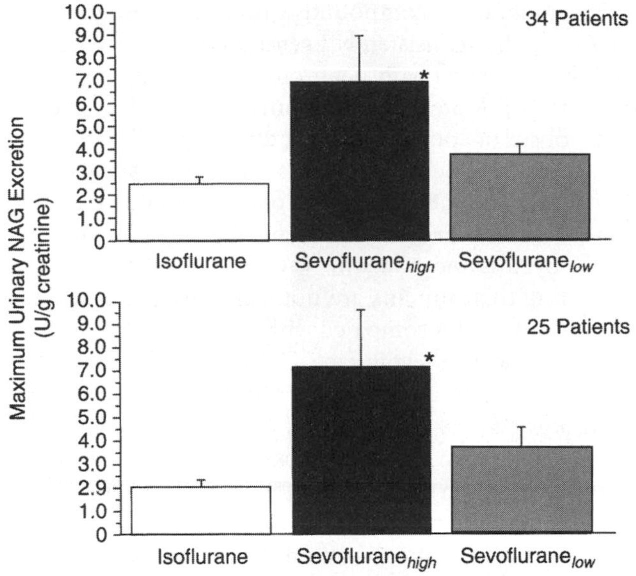

Figure 2-50. Urinary excretion of the renal enzyme beta-*N*-acetylglucosaminidase (NAG) was significantly greater (**P* <.05) in the sevoflurane$_{high}$ patients (peak plasma inorganic fluoride concentration >50 μm/liter) compared with the other anesthesia groups. (From Higuchi H, Sumikura H, Sumita S, et al. Renal function in patients with high serum fluoride concentrations after prolonged sevoflurane anesthesia. *Anesthesiology* 1995;83:449–458; with permission.)

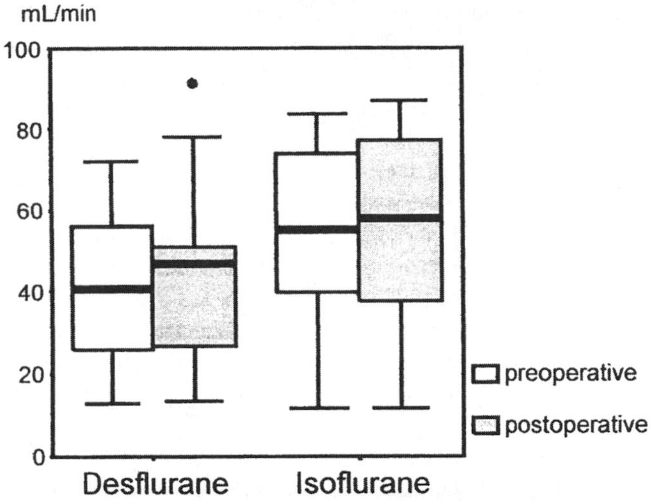

Figure 2-51. Preoperative and postoperative creatinine clearance values (mL/min). Thick lines represent median values, the box boundaries represent 25th to 75th percentiles, and the bar lines represent the 10th to 90th percentiles. The single outlier beyond the 90th percentile is shown as an individual data point (*). There were no differences between desflurane and isoflurane. (From Litz RJ, Hubler M, Lorenz W, et al. Renal responses to desflurane and isoflurane in patients with renal insufficiency. *Anesthesiology* 2002;97:1133-1136; with permission.)

It has been postulated that intrarenal production of inorganic fluoride may be a more important factor for nephrotoxicity than hepatic metabolism that causes increased plasma fluoride concentrations (Brown, 1995; Kharasch et al., 1995a). This would explain why patients with increased plasma concentrations of fluoride after administration of sevoflurane occasionally experience less renal dysfunction than patients receiving enflurane and manifesting lower plasma fluoride concentrations (see Figs. 2-47 and 2-48) (Conzen et al., 1995; Frink et al., 1994; Mazze et al., 1977). Presumably, inhaled anesthetics such as methoxyflurane and enflurane undergo greater intrarenal metabolism to fluoride than sevoflurane whereas sevoflurane undergoes greater hepatic metabolism, thus accounting for the higher plasma concentrations of fluoride.

Vinyl Halide Nephrotoxicity

Carbon dioxide absorbents containing potassium and sodium hydroxide react with sevoflurane and eliminate hydrogen fluoride from its isopropyl moiety to form breakdown products (see Fig. 2-4) (Smith et al., 1996; Yamakage et al., 2000). The degradation product produced in greatest amounts is fluoromethyl-2,2-difluro-1-(trifluoromethyl) vinyl ether (compound A). Compound A is a dose-dependent nephrotoxin in rats causing proximal renal tubular injury at concentrations of 50 to 100 ppm (Morio et al., 1992). The concentration of compound A fatal to 50% of rats after a 3-hour exposure is about 400 ppm (Gonsowski et al., 1994). In patients, the mean maximum concentration of compound A in the anesthesia breathing circuit averages 19.7, 8.1, and 2.1 ppm during fresh gas flows of 1, 3, and 6 liters per minute, respectively (Fig. 2-52) (Bito and Ikeda, 1995; Bito et al., 1997). During closed-circuit anesthesia with sevoflurane administered to patients undergoing operations lasting longer than 5 hours, the average concentration of compound A in the anesthesia circuit was <20 ppm and no evidence of renal dysfunction occurred based on measurements of blood urea nitrogen and plasma creatinine concentrations (Fig. 2-53) (Bito and Ikeda, 1994). Higher concentrations of compound A occurred in the presence of

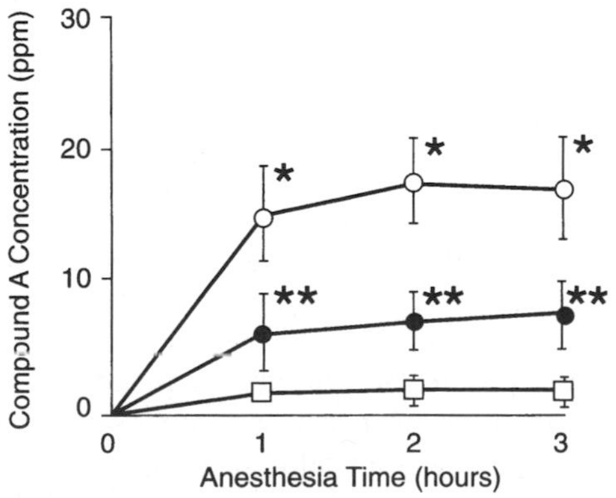

Figure 2-52. Inhaled compound A concentrations during administration of sevoflurane at fresh gas flow rates of 1 liter/minute (*open circles*), 3 liters/minute (*solid circles*), and 6 liters/minute (*squares*). (**P* <.05 versus 3 liters/minute; ***P* <.05 versus 6 liters/minute.) (From Bito H, Ikeda K. Effect of total flow rate on the concentration of degradation products generated by reaction between sevoflurane and soda lime. *Br J Anaesth* 1995;74:667–669; with permission.)

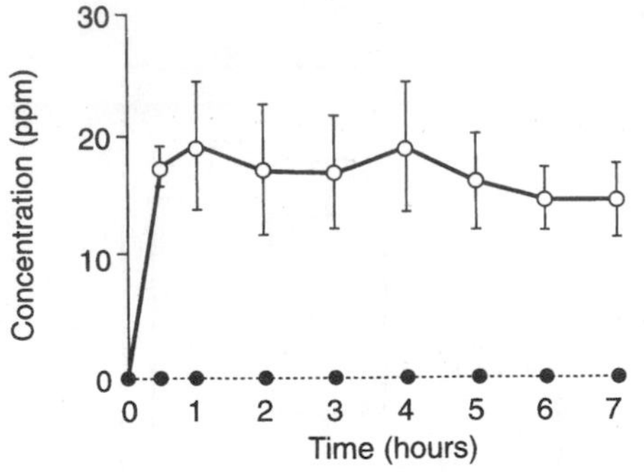

Figure 2-53. Inhaled compound A concentrations (*open circles*) and compound B concentrations (*solid circles*) during closed-circuit sevoflurane anesthesia. (Mean ± SD.) (From Bito H, Ikeda K. Closed-circuit anesthesia with sevoflurane in humans: effects on renal and hepatic function and concentrations of breakdown products with soda lime in the circuit. *Anesthesiology* 1994;80:71–76; with permission.)

Baralyme (no longer clinically available) probably as a result of higher absorbent temperatures compared with soda lime (Eger et al., 1997b; Smith et al., 1996). Similarly, carbon dioxide production increases the absorbent temperature and thus the production of compound A. Probenecid is a selective inhibitor of organic anion transport and pretreatment with this drug prevents compound A-induced renal injury in rats and may provide similar protection in humans (Higuchi et al., 2001a).

The rationale for utilizing at least a 2 liters/minute fresh gas flow rate when administering sevoflurane is intended to minimize the concentration of compound A that may accumulate in the anesthesia breathing circuit. To assess the adequacy of this recommendation, the nephrotoxicity of 2, 4, or 8 hours of anesthesia with 1.25 MAC sevoflurane has been compared with a similar exposure to desflurane (Eger et al., 1997a; Eger et al., 1997d). Compound A concentrations ranged from 40 to 42 ppm during the three different durations of sevoflurane administration. In patients receiving 1.25 MAC sevoflurane for 8 hours or 4 hours, there was transient evidence of injury to the glomeruli (albuminuria), proximal renal tubules (glucosuria and increased urinary excretion of glutathione-S-transferase), and distal renal tubules (increased urinary excretion of glutathione-S-transferase) that was greater in the 8-hour group. Urine-concentrating ability and plasma creatinine were not altered despite these findings in the patients receiving sevoflurane. Desflurane administered at 1.25 MAC for 2, 4, or 8 hours or sevoflurane exposure for 2 hours did not produce any evidence of renal injury. Conversely, comparisons of the renal effects of sevoflurane and isoflurane using fresh gas flows of 1 liter per minute or less demonstrated no difference between these drugs based on measurement of indices of renal function (Conzen et al., 2002; Kharasch et al. 2001). In children, sevoflurane anesthesia lasting 4 hours using total fresh gas flows of 2 liters per minute produced concentrations of compound A of <15 ppm, and there was no evidence of renal dysfunction (Frink et al., 1996).

The amount of compound A produced under clinical conditions has consistently been far below those concentrations associated with nephrotoxicity in animals (Smith et al., 1996). A proposed mechanism for nephrotoxicity is metabolism of compound A via the beta-lyase pathway to a reactive thiol. Because humans have less than one-tenth of the enzymatic activity for this pathway compared to rats, it is possible that humans should be less vulnerable to injury by this mechanism. Nevertheless, there are data indicating that humans are not less vulnerable to injury from compound A compared with rats (Eger et al., 1997a).

Halothane, like sevoflurane, is degraded by carbon dioxide absorbents to unsaturated volatile compounds that are nephrotoxic to rats. Based on the long history of halothane use without evidence of nephrotoxicity, it has been suggested the same may also be true for sevoflurane. There is evidence, however, that the product of halothane breakdown ($CF_2 = CBrCl$) from exposure to carbon dioxide absorbents is less nephrotoxic than compound A (Eger et al., 1997c). For this reason, the clinical absence of halothane nephrotoxicity does not necessarily indicate a similar absence for sevoflurane.

SKELETAL MUSCLE EFFECTS

Neuromuscular Junction

Ether derivative fluorinated volatile anesthetics produce skeletal muscle relaxation that is about twofold greater than that associated with a comparable dose of halothane. Nitrous oxide does not relax skeletal muscles, and in doses of >1 MAC (delivered in a hyperbaric chamber), it may produce skeletal muscle rigidity (Hornbein et al., 1982). This effect of nitrous oxide is consistent with enhancement of skeletal muscle rigidity produced by opioids when low concentrations of nitrous oxide are administered. The ability of skeletal muscles to sustain contractions in response to continuous stimulation is impaired in the presence of increasing concentrations of ether derivative volatile anesthetics but not in the presence of halothane or nitrous oxide (Fig. 2-54) (Eger, 1993).

Volatile anesthetics produce dose-dependent enhancement of the effects of neuromuscular-blocking drugs, with the effects of enflurane, isoflurane, desflurane, and sevoflurane being similar and greater than halothane (see Chapter 8). In vitro, isoflurane and halothane produce similar potentiation of the effects of neuromuscular-blocking drugs (Vitez et al., 1974). Nitrous oxide does not significantly potentiate the in vivo effects of neuromuscular-blocking drugs.

Malignant Hyperthermia

Volatile anesthetics including desflurane and sevoflurane can trigger malignant hyperthermia in genetically susceptible patients even in the absence of concomitant administration of succinylcholine (Papadimos et al., 2003; Ducart

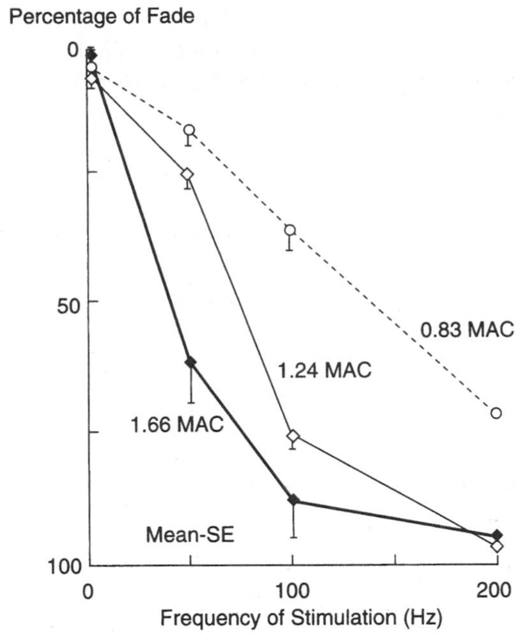

Figure 2-54. Increases in fade with tetanic stimulation accompany increasing doses of desflurane or increasing frequency of stimulation. [From Eger EI. *Desflurane (Suprane): a compendium and reference*. Nutley, NJ: Anaquest, 1993:1–119; with permission.]

et al., 1995; Ochiai et al., 1992). In one report, malignant hyperthermia did not manifest until 3 hours following uneventful desflurane anesthesia (Hoenemann et al., 2003). Among the volatile anesthetics, however, halothane is the most potent trigger. Nitrous oxide compared with volatile anesthetics is a weak trigger for malignant hyperthermia. For example, augmentation of caffeine-induced contractures of frog sartorius muscle by nitrous oxide is 1.3 times, whereas that for isoflurane is 3 times, enflurane 4 times, and halothane 11 times (Reed and Strobel, 1978).

OBSTETRIC EFFECTS

Volatile anesthetics produce similar and dose-dependent decreases in uterine smooth muscle contractility and blood flow (Fig. 2-55) (Eger, 1985a; Munson and Embro, 1977; Palahniuk and Shnider, 1974). These changes are modest at 0.5 MAC (analgesic concentrations) and become substantial at concentrations of >1 MAC. Nitrous oxide does not alter uterine contractility in doses used to provide analgesia during vaginal delivery.

Anesthetic-induced uterine relaxation may be desirable to facilitate removal of retained placenta. Conversely, uterine relaxation produced by volatile anesthetics may contribute to blood loss due to uterine atony. Indeed, blood loss during therapeutic abortion is greater in patients anesthetized with a volatile anesthetic compared with that in patients receiving nitrous oxide–barbiturate-opioid anesthesia (Cullen et al., 1970; Dolan et al., 1972).

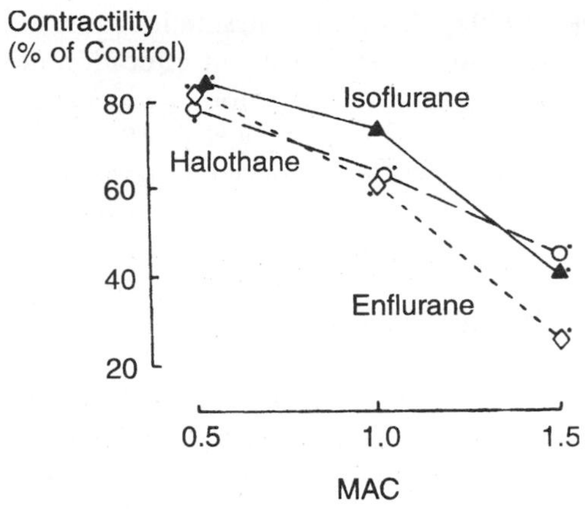

Figure 2-55. Impact of volatile anesthetics on contractility of uterine smooth muscle strips studied in vitro. (*P >.05.) [From Eger EI. *Isoflurane (Forane): a compendium and reference*. Madison, WI: Ohio Medical Products, 1985:1–110; with permission.]

In animals, evidence of fetal distress does not accompany anesthetic-induced decreases in maternal uterine blood flow as long as the anesthetic concentration is <1.5 MAC (Biehl et al., 1983). Furthermore, volatile anesthetics at about 0.5 MAC concentrations combined with 50% nitrous oxide ensure amnesia during cesarean section and do not produce detectable effects in the neonate (Warren et al., 1983). Inhaled anesthetics rapidly cross the placenta to enter the fetus, but these drugs are likewise rapidly exhaled by the newborn infant. Nitrous oxide–induced analgesia for vaginal delivery develops more rapidly than with most volatile anesthetics (desflurane and sevoflurane may be exceptions), but, after about 10 minutes, all inhaled drugs provide comparable analgesia.

RESISTANCE TO INFECTION

Many normal functions of the immune system are depressed after patient exposure to the combination of anesthesia and surgery (Stevenson et al., 1990). It would seem that many of the immune changes seen in surgical patients are primarily the result of surgical trauma and endocrine responses (increased catecholamines and corticosteroids) rather than the result of the anesthetic exposure itself. Inhaled anesthetics, particularly nitrous oxide, produce dose-dependent inhibition of polymorphonuclear leukocytes and their subsequent migration (chemotaxis) for phagocytosis, which is necessary for the inflammatory response to infection. Nevertheless, decreased resistance to bacterial infection due to inhaled anesthetics seems unlikely, considering the duration of administration and dose of these drugs. Furthermore, when leukocytes reach the site of infection, their ability to phagocytize bacteria appears to be normal.

Inhaled anesthetics do not have bacteriostatic effects at clinically useful concentrations. Conversely, the liquid form of volatile anesthetics may be bactericidal (Johnson and Eger, 1979). All volatile anesthetics (doses as low as 0.2 MAC) produce dose-dependent inhibition of measles virus replication and decrease mortality in mice receiving intranasal influenza virus (Knight et al., 1983). This inhibition may reflect anesthetic-induced decreases in DNA synthesis.

GENETIC EFFECTS

The Ames test, which identifies chemicals that act as mutagens and carcinogens, is negative for enflurane, isoflurane, desflurane, sevoflurane, and nitrous oxide, including their known metabolites (Baden et al., 1987; Baden et al., 1982; Kharasch, 1995). Compound A formed from sevoflurane degradation by carbon dioxide absorbents might be expected to be an alkylating agent (and thus a mutagen), but tests of this product do not reveal mutagenicity (Morio et al., 1992). Halothane also results in a negative Ames test, but potential metabolites may be positive (Sachder et al., 1980). In animals, nitrous oxide administered during vulnerable periods of gestation may result in adverse reproductive effects manifesting as an increased incidence of fetal resorptions (abortions) (Bussard et al., 1974; Lane et al., 1980). Conversely, administration of volatile anesthetics during these vulnerable periods does not increase the incidence of fetal resorptions (Mazze et al., 1986). Learning function may be impaired in newborn animals exposed in utero to inhaled anesthetics (Chalon et al., 1982; Mazze et al., 1984).

The increased incidence of spontaneous abortions in operating room personnel may reflect a teratogenic effect from chronic exposure to trace concentrations of inhaled anesthetics, especially nitrous oxide (Lane et al., 1980). Nitrous oxide irreversibly oxidizes the cobalt atom of vitamin B_{12} such that the activity of vitamin B_{12}–dependent enzymes (methionine synthetase and thymidylate synthetase) is decreased. In patients undergoing laparotomy with general anesthesia including 70% nitrous oxide, the half-time for inactivation of methionine synthetase is about 46 minutes (Fig. 2-56) (Nunn et al., 1988). Inactivation of methionine synthetase is more rapid in rats exposed to 50% nitrous oxide, with a half-time of 5.4 minutes. Therefore, it is probably not valid to extrapolate time frames established in rodents to humans. Volatile anesthetics do not alter activity of vitamin B_{12}–dependent enzymes.

Methionine synthetase converts homocysteine to methionine, which is necessary for the formation of myelin. Thymidylate synthetase is important in the conversion of DNA to thymidine and the subsequent formation of DNA. Interference with myelin formation and DNA synthesis could have significant effects on the rapidly growing fetus, manifesting as spontaneous abortions or congenital anomalies. Inhibition of these enzymes could also manifest as depression of bone marrow function and neurologic disturbances. The speculated but undocumented role of trace

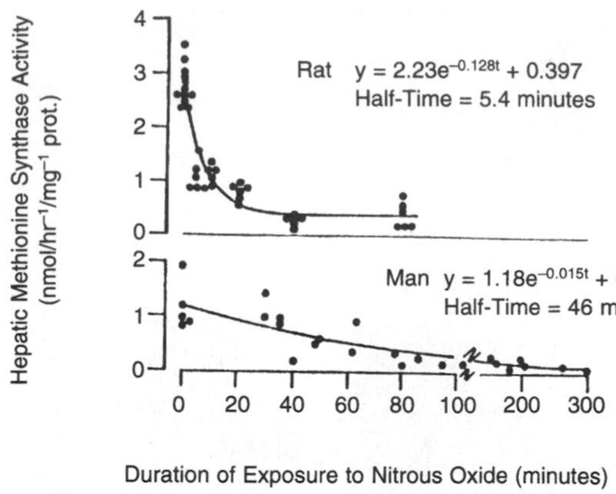

Figure 2-56. Time course of inactivation of hepatic methionine synthase (synthetase) activity during administration of 50% nitrous oxide to rats or 70% nitrous oxide to humans. (From Nunn JF, Weinbran HK, Royston D, et al. Rate of inactivation of human and rodent hepatic methionine synthase by nitrous oxide. *Anesthesiology* 1988;68:213–216; with permission.)

concentrations of nitrous oxide in the production of spontaneous abortions has led to the use of scavenging systems designed to remove waste anesthetic gases, including nitrous oxide, from the ambient air of the operating room. Nevertheless, animal studies using intermittent exposure to trace concentrations of nitrous oxide, halothane, enflurane, and isoflurane have not revealed harmful reproductive effects (Mazze, 1985).

BONE MARROW FUNCTION

Interference with DNA synthesis is responsible for the megaloblastic changes and agranulocytosis that may follow prolonged administration of nitrous oxide. Megaloblastic changes in bone marrow are consistently found in patients who have been exposed to anesthetic concentrations of nitrous oxide for 24 hours (Nunn, 1987). Exposure to nitrous oxide lasting 4 days or longer results in agranulocytosis. These bone marrow effects occur as a result of nitrous oxide–induced interference with activity of vitamin B_{12}–dependent enzymes, which are necessary for synthesis of DNA and the subsequent formation of erythrocytes (see the section on Genetic Effects). Despite these potential adverse effects on bone marrow function, the administration of nitrous oxide to patients undergoing bone marrow transplantation does not influence bone marrow viability (Fig. 2-57) (Lederhaas et al., 1995).

It is presumed that a healthy surgical patient could receive nitrous oxide for 24 hours without harm. Because the inhibition of methionine synthetase is rapid and its recovery is slow, it is to be expected that repeated exposures at intervals of <3 days may result in a cumulative effect. This relationship may be further complicated by other factors influencing levels of methionine synthetase and tetrahydrofolate (necessary for the transmethylation reaction) that might be important in critically ill patients

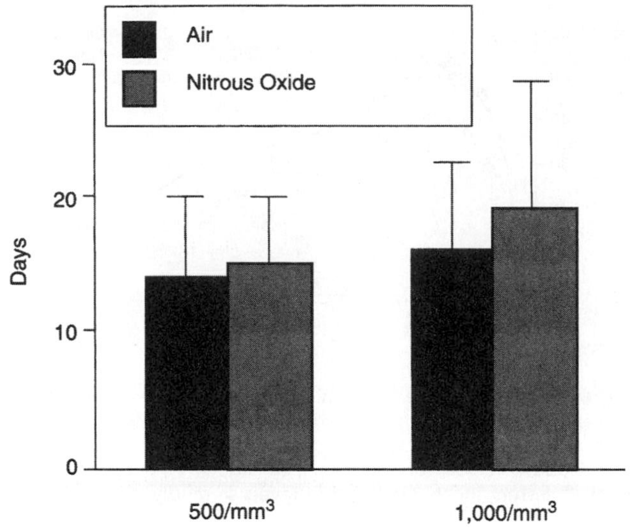

Figure 2-57. Nitrous oxide administered during bone marrow harvest did not alter the subsequent number of days needed for cultures to grow 500 to 1,000 cells/mm^3. (Mean ± SD.) (From Lederhaas G, Brock-Utne JG, Negrin RS, et al. Is nitrous oxide safe for bone marrow harvest? *Anesth Analg* 1995;80:770–772; with permission.)

receiving nitrous oxide. Nevertheless, the contradiction between the serious biochemical effects of nitrous oxide and the apparent absence of adverse clinical effects in routine use of this inhaled anesthetic makes it difficult to draw firm conclusions.

PERIPHERAL NEUROPATHY

Animals exposed to 15% nitrous oxide for up to 15 days develop ataxia and exhibit evidence of spinal cord and peripheral nerve degeneration. Humans who chronically inhale nitrous oxide for nonmedical purposes may develop a neuropathy characterized by sensorimotor polyneuropathy that is often combined with signs of posterior lateral spinal cord degeneration resembling pernicious anemia (Layzer et al., 1978). The speculated mechanism of this neuropathy is the ability of nitrous oxide to oxidize irreversibly the cobalt atom of vitamin B_{12} such that activity of vitamin B_{12}–dependent enzymes is decreased (see the section on Genetic Effects).

TOTAL BODY OXYGEN REQUIREMENTS

Total body oxygen requirements are decreased by similar amounts by volatile anesthetics. The oxygen requirements of the heart decrease more than those of other organs, reflecting drug-induced decreases in cardiac work associated with decreases in systemic blood pressure and myocardial contractility. Therefore, decreased oxygen requirements would protect tissues from ischemia that might result from decreased oxygen delivery due to drug-induced decreases in perfusion pressure. Decreases in total body oxygen requirements probably reflect metabolic depressant effects as well as decreased functional needs in the presence of anesthetic-produced depression of organ function.

METABOLISM

Metabolism of inhaled anesthetics is important for two reasons. First, intermediary metabolites, end-metabolites, or breakdown products from exposure to carbon dioxide absorbents may be toxic to the kidneys, liver, or reproductive organs. Second, the degree of metabolism may influence the rate of decrease in the alveolar partial pressure at the conclusion of the anesthetic. Conversely, the rate of increase in the alveolar partial pressure during induction of anesthesia is unlikely to be influenced by metabolism because inhaled anesthetics are administered in great excess to the amount metabolized.

Assessment of the magnitude of metabolism of inhaled anesthetics is by (a) measurement of metabolites or (b) comparison of the total amount of anesthetic recovered in the exhaled gases with the amount taken up during administration (mass balance). The advantages of the mass balance technique are that knowledge of metabolite pharmacokinetics and identification and collection of metabolites are not necessary. Indeed, recovery of metabolites may be incomplete, leading to an underestimation of the magnitude of metabolism. A disadvantage of the mass balance approach is that loss of anesthetic through the surgical skin incision, across the intact skin, in urine, and in feces may prevent complete recovery, and these losses would be construed as due to metabolism. Nevertheless, the error introduced by these losses is likely to be insignificant, with the occasional exception of large and highly perfused wound surfaces.

Comparison of metabolite recovery and mass balance studies results in greatly different estimates of the magnitude of metabolism of volatile anesthetics (Table 2-4) (Carpenter et al., 1986). For example, mass balance estimates of the magnitude of metabolism are 1.5 to 3 times greater than estimates determined by the recovery of metabolites. This is not surprising because recovery of metabolites will underestimate the magnitude of metabolism unless all metabolites are recovered. Based on mass balance studies, it is concluded that alveolar ventilation is principally responsible for the elimination of enflurane and isoflurane (presumably also desflurane and sevoflurane), that alveolar ventilation and metabolism are equally important for elimination of halothane, and that metabolism is the most important mechanism for the elimination of methoxyflurane (Carpenter et al., 1986).

Determinants of Metabolism

The magnitude of metabolism of inhaled anesthetics is determined by the (a) chemical structure, (b) hepatic

TABLE 2-4.
METABOLISM OF VOLATILE ANESTHETICS AS ASSESSED BY METABOLITE RECOVERY VERSUS MASS BALANCE STUDIES

	Magnitude of Metabolism	
Anesthetic	Metabolite Recovery (%)	Mass Balance (%)
Nitrous oxide	0.004	
Halothane	15–20	46.1
Enflurane	3	8.5
Isoflurane	0.2	0*
Desflurane	0.02	
Sevoflurane	5	

*Metabolism of isoflurane assumed to be 0 for this calculation.
Source: Data adapted from Carpenter RL, Eger EI, Johnson BH, et al. The extent of metabolism of inhaled anesthetics in humans. *Anesthesiology* 1986;65:201–205.

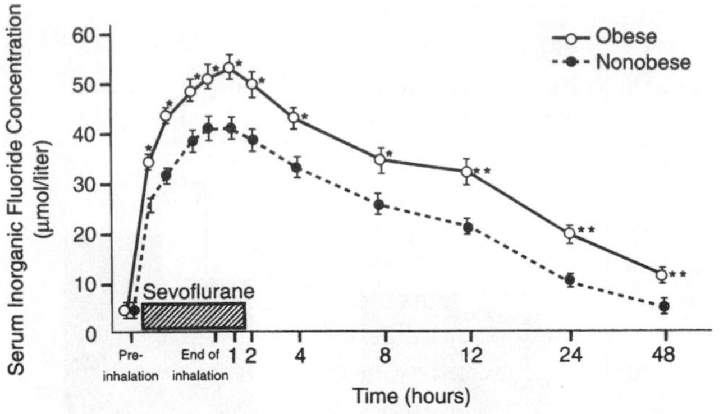

Figure 2-58. Plasma inorganic fluoride concentrations during and after sevoflurane administration are higher in obese compared with nonobese patients. (**P* <.01 obese versus nonobese. ***P* <.001 obese versus nonobese.) (From Higuchi H, Satoh T, Arimura S, et al. Serum inorganic fluoride levels in mildly obese patients during and after sevoflurane anesthesia. *Anesth Analg* 1993;77: 1018–1021; with permission.)

enzyme activity, (c) blood concentration of the anesthetic, and (d) genetic factors.

Chemical Structure

The ether bond and carbon-halogen bond are the sites in the anesthetic molecule most susceptible to oxidative metabolism. Oxidation of the ether bond is less likely when hydrogen atoms on the carbons surrounding the oxygen atom of this bond are replaced by halogen atoms. Two halogen atoms on a terminal carbon represent the optimal arrangement for dehalogenation, whereas a terminal carbon with fluorine atoms is very resistant to oxidative metabolism. The bond energy for carbon-fluorine is twice that for carbon-bromine or carbon-chlorine. The absence of ester bonds in inhaled anesthetics negates any role of metabolism by hydrolysis.

Hepatic Enzyme Activity

The activity of hepatic cytochrome P-450 enzymes responsible for metabolism of volatile anesthetics may be increased by a variety of drugs, including the anesthetics themselves. Phenobarbital, phenytoin, and isoniazid may increase defluorination of volatile anesthetics, especially enflurane. There is evidence in patients that brief (1 hour) exposures during surgical stimulation increase hepatic microsomal enzyme activity independently of the anesthetic drug (halothane or isoflurane) or technique (spinal) used (Loft et al., 1985). Conversely, surgery lasting >4 hours can lead to depressed microsomal enzyme activity.

For unknown reasons, obesity predictably increases defluorination of halothane, enflurane, and isoflurane (Strube et al., 1987). Peak plasma fluoride concentrations after administration of sevoflurane are higher in obese compared with nonobese patients (Fig. 2-58) (Higuchi et al., 1993). Conversely, another report describes no difference in peak plasma fluoride concentrations based on body weight (Frink et al., 1993).

Blood Concentration

The fraction of anesthetic that is metabolized on passing through the liver is influenced by the blood concentration of the anesthetic (Fig. 2-59) (Sawyer et al., 1971; White et al., 1979). For example, a 1 MAC concentration saturates hepatic enzymes and decreases the fraction of anesthetic that is removed (metabolized) during a single passage through the liver. Conversely, subanesthetic concentrations (≤0.1 MAC) undergo extensive metabolism on passage through the liver. Disease states such as cirrhosis of the liver or congestive heart failure could theoretically alter metabolism by decreasing hepatic blood flow and drug delivery or by decreasing the amount of viable liver and thus enzyme activity.

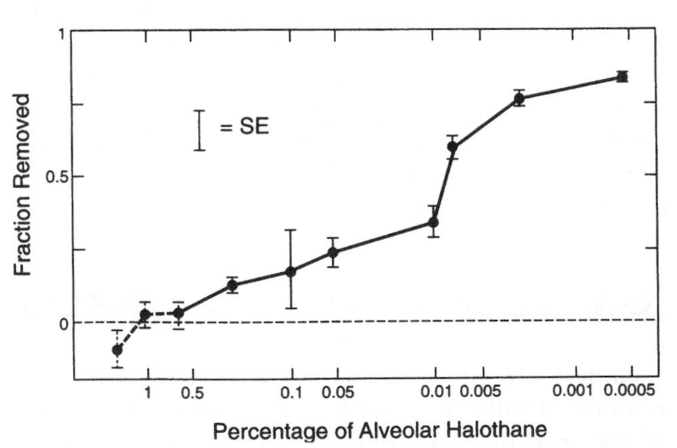

Figure 2-59. Fraction of halothane removed during passage through the liver at progressively decreasing alveolar concentrations. (From Sawyer DC, Eger EI, Bahlam SH, et al. Concentration dependence of hepatic halothane metabolism. *Anesthesiology* 1971;34:230–235; with permission.)

Inhaled anesthetics that are not highly soluble in blood and tissues (nitrous oxide, enflurane, isoflurane, desflurane, sevoflurane) tend to be exhaled rapidly via the lungs at the conclusion of an anesthetic. As a result, less drug is available to pass through the liver continually at low blood concentrations conducive to metabolism. This is reflected in the magnitude of metabolism of these drugs (see Table 2-4) (Carpenter et al., 1986). Halothane and methoxyflurane are more soluble in blood and lipids and thus likely to be stored in tissues that act as a reservoir to maintain subanesthetic concentrations conducive to metabolism for prolonged periods of time after discontinuation of their administration.

Genetic Factors

Overall, genetic factors appear to be the most important determinant of drug-metabolizing enzyme activity. In this regard, humans are active metabolizers of drugs compared with lower animal species such as the rat.

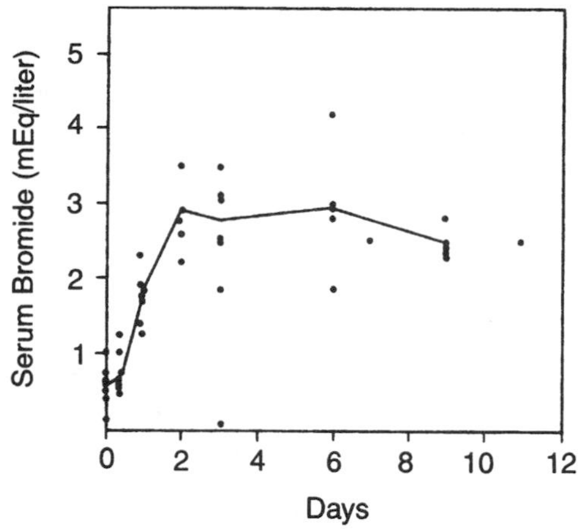

Figure 2-60. Serum bromide concentrations in volunteers after prolonged (about 7 hours) exposure to halothane. (From Johnstone RE, Kennell EM, Behar MG, et al. Increased serum bromide concentration after halothane anesthesia in man. *Anesthesiology* 1975;42:598–601; with permission.)

Metabolism of Inhaled Anesthetics

Nitrous Oxide

An estimated 0.004% of an absorbed dose of nitrous oxide undergoes reductive metabolism to nitrogen in the gastrointestinal tract (Hong et al., 1980a; Trudell, 1985). Anaerobic bacteria, such as *Pseudomonas*, are responsible for this reductive metabolism. Reductive products of some nitrogen compounds include free radicals that could produce toxic effects on cells. The potential toxic role of these metabolites, however, remains undocumented. Oxygen concentrations of >10% in the gastrointestinal tract and antibiotics inhibit metabolism of nitrous oxide by anaerobic bacteria. There is no evidence that nitrous oxide undergoes oxidative metabolism in the liver (Hong et al., 1980b).

Halothane

An estimated 15% to 20% of absorbed halothane undergoes metabolism (see Table 2-4) (Cascorbi et al., 1970). Halothane is uniquely metabolized because it undergoes oxidation by cytochrome P-450 enzymes when ample oxygen is present but reductive metabolism when hepatocyte Po_2 decreases.

Oxidative Metabolism

The principal oxidative metabolites of halothane resulting from metabolism by cytochrome P-450 enzymes are trifluoroacetic acid, chloride, and bromide. In genetically susceptible patients, a reactive trifluoroacetyl halide oxidative metabolite of halothane may interact with (acetylate) hepatic microsomal proteins on the surfaces of hepatocytes (neoantigens) to stimulate the formation of antibodies against this new foreign protein (see Fig. 2-44) (Martin et al., 1995).

The energy bond for carbon-fluorine is strong, accounting for the absence of detectable amounts of inorganic fluoride as an oxidative metabolite of halothane. It is estimated that the plasma concentration of bromide increases 0.5 mEq/liter for every MAC hour of halothane administration (Fig. 2-60) (Johnstone et al., 1975). Because signs of bromide toxicity, such as somnolence and confusion, do not occur until plasma concentrations of bromide are >6 mEq/liter, the likelihood of symptoms from metabolism of halothane to bromide seems remote. Nevertheless, prolonged halothane anesthesia may more likely be associated with intellectual impairment than a similar dose of an anesthetic that is not metabolized to bromide.

Reductive Metabolism

Reductive metabolism, which, among the volatile anesthetics, has been documented to occur only during metabolism of halothane, is most likely to occur in the presence of hepatocyte hypoxia and enzyme induction. Reductive metabolites of halothane include fluoride and volatile products, some of which result from the reaction of halothane with carbon dioxide absorbents. In the past, reductive metabolites were considered to be potentially hepatotoxic. Nevertheless, data do not support a role for reductive metabolism in the initiation of halothane hepatitis (see the section on Halothane Hepatitis). Increased plasma fluoride concentrations reflect reductive metabolism of halothane in obese patients and children with cyanotic congenital heart disease (Fig. 2-61) (Moore et al., 1986; Nawaf and Stoelting, 1979). The level of plasma fluoride (<10 μm/liter) is far below the level likely to produce even subclinical nephrotoxicity (50 μm/liter), and changes in liver transaminase enzymes as evidence of hepatotoxicity due to reductive metabolism are not seen in these patients.

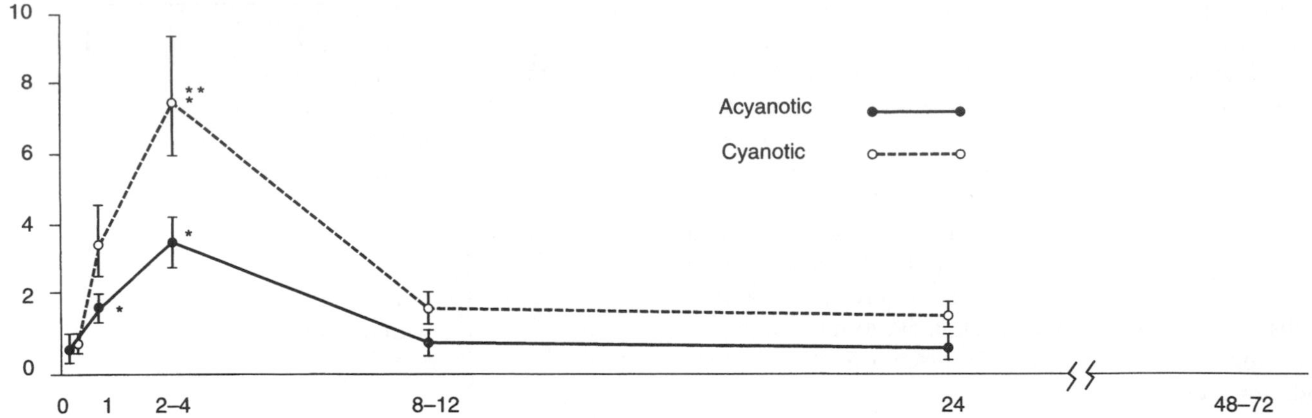

Figure 2-61. Plasma concentrations of fluoride are higher after administration of halothane in cyanotic patients than in acyanotic patients. (*$P < .05$ within groups compared to prehalothane level; **$P < .05$ between groups.) (Modified from Moore RA, McNicholas KW, Gallagher JD, et al. Halothane metabolism in acyanotic and cyanotic patients undergoing open heart surgery. *Anesth Analg* 1986;65:1257–1262; with permission.)

Enflurane

An estimated 3% of absorbed enflurane undergoes oxidative metabolism by cytochrome P-450 enzymes to form inorganic fluoride and organic fluoride compounds (see Table 2-4) (Chase et al., 1971). Like halothane, enflurane also undergoes P-450–mediated oxidative metabolism to adducts, which may cause the formation of neoantigens in susceptible patients (see Fig. 2-44) (Martin et al., 1995) (see the section on Hepatic Effects). Fluoride results from dehalogenation of the terminal carbon atom. Oxidation of the ether bond and release of additional fluoride does not occur, reflecting the chemical stability imparted to this bond by the surrounding halogens. As with isoflurane, the methyl portion of the molecule seems to be resistant to oxidation, and reductive metabolism does not occur. Minimal metabolism of enflurane reflects its chemical stability and low solubility in tissues such that the drug is exhaled unchanged rather than repeatedly passing through the liver at low plasma concentrations conducive to metabolism.

Enzyme induction with phenobarbital or phenytoin increases the liberation of fluoride from enflurane in vitro but not in vivo (Mazze et al., 1982). This observation is most likely due to low tissue solubility of enflurane such that, in vivo, the availability of substrate (enflurane) becomes the rate-limiting factor, whereas in vitro, the substrate concentration is controlled and the effect of enzyme induction manifests as increased metabolism of enflurane to inorganic fluoride (Greenstein et al., 1975). For these reasons, it seems unlikely that the nephrotoxic potential of enflurane would be increased by enzyme induction. An exception may be patients who are being treated with isoniazid, because this drug can increase defluorination of enflurane in genetically determined patients who are rapid acetylators.

Isoflurane

An estimated 0.2% of absorbed isoflurane undergoes oxidative metabolism by cytochrome P-450 enzymes (see Table 2-4) (Holaday et al., 1975). Metabolism begins with oxidation of the carbon-halogen link of the alpha carbon atom, leading to an unstable compound that subsequently decomposes to difluoromethanol and trifluoroacetic acid (Fig. 2-62) (Eger, 1993). Trifluoroacetic acid is the principal organic fluoride metabolite of isoflurane. Like halothane, isoflurane also undergoes P-450–mediated oxidative metabolism to adducts, which may cause formation of neoantigens in susceptible patients (see Fig. 2-44) (Martin et al., 1995) (see the section on Hepatic Effects). Reductive metabolism of isoflurane does not occur.

Minimal metabolism of isoflurane reflects the drug's chemical stability and low solubility in tissues such that the drug is exhaled unchanged rather than repeatedly passing through the liver at low plasma concentrations conducive to metabolism. The chemical stability of isoflurane is ensured by the trifluorocarbon molecule and the presence of halogen atoms on three sides of the ether bond.

Minimal changes in plasma concentrations of fluoride (peak <5 μm/liter) resulting from metabolism of isoflurane plus the absence of other toxic metabolites render nephrotoxicity or hepatotoxicity after administration unlikely. Enzyme induction with phenobarbital or phenytoin increases the liberation of fluoride from isoflurane in vivo (Mazze et al., 1982). Even in the presence of enzyme induction, however, the metabolism of isoflurane and resulting plasma concentrations of fluoride remain much less than with enflurane. Likewise, isoniazid, which dramatically increases metabolism of enflurane in susceptible patients, fails to significantly alter metabolism of isoflurane.

Desflurane

An estimated 0.02% of absorbed desflurane undergoes oxidative metabolism by cytochrome P-450 enzymes (see Table 2-4) (Sutton et al., 1991). The metabolic pathways for desflurane likely parallel those for isoflurane

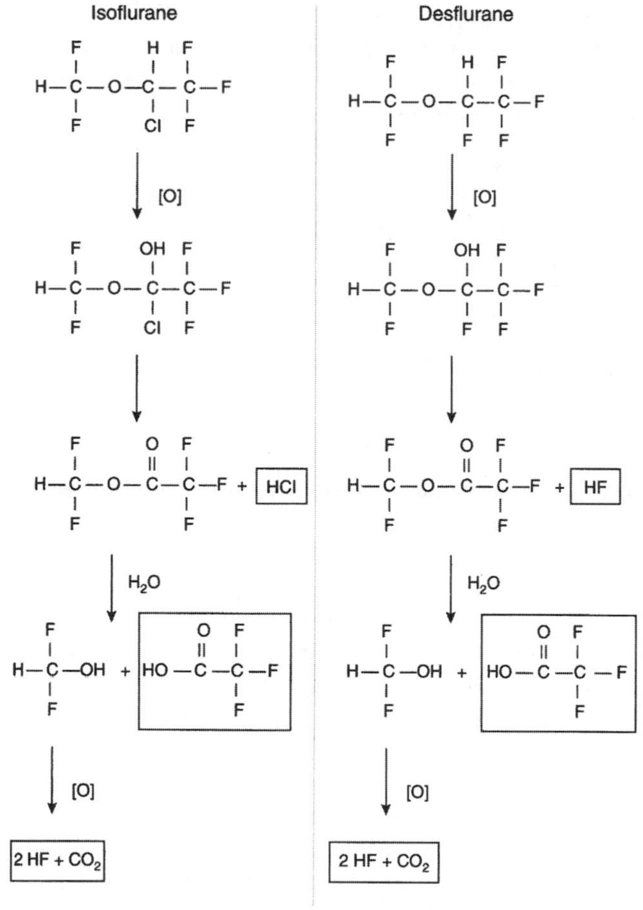

Figure 2-62. The proposed metabolic pathways for isoflurane and desflurane are similar. [From Eger EI. *Desflurane (Suprane): a compendium and reference.* Nutley, NJ: Anaquest, 1993:1–119; with permission.]

although the greater strength of the carbon-fluorine bond renders desflurane less vulnerable to metabolism than its chlorinated analog, isoflurane (see Fig. 2-62) (Eger, 1993). Metabolism begins with the insertion of an active oxygen atom between the alpha ethyl carbon of desflurane and its hydrogen. The resulting unstable molecule degrades ultimately to inorganic fluoride, trifluoroacetic acid, carbon dioxide, and water. The only evidence of metabolism of desflurane is the presence of measurable concentrations of urinary trifluoroacetic acid equal to about one-fifth to one-tenth that produced by metabolism of isoflurane (Sutton et al., 1991). Neither plasma fluoride concentrations nor urinary organic fluoride excretion increase significantly after even prolonged administration of desflurane (7.4 MAC hours) to humans (Sutton et al., 1991). Enzyme induction with phenobarbital or ethanol does not influence the magnitude of metabolism of desflurane in animals (Koblin et al., 1988). Kinetic studies in humans indicate that all the desflurane absorbed during its administration can be recovered during elimination, emphasizing both the molecular stability of this compound as well as its poor blood and tissue solubility (Yasuda et al., 1991). Like halothane, desflurane also undergoes P-450 mediated oxidative metabolism to adducts, which may cause formation of neoantigens in susceptible patients (see Fig. 2-44) (Martin et al., 1995) (see the section on Hepatic Effects).

Carbon Monoxide Toxicity

Carbon monoxide formation reflects the degradation of volatile anesthetics that contain a CHF_2moiety (desflurane, enflurane, and isoflurane) by the strong bases present in desiccated carbon dioxide absorbents (Baum et al., 1995). Indeed, increases in intraoperative carboxyhemoglobin concentrations have been attributed to this degradation. Factors that influence the magnitude of carbon monoxide production from volatile anesthetics include (a) dryness of the carbon dioxide absorbent with hydration preventing formation, (b) high temperatures of the carbon dioxide absorbent as during low fresh gas flows and/or increased metabolic production of carbon dioxide, (c) prolonged high fresh gas flows that cause desiccation (dryness) of the carbon dioxide absorbent, and (d) type of carbon dioxide absorbent. (Baxter et al., 1998; Baxter and Kharasch, 1997; Fang et al., 1995). Desflurane produces the highest carbon monoxide concentration (package insert for desflurane describes this risk) followed by enflurane and isoflurane. A carboxyhemoglobin concentration of 36% has been described in a patient receiving desflurane (Berry et al., 1999).

Halothane and sevoflurane do not possess a vinyl group and thus carbon monoxide production on exposure to carbon dioxide absorbants has been considered unlikely. Nevertheless, carbon monoxide formation is a risk of sevoflurane administration in the presence of desiccated carbon dioxide absorbent especially when an exothermic reaction between the volatile anesthetic and desiccated absorbent occurs (see the section on Carbon Dioxide Absorber Fires) (Wissing et al., 2001). In the presence of carbon dioxide absorbent temperatures $>70\,°C$, hexafluoroisopropanol, an intermediate of sevoflurane metabolism, degradates to carbon monoxide.

It is not possible to completely avoid hazards of carbon monoxide by using sevoflurane. It is concluded that the potential for carbon monoxide formation is a property of all modern volatile anesthetics contacting dry carbon dioxide absorbents that contain potassium hydroxide and/or sodium hydroxide (Versichelen et al., 2001; Wissing et al., 2001). Patients with low hemoglobin quantities (anemia, pediatric patients) are at greater risk for high carboxyhemoglobin concentrations in response to exposure to carbon monoxide (Woehlck et al., 2001). Precautions to insure carbon dioxide absorbents that contain strong bases have not become desiccated is important for preventing the formation of carbon monoxide during administration of volatile anesthetics. Current Environmental Protection

Agency limits for carbon monoxide exposure are 35 ppm for 1 hour.

Intraoperative Diagnosis

Intraoperative detection of carbon monoxide is difficult because pulse oximetry cannot differentiate between carboxyhemoglobin and oxyhemoglobin. Moderately decreased pulse oximetry readings despite adequate arterial partial pressures of oxygen (especially during the first case of the day, "Monday morning phenomena") should suggest the possibility of carbon monoxide exposure and the need to measure carboxyhemoglobin (Woehlck et al., 2001). Furthermore, there is no routinely available means to reliably identify the presence of carbon monoxide in the breathing circuit, nor to detect when carbon dioxide absorbent has become desiccated (absorbent color change does not occur in response to desiccation or carbon monoxide formation). In addition to decreased pulse oximeter readings, an erroneous gas analyzer reading (indicates mixed gas readings or enflurane when desflurane is being administered) has been described as an early indirect warning of carbon monoxide formation (Berry et al., 1999; Holak et al., 2003). This erroneous gas analyzer reading was attributed to trifluoromethane, which is produced along with carbon monoxide by degradation of isoflurane, enflurane, and desflurane, but not sevoflurane. Trifluoromethane has an infrared absorption profile similar to enflurane resulting in the gas analyzer indicating administration of this volatile anesthetic when the vaporizer is known to contain desflurane or isoflurane. An erroneous gas analyzer reading as an early warning of carbon monoxide exposure does not occur during administration of sevoflurane (Holak et al. 2003). Delayed neurophysiologic sequelae due to carbon monoxide (cognitive defects, personality changes, gait disturbances) may occur as late as 3 to 21 days after anesthesia. Intraoperative hemolysis has the potential to result in carbon monoxide exposure which can mimic carbon monoxide production from degradation of volatile anesthetics (Wohlfeil et al., 2001).

Endogenous Carbon Monoxide

Endogenous carbon monoxide production reflects heme catabolism. The rate-limiting enzyme in formation of carbon monoxide from heme is heme oxygenase-1. This enzyme is induced by its substrate (heme) and by various oxidative stresses. Heme oxygenase-1 is thought to confer protection against oxidative tissue injuries. Conversion of the heme moiety of hemeproteins (hemoglobin, myoglobin, cytochrome P-450) to biliverdin results in liberation of carbon monoxide. This endogenous carbon monoxide diffuses from cells into the circulation to form carboxyhemoglobin and is also transported to the lungs where it is exhaled. Independent of volatile anesthetics and carbon dioxide absorbents, the exhaled carbon monoxide and carboxyhemoglobin concentrations are increased on the day following surgery (Hayashi et al., 2004). This suggests that oxidative stress associated with anesthesia and surgery may induce heme oxygenase-1 which catalyzes heme to produce carbon monoxide.

Sevoflurane

An estimated 5% of absorbed sevoflurane undergoes oxidative metabolism by cytochrome P-450 enzymes to form organic and inorganic fluoride metabolites (see Table 2-4 and Fig. 2-44) (Kharasch et al., 1995b). In addition, sevoflurane is degraded by desiccated carbon dioxide absorbents containing strong bases to potentially toxic compounds (see the section on Vinyl Halide Nephrotoxicity) (Smith et al., 1996). Unlike all the other fluorinated volatile anesthetics, sevoflurane does not undergo metabolism to acetyl halide that could result in formation of trifluoatated liver proteins. As a result, sevoflurane cannot stimulate the formation of antitrifluoroacetylated protein antibodies leading to hepatotoxicity by this mechanism (Kharasch, 1995) (see the section on Hepatic Effects).

Cytochrome P-450–mediated sevoflurane oxidation at the fluoromethoxy carbon produces a transient intermediate that decomposes to inorganic fluoride and the organic fluoride metabolite hexafluoroisopropanol. Hexafluoroisopropanol undergoes conjugation with glucuronic acid and this conjugate is excreted in the urine. There is no evidence that hexafluoroisopropanol is toxic.

Peak plasma fluoride concentrations are higher after administration of sevoflurane than after comparable doses of enflurane (Conzen et al., 1995; Frink et al., 1994). Nevertheless, the duration of exposure of renal tubules to fluoride that results from sevoflurane metabolism is limited because of the rapid pulmonary elimination of this poorly blood-soluble anesthetic. Furthermore, hepatic production of fluoride from sevoflurane may be less of a nephrotoxic risk than is intrarenal production of fluoride from enflurane (Brown, 1995).

Sevoflurane is absorbed and degraded by desiccated carbon dioxide absorbents, especially when the temperature of the absorbent is increased (see Fig. 2-4) (Smith et al., 1996). Among these compounds, only compound A (and to a lesser extent compound B) is produced under conditions likely to be encountered clinically. The type of carbon dioxide absorbent may influence the magnitude of compound A production. (Eger et al., 1997b). Compound A is nephrotoxic and hepatotoxic in animals (see the sections on Hepatic Effects and Renal Effects). Nevertheless, the amount of compound A produced under clinically relevant circumstances has always been substantially lower than that which produces toxicity in animals (Smith et al., 1996).

Carbon Dioxide Absorber Fires

Sevoflurane reacts chemically with desiccated carbon dioxide absorbents (especially Baralyme® which is no longer clinically available) to produce carbon monoxide and flammable organic compounds, including methanol and formaldehyde. The reaction produces heat and heat increases the reaction speed so the rate of sevoflurane breakdown can accelerate rapidly. Sevoflurane may be so extensively consumed that maintaining anesthesia is difficult. At high temperatures flammable metabolites can spontaneously combust (formaldehyde gas). A peak absorbent canister temperature of 120° to 140°C is generally reached 10 to 50 minutes after the start of the reaction followed by a rapid decrease in the canister temperature. In nonhuman trials utilizing anesthesia machines the carbon dioxide absorbent temperatures increased rapidly to greater than 300°C and parts of the absorbent canister melted (Holak et al., 2003).

In the presence of desiccated carbon dioxide absorbent, temperature increases are greater with sevoflurane than with other volatile anesthetics and at absorbent temperatures >70°C there is increased likelihood of degradation of sevoflurane to flammable products and carbon monoxide (Figs. 2-63 and 2-64) (Lester et al., 2004; Holak et al., 2003; Wissing et al., 2001). For example, temperatures of desiccated soda lime exposed to 1.5 MAC isoflurane and desflurane peaked at about 100°C and then decreased progressively, whereas temperatures in desiccated carbon dioxide absorbents exposed to 1.5 MAC increased progressively to nearly 200°C and spontaneous combustion in the anesthesia circuit occurred in some instances (Fig. 2-64) (Lester et al, 2004). Spontaneous combustion and even explosions involving the carbon dioxide absorber and anesthesia breathing circuit have been described clinically and are most often (perhaps always) associated with Baralyme® carbon dioxide absorbent (no longer clinically available), anesthesia machine use factors that contribute to desiccation of the absorbent (flow of dry gases through the absorber during a weekend, "Monday morning phenomena") and administration of sevoflurane (Castro et al., 2004; Holak et al, 2003; Hazard Report, 2003; Woehlck, 2004; Wu et al., 2004). Apparently, under certain conditions, exothermic chemical reactions between sevoflurane and desiccated carbon dioxide absorbent creates high temperatures with production of flammable gases (formaldehyde, methanol) and autoignition of plastics and gases in the absorber. The critical observation regarding fires and production of carbon monoxide is that desiccated carbon dioxide absorbents containing strong bases allows these reactions to occur. Clinically, delayed increases or unexpected sudden decreases in inspired sevoflurane concentrations relative to the vaporizer setting may reflect excessive heating of the carbon dioxide absorber canister. Pulmonary injury

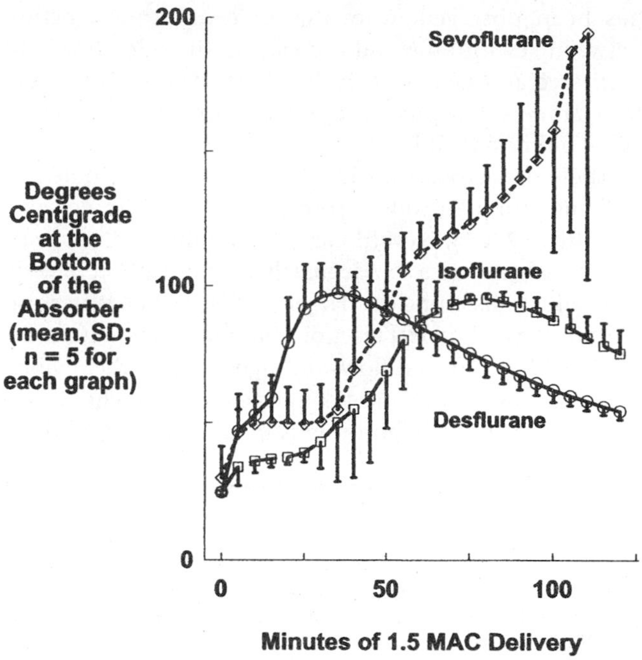

Figure 2-64. Temperatures recorded from the bottom of the desiccated carbon dioxide absorbent canister peaked at about 100C° when exposed to 1.5 MAC desflurane and isoflurane and then decreased. Temperatures in the desiccated carbon dioxide absorbent canister increased progressively to over 200C° when exposed to 1.5 MAC sevoflurane and spontaneous flames occurred in some of the anesthesia circuits (From Lester M, Roth P, Eger, EI. Fires from the interaction of anesthetics with desiccated absorbent. *Anesth Analg* 2004;99:769-774; with permission.)

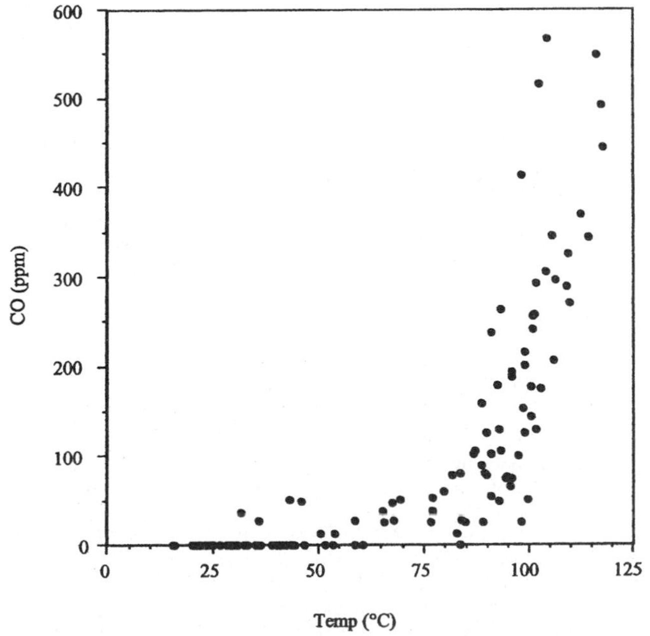

Figure 2-63. Carbon monoxide (CO) concentrations in parts per million (ppm) are plotted against absorbent temperatures measured in the center of the canister. Most clinically relevant CO concentrations do not occur until the absorbent temperature exceeds 70°C. (From Holak E, Mei DA, Dunning MB, et al. Carbon monoxide production from sevoflurane breakdown: Modeling of exposures under clinical conditions. *Anesth Analg* 2003;96:757-764; with permission.)

has been observed following an exothermic reaction between sevoflurane and the carbon dioxide absorbent (Fatheree and Leighton, 2004). Furthermore, formaldehyde alone as a byproduct of sevoflurane breakdown may cause pulmonary injury.

These dangerous chemical reactions can be avoided by utilizing carbon dioxide absorbents devoid of strong bases (Woehlck, 2004). Nevertheless, the ability of absorbents lacking strong bases to adequately absorb carbon dioxide in all situations is unclear (Higuchi et al., 2001). Water also inhibits these chemical reactions but may evaporate particularly with prolonged flows through the absorbent when the breathing circuit is not connected to a patient. Strong bases are included in absorbents to enhance carbon dioxide absorption.

REFERENCES

Adams RW, Cucchiari RF, Gronert GA, et al. Isoflurane and cerebrospinal fluid pressure in neurosurgical patients. *Anesthesiology* 1981;54: 97–99.

Albrecht RF, Miletich DJ, Madala LR. Normalization of cerebral blood flow during prolonged anesthesia. *Anesthesiology* 1983;58: 26–31.

Artru AA. Anesthetics produce prolonged alterations of CSF dynamics. *Anesthesiology* 1982;57:A356.

Artru AA. Effects of halothane, enflurane, isoflurane and fentanyl on resistance to reabsorption of cerebrospinal fluid. *Anesth Analg* 1984a;63:180.

Artru AA. Isoflurane does not increase the rate of CSF production in the dog. *Anesthesiology* 1984b;60:193–197.

Atlee JL, Bosnjak ZJ. Mechanisms for cardiac dysrhythmias during anesthesia. *Anesthesiology* 1990;72:347–374.

Baden J, Kelley M, Mazze R. Mutagenicity of experimental inhalational anesthetic agents: sevoflurane, synthane, diozychlorane, and dioxyflurane. *Anesthesiology* 1982;56:462–463.

Baden JM, Serra M, Fujinaga M, Mazze RI. Halothane metabolism in cirrhotic rats. *Anesthesiology* 1987;67:660–664.

Bahlman SH, Eger EI, Halsey MJ, et al. The cardiovascular effects of halothane in man during spontaneous ventilation. *Anesthesiology* 1972;36:494–502.

Baum J, Sachs G, Driesch CVD, et al. Carbon monoxide generation in carbon dioxide absorbents. *Anesth Analg* 1995;81:144–146.

Baxter PJ, Garton K, Kaharasch ED. Mechanistic aspects of carbon monoxide formation from volatile anesthetics. *Anesthesiology* 1998;89:929–941.

Baxter PJ, Kharasch ED. Rehydration of desiccated Baralyme prevents carbon monoxide formation from desflurane in an anesthesia machine. *Anesthesiology* 1997;86:1061–1065.

Beck DH, Doepfmer UR, Sinemus C, et al. Effects of sevoflurane and propofol on pulmonary shunt fraction during one-lung ventilation for thoracic surgery. *Br J Anaesth* 2001;86:38–43

Bedforth NM, Girling KJ, Skinner HJ, et al. Effects of desflurane on cerebral regulation. *Br J Anaesth* 2001;87:193–197.

Benumof JL, Bookstein JJ, Saidman LJ, et al. Diminished hepatic arterial flow during halothane administration. *Anesthesiology* 1976;45:545–551.

Berry PD, Sessler DI, Larson MD. Severe carbon monoxide poisoning during desflurane anesthesia. *Anesthesiology* 1999;90: 613–616.

Biehl DR, Yarnell R, Wade JG, et al. The uptake of isoflurane by the fetal lamb in utera: effect on regional blood flow. *Can Anaesth Soc J* 1983;30:581–586.

Bito H, Ikeda K. Closed-circuit anesthesia with sevoflurane in humans: effects of renal and hepatic function and concentrations of breakdown products with soda lime in the circuit. *Anesthesiology* 1994;80:71–76.

Bito H, Ikeda K. Effect of total flow rate on the concentration of degradation products generated by reaction between sevoflurane and soda lime. *Br J Anaesth* 1995;74:667–669.

Boisseau N, Madany M, Staccini P, et al. Comparison of the effects of sevoflurane and propofol on cortical somatosensory evoked potentials. *Br J Anaesth* 2002;88:785–789.

Brown BR. Sibboleths and jigsaw puzzles: the fluoride nephrotoxicity enigma. *Anesthesiology* 1995;82:607–608.

Brunt EM, White H, Marsh JW, et al. Fulminant hepatic failure after repeated exposure to isoflurane anesthesia: a case report. *Hepatology* 1991;13:1017–1021.

Burke D, Henderson DJ. Chirality: A blueprint for the future. *Br J Anaesth* 2002;88:563–576.

Bussard DA, Stoelting RK, Peterson C, et al. Fetal changes in hamsters anesthetized with nitrous oxide and halothane. *Anesthesiology* 1974;41:275–278.

Cahalan MK, Lurz FW, Eger EI, et al. Narcotics decrease heart rate during inhalational anesthesia. *Anesth Analg* 1987;66:166–170.

Cahalan MK. Hemodynamic effects of inhaled anesthetics [review courses]. Cleveland: *International Anesthesia Research Society*, 1996:14–18.

Calverley RK, Smith NT, Jones CW, et al. Ventilatory and cardiovascular effects of enflurane anesthesia during spontaneous ventilation in man. *Anesth Analg* 1978a;57:610–618.

Calverley RK, Smith NT, Prys-Roberts C, et al. Cardiovascular effects of enflurane anesthesia during controlled ventilation in man. *Anesth Analg* 1978b;57:619–628.

Canet J, Sanchis J, Zegri A, et al. Effects of halothane and sevoflurane on ventilation and occlusion pressure. *Anesthesiology* 1994;81:563–571.

Carpenter RL, Eger EI, Johnson BH, et al. The extent of metabolism of inhaled anesthetics in humans. *Anesthesiology* 1986;65: 201–205.

Castro BA, Freedman LA, Craig WL, et al. Explosion within an anesthesia machine: Baralyme®, high fresh gas flows and sevoflurance concentration. *Anesthesiology* 2004;101:537–539.

Chalon J, Ramanathan S, Turndorf H. Exposure to isoflurane affects learning function of murine progeny. *Anesthesiology* 1982;57:A360.

Chase RE, Holaday DA, Fiserova-Bergerova V, et al. The biotransformation of Ethrane in man. *Anesthesiology* 1971;35:262–267.

Cho S, Fujigake T, Uchiyama Y, et al. Effects of sevoflurane with and without nitrous oxide on human cerebral circulation. *Anesthesiology* 1996;85:755–760.

Christ DD, Kenna JG, Kammerer W, et al. Enflurane metabolism produces covalently bound live adducts recognized by antibodies from patients with halothane hepatitis. *Anesthesiology* 1988;69:833–838.

Conzen PF, Fischer S, Detter C, et al. Sevoflurane provides greater protection of the myocardium than propofol in patients undergoing off-pump coronary artery bypass surgery. *Anesthesiology* 2003;99: 826–833.

Conzen PF, Habazettl, Vollmar B, et al. Coronary microcirculation during halothane, enflurane, isoflurane, and adenosine in dogs. *Anesthesiology* 1992;76:261–270.

Conzen PF, Kaharasch ED, Czerner SFA, et al. Low-flow sevoflurane compared with low-flow isoflurane anesthesia in patients with stable renal insufficiency. *Anesthesiology* 2002;97:578–584.

Conzen PF, Nuscheler M, Melotte A, et al. Renal function and serum fluoride concentrations in patients with stable renal insufficiency after anesthesia with sevoflurane or enflurane. *Anesth Analg* 1995;81:569–575.

Cromwell TH, Stevens WC, Eger EI, et al. The cardiovascular effects of compound 469 (Forane) during spontaneous ventilation and CO_2 challenge in man. *Anesthesiology* 1971;35:17–25.

Cronnelly R, Salvatierra O, Feduska NJ. Renal allograft function following halothane, enflurane, or isoflurane anesthesia. *Anesth Analg* 1984;63:202.

DeHert, SG, ten Broecke PW, Mertens E, et al. Sevoflurane but not propofol preserves myocardial function in coronary surgery patients. *Anesthesiology* 2002;97:42–49.

DeHert, Van der Linden PJ, Cromheecke S, et al. Cardioprotective properties of sevoflurane in patients undergoing coronary surgery with cardiopulmonary bypass are related to its modalities of its administration. *Anesthesiology* 2004;101:299–310.

Divatia JV, Vaidya JA, Badwe RA, et al. Omission of nitrous oxide during anesthesia reduces the incidence of postoperative nausea and vomiting: a meta-analysis. *Anesthesiology* 1996;85: 1055–1062.

Drummond JC, Todd MM, Shapiro HM. CO_2 responsiveness of the cerebral circulation during isoflurane anesthesia and N_2O sedation in cats. *Anesthesiology* 1982;57:A333.

Ducart A, Adnet P, Renaud B, et al. Malignant hyperthermia during sevoflurane administration. *Anesth Analg* 1995;80:609–611.

Ebert TJ, Muzi M, Lopatka CW. Neurocirculatory responses to sevoflurane in humans: a comparison to desflurane. *Anesthesiology* 1995;83:88–95.

Ebert TJ, Robinson BJ, Uhrich TD, et al. Recovery from sevoflurane anesthesia: A comparison to isoflurane and propofol anesthesia. *Anesthesiology* 1998;89:1524–1531.

Eger EI, Gong D, Koblin DD, et al. Dose-related biochemical markers on renal injury after sevoflurane versus desflurane anesthesia in volunteers. *Anesth Analg* 1997a;85:1154–1163.

Eger EI, Ionescu P, Laster MJ, et al. Baralyme dehydration increases and soda lime dehydration decreases the concentration of compound A resulting from sevoflurane degradation in a standard anesthetic circuit. *Anesth Analg* 1997b;85:892–898.

Eger EI, Ionescu P, Laster MJ, et al. Quantitative differences in the production and toxicity of $CF_2{=}BrCl$ versus $Ch_2F\text{-}O\text{-}C({=}CF_2)(CF_3)$ (Compound A): the safety of halothane does not indicate the safety of sevoflurane. *Anesth Analg* 1997c;85: 1164–1170.

Eger EI, Koblin DD, Bowland T, et al. Nephrotoxicity of sevoflurane versus desflurane anesthesia in volunteers. *Anesth Analg* 1997d;84: 160–168.

Eger EI, Smuckler EA, Ferrell LD, et al. Is enflurane hepatotoxic? *Anesth Analg* 1986;65:21–30.

Eger EI, Stevens WC, Cromwell TH. The electroencephalogram in man anesthetized with Forane. *Anesthesiology* 1971;35:504–508.

Eger EI. *Desflurane (Suprane): a compendium and reference*. Nutley, NJ: Anaquest, 1993:1–119.

Eger EI. Good news, bad news. *Anesth Analg* 2002;94:239–240.

Eger EI. *Isoflurane (Forane): a compendium and reference*, 2nd ed. Madison, WI: Ohio Medical Products, 1985a:1–110.

Eger EI. *Nitrous oxide*. New York: Elsevier Science, 1985b.

Eisele JH, Milstein JM, Goetzman BW. Pulmonary vascular responses to nitrous oxide in newborn lambs. *Anesth Analg* 1986;65:62–64.

Eisele JH, Smith NT. Cardiovascular effects of 40 percent nitrous oxide in man. *Anesth Analg* 1972;51:956–963.

Elliott RH, Strunin L. Hepatotoxicity of volatile anesthetics. *Br J Anaesth* 1993;70:339–348.

Fang ZX, Eger EI, Laster MJ, et al. Carbon monoxide production from degradation of desflurane, enflurane, isoflurane, halothane, and sevoflurane by soda lime and Baralyme. *Anesth Analg* 1995;80: 1187–1193.

Farrell G, Prendergast D, Murray M. Halothane hepatitis. Detection of a constitutional susceptibility factor. *N Engl J Med* 1985;313: 1310–1314.

Fatheree RS, Leighton BL. Acute respiratory distress syndrome after an exothermic Baralyme®-sevoflurane reaction. *Anesthesiology* 2004; 101;531–533.

Fisher DM. Does nitrous oxide cause vomiting? *Anesth Analg* 1996;83:4–5.

Frankhuizen JL, Vlek CAJ, Burm AGL, et al. Failure to replicate negative effects of trace anesthetics on mental performance. *Br J Anaesth* 1978;50:229–234.

Frink EJ, Ghantous H, Malan TP, et al. Plasma inorganic fluoride with sevoflurane anesthesia: correlation with indices of hepatic and renal function. *Anesth Analg* 1992a;74:231–235.

Frink EJ, Green WB, Brown EA, et al. Compound A concentrations during sevoflurane anesthesia in children. *Anesthesiology* 1996;84: 566–571.

Frink EJ, Malan TP, Brown EA, et al. Plasma inorganic fluoride levels with sevoflurane anesthesia in morbidly obese and nonobese patients. *Anesth Analg* 1993;76:1133–1137.

Frink EJ, Malan TP, Isner RJ, et al. Renal concentrating function with prolonged sevoflurane or enflurane anesthesia in volunteers. *Anesthesiology* 1994;80:1019–1025.

Frink EJ, Morgan S, Coetzee A, et al. The effect of sevoflurane, halothane, enflurane, and isoflurane on hepatic blood flow and oxygenation in chronically instrumented greyhound dogs. *Anesthesiology* 1992b;76:85–92.

Froeba G, Marx T, Pazhur J, et al. Xenon does not trigger malignant hyperthermia in susceptible swine. *Anesthesiology* 1999;91: 1047–1052.

Fukunaga AF, Epstein RM. Sympathetic excitation during nitrous-oxide-halothane anesthesia in the cat. *Anesthesiology* 1973;39:23–36.

Funk W, Gruber M, Wild K, et al. Dry soda lime markedly degrades sevoflurane during simulated inhalation induction. *Br J Anaesth* 1999;82:193–198.

Gallagher JD, Weindling SN, Anderson G, et al. Effects of sevoflurane on QT interval in a patient with congenital long QT syndrome. *Anesthesiology* 1998;89:1569–1573.

Garfield JM, Garfield FB, Sampson J. Effects of nitrous oxide on decision strategy and sustained attention. *Psycopharmacologia* 1975;42:5–10.

Gatecel C, Losser M-R, Didier P. The postoperative effects of halothane versus isoflurane on hepatic artery and portal vein blood flow in humans. *Anesth Analg* 2003;96:740–745.

Ghoneim MM, Block RI. Learning and memory during general anesthesia. An update. *Anesthesiology*1997;87:387–395.

Goff MJ, Arain SR, Ficke DJ, et al. Absence of bronchodilation during desflurane anesthesia. *Anesthesiology* 2000;93:404–408.

Gold MI, Schwam SJ, Goldberg M. Chronic obstructive pulmonary disease and respiratory complications. *Anesth Analg* 1983;62:975–981.

Goldfarb G, Debaene B, Ang ET, et al. Hepatic blood flow in humans during isoflurane N_2O and halothane N_2O anesthesia. *Anesth Analg* 1990;71:349–353.

Gonsowski CT, Laster MJ, Eger EI, et al. Toxicity of compound A in rats: effect of a 3-hour administration. *Anesthesiology* 1994;80:556–565.

Goto T, Nakata Y, Ishiguro Y, et al. Minimum alveolar concentration-awake of xenon alone and in combination with isoflurane or sevoflurane. *Anesthesiology* 2000;93:1188–1193.

Goto T, Nakata Y, Morita S. The minimum alveolar concentration of xenon in the elderly is sex-dependent. *Anesthesiology* 2002;97: 1129–1132.

Goto T, Nakata Y, Morita S. Will xenon be a stranger or a friend? The cost, benefit, and future of xenon anesthesia. *Anesthesiology* 2003;98:1–2.

Gourlay GK, Adams JF, Cousins MJ, et al. Genetic differences in reductive metabolism and hepatotoxicity of halothane in three rat strains. *Anesthesiology* 1981;55:96–103.

Greenstein LR, Hitt BA, Mazze RI. Metabolism in vitro of enflurane, isoflurane, and methoxyflurane. *Anesthesiology* 1975;42:420–424.

Hanouz J-L, Yvon A, Massetti M, et al. Mechanisms of desflurane-induced preconditioning in isolated human right atria in vitro. *Anesthesiology* 2002;97:33–41.

Hartung J. Twenty-four of twenty-seven studies show a greater incidence of emesis associated with nitrous oxide than with alternative anesthetics. *Anesth Analg* 1996;83:114–116.

Hayashi M, Takahashi T, Morimatsu H, et al. Increased carbon monoxide concentration in exhaled air after surgery and anesthesia. *Anesth Analg* 2004;99:444–448.

Hazard Report. Anesthesia carbon dioxide absorber fires. Health Devices 2003;32:436–440.

Henderson JM, Spence DG, Komocar LM, et al. Administration of nitrous oxide to pediatric patients provides analgesia for venous cannulation. *Anesthesiology* 1990;72:269–271.

Higuchi H, Adachi Y Arimura S, et al. The carbon dioxide absorption capacity of Amsorb® is half that of soda lime. *Anesth Analg* 2001b;93:2212–2225

Higuchi H, Satoh T, Arimura S, et al. Serum inorganic fluoride levels in mildly obese patients during and after sevoflurane anesthesia. *Anesth Analg* 1993;77:1018–1021.

Higuchi H, Sumikura H, Sumita S, et al. Renal function in patients with high serum fluoride concentrations after prolonged sevoflurane anesthesia. *Anesthesiology* 1995;83:449–458.

Higuchi H, Wada H, Usua Y, et al. Effects of probenecid on renal function in surgical patients anesthetized with low-flow sevoflurane. *Anesthesiology* 2001a;94:21–31.

Hilgenberg JC, McCammon RL, Stoelting RK. Pulmonary and systemic vascular responses to nitrous oxide in patients with mitral stenosis and pulmonary hypertension. *Anesth Analg* 1980;59:323–326.

Hoenemann CW, Halene-Holtgraeve TB, Booke M, et al. Delayed onset of malignant hyperthermia in desflurane anesthesia. *Anesth Analg* 2003;96:165–167.

Holaday DA, Fiserova-Bergerova V, Latto IP, Zumbiel MA. Resistance of isoflurane to biotransformation in man. *Anesthesiology* 1975;43: 325–332.

Holak E, Mei DA, Dunning MB, et al. Carbon monoxide production from sevoflurane breakdown: Modeling of exposures under clinical conditions. *Anesth Analg* 2003;96:757–764.

Hong K, Trudell JR, O'Neil JR, et al. Biotransformation of nitrous oxide. *Anesthesiology* 1980b;53:354–355.

Hong K, Trudell JR, O'Neil JR, et al. Metabolism of nitrous oxide by human and rat intestinal contents. *Anesthesiology* 1980a;52:16–19.

Horrigan RW, Eger EI, Wilson EI, et al. Epinephrine-induced arrhythmias during enflurane anesthesia in man: a non-linear dose response relationship and dose-dependent protection from lidocaine. *Anesth Analg* 1978;57:547–550.

Ide T, Kochi T, Isono S, Mizuguchi T. Effect of sevoflurane on diaphragmatic contractility in dogs. *Anesth Analg* 1992;74:739–764.

Iohom G, Collins I, Murphy D, et al. Postoperative changes in visual evoked potentials and cognitive function tests following sevoflurane anaesthesia. *Br J Anaesth* 2001;87:855–859.

Johnson BH, Eger EI. Bactericidal effects of anesthetics. *Anesth Analg* 1979;58:136–138.

Johnston RR, Cromwell TH, Eger EI, et al. The toxicity of fluroxene in animals and man. *Anesthesiology* 1973;38:313–319.

Johnston RR, Eger ET, Wilson C. A comparative interaction of epinephrine with enflurane, isoflurane and halothane in man. *Anesth Analg* 1976;55:709–712.

Johnstone RE, Kennell EM, Behar MG, et al. Increased serum bromide concentration after halothane anesthesia in man. *Anesthesiology* 1975;42:598–601.

Kaisti KK, Jaaskelainen SK, Rinne JO, et al. Epileptiform discharges during 2 MAC sevoflurane anesthesia in two healthy volunteers. *Anesthesiology* 1998;91:1952–1955.

Kaisti KK, Lansjo J, Aalto S, et al. Effects of sevoflurane, propofol, and adjunct nitrous oxide on regional cerebral blood flow, oxygen consumption, and blood volume in humans. *Anesthesiology* 2003;99: 603–613.

Kambam JR, Holaday DA. Effect of nitrous oxide on the oxyhemoglobin dissociation curve and PO_2 measurements. *Anesthesiology* 1987;66:208–209.

Karl HW, Swedlow DB, Lee KW, et al. Epinephrine-halothane interactions in children. *Anesthesiology* 1983;58:142–145.

Kehl F, Krolikowski JG, Mravoic B, et al. Is isoflurane-induced preconditioning dose related? *Anesthesiology* 2002;96:675–680.

Kenna JG, Neuberger J, Mieli-Vergani G, et al. Halothane hepatitis in children. *BMJ* 1987;294:1209–1210.

Kevin LE, Katz P, Camara AKS, et al. Anesthetic preconditioning: Effects of latency to ischemic injury in isolated hearts. *Anesthesiology* 2003; 99:385–391.

Kharasch ED, Frink EJ, Artru A, et al. Long-duration low-flow sevoflurane and isoflurane effects on postoperative renal and hepatic function. *Anesth Analg* 2001;93:1511–1520.

Kharasch ED, Hankins DC, Thummel KE. Human kidney methoxyflurane and sevoflurane metabolism: intrarenal fluoride productions as a possible mechanism of methoxyflurane nephrotoxicity. *Anesthesiology* 1995a;82:689–699.

Kharasch ED, Karol MD, Lanni C, et al. Clinical sevoflurane metabolism and disposition. I. Sevoflurane and metabolite pharmacokinetics. *Anesthesiology* 1995b;82:1369–1378.

Kharasch ED. Biotransformation of sevoflurane. *Anesth Analg* 1995;81: S27–38.

Kitaguchi K, Ohsumi H, Juro M, et al. Effects of sevoflurane on cerebral circulation and metabolism in patients with ischemic cerebrovascular disease. *Anesthesiology* 1993;79:704–709.

Kleinsasser A, Kuenszberg E, Loeckinger A, et al. Sevoflurane, but not propofol, significantly prolongs the Q-T interval. *Anesth Analg* 2000;90:25–27.

Klock PA, Czeslick EG, Klafta JM, et al. The effect of sevoflurane and desflurane on upper airway reactivity. *Anesthesiology* 2001;94:963–967.

Knight PR, Bedows E, Nahrwold ML, et al. Alterations in influenza virus pulmonary pathology induced by diethyl ether, halothane, enflurane and pentobarbital in mice. *Anesthesiology* 1983;58:209–215.

Knill RL, Clement JL. Variable effects of anaesthetics on the ventilatory response to hypoxemia in man. *Can Anaesth Soc J* 1982;29: 93–99.

Koblin DD, Eger EI, Johnson BH, et al. Are convulsant gases also anesthetics? *Anesthesiology* 1980;53:S47.

Koblin DD, Eger EI, Johnson BH, et al. I-653 resists degradation in rats. *Anesth Analg* 1988;67:534–538.

Komatsu H, Taie S, Endo S, et al. Electrical seizures during sevoflurane anesthesia in two pediatric patients with epilepsy. *Anesthesiology* 1994;81:1535–1537.

Kong CF, Chew STH, Ip-Yam PC. Intravenous opioids reduce airway irritation during induction of anaesthesia with desflurane in adults. *Anesthesiology* 1999;91:A431.

Kunitz O, Baumert J-H, Hecker K, et al. Xenon does not prolong neuromuscular block of rocuronium. *Anesth Analg* 2004;99:1398–1401.

Kuroda Y, Murakami M, Tsuruta J, et al. Preservation of the ratio of cerebral blood flow/metabolic rate for oxygen during prolonged anesthesia with isoflurane, sevoflurane, and halothane in humans. *Anesthesiology* 1996;84:555–561.

Lam AM, Clement JL, Chung DC, et al. Respiratory effects of nitrous oxide during enflurane anesthesia in humans. *Anesthesiology* 1982; 56:298–303.

Lam AM, Mayberg TS, Eng CC, et al. Nitrous oxide-isoflurane anesthesia causes more cerebral vasodilation than an equipotent dose of isoflurane in humans. *Anesth Analg* 1994;78:462–468.

Lane GA, Nahrwold ML, Tait AR. Anesthetics as teratogens: nitrous oxide is fetotoxic, xenon is not. *Science* 1980;210:899–901.

Lannes M, Desparmet JF, Zifkin BG. Generalized seizures associated with nitrous oxide in an infant. *Anesthesiology* 1997;87:705–708.

Lappas DG, Buckey MJ, Laver MB, et al. Left ventricular performance and pulmonary circulation following addition of nitrous oxide to morphine during coronary artery surgery. *Anesthesiology* 1975;43: 61–69.

Layzer RB, Fishman RA, Schafer JA. Neuropathy following use of nitrous oxide. *Neurology* 1978;28:504–506.

Lederhaas G, Brock-Utne JG, Negrin RS, et al. Is nitrous oxide safe for bone marrow harvest? *Anesth Analg* 1995;80:770–772.

Lester M, Roth P, Eger, EI. Fires from the interaction of anesthetics with desiccated absorbent. *Anesth Analg* 2004;99:769–774.

Litz RJ, Hubler M, Lorenz W, et al. Renal responses to desflurane and isoflurane in patients with renal insufficiency. *Anesthesiology* 2002; 97:1133–1136.

Lockhart SH, Rampil IJ, Yasuda N, et al. Depression of ventilation by desflurane in humans. *Anesthesiology* 1991;74:484–488.

Loft S, Boel J, Kyst A, et al. Increased hepatic microsomal enzyme activity after surgery under halothane or spinal anesthesia. *Anesthesiology* 1985;62:11–16.

Ludwig LM, Patel HH, Gross GJ, et al. Morphine enhances pharmacological preconditioning by isoflurane. *Anesthesiology* 2003;98:705–711.

Lynch C, Vogel S, Sperelakis N. Halothane depression of myocardial slow action potentials. *Anesthesiology* 1981;55:360–368.

Lynch C. Anesthetic preconditioning: Not just for the heart? *Anesthesiology* 1999;91:606–608.

Ma D, Wilhelm S, Maze M, et al. Neuroprotective and neurotoxic properties of the "inert" gas, xenon. *Br J Anaesth* 2002;89:739–746.

Malan TP, DiNardo JA, Isner RJ, et al. Cardiovascular effects of sevoflurane compared with those of isoflurane in volunteers. *Anesthesiology* 1995;83:918–928.

Maria NS, Eckmann DM. Model predictions of gas embolism growth and reabsorption during xenon anesthesia. *Anesthesiology* 2003; 99:638–645.

Martin JL, Keegan MT, Vasdev GMS, et al. Fatal hepatitis associated with isoflurane exposure and CYP2A6 autoantibodies. *Anesthesiology* 2001;95:551–553.

Martin JL, Plevak DJ, Flannery KD, et al. Hepatotoxicity after desflurane anesthesia. *Anesthesiology* 1995;83:1125–1129.

Matta BF, Heath KJ, Tipping K, et al. Direct cerebral vasodilatory effects of sevoflurane and isoflurane. *Anesthesiology* 1999;91:677–680.

Mazze RI, Calverley RK, Smith NT. Inorganic fluoride nephrotoxicity: prolonged enflurane and halothane anesthesia in volunteers. *Anesthesiology* 1977;46:265–271.

Mazze RI, Fujinaga M, Rice SA, et al. Reproductive and teratogenic effects of nitrous oxide, halothane, isoflurane and enflurane in Sprague-Dawley rats. *Anesthesiology* 1986;64:339–344.

Mazze RI, Wilson AI, Rice SA, et al. Effects of isoflurane on reproduction and fetal development in mice. *Anesth Analg* 1984;63:249.

Mazze RI, Woodruff RE, Heerdt ME. Isoniazid-induced enflurane defluorination in humans. *Anesthesiology* 1982;57:5–8.

Mazze RI. Fertility, reproduction, and postnatal survival in mice chronically exposed to isoflurane. *Anesthesiology* 1985;63:663–667.

Metz S, Maze M. Halothane concentration does not alter the threshold for epinephrine-induced arrhythmias in dogs. *Anesthesiology* 1985;62:470–474.

Michenfelder JD, Sundt TM, Fode N, et al. Isoflurane when compared to enflurane and halothane decreases the frequency of cerebral ischemia during carotid endarterectomy. *Anesthesiology* 1987;67: 336–340.

Mielck F, Stephan H, Buhre W, et al. Effects of 1 MAC desflurane on cerebral metabolism, blood flow and carbon dioxide reactivity in humans. *Br J Anaesth* 1998;81:155–160.

Milde LN, Milde JH, Lanier WL, Michenfelder JD. Comparison of the effects of isoflurane and thiopental on neurologic outcome and neuropathology after temporary focal cerebral ischemia in primates. *Anesthesiology* 1988;69:905–913.

Moore MA, Weiskopf RB, Eger EI, et al. Arrhythmogenic doses of epinephrine are similar during desflurane or isoflurane anesthesia in humans. *Anesthesiology* 1993;79:943–947.

Moore MA, Weiskopf RB, Eger EI, et al. Rapid 1% increases of end-tidal desflurane concentration to greater than 5% transiently increase heart rate and blood pressure in humans. *Anesthesiology* 1994;81:94–98.

Moore RA, McNicholas KW, Gallagher JD, et al. Halothane metabolism in acyanotic and cyanotic patients undergoing open heart surgery. *Anesth Analg* 1986;65:1257–1262.

Morio M, Fujii K, Satoh N, et al. Reaction of sevoflurane and its degradation products with soda lime: toxicity of the byproducts. *Anesthesiology* 1992;77:1155–1164.

Moult PJ, Sherlock S. Halothane-related hepatitis. A clinical study of twenty-six cases. *Q J Med* 1975;44:99–114.

Munday IT, Stoddart PA, Jones RM, et al. Serum fluoride concentration and urine osmolality after enflurane and sevoflurane anesthesia in male volunteers. *Anesth Analg* 1995;81:353–359.

Munson ES, Embro WJ. Enflurane, isoflurane and halothane and isolated human uterine muscle. *Anesthesiology* 1977;46:11–14.

Murat I, Lapeyre G, Saint-Maurice C. Isoflurane attenuates baroreflex control of heart rate in human neonates. *Anesthesiology* 1989;70: 395–400.

Muzi M, Ebert TJ, Hope WG, et al. Site(s) mediating sympathetic activation with desflurane. *Anesthesiology* 1996;85:737–747.

Muzi M, Ebert TJ. A comparison of baroreflex sensitivity during isoflurane and desflurane anesthesia in humans. *Anesthesiology* 1995;82:919–925.

Muzzi D, Losasso T, Dietz N, et al. The effect of desflurane and isoflurane on cerebrospinal fluid pressure in humans with supratentorial mass lesions. *Anesthesiology* 1992;76:720–724.

Nagyova B, Dorrington KL, Poulin MJ, et al. Influence of 0.2 minimum alveolar concentration of enflurane on the ventilatory response to sustained hypoxia in humans. *Br J Anaesth* 1997;78: 707–713.

Naito H, Gillis CN. Effects of halothane and nitrous oxide on removal of norepinephrine from the pulmonary circulation. *Anesthesiology* 1973;39:575–580.

Nakata Y, Goto T, Ishiguro Y, et al. Minimum alveolar concentration (MAC) of xenon with sevoflurane in humans. *Anesthesiology* 2001;94:611–614.

Nau C, Strichartz GR. Drug chirality in anesthesia. *Anesthesiology* 2002;97:497–502.

Navarro R, Weiskopf RB, Moore MA, et al. Humans anesthetized with sevoflurane or isoflurane have similar arrhythmic response to epinephrine. *Anesthesiology* 1994;80:545–549.

Nawaf K, Stoelting RK. SGOT values following evidence of reductive biotransformation of halothane in man. *Anesthesiology* 1979;51: 185–186.

Neuman GG, Sidebotham G, Negoianu E, et al. Laparoscopy explosive hazards with nitrous oxide. *Anesthesiology* 1993;78: 875–879.

Newman B, Gelb AW, Lam AM. The effect of isoflurane induced hypotension on cerebral blood flow and cerebral metabolic rate for oxygen in humans. *Anesthesiology* 1986;64:307–310.

Njoku D, Laster MJ, Gong DH, et al. Biotransformation of halothane, enflurane, isoflurane, and desflurane to trifluoroacetylated liver proteins: association between protein acylation and hepatic injury. *Anesth Analg* 1997;84:173–178.

Njoku DB, Greenberg RS, Bourdi M, et al. Autoantibodies associated with volatile anesthetic hepatitis found in the sera of a large cohort of pediatric anesthesiologists. *Anesth Analg* 2002b;94: 243–249.

Njoku DB, Shrestha S, Soloway R, et al. Subcellular localization of trifluoroacetylated liver proteins in association with hepatitis following isoflurane. *Anesthesiology* 2002a;96:757–761.

Nunn JF, Weinbran HK, Royston D, et al. Rate of inactivation of human and rodent hepatic methionine synthase by nitrous oxide. *Anesthesiology* 1988;68:213–216.

Nunn JF. Clinical aspects of the interaction between nitrous oxide and vitamin B_{12}. *Br J Anaesth* 1987;59:3–13.

Ochiai R, Toyoda Y, Nishio I, et al. Possible association of malignant hyperthermia with sevoflurane anesthesia. *Anesth Analg* 1992;74:616–618.

Orhan H, Vermeulen NPE, Sahin G, et al. Characterization of thioether compounds formed from alkaline degradation products of enflurane. *Anesthesiology* 2001;95:165–175.

Ornstein E, Young WL, Fleischer LH, et al. Desflurane and isoflurane have similar effects on cerebral blood flow in patients with intracranial mass lesions. *Anesthesiology* 1993;79:498–502.

Oshima E, Urabe N, Shingu K, et al. Anticonvulsant actions of enflurane on epilepsy models in cats. *Anesthesiology* 1985;63:29–40.

Palahniuk RJ, Shnider SM. Maternal and fetal cardiovascular and acid-base changes during halothane and isoflurane anesthesia in the pregnant ewe. *Anesthesiology* 1974;41:462–472.

Papadimos TJ, Almasri M, Padgett JC, et al. A suspected case of delayed onset malignant hyperthermia with desflurane anesthesia. *Anesth Analg* 2004;98:548–549.

Pathak KS, Ammadio M, Kalamchi A, et al. Effects of halothane, enflurane, and isoflurane on somatosensory evoked potentials during nitrous oxide anesthesia. *Anesthesiology* 1987;66:753–757.

Philbin DM, Lowenstein E. Lack of beta-adrenergic activity of isoflurane in the dog: a comparison of circulatory effects of halothane and isoflurane after propranolol administration. *Br J Anaesth* 1976;48:1165–1170.

Pietak S, Weenig CS, Hickey RF, et al. Anesthetic effects of ventilation in patients with chronic obstructive pulmonary disease. *Anesthesiology* 1975;42:160–166.

Price HL, Skovsted P, Pauca AW, et al. Evidence for a receptor activation produced by halothane in normal man. *Anesthesiology* 1970;32:389–395.

Ravin MB, Olsen MB. Apneic thresholds in anesthetized subjects with chronic obstructive pulmonary disease. *Anesthesiology* 1972;37: 450–454.

Reed SB, Strobel GE. An in vitro model of malignant hyperthermia: differential effects of inhalation anesthetics on caffeine-induced muscle contractures. *Anesthesiology* 1978;48:254–259.

Reich A, Everding AS, Bulla M, et al. Hepatitis after sevoflurane exposure in an infant suffering from primary hyperoxaluria type 1. *Anesth Analg* 2004;99:370–372.

Reilly CS, Wood AJJ, Koshaji RP, et al. The effect of halothane on drug disposition in intrinsic drug metabolizing capacity and hepatic blood flow. *Anesthesiology* 1985;63:70–76.

Reinelt H, Schirmer U, Marx T, et al. Diffusion of xenon and nitrous oxide into the blood. *Anesthesiology* 2001;94:475–7.

Rooke GA, Choi JH, Bishop MJ. The effect of isoflurane, halothane, sevoflurane, and thiopental/nitrous oxide on respiratory system resistance after tracheal intubation. *Anesthesiology* 1997;86: 1294–1299.

Ross S, Foex P. Protective effects of anaesthetics in reversible and irreversible ischaemia-reperfusion injury. *Br J Anaesth* 1999;82: 622–632.

Rossaint R, Reyle-Hahn M, Esch JS, et al. Multicenter randomized comparison of the efficacy and safety of xenon and isoflurane in patients undergoing elective surgery. *Anesthesiology* 2003;98: 6–13.

Russell GB, Snider MT, Richard RB, et al. Hyperbaric nitrous oxide as a sole anesthetic agent in humans. *Anesth Analg* 1990;70: 289–295.

Sachder K, Cohen EN, Simmou VF. Genotoxic and mutagenic assays of halothane metabolites in *Bacillus subtilis* and *Salmonella typbimurium*. *Anesthesiology* 1980;53:31–39.

Sarton E, van der Wal M, Nieuwenhuijs D, et al. Sevoflurane-induced reduction of hypoxic drive is sex-independent. *Anesthesiology* 1999;90:1288–1293.

Sawyer DC, Eger EI, Bahlman SH, et al. Concentration dependence of hepatic halothane metabolism. *Anesthesiology* 1971;34: 230–235.

Schmeling WT, Warltier DC, McDonald DJ, et al. Prolongation of the QT interval by enflurane, isoflurane, and halothane in humans. *Anesth Analg* 1991;72:137–144.

Schulte-Sasse U, Hesse W, Tarnow J. Pulmonary vascular responses to nitrous oxide in patients with normal and high pulmonary vascular resistance. *Anesthesiology* 1982;57:9–13.

Sharpe MD, Cuillerier DJ, Lee JK, et al. Sevoflurane has no effect on sinoatrial node function or on normal atrioventricular and accessory pathway conduction in Wolff-Parkinson-White syndrome during alfentanil/midazolam anesthesia. *Anesthesiology* 1999;90: 60–65.

Shingu K, Eger EI, Johnson BH, et al. Effect of oxygen concentration, hyperthermia, and choice of vendor on anesthetic induced hepatic injury rats. *Anesth Analg* 1983;62:146–150.

Sigurdsson J, Hreidarson AB, Thjodleifsson B. Enflurane hepatitis: a report of a case with a previous history of halothane hepatitis. *Acta Anaesthesiol Scand* 1985;29:495–496.

Smith I, Nathanson M, White PF. Sevoflurane—a long awaited volatile anesthetic. *Br J Anaesth* 1996;76:435–445.

Smith NT, Calverley RK, Prys-Roberts C, et al. Impact of nitrous oxide on the circulation during enflurane anesthesia in man. *Anesthesiology* 1978;48:345–349.

Smith RA, Winter PM, Smith M, et al. Convulsion in mice after anesthesia. *Anesthesiology* 1979;50:501–504.

Stevens WC, Cromwell TH, Halsey MJ, et al. The cardiovascular effects of a new inhalation anesthetic, Forane, in human volunteers at constant arterial carbon dioxide tension. *Anesthesiology* 1971;35:8–16.

Stevenson GW, Hall SC, Rudnick S, et al. The effect of anesthetic agents on the human immune response. *Anesthesiology* 1990;72:542–552.

Stoelting RK, Blitt CD, Cohen PJ, et al. Hepatic dysfunction after isoflurane anesthesia. *Anesth Analg* 1987;66:147–154.

Stoelting RK, Gibbs PS. Hemodynamic effects of morphine and morphine-nitrous oxide in valvular heart disease and coronary artery disease. *Anesthesiology* 1973;38:45–52.

Stoelting RK. Plasma lidocaine concentrations following subcutaneous or submucosal epinephrine-lidocaine injection. *Anesth Analg* 1978;57:724–726.

Strube PJ, Hulands GH, Halsey MJ. Serum fluoride levels in morbidly obese patients: enflurane compared with isoflurane anaesthesia. *Anaesthesia* 1987;42:685–689.

Sutton TS, Koblin DD, Gruenke LD, et al. Fluoride metabolites after prolonged exposure of volunteers and patients to desflurane. *Anesth Analg* 1991;73:180–185.

Tanaka K, Ludwig LM, Kersten JR, et al. Mechanisms of cardioprotection by volatile anesthetics. *Anesthesiology* 2004;100:707–721.

Tiainen P, Lindgren L, Rosenberg PH. Changes in hepatocellular integrity during and after desflurane or isoflurane anaesthesia in patients undergoing breast surgery. *Br J Anaesth* 1998;80:87–89.

Tinker JH, Sharbrough FW, Michenfelder JD. Anterior shift of the dominant EEG rhythm during anesthesia in the JAVA monkey: correlation with anesthetic potency. *Anesthesiology* 1977;46: 252–259.

Todd MM, Drummond JC. A comparison of the cerebrovascular and metabolic effects of halothane and isoflurane in the cat. *Anesthesiology* 1984;60:276–282.

Trudell JR. Metabolism of nitrous oxide. In: Eger EI, ed. *Nitrous oxide*. New York: Elsevier Science, 1985.

Tusiewicz K, Bryan AC, Froese AB. Contributions of chaining rib cage-diaphragm interactions to the ventilatory depression of halothane anesthesia. *Anesthesiology* 1977;47:327–337.

Ueda W, Hirakawa M, Mae O. Appraisal of epinephrine administration to patients under halothane anesthesia for closure of cleft palate. *Anesthesiology* 1983;58:574–576.

Versichelen LFM, Bouche M-P LA, Rolly G, et al. Only carbon dioxide absorbents free of both *NaOH* and *KOH* do not generate compound A during in vitro closed-system sevoflurane: Evaluation of five absorbents. *Anesthesiology* 2001;95:750–755.

Vitez TS, Miller RD, Eger EI, et al. Comparison in vitro of isoflurane and halothane potentiation of d-tubocurarine and succinylcholine neuromuscular blockades. *Anesthesiology* 1974;41: 53–56.

Volta CA, Alvisi V, Petrini S, et al. The effect of volatile anesthetics on respiratory system resistance in patients with chronic obstructive pulmonary disease. *Anesth Analg* 2005;100:348–353.

Warltier DC, Kersten JR, Pagel PS, et al. Anesthetic preconditioning: Serendipity and science. *Anesthesiology* 2002;97:1–3.

Warner DS, Boarini DJ, Kassell NE. Cerebrovascular adaptation to prolonged halothane anesthesia is not related to cerebrovascular fluid pH. *Anesthesiology* 1985;63:243–248.

Warner DS. Isoflurane neuroprotection. A passing fantasy, again? *Anesthesiology* 2000;92:1126–1128.

Warner LO, Beach TJ, Garvin JP, et al. Halothane and children: the first quarter century. *Anesth Analg* 1984;63:838–840.

Warren TM, Datta S, Ostheimer GW, et al. Comparison of the maternal and neonatal effects of halothane, enflurane and isoflurane for cesarean delivery. *Anesth Analg* 1983;62:516–520.

Weiskopf RB, Eger EI, Ionescu P, et al. Desflurane does not produce hepatic or renal injury in human volunteers. *Anesth Analg* 1992;74: 570–574.

Weiskopf RB, Eger EI, Noorani M, et al. Fentanyl, esmolol, and clonidine blunt the transient cardiovascular stimulation induced by desflurane in humans. *Anesthesiology* 1994a;81:1350–1355.

Weiskopf RB, Eger EI. Comparing the costs of inhaled anesthetics. *Anesthesiology* 1993;79:1413–1418.

Weiskopf RB, Moore MA, Eger EI, et al. Rapid increase in desflurane concentration is associated with greater transient cardiovascular stimulation than with rapid increases in isoflurane concentration in humans. *Anesthesiology* 1994b;80:1035–1045.

Whelan E, Wood AJJ, Koshakji R, et al. Halothane inhibition of propranolol metabolism is stereoselective. *Anesthesiology* 1989;71: 561–564.

White AE, Stevens WC, Eger EI, et al. Enflurane and methoxyflurane metabolism at anesthetic and subanesthetic concentrations. *Anesth Analg* 1979;58:221–224.

Williamson DC, Munson ES. Correlation of peripheral venous and arterial blood gas values during general anesthesia. *Anesth Analg* 1982;61:950–952.

Wissing H, Kuhn K, Warnken U, et al. Carbon monoxide production from desflurane, enflurane, halothane, and sevoflurane with dry soda lime. *Anesthesiology* 2001;95:1205–1212.

Wodey E, Pladys P, Copin C, et al. Comparative hemodynamic depression of sevoflurane versus halothane in infants: an echocardiographic study. *Anesthesiology* 1997;87:795–800.

Woehlck HJ, Mei D, Duning MB, et al. Mathematical modeling of carbon monoxide exposures from anesthetics from anesthetic breakdown. Effect of subject size, hematocrit, fraction of inspired oxygen, and quantity of carbon monoxide. *Anesthesiology* 2001;94: 457–460.

Woehlck HJ. Sleeping with uncertainty: Anesthetics and desiccated absorbent. *Anesthesiology* 2004;101;276–278.

Wohlfeil ER, Woehlck HJ, Gottschall, et al. Increased carboxyhemoglobin from hemolysis mistaken as intraoperative desflurane breakdown. *Anesth Analg* 2001;92:1609–1610.

Wolfson B, Hetrick WD, Lake CL, et al. Anesthetic indices: further data. *Anesthesiology* 1978;48:187–190.

Wright R, Eade OE, Chilsom M, et al. Controlled prospective study of the effect of liver function on multiple exposure to halothane. *Lancet* 1975;1:817–820.

Wu J, Previte JP, Adler E, et al. Spontaneous ignition, explosion, and fire with sevoflurane and barium hydroxide lime. *Anesthesiology* 2004;101:534–537.

Yamakage M, Yamada S, Chen X, et al. Carbon dioxide absorbents containing potassium hydroxide produce much larger concentrations of compound A from sevoflurane in clinical practice. *Anesth Analg* 2000;91:220–224.

Yasuda N, Lockhart SH, Eger EI, et al. Kinetics of desflurane, isoflurane, and halothane in humans. *Anesthesiology* 1991;74:489–498.

Yonker-Sell AE, Muzi M, Hope WG, et al. Alfentanil modifies the neurocirculatory responses to desflurane. *Anesth Analg* 1996;82: 162–166.

Yvon A, Hanouz J-C, Haelewyn B, et al. Mechanisms of sevoflurane-induced myocardial preconditioning in isolated human right atria in vitro. *Anesthesiology* 2003;99:27–33.

Zaugg M, Lucchinetti E, Spahn DR, et al. Volatile anesthetics mimic cardiac preconditioning by priming the activation of mitochondrial K_{ATP} channels via multiple signaling pathways. *Anesthesiology* 2002;97:4–14.

Opioid Agonists and Antagonists

3

The word *opium* is derived from the Greek word for juice; the juice of the poppy is the source of 20 distinct alkaloids of opium. *Opiate* is the term used for drugs derived from opium. Morphine was isolated in 1803, followed by codeine in 1832 and papaverine in 1848. Morphine can be synthesized, but it is more easily derived from opium. The term *narcotic* is derived from the Greek word for stupor and traditionally has been used to refer to potent morphine-like analgesics with the potential to produce physical dependence. The development of synthetic drugs with morphine-like properties has led to the use of the term *opioid* to refer to all exogenous substances, natural and synthetic, that bind specifically to any of several subpopulations of opioid receptors and produce at least some agonist (morphine-like) effects. Opioids are unique in producing analgesia without loss of touch, proprioception, or consciousness. A convenient classification of opioids includes opioid agonists, opioid agonist-antagonists, and opioid antagonists (Table 3-1).

STRUCTURE ACTIVITY RELATIONSHIPS

The alkaloids of opium can be divided into two distinct chemical classes: phenanthrenes and benzylisoquinolines. The principal phenanthrene alkaloids present in opium are morphine, codeine, and thebaine (Fig. 3-1). The principal benzylisoquinoline alkaloids present in opium, which lack opioid activity, are papaverine and noscapine (Fig. 3-2).

The three rings of the phenanthrene nucleus are composed of 14 carbon atoms (see Fig. 3-1). The fourth piperidine ring includes a tertiary amine nitrogen and is present in most opioid agonists. At pH 7.4, the tertiary amine nitrogen is highly ionized, making the molecule water soluble. A close relationship exists between stereochemical structure and potency of opioids, with levorotatory isomers being the most active.

Semisynthetic Opioids

Semisynthetic opioids result from relatively simple modification of the morphine molecule (see Fig. 3-1). For example, substitution of a methyl group for the hydroxyl group on carbon 3 results in methylmorphine (codeine). Substitution of acetyl groups on carbons 3 and 6 results in diacetylmorphine (heroin). Thebaine has insignificant analgesic activity but serves as the precursor for etorphine (analgesic potency >1,000 times morphine).

Synthetic Opioids

Synthetic opioids contain the phenanthrene nucleus of morphine but are manufactured by synthesis rather than chemical modification of morphine. Morphine derivatives (levorphanol), methadone derivatives, benzomorphan derivatives (pentazocine), and phenylpiperidine derivatives (meperidine, fentanyl) are examples of groups of synthetic opioids. There are similarities in the molecular weights (236 to 326) and pKs of phenylpiperidine derivatives and amide local anesthetics.

Fentanyl, sufentanil, alfentanil, and remifentanil are semisynthetic opioids that are widely used to supplement general anesthesia or as primary anesthetic drugs in very high doses during cardiac surgery. There are important pharmacokinetic and pharmacodynamic differences between these opioids (Burkle et al., 1996; Egan et al., 1993; Shafer and Varvel, 1991). The major pharmacodynamic differences between these drugs are potency and rate of equilibration between the plasma and the site of drug effect (biophase).

MECHANISM OF ACTION

Opioids act as agonists at stereospecific opioid receptors at presynaptic and postsynaptic sites in the central nervous

TABLE 3-1.
CLASSIFICATION OF OPIOID AGONISTS AND ANTAGONISTS

Opioids
Morphine
Morphine-6-glucuronide
Meperidine
Sufentanil
Fentanyl
Alfentanil
Remifentanil
Codeine
Hydromorphone
Oxymorphone
Oxycodone
Hydrocodone
Propoxyphene
Methadone
Tramadol
Heroin
Opioid Agonists-Antagonists
Pentazocine
Butorphanol
Nalbuphine
Buprenorphine
Nalorphine
Bremazocine
Dezocine
Meptazinol
Opioid Antagonists
Naloxone
Naltrexone
Nalmefene

system (CNS) (principally the brainstem and spinal cord) and outside the CNS in peripheral tissues (Pleuvry, 1993; Stein, 1993; Stein, 1995). Inflammatory hyperalgesic conditions appear to be especially amenable to peripheral opioid antinociceptive actions. The most likely mechanism of these peripheral actions appears to be activation of opioid receptors located on primary afferent neurons. These same opioid receptors normally are activated by three endogenous peptide opioid receptor ligands known as enkephalins, endorphins, and dynorphins. Opioids mimic the actions of these endogenous ligands by binding to opioid receptors, resulting in activation of pain-modulating (antinociceptive) systems.

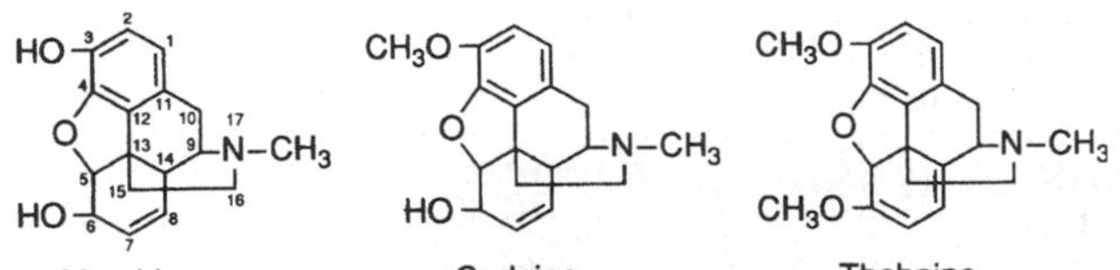

Figure 3-1. Phenanthrene alkaloids.

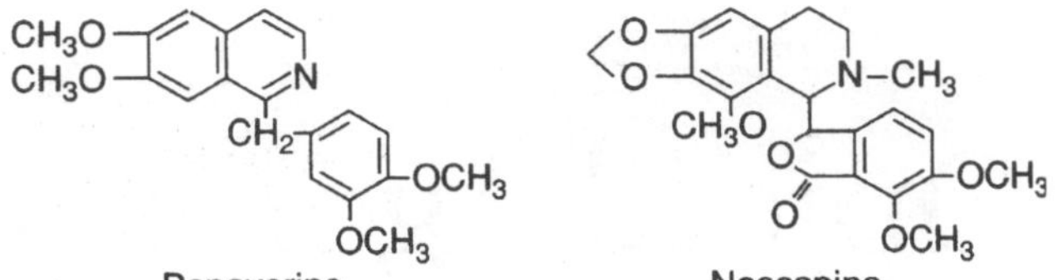

Figure 3-2. Benzylisoquinoline alkaloids.

Existence of the opioid in the ionized state appears to be necessary for strong binding at the anionic opioid receptor site. Only levorotatory forms of the opioid exhibit agonist activity. Indeed, the naturally occurring form of morphine is the levorotatory isomer. The affinity of most opioid agonists for receptors correlates well with their analgesic potency.

The principal effect of opioid receptor activation is a decrease in neurotransmission (Atcheson and Lambert, 1994; de Leon-Casasola and Lema, 1996). This decrease in neurotransmission occurs largely by presynaptic inhibition of neurotransmitter (acetylcholine, dopamine, norepinephrine, substance P) release, although postsynaptic inhibition of evoked activity may also occur. The intracellular biochemical events initiated by occupation of opioid receptors with an opioid agonist are characterized by increased potassium conductance (leading to hyperpolarization), calcium channel inactivation, or both, which produce an immediate decrease in neurotransmitter release. Opioid receptor-mediated inhibition of adenylate cyclase is not responsible for an immediate effect but may have a delayed effect, possibly via a reduction in cyclic adenosine monophosphate (cAMP)–responsive neuropeptide genes and reduction in neuropeptide messenger RNA concentrations. Opioid receptors exist on the peripheral ends of primary afferent neurons and their activation may either directly decrease neurotransmission or inhibit the release of excitatory neurotransmitters, such as substance P. In this regard, intraarticular morphine (3 mg) produces prolonged analgesia after arthroscopic knee surgery (Heine et al., 1994). Depression of cholinergic transmission in the CNS as a result of opioid-induced inhibition of acetylcholine release from nerve endings may play a prominent role in the analgesic and other side effects of opioid agonists. Opioids do not alter responsiveness of afferent nerve endings to noxious stimulation, nor do they impair conduction of nerve impulses along peripheral nerves. It is assumed that increasing opioid receptor occupancy parallels opioid effects.

OPIOID RECEPTORS

Opioid receptors are classified as mu, delta, and kappa receptors (MOR, DOR, and KOR respectively) (Atcheson and Lambert, 1994; Lambert 1998) (Table 3-2). These opi-

TABLE 3-2.
CLASSIFICATION OF OPIOID RECEPTORS

	Mu_1#	Mu_2#	Kappa	Delta
Effect	Analgesia (supraspinal, spinal)	Analgesia (spinal)	Analgesia (supraspinal, spinal)	Analgesia (supraspinal, spinal)
	Euphoria	Depression of ventilation	Dysphoria, sedation	Depression of ventilation
	Low abuse potential	Physical dependence	Low abuse potential	Physical dependence
	Miosis		Miosis	
		Constipation (marked)		Constipation (minimal)
	Bradycardia			
	Hypothermia			
	Urinary retention		Diuresis	Urinary retention
Agonists	Endorphins*	Endorphins*	Dynorphins	Enkephalins
	Morphine	Morphine		
	Synthetic opioids	Synthetic opioids		
Antagonists	Naloxone	Naloxone	Naloxone	Naloxone
	Naltrexone	Naltrexone	Naltrexone	Naltrexone
	Nalmefene	Nalmefene	Nalmefene	Nalmefene

#The existence of specific mu_1 and mu_2 receptors is not supported based on cloning studies of mu receptors.
*Mu receptors seem to be a universal site of action for all endogenous opioid receptors.
Source: Adapted from Atcheson R, Lambert DG. Update on opioid receptors. *Br J Anaesth* 1994;73:132–134.

oid receptors belong to a superfamily of guanine (G) protein–coupled receptors that constitute 80% of all known receptors and includes muscarinic, adrenergic, gamma-aminobutyric acid, and somatostatin receptors. The opioid receptors have been cloned and their amino acid sequence defined (Chen et al., 1993). A single mu-receptor gene has been identified and six distinct mu receptors have been identified. It is likely that distinct morphine-6-glucuronide receptors exist as variants of the mu-receptor gene. Cloning of opioid receptors introduces the possibility for the development of highly selective and subtype-specific receptor agonists. An ideal opioid agonist would have a high specificity for receptors, producing desirable responses (analgesia) and little or no specificity for receptors associated with side effects (hypoventilation, nausea, physical dependence).

All three opioid receptor classes couple to G proteins and subsequently inhibit adenyl cyclase, decrease the conductance of voltage-gated calcium channels, or open inward flowing potassium channels. Any of these effects ultimately results in decreased neuronal activity. Opioid receptors also modulate the phosphoinositide-signaling cascade and phospholipase C. The prevention of calcium ion inflow results in suppression of neurotransmitter release (substance P) in many neuronal systems. Hyperpolarization results from actions at potassium channels thus preventing excitation or propagation of action potentions. Opioid receptors may regulate the functions of other ion channels including excitatory postsynaptic currents evoked by *N*-methyl-D-aspartate (NMDA) receptors.

Mu or morphine-preferring receptors are principally responsible for supraspinal and spinal analgesia. Activation of a subpopulation of mu receptors (mu_1) is speculated to produce analgesia, whereas mu_2 receptors are responsible for hypoventilation, bradycardia, and physical dependence. Nevertheless, cloning of the mu receptors does not support the existence of separate mu_1 and mu_2 receptor subtypes (Lambert, 1998). It is possible that such subtypes result from posttranslation modification of a common protein. Whether beta-endorphins or even morphine itself is the endogenous ligand for mu receptors is speculative (Kosterlitz, 1987). Endomorphins are peptides with high affinity and selectivity for mu receptors that are present in the brain. Exogenous mu receptor agonists include morphine, meperidine, fentanyl, sufentanil, alfentanil, and remifentanil. Naloxone is a specific mu receptor antagonist, attaching to but not activating the receptor.

Agonists, including the endogenous ligand dynorphin, act at kappa receptors, resulting in inhibition of neurotransmitter release via type N calcium channels. Respiratory depression characteristic of mu receptor activation is less with kappa receptor activation although dysphoria and diuresis may accompany activation of these calcium channel–linked receptors. In addition, high-intensity painful stimulation may be resistant to the analgesic effect of kappa receptors. Opioid agonist-antagonists often act principally on kappa receptors. Delta receptors respond to the endogenous ligands known as *enkephalins,* and these opioid receptors may serve to modulate the activity of the mu receptors.

Endogenous Pain Suppression System

The obvious role of opioid receptors and endorphins is to function as an endogenous pain suppression system (see Chapter 43). Opioid receptors are located in areas of the brain (periaqueductal gray matter of the brainstem, amygdala, corpus striatum, and hypothalamus) and spinal cord (substantia gelatinosa) that are involved with pain perception, integration of pain impulses, and responses to pain. It is speculated that endorphins inhibit the release of excitatory neurotransmitters from terminals of nerves carrying nociceptive impulses. As a result, neurons are hyperpolarized, which suppresses spontaneous discharges and evoked responses. Analgesia induced by electrical stimulation of specific sites in the brain or mechanical stimulation of peripheral areas (acupuncture) most likely reflects release of endorphins (Pomeranz and Chiu, 1976). Even the analgesic response to a placebo may also involve the release of endorphins. After about 60 years of age, patients experience a decrease in sensitivity to pain and an enhanced analgesic response to opioids (Bellville et al., 1971).

NEURAXIAL OPIOIDS

Placement of opioids in the epidural or subarachnoid space to manage acute or chronic pain is based on the knowledge that opioid receptors (principally mu receptors) are present in the substantia gelatinosa of the spinal cord (Cousins and Mather, 1984). Analgesia produced by neuraxial opioids, in contrast to intravenous (IV) administration of opioids or regional anesthesia with local anesthetics, is not associated with sympathetic nervous system denervation, skeletal muscle weakness, or loss of proprioception. Analgesia is dose related (epidural dose is 5 to 10 times the subarachnoid dose) and specific for visceral rather than somatic pain. Neuraxial morphine may decrease the minimum alveolar concentration (MAC) for volatile anesthetics, although not all investigators have demonstrated this effect (Drasner et al., 1988; Licina et al., 1991; Schwieger et al., 1992).

Analgesia that follows epidural placement of opioids reflects diffusion of the drug across the dura to gain access to mu opioid receptors on the spinal cord as well as systemic absorption to produce effects similar to those that would follow IV administration of the opioid. For example, the mechanism of postoperative analgesia produced by epidural administration of highly lipophilic opioids (fentanyl, sufentanil) is primarily a reflection of systemic absorption (de Leon-Casasola and Lema, 1996). In fact, it has been proposed that epidural administration of lipophilic opioids may offer no clinical advantages over IV administration (de Leon-Casasola and Lema, 1996). Poorly lipid-soluble opioids such as morphine result in a slower onset of analgesia but a longer duration of action than lipid-soluble opioids when administered via the neuraxial route.

Pharmacokinetics

Opioids placed in the epidural space may undergo uptake into epidural fat, systemic absorption, or diffusion across the dura into the cerebrospinal fluid (CSF) (Chaney, 1995). Epidural administration of opioids produces considerable CSF concentrations of drug. Penetration of the dura is considerably influenced by lipid solubility, but molecular weight may also be important. Fentanyl and sufentanil are, respectively, approximately 800 and 1,600 times as lipid soluble as morphine. After epidural administration, CSF concentrations of fentanyl peak in about 20 minutes and sufentanil in about 6 minutes. In contrast, CSF concentrations of morphine, after epidural administration, peak in 1 to 4 hours. Furthermore, only about 3% of the dose of morphine administered epidurally crosses the dura to enter the CSF (Ionescu et al., 1989).

The epidural space contains an extensive venous plexus, and vascular absorption of opioids from the epidural space is extensive. After epidural administration, fentanyl blood concentrations peak in 5 to 10 minutes, whereas blood concentrations of the more lipid-soluble sufentanil peak even sooner (Ionescu et al., 1991). In contrast, blood concentrations of morphine after epidural administration peak after 10 to 15 minutes. Epidural administration of morphine, fentanyl, and sufentanil produces opioid blood concentrations that are similar to those produced by an intramuscular (IM) injection of an equivalent dose (Chaney, 1995). The addition of epinephrine to the solution placed into the epidural space decreases systemic absorption of the opioid but does not influence the diffusion of morphine across the dura into the CSF. The addition of epinephrine to intrathecal morphine solutions enhances postoperative analgesia compared with intrathecal morphine alone (Goyagi and Nishikawa, 1995). Vascular absorption after intrathecal administration of opioids is clinically insignificant.

Cephalad movement of opioids in the CSF principally depends on lipid solubility. For example, lipid-soluble opioids such as fentanyl and sufentanil are limited in their cephalad migration by uptake into the spinal cord, whereas less lipid-soluble morphine remains in the CSF for transfer to more cephalad locations. After lumbar intrathecal morphine administration, appreciable cervical CSF concentrations occur 1 to 5 hours after injection, whereas cervical CSF concentrations of highly lipid-soluble opioids are minimal after their epidural administration. The underlying cause of ascension of morphine is bulk flow of CSF. CSF ascends in a cephalad direction from the lumbar region, reaching the cisterna magna in 1 to 2 hours and the fourth and lateral ventricles by 3 to 6 hours (Chaney, 1995). Coughing or straining, but not body position, can affect movement of CSF. The elimination half-time of morphine in CSF is similar to that in plasma (Sjöström et al., 1987).

Side Effects

Side effects of neuraxial opioids are caused by the presence of drug in either the CSF or systemic circulation (Table 3-3) (Chaney, 1995). In general, most side effects are dose

TABLE 3-3.
SIDE EFFECTS OF NEURAXIAL (EPIDURAL AND SPINAL) OPIOIDS

Pruritus
Nausea and vomiting
Urinary retention
Depression of ventilation
Sedation
Central nervous system excitation
Viral reactivation
Neonatal morbidity
Sexual dysfunction
Ocular dysfunction
Gastrointestinal dysfunction
Thermoregulatory dysfunction
Water retention

dependent. Some side effects are mediated via interaction with specific opioid receptors, whereas others are not due to this interaction. Side effects are less common in patients chronically exposed to opioids. The four classic side effects of neuraxial opioids are pruritus, nausea and vomiting, urinary retention, and depression of ventilation.

Pruritus

Pruritus is the most common side effect with neuraxial opioids. It may be generalized but is more likely to be localized to the face, neck, or upper thorax. The incidence of pruritus varies widely and is often elicited only after direct questioning. Severe pruritus is rare, occurring in about 1% of patients. Pruritus is more likely to occur in obstetric patients, perhaps due to the interaction of estrogen with opioid receptors. The incidence may or may not be dose related. Pruritus usually occurs within a few hours of injection and may precede the onset of analgesia.

Although opioids may liberate the release of histamine from mast cells, this does not appear to be the mechanism for pruritus. Instead, pruritus induced by neuraxial opioids is likely due to cephalad migration of the opioid in CSF and subsequent interaction with opioid receptors in the trigeminal nucleus. An opioid antagonist such as naloxone is effective in relieving opioid-induced pruritus. Paradoxically, antihistamines may be an effective treatment for pruritus, likely secondary to their sedative effect.

Urinary Retention

The incidence of urinary retention varies widely and is most common in young males. Urinary retention with neuraxial opioids is more common than after IV or IM administration of equivalent doses of the opioid. The incidence of this side effect is not dose dependent or related to systemic absorption of the opioid. Urinary retention is most likely due to interaction of the opioid with opioid receptors located in the sacral spinal cord. This interaction promotes inhibition of sacral parasympathetic nervous system outflow, which causes detrusor muscle relaxation and an increase in maximum bladder capacity, leading to urinary retention. In humans, epidural morphine causes marked detrusor muscle relaxation within 15 minutes of injection that persists for up to 16 hours; it is readily reversed with naloxone (Rawal et al., 1986).

Depression of Ventilation

The most serious side effect of neuraxial opioids is depression of ventilation, which may occur within minutes of administration or may be delayed for hours. The incidence of ventilatory depression requiring intervention after conventional doses of neuraxial opioids is about 1%, which is the same as that after conventional doses of IV or IM opioids (Chaney, 1995).

Early depression of ventilation occurs within 2 hours of neuraxial injection of the opioid. Most reports of clinically important depression of ventilation involve epidural administration of fentanyl or sufentanil. This depression of ventilation most likely results from systemic absorption of the lipid-soluble opioid, although cephalad migration of opioid in the CSF may also be responsible. Clinically significant early depression of ventilation after intrathecal injection of morphine is unlikely.

Delayed depression of ventilation occurs more than 2 hours after neuraxial opioid administration and reflects cephalad migration of the opioid in the CSF and subsequent interaction with opioid receptors located in the ventral medulla. All reports of clinically significant delayed depression of ventilation involve morphine (Chaney, 1995). Delayed depression of ventilation characteristically occurs 6 to 12 hours after epidural or intrathecal administration of morphine. Clinically important depression of ventilation has not been described more than 24 hours after the epidural or intrathecal injection of morphine.

Factors that increase the risk of delayed depression of ventilation, especially concomitant use of any IV opioid or sedative, must be considered in determining the dose of neuraxial opioid (Table 3-4) (Chaney, 1995). Coughing may affect the movement of CSF and increase the likelihood of depression of ventilation. Obstetric patients appear to be at less risk for ventilatory depression, perhaps

TABLE 3-4.
FACTORS THAT INCREASE THE RISK OF DEPRESSION OF VENTILATION

High opioid dose
Low lipid solubility of opioids
Concomitant administration of parenteral opioids or other sedatives
Lack of opioid tolerance
Advanced age
Patient position (?)
Increased intrathoracic pressure

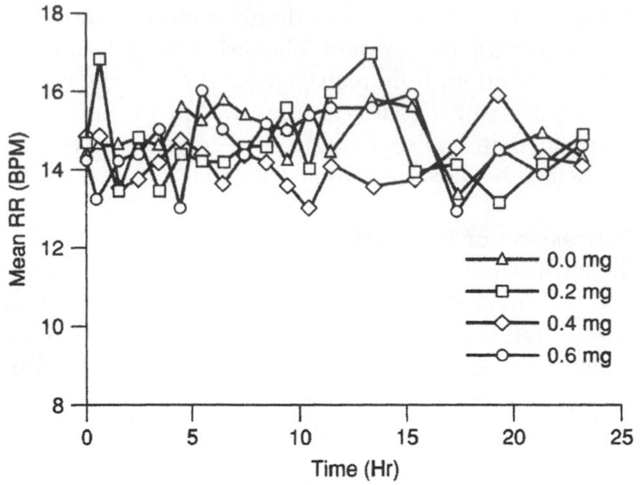

Figure 3-3. Mean respiratory rate (RR) versus times before (time 0) and after three different doses of intrathecal morphine. (From Bailey PL, Rhondeau S, Schafer PG, et al. Dose-response pharmacology of intrathecal morphine in human volunteers. *Anesthesiology* 1993;79:49–59; with permission.)

because of the increased stimulation to ventilation provided by progesterone.

Detection of depression of ventilation induced by neuraxial opioids may be difficult. Arterial hypoxemia and hypercarbia may develop despite a normal breathing rate (Figs. 3-3 and 3-4) (Bailey et al., 1993). Pulse oximetry reliably detects opioid-induced arterial hypoxemia, and supplemental oxygen (2 liters/minute) is an effective treatment (Bailey et al., 1993). The most reliable clinical sign of depression of ventilation appears to be a depressed level of consciousness, possibly caused by hypercarbia (Chaney, 1995). Prophylactic infusions of naloxone are of variable efficacy in protecting against depression of ventilation (Morgan, 1989; Rawal et al., 1986). Naloxone (0.25 μg/kg/hour IV) is effective in attenuating the side effects (nausea and vomiting, pruritus) associated with morphine-induced analgesia delivered by a patient-controlled IV delivery system (Gan et al., 1997).

Sedation

Sedation after administration of neuraxial opioids appears to be dose related and occurs with all opioids but is most commonly associated with the use of sufentanil. When sedation occurs with neuraxial opioids, depression of ventilation must be considered. Mental status changes other than sedation may also occur with neuraxial opioids. Naloxone-reversible paranoid psychoses, catatonia, and hallucinations have been described (Chaney, 1995).

Central Nervous System Excitation

Tonic skeletal muscle rigidity resembling seizure activity is a well-known side effect of large IV doses of opioids, but this response is rarely observed after neuraxial administration. Myoclonic activity has been observed after neuraxial opioids, and, in one report, progressed to a grand mal seizure (Rozan et al., 1995). Although large doses of opioids reliably produce seizures in animals, clinically relevant doses of IV or neuraxial opioids are unlikely to be associated with generalized cortical seizure activity in humans (Chaney, 1995). Cephalad migration of the opioid in CSF and subsequent interaction with nonopioid receptors in the brainstem or basal ganglia is the most likely explanation for opioid-induced CNS excitation. In this regard, opioids may block glycine or gamma-aminobutyric acid–mediated inhibition.

Viral Reactivation

A link exists between the use of epidural morphine in obstetric patients and reactivation of herpes simplex labialis virus. Reactivation of the herpes virus occurs 2 to 5 days after epidural administration of the opioid (Crone et al., 1990). Manifestation of symptoms of herpes labialis (cold sores) characteristically occurs in the same sensory innervation as the primary infection, which are usually facial areas innervated by the trigeminal nerve. The underlying mechanism causing herpes virus reactivation likely involves cephalad migration of opioid in CSF and subsequent interaction with the trigeminal nucleus.

Neonatal Morbidity

Systemic absorption after epidural administration of an opioid results in predictable blood levels of the drug in the neonate immediately after birth. Clinically important depression of ventilation has been observed in the newborns of mothers receiving epidural opioids (Chaney, 1995). The progress of labor has been both inhibited and enhanced by intrathecal morphine. After administration of epidural fentanyl or sufentanil to parturients, the concentration of opioid in breast milk is negligible.

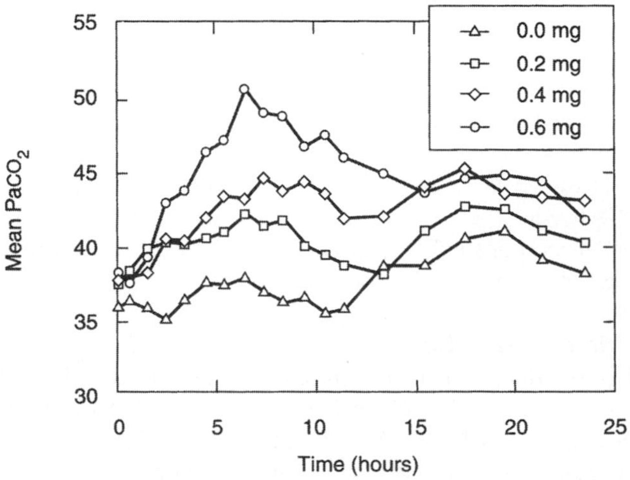

Figure 3-4. Mean arterial carbon dioxide partial pressure (mm Hg) versus times before (time 0) and after three different doses of intrathecal morphine. (From Bailey PL, Rhondeau S, Schafer PG, et al. Dose-response pharmacology of intrathecal morphine in human volunteers. *Anesthesiology* 1993;79:49–59; with permission.)

Miscellaneous Side Effects

Epidural morphine has been associated with sustained erection and inability to ejaculate in male volunteers. Naloxone-reversible miosis, nystagmus, and vertigo may occur after neuraxial opioids, most commonly morphine. Neuraxial opioids may delay gastric emptying, most likely reflecting an interaction of the opioid with a spinal cord opioid receptor (Kelly et al., 1997). Neuraxial opioids, by inhibiting shivering, may cause decreased body temperature. Oliguria and water retention leading to peripheral edema have been reported after neuraxial opioid administration. Water retention is likely caused by release of vasopressin, stimulated by cephalad migration of the opioid in the CSF. Neuraxial opioids have been implicated as possible causes of spinal cord damage, especially following accidental use of opioids containing toxic preservatives (Chaney, 1995). Clinical manifestations in these patients include sensory and motor neurologic dysfunction, myoclonic spasms, paresis, and paralysis. On the other hand, neuraxial opioids have been administered chronically without adverse sequelae.

OPIOID AGONISTS

Opioid agonists include but are not limited to morphine, meperidine, fentanyl, sufentanil, alfentanil, and remifentanil (see Table 3-1) (Cherny, 1996). These are the opioids most likely to be used with inhaled anesthetics during general anesthesia. Large doses of morphine, fentanyl, and sufentanil have been used as the sole anesthetic in critically ill patients. The most notable feature of the clinical use of opioids is the extraordinary variation in dose requirements for pain management (Auburn et al., 2002). This interindividual variation emphasizes that usual doses of opioids may produce inadequate or excessive opioid effects. Opioid rotation may be useful when dose escalation is not effective in treating pain.

Morphine

Morphine is the prototype opioid agonist to which all other opioids are compared. In humans, morphine produces analgesia, euphoria, sedation, and a diminished ability to concentrate. Other sensations include nausea, a feeling of body warmth, heaviness of the extremities, dryness of the mouth, and pruritus, especially in the cutaneous areas around the nose. The cause of pain persists, but even low doses of morphine increase the threshold to pain and modify the perception of noxious stimulation such that it is no longer experienced as pain. Continuous, dull pain is relieved by morphine more effectively than is sharp, intermittent pain. In contrast to nonopioid analgesics, morphine is effective against pain arising from the viscera as well as from skeletal muscles, joints, and integumental structures. Analgesia is most prominent when morphine is administered before the painful stimulus occurs (Woolf and Wall, 1986). This is a pertinent consideration in administering an opioid to patients before the acute surgical stimulus. In the absence of pain, however, morphine may produce dysphoria rather than euphoria.

Pharmacokinetics

Morphine is well absorbed after IM administration, with onset of effect in 15 to 30 minutes and a peak effect in 45 to 90 minutes. The duration of action is about 4 hours. Morphine can be administered orally for treatment of chronic pain recognizing that absorption from the gastrointestinal tract may be limited. Morphine is usually administered IV in the perioperative period, thus eliminating the unpredictable influence of drug absorption. The peak effect (equilibration time between the blood and brain) after IV administration of morphine is delayed compared with opioids such as fentanyl and alfentanil, requiring about 15 to 30 minutes (Table 3-5). Morphine, 5 mg in 4.5 ml of saline and inhaled as an aerosol from a nebulizer, may act on afferent nerve pathways in the airways to

TABLE 3-5.
PHARMACOKINETICS OF OPIOID AGONISTS

	pK	Percent Nonionized (pH 7.4)	Protein Binding (%)	Clearance (ml/min)	Volume of Distribution (liters)	Partition Coefficient	Elimination Half-Time (hrs)	Context Sensitive Half-Time: 4-Hour Infusion (mins)	Effect-Site (Blood/Brain) Equilibration Time (mins)
Morphine	7.9	23	35	1,050	224	1	1.7–3.3		
Meperidine	8.5	7	70	1,020	305	32	3–5		
Fentanyl	8.4	8.5	84	1,530	335	955	3.1–6.6	260	6.8
Sufentanil	8.0	20	93	900	123	1,727	2.2–4.6	30	6.2
Alfentanil	6.5	89	92	238	27	129	1.4–1.5	60	1.4
Remifentanil	7.3	58	66–93	4,000	30		0.17–0.33	4	1.1

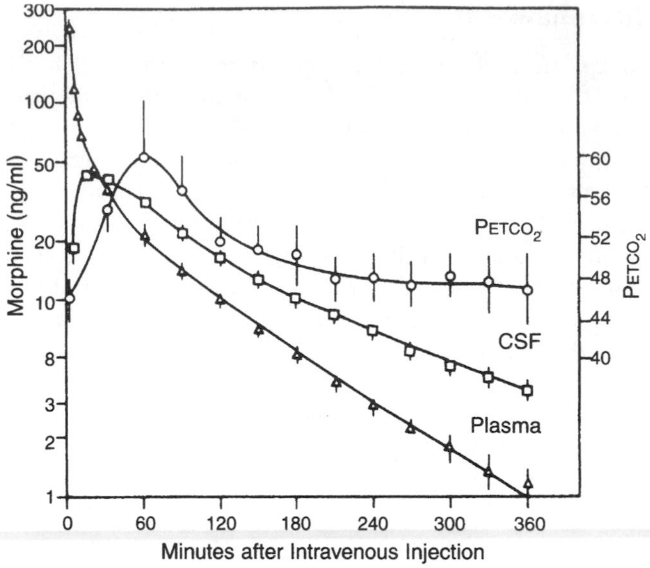

Figure 3-5. Cerebrospinal fluid (CSF) concentrations following intravenous administration of morphine decay more slowly than plasma concentrations. The end-tidal CO_2 concentration ($PETCO_2$) remains increased despite a decreasing plasma concentration of morphine. (Mean ± SE.) (From Murphy MR, Hug CC. Pharmacokinetics of intravenous morphine in patients anesthetized with enflurane-nitrous oxide. *Anesthesiology* 1981;54:187–192; with permission.)

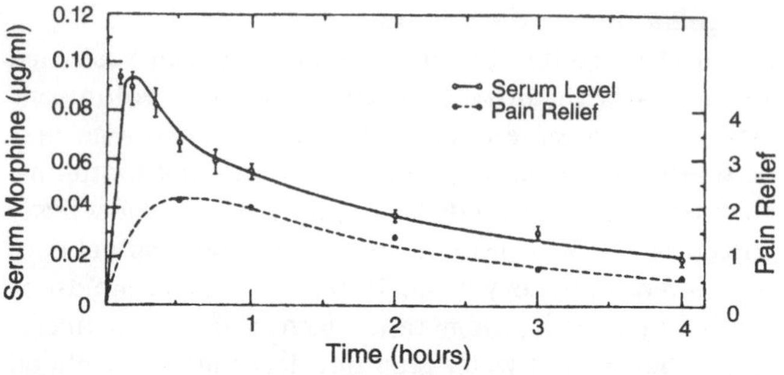

Figure 3-6. Moderate analgesia probably requires maintenance of plasma (serum) concentrations of morphine of at least 0.05 µg/mL. (Mean ± SE.) (From Berkowitz BA, Ngai SH, Yang JC, et al. The disposition of morphine in surgical patients. *Clin Pharmacol Ther* 1975;17:629–635; with permission.)

relieve dyspnea as associated with lung cancer and associated pleural effusion (Tooms and McKenzie, 1993). Profound depression of ventilation may follow aerosol administration of morphine (Lang and Jedeikin, 1998). The onset and duration of the analgesic effects of morphine are similar after IV administration or inhalation via a pulmonary drug delivery system that produces a fine monodisperse aerosol (Dershwitz et al., 2000; Thipphawong et al., 2003).

Plasma morphine concentrations after rapid IV injections do not correlate closely with the opioid's pharmacologic activity. Presumably, this discrepancy reflects a delay in penetration of morphine across the blood-brain barrier. CSF concentrations of morphine peak 15 to 30 minutes after IV injection and decay more slowly than plasma concentrations (Fig. 3-5) (Murphy and Hug, 1981). As a result, the analgesic and ventilatory depressant effects of morphine may not be evident during the initial high plasma concentrations after IV administration of the opioid. Likewise, these same drug effects persist despite decreasing plasma concentrations of morphine. Moderate analgesia probably requires maintenance of plasma morphine concentrations of at least 0.05 µg/mL (Fig. 3-6) (Berkowitz et al., 1975). Patient-controlled demand delivery systems usually provide acceptable postoperative analgesia, with total doses of morphine ranging from 1.3 to 2.7 mg/hour (White, 1985).

Only a small amount of administered morphine gains access to the CNS. For example, it is estimated that <0.1% of morphine that is administered IV has entered the CNS at the time of peak plasma concentrations. Reasons for poor penetration of morphine into the CNS include (a) relatively poor lipid solubility, (b) high degree of ionization at physiologic pH, (c) protein binding, and (d) rapid conjugation with glucuronic acid. Alkalinization of the blood, as produced by hyperventilation of the patient's lungs, will increase the nonionized fraction of morphine and thus enhance its passage into the CNS. Nevertheless, respiratory acidosis, which decreases the nonionized fraction of morphine, results in higher plasma and brain concentrations of morphine than are present during normocarbia (Fig. 3-7) (Finck et al., 1977). This suggests that carbon dioxide-induced increases in cerebral blood flow and enhanced delivery of morphine to the brain are more important than the fraction of drug that exists in either the ionized or nonionized fraction. In contrast to the CNS, morphine accumulates rapidly in the kidneys, liver, and skeletal muscles. Morphine, unlike fentanyl, does not undergo significant first-pass uptake into the lungs (Roerig et al., 1987).

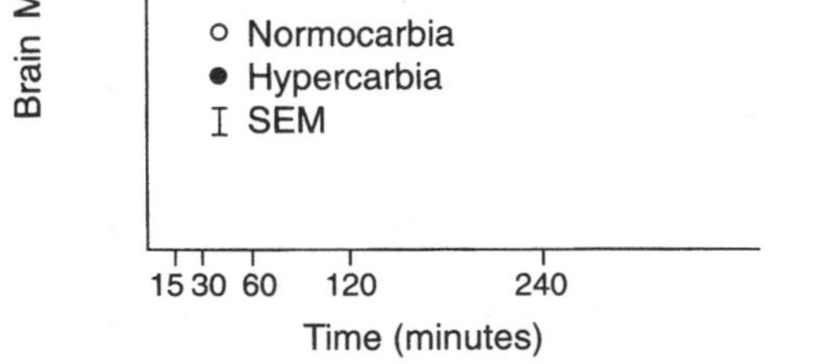

Figure 3-7. Hypercarbia, which decreases the nonionized fraction of morphine, results in a higher brain concentration and longer elimination half-time ($t1/2_\beta$) than occurs in the presence of normocarbia. (*P <.05.) (From Finck AD, Ngai SH, Berkowitz BA. Antagonism of general anesthesia by naloxone in the rat. *Anesthesiology* 1977;46:241–245; with permission.)

Metabolism

The principal pathway of metabolism of morphine is conjugation with glucuronic acid in hepatic and extrahepatic sites, especially the kidneys. About 75% to 85% of a dose of morphine appears as morphine-3-glucuronide, and 5% to 10% as morphine-6-glucuronide (a ratio of 9:1). Morphine-3-glucuronide is detectable in the plasma within 1 minute after IV injection, and its concentration exceeds that of unchanged drug by almost tenfold within 90 minutes (Fig. 3-8) (Murphy and Hug, 1981). An estimated 5% of morphine is demethylated to normorphine, and a small amount of codeine may also be formed. Metabolites of morphine are eliminated principally in the urine, with only 7% to 10% undergoing biliary excretion. Morphine-3-glucuronide is detectable in the urine for up to 72 hours after the administration of morphine. A small fraction (1% to 2%) of injected morphine is recovered unchanged in the urine.

Morphine-3-glucuronide is pharmacologically inactive, whereas morphine-6-glucuronide produces analgesia and depression of ventilation via its agonist actions at mu receptors (Vaughn and Connor, 2003). In fact, the ventilatory response to carbon dioxide is impacted similarly by morphine and morphine-6-glucuronide (Fig. 3-9) (Romberg et al., 2003).

Renal metabolism makes a significant contribution to the total metabolism of morphine, which offers a possible explanation for the absence of any decrease in systemic clearance of morphine in patients with hepatic cirrhosis or during the anhepatic phase of orthotopic liver transplantation (Sear, 1991). In fact, increased rates of renal metabolism of morphine may be possible when liver metabolism is impaired.

Elimination of morphine glucuronides may be impaired in patients with renal failure, causing an accumulation of metabolites and unexpected ventilatory depressant effects of small doses of opioids (Fig. 3-10) (Chauvin et al., 1987b). Indeed, prolonged depression of ventilation (<7 days) has been observed in patients in renal failure after administration of morphine (Don et al., 1975). Formation of glucuronide conjugates may be impaired by monoamine oxidase inhibitors, which is consistent with exaggerated effects of morphine when administered to patients being treated with these drugs.

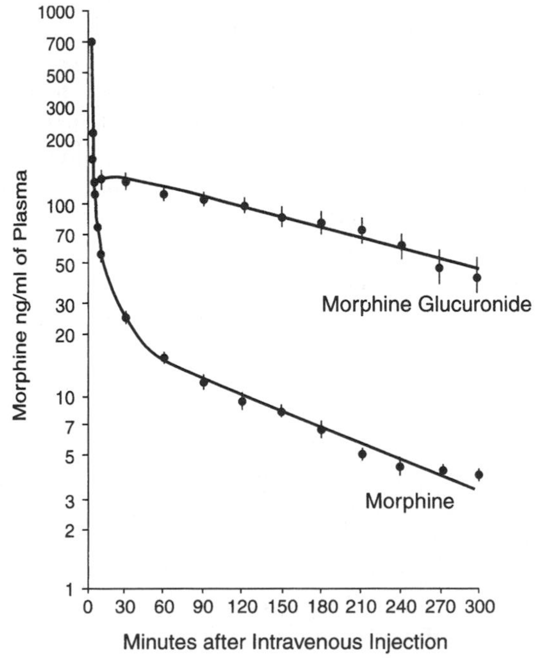

Figure 3-8. Morphine glucuronide is detectable in the plasma within 1 minute after intravenous injection, and its concentration exceeds that of unchanged morphine by almost tenfold within 90 minutes. (Mean ± SE.) (From Murphy MR, Hug CC. Pharmacokinetics of intravenous morphine in patients anesthetized with enflurane-nitrous oxide. *Anesthesiology* 1981;54:187–192; with permission.)

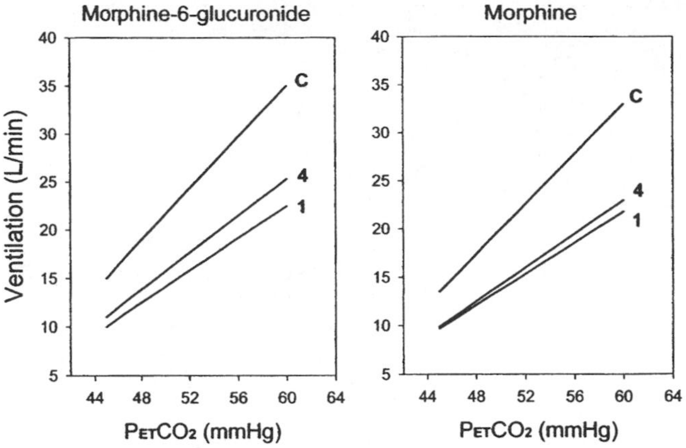

Figure 3-9. Influence of 0.2 mg/kg morphine-6-glucuronide IV and 0.13 mg/kg morphine IV on the ventilatory response to carbon dioxide. The effects of both opioids were similar over the 4 hour period of study. $P_{ET}CO_2$ = end-tidal partial pressure of carbon dioxide. (From Romberg R, Olofsen E, Satron E, et al. Pharmacodynamic effect of morphine-6-glucuronide versus morphine on hypoxic and hypercapnic breathing in healthy volunteers. *Anesthesiology* 2003;99:788–798; with permission.)

Elimination Half-Time

After IV administration of morphine, the elimination of morphine-3-glucuronide is somewhat longer than for morphine (see Table 3-5 and Fig. 3-8) (Murphy and Hug, 1981). The decrease in the plasma concentration of morphine after initial distribution of the drug is principally due to metabolism, because only a small amount of unchanged opioid is excreted in the urine. Plasma morphine concentrations are higher in the elderly than in young adults (Fig. 3-11) (Berkowitz et al., 1975). In the first 4 days of life, the clearance of morphine is decreased and its elimination half-time is prolonged compared with that found in older infants (Lynn and Slattery, 1987). This is consistent with the clinical observation that neonates are more sensitive than older children to the ventilatory depressant effects of morphine.

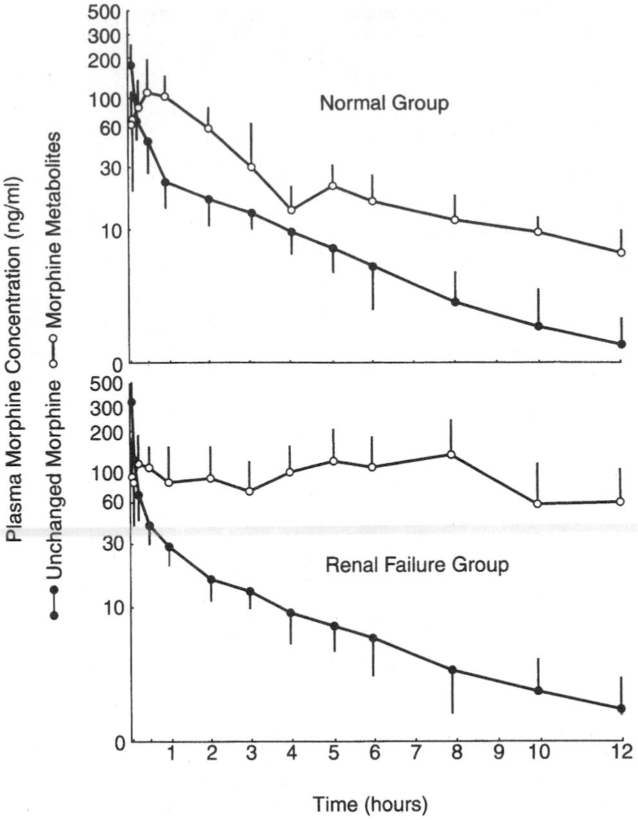

Figure 3-10. Plasma concentrations of unchanged morphine (*closed circles*) and morphine metabolites (*open circles*) in normal and renal failure patients. (From Chauvin M, Sandouk P, Scherrman JM, et al. Morphine pharmacokinetics in renal failure. *Anesthesiology* 1987;66:327–331; with permission.)

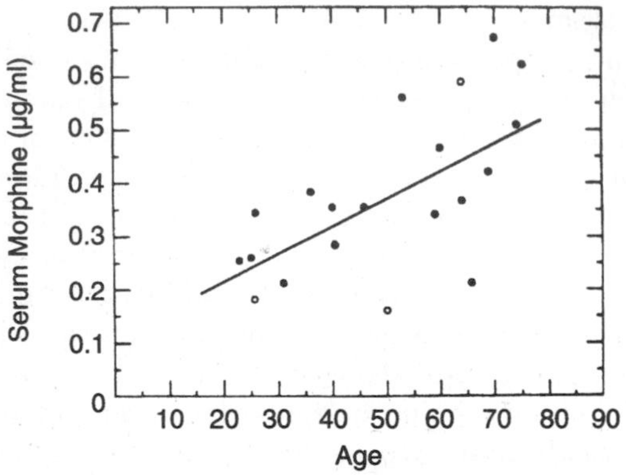

Figure 3-11. The plasma (serum) concentration of morphine increases progressively with advancing age. (From Berkowitz BA, Ngai SH, Yang JC, et al. The disposition of morphine in surgical patients. *Clin Pharmacol Ther* 1975;17:629–635; with permission.)

Patients with renal failure exhibit higher plasma and CSF concentrations of morphine and morphine metabolites than do normal patients, reflecting a smaller volume of distribution (Vd) (Hanna et al., 1993). Possible accumulation of morphine-6-glucuronide suggests the need for caution when administering morphine to patients with renal dysfunction. Anesthesia alone does not alter the elimination half-time of morphine. Concentrations of morphine in colostrums of parturients receiving patient controlled analgesia with morphine are small and it is unlikely that significant amounts of drug will be transferred to the breast-fed neonate (Baka et al., 2002).

Gender

Gender may affect opioid analgesia but the direction and magnitude of these differences depend on many interacting variables including the opioid used (Kest et al., 2000). Morphine exhibits greater analgesic potency and slower speed of offset in women than men (Sarton et al., 2000). This observation is consistent with higher postoperative opioid consumption in men compared with women. Likewise, morphine decreases the slope of the ventilatory response to carbon dioxide in women whereas in men there was no significant effect (Dahan et al., 1998). Morphine had no effect on the apneic threshold in women but caused an increase in men. Hypoxic sensitivity was decreased by morphine in women but not men.

Side Effects

Side effects described for morphine are also characteristic of other opioid agonists, although the incidence and magnitude may vary.

Cardiovascular System

The administration of morphine, even in large doses (1 mg/kg IV), to supine and normovolemic patients is unlikely to cause direct myocardial depression or hypotension. The same patients changing from a supine to a standing position, however, may manifest orthostatic hypotension and syncope, presumably reflecting morphine-induced impairment of compensatory sympathetic nervous system responses. For example, morphine decreases sympathetic nervous system tone to peripheral veins, resulting in venous pooling and subsequent decreases in venous return, cardiac output, and blood pressure (Lowenstein et al., 1972).

Morphine can also evoke decreases in systemic blood pressure due to drug-induced bradycardia or histamine release. Morphine-induced bradycardia results from increased activity over the vagal nerves, which probably reflects stimulation of the vagal nuclei in the medulla. Morphine may also exert a direct depressant effect on the sinoatrial node and acts to slow conduction of cardiac impulses through the atrioventricular node. These actions, may, in part, explain decreased vulnerability to ventricular fibrillation in the presence of morphine. Administration of opioids (morphine) in the preoperative medication or before the induction of anesthesia (fentanyl) tends to slow heart rate during exposure to volatile anesthetics with or without surgical stimulation (Cahalan et al., 1987).

Opioid-induced histamine release and associated hypotension are variable in both incidence and degree. The magnitude of morphine-induced histamine release and subsequent decrease in systemic blood pressure can be minimized by (a) limiting the rate of morphine infusion to 5 mg/minute IV, (b) maintaining the patient in a supine to slightly head-down position, and (c) optimizing intravascular fluid volume. Conversely, administration of morphine, 1 mg/kg IV, over a 10-minute period produces substantial increases in the plasma concentrations of histamine that are paralleled by significant decreases in systemic blood pressure and systemic vascular resistance (Figs. 3-12 and 3-13) (Rosow et al., 1982). It is important to recognize, however, that not all patients respond to this rate of morphine infusion with the release of histamine, emphasizing the individual variability associated with the administration of this drug (see Fig. 3-12) (Rosow et al., 1982). In contrast to morphine, the infusion of fentanyl, 50 μg/kg IV over a 10-minute period, does not evoke release of histamine in any patient (see Fig. 3-12) (Rosow et al., 1982). Sufentanil, like fentanyl, does not evoke the release of histamine.

Pretreatment of patients with H_1 and H_2 receptor antagonists does not alter release of histamine evoked by morphine but does prevent changes in systemic blood pressure and systemic vascular resistance (Philbin et al., 1981).

Morphine does not sensitize the heart to catecholamines or otherwise predispose to cardiac dysrhythmias as long as hypercarbia or arterial hypoxemia does not result from ventilatory depressant effects of the opioid. Tachycardia and hypertension that occur during anesthesia with morphine are not pharmacologic effects of the opioid but rather are responses to painful surgical stimulation that are not suppressed by morphine. Both the sympathetic nervous system and the renin-angiotensin mechanism contribute to these cardiovascular responses. Large doses of morphine or other opioid agonists may decrease the likelihood that tachycardia and hypertension will occur in response to painful stimulation, but once this response has occurred, administration of additional opioid is unlikely to be effective. During anesthesia, opioid agonists are commonly administered with inhaled anesthetics to ensure complete amnesia for the painful surgical stimulus. The combination of an opioid agonist such as morphine or fentanyl with nitrous oxide results in cardiovascular depression (decreased cardiac output and systemic blood pressure plus increased cardiac filling pressures), which does not occur when either drug is administered alone (Stoelting and Gibbs, 1973). Likewise, decreases in systemic vascular resistance and systemic blood pressure may accompany the combination of an opioid and a benzodiazepine, whereas these effects do not accompany the

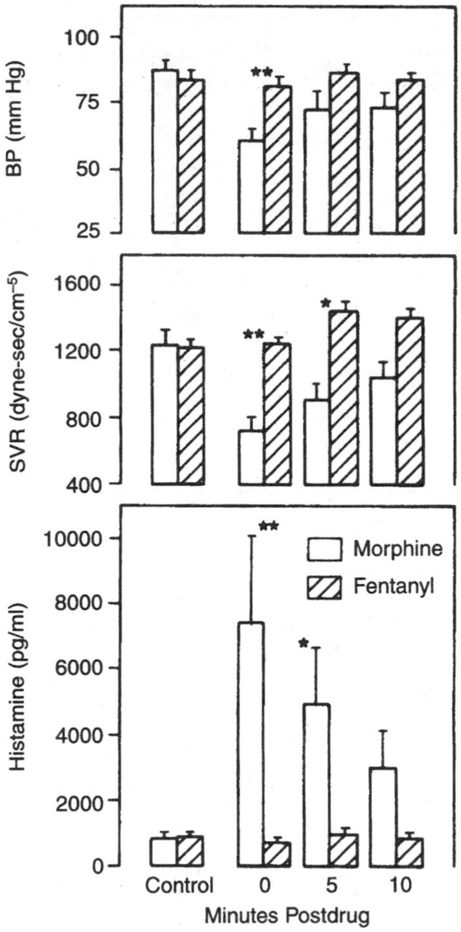

Figure 3-13. Morphine-induced decreases in systemic blood pressure (BP) and systemic vascular resistance (SVR) are accompanied by increases in the plasma concentration of histamine. Similar changes do not accompany the intravenous administration of fentanyl. (*$P < .05$; **$P < .005$; mean ± SE.) (From Rosow CE, Moss J, Philbin DM, et al. Histamine release during morphine and fentanyl anesthesia. *Anesthesiology* 1982;56:93–96; with permission.)

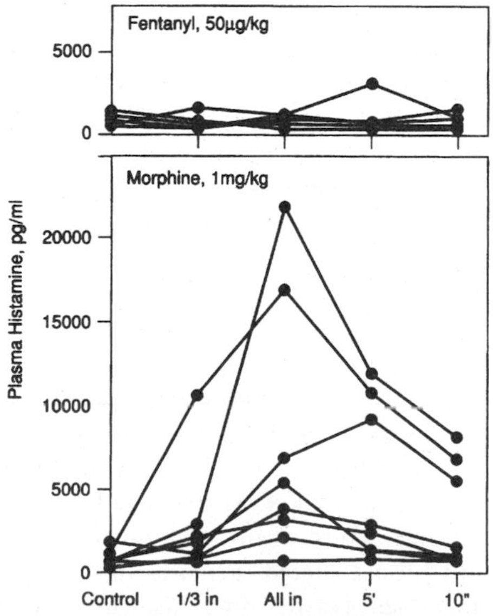

Figure 3-12. Intravenous administration of morphine, but not fentanyl, is associated with an unpredictable increase in the plasma concentration of histamine. (From Rosow EC, Moss J, Philbin DM, et al. Histamine release during morphine and fentanyl anesthesia. *Anesthesiology* 1982:93–96; with permission.)

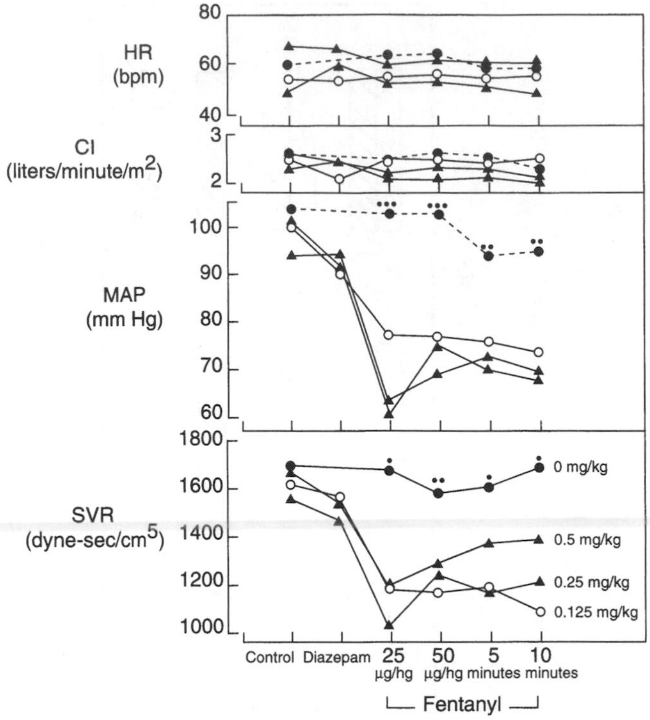

Figure 3-14. Administration of fentanyl (50 µg/kg IV at 400 µg/minute) after injection of diazepam (0.125 to 0.50 mg/kg IV) is associated with significant decreases in mean arterial pressure (MAP) and systemic vascular resistance (SVR), whereas heart rate (HR) and cardiac index (CI) do not change. Administration of fentanyl in the absence of prior injection of diazepam (0 mg/kg) is devoid of circulatory effects. (From Tomicheck RC, Rosow CE, Philbin DM, et al. Diazepam-fentanyl interaction: hemodynamic and hormonal effects in coronary artery surgery. *Anesth Analg* 1983;62: 881–884; with permission.)

administration of either drug alone (Fig. 3-14) (Tomicheck et al., 1983).

Ventilation

All opioid agonists produce dose-dependent and gender-specific depression of ventilation, primarily through an agonist effect at mu_2 receptors leading to a direct depressant effect on brainstem ventilation centers (Atcheson and Lambert, 1995) (see the section on Gender and Chapter 49). Because analgesic and ventilatory effects of opioids occur by similar mechanisms it is assumed that equianalgesic doses of all opioids will produce some degree of ventilatory depression and reversal of ventilatory depression with an opioid antagonist always involves some reversal of analgesia. Opioid-induced depression of ventilation is characterized by decreased responsiveness of these ventilation centers to carbon dioxide as reflected by an increase in the resting $Paco_2$ and displacement of the carbon dioxide response curve to the right. Opioid agonists also interfere with pontine and medullary ventilatory centers that regulate the rhythm of breathing, leading to prolonged pauses between breaths and periodic breathing. It is possible that opioid agonists diminish sensitivity to carbon dioxide by decreasing the release of acetylcholine from neurons in the area of the medullary ventilatory center in response to hypercarbia. In this regard, physostigmine, which increases CNS levels of acetylcholine, may antagonize depression of ventilation but not analgesia produced by morphine (see Chapter 9).

Depression of ventilation produced by opioid agonists is rapid and persists for several hours, as demonstrated by decreased ventilatory responses to carbon dioxide. High doses of opioids may result in apnea, but the patient remains conscious and able to initiate a breath if asked to do so. Death from an opioid overdose is almost invariably attributable to depression of ventilation.

Clinically, depression of ventilation produced by opioid agonists manifests as a decreased frequency of breathing that is often accompanied by a compensatory increase in tidal volume. The incompleteness of this compensatory increase in tidal volume is evidenced by predictable increases in the $Paco_2$. Many factors influence the magnitude and duration of depression of ventilation produced by opioid agonists. For example, advanced age and the occurrence of natural sleep increases the ventilatory depressant effects of opioids. Conversely, pain from surgical stimulation counteracts depression of ventilation produced by opioids. Likewise, the analgesic effect of opioids slows breathing that has been rapid and shallow due to pain.

Opioids produce dose-dependent depression of ciliary activity in the airways. Increases in airway resistance after administration of an opioid are probably due to a direct effect on bronchial smooth muscle and an indirect action due to release of histamine.

Cough Suppression

Opioids depress cough by effects on the medullary cough centers that are distinct from the effects of opioids on ventilation. The greatest cough suppression occurs with opioids that have bulky substitutions at the number 3 carbon position (codeine). Cough suppression is produced by dextrotatory isomers of opioids (dextromethorphan) that do not produce analgesia.

Nervous System

Opioids in the absence of hypoventilation decrease cerebral blood flow and possibly intracranial pressure (ICP). These drugs must be used with caution in patients with head injury because of their (a) associated effects on wakefulness, (b) production of miosis, and (c) depression of ventilation with associated increases in ICP if the $Paco_2$ becomes increased. Furthermore, head injury may impair the integrity of the blood-brain barrier, with resultant increased sensitivity to opioids.

The effect of morphine on the electroencephalogram (EEG) resembles changes associated with sleep. For example, there is replacement of rapid alpha waves by slower delta waves. Recording of the EEG fails to reveal any evidence of seizure activity after administration of large doses of opioids (see the section on Fentanyl). Opioids do not alter the responses to neuromuscular blocking drugs. Skeletal muscle rigidity, especially of the thoracic and abdominal muscles, is common when large doses of opioid agonists are administered rapidly and intravenously (Bowdle and Rooke, 1994). Clonic skeletal muscle activity (myoclonus) occurring during administration of opioids may resemble grand mal seizures, but the EEG does not reflect seizure activity. Skeletal muscle rigidity may be related to actions at opioid receptors and involve interactions with dopaminergic and gamma-aminobutyric acid–responsive neurons.

Rapid IV administration of an opioid, as for induction of anesthesia, may be associated with thoracic and abdominal skeletal muscle rigidity sufficient to interfere with adequate ventilation of the lungs. Attempts to manually inflate the lungs in the presence of this skeletal muscle rigidity may result in airway pressures that interfere with venous return. Conversely, there is evidence that the major cause of difficult ventilation after induction of anesthesia with sufentanil (and presumably other opioids) is closure of the vocal cords (Bennett et al., 1997a). The incidence of opioid-induced skeletal muscle rigidity (generalized hypertonus of skeletal muscles) depends on the opioid (most common with fentanyl) and dose used and the rate of administration. Inhibition of striatal release of gamma-aminobutyric acid and increased dopamine production are the likely explanations for opioid-induced increased skeletal muscle tone. The reported incidence of difficult ventilation after a moderate dose of sufentanil ranges from 84% to 100% (Bennett et al., 1997a).

Miosis is due to an excitatory action of opioids on the autonomic nervous system component of the Edinger-Westphal nucleus of the oculomotor nerve. Tolerance to the miotic effect of morphine is not prominent. Miosis can be antagonized by atropine, and profound arterial hypoxemia in the presence of morphine can still result in mydriasis.

Sedation

Postoperative titration of morphine frequently induces sedation that precedes the onset of analgesia (Paqueron et al., 2002). The usual recommendation for morphine titration includes a short interval between boluses (5 to 7 minutes) to allow evaluation of its clinical effect. Sedation occurs in up to 60% of patients during morphine titration and represents a common reason to discontinue morphine titration for postoperative analgesia. The assumption that sleep occurs when pain is relieved is not necessarily accurate and morphine-induced sedation should not be considered as an indicator of appropriate analgesia during intravenous morphine titration.

Biliary Tract

Opioids can cause spasm of biliary smooth muscle, resulting in increases in intrabiliary pressure that may be associated with epigastric distress or biliary colic. This pain may be confused with angina pectoris. Naloxone will relieve pain caused by biliary spasm but not myocardial ischemia. Conversely, nitroglycerin will relieve pain due to biliary spasm or myocardial ischemia. Equal analgesic doses of fentanyl, morphine, meperidine, and pentazocine increase common bile duct pressure 99%, 53%, 61%, and 15% above predrug levels, respectively (Radnay et al., 1980). During surgery, opioid-induced spasm of the sphincter of Oddi may appear radiologically as a sharp constriction at the distal end of the common bile duct and be misinterpreted as a common bile duct stone. It may be necessary to reverse opioid-induced biliary smooth muscle spasm with naloxone so as to correctly interpret the cholangiogram. Glucagon, 2 mg IV, also reverses opioid-induced biliary smooth muscle spasm and, unlike naloxone, does not antagonize the analgesic effects of the opioid (Jones et al., 1980). Nevertheless, biliary muscle spasm does not occur in most patients who receive opioids. Indeed, the incidence of spasm of the sphincter of Oddi is about 3% in patients receiving fentanyl as a supplement to inhaled anesthetics (Jones et al., 1981).

Contraction of the smooth muscles of the pancreatic ducts is probably responsible for increases in plasma amylase and lipase concentrations that may be present after the administration of morphine. Such increases may confuse the diagnosis when acute pancreatitis is a possibility.

Gastrointestinal Tract

Commonly used opioids such as morphine, meperidine, and fentanyl can produce spasm of the gastrointestinal smooth muscles, resulting in a variety of side effects including constipation, biliary colic, and delayed gastric emptying.

Morphine decreases the propulsive peristaltic contractions of the small and large intestines and enhances the tone of the pyloric sphincter, ileocecal valve, and anal sphincter. The delayed passage of intestinal contents through the colon allows increased absorption of water. As a result, constipation often accompanies therapy with opioids and may become a debilitating problem in patients who require chronic opioid therapy, as little tolerance develops to this effect. Of interest, opium (morphine) was used to treat diarrhea before its use as an analgesic was popularized.

Increased biliary pressure occurs when the gallbladder contracts against a closed or narrowed sphincter of Oddi. Passage of gastric contents into the proximal duodenum is delayed because there is increased tone at the gastroduodenal junction. In this regard, preoperative medication that includes an opioid could slow gastric emptying (potentially increase the risk of aspiration) or delay the absorption of orally administered drugs. All these effects may be reversed or prevented by a peripheral-acting opioid antagonist (see the section on Methylnaltrexone).

Nausea and Vomiting

Opioid-induced nausea and vomiting are caused by direct stimulation of the chemoreceptor trigger zone in the floor of the fourth ventricle (see Fig. 41-16). This may reflect the role of opioid agonists as partial dopamine agonists at dopamine receptors in the chemoreceptor trigger zone. Indeed, apomorphine is a profound emetic and is also the most potent of the opioids at dopamine receptors. Stimulation of dopamine receptors as a mechanism for opioid-induced nausea and vomiting is consistent with the antiemetic efficacy of butyrophenones. Morphine may also cause nausea and vomiting by increasing gastrointestinal secretions and delaying passage of intestinal contents towards the colon.

Morphine depresses the vomiting center in the medulla (see Fig. 41-16). As a result, IV administration of morphine produces less nausea and vomiting than the IM administration of morphine, presumably because opioid administered intravenously reaches the vomiting center as rapidly as it reaches the chemoreceptor trigger zone. Nausea and vomiting are relatively uncommon in recumbent patients given morphine, suggesting that a vestibular component may contribute to opioid-induced nausea and vomiting.

Genitourinary System

Morphine can increase the tone and peristaltic activity of the ureter. In contrast to similar effects on biliary tract smooth muscle, the same opioid-induced effects on the ureter can be reversed by an anticholinergic drug such as atropine. Urinary urgency is produced by opioid-induced augmentation of detrusor muscle tone, but, at the same time, the tone of the vesicle sphincter is enhanced, making voiding difficult.

Antidiuresis that accompanies administration of morphine to animals has been attributed to opioid-induced release of arginine vasopressin hormone (antidiuretic hormone). In humans, however, administration of morphine in the absence of painful surgical stimulation does not evoke the release of this hormone (Philbin et al., 1976). Furthermore, when morphine is administered in the presence of an adequate intravascular fluid volume, there is no change in urine output.

Cutaneous Changes

Morphine causes cutaneous blood vessels to dilate. The skin of the face, neck, and upper chest frequently becomes flushed and warm. These changes in cutaneous circulation are in part caused by the release of histamine. Histamine release probably accounts for urticaria and erythema commonly seen at the morphine injection site. In addition, morphine-induced histamine release probably accounts for conjunctival erythema and pruritus.

Localized cutaneous evidence of histamine release, especially along the vein into which morphine is injected, does not represent an allergic reaction. Overall, the incidence of true allergy to opioids is uncommon, although there have been documented cases (Bennett et al., 1986). More often, predictable side effects of opioids such as localized histamine release, orthostatic hypotension, nausea and vomiting are misinterpreted as an allergic reaction.

Placenta

The placenta offers no real barrier to the transfer of opioids from mother to fetus. Therefore, depression of the neonate can occur as a consequence of administration of opioids to the mother during labor. In this regard, maternal administration of morphine may produce greater neonatal depression than meperidine does (Way et al., 1965). This may reflect immaturity of the neonate's blood-brain barrier. Chronic maternal use of an opioid can result in the development of physical dependence (intrauterine addiction) in the fetus. Subsequent administration of naloxone to the neonate can precipitate a life-threatening neonatal abstinence syndrome.

Drug Interactions

The ventilatory depressant effects of some opioids may be exaggerated by amphetamines, phenothiazines, monoamine oxidase inhibitors, and tricyclic antidepressants. For example, patients receiving monoamine oxidase inhibitors may experience exaggerated CNS depression and hyperpyrexia after administration of an opioid agonist, especially meperidine. This exaggerated response may reflect alterations in the rate or pathway of metabolism of the opioid. Sympathomimetic drugs appear to enhance analgesia produced by opioids. The cholinergic nervous system seems to be a positive modulator of opioid-induced analgesia in that physostigmine enhances and atropine antagonizes analgesia.

Pharmacodynamic Tolerance and Physical Dependence

Pharmacodynamic tolerance and physical dependence with repeated opioid administration are characteristic features of all opioid agonists and are among the major limitations of their clinical use. Cross-tolerance develops between all the opioids. Tolerance can occur without physical dependence, but the reverse does not seem to occur.

Tolerance is the development of the need to increase the dose of opioid agonist to achieve the same analgesic effect previously achieved with a lower dose. Such acquired tolerance usually takes 2 to 3 weeks to develop with analgesic doses of morphine. Tolerance develops to analgesic, euphoric, sedative, depression of ventilation and emetic effects of opioids but not to their effects on miosis and bowel motility (constipation). The potential for physical dependence (addiction) is an agonist effect of opioids. Indeed, physical dependence does not occur with opioid antagonists and is unlikely with opioid agonist-antagonists. When opioid agonist actions predominate, there often develops, with repeated use, a compulsive desire (psychological) and continuous need (physiologic) for the drug. Physical dependence on morphine usually requires about 25 days to develop but may occur sooner in emotionally unstable persons. Some degree of physical dependence, however, occurs after only 48 hours of continuous medication. When physical dependence is established, discontinuation of the opioid agonist produces a typical withdrawal abstinence syndrome (Table 3-6) (Mitra and Sinatra, 2004). Initial symptoms of withdrawal include yawning, diaphoresis, lacrimation, or coryza. Insomnia and restlessness are prominent. Abdominal cramps, nausea, vomiting, and diarrhea reach their peak in 72 hours and then decline over the next 7 to 10 days. During withdrawal, tolerance to morphine is rapidly lost, and the syndrome can be terminated by a modest dose of opioid agonist. The longer the period of abstinence, the smaller the dose of opioid agonist that will be required.

Pharmacodynamic tolerance has been related to neuroadaptive changes that take place after long-term expsoure to the opioid (Mitra and Sinatra, 2004). These changes occur at the level of opioid receptors and involve receptor desensitization. Opioid receptors on the cell membrane surfaces become gradually desensitized by reduced transcription and subsequent decreases in the absolute numbers of opioid receptors (down-regulation). This classic hypothesis of pharamacodynamic tolerance remains unproven.

TABLE 3-6.
TIME COURSE OF OPIOID WITHDRAWAL

	Onset	Peak Intensity	Duration
Morphine	6–18 hrs	36–72 hrs	7–10 days
Heroin	6–18 hrs	36–72 hrs	7–10 days
Meperidine	2–6 hrs	8–12 hrs	4–5 days
Fentanyl	2–6 hrs	8–12 hrs	4–5 days
Methadone	24–48 hrs	3–21 days	6–7 weeks

Adapted from Mitra S, Sinatra RS. Perioperative management of acute pain in the opioid-dependent patient. *Anesthesiology* 2004; 101:212–227.

A second mechanism proposed to explain pharmacodynamic tolerance involves up-regulation of the cyclic adenosine mononphosphate (cAMP) system. Acutely, opioids inhibit functional activity of cAMP pathways by blocking adenyl cyclase, the enzyme that catalyzes the synthesis of cAMP. Long-term opioid exposure is associated with gradual recovery of cAMP pathways and tolerance develops. Increased synthesis of cAMP may be responsible for physical dependence and physiololgic changes associated with withdrawal. Up-regulation of cAMP has been most clearly demonstrated in the locus ceruleus of the brain. Clonidine, a centrally acting alpha$_2$-adrenergic agonist that diminishes transmission in sympathetic pathways in the CNS, is an effective drug in suppressing withdrawal signs in persons who are physically dependent on opioids. Tolerance is not due to enzyme induction, because no increase in the rate of metabolism of opioid agonists occurs.

Long-term pharmacodynamic tolerance characterized by opioid insensitivity may persist for months or years in some individuals and most likely represents persistent neural adaptation (Mitra and Sinatra, 2004). In this regard, glutamate and *N*-methyl-D-aspartate (NMDA) receptors are important in the development of opioid tolerance and increased pain sensitivity. Prolonged exposure to opioids activates NMDA receptors via second messenger mechansims and also down-regulates spinal glutamate transporters. The resultant high synaptic concentrations of glutamate and NMDA activation contributes to opioid tolerance and abnormal pain sensitivity (pronociceptive or sensitization process).

Hormonal Changes

Prolonged opioid therapy may influence the hypothalamic-pituitary-adrenal axis and the hypothalamic-pituitary-gonadal axis (Ballantyne and Mao, 2003). Morphine may cause a progressive decrease in plasma corisol concentrations. The main effects of opioids on the hypothalamic-pituitary-gonadal axis involve modulation of hormone release including increased prolactin and decreased luteinizing hormone, follicle stimulating hormone, testosterone, and estrogen concentrations.

Immune Modulation

Opioid therapy may alter immunity through neuroendocrine effects or via direct effects on the immune system (Ballantyne and Mao, 2004; Webster 1998). Prolonged exposure to opioids appears more likely than short term exposure to produce immunosuppression especially in susceptible persons and abrupt withdrawal may also induce immunosuppression. Opioids alter the development, differentiation, and function of immune cells (bone marrow progenitor cells, macrophages, T cells). Opioid-related receptors are present on immune cells. Although immunosuppressant effects of opioids raise concerns (incidence of postoperative infections) it is equally important to recognize that pain itself can impair immune function.

Overdose

The principal manifestation of opioid overdose is depression of ventilation manifesting as a slow breathing frequency, which may progress to apnea. Pupils are symmetric and miotic unless severe arterial hypoxemia is present, which results in mydriasis. Skeletal muscles are flaccid, and upper airway obstruction may occur. Pulmonary edema commonly occurs, but the mechanism is not known. Hypotension and seizures develop if arterial hypoxemia persists. The triad of miosis, hypoventilation, and coma should suggest overdose with an opioid. Treatment of opioid overdose is mechanical ventilation of the patient's lungs with oxygen and administration of an opioid antagonist such as naloxone. Administration of an opioid antagonist to treat opioid overdose may precipitate acute withdrawal.

Morphine-6-Glucuronide

The duration of action of morphine-6-glucuronide is greater than that of morphine, and it is possible that the majority of analgesic activity attributed to morphine is actually due to morphine-6-glucuronide especially with long-term administration of morphine (Hanna et al., 1990). Morphine and morphine-6-glucuronide bind to mu opioid receptors with comparable affinity whereas the analgesic potency of morphine-6-glucuronide is 650-fold higher than morphine (Paul et al., 1989). Accumulation of morphine-6-glucuronide during long-term infusion of morphine may contribute to both analgesia and depression of ventilation. Likewise, in the presence of acute renal failure, severe opioid side effects may occur many hours after plasma morphine concentrations have peaked, reflecting the peak plasma concentrations of morphine-6-glucuronide (Angst et al., 2000). Morphine-6-glucuronide does not produce clinical or analgesic effects when administered as a single intravenous bolus or an intravenous bolus followed by a 4 hour infusion (Lotsch et al., 1999; Motamed et al., 2000). This most likely reflects the low permeability of the blood-brain barrier for morphine-6-glucuronide and emphasizes that short term infusion may not produce sufficient central nervous system concentrations of morphine-6-glucuronide to produce detectable pharmacologic effects. Under conditions of long-term administration, CNS concentrations of morphine-6-glucuronide become more relevant (Lotsch et al., 1999). Nevertheless, morphine-6-glucuronide administered over 1 hour has been reported to produce prolonged analgesia, suggesting this drug has value as an intravenous analgesic for postoperative pain relief (Romberg et al., 2004). Intrathecal administration of morphine-6-glucuronide produces analgesia similar to that produced by morphine (Grace and Fee, 1996).

Meperidine

Meperidine is a synthetic opioid agonist at mu and kappa opioid receptors and is derived from phenylepiperidine (Fig. 3-15). There are several analogues of meperidine, including fentanyl, sufentanil, alfentanil, and remifentanil (see Fig. 3-15). Meperidine shares several structural features that are present in local anesthetics including a tertiary amine, an ester group and a lipophilic phenyl group. Indeed, meperidine administered intrathecally blocks sodium channels to a degree comparable with lidocaine. Structurally, meperidine is similar to atropine, and it possesses a mild atropine-like antispasmodic effect.

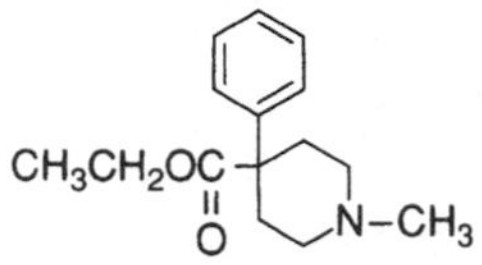

Meperidine

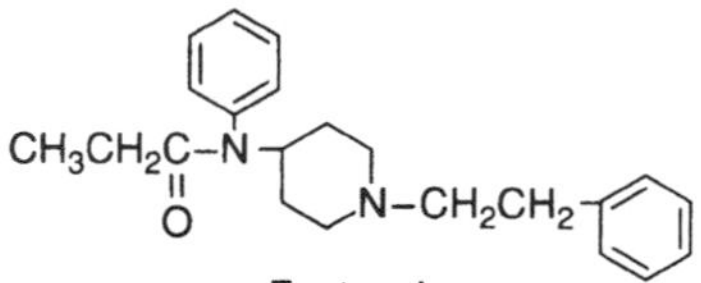

Fentanyl

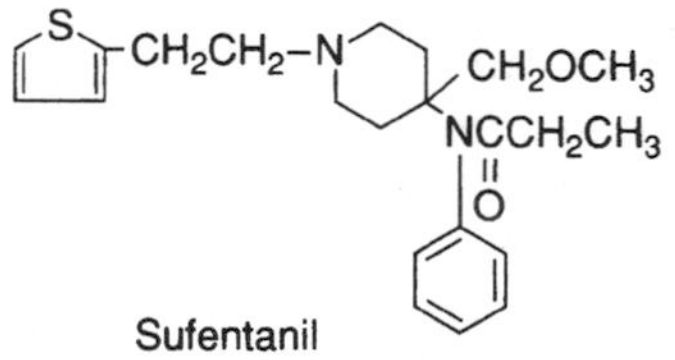

Sufentanil

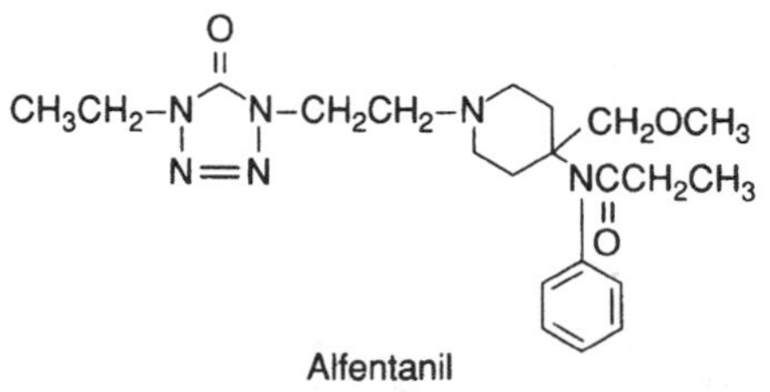

Alfentanil

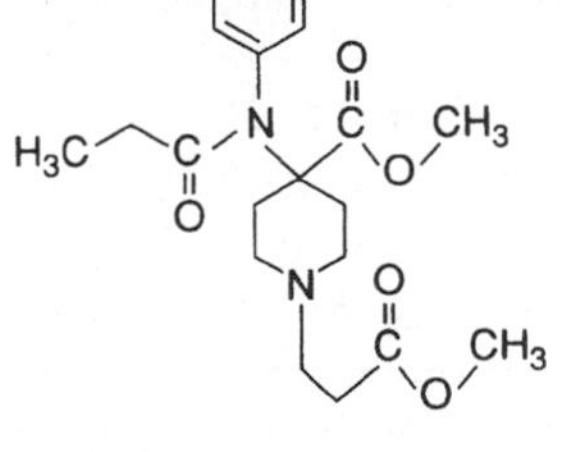

Remifentanil

Figure 3-15. Synthetic opioid agonists.

Nevertheless, the principal pharmacologic effects of meperidine resemble morphine.

Pharmacokinetics

Meperidine is about one-tenth as potent as morphine, with 80 to 100 mg IM being equivalent to about 10 mg IM of morphine. The duration of action of meperidine is 2 to 4 hours, making it a shorter-acting opioid agonist than morphine. In equal analgesic doses, meperidine produces as much sedation, euphoria, nausea, vomiting, and depression of ventilation as does morphine. Unlike morphine, meperidine is well absorbed from the gastrointestinal tract, but nevertheless, it is only about one-half as effective orally as when administered IM.

Metabolism

Hepatic metabolism of meperidine is extensive, with about 90% of the drug initially undergoing demethylation to normeperidine and hydrolysis to meperidinic acid (Stone et al., 1993). Normeperidine subsequently undergoes hydrolysis to normeperidinic acid. Urinary excretion is the principal elimination route and is pH dependent. For example, if the urinary pH is <5, as much as 25% of meperidine is excreted unchanged. Indeed, acidification of the urine can be considered in an attempt to speed elimination of meperidine. Decreased renal function can predispose to accumulation of normeperidine.

Normeperidine has an elimination half-time of 15 hours (<35 hours in patients in renal failure) and can be detected in urine for as long as 3 days after administration of meperidine. This metabolite is about one-half as active as meperidine as an analgesic. In addition, normeperidine produces CNS stimulation. Normeperidine toxicity manifesting as myoclonus and seizures is most likely during prolonged administration of meperidine as during patient-controlled analgesia, especially in the presence of impaired renal function (Stone et al., 1993). Normeperidine may also be important in meperidine-induced delirium (confusion, hallucinations), which has been observed in patients receiving the drug for longer than 3 days, corresponding to accumulation of this active metabolite.

Elimination Half-Time

The elimination half-time of meperidine is 3 to 5 hours (see Table 3-5). Because clearance of meperidine primarily depends on hepatic metabolism, it is possible that large doses of opioid would saturate enzyme systems and result in prolonged elimination half-times. Nevertheless, elimination half-time is not altered by doses of meperidine up to 5 mg/kg IV. About 60% of meperidine is bound to plasma proteins. Elderly patients manifest decreased plasma protein binding of meperidine, resulting in increased plasma concentrations of free drug and an apparent increased sensitivity of the opioid. The increased tolerance of alcoholics to meperidine and other opioids presumably reflects an increased Vd, resulting in lower plasma concentrations of meperidine.

Clinical Uses

The principal use of meperidine is for analgesia during labor and delivery and after surgery. Meperidine is the only opioid considered adequate for surgery when administered intrathecally (Cozian et al., 1986). An IM injection of meperidine for postoperative analgesia results in peak plasma concentrations that vary three- to fivefold as well as a time required to achieve peak concentrations that varies three- to sevenfold among patients (Austin et al., 1980a). The minimum analgesic plasma concentration of meperidine is highly variable among patients; however, in the same patient, differences in concentrations as small as 0.05 μg/mL can represent a margin between no relief and complete analgesia. A plasma meperidine concentration of 0.7 μg/mL would be expected to provide postoperative analgesia in about 95% of patients (Austin et al., 1980b). Patient-controlled analgesia delivery systems usually provide acceptable postoperative analgesia, with total doses of meperidine ranging from 12 to 36 mg/hour (White, 1985). Normeperidine toxicity has been described in patients receiving meperidine for patient-controlled analgesia (Stone et al., 1993).

Meperidine may be effective in suppressing postoperative shivering that may result in detrimental increases in metabolic oxygen consumption. The antishivering effects of meperidine may reflect stimulation of kappa receptors (estimated to represent 10% of its activity) and a drug-induced decrease in the shivering threshold (not present with alfentanil, clonidine, propofol, or volatile anesthetics) (Fig. 3-16) (Alfonsi et al., 1998; Ikeda et al., 1998, Kurz et al., 1997). In addition, meperidine is a potent agonist at $alpha_2$ receptors which might contribute to antishivering effects (Takada et al, 2002). Indeed, clonidine is even more effective than meperidine in reducing postoperative shivering. Butorphanol (a kappa receptor agonist-antagonist) stops shivering more effectively than opioids with a predominant mu opioid receptor agonist effect. Evidence for a role of kappa receptors in the antishivering effects of meperidine and butorphanol is the failure of naloxone to completely inhibit this drug-induced effect.

Oral absorption may make meperidine more useful than morphine for the treatment of many forms of pain. Unlike morphine, meperidine is not useful for the treatment of diarrhea and is not an effective antitussive. During bronchoscopy, the relative lack of antitussive activity of meperidine makes this opioid less useful. Meperidine is not used in high doses because of significant negative cardiac inotropic effects plus histamine release in a substantial number of patients (Flacke et al., 1987).

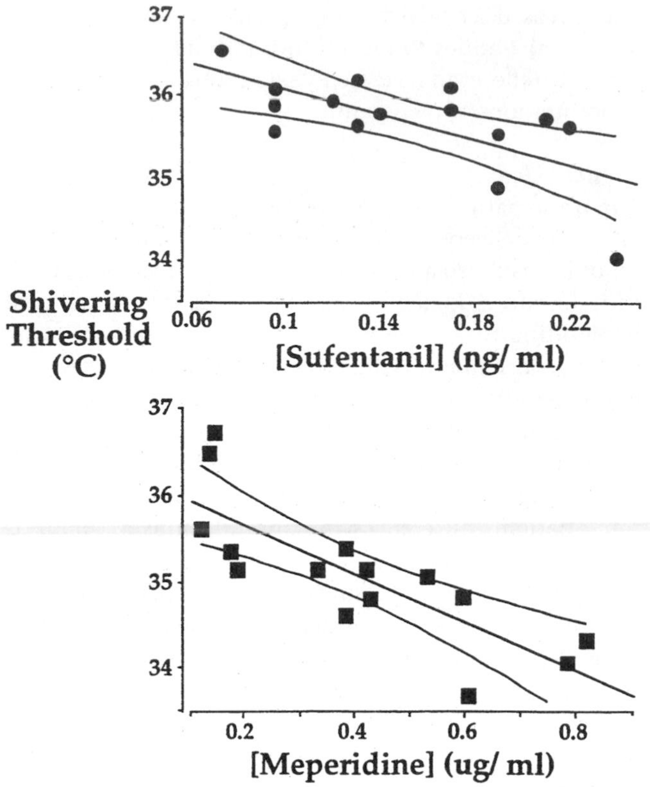

Figure 3-16. Sufentanil and meperidine decrease the shivering threshold. (From Alfonsi P, Sessler DI, Du Manoir B, et al. The effects of meperidine and sufentanil on the shivering threshold in postoperative patients. *Anesthesiology* 1998;89:43–48; with permission.)

Side Effects

The side effects of meperidine resemble those described for morphine. In therapeutic doses, meperidine is associated with orthostatic hypotension. In fact, hypotension after meperidine injection is more frequent and more profound than after comparable doses of morphine. Orthostatic hypotension suggests that meperidine, like morphine, interferes with compensatory sympathetic nervous system reflexes. Meperidine, in contrast to morphine, rarely causes bradycardia but instead may increase heart rate, reflecting its modest atropine-like qualities. Large doses of meperidine result in decreases in myocardial contractility, which, among opioids, is unique for this drug. Delirium and seizures, when they occur, presumably reflect accumulation of normeperidine, which has stimulating effects on the CNS.

Serotonin syndrome (autonomic instability with hypertension, tachycardia, diaphoresis, hyperthermia, behavioral changes including confusion and agitation, and neuromuscular changes manifesting as hyperreflexia) occurs when drugs capable of increasing serotonin administration are administered. In severe cases, coma, seizures, coagulopathy, and metabolic acidosis may develop. Administration of meperidine to patients receiving antidepressant drugs (monoamine oxidase inhibitors, fluoxetine) may elicit this syndrome (Tissot, 2003).

Meperidine readily impairs ventilation and may be even more of a ventilatory depressant than morphine. This opioid promptly crosses the placenta, and concentrations of meperidine in umbilical cord blood at birth may exceed maternal plasma concentrations (Way et al., 1965). Meperidine may produce less constipation and urinary retention than morphine. After equal analgesic doses, biliary tract spasm is less after meperidine injection than after morphine injection but greater than that caused by codeine (Radnay et al., 1980). Meperidine does not cause miosis but rather tends to cause mydriasis, reflecting its modest atropine-like actions. A dry mouth and an increase in heart rate are further evidence of the atropine-like effects of meperidine. Transient neurologic symptoms have been described following the administration of intrathecal meperidine for surgical anesthesia (Lewis and Perrino, 2002).

The pattern of withdrawal symptoms after abrupt discontinuation of meperidine differs from that of morphine in that there are few autonomic nervous system effects. In addition, symptoms of withdrawal develop more rapidly and are of a shorter duration compared with those of morphine.

Fentanyl

Fentanyl is a phenylpiperidine-derivative synthetic opioid agonist that is structurally related to meperidine (see Fig. 3-15). As an analgesic, fentanyl is 75 to 125 times more potent than morphine.

Pharmacokinetics

A single dose of fentanyl administered IV has a more rapid onset and shorter duration of action than morphine. Despite the clinical impression that fentanyl produces a rapid onset, there is a distinct time lag between the peak plasma fentanyl concentration and peak slowing on the EEG. This delay reflects the effect-site equilibration time between blood and the brain for fentanyl, which is 6.4 minutes. The greater potency and more rapid onset of action reflect the greater lipid solubility of fentanyl compared with that of morphine, which facilitates its passage across the blood-brain barrier. Likewise, the short duration of action of a single dose of fentanyl reflects its rapid redistribution to inactive tissue sites such as fat and skeletal muscles, with an associated decrease in the plasma concentration of the drug (Fig. 3-17) (Hug and Murphy, 1981). The lungs also serve as a large, inactive storage site, with an estimated 75% of the initial fentanyl dose undergoing first-pass pulmonary uptake (Roerig et al., 1987). This nonrespiratory function of the lungs limits the initial amount of drug that reaches the systemic circulation and may play an important role in determining the pharmacokinetic profile of fentanyl. When multiple IV doses of fentanyl are administered or when there is continuous infusion of the drug,

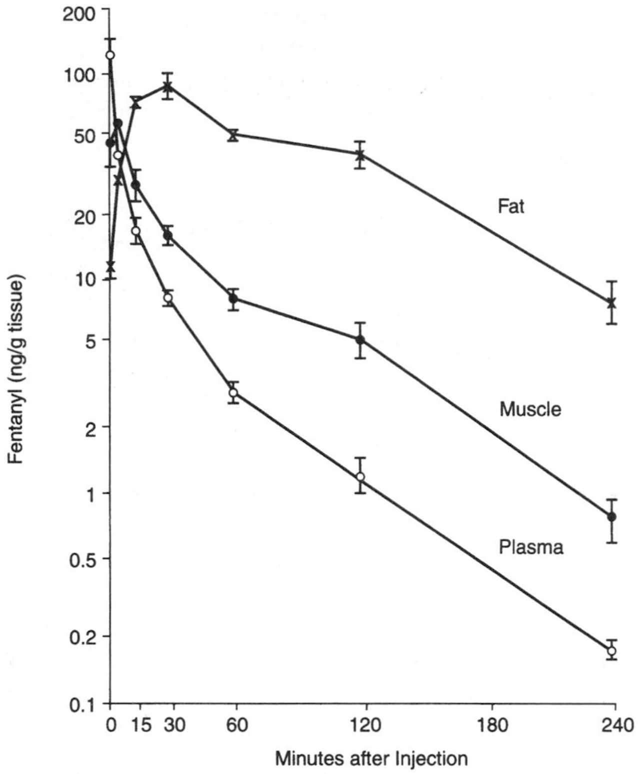

Figure 3-17. The short duration of action of a single intravenous dose of fentanyl reflects its rapid redistribution to inactive tissue sites such as fat and skeletal muscles, with associated decreases in the plasma concentration of drug. (Mean ± SE.) (From Hug CC, Murphy MR. Tissue redistribution of fentanyl and termination of its effects in rats. *Anesthesiology* 1981;55:369–375; with permission.)

progressive saturation of these inactive tissue sites occurs. As a result, the plasma concentration of fentanyl does not decrease rapidly, and the duration of analgesia, as well as depression of ventilation, may be prolonged (see the section on Context-Sensitive Half-Time). Cardiopulmonary bypass causes clinically insignificant effects on the pharmacokinetics of fentanyl despite associated hemodilution, hypothermia, nonphysiologic blood flow and cardiopulmonary bypass-induced systemic inflammatory responses (Hudson et al., 2003).

Metabolism

Fentanyl is extensively metabolized by *N*-demethylation, producing norfentanyl, hydroxyproprionyl-fentanyl, and hydroxyproprionyl-norfentanyl. Norfentanyl is structurally similar to normeperidine and is the principal metabolite of fentanyl in humans. It is excreted by the kidneys and can be detected in the urine for 72 hours after a single IV dose of fentanyl. Less than 10% of fentanyl is excreted unchanged in the urine. The pharmacologic activity of fentanyl metabolites is believed to be minimal (Peng and Sandler, 1999). Fentanyl is a substrate for hepatic P-450 enzymes (CYP3A) and is susceptible to drug interactions that reflect interference with enzyme activity (less likely than with alfentanil) (Ibrahim et al., 2003).

Elimination Half-Time

Despite the clinical impression that fentanyl has a short duration of action, its elimination half-time is longer than that for morphine (see Table 3-5). This longer elimination half-time reflects a larger Vd of fentanyl because clearance of both opioids is similar (see Table 3-5). The larger Vd of fentanyl is due to its greater lipid solubility and thus more rapid passage into tissues compared with the less lipid-soluble morphine. After an IV bolus, fentanyl distributes rapidly from the plasma to highly vascular tissues (brain, lungs, heart). More than 80% of the injected dose leaves the plasma in <5 minutes. The plasma concentrations of fentanyl are maintained by slow reuptake from inactive tissue sites, which accounts for persistent drug effects that parallel the prolonged elimination half-time. In animals, the elimination half-time, Vd, and clearance of fentanyl are independent of the dose of opioid between 6.4 and 640 μg/kg IV (Murphy et al., 1983).

A prolonged elimination half-time for fentanyl in elderly patients is due to decreased clearance of the opioid because Vd is not changed in comparison with younger adults (Bentley et al., 1982). This change may reflect age-related decreases in hepatic blood flow, microsomal enzyme activity, or albumin production, as fentanyl is highly bound (79% to 87%) to protein. For these reasons, it is likely that a given dose of fentanyl will be effective for a longer period of time in elderly patients than in younger patients. A prolonged elimination half-time of fentanyl has also been observed in patients undergoing abdominal aortic surgery requiring infrarenal aortic cross-clamping (Hudson et al., 1986). Somewhat surprising, however, is the failure of hepatic cirrhosis to prolong significantly the elimination half-time of fentanyl (Haberer et al., 1982).

Context-Sensitive Half-Time

As the duration of continuous infusion of fentanyl increases beyond about 2 hours, the context-sensitive half-time of this opioid becomes greater than sufentanil (Fig. 3-18) (Egan et al., 1993; Hughes et al., 1992). This reflects saturation of inactive tissue sites with fentanyl during prolonged infusions and return of the opioid from peripheral compartments to the plasma. This tissue reservoir of fentanyl replaces fentanyl eliminated by hepatic metabolism so as to slow the rate of decrease in the plasma concentration of fentanyl when the infusion is discontinued.

Cardiopulmonary Bypass

All opioids show a decrease in plasma concentration with initiation of cardiopulmonary bypass (Gedney and Ghosh, 1995). The degree of this decrease is greater with fentanyl

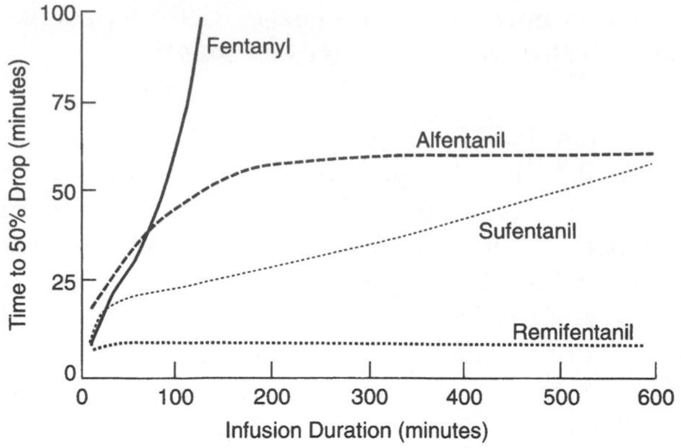

Figure 3-18. Computer simulation–derived context-sensitive half-times (time necessary for the plasma concentration to decrease 50% after discontinuation of the infusion) as a function of the duration of the intravenous infusion. (From Egan TD, Lemmens HJM, Fiset P, et al. The pharmacokinetics of the new short-acting opioid remifentanil (GI87084B) in healthy adult male volunteers. *Anesthesiology* 1993;79:881–892; with permission.)

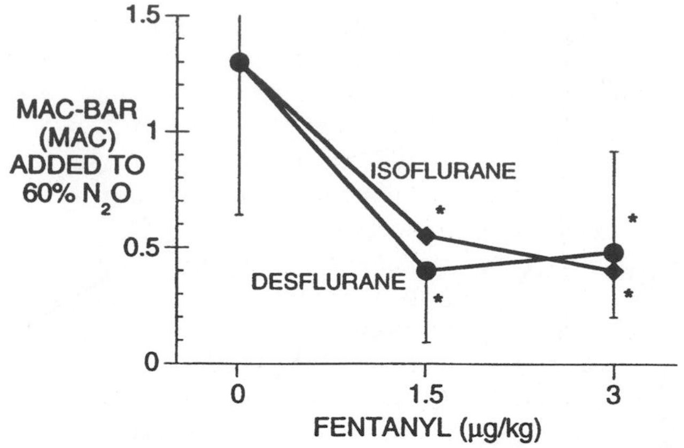

Figure 3-19. The anesthetic dose of desflurane and isoflurane required to block the adrenergic response (MAC-BAR) to incision in 50% of patients without and with fentanyl. There was no significant difference between the inhaled anesthetics at any fentanyl dose and both does of fentanyl significantly and similarly decreased MAC-BAR. *P<0.05. Mean ≠ SD. (From Daniel M, Weiskopf RB, Noorani M, et al. Fentanyl augments the blockade of the sympathetic response to incision (MAC-BAR) produced by desflurane and isoflurane. Desflurane and isoflurane MAC-BAR without and with fentanyl. *Anesthesiology* 1998;88:43–49; with permission.)

because a significant proportion of the drug adheres to the surface of the cardiopulmonary bypass circuit. The decrease is least with opioids that have a large Vd such that the addition of prime volume is less important. In this respect, sufentanil and alfentanil may provide more stable plasma concentrations during cardiopulmonary bypass. Elimination of fentanyl and alfentanil has been shown to be prolonged by cardiopulmonary bypass.

Clinical Uses

Fentanyl is administered clinically in a wide range of doses. For example, low doses of fentanyl, 1 to 2 μg/kg IV, are injected to provide analgesia. Fentanyl, 2 to 20 μg/kg IV, may be administered as an adjuvant to inhaled anesthetics in an attempt to blunt circulatory responses to (a) direct laryngoscopy for intubation of the trachea, or (b) sudden changes in the level of surgical stimulation. Timing of the IV injection of fentanyl to prevent or treat such responses should consider the effect-site equilibration time, which for fentanyl is prolonged compared with alfentanil and remifentanil. Injection of an opioid such as fentanyl before painful surgical stimulation may decrease the subsequent amount of opioid required in the postoperative period to provide analgesia (Woolf and Wall, 1986). Administration of fentanyl 1.5 or 3 μg/kg IV 5 minutes before induction of anesthesia decreases the subsequent doses of isoflurane or desflurane with 60% nitrous oxide needed to block the sympathetic nervous system response to surgical stimulation (Fig. 3-19) (Daniel et al., 1998). Large doses of fentanyl, 50 to 150 μg/kg IV, have been used alone to produce surgical anesthesia. Large doses of fentanyl as the sole anesthetic have the advantage of stable hemodynamics due principally to the (a) lack of direct myocardial depressant effects, (b) absence of histamine release, and (c) suppression of the stress responses to surgery. Disadvantages of using fentanyl as the sole anesthetic include (a) failure to prevent sympathetic nervous system responses to painful surgical stimulation at any dose, especially in patients with good left ventricular function, (b) possible patient awareness, and (c) postoperative depression of ventilation (Hilgenberg, 1981; Sprigge et al., 1982; Wynands et al., 1983). Intrathecal fentanyl (maximal benefit achieved with 25 μg) produces rapid, profound labor analgesia with minimal side effects (Fig. 3-20) (Palmer et al., 1998).

Fentanyl may be administered as a transmucosal preparation (oral transmucosal fentanyl) in a delivery device (lozenge mounted on a handle) designed to deliver 5 to

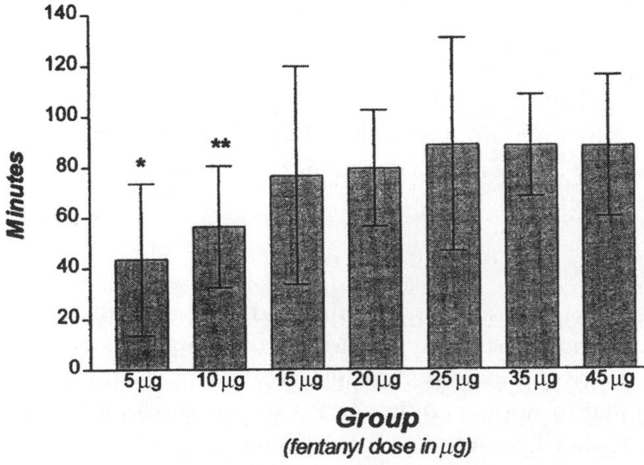

Figure 3-20. Duration of analgesia as reflected by the time to the first request for additional analgesia with varying doses of intrathecal fentanyl. Mean ≠ SD *P <0.05 versus groups 15–45 μg. **P <0.05 versus groups 25 through 45 μg. (From Palmer CM, Cork RC, Hays R, et al. The dose-response relation of intrathecal fentanyl for labor analgesia. *Anesthesiology* 1998;88:355–361; with permission.)

20 μg/kg of fentanyl. The goal is to decrease preoperative anxiety and facilitate the induction of anesthesia, especially in children (Macaluso et al., 1996; Stanley et al., 1989). In children 2 to 8 years of age, the preoperative administration of oral transmucosal fentanyl, 15 to 20 μg/kg 45 minutes before the induction of anesthesia, reliably induces preoperative sedation and facilitates induction of inhalation anesthesia (Friesen and Lockhart, 1992). These same patients, however, are likely to experience decreases in breathing frequency and arterial oxygenation and an increased incidence of postoperative nausea and vomiting that is not influenced by prophylactic administration of droperidol. In children 6 years of age and younger, the preoperative administration of oral transmucosal fentanyl, 15 μg/kg, is associated with an unacceptably high incidence of preoperative vomiting (Epstein et al., 1996). Conversely, another report did not observe an increased incidence of vomiting or arterial oxygen desaturation after premedication with oral transmucosal fentanyl (Dsida et al., 1998). For treatment of postoperative pain after orthopedic surgery, 1 mg of oral transmucosal fentanyl is equivalent to 5 mg of IV morphine (Ashburn et al., 1993). Patients experiencing pain due to cancer may self-administer this opioid to the extent necessary to produce a desirable level of analgesia.

Transdermal fentanyl preparations delivering 75 to 100 μg/hour result in peak plasma fentanyl concentrations in about 18 hours that tend to remain stable during the presence of the patch, followed by a decreasing plasma concentration for several hours after removal of the delivery system, reflecting continued absorption from the cutaneous depot. The Transdermal fentanyl systems applied before the induction of anesthesia and left in place for 24 hours decrease the amount of parenteral opioid required for postoperative analgesia (Caplan et al., 1989). Acute toxic delirium has been observed in patients with chronic pain due to cancer being treated with transdermal fentanyl for prolonged periods of time (Kuzma et al., 1995). It is possible that renal failure and accumulation of norfentanyl contributes to the possible toxic effects of prolonged use of transdermal fentanyl.

In dogs, maximal analgesic, ventilatory, and cardiovascular effects are present when the plasma concentration of fentanyl is about 30 ng/mL (Arndt et al., 1984). This confirms that the analgesic actions of fentanyl cannot be separated from its effects on ventilation and heart rate. The fact that all receptor-mediated effects are similar at the same plasma concentration of fentanyl suggests saturation of the opioid receptors. Evidence of opioid overdose has been observed when an upper body warming blanket was placed intraoperatively and came into contact with the fentanyl patch (Frolich et al., 2001).

Side Effects

The side effects of fentanyl resemble those described for morphine. Persistent or recurrent depression of ventilation

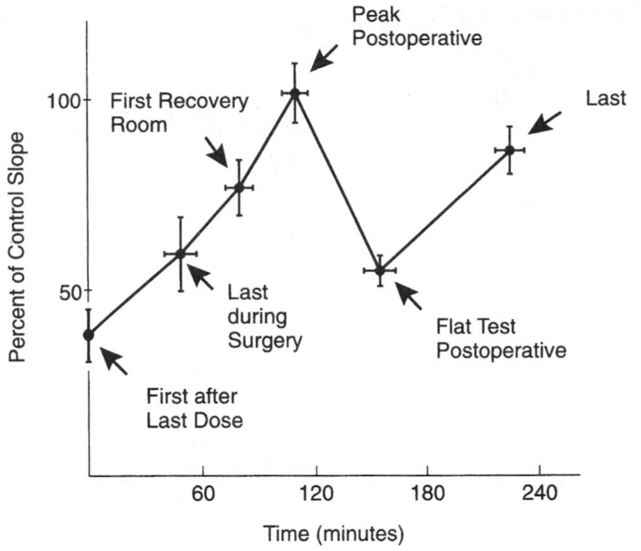

Figure 3-21. Recurrent fentanyl-induced depression of ventilation is evidenced by changes in the slope of the carbon dioxide ventilatory response curve. (Mean ± SE.) (From Becker LD, Paulson BA, Miller RD, et al. Biphasic respiratory depression after fentanyl-droperidol or fentanyl alone used to supplement nitrous oxide anesthesia. *Anesthesiology* 1976;44:291–296; with permission.)

due to fentanyl is a potential postoperative problem (Fig. 3-21) (Becker et al., 1976). Secondary peaks in plasma concentrations of fentanyl and morphine have been attributed to sequestration of fentanyl in acidic gastric fluid (ion trapping). Sequestered fentanyl could then be absorbed from the more alkaline small intestine back into the circulation to increase the plasma concentration of opioid and cause depression of ventilation to recur. This, however, may not be the mechanism for the secondary peak of fentanyl, because reabsorbed opioid from the gastrointestinal tract or skeletal muscles, as evoked by movement associated with transfer from the operating room, would be subject to first-pass hepatic metabolism. An alternative explanation for the secondary peak of fentanyl is washout of opioid from the lungs as ventilation to perfusion relationships are reestablished in the postoperative period.

Cardiovascular Effects

In comparison with morphine, fentanyl even in large doses (50 μg/kg IV) does not evoke the release of histamine (see Fig. 3-12) (Rosow et al., 1982). As a result, dilatation of venous capacitance vessels leading to hypotension is unlikely. Carotid sinus baroreceptor reflex control of heart rate is markedly depressed by fentanyl, 10 μg/kg IV, administered to neonates (Fig. 3-22) (Murat et al., 1988). Therefore, changes in systemic blood pressure occurring during fentanyl anesthesia have to be carefully considered because cardiac output is principally rate dependent in neonates. Bradycardia is more prominent with fentanyl than morphine and may lead to occasional decreases in blood pressure and cardiac output. Allergic reactions occur rarely in

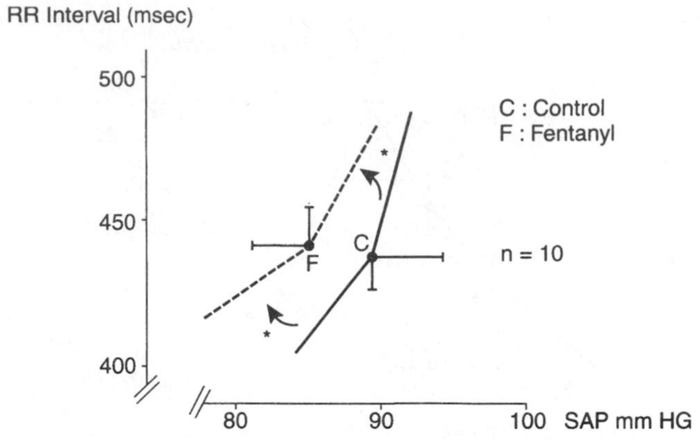

Figure 3-22. Fentanyl depresses the carotid sinus reflex–mediated heart rate response to changes in blood pressure in neonates. (*P <.02.) (From Murat I, Levron JB, Berg A, et al. Effects of fentanyl on baroreceptor reflex control of heart rate in newborn infants. *Anesthesiology* 1988;68:717–722, with permission.)

response to administration of fentanyl (Bennett et al., 1986). In this regard, latex anaphylaxis has been erroneously attributed to fentanyl allergy (Zucker-Pinchoff and Chandler, 1993).

Seizure Activity

Seizure activity has been described to follow rapid IV administration of fentanyl, sufentanil, and alfentanil (Manninen, 1997). In the absence of EEG evidence of seizure activity, however, it is difficult to distinguish opioid-induced skeletal muscle rigidity or myoclonus from seizure activity. Indeed, recording of the EEG during periods of opioid-induced skeletal muscle rigidity fails to reveal evidence of seizure activity in the brain (Smith et al., 1989). Even plasma concentrations as high as 1,750 ng/mL after rapid administration of fentanyl, 150 μg/kg IV, do not produce EEG evidence of seizure activity (Murkin et al., 1984). Conversely, opioids might produce a form of myoclonus secondary to depression of inhibitory neurons that would produce a clinical picture of seizure activity in the absence of EEG changes.

Somatosensory Evoked Potentials and Electroencephalogram

Fentanyl in doses exceeding 30 μg/kg IV produces changes in somatosensory evoked potentials that, although detectable, do not interfere with the use and interpretation of this monitor during anesthesia (Schubert et al., 1987). Opioids, including fentanyl, attenuate skeletal muscle movement at doses that have little effect on the EEG. This suggests that movement in response to surgical skin incision (used to measure MAC) primarily reflects the ability of a drug to obtund noxious reflexes and may not be the most appropriate measure for assessing consciousness or loss of consciousness (Glass et al., 1997). This opioid effect confounds the use of bispectral analysis as a measure of anesthetic adequacy when lack of movement with surgical skin incision is used to define efficacy (Sebel et al., 1997).

Intracranial Pressure

Administration of fentanyl and sufentanil to head injury patients has been associated with modest increases (6 to 9 mm Hg) in ICP despite maintenance of an unchanged Pa_{CO_2} (Albanese et al., 1993; Sperry et al., 1992). These increases in ICP are typically accompanied by decreases in mean arterial pressure and cerebral perfusion pressure. In fact, increases in ICP do not accompany the administration of sufentanil when changes in mean arterial pressure are prevented (Fig. 3-23) (Werner et al., 1995). This suggests that increases in ICP evoked by sufentanil (and presumably fentanyl) may have been due to autoregulatory decreases in cerebral vascular resistance due to decreases in systemic blood pressure resulting in vasodilation,

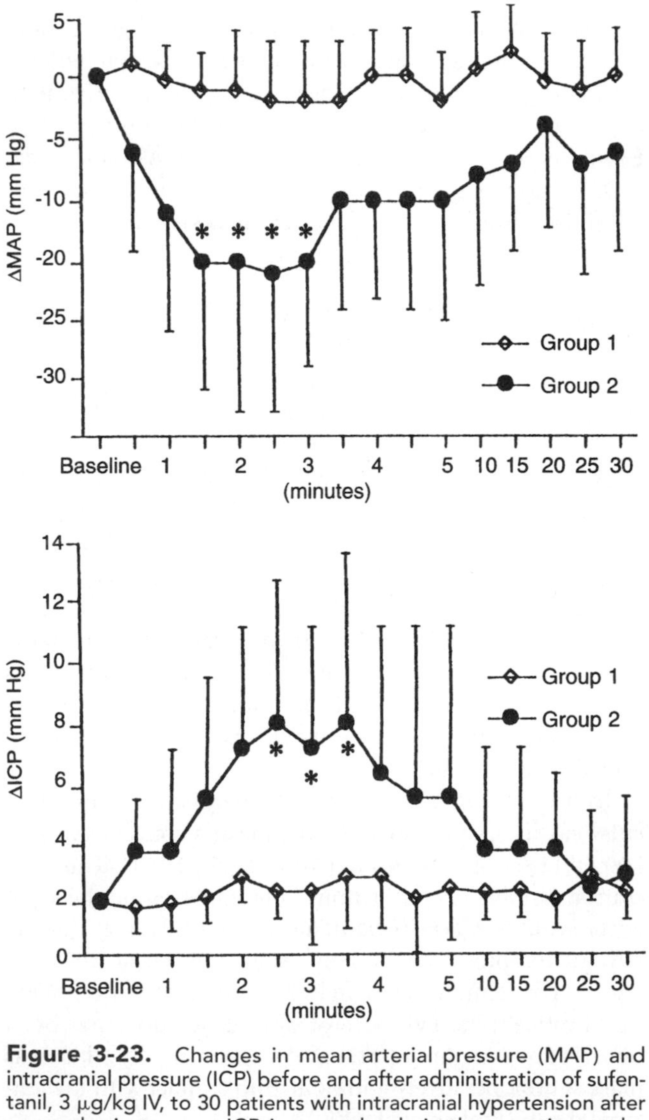

Figure 3-23. Changes in mean arterial pressure (MAP) and intracranial pressure (ICP) before and after administration of sufentanil, 3 μg/kg IV, to 30 patients with intracranial hypertension after severe brain trauma. ICP increased only in those patients who experienced a decrease in MAP after administration of sufentanil. (Mean ± SD; *P <.05 vs. group I.) (From Werner C, Kochs E, Bause H, et al. Effects of sufentanil on cerebral hemodynamics and intracranial pressure in patients with brain injury. *Anesthesiology* 1995;83:721–726; with permission.)

increased blood volume and increased ICP. Nevertheless, opioid-induced increases in ICP are similar in the presence of intact or impaired autoregulation suggesting that mechanisms other than activation of the vasodilatory cascade need to be considered (de Nadal et al., 2000).

Drug Interactions

Analgesic concentrations of fentanyl greatly potentiate the effects of midazolam and decrease the dose requirements of propofol. The opioid-benzodiazepine combination displays marked synergism with respect to hypnosis and depression of ventilation (Bailey et al., 1990a). In clinical practice, the advantage of synergy between opioids and benzodiazepines for the maintenance of patient comfort is carefully weighed against the disadvantages of the potentially adverse depressant effects of this combination. Preinduction administration of fentanyl IV (also sufentanil and alfentanil) may be associated with reflex coughing (Tweed and Dakin, 2001).

Sufentanil

Sufentanil is a thienyl analogue of fentanyl (see Fig. 3-15). The analgesic potency of sufentanil is five to ten times that of fentanyl, which parallels the greater affinity of sufentanil for opioid receptors compared with that of fentanyl. Based on the plasma concentration necessary to cause 50% of the maximum slowing on the EEG (EC50), sufentanil is 12 times more potent than fentanyl (Scott et al., 1991). An important distinction from fentanyl is the 1,000-fold difference between the analgesic dose of sufentanil and the dose that produces seizures in animals. This difference is 160-fold for fentanyl and may be important when large doses of opioid agonists are used to produce anesthesia. Transient skeletal muscle spasm has been described after the accidental intrathecal injection of a large dose of sufentanil (40 μg), suggesting an irritative effect produced by the opioid (Malinovsky et al., 1996).

Pharmacokinetics

The elimination half-time of sufentanil is intermediate between that of fentanyl and alfentanil (see Table 3-5) (Bovill et al., 1984). A single IV dose of sufentanil has a similar elimination half-time in patients with or without cirrhosis of the liver (Chauvin et al., 1989). A prolonged elimination half-time has been observed in elderly patients receiving sufentanil for abdominal aortic surgery (Hudson et al., 1989). The Vd and elimination half-time of sufentanil is increased in obese patients, which most likely reflects the high lipid solubility of this opioid (Schwartz et al., 1991).

A high tissue affinity is consistent with the lipophilic nature of sufentanil, which permits rapid penetration of the blood-brain barrier and onset of CNS effects (effect-site equilibration time of 6.2 minutes is similar to that of 6.8 minutes for fentanyl) (Scott et al., 1991). A rapid redistribution to inactive tissue sites terminates the effect of small doses, but a cumulative drug effect can accompany large or repeated doses of sufentanil. Sufentanil undergoes significant first-pass pulmonary uptake (approximately 60%) after rapid IV injection (Boer et al., 1996). This pulmonary first-pass uptake is similar to fentanyl and greater than morphine (about 7%) and alfentanil (about 10%).

The extensive protein binding of sufentanil (92.5%) compared with that of fentanyl (79% to 87%) contributes to a smaller Vd, which is characteristic of sufentanil. Binding to alpha$_1$-acid glycoprotein constitutes a principal proportion of the total plasma protein binding of sufentanil. Levels of alpha$_1$-acid glycoprotein vary over a threefold range in healthy volunteers and are increased after surgery, which could result in a decrease in the plasma concentration of pharmacologically active unbound sufentanil. Lower concentrations of alpha$_1$-acid glycoprotein in neonates and infants probably account for decreases in protein binding of sufentanil in these age groups compared with that in older children and adults (Meistelman et al., 1990). The resulting increased free fraction of sufentanil in the neonate might contribute to enhanced effects of this opioid. Indeed, fentanyl and its derivatives produce anesthesia and depression of ventilation at lower doses in neonates than in adults (Greeley et al., 1987; Yaster, 1987).

Metabolism

Sufentanil is rapidly metabolized by *N*-dealkylation at the piperidine nitrogen and by O-demethylation. The products of *N*-dealkylation are pharmacologically inactive, whereas desmethyl sufentanil has about 10% of the activity of sufentanil. Less than 1% of an administered dose of sufentanil appears unchanged in urine. Indeed, the high lipid solubility of sufentanil results in maximal renal tubular reabsorption of free drug as well as its enhanced access to hepatic microsomal enzymes. Extensive hepatic extraction means that clearance of sufentanil will be sensitive to changes in hepatic blood flow but not to alterations in the drug-metabolizing capacity of the liver. Sufentanil metabolites are excreted almost equally in urine and feces, with about 30% appearing as conjugates. The production of a weakly active metabolite and the substantial amount of conjugated metabolite formation imply the possible importance of normal renal function for the clearance of sufentanil. Indeed, prolonged depression of ventilation in association with an abnormally increased plasma concentration of sufentanil has been observed in a patient with chronic renal failure (Waggum et al., 1985).

Context-Sensitive Half-Time

The context-sensitive half-time of sufentanil is actually less than that for alfentanil for continuous infusions of up to 8 hours in duration (see Fig. 3-18) (Egan et al., 1993;

Hughes et al., 1992). This shorter context-sensitive half-time can be explained in part by the large Vd of sufentanil compared to alfentanil. After termination of a sufentanil infusion, the decrease in the plasma drug concentration is accelerated not only by metabolism but by continued redistribution of sufentanil into peripheral tissue compartments. Compared with alfentanil, sufentanil may have a more favorable recovery profile when used over a longer period of time. Conversely, alfentanil has a pharmacokinetic advantage for the treatment of discrete and transient noxious stimuli because its short effect-site equilibration time allows rapid access of the drug to the brain and facilitates titration.

Clinical Uses

In volunteers, a single dose of sufentanil, 0.1 to 0.4 μg/kg IV, produces a longer period of analgesia and less depression of ventilation than does a comparable dose of fentanyl (1 to 4 μg/kg IV) (Bailey et al., 1990b). Compared with large doses of morphine or fentanyl, sufentanil, 18.9 μg/kg IV, results in more rapid induction of anesthesia, earlier emergence from anesthesia, and earlier tracheal extubation (Fig. 3-24) (Sanford et al., 1986). As observed with other opioids, sufentanil causes a decrease in cerebral metabolic oxygen requirements and cerebral blood flow is also decreased or unchanged (Mayer et al., 1990). Bradycardia produced by sufentanil may be sufficient to decrease cardiac output. As observed with fentanyl, delayed depression of ventilation has also been described after the administration of sufentanil (Chang and Fish, 1985).

Although large doses of sufentanil (10 to 30 μg/kg IV) or fentanyl (50 to 150 μg/kg IV) produce minimal hemodynamic effects in patients with good left ventricular function, the systemic blood pressure and hormonal (catecholamine) responses to painful stimulation such as median sternotomy are not predictably prevented (Philbin et al., 1990). It seems unlikely that any clinically useful dose of sufentanil or fentanyl will abolish such responses in all patients. Use of large doses of opioids, including sufentanil or fentanyl, to produce the IV induction of anesthesia may result in rigidity of chest and abdominal musculature. This skeletal muscle rigidity makes ventilation of the patient's lungs with positive airway pressure difficult. Difficult ventilation during sufentanil-induced skeletal muscle rigidity may reflect obstruction at the level of the glottis or above, which can be overcome by tracheal intubation (Abrams et al., 1996).

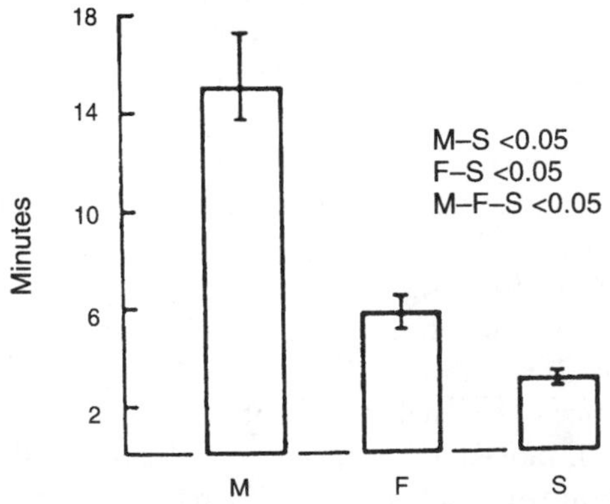

Figure 3-24. The time between the beginning of opioid administration and the patient's ability to respond to verbal command was defined as induction time. Sufentanil resulted in a significantly more rapid induction of anesthesia than did morphine or fentanyl. (Mean ± SE.) (F, fentanyl; M, morphine; S, sufentanil.) (From Sanford TJ, Smith NT, Dee-Silver H, et al. A comparison of morphine, fentanyl, and sufentanil anesthesia for cardiac surgery: induction, emergence, and extubation. *Anesth Analg* 1986;65: 259–266; with permission.)

Alfentanil

Alfentanil is an analogue of fentanyl that is less potent (one-fifth to one-tenth) and has one-third the duration of action of fentanyl (see Fig. 3-15). A unique advantage of alfentanil compared with fentanyl and sufentanil is the more rapid onset of action (rapid effect-site equilibration) after the IV administration of alfentanil. For example, the effect-site equilibration time for alfentanil is 1.4 minutes compared with 6.8 and 6.2 minutes for fentanyl and sufentanil, respectively (see Table 3-5) (Scott et al., 1985; Scott and Stanski, 1987; Shafer and Varvel, 1991).

Pharmacokinetics

Alfentanil has a short elimination half-time compared with fentanyl and sufentanil (see Table 3-5). Cirrhosis of the liver, but not cholestatic disease, prolongs the elimination half-time of alfentanil (Davis et al., 1989). Renal failure does not alter the clearance or elimination half-time of alfentanil (Chauvin et al., 1987a). The elimination half-time of alfentanil is shorter in children (4 to 8 years old) than adults, reflecting a smaller Vd in these younger patients (Meistelman et al., 1987).

The rapid effect-site equilibration characteristic of alfentanil is a result of the low pK of this opioid such that nearly 90% of the drug exists in the nonionized form at physiologic pH. It is the nonionized fraction that readily crosses the blood-brain barrier. The rapid peak effect of alfentanil at the brain is useful when an opioid is required to blunt the response to a single, brief stimulus such as tracheal intubation or performance of a retrobulbar block.

The Vd of alfentanil is four to six times smaller than that of fentanyl (see Table 3-5) (Camu et al., 1982; Stanski and Hug, 1982). This smaller Vd compared with that of fentanyl reflects lower lipid solubility and higher protein binding. Despite this lesser lipid solubility, penetration of the blood-brain barrier by alfentanil is rapid because of its high degree of nonionization at physiologic pH. Alfentanil is principally bound to alpha$_1$-acid glycoprotein, a protein whose plasma concentration is not altered by liver disease. Because protein binding is similar, it is likely that a decreased percentage of adipose tissue in children is responsible for the short elimination half-time.

Metabolism

Alfentanil is metabolized predominantly by two independent pathways, piperidine *N*-dealkylation to noralfentanil and amide *N*-dealkylation to *N*-phenylpropionamide. Noralfentanil is the major metabolite recovered in urine, with <0.5% of an administered dose of alfentanil being excreted unchanged. The efficiency of hepatic metabolism is emphasized by clearance of about 96% of alfentanil from the plasma within 60 minutes of its administration.

Confounding attempts to develop reliable infusion regimens to attain and maintain specific plasma concentrations of alfentanil is the wide interindividual variability in alfentanil pharmacokinetics. The most significant factor responsible for unpredictable alfentanil disposition is the tenfold interindividual variability in alfentanil systemic clearance, presumably reflecting variability in hepatic intrinsic clearance. In this regard, it is likely that population variability in P-450 3A4 (CYP3A) activity (most abundant P-450 hepatic enzyme and the major isoform of P-450 responsible for alfentanil metabolism and clearance) is the mechanistic explanation for the interindividual variability in alfentanil disposition (Kharasch et al., 1997). Alfentanil clearance is markedly influenced by CYP3A activity and alfentanil is a sensitive and validated probe for CYP3A activity (Ibrahim et al., 2003). Alterations in P-450 activity may be responsible for the ability of erythromycin to inhibit the metabolism of alfentanil and a resulting prolonged opioid effect (Bartkowski and McDonnell, 1990).

Context-Sensitive Half-Time

The context-sensitive half-time of alfentanil is actually longer than that of sufentanil for infusions up to 8 hours in duration (see Fig. 3-18) (Egan et al., 1993; Hughes et al., 1992). This phenomenon can be explained in part by the large Vd of sufentanil. After termination of a continuous infusion of sufentanil, the decrease in the plasma drug concentration is accelerated not only by metabolism but also by continued redistribution of sufentanil into peripheral compartments. Conversely, the Vd of alfentanil equilibrates rapidly; therefore peripheral distribution of drug away from the plasma is not a significant contributor to the decrease in the plasma concentration after discontinuation of the alfentanil infusion. Thus, despite the short elimination half-time of alfentanil, it may not necessarily be a superior choice to sufentanil for ambulatory sedation techniques.

Clinical Uses

Alfentanil has a rapid onset and offset of intense analgesia reflecting its very prompt effect-site equilibration. This characteristic of alfentanil is used to provide analgesia when the noxious stimulation is acute but transient as associated with laryngoscopy and tracheal intubation and performance of a retrobulbar block. For example, administration of alfentanil, 15 μg/kg IV, about 90 seconds before beginning direct laryngoscopy is effective in blunting the systemic blood pressure and heart rate response to tracheal intubation (Fig. 3-25) (Miller et al., 1993). The catecholamine response to this noxious stimulation is also blunted by alfentanil, 30 μg/kg IV (Fig. 3-26) (Miller et al., 1993). Alfentanil in doses of 10 to 20 μg/kg IV blunts the circulatory but not the catecholamine release response to the sudden exposure to high inhaled concentrations of desflurane (Yonker-Sell et al., 1996). Alfentanil, 150 to 300 μg/kg IV, administered rapidly, produces unconsciousness in about 45 seconds. After this induction, maintenance of anesthesia can be provided with a continuous infusion of alfentanil, 25 to 150 μg/kg/hour IV, combined with an inhaled drug (Ausems et al., 1983). Unlike other opioids, supplemental

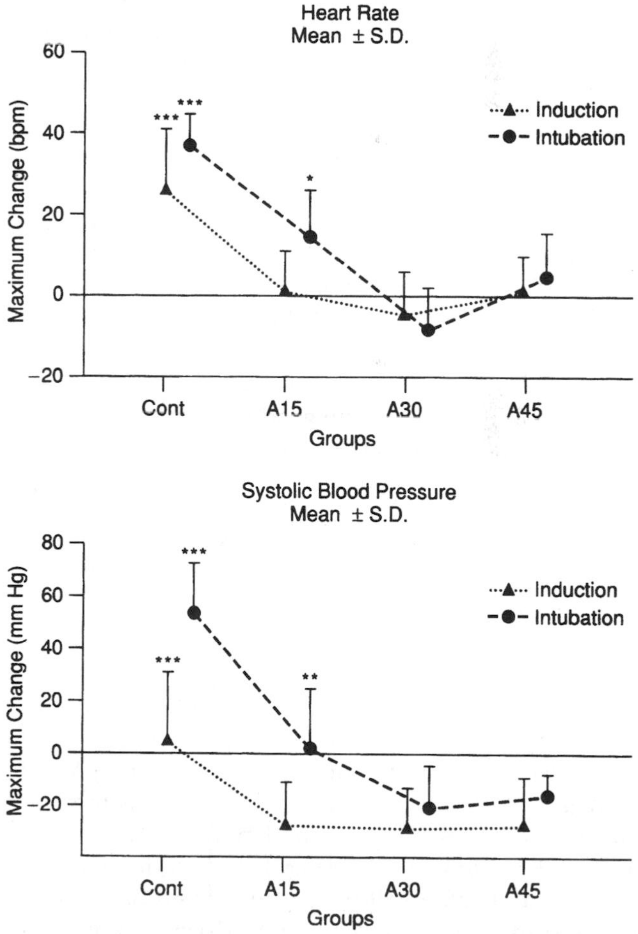

Figure 3-25. Dose-response curves of the maximum (%) changes in heart rate and systolic blood pressure in response to induction of anesthesia and tracheal intubation. (A15, 15 μg/kg IV of alfentanil; A30, 30 μg/kg IV of alfentanil; A45, 45 μg/kg IV of alfentanil; Cont, control; *different from A30; **different from A30, A45; ***different from A15, A30, A45; $P < .05$ by ANOVA.) (From Miller DR, Martineau RJ, O'Brien H, et al. Effect of alfentanil on the hemodynamic and catecholamine response to tracheal intubation. *Anesth Analg* 1993;76:1040–1046; with permission.)

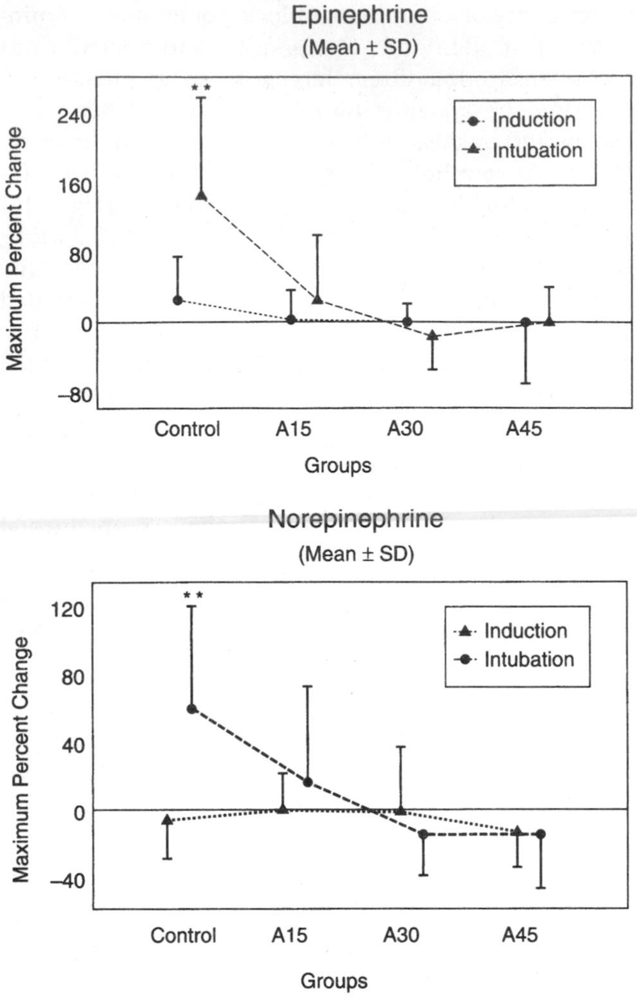

Figure 3-26. Dose-response curves of the maximum (%) changes in the plasma concentrations of epinephrine and norepinephrine in response to induction of anesthesia and tracheal intubation. (A15, 15 μg/kg IV of alfentanil; A30, 30 μg/kg IV of alfentanil; A45, 45 μg/kg IV of alfentanil; **different from A30, A45; $P < .05$ by ANOVA.) (From Miller DR, Martineau RJ, O'Brien H, et al. Effect of alfentanil on the hemodynamic and catecholamine response to tracheal intubation. *Anesth Analg* 1993;76:1040–1046; with permission.)

doses of alfentanil seem to be more likely to decrease systemic blood pressure that is increased after painful stimulation. Alfentanil increases biliary tract pressures similarly to fentanyl, but the duration of this increase is shorter than that produced by fentanyl (Hynyen et al., 1986). Alfentanil, compared with equipotent doses of fentanyl and sufentanil, is associated with a lower incidence of postoperative nausea and vomiting in outpatients (Fig. 3-27) (Langevin et al., 1999). Acute dystonia has been described after administration of alfentanil to a patient with untreated Parkinson's disease (Mets, 1991). This may reflect an ability of opioids to decrease central dopaminergic transmission and suggests caution in administration of this opioid to patients with untreated Parkinson's disease.

Remifentanil

Remifentanil is a selective mu opioid agonist with an analgesic potency similar to that of fentanyl (15 to 20 times as potent as alfentanil) and a blood-brain equilibration (effect-site equilibration) time similar to that of alfentanil (see Table 3-5) (Burkle et al., 1996; Egan et al., 1993; Jhaveri et al., 1997; Rosow, 1993; Thompson and Rowbotham, 1996). Although chemically related to the fentanyl family of short-acting phenylpiperidine derivatives, remifentanil is structurally unique because of its ester linkage (see Fig. 3-15). Remifentanil's ester structure renders it susceptible to hydrolysis by nonspecific plasma and tissue esterases to inactive metabolites (Fig. 3-28) (Egan et al., 1993). This unique pathway of metabolism imparts to remifentanil (a) brevity of action, (b) precise and rapidly titratable effect due to its rapid onset (similar to that of alfentanil) and offset, (c) noncumulative effects, and (d) rapid recovery after discontinuation of its administration.

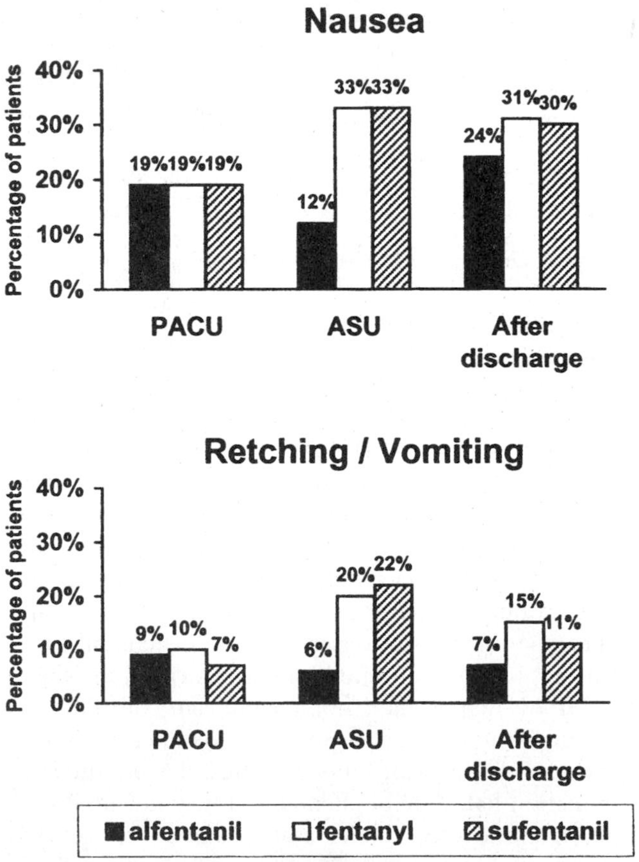

Figure 3-27. Incidence of nausea and retching/vomiting in the postanesthesia care unit (PACU), in the ambulatory surgery unit (ASU) and after discharge from the hospital. In the PACU there was no difference between the opioid groups. In the ASU, the incidence of nausea and retching/vomiting was significantly lower with alfentanil compared with fentanyl ($P < 0.05$) and sufentanil ($P < 0.01$). (From Langevin S, Lessard MR, Trepanier CA, et al. Alfentanil causes less postoperative nausea and vomiting than equipotent doses of fentanyl or sufentanil in outpatients. *Anesthesiology* 1999:91:1666–1673; with permission.)

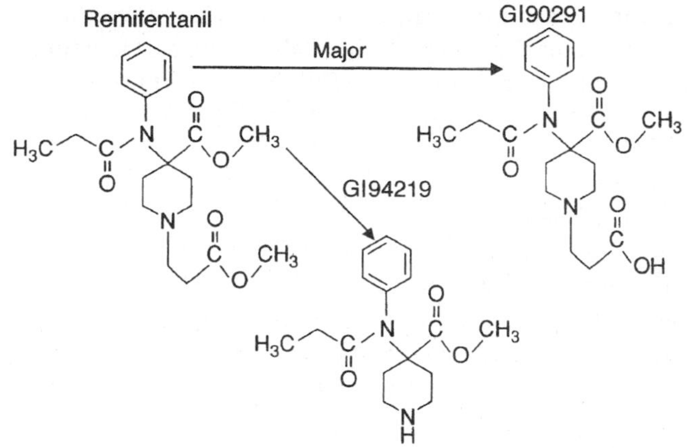

Figure 3-28. Remifentanil undergoes hydrolysis by nonspecific plasma and tissue esterases (major pathway) to a carboxylic acid metabolite (GI90291) that has no clinically significant agonist activity at opioid receptors. *N*-dealkylation of remifentanil to GI94219 is a minor pathway of metabolism. (From Egan TD, Lemmens HJM, Fiset P, et al. The pharmacokinetics of the new short-acting opioid remifentanil (GI87084B) in healthy adult male volunteers. *Anesthesiology* 1993;79:881–892; with permission.)

Ventilation

After administration of 0.5 μg/kg IV remifentanil there is a decrease in the slope and downward shift of the carbon dioxide ventilatory response curve that reaches its nadir after about 150 seconds following injection (Fig. 3-29) (Babenco et al., 2000). Recovery after this small dose of remifentanil was complete within about 15 minutes. The combination of remifentanil and propofol is synergistic resulting in severe depression of ventilation (Fig 3-30) (Nieuwenhuijs et al., 2003).

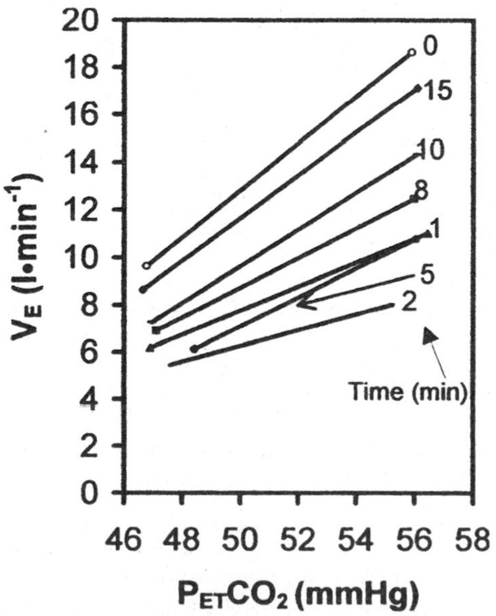

Figure 3-29. Carbon dioxide response curves before (time = 0) and at selected times after administration of 0.5 μg/kg IV remifentanil. (From Babenco HD, Conard PF, Gross JB. The pharmacodynamic effect of a remifentanil bolus on ventilatory control. *Anesthesiology* 2000;92:393–398; with permission.)

Pharmacokinetics

The pharmacokinetics of remifentanil are characterized by small Vd, rapid clearance, and low interindividual variability compared to other IV anesthetic drugs. The rapid metabolism of remifentanil and its small Vd mean that remifentanil will accumulate less than other opioids. Because of its rapid systemic clearance, remifentanil provides pharmacokinetic advantages in clinical situations requiring predictable termination of drug effect. Remifentanil's pharmacokinetics are similar in obese and lean patients confirming that clinical dosing regimens should be based on ideal (lean) body mass rather than total body weight (Egan et al., 1998).

The most salient pharmacokinetic feature of remifentanil is the extraordinary clearance of nearly 3 liters/minute, which is about eight times more rapid than that of alfentanil. Remifentanil has a smaller Vd than alfentanil. The combination of rapid clearance and small Vd produces a drug with a uniquely evanescent effect. In fact, the rate of decline (context-sensitive half-time) of the remifentanil plasma concentration will be nearly independent of the infusion duration (see Fig. 3-18) (Burkle et al., 1996; Egan et al., 1993). The rapid effect-site equilibration means that a remifentanil infusion rate will promptly approach steady-state in the plasma and its effect site. It is estimated that remifentanil plasma concentrations will reach a steady state within 10 minutes of beginning an infusion. The relationship between infusion rate and opioid concentration will be less variable for remifentanil than for other opioids. Furthermore, the rapid clearance of remifentanil,

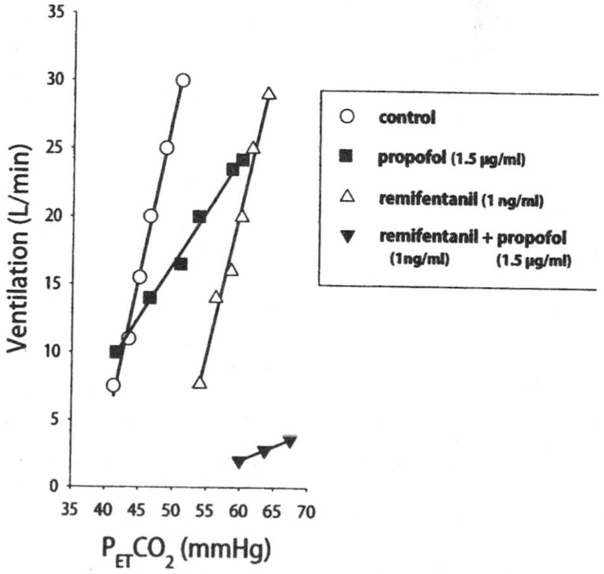

Figure 3-30. Ventilatory response curves from one individual. The combined administration of remifentanil and propofol decreased the slope of the carbon dioxide response curve and caused a rightward shift. (From Niewenhuijs DJF, Olofsen E, Romberd RR, et al. Response surface modeling of remifentanil-propofol interaction on cardiorespiratory control and bispectral index. *Anesthesiology* 2003;98:312–322; with permission.)

combined with the rapid blood-brain equilibration, means changes in infusion rates will be paralleled by prompt changes in drug effect.

Based on analysis of the EEG response, it is concluded that remifentanil is about 19 times more potent than alfentanil (EC_{50} for EEG depression 20 ng/mL versus 376 ng/mL) (Egan et al., 1993). The effect-site equilibration time, however, is similar for both opioids, suggesting that remifentanil will have an alfentanil-like onset (see Table 3-5). For example, after a rapid IV injection, the peak effect-site concentration of remifentanil will be present within 1.1 minutes, compared with 1.4 minutes for alfentanil. The effect, however, will be more transient after administration of remifentanil than alfentanil.

Metabolism

Remifentanil is unique among the opioids in undergoing metabolism by nonspecific plasma and tissue esterases to inactive metabolites (see Fig. 3-26) (Egan et al., 1993). The principal metabolite, remifentanil acid, is 300 to 4,600-fold less potent than remifentanil as a mu agonist and is excreted primarily by the kidneys. This and the other inactive metabolites undergo renal excretion. *N*-dealkylation of remifentanil is a minor metabolic pathway in humans. Remifentanil does not appear to be a substrate for butyrylcholinesterases (pseudocholinesterase), and thus its clearance should not be affected by cholinesterase deficiency or anticholinergics (Burkle et al., 1996). Additionally, it is likely that remifentanil's pharmacokinetics will be unchanged by renal or hepatic failure because esterase metabolism is usually preserved in these states (Hoke et al., 1997). In this regard, the clearance of remifentanil is not altered during the anhepatic phase of liver transplantation. Hypothermic cardiopulmonary bypass decreases clearance of remifentanil by an average of 20%, presumably reflecting the effect of temperature on blood and tissue esterase activity. Esterase metabolism appears to be a very well-preserved metabolic system with little variability between individuals, which contributes to the predictability of drug effect associated with the infusion of remifentanil (Rosow, 1993).

Elimination Half-Time

An estimated 99.8% of remifentanil is eliminated during the distribution (0.9 minute) and elimination (6.3 minutes) half-time. Clinically, remifentanil behaves like a drug with an elimination half-time of 6 minutes or less.

Context-Sensitive Half-Time

Context-sensitive half-time for remifentanil is independent of the duration of infusion and is estimated to be about 4 minutes (see Fig. 3-18) (Burkle et al., 1996; Egan et al., 1993; Kapila et al., 1995). This drug's rapid clearance is responsible for the lack of accumulation even during prolonged periods of infusion. In contrast, the context-sensitive half-time for sufentanil, alfentanil, and fentanyl is longer and dependent on the duration of the infusion (see Table 3-5) (see Fig. 3-18) (Burkle et al., 1996; Egan et al., 1993).

Clinical Uses

The clinical uses of remifentanil reflect the unique pharmacokinetic profile of this opioid, which allows rapid onset of drug effect, precise titration to the desired effect, the ability to maintain a sufficient plasma opioid concentration to suppress the stress response, and rapid recovery from the drug's effects. In cases where a profound analgesic effect is desired transiently (performance of a retrobulbar block), remifentanil may be useful. Prompt onset and short duration of action make remifentanil a useful selection for suppression of the transient sympathetic nervous system response to direct laryngoscopy and tracheal intubation in at risk patients (Thompson et al., 1998). Intermittent remifentanil administered as patient controlled analgesia is an effective and reliable analgesic during labor and delivery (Evron et al., 2005). Conceivably, remifentanil could be used for long operations, when a quick recovery time is desired (neurologic assessment, wake-up test). High-dose remifentanil anesthetic techniques will be associated with a more rapid recovery and less risk of postoperative depression of ventilation than similar techniques with other opioids. The rapid onset and offset of action of remifentanil makes it possible to quickly adjust the required level of sedation in mechanically ventilated critically ill patients (Dahaba et al., 2004).

Anesthesia can be induced with remifentanil, 1 μg/kg IV administered over 60 to 90 seconds, or with a gradual initiation of the infusion at 0.5 to 1.0 μg/kg IV for about 10 minutes, before administration of a standard hypnotic prior to tracheal intubation (Hogue et al., 1996). The dose of hypnotic drug may need to be decreased to compensate for the synergistic effect with remifentanil. Remifentanil can be used as the analgesic component of a general anesthetic (0.25 to 1.00 μg/kg IV or 0.05 to 2.00 μg/kg/minute IV) or sedation techniques with the ability to rapidly recover from undesirable effects such as opioid-induced depression of ventilation or excessive sedation (Burkle et al., 1996). Remifentanil, 0.05 to 0.10 μg/kg/minute in combination with midazolam, 2 mg IV, provides effective sedation and analgesia during monitored anesthesia care in otherwise healthy adult patients (Avramov et al., 1996). Midazolam also produces a dose-dependent potentiation of remifentanil's depressant effect on breathing rate. Changes in remifentanil drug effect predictably follow changes in the infusion rate, making it possible to more precisely titrate to the desired response than with other opioids. Before cessation of the remifentanil infusion, a longer-acting opioid may be administered to ensure analgesia when the patient awakens. The spinal or epidural administration of remifentanil is not recommended, as the safety of the vehicle (glycine, which acts as an inhibitory neurotransmitter) or opioid have not been determined (Burkle et al., 1996). Remifentanil, 100 μg IV, attenuates the acute hemodynamic responses to electroconvulsive therapy and does not alter the duration of electroconvulsive-induced seizure activity (Recart et al., 2003).

Side Effects

The advantage of remifentanil possessing a short recovery period may be considered a disadvantage if the infusion is stopped suddenly, whether it be deliberate or accidental. It is important to administer a longer-acting opioid for post-operative analgesia when remifentanil has been administered for this purpose intraoperatively. All fentanyl analogs, including remifentanil, have been reported to induce "seizure-like" activity (Haber and Litman, 2001).

Nausea and vomiting, depression of ventilation and mild decreases in systemic blood pressure and heart rate may accompany the administration of remifentanil. Depression of ventilation produced by remifentanil is not altered by renal or liver dysfunction. Histamine release does not accompany the administration of remifentanil. ICP and intraocular pressure are not changed by remifentanil (Guy et al., 1997; Warner et al., 1996). High-dose remifentanil decreases cerebral blood flow and cerebral metabolic oxygen requirements without impairing cerebrovascular carbon dioxide reactivity (Klimscha et al., 2003). Remifentanil delays drainage of dye from the gallbladder into the duodenum but the delay is shorter than with other opioids (Fragen et al., 1999). Placental passage of remifentanil is prompt but neonatal effects do not seem to occur (Kan et al., 1998).

Acute Opioid Tolerance

Postoperative analgesic requirements in patients receiving relatively large doses of remifentanil intraoperatively are often surprisingly high suggesting remifentanil may be associated with acute opioid tolerance (Fig. 3-31) (Guignard et al., 2000). In addition, delayed hyperalgesia may be produced by acute exposure to large doses of opioids. Tolerance to opioids is pharmacodynamic and tolerance is dose-dependent. Possible mechanisms for tolerance include alterations of the NDMA receptors and its intracellular second messenger systems. In this regard, NMDA receptor antagonists such as ketamine and magnesium block opioid tolerance. Not all data supports the development of acute opioid tolerance following remifentanil-based anesthesia (Cortinez et al., 2001; Gustorff et al., 2002).

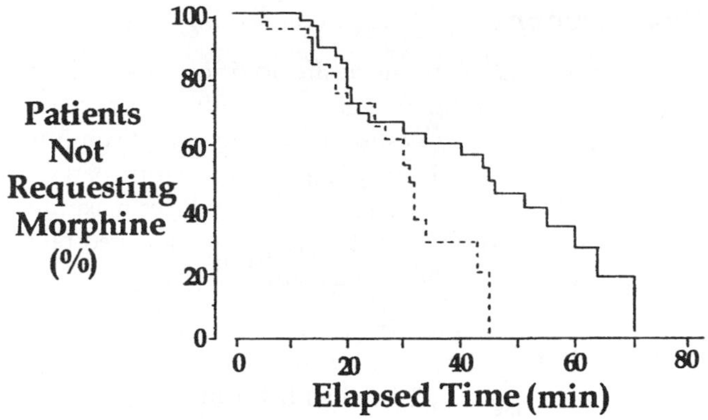

Figure 3-31. Cumulative curves for patients who did not request an additional morphine injection following discontinuation of remifentanil (dashed line) or desflurane (solid line). (From Guignard B, Bossard AE, Coste C, et al. Acute opioid tolerance. Intraoperative remifentanil increases postoperative pain and morphine requirement. *Anesthesiology* 2000;93:409–417; with permission.)

Codeine

Codeine is the result of the substitution of a methyl group for the hydroxyl group on the number 3 carbon of morphine (see Fig. 3-1). The presence of this methyl group limits its first-pass hepatic metabolism and accounts for the efficacy of codeine when administered orally. The elimination half-time of codeine after oral or IM administration is 3.0 to 3.5 hours. About 10% of administered codeine is demethylated in the liver to morphine, which may be responsible for the analgesic effect of codeine. Any remaining codeine is demethylated to inactive norcodeine, which is conjugated or excreted unchanged by the kidneys.

Codeine is an effective antitussive at oral doses of 15 mg. Maximal analgesia, equivalent to that produced by 650 mg of aspirin, occurs with 60 mg of codeine. When administered IM, 120 mg of codeine is equivalent in analgesic effect to 10 mg of morphine. Most often, codeine is included in medications as an antitussive or is combined with nonopioid analgesics for the treatment of mild to moderate pain. The liability of physical dependence on codeine appears to be less than that of morphine and occurs only rarely after oral analgesic use. Codeine produces minimal sedation, nausea, vomiting, and constipation. Dizziness may occur in ambulatory patients. Even in large doses, codeine is unlikely to produce apnea. Administration of codeine IV is not recommended, because histamine-induced hypotension is likely.

Hydromorphone

Hydromorphone is a derivative of morphine that is about five times as potent as morphine but has a slightly shorter duration of action. This opioid produces somewhat more sedation and evokes less euphoria than morphine. Because of rapid elimination and redistribution, oral dosing every 4 hours is needed to maintain adequate plasma concentrations for analgesia. Hydromorphone is an effective alternative to morphine in the treatment of opioid-responsive moderate to severe pain (Angst et al., 2001). This drug's medium duration of action and high water solubility make it possible to utilize a nasal transmucosal delivery system (Coda et al., 2003). The uses and side effects of hydromorphone are the same as those of morphine.

Oxymorphone

Oxymorphone is the result of the addition of a hydroxyl group to hydromorphone. It is about 10 times as potent as morphine and seems to cause more nausea and vomiting. Physical dependence liability is great. An oral preparation of oxymorphone (immediate release) produces maximum plasma concentrations in 0.5 hour with associated rapid onset of analgesia (Gimbel and Ahdieh, 2004).

Oxycodone

Sustained-release oral oxycodone preparations (Oxy Contin®; Percocet®; Percodan®) provide stable plasma concentrations for the treatment of moderate to severe pain. Abuse potential is great including tampering (crushing and powdering) for intravenous or intranasal injection to obtain a rapid and powerful opioid effect.

Hydrocodone

Hydrocodone is available as an oral preparation (Vicodan®) for the treatment of chronic pain. Abuse potential is high for patients being treated with hydrocodone.

Methadone

Methadone is a synthetic opioid agonist that produces analgesia in the setting of chronic pain syndromes and is highly effective by the oral route (Fig. 3-32). The efficient oral absorption, prompt onset of action, and prolonged duration of action of methadone render this an attractive drug for suppression of withdrawal symptoms in physically dependent persons such as heroin addicts.

Opioid Withdrawal

Methadone can substitute for morphine in addicts at about one-fourth the dosage. Controlled withdrawal from opioids using methadone is milder and less acute than that from morphine. Methadone, 20 mg IV, produces postoperative analgesia lasting >24 hours, reflecting its prolonged (35 hours) elimination half-time. This drug is metabolized in the liver to inactive substances that are excreted in the urine and bile with small amounts of unchanged drug.

The side effects of methadone (depression of ventilation, miosis, constipation, biliary tract spasm) resemble those of morphine. Its sedative and euphoric actions are less than those produced by morphine. Methadone-induced miosis is less prominent than that caused by morphine, and the addict develops complete tolerance to this action.

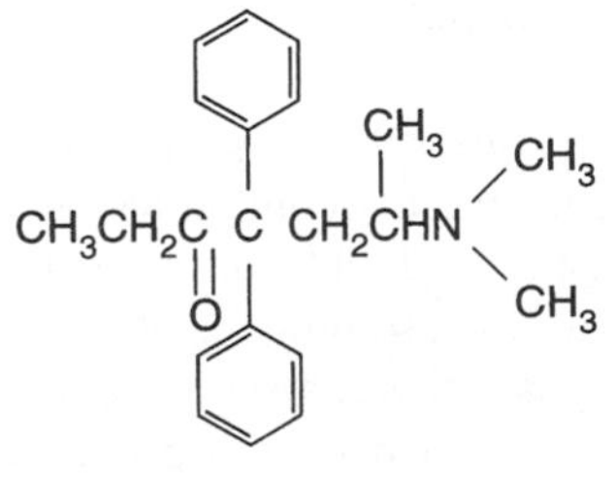

Figure 3-32. Methadone.

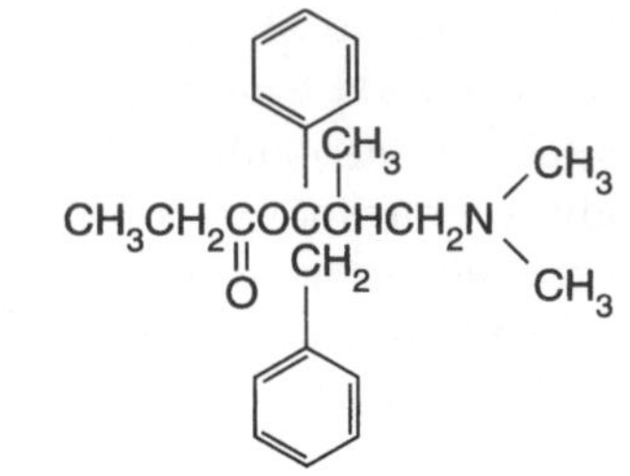

Figure 3-33. Propoxyphene.

Treatment of Chronic Pain

Methadone has been proposed as an alternative to slow-release formulations for treatment of chronic pain because of its low abuse potential. In addition, NMDA receptor antagonist activity may be useful in treatment of neuropathic pain and minimize the potential for development of tolerance. The principal disadvantage for use of methadone to treat chronic pain is it prolonged and unpredictable half-time. When methadone is administered more than once daily, as is common in treatment of chronic pain syndromes, the drug may accumulate and result in high plasma concentrations and associated depression of ventilation (Fishman et al., 2002). For this reason, slow-release formulations (oxycodone) may be preferable to methadone for the treatment of outpatient postoperative pain (Wilson, 2002).

Propoxyphene

Propoxyphene is structurally similar to methadone and binds to opioid receptors as reflected by antagonism of its pharmacologic effects by naloxone (Fig. 3-33). Oral doses of 90 to 120 mg of propoxyphene produce analgesia and CNS effects similar to those produced by 60 mg of codeine and 650 mg of aspirin. The only clinical use of propoxyphene is treatment of mild to moderate pain that is not adequately relieved by aspirin. Propoxyphene does not possess antipyretic or anti-inflammatory effects, and antitussive activity is not significant.

Propoxyphene is completely absorbed after oral administration, but because of extensive first-pass hepatic metabolism (demethylation to norpropoxyphene); the systemic availability is greatly decreased. The elimination half-time after oral administration is about 14.5 hours. The most common side effects of propoxyphene are vertigo, sedation, nausea, and vomiting. Propoxyphene is about one-third as potent as codeine in depressing ventilation. Overdose, however, is complicated by seizures and depression of ventilation.

Abrupt discontinuation of chronically administered propoxyphene results in a mild withdrawal syndrome. The incidence of abuse of propoxyphene is similar to that of codeine. Administration of this drug IV produces severe damage to veins and limits abuse by this route. Administration of propoxyphene in combination with alcohol and other CNS depressants may result in excessive drug-induced depression of ventilation.

Tramadol

Tramadol is a centrally acting analgesic that has moderate affinity for mu receptors and weak kappa and delta opioid receptor affinity but is 5 to 10 times less potent than morphine as an analgesic (Budd and Landlord, 1999). In addition to mu opioid agonist effects, tramadol enhances the function of the spinal descending inhibitory pathways by inhibition of neuronal reuptake of norepinephrine and 5-hydroxytryptamine (serotonin) as well as presynaptic stimulation of 5-hydroxytryptamine release. In volunteers, naloxone antagonized only an estimated 30% of the effect of tramadol (Collart et al., 1993).

Tramadol is a racemic mixture of two enantiomers, one of which is responsible for inhibition of norepinephrine uptake, whereas the other is responsible for inhibition of 5-hydroxytryptamine reuptake and facilitation of its release, plus the actions of this drug at mu receptors. In this regard, tramadol may be an exception to the argument that chiral mixtures should be avoided when technology exists to prepare a single, pure isomer (Calvey, 1992). For example, the production of analgesia by tramadol with the absence of depression of ventilation and a low potential for the development of tolerance, dependence, and abuse may be a result of the complementary and synergistic antinociceptive interaction of the two enantiomers. Tramadol is metabolized by hepatic P-450 enzyme systems to the major metabolite is O-desmethyltramadol, which also exerts modest stereoselective analgesic effects.

Tramadol 3 mg/kg administered orally, IM, or IV is effective for the treatment of moderate to severe pain. A marked decrease in postoperative shivering has been noted in treated patients and the minimal depressant effects on breathing are useful (Nieuwenhuijs et al., 2001). Tramadol slows gastric emptying although the effect is small compared with other opioids (Crighton et al., 1998). Tramadol is useful for the treatment of chronic pain because it does not cause tolerance or addiction and is not associated with major organ toxicity or significant sedative effects. This drug is useful in patients who do not tolerate nonsteroidal anti-inflammatory drugs. Disadvantages of tramadol include its interaction with coumadin anticoagulants (not all reports confirm this interaction) and the occurrence of drug-related seizures (avoid in patients with epilepsy or those being treated with drugs that lower the seizure threshold such as antidepressants) (Budd and Langford, 1999; Kahn et al., 1997). A further drawback to the perioperative use of this drug as an analgesic is a high incidence of associated nausea and vomiting. Ondansetron may interfere with the analgesic component of tramadol that is due to effects on the reuptake and release of 5-hydroxytryptamine.

Heroin

Heroin (diacetylmorphine) is a synthetic opioid produced by acetylation of morphine. When administered parenterally, heroin acts in a markedly different way than morphine. For example, there is rapid penetration of heroin into the brain, where it is hydrolyzed to the active metabolites monoacetylmorphine and morphine. The unique rapid entrance into the CNS is most likely caused by the lipid solubility and chemical structure of heroin. Compared with morphine, parenteral heroin has a (a) more rapid onset, (b) lack of a nauseating effect, and (c) greater potential for physical dependency. This greater liability for physical dependence is the reason that heroin is not available legally in the United States (Angell, 1984; Mondzac, 1984).

OPIOID AGONIST-ANTAGONISTS

Opioid agonist-antagonists include, but are not limited to, pentazocine, butorphanol, nalbuphine, buprenorphine, nalorphine, bremazocine, and dezocine (Fig. 3-34). These drugs bind to mu receptors, where they produce limited responses (partial agonists) or no effect (competitive antagonists). In addition, these drugs often exert partial

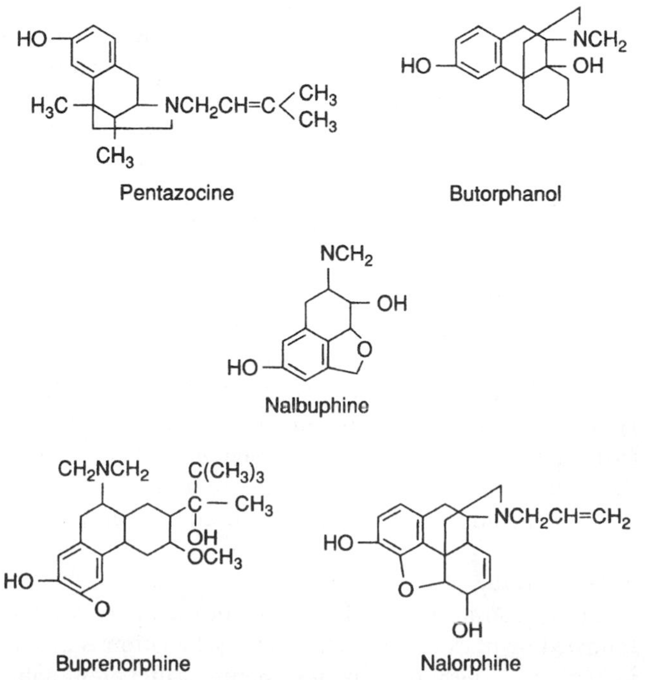

Figure 3-34. Opioid agonist-antagonists.

agonist actions at other receptors, including kappa and delta receptors. Antagonist properties of these drugs can attenuate the efficacy of subsequently administered opioid agonists. The side effects are similar to those of opioid agonists, and, in addition, these drugs may cause dysphoric reactions. The advantages of opioid agonist-antagonists are the ability to produce analgesia with limited depression of ventilation and a low potential to produce physical dependence. Furthermore, these drugs have a ceiling effect such that increasing doses do not produce additional responses. This ceiling effect on depression of ventilation, however, is often accompanied by an equally modest ability to decrease anesthetic requirements. In general, agonist-antagonist drugs should be reserved for patients who are unable to tolerate a pure agonist.

Pentazocine

Pentazocine is a benzomorphan derivative that possesses opioid agonist actions as well as weak antagonist actions. It is presumed to exert its agonist effects at delta and kappa receptors. Concomitant opioid antagonist activity is weak, being only about one-fifth as potent as nalorphine. Nevertheless, antagonist effects of pentazocine are sufficient to precipitate withdrawal symptoms when administered to patients who have been receiving opioids on a regular basis. The agonist effects of pentazocine are antagonized by naloxone. Indeed, physical dependence to pentazocine can be demonstrated by abrupt withdrawal precipitated by naloxone.

Pharmacokinetics

Pentazocine is well absorbed after oral or parenteral administration. First-pass hepatic metabolism is extensive, with only about 20% of an oral dose entering the circulation. Metabolism of pentazocine occurs by oxidation of terminal methyl groups, and resulting inactive glucuronide conjugates are excreted in the urine. An estimated 5% to 25% of an administered dose of pentazocine is excreted unchanged in the urine, and $<$2% undergoes biliary excretion. The elimination half-time is 2 to 3 hours.

Clinical Uses

Pentazocine, 10 to 30 mg IV or 50 mg orally, is used most often for the relief of moderate pain. An oral dose of 50 mg is equivalent in analgesic potency to 60 mg of codeine. Pentazocine is useful for treatment of chronic pain when there is a high risk of physical dependence. Placement in the epidural space produces a rapid onset of analgesia that is of shorter duration than that produced by morphine.

Side Effects

The most common side effect of pentazocine is sedation, followed by diaphoresis and dizziness. Sedation is prominent after epidural placement of pentazocine, presumably reflecting activation of kappa receptors. Nausea and vomiting are less common than with morphine. Dysphoria, including fear of impending death, is associated with high doses of pentazocine. This tendency to dysphoria limits the physical dependence liability of pentazocine. Pentazocine produces an increase in the plasma concentrations of catecholamines, which may account for increases in heart rate, systemic blood pressure, pulmonary artery blood pressure, and left ventricular end-diastolic pressure that accompany administration of this drug. Pentazocine, 20 to 30 mg IM, produces analgesia, sedation, and depression of ventilation similar to 10 mg of morphine. Increasing the IM dose above 30 mg does not produce proportionate increases in these responses. The increase in biliary tract pressure is less than that produced by equal analgesic doses of morphine, meperidine, or fentanyl (Radnay et al., 1980). Pentazocine crosses the placenta and may cause fetal depression. In contrast to morphine, miosis does not occur after administration of pentazocine.

Butorphanol

Butorphanol is an agonist-antagonist opioid that resembles pentazocine. Compared with pentazocine, its agonist effects are about 20 times greater, whereas its antagonist actions are 10 to 30 times greater. It is speculated that butorphanol has a (a) low affinity for mu receptors to produce antagonism, (b) moderate affinity for kappa receptors to produce analgesia and antishivering effects, and (c) minimal affinity for sigma receptors, so the incidence of dysphoria is low.

Butorphanol is rapidly and almost completely absorbed after IM injection. In postoperative patients, 2 to 3 mg IM produces analgesia and depression of ventilation similar to 10 mg of morphine. Intranasal butorphanol is used for the treatment of postoperative pain and migraine pain. The intraoperative use of butorphanol, like pentazocine, seems to be limited. The elimination half-time of butorphanol is 2.5 to 3.5 hours. Metabolism is principally to inactive hydroxybutorphanol, which is eliminated largely in the bile and to a lesser extent in the urine.

Side Effects

Common side effects of butorphanol include sedation, nausea, and diaphoresis. Dysphoria, reported frequently with other opioid agonist-antagonists, is infrequent after administration of butorphanol. Depression of ventilation is similar to that produced by similar doses of morphine. Like pentazocine, analgesic doses of butorphanol increase systemic blood pressure, pulmonary artery blood pressure, and cardiac output. Also, similar to pentazocine, the effects of butorphanol on the biliary and gastrointestinal tract seem to be milder than those produced by morphine. It may be difficult to use an opioid agonist effectively as an analgesic in the presence of butorphanol. This must be remembered when considering the use of butorphanol or any other opioid-agonist for preoperative medication.

Withdrawal symptoms do occur after acute discontinuation of chronic therapy with butorphanol, but symptoms are mild.

Nalbuphine

Nalbuphine is an agonist-antagonist opioid that is related chemically to oxymorphone and naloxone. It is equal in potency as an analgesic to morphine, and is about one-fourth as potent as nalorphine as an antagonist. Nalbuphine is metabolized in the liver and has an elimination half-time of 3 to 6 hours. Naloxone reverses the agonist effects of nalbuphine. Nalbuphine, 10 mg IM, produces analgesia with an onset of effect and duration of action similar to those of morphine. Depression of ventilation is similar to that of morphine until 30 mg IM of nalbuphine is exceeded, after which no further depression of ventilation occurs (ceiling effect) (Gal et al., 1982). Sedation is the most common side effect, occurring in about one-third of patients treated with nalbuphine. The incidence of dysphoria is less than that with pentazocine or butorphanol but is qualitatively similar and increases in frequency as the dose of nalbuphine is increased. In contrast to pentazocine and butorphanol, nalbuphine does not increase systemic blood pressure, pulmonary artery blood pressure, heart rate, or atrial filling pressures. For this reason, nalbuphine may be useful to provide sedation and analgesia in patients with heart disease, as during cardiac catheterization. Abrupt withdrawal of nalbuphine after chronic administration produces withdrawal symptoms that are milder than those of morphine and more severe than those of pentazocine. The abuse potential of nalbuphine is low.

The antagonist effects of nalbuphine are speculated to occur at mu receptors. As a result, the subsequent use of morphine-like drugs for anesthesia after preoperative medication with nalbuphine may not provide adequate analgesia. Likewise, the efficacy of opioid agonists to provide analgesia may be compromised by nalbuphine, which has previously been administered and found to be inadequate in controlling postoperative pain. Conversely, the antagonist effects of nalbuphine at mu receptors could be an advantage in the postoperative period to reverse lingering ventilatory depressant effects of opioid agonists while still maintaining analgesia. Nalbuphine, 10 to 20 mg IV, reverses postoperative depression of ventilation caused by fentanyl but maintains analgesia (Bailey et al., 1987). Evidence of recurrent hypoventilation often occurs 2 to 3 hours after administration of nalbuphine to antagonize the effects of fentanyl.

Buprenorphine

Buprenorphine is an agonist-antagonist opioid derived from the opium alkaloid thebaine. Its analgesic potency is great, with 0.3 mg IM being equivalent to 10 mg of morphine. After IM administration, the onset of buprenorphine effect occurs in about 30 minutes, and the duration of action is at least 8 hours. It is estimated that the affinity of buprenorphine for mu receptors is 50 times greater than that of morphine, and subsequent slow dissociation from these receptors accounts for its prolonged duration of action and resistance to antagonism with naloxone. After IM administration, nearly two-thirds of the drug appears unchanged in the bile and the remainder is excreted in urine as inactive metabolites.

Buprenorphine is effective in relieving moderate to severe pain such as that present in the postoperative period and that associated with cancer, renal colic, and myocardial infarction. Placed in the epidural space, the high lipid solubility (five times that of morphine) and affinity for opioid receptors limits cephalad spread and the likelihood of delayed depression of ventilation (Lanz et al., 1984). The antagonist effects of buprenorphine reflect the ability of this drug to displace opioid agonists from mu receptors.

Side Effects

The side effects of buprenorphine include drowsiness, nausea, vomiting, and depression of ventilation that are similar in magnitude to the side effects of morphine but may be prolonged and resistant to antagonism with naloxone. Pulmonary edema has been observed after administration of buprenorphine (Gould, 1995). In contrast to other opioid agonist-antagonists, dysphoria is unlikely to occur in association with administration of this drug. Because of its antagonist properties, buprenorphine can precipitate withdrawal in patients who are physically dependent on morphine. Conversely, withdrawal symptoms in patients who are physically dependent on buprenorphine develop slowly and are of lesser intensity than those associated with morphine. In this respect, withdrawal from buprenorphine resembles that from other opioid agonist-antagonists, and the risk of abuse is low.

Nalorphine

Nalorphine is equally potent with morphine as an analgesic but is not clinically useful because of a high incidence of dysphoria. The high incidence of dysphoria may reflect activity of this drug at sigma receptors. The antagonist actions of nalorphine reflect its ability to displace opioid agonists from mu receptors.

Bremazocine

Bremazocine is a benzomorphan derivative that is twice as potent as morphine as an analgesic but, in animals, does not produce depression of ventilation or evidence of physical dependence. It is speculated that bremazocine interacts selectively with kappa receptors. Failure of naloxone to reverse sedation produced by bremazocine is further evidence that this drug is acting at sites other than mu receptors.

Dezocine

Dezocine, 0.15 mg/kg IM, is an opioid agonist-antagonist with the analgesic potency, onset, and duration of action in the relief of postoperative pain comparable to morphine. Absorption of dezocine, 10 to 15 mg, after IM administration is rapid and complete, with analgesia occurring after about 30 minutes. After IV administration of dezocine, 5 to 10 mg, the onset of analgesia occurs in about 15 minutes. Elimination of dezocine is principally in the urine as a glucuronide conjugate. Like other opioid agonist-antagonists, dezocine exhibits a ceiling effect for depression of ventilation that parallels its analgesic activity (Gal and DiFazio, 1984). Large doses of dezocine administered IV to humans do not produce significant changes in systemic blood pressure, pulmonary artery pressure, or cardiac output.

Dezocine has a high affinity for mu receptors and a moderate affinity for delta receptors. The interaction at delta receptors serves to facilitate the effect of agonist activity at mu receptors. The incidence of dysphoria is minimal after administration of dezocine, presumably reflecting the low affinity of this drug for sigma receptors.

Meptazinol

Meptazinol is a partial opioid agonist with relative selectivity at mu_1 receptors. As a result, depression of ventilation does not occur with analgesic doses of meptazinol (100 mg IM is equivalent to morphine, 8 mg IM). The onset of analgesia is rapid, but the duration of action is <2 hours. Bioavailability after oral administration is <10%. Metabolism is to inactive glucuronide conjugates that are excreted by the kidneys. Protein binding is 20% to 25%, and the elimination half-time is about 2 hours. Physical dependence does not occur, miosis is slight, and constipation is absent. Nausea and vomiting are common side effects. Meptazinol cannot be substituted for an opioid agonist in patients physically dependent on opioids.

OPIOID ANTAGONISTS

Minor changes in the structure of an opioid agonist can convert the drug into an opioid antagonist at one or more of the opioid receptor sites (Fig. 3-35) (Glass et al., 1994). The most common change is substitution of an alkyl group for a methyl group on an opioid agonist. For example, naloxone is the *N*-alkyl derivative of oxymorphone (see Fig. 3-34).

Naloxone, naltrexone, and nalmefene are pure mu opioid receptor antagonists with no agonist activity. These antagonists have replaced nalorphine and levorphanol, each of which possesses opioid agonist as well as antagonist activity. The high affinity for opioid receptors characteristic of pure opioid antagonists results in displacement of the

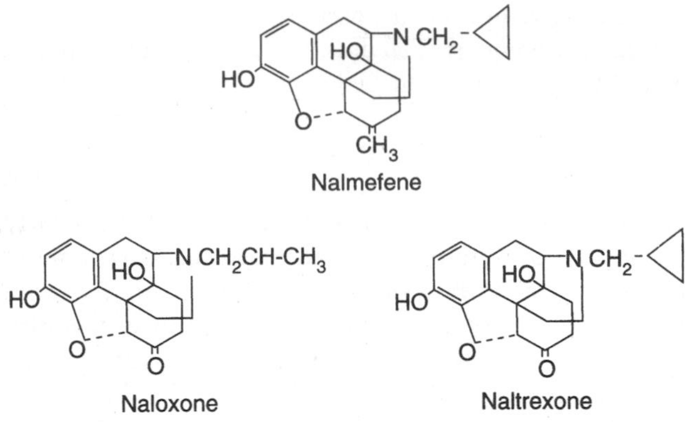

Figure 3-35. Opioid antagonists.

opioid agonist from mu receptors. After this displacement, the binding of the pure antagonist does not activate mu receptors and antagonism occurs.

Naloxone

Naloxone is a nonselective antagonist at all three opioid receptors. Naloxone is selective when used to (a) treat opioid-induced depression of ventilation as may be present in the postoperative period, (b) treat opioid-induced depression of ventilation in the neonate due to maternal administration of an opioid, (c) facilitate treatment of deliberate opioid overdose, and (d) detect suspected physical dependence. Naloxone, 1 to 4 μg/kg IV, promptly reverses opioid-induced analgesia and depression of ventilation. The short duration of action of naloxone (30 to 45 minutes) is presumed to be due to its rapid removal from the brain. This emphasizes that supplemental doses of naloxone will likely be necessary for sustained antagonism of opioid agonists. In this regard, a continuous infusion of naloxone, 5 μg/kg/hour, prevents depression of ventilation without altering analgesia produced by neuraxial opioids (Rawal et al., 1986).

Naloxone is metabolized primarily in the liver by conjugation with glucuronic acid to form naloxone-3-glucuronide. The elimination half-time is 60 to 90 minutes. Naloxone is absorbed orally, but metabolism during its first pass through the liver renders it only one-fifth as potent as when administered parenterally.

Side Effects

Antagonism of opioid-induced depression of ventilation is accompanied by an inevitable reversal of analgesia. It may be possible, however, to titrate the dose of naloxone such that depression of ventilation is partially but acceptably antagonized to also maintain partial analgesia.

Nausea and vomiting appear to be closely related to the dose and speed of injection of naloxone. Administration of naloxone slowly over 2 to 3 minutes rather than as a bolus seems to decrease the incidence of nausea and vomiting.

Awakening occurs either before or simultaneously with vomiting, which ensures that the patient's protective upper airway reflexes have returned and the likelihood of pulmonary aspiration is minimized.

Cardiovascular stimulation after administration of naloxone manifests as increased sympathetic nervous system activity, presumably reflecting the abrupt reversal of analgesia and the sudden perception of pain. This increased sympathetic nervous system activity may manifest as tachycardia, hypertension, pulmonary edema, and cardiac dysrhythmias (Partridge and Ward, 1986). Even ventricular fibrillation has occurred after the IV administration of naloxone and the associated sudden increase in sympathetic nervous system activity (Andree, 1980).

Naloxone can easily cross the placenta. For this reason, administration of naloxone to an opioid-dependent parturient may produce acute withdrawal in the neonate.

Role in Treatment of Shock

Naloxone produces dose-related improvement in myocardial contractility and survival in animals subjected to hypovolemic shock and, to a lesser extent, in those subjected to septic shock (Faden, 1984). The beneficial effects of naloxone in the treatment of shock occur only with doses >1 mg/kg IV, suggesting that the beneficial effects of this drug are not opioid receptor–mediated or, alternatively, are mediated by opioid receptors other than mu receptors—possibly delta and kappa receptors.

Antagonism of General Anesthesia

The occasional observation that high doses of naloxone seem to antagonize the depressant effect of inhaled anesthetics may represent drug-induced activation of the cholinergic arousal system in the brain, independent of any interaction with opioid receptors (Kraynack and Gintautas, 1982). A role of endorphins in the production of general anesthesia is not supported by data demonstrating a failure of naloxone to alter anesthetic requirements (MAC) in animals.

Naltrexone

Naltrexone, in contrast to naloxone, is highly effective orally, producing sustained antagonism of the effects of opioid agonists for as long as 24 hours.

Nalmefene

Nalmefene is a pure opioid antagonist that is a 6-methylene analogue of naltrexone (see Fig. 3-35) (Dougherty et al., 2000). Nalmefene is equipotent to naloxone. The recommended dose is 15 to 25 μg IV administered every 2 to 5 minutes until the desired effect is achieved, with the total dose not exceeding 1 μg/kg (Abramowicz, 1995). Prophylactic administration of nalmefene significantly decreases the need for antiemetics and antipruritic medications in patients receiving intravenous patient-controlled analgesia with morphine (Joshi et al., 1999). The primary advantage of nalmefene over naloxone is its longer duration of action, which might provide a greater degree of protection from delayed depression of ventilation due to residual effects of the opioid as the antagonist is cleared. Compared with the brief elimination half-time of naloxone, the half-time of nalmefene is about 10.8 hours. This longer duration of action is likely due to the slower clearance of nalmefene compared with naloxone. Nalmefene is metabolized by hepatic conjugation, with <5% excreted unchanged in the urine. As with naloxone, acute pulmonary edema has occurred after the IV administration of nalmefene (Henderson and Reynolds, 1997).

Methylnaltrexone

Methylnaltrexone is a quaternary opioid receptor antagonist. The highly ionized quaternary methyl group limits the transfer of methylnatrexone across the blood-brain barrier. As a result, methylnaltrexone is active at peripheral rather than central opioid receptors as demonstrated by its failure to penetrate the CNS sufficiently to promote withdrawal in morphine-dependent animals.

In humans, methylnaltrexone attenuates morphine-induced changes in the rate of gastric emptying and also decreases the incidence of nausea (see Chapter 26) (Murphy et al., 1997). The attenuation of morphine-induced nausea may be due to antagonism of morphine at the chemoreceptor trigger zone (located outside the blood-brain barrier) or through limitation of the delay in gastric emptying, which, in itself, may cause nausea. Presumably, methylnaltrexone could prevent the undesirable effects of opioids on gastric emptying and possibly vomiting without altering centrally mediated analgesia.

ANESTHETIC REQUIREMENTS

The contribution of opioids to total anesthetic requirements can be quantitated by determining the decrease in MAC of a volatile anesthetic in the presence of opioids. In animals, morphine decreases the MAC of volatile anesthetics in a dose-dependent manner, but there appears to be a ceiling effect to the anesthetic-sparing ability of morphine, with a plateau at 65% MAC (Steffey et al., 1993). A single dose of fentanyl, 3 μg/kg IV 25 to 30 minutes before surgical skin incision, decreases isoflurane or desflurane MAC by about 50% (Sebel et al., 1992). In animals, sufentanil decreases enflurane MAC by 70% to 90% (Fig. 3-36) (Hall et al., 1987). In patients, a sufentanil plasma concentration of 0.145 ng/mL produced a 50% decrease in isoflurane MAC, whereas plasma sufentanil concentrations of >0.5 ng/mL exhibited a ceiling effect (Brunner et al., 1994; Schwartz et al., 1994). As with other opioids, alfentanil administered to animals decreases MAC in a dose-dependent manner

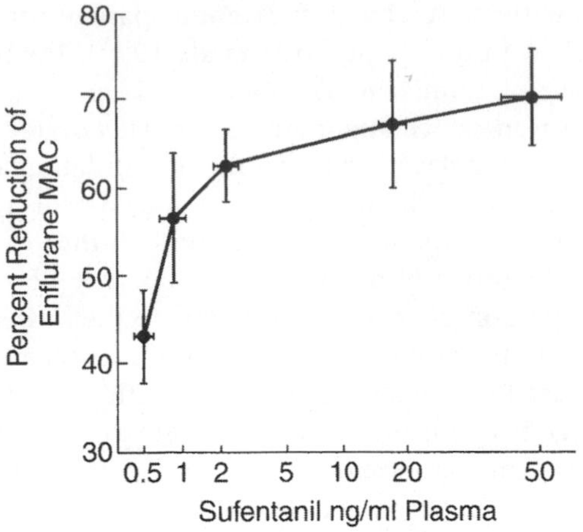

Figure 3-36. The decrease in enflurane minimum alveolar concentration (MAC) was determined during continuous intravenous infusion of sufentanil to maintain an unchanging plasma concentration of opioid. (Mean ± SE.) (From Hall RI, Murphy MR, Hug CC. The enflurane sparing effect of sufentanil in dogs. *Anesthesiology* 1987;67:518–525; with permission.)

until a plateau is reached at about a 70% decrease in MAC. The decrease in MAC produced by remifentanil is similar to that produced by other opioids and ranges from 50% to 91%, depending on the plasma concentration of remifentanil (Lang et al., 1996). These data cast doubt on the ability of opioid agonists to provide total amnesia reliably in every patient, even with high doses.

Opioid agonist-antagonists are less effective than opioid agonists in decreasing MAC. For example, butorphanol, nalbuphine, and pentazocine maximally decrease MAC 11%, 8%, and 20%, respectively, even when the dose of these drugs is increased 40-fold (Murphy and Hug, 1982). The ceiling effect for MAC parallels the ceiling effect for depression of ventilation and is consistent with the clinical impression that even large doses of opioid agonist-antagonists do not produce unconsciousness or prevent patient movement in response to painful stimulation. For this reason, the use of large doses of opioid agonist-antagonists for anesthesia does not seem logical.

REFERENCES

Abramowicz M. Nalmefene—a long acting injectable opioid antagonist. *Med Lett Drugs Ther* 1995;37:97–98.

Abrams JT, Horrow JC, Bennett, et al. Upper airway closure: a primary source of difficult ventilation with sufentanil induction of anesthesia. *Anesth Analg* 1996;83:629–632.

Albanese J, Durbec O, Viviand X, et al. Sufentanil increases intracranial pressure in patients with head trauma. *Anesthesiology* 1993; 79:493–497.

Alfonsi P, Sessler DI, Du Manoir B, et al. The effects of meperidine and sufentanil on the shivering threshold in postoperative patients. *Anesthesiology* 1998;89:43–48.

Andree RA. Sudden death following naloxone administration. *Anesth Analg* 1980;59:782–784.

Angell M. Should heroin be legalized for the treatment of pain? *N Engl J Med* 1984;311:529–530.

Angst MS, Buhrer M, Lotsch J. Insidious intoxication after morphine treatment in renal failure: Delayed onset of morphine-6-glucuronide action. *Anesthesiology* 2000:92:1473–1476.

Angst MS, Drover DR, Lotsch J, et al. Pharmacodynamics of orally administered sustained-release hydromorphone in humans. *Anesthesiology* 2001;94:63–73.

Arndt JO, Mikat M, Parasher C. Fentanyl's analgesic, respiratory, and cardiovascular actions in relation to dose and plasma concentration in unanesthetized dogs. *Anesthesiology* 1984;61:355–361.

Ashburn MA, Lind GH, Gillie MH, et al. Oral transmucosal fentanyl citrate (OTFC) for the treatment of postoperative pain. *Anesth Analg* 1993;76:377–381.

Atcheson R, Lambert DG. Update on opioid receptors. *Br J Anaesth* 1994;73:132–134.

Auburn F, Monsel S, Langeron O, et al. Postoperative titration of intravenous morphine in the elderly patient. *Anesthesiology* 2002;96:17–23.

Ausems ME, Hug CC, deLange S. Variable rate infusion of alfentanil as a supplement to nitrous oxide anesthesia for general surgery. *Anesth Analg* 1983;62:982–986.

Austin KL, Stapleton JV, Mather LE. Multiple intramuscular injections—a major source of variability in analgesic response to meperidine. *Pain* 1980a;8:47–62.

Austin KL, Stapleton JV, Mather LE. Relationship between blood meperidine concentrations and analgesic response. *Anesthesiology* 1980b;53:460–466.

Avramov MN, Smith I, White PF. Interactions between midazolam and remifentanil during monitored anesthesia care. *Anesthesiology* 1996;85:1283–1289.

Babenco HD, Conard PF, Gross JB. The pharmacodynamic effect of a remifentanil bolus on ventilatory control. *Anesthesiology* 2000;92: 393–398.

Bailey PL, Clark NJ, Pace NL, et al. Antagonism of post-operative opioid-induced respiratory depression: nalbuphine versus naloxone. *Anesth Analg* 1987;66:1109–1114.

Bailey PL, Pace NL, Ashburn MA, et al. Frequent hypoxemia and apnea after sedation with midazolam and fentanyl. *Anesthesiology* 1990a;73:826–830.

Bailey PL, Rhondeau S, Schafer PG, et al. Dose-response pharmacology of intrathecal morphine in human volunteers. *Anesthesiology* 1993;79:49–59.

Bailey PL, Streisand JB, East KA, et al. Differences in magnitude and duration of opioid-induced respiratory depression and analgesia with fentanyl and sufentanil. *Anesth Analg* 1990b;70:8–15.

Baka N-E, Bayoumeu F, Boutroy M-J, et al. Colostrum morphine concentrations during postcesarean intravenous patient-controlled analgesia. *Anesth Analg* 2002;94:184–187.

Ballantyne JC, Mao J. Opioid therapy for chronic pain. *N Engl J Med* 2003;349:1943–1953.

Bartkowski RR, McDonnell TE. Prolonged alfentanil effect following erythromycin administration. *Anesthesiology* 1990;73:566–568.

Becker LD, Paulson BA, Miller RD, et al. Biphasic respiratory depression after fentanyldroperidol or fentanyl alone used to supplement nitrous oxide anesthesia. *Anesthesiology* 1976;44:291–296.

Bellville JW, Forrest WH, Miller E, et al. Influence of age on pain relief from analgesics. *JAMA* 1971;217:1835–1841.

Bennett JA, Abrams JT, Van Riper DF, et al. Difficult or impossible ventilation after sufentanil-induced anesthesia is caused primarily by vocal cord closure. *Anesthesiology* 1997;87:1070–1074.

Bennett MJ, Anderson LK, McMillan JC, et al. Anaphylactic reaction during anesthesia associated with positive intradermal skin test to fentanyl. *Can Anaesth Soc J* 1986;33:75–78.

Bentley JB, Borel JD, Nenad RE, et al. Age and fentanyl pharmacokinetics. *Anesth Analg* 1982;61:968–971.

Berkowitz BA, Ngai SH, Yang JC, et al. The disposition of morphine in surgical patients. *Clin Pharmacol Ther* 1975;17:629–635.

Boer F, Olofsen E, Bovill JG, et al. Pulmonary uptake of sufentanil during and after constant rate infusion. *Br J Anaesth* 1996;76: 203–208.

Bovill JG, Sebel PS, Blackburn CL, et al. The pharmacokinetics of sufentanil in surgical patients. *Anesthesiology* 1984;61:502–506.

Bowdle TA, Rooke GA. Postoperative myoclonus and rigidity after anesthesia with opioids. *Anesth Analg* 1994;78:783–786.

Brunner MD, Braithwaite P, Jhaveri R, et al. MAC reduction of isoflurane by sufentanil. *Br J Anaesth* 1994;72:42–46.

Budd K, Langford R. Tramadol revisited. *Br J Anaesth* 1999;82: 493–495.

Burkle H, Dunbar S, Van Aken H. Remifentanil: a novel, short-acting, mu opioid. *Anesth Analg* 1996;83:646–651.

Cahalan MK, Lurz FW, Eger EI II, et al. Narcotics decrease heart rate during inhalational anesthesia. *Anesth Analg* 1987;66:166–170.

Calvey TN. Chirality in anaesthesia. *Anaesthesia* 1992;47:93–94.

Camu F, Gepts E, Rucquoi M, et al. Pharmacokinetics of alfentanil in man. *Anesth Analg* 1982;61:657–661.

Caplan RA, Ready LB, Oden RV, et al. Transdermal fentanyl for post-operative pain management. A double-blind placebo study. *JAMA* 1989;260:1036–1039.

Chaney MA. Side effects of intrathecal and epidural opioids. *Can J Anaesth* 1995;42:891–903.

Chang J, Fish KJ. Acute respiratory arrest and rigidity after anesthesia with sufentanil: a case report. *Anesthesiology* 1985;63:710–711.

Chauvin M, Ferrier C, Haberer JP, et al. Sufentanil pharmacokinetics in patients with cirrhosis. *Anesth Analg* 1989;68:1–4.

Chauvin M, Lebrault C, Levron JC, et al. Pharmacokinetics of alfentanil in chronic renal failure. *Anesth Analg* 1987a;66:53–56.

Chauvin M, Sandouk P, Scherrman JM, et al. Morphine pharmacokinetics in renal failure. *Anesthesiology* 1987b;66:327–331.

Chen Y, Mestek A, Liu J, et al. Molecular cloning and functional expression of an μ-opioid from rat brain. *Mol Pharmacol* 1993;44:8–12.

Cherny NI. Opioid analgesics: comparative features and prescribing guidelines. *Drugs* 1996;51:713–737.

Coda BA, Rudy AC, Archer SM, et al. Pharmacokinetics and bioavailability of single-dose intranasal hydromorphone hydrochloride in healthy volunteers. *Anesth Analg* 2003;97:117–23.

Collart L, Luthy C, Dayer P. Multimodal analgesic effects of tramadol. *Clin Pharmacol Ther* 1993;53:223–226.

Cortinez LI, Brandes V, Munoz HR, et al. No clinical evidence of acute opioid tolerance after remifentanil-based anaesthesia. *Br J Anaesth* 2001;87:866–869.

Cousins MJ, Mather LE. Intrathecal and epidural administration of opioids. *Anesthesiology* 1984;61:276–310.

Cozian A, Pinaud M, Lepage JY, et al. Effects of meperidine spinal anesthesia on hemodynamics, plasma catecholamines, angiotensin I, aldosterone, and histamine concentrations in elderly men. *Anesthesiology* 1986;64:815–819.

Crighton I, Martin PH, Hobbs GJ, et al. A comparison of the effects of intravenous tramadol, codeine, and morphine on gastric emptying in human volunteers. *Anesth Analg* 1988;87:445–449.

Crone LA, Conly JM, Storgard C, et al. Herpes labialis in parturients receiving morphine following cesarean section. *Anesthesiology* 1990;73:208–213.

Dahaba AA, Grabner T, Rehak PH, et al. Remifentanil versus morphine analgesia and sedation for mechanically ventilated critically ill patients. A randomized double blind study. *Anesthesiology* 2004;101:640–646.

Dahan A, Sarton E, Teppema L, et al. Sex-related differences in the influence of morphine on ventilatory control in humans. *Anesthesiology* 1998;88:901–913.

Daniel M, Weiskopf RB, Noorani M, et al. Fentanyl augments the blockade of the sympathetic response to incision (MAC-BAR) produced by desflurane and isoflurane. Desflurane and isoflurane MAC-BAR without and with fentanyl. *Anesthesiology* 1998;88:43–49.

Davis PJ, Stiller RL, Cook DR, et al. Effects of cholestatic hepatic disease and chronic renal failure on alfentanil pharmacokinetics in children. *Anesth Analg* 1989;68:579–583.

de Leon-Casasola OA, Lema MJ. Postoperative epidural opioid analgesia: what are the choices? *Anesth Analg* 1996;83:867–875.

de Nadal M, Munar F, Poca MA, et al. Cerebral hemodynamic effects of morphine and fentanyl in patient with severe head injury: Absence of correlation to cerebral autoregulation. *Anesthesiology* 2000;92:11–19.

De Witte JL, Schoenmaekers B, Sessler DI, et al. The analgesic efficacy of tramadol is impaired by concurrent administration of ondansetron. *Anesth Analg* 2001;92:1319–1321.

Dershwitz M, Walsh JL, Morishige RJ, et al. Pharmacokinetics and pharmacodynamics of inhaled versus intravenous morphine in healthy volunteers. *Anesthesiology* 2000;93:619–628.

Don HF, Dieppa RD, Taylor P. Narcotic analgesics in anuric patients. *Anesthesiology* 1975;42:745–747.

Dougherty TB, Porche VH, Thall PF. Maximum tolerated dose of nalmefene in patients receiving epidural fentanyl and dilute bupivacaine for postoperative analgesia. *Anesthesiology* 2000;92: 1010–1016.

Drasner K, Bernards CM, Ozanne GM. Intrathecal morphine reduces the minimum alveolar concentration of halothane in humans. *Anesthesiology* 1988;69:310–312.

Dsida, RM, Wheeler M, Birmingham PK, et al. Premedication of pediatric patients with oral transmucosal fentanyl citrate. *Anesth Analg* 1998;86:66–70.

Egan TD, Huizinga B, Gupta SK, et al. Remifentanil pharmacokinetics in obese versus lean patients. *Anesthesiology* 1998;89:562–573.

Egan TD, Lemmens JHM, Fiset P, et al. The pharmacokinetics of the new short-acting opioid remifentanil (GI87084B) in healthy adult male volunteers. *Anesthesiology* 1993;79:881–892.

Epstein RH, Mendel HG, Witkowski TA, et al. The safety and efficacy of oral transmucosal fentanyl citrate for preoperative sedation in young children. *Anesth Analg* 1996;83:1200–1205.

Evron S, Glezerman M, Sadan O, et al. Remifentanil: A novel systemic analgesic for labor pain. *Anesth Analg* 2005;100:233–238.

Faden AI. Opiate antagonists and thyrotropin-releasing hormone. I. Potential role in the treatment of shock. *JAMA* 1984;252:1177–1180.

Finck AD, Ngai SH, Berkowitz BA. Antagonism of general anesthesia by naloxone in the rat. *Anesthesiology* 1977;46:241–245.

Fishman SM, Wilsey B, Mahajan G, et al. Methadone reincarnated: Novel clinical applications and related concerns. *Pain Med* 2002; 3:339–348.

Flacke JW, Flacke WE, Bloor BC, VanEtten AP, Kripke BJ. Histamine release by four narcotics: a double-blind study in humans. *Anesth Analg* 1987;66:723–730.

Fragen RJ, Vilich F, Spies SM, et al. The effect of remifentanil on biliary tract drainage into the duodenum. *Anesth Analg* 1999;89: 1561–1564.

Friesen RH, Lockhart CH. Oral transmucosal fentanyl citrate for preanesthetic medication of pediatric day surgery patients with and without droperidol as a prophylactic anti-emetic. *Anesthesiology* 1992;76:46–51.

Frolich M, Giannotti A, Modell JH. Opioid overdose in a patient using a fentanyl patch during treatment with a warming blanket. *Anesth Analg* 2001;93:647–648.

Gal TJ, DiFazio CA, Moscicki J. Analgesic and respiratory depressant activity of nalbuphine: a comparison with morphine. *Anesthesiology* 1982;57:367–374.

Gal TJ, DiFazio CA. Ventilatory and analgesic effects of dezocine in humans. *Anesthesiology* 1984;61:716–722.

Gan TJ, Ginsberg B, Glass PSA, et al. Opioid-sparing effects of a low-dose infusion of naloxone in patient-administered morphine sulfate. *Anesthesiology* 1997;87:1075–1081.

Gedney JA, Ghosh S. Pharmacokinetics of analgesics, sedatives and anaesthetic agents during cardiopulmonary bypass. *Br J Anaesth* 1995;75: 344–351.

Gimbel J, Ahdieh H. The efficacy and safety of oral immediate-release oxymorphone for postsurgical pain. *Anesth Analg* 2004;99: 1472–1477.

Glass PSA, Bloom M, Kearse L, et al. Bispectral analysis measures sedation and memory effects of propofol, midazolam, isoflurane, and alfentanil in healthy volunteers. *Anesthesiology* 1997;86:836–847.

Glass PSA, Jhaveri RM, Smith LR. Comparison of potency and duration of action of nalmefene and nalaxone. *Anesth Analg* 1994; 78:536–541.

Gould DB. Buprenorphine causes pulmonary edema just like all other μ-opioid narcotics. Upper airway obstruction, negative alveolar pressure. *Chest* 1995;107:1478–1479.

Goyagi T, Nishikawa T. The addition of epinephrine enhances postoperative analgesia by intrathecal morphine. *Anesth Analg* 1995;81: 508–513.

Grace D, Fee JPH. A comparison of intrathecal morphine-6-glucuronide and intrathecal morphine sulfate as analgesics for total hip replacement. *Anesth Analg* 1996;83:1055–1059.

Greeley WJ, DeBruijn NP, Davis DP. Sufentanil pharmacokinetics in pediatric cardiovascular patients. *Anesth Analg* 1987;66:1067– 1072.

Guignard B, Bossard AE, Coste C, et al. Acute opioid tolerance. Intraoperative remifentanil increases postoperative pain and morphine requirement. *Anesthesiology* 2000;93:409–417.

Gustorff B, Nahlik G, Hoerauf KH, et al. The absence of acute tolerance during remifentanil infusion in volunteers. *Anesth Analg* 2002;94:1223–1228.

Guy J, Hindman BJ, Baker KZ, et al. Comparison of remifentanil and fentanyl in patients undergoing craniotomy for supratentorial space-occupying lesions. *Anesthesiology* 1997;86:514–524.

Haber GW, Litman RS. Generalized tonic-clonic activity after remifentanil administration. *Anesth Analg* 2001;93:1532–1533.

Haberer JP, Schoeffler P, Couderc E, et al. Fentanyl pharmacokinetics in anaesthetized patients with cirrhosis. *Br J Anaesth* 1982;54: 1267–1270.

Hall RI, Murphy MR, Hug CC. The enflurane sparing effect of sufentanil in dogs. *Anesthesiology* 1987;67:518–525.

Hanna MH, D'Costa F, Peat SJ, et al. Morphine-6-glucuronide disposition in renal impairment. *Br J Anaesth* 1993;70:511–514.

Hanna MH, Peat SJ, Woodham M, Knibb A, Fung C. Analgesic efficacy and CSF pharmacokinetics of intrathecal morphine-6-glucuronide: comparison with morphine. *Br J Anaesth* 1990;64:547–550.

Heine MF, Tillet ED, Tseuda K, et al. Intra-articular morphine after arthroscopic knee operation. *Br J Anaesth* 1994;73:413–415.

Henderson CA, Reynolds JE. Acute pulmonary edema in a young male after intravenous nalmefene. *Anesth Analg* 1997;84:218–219.

Hilgenberg JC. Intraoperative awareness during high-dose fentanyl-oxygen anesthesia. *Anesthesiology* 1981;54:341–343.

Hogue CW, Bowdle TA, O'Leary C, et al. A multicenter evaluation of total intravenous anesthesia with remifentanil and propofol for elective inpatient surgery. *Anesth Analg* 1996;83:279–285.

Hoke JF, Shlugman D, Dershwitz M, et al. Pharmacokinetics and pharmacodynamics of remifentanil in persons with renal failure compared with healthy volunteers. *Anesthesiology* 1997;87:533–541.

Hudson RJ, Bergstrom RG, Thomson IR, et al. Pharmacokinetics of sufentanil in patients undergoing abdominal aortic surgery. *Anesthesiology* 1989;70:426–431.

Hudson RJ, Thomson IR, Cannon JE, et al. Pharmacokinetics of fentanyl in patients undergoing abdominal aortic surgery. *Anesthesiology* 1986; 64:334–338.

Hudson RJ, Thomson IR, Jassal R, et al. Cardiopulmonary bypass has minimal effects on the pharmacokinetics of fentanyl in adults. *Anesthesiology* 2003;99:847–854.

Hug CC, Murphy MR. Tissue redistribution of fentanyl and termination of its effects in rats. *Anesthesiology* 1981;55:369–375.

Hughes MA, Glass PSA, Jacobs JR. Context-sensitive half-time in multicompartment pharmacokinetic models for intravenous anesthetic drugs. *Anesthesiology* 1992;76:334–341.

Hynyen MJ, Turunen MT, Korttila KT. Effects of alfentanil and fentanyl on common bile duct pressure. *Anesth Analg* 1986;65:370–372.

Ibrahim AE, Feldman J, Darim A, et al. Simultaneous assessment of drug interactions with low- and high-extraction opioids: application to parecoxib effects on the pharmacokinetics and pharmacodynamics of fentanyl and alfentanil. *Anesthesiology* 2003;98:853–861.

Ikeda T, Sessler DI, Tayefeh F, et al. Meperidine and alfentanil do not reduce the gains or maximum intensity of shivering. *Anesthesiology* 1998;88:858–865.

Ionescu TI, Taverne RHT, Drost RH, et al. Epidural morphine anesthesia for abdominal aortic surgery-pharmacokinetics. *Reg Anesth* 1989; 14:107–114.

Ionescu TI, Taverne RHT, Houweling PL, et al. Pharmacokinetic study of extradural and intrathecal sufentanil anaesthesia for major surgery. *Br J Anaesth* 1991;66:458-464.

Jhaveri R, Joshi P, Batenhorst R, et al. Dose comparison of remifentanil and alfentanil for loss of consciousness. *Anesthesiology* 1997;87:253–259.

Jones RM, Detmer M, Hill AB, et al. Incidence of choledochoduodenal sphincter spasm during fentanyl-supplemented anesthesia. *Anesth Analg* 1981;60:638–640.

Jones RM, Fiddian-Green R, Knight PR. Narcotic-induced choledochoduodenal sphincter spasm reversed by glucagon. *Anesth Analg* 1980;59:946–947.

Joshi G, Duffy L, Chehade J, et al. Effects of prophylactic nalmefene on the incidence of morphine-related side effects in patients receiving intravenous patient-controlled analgesia. *Anesthesiology* 1999;90:1007–1011.

Kahn LH, Alderfer RJ, Graham DJ. Seizures associated with tramadol. *JAMA* 1997;278:1661.

Kan RE, Hughes SC, Rosen MA, et al. Intravenous remifentanil. Placental transfer, maternal and neonatal effects. *Anesthesiology* 1998;88:1467–1474.

Kapila A, Glass PSA, Jacobs JR, et al. Measured context-sensitive half-times of remifentanil and alfentanil. *Anesthesiology* 1995;83: 968–975.

Kelly MC, Carabine UA, Hill DA, et al. A comparison of the effect of intrathecal and extradural fentanyl on gastric emptying in laboring women. *Anesth Analg* 1997;85:834.

Kest B, Sarton e, Dahan A. Gender differences in opioid-mediated analgesia: animal and human studies. *Anesthesiology* 2000;93: 539–547.

Kharasch ED, Russell M, Mautz D, et al. The role of cytochrome P450 3A4 in alfentanil clearance: implications for interindividual variability in disposition and perioperative drug interactions. *Anesthesiology* 1997;87:36–50.

Klimscha W, Ullrich R, Nasel C, et al. High-dose remifentanil does not impair cerebrovascular carbon dioxide reactivity in healthy male volunteers. *Anesthesiology* 2003;99:834–840.

Kosterlitz HW. Biosynthesis of morphine in the animal kingdom. *Nature* 1987;330:606.

Kraynack BJ, Gintautas JG. Naloxone: analeptic action unrelated to opiate receptor antagonism? *Anesthesiology* 1982;56:251–253.

Kuzma PJ, Kline MD, Stamatos JM, et al. Acute toxic delirium: an uncommon reaction to transdermal fentanyl. *Anesthesiology* 1995; 83:869–871.

Lambert DG. Recent advances in opioid pharmacology. *Br J Anaesth* 1998;81:1–2.

Lang E, Jedeikin R. Acute respiratory depression as a complication of nebulized morphine. *Can J Anaesth* 1998;45:60–62.

Lang E, Kapila A, Shlugman D, et al. Reduction of isoflurane minimal alveolar concentration by remifentanil. *Anesthesiology* 1996;85: 721–728.

Langevin S, Lessard MR, Trepanier CA, et al. Alfentanil causes less postoperative nausea and vomiting than equipotent doses of fentanyl or sufentanil in outpatients. *Anesthesiology* 1999:91: 1666–1673.

Lanz E, Simko G, Theiss D, et al. Epidural buprenorphine: a double-blind study of postoperative analgesia and side effects. *Anesth Analg* 1984;63:593–598.

Lewis WR, Perrino AC. Transient neurological symptoms after subarachnoid meperidine. *Anesth Analg* 2002;94:213–214.

Licina MG, Schubert A, Tobin JE, et al. Intrathecal morphine does not reduce minimum alveolar concentration of halothane in humans: results of a double-blind study. *Anesthesiology* 1991;74: 660–663.

Lotsch J, Weiss M, Ahne G, et al. Pharmacokinetic modeling of M6G formation after oral administration of morphine in healthy volunteers. *Anesthesiology* 1999;90:1026–1038.

Lowenstein E, Whiting RB, Bittar DA, et al. Locally and neurally mediated effects of morphine on skeletal muscle vascular resistance. *J Pharmacol Exp Ther* 1972;180:359–367.

Lynn AM, Slattery JT. Morphine pharmacokinetics in early infancy. *Anesthesiology* 1987;66:136–139.

Macaluso AD, Connelly AM, Hayes B, et al. Oral transmucosal fentanyl citrate for premedication in adults. *Anesth Analg* 1996;82: 158–161.

Malinovsky JM, Lepage JY, Cozian A, et al. Transient muscular spasm after a large dose of intrathecal sufentanil. *Anesthesiology* 1996; 84:1513–1515.

Manninen PH. Opioids and seizures. *Can J Anaesth* 1997;44:463–466.

Mayer N, Weinstabl C, Podreka I, et al. Sufentanil does not increase cerebral blood flow in healthy human volunteers. *Anesthesiology* 1990;73:240–243.

Meistelman C, Benhamou D, Barre J, et al. Effects of age on plasma protein binding of sufentanil. *Anesthesiology* 1990;72:470–473.

Meistelman C, Saint-Maurice C, Lepaul M, et al. A comparison of alfentanil pharmacokinetics in children and adults. *Anesthesiology* 1987;66:13–16.

Mets B. Acute dystonia after alfentanil in untreated Parkinson's disease. *Anesth Analg* 1991;72:557–558.

Miller DR, Martineau RJ, O'Brien H, et al. Effects of alfentanil on the hemodynamic and catecholamine response to tracheal intubation. *Anesth Analg* 1993;76:1040–1046.

Mitra S, Sinatra RS. Perioperative management of acute pain in the opioid-dependent patient. *Anesthesiology* 2004;101:212–227.
Mondzac AM. Compassionate pain relief: is heroin the answer? *N Engl J Med* 1984;311:530–535.
Morgan M. The rational use of intrathecal and extradural opioids. *Br J Anaesth* 1989;63:165–188.
Motamed C, Mazoit X, Ghanouchi K, et al. Preemptive intravenous morphine-6-glucuronide is ineffective for postoperative pain relief. *Anesthesiology* 2000;92:355–360.
Murat I, Levron JB, Berg A, et al. Effects of fentanyl on baroreceptor reflex control of heart rate in newborn infants. *Anesthesiology* 1988;68:717–722.
Murkin JM, Moldenhauer CC, Hug CC, et al. Absence of seizures during induction of anesthesia with high dose fentanyl. *Anesth Analg* 1984;63:489–494.
Murphy DB, Sutton JA, Prescott LF, et al. Opioid-induced delay in gastric emptying: a peripheral mechanism in humans. *Anesthesiology* 1997;87:765–770.
Murphy MR, Hug CC, McClain DD. Dose-dependent pharmacokinetics of fentanyl. *Anesthesiology* 1983;59:537–540.
Murphy MR, Hug CC. Pharmacokinetics of intravenous morphine in patients anesthetized with enflurane-nitrous oxide. *Anesthesiology* 1981;54:187–192.
Murphy MR, Hug CC. The enflurane sparing effect of morphine, butorphanol, and nalbuphine. *Anesthesiology* 1982;57:489–492.
Nieuwenhuijs D, Bruce J, Drummond GB, et al. Influence of oral tramadol on the dynamic ventilatory response to carbon dioxide in healthy volunteers. *Br J Anaesth* 2001;87:860–865.
Niewenhuijs DJF, Olofsen E, Romberd RR, et al. Response surface modeling of remifentanil-propofol interaction on cardiorespiratory control and bispectral index. *Anesthesiology* 2003;98:312–322.
Palmer CM, Cork RC, Hays R, et al. The dose-response relation of intrathecal fentanyl for labor analgesia. *Anesthesiology* 1998;88: 355–361.
Paqueron X, Lumbroso A, Mergoni P, et al. Is morphine-induced sedation synonymous with analgesia during intravenous morphine titration? *Br J Anaesth* 2002;89:697–701.
Partridge BL, Ward CF. Pulmonary edema following low-dose naloxone administration. *Anesthesiology* 1986;65:710–711.
Paul D, Standifer KM, Inturrisi CE, et al. Pharmacological characterization of morphine-6 beta-glucuronide: a very potent morphine metabolite. *J Pharmacol Exp Ther* 1989;251:477–483.
Peng P, Sandler AN. A review of the use of fentanyl analgesia in the management of acute pain in adults. *Anesthesiology* 1999;90: 576–599.
Philbin DM, Moss J, Akins CW, et al. The use of H_1 and H_2 histamine antagonists with morphine anesthesia: a double blind study. *Anesthesiology* 1981;55:292–296.
Philbin DM, Rosow CE, Schneider RC, et al. Fentanyl and sufentanil anesthesia revisited: how much is enough? *Anesthesiology* 1990; 73:5–11.
Philbin DM, Wilson NE, Sokoloshi I, et al. Radioimmunoassay of antidiuretic hormone during morphine anesthesia. *Can Anaesth Soc J* 1976;23:290–295.
Pleuvry BJ. Opioid receptors and their relevance to anaesthesia. *Br J Anaesth* 1993;71:119–126.
Pomeranz B, Chiu D. Naloxone blockade of acupuncture analgesia: endorphin implicated. *Life Sci* 1976;19:1757–1762.
Radnay PA, Brodman E, Mankikar D, et al. The effect of equi-analgesic doses of fentanyl, morphine, meperidine, and pentazocine on common bile duct pressure. *Anaesthetist* 1980;29:26–29.
Rawal N, Schott U, Dahlstrom B, et al. Influence of naloxone infusion on analgesia and respiratory depression following epidural morphine. *Anesthesiology* 1986;64:194–201.
Recart A, Rawal S, White PF, et al. The effect of remifentanil on seizure duration and acute hemodynamic responses to electroconvulsive therapy. *Anesth Analg* 2003;96:1047–1050.
Roerig DL, Kotrly KJ, Vucins EJ, et al. First pass uptake of fentanyl, meperidine, and morphine in the human lung. *Anesthesiology* 1987;67:466–472.
Romberg R, Olofsen E, Sarton E, et al. Pharmacokinetic-pharmacodynamic modeling of morphine-6-glucuronide-induced analgesia in healthy volunteers: absence of sex differences. *Anesthesiology* 2004; 100:120–133.
Romberg R, Olofsen E, Satron E, et al. Pharmacodynamic effect of morphine-6-glucuronide versus morphine on hypoxic and hypercapnic breathing in healthy volunteers. *Anesthesiology* 2003;99: 788–798.
Rose JB, Finkel JC, Arquedas-Mohs A, et al. Oral tramadol for the treatment of pain 7-3-days' duration in children. *Anesth Analg* 2003; 96:78–81.
Rosow C. Remifentanil: a unique opioid analgesic. *Anesthesiology* 1993;79:875–876.
Rosow CE, Moss J, Philbin DM, et al. Histamine release during morphine and fentanyl anesthesia. *Anesthesiology* 1982;56:93–96.
Rozan JP, Kahn CH, Warfield CA. Epidural and intravenous opioid-induced neuroexcitation. *Anesthesiology* 1995;83:860–863.
Sanford TJ, Smith NT, Dee-Silver H, et al. A comparison of morphine, fentanyl, and sufentanil anesthesia for cardiac surgery: induction, emergency and extubation. *Anesth Analg* 1986;65:259–266.
Sarton E, Olofsen E, Romberg R, et al. Sex differences in morphine analgesia: an experimental study in healthy volunteers. *Anesthesiology* 2000;93:1245–1254.
Schubert A, Drummond JC, Peterson DO, Saidman LJ. The effect of high-dose fentanyl on human median nerve somatosensory-evoked responses. *Can J Anaesth* 1987;34:35–40.
Schwartz AE, Matteo RS, Ornstein E, et al. Pharmacokinetics of sufentanil in obese patients. *Anesth Analg* 1991;73:790–793.
Schwartz AE, Matteo RS, Ornstein R, et al. MAC reduction of isoflurane by sufentanil. *Br J Anaesth* 1994;72:42–46.
Schwieger IM, Klopfenstein CE, Forster A. Epidural morphine reduces halothane MAC in humans. *Can J Anaesth* 1992;39:911–914.
Scott JC, Cooke JE, Stanski DR. Electroencephalographic quantitation of opioid effect: comparative pharmacodynamics of fentanyl and sufentanil. *Anesthesiology* 1991;74:34–42.
Scott JC, Ponganis KV, Stanski DR. EEG quantitation of narcotic effect: the comparative pharmacodynamics of fentanyl and alfentanil. *Anesthesiology* 1985;62:234–241.
Scott JC, Stanski DR. Decreased fentanyl and alfentanil dose requirements with age. A simultaneous pharmacokinetic and pharmacodynamic evaluation. *J Pharmacol Exp Ther* 1987;240:159–166.
Sear JW. Drug biotransformation by the kidney: how important is it, and how much do we really know? *Br J Anaesth* 1991;67:169–172.
Sebel PS, Glass PSA, Fletcher JE, et al. Reduction of the MAC of desflurane with fentanyl. *Anesthesiology* 1992;76:52–59.
Sebel PS, Lang E, Rampil IJ, et al. A multicenter study of bispectral electroencephalogram analysis for monitoring anesthetic effect. *Anesth Analg* 1997;84:891–899.
Shafer SL, Varvel JR. Pharmacokinetics, pharmacodynamics, and rational opioid selection. *Anesthesiology* 1991;74:53–63.
Sjöström S, Tamsen A, Persson MP, et al. Pharmacokinetics of intrathecal morphine and meperidine in humans. *Anesthesiology* 1987;67:889–895.
Smith NT, Benthuysen JL, Bickford RG, et al. Seizures during opioid anesthetic induction: are they opioid-induced rigidity? *Anesthesiology* 1989;71:852–862.
Sperry RJ, Bailey PL, Reichman MV, et al. Fentanyl and sufentanil increase intracranial pressure in head trauma patients. *Anesthesiology* 1992;77:416–420.
Sprigge JS, Wynands JE, Whalley DG, et al. Fentanyl infusion anesthesia for aortocoronary bypass surgery: plasma levels and hemodynamic response. *Anesth Analg* 1982;61:1972–1978.
Stanley TH, Hague B, Mock DL, et al. Oral transmucosal fentanyl citrate (lollipop) premedication in human volunteers. *Anesth Analg* 1989;69:21–27.
Stanski DR, Hug CC. Alfentanil: a kinetically predictable narcotic analgesic. *Anesthesiology* 1982;57:435–438.
Steffey EP, Eisele JH, Baggot JD, et al. Influence of inhaled anesthetics on the pharmacokinetics and pharmacodynamics of morphine. *Anesth Analg* 1993;77:346–351.
Stein C. The control of pain in peripheral tissue by opioids. *N Engl J Med* 1995;332:1685–1690.
Stoeckel H, Hengstmann JH, Schuttler J. Pharmacokinetics of fentanyl as a possible explanation for recurrence of respiratory depression. *Br J Anaesth* 1979;51:741–745.
Stoelting RK, Gibbs PS. Hemodynamic effects of morphine and morphine-nitrous oxide in valvular heart disease and coronary artery disease. *Anesthesiology* 1973;38:45–52.

Stone PA, Macintyre PE, Jarvis DA. Norpethidine toxicity and patient controlled analgesia. *Br J Anaesth* 1993;71:738–740.

Takada K, Clark DJ, Davies MF, et al. Meperidine exerts agonist activity at the alpha$_{2B}$-adrenoceptor subtype. *Anesthesiology* 2002;96: 1420–1426.

Thipphawong JB, Babul N, Morishige RJ, et al. Analgesic efficacy of inhaled morphine in patients after bunionectomy surgery. *Anesthesiology* 2003;99:693–700.

Thompson JP, Hall AP, Russell J, et al. Effect of remifentanil on the haemodynamic response to orotracheal intubation. *Br J Anaesth* 1998;80:467–469.

Thompson JP, Rowbotham DJ. Remifentanil—an opioid for the 21st century. *Br J Anaesth* 1996;76:341–343.

Tissot TA. Probable meperidine-induced serotoninic syndrome in a patient with a history of fluoxetine use. *Anesthesiology* 2003;98: 1511–1512.

Tomicheck RC, Rosow CE, Philbin DM, et al. Diazepam-fentanyl interaction: hemodynamic and hormonal effects in coronary artery surgery. *Anesth Analg* 1983;62:881–884.

Tooms A, McKenzie A. Nebulized morphine. *Lancet* 1993;342:1 123–1124.

Tweed WA, Dakin D. Explosive coughing after bolus fentanyl injection. *Anesth Analg* 2001;92:1442–1443.

Vaughn CW, Connor M. In search of a role for the morphine metabolite morphine-3-glucuronide. *Anesth Analg* 2003;97: 311–312.

Waggum DC, Cork RC, Weldon ST, et al. Postoperative respiratory depression and elevated sufentanil levels in a patient in chronic renal failure. *Anesthesiology* 1985;63:708–710.

Warner DS, Hindman BJ, Todd MM, et al. Intracranial pressure and hemodynamic effects of remifentanil versus alfentanil in patients undergoing supratentorial craniotomy. *Anesth Analg* 1996;83:348–353.

Way WL, Costley EC, Way EL. Respiratory sensitivity of the newborn infant to meperidine and morphine. *Clin Pharmacol Ther* 1965;6:454–461.

Webster NR. Opioids and the immune system. *Br J Anaesth* 1998; 81:835–836.

Werner C, Kochs E, Bause H, et al. Effects of sufentanil on cerebral hemodynamics and intracranial pressure in patients with brain injury. *Anesthesiology* 1995;83:721–726.

White PF. Patient-controlled analgesia: a new approach to the management of postoperative pain. *Semin Anesth* 1985;4:255–266.

Wilson PR. Opioid use and diversion: Report on hearing by FDA and DEA. ASA statement to FDA committee. *ASA Newsletter* 2002; 66:9–10.

Woolf CJ, Wall PD. Morphine-sensitive and morphine-insensitive actions of C-fibres input on the rat spinal cord. *Neurosci Lett* 1986;64:221–225.

Wynands JE, Wong P, Whalley DG, et al. Oxygen-fentanyl anesthesia in patients with poor left ventricular function: hemodynamics and plasma fentanyl concentrations. *Anesth Analg* 1983;62:476–482.

Yaster M. The dose response of fentanyl in neonatal anesthesia. *Anesthesiology* 1987;66:433–435.

Yonker-Sell AE, Muzi M, Hope WG, et al. Alfentanil modifies the neurocirculatory responses to desflurane. *Anesth Analg* 1996;82: 162–166.

Zucker-Pinchoff B, Chandler MJ. Latex anaphylaxis masquerading as fentanyl anaphylaxis: retraction of a case report. *Anesthesiology* 1993;79:1152–1153.

Barbiturates

4

Classification of barbiturates as long, intermediate, short, and ultrashort acting is not recommended, as it incorrectly suggests that the action of these drugs ends abruptly after specified time intervals. This is clearly not the case for barbiturates; residual plasma concentrations and drug effects persist for several hours, even after administration of "ultrashort-acting" drugs for induction of anesthesia.

COMMERCIAL PREPARATIONS

Barbiturates are prepared commercially from highly alkaline solutions as sodium salts that are readily soluble in water or saline. For example, the pH of a 2.5% solution of thiopental is 10.5. These highly alkaline solutions are incompatible for mixture with drugs such as opioids, catecholamines, and neuromuscular-blocking drugs, which are acidic in solution. The bacteriostatic properties of commercial preparations of barbiturates are due to their highly alkaline pH. Commercial preparations of barbiturates often contain a mixture of six parts anhydrous sodium carbonate to prevent precipitation of the insoluble acid form of the barbiturate by atmospheric carbon dioxide.

Although the S(−) isomers of thiopental and thiamylal are twice as potent as the R(+) isomers, both drugs are commercially available only as racemic mixtures (Sueyasu et al., 2000). Methohexital is also marketed as the racemic mixture of the S(−) and R(+) isomers with the S(−) isomers being four to five times more potent than the R(+) isomers. Alone, the S(−) isomers of methohexital cause excessive skeletal muscle activity. Thiopental and thiamylal are usually prepared for clinical use in 2.5% solutions. A 5% solution is not recommended. Methohexital is used most often as a 1% solution. The powder form of thiopental is stable at room temperature indefinitely. Refrigerated solutions of thiobarbiturates are stable for up to 2 weeks, and solutions of methohexital are stable for up to 6 weeks. At room temperature (22°C), reconstituted solutions of thiopental remain stable and sterile for at least 6 days (Haws et al., 1998).

STRUCTURE ACTIVITY RELATIONSHIPS

Barbiturates are defined as any drug derived from barbituric acid. Barbituric acid, which lacks central nervous system (CNS) activity, is a cyclic compound obtained by the combination of urea and malonic acid (Fig. 4-1). Barbiturates with sedative-hypnotic properties result from substitutions at the number 2 and 5 carbon atoms of barbituric acid (Fig. 4-2). A barbiturate with a branched-chain substitution on the number 5 carbon atom usually has greater hypnotic activity than the corresponding drug with a straight chain. Drugs with a phenyl group in the number 5 carbon position, such as phenobarbital, have enhanced anticonvulsant activity. Sedative and anticonvulsant properties are separate effects of barbiturates. A methyl radical, as present with methohexital, confers convulsive activity manifesting as involuntary skeletal muscle movement.

Barbiturates that retain an oxygen atom on the number two carbon atom of the barbituric acid ring are designated as oxybarbiturates. Replacement of this oxygen atom with a sulfur atom results in thiobarbiturates, which are more lipid soluble than oxybarbiturates. In general, a structural change such as sulfuration that increases lipid solubility is associated with greater hypnotic potency and a more rapid onset but shorter duration of action. For example, thiopental has a more rapid onset and shorter duration of action than its oxybarbiturate analogue pentobarbital. Thiamylal is the thioanalogue of the oxybarbiturate secobarbital. Addition of a methyl group to the nitrogen atom of the barbituric acid ring, as with methohexital, results in a compound with a short duration of action.

MECHANISM OF ACTION

Barbiturates most likely produce their sedative-hypnotic effects through an interaction with the inhibitory neurotransmitter gamma-aminobutyric acid (GABA) in the CNS. $GABA_A$ receptors consist of up to five glycoprotein subunits. When $GABA_A$ receptors are activated, transmembrane chloride conductance increases, resulting in

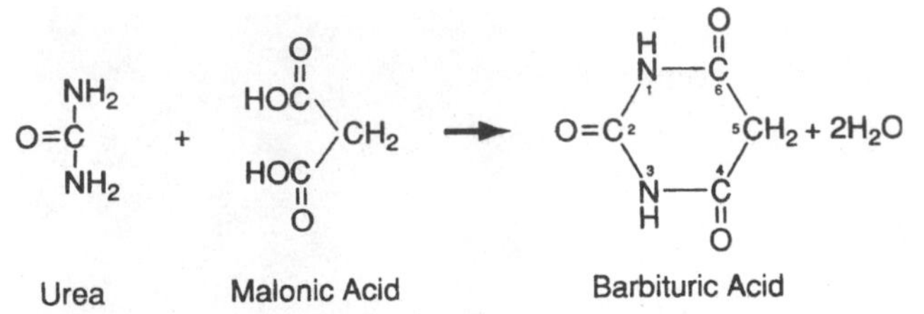

Figure 4-1. Barbituric acid is formed by the combination of urea and malonic acid.

hyperpolarization of postsynaptic cell membranes and functional inhibition of postsynaptic neurons. The interaction of barbiturates (and propofol) with specific membrane components of $GABA_A$ receptors appears to decrease the rate of dissociation of GABA from these receptors, thereby increasing the duration of the $GABA_A$-activated opening of chloride channels (see Fig. 3-2). The ability of barbiturates to uniquely depress the reticular activating system, which is presumed to be important in the maintenance of wakefulness, may reflect the ability of barbiturates to decrease the rate of dissociation of GABA from its receptors. Barbiturates can also mimic the action of GABA by directly activating $GABA_A$ receptors. In addition to acting at $GABA_A$ receptors, barbiturates target glutamate receptors, adenosine receptors and neuronal nicotinic acetylcholine receptors (nAChRs) at concentrations that are achieved with clinical use of these drugs. Although nAChRs belong to the same superfamily of fast neurotransmitter-gated receptors as do $GABA_A$ receptors, there is evidence that nAChRs are not critical targets for barbiturates (Downie et al., 2000). Glycine and *N*-methyl-D-aspartate receptors are not responsive to barbiturates.

Barbiturates selectively depress transmission in sympathetic nervous system ganglia in concentrations that have no detectable effect on nerve conduction. This effect may contribute to decreases in systemic blood pressure that may accompany intravenous (IV) administration of barbiturates or that occur in association with a barbiturate overdose. At the neuromuscular junction, high doses of barbiturates decrease sensitivity of postsynaptic membranes to the depolarizing actions of acetylcholine.

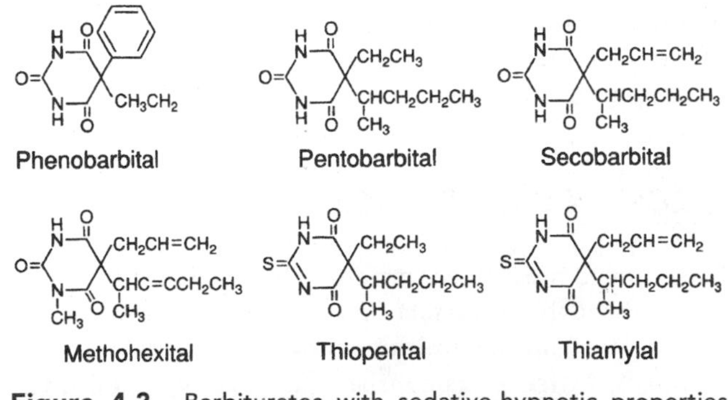

Figure 4-2. Barbiturates with sedative-hypnotic properties result from substitutions at the number two and five carbon atoms of barbituric acid (see Fig. 4-1).

PHARMACOKINETICS

Prompt awakening after a single IV dose of thiopental, thiamylal, or methohexital reflects redistribution of these drugs from the brain to inactive tissues (Fig. 4-3) (Saidman, 1974). Ultimately, however, elimination from the body depends almost entirely on metabolism, because <1% of these drugs are recovered unchanged in urine (Saidman and Eger, 1966). The time required for equilibration of the brain with the thiopental concentration in the blood (effect-site equilibration time) is rapid. Conversely, the time necessary for the plasma concentration of thiopental to decrease 50% after discontinuation of a prolonged infusion (context-sensitive half-time) is prolonged as drug sequestered in fat and skeletal muscle reenters the circulation to maintain a plasma concentration (see Fig. 1-3) (Hughes et al., 1992).

Protein Binding

Protein binding of barbiturates parallels lipid solubility. The lipid solubility of a barbiturate is determined almost entirely by the solubility of the nonionized molecule; the ionized molecule is poorly soluble in lipid. Thiobarbiturates are bound to a greater extent than their oxybarbiturate analogues. This difference probably relates to the effect of the sulfur substitution on the affinity for a hydrophobic portion of the protein.

Thiopental, as a highly lipid-soluble barbiturate, is the most avidly bound to plasma proteins, with binding to

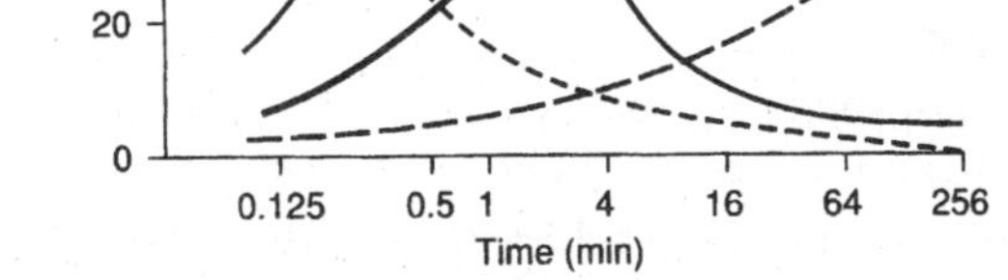

Figure 4-3. After a rapid intravenous injection, the percentage of thiopental remaining in the blood rapidly decreases as drug moves from the blood to tissues. Time to achievement of peak levels is a direct function of tissue capacity for barbiturate relative to blood flow. Initially, most thiopental is taken up by the vessel-rich group tissues because of their high blood flow. Subsequently, drug is redistributed to skeletal muscles and, to a lesser extent, to fat. The rate of metabolism equals the early rate of removal by fat, and the sum of these two events is similar to uptake of drug by skeletal muscles. (From Saidman LJ. Uptake, distribution, and elimination of barbiturates. In: Eger EI, ed. *Anesthetic uptake and action*. Baltimore: Williams & Wilkins, 1974; with permission.)

albumin ranging from 72% to 86%. The higher percentage of protein binding occurs at lower plasma concentrations of thiopental. Changes in pH between 7.35 to 7.5 do not alter the degree of protein binding. Decreased protein binding of thiopental as a result of displacement from binding sites by other drugs, such as aspirin and phenylbutazone, can lead to enhanced drug effects. Decreased protein binding of thiopental may explain, in part, increased drug sensitivity demonstrated by patients with uremia or cirrhosis of the liver. Decreased protein binding in patients with uremia may be partially a result of competitive binding inhibitors such as nitrogenous waste products. Hypoalbuminemia may account for decreased protein binding of barbiturates in patients with cirrhosis of the liver. Protein binding of thiopental in neonatal plasma (placental blood) is about half that measured in adults, suggesting a possible increased sensitivity to thiopental in neonates (Kingston et al., 1990). This unbound fraction of thiopental could be increased further by fetal acidosis that may accompany a stressful delivery. There is a possibility of a drug/drug binding interaction in patients being treated with coumarin anticoagulants.

Distribution

Distribution of barbiturates in the body is determined by their lipid solubility, protein binding, and degree of ionization. Of the factors that influence distribution of thiopental, thiamylal, and methohexital, lipid solubility is the most important. Tissue blood flow is a major determinant in delivery of barbiturates to tissues and their ultimate distribution in the body. Alterations in blood volume or distribution of blood flow to tissues may alter the distribution of thiopental or similar drugs. For example, hypovolemia may decrease blood flow to skeletal muscles, whereas blood flow to the brain and heart are maintained. Thiopental plasma concentrations are increased because of less dilution, resulting in the potential for exaggerated cerebral and cardiac depression in the presence of hypovolemia.

Brain

Thiopental, thiamylal, and methohexital undergo maximal brain uptake within 30 seconds (rapid effect-site equilibration), accounting for the prompt onset of CNS depression (see Fig. 4-3) (Saidman, 1974). The brain receives about 10% of the total dose of thiopental in the first 30 to 40 seconds. This maximal brain concentration is followed by a decrease over the next 5 minutes to one-half the initial peak concentration, due to redistribution of the drug from the brain to other tissues. Indeed, redistribution is the principal mechanism, accounting for early awakening after a single IV dose of these drugs. After about 30 minutes, the barbiturate has been further redistributed and as little as 10% remains in the brain. Redistribution occurs promptly because initial high uptake of lipid-soluble drug into the brain and other highly perfused tissues causes the plasma concentration of barbiturate to decrease, resulting in reversal of the concentration gradient for the movement of drug between blood and tissues.

Skeletal Muscles

Skeletal muscles are the most prominent sites for initial redistribution of highly lipid-soluble barbiturates such as thiopental (see Fig. 4-3) (Saidman, 1974). Indeed, the initial decrease in the plasma concentration of thiopental is principally a result of uptake of drug into skeletal muscles, with only a modest contribution from metabolism. Equilibrium with skeletal muscles is reached in about 15 minutes after IV injection of thiopental emphasizing the need to decrease the dose of thiopental when skeletal muscle perfusion is reduced (shock) or when skeletal muscle mass is decreased (elderly).

Fat

Fat is the only compartment in which thiopental content continues to increase 30 minutes after injection (see Fig. 4-3) (Saidman, 1974). With a fat:blood partition coefficient of about 11, thiopental will move from blood to fat as long as the concentration in fat is less than 11 times that in blood. Despite the affinity for fat, the initial uptake of drug into adipose tissue is slow, emphasizing the role of low blood flow to fat in limiting delivery of barbiturate to this tissue. Indeed, redistribution of drug to fat will not significantly affect early awakening from a single intravenous (IV) dose of barbiturate. Maximal deposition of thiopental in fat is present after about 2.5 hours, and this tissue becomes a potential reservoir for maintaining plasma concentrations of the drug. For example, large or repeated doses of lipid-soluble barbiturates produce a cumulative effect because of the storage capacity of fat. When this occurs, the usual rapid awakening characteristic of these drugs is absent. For this reason, the dose of thiopental is best calculated according to lean body mass to avoid an overdose.

Cardiopulmonary Bypass

Administration of thiopental during cardiopulmonary bypass and in the presence of hypothermia is associated with a significant decrease in systemic clearance (Gedney and Ghosh, 1995). In the presence of an existing steady plasma concentration of thiopental, the institution of cardiopulmonary bypass results in an abrupt 50% decrease in the plasma concentration followed by a gradual increase to 70% of the prebypass concentration. There is a strong correlation between the binding ratio of thiopental and the plasma albumin concentration before and after cardiopulmonary bypass, suggesting that the decrease in plasma protein binding during cardiopulmonary bypass is largely dilutional.

Ionization

The distribution of thiopental from blood to tissues will be influenced by the state of ionization of the drug and its binding to plasma proteins. Because the pK of thiopental

(7.6) is near blood pH, acidosis will favor the nonionized fraction of drug, whereas alkalosis has the opposite effect. The nonionized form of drug has greater access to the CNS because of its higher lipid solubility. Acidosis will thus increase and alkalosis will decrease the intensity of the barbiturate effect. Evidence of increased brain penetration of barbiturate is the decrease in plasma concentration of thiopental associated with an acute decrease in blood pH.

Metabolism-induced alterations in blood pH produce more pronounced effects on drug distribution than do changes in pH due to alterations in ventilation. For example, in the presence of metabolic changes, the intracellular pH in the brain may remain relatively unchanged, reflecting the inability of hydrogen ions to cross the lipid barrier easily. As a result, movement of drug across the blood-brain barrier is favored. In contrast, ventilation-induced changes in blood pH are associated with rapid diffusion of carbon dioxide and similar changes in intracellular and extracellular pH, resulting in less net movement of drug.

Metabolism

Oxybarbiturates are metabolized only in hepatocytes, whereas thiobarbiturates also break down to a small extent in extrahepatic sites such as the kidneys and possibly the CNS. Metabolites are usually inactive and are always more water soluble than the parent compound, which facilitates renal excretion. Side chain oxidation at the number 5 carbon atom of the benzene ring to yield carboxylic acid is the most important initial step in terminating pharmacologic activity of barbiturates by metabolism. This oxidation occurs primarily in the endoplasmic reticulum of hepatocytes. The reserve capacity of the liver to carry out oxidation of barbiturates is large, and hepatic dysfunction must be extreme before a prolonged duration of action of barbiturates as a result of decreased metabolism occurs.

Thiopental

Redistribution of thiopental to inactive tissue sites rather than metabolism is the most important determinant of early awakening following a single intravenous injection. Data based on measurements obtained several hours after injection of thiopental suggest that metabolism of thiopental occurs at a slow rate, with 10% to 24% being metabolized by the liver each hour (Mark et al., 1965). These data do not reflect the magnitude of metabolism early after drug administration and thus underestimate the role of metabolism of thiopental in prompt awakening after a single IV injection of the drug (see Fig. 4-3) (Saidman, 1974). For example, after several hours, most of the thiopental body stores are in fat and the fraction of drug delivered to the liver is far less than in the first few minutes after injection. Thiopental is metabolized in the liver to hydroxythiopental and carboxylic acid derivatives, which are more water soluble and have little CNS activity. Ultimately, metabolism of thiopental is almost complete (99%), with the principal sites of metabolism being oxidation of substituents on the number five carbon atom, desulfuration on the number two carbon atom, and hydrolytic opening of the barbituric acid ring. When large doses of thiopental are administered, a desulfuration reaction can occur with the production of pentobarbital (Chan et al., 1985; Nguyen et al., 1996).

Hepatic clearance of thiopental is characterized by a low hepatic extraction ratio and capacity-dependent elimination influenced by hepatic enzyme activity but not hepatic blood flow. Nevertheless, enzyme induction or inhibition does not modify the duration of action of thiopental as observed in animals. In patients with cirrhosis of the liver, clearance of thiopental from the plasma is not different from that in normal patients (Pandele et al., 1983). Therefore, it is unlikely that a prolonged effect of a single dose of thiopental will occur in patients with cirrhosis of the liver. Conversely, enzyme induction from chronic exposure to environmental pollution is presumed to be the explanation for increased thiopental dose requirements in patients from urban compared with rural areas.

Methohexital

Methohexital is metabolized more rapidly than thiopental, reflecting its lesser lipid solubility; thus, more methohexital remains in the plasma to become available for metabolism. Side chain oxidation of methohexital results in the formation of an inactive metabolite, 4-hydroxymethohexital. Overall, the hepatic clearance of methohexital is three to four times that of thiopental. Despite this greater hepatic clearance, early awakening from a single IV dose of methohexital depends primarily on its redistribution to inactive tissue sites (Hudson et al., 1983). Nevertheless, metabolism will exert a greater role in terminating the effect of methohexital than of thiopental. For example, metabolism may be an important determinant of the time required for complete psychomotor recovery. Indeed, many psychomotor functions recover more quickly after administration of methohexital compared with thiopental (Korttila et al., 1975). Recovery from methohexital is predictably more rapid than that from thiopental when repeated doses of drug are administered, reflecting the greater role of metabolism in the clearance of methohexital from the plasma. The hepatic clearance of methohexital is more dependent on changes in cardiac output and hepatic blood flow than is the hepatic clearance of thiopental.

Renal Excretion

All barbiturates are filtered by the renal glomeruli, but the high degree of protein binding limits the magnitude of filtration, whereas high lipid solubility favors reabsorption of any filtered drug back into the circulation. Indeed, <1% of administered thiopental, thiamylal, or methohexital is excreted unchanged in urine. Among the barbiturates, phenobarbital is the only one that undergoes significant renal excretion in the unchanged form, reflecting the lesser protein binding and lipid solubility of this barbiturate compared with that of thiopental. Renal excretion of phenobarbital can be significantly increased by osmotic diuresis. Alkalinization of urine also hastens renal excretion of phenobarbital because of the shift toward the ionized state caused by this pH change.

Elimination Half-Time

The distribution half-time and volume of distribution (Vd) of thiopental and methohexital is similar (Table 4-1) (Hudson et al., 1983). Conversely, elimination half-time and clearance of these two drugs differ (see Table 4-1) (Fig. 4-4) (Hudson et al., 1983). The shorter elimination half-time of methohexital compared with that of thiopental results from the greater hepatic clearance of methohexital.

The elimination half-time of thiopental is prolonged in obese patients compared with nonobese patients, reflecting an increased Vd resulting from excess fat storage sites (Jung et al., 1982). Increasing age is associated with a slower passage of thiopental from the central compartment to peripheral compartments (approximately 30% slower in 80-year-old patients compared with young adults), whereas the initial Vd is unchanged (Fig. 4-5) (Avram et al., 1990; Stanski and Maitre, 1990). This slower rate of intercompartmental clearance results in higher plasma concentrations of thiopental for distribution into the brain to create a greater anesthetic effect in the elderly. Evidence that pharmacokinetics (intercompartmental clearance) are responsible for the decreased thiopental dose requirements in elderly patients is the similar plasma concentration of thiopental in all adult-age patients required to suppress the electroencephalogram (EEG) to a similar degree (Fig. 4-6) (Avram et al., 1990; Homer and Stanski, 1985; Stanski and Maitre, 1990).

TABLE 4-1.
COMPARATIVE PHARMACOKINETICS

	Thiopental	Methohexital
Rapid distribution half-time (mins)	8.5	5.6
Slow distribution half-time (mins)	62.7	58.3
Elimination half-time (hrs)	11.6	3.9*
Clearance (mL/kg/min)	3.4	10.9
Volume of distribution (liters/kg)	2.5	2.2

*Significantly different from thiopental.
Source: Data from Hudson RJ, Stanski DR, Burch PG. Pharmacokinetics of methohexital and thiopental in surgical patients. *Anesthesiology* 1983;59:215–219.

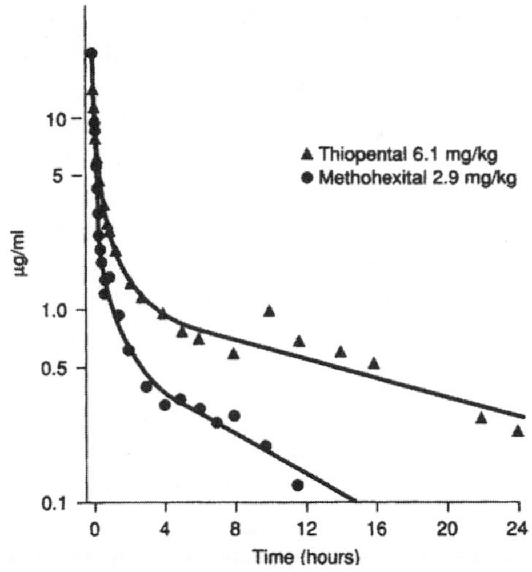

Figure 4-4. The rate of decline of the plasma concentration and thus the elimination half-time is shorter after the IV administration of methohexital than after the administration of thiopental. (From Hudson RJ, Stanski DR, Burch PG. Pharmacokinetics of methohexital and thiopental in surgical patients. *Anesthesiology* 1983;59:215–219; with permission.)

In pediatric patients, the elimination half-time of thiopental is shorter than in adults (Sorbo et al., 1984). This shorter elimination half-time is due to more rapid hepatic clearance of thiopental by pediatric patients. Therefore, recovery after large or repeated doses of thiopental may be more rapid for infants and children than for adults. Protein binding and Vd of thiopental are not different in pediatric and adult patients. Elimination half-time is prolonged during pregnancy because of the increased protein binding of thiopental.

CLINICAL USES

The principal clinical uses of barbiturates are for (a) induction of anesthesia and (b) treatment of increased intracranial

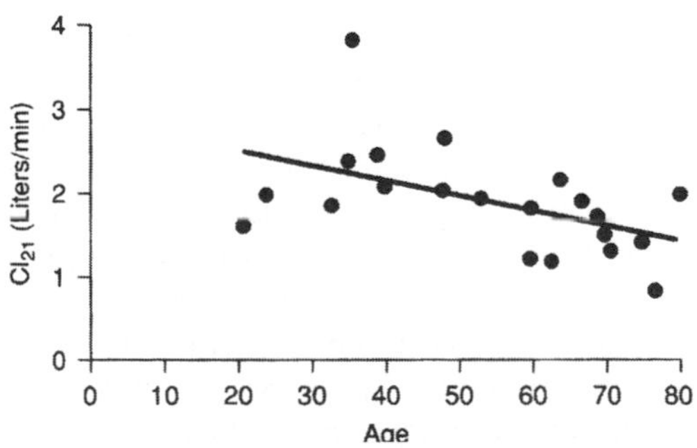

Figure 4-5. The rate of intercompartmental clearance of thiopental from the central compartment to the peripheral compartment slows with increasing age. (From Avram JJ, Krejcie TC, Henthorn TK. The relationship of age to the pharmacokinetics to early drug distribution: The concurrent disposition of thiopental and indocyanine green. *Anesthesiology* 1990;72:403–411; with permission.)

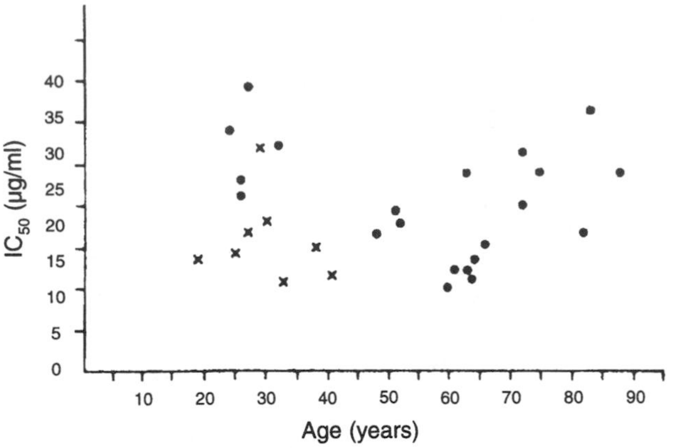

Figure 4-6. The plasma concentration of thiopental needed to slow activity on the electroencephalogram 50% (IC_{50}) is independent of age. Blood sampling was either arterial (X) or venous (•). (From Homer TD, Stanski DR. The effect of increasing age on thiopental disposition and anesthetic requirement. *Anesthesiology* 1985;62:714–724; with permission.)

pressure (ICP). Use of phenobarbital to treat hyperbilirubinemia and kernicterus reflects barbiturate-induced increases in hepatic glucuronyl transferase enzyme activity. Other clinical uses of barbiturates are declining in frequency because these drugs (a) lack specificity of effect in the central nervous system (CNS), (b) have a lower therapeutic index than do benzodiazepines, (c) result in tolerance more often than do benzodiazepines, (d) have a greater liability for abuse, and (e) have a high risk for drug interactions. Other undesirable features of barbiturates include paradoxical excitement instead of sedation, especially in elderly patients or in the presence of pain. Barbiturate-induced paradoxical excitement suggests depression of CNS inhibitory centers as the mechanism. Small doses of barbiturates seem to lower the pain threshold, accounting for the clinical impression that these drugs are antianalgesic. Therefore, barbiturates cannot be relied on to produce sedation in the presence of pain. Nevertheless, the concept that barbiturates are antianalgesic has never been confirmed (Kitahata and Saberski, 1992).

Skeletal muscle relaxation does not occur, and there is no clinically significant effect of barbiturates on the neuromuscular junction. Drowsiness may last for only a short time after a sedative-hypnotic dose of a barbiturate administered orally, but residual CNS effects characterized as "hangover" may persist for several hours. Barbiturates have been replaced by benzodiazepines for preanesthetic medication. The rapid onset of action of barbiturates renders these drugs useful for treatment of grand mal seizures, but, again, benzodiazepines are probably superior, providing a more specific site of action in the CNS.

Induction of Anesthesia

The supremacy of barbiturates for IV induction of anesthesia remained virtually unchallenged from 1934 with the introduction of thiopental until the approval of propofol for clinical use in 1989. Propofol, although more expensive than thiopental, has replaced barbiturates for induction of anesthesia in many patients, especially in those where rapid awakening is considered desirable. Thiamylal is indistinguishable from thiopental when used for IV induction of anesthesia.

The oxybarbiturate methohexital is the only barbiturate with actions sufficiently different from the thiobarbiturates to offer an alternative to these drugs for the IV induction of anesthesia. The most important advantage of methohexital compared with thiopental is a more rapid recovery of consciousness, which is considered to be of greatest importance for outpatient procedures (Beskow et al., 1995). The principal disadvantage of methohexital is the associated increased incidence of excitatory phenomena, such as involuntary skeletal muscle movements (myoclonus) and other signs of excitatory activity including hiccoughs. The incidence of these excitatory phenomena is dose dependent and may be decreased by inclusion of opioids in the preoperative medication and by use of optimum doses of methohexital (1.0 to 1.5 mg/kg IV). Indeed, high doses of methohexital, as administered in a continuous infusion for neuroanesthesia, are associated with postoperative seizures in about one-third of patients (Todd et al., 1984). Thiopental infusion is seldom used to maintain anesthesia because of its long context-sensitive half-time and prolonged recovery period (see Fig. 1-3) (Hughes et al., 1992).

The relative potency of barbiturates used for IV induction of anesthesia assumes that thiopental is 1, thiamylal is 1.1, and methohexital is 2.5. At a blood pH of 7.4, methohexital is 76% nonionized compared with 61% for thiopental, which is consistent with the greater potency of methohexital. The CNS is exquisitely sensitive to IV doses of these barbiturates, which produce minimal to no effect on skeletal, cardiac, or smooth muscles. For example, thiopental, 3 to 5 mg/kg IV, rapidly enters the CNS and produces unconsciousness within 30 seconds. Induction dose requirements for thiopental vary with patient age, weight, and most importantly with cardiac output. The dose of thiopental required to induce anesthesia decreases with age, reflecting a slower passage of barbiturate from the central compartment to peripheral compartments (see Fig. 4-5) (Avram et al., 1990; Stanski and Maitre, 1990). The dose of thiopental needed to produce anesthesia in early pregnancy (7 to 13 weeks' gestation) is decreased about 18% compared with that for nonpregnant females (Fig. 4-7) (Gin et al., 1997). A similar decrease in dose requirements for isoflurane has also been described (see Chapter 2). Thiopental requirements, for unknown reasons, seem to be increased in children more than 1 year after thermal injury (Cote and Petkau, 1985). Despite a contrary clinical impression, thiopental dose requirements (with EEG suppression as the end point) are not different between nonalcoholics and alcoholics with abstinence of 9 to 17 days and 30 days (Fig. 4-8) (Swerdlow et al., 1990).

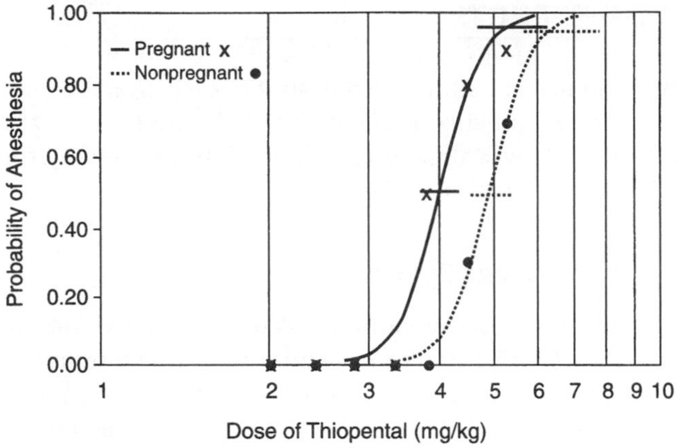

Figure 4-7. Dose-response curves for anesthesia in pregnant and nonpregnant females demonstrate a decreased dose requirement during 7 to 13 weeks of gestation. (From Gin T, Mainland P, Chan MT, et al. Decreased thiopental requirements in early pregnancy. *Anesthesiology* 1997;86:73–78; with permission.)

Rectal administration of barbiturates, especially methohexital, 20 to 30 mg/kg, has been used to induce anesthesia in uncooperative or young patients (Manuli and Davies, 1993). Loss of consciousness after rectal administration of methohexital correlates with a plasma concentration >2 μg/ml (Liu et al., 1985).

Occasionally, IV administration of a barbiturate is used as a supplement to inhaled anesthetics or as the sole anesthetic for brief and usually pain-free procedures such as cardioversion or electroconvulsive therapy. Methohexital, but not thiopental, is effective in inducing seizure activity in patients with psychomotor epilepsy undergoing temporal lobe resection of seizure-producing areas (Ford et al., 1982; Rockoff and Goudsouzian, 1981). A generalized anticonvulsant effect of barbiturates, however, may be undesirable if the therapeutic value of the electroconvulsive therapy is related to the duration of the seizure. Indeed, methohexital or propofol administered in doses of >1 mg/kg IV to patients before electroconvulsive therapy results in a 35% to 45% decrease in the duration of the electrically induced seizure compared with etomidate (Avramov et al., 1995).

Treatment of Increased Intracranial Pressure

Barbiturates are administered to decrease ICP that remains increased despite deliberate hyperventilation of the patient's lungs and drug-induced diuresis. Barbiturates decrease ICP by decreasing cerebral blood volume through drug-induced cerebral vascular vasoconstriction and an associated decrease in cerebral blood flow. The decrease in cerebral blood flow and associated increase in the perfusion-to-metabolism ratio render thiopental an attractive drug for induction of anesthesia in patients with increased ICP (Fig. 4-9) (Bedford et al., 1980). An isoelectric EEG confirms the presence of maximal barbiturate-induced depression of cerebral metabolic oxygen requirements by about 55%. Improved outcome after head trauma has not, however, been demonstrated in patients treated with barbiturates, despite the ability of these drugs to decrease and control ICP (Ward et al., 1985).

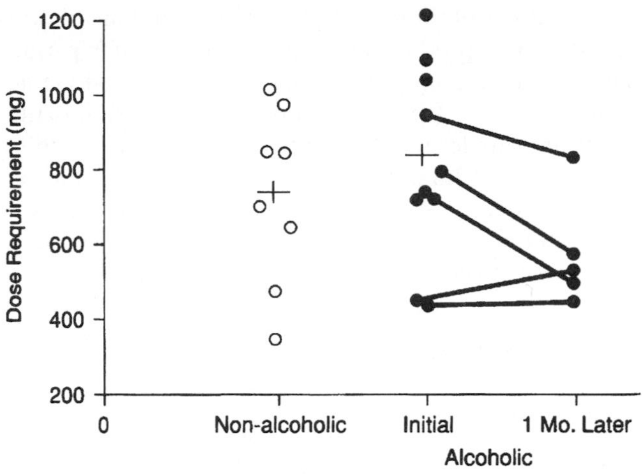

Figure 4-8. Thiopental doses needed to achieve burst suppression with 3 seconds of an isoelectric electroencephalogram are similar in nonalcoholics and alcoholic patients with abstinence of 9 to 17 days (initial) and 30 days (1 month later). (From Swerdlow BN, Holley FO, Maitre PO, et al. Chronic alcohol intake does not change thiopental anesthetic requirements, pharmacokinetics, or pharmacodynamics. *Anesthesiology* 1990;72:455–461; with permission.)

A hazard of high-dose barbiturate therapy used to lower ICP is hypotension, which can jeopardize the maintenance of an adequate cerebral perfusion pressure. Doses of thiopental sufficient to suppress EEG activity in animals are more likely than pentobarbital to lead to hypotension and ventricular fibrillation (Roesch et al., 1983). In

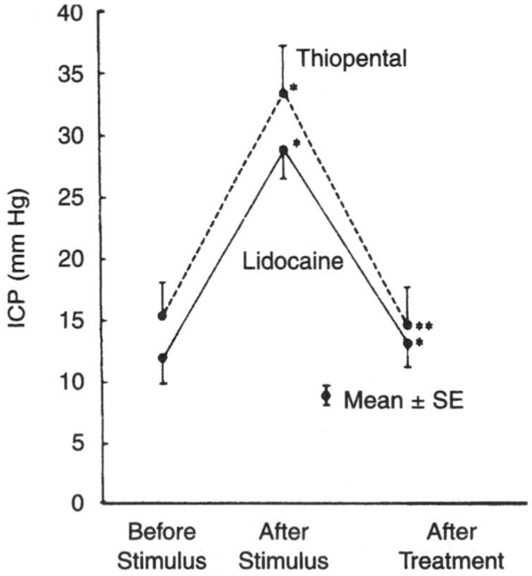

Figure 4-9. The administration of thiopental, 3 mg/kg IV, is as effective as lidocaine, 1.5 mg/kg IV, in decreasing intracranial pressure (ICP) after surgical stimulation in patients with brain tumors. (*P <.025 versus preceding value; **P <.02 versus preceding value.) (From Bedford RF, Persing JA, Poberskin L, et al. Lidocaine or thiopental for rapid control of intracranial hypertension. *Anesth Analg* 1980;59:435–437; with permission.)

patients, doses of thiopental (37.5 mg/kg) and methohexital sufficient to produce an isoelectric EEG result in peripheral vasodilation and myocardial depression (Todd et al., 1984, Todd et al., 1985). Nevertheless, these cardiovascular effects are smaller in magnitude than those produced by the dose of isoflurane (2 MAC) required to produce an equivalent degree of suppression of the EEG. This suggests that barbiturates may be hemodynamically preferable to isoflurane if profound EEG depression is desired.

Cerebral Protection

The ability of barbiturate therapy to improve brain survival after global cerebral ischemia due to cardiac arrest is unlikely, because these drugs are effective only when the EEG remains active and metabolic suppression is possible (Michenfelder, 1986). During cardiac arrest, the EEG becomes flat in 20 to 30 seconds, and barbiturates would not be expected to improve outcome. Indeed, administration of thiopental, 30 mg/kg IV, as a single injection to comatose survivors of cardiac arrest does not increase survival or improve neurologic outcome (Brain Resuscitation Clinical Trial I Study Group, 1986).

In contrast to global cerebral ischemia, animal studies consistently show improved outcome with barbiturate therapy of incomplete (focal) cerebral ischemia that permits drug-induced metabolic suppression (Todd et al., 1982). In this regard, barbiturate-induced decreases in cerebral metabolic oxygen requirements exceed decreases in cerebral blood flow, which may provide protection to poorly perfused areas of the brain. Consistent with these animal data showing protection against focal ischemic effects is the observation that neuropsychiatric complications after cardiopulmonary bypass (presumably due to embolism) clear more rapidly in patients treated prospectively with thiopental (average dose 39.5 mg/kg IV) to maintain an isoelectric EEG (Nussmeier et al., 1986). This beneficial effect is accompanied by an increased need for inotropic support at the conclusion of cardiopulmonary bypass and a delayed awakening. The routine use of barbiturates during cardiac surgery is not recommended because moderate degrees of hypothermia (33° to 34°C) may provide superior neuroprotection without prolonging the recovery phase. There are also data from patients in which thiopental did not decrease the risk of stroke after cardiac surgery (Todd et al., 1991; Zaidan et al., 1991). In patients with good preoperative cardiac function, doses of thiopental necessary to produce an isoelectric EEG have been reported to cause negligible cardiac impairment and not to impede separation from cardiopulmonary bypass (Stone et al., 1993). Other patients at risk for incomplete cerebral ischemia who might benefit from prior production of an isoelectric EEG (metabolic suppression) with barbiturates include those scheduled for carotid endarterectomy or thoracic aneurysm resection, and those managed with profound controlled hypotension.

SIDE EFFECTS

Barbiturates are administered almost exclusively to produce depressant effects on the CNS. Side effects, especially on the cardiovascular system, inevitably accompany the clinical use of barbiturates.

Cardiovascular System

Oral sedative doses of barbiturates do not produce cardiovascular effects different from the slight decrease in systemic blood pressure and heart rate that accompany physiologic sleep. The hemodynamic effects of equivalent doses of methohexital, thiamylal, and thiopental as administered for the IV induction of anesthesia are similar (Todd et al., 1984). In normovolemic subjects, thiopental, 5 mg/kg IV, produces a transient 10- to 20-mm Hg decrease in blood pressure that is offset by a compensatory 15 to 20 beats/minute increase in heart rate (Fig. 4-10) (Filner and Karliner, 1976). This dose of thiopental produces minimal to no evidence of myocardial depression. When decreases in myocardial contractility are demonstrated after induction of anesthesia with barbiturates, the magnitude of this decrease is far less than that produced by volatile anesthetics (Becker and Tonnesen, 1978; Kaplan et al., 1976). Cardiac dysrhythmias after induction of anesthesia with barbiturates are unlikely in the presence of adequate ventilation and oxygenation.

The most likely explanation for compensatory tachycardia and unchanged myocardial contractility associated with IV administration of thiopental is a carotid sinus baroreceptor–mediated increase in peripheral sympathetic nervous system activity. In the absence of compensatory increases in sympathetic nervous system activity, as in isolated heart preparations, a negative inotropic effect of barbiturates is readily demonstrated. Direct myocardial depression may also accompany overdoses of barbiturates or the large doses of barbiturates administered to lower ICP.

The mild and transient decrease in systemic blood pressure that accompanies induction of anesthesia with barbiturates is principally due to peripheral vasodilation, reflecting

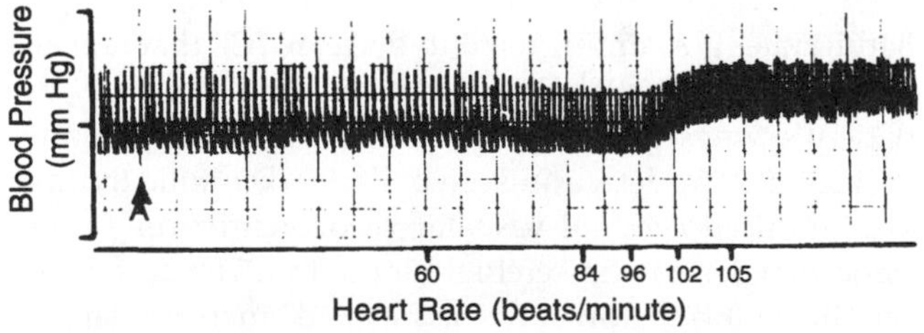

Figure 4-10. In normovolemic patients, the rapid administration of thiopental, 5 mg/kg IV (A), is followed by a modest decrease in blood pressure, which is subsequently offset by a compensatory increase in heart rate. (From Filner BF, Karliner JS. Alterations of normal left ventricular performance by general anesthesia. *Anesthesiology* 1976;45:610–620; with permission.)

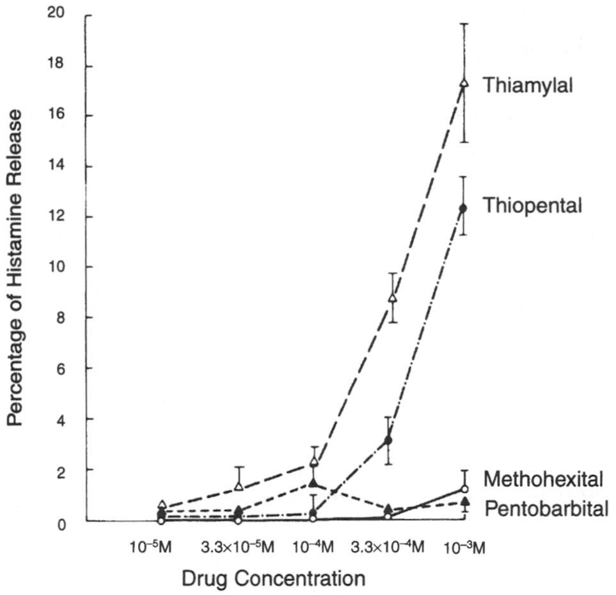

Figure 4-11. Thiamylal and thiopental produce dose-dependent release of histamine from human skin mast cell preparations, whereas methohexital and pentobarbital are devoid of this effect. (Mean ± SEM.) (From Hirshman CA, Edelstein RA, Ebertz JM, et al. Thiobarbiturate-induced histamine release in human skin mast cells. *Anesthesiology* 1985;63:353–356; with permission.)

depression of the medullary vasomotor center and decreased sympathetic nervous system outflow from the CNS. The resulting dilatation of peripheral capacitance vessels leads to pooling of blood, decreased venous return, and the potential for decreases in cardiac output and blood pressure (Yamamura et al., 1983). Histamine release can occur in response to rapid IV administration of barbiturates, but this is rarely of clinical significance. Nevertheless, profound hypotension simulating an allergic reaction has been attributed to nonimmunologically mediated histamine release evoked by thiopental (Sprung et al., 1997). In an in vitro model, thiopental and thiamylal, but not methohexital, evoke histamine release (Fig. 4-11) (Hirshman et al., 1985).

Vasodilation of cutaneous and skeletal muscle blood vessels may also contribute to heat loss and decreases in body temperature. The fact that blood pressure and cardiac output are minimally altered by the IV induction of anesthesia with barbiturates reflects the ability of carotid sinus–mediated baroreceptor reflex responses to offset the effects of peripheral vasodilation. In the absence of compensatory baroreceptor-mediated increases in peripheral sympathetic nervous system activity, peripheral pooling of blood can result in sustained decreases in venous return, cardiac output, and systemic blood pressure. Indeed, hypovolemic patients, who are less able to compensate for peripheral vasodilating effects of barbiturates, are highly vulnerable to marked decreases in systemic blood pressure when these drugs are administered rapidly for the IV induction of anesthesia. Treatment with beta-adrenergic antagonists or centrally acting antihypertensive drugs could theoretically accentuate blood pressure decreases evoked by barbiturates by impairing the activity of compensatory baroreceptor responses.

Conceptually, the slow IV administration of thiopental should be more likely to permit compensatory reflex responses and thus minimize systemic blood pressure decreases compared with rapid IV injection. This would be most important in the presence of hypovolemia. Nevertheless, rapid or slow IV administration of thiopental to normovolemic patients produces similar decreases in blood pressure and increases in heart rate (Table 4-2) (Seltzer et al., 1980). Furthermore, the dose administered slowly in 50-mg increments to achieve a predetermined clinical endpoint (loss of lash reflex) was more than the single dose administered intravenously (see Table 4-2) (Seltzer et al., 1980).

Ventilation

Barbiturates administered IV for the induction of anesthesia produce dose-dependent depression of medullary and pontine ventilatory centers. For example, thiopental decreases the sensitivity of the medullary ventilatory center to stimulation of carbon dioxide. Apnea is especially likely in the presence of other depressant drugs used for preoperative medication. Resumption of spontaneous ventilation after a single IV induction dose of barbiturate is characterized by a slow frequency of breathing and decreased tidal volume. Laryngeal reflexes and the cough reflex are not depressed until large doses of barbiturates have been administered. Stimulation of the upper airway as by laryngoscopy, intubation of the trachea, or secretions in the presence of inadequate depression of laryngeal reflexes by barbiturate may result in laryngospasm or bronchospasm.

TABLE 4-2.
INCREMENTAL VERSUS RAPID INJECTION OF THIOPENTAL

	Rapid	Incremental (50 mg Every 15 Seconds Until Loss of Lash Reflex)
Total dose (mg/kg)	5.58	4
Systolic blood pressure decrease (mm Hg)	14	16
Diastolic blood pressure decrease (mm Hg)	6	9
Heart rate increase (beats/min)	12	16
Measure of myocardial contractility	17.5	22.5

Source: Data from Seltzer JL, Gerson JI, Allen FB. Comparison of the cardiovascular effects of bolus vs. incremental administration of thiopentone. *Br J Anaesth* 1980;52:527–529.

Increased irritability of the larynx because of a parasympathomimetic action of thiopental is an unlikely explanation for laryngospasm or bronchospasm. Indeed, thiopental is not likely to selectively alter parasympathetic nervous system activity, although depression of sympathetic nervous system outflow from the CNS could theoretically result in a predominance of vagal tone.

Electroencephalogram

Small IV doses of barbiturates increase low-voltage, fast-wave activity (1 to 5 cycles/s) on the EEG. This activation of the EEG is accompanied by clouding of the consciousness. As the dose of barbiturate is increased, high-voltage, slow-wave activity (<4 cycles/s) similar to physiologic sleep appears on the EEG and consciousness is lost, although arousal may accompany intense painful stimulation. A further increase in the dose of barbiturate causes the frequency of activity on the EEG to decrease to 1 to 3 cycles/s, followed by electrical silence on the EEG if the plasma concentration of barbiturate continues to increase. A continuous infusion of thiopental, 4 mg/kg, produces an isoelectric EEG that is consistent with near-maximal decreases in cerebral metabolic oxygen requirements (Turcant et al., 1985). Alternatively, pentobarbital administered as a continuous infusion to maintain the plasma concentration between 3 and 6 mg/dL is also associated with an isoelectric EEG (Rockoff et al., 1979). Barbiturate-induced depression of cerebral metabolic oxygen requirements when the EEG is isoelectric is about 55%, reflecting a decrease in neuronal, but not metabolic, needs for oxygen. Hypothermia is the only reliable method for decreasing the basal cellular metabolic requirements for oxygen.

Somatosensory Evoked Responses

Thiopental produces dose-dependent changes in median nerve somatosensory evoked responses and brainstem auditory evoked responses. Nevertheless, even doses of thiopental sufficient to produce an isoelectric EEG fail to render any component of these responses unobtainable (Drummond et al., 1985). Therefore, thiopental is an acceptable drug to administer when the ability to monitor somatosensory evoked potentials is desirable.

Liver

Thiopental, in the absence of other drugs, produces only modest decreases in hepatic blood flow. Induction doses of thiopental do not alter postoperative liver function tests. Continuous infusion of methohexital for up to 4 hours does not produce laboratory evidence of hepatocellular damage (Prys-Roberts et al., 1983). In the hypoxic rat model, thiopental has a detectable but minimal potential to produce hepatocellular damage (Shingu et al., 1983).

Enzyme Induction

Barbiturates stimulate an increase in liver microsomal protein content (enzyme induction) after 2 to 7 days of sustained drug administration. Phenobarbital is the most potent of the barbiturates for producing enzyme induction, leading to a 20% to 40% increase in the protein content of hepatic microsomal enzymes. At maximal induction of enzyme activity, rates of metabolism are approximately doubled. After discontinuation of a barbiturate, enzyme induction may persist for up to 30 days.

Altered drug responses and drug interactions may reflect barbiturate-induced enzyme induction, resulting in accelerated metabolism of (a) other drugs, such as oral anticoagulants, phenytoin, and tricyclic antidepressants; or (b) endogenous substances, including corticosteroids, bile salts, and vitamin K. Indeed, glucuronyl transferase activity is increased by barbiturates. Barbiturates also stimulate the activity of a mitochondrial enzyme (in contrast to a microsomal enzyme) known as *D-aminolevulinic acid synthetase*. As a result, the production of heme is accelerated, and acute intermittent porphyria may be exacerbated in susceptible patients who receive barbiturates. Barbiturates can also enhance their own metabolism, which contributes to tolerance.

Kidneys

Renal effects of thiopental may include modest decreases in renal blood flow and glomerular filtration rate. The most likely explanation is drug-induced decreases in systemic blood pressure and cardiac output. Histologic evidence of renal damage is not detectable after use of barbiturates for induction of anesthesia.

Placental Transfer

Barbiturates used for IV induction of anesthesia readily cross the placenta, as evidenced by peak umbilical vein concentrations within 1 minute after administration. Nevertheless, fetal plasma concentrations of barbiturates are substantially less than those in maternal plasma (Christensen et al., 1981; Mark and Poppers, 1982). Clearance by the fetal liver and dilution by blood from the fetal viscera and extremities result in the fetal brain being exposed to lower barbiturate concentrations than are measured in the umbilical vein. Indeed, maternal doses of thiopental up to 4 mg/kg IV probably do not result in excessive concentrations of barbiturate in the fetal brain.

The elimination half-time of thiopental in neonates after maternal administration at cesarean section is 11.0 to 42.7 hours (Christensen et al., 1981). Nevertheless, these residual drug concentrations seem to be innocuous, as evidenced by unchanged neurobehavioral scores measured 48 hours after delivery (Hodgkinson et al., 1978).

Tolerance and Physical Dependence

Acute tolerance to barbiturates occurs earlier than does barbiturate-induced induction of microsomal enzymes. When barbiturate tolerance becomes maximal, the required effective dose of barbiturate may be increased sixfold. This magnitude of increase is at least double that which could be accounted for by increased metabolism resulting from enzyme induction. The observation that plasma concentrations of thiopental present on awakening are higher after a single large sleep dose than after a single small sleep dose may be an artifact of rapid IV injection, resulting in a transient distortion of drug distribution between the brain and peripheral circulation.

Tolerance to the sedative effects of barbiturates occurs sooner and is greater than what occurs for the anticonvulsant and lethal effects. Thus, as tolerance to barbiturate-induced sedation increases, the therapeutic index decreases. Acute tolerance also applies to the effect of barbiturates on metabolic oxygen consumption, with supplemental doses of thiopental having less effect than the initial dose. The development of tolerance may be less for barbiturates that produce short-term depression of the CNS.

Tolerance and physical dependence on barbiturates are closely related. The severity of the barbiturate withdrawal syndrome relates to the degree of tolerance and the rate of elimination of the barbiturates. Slow elimination of the barbiturate allows time for the CNS to diminish its compensatory excitatory responses more nearly in phase with the diminution in barbiturate-induced depression of the CNS. For example, persons who are physiologically dependent on barbiturates may be withdrawn more safely if long-acting phenobarbital is substituted for the shorter-acting barbiturates on which the individual is dependent. Nevertheless, abrupt discontinuation of phenobarbital in patients being treated for epilepsy may result in status epilepticus, even when the patient has been taking relatively small doses of the drug.

Intraarterial Injection

Intraarterial injection of thiopental usually results in immediate, intense vasoconstriction and excruciating pain that radiates along the distribution of the artery. Vasoconstriction may obscure distal arterial pulses, and blanching of the extremity is followed by cyanosis. Gangrene and permanent nerve damage may occur. It is generally accepted that the risk of initiating vascular damage with intraarterial thiopental increases with increasing concentrations of the drug, and the use of a 2.5% solution is relatively safe (Mark, 1983).

Mechanism of Damage

The pathogenesis of arterial occlusion, ischemia, and tissue necrosis that may follow accidental intraarterial injection of thiopental (also thiamylal and methohexital) is not fully resolved (Dohi and Naito, 1983; MacPherson et al., 1991). Of the many theories advanced, the most likely mechanism of damage seems to be precipitation of thiopental crystals in the arterial vessels leading to an inflammatory response and arteritis, which, coupled with the microembolization that follows, eventually results in occlusion of the distal arterial circulation. After accidental intraarterial thiopental injection, endothelial cell destruction and subsequent exposure of the intimal surface may be an important process in decreasing vessel diameter, by attenuating the local release of nitric oxide and initiating or promoting thrombus formation. The adverse response is not due to the alkalinity of thiopental as emphasized by the absence of vascular damage when isotonic solutions buffered to a pH >10 are injected into animal models (MacPherson et al., 1991).

Treatment

Treatment of accidental intraarterial injection of a barbiturate includes immediate attempts to dilute the drug, prevention of arterial spasm, and general measures to sustain adequate blood flow. Dilution of the barbiturate is best accomplished by injection of saline through the needle or catheter that still remains in the artery. At the same time, injection of lidocaine, papaverine, or phenoxybenzamine may be administered to produce vasodilation (Guerra, 1980). A strategy that uses endothelium-dependent vasodilation to enhance flow in thiopental-damaged vessels may be less effective than drugs that are not dependent on an intact and functional endothelium (MacPherson et al., 1991). If the needle or catheter has been removed from the artery before recognition of the accidental injection, the injection of a vasodilator drug may be made into a more proximal artery because the affected artery will be in spasm. Direct injection of heparin into the artery may be considered. Sympathectomy of the upper extremity produced by a stellate ganglion block or brachial plexus block may relieve vasoconstriction. Urokinase may improve distal blood flow after accidental intraarterial injection of thiopental (Vangerven et al., 1989).

Venous Thrombosis

Venous thrombosis after IV administration of a barbiturate for induction of anesthesia presumably reflects deposition of barbiturate crystals in the vein. Crystal formation in veins, however, is less hazardous than in arteries because of the ever-increasing diameter of the veins. The importance of administering a dilute solution of barbiturate for IV induction of anesthesia is suggested by the decreased incidence of venous thrombosis after the use of 2.5% thiopental and

1% methohexital, compared with 5% and 2% solutions, respectively.

Allergic Reactions

Allergic reactions in association with IV administration of barbiturates for induction of anesthesia most likely represent anaphylaxis (antigen-antibody interaction). Nevertheless, thiopental can also produce signs of an allergic reaction in the absence of prior exposure, suggesting an anaphylactoid response (Hirshman et al., 1982). The incidence of allergic reactions to thiopental is estimated to be 1 per 30,000 patients (Clarke, 1981). The majority of reported cases are in patients with a history of chronic atopy who often have received thiopental previously without adverse responses (Etter et al., 1980; Hirshman et al., 1982; Lilly and Hoy, 1980). Treatment of an allergic reaction after IV administration of thiopental, thiamylal, or methohexital must be aggressive, including the IV administration of epinephrine and prompt intravascular fluid replacement. Despite appropriate therapy, mortality after an allergic reaction to barbiturates such as thiopental is unusually high (Stoelting, 1983).

Immunosuppression

Long-term administration of high doses of thiopental is associated with an increased incidence of nosocomial infections and associated mortality. Bone marrow suppression and leukopenia may accompany long-term administration of thiopental to treat increased ICP. It is possible that thiopental could exert its permissive effect on nosocomial infections, in part by inhibiting the function of immune cells. In this regard, thiopental inhibits the nuclear transcription factor κB which is a central regulator of the immune response (Loop et al., 2002). Furthermore, at clinically relevant concentrations, thiopental and midazolam, but not ketamine, impair neutrophil functions (Nishina et al., 1998). Neutrophils play a central role in the antibacterial host defense mechanism as a component of nonspecific cell-mediated immunity. Impairment of neutrophil function is potentially a disadvantage (allows bacterial infection to develop) and an advantage (decreases autotissue injury and subsequent organ dysfunction).

REFERENCES

Avram MJ, Krejcie TC, Henthorn TK. The relationship of age to the pharmacokinetics of early drug distribution: the concurrent disposition of thiopental and indocyanine green. *Anesthesiology* 1990;72:403–411.

Avramov MN, Husain MM, White PF. The comparative effects of methohexital, propofol, and etomidate for electroconvulsive therapy. *Anesth Analg* 1995;81:596–602.

Becker KE, Tonnesen AS. Cardiovascular effects of plasma levels of thiopental necessary for anesthesia. *Anesthesiology* 1978;49: 197–208.

Bedford RF, Persing JA, Pobereskin L, et al. Lidocaine or thiopental for rapid control of intracranial hypertension. *Anesth Analg* 1980;59: 435–437.

Beskow A, Werner O, Westrin P. Faster recovery after anesthesia in infants after intravenous induction with methohexital instead of thiopental. *Anesthesiology* 1995;83:976–979.

Brain Resuscitation Clinical Trial I Study Group. Randomized clinical study of thiopental loading in comatose survivors of cardiac arrest. *N Engl J Med* 1986;314:397–403.

Brodie BB, Mark LC, Papper EM, et al. The fate of thiopental in man and a method for its estimation in biological material. *J Pharmacol Exp Ther* 1950;98:85–96.

Christensen JH, Andreasen F, Jansen JA. Pharmacokinetics of thiopental in cesarean section. *Acta Anaesthesiol Scand* 1981;25:174–179.

Clarke RSJ. Adverse effects of intravenously administered drugs in anaesthetic practice. *Drugs* 1981;22:26–41.

Cote CJ, Petkau AJ. Thiopental requirements may be increased in children reanesthetized at least one year after recovery from extensive thermal injury. *Anesth Analg* 1985;64:1156–1160.

Dohi S, Naito H. Intraarterial injection of 2.5% thiamylal does cause gangrene [letter]. *Anesthesiology* 1983;59:154.

Downie DL, Franks NP, Lieb WR. Effects of thiopental and its optical isomers on nicotinic acetylcholine receptors. *Anesthesiology* 2000;93:774–783.

Drummond JC, Todd MM, U HS. The effect of high dose sodium thiopental on brain stem auditory and median nerve somatosensory evoked responses in humans. *Anesthesiology* 1985;63; 249–254.

Etter MS, Helrich M, Mackenzie CF. Immunoglobulin E fluctuation in thiopental anaphylaxis. *Anesthesiology* 1980;52:181–183.

Filner BF, Karliner JS. Alterations of normal left ventricular performance by general anesthesia. *Anesthesiology* 1976;45:610–620.

Ford FV, Morrell F, Whisler WW. Methohexital anesthesia in the surgical treatment of uncontrollable epilepsy. *Anesth Analg* 1982;61: 997–1001.

Gedney JA, Ghosh S. Pharmacokinetics of analgesics, sedatives and anaesthetic agents during cardiopulmonary bypass. *Br J Anaesth* 1995;74: 344–351.

Gin T, Mainland P, Chan MT, et al. Decreased thiopental requirements in early pregnancy. *Anesthesiology* 1997;86:73–78.

Guerra F. Thiopental forever after. In: Aldrete JA, Stanley TH, eds. *Trends in intravenous anesthesia.* Chicago: Mosby–Year Book, 1980:143.

Haws JL, Herman N, Clark Y, et al. The chemical stability and sterility of sodium thiopental after preparation. *Anesth Analg* 1998;86: 208–213.

Hirshman CA, Edelstein RA, Ebertz JM, et al. Thiobarbiturate-induced histamine release in human skin mast cells. *Anesthesiology* 1985;63:353–356.

Hirshman CA, Peters J, Cartwright-Lee I. Leukocyte histamine release of thiopental. *Anesthesiology* 1982;56:64–67.

Hodgkinson R, Bhatt M, Kim SS, et al. Neonatal neurobehavioral tests following cesarean section under general and spinal anesthesia. *Am J Obstet Gynecol* 1978;132:670–674.

Homer TD, Stanski DR. The effect of increasing age on thiopental disposition and anesthetic requirement. *Anesthesiology* 1985;62: 714–724.

Hudson RJ, Stanski DR, Burch PG. Pharmacokinetics of methohexital and thiopental in surgical patients. *Anesthesiology* 1983;59:215–219.

Hughes MA, Glass PSA, Jacobs JR. Context-sensitive half-time in multicompartment pharmacokinetic models for intravenous anesthetic drugs. *Anesthesiology* 1992;76:334–341.

Jung D, Mayersohn M, Perrier D, et al. Thiopental disposition in lean and obese patients undergoing surgery. *Anesthesiology* 1982;56: 269–274.

Kaplan JA, Miller ED, Bailey DR. A comparative study of enflurane and halothane using systolic time intervals. *Anesth Analg* 1976;55:263–268.

Kingston HGG, Kendrick A, Sommer KM, et al. Binding of thiopental in neonatal serum. *Anesthesiology* 1990;72:428–431.

Kitahata LM, Saberski L. Are barbiturates hyperalgesic? *Anesthesiology* 1992;77:1059–1061.

Korttila K, Linnoila M, Ertama P, et al. Recovery and simulated driving after intravenous anesthesia with thiopental, methohexital, propanidid or alphadione. *Anesthesiology* 1975;43:291–299.

Lilly JK, Hoy RH. Thiopental anaphylaxis and reagin involvement. *Anesthesiology* 1980;53:335–337.

Liu LMP, Gaudreault P, Friedman PA, et al. Methohexital plasma concentrations in children following rectal administration. *Anesthesiology* 1985;62:567–570.

Loop T, Liu Z, Humar M, et al. Thiopental inhibits the activation of nuclear factor κB. *Anesthesiology* 2002;96:1202–1213.

MacPherson RD, McLeod LJ, Grove AJ. Intra-arterial thiopentone is directly toxic to vascular endothelium. *Br J Anaesth* 1991;67: 546–552.

Manuli MA, Davies L. Rectal methohexital for sedation of children during imaging procedures. *AJR Am J Roentgenol* 1993;160: 577–580.

Mark LC, Brand L, Kamvyssi S, et al. Thiopental metabolism by human liver in vivo and in vitro. *Nature* 1965;206:1117–1119.

Mark LC, Poppers PJ. The dilemma of general anesthesia for cesarean section: adequate fetal oxygenation vs. maternal awareness during operation. *Anesthesiology* 1982;56:405–406.

Mark LC. A lone case of gangrene following intraarterial thiopental 2.5%. *Anesthesiology* 1983;59:153.

Michenfelder JD. A valid demonstration of barbiturate-induced brain protection in man—at last. *Anesthesiology* 1986;64:140–142.

Nguyen KT, Stephens DP, McLeish MJ, et al. Pharmacokinetics of thiopental and pentobarbital enantiomers after intravenous administration of racemic thiopental. *Anesth Analg* 1996;83: 552–558.

Nishina K, Akamatsu H, Mikawa K, et al. The inhibitory effects of thiopental, midazolam, and ketamine on human neutrophil functions. *Anesth Analg* 1998;86:159–165.

Nussmeier NA, Arlund C, Slogoff S. Neuropsychiatric complications after cardiopulmonary bypass: cerebral protection by a barbiturate. *Anesthesiology* 1986;64:165–170.

Pandele G, Chaux F, Salvadori C, et al. Thiopental pharmacokinetics in patients with cirrhosis. *Anesthesiology* 1983;59:123–126.

Prys-Roberts C, Sear JW, Low JM, et al. Hemodynamic and hepatic effects of methohexital infusion during nitrous oxide anesthesia in humans. *Anesth Analg* 1983;62:317–323.

Rockoff MA, Goudsouzian NG. Seizures induced by methohexital. *Anesthesiology* 1981;54:333–335.

Rockoff MA, Marshall LF, Shapiro HM. High dose barbiturate therapy in humans: a clinical review of 60 patients. *Ann Neurol* 1979;6:194–199.

Roesch C, Haselby KA, Paradise RP, et al. Comparison of cardiovascular effects of thiopental and pentobarbital at equivalent levels of CNS depression. *Anesth Analg* 1983;62:749–753.

Saidman LJ, Eger EI. The effect of thiopental metabolism on duration of anesthesia. *Anesthesiology* 1966;27:118–126.

Saidman LJ. Uptake, distribution, and elimination of barbiturates. In: Eger EI, ed. *Anesthetic uptake and action.* Baltimore: Williams & Wilkins, 1974.

Seltzer JL, Gerson JI, Allen FB. Comparison of the cardiovascular effects of bolus vs. incremental administration of thiopentone. *Br J Anaesth* 1980;52:527–529.

Shingu K, Eger EI, Johnson BH, et al. Hepatic injury induced by anesthetic agents in rats. *Anesth Analg* 1983;62:140–145.

Sorbo S, Hudson RJ, Loomis JC. The pharmacokinetics of thiopental in pediatric surgical patients. *Anesthesiology* 1984;61:666–670.

Sprung J, Schoenwald PK, Schwartz LB. Cardiovascular collapse resulting from thiopental-induced histamine release. *Anesthesiology* 1997;86:106–107.

Stanski DR, Maitre PO. Population pharmacokinetics and pharmacodynamics of thiopental: the effect of age revisited. *Anesthesiology* 1990; 72:412–422.

Stoelting RK. Allergic reactions during anesthesia. *Anesth Analg* 1983; 62:341–356.

Stone JG, Young WL, Marans ZS, et al. Cardiac performance preserved despite thiopental loading. *Anesthesiology* 1993;799:36–41.

Sueyasu M, Fujito K, Shuto H, et al., Protein binding and the metabolism of thiamylal enantiomers in vitro. *Anesth Analg* 2000;91: 736–740.

Swerdlow BN, Holley FO, Maitre PO, et al. Chronic alcohol intake does not change thiopental anesthetic requirements, pharmacokinetics, or pharmacodynamics. *Anesthesiology* 1990;72:455–461.

Todd MM, Chadwick HS, Shapiro HM, et al. The neurologic effects of thiopental therapy following experimental cardiac arrest in cats. *Anesthesiology* 1982;57:76–86.

Todd MM, Drummond JC, Sang H. The hemodynamic consequences of high-dose methohexital anesthesia in humans. *Anesthesiology* 1984; 61:495–501.

Todd MM, Drummond JC, Sang H. The hemodynamic consequences of high-dose thiopental anesthesia. *Anesth Analg* 1985;64:681–687.

Todd MM, Hindman BJ, Warner DS. Barbiturate protection and cardiac surgery: a different result. *Anesthesiology* 1991;74:402–405.

Turcant A, Delhumeau A, Premel-Cabic A, et al. Thiopental pharmacokinetics under conditions of long-term infusion. *Anesthesiology* 1985;63: 50–54.

Vangerven M, Delrue G, Brugman E, et al. A new therapeutic approach to accidental intra-arterial injection of thiopentone. *Br J Anaesth* 1989; 62:98–100.

Ward JD, Becker DP, Miller DJ, et al. Failure of prophylactic barbiturate coma in the treatment of severe head trauma. *J Neurosurg* 1985;62: 383–388.

Yamamura T, Kimura T, Furukawa K. Effects of halothane, thiamylal, and ketamine on central sympathetic and vagal tone. *Anesth Analg* 1983; 62:129–134.

Zaidan JR, Klohany A, Martin WM, et al. Effect of thiopental on neurologic outcome following coronary artery bypass grafting. *Anesthesiology* 1991;74:406–411.

Benzodiazepines

5

Benzodiazepines are drugs that exert, in slightly varying degrees, five principal pharmacologic effects: anxiolysis, sedation, anticonvulsant actions, spinal cord-mediated skeletal muscle relaxation, and anterograde (acquisition or encoding of new information) amnesia (Ashton, 1994). The amnestic potency of benzodiazepines is greater than their sedative effects resulting in a longer duration of amnesia than sedation. Stored information (retrograde amnesia) is not altered by benzodiazepines (Ghoneim and Mewaldt, 1990). Benzodiazepines do not produce adequate skeletal muscle relaxation for surgical procedures, nor does their use influence the dose requirements for neuromuscular-blocking drugs. The efficacy of benzodiazepines, combined with the frequency of anxiety and insomnia in clinical practice, has led to widespread use of these drugs. For example, it is estimated that 4% of the population uses "sleeping pills" sometime during a given year, and 0.4% of the population uses hypnotics for more than a year (Nowell et al., 1997). Although benzodiazepines are effective for the treatment of acute insomnia, their use for management of chronic insomnia is decreasing. Compared with barbiturates, benzodiazepines have less tendency to produce tolerance, less potential for abuse, a greater margin of safety after an overdose, and elicit fewer and less serious drug interactions. Unlike barbiturates, benzodiazepines do not induce hepatic microsomal enzymes. Benzodiazepines are intrinsically far less addicting than opioids, cocaine, amphetamines, or barbiturates.

Benzodiazepines have replaced barbiturates for preoperative medication and production of sedation during monitored anesthesia care. In this regard, midazolam has replaced diazepam as the most commonly administered benzodiazepine in the perioperative period for preoperative medication and intravenous (IV) ("conscious") sedation. Furthermore, the context-sensitive half-times for diazepam and lorazepam are prolonged; therefore, only midazolam is likely to be used for prolonged administration when prompt recovery is desired. However, the longer context-sensitive half-time of lorazepam makes this drug an attractive choice to facilitate sedation of patients in critical care environments. Unlike other drugs administered IV to produce central nervous system (CNS) effects, benzodiazepines, as a class of drugs, are unique in the availability of a specific pharmacologic antagonist, flumazenil.

STRUCTURE ACTIVITY RELATIONSHIPS

Structurally, benzodiazepines are similar and share many active metabolites (Fig. 5-1). The term *benzodiazepine* refers to the portion of the chemical structure composed of a benzene ring fused to a seven-membered diazepine ring. Because all important benzodiazepines contain a 5-aryl substituent and a 1,4-diazepine ring, the term has come to mean the 5-aryl-1,4-benzodiazepine structure.

MECHANISM OF ACTION

Benzodiazepines appear to produce all their pharmacologic effects by facilitating the actions of gamma-aminobutyric acid (GABA), the principal inhibitory neurotransmitter in the CNS (Goodchild, 1993). Benzodiazepines do not activate the $GABA_A$ receptors but rather enhance the affinity of the receptors for GABA (Fig. 5-2) (Mohler and Richards, 1988). As a result of this drug-induced increased affinity of the GABA receptor for the inhibitory neurotransmitter, there is enhanced opening of chloride gating channels resulting in increased chloride conductance, producing hyperpolarization of the postsynaptic cell membrane, and rendering postsynaptic neurons more resistant to excitation. This resistance to excitation is presumed to be the mechanism by which benzodiazepines produce anxiolysis, sedation, anterograde amnesia, alcohol potentiation, and anticonvulsant and skeletal muscle relaxant effects.

It is likely that sedative effects of benzodiazepines reflect activation of alpha-1 subunits of $GABA_A$ receptors, whereas anxiolytic activity is due to alpha-2 subunit activity (Low et al., 2000; McKernan et al., 2000). Alpha-1 containing $GABA_A$ receptors are the most abundant receptor subtypes (cerebral cortex, cerebellar cortex, thalamus) accounting for approximately 60% of $GABA_A$ receptors in the brain. Alpha-2 subunits are less abundant and present principally in the hippocampus, and amygdala. This anatomic distribution of receptors is consistent with the minimal

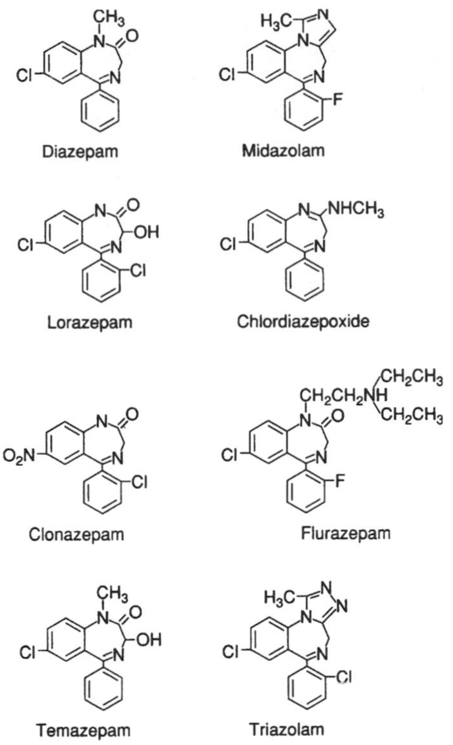

Figure 5-1. Benzodiazepines.

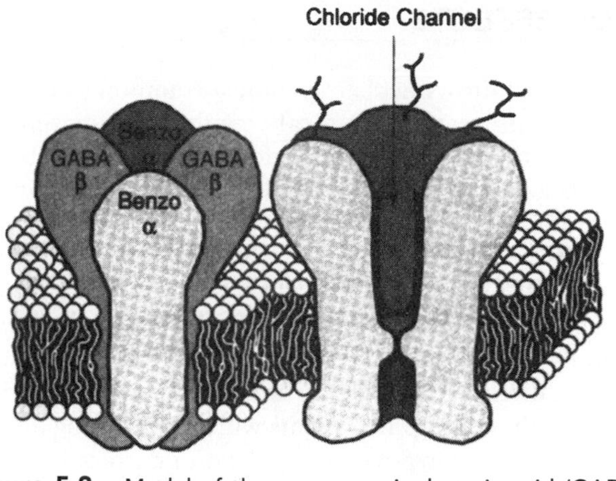

Figure 5-2. Model of the gamma-aminobutyric acid (GABA) receptor forming a chloride channel. Benzodiazepines (Benzo) attach selectively to alpha subunits and are presumed to facilitate the action of the inhibitory neurotransmitter GABA on alpha subunits. (From Mohler H, Richards JG. The benzodiazepine receptor: a pharmacologic control element of brain function. *Eur J Anesthesiol Suppl* 1988;2:15–24; with permission.)

effects of these drugs outside the CNS (minimal circulatory effects). In the future, it may be possible to design benzodiazepines that selectively activate alpha-2 subunits and thus produce anxiolysis without sedation. The physiologic significance of presumed endogenous substances that act on the $GABA_A$ receptor is unclear.

The $GABA_A$ receptor is a large macromolecule that contains physically separate binding sites (principally alpha, beta, and gamma subunits) not only for GABA and the benzodiazepines but also barbiturates, etomidate, propofol, neurosteroids, and alcohol. Acting on a single receptor by different mechanisms, the benzodiazepines, barbiturates, and alcohol can produce synergistic effects to increase $GABA_A$ receptor–mediated inhibition in the CNS. This property explains the pharmacologic synergy of these substances and, likewise, the risks of combined overdose, which can produce life-threatening CNS depression. This synergy is also the basis for pharmacologic cross-tolerance between these different classes of drugs and is consistent with the clinical use of benzodiazepines as the first-choice drugs for detoxication from alcohol. Conversely, benzodiazepines have a built-in ceiling effect that prevents them from exceeding the physiologic maximum of GABA inhibition. The low toxicity of the benzodiazepines and their corresponding clinical safety is attributed to this limitation of their effect on GABAergic neurotransmission.

Differences in the onset and duration of action among commonly administered benzodiazepines reflect differences in potency (receptor binding affinity), lipid solubility (ability to cross the blood-brain barrier and redistribute to peripheral tissues) and pharmacokinetics (uptake, distribution, metabolism, and elimination). All benzodiazepines are highly lipid soluble and are highly bound to plasma proteins, especially albumin. Hypoalbuminemia owing to hepatic cirrhosis or chronic renal failure may increase the unbound fraction of benzodiazepines, resulting in enhanced clinical effects produced by these drugs. Following oral administration, benzodiazepines are highly absorbed from the gastrointestinal tract and after IV injection they rapidly enter the CNS and other highly perfused organs.

Nucleoside Transporter Systems

Benzodiazepines decrease adenosine degradation by inhibiting the nucleoside transporter, which is the principal mechanism whereby the effect of adenosine is terminated through reuptake into cells (Seubert et al., 2000). Adenosine is an important regulator of cardiac function (reduces cardiac oxygen demand by slowing heart rate and increases oxygen delivery by causing coronary vasodilation) and its physiologic effects convey cardioprotection during myocardial ischemia.

Electroencephalogram

The effects of benzodiazepines that appear on the electroencephalogram (EEG) resemble those of barbiturates in that alpha activity is decreased and low-voltage rapid beta activity is increased. This shift from alpha to beta activity occurs more in the frontal and rolandic areas with benzodiazepines, which, unlike the barbiturates, do not cause posterior spread. In common with the barbiturates, however, tolerance to the effects of benzodiazepines on the EEG does not occur. Midazolam, in contrast to barbiturates and propofol, is unable to produce an isoelectric EEG.

SIDE EFFECTS

Fatigue and drowsiness are the most common side effects in patients treated chronically with benzodiazepines. Sedation that could impair performance usually subsides within 2 weeks. Patients should be instructed to ingest benzodiazepines before meals and in the absence of antacids because meals and antacids may decrease absorption from the gastrointestinal tract. Chronic administration of benzodiazepines does not adversely affect systemic blood pressure, heart rate, or cardiac rhythm. Although effects on ventilation seem to be absent, it may be prudent to avoid these drugs in patients with chronic lung disease characterized by hypoventilation and/or decreased arterial oxygenation. Decreased motor coordination and impairment of cognitive function may occur, especially when benzodiazepines are used in combination with other CNS depressant drugs. Acute administration of benzodiazepines may produce transient anterograde amnesia, especially if there is concomitant ingestion of alcohol. For example, there have been reports of profound amnesia in travelers who have ingested triazolam combined with alcohol to facilitate sleep on airline flights across several time zones (Morris and Estes, 1987).

Drug Interactions

Benzodiazepines exert synergistic sedative effects with other CNS depressants including alcohol, inhaled and injected anesthetics, opioids and alpha-2 agonists. Anesthetic requirements for inhaled and injected anesthetics are decreased by benzodiazepines. Although benzodiazepines, especially midazolam, potentiate the ventilatory depressant effects of opioids, the analgesic actions of opioids are reduced by benzodiazepines (Gear et al., 1997; Gross et al, 1996). Indeed, antagonism of benzodiazepine effects with flumazenil results in enhanced analgesic effects of opioids.

Hypothalamic-Pituitary Adrenal Axis

Benzodiazepine-induced suppression of the hypothalamic-pituitary adrenal axis is supported by evidence of suppression of cortisol levels in treated patients (Petraglia et al., 1986). In animals, alprazolam produces dose-dependent inhibition of adrenocorticotrophic hormone and cortisol secretion (Kalogeras et al., 1990). This suppression is enhanced compared with other benzodiazepines and may contribute to the unique efficacy of alprazolam in the treatment of major depression.

Dependence

Even therapeutic doses of benzodiazepines may produce dependence as evidenced by the onset of physical or psychologic symptoms after the dosage is decreased or the drug is discontinued. Symptoms of dependence may occur after >6 months use of commonly prescribed low-potency benzodiazepines. It is misleading to consider dependence as evidence of addiction in the absence of inappropriate drug-seeking behaviors. Withdrawal symptoms (irritability, insomnia, tremulousness) have a time of onset that reflects the elimination half-time of the drug being discontinued. Typically, symptoms of withdrawal appear within 1 to 2 days for short-acting benzodiazepines and within 2 to 5 days for longer-acting drugs.

Aging

Aging and liver disease affect glucuronidation less than oxidative metabolic pathways. In this regard, lorazepam, oxazepam, and temazepam are metabolized only by glucuronidation and have no active metabolites. For this reason, these benzodiazepines may be preferentially selected in elderly patients over benzodiazepines, such as diazepam, and that is metabolized by hepatic microsomal enzymes to form active metabolites. Elderly patients may also be intrinsically sensitive to benzodiazepines, suggesting that the enhanced response to these drugs that occurs with aging has pharmacodynamic as well as pharmacokinetic components. Oxidation reactions are more likely to be influenced by other drugs administered in the perioperative period.

Long-term benzodiazepine administration may accelerate cognitive decline in elderly patients. Benzodiazepine withdrawal symptoms in the elderly include confusion. Postoperative confusion is more common in elderly long-term benzodiazepine users (daily use for >1 year) than in short-term users or nonusers of benzodiazepines (Kudoh et al., 2004).

Platelet Aggregation

Benzodiazepines may inhibit platelet-activating factor-induced aggregation resulting in drug-induced inhibition of platelet aggregation. Midazolam-induced inhibition of platelet aggregation may reflect conformational changes in platelet membranes (Sheu et al., 2002).

MIDAZOLAM

Midazolam is a water-soluble benzodiazepine with an imidazole ring in its structure that accounts for stability in aqueous solutions and rapid metabolism (Reves et al., 1985). This benzodiazepine has replaced diazepam for use in preoperative medication and conscious sedation. Compared with diazepam, midazolam is two to three times as potent. Indeed, midazolam has an affinity for the benzodiazepine receptor that is approximately twice that of diazepam. As with other benzodiazepines, the amnestic effects of midazolam are more potent than its sedative effects. Thus, patients may be awake following administration of midazolam but

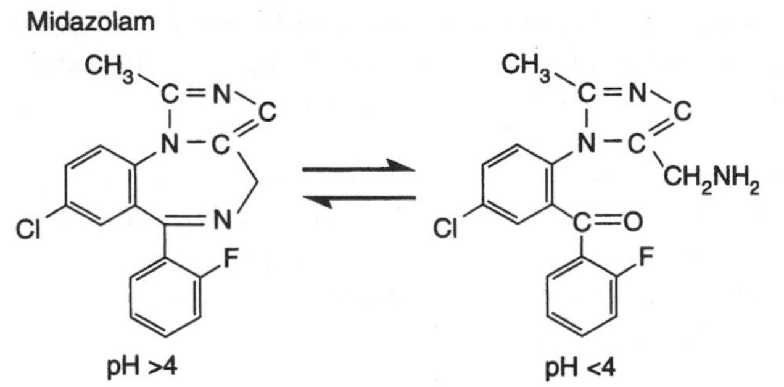

Figure 5-3. Reversible ring opening of midazolam above and below a pH of 4. The ring closes at a pH >4, converting midazolam from a water-soluble to a lipid-soluble drug.

remain amnestic for events and conversations (postoperative instructions) for several hours.

Commercial Preparation

The pK of midazolam is 6.15, which permits the preparation of salts that are water soluble. The parenteral solution of midazolam used clinically is buffered to an acidic pH of 3.5. This is important because midazolam is characterized by a pH-dependent ring-opening phenomenon in which the ring remains open at pH values of <4, thus maintaining water solubility of the drug (Fig. 5-3). The ring closes at pH values of >4, as when the drug is exposed to physiologic pH, thus converting midazolam to a highly lipid-soluble drug (see Fig. 5-3).

The water solubility of midazolam obviates the need for a solubilizing preparation, such as propylene glycol, that can produce venoirritation or interfere with absorption after intramuscular (IM) injection. Indeed, midazolam causes minimal to no discomfort during or after IV or IM injection. Midazolam is compatible with lactated Ringer solution and can be mixed with the acidic salts of other drugs, including opioids and anticholinergics.

Pharmacokinetics

Midazolam undergoes rapid absorption from the gastrointestinal tract and prompt passage across the blood-brain barrier. Despite this prompt passage into the brain, midazolam is considered to have a slow effect-site equilibration time (0.9 to 5.6 minutes) compared with other drugs such as propofol and thiopental. In this regard, IV doses of midazolam should be sufficiently spaced to permit the peak clinical effect to be appreciated before a repeat dose is considered. Only about 50% of an orally administered dose of midazolam reaches the systemic circulation, reflecting a substantial first-pass hepatic effect. As for most benzodiazepines, midazolam is extensively bound to plasma proteins; this binding is independent of the plasma concentration of midazolam (Table 5-1) (Greenblatt et al., 1984; Reves et al., 1985). The short duration of action of a single dose of midazolam is due to its lipid solubility, leading to rapid redistribution from the brain to inactive tissue sites as well as rapid hepatic clearance. The context-sensitive half-times for diazepam and lorazepam are prolonged compared with midazolam, emphasizing the rationale in selecting midazolam when continuous infusion of a benzodiazepine is chosen.

The elimination half-time of midazolam is 1 to 4 hours, which is much shorter than that of diazepam (see Table 5-1) (Reves et al., 1985). The elimination half-time may be doubled in elderly patients, reflecting age-related decreases in hepatic blood flow and possibly enzyme activity. The volume of distribution (Vd) of midazolam and diazepam are similar, probably reflecting their similar lipid solubility and high degree of protein binding. Elderly and morbidly obese patients have an increased Vd of midazolam resulting from enhanced distribution of the drug into peripheral adipose tissues. The clearance of midazolam is more rapid than that of diazepam, as reflected by the context-sensitive half-time. As a result of these differences, the CNS effects of midazolam would be expected to be shorter than those of diazepam. Indeed, tests of mental function return to normal within 4 hours after the administration of midazolam.

The institution of cardiopulmonary bypass is associated with a decrease in the plasma concentration of midazolam and an increase on termination of cardiopulmonary bypass (Gedney and Ghosh, 1995). These changes are attributed to redistribution of priming fluid into body tissues. In addition, benzodiazepines are extensively bound to protein, and changes in protein concentrations and pH that accompany institution and termination of cardiopulmonary bypass may have significant effects on the unbound and pharmacologically active fractions of these drugs. The elimination half-time of midazolam is prolonged after

TABLE 5-1.
COMPARATIVE PHARMACOLOGY OF BENZODIAZEPINES

	Equivalent Dose (mg)	Volume of Distribution (liters/kg)	Protein Binding (%)	Clearance (mL/kg/min)	Elimination Half-Time (hrs)
Midazolam	0.15–0.3	1.0–1.5	96–98	6–8	1–4
Diazepam	0.3–0.5	1.0–1.5	96–98	0.2–0.5	21–37
Lorazepam	0.05	0.8–1.3	96–98	0.7–1.0	10–20

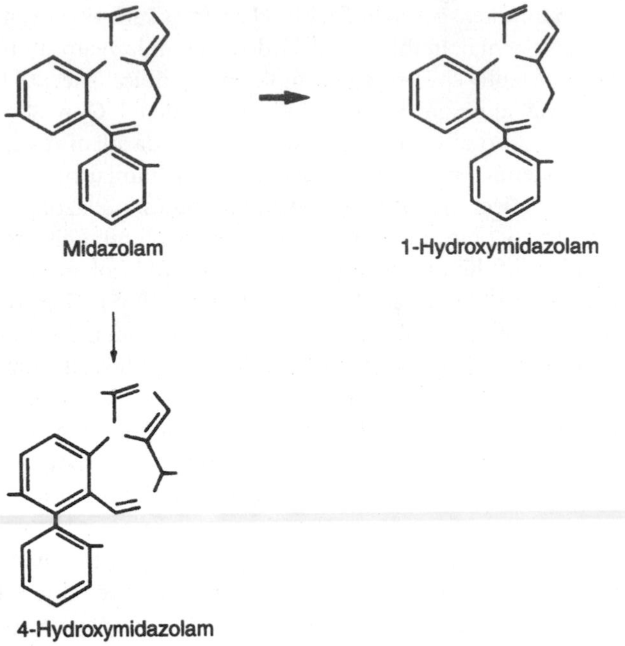

Figure 5-4. The principal metabolite of midazolam is 1-hydroxymidazolam. A lesser amount of midazolam is metabolized to 4-hydroxymidazolam. (From Reves JG, Fragen RJ, Vinik HR, et al. Midazolam: pharmacology and uses. *Anesthesiology* 1985;62:310–324; with permission.)

cardiopulmonary bypass compared with values obtained from patients not undergoing this procedure.

Metabolism

Midazolam is rapidly metabolized by hepatic and small intestine cytochrome P-450 (CYP3A4) enzymes to active and inactive metabolites (Fig. 5-4) (Reves et al., 1985). The principal metabolite of midazolam, 1-hydroxymidazolam, has approximately half the activity of the parent compound (Johnson et al., 2002). This active metabolite is rapidly conjugated to 1-hydroxymidazolam glucuronide and is subsequently cleared by the kidneys. This glucuronide metabolite has substantial pharmacologic activity when present in high concentrations, as may occur in critically ill patients with renal insufficiency who are receiving continuous intravenous infusions of midazolam over prolonged periods of time. In these patients, the glucuronide metabolite may have synergistic sedative effects with the parent compound (Bauer et al., 1995). The other pharmacologically active metabolite of midazolam, 4-hydroxymidazolam, is not present in detectable concentrations in the plasma following IV administration of midazolam.

Metabolism of midazolam is slowed in the presence of drugs (cimetidine, erythromycin, calcium channel blockers, antifungal drugs) that inhibit cytochrome P-450 enzymes resulting in unexpected CNS depression (Hiller et al., 1990). Cytochrome P-450 3A enzymes also influence the metabolism of fentanyl. In this regard, the hepatic clearance of midazolam is inhibited by fentanyl as administered during general anesthesia (Hase et al., 1997). Overall, the hepatic clearance rate of midazolam is five times greater than that of lorazepam and ten times greater than that of diazepam.

Renal Clearance

The elimination half-time, Vd, and clearance of midazolam are not altered by renal failure (Vinik et al., 1983). This is consistent with the extensive hepatic metabolism of midazolam.

Effects on Organ Systems

Central Nervous System

Midazolam, like other benzodiazepines, produces decreases in cerebral metabolic oxygen requirements ($CMRO_2$) and cerebral blood flow analogous to barbiturates and propofol. In contrast to these drugs, however, midazolam is unable to produce an isoelectric EEG, emphasizing that there is a ceiling effect with respect to the decrease in $CMRO_2$ produced by increasing doses of midazolam. Midazolam causes dose-related changes in regional cerebral blood flow in brain regions associated with the normal functioning of arousal, attention, and memory (Veselis et al., 1997). Cerebral vasomotor responsiveness to carbon dioxide is preserved during midazolam anesthesia (Strebel et al., 1994). Patients with decreased intracranial compliance show little or no change in intracranial pressure (ICP) when given midazolam doses of 0.15 to 0.27 mg/kg IV. Thus, midazolam is an acceptable alternative to barbiturates for induction of anesthesia in patients with intracranial pathology. There is some evidence, however, that patients with severe head trauma but ICP of <18 mm Hg may experience an undesirable increase in ICP when midazolam (0.15 mg/kg IV) is administered rapidly (Fig. 5-5) (Papazian et al., 1993). Similar to thiopental, induction of anesthesia with midazolam does not prevent increases in ICP associated with

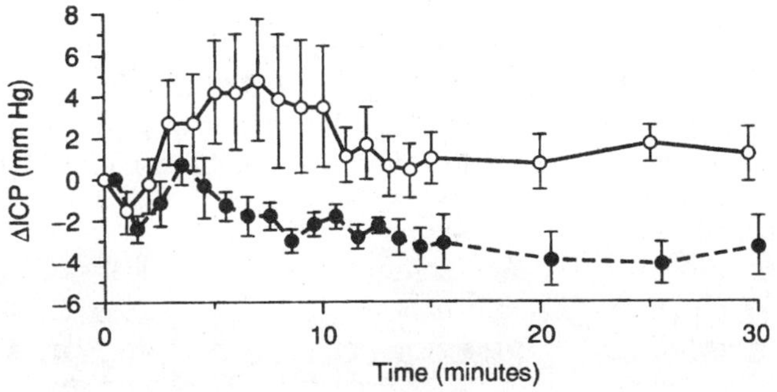

Figure 5-5. Administration of midazolam, 0.15 mg/kg IV, to patients with severe head injury (Glasgow Coma Score ≤6) was associated with an increase in intracranial pressure (ICP) when the control ICP was <18 mm Hg (*open circles*) but not when the control ICP was ≥18 mm Hg (*closed circles*). (From Papazian L, Albanese J, Thirion X, et al. Effect of bolus doses of midazolam on intracranial pressure and cerebral perfusion pressure in patients with severe head injury. *Br J Anaesth* 1993;71:267–271; with permission.)

direct laryngoscopy for tracheal intubation (Giffin et al., 1984). Although midazolam may improve neurologic outcome after incomplete ischemia, benzodiazepines have not been shown to possess neuroprotective activity in humans. Midazolam is a potent anticonvulsant effective in the treatment of status epilepticus. Prolonged sedation of infants in critical care units (4 to 11 days) with midazolam and fentanyl has been associated with encephalopathy on withdrawal of the benzodiazepine (Bergman et al., 1991). Parodoxical excitement occurs in <1% of all patients receiving midazolam and is effectively treated with a specific benzodiazepine antagonist, flumazenil (Thurston et al., 1996).

Ventilation

Midazolam produces dose-dependent decreases in ventilation with 0.15 mg/kg IV producing effects similar to diazepam, 0.3 mg/kg IV (Forster et al., 1980). Patients with chronic obstructive pulmonary disease experience even greater midazolam-induced depression of ventilation (Gross et al., 1983). Transient apnea may occur after rapid injection of large doses of midazolam (>0.15 mg/kg IV), especially in the presence of preoperative medication that includes an opioid (Kanto et al., 1982). In healthy volunteers, midazolam alone produced no ventilatory depressant effects, whereas the combination of midazolam, 0.05 mg/kg IV, and fentanyl, 2 μg/kg IV, resulted in arterial hypoxemia and/or hypoventilation (Bailey et al., 1990). Midazolam, 0.05 or 0.075 mg/kg IV, was shown to depress resting ventilation in healthy volunteers, whereas spinal anesthesia (mean sensory level T6) stimulated resting ventilation, and the combination had a modest synergistic effect for depressing resting ventilation (Gauthier et al., 1992). Benzodiazepines also depress the swallowing reflex and decrease upper airway activity.

Cardiovascular System

Midazolam, 0.2 mg/kg IV, for induction of anesthesia produces a greater decrease in systemic blood pressure and increase in heart rate than does diazepam, 0.5 mg/kg IV (Samuelson et al., 1981). Conversely, these midazolam-induced hemodynamic changes are similar to the changes produced by thiopental, 3 to 4 mg/kg IV (Lebowitz et al., 1982). Cardiac output is not altered by midazolam, suggesting that blood pressure changes are due to decreases in systemic vascular resistance. In this regard, benzodiazepines may be beneficial in improving cardiac output in the presence of congestive heart failure. In the presence of hypovolemia, administration of midazolam results in enhanced blood pressure–lowering effects similar to those produced by other IV induction drugs (Adams et al., 1985). Midazolam does not prevent blood pressure and heart rate responses evoked by intubation of the trachea. In fact, this mechanical stimulus may offset the blood pressure–lowering effects of large doses of midazolam administered IV. The effects of midazolam on systemic blood pressure are directly related to the plasma concentration of the benzodiazepine. However, a plateau plasma concentration appears to exist (ceiling effect) above which little further change in systemic blood pressure occurs.

Clinical Uses

Midazolam is the most commonly used benzodiazepine for preoperative medication in pediatric patients, IV ("conscious") sedation, and induction of anesthesia. In combination with other drugs, midazolam may be used for maintenance of anesthesia. Like diazepam, midazolam is a potent anticonvulsant for the treatment of grand mal seizures, which may occur with systemic toxicity produced by local anesthetics.

Preoperative Medication

Midazolam is the most commonly used oral preoperative medication for children. Oral midazolam syrup (2 mg/mL) is effective for producing sedation and anxiolyis at a dose of 0.25 mg/kg with minimal effects on ventilation and oxygen saturation even when administered at doses as large as 1 mg/kg (maximum, 20 mg) (Cote et al., 2002). Midazolam, 0.5 mg/kg administered orally 30 minutes before induction of anesthesia, provides reliable sedation and anxiolysis in children without producing delayed awakening (Fig. 5-6) (McMillan et al., 1992). Although it is recommended that oral midazolam be administered at least 20 minutes before surgery, there is evidence that

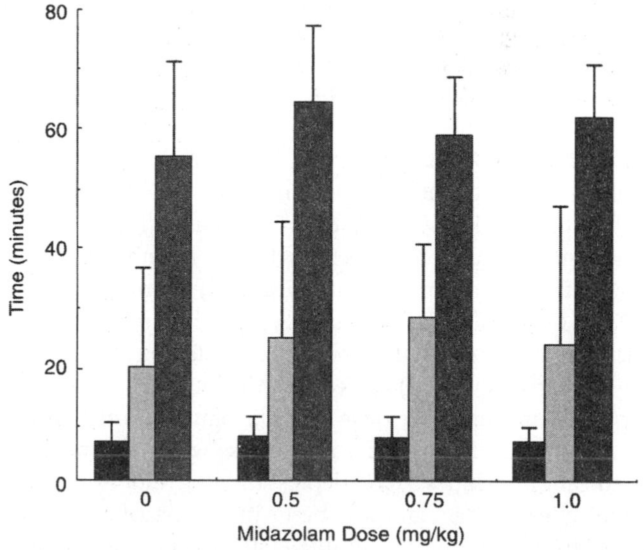

Figure 5-6. Increasing doses of oral midazolam premedication administered 30 minutes before the induction of anesthesia did not produce different effects on the interval from the end of surgery until transported to the postanesthesia care unit (*solid bars*), interval from arrival in the postanesthesia care unit until spontaneous eye opening (*light gray bars*), and time in the postanesthesia care unit (*dark gray bars*). (From McMillan CO, Spahr-Schopfer IA, Sikich N, et al. Premedication of children with oral midazolam. *Can J Anaesth* 1992; 39:545–550; with permission.)

significant anterograde amnesia is present when 0.5 mg/kg orally is administered 10 minutes before surgery (Kain et al., 2000).

Intravenous Sedation

Midazolam in doses of 1.0 to 2.5 mg IV (onset within 30 to 60 seconds, time to peak effect 3 to 5 minutes, duration of sedation 15 to 80 minutes) is effective for sedation during regional anesthesia as well as for brief therapeutic procedures. Compared with diazepam, midazolam produces a more rapid onset, with greater amnesia and less postoperative sedation, but the time to complete recovery is no shorter (McClure et al., 1983). The effect-site equilibrium time for midazolam must be considered in recognizing the likely time of peak clinical effect and the need for supplemental doses of midazolam. Pain on injection and subsequent venous thrombosis are less likely after administration of midazolam than diazepam.

The most significant side effect of midazolam administration to produce sedation is depression of ventilation caused by a decrease in the hypoxic drive. The ventilatory depressant effects of midazolam are greater than lorazepam and diazepam. Midazolam-induced depression of ventilation is exaggerated (synergistic effects) in the presence of opioids and other CNS depressant drugs (Gross et al., 1996). Patients with chronic obstructive pulmonary disease may also manifest exaggerated depression of ventilation following administration of benzodiazepines to produce sedation. It is important to appreciate that increasing age greatly increases the pharmacodynamic sensitivity to the hypnotic effects of midazolam (Jacobs et al., 1995). Patient-controlled administration of midazolam during procedures performed under local anesthesia is an alternative to continuous IV infusion (about 4 μg/kg/minute IV) techniques (Ghouri et al., 1992).

Induction of Anesthesia

Anesthesia can be induced by administration of midazolam, 0.1 to 0.2 mg/kg IV, over 30 to 60 seconds. Nevertheless, thiopental usually produces induction of anesthesia 50% to 100% faster than midazolam (Fig. 5-7) (Sarnquist et al., 1980). Onset of unconsciousness (synergistic interaction) is facilitated when a small dose of opioid (fentanyl, 50 to 100 μg IV or its equivalent) precedes the injection of midazolam by 1 to 3 minutes. The dose of midazolam required for the IV induction of anesthesia is also less when preoperative medication includes a CNS depressant drug. Elderly patients require less midazolam for the IV induction of anesthesia than do young adults (Gamble et al., 1981). The explanation for this is not clear, because a prolonged elimination half-time should not alter the acute hypnotic effect of a single IV dose of midazolam. A possible explanation is the increased sensitivity of the CNS to the effects of midazolam with increasing age (Greenblatt et al., 1982).

In healthy patients receiving small doses of benzodiazepines, the cardiovascular depression associated with these drugs is minimal. When significant cardiovascular responses occur, it is most likely a reflection of benzodiazepine-induced peripheral vasodilation. As with depression of ventilation, cardiovascular changes produced by benzodiazepines may be exaggerated in the presence of other CNS depressant drugs such as propofol and thiopental.

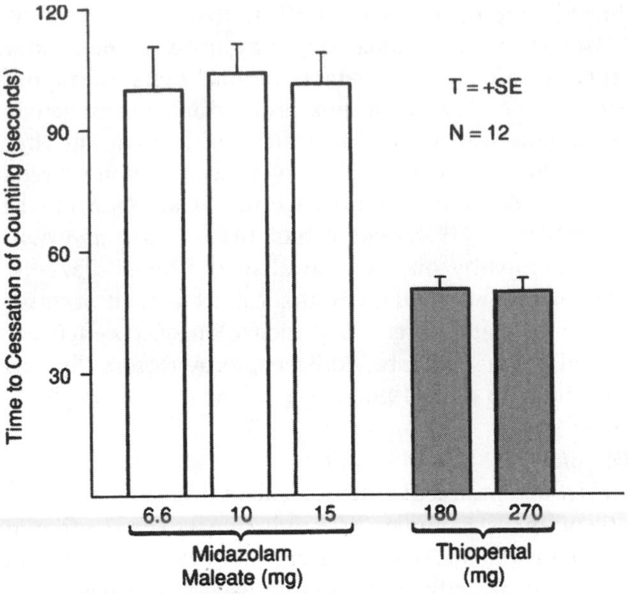

Figure 5-7. Induction of anesthesia as depicted by time to cessation of counting occurs in about 110 seconds after the intravenous administration of midazolam compared with about 50 seconds after injection of thiopental. (From Sarnquist FH, Mathers WD, Brock-Utne J, et al. A bioassay of water-soluble benzodiazepine against sodium thiopental. *Anesthesiology* 1980;52:149–153; with permission.)

Maintenance of Anesthesia

Midazolam may be administered to supplement opioids, propofol, and/or inhaled anesthetics during maintenance of anesthesia. The context-sensitive half-time for midazolam increases modestly with an increasing duration of administration of a continuous infusion of this benzodiazepine (see Fig. 1-3) (Hughes et al., 1992). Anesthetic requirements for volatile anesthetics are decreased in a dose-dependent manner by midazolam. Awakening after general anesthesia that includes induction of anesthesia with midazolam is 1.0 to 2.5 times longer than that observed when thiopental is used for the IV induction of anesthesia (Jensen et al., 1982). Gradual awakening in patients who receive midazolam is rarely associated with nausea, vomiting, or emergence excitement. One hour after surgery, patients are equally alert with either midazolam or thiopental, and discharge time from an outpatient recovery room is similar with both drugs (Crawford et al., 1984).

Postoperative Sedation

Long-term intravenous administration of midazolam (loading dose 0.5 to 4 mg IV and maintenance dose 1 to

7 mg/hr IV) to produce sedation in intubated patients results in relative saturation of peripheral tissues with midazolam and clearance from the systemic circulation becomes less dependent on redistribution into peripheral tissues and more dependent on hepatic metabolism (Barr et al., 2001). In addition, pharmacologically active metabolites may accumulate with prolonged IV administration of the parent drug. Under these conditions, plasma concentrations of midazolam decrease more slowly (emergence delayed) after discontinuation of the IV infusion compared with single IV injections. Emergence time is also a function of the plasma concentrations of midazolam at the the time the IV infusion is discontinued. Patients maintained at higher plasma concentrations of midazolam take longer to awaken than patients maintained at lower plasma concentrations for comparable periods of time. The concomitant administration of analgesic doses of opioids greatly decreases the needed dose of midazolam and results in a more rapid recovery from sedation following discontinuation of the IV infusion of midazolam (Barr et al., 2001). Emergence time from midazolam is increased in elderly patients, obese patients, and in the presence of severe liver disease.

Paradoxical Vocal Cord Motion

Paradoxical vocal cord motion is a cause of nonorganic upper airway obstruction and stridor that may manifest postoperatively. Midazoalm 0.5 to 1 mg IV may be an effective treatment for paradoxical vocal cord motion (Roberts et al., 1998).

DIAZEPAM

Diazepam is a highly lipid-soluble benzodiazepine with a more prolonged duration of action compared with midazolam.

Commercial Preparation

Diazepam is dissolved in organic solvents (propylene glycol, sodium benzoate) because it is insoluble in water. The solution is viscid, with a pH of 6.6 to 6.9. Dilution with water or saline causes cloudiness but does not alter the potency of the drug. Injection by either the IM or IV route may be painful. Diazepam is also available in a unique soybean formulation for IV injection. This formulation is associated with a lower incidence of pain on injection and thrombophlebitis.

Pharmacokinetics

Diazepam is rapidly absorbed from the gastrointestinal tract after oral administration, reaching peak concentrations in about 1 hour in adults but as quickly as 15 to 30 minutes in children. There is rapid uptake of diazepam into the brain, followed by redistribution to inactive tissue sites, especially fat, as this benzodiazepine is highly lipid soluble. The Vd of diazepam is large, reflecting extensive tissue uptake of this lipid-soluble drug (see Table 5-1). Women, with a greater body fat content, are likely to have a larger Vd for diazepam than men. Diazepam rapidly crosses the placenta, achieving fetal concentrations equal to and sometimes greater than those present in the maternal circulation (Dawes, 1973). The duration of action of benzodiazepines is not linked to receptor events but rather is determined by the rate of metabolism and elimination.

Protein Binding

The protein binding of benzodiazepines parallels their lipid solubility. As such, highly lipid-soluble diazepam is extensively bound, presumably to albumin (see Table 5-1). Cirrhosis of the liver or renal insufficiency, with associated decreases in plasma concentrations of albumin, may manifest as decreased protein binding of diazepam and an increased incidence of drug-related side effects (Greenblatt and Koch-Weser, 1974). The high degree of protein binding limits the efficacy of hemodialysis in the treatment of diazepam overdose.

Metabolism

Diazepam is principally metabolized by hepatic microsomal enzymes using an oxidative pathway of *N*-demethylation. The two principal metabolites of diazepam are desmethyldiazepam and oxazepam, with a lesser amount metabolized to temazepam (Fig. 5-8). Desmethyldiazepam is metabolized more slowly than oxazepam and is only slightly less potent than diazepam. Therefore, it is likely that this metabolite contributes to the return of drowsiness that manifests 6 to 8 hours after administration of diazepam, as well as to sustained effects usually attributed to the parent drug. Alternatively, enterohepatic recirculation

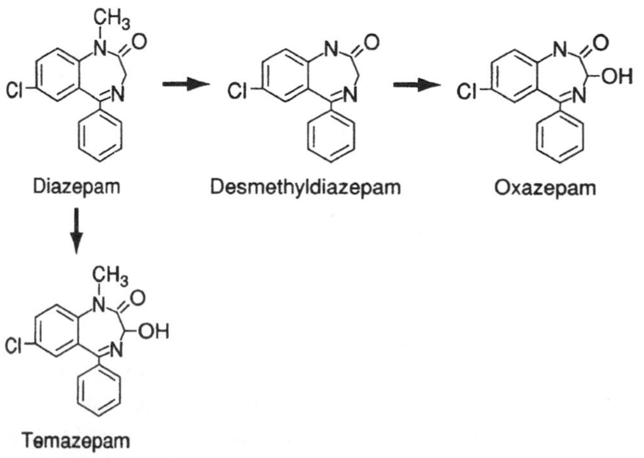

Figure 5-8. The principal metabolites of diazepam are desmethyldiazepam and oxazepam. A lesser amount of diazepam is metabolized to temazepam.

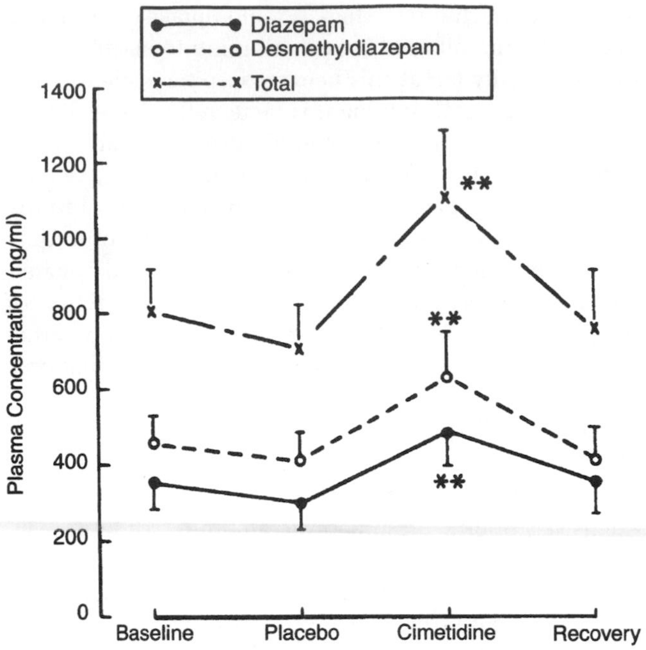

Figure 5-9. The plasma concentrations of diazepam and its active metabolite, desmethyldiazepam, are increased when the parent drug is administered during cimetidine therapy. (Mean ± SE.) (From Greenblatt DJ, Abernathy DR, Morse DS, et al. Clinical importance of the interaction of diazepam and cimetidine. *N Engl J Med* 1984;310: 1639–1643; with permission.)

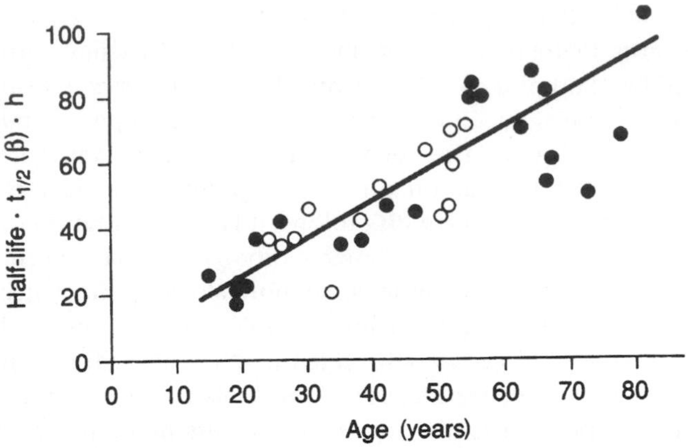

Figure 5-10. The elimination half-time of diazepam increases progressively with increasing age. (From Klotz U, Avant GR, Hoyumpa A, et al. The effects of age and liver disease on the deposition and elimination of diazepam in adult man. *J Clin Invest* 1975;55:347–359; with permission.)

may contribute to recurrence of sedation (Eustace et al., 1975). The plasma concentration of diazepam at this time is clinically insignificant and probably reflects its rapid removal as a conjugate of glucuronic acid. Ultimately, desmethyldiazepam is excreted in urine in the form of oxidized and glucuronide conjugated metabolites. Unchanged, diazepam is not appreciably excreted in urine. Benzodiazepines do not produce enzyme induction.

Cimetidine

Cimetidine inhibits P-450 hepatic microsomal enzymes and thus prolongs the elimination half-time of both diazepam and desmethyldiazepam (Fig. 5-9) (Greenblatt et al., 1984). Indeed, sedation is increased when diazepam is administered with cimetidine compared with that when diazepam is administered alone. Presumably, this delayed clearance reflects cimetidine-induced inhibition of microsomal enzymes necessary for the oxidation of diazepam and desmethyldiazepam.

Elimination Half-Time

The elimination half-time of diazepam is prolonged, ranging from 21 to 37 hours in healthy volunteers (see Table 5-1). Cirrhosis of the liver is accompanied by up to fivefold increases in the elimination half-time of diazepam (Klotz et al., 1975). Likewise, the elimination half-time of diazepam increases progressively with increasing age, which is consistent with the increased sensitivity of these patients to the drug's sedative effects (Fig. 5-10) (Klotz et al., 1975). Prolongation of the elimination half-time of diazepam in the presence of cirrhosis of the liver is due to decreased protein binding of the drug, leading to an increased Vd. In addition, hepatic clearance of diazepam is likely to be decreased, reflecting decreased hepatic blood flow characteristic of cirrhosis of the liver. The explanation for the prolonged elimination half-time of diazepam in elderly patients is also an increased Vd. Presumably, increased total body fat content that accompanies aging results in an increased Vd of a highly lipid-soluble drug such as diazepam. Hepatic clearance of diazepam is not changed by aging. Compared with lorazepam, diazepam has a longer elimination half-time but shorter duration of action because it dissociates more rapidly than lorazepam from $GABA_A$ receptors, permitting more rapid redistribution to inactive tissue sites.

Desmethyldiazepam, the principal metabolite of diazepam, has an elimination half-time of 48 to 96 hours. As such, the elimination half-time of the metabolite may exceed that of the parent drug. Indeed, plasma concentrations of diazepam often decline more rapidly than plasma concentrations of desmethyldiazepam. This pharmacologically active metabolite can accumulate in plasma and tissues during chronic use of diazepam. Prolonged somnolence associated with high doses of diazepam is likely to be caused by sequestration of the parent drug and its active metabolite, demethyldiazepam, in tissues, presumably fat, for subsequent release back into the circulation. A week or more is often required for elimination of these compounds from plasma after discontinuation of chronic diazepam therapy.

Effects on Organ Systems

Diazepam, like other benzodiazepines, produces minimal effects on ventilation and the systemic circulation. Hepatic and renal function are not altered appreciably. Diazepam does not increase the incidence of nausea and vomiting. There is no change in the circulating plasma concentrations of stress-responding hormones (catecholamines, arginine vasopressin, cortisol).

Ventilation

Diazepam produces minimal depressant effects on ventilation, with detectable increases in Pa_{CO_2} not occurring until 0.2 mg/kg IV is administered. This slight increase in Pa_{CO_2} is due primarily to a decrease in tidal volume. Nevertheless, rarely, small doses of diazepam (<10 mg IV) have produced apnea (Braunstein, 1979). Combination of diazepam with other CNS depressants (opioids, alcohol) or administration of this drug to patients with chronic obstructive airway disease may result in exaggerated or prolonged depression of ventilation.

The slope of the line depicting the ventilatory response to carbon dioxide is decreased nearly 50% within 3 minutes after the administration of diazepam, 0.4 mg/kg IV (Fig. 5-11) (Gross et al., 1982). This depression of the slope persists for about 25 minutes and parallels the level of consciousness. Despite the decrease in slope, the carbon dioxide response curve is not shifted to the right as observed with depression of ventilation produced by opioids. These depressant effects on ventilation seem to be a CNS effect, because the mechanics of respiratory muscles are unchanged. The ventilatory depressant effects of benzodiazepines are reversed by surgical stimulation but not by naloxone.

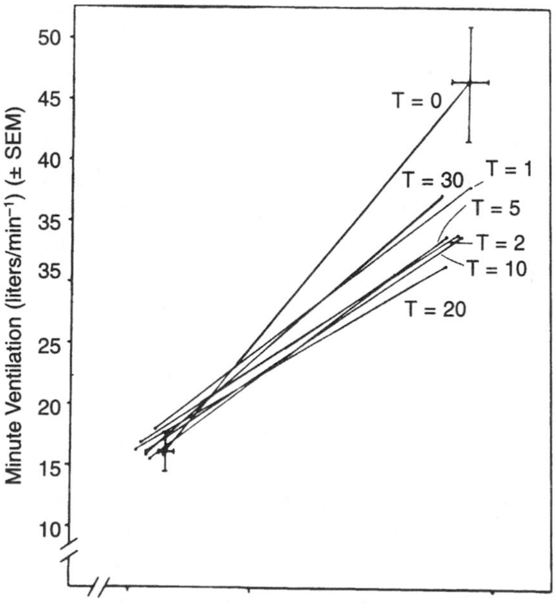

Figure 5-11. The slope of the line depicting the ventilatory response to carbon dioxide is decreased (T = minutes) following administration of diazepam, 0.4 mg/kg IV. (From Gross JB, Smith L, Smith TC. Time course of ventilatory response to carbon dioxide after intravenous diazepam. *Anesthesiology* 1982;57:18–21; with permission.)

TABLE 5-2.
CARDIOVASCULAR EFFECTS OF DIAZEPAM (0.5 mg/kg IV) AND DIAZEPAM-NITROUS OXIDE

	Awake	Diazepam	Diazepam-Nitrous oxide
Systolic blood pressure (mm Hg)	144	125*	121*
Diastolic blood pressure (mm Hg)	81	74	75
Mean arterial pressure (mm Hg)	102	91*	91*
Heart rate (beats/minute)	66	68	65
Pulmonary artery pressure (mm Hg)	18.4	16.3	17.2
Pulmonary artery occlusion pressure (mm Hg)	11.5	10.6	11.9
Cardiac output (liters/minute)	5.3	5.1	4.8*
Systemic vascular resistance (dynes/sec/cm^{-5})	1391	1344	1377

*P <.05 compared with the awake value.
Source: Data from McCammon RL, Hilgenberg JC, Stoelting RK. Hemodynamic effects of diazepam-nitrous oxide in patients with coronary artery disease. *Anesth Analg* 1980;59:438–441.

Cardiovascular System

Diazepam administered in doses of 0.5 to 1 mg/kg IV for induction of anesthesia typically produces minimal decreases in systemic blood pressure, cardiac output, and systemic vascular resistance that are similar in magnitude to those observed during natural sleep (10% to 20% decreases) (Table 5-2) (McCammon et al., 1980). There is a transient depression of baroreceptor-mediated heart rate responses that is less than the depression evoked by volatile anesthetics but that could, in hypovolemic patients, interfere with optimal compensatory changes (Marty et al., 1986). In patients with increased left ventricular end-diastolic pressure, a small dose of diazepam significantly decreases this pressure. Diazepam appears to have no direct action on the sympathetic nervous system, and it does not cause orthostatic hypotension.

The incidence and magnitude of systemic blood pressure decreases produced by diazepam seem to be less than those associated with barbiturates administered IV for the induction of anesthesia (Knapp and Dubow, 1970). Nevertheless, occasionally, a patient may unpredictably experience hypotension with even small doses of diazepam (Falk et al., 1978). The addition of nitrous oxide after induction of anesthesia with diazepam is not associated with adverse cardiac changes (see Table 5-2) (McCammon et al., 1980). Therefore, nitrous oxide can be administered in the presence of diazepam to ensure absence of patient awareness during surgery. This contrasts with direct myocardial depression and decreases in systemic blood pressure that occur when nitrous oxide is administered in the presence of opioids (see Chapter 3). Likewise, prior administration of diazepam, 0.125 to 0.5 mg/kg IV, followed by injection of fentanyl, 50 μg/kg IV, is associated with decreases in systemic vascular resistance and systemic blood pressure that do not accompany administration of the opioid alone (see Fig. 3-12).

Skeletal Muscle

Skeletal muscle relaxant effects reflect actions of diazepam on spinal internuncial neurons and not actions at the neuromuscular junction (Dretchen et al., 1971). Presumably, diazepam diminishes the tonic facilitatory influence on spinal gamma neurons, and, thus, skeletal muscle tone is decreased. Tolerance occurs to the skeletal muscle relaxant effects of benzodiazepines.

Overdose

CNS intoxication can be expected at diazepam plasma concentrations of >1,000 ng/mL. Despite massive overdoses of diazepam, serious sequelae (coma) are unlikely to occur if cardiac and pulmonary function are supported and other drugs such as alcohol are not present.

Clinical Uses

Diazepam remains a popular oral drug for preoperative medication of adults and is the benzodiazepine most likely to be selected for management of delirium tremens and treatment of local anesthetic–induced seizures. Production of skeletal muscle relaxation by diazepam is often used in the management of lumbar disc disease and may be of value in the rare patient who develops tetany. Midazolam has largely replaced diazepam for IV sedation and the preoperative medication of children.

Anticonvulsant Activity

The prior administration of diazepam, 0.25 mg/kg IV, to animals protects against the development of seizures due to local anesthetic toxicity. Evidence for this protection is an increased convulsant dose of lidocaine in benzodiazepine-pretreated animals (Fig. 5-12) (De Jong and Heavner, 1974). Diazepam, 0.1 mg/kg IV, is effective in abolishing seizure activity produced by lidocaine, delirium tremens, and status epilepticus.

The efficacy of diazepam as an anticonvulsant may reflect its ability to facilitate the actions of the inhibitory neurotransmitter GABA. In contrast to barbiturates, which inhibit seizures by nonselective depression of the CNS, diazepam selectively inhibits activity in the limbic system, particularly the hippocampus. If diazepam is administered to terminate seizures, a longer acting antiepileptic drug such as fosphenytoin is also administered.

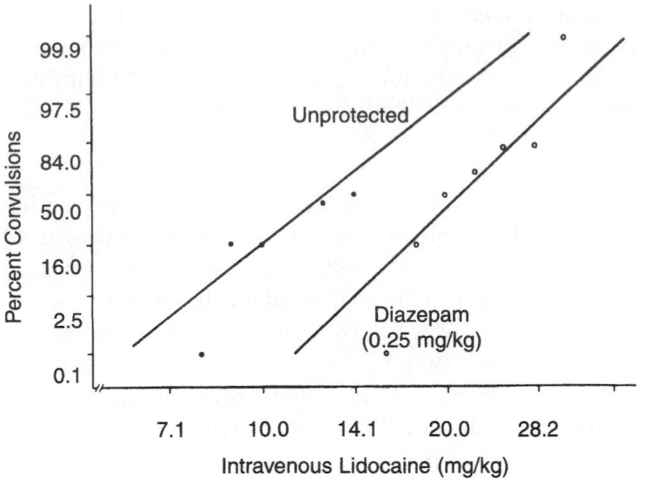

Figure 5-12. Prior administration of diazepam, 0.25 mg/kg IV, increases the intravenous dose of lidocaine required to produce seizures compared with untreated (unprotected) animals. (From De Jong RH, Heavner JE. Diazepam prevents and aborts lidocaine convulsions in monkeys. *Anesthesiology* 1974;49:226–230; with permission.)

LORAZEPAM

Lorazepam resembles oxazepam, differing only in the presence of an extra chloride atom on the ortho position of the 5-phenyl moiety (see Fig. 5-1). Lorazepam is a more potent sedative and amnesic than midazolam and diazepam, whereas its effects on ventilation, the cardiovascular system, and skeletal muscles resemble those of other benzodiazepines.

Pharmacokinetics

Lorazepam is conjugated with glucuronic acid in the liver to form pharmacologically inactive metabolites that are excreted by the kidneys. This contrasts with formation of pharmacologically active metabolites after the administration of midazolam and diazepam. The elimination half-time is 10 to 20 hours, with urinary excretion of lorazepam glucuronide accounting for >80% of the injected dose (see Table 5-1). Compared with midazolam, lorazepam has a much slower metabolic clearance. This may be explained by the slower hepatic glucuronidation of lorazepam compared with more rapid oxidative hydroxylation of midazolam. Because formation of glucuronide metabolites of lorazepam is not entirely dependent on hepatic microsomal enzymes, the metabolism of lorazepam is less likely than that of diazepam to be influenced by alterations in hepatic function, increasing age, or drugs that inhibit P-450 enzymes such as cimetidine. Indeed, the elimination half-time of lorazepam is not prolonged in elderly patients or in those treated with cimetidine. Lorazepam has a slower onset of action than midazolam or diazepam because of its lower lipid solubility and slower entrance into the CNS.

Clinical Uses

Lorazepam undergoes reliable absorption after oral and IM injection, which contrasts with diazepam. After oral administration, maximal plasma concentrations of lorazepam occur in 2 to 4 hours and persist at therapeutic levels for up to 24 to 48 hours. The recommended oral dose of lorazepam for preoperative medication is 50 μg/kg, not to exceed 4 mg (Fragen and Caldwell, 1976). With this dose, maximal anterograde amnesia lasting up to 6 hours occurs, and sedation is not excessive. Larger oral doses produce additional sedation without increasing amnesia. The prolonged duration of action of lorazepam limits its usefulness for preoperative medication when rapid awakening at the end of surgery is desirable.

After a single IV dose (1 to 4 mg) the onset of effect occurs within 1 to 2 minutes, with a time-to-peak effect of 20 to 30 minutes, and a duration of sedative effects ranging from 6 to 10 hours (Greenblatt et al., 1989). Infusions of lorazepam to produce postoperative sedation result in significant delays in emergence from sedation compared with midazolam (Barr et al., 2001). Obesity prolongs the sedative effects of lorazepam reflecting the larger volume of distribution and longer elimination half-time.

A slow onset limits the usefulness of lorazepam for (a) IV induction of anesthesia, (b) IV sedation during regional anesthesia, or (c) use as an anticonvulsant. Like diazepam, lorazepam is effective in limiting the incidence of emergence reactions after administration of ketamine. Although it is insoluble in water and thus requires use of solvents such as polyethylene glycol or propylene glycol, lorazepam is alleged to be less painful on injection and to produce less venous thrombosis than diazepam.

Lorazepam may be used as an economic alternative to midazolam for postoperatvie sedation of intubated patients. The risk of delayed emergence from sedation is increased when lorazepam is used for postoperative sedation and amnestic effects may last for several days. Delayed emergence from sedation may delay weaning from mechanical ventilation.

OXAZEPAM

Oxazepam, a pharmacologically active metabolite of diazepam, is commercially available (see Fig. 5-9). Its duration of action is slightly shorter than that of diazepam because oxazepam is converted to pharmacologically inactive metabolites by conjugation with glucuronic acid. The elimination half-time is 5 to 15 hours. Like lorazepam, the duration of action of oxazepam is unlikely to be influenced by hepatic dysfunction or administration of cimetidine.

Oral absorption of oxazepam is relatively slow. As a result, this drug may not be useful for the treatment of insomnia characterized by difficulty falling asleep. Conversely, oxazepam may be used for treatment of insomnia characterized by nightly awakenings or shortened total sleep time.

ALPRAZOLAM

Alprazolam has significant anxiety reducing effects in patients with primary anxiety and panic attacks. Based on these effects, alprazolam may be an alternative to midazolam for preoperative medication (Witte et al., 2002). Inhibition of adrenocorticotrophic hormone and cortisol secretion may be more prominent with aprazolam than with other benzodiazepines.

CLONAZEPAM

Clonazepam is a highly lipid-soluble benzodiazepine that is well absorbed after oral administration. Clonazepam is metabolized to inactive conjugated and unconjugated metabolites that appear in the urine. The elimination half-time is 24 to 48 hours. Clonazepam is particularly effective in the control and prevention of seizures, especially myoclonic and infantile spasms (see Chapter 30).

FLURAZEPAM

Flurazepam is chemically and pharmacologically similar to other benzodiazepines but is used exclusively to treat insomnia (see Fig. 5-1). After administration of 15 to 30 mg orally to adults, a hypnotic effect occurs in 15 to 25 minutes and lasts 7 to 8 hours. The period of rapid eye movement sleep is decreased by this drug. The principal metabolite of flurazepam is desalkylflurazepam. This metabolite is pharmacologically active and has a prolonged elimination half-time that may manifest as daytime sedation (hangover). Furthermore, repeated doses of flurazepam may result in accumulation of this metabolite, producing cumulative sedation. Elderly patients are susceptible to the adverse effects of flurazepam and other benzodiazepines with long elimination half-times.

TEMAZEPAM

Temazepam is an orally active benzodiazepine administered exclusively for the treatment of insomnia (see Figs. 5-1 and 5-3). Oral absorption is complete, but peak plasma concentrations do not reliably occur until about 2.5 hours after its administration. Metabolism in the liver results in weakly active to inactive metabolites that are conjugated with glucuronic acid. The elimination half-time is about 15 hours. Temazepam, 15 to 30 mg orally, does not alter the proportion of rapid eye movement sleep to total sleep in adults. Despite the relatively long elimination half-time, temazepam, as used to treat insomnia, is unlikely to be accompanied by residual drowsiness the following morning. Tolerance or signs of withdrawal do not occur, even after nightly administration for 30 consecutive days.

TRIAZOLAM

Triazolam is an orally absorbed benzodiazepine that is effective in the treatment of insomnia (see Fig. 5-1). Peak plasma concentrations after oral administration of 0.25 to 0.50 mg to adults occur in about 1 hour. The elimination half-time is 1.7 hours, rendering triazolam one of the shortest-acting benzodiazepines. The two principal metabolites of triazolam have little if any hypnotic activity, and their elimination half-time is <4 hours. For these reasons, residual daytime effects or cumulative sedation effects with repeated doses of triazolam seem less likely than with other benzodiazepines.

Triazolam does not change the proportion of rapid eye movement to total sleep time. Rebound insomnia, however, may occur when this drug is discontinued. Marked anterograde amnesia has developed when this drug has been self-administered in attempts to facilitate sleep when traveling through several time zones (Morris and Estes, 1987). In otherwise healthy elderly patients, triazolam causes a greater degree of sedation or psychomotor impairment than in young persons (Greenblatt et al., 1991). These effects are due to decreased clearance and higher plasma concentrations rather than from an increased sensitivity to the drug. For these reasons, it is recommended that the dose of triazolam be decreased 50% in elderly persons.

FLUMAZENIL

Flumazenil, a 1,4-imidazobenzodiazepine derivative, is a specific and exclusive benzodiazepine antagonist with a high affinity for benzodiazepine receptors, where it exerts minimal agonist activity (Fig. 5-13) (Brogden and Goa, 1991; Ghoneim et al., 1993). As a competitive antagonist, flumazenil prevents or reverses, in a dose-dependent manner, all the agonist effects of benzodiazepines. Flumazenil also effectively antagonizes the benzodiazepine component of ventilatory depression that is present during combined administration of a benzodiazepine and opioid (Gross et al., 1996). Metabolism of flumazenil is by hepatic microsomal enzymes to inactive metabolites.

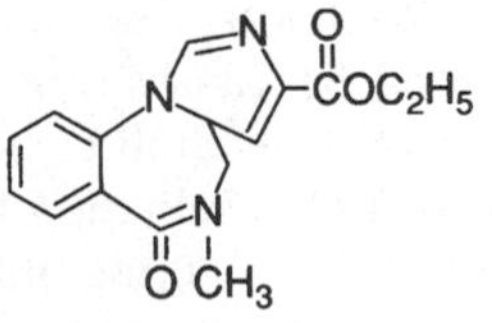

Figure 5-13. Flumazenil.

Dose and Administration

The dose of flumazenil should be titrated individually to obtain the desired level of consciousness. The recommended initial dose is 0.2 mg IV (8 to 15 μg/kg IV), which typically reverses the CNS effects of benzodiazepine agonists within about 2 minutes. If required, further doses of 0.1 mg IV (to a total of 1 mg IV) may be administered at 60-second intervals. Generally, total doses of 0.3 to 0.6 mg IV have been adequate to decrease the degree of sedation to the required extent in patients sedated or anesthetized with benzodiazepines, whereas total doses of 0.5 to 1.0 mg IV are usually sufficient to completely abolish the effect of a therapeutic dose of a benzodiazepine. In patients who are unconscious due to an overdose with an unknown drug or drugs, failure to respond to IV doses of flumazenil of more than 5 mg probably indicates the involvement of intoxicants other than benzodiazepines, or the presence of functional organic disorders. The duration of action of flumazenil is 30 to 60 minutes, and supplemental doses of the antagonist may be needed to maintain the desired level of consciousness. An alternative to repeated doses of flumazenil to maintain wakefulness is a continuous low-dose infusion of flumazenil, 0.1 to 0.4 mg/hour (Brogden and Goa, 1991). The administration of flumazenil to patients being treated with antiepileptic drugs for control of seizure activity is not recommended as it could precipitate acute withdrawal seizures (Spivey, 1992).

Side Effects

Flumazenil-induced antagonism of excess benzodiazepine agonist effects is not followed by acute anxiety, hypertension, tachycardia, or neuroendocrine evidence of a stress response in postoperative patients (White et al., 1989; Kaukinen et al., 1990). Reversal of benzodiazepine agonist effects with flumazenil is not associated with alterations in left ventricular systolic function or coronary hemodynamics in patients with coronary artery disease (Marty et al., 1991). The weak intrinsic agonist activity of flumazenil most likely attenuates evidence of abrupt reversal of agonist effects. Flumazenil does not alter anesthetic requirements (MAC) for volatile anesthetics, suggesting that these drugs do not exert any of their depressant effects on the CNS at benzodiazepine receptors (Schwieger et al., 1989). Flumazenil, administered at about ten times the clinically recommended dose, has no agonist effects on resting ventilation or psychomotor performance in normal individuals (Forster et al., 1993).

SHORT-ACTING HYPNOSEDATIVES

Zaleplon, zolpidem, and zopiclone are similar to benzodiazepines in exerting activity at the GABA receptor complex

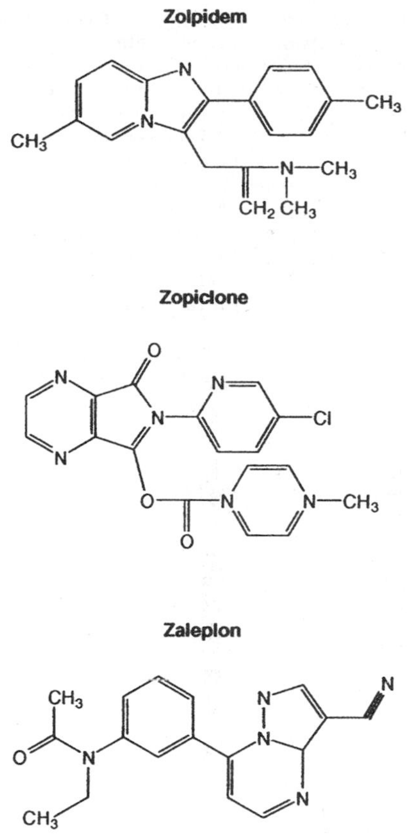

Figure 5-14. Chemical structures of short-acting hypnosedatives.

(Fig. 5-14) (Drover, 2004). These drugs seem to have more selectivity for certain subunits of GABA receptors, resulting in a clinical profile for treatment of sleeping disorders that is more efficacious with fewer side effects than occur with conventional benzodiazepines. Due to variations in binding to GABA receptor subunits, these three drugs show differences in their effect on sleep stages. Zalepoln (10 mg orally) has a rapid elimination so there are few residual side effects after taking a single dose at bedtime. By comparison, zolpidem (10 mg orally) and zopiclone (7.5 mg orally) have a more delayed elimination so there may be a prolonged drug effect. This may result in residual sedation and side effects but may be used for sustained treatment of insomnia with less waking during the night. Conversely, zaleplon is better utilized for patients who experience delayed onset of sleep.

REFERENCES

Adams P, Gelman S, Reves JG, et al. Midazolam pharmacodynamics and pharmacokinetics during acute hypovolemia. *Anesthesiology* 1985;63:140–146.

Ashton A. Guidelines for the rational use of benzodiazepines: when and what to use. *Drugs* 1994;48:25–40.

Bailey PL, Pace NL, Ashburn MA, et al. Frequent hypoxemia and apnea after sedation with midazolam and fentanyl. *Anesthesiology* 1990;73:826–830.

Barr J, Zomorodi K, Bertaccini E, et al. A double-blind, randomized comparison of IV lorazepam vs. midazolam for sedation of ICU patients via a pharmacologic model. *Anesthesiology* 2001;95:286–291.

Bauer TM, Ritz R, Haberthur C, et al. Prolonged sedation due to accumulation of conjugated metabolites of midazolam. *Lancet* 1995;346:145–150.

Bergman I, Steeves M, Burckart G, et al. Reversible neurologic abnormalities associated with prolonged intravenous midazolam and fentanyl administration. *J Pediatr* 1991;119:644–649.

Braunstein MC. Apnea with maintenance of consciousness following intravenous diazepam. *Anesth Analg* 1979;58:52–53.

Brogden RN, Goa KL. Flumazenil: a reappraisal of its pharmacological properties and therapeutic efficacy as a benzodiazepine antagonist. *Drugs* 1991;42:1061–1089.

Cote CJ, Cohen IT, Suresh S, et al. A comparison of three doses of a commercially prepared oral midazolam syrup in children. *Anesth Analg* 2002;94:37–43.

Crawford ME, Carl P, Andersen RS, et al. Comparison between midazolam and thiopentone-based balanced anaesthesia for day-care surgery. *Br J Anaesth* 1984;56:165–169.

Dawes GS. The distribution and action of drugs on the fetus in utero. *Br J Anaesth* 1973;45:766–769.

De Jong RH, Heavner JE. Diazepam prevents and aborts lidocaine convulsions in monkeys. *Anesthesiology* 1974;41:226–230.

Dretchen K, Ghoneim MM, Long JP. The interaction of diazepam with myoneural blocking agents. *Anesthesiology* 1971;34:463–468.

Drover DR. Comparative pharmacokinetics and pharmacodynamics of short-acting hypnosedatives: zaleplon, zolpidem and zopiclone. *Clin Pharmacokinet* 2004;43:227–238.

Eustace PW, Hailey DM, Cox AG, Baird ES. Biliary excretion of diazepam in man. *Br J Anaesth* 1975;47:983–985.

Falk RB, Denlinger JK, Nahrwold ML, et al. Acute vasodilation following induction of anesthesia with intravenous diazepam and nitrous oxide. *Anesthesiology* 1978;49:149–150.

Forster A, Crettenand G, Klopfenstein CE, et al. Absence of agonist effects of high-dose flumazenil on ventilation and psychometric performance in human volunteers. *Anesth Analg* 1993;77:980–984.

Forster A, Gardaz JP, Suter PM, et al. Respiratory depression of midazolam and diazepam. *Anesthesiology* 1980;53:494–499.

Fragen RJ, Caldwell N. Lorazepam premedication: lack of recall and relief of anxiety. *Anesth Analg* 1976;55:792–796.

Frumin MJ, Herekar VR, Jarvik ME. Amnesic actions of diazepam and scopolamine in man. *Anesthesiology* 1976;45:406–412.

Gamble JAS, Kawar P, Dundee JW, et al. Evaluation of midazolam as an intravenous induction agent. *Anesthesia* 1981;36:868–873.

Gauthier RA, Dyck B, Chung F, et al. Respiratory interaction after spinal anesthesia and sedation with midazolam. *Anesthesiology* 1992;77:909–914.

Gear RW, Miaskowski C, Heller PH et al. Benzodiazepine mediated antagonism of opioid analgesia. *Pain* 1997;71:25–29.

Gedney JA, Ghosh S. Pharmacokinetics of analgesics, sedatives and anaesthetic agents during cardiopulmonary bypass. *Br J Anaesth* 1995;75:344–351.

Ghoneim MM, Block RI, Ping Sum ST, et al. The interactions of midazolam and flumazenil on human memory and cognition. *Anesthesiology* 1993;79:1183–1192.

Ghoneim MM, Mewaldt SP. Benzodiazepines and human memory: a review. *Anesthesiology* 1990;72:926–938.

Ghouri A, Taylor E, White PF. Patient-controlled drug administration during local anesthesia: a comparison of midazolam, propofol, and alfentanil. *J Clin Anesth* 1992;4:476–480.

Giffin JP, Cottrell JE, Shwiry B, et al. Intracranial pressure, mean arterial pressure, and heart rate following midazolam or thiopental in humans with brain tumors. *Anesthesiology* 1984;60:491–494.

Goodchild CS. GABA receptors and benzodiazepines. *Br J Anaesth* 1993;71:127–133.

Greenblatt DJ, Abernathy DR, Locniskar A, et al. Effect of age, gender, and obesity on midazolam kinetics. *Anesthesiology* 1984;61:27–35.

Greenblatt DJ, Ehrenberg BL, Gunderman J et al. Kinetic and dynamic study of intravenous lorazepam: Comparison with intravenous diazepam. *J Pharmacol Exp Ther* 1989;250:134–139.

Greenblatt DJ, Harmatz JS, Shapiro L, et al. Sensitivity to triazolam in the elderly. *N Engl J Med* 1991;324:1691–1698.

Greenblatt DJ, Koch-Weser J. Clinical toxicity of chlordiazepoxide and diazepam in relation to serum albumin concentration: a report from the Boston Collaborative Drug Surveillance Program. *Eur J Clin Pharmacol* 1974;7:259–262.

Greenblatt DJ, Sellers EM, Shader RI. Drug disposition in old age. *N Engl J Med* 1982;306:1081–1088.

Gross JB, Blouin RT, Zandsberg S, et al. Effect of flumazenil on ventilatory drive during sedation with midazolam and alfentanil. *Anesthesiology* 1996;85:713–720.

Gross JB, Smith L, Smith TC. Time course of ventilatory response to carbon dioxide after intravenous diazepam. *Anesthesiology* 1982; 57;18–21.

Gross JB, Zebroski ME, Carel WD, et al. Time course of ventilatory depression after thiopental and midazolam in normal subjects and in patients with chronic obstructive pulmonary disease. *Anesthesiology* 1983;58:540–544.

Hase I, Oda Y, Tanaka K, et al. I.V. fentanyl decreases the clearance of midazolam. *Br J Anaesth* 1997;79:740–743.

Hiller A, Olkkola KT, Isohanni P, Saarnivaara L. Unconsciousness associated with midazolam and erythromycin. *Br J Anaesth* 1990;65:826–828.

Hughes MA, Glass PSA, Jacobs JR. Context-sensitive half-time in multicompartment pharmacokinetic models for intravenous anesthetic drugs. *Anesthesiology* 1992;76:334–341.

Jacobs JR, Reves JG, Marty J, et al. Aging increases pharmacodynamic sensitivity to the hypnotic effects of midazolam. *Anesth Analg* 1995;80:143–148.

Jensen S, Schou-Olesen A, Huttel MS. Use of midazolam as an induction agent: comparison with thiopental. *Br J Anaesth* 1982;54: 605–607.

Johnson TN, Rostami-Hodjegan A, Goddard JM, et al. Contribution of midazolam and its 1-hydroxy metabolite to preoperative sedation in children: a pharmacokinetic-pharmacodynamic analysis. *Br J Anaesth* 2002;89:428–437.

Kain ZN, Hofstadter MB, Mayes LC et al. Midazolam. Effects on amnesia and anxiety in children. *Anesthesiology* 2000;93:676–684.

Kalogeras KT, Calogero AE, Kuribayiashi T, et al. In vitro and in vivo effects of the triazolobenzodiazepine alprazolam on hypothalamic-pituitary adrenal function: pharmacological and clinical implications. *J Clin Endocrinol Metab* 1990;70:1462–1471.

Kanto J, Sjovall S, Buori A. Effect of different kinds of premedication of the induction properties of midazolam. *Br J Anaesth* 1982; 54:507–511.

Kaukinen S, Kataja J, Kaukinen L. Antagonism of benzodiazepine-fentanyl anesthesia with flumazenil. *Can J Anaesth* 1990;37:40–45.

Klotz U, Avant GR, Hoyumpa A, et al. The effects of age and liver disease on the disposition and elimination of diazepam in adult man. *J Clin Invest* 1975;55:347–359.

Knapp RB, Dubow H. Comparison of diazepam with thiopental as an induction agent in cardiopulmonary disease. *Anesth Analg* 1970; 49:722–726.

Kudoh A, Takase H, Takahira Y, et al. Postoperative confusion increases in elderly long-term benzodiazepine users. *Anesth Analg* 2004;99:1674–1678.

Lebowitz PW, Cote ME, Daniels AL, et al. Comparative cardiovascular effects of midazolam and thiopental in healthy patients. *Anesth Analg* 1982;61:661–665.

Low K, Crestani F, Keist R, et al. Molecular and neuronal substrate for the selective attenuation of anxiety. *Science* 2000;290: 131–134.

Marty J, Gauzit R, Lefevre P, et al. Effects of diazepam and midazolam on baroreflex control of heart rate and on sympathetic activity in humans. *Anesth Analg* 1986;65:113–119.

Marty J, Nitenberg A, Philip I, et al. Coronary and left ventricular hemodynamic responses following reversal of flunitrazepam-induced sedation with flumazenil in patients with coronary artery disease. *Anesthesiology* 1991;74:71–76.

McCammon RL, Hilgenberg JC, Stoelting RK. Hemodynamic effects of diazepam-nitrous oxide in patients with coronary artery disease. *Anesth Analg* 1980;59:438–441.

McClure JH, Brown DT, Wildsmith JAW. Comparison of the IV administration of midazolam and diazepam as sedation during spinal anesthesia. *Br J Anaesth* 1983;55:1089–1093.

McKernan RM, Rosahl TW, Reynolds DS, et al. Sedative but not anxiolytic properties of benzodiazepines are mediated by $GABA_A$ receptor $alpha_1$ subtype. *Nat Neurosci* 2000;3:587–592.

McMillan CO, Spahr-Schopfer IA, Sikich N, et al. Premedication of children with oral midazolam. *Can J Anaesth* 1992;39:545–550.

Mohler H, Richards JG. The benzodiazepine receptor: a pharmacological control element of brain function. *Eur J Anaesthesiol Suppl* 1988;2:15–24.

Morris HH, Estes ML. Traveler's amnesia. Transient global amnesia secondary to triazolam. *JAMA* 1987;258:945–946.

Nowell PD, Mazumdar S, Buysse DJ, et al. Benzodiazepines and zolpidem for chronic insomnia: a meta-analysis of treatment efficacy. *JAMA* 1997;278:2170–2177.

Papazian L, Albanese J, Thirion X, et al. Effect of bolus doses of midazolam on intracranial pressure and cerebral perfusion pressure in patients with severe head injury. *Br J Anaesth* 1993;71:267–271.

Petraglia F, Bakalakis S, Facchinetti F, et al. Effects of sodium valproate and diazepam on beta-endorphin, beta-lipotropin and cortisol secretion induced by hypoglycemic stress in humans. *Neuroendocrinology* 1986;44:320–325.

Reves JG, Fragen RJ, Vinik HR, et al. Midazolam: pharmacology and uses. *Anesthesiology* 1985;62:310–324.

Roberts KW, Crnkovic A, Steiniger JR. Post-anesthesia paradoxical vocal cord motion successfully treated with midazolam. *Anesthesiology* 1998;89:517–519.

Samuelson PN, Reves JG, Kouchoukos NT, et al. Hemodynamic responses to anesthetic induction with midazolam or diazepam in patients with ischemic heart disease. *Anesth Analg* 1981;60: 802–809.

Sarnquist FH, Mathers WD, Brock-Utne J, et al. A bioassay of a water-soluble benzodiazepine against sodium thiopental. *Anesthesiology* 1980;52:149–153.

Schwieger IM, Szlam F, Hug CC. Absence of agonistic or antagonistic effect of flumazenil (Ro 15–7088) in dogs anesthetized with enflurane, isoflurane, or fentanyl-enflurane. *Anesthesiology* 1989;70: 477–480.

Seubert CN, Morey TE, Martynuk AE et al. Midazolam selectively potentiates the A_{2a}- but not the A_1- receptor-mediated effects of adenosine. *Anesthesiology* 2000;92:567–577.

Sheu JR, Hsiao G, Luk HN, et al. Mechanisms involved in the antiplatelet activity of midazolam in human platelets. *Anesthesiology* 2002;96:651–658.

Spivey WH. Flumazenil and seizures: analysis of 43 cases. *Clin Ther* 1992;14:292–297.

Strebel S, Kaufmann M, Guardiola PM, et al. Cerebral vasomotor responsiveness to carbon dioxide is preserved during propofol and midazolam anesthesia in humans. *Anesth Analg* 1994;78:884–888.

Thurston TA, Williams CGS, Foshee SL. Reversal of a paradoxical reaction to midazolam with flumazenil. *Anesth Analg* 1996;83:192.

Veselis RA, Reinsel RA, Beattie BJ, et al. Midazolam changes regional cerebral blood flow in discrete brain regions: an $H_2{}^{15}O$ positron tomography study. *Anesthesiology* 1997;87:1106–1117.

Vinik HR, Reves JG, Greenblatt DJ, et al. The pharmacokinetics of midazolam in chronic renal failure patients. *Anesthesiology* 1983; 59:390–394.

White PF, Shafer A, Boyle WA, et al. Benzodiazepine antagonism does not provoke a stress response. *Anesthesiology* 1989;70:636–639.

Witte JL, Alegret C, Sessler DI et al. Preopeative alprazolam reduces anxiety in ambulatory surgery patients: A comparison with oral midazolam. *Anesth Analg* 2002;95:1601–1606.

6

Nonbarbiturate Intravenous Anesthetic Drugs

PROPOFOL

Propofol is a substituted isopropylphenol (2,6-diisopropylphenol) that is administered intravenously as 1% solution in an aqueous solution of 10% soybean oil, 2.25% glycerol, and 1.2% purified egg phosphatide (Fig. 6-1) (Bryson et al., 1995; Fulton and Sorkin, 1995; Smith et al., 1994). This drug is chemically distinct from all other drugs that act as intravenous (IV) sedative-hypnotics. Administration of propofol, 1.5 to 2.5 mg/kg IV (equivalent to thiopental, 4 to 5 mg/kg IV, or methohexital, 1.5 mg/kg IV) as a rapid IV injection (<15 s), produces unconsciousness within about 30 seconds. Awakening is more rapid and complete than that after induction of anesthesia with all other drugs used for rapid IV induction of anesthesia. The more rapid return of consciousness with minimal residual central nervous system (CNS) effects is one of the most important advantages of propofol compared with alternative drugs administered for the same purp<None>ose. Pain on injection occurs in a high proportion of patients when propofol is injected into small hand veins. This discomfort can be decreased by selecting larger veins or by prior administration of 1% lidocaine (using same injection site as for propofol) or a potent short-acting opioid.

Commercial Preparations

Propofol is an insoluble drug that requires a lipid vehicle for emulsification. Current formulations of propofol use a soybean oil as the oil phase and egg lecithin as the emulsifying agent that is composed of long-chain triglycerides (Ward et al., 2002). This formulation supports bacterial growth and causes increased plasma triglyceride concentrations especially when prolonged IV infusions are utilized. Diprivan® and generic propofol differ with respect to the preservatives utilized and the pH of the formulation. Diprivan® utilizes the preservative disodium edenate (0.005%) with sodium hydroxide to adjust the pH to 7 to 8.5. The generic formulation of propofol incorporates sodium metabisulfite (0.25 mg/mL) as the preservative and has a lower pH (4.5 to 6.4). Propofol, unlike thiopental, etomidate and ketamine, is not a chiral compound.

The mixing of propofol with any other drug is not recommended although lidocaine has been frequently added to propofol in attempts to prevent pain with intravenous injection. However, mixing of lidocaine with propofol may result in coalescence of oil droplets which may pose the risk of pulmonary embolism (Masaki et al., 2003).

A low-lipid emulsion of propofol (Ampofol®) contains 5% soybean oil and 0.6% egg lecithin but does not require a preservative or microbial growth retardant (Song et al., 2004). This formulation is equipotent to Diprivan® but is associated with a higher incidence of pain on injection.

An alternative to emulsion formulations of propofol and associated side effects (pain on injection, risk of infection, hypertriglyceridemia, pulmonary embolism) is creation of a prodrug (Aqauvan®) by cleaving groups to the parent compound that increase its water solubility (phosphate monoesters, hemisuccinates). Propofol is liberated after hydrolysis by endothelial cell surface alkaline phosphatases. In this regard, injection of the water-soluble propofol phosphate prodrug results in propofol and dose-dependent sedative effects (Banaszczyk et al., 2003; Fechner et al., 2003). Compared with propofol, this prodrug has a larger volume of distribution and higher potency (Fechner et al., 2004).

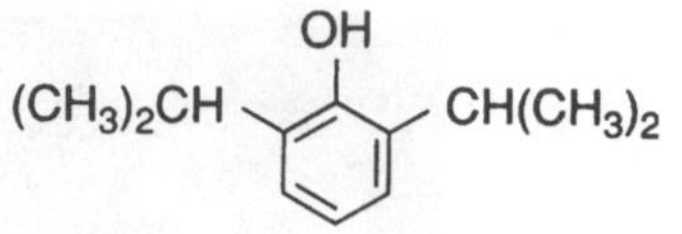

Figure 6-1. Propofol.

A nonlipid formulation of propofol uses cyclodextrins as a solublilizing agent (Sneyd, 2004). Cyclodextrins are ring sugar molecules that form guest (propofol)–host complexes migrating between the hydrophilic center of the cyclodextrin molecule and the water-soluble phase. This allows propofol, which is poorly soluble in water, to be presented in an injectable form. After injection, propofol migrates out of the cyclodextrin into the blood.

Mechanism of Action

Propofol is a relatively selective modulator of gamma aminobutyric acid ($GABA_A$) receptors and does not appear to modulate other ligand-gated ion channels at clinically relevant concentrations (Yamakura et al. 2001). Propofol is presumed to exert its sedative-hypnotic effects through a $GABA_A$ receptor interaction. GABA is the principal inhibitory neurotransmitter in the CNS. When $GABA_A$ receptors are activated, transmembrane chloride conductance increases, resulting in hyperpolarization of the postsynaptic cell membrane and functional inhibition of the postsynaptic neuron. The interaction of propofol (also etomidate and barbiturates) with specific components of $GABA_A$ receptors appears to decrease the rate of dissociation of the inhibitory neurotransmitter, GABA from the receptor, thereby increasing the duration of the GABA-activated opening of the chloride channel with resulting hyperpolarization of cell membranes.

In contrast to volatile anesthetics, spinal motorneuron excitability, as measured by H-reflexes, is not altered by propofol, suggesting that immobility during propofol anesthesia is not caused by drug-induced spinal cord depression (Kerz et al., 2001).

Pharmacokinetics

Clearance of propofol from the plasma exceeds hepatic blood flow, emphasizing that tissue uptake (possibly into the lungs), as well as hepatic oxidative metabolism by cytochrome P-450, is important in removal of this drug from the plasma (Fig. 6-2) (Table 6-1) (Court et al., 2001). Indeed, propofol metabolism in humans is considered to be both hepatic and extrahepatic. Hepatic metabolism is rapid and extensive, resulting in inactive, water-soluble sulfate and glucuronic acid metabolites that are excreted by the kidneys. Propofol may also undergo ring hydroxylation by cytochrome P-450 to form 4-hydroxypropofol which is then glucuronidated or sulfated. Although the glucuronide and sulfate conjugates of propofol appear to be pharmacologically inactive, 4-hydroxypropofol has about one-third the hypnotic activity of propofol. Less than 0.3% of a dose is excreted unchanged in urine. The elimination half-time is 0.5 to 1.5 hours, but more important, the context-sensitive half-time for propofol infusions lasting up to 8 hours is <40 minutes (see Fig. 1-3) (Hughes et al., 1992). The context-sensitive half-time of propofol is minimally influenced by the duration of the infusion because of rapid metabolic clearance when the infusion is discontinued so that the drug that returns from tissue storage sites to the circulation is not available to retard the decrease in plasma concentrations of the drug. Propofol, like thiopental and

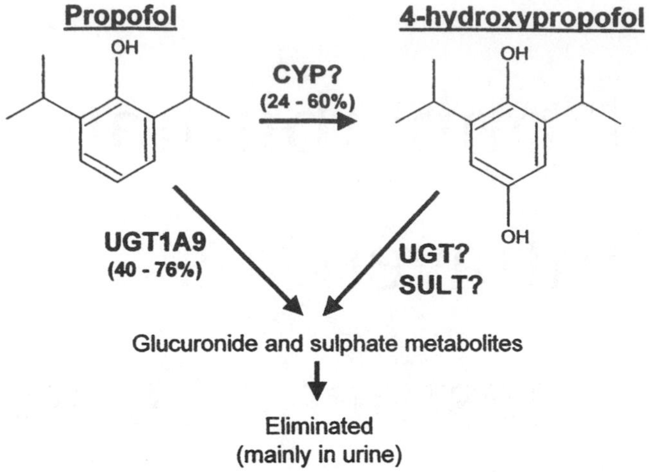

Figure 6-2. Major metabolic pathways for propofol. (From Court MH, Duan SX, Hesse LM, et al. Cytochrome P-450 2B6 is responsible for interindividual variability of propofol hydroxylation by human liver microsomes. *Anesthesiology* 2001;94:110–119; with permission.)

TABLE 6-1.
COMPARATIVE CHARACTERISTICS OF NONBARBITURATE INDUCTION DRUGS

	Elimination Half-Time (hrs)	Volume of Distribution (liters/kg)	Clearance (mL/kg/min)	Systemic Blood Pressure	Heart Rate
Propofol	0.5–1.5	3.5–4.5	30–60	Decreased	Decreased
Etomidate	2–5	2.2–4.5	10–20	No change to decreased	No change
Ketamine	2–3	2.5–3.5	16–18	Increased	Increased

alfentanil, has a short effect-site equilibration time such that effects on the brain occur promptly after IV administration.

The fact that total body clearance of propofol exceeds hepatic blood flow is consistent with extrahepatic clearance (pulmonary uptake and first pass elimination, renal excretion) of propofol (Kuipers et al., 1999; Takizawa et al., 2005). Pulmonary uptake of propofol is significant and influences the initial availability of propofol. Although propofol can be transformed in the lungs to 2,6-diisopropyl-1,4-quiniol, most of the drug that undergoes pulmonary uptake during the first pass is released back into the circulation (Dawidowicz et al., 2000; He et al., 2000). Glucuronidation is the major metabolic pathway for propofol and UDP-glucuronosyltransferase isoforms are expressed in the kidneys and brain. Indeed, human kidneys play an important role in the elimination of propofol (Takizawa et al., 2005).

Despite the rapid clearance of propofol by metabolism, there is no evidence of impaired elimination in patients with cirrhosis of the liver. Plasma concentrations of propofol at the time of awakening are similar in alcoholic and normal patients (Servin et al., 2003). Extrahepatic elimination of propofol occurs during the anhepatic phase of orthotopic liver transplantation. Renal dysfunction does not influence the clearance of propofol despite the observation that nearly three-fourths of propofol metabolites are eliminated in urine in the first 24 hours (Masuda et al., 1997). Patients older than 60 years of age exhibit a decreased rate of plasma clearance of propofol compared with younger adults. The rapid clearance of propofol confirms this drug can be administered as a continuous infusion without an excessive cumulative effect. Propofol readily crosses the placenta but is rapidly cleared from the neonatal circulation (Dailland et al., 1989). The effect of instituting cardiopulmonary bypass on the plasma propofol concentration is unpredictable, with some studies reporting a decrease whereas other observations fail to document any change (Gedney and Ghosh, 1995).

Clinical Uses

Propofol has become the induction drug of choice for many forms of anesthesia, especially when rapid and complete awakening is considered desirable (Smith et al., 1994). Continuous IV infusion of propofol, with or without other anesthetic drugs, has become a commonly used method for producing IV "conscious" sedation or as part of a balanced or total IV anesthetic (Bryson et al., 1995; Smith et al., 1994). Administration of propofol as a continuous infusion may be used for sedation of patients in the intensive care unit (ICU) (Fulton and Sorkin, 1995). In this regard, a 2% solution may be useful to decrease the volume of lipid emulsion administered with long-term sedation. A computer-controlled infusion pump is available to allow the clinician to select the propofol target concentration and the computer calculates the infusion rates that are necessary to achieve this target concentration based on the pharmacokinetics of propofol (Short et al., 1996).

Induction of Anesthesia

The induction dose of propofol in healthy adults is 1.5 to 2.5 mg/kg IV, with blood levels of 2 to 6 μg/mL producing unconsciousness depending on associated medications and the patient's age. As with barbiturates, children require higher induction doses of propofol on a milligram per kilogram basis, presumably reflecting a larger central distribution volume and higher clearance rate. Elderly patients require a lower induction dose (25% to 50% decrease) as a result of a smaller central distribution volume and decreased clearance rate (Smith et al., 1994). Awakening typically occurs at plasma propofol concentrations of 1.0 to 1.5 μg/mL. The complete awakening without residual CNS effects that is characteristic of propofol is the principal reason this drug has replaced thiopental for induction of anesthesia in many clinical situations. Although propofol is more expensive than thiopental, the additional expense may be offset by decreased costs made possible by prompt awakening.

Intravenous Sedation

The short context-sensitive half-time of propofol, even with prolonged periods of infusion, combined with the short effect-site equilibration time, make this a readily titratable drug for production of IV sedation (Bryson et al., 1995). The prompt recovery without residual sedation and low incidence of nausea and vomiting make propofol particularly well suited to ambulatory conscious sedation techniques. The typical conscious sedation dose of 25 to 100 μg/kg/minute IV produces minimal analgesic and amnestic effects (Smith et al., 1994). In selected patients, midazolam or an opioid may be added to propofol for continuous IV sedation. A sense of well-being may accompany recovery from conscious sedation with propofol, although this may be related more to the patient's relief that the procedure is over than to a specific pharmacologic effect of propofol. Indeed, pain intensity and unpleasantness of pain have been rated as lessened by patients sedated with propofol (Frolich et al., 2005). A conventional patient-controlled analgesia delivery system set to deliver 0.7 mg/kg doses of propofol with a 3-minute lockout period is an alternative to continuous IV sedation techniques.

Propofol has been administered as a sedative during mechanical ventilation in the ICU in a variety of patient populations including postoperative patients (cardiac surgery, neurosurgery) and patients with head injury (Fulton and Sorkin, 1995). Propofol also provides control of stress responses and has anticonvulsant and amnestic properties. After cardiac surgery, propofol sedation appears to modulate postoperative hemodynamic responses by decreasing the incidence and severity of tachycardia and hypertension (Wahr et al., 1996). Increasing metabolic acidosis, lipemic plasma, bradycardia, and progressive myocardial failure has been described in a few children who were sedated with propofol during management of acute respiratory failure in the ICU (Parke et al., 1992).

Maintenance of Anesthesia

The typical dose of propofol for maintenance of anesthesia is 100 to 300 μg/kg/minute IV, often in combination with a short-acting opioid (Smith et al., 1994). Although propofol has proved to be a valuable adjuvant during short ambulatory procedures, its use for more prolonged operations (>2 hours) is questionable based on the cost of the drug and only modest differences in recovery times compared with those of standard inhalation or balanced anesthetic techniques (Smith et al., 1994). General anesthesia that includes propofol is typically associated with minimal postoperative nausea and vomiting, and awakening is prompt, with minimal residual sedative effects.

Nonhypnotic Therapeutic Applications

In addition to its clinical application as an IV induction drug, propofol has been shown to have beneficial effects that were not anticipated when the drug was initially introduced in 1989 (Borgeat et al., 1994).

Antiemetic Effects

The incidence of postoperative nausea and vomiting is decreased when propofol is administered, regardless of the anesthetic technique or anesthetic drugs used (Borgeat et al., 1994). Subhypnotic doses of propofol (10 to 15 mg IV) may be used in the postanesthesia care unit to treat nausea and vomiting, particularly if it is not of vagal origin. In the postoperative period, the advantage of propofol is its rapid onset of action and the absence of serious side effects. Propofol is generally efficacious in treating postoperative nausea and vomiting at plasma concentrations that do not produce increased sedation. Simulations indicate that antiemetic plasma concentrations of propofol are achieved by a single IV dose of 10 mg followed by 10 μg/kg/minute (Gan et al., 1997). Propofol in subhypnotic doses is effective against chemotherapy-induced nausea and vomiting. When administered to induce and maintain anesthesia, it is more effective than ondansetron in preventing postoperative nausea and vomiting (Gan et al., 1996). Despite the large number of clinical studies suggesting an antiemetic effect of propofol, metaanalysis of published studies has suggested that (a) there is insufficient evidence that total IV anesthesia with propofol is an anesthetic technique with a low emetogenic potency, and (b) it is overly optimistic to expect propofol to act as an antiemetic in every clinical setting, especially if the event rate without prophylaxis is low (Tramer et al., 1997a; Tramer et al., 1997b).

Propofol has a profile of CNS depression that differs from other anesthetic drugs. In contrast to thiopental, for example, propofol uniformly depresses CNS structures, including subcortical centers. Most drugs of known antiemetic efficacy exert this effect via subcortical structures, and it is possible that propofol modulates subcortical pathways to inhibit nausea and vomiting or produces a direct depressant effect on the vomiting center. Nevertheless, the mechanisms mediating the antiemetic effects of propofol remain unknown. An antiemetic effect of propofol based on inhibition of the dopaminergic system is unlikely in view of the observation that subhypnotic doses of propofol fail to increase plasma prolactin concentrations (Borgeat, 1997). A rapid and distinct increase in plasma prolactin concentrations is characteristic of drugs that block the dopaminergic system. The antiemetic effect of propofol is not due to the intralipid emulsion in the formulation (Gan et al., 1997). Subhypnotic doses of propofol that are effective as an antiemetic do not inhibit gastric emptying and propofol is not considered a prokinetic drug (Chassard et al, 2002).

Antipruritic Effects

Propofol, 10 mg IV, is effective in the treatment of pruritus associated with neuraxial opioids or cholestasis (Borgeat et al., 1992). The quality of analgesia is not affected by propofol. The mechanism of the antipruritic effect may be related to the drug's ability to depress spinal cord activity. In this regard, there is evidence that intrathecal opioids produce pruritus by segmental excitation within the spinal cord.

Anticonvulsant Activity

Propofol possesses antiepileptic properties, presumably reflecting GABA-mediated presynaptic and postsynaptic inhibition of chloride ion channels. In this regard, propofol in doses of >1 mg/kg IV decreases seizure duration 35% to 45% in patients undergoing electroconvulsive therapy (Avramov et al., 1995).

Attenuation of Bronchoconstriction

Compared with thiopental, propofol decreases the prevalence of wheezing after induction of anesthesia and tracheal intubation in healthy and asthmatic patients (Fig. 6-3) (Eames et al., 1996). However, a newer formulation of propofol utilizes metabisulfite as a preservative. Metabisulfite may cause bronchoconstriction in asthmatic patients. In an animal model, propofol without metabisulfite attenuated vagal nerve stimulation-induced bronchoconstriction, whereas propofol with metabisulfite did not attenuate vagally or methacholine-induced bronchoconstriction and metabisulfite alone caused increases in airway responsiveness (Brown et al., 2001). Following tracheal intubation, in patients with a history of smoking, airway resistance was increased more following the administration of propofol containing metabisulfite than ethylenediaminetetraacetic acid (EDTA) (Rieschke et al., 2003). Therefore, the preservative used for propofol can have effects on its ability to attenuate bronchoconstriction.

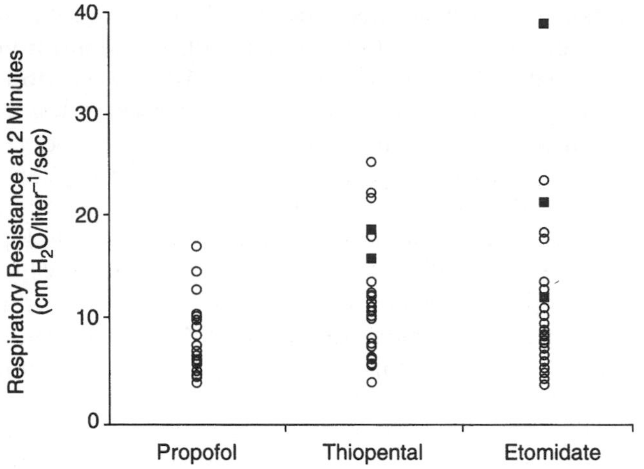

Figure 6-3. Respiratory resistance after tracheal intubation is less after induction of anesthesia with propofol than after induction of anesthesia with thiopental or etomidate. The solid squares represent four patients in whom audible wheezing was present. (From Eames WO, Rooke GA, Sai-Chuen R, et al. Comparison of the effects of etomidate, propofol, and thiopental on respiratory resistance after tracheal intubation. *Anesthesiology* 1996;84: 1307–1311; with permission.)

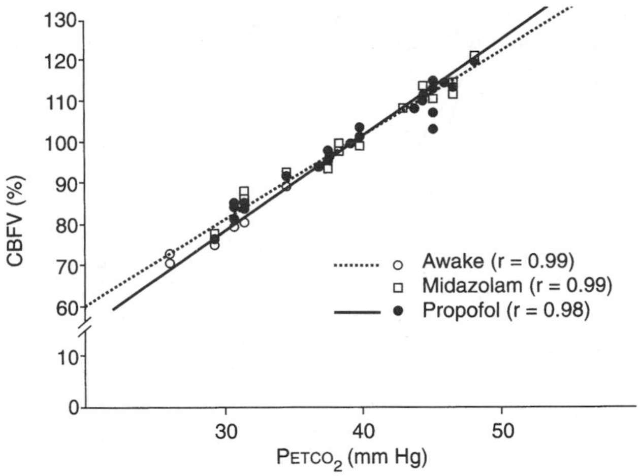

Figure 6-4. Changes in the end-tidal P_{CO_2} (P_{ETCO_2}) produce corresponding changes in the cerebral blood flow velocity (CBFV) during infusion of propofol or midazolam. (From Strebel S, Kaufmann M, Guardiola PM, Schaefer HG. Cerebral vasomotor responsiveness to carbon dioxide is preserved during propofol and midazolam anesthesia in humans. *Anesth Analg* 1994;78:884–888; with permission.)

Nevertheless, propofol-induced bronchoconstriction has been described in patients with allergy histories and the formulation of propofol administered to these patients was Diprivan® containing soybean oil, glycerin, yolk lecithin, and sodium edetate (Nishiyama and Hanaoka, 2001).

Effects on Organ Systems

Central Nervous System

Propofol decreases cerebral metabolic rate for oxygen ($CMRO_2$), cerebral blood flow, and intracranial pressure (ICP) (Kaisti et al., 2003; Pinaud et al., 1990). Administration of propofol to produce sedation in patients with intracranial space-occupying lesions does not increase ICP (Girard et al., 2004). Large doses of propofol may decrease systemic blood pressure sufficiently to also decrease cerebral perfusion pressure. Cerebrovascular autoregulation in response to changes in systemic blood pressure and reactivity of the cerebral blood flow to changes in Pa_{CO_2} are not affected by propofol. Indeed, cerebral blood flow velocity changes in parallel with changes in Pa_{CO_2} in the presence of propofol and midazolam (Fig. 6-4) (Strebel et al., 1994). Propofol produces cortical electroencephalographic (EEG) changes that are similar to those of thiopental, including the ability of high doses to produce burst suppression (Hewitt et al., 1999). Cortical somatosensory evoked potentials as utilized for monitoring spinal cord function are not significantly modified in the presence of propofol alone but the addition of nitrous oxide or a volatile anesthetic results in decreased amplitude (Boisseau et al., 2002). Propofol does not interfere with the adequacy of electrocorticographic recordings during awake craniotomy performed for the management of refractory epilepsy, provided administration is discontinued at least 15 minutes before recording (Herrick et al., 1997). At equal levels of sedation, propofol produces the same degree of memory impairment as midazolam, whereas thiopental has mild memory effects and fentanyl has none (Veselis et al., 1997).

Development of tolerance to drugs that depress the central nervous system (CNS) is a common finding occurring with repeated exposure to opioids, sedative-hypnotic drugs, ketamine, and nitrous oxide. However, tolerance to propofol does not develop in children undergoing repeated exposure to the drug during radiation therapy (Keidan et al., 2004).

Cardiovascular System

Propofol produces decreases in systemic blood pressure that are greater than those evoked by comparable doses of thiopental (Fig. 6-5) (Rouby et al., 1991). These decreases in blood pressure are often accompanied by corresponding changes in cardiac output and systemic vascular resistance. The relaxation of vascular smooth muscle produced by propofol is primarily due to inhibition of sympathetic vasoconstrictor nerve activity (Robinson et al., 1997). A negative inotropic effect of propofol may result from a decrease in intracellular calcium availability secondary to inhibition of trans-sarcolemmal calcium influx. Stimulation produced by direct laryngoscopy and intubation of the trachea reverses the blood pressure effects of propofol, although this drug is more effective than thiopental in blunting the magnitude of this pressor response. Propofol also effectively blunts the hypertensive response to placement of a laryngeal mask airway. The impact of propofol

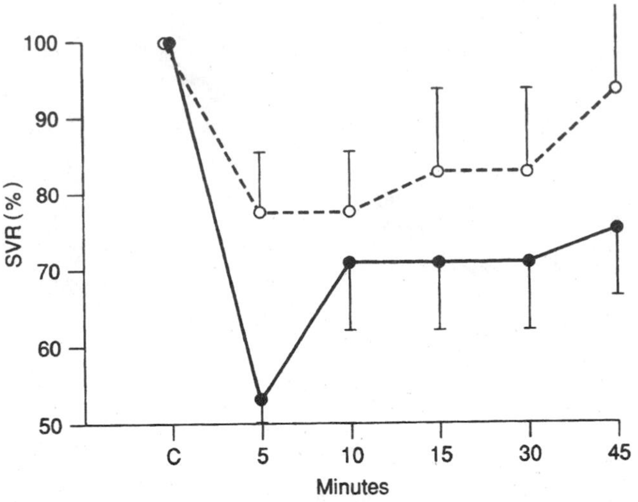

Figure 6-5. Comparative changes [expressed in % changes (mean ± SD)] from control values (C) in systemic vascular resistance (SVR) in the 45 minutes after the administration of thiopental, 5 mg/kg IV (*open circles*), or propofol, 2.5 mg/kg IV (*solid circles*). (From Rouby JJ, Andreev A, Leger P, et al. Peripheral vascular effects of thiopental and propofol in humans with artificial hearts. *Anesthesiology* 1991;75:32–42; with permission.)

on desflurane-mediated sympathetic nervous system activation is unclear. In one report, propofol 2 mg/kg IV blunted the increase in epinephrine concentration that accompanied a sudden increase in the delivered desflurane concentration but did not attenuate the transient cardiovascular response to a rapid increase in the concentration of this volatile anesthetic to >1 MAC (Daniel et al., 1996). Conversely, in another report, induction of anesthesia with propofol, but not etomidate, blunted the sympathetic nervous system activation and systemic hypertension associated with the introduction of rapidly increasing inhaled concentrations of desflurane (Lopatka et al., 1999). The blood pressure effects of propofol may be exaggerated in hypovolemic patients, elderly patients, and patients with compromised left ventricular function due to coronary artery disease. Adequate hydration before rapid IV administration of propofol is recommended to minimize the blood pressure effects of this drug.

Addition of nitrous oxide does not alter the cardiovascular effects of propofol. The pressor response to ephedrine is augmented by propofol (Fig. 6-6) (Kanaya et al., 2002).

Despite decreases in systemic blood pressure, heart rate often remains unchanged in contrast to the modest increases that typically accompany the rapid IV injection of thiopental. Bradycardia and asystole have been observed after induction of anesthesia with propofol, resulting in the occasional recommendation that anticholinergic drugs be administered when vagal stimulation is likely to occur in association with administration of propofol (see the section on Bradycardia-Related Death). Propofol may decrease sympathetic nervous system activity to a greater extent than parasympathetic nervous system activity, resulting in a predominance of parasympathetic activity (Bryson et al., 1995). There is also evidence that propofol does not alter sinoatrial or atrioventricular node function in normal patients or in patients with Wolff-Parkinson-White syndrome, thus making it an acceptable drug to administer during ablative procedures (Lavoie et al., 1995; Sharpe et al., 1995). Nevertheless, there is a report of a patient with Wolff-Parkinson-White syndrome in whom delta waves on the electrocardiogram disappeared during infusion of propofol (Seki et al., 1999). Unlike sevoflurane, propofol does not prolong the QTc interval on the electrocardiogram (Kleinsasser et al., 2000). Baroreceptor reflex control of heart rate may be depressed by propofol (Deutschman et al., 1994).

Bradycardia-Related Death

Profound bradycardia and asystole after administration of propofol have been described in healthy adult patients, despite prophylactic anticholinergics (Egan and Brock, 1991; Freysz et al., 1991; James et al., 1989; Tramer et al., 1997c). The risk of bradycardia-related death during propofol anesthesia has been estimated to be 1.4 in 100,000. Severe, refractory, and fatal bradycardia in children in the ICU has been observed with long-term propofol sedation (Bray, 1995; Dearlove and Dobson, 1995). Propofol anesthesia, compared with other anesthetics, increases the incidence of the oculocardiac reflex in pediatric strabismus surgery, despite prior administration of anticholinergics (Tramer et al., 1995c).

Heart rate responses to IV administration of atropine are attenuated in patients receiving propofol compared with awake patients (Fig. 6-7) (Horiguchi and Nishikawa, 2002). This decreased responsiveness to atropine cannot be

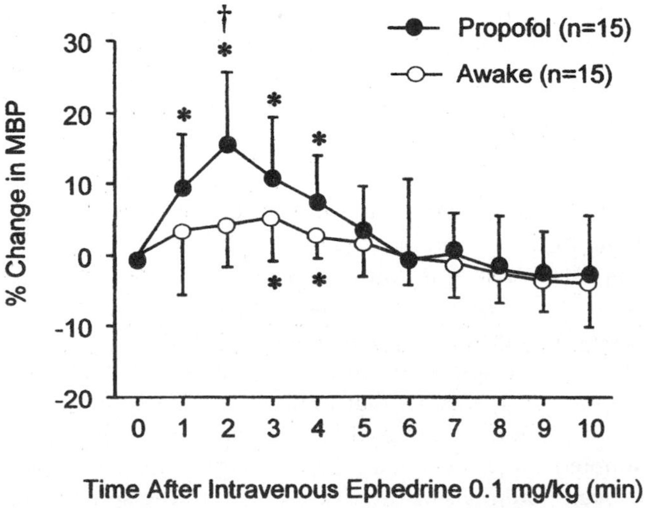

Figure 6-6. Mean blood pressure (MBI) increased more following administration of ephedrine (0.1 mg/kg IV) to patients during propofol anesthesia than when awake. (From Kanaya N, Satoh H, Seki S, et al. Propofol anesthesia enhances the pressor response to intravenous ephedrine. *Anesth Analg* 2002;94:1207–1213; with permission.)

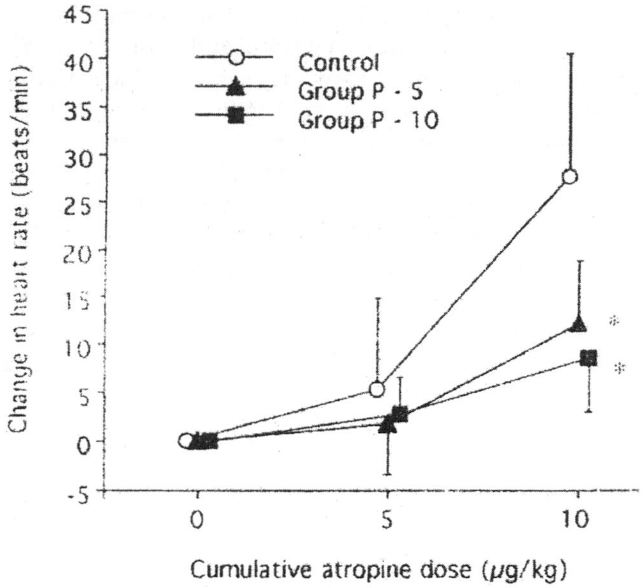

Figure 6-7. Heart rate responses to cumulative IV atropine doses in patients receiving no propofol, patients receiving 5 mg/kg/hour IV (Group P-5), and patients receiving 10 mg/kg/hour IV (Group P-10). Mean ≠ SD. *P <0.05 compared with the control group. (From Horiguchi T, Nishikawa T. Heart rate response to intravenous atropine during propofol anesthesia. *Anesth Analg* 2002;95:389–392; with permission.)

effectively overcome by large doses of atropine suggesting that propofol may induce suppression of sympathetic nervous system activity. Treatment of propofol-induced bradycardia may require treatment with a beta-agonist such as insoproterenol.

Lungs

Propofol produces dose-dependent depression of ventilation, with apnea occurring in 25% to 35% of patients after induction of anesthesia with propofol (Bouillon et al., 2004). Opioids administered with the preoperative medication may enhance this ventilatory depressant effect. Painful surgical stimulation is likely to counteract the ventilatory depressant effects of propofol. A maintenance infusion of propofol decreases tidal volume and frequency of breathing. The ventilatory response to carbon dioxide and arterial hypoxemia are decreased by propofol (Blouin et al., 1993). Propofol can produce bronchodilation and decrease the incidence of intraoperative wheezing in patients with asthma (Fig. 6-3) (Eames et al., 1996; Pizov et al., 1995). Sedative concentrations of propofol depress the ventilatory response to hypercapnia due to an effect at the central chemoreceptors (Nieuwenhuijs et al., 2001). In contrast to low-dose volatile anesthetics, the periperal chemoreflex response to carbon dioxide remains intact when stimulated by carbon dioxide in the presence of propofol. Likewise, propofol infusion to produce sedation significantly decreases the slope and causes a downward shift of the ventilatory response curve to hypoxia (Blouin et al., 1993). Hypoxic pulmonary vasoconstriction seems to remain intact in patients receiving propofol.

Hepatic and Renal Function

Propofol does not adversely affect hepatic or renal function as reflected by measurements of liver transaminase enzymes or creatinine concentrations. Prolonged infusions of propofol have been associated with hepatocellular injury accompanied by lactic acidosis, bradydysrhythmias, and rhabdomyolysis. In rare instances, propofol-induced hepatocellular injury following uneventful anesthesia and surgery has been described (Anand et al., 2001). Prolonged infusions of propofol may also result in excretion of green urine, reflecting the presence of phenols in the urine. This discoloration does not alter renal function. Urinary uric acid excretion is increased after administration of propofol and may manifest as cloudy urine when the uric acid crystallizes in the urine under conditions of low pH and temperature (Masuda et al., 1997). This cloudy urine is not considered to be detrimental or indicative of adverse renal effects of propofol.

Intraocular Pressure

Laparoscopic surgery is associated with increased intraocular pressure and some consider laparoscopic surgery with the head down position a risk in the presence of preexisting ocular hypertension. In this regard, propofol is associated with significant decreases in intraocular pressure that occur immediately after induction of anesthesia and are sustained during tracheal intubation (Bryson et al., 1995). Total IV anesthesia with propofol for laparoscopic surgery was associated with lower intraocular pressures than in patients undergoing similar surgery with isoflurane anesthesia (Fig. 6-8) (Mowafi et al., 2003).

Coagulation

Propofol does not alter tests of coagulation or platelet function. This is reassuring because the emulsion in which propofol is dispensed resembles intralipid, which has been associated with alterations in blood coagulation. Propofol inhibits platelet aggregation that is induced by proinflammatory lipid mediators including thromboxane A_2 and platelet-activating factor (Fourcade et al., 2004).

Side Effects

Side effects of propofol may reflect the parent drug or actions attributed to the oil-in-water emulsion formulation. For example, some of the side effects of propofol (bradycardia, risk of infection, pain on injection, hypertriglyceridemia with prolonged administration, potential for pulmonary embolism) are believed to be due in large part to the lipid emulsion formulation (Banaszczyk et al., 2002; Fechner et al., 2003).

Allergic Reactions

Allergenic components of propofol include the phenyl nucleus and diisopropyl side chain (de Leon-Casasola

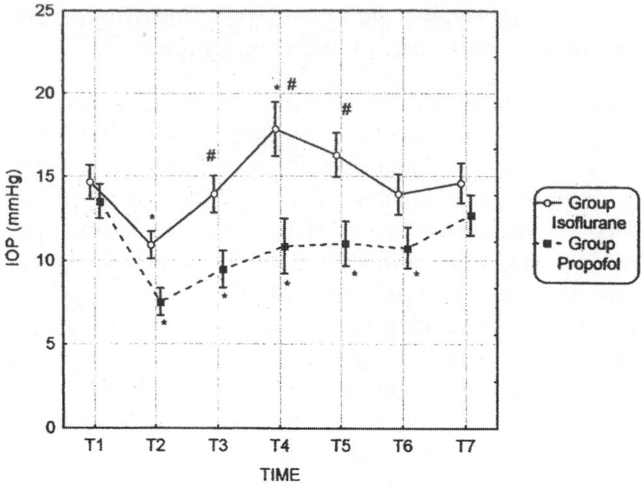

Figure 6-8. Changes in intraocular pressure (IOP) in patients receiving isoflurane or propofol. Measurements were made before induction of anesthesia (T1), after induction of anesthesia (T2), after pneumoperitoneum (T3), after head-down position (T4), after return to neutral supine position (T5), after evacuation of pneumoperitoneum (T6), and in the postanaesthesia care unit (T7). *Significant difference compared with T1. #Significant difference between the isoflurane and propofol groups. (From Mowafi HA, Al-Ghamdi A, Rushood A. Intraocular pressure changes during laparoscopy in patients anesthetized with propofol total intravenous anesthesia versus isoflurane inhaled anesthesia. *Anesth Analg* 2003;97:471–474; with permission.)

et al., 1992). Patients who develop evidence of anaphylaxis on first exposure to propofol may have been previously sensitized to the diisopropyl radical, which is present in many dermatologic preparations. Likewise, the phenol nucleus is common to many drugs. Indeed, anaphylaxis to propofol during the first exposure to this drug has been observed, especially in patients with a history of other drug allergies, often to neuromuscular-blocking drugs (Laxenaire et al., 1992). Propofol-induced bronchoconstriction has been described in patients with allergy histories (Nishiyama and Hanaoka, 2001). The formulation of propofol administered to these patients was Diprivan® containing soybean oil, glycerin, yolk lecithin, and sodium edetate.

Lactic Acidosis

Lactic acidosis ("propofol infusion syndrome") has been described in pediatric and adult patients receiving prolonged high-dose infusions of propofol (>75 μg/kg/minute) for longer than 24 hours (Badr et al., 2001; Cremer et al., 2001). Even short-term infusions of propofol (Diprivan®) for surgical anesthesia have been associated with development of metabolic acidosis (Burow et al., 2004; Salengros et al., 2004). Unexpected tachycardia occurring during propofol anesthesia should prompt laboratory evaluation for possible metabolic (lactic) acidosis. Measurement of arterial blood gases and serum lactate concentrations is recommended. Documentation of an increased ion gap is useful but will take time and delay treatment which includes prompt discontinuation of propofol administration (Funston and Prough, 2004). Metabolic acidosis in its early stages is reversible with discontinuation of propofol administration although cardiogenic shock requiring assistance with extracorporeal membrane oxygenation has been described in a patient receiving a prolonged propofol infusion (Diprivan®) for a craniotomy (Culp et al., 2004).

The mechanism for sporadic propofol-induced metabolic acidosis is unclear but may reflect poisoning (cytopathic hypoxia) of the electron transport chain and impaired oxidation of long-chain fatty acids by propofol or a propofol metabolite in uniquely susceptible patients (Wolf et al., 2001). Indeed, this propofol infusion syndrome mimics the mitochondrial myopathies, in which there are specific defects in the mitochondrial respiratory chain associated with specific mitochondrial DNA abnormalities, resulting in abnormal lipid metabolism in cardiac and skeletal muscles. These individuals, who are probably genetically susceptible, remain asymptomatic until a triggering event (sepsis, malnutrition) intervenes.

The differential diagnosis when propofol-induced lactic acidosis is suspected includes hyperchloremic metabolic acidosis associated with large volume infusions of 0.9% saline and metabolic acidosis associated with excessive generation of organic acids, such as lactate and ketones (diabetic acidosis, release of a tourniquet). Measurement of the anion gap and individual measurements of anions and organic acids will differentiate hyperchloremic metabolic acidosis from lactic acidosis.

Proconvulsant Activity

The majority of reported propofol-induced seizures during induction of anesthesia or emergence from anesthesia reflect spontaneous excitatory movements of subcortical origin (Borgeat et al., 1994). These responses are not thought to be due to cortical epileptic activity, although some recommend caution in administering propofol to patients with poorly controlled epilepsy (Cochran et al., 1996). Prolonged myoclonus associated with meningismus has been associated with propofol administration (Hughes and Lyons, 1995).

The incidence of excitatory movements and associated ECG changes are low after the administration of propofol (Reddy et al., 1993). Propofol resembles thiopental in that it does not produce seizure activity on the EEG when administered to patients with epilepsy, including those undergoing cortical resection (Hewitt et al., 1999). There appears to be no reason to avoid propofol for sedation, induction, and maintenance of anesthesia in patients with known seizures (Snyed, 1999).

Abuse Potential

Intense dreaming activity, amorous behavior, and hallucinations have been reported during recovery from the effects of propofol (Borgeat et al., 1994). Addiction to virtually all opioids and hypnotics, including propofol, has been described (Follette and Farley, 1992).

Bacterial Growth

Propofol strongly supports the growth of *Escherichia coli* and *Pseudomonas aeruginosa,* whereas the solvent (Intralipid) appears to be bactericidal for these same organisms and bacteriostatic for *Candida albicans* (Crowther et al., 1996). Clusters of postoperative surgical infections manifesting as temperature elevations have been attributed to extrinsic contamination of propofol (Kuehnert et al., 1997; Nichols and Smith, 1995). For this reason, it is recommended that (a) an aseptic technique be used in handling propofol as reflected by disinfecting the ampule neck surface or vial rubber stopper with 70% isopropyl alcohol; (b) the contents of the ampule containing propofol should be withdrawn into a sterile syringe immediately after opening and administered promptly; and (c) the contents of an opened ampule must be discarded if they are not used within 6 hours. In the ICU, the tubing and any unused portion of propofol must be discarded after 12 hours. Despite these concerns, there is evidence that when propofol is aseptically drawn into an uncapped syringe, it will remain sterile at room temperature for several days (Warwick and Bladke, 1994). Given the cost of propofol, some have questioned the logic of discarding unused drug at the end of an anesthetic or 6 hours, whichever occurs sooner (Smith et al., 1994).

Antioxidant Properties

Propofol has potent antioxidant properties that resemble those of the endogenous antioxidant vitamin E (Daskalopoulos et al., 2001; Peters et al., 2001). Like vitamin E, propofol contains a phenolic hydroxyl group that scavenges free radicals and inhibits lipid peroxidation. A neuroprotective effect of propofol may be at least partially related to the antioxidant potential of propofol's phenol ring structure. For example, propofol reacts with lipid peroxyl radicals and thus inhibits lipid peroxidation by forming relatively stable propofol phenoxyl radicals. In addition, propofol also scavenges peroxynitrite, which is one of the most potent reactive metabolites for the initiation of lipid peroxidation. Because peroxynitrite is a potent bactericidal agent, it is likely that the peroxynitrite-scavenging activity of propofol contributes to this anesthetic's known ability to suppress phagocytosis (Krumholz et al., 1994). Conversely, propofol might be beneficial in disease states, such as acute lung injury, in which peroxynitrite formation is thought to play an important role (Kooy et al., 1995).

Reintroduction of molecular oxygen into previously ischemic tissues (removal of an aortic cross-clamp) can further damage partially injured cells (reperfusion injury). Oxygen leads to the formation of free oxygen radicals which react with polyunsaturated fatty acids of cell membranes resulting in disruption of cell membranes. Myocardial cell injury can cause postischemic dysfunction, myocardial stunning, and reperfusion cardiac dysrhythmias. Propofol strongly attenuates lipid peroxidation during coronary artery bypass graft surgery (Sayin et al., 2002).

Pain on Injection

Pain on injection is the most commonly reported adverse event associated with propofol administration to awake patients. This unpleasant side effect of propofol occurs in <10% of patients when the drug is injected into a large vein rather than a dorsum vein on the hand. Preceding the propofol with (using the same injection site as for propofol) 1% lidocaine or by prior administration of a potent short-acting opioid decreases the incidence of discomfort experienced by the patient. The incidence of thrombosis or phlebitis is usually <1%. Changing the composition of the carrier fat emulsion for propofol to long- and medium-chain triglycerides decreases the incidence of pain on injection (Doenicke et al., 1997).

Accidental intraarterial injection of propofol has been described as producing severe pain but no vascular compromise (Holley and Cuthrell, 1990). In an animal model, propofol-exposed arteries showed no changes in the vascular smooth muscle, and the endothelium was not damaged (MacPherson et al., 1992).

Airway Protection

Inhaled and injected anesthetic drugs alter pharyngeal function with the associated risk of impaired upper airway protection and pulmonary aspiration. Subhypnotic concentrations of propofol, isoflurane and sevoflurane cause decreased pharyngeal contraction force that is most marked in patients receiving propofol (Sundman et al., 2001).

Miscellaneous Effects

Propofol does not trigger malignant hyperthermia and has been administered to patients with hereditary coproporphyria without incident (Kasraie and Cousins, 1993; Raff and Harrison, 1989; Sebel and Lowdon, 1989). Secretion of cortisol is not influenced by propofol, even when administered for prolonged periods in the ICU. Temporary abolition of tremors in patients with Parkinson's disease may occur after the administration of propofol (Krauss et al., 1996). For this reason, propofol may not be ideally suited for patients undergoing stereotactic neurosurgery, such as pallidotomy.

ETOMIDATE

Etomidate is a carboxylated imidazole–containing compound that is chemically unrelated to any other drug used for the IV induction of anesthesia (Fig. 6-9) (Tomlin et al., 2003). The imidazole nucleus renders etomidate, like midazolam, water soluble at an acidic pH and lipid soluble at physiologic pH.

Commercial Preparation

The original formulation of etomidate included 35% propylene glycol (pH 6.9) contributing to a high incidence of pain during IV injection and occasional venous irritation. This has been changed to a fat emulsion which has virtually abolished pain on injection and venous irritation, whereas the incidence of myoclonus remains unchanged. An oral formulation of etomidate for transmucosal delivery has been shown to produce dose-dependent sedation (Streisand et al., 1998). Administration through the oral mucosa results in direct systemic absorption while bypassing hepatic metabolism. The result is achievement of higher blood concentrations more rapidly compared with drug that is administered by mouth for delivery to the gastrointestinal tract.

Mechanism of Action

Etomidate is unique among injected and inhaled anesthetics in being administered as a single isomer. (Fig. 6-9) (Tomlin et al., 2003). The anesthetic effect of etomidate resides predominantly in the R(+) isomer, which is approximately five times as potent as the S(−) isomer. In contrast to barbiturates, etomidate appears to be relatively selective as a modulator of $GABA_A$ receptors. Stereoselectivity of etomidate supports the concept that $GABA_A$ receptors are the site of action of etomidate. Etomidate is believed to exert its effects on $GABA_A$ receptors by binding directly to a specific site or sites on the protein and enhancing the affinity of the inhibitory neurotransmitter (GABA) for these receptors (Tomlin et al., 1998). Antagonism of steroid-induced psychosis by etomidate is consistent with enhancement of GABA receptor function by this anesthetic drug (Iibeigi et al., 1998). Etomidate does not modulate other ligand-gated ion channels at clinically relevant concentrations.

Pharmacokinetics

The volume of distribution (Vd) of etomidate is large, suggesting considerable tissue uptake (see Table 6-1).

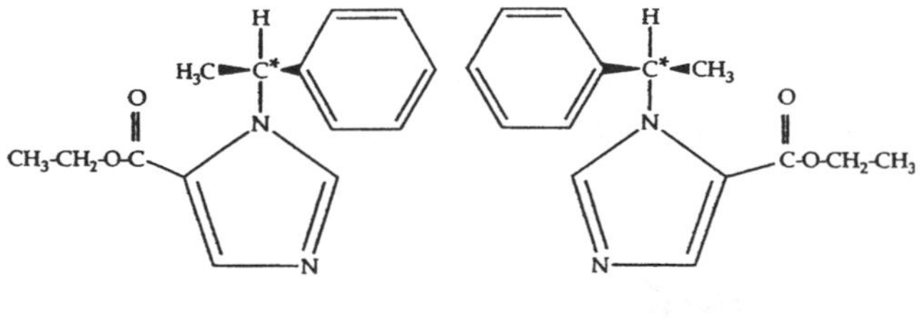

S(-) R(+)

Figure 6-9. Structural isomers of etomidate. The asymmetric carbon atom is marked by an asterisk. R(+)-etomidate is the clinically useful isomer. (From Tomlin SL, Jenkins A, Lieb WR, et al. Stereoselective effects of etomidate optical isomers on gamma-aminobutyric acid type A receptors and animals. *Anesthesiology* 1998;88:708–717; with permission.)

Distribution of etomidate throughout body water is favored by its moderate lipid solubility and existence as a weak base (pK 4.2, pH 8.2, 99% unionized at physiologic pH). Etomidate penetrates the brain rapidly, reaching peak levels within 1 minute after IV injection. About 76% of etomidate is bound to albumin independently of the plasma concentration of the drug. Decreases in plasma albumin concentrations, however, result in dramatic increases in the unbound pharmacologically active fraction of etomidate in the plasma. Prompt awakening after a single dose of etomidate principally reflects the redistribution of the drug from brain to inactive tissue sites. Rapid metabolism is also likely to contribute to prompt recovery.

Metabolism

Etomidate is rapidly metabolized by hydrolysis of the ethyl ester side chain to its carboxylic acid ester, resulting in a water-soluble, pharmacologically inactive compound. Hepatic microsomal enzymes and plasma esterases are responsible for this hydrolysis. Hydrolysis is nearly complete, as evidenced by recovery of <3% of an administered dose of etomidate as unchanged drug in urine. About 85% of a single IV dose of etomidate can be accounted for as the carboxylic acid ester metabolite in urine, whereas another 10% to 13% is present as this metabolite in the bile. Overall, the clearance of etomidate is about five times that for thiopental; this is reflected as a shorter elimination half-time of 2 to 5 hours. Likewise, the context-sensitive half-time of etomidate is less likely to be increased by continuous infusion as compared with thiopental.

Cardiopulmonary Bypass

Institution of hypothermic cardiopulmonary bypass causes an initial decrease of about 34% in the plasma etomidate concentration that then returns to within 11% of the prebypass value only to be followed by a further decrease with rewarming (Gedney and Ghosh, 1995). The return of the plasma concentration toward prebypass levels is attributed to decreased metabolism, and the subsequent decrease on rewarming is attributed to increased metabolism. In addition, hepatic blood flow changes during cardiopulmonary bypass may be important, as etomidate is a high hepatic-extraction drug.

Clinical Uses

Etomidate may be viewed as an alternative to propofol or barbiturates for the IV induction of anesthesia, especially in the presence of an unstable cardiovascular system. After a standard induction dose of 0.2 to 0.4 mg/kg IV, the onset of unconsciousness occurs within one arm-to-brain circulation time. Involuntary myoclonic movements are common during the induction period as a result of alteration in the balance of inhibitory and excitatory influences on the thalamocortical tract. The frequency of this myoclonic-like activity can be attenuated by prior administration of an opioid. Awakening after a single IV dose of etomidate is more rapid than after barbiturates, and there is little or no evidence of a hangover or cumulative drug effect. Recovery of psychomotor function after administration of etomidate is intermediate between that of methohexital and thiopental. The duration of action is prolonged by increasing the dose of etomidate or administering the drug as a continuous infusion. As with barbiturates, analgesia is not produced by etomidate. For this reason, administration of an opioid before induction of anesthesia with etomidate may be useful to blunt the hemodynamic responses evoked by direct laryngoscopy and tracheal intubation. Etomidate, 0.15 to 0.3 mg/kg IV, has minimal effects on the duration of electrically induced seizures and thus may serve as an alternative to drugs that decrease the duration of seizures (propofol, thiopental) in patients undergoing electroconvulsive therapy (Avramov et al., 1995).

The principal limiting factor in the clinical use of etomidate for induction of anesthesia is the ability of this drug to transiently depress adrenocortical function (see the section on Adrenocortical Suppression). It is widely viewed that postoperative nausea and vomiting is increased in patients receiving etomidate for induction of anesthesia (Holdcroft et al., 1976). Nevertheless, comparison of etomidate with propofol did not document an increased incidence of nausea and vomiting in the first 24 hours after surgery in patients receiving etomidate (St. Pierre et al., 2000).

Side Effects

Central Nervous System

Etomidate is a potent direct cerebral vasoconstrictor that decreases cerebral blood flow and $CMRO_2$ 35% to 45% (Milde et al., 1985). As a result, previously increased ICP is lowered by etomidate. These effects of etomidate are similar to those changes produced by comparable doses of thiopental. Suppression of adrenocortical function limits the clinical usefulness for long-term treatment of intracranial hypertension (see the section on Adrenocortical Suppression).

Etomidate produces a pattern on the EEG that is similar to thiopental. However, the frequency of excitatory spikes on the EEG is greater with etomidate than with thiopental and methohexital, suggesting caution in administration of etomidate to patients with a history of seizures (Reddy et al., 1993). Like methohexital, etomidate may activate seizure foci, manifesting as fast activity on the EEG (Ebrahim et al., 1986). For this reason, etomidate should be used with caution in patients with focal epilepsy. Conversely, this characteristic has been observed to facilitate localization of seizure foci in patients undergoing cortical resection of epileptogenic tissue. Etomidate also possesses anticonvulsant properties and has been used to terminate status epilepticus. Etomidate has been observed to augment the amplitude of somatosensory evoked potentials, making monitoring of these responses more reliable (Sloan et al., 1988).

Cardiovascular System

Cardiovascular stability is characteristic of induction of anesthesia with 0.3 mg/kg IV of etomidate. After this dose of etomidate, there are minimal changes in heart rate, stroke volume, or cardiac output, whereas mean arterial blood pressure may decrease up to 15% because of decreases in systemic vascular resistance. The decrease in systemic blood pressure in parallel with changes in systemic vascular resistance suggests that administration of etomidate to acutely hypovolemic patients could result in sudden hypotension. When an induction dose of etomidate is 0.45 mg/kg IV, significant decreases in systemic blood pressure and cardiac output may occur (Craido et al., 1980). The cardiovascular effects of etomidate and thiopental are similar when continuously infused in patients with severe valvular heart disease (Karliczek et al., 1982).

Effects of etomidate on myocardial contractility are important to consider, as this drug has been proposed for induction of anesthesia in patients with little or no cardiac reserve. It is difficult to document anesthetic-induced negative inotropic effects in vivo because of concurrent changes in preload, afterload, sympathetic nervous system activity, and baroreceptor reflex activity. Therefore, direct effects of anesthetics on intrinsic myocardial contractility may be more accurately assessed in vitro. In this regard, etomidate causes dose-dependent decreases in developed tension in isolated cardiac muscle obtained from patients undergoing coronary artery bypass graft operations or cardiac transplantation (Fig. 6-10) (Sprung et al., 2000). This depression was reversible with beta-adrenergic stimulation. Nevertheless, concentrations required to produce these negative inotropic effects are in excess of those achieved with clinical use. In this regard, etomidate may differ from most other IV anesthetics in that depressive effects on myocardial contractility are minimal at concentrations needed for the production of anesthesia. In contrast to other IV anesthetics, etomidate does not greatly decrease renal blood flow. Hepatic and renal functions tests are not altered by etomidate. Intraocular pressure is decreased by etomidate to a similar degree as by thiopental. Etomidate does not result in detrimental effects when accidentally injected into an artery.

Ventilation

The depressant effects of etomidate on ventilation seem to be less than those of barbiturates, although apnea may occasionally accompany a rapid IV injection of the drug (Choy et al., 1985). In the majority of patients, etomidate-induced decreases in tidal volume are offset by compensatory increases in the frequency of breathing. These effects on ventilation are transient, lasting only 3 to 5 minutes. Etomidate may stimulate ventilation independently of the

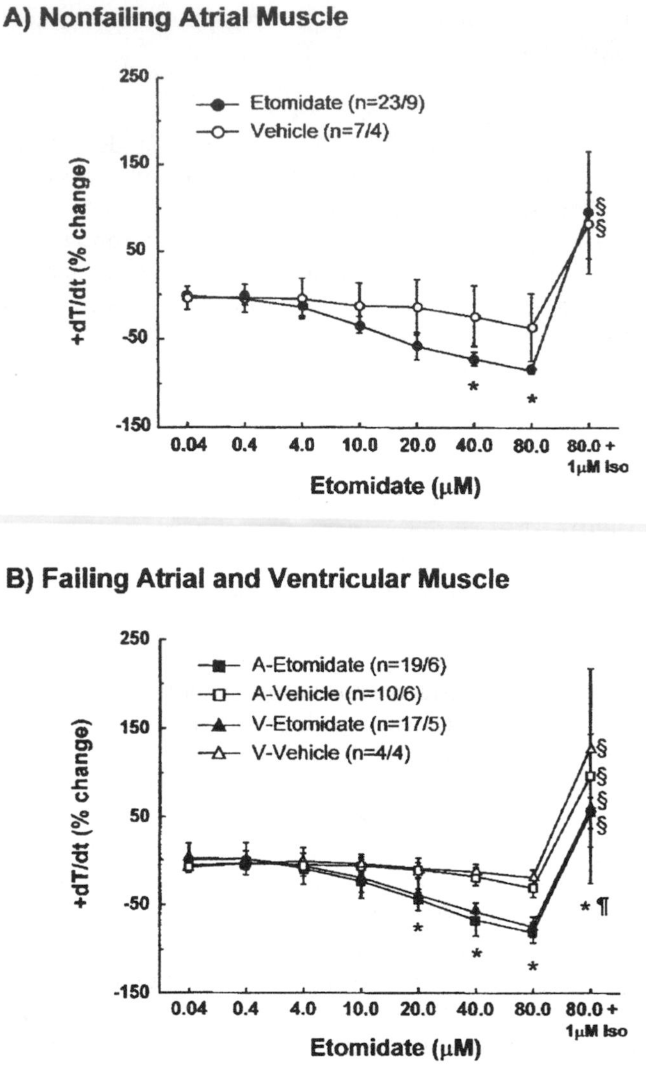

Figure 6-10. Effects of etomidate on maximal rate of contraction (+dT/dt) in nonfailing atrial muscle (A) and in failing atrial and ventricular muscle (B) Mean ≠ SD *P <0.05 vs vehicle. (From Sprung J, Ogletree-Hughes ML, Moravec CS. The effects of etomidate on the contractility of failing and nonfailing human heart muscle. *Anesth Analg* 2000;91:68–75; with permission.)

medullar centers that normally respond to carbon dioxide. For this reason, etomidate may be useful when maintenance of spontaneous ventilation is desirable. Depression of ventilation may be exaggerated when etomidate is combined with inhaled anesthetics or opioids during continuous infusion techniques.

Pain on Injection

Pain on injection and venous irritation has been virtually eliminated with use of etomidate utilizing a lipid emulsion vehicle rather than propylene glycol.

Myoclonus

Commonly administered IV anesthetics can cause excitatory effects that may manifest as spontaneous movements, such as myoclonus, dystonia, and tremor. These spontaneous movements, particularly myoclonus, occur in 50% to 80% of patients receiving etomidate in the absence of premedication (Reddy et al., 1993). In one report, 87% of patients receiving etomidate developed excitatory effects, of which 69% were myoclonic. Multiple spikes appeared on the EEG of 22% of these patients (Reddy et al., 1993). In this same report, the frequency of excitatory effects was 17% after thiopental, 13% after methohexital, and 6% after propofol, and none of these patients developed myoclonus with spike activity on the EEG (Reddy et al., 1993). Inclusion of atropine in the preoperative medication may suppress spike activity on the EEG associated with the administration of etomidate. Prior administration of an opioid (fentanyl, 1 to 2 μg/kg IV) or a benzodiazepine may decrease the incidence of myoclonus associated with administration of etomidate. Furthermore, the incidence and intensity of myoclonus following the administration of etomidate is dose-related and suppressed by pretreatment with small doses of etomidate (0.03 to 0.075 mg/kg IV) before administration of the induction dose (Doenicke et al., 1999).

The mechanism of etomidate-induced myoclonus appears to be disinhibition of subcortical structures that normally suppress extrapyramidal motor activity. In many patients, excitatory movements are coincident with the early slow phase of the EEG, which corresponds to the beginning of deep anesthesia (Reddy et al., 1993). It is possible that myoclonus could occur on awakening if the extrapyramidal system emerged more quickly than the cortex that inhibits it (Laughlin and Newberg, 1985). The fact that etomidate-induced myoclonic activity may be associated with seizure activity on the EEG suggests caution in the use of this drug for the induction of anesthesia in patients with a history of seizure activity (Reddy et al., 1993). Conversely, others have not documented seizure-like activity on the EEG in association with etomidate-induced myoclonus (Doenicke et al., 1999).

Adrenocortical Suppression

Etomidate causes adrenocortical suppression by producing a dose-dependent inhibition of the conversion of cholesterol to cortisol (Fig. 6-11) (Fragen et al., 1984; Wagner et al., 1984). The specific enzyme inhibited by etomidate appears to be 11-beta-hydroxylase as evidenced by the accumulation of 11-deoxycorticosterone (Owen and Spence, 1984). This enzyme inhibition lasts 4 to 8 hours after an induction dose of etomidate. Conceivably, patients experiencing sepsis or hemorrhage and who might require an intact cortisol response would be at a disadvantage should etomidate be administered (Longnecker, 1984). Conversely, suppression of adrenocortical function could be considered desirable from the standpoint of "stress-free" anesthesia. Nevertheless, in at least one report, it was not possible to demonstrate a difference in the plasma concentrations of cortisol, corticos-

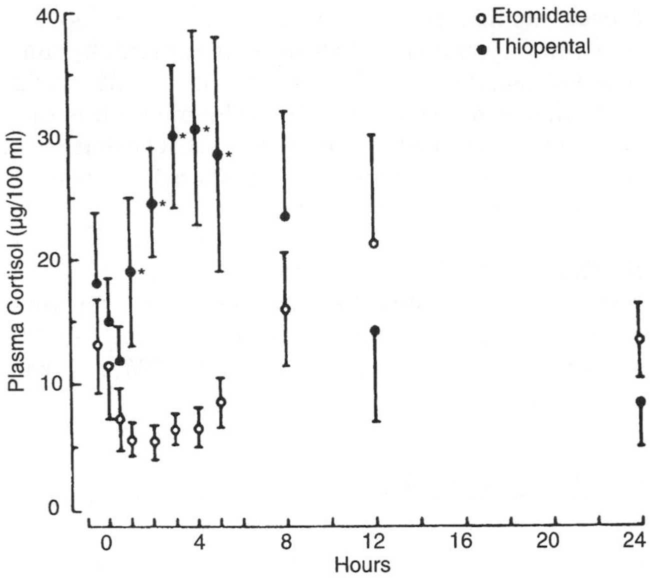

Figure 6-11. Etomidate, but not thiopental, is associated with decreases in the plasma concentrations of cortisol. (*$P < .05$ compared with thiopental; mean ± SD.) (From Fragen RJ, Shanks CA, Molteni A, et al. Effects of etomidate on hormonal responses to surgical stress. *Anesthesiology* 1984; 61:652–656; with permission.)

terone, or adrenocorticotrophic hormone in patients receiving a single dose of etomidate or thiopental (Duthie et al., 1985).

Allergic Reactions

The incidence of allergic reactions following administration of etomidate is very low (Watkins, 1983). When reactions have occurred, it is difficult to separate the role of etomidate from other concomitantly administered drugs (neuromuscular blocking drugs) that are more likely to evoke histamine release than etomidate.

KETAMINE

Ketamine is a phencyclidine derivative that produces "dissociative anesthesia," which is characterized by evidence on the EEG of dissociation between the thalamocortical and limbic systems (Kohrs and Durieux, 1998; Reich and Silvay, 1989). Dissociative anesthesia resembles a cataleptic state in which the eyes remain open with a slow nystagmic gaze. The patient is noncommunicative, although wakefulness may appear to be present. Varying degrees of hypertonus and purposeful skeletal muscle movements often occur independently of surgical stimulation. The patient is amnesic, and analgesia is intense. Ketamine has advantages over propofol and etomidate in being water soluble (does not require a lipid emulsion vehicle) and in producing profound analgesia at subanesthetic doses. However, the possibility of emergence delirium limits the clinical usefulness of ketamine. Ketamine is considered a drug with abuse potential, emphasizing the need to take appropriate precautions against unauthorized nonmedical use.

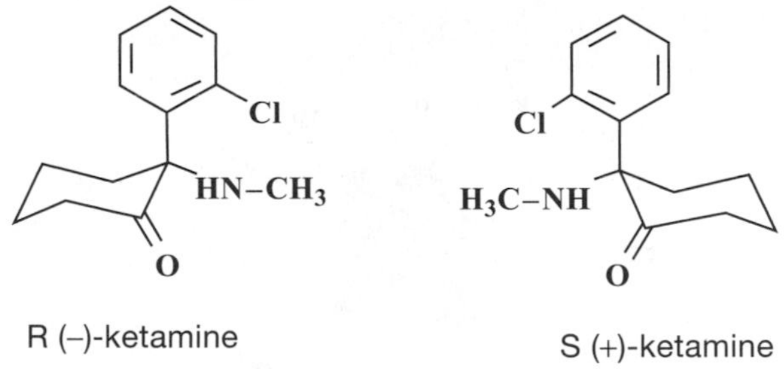

Figure 6-12. Structural formula of the two isomers of ketamine. (From Kohrs R, Durieux ME. Ketamine: Teaching an old drug new tricks. *Anesth Analg* 1998;87;1186–1193; with permission.)

Structure Activity Relationships

Ketamine is a water-soluble molecule that structurally resembles phencyclidine. The presence of an asymmetric carbon atom results in the existence of two optical isomers of ketamine (Fig. 6-12) (Kohrs and Durieux, 1998). The left-handed optical ismomer of ketamine is designated S(+)-ketamine and the right-handed optical isomer is designated *R(−)-ketamine.* The racemic form of ketamine has been the most frequently used preparation although S(+)-ketamine is clinically available. When studied separately, S(+)-ketamine produces (a) more intense analgesia, (b) more rapid metabolism and thus recovery, and (c) less salivation, and (d) a lower incidence of emergence reactions than R(−)-ketamine (Kienbaum et al., 2001; White et al., 1980). For example, the analgesic potency of S(+)-ketamine is approximately twice that of racemic ketamine and four times greater than R(−)-ketamine. Ketamine isomers induce less fatigue and cognitive impairment than equianalgesic small-dose racemic ketamine (Pfenninger et al., 2002). Both isomers of ketamine appear to inhibit uptake of catecholamines back into postganglionic sympathetic nerve endings (cocaine-like effect). The fact that individual optical isomers of ketamine differ in their pharmacologic properties suggests that this drug interacts with specific receptors. The preservative utilized for ketamine is benzethonium chloride.

Mechanism of Action

Ketamine binds noncompetitively to the phencyclidine recognition site on *N*-methyl-D-aspartate (NMDA) receptors. In addition, ketamine may exert effects at other sites including opioid receptors, monoaminergic receptors, muscarinic receptors, and voltage-sensitive sodium and L-type calcium channels (Hirota and Lambert, 1996; Wagner et al., 2001). Unlike propofol and etomidate, ketamine has only weak actions at $GABA_A$ receptors. Inflammatory mediators produced locally by compression of

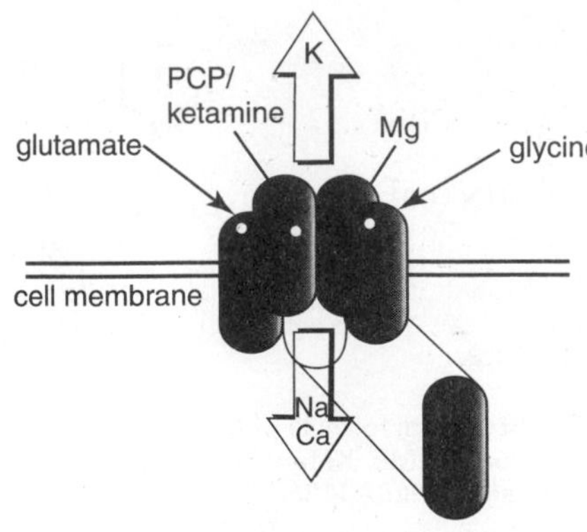

Figure 6-13. Schematic diagram of the *N*-methyl-D-aspartate (NMDA) glutamate receptor-channel complex. The receptor consists of five subunits surrounding a central ion channel that is permeable to calcium, potassium, and sodium. Binding sites for the agonist glutamate and the obligatory coagonist glycine are indicated. NMDA receptors are ligand-gated ion channels that are activated by the excitatory neurotransmitter, glutamate. Glutamate is the most abundant neurotransmitter in the central nervous system. One of the subunits has been removed to show the interior of the ion channel and binding sites for magnesium and ketamine, which produce noncompetitive NMDA receptor blockade. (From Kohrs R, Durieux ME. Ketamine: Teaching an old drug new tricks. *Anesth Analg* 1998;87;1186–1193; with permission.)

nerve roots can activate neutrophils that then adhere to blood vessels and impair blood flow. Ketamine suppresses neutrophil production of inflammatory mediators and improves blood flow (Weigand et al., 2000). Direct inhibition of cytokines in blood by ketamine may contribute to the analgesic effects of this drug.

N-Methyl-D-Aspartate Receptor Antagonism

NMDA receptors (members of the glutamate receptors family) are ligand-gated ion channels that are unique in that channel activation requires binding of the excitatory neurotransmitter, glutamate with glycine as an obligatory coagonist (Fig. 6-13) (Kohrs and Durieux, 1998). Ketamine inhibits activation of NMDA receptors by glutamate, decreases presynaptic release of glutamate, and potentiates the effects of the inhibitory neurotransmitter, gamma aminobutyric acid. This interaction with phencyclidine binding sites appears to be stereoselective, with the S(+) isomer of ketamine having the greatest affinity.

Opioid Receptors

Ketamine has been reported to interact with mu, delta, and kappa opioid receptors (Hurstveit et al., 1995). In contrast, other studies have suggested ketamine may be an antagonist at mu receptors and an agonist at kappa receptors. Ketamine also interacts with sigma receptors, although this receptor is no longer classified as an opioid receptor and the interaction with ketamine is weak.

Monoaminergic Receptors

The antinociceptive action of ketamine may involve descending inhibitory monoaminergic pain pathways.

Muscarinic Receptors

Ketamine anesthesia is partially antagonized by anticholinesterase drugs. The fact that ketamine produces anticholinergic symptoms (emergence delirium, bronchodilation, sympathomimetic action) suggests that an antagonist effect of ketamine at muscarinic receptors is more likely than an agonist effect.

Sodium Channels

Consistent with its mild local anesthetic-like properties, ketamine interacts with voltage-gated sodium channels, sharing a binding site with local anesthetics (Wagner et al., 2001).

Pharmacokinetics

The pharmacokinetics of ketamine resemble that of thiopental in rapid onset of action, relatively short duration of action, and high lipid solubility (see Table 6-1). Ketamine has a pK of 7.5 at physiologic pH. Peak plasma concentrations of ketamine occur within 1 minute after IV administration and within 5 minutes after intramuscular (IM) injection. Ketamine is not significantly bound to plasma proteins and leaves the blood rapidly to be distributed into tissues. Initially, ketamine is distributed to highly perfused tissues such as the brain, where the peak concentration may be 4 to 5 times that present in plasma. The extreme lipid solubility of ketamine (five to ten times that of thiopental) ensures its rapid transfer across the blood-brain barrier. Furthermore, ketamine-induced increases in cerebral blood flow could facilitate delivery of drug and thus enhance rapid achievement of high brain concentrations. Subsequently, ketamine is redistributed from the brain and other highly perfused tissues to less well-perfused tissues. Ketamine has a high hepatic clearance rate (1 liter/minute) and a large Vd (3 liters/kg), resulting in an elimination half-time of 2 to 3 hours. The high hepatic extraction ratio suggests that alterations in hepatic blood flow could influence ketamine's clearance rate.

Metabolism

Ketamine is metabolized extensively by hepatic microsomal enzymes. An important pathway of metabolism is demethylation of ketamine by cytochrome P-450 enzymes to form norketamine (Fig. 6-14) (White et al., 1982). In animals, norketamine is one-fifth to one-third as potent as ketamine. This active metabolite may contribute to prolonged effects of ketamine (analgesia), especially with repeated doses or a continuous IV infusion. Norketamine is eventually hydroxylated and then conjugated to form more water-soluble and inactive glucuronide metabolites that are excreted by the kidneys. After IV administration, $<4\%$ of a dose of ketamine can be recovered from urine as unchanged drug. Fecal excretion accounts for $<5\%$ of an injected dose of ketamine. Chronic administration of ketamine stimulates the activity of enzymes responsible for its

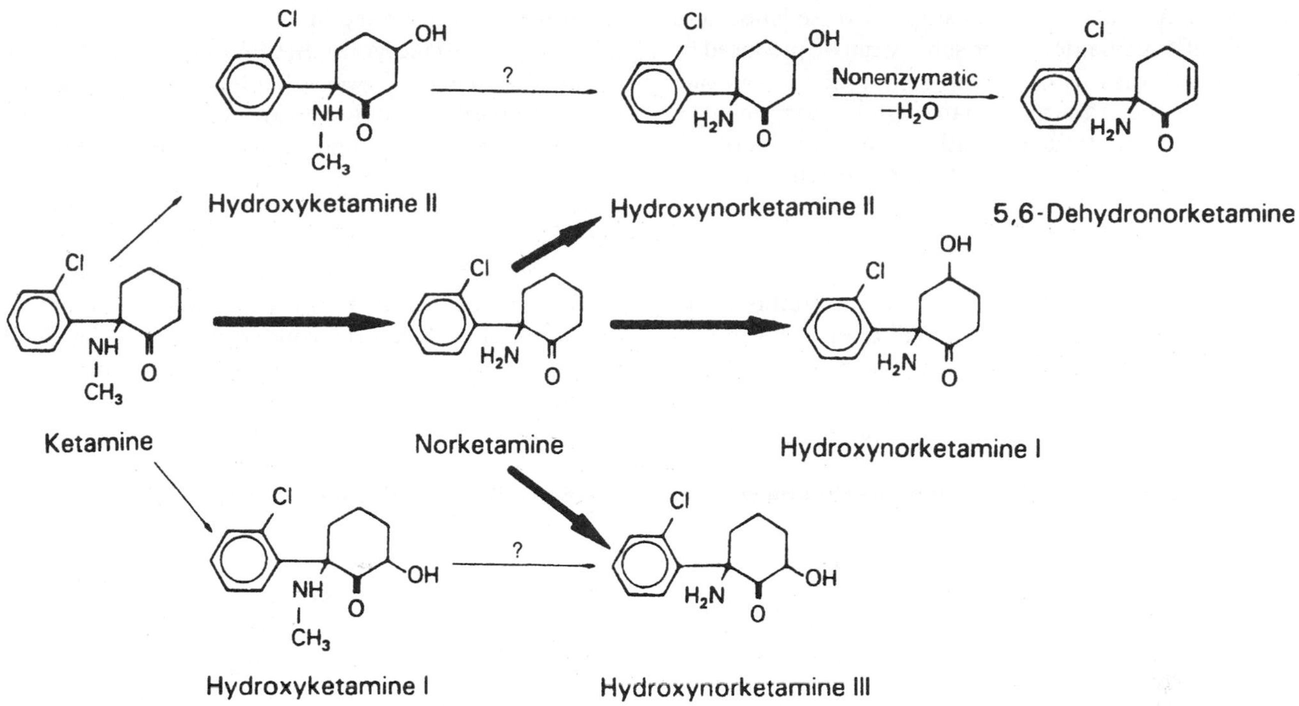

Figure 6-14. Metabolism of ketamine. (From White PF, Way WL, Trevor AJ. Ketamine: its pharmacology and therapeutic uses. *Anesthesiology* 1982;56:119–136; with permission.)

metabolism. Accelerated metabolism of ketamine as a result of enzyme induction could explain, in part, the observation of tolerance to the analgesic effects of ketamine that occurs in patients receiving repeated doses of this drug. Indeed, tolerance may occur in burn patients receiving more than two short-interval exposures to ketamine (Demling et al., 1978). Development of tolerance is also consistent with reports of ketamine dependence (White et al., 1982).

Clinical Uses

Ketamine is a unique drug evoking intense analgesia at subanesthetic doses and producing prompt induction of anesthesia when administered IV at higher doses. Inclusion of an antisialagogue in the preoperative medication is often recommended to decrease the likelihood of coughing and laryngospasm due to ketamine-induced salivary secretions. Glycopyrrolate may be preferable, as atropine or scopolamine can easily cross the blood-brain barrier and could theoretically increase the incidence of emergence delirium (see the section on Emergence Delirium).

Analgesia

Intense analgesia can be achieved with subanesthetic doses of ketamine, 0.2 to 0.5 mg/kg IV (Himmelseher and Durieux, 2005). Plasma concentrations of ketamine that produce analgesia are lower after oral than IM administration, presumably reflecting a higher norketamine concentration due to hepatic first-pass metabolism that occurs after oral administration. Analgesia is thought to be greater for somatic than for visceral pain. The analgesic effects of ketamine are primarily due to its activity in the thalamic and limbic systems, which are responsible for the interpretation of painful signals. Small doses of ketamine are also useful adjuvants to opioid analgesia (Subramaniam et al., 2004).

Spinal cord sensitization is reponsible for pain associated with touching or moving an injured body part. Central to the development of spinal cord sensitization is activation of NMDA receptors which are located in the spinal cord dorsal horn. NMDA receptors are excitatory amino acid receptors that are important in pain processing and the modulation of pain (Liu et al., 2001). Excitatory amino acids, particularly glutamate, acting at NMDA receptors play an important role in spinal nociceptive pathways. Inhibition of spinal NMDA receptors by drugs such as ketamine, magnesium, and dextromethorphan is useful in the management of postoperative pain including decreases in analgesic consumption. S(+)-ketamine has a fourfold higher affinity for NMDA receptors than its R(−) isomer and the analgesic potency of S(+)-ketamine is about twice that of racemic ketamine. Analgesia can be produced during labor without associated depression of the neonate (Akamatsu et al., 1974; Janeczko et al., 1974). Neonatal neurobehavioral scores of infants born by vaginal delivery with ketamine analgesia are lower than those for infants born with epidural anesthesia, but higher than the scores in infants delivered with thiopental–nitrous oxide anesthesia

(Hodgkinson et al., 1977). Postoperative sedation and analgesia after pediatric cardiac surgery can be produced by continuous infusions of ketamine, 1 to 2 mg/kg/hour. Evidence for the efficacy of ketamine for management of chronic pain is moderate to weak and ketamine is not recommended as a first-option intervention (Hocking and Cousins, 2003).

Neuraxial Analgesia

The efficacy of extradural ketamine is controversial. Although ketamine has been reported to interact with opioid receptors, the affinity for spinal opioid receptors may be 10,000-fold weaker than that of morphine (Salt et al., 1988). It seems likely that extradural effects of ketamine (30 mg) are due to both spinal and systemic effects and possibly interaction with local anesthetic binding sites on voltage-gated sodium ion channels. Overall, the epidural effects of ketamine are relatively small but in combination with other epidural analgesics (opioids, local anesthetics) an additive or synergistic effect may occur (Sandler et al., 1998). Intrathecal administration of ketamine (5 to 50 mg in 3 mL of saline) produces variable and brief analgesia, unless the ketamine is also combined with epinephrine to slow systemic absorption. The neuraxial use of ketamine to produce analgesia is of limited value (Hirota and Lambert, 1996).

Induction of Anesthesia

Induction of anesthesia is produced by administration of ketamine, 1 to 2 mg/kg IV or 4 to 8 mg/kg IM. Injection of ketamine IV does not produce pain or venous irritation. The need for large IV doses reflects a significant first-pass hepatic effect for ketamine. Consciousness is lost in 30 to 60 seconds after IV administration and in 2 to 4 minutes after IM injection. Unconsciousness is associated with maintenance of normal or only slightly depressed pharyngeal and laryngeal reflexes. Return of consciousness usually occurs in 10 to 20 minutes after an injected induction dose of ketamine, but return to full orientation may require an additional 60 to 90 minutes. Emergence times are even longer after repeated IV injections or a continuous infusion of ketamine. Amnesia persists for about 60 to 90 minutes after recovery of consciousness, but ketamine does not produce retrograde amnesia.

Because of its rapid onset of action, ketamine has been used as an IM induction drug in children and difficult-to-manage mentally retarded patients regardless of age. Ketamine has been used extensively for burn dressing changes, débridements, and skin-grafting procedures. The excellent analgesia and ability to maintain spontaneous ventilation in an airway that might otherwise be altered by burn-scar contractures are important advantages of ketamine in these patients. Tolerance may develop, however, in burn patients receiving repeated, short-interval anesthesia with ketamine (Demling et al., 1978).

Induction of anesthesia in acutely hypovolemic patients is often accomplished with ketamine, taking advantage of the drug's cardiovascular-stimulating effects. In this regard, it is important to recognize that ketamine, like all injected anesthetics, may be a myocardial depressant, especially if endogenous catecholamine stores are depleted and sympathetic nervous system compensatory responses are impaired (Waxman et al., 1980).

The administration of ketamine to patients with coronary artery disease is influenced by increased myocardial oxygen requirements that may accompany this drug's sympathomimetic effects on the heart. Furthermore, the loss of cardioprotective effects (preconditioning) associated with racemic ketamine is a consideration when this drug is administered to patients with known coronary artery disease (see the section on Preconditioning). Nevertheless, induction of anesthesia with administration of diazepam, 0.5 mg/kg IV, and ketamine, 0.5 mg/kg IV, followed by a continuous infusion of ketamine, 15 to 30 μg/kg/minute IV, has been proposed for anesthesia in patients with coronary artery disease (White et al., 1982). The combination of subanesthetic doses of ketamine with propofol for production of total IV anesthesia has been reported to produce more stable hemodynamics than propofol and fentanyl while avoiding the undesirable emergence reactions that may accompany administration of higher doses of ketamine (Guit et al., 1991).

The beneficial effects of ketamine on airway resistance due to drug-induced bronchodilation make this a potentially useful drug for rapid IV induction of anesthesia in patients with asthma (Hirshman et al., 1979).

Ketamine should be used cautiously or avoided in patients with systemic or pulmonary hypertension or increased ICP, although this recommendation may deserve reevaluation based on more recent data (see the sections on Central Nervous System and Cardiovascular System). Nystagmus associated with administration of ketamine may be undesirable in operations or examinations of the eye performed under anesthesia.

Ketamine has been administered safely to patients with malignant hyperthermia and does not trigger the syndrome in susceptible swine (Dershwitz et al., 1989). This drug has also been administered without incident to a patient with acute intermittent porphyria, but caution is recommended because ketamine can increase aminolevulinic acid synthetase activity in animals (Kostrzewski and Gregor, 1978). Extensive experience with ketamine for pediatric cardiac catheterization has shown the drug to be useful, but its possible cardiac-stimulating effects must be considered in the interpretation of catheterization data.

Reversal of Opioid Tolerance

Subanesthetic doses of ketamine are effective in preventing and reversing morphine-induced tolerance (Eilers et al., 2001). Although the mechanism of opioid-induced tolerance is unknown, it is believed to involve interaction between NMDA receptors, the nitric oxide pathway, and μ-opioid receptors. Administration of subanesthetic doses of ketamine (0.3 mg/kg/hour) reduces the likelihood of opioid tolerance and improves analgesia.

Improvement of Mental Depression

NMDA receptors for glutamate are involved in the pathophysiology of mental depression and the mechanism of action of antidepressants. As a NMDA antagonist, ketamine in small doses improved the postoperative depressive state in patients with mental depression (Kudoh et al., 2002).

Restless Leg Syndrome

A single case report describes symptomatic improvement in two patients with restless leg syndrome treated with oral ketamine (Kapur and Friedman, 2002). It is possible that ketamine inhibits neuroinflammation in the spinal cord or higher centers. Within the spinal cord, restless leg syndrome may reflect NMDA receptor activation and production of inflammatory mediators that impair spinal cord blood flow.

Side Effects

Ketamine is unique among injected anesthetics in its ability to stimulate the cardiovascular system and produce emergence delirium (Reich and Silvay, 1989). Although generally considered contraindicated in patients with increased ICP, it must be recognized that many of the early studies of ketamine's effects on ICP were conducted on spontaneously breathing subjects (Reich and Silvay, 1989).

Central Nervous System

Ketamine is traditionally considered to increase cerebral blood flow and $CMRO_2$, although there is also evidence suggesting that this may not be a valid generalization (Reich and Silvay, 1989).

Intracranial Pressure

Ketamine is reported to be a potent cerebral vasodilator capable of increasing cerebral blood flow by 60% in the presence of normocapnia (Takeshita et al., 1972). As a result, patients with intracranial pathology are commonly considered vulnerable to sustained increases in ICP after administration of ketamine. Nevertheless, in mechanically ventilated animals with increased ICP, there was no further increase in ICP after administration of ketamine, 0.5 to 2.0 mg/kg IV (Pfenninger et al., 1985). Furthermore, anterior fontanelle pressure, an indirect monitor of ICP, decreases in mechanically ventilated preterm neonates after administration of ketamine, 2 mg/kg IV (Friesen et al., 1987). In patients requiring craniotomy for brain tumor or cerebral aneurysm resection, administration of ketamine, 1 mg/kg IV, did not increase middle cerebral artery blood flow velocity, and ICP decreased modestly (Fig. 6-15) (Mayberg et al., 1995). In patients with traumatic brain injury, the administration of ketamine, 1.5, 3.0, and 5.0 mg/kg IV, during mechanical ventilation of the lungs resulted in significant decreases in ICP regardless of the dose of ketamine (Albanese et al., 1997). These results in patients suggest that ketamine can be administered to anesthetized and mechanically ventilated patients with mildly increased ICP without adversely altering cerebral hemodynamics. Prior administration of thiopental, diazepam, or midazolam has been shown to blunt ketamine-induced increases in cerebral blood flow.

Neuroprotective Effects

Activation of NMDA receptors has been implicated in cerebral ischemic damage (Hirota and Lambert, 1996). The antagonist effect of ketamine on NMDA receptors suggests a possible neuroprotective role for this drug although this remains an unproved hypothesis. Indeed, S(+) ketamine offers no greater neuroprotection than remifentanil (Nagels et al., 2004).

Electroencephalogram

Ketamine's effects on the EEG are characterized by abolition of alpha rhythm and dominance of theta activity. Onset of delta activity coincides with loss of consciousness. At high doses, ketamine produces a burst suppression pattern. Ketamine-induced excitatory activity occurs in both the thalamus and limbic systems without evidence of subsequent spread of seizure activity to cortical areas (Ferrer-Allado et al., 1973). As such, ketamine would be unlikely to precipitate generalized convulsions in patients with seizure disorders. Indeed, ketamine does not alter the seizure threshold in epileptic patients (Celesia et al., 1975). Although myoclonic- and seizure-like activity may occur in normal patients, EEG evidence of cortical epileptic

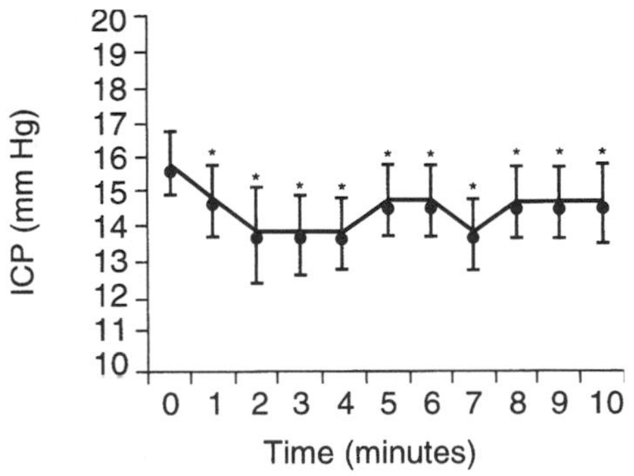

Figure 6-15. In patients with a brain tumor or cerebral aneurysm, the administration of ketamine, 1 mg/kg IV, during mechanical ventilation of the lungs with nitrous oxide and isoflurane was associated with a modest decrease in intracranial pressure (ICP). This decrease in ICP was accompanied by a corresponding decrease in cerebral artery blood flow velocity. (From Mayberg TS, Lam AM, Matta BF, et al. Ketamine does not increase cerebral blood flow velocity or intracranial pressure during isoflurane/nitrous oxide anesthesia in patients undergoing craniotomy. *Anesth Analg* 1995;81:84–89; with permission.)

activity is absent and ketamine is considered to possess anticonvulsant activity (Modica et al., 1990).

Somatosensory Evoked Potentials

Ketamine increases the cortical amplitude of somatosensory evoked potentials (Schubert et al., 1990). This ketamine-induced increase in amplitude is attenuated by nitrous oxide. Auditory and visual evoked responses are decreased by ketamine.

Cardiovascular System

Ketamine produces cardiovascular effects that resemble sympathetic nervous system stimulation. Indeed, a direct negative cardiac inotropic effect is usually overshadowed by central sympathetic stimulation.

Hemodynamic Effects

Systemic and pulmonary arterial blood pressure, heart rate, cardiac output, cardiac work, and myocardial oxygen requirements are increased after IV administration of ketamine (Table 6-2) (Tweed et al., 1972). The increase in systolic blood pressure in adults receiving clinical doses of ketamine is 20 to 40 mm Hg, with a slightly smaller increase in diastolic blood pressure. Typically, systemic blood pressure increases progressively during the first 3 to 5 minutes after IV injection of ketamine and then decreases to predrug levels over the next 10 to 20 minutes. The cardiovascular-stimulating effects on the systemic and pulmonary circulations are blunted or prevented by prior administration of benzodiazepines or concomitant administration of inhaled anesthetics, including nitrous oxide (Balfors et al., 1983; Reich and Silvay, 1989). Likewise, ketamine administered to mildly sedated infants fails to produce hemodynamic changes in either the systemic or pulmonary circulation (Hickey et al., 1985).

Critically ill patients occasionally respond to ketamine with unexpected decreases in systemic blood pressure and cardiac output, which may reflect depletion of endogenous catecholamine stores and exhaustion of sympathetic nervous system compensatory mechanisms, leading to an unmasking of ketamine's direct myocardial depressant effects (Hoffman et al., 1992; Waxman et al., 1980). Conversely, ketamine has been shown to decrease the need for inotropic support in septic patients, perhaps reflecting an inhibition of catecholamine reuptake (Lundy et al., 1986; Yli-Hankala et al., 1992).

In shocked animals, ketamine is associated with an increased survival rate compared with animals anesthetized with halothane (Longnecker and Sturgill, 1976). [Blood pressure may be better maintained in hemorrhaged animals anesthetized with ketamine. However, ketamine administration is associated with greater increases in arterial lactate concentrations than occur in animals with lower systemic blood pressures anesthetized with a volatile anesthetic (Weiskopf et al., 1981).] This suggests inadequate tissue perfusion despite maintenance of systemic blood pressure by ketamine. Presumably, ketamine-induced vasoconstriction maintains systemic blood pressure at the expense of tissue perfusion.

TABLE 6-2.
CIRCULATORY EFFECTS OF KETAMINE

	Control	Ketamine (2 mg/kg IV)	Percent Change
Heart rate (beats/min)	74	98	+33
Mean arterial pressure (mm Hg)	93	119	+28
Stroke volume index (mL/m^2)	43	44	
Systemic vascular resistance (units)	16.2	15.9	
Right atrial pressure (mm Hg)	7.0	8.9	
Left ventricular end-diastolic pressure (mm Hg)	13.0	13.1	
Pulmonary artery pressure (mm Hg)	17.0	24.5	+44
Minute work index (kg/min/m^2)	5.4	8.9	+40
Tension-time index (mm Hg/sec)	2,700	4,600	+68

Cardiac Rhythm

The effect of ketamine on cardiac rhythm is inconclusive. There is evidence that ketamine enhances the dysrhythmogenicity of epinephrine (Koehntop et al., 1977). Conversely, ketamine may abolish epinephrine-induced cardiac dysrhythmias.

Mechanisms of Cardiovascular Effects

The mechanisms for ketamine-induced cardiovascular effects are complex. Direct stimulation of the CNS leading to increased sympathetic nervous system outflow seems to be the most important mechanism for cardiovascular stimulation (Wong and Jenkins, 1974). Evidence for this mechanism is the ability of inhaled anesthetics, ganglionic blockade, cervical epidural anesthesia, and spinal cord transection to prevent ketamine-induced increases in systemic blood pressure and heart rate (Stanley, 1973; Traber et al., 1970). Furthermore, increases in plasma concentrations of epinephrine and norepinephrine occur as early as 2 minutes after IV administration of ketamine and return to control levels 15 minutes later (Baraka et al., 1973). In vitro, ketamine produces direct myocardial depression, emphasizing the importance of an intact sympathetic nervous system for the cardiac-stimulating effects of this drug (Schwartz and

Horwitz, 1975). Depression of the baroreceptor reflex via an effect of ketamine on CNS NMDA receptors could lead to activation of the sympathetic nervous system. The role of ketamine-induced inhibition of norepinephrine uptake (reuptake) into postganglionic sympathetic nerve endings and associated increases of plasma catecholamine concentrations on the drug's cardiac-stimulating effects are not known (Koehntop et al., 1977).

Ventilation and Airway

Ketamine does not produce significant depression of ventilation. The ventilatory response to carbon dioxide is maintained during ketamine anesthesia and the $Pa{CO_2}$ is unlikely to increase >3 mm Hg (Soliman et al., 1975). Breathing frequency typically decreases for 2 to 3 minutes after administration of ketamine. Apnea, however, can occur if the drug is administered rapidly IV or an opioid is included in the preoperative medication.

Upper airway skeletal muscle tone is well maintained, and upper airway reflexes remain relatively intact after administration of ketamine (Taylor and Towey, 1971). Despite continued presence of upper airway reflexes, ketamine anesthesia does not negate the need for protection of the lungs against aspiration by placement of a cuffed tube in the patient's trachea. Salivary and tracheobronchial mucous gland secretions are increased by IM or IV administration of ketamine, leading to the frequent recommendation that an antisialagogue be included in the preoperative medication when use of this drug is anticipated.

Bronchomotor Tone

Ketamine has bronchodilatory activity and is as effective as halothane or enflurane in preventing experimentally induced bronchospasm in dogs (Hirshman et al., 1979). Ketamine has been used in subanesthetic doses to treat bronchospasm in the operating room and ICU. Successful treatment of status asthmaticus with ketamine has been reported (Sarma, 1992). In the presence of active bronchospasm, ketamine may be recommended as the IV induction drug of choice. The mechanism by which ketamine produces airway relaxation is unclear, although several mechanisms have been suggested, including increased circulating catecholamine concentrations, inhibition of catecholamine uptake, voltage-sensitive calcium channel block, and inhibition of postsynaptic nicotinic or muscarinic receptors (Hirota and Lambert, 1996).

Hepatic or Renal Function

Ketamine does not significantly alter laboratory tests that reflect hepatic or renal function.

Allergic Reactions

Ketamine does not evoke the release of histamine and rarely, if ever, causes allergic reactions (Laxenaiore et al., 1985).

Platelet Aggregation

Ketamine inhibits platelet aggregation possibly by suppressed formation of inositol 1,4,5-triphosphate and subsequent inhibition of cytosolic free calcium concentrations (Nakagawa et al., 2002). Drug-induced effects on platelet aggregation are a consideration in patients with known bleeding disorders undergoing surgery.

Drug Interactions

The importance of an intact and normally functioning CNS in determining the cardiovascular effects of ketamine is emphasized by hemodynamic depression rather than stimulation that occurs when ketamine is administered in the presence of inhaled anesthetics. For example, depression by inhaled anesthetics of sympathetic nervous system outflow from the CNS prevents the typical increases in systemic blood pressure and heart rate that occur when ketamine is administered alone (Stanley, 1973). Ketamine administered in the presence of volatile anesthetics may result in hypotension (Bidwai et al., 1975). Presumably, volatile anesthetics depress sympathetic nervous system outflow from the CNS, thus unmasking the direct cardiac-depressant effects of ketamine. Diazepam, 0.3 to 0.5 mg/kg IV, or an equivalent dose of midazolam, is also effective in preventing the cardiac-stimulating effects of ketamine. In the presence of verapamil, the blood pressure-elevating effects of ketamine may be attenuated, whereas drug-induced increases in heart rate are enhanced (Fragen and Avram, 1986).

Ketamine-induced enhancement of nondepolarizing neuromuscular-blocking drugs may reflect interference by ketamine with calcium ion binding or its transport (Johnston et al., 1974). Alternatively, ketamine may decrease sensitivity of postjunctional membranes to neuromuscular-blocking drugs. The duration of apnea after administration of succinylcholine is prolonged, possibly reflecting inhibition of plasma cholinesterase activity by ketamine. Pancuronium may enhance the cardiac-stimulating effects of ketamine.

Seizures have been described in asthmatic patients receiving aminophylline followed by administration of ketamine (Hirshman et al., 1982). Furthermore, in animals, aminophylline or ketamine alone does not alter the seizure threshold, but the combination of these two drugs decreases the seizure threshold.

Emergence Delirium (Psychedelic Effects)

Emergence from ketamine anesthesia in the postoperative period may be associated with visual, auditory, proprioceptive, and confusional illusions, which may progress to delirium. Cortical blindness may be transiently present. Dreams and hallucinations can occur up to 24 hours after administration of ketamine. The dreams frequently have a morbid content and are often experienced in vivid color. Dreams and hallucinations usually disappear within a few hours.

Mechanisms

Emergence delirium probably occurs secondary to ketamine-induced depression of the inferior colliculus and medial geniculate nucleus, leading to misinterpretation of auditory and visual stimuli (White et al., 1982). Furthermore, the loss of skin and musculoskeletal sensations results in decreased ability to perceive gravity, thereby producing a sensation of bodily detachment or floating in space. Opioids that act as kappa-agonists produce similar psychedelic effects suggesting a role for ketamine interaction with kappa receptors.

Incidence

The observed incidence of emergence delirium after ketamine ranges from 5% to 30% (White et al., 1982). Factors associated with an increased incidence of emergence delirium include (a) age >15 years, (b) female gender, (c) doses of ketamine of >2 mg/kg IV, and (d) a history of personality problems or frequent dreaming (White et al., 1982). In healthy volunteers, the incidence of psychedelic effects is related to the plasma concentration of ketamine (Fig. 6-16) (Bowdel et al., 1998). It is possible that the incidence of dreaming is similar in children, but this age group is unable to communicate the dream's occurrence. Indeed, there are reports of recurrent hallucinations in children as well as in adults receiving ketamine (Fine and Finestone, 1973; Meyers and Charles, 1978). Nevertheless, psychological changes in children after anesthesia with ketamine or inhaled drugs are not different (Modvig and Nielsen, 1977). Likewise, no significant long-term personality differences are present in adults receiving ketamine compared with thiopental (Moretti et al., 1984).

Emergence delirium occurs less frequently when ketamine is used repeatedly. For example, it is rare for emergence delirium to occur after three or more anesthetics with ketamine. Finally, inhaled anesthetics can also produce auditory, visual, proprioceptive, and confusional illusions, but the incidence of such phenomena, especially unpleasant experiences, is indeed greater after anesthesia that includes administration of ketamine.

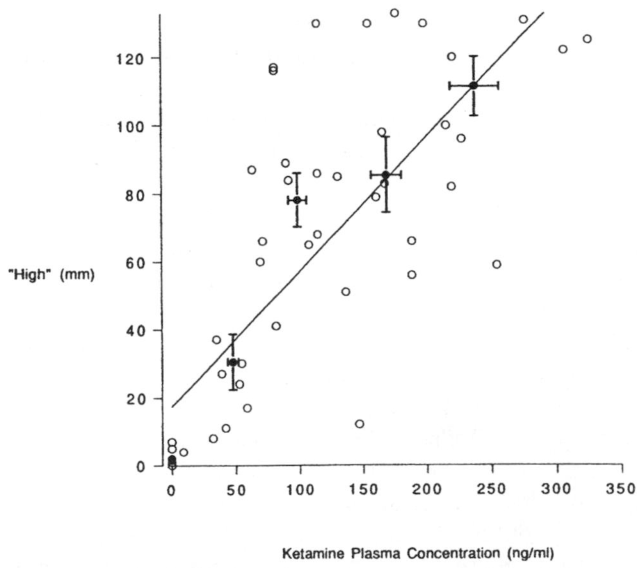

Figure 6-16. Visual analog scores for those patients experiencing ketamine-induced psychedelic effects ("High") versus venous plasma concentrations of ketamine. (From Bowdle TA, Radant AD, Cowley DS, et al. Psychedelic effects of ketamine in healthy volunteers: Relationship to steady-state plasma concentrations. *Anesthesiology* 1998;88:82–88; with permission.)

Prevention

A variety of drugs used in preoperative medication or as adjuvants during maintenance of anesthesia have been evaluated in attempts to prevent emergence delirium after administration of ketamine. Benzodiazepines have proved the most effective in prevention of this phenomenon, with midazolam being more effective than diazepam (Cartwright and Pingel, 1984; Toft and Romer, 1987). A common approach is to administer the benzodiazepine IV about 5 minutes before induction of anesthesia with ketamine. Inclusion of thiopental or inhaled anesthetics may decrease the incidence of emergence delirium attributed to ketamine. Conversely, the inclusion of atropine or droperidol in the preoperative medication may increase the incidence of emergence delirium (Erbguth et al., 1972).

Despite contrary opinions, there is no evidence that permitting patients to awaken from ketamine anesthesia in quiet areas alters the incidence of emergence delirium (Hejja and Galloon, 1975). Prospective discussion with the patient of the common side effects of ketamine (dreams, floating sensations, blurred vision) is likely to decrease the incidence of emergence delirium as much as any other approach (White et al., 1982).

Preconditioning

Pharmacologic activation of adenosine triphosphate-regulated potassium (K_{ATP}) channels mimics ischemic preconditioning and decreases infarct size or improves functional recovery of ischemic-reperfused viable (stunned) myocardium. Conversely, pharmacologic blockade of K_{ATP} channels can antagonize the cardioprotective effects of ischemic preconditioning. In an animal model, ketamine blocked the cardioprotective effects of ischemic preconditioning and this effect was due to the R(−) isomer (Molojavyi et al., 2001). Conversely, S(+)-ketamine does not block the cardioprotective effects of preconditioning or alter myocardial infarct size (Fig. 6-17) (Mullenheim et al., 2001). In patients at risk for myocardial infarction during the perioperative period, drugs known to block preconditioning should be used with caution, whereas drugs known to elicit early and late preconditioning (opioids, volatile anesthetics) may be beneficial.

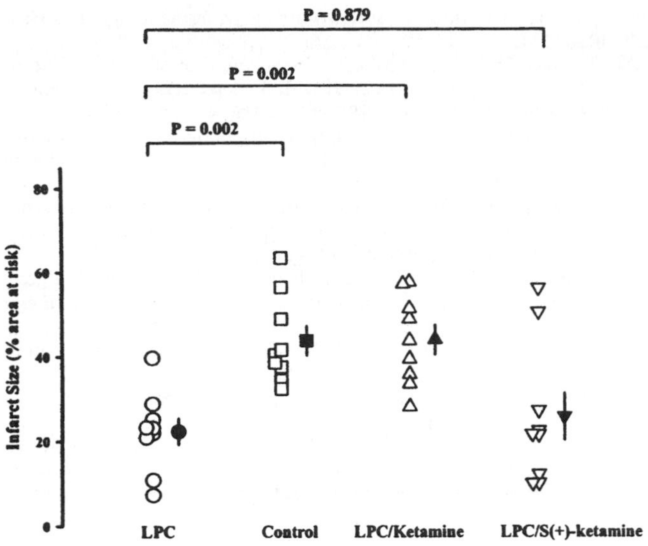

Figure 6-17. Infarct size as a percentage of the area at risk in late preconditioning (LPC), control, LPC/ketamine and LPS/S(+)-ketamine. Solid symbols represent Mean ≠ SEM. (From Mullenheim J, Rulands R, Wietschorke T, et al. Late preconditioning is blocked by racemic ketamine, but not by S(+)-ketamine. *Anesth Analg* 2001;93:265–270; with permission.)

DEXTROMETHORPHAN

Dextromethorphan (*d*-isomer of levorphanol) is a low affinity NMDA antagonist that is a common ingredient in over-the-counter cough suppressants. It is equal in potency to codeine as an antitussive but lacks analgesic or physical dependence properties. Unlike codeine, this drug rarely produces sedation or gastrointestinal disturbances. Its euphoric effects lead to a significant abuse potential. Signs and symptoms of intentional excessive intake of dextromethorphan include systemic hypertension, tachycardia, somnolence, agitation, slurred speech, ataxia, diaphroesis, skeletal muscle rigidity, seizures, coma, and decreased core body temperature. Hepatotoxicity may be a consideration when dextromethorphan with acetaminophen is ingested in excessive amounts.

REFERENCES

Akamatsu TJ, Bonica JJ, Rhemet R. Experiences with the use of ketamine for parturition. I: Primary anesthetic for vaginal delivery. *Anesth Analg* 1974;53:284–287.

Albanese J, Arnaud S, Rey M, et al. Ketamine decreases intracranial pressure and electroencephalographic activity in traumatic brain injury patients during propofol sedation. Anesthesiology 1997; 87:1328–1334.

Anand K, Ramsay MA, Crippin JS. Hepatocellular injury following the administration of propofol. *Anesthesiology* 2001;95: 1523–1524.

Avramov MN, Husain MM, White PF. The comparative effects of methohexital, propofol, and etomidate for electroconvulsive therapy. *Anesth Analg* 1995;81:596–602.

Badr AE, Mychaskiw GH, Eichhorn JH. Metabolic acidosis associated with a new formulation of propofol. *Anesthesiology* 2001;94: 536–538.

Balfors E, Haggmark S, Nyhman H, et al. Droperidol inhibits the effects of intravenous ketamine on central hemodynamics and myocardial O_2 consumption in patients with generalized atherosclerotic disease. *Anesth Analg* 1983;62:193–197.

Banaszczyk M, Carlo AT, Millan V, et al. Propofol phosphate, a water-soluble propofol prodrug: In vivo evaluation. *Anesth Analg* 2002;95:1285–1292.

Baraka A, Harrison T, Kachachi T. Catecholamine levels after ketamine anesthesia in man. *Anesth Analg* 1973;52:198–200.

Blouin RT, Seifert HA, Babenco HD, et al. Propofol decreases the hypoxic ventilatory response during conscious sedation and isohypercapnia. *Anesthesiology* 1993;79:1177–1182.

Boisseau N, Madany M, Staccini P, et al. Comparison of the effects of sevoflurane and propofol on cortical somatosensory evoked potentials. *Br J Anaesth* 2002;88:785–789.

Borgeat A, Wilder-Smith OHG, Saiah M, et al. Subhypnotic doses of propofol relieve pruritus induced by epidural and intrathecal morphine. *Anesthesiology* 1992;76:510–512.

Borgeat A, Wilder-Smith OHG, Suter PM. The nonhypnotic therapeutic applications of propofol. *Anesthesiology* 1994;80:642–656.

Borgeat A. Subhypnotic doses of propofol do not possess antidopaminergic properties. *Anesth Analg* 1997;84:196–198.

Bouillon T, Bruhn J, Radu-Radulescu L, et al. Mixed-effects modeling of the intrinsic ventilatory depressant potency of propofol in the non-steady state. *Anesthesiology* 2004;100:240–250.

Bowdle TA, Radant AD, Cowley DS, et al. Psychedelic effects of ketamine in healthy volunteers: relationship to steady-state plasma concentrations. *Anesthesiology* 1998;88:82–88.

Bray RJ. Fatal myocardial failure associated with a propofol infusion in a child. *Anaesthesia* 1995;50:94.

Brown RH, Greenberg RS, Wagner EM. Efficacy of propofol to prevent bronchoconstriction: Effects of preservative. *Anesthesiology* 2001; 94:851–855.

Bryson HM, Fulton BR, Faulds D. Propofol: an update of its use in anaesthesia and conscious sedation. *Drugs* 1995;50:513–559.

Burow BK, Johnson ME, Packer DL. Metabolic acidosis associated with propofol in the absence of other causative factors. *Anesthesiology* 2004;101:239–241

Cartwright PD, Pingel SM. Midazolam and diazepam in ketamine anaesthesia. *Anaesthesia* 1984;59:439–442.

Celesia GG, Chen RC, Bamforth BJ. Effects of ketamine in epilepsy. *Neurology* 1975;25:169–172.

Chassard D, Lansiaux S, Duflo F, et al. Effects of subhypnotic doses of propofol on gastric emptying in volunteers. *Anesthesiology* 2002; 97:96–101.

Choi SD, Spulding BC, Gross JB, et al. Comparison of the ventilatory effects of etomidate and methohexital. *Anesthesiology* 1985;62: 442–447.

Cochran D, Price W, Gwinnutt CL. Unilateral convulsion after induction of anesthesia with propofol. *Br J Anaesth* 1996;76: 570–572.

Court MH, Duan SX, Hesse LM, et al. Cytochrome P-450 2B6 is responsible for interindividual variability of propofol hydroxylation by human liver microsomes. *Anesthesiology* 2001;94: 110–119.

Craido A, Maseda J, Navarro E, et al. Induction of anaesthesia with etomidate: haemodynamic study of 36 patients. *Br J Anaesth* 1980;52:803–809.

Crowther J, Hrazdil J, Jolly DT, et al. Growth of microorganisms in propofol, thiopental, and a 1:1 mixture of propofol and thiopental. *Anesth Analg* 1996;82:475–478.

Culp KE, Augoustides JG, Ochroch AE, et al. Clinical management of cardiogenic shock associated with prolonged propofol infusion. *Anesth Analg* 2004;99:221–226.

Dailland P, Cockshott ID, Lirzin JD, et al. Intravenous propofol during cesarean section: placental transfer, concentrations in breast milk, and neonatal effects. A preliminary study. *Anesthesiology* 1989; 71:827–834.

Daniel M, Eger IE, Weiskopf RB, et al. Propofol fails to attenuate the cardiovascular response to rapid increases in desflurane concentration. *Anesthesiology* 1996;84:75–80.

Daskalopoulos R, Korcok J, Farhangkhgoee P, et al. Propofol protection of sodium-hydrogen activity sustains glutamate uptake during oxidative stress. *Anesth Analg* 2001;93:1199–1204.

Dawidowicz AL, Fornal E, Mardarowicz M et al. The role of human lungs in the biotransformation of propofol. *Anesthesiology* 2000; 93:992–997.

de Leon-Casasola, Weiss A, Lema MJ. Anaphylaxis due to propofol. *Anesthesiology* 1992;77:384–386.

Dearlove O, Dobson A. Does propofol cause death in children? *Anaesthesia* 1995;50:916.

Demling RH, Ellerbee S, Jarrett F. Ketamine anesthesia for tangential excision of burn eschar: a burn unit procedure. *J Trauma* 1978;18:269–270.

Dershwitz M, Sreter FA, Ryan JF. Ketamine does not trigger malignant hyperthermia in susceptible swine. *Anesth Analg* 1989;69:501–503.

Deutschman CS, Harris AP, Fleisher LA. Changes in heart rate variability under propofol anesthesia: a possible explanation for propofol-induced bradycardia. *Anesth Analg* 1994;79:373–377.

Doenicke AW, Roizen MF, Kugler J, et al. Reducing myoclonus after etomidate. *Anesthesiology* 1999;90:113–119.

Doenicke AW, Roizen MF, Rau J, et al. Pharmacokinetics and pharmacodynamics of propofol in a new solvent. *Anesth Analg* 1997;85: 1399–1403.

Duthie DJR, Fraser R, Nimmo WS. Effect of induction of anaesthesia with etomidate on corticosteroid synthesis in man. *Br J Anaesth* 1985;57: 156–159.

Eames WO, Rooke GA, Sai-Chuen R, et al. Comparison of the effects of etomidate, propofol, and thiopental on respiratory resistance after tracheal intubation. *Anesthesiology* 1996;84:1307–1311.

Ebrahim ZY, DeBoer GE, Luders H, et al. Effect of etomidate on the electroencephalogram of patients with epilepsy. *Anesth Analg* 1986;65:1004–1006.

Egan TD, Brock UJG. Asystole after anesthesia induction with a fentanyl, propofol, and succinylcholine sequence. *Anesth Analg* 1991; 73:818–820.

Eilers H, Philip LA, Bickler PE, et al. The reversal of fentanyl-induced tolerance by administration of "small-dose" ketamine. *Anesth Analg* 2001;93:213–214.

Erbguth PH, Reiman B, Klein RL. The influence of chlorpromazine, diazepam and droperidol on emergence from ketamine. *Anesth Analg* 1972;51:693–700.

Fechner J, Ihmsen H, Hatterscheid D, et al. Comparative pharmacokinetics and pharmacodynamics of the new propofol prodrug GPI 15715 and propofol emulsion. *Anesthesiology* 2004;101: 626–639.

Fechner J, Ihmsen H, Hatterscheid D, et al. Pharmacokinetics and clinical pharmacodynamics of the new propofol prodrug GPI 15715 in volunteers. *Anesthesiology* 2003;99:303–313.

Ferrer-Allado T, Brechner VL, Diamond A, et al. Ketamine-induced electroconvulsive phenomena in the human limbic and thalamic regions. *Anesthesiology* 1973;38:333–344.

Fine J, Finestone SC. Sensory disturbances following ketamine anesthesia: recurrent hallucinations. *Anesth Analg* 1973;52:428–430.

Follette JW, Farley WJ. Anesthesiologist addicted to propofol. *Anesthesiology* 1992;77:817–818.

Fourcade O, Simon M-F, Litt L, et al. Propofol inhibits human platelet aggregation induced by proinflammatory lipid mediators. *Anesth Analg* 2004;99:393–398.

Fragen RJ, Avram MJ. Comparative pharmacology of drugs used for the induction of anesthesia. In: Stoelting RK, Barash PG, Gallagher TJ, eds. *Advances in anesthesia*. Chicago: Year Book Medical Publishers, 1986:103–132.

Fragen RJ, Shanks CA, Molteni A, et al. Effects of etomidate on hormonal responses to surgical stress. *Anesthesiology* 1984;61: 652–656.

Freysz M, Timourt Q, Betrix L, et al. Propofol and bradycardia. *Can J Anaesth* 1991;28:137–138.

Friesen RH, Thieme RE, Honda AT, et al. Changes in anterior fontanel pressure in preterm neonates receiving isoflurane, halothane, fentanyl, or ketamine. *Anesth Analg* 1987;66:431–434.

Fulton B, Sorkin EM. Propofol: an overview of its pharmacology and a review of its clinical efficacy in intensive care sedation. *Drugs* 1995; 50:636–657.

Funston JS, Prough DS. Two reports of propofol anesthesia associated with metabolic acidosis in adults. *Anesthesiology* 2004;101:6–8.

Gan TJ, Ginsberg B, Grant BS, et al. Double-blind, randomized comparison of ondansetron and intraoperative propofol to prevent postoperative nausea and vomiting. *Anesthesiology* 1996;85: 1036–1042.

Gan TJ, Glass PSA, Howell ST, et al. Determination of plasma concentrations of propofol associated with 50% reduction in postoperative nausea. *Anesthesiology* 1997;87:779–784.

Gedney JA, Ghosh S. Pharmacokinetics of analgesics, sedatives and anaesthetic agents during cardiopulmonary bypass. *Br J Anaesth* 1995;75:344–351.

Girard F, Moumdjian R, Boudreault D, et al. The effect of propofol sedation on the intracranial pressure of patients with space-occupying lesion. *Anesth Analg* 2004;99:573–577.

Guit JBM, Koning HM, Niemeijer RPE, et al. Ketamine as an analgesic for total intravenous anaesthesia with propofol. *Anaesthesia* 1991;46: 24–31.

He Y-L, Ueyama H, Tashiro c, et al. Pulmonary disposition of propofol in surgical patients. *Anesthesiology* 2000;93:986–991.

Hejja P, Galloon S. A consideration of ketamine dreams. *Can Anaesth Soc J* 1975;22:100–105.

Herrick IA, Craen RA, Gelb AW, et al. Propofol sedation during awake craniotomy for seizures: electrocorticographic and epileptogenic effects. *Anesth Analg* 1997;84:1280–1284.

Hewitt PB, Chu DKL, Polkey CE, et al. Effect of propofol on the electrocorticogram in epileptic patients undergoing cortical resection. *Br J Anaesth* 1999;82:199–202.

Hickey PR, Hansen DD, Cramoline GM, et al. Pulmonary and systemic hemodynamic responses to ketamine in infants with normal and elevated pulmonary vascular resistance. *Anesthesiology* 1985; 62:287–293.

Himmelseher S, Durieux ME. Ketamine for perioperative pain management. *Anesthesiology* 2005;102:211–220.

Hirota K, Lambert DG. Ketamine: its mechanism(s) of action and unusual clinical uses. *Br J Anaesth* 1996;77:441–444.

Hirshman CA, Downes H, Farbood A, et al. Ketamine block of bronchospasm in experimental canine asthma. *Br J Anaesth* 1979;51:713–718.

Hirshman CA, Krieger W, Littlejohn G, et al. Ketamine-aminophylline-induced decreased in seizure threshold. *Anesthesiology* 1982;56: 464–467.

Hocking G, Cousins MJ. Ketamine in chronic pain management: an evidence-based review. *Anesth Analg* 2003;97:1730–1739.

Hodgkinson K, Marx GF, Kim SS, et al. Neonatal neurobehavioral tests following vaginal delivery under ketamine, thiopental, and extradural anesthesia. *Anesth Analg* 1977;56:548–553.

Hoffman WE, Pelligrino D, Werner C, et al. Ketamine decreases plasma catecholamines and improves outcome from incomplete cerebral ischemia in rats. *Anesthesiology* 1992;76:755–762.

Holley HS, Cuthrell L. Intraarterial injection of propofol. *Anesthesiology* 1990;73:183–184.

Horiguchi T, Nishikawa T. Heart rate response to intravenous atropine during propofol anesthesia. *Anesth Analg* 2002;95:389–392.

Hughes MA, Glass PSA, Jacobs JR. Context-sensitive half-time in multicompartment pharmacokinetic models for intravenous anesthetic drugs. *Anesthesiology* 1992;76:334–341.

Hughes NJ, Lyons JB. Prolonged myoclonus and meningismus following propofol. *Can J Anaesth* 1995;42:744–746.

Hurstveit O, Maurset A, Oye I. Interaction of the chiral forms of ketamine with opioid, phencyclidine, and muscarinic receptors. *Pharmacol Toxicol* 1995;77:355–359.

Iibeigi MS, Davidson ML, Yarmush JM. An unexpected arousal effect of etomidate in a patient on high-dose steroids. *Anesthesiology* 1998;89:1587–1589.

James MFM, Reyneke CJ, Whiffler K. Heart block following propofol: a case report. *Br J Anaesth* 1989;62:213–215.

Janeczko GF, El-Etr AA, Youngest S. Low-dose ketamine anesthesia for obstetrical delivery. *Anesth Analg* 1974;53:828–831.

Johnston RR, Miller RD, Way WL. The interaction of ketamine with *d*-tubocurarine, pancuronium, and succinylcholine in man. *Anesth Analg* 1974;53:496–501.

Kaisti KK, Langsjo JW, Aalto S, et al. Effects of sevoflurane, propofol, and adjunct nitrous oxide on regional cerebral blood flow, oxygen consumption, and blood volume in humans. *Anesthesiology* 2003;99:603–613.

Kapur N, Friedman R. Oral ketamine: a promising treatment for restless legs syndrome. *Anesth Analg* 2002;94:1558–1559.

Karliczek GF, Brenken U, Schokkenbrock R, et al. Etomidate-analgesic combinations for the induction of anesthesia in cardiac patients. *Anaesthesist* 1982;31:213–220.
Kasraie N, Cousins TB. Propofol and the patient with hereditary coproporphyria. *Anesth Analg* 1993;77:862–863.
Keidan I, Perel A, Shabtai EL, et al. Children undergoing repeated exposures for radiation therapy do not develop tolerance to propofol. *Anesthesiology* 2004;100:251–254.
Kerz T, Hennes H-J, Feve A, et al. Effects of propofol on H-reflex in humans. *Anesthesiology* 2001;94:32–37.
Kienbaum P, Heuter T, Paviakovic G, et al. S(+)-ketamine increases muscle sympathetic activity and maintains the neural response to hypotensive challenges in humans. *Anesthesiology* 2001;94: 252–258.
Kleinsasser A, Kuenszberg E, Loeckinger A, et al. Sevoflurane, but not propofol, significantly prolongs the Q-T interval. *Anesth Analg* 2000;90:25–27.
Koehntop DE, Liao JC, Van Bergen FH. Effects of pharmacologic alterations of adrenergic mechanisms by cocaine, tropolene, aminophylline and ketamine on epinephrine-induced arrhythmias during halothane nitrous oxide anesthesia. *Anesthesiology* 1977;46: 83–93.
Kohrs R, Durieux ME. Ketamine: Teaching an old drug new tricks. *Anesth Analg* 1998;87;1186–1193.
Kooy NW, Royall JA, Ye YZ, et al. Evidence for in vivo peroxynitrite production in human acute lung injury. *Am J Respir Crit Care Med* 1995;151:1250–1254.
Kostrzewski E, Gregor A. Ketamine in acute intermittent porphyria—dangerous or safe? *Anesthesiology* 1978;49:376–377.
Krauss JK, Akeyson EW, Giam P, et al. Propofol-induced dyskinesias in Parkinson's disease. *Anesth Analg* 1996;83:420–422.
Krumholz W, Endrass J, Hempelmann G. Propofol inhibits phagocytosis and killing of *Staphylococcus aureus* and *Escherichia coli* by polymorphonuclear leukocytes in vitro. *Can J Anaesth* 1994; 41:446–449.
Kudoh A, Takahira Y, Katagai H, et al. Small-dose ketamine improves the postoperative state of depressed patients. *Anesth Analg* 2002; 95:114–118.
Kuehnert MJ, Webb RM, Jochimsen EM, et al. *Staphylococcus aureus* bloodstream infections among patients undergoing electroconvulsive therapy traced to breaks in infection control and possible extrinsic contamination by propofol. *Anesth Analg* 1997;85: 420–425.
Kuipers JA, Boer F, Olieman W, et al. First-pass lung uptake and pulmonary clearance of propofol: assessment with a recirculatory indocyanine green pharmacokinetic model. *Anesthesiology* 1999;91:1780–1787.
Laughlin TP, Newberg LA. Prolonged myoclonus after etomidate anesthesia. *Anesth Analg* 1985;64:80–82.
Lavoie J, Walsh EP, Burrows FA, et al. Effects of propofol or isoflurane anesthesia on cardiac conduction in children undergoing radiofrequency catheter ablation for tachydysrhythmias. *Anesthesiology* 1995;82:884–887.
Laxenaire MC, Mata-Bremejo E, Moneret-Vautrin DA, et al. Life-threatening anaphylactoid reactions to propofol (Diprivan). *Anesthesiology* 1992;77:275–280.
Laxenaire MC, Moneret-Vautrin D, Vervloet D. The French experience of anaphylactoid reactions. *Int Anesthesiol Clin* 1985;23:145–160.
Liu H-T, Hollmann MW, Liu W-H, et al. Modulation of NMDA receptor function by ketamine and magnesium: Part I. *Anesth Analg* 2001;92:1173–1181.
Longnecker DE, Sturgill BC. Influence of anesthetic agents on survival following hemorrhage. *Anesthesiology* 1976;45:516–521.
Longnecker DE. Stress free: to be or not to be? *Anesthesiology* 1984;61: 643–644.
Lopatka CW, Muzi M, Eberft JT. Propofol, but not etomidate, reduces desflurane-mediated sympathetic activation in humans. *Can J Anesth* 1999;46:342–347.
Lundy PM, Lockwood PA, Thompson G, et al. Differential effects of ketamine isomers on neuronal and extraneuronal catecholamine uptake mechanisms. *Anesthesiology* 1986;64:359–363.
MacPherson RD, Rasiah RL, McLeod LJ. Intraarterial propofol is not directly toxic to vascular endothelium. *Anesthesiology* 1992;76: 967–971.
Masaki Y, Tanaka M, Nishikawa T. Physicochemical compatibility of propofol-lidocaine mixture. *Anesth Analg* 2003;97:1646–1651.
Masuda A, Asahi T, Sakamaki M, et al. Uric acid excretion increases during propofol anesthesia. *Anesth Analg* 1997;85:144–148.
Mayberg TS, Lam AM, Matta BF, et al. Ketamine does not increase cerebral blood flow velocity or intracranial pressure during isoflurane/nitrous oxide anesthesia in patients undergoing craniotomy. *Anesth Analg* 1995;81:84–89.
Meyers EF, Charles P. Prolonged adverse reactions to ketamine in children. *Anesthesiology* 1978;49:39–40.
Milde LN, Milde JH, Michenfelder JD. Cerebral functional, metabolic, and hemodynamic effects of etomidate in dogs. *Anesthesiology* 1985;63:371–377.
Modica PA, Tempelhoff R, White PF. Pro- and anticonvulsant effects of anesthetics (part II). *Anesth Analg* 1990;70:433–444.
Modvig KM, Nielsen SF. Psychological changes in children after anesthesia: a comparison between halothane and ketamine. *Acta Anaesthesiol Scand* 1977;21:541–544.
Molojavyi A, Preckel B, Cofmere T, et al. Effects of ketamine and its isomers on ischemic preconditioning in the isolated rat heart. *Anesthesiology* 2001;94:623–628.
Moretti RJ, Hassan SZ, Goodman LI, et al. Comparison of ketamine and thiopental in healthy volunteers: effects on mental status, mood, and personality. *Anesth Analg* 1984;63:1087–1096.
Mowafi HA, Al-Ghamdi A, Rushood A. Intraocular pressure changes during laparoscopy in patients anesthetized with propofol total intravenous anesthesia versus isoflurane inhaled anesthesia. *Anesth Analg* 2003;97:471–474.
Mullenheim J, Rulands R, Wietschorke T, et al. Late preconditioning is blocked by racemic ketamine, but not by S(+)-ketamine. *Anesth Analg* 2001;93:265–270.
Nagels W, Demeyere R, Van Hemelrijck J, et al. Evaluation of the neuroprotective effects of S(+)-ketamine during open-heart surgery. *Anesth Analg* 2004;98:1595–1603.
Nakagawa T, Hirakata H, Sato M et al. Ketamine suppresses platelet aggregation possibly by suppressed inositol triphosphate formation and subsequent suppression of cytosolic calcium increase. *Anesthesiology* 2002;96:1147–1152.
Nichols RL, Smith JW. Bacterial contamination of an anesthetic agent. *N Engl J Med* 1995;333:184–185.
Nieuwenhuijs D, Sarton E, Teppema LJ, et al. Respirator sites of action of propofol: Absence of depression of peripheral chemoreflex loop by low-dose propofol. *Anesthesiology* 2001;95:889–895.
Nishiyama T, Hanaoka K. Propofol-induced bronchoconstriction: Two case reports. *Anesth Analg* 2001;93:645–646.
Owen H, Spence AA. Etomidate. *Br J Anaesth* 1984;56:555–557.
Parke TJ, Steven JE, Rice ASC, et al. Metabolic acidosis and fatal myocardial failure after propofol infusion in children: five case reports. *BMJ* 1992;305:613–616.
Peters CE, Korcok J, Gelb AW, et al. Anesthetic concentrations of propofol protect against oxidative stress in primary astrocyte cultures: Comparison with hypothermia. *Anesthesiology* 2001;94: 313–321.
Pfenninger E, Dick W, Ahnefeld FW. The influence of ketamine on both normal and raised intracranial pressure of artificially ventilated animals. *Eur J Anaesthesiol* 1985;2:297–307.
Pfenninger EG, Durieux ME, Himmelseher S. Cognitive impairment after small-dose ketamine isomers in comparison to equianalgesic racemic ketamine in human volunteers. *Anesthesiology* 2002;96: 357–366.
Pinaud M, Leausque JN, Chetanneau A, et al. Effects of propofol on cerebral hemodynamics and metabolism in patients with brain trauma. *Anesthesiology* 1990;73:404–409.
Pizov R, Brown RH, Weiss YS, et al. Wheezing during induction of general anesthesia in patients with and without asthma. A randomized, blinded trial. *Anesthesiology* 1995;82:1111–1116.
Raff M, Harrison GG. The screening of propofol in MHS swine. *Anesth Analg* 1989;68:750–751.
Reddy RV, Moorthy SS, Dierdorf SF, et al. Excitatory effects and electroencephalographic correlation of etomidate, thiopental, methohexital, and propofol. *Anesth Analg* 1993;77:1008–1011.
Reich DL, Silvay G. Ketamine: an update on the first twenty-five years of clinical experience. *Can J Anaesth* 1989;36:186–197.
Rieschke P, LaFleur BJ, Janicki PK. Effects of EDTA- and sulfite-containing formulations of propofol on respiratory system

resistance after tracheal intubation in smokers. *Anesthesiology* 2003;98: 323–328.

Robinson BJ, Ebert TJ, O'Brien TJ, et al. Mechanisms whereby propofol mediates peripheral vasodilation in humans. Sympathoinhibition or direct vascular relaxation? *Anesthesiology* 1997;86: 64–72.

Rouby JJ, Andreev A, Leger P, et al. Peripheral vascular effects of thiopental and propofol in humans with artificial hearts. *Anesthesiology* 1991;75:32–42.

Salengros J-C, Velghe-Lenelle C-E, Bollens R, et al. Lactic acidosis during propofol-remifentanil anesthesia in an adult. *Anesthesiology* 2004;101:241–243.

Salt TE, Wilson DG, Prasad SK. Antagonism of N-methylaspartate and synaptic responses of neurones in the rat ventrobasal thalamus by ketamine and MK-801. *Br J Pharmacol* 1988;94:443–448.

Sandler AN, Schmid R, Katz J. Epidural ketamine for postoperative analgesia. *Can J Anaesth* 1998;45:99–102.

Sarma VJ. Use of ketamine in acute severe asthma. *Acta Anaesthesiol Scand* 1992;36:106–107.

Sayin MM, Ozatamer O, Tasoz R, et al. Propofol attenuates myocardial lipid peroxiidation during coronary artery bypass grafting surgery *Br J Anaesth* 2002;89:242–246.

Schubert A, Licine MG, Lineberry PJ. The effect of ketamine on human somatosensory evoked potentials and its modification by nitrous oxide. *Anesthesiology* 1990;72:33–39.

Schwartz DA, Horwitz LD. Effects of ketamine on left ventricular performance. *J Pharmacol Exp Ther* 1975;194:410–414.

Sebel PS, Lowdon JD. Propofol: a new intravenous anesthetic. *Anesthesiology* 1989;71:260–277.

Servin FS, Bourgeois B, Gomeni R, et al. Pharmacokinetics of propofol administered by target controlled infusion to alcoholic patients. *Anesthesiology* 2003;99:576–585.

Sharpe MD, Dobkowski WB, Murkin JM, et al. Propofol has no direct effect on sinoatrial node function or on normal atrioventricular and accessory pathway conduction in Wolff-ParkinsonWhite syndrome during alfentanil/midazolam anesthesia. *Anesthesiology* 1995;82:888–895.

Short TG, Lim TA, Tam YH. Prospective evaluation of pharmacokinetic model-controlled infusion of propofol in adult patients. *Br J Anaesth* 1996;76:313–315.

Skei S, Ichimiya T, Hideaki T, et al. A case of normalization of Wolff-Parkinson-White syndrome conduction during propofol anesthesia. *Anesthesiology* 1999;90:1779–1781.

Sloan TB, Ronai AK, Toleikis R, et al. Improvement of intraoperative somatosensory evoked potentials by etomidate. *Anesth Analg* 1988; 67:582–585.

Smith I, White PF, Nathanson M, et al. Propofol: an update on its clinical use. *Anesthesiology* 1994;81:1005–1043.

Sneyd JR. Propofol and epilepsy. *Br J Anaesth* 1999;82:168–169.

Soliman MG, Brinale GF, Kuster G. Response to hypercapnia under ketamine anesthesia. *Can Anaesth Soc J* 1975;22:486–494.

Song D, Hamza MA, White PF, et al. Comparison of a lower-lipid propofol emulsion with the standard emulsion for sedation during monitored anesthesia care. *Anesthesiology* 2004;100: 1072–1075.

Sprung J, Ogletree-Hughes ML, Moravec CS. The effects of etomidate on the contractility of failing and nonfailing human heart muscle. *Anesth Analg* 2000;91:68–75.

St Pierre M, Dunkel M, Rutherford A, et al. Does etomidate increase postoperative nausea? A double-blind controlled comparison of etomidate in lipid emulsion with propofol for balanced anaesthesia. *Eur J Anaesthesiol* 2000;17:634–641.

Stanley TH. Blood pressure and pulse rate responses to ketamine during general anesthesia. *Anesthesiology* 1973;39:648–649.

Strebel S, Kaufmann M, Guardiola PM, Schaefer HG. Cerebral vasomotor responsiveness to carbon dioxide is preserved during propofol and midazolam anesthesia in humans. *Anesth Analg* 1994;78:884–888.

Streisand JB, Jaarsma RL, Jay MA, et al. Oral transmucosal etomidate in volunteers. Anesthesiology 1998;88:89–95.

Subramaniam K, Balachundar S, Steinbrook RA. Ketamine as adjuvant analgesic to opioids: a quantitative and qualitative systematic review. *Anesth Analg* 2004;99:482–495.

Sundman E, Witt HR, Sandin R, et al. Pharyngeal function and airway protection during subhypnotic concentrations of propofol, isoflurane, and sevoflurane: volunteers examined by pharyngeal videoradiography and simultaneous manometry. *Anesthesiology* 2001;95:1125–1132.

Takeshita H, Okuda Y, Sari A. The effects of ketamine on cerebral circulation and metabolism in man. *Anesthesiology* 1972;36:69–75.

Takizawa D, Hiraoka H, Gota F, et al. Human kidneys plan an important role in the elimination of propofol. *Anesthesiology* 2005; 102:327–330.

Taylor PA, Towey RM. Depression of laryngeal reflexes during ketamine anesthesia. *Br Med J* 1971;2:688–689.

Toft P, Romer U. Comparison of midazolam and diazepam to supplement total intravenous anaesthesia with ketamine for endoscopy. *Can J Anaesth* 1987;34:466–469.

Tomlin SL, Jenkins A, Lieb WR, et al. Stereoselective effects of etomidate optical isomers on gamma-aminobutyric acid type A receptors and animals. *Anesthesiology* 1998;88:708–717.

Traber DL, Wilson RD, Priano LL. Blockade of the hypertensive response to ketamine. *Anesth Analg* 1970;49:420–426.

Tramer M, Moore A, McQuay H. Meta-analytic comparison of prophylactic antiemetic efficacy for postoperative nausea and vomiting: propofol anaesthesia vs omitting nitrous oxide vs total i.v. anaesthesia with propofol. *Br J Anaesth* 1997b;78:256–259.

Tramer M, Moore A, McQuay H. Prevention of vomiting after paediatric strabismus surgery: a systematic review using the numbers-needed-to-treat method. *Br J Anaesth* 1995;75:556–561.

Tramer M, Moore A, McQuay H. Propofol anaesthesia and postoperative nausea and vomiting: quantitative systematic review of randomized controlled studies. *Br J Anaesth* 1997a;78:247–255.

Tramer MR, Moore RA, McQuay HJ. Propofol and bradycardia: causation, frequency and severity. *Br J Anaesth* 1997c;78:642–651.

Tweed WA, Minuck MS, Mymin D. Circulatory response to ketamine anesthesia. *Anesthesiology* 1972;37:613–619.

Veselis RA, Reinsel RA, Feshchenko VA, et al. The comparative amnestic effects of midazolam, propofol, thiopental, and fentanyl at equisedative concentrations. *Anesthesiology* 1997;87:749–764.

Wagner LE, Gingrich KJ, Kulli JC, et al. Ketamine blockade of voltage-gated sodium channels: Evidence for a shared receptor site with local anesthetics. *Anesthesiology* 2001;95:1406–1413.

Wagner RL, White PF, Kan PB, et al. Inhibition of adrenal steroidogenesis by the anesthetic etomidate. *N Engl J Med* 1984;310: 1415–1421.

Wahr JA, Plunkett JJ, Ramsay JG, et al. Cardiovascular responses during sedation after coronary revascularization: incidence of myocardial ischemia and hemodynamic episodes with propofol versus midazolam. *Anesthesiology* 1996;84:1350–1360.

Ward DS, Norton JR, Guivarc'h P-H, et al. Pharmacodynamics and pharmacokinetics of propofol in a medium-chain triglyceride emulsion. *Anesthesiology* 2002;97:1401–1408.

Warwick JP, Bladke D. Drawing up propofol [letter]. *Anaesthesia* 1994; 49:172.

Watkins JA. Etomidate: An "immunologically safe" anaesthetic agent. *Anaesthesia* 1983;34:208–210.

Weigand MA, Schmidt H, Zhao Q, et al. Ketamine modulates the stimulated adhesion molecule expression on human neutrophils in vitro. *Anesth Analg* 2000;90:206–212.

Weiskopf RB, Townley MI, Riordan KK, et al. Comparison of cardiopulmonary responses to graded hemorrhage during enflurane, halothane, isoflurane and ketamine anesthesia. *Anesth Analg* 1981;60:481–492.

White PF, Ham J, Way WL, et al. Pharmacology of ketamine isomers in surgical patients. *Anesthesiology* 1980;52:231–239.

White PF, Way WL, Trevor AJ. Ketamine: its pharmacology and therapeutic uses. *Anesthesiology* 1982;56:119–136.

Wolf A, Weir P, Setage P, et al. Impaired fatty acid oxidation in propofol infusion syndrome. *Lancet* 2001;357:606–607.

Wong DHW, Jenkins LC. An experimental study of the mechanism of action of ketamine on the central nervous system. *Can Anaesth Soc J* 1974;21:57–67.

Yamakura T, Bertaccini E, Trudell JR, et al. Anesthetics and ion channels: molecular models and sites of action. *Annu Rev Pharmacol Toxicol* 2001;41:23–51.

Yli-Hankala A, Kirvela M, Randell T, Lindgren L. Ketamine anaesthesia in a patient with septic shock. *Acta Anaesthesiol Scand* 1992;36: 483–485.

Local Anesthetics

7

Local anesthetics are drugs that produce reversible conduction blockade of impulses along central and peripheral nerve pathways after regional anesthesia. With progressive increases in concentrations of local anesthetics, the transmission of autonomic, somatic sensory, and somatic motor impulses is interrupted, producing autonomic nervous system blockade, sensory anesthesia, and skeletal muscle paralysis in the area innervated by the affected nerve. Removal of the local anesthetic is followed by spontaneous and complete return of nerve conduction, with no evidence of structural damage to nerve fibers as a result of the drug's effects.

Cocaine was introduced as the first local anesthetic in 1884, by Kollar, for use in ophthalmology. Halsted recognized the ability of injected cocaine to interrupt nerve impulse conduction, leading to the introduction of peripheral nerve block anesthesia and spinal anesthesia. As an ester of benzoic acid, cocaine is present in large amounts in the leaves of *Erythroxylon coca*, a plant growing in the Andes mountains, where its cerebral-stimulating qualities are well known. Another unique feature of cocaine is its ability to produce localized vasoconstriction, making it useful to shrink the nasal mucosa in rhinolaryngologic procedures and nasotracheal intubation. The abuse potential of cocaine limits its legitimate medical uses, whereas irritant properties of cocaine preclude its use for topical anesthesia of the cornea or any form of injection to produce anesthesia (see the section on Cocaine Toxicity).

The first synthetic local anesthetic was the ester derivative procaine, introduced by Einhorn in 1905. Lidocaine was synthesized as an amide local anesthetic by Lofgren in 1943. It produces more rapid, intense, and longer-lasting conduction blockade than procaine. Unlike procaine, lidocaine is effective topically and is a highly efficacious cardiac antidysrhythmic drug. For these reasons, lidocaine is the standard to which all other anesthetics are compared.

COMMERCIAL PREPARATIONS

Local anesthetics are poorly soluble in water and therefore are marketed most often as water-soluble hydrochloride salts. These hydrochloride salt solutions are acidic (pH 6), contributing to the stability of the local anesthetic. An acidic pH is also important if epinephrine is present in the local anesthetic solution, because this catecholamine is unstable at an alkaline pH. Sodium bisulfite, which is strongly acidic, may be added to commercially prepared local anesthetic–epinephrine solutions (pH 4) to prevent oxidative decomposition of epinephrine.

Liposomal Local Anesthetics

Drugs such as lidocaine, tetracaine, and bupivacaine have been incorporated into liposomes to prolong the duration of action and decrease toxicity (Mowat et al., 1996). Liposomes are vesicles consisting of bilayers of phospholipid surrounding an aqueous phase. The phospholipid can act as a barrier to drug diffusion from the liposome, effectively providing a slow-release preparation with a prolonged duration of action (Duncan and Wildsmith, 1995). Extended-duration local anesthetics could have clinical use for prolonged postoperative analgesia and treatment of chronic pain when infiltrated or applied topically. Unlike systemic analgesics, local anesthetics reliably relieve pain without associated systemic side effects characteristic of opioids. Bupivacaine incorporated into biodegradable microcapsules provided analgesia for 96 hours after subcutaneous infiltration (Pedersen et al., 2004).

Alkalinization of Local Anesthetic Solutions

Alkalinization of local anesthetic solutions shortens the onset of neural blockade, enhances the depth of sensory and motor blockade, and increases the spread of epidural blockade (Curatolo et al., 1998). The pH of commercial preparations of local anesthetic solutions ranges from 3.9 to 6.5 and is especially acidic if prepackaged with epinephrine (increased acidity prolongs the shelf life of epinephrine). The pKa of local anesthetics used clinically is near 8, so that only a small fraction (about 3%) of the local anesthetic exists in the lipid-soluble form. Alkalinization increases the percentage of local anesthetic existing in the lipid-soluble form that is available to diffuse across lipid cellular barriers. Adding sodium bicarbonate will speed the onset of peripheral nerve block and epidural block by 3 to 5 minutes.

STRUCTURE–ACTIVITY RELATIONSHIPS

Local anesthetics consist of a lipophilic and a hydrophilic portion separated by a connecting hydrocarbon chain (Fig. 7-1). The hydrophilic group is usually a tertiary amine, such as diethylamine, whereas the lipophilic portion is usually an unsaturated aromatic ring, such as paraaminobenzoic acid. The lipophilic portion is essential for anesthetic activity, and therapeutically useful local anesthetics require a delicate balance between lipid solubility and water solubility. In almost all instances, an ester (–CO–) or an amide (–NHC–) bond links the hydrocarbon chain to the lipophilic aromatic ring. The nature of this bond is the basis for classifying drugs that produce conduction blockade of nerve impulses as ester local anesthetics or amide local anesthetics (Fig. 7-2). The important differences between ester and amide local anesthetics relate to the site of metabolism and the potential to produce allergic reactions.

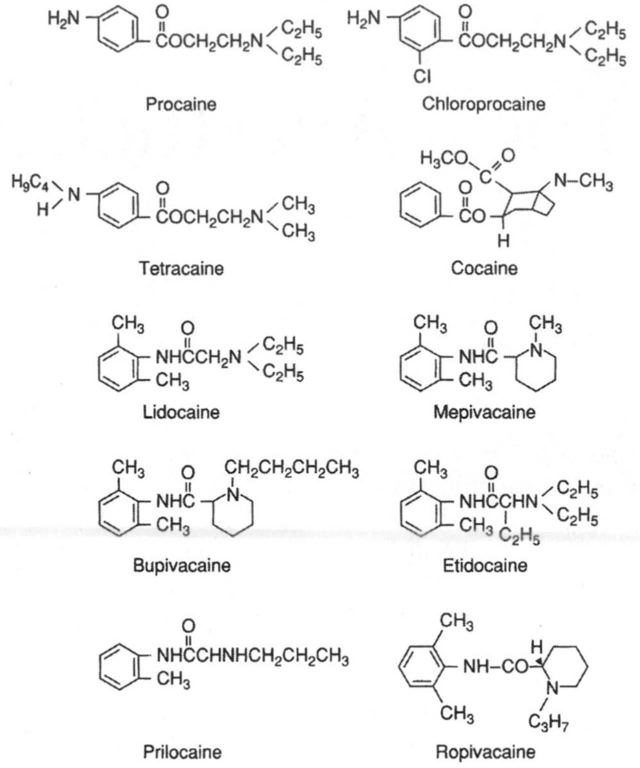

Figure 7-2. Ester and amide local anesthetics. Mepivacaine, bupivacaine, and ropivacaine are chiral drugs because the molecules possess an asymmetric carbon atom.

Modification of Chemical Structure

Modifying the chemical structure of a local anesthetic alters its pharmacologic effects. For example, lengthening the connecting hydrocarbon chain or increasing the number of carbon atoms on the tertiary amine or aromatic ring often results in a local anesthetic with a different lipid solubility, potency, rate of metabolism, and duration of action (Table 7-1). Indeed, substituting a butyl group for the amine group on the benzene ring of procaine results in tetracaine. Compared with procaine, tetracaine is more lipid soluble, is ten times more potent, and has a longer duration of action corresponding to a four- to fivefold decrease in the rate of metabolism. Halogenation of procaine to chloroprocaine results in a three- to fourfold increase in the hydrolysis rate of chloroprocaine by plasma cholinesterase. This rapid hydrolysis rate of chloroprocaine limits the duration of action and systemic toxicity of this local anesthetic. Etidocaine resembles lidocaine, but substituting a propyl group for an ethyl group at the amine end and adding an ethyl group on the alpha carbon of the connecting hydrocarbon chain produces a 50-fold increase in lipid solubility and a two- to threefold increase in the duration of action.

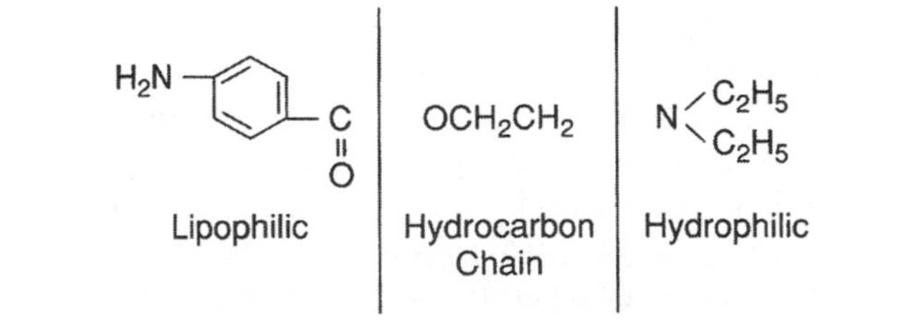

Figure 7-1. Local anesthetics consist of a lipophilic and hydrophilic portion separated by a connecting hydrocarbon chain.

Mepivacaine, bupivacaine, and ropivacaine are characterized as pipecoloxylidides (see Fig. 7-2). Mepivacaine has a methyl group on the piperidine nitrogen atom (amine end) of the molecule. Addition of a butyl group to the piperidine nitrogen of mepivacaine results in bupivacaine, which is 35 times more lipid soluble and has a potency and duration of action three to four times that of mepivacaine. Ropivacaine structurally resembles bupivacaine and mepivacaine, with a propyl group on the piperidine nitrogen atom of the molecule.

Racemic Mixtures or Pure Isomers

The pipecoloxylidide local anesthetics (mepivacaine, bupivacaine, ropivacaine, levobupivacaine) are chiral drugs because their molecules possess an asymmetric carbon atom (see Fig. 7-2). As such, these drugs may have a left- (S) or right- (R) handed configuration.

TABLE 7-1.
COMPARATIVE PHARMACOLOGY OF LOCAL ANESTHETICS

Classification	Potency	Onset	Duration after Infiltration (mins)	Maximum Single Dose for Infiltration (mg)	Toxic Plasma Concentration (μg/ml)	pK	Protein Binding (%)
Esters							
Procaine	1	Slow	45–60	500		8.9	6
Chloroprocaine	4	Rapid	30–45	600		8.7	
Tetracaine	16	Slow	60–180	100 (topical)		8.5	76
Amides							
Lidocaine	1	Rapid	60–120	300	>5	7.9	70
Etidocaine	4	Slow	240–480	300	~2	7.7	94
Prilocaine	1	Slow	60–120	400	>5	7.9	55
Mepivacaine	1	Slow	90–180	300	>5	7.6	77
Bupivacaine	4	Slow	240–480	175	>3	8.1	95
Levobupivacaine	4	Slow	240–480	175		8.1	>97
Ropivacaine	4	Slow	240–480	200	>4	8.1	94

Classification	Fraction Nonionized (%) at pH 7.2	Fraction Nonionized (%) at pH 7.4	Fraction Nonionized (%) at pH 7.6	Lipid Solubility	Volume of Distribution (liters)	Clearance (liters/min)	Elimination Half-Time (mins)
Esters							
Procaine	2	3	5	0.6	65		9
Chloroprocaine	3	5	7		35		7
Tetracaine	5	7	11	80			
Amides							
Lidocaine	17	25	33	2.9	91	0.95	96
Etidocaine	24	33	44	141	133	1.22	156
Prilocaine	17	24	33	0.9	191		96
Mepivacaine	28	39	50	1	84	9.78	114
Bupivacaine	11	17	24	28	73	0.47	210
Levobupivacaine	11	17	24		55		156
Ropivacaine		17			59	0.44	108

Adapted from Denson DD. Physiology and pharmacology of local anesthetics. In: Sinatra RS, Hord AH, Ginsberg B, Preble LM (eds): *Acute pain. Mechanisms and management.* St Louis, Mosby Year Book, 1992:124; and Burm AG, van der Meer AD, van Kleef JW, et al. Pharmacokinetics of the enantiomers of bupivacaine following intravenous administration of the racemate. *Br J Clin Pharmacol* 1994;38:125–129.

Mepivacaine and bupivacaine are available for clinical use as racemic mixtures (50:50 mixture) of the enantiomers. The enantiomers of a chiral drug may vary in their pharmacokinetics, pharmacodynamics, and toxicity. Administering a racemic drug mixture is, in reality, the administration of two different drugs (Ehrlich, 1992). These differences in pharmacologic activity reflect the fact that individual enantiomers bind to receptors or enzymes that are chiral amino acids with stereoselective properties. The S enantiomers of bupivacaine and mepivacaine appear to be less toxic than the commercially available racemic mixtures of these local anesthetics (Burm et al., 1997). In contrast to mepivacaine and bupivacaine, ropivacaine and levobupivacaine have been developed as a pure S enantiomers (McClure, 1996). These S enantiomers are considered to produce less neurotoxicity and cardiotoxicity than racemic mixtures or the R enantiomers of local anesthetics, perhaps reflecting decreased potency at sodium ion channels (Vladimirov et al., 2000).

MECHANISM OF ACTION

Local anesthetics prevent transmission of nerve impulses (conduction blockade) by inhibiting passage of sodium ions through ion-selective sodium channels in nerve membranes (Butterworth and Strichartz, 1990). The sodium channel itself is a specific receptor for local anesthetic molecules. Occlusion of open sodium channels by local anesthetic molecules contributes little to overall inhibition of sodium permeability. Failure of sodium ion channel permeability to increase slows the rate of depolarization such that threshold potential is not reached and thus an action potential is not propagated (Fig. 7-3). Local anesthetics do not alter the resting transmembrane potential or threshold potential.

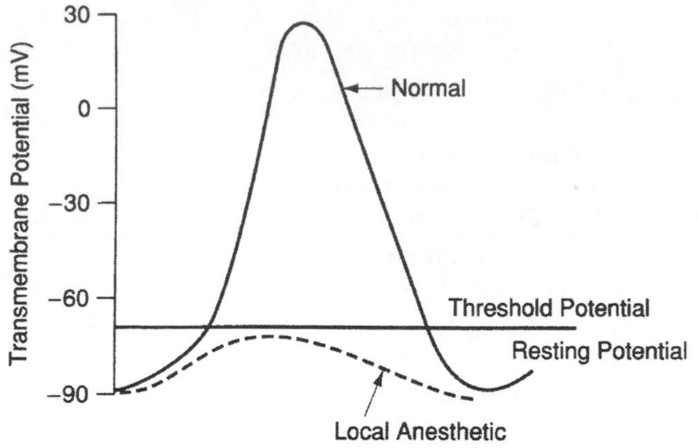

Figure 7-3. Local anesthetics slow the rate of depolarization of the nerve action potential such that the threshold potential is not reached. As a result, an action potential cannot be propagated in the presence of local anesthetic, and conduction blockade results.

Sodium Channels

The sodium channel consists of the large sodium-conducting pore (alpha-subunit) and varying numbers of adjacent smaller beta subunits. The large polypeptide that forms the alpha-subunit is further divided into four subunits (DI-IV). H is the alpha subunit that allows ion conduction and binds to local anesthetics. However, beta subunits may modulate local anesthetic binding to the alpha subunit. Binding affinities of local anesthetics to the sodium ion channels are stereospecific and depend on the conformational state of the sodium channel (Lee-Son et al., 1992). Sodium channels exist in activated-open, inactivated-closed, and rested-closed states during various phases of the action potential. In the resting nerve membrane, sodium channels are distributed in equilibrium between the rested-closed and inactivated-closed states. By selectively binding to sodium channels in inactivated-closed states, local anesthetic molecules stabilize these channels in this configuration and prevent their change to the rested-closed and activated-open states in response to nerve impulses. Sodium channels in the inactivated-closed state are not permeable to sodium, and thus conduction of nerve impulses in the form of propagated action potentials cannot occur. It is speculated that local anesthetics bind to specific sites located on the inner portion of sodium channels (internal gate or H gate) as well as obstructing sodium channels near their external openings to maintain these channels in inactivated-closed states (Butterworth and Strichartz, 1990). This binding appears to be weak and to reflect a relatively poor fit of the local anesthetic molecule with the receptor. This is consistent with the broad variety of chemical structures that exhibit local anesthetic activity on sodium channels (Lee-Son et al., 1992).

Frequency-Dependent Blockade

Sodium ion channels tend to recover from local anesthetic-induced conduction blockade between action potentials and to develop additional conduction blockade each time sodium channels open during an action potential (frequency-dependent blockade). Therefore, local anesthetic molecules can gain access to receptors only when sodium channels are in activated-open states. For this reason, selective conduction blockade of nerve fibers by local anesthetics may be related to the nerve's characteristic frequencies of activity as well as to its anatomic properties, such as diameter. Indeed, a resting nerve is less sensitive to local anesthetic-induced conduction blockade than is a nerve that has been repetitively stimulated. Etidocaine characteristically blocks motor nerves before sensory nerves because of frequency-dependent blockade (Bromage et al., 1974). The pharmacologic effects of other drugs, including anticonvulsants and barbiturates in addition to local anesthetics, may reflect frequency-dependent blockade.

Other Site of Action Targets

In addition to sodium ion channels, local anesthetics block voltage-dependent potassium ion channels. Compared with sodium ion channels, local anesthetics exhibit a much lower affinity. However, blockade of potassium ion channels might explain broadening of the action potential in the presence of local anesthetics. Considering the structural similarity between voltage-dependent calcium ion channels and sodium ion channels, it is not surprising that calcium ion currents (L-type most sensitive) may also be blocked by local anesthetics (Sugiyama and Muteki, 1994). Although local anesthetics are considered principally ion channel blockers, there is evidence these drugs may also act on G-protein coupled receptors (Hollmann et al., 2001a).

MINIMUM CONCENTRATION

The minimum concentration of local anesthetic necessary to produce conduction blockade of nerve impulses is termed the *Cm*. The Cm is analogous to the minimum alveolar concentration (MAC) for inhaled anesthetics. Nerve fiber diameter influences Cm, with larger nerve fibers requiring higher concentrations of local anesthetic for production of conduction blockade. An increased tissue pH or high frequency of nerve stimulation decreases Cm.

Each local anesthetic has a unique Cm, reflecting differing potencies of each drug. The Cm of motor fibers is approximately twice that of sensory fibers; thus, sensory anesthesia may not always be accompanied by skeletal muscle paralysis. Despite an unchanged Cm, less local anesthetic is needed for subarachnoid anesthesia than for epidural anesthesia, reflecting greater access of local anesthetics to unprotected nerves in the subarachnoid space.

Peripheral nerves are comprised of myelinated A and B fibers and unmyelinated C fibers (see Chapter 41). A minimal length of myelinated nerve fiber must be exposed to an adequate concentration of local anesthetic for conduction blockade of nerve impulses to occur. For example, if only one node of Ranvier is blocked (site of change in sodium permeability), the nerve impulse can jump (skip) across this node and conduction blockade does not occur. For conduction blockade to occur in an A fiber, it is necessary to expose at least two and preferably three successive nodes of Ranvier (approximately 1 cm) to an adequate concentration of local anesthetic. Both types of pain-conducting fibers (myelinated A-delta and nonmyelinated C fibers) are blocked by similar concentrations of local anesthetics, despite the differences in the diameters of these fibers. Preganglionic B fibers are more readily blocked by local anesthetics than any fiber, even though these fibers are myelinated.

Differential Conduction Blockade

Differential conduction blockade is illustrated by selective blockade of preganglionic sympathetic nervous system B fibers using low concentrations of local anesthetics. Slightly higher concentrations of local anesthetics interrupt conduction in small C fibers and small- and medium-sized A fibers, with loss of sensation for pain and temperature. Nevertheless, touch, proprioception, and motor function are still present such that the patient will sense pressure but not pain with surgical stimulation. In an anxious patient, however, any sensation may be misinterpreted as failure of the local anesthetic.

Changes during Pregnancy

Increased sensitivity (more rapid onset of conduction blockade) may be present during pregnancy (Datta et al., 1983). Alterations in protein-binding characteristics of bupivacaine may result in increased concentrations of pharmacologically active unbound drug in the parturient's plasma (Denson et al., 1984). Nevertheless, progesterone, which binds to the same alpha$_1$-acid glycoprotein as bupivacaine, does not influence protein binding of this local anesthetic (Denson et al., 1984). This evidence suggests that bupivacaine and progesterone bind to discrete but separate sites on protein molecules.

PHARMACOKINETICS

Local anesthetics are weak bases that have pK values somewhat above physiologic pH (see Table 7-1). As a result, <50% of the local anesthetic exists in a lipid-soluble nonionized form at physiologic pH. For example, at pH 7.4, only 5% of tetracaine exists in a nonionized form. Acidosis in the environment into which the local anesthetic is injected (as is present with tissue infection) further increases the ionized fraction of drug. This is consistent with the poor quality of local anesthesia that often results when a local anesthetic is injected into an acidic infected area. Local anesthetics with pKs nearest to physiologic pH have the most rapid onset of action, reflecting the presence of an optimal ratio of ionized to nonionized drug fraction (see Table 7-1).

Intrinsic vasodilator activity will also influence apparent potency and duration of action. For example, the enhanced vasodilator action of lidocaine compared with mepivacaine results in the greater systemic absorption and shorter duration of action of lidocaine. Bupivacaine and etidocaine produce similar vasodilation, but plasma concentrations of bupivacaine after epidural placement exceed those of etidocaine. Presumably, the greater lipid solubility of etidocaine results in tissue sequestration and less available drug for systemic absorption. Occasional prolonged sensory blockade after injection of etidocaine has been attributed to tissue sequestration.

Absorption and Distribution

Absorption of a local anesthetic from its site of injection into the systemic circulation is influenced by the site of injection and dosage, use of epinephrine, and pharmacologic characteristics of the drug (Fig. 7-4) (Covino and Vassallo, 1976). The ultimate plasma concentration of a local anesthetic is determined by the rate of tissue distribution and the rate of clearance of the drug. For example, the infusion of lidocaine for 1 minute is followed by a rapid decrease in the drug's plasma concentration that is paralleled by an initial high uptake into the lungs and distribution of the local anesthetic to highly perfused tissues

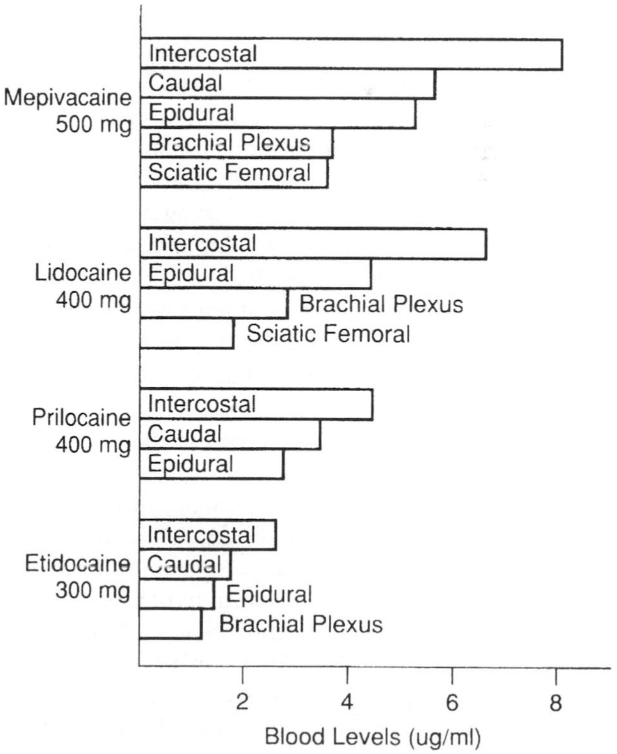

Figure 7-4. Peak plasma concentrations of local anesthetic are influenced by the site of injection for accomplishment of regional anesthesia. (From Covino BG, Vassallo HL. *Local anesthetics: mechanisms of action and clinical use*. New York: Grune & Stratton, 1976; with permission.)

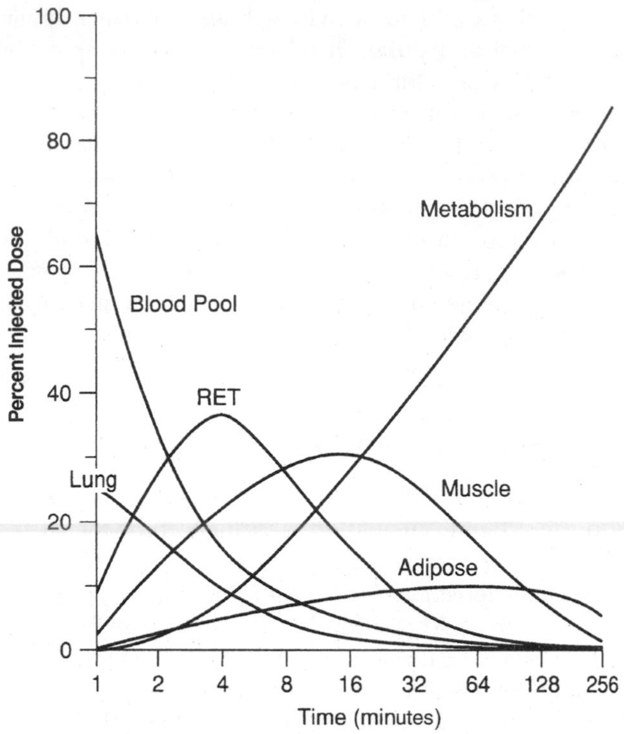

Figure 7-5. Perfusion model for the distribution of lidocaine in various tissues and its elimination after an intravenous infusion for 1 minute. (RET, rapidly equilibrating [highly perfused] tissues.) (From Benowitz N, Forsyth RP, Melmon KL, et al. Lidocaine disposition kinetics in monkey and man. I: Prediction by a perfusion model. *Clin Pharmacol Ther* 1974;16: 87–92; with permission.)

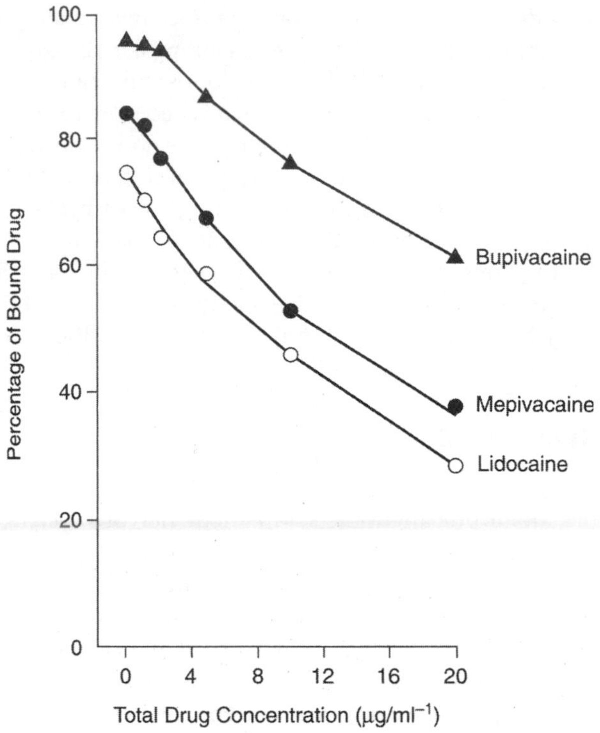

Figure 7-6. The percentage of local anesthetic bound to protein is inversely related to the plasma concentration of drug. (From Tucker GT, Boyes RN, Bridenbaugh PO, et al. Binding of anilide-type local anesthetics in human plasma: I. Relationships between binding, physiochemical properties, and anesthetic activity. *Anesthesiology* 1970;33:287–293; with permission.)

(brain, heart, and kidneys) (Fig. 7-5) (Benowitz et al., 1974). Lipid solubility of the local anesthetic is important in this redistribution, as well as being a primary determinant of intrinsic local anesthetic potency. After distribution to highly perfused tissues, the local anesthetic is redistributed to less well perfused tissues, including skeletal muscles and fat. Consideration of cardiac output is important for describing the overall tissue distribution of local anesthetics and presumably their intercompartmental clearance (Kuipers et al., 2001). Ultimately, the local anesthetic is eliminated from the plasma by metabolism and excretion.

In addition to the tissue blood flow and lipid solubility of the local anesthetic, patient-related factors such as age, cardiovascular status, and hepatic function will also influence the absorption and resultant plasma concentrations of local anesthetics. Protein binding of local anesthetics will influence their distribution and excretion. In this regard, protein binding parallels lipid solubility of the local anesthetic and is inversely related to the plasma concentration of drug (see Table 7-1) (Fig. 7-6) (Tucker et al., 1970). Overall, after systemic absorption, amide local anesthetics are more widely distributed in tissues than ester local anesthetics.

Lung Extraction

The lungs are capable of extracting local anesthetics such as lidocaine, bupivacaine, and prilocaine from the circulation (Jorfeldt et al., 1980). After rapid entry of local anesthetics into the venous circulation, this pulmonary extraction will limit the concentration of drug that reaches the systemic circulation for distribution to the coronary and cerebral circulations. For bupivacaine, this first-pass pulmonary extraction is dose dependent, suggesting that the uptake process becomes saturated rapidly (Rothstein et al., 1984). Propranolol impairs bupivacaine extraction by the lungs, perhaps reflecting a common receptor site for the two drugs (Rothstein and Pitt, 1983). Furthermore, propranolol decreases plasma clearance of lidocaine and bupivacaine, presumably reflecting propranolol-induced decreases in hepatic blood flow or inhibition of hepatic metabolism (Bowdle et al., 1987).

Placental Transfer

There may be clinically significant transplacental transfer of local anesthetics between the mother and fetus. Plasma protein binding influences the rate and degree of diffusion of local anesthetics across the placenta (see Table 7-1). Bupivacaine, which is highly protein bound (approximately 95%), has an umbilical vein–maternal arterial concentration ratio of about 0.32 compared with a ratio of 0.73 for lidocaine (approximately 70% protein bound) and a ratio of 0.85 for prilocaine (approximately 55% protein bound) (Thomas et al., 1976). Ester local anesthetics, because of their rapid hydrolysis, are not available to cross

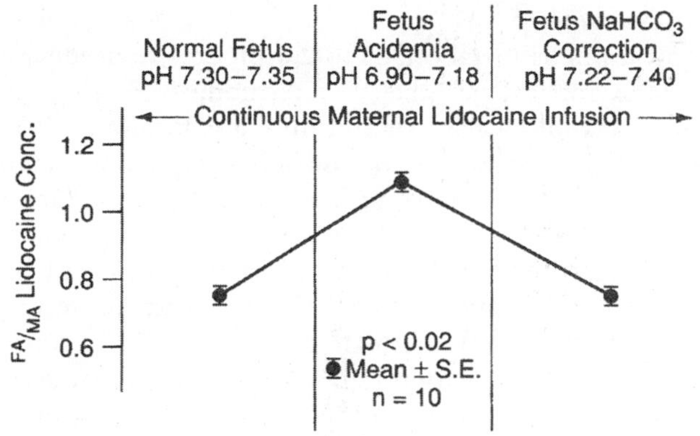

Figure 7-7. Fetal–maternal arterial (FA/MA) lidocaine ratios are greater during acidemia compared with a normal pH. (From Biehl D, Shnider SM, Levinson G, et al. Placental transfer of lidocaine: effects of fetal acidosis. *Anesthesiology* 1978;48: 409–412; with permission.)

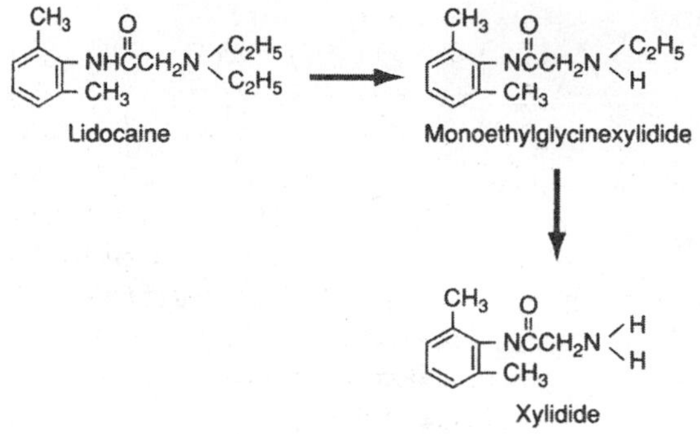

Figure 7-8. Metabolism of lidocaine.

the placenta in significant amounts. Acidosis in the fetus, which may occur during prolonged labor, can result in accumulation of local anesthetic molecules in the fetus (ion trapping) (Fig. 7-7) (Biehl et al., 1978).

Clearance

Clearance values and elimination half-times for amide local anesthetics probably represent mainly hepatic metabolism, because renal excretion of unchanged drug is minimal (see Table 7-1). Pharmacokinetic studies of ester local anesthetics are limited because of a short elimination half-time due to their rapid hydrolysis in the plasma and liver.

Metabolism of Amide Local Anesthetics

Amide local anesthetics undergo varying rates of metabolism by microsomal enzymes located primarily in the liver. Prilocaine undergoes the most rapid metabolism; lidocaine and mepivacaine are intermediate; and etidocaine, bupivacaine, and ropivacaine undergo the slowest metabolism among the amide local anesthetics. The initial step is conversion of the amide base to aminocarboxylic acid and a cyclic aniline derivative. Complete metabolism usually involves additional steps, such as hydroxylation of the aniline moiety and *N*-dealkylation of the aminocarboxylic acid.

Compared with that of ester local anesthetics, the metabolism of amide local anesthetics is more complex and slower. This slower metabolism means that sustained increases of the plasma concentrations of amide local anesthetics, and thus systemic toxicity, are more likely than with ester local anesthetics. Furthermore, cumulative drug effects of amide local anesthetics are more likely than with ester local anesthetics.

Lidocaine

The principal metabolic pathway of lidocaine is oxidative dealkylation in the liver to monoethylglycinexylidide followed by hydrolysis of this metabolite to xylidide (Fig. 7-8). Monoethylglycinexylidide has approximately 80% of the activity of lidocaine for protecting against cardiac dysrhythmias in an animal model. This metabolite has a prolonged elimination half-time, accounting for its efficacy in controlling cardiac dysrhythmias after the infusion of lidocaine is discontinued. Xylidide has only approximately 10% of the cardiac antidysrhythmic activity of lidocaine. In humans, approximately 75% of xylidide is excreted in the urine as 4-hydroxy-2,6-dimethylaniline.

Hepatic disease or decreases in hepatic blood flow, which may occur during anesthesia, can decrease the rate of metabolism of lidocaine. For example, the elimination half-time of lidocaine is increased more than fivefold in patients with liver dysfunction compared with normal patients. Decreased hepatic metabolism of lidocaine should be anticipated when patients are anesthetized with volatile anesthetics (Fig. 7-9) (Adejepon-Yamoah et al., 1973). Maternal clearance of lidocaine is prolonged in the presence of pregnancy-induced hypertension, and repeated administration of lidocaine can result in higher plasma concentrations than in normotensive parturients (Ramanathan et al., 1986).

Etidocaine

A small amount (<1%) of etidocaine is excreted unchanged in the urine. Despite its structural similarity to lidocaine, the metabolites of etidocaine differ from those of lidocaine.

Prilocaine

Prilocaine is an amide local anesthetic that is metabolized to orthotoluidine. Orthotoluidine is an oxidizing compound capable of converting hemoglobin to its oxidized form, methemoglobin, resulting in a potentially life-threatening complication, methemoglobinemia (see the section, Methemoglobinemia). When the dose of prilocaine is >600 mg, there may be sufficient methemoglobin present (3 to 5 g/dL) to cause the patient to appear cyanotic, and oxygen-carrying capacity is decreased. Methemoglobinemia is readily reversed by the administration of methylene blue, 1 to 2 mg/kg intravenously (IV), over 5 minutes (total dose should not exceed 7 to 8 mg/kg). The ability of

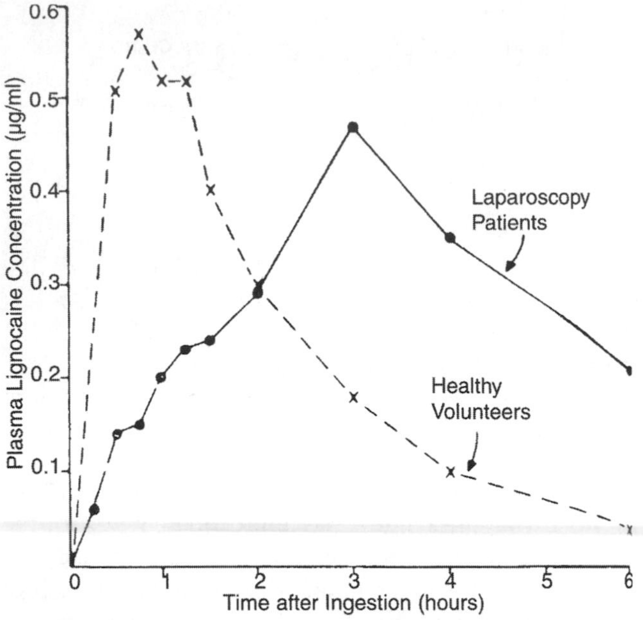

Figure 7-9. Plasma lidocaine (lignocaine) concentrations are higher during general anesthesia (laparoscopy patients) than in the absence of general anesthesia (healthy volunteers). (From Adejepon-Yamoah KK, Scott DB, Prescott LF. Impaired absorption and metabolism of oral lignocaine in patients undergoing laparoscopy. *Br J Anaesth* 1973;45: 143–147; with permission.)

prilocaine to cause dose-related methemoglobinemia limits its clinical usefulness, with the exception of IV regional anesthesia. Prilocaine causes less vasodilation than other local anesthetics and thus can be utilized without epinephrine added to the local anesthetic solution.

Mepivacaine

Mepivacaine has pharmacologic properties similar to those of lidocaine, although the duration of action of mepivacaine is somewhat longer. Clearance of mepivacaine is decreased in neonates, leading to a prolonged elimination half-time. In contrast to lidocaine, mepivacaine lacks vasodilator activity. As such, mepivacaine is an alternate selection when addition of epinephrine to the local anesthetic solution is not recommended.

Bupivacaine

Possible pathways for metabolism of bupivacaine include aromatic hydroxylation, *N*-dealkylation, amide hydrolysis, and conjugation (Pihlajamaki et al., 1990). Only the *N*-dealkylated metabolite *N*-desbutylbupivacaine, has been measured in blood or urine after epidural or spinal anesthesia. The mean total urinary excretion of bupivacaine and its dealkylation and hydroxylation metabolites account for >40% of the total anesthetic dose (Pihlajamaki et al., 1990). Alpha$_1$-acid glycoprotein is the most important plasma protein binding site of bupivacaine, and its concentration is increased in many clinical situations, including postoperative trauma (Dauphin et al., 1997).

Ropivacaine

Ropivacaine is metabolized to 2,6-pipecoloxylidide and 3-hydroxyropivacaine by hepatic cytochrome P-450 enzymes. Both metabolites have significantly less local anesthetic potency than ropivacaine. Becuse only a very small fraction of ropivacaine is excreted unchanged in the urine (about 1%) when the liver is functioning normally, dosage adjustments based on renal function do not seem necessary. However, in uremic patients, 2,6-pipecoloxylidide may accumulate and produce toxic effects (Pere et al., 2003). Overall, clearance of ropivacaine is higher than that determined for bupivacaine, and its elimination half-time is shorter (McClure, 1996). The higher clearance of ropivacaine may offer an advantage over bupivacaine in terms of systemic toxicity. The lipid solubility of ropivacaine is intermediate between lidocaine and bupivacaine. Ropivacaine is highly bound to alpha$_1$-acid glycoprotein.

Dibucaine

Dibucaine is a quinoline derivative with an amide bond in the connecting hydrocarbon chain. This local anesthetic is metabolized in the liver and is the most slowly eliminated of all the amide derivatives.

Metabolism of Ester Local Anesthetics

Ester local anesthetics undergo hydrolysis by cholinesterase enzyme, principally in the plasma and to a lesser extent in the liver. The rate of hydrolysis varies, with chloroprocaine being most rapid, procaine being intermediate, and tetracaine being the slowest. The resulting metabolites are pharmacologically inactive, although paraaminobenzoic acid may be an antigen responsible for subsequent allergic reactions. The exception to hydrolysis of ester local anesthetics in the plasma is cocaine, which undergoes significant metabolism in the liver.

Systemic toxicity is inversely proportional to the rate of hydrolysis; thus, tetracaine is more likely than chloroprocaine to result in excessive plasma concentrations. Because cerebrospinal fluid contains little to no cholinesterase enzyme, anesthesia produced by subarachnoid placement of tetracaine will persist until the drug has been absorbed into the systemic circulation. Plasma cholinesterase activity and the hydrolysis rate of ester local anesthetics are slowed in the presence of liver disease or an increased blood urea nitrogen concentration. Plasma cholinesterase activity may be decreased in parturients and in patients being treated with certain chemotherapeutic drugs. Patients with atypical plasma cholinesterase may be at increased risk for developing excess systemic concentrations of an ester local anesthetic due to absent or limited plasma hydrolysis.

Procaine

Procaine is hydrolyzed to paraaminobenzoic acid, which is excreted unchanged in urine, and to diethylaminoethanol, which is further metabolized because only 30% is recovered in urine. Overall, <50% of procaine is excreted unchanged in urine. Increased plasma concentrations of paraaminobenzoic acid do not produce symptoms of systemic toxicity.

Chloroprocaine

Addition of a chlorine atom to the benzene ring of procaine to form chloroprocaine increases by 3.5 times the rate of hydrolysis of the local anesthetic by plasma cholinesterase, as compared with procaine. Resulting pharmacologically inactive metabolites of chloroprocaine are 2-chloroaminobenzoic acid and 2-diethylaminoethanol. Maternal and neonatal plasma cholinesterase activity may be decreased up to 40% at term, but minimal placental passage of chloroprocaine confirms that even this decreased activity is adequate to hydrolyze most of the chloroprocaine that is absorbed from the maternal epidural space (Kuhnert et al., 1986a).

Tetracaine

Tetracaine undergoes hydrolysis by plasma cholinesterase, but the rate is slower than for procaine.

Benzocaine

Benzocaine (ethyl aminobenzoate) is unique among clinically useful local anesthetics because it is a weak acid (pKa 3.5), so that it exists only in the nonionized form at physiologic pH. As such, benzocaine is ideally suited for topical anesthesia of mucous membranes prior to tracheal intubation, endoscopy, transesophageal echocardiography, and bronchoscopy. Onset of topical anesthesia is rapid and lasts 30 to 60 minutes. A brief spray of 20% benzocaine delivers the recommended dose of 200 to 300 mg. Systemic absorption of topical benzocaine is enhanced by defects in the skin and mucosa as well as from the gastrointestinal tract should any of the local anesthetic be swallowed. Cetacaine is a combination of 14% benzocaine, 2% tetracaine, and 2% butamben. Methemoglobinemia is a rare but potentially life-threatening complication following topical application of benzocaine, especially when the dose exceeds 200 to 300 mg (see the section, Methemoglobinemia).

Cocaine

Cocaine is metabolized by plasma and liver cholinesterases to water-soluble metabolites that are excreted in urine. Plasma cholinesterase activity is decreased in parturients, neonates, the elderly, and patients with severe underlying hepatic disease. Cocaine may be present in urine for 24 to 36 hours, depending on the route of administration and cholinesterase activity. Assays for the metabolites of cocaine in urine are useful markers of cocaine use or absorption (see the section, Cocaine Toxicity).

Renal Elimination

The poor water solubility of local anesthetics usually limits renal excretion of unchanged drug to <5% (Tucker and Mather, 1979). The exception is cocaine, of which 10% to 12% of unchanged drug can be recovered in urine. Water-soluble metabolites of local anesthetics, such as paraaminobenzoic acid resulting from metabolism of ester local anesthetics, are readily excreted in urine.

Use of Vasoconstrictors

The duration of action of a local anesthetic is proportional to the time the drug is in contact with nerve fibers. For this reason, epinephrine (1:200,000 or 5 μg/mL) may be added to local anesthetic solutions to produce vasoconstriction, which limits systemic absorption and maintains the drug concentration in the vicinity of the nerve fibers to be anesthetized. Indeed, addition of epinephrine to a lidocaine solution prolongs the duration of conduction blockade and decreases systemic absorption of local anesthetics by approximately one-third (Table 7-2) (Fig. 7-10) (Liu 1997; Scott et al., 1972). Most local anesthetics, with the exception of ropivacaine, possess intrinsic vasodilator properties, and it is possible that epinephrine-induced vasoconstriction will slow clearance from the injection site, thus prolonging the time the drug is in contact with nerve fibers.

The impact of adding epinephrine to the local anesthetic solution is influenced by the specific local anesthetic selected and the level of sensory blockade required if a spinal or epidural anesthetic is chosen. For example, the impact of epinephrine in prolonging the duration of

TABLE 7-2.
EFFECTS OF ADDITION OF EPINEPHRINE (1:200,000) TO LOCAL ANESTHETIC SOLUTIONS

	Increase Duration	Decrease Blood Levels (%)
Peripheral nerve block		
Lidocaine	++	20–30
Mepivacaine	++	20–30
Bupivacaine	++	10–20
Ropivacaine	−−	0
Epidural		
Chloroprocaine	++	
Lidocaine	++	20–30
Mepivacaine	++	20–30
Bupivacaine	++	10–20
Levobupivacaine	−−	0
Ropivacaine	−−	0
Spinal*		
Lidocaine	++	
Tetracaine	++	
Bupivacaine	++	

*Epinephrine dose, 0.2 mg
Adapted from Liu SS. Local anesthetics and analgesia. In: Ashburn MA, Rice LJ (eds). *The management of pain*. New York. Churchill Livingstone, 1997;141–170.

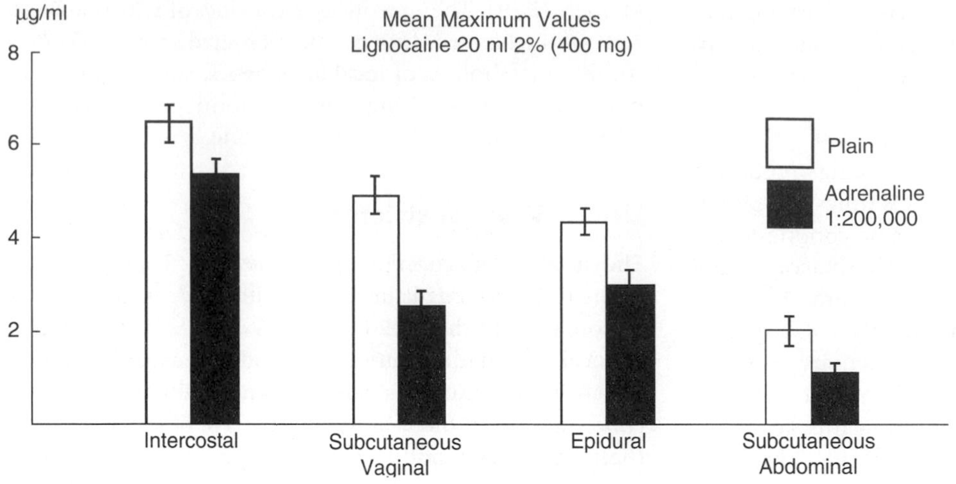

Figure 7-10. Addition of epinephrine (adrenaline) to the solution containing lidocaine (lignocaine) or prilocaine decreases systemic absorption of the local anesthetic by about one-third. (From Scott DB, Jebson PJR, Braid B, et al. Factors affecting plasma levels of lignocaine and prilocaine. *Br J Anaesth* 1972;44:1040–1049; with permission.)

conduction blockade and decreasing systemic absorption of bupivacaine and etidocaine is less than that observed with lidocaine, presumably because the greater lipid solubility of bupivacaine and etidocaine causes them to bind avidly to tissues. The duration of sensory anesthesia in the lower extremities, but not the abdominal region, is extended when epinephrine (0.2 mg) or phenylephrine (2 mg) is added to local anesthetic solutions of bupivacaine or lidocaine placed into the subarachnoid space. Vasoconstrictors prolong the effect of tetracaine for spinal anesthesia. Epinephrine added to a low dose of tetracaine (6 mg) increases the success rate of spinal anesthesia, whereas the success rate is not altered by epinephrine when the subarachnoid dose of tetracaine is 10 mg (Carpenter et al., 1989). In addition to decreasing systemic absorption to prolong conduction blockade, epinephrine may also enhance conduction blockade by increasing neuronal uptake of the local anesthetic. The alpha-adrenergic effects of epinephrine may be associated with some degree of analgesia that could contribute to the effects of the conduction blockade. The addition of epinephrine to local anesthetic solutions has little, if any, effect on the onset rate of local anesthesia.

Decreased systemic absorption of local anesthetic due to vasoconstriction produced by epinephrine increases the likelihood that the rate of metabolism will match that of absorption, thus decreasing the possibility of systemic toxicity. Whenever local anesthetic solutions containing epinephrine are administered in the presence of inhaled anesthetics, the possibility of enhanced cardiac irritability should be considered. Systemic absorption of epinephrine may accentuate systemic hypertension in vulnerable patients.

Low-molecular-weight dextran added to local anesthetic solutions, as used for peripheral nerve block anesthesia, prolongs the duration of action of the anesthetic. Presumably, dextran decreases the systemic absorption rate of local anesthetic (Kaplan et al., 1975).

Combinations of Local Anesthetics

Local anesthetics may be combined in an effort to produce a rapid onset (chloroprocaine) and prolonged duration (bupivacaine) of action. Nevertheless, placement of chloroprocaine in the epidural space may decrease the efficacy of subsequent epidural bupivacaine-induced analgesia during labor. It is speculated that the low pH of the chloroprocaine solution could decrease the nonionized pharmacologically active fraction of bupivacaine. Tachyphylaxis to the local anesthetic mixture could also reflect local acidosis due to the low pH of the bathing solution. For these reasons, adjustment of the pH of the chloroprocaine solution with the addition of 1 mL of 8.4% sodium bicarbonate added to 30 mL of chloroprocaine solution just before placement into the epidural space may improve the efficacy of the chloroprocaine-bupivacaine combination (Chestnut et al., 1989). Local anesthetic toxicity of combinations of drugs are additive rather than synergistic (Munson et al., 1977).

SIDE EFFECTS

The principal side effects related to the use of local anesthetics are allergic reactions and systemic toxicity due to excessive plasma and tissue concentrations of the local anesthetic. Systemic toxicity in association with regional anesthesia is estimated to result in seizures in 1 to 4 per 1,000 patient exposures to local anesthetics, with bupivacaine being the drug most likely to be associated with this adverse response (Brown et al., 1995).

Allergic Reactions

Allergic reactions to local anesthetics are rare despite the frequent use of these drugs. It is estimated that less than 1% of all adverse reactions to local anesthetics are due to an allergic mechanism (Brown et al., 1981). Instead, the overwhelming majority of adverse responses that are often attributed to an allergic reaction are instead manifestations of excess plasma concentrations of the local anesthetic.

Esters of local anesthetics that produce metabolites related to paraaminobenzoic acid are more likely than amide local anesthetics, which are not metabolized to paraaminobenzoic acid, to evoke an allergic reaction. An allergic reaction after the use of a local anesthetic may be due to methylparaben or similar substances used as preservatives in commercial preparations of ester and amide local anesthetics. These preservatives are structurally similar to paraaminobenzoic acid. As a result, an allergic reaction may reflect prior stimulation of antibody production by the preservative and not a reaction to the local anesthetic.

Cross-Sensitivity

Cross-sensitivity between local anesthetics reflects the common metabolite paraaminobenzoic acid. A similar cross-sensitivity, however, does not exist between classes of local anesthetics. Therefore, a patient with a known allergy to an ester local anesthetic can receive an amide local anesthetic without an increased risk of an allergic reaction. Likewise, an ester local anesthetic can be administered to a patient with a known allergy to an amide local anesthetic. It is important that the "safe" local anesthetic be preservative-free.

Documentation of Allergy

Documentation of allergy to a local anesthetic is based on the clinical history and perhaps the use of intradermal testing. The occurrence of rash, urticaria, and laryngeal edema, with or without hypotension and bronchospasm, is highly suggestive of a local anesthetic–induced allergic reaction. Conversely, hypotension associated with syncope or tachycardia when an epinephrine-containing local anesthetic solution is administered suggests an accidental intravascular injection of drug. Use of an intradermal test requires injection of preservative-free preparations of local anesthetic solutions to eliminate the possibility that the allergic reaction was caused by a substance other than the local anesthetic.

Systemic Toxicity

Systemic toxicity of a local anesthetic is due to an excess plasma concentration of the drug. Plasma concentrations of local anesthetics are determined by the rate of drug entrance into the systemic circulation relative to their redistribution to inactive tissue sites and clearance by metabolism. Accidental direct intravascular injection of local anesthetic solutions during performance of peripheral nerve block anesthesia or epidural anesthesia is the most common mechanism for production of excess plasma concentrations of local anesthetics. Less often, excess plasma concentrations of local anesthetics result from absorption of the local anesthetic from the injection site. The magnitude of this systemic absorption depends on the (a) dose administered into the tissues, (b) vascularity of the injection site, (c) presence of epinephrine in the solution, and (d) physicochemical properties of the drug (see Table 7-1). For example, systemic absorption of local anesthetics is greatest after injection for an intercostal nerve bock, intermediate for epidural anesthesia, and least for a brachial plexus block (see Fig. 7-4) (Covino and Vassallo, 1976). Addition of 5 μg of epinephrine to every milliliter of local anesthetic solution (1:200,000 dilution) decreases systemic absorption of local anesthetics by approximately one-third (Scott et al., 1972) (see the section, Use of Vasoconstrictors). Systemic toxicity of local anesthetics involves the central nervous system (CNS) and cardiovascular system.

Central Nervous System

Low plasma concentrations of local anesthetics are likely to produce numbness of the tongue and circumoral tissues, presumably reflecting delivery of drug to these highly vascular tissues. As the plasma concentrations continue to increase, local anesthetics readily cross the blood-brain barrier and produce a predictable pattern of CNS changes. Restlessness, vertigo, tinnitus, and difficulty in focusing occur initially. Further increases in the CNS concentration of local anesthetic result in slurred speech and skeletal muscle twitching. Skeletal muscle twitching is often first evident in the face and extremities and signals the imminence of tonic-clonic seizures. Lidocaine and other amide local anesthetics may cause drowsiness before the onset of seizures. Seizures are classically followed by CNS depression, which may be accompanied by hypotension and apnea. The onset of seizures may reflect selective depression of inhibitory cortical neurons by local anesthetics, leaving excitatory pathways unopposed. An alternative explanation for seizures is local anesthetic-induced inhibition of the release of neurotransmitters, particularly gamma-aminobutyric acid. The precise site of local anesthetic-induced seizures is not known, although it appears to be in the temporal lobe or the amygdala.

Plasma concentrations of local anesthetics producing signs of central nervous system (CNS) toxicity depend on the specific drug involved. Lidocaine, mepivacaine, and prilocaine demonstrate effects on the CNS at plasma concentrations of 5 to 10 μg/mL. The typical plasma concentration of bupivacaine associated with seizures is 4.5 to 5.5 μg/mL (Covino and Vassallo, 1976). Ropivacaine and bupivacaine produce convulsions in awake animals at similar doses (McClure, 1996). The threshold plasma concentration at which CNS toxicity occurs may be related more to the rate of increase of the serum concentration than to the total amount of drug injected (Tucker and Mather, 1979).

The active metabolites of lidocaine, including monoethylglycinexylidide, may exert an additive effect in causing systemic toxicity after epidural administration of lidocaine. For this reason, it has been recommended that the plasma venous concentration of lidocaine be monitored when the cumulative epidural dose of lidocaine is >900 mg (Inoue et al., 1985). The seizure threshold for lidocaine may be related to CNS levels of serotonin (5-hydroxytryptophan). For example, accumulation of serotonin decreases the seizure threshold of lidocaine and prolongs the duration of seizure activity.

There is an inverse relationship between the $PaCO_2$ and seizure thresholds of local anesthetics, presumably reflecting variations in cerebral blood flow and resultant delivery of drugs to the brain. Increases in the serum potassium concentration can facilitate depolarization and thus markedly increase local anesthetic toxicity. Conversely, hypokalemia, by creating hyperpolarization, can greatly decrease local anesthetic toxicity. The threshold for neurotoxicity of lidocaine may be decreased when patients being treated with the antidysrhythmic drug mexiletine receive lidocaine during the perioperative period (Christie et al., 1993).

Treatment

Treatment of local anesthetic-induced seizures includes ventilation of the patient's lungs with oxygen because arterial hypoxemia and metabolic acidosis occur within seconds (Moore et al., 1980). Equally important is the delivery of supplemental oxygen at the earliest sign of local anesthetic toxicity. Hyperventilation of the patient's lungs seems logical in an attempt to decrease the delivery of local anesthetic to the brain. Conversely, this maneuver could theoretically slow removal of local anesthetic from the brain. IV administration of a benzodiazepine such as midazolam or diazepam is effective in suppressing local anesthetic–induced seizures (see Chapter 5).

Neurotoxicity

Neurotoxicity from placement of local anesthetic–containing solutions into the epidural or subarachnoid space is an increasingly recognized phenomenon. The spectrum of this neurotoxicity may range from patchy groin numbness and persistent isolated myotomal weakness to cauda equina syndrome (Horlocker et al., 1997). An intermediate manifestation of this continuous dose-dependent neurotoxic effect of local anesthetics placed in the subarachnoid space are symptoms characterized clinically as transient neurologic symptoms (see the section, Transient Neurologic Symptoms). In the past, symptoms of neurotoxicity were likely to have been erroneously attributed to myoskeletal discomfort secondary to positioning. Likewise, myofascial pain may be erroneously diagnosed as transient neurologic symptoms after intrathecal placement of local anesthetics (Naveira et al., 1998). Overall, permanent neurologic injury after regional anesthesia remains a very rare event (Eisenach, 1997; Lee et al., 2004).

Clinical studies and animal models suggests that lidocaine is neurotoxic to sensory neurons, and this toxicity results from direct action on sensory neurons. Lidocaine-induced increases in intracellular calcium ion concentrations may be the mechanism for this toxicity (Kuboyoma et al, 1997). It is likely that other local anesthetics act similarly.

Transient Neurologic Symptoms

Transient neurologic symptoms manifest as moderate to severe pain in the lower back, buttocks, and posterior thighs that appears within 6 to 36 hours after complete recovery from uneventful single-shot spinal anesthesia (Schneider et al., 1993). Previous description of these symptoms as transient radicular irritation is no longer used, as the etiology of transient neurologic symptoms is not known. For example, sensory and motor neurologic examination is not abnormal, and relief of pain with trigger point injections and nonsteroidal antiinflammatory drugs suggests a musculoskeletal component. In some patients, the pain is sufficiently intense to require treatment with opioids. Full recovery from transient neurologic symptoms usually occurs within 1 to 7 days.

The incidence of transient neurologic symptoms is greatest following the intrathecal injection of lidocaine (as high as 30%) (Hodgson et al., 1999). Initial reports of transient neurologic symptoms involved spinal anesthesia produced by hyperbaric 5% lidocaine, suggesting that the observed neurotoxicity might be, at least in part, concentration dependent. Nevertheless, the incidence of transient neurologic symptoms is similar after intrathecal placement of 1 mg/kg of either 5% or 2% lidocaine in 7.5% glucose (Hampl et al., 1996; Liu et al., 1996). For ambulatory patients undergoing arthroscopy, the incidence of transient neurologic symptoms is not altered by decreasing spinal lidocaine concentrations from 2% to 1% or 0.5% and are similar to the incidence of symptoms described with 5% lidocaine (Pollock et al., 1999). The risk of transient neurologic symptoms associated with bupivacaine, tetracaine, mepivacaine, prilocaine, or procaine is significantly less than with lidocaine (Schneider and Birnbach, 2001).

Mepivacaine 4%, placed in the subarachnoid space, has also been associated with transient neurologic symptoms (Hiller and Rosenberg, 1997; Lynch et al., 1997). However, the incidence of transient neurologic symptoms is lower with 1.5% mepivacaine than 2% lidocaine in patients undergoing unilateral knee arthroscopy (Liguori et al., 1998). Spinal anesthesia produced with 0.5% bupivacaine or 0.5% tetracaine is associated with a lower incidence of transient neurologic symptoms compared with lidocaine (Hiller and Rosenberg, 1997; Tarkkila et al., 1996; Sakura et al., 1997; Sumi et al., 1996).

Lumbosacral nerve root irritation by local anesthetics may be exaggerated when the nerves are stretched by placement of the patient in the lithotomy position (de Jong, 1994; Douglas, 1995). Conversely, other data do not support the concept that patient positioning influences the incidence of transient neurologic symptoms (Sakura et al., 1997). Early ambulation was not found to be a risk factor for transient neurologic symptoms after spinal anesthesia with 2% lidocaine (Silvanto et al, 2004). Likewise, the glucose concentration and osmolarity of the anesthetic solution do not influence the incidence of transient neurologic symptoms (Sakura et al., 1997).

Epinephrine and phenylephrine are commonly added to local anesthetic solutions to prolong the duration of spinal anesthesia. Prolongation is thought to result, at least in part, from a decrease in nerve blood flow resulting in decreased systemic uptake of the local anesthetic. Therefore, it is theoretically possible that these vasoconstrictor drugs could contribute to the development of transient neurologic symptoms directly, or indirectly by inducing ischemia or by increasing exposure to the local anesthetic. There is evidence that adding phenylephrine to the local anesthetic solution increases the incidence of transient neurologic symptoms after spinal anesthesia with tetracaine (Sakura et al., 1997). There are some clinical data suggesting that addition of epinephrine to local anesthetic solutions does not alter the incidence of transient neurologic symptoms (Pollack et al., 1996).

Cauda Equina Syndrome

Cauda equina syndrome occurs when diffuse injury across the lumbosacral plexus produces varying degrees of (a) sensory anesthesia, (b) bowel and bladder sphincter dysfunction, and (c) paraplegia. Initial reports of cauda equina syndrome were associated with the use of hyperbaric 5% lidocaine for continuous spinal anesthesia (Lambert and Hurley, 1991; Rigler et al., 1991). In these cases, it was postulated that microcatheters used during continuous spinal anesthesia (28 gauge or smaller) contributed to nonhomogeneous distribution of the local anesthetic solution, with pooling of high concentrations of the local anesthetic solution on certain dependent or stretched (lithotomy position) nerves. Nevertheless, this same complication has also been reported after intrathecal injection of 100 mg of 5% lidocaine through a 25-gauge needle (Gerancher, 1997). Intended epidural anesthesia has also been implicated as a cause of cauda equina syndrome (Cheng, 1994).

Anterior Spinal Artery Syndrome

Anterior spinal artery syndrome consists of lower-extremity paresis with a variable sensory deficit that is usually diagnosed as the neural blockade resolves. The etiology of this syndrome is uncertain, although thrombosis or spasm of the anterior spinal artery is possible, as well as effects of hypotension or vasoconstrictor drugs. Although the addition of epinephrine to local anesthetic solutions has been implicated as a theoretical cause, spinal cord perfusion studies do not show a deleterious effect of the catecholamine (Kozody et al., 1984). Advanced age and the presence of peripheral vascular disease may predispose patients to development of anterior spinal artery syndrome. It may be difficult to distinguish symptoms due to anterior spinal artery syndrome from those caused by spinal cord compression produced by an epidural abscess or hematoma.

Cardiovascular System

The cardiovascular system is more resistant to the toxic effects of high plasma concentrations of local anesthetics than is the CNS. For example, lidocaine in plasma concentrations of <5 μg/mL is devoid of adverse cardiac effects, producing only a decrease in the rate of spontaneous phase 4 depolarization (automaticity). Nevertheless, plasma lidocaine concentrations of 5 to 10 μg/mL, and equivalent plasma concentrations of other local anesthetics, may produce profound hypotension due to relaxation of arteriolar vascular smooth muscle and direct myocardial depression (Table 7-3). As a result, hypotension reflects both decreased systemic vascular resistance and cardiac output.

Part of the cardiac toxicity that results from high plasma concentrations of local anesthetics occurs because these drugs also block cardiac sodium channels. At low concentrations of local anesthetics, this effect on sodium channels probably contributes to cardiac antidysrhythmic properties of these drugs. However, when the plasma concentrations of local anesthetics are excessive, sufficient cardiac sodium channels become blocked so that conduction and automaticity become adversely depressed. For example, excessive plasma concentrations of lidocaine may slow conduction of cardiac impulses through the heart, manifesting as prolongation of the P-R interval and QRS complex on the electrocardiogram. Effects of local anesthetics on calcium ion and potassium ion channels and local anesthetic-induced inhibition of cyclic adenosine monophosphate (cAMP) production may also contribute to cardiac toxicity (Butterworth et al., 1997).

Selective Cardiac Toxicity

Accidental IV injection of bupivacaine may result in precipitous hypotension, cardiac dysrhythmias, and atrioventricular

TABLE 7-3.
DOSE-DEPENDENT EFFECTS OF LIDOCAINE

Plasma Lidocaine Concentration (μg/ml)	Effect
1–5	Analgesia
5–10	Circumoral numbness
	Tinnitus
	Skeletal muscle twitching
	Systemic hypotension
	Myocardial depression
10–15	Seizures
	Unconsciousness
15–25	Apnea
	Coma
>25	Cardiovascular depression

TABLE 7-4.
ANIMALS MANIFESTING ADVERSE CARDIAC CHANGES AFTER ADMINISTRATION OF BUPIVACAINE OR LIDOCAINE

Cardiac Change	Bupivacaine (% of Animals)	Lidocaine (% of Animals)
Sinus tachycardia	0	100
Supraventricular tachycardia	60	9
Atrioventricular heart block	60	0
Ventricular tachycardia	80	0
Premature ventricular contractions	100	0
Wide QRS complexes	100	0
ST-T wave changes	60	40

Source: Kotelko DM, Shnider SM, Dailey PA, et al. Bupivacaine-induced cardiac arrhythmias in sheep. *Anesthesiology* 1984;60:10–18; with permission.

heart block (Albright, 1979). After accidental IV injection, the protein-binding sites (alpha$_1$-acid glycoprotein and albumin) for bupivacaine are quickly saturated, leaving a significant mass of unbound drug available for diffusion into the conducting tissue of the heart. IV injection of bupivacaine or lidocaine to awake animals produces serious cardiac dysrhythmias only in animals receiving bupivacaine (Table 7-4) (Kotelko et al., 1984). Cardiotoxic plasma concentrations of bupivacaine are 8 to 10 μg/mL (Timour et al., 1990).

Physiologic changes and concomitant drug therapy may make patients more vulnerable to bupivacaine cardiac toxicity. For example, pregnancy may increase sensitivity to cardiotoxic effects of bupivacaine, but not ropivacaine, as emphasized by occurrence of cardiopulmonary collapse with a smaller dose of bupivacaine in pregnant compared with nonpregnant animals (Fig. 7-11) (McClure, 1996; Morishima et al., 1985). The threshold for cardiac toxicity produced by bupivacaine may be decreased in patients being treated with drugs that inhibit myocardial impulse propagation (beta-adrenergic blockers, digitalis preparations, calcium channel blockers) (Roitman et al., 1993). Indeed, in the presence of propranolol, atrioventricular heart block and cardiac dysrhythmias occurred at plasma bupivacaine concentrations of 2 to 3 μg/ml (Timour et al., 1990). This suggests that caution must be taken in the use of bupivacaine in patients who are on antidysrhythmic drugs or other cardiac medications known to depress impulse propagation. Epinephrine and phenylephrine may increase bupivacaine cardiotoxicity, reflecting bupivacaine-induced inhibition of catecholamine-stimulated production of cAMP (Butterworth et al., 1993). The cardiac toxicity

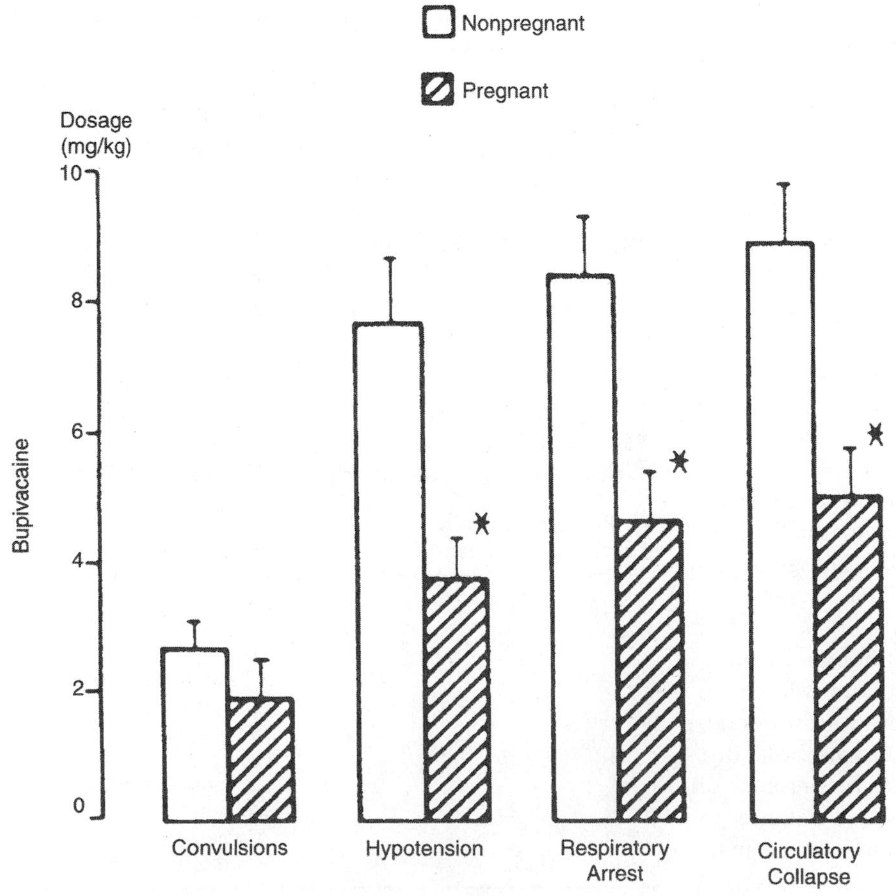

Figure 7-11. The dose of bupivacaine required to evoke toxic effects is less in pregnant than in nonpregnant ewes. (Mean ± SE; *$P < .05$.) (From Morishima HO, Pedersen H, Finster M, et al. Bupivacaine toxicity in pregnant and nonpregnant ewes. *Anesthesiology* 1985;63:134–139; with permission.)

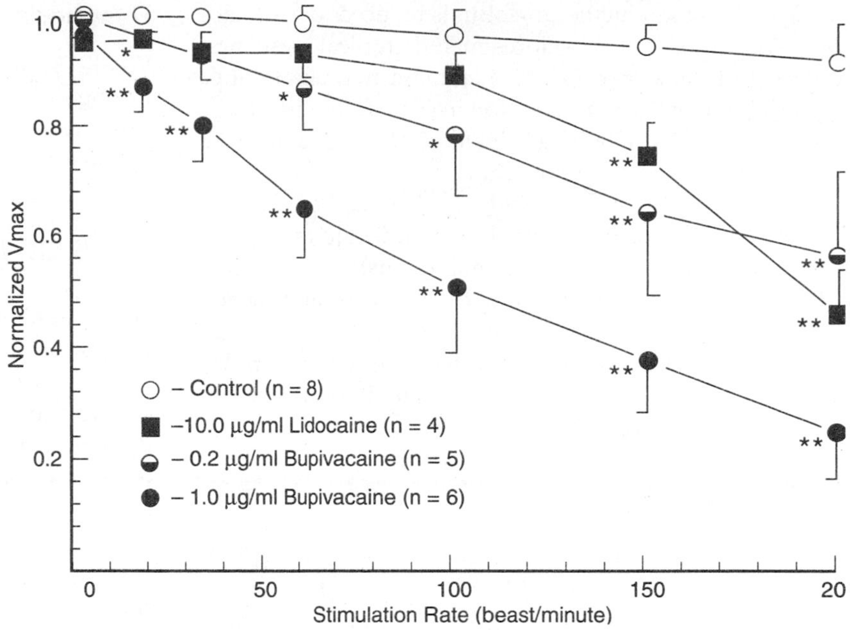

Figure 7-12. In an isolated papillary muscle preparation, V_{max} is depressed more by bupivacaine than by lidocaine. (*$P < .05$; **$P < .01$.) (From Clarkson CW, Hondeghem LM. Mechanism for bupivacaine depression of cardiac conduction: fast block of sodium channels during the action potential with slow recovery from block during diastole. *Anesthesiology* 1985;62:396–405; with permission.)

of bupivacaine in animals is enhanced by arterial hypoxemia, acidosis, or hypercarbia.

All local anesthetics depress the maximal depolarization rate of the cardiac action potential (V_{max}) by virtue of their ability to inhibit sodium ion influx via sodium channels. In isolated papillary muscle preparations, bupivacaine depresses V_{max} considerably more than lidocaine, whereas ropivacaine is intermediate in its depressant effect on V_{max} (Fig. 7-12) (Clarkson and Hondeghem, 1985; McClure, 1996). The resulting slowed conduction of the cardiac action potential manifests on the electrocardiogram as prolongation of the P-R and QRS intervals and reentry ventricular cardiac dysrhythmias. Both bupivacaine and lidocaine block cardiac sodium ion channels during systole, whereas during diastole, highly lipid soluble bupivacaine dissociates off these channels at a slow rate compared with lidocaine, thus accounting for the drug's persistent depressant effect on V_{max} and subsequent cardiac toxicity (Atlee and Bosnjak, 1990). At normal heart rates, diastolic time is sufficiently long for lidocaine dissociation but bupivacaine block intensifies and depresses electrical conduction, causing reentrant-type ventricular dysrhythmias, Less lipid-soluble lidocaine dissociates rapidly from cardiac sodium channels and cardiac toxicity is low. Furthermore, high plasma concentrations of bupivacaine may cause ventricular cardiac dysrhythmias through a direct brainstem effect. The R enantiomer of bupivacaine is more toxic than the S enantiomer. For example, seizure activity following an interscalent block with levobupivacaine was not associated with cardiac dysrhythmias or other signs of cardiovascular toxicity (Crews and Rothman, 2003). In animals, levobupivacaine compared with bupivacaine was associated with a lower incidence of ventricular cardiac dysrhythmias, and successful resuscitation was more likely in the presence of levobupivacaine (Groban et al., 2001; Huang et al., 1998). Ropivacaine is a pure S enantiomer that is less lipid soluble and less cardiotoxic than bupivacaine but more cardiotoxic than lidocaine (Moller and Covino, 1990; Scott et al., 1989). Although, ropivacaine-induced cardiac arrest has been described following peripheral nerve block anesthesia, in contrast to bupivacaine, cardiac resuscitation is more likely to be successful (Chazalon et al., 2003; Klein et al., 2003; Polley and Santos, 2003a).

Tachycardia can enhance frequency-dependent blockade of cardiac sodium channels by bupivacaine, further contributing to the selective cardiac toxicity of this local anesthetic (Kendig, 1985). Conversely, a low degree of frequency-dependent blockade may contribute to the antidysrhythmic properties of lidocaine. In anesthetized dogs, bretylium, 20 mg/kg IV, reverses bupivacaine-induced cardiac depression and increases the threshold for ventricular tachycardia (Kasten and Martin, 1985). In an effort to decrease the potential for cardiotoxicity should accidental intravascular injection occur, it may be prudent to limit the concentration of bupivacaine to be used for epidural anesthesia to 0.5%. In addition, slow or fractionated administration of all local anesthetics, but particularly bupivacaine, so as to detect systemic toxicity from accidental intravascular injection, should help decrease the risk of cardiotoxicity (Xuecheng et al., 1997).

Methemoglobinemia

Methemoglobinemia is a rare but potentially life-threatening complication (decreased oxygen-carrying capacity) that may follow the administration of certain drugs or chemicals that cause oxidation of hemoglobin to methemoglobin more rapidly than methemoglobin is reduced to hemoglobin. Known oxidant substances include topical local anesthetics (prilocaine, benzocaine, Cetacaine, lidocaine), nitroglycerin, phenytoin, and sulfonamides (Nguyen et al., 2000). Neonates may be at greater risk because of more readily oxidized fetal hemoglobin.

Methemoglobin cannot bind oxygen or carbon dioxide, resulting in loss of the hemoglobin molecule's transport function. Methemoglobin normally constitutes <1% of the total hemoglobin. Central cyanosis usually occurs when methemoglobin concentrations exceed 15%. The presence of methemoglobinemia is suggested by a difference between the calculated and measured arterial oxygen saturation. The diagnosis is confirmed by qualitative measurements of methemoglobin by cooximetry.

Methemoglobinemia is readily reversed by the administration of methylene blue, 1 to 2 mg/kg IV, over 5 minutes (total dose should not exceed 7 to 8 mg/kg). Methylene blue is reduced to leukomethylene blue, which then acts as an electron donor and nonenzymatically reduces methemoglobin to hemoglobin. Normal levels of methemoglobin should be achieved within 20 to 60 minutes after the administration of methylene blue. This therapeutic effect, however, is short-lived because methylene blue may be cleared before conversion of all the methemoglobin to hemoglobin. Furthermore, continued absorption of highly lipophilic local anesthetics such as benzocaine from adipose tissue stores may continue to occur after methylene blue plasma concentrations are no longer therapeutic.

Ventilatory Response to Hypoxia

Lidocaine at clinically useful plasma concentrations depresses the ventilatory responses to arterial hypoxemia (Gross et al., 1984). In this regard, patients with carbon dioxide retention whose resting ventilation depends on hypoxic drive may be at risk of ventilatory failure when lidocaine is administered for treatment of cardiac dysrhythmias. Conversely, systemic absorption of bupivacaine, such as follows a brachial plexus block, stimulates the ventilatory response to carbon dioxide.

Hepatotoxicity

Continous or intermittent epidural administration of bupivacaine to treat postherpetic neuralgia has been associated with increased plasma concentrations of liver transaminase enzymes that normalized when bupivacaine infusion was discontinued or lidocaine was substitued for bupivacaine (Yokoyama et al., 2001). The preservative present in both local anesthetics was the same. Drug-induced liver injury can be a direct toxic injury, an allergic reaction, or idosyncratic metabolic abnormality. The hepatic dysfunction described seems most likely to represent an allergic reaction (Craft and Good, 1994).

Dysphoria

Vivid fear of imminent death and a delusional belief of having died have been described in patients experiencing toxic reactions to local anesthetics administered for regional anesthesia and pain relief (Marsch et al., 1998).

USES OF LOCAL ANESTHETICS

Local anesthetics are most often used to produce topical, infiltration, and regional anesthesia (Table 7-5) (Covino et al., 1998; Foster and Markham, 2000). Less common reasons to select local anesthetics are to prevent or treat cardiac dysrhythmias (see Chapter 17), prevent or treat increases in intracranial pressure, provide analgesia, and treat grand mal seizures.

Antiinflammatory effects of local anesthetics may be responsible for benefical effects in the perioperative period that are attributed to spinal or epidural anesthesia (Hollmann and Durieux, 2000).

Regional Anesthesia

Regional anesthesia is classified according to the following six sites of placement of the local anesthetic solution: (a) topical or surface anesthesia, (b) local infiltration, (c) peripheral nerve block, (d) IV regional anesthesia (Bier block), (e) epidural anesthesia, and (f) spinal (subarachnoid) anesthesia (see Table 7-3). *Spinal anesthesia* rather than "subarachnoid anesthesia" or "spinal block" is the preferred terminology because it is understood by nonanesthesiologists. Furthermore, the term *block* implies an obstruction. Maximum doses of local anesthetics (based on body weight) as recommended for topical or peripheral nerve block anesthesia must be viewed as imprecise guidelines that often do not consider the pharmacokinetics of the drugs (Scott, 1989).

Topical Anesthesia

Local anesthetics are used to produce topical anesthesia by placement on the mucous membranes of the nose, mouth, tracheobronchial tree, esophagus, or genitourinary tract. Cocaine (4% to 10%), tetracaine (1% to 2%), and lidocaine (2% to 4%) are most often used. It is estimated that topical cocaine anesthesia is used in >50% of rhinolaryngologic procedures performed annually in the United States (Lange et al., 1989) (see the section on Cocaine Toxicity). Cocaine's popularity for topical anesthesia reflects its unique ability to produce localized vasoconstriction, thus decreasing blood loss and improving surgical visualization. There is no difference between the intranasal anesthetic or vasoconstrictive effects of cocaine and those of a lidocaine-oxymetazoline or tetracaine-oxymetazoline mixture, emphasizing the usefulness of these combinations

TABLE 7-5.
CLINICAL USES OF LOCAL ANESTHETICS

	Clinical Use	Concentration (%)	Onset	Duration (min)	Recommended Maximum Single Dose (mg)
Lidocaine	Topical	4	Fast	30–60	300
	Infiltration	0.5–1	Fast	60–240	300 or 500 with epinephrine
	IVRA	0.25–0.5	Fast	30–60`	300
	PNB	1–1.5	Fast	60–180	300 or 500 with epinephrine
	Epidural	1.5–2	Fast	60–120	300 or 500 with epinephrine
	Spinal	1.5–5	Fast	30–60	100
Mepivacaine	Infiltration	0.5–1	Fast	60–240	400 or 500 with epinephrine
	PNB	1–1.5	Fast	120–240	400 or 500 with epinephrine
	Epidural	1.5–2	Fast	60–180	400 or 500 with epinephrine
	Spinal	2–4	Fast	60–120	100
Etidocaine	Infiltration	0.5	Fast	120–480	300 or 400 with epinephrine
	PNB	0.5–1	Fast	180–720	300 or 400 with epinephrine
	Epidural	1–1.5	Fast	120–480	300 or 400 with epinephrine
Prilocaine	Infiltration	0.5–1	Fast	60–120	600
	IVRA	0.25–0.5	Fast	30–60	600
	PNB	1.5–2	Fast	90–180	600
	Epidural	2–3	Fast	60–180	600
Bupivacaine	Infiltration	0.25	Fast	120–480	175 or 225 with epinephrine
	PNB	0.25–0.5	Slow	240–960	175 or 225 with epinephrine
	Epidural	0.5–0.75	Moderate	120–300	175 or 225 with epinephrine
	Spinal	0.5–0.75	Fast	60–240	20
Levobupivacaine	Infiltration	0.25	Fast	120–480	150
	PNB	0.25–0.5	Slow	840–1,020	150
	Epidural	0.5–0.75	Moderate	300–540	150
	Spinal	0.5–0.75	Fast	60–360	20
Ropivacaine	Infiltration	0.2–0.5	Fast	120–360	200
	PNB	0.5–1	Slow	300–480	250
	Epidural	0.5–1	Moderate	120–360	200
	SPINAL?				
Chloroprocaine	Infiltration	1	Fast	30–60	800 or 1,000 with epinephrine
	PNB	2	Fast	30–60	800 or 1,000 with epinephrine
	Epidural	2–3	Fast	30–60	800 or 1,000 with epinephrine
	Spinal	2–3	Fast	30–60	Preservative free*
Procaine	Spinal	10	Fast	30–60	1,000
Tetracaine	Topical	2	Fast	30–60	20
	Spinal	0.5	Fast	120–360	20
Benzocaine	Topical	Up to 20%	Fast	30–60	200
Cocaine	Topical	4–10	Fast	30–60	150

*Off label use

Adapted from Covino BG, Wildsmith JAW. Clinical pharmacology of local anesthetic agents. In: Cousins MJ, Bridenbaugh PO (eds). *Neural blockade in clinical anesthesia and management of pain.* Philadelphia. Lippincott-Raven, 1998:97–128; and Foster RH, Markham A. Levobupivacaine: A review of its pharmacology and use as a local anesthetic. *Drugs* 2000;59:551–559.

as substitutes for cocaine (Noorily et al., 1995). Procaine and chloroprocaine penetrate mucous membranes poorly and are ineffective for topical anesthesia.

Nebulized lidocaine is used to produce surface anesthesia of the upper and lower respiratory tract before fiberoptic laryngoscopy and/or bronchoscopy and as a treatment for patients experiencing intractable coughing (McAlpine and Thomson, 1989). The inhalation of local anesthetics by normal subjects does not alter airway resistance and may even produce mild bronchodilation (Kirkpatrick et al., 1987). In contrast, inhalation of nebulized lidocaine can cause bronchoconstriction in some patients with asthma, which may become an important consideration when bronchoscopy is planned in these patients (McAlpine and Thomson, 1989). Local anesthetics are absorbed into the systemic circulation after topical application to mucous membranes. Systemic absorption of tetracaine, and to a lesser extent lidocaine, after placement on the tracheobronchial mucosa produces plasma concentrations similar to those present after IV injection of the local anesthetic. For example, plasma lidocaine concentrations 15 minutes after laryngotracheal spray of the local anesthetic are similar to those concentrations present at the same time after an IV injection of lidocaine (Viegas and Stoelting, 1975). This systemic absorption reflects the high vascularity of the tracheobronchial tree and the injection of the local anesthetic as a spray that spreads the solution over a wide surface area.

Eutectic Mixture of Local Anesthetics

The keratinized layer of the skin provides an effective barrier to diffusion of topical drugs, making it difficult to achieve anesthesia of intact skin by topical application. A popular use of prilocaine is for topical anesthesia when used in an eutectic mixture. A 5% lidocaine-prilocaine cream (2.5% lidocaine and 2.5% prilocaine) allows the use of high concentrations of the anesthetic bases without concern about local irritation, uneven absorption, or systemic toxicity (Gajraj et al., 1994; Taddio et al., 1997). This combination of local anesthetics is considered a eutectic mixture of local anesthetics (EMLA), as the melting point of the combined drugs is lower than lidocaine or prilocaine alone. EMLA cream acts by diffusing through intact skin to block neuronal transmission from dermal receptors. Usually 1 to 2 g of EMLA cream are applied per a 10-cm^2 area of skin and covered with an occlusive dressing. The duration of application varies according to the type of procedure being undertaken and the site of application. For example, skin-graft harvesting requires 2 hours, whereas cautery of genital warts can be undertaken after only a 10-minute application. EMLA cream is effective in relieving the pain of venipuncture, arterial cannulation, lumbar puncture, and myringotomy in children and adults. Pain during circumcision in neonates is attenuated by this topical anesthetic (Taddio et al., 1997). Although 45 minutes has been suggested as the minimum effective onset time for decreasing the pain of IV cannulation, a significant decrease in pain scores may be noted after only 5 minutes. Low-frequency ultrasound pretreatment is effective in accelerating the onset of EMLA cream (Katz et al., 2004). The addition of nitroglycerin ointment to EMLA cream increases the ease of venous cannulation by promoting venodilation (Teillol-Foo and Kassab, 1991). If EMLA cream is used to anesthetize the skin before blood sampling, the results of the analyses of the blood are not distorted. However, the use of EMLA cream to prevent the pain of intradermal skin tests decreases the flare response and may lead to false-negative interpretation of weakly positive tests.

Skin blood flow, epidermal and dermal thickness, duration of application, and the presence of skin pathology are important factors affecting the onset, efficacy, and duration of EMLA analgesia. African-Americans may be less responsive than whites, presumably because of increased density of the stratum corneum (Hymes and Spraker, 1986). Blanching of the skin may be seen after 30 to 60 minutes, probably due to vasoconstriction. Plasma levels of lidocaine and prilocaine are below toxic levels, although methemoglobin concentrations reflecting the metabolism of prilocaine may be increased in children <3 months of age, reflecting immature reductase pathways. The enzyme capacity for red blood cell methemoglobin reductase in children <3 months of age can be overloaded when EMLA cream is administered concurrently with other methemoglobin-inducing drugs (sulfonamides, acetaminophen, phenytoin, nitroglycerin, nitroprusside) (Jakobsen and Nilsson, 1985). Likewise, EMLA cream should not be used in those rare patients with congenital or idiopathic methemoglobinemia. Local skin reactions, such as pallor, erythema, and alterations in temperature sensation, edema, pruritus, and rash are common after EMLA cream application.

EMLA cream is not recommended for use on mucous membranes because of the faster absorption of lidocaine and prilocaine than through intact skin (Gajraj et al., 1994). Similarly, EMLA cream is not recommended for skin wounds, and the risk of wound infection may be increased (Powell et al., 1991). Patients being treated with certain antidysrhythmic drugs (mexiletine) may experience additive and potentially synergistic effects when exposed to EMLA cream. EMLA cream is contraindicated in patients with a known history of allergy to amide local anesthetics.

Amethocaine, like EMLA cream, requires several minutes to become effective, and the cream must be covered with an occlusive dressing. A microemulsion of amethocaine increases skin penetration and shortens the time until cutaneous anesthesia is achieved (Arevalo et al., 2004).

Other Topically Effective Local Anesthetics (see the section, Benzocaine)

Dyclonine (0.5% to 1.0%), hexylcaine, and piperocaine are effective topically for producing anesthesia of the mucous membranes (onset is 2 to 10 minutes and duration is 20 to 30 minutes), as required before direct laryngoscopy. Dyclonine has been used to provide topical anesthesia of the airway in a patient presumed to be allergic to bupivacaine and procaine (Bacon et al., 1997). The unique ketone structure of dyclonine makes cross-sensitivity with amide or ester local anesthetics unlikely.

Local Infiltration

Local infiltration anesthesia involves extravascular placement of local anesthetic in the area to be anesthetized. Subcutaneous injection of the local anesthetic in the area to be traversed for placement of an intravascular cannula is one example. Lidocaine is the local anesthetic most often selected for infiltration anesthesia. Infiltration of 0.25% ropivacaine or bupivacaine is equally effective in the management of pain at an inguinal operative site (Erichsen et al., 1995).

The duration of infiltration anesthesia can be approximately doubled by adding 1:200,000 epinephrine to the local anesthetic solution. Epinephrine-containing solutions, however, should not be injected intracutaneously or into tissues supplied by end-arteries (fingers, ears, and nose) because resulting vasoconstriction can produce ischemia and even gangrene.

Peripheral Nerve Block Anesthesia

Peripheral nerve block anesthesia is achieved by injection of local anesthetic solutions into tissues surrounding individual peripheral nerves or nerve plexuses such as the brachial plexus. When local anesthetic solutions are deposited in the vicinity of a peripheral nerve, they diffuse from the outer surface (mantle) toward the center (core) of the nerve along a concentration gradient (Winnie et al., 1977b). Consequently, nerve fibers located in the mantle of the mixed nerve are anesthetized first. These mantle fibers usually are distributed to more proximal anatomic structures in contrast to distal structures innervated by nerve fibers near the core of the nerve. This explains the initial development of anesthesia proximally, with subsequent distal spread as local anesthetic solution diffuses to reach more central core nerve fibers. Conversely, recovery of sensation occurs in a reverse direction; nerve fibers in the mantle that are exposed to extraneural fluid are the first to lose local anesthetic, so that sensation returns initially to the proximal and last to the distal parts of the limb.

Skeletal muscle paralysis may precede the onset of sensory anesthesia if motor nerve fibers are distributed peripheral to sensory fibers in the mixed peripheral nerve (Winnie et al., 1977a). Indeed, the sequence of onset and recovery from blockade of sympathetic, sensory, and motor nerve fibers in a mixed peripheral nerve depends as much on anatomic location of the nerve fibers within the mixed nerve as on their sensitivity to local anesthetics. This differs from results of in vitro studies on single nerve fibers, in which diffusion distance does not play a role. In an in vitro model, nerve fiber size is most important, with the onset of conduction blockade being inversely proportional to fiber size. For example, the smallest sensory and autonomic nervous system fibers are anesthetized first, followed by larger motor and proprioceptive axons.

The rapidity of onset of sensory anesthesia after injection of a local anesthetic solution into tissues around a peripheral nerve depends on the pK of the drug. The pK determines the amount of local anesthetic that exists in the active nonionized form at the pH of the tissue (see Table 7-1). For example, the onset of action of lidocaine occurs in approximately 3 minutes, whereas onset after injection of bupivacaine, levobupivacaine, or ropivacaine requires approximately 15 minutes, reflecting the greater fraction of lidocaine that exists in the lipid-soluble nonionized form. The onset and duration of sensory anesthesia for brachial plexus block produced by 0.5% bupivacaine, levobupivacaine, or ropivacaine is similar. Ropivacaine, 33 mL of a 0.5% solution used for performance of a subclavian perivascular block, produces a rapid onset of sensory anesthesia (about 4 minutes) with prolonged sensory (>13 hours) and motor blockade (Hickey et al., 1990). For ulnar nerve block, ropivacaine was found to be maximally effective at concentrations between 0.5% and 0.75%, and its onset and duration of action resembled those of bupivacaine (Nolte et al., 1990). Tetracaine, with a slow onset of anesthesia and a high potential to cause systemic toxicity, is not recommended for local infiltration or peripheral nerve block anesthesia.

Duration of peripheral nerve block anesthesia depends on the dose of local anesthetic, its lipid solubility, its degree of protein binding, and concomitant use of a vasoconstrictor such as epinephrine. The duration of action is prolonged more safely by epinephrine than by increasing the dose of local anesthetic, which also increases the likelihood of systemic toxicity. Bupivacaine combined with epinephrine may produce peripheral nerve block anesthesia lasting up to 14 hours. Conversely, not all reports document a prolongation of the duration of action when epinephrine is added to bupivacaine or ropivacaine (Niesel et al., 1993).

Intravenous Regional Anesthesia (Bier Block)

The IV injection of a local anesthetic solution into an extremity isolated from the rest of the systemic circulation by a tourniquet produces a rapid onset of anesthesia and skeletal muscle relaxation. The duration of anesthesia is independent of the specific local anesthetic and is determined by how long the tourniquet is kept inflated. The mechanism by which local anesthetics produce IV regional anesthesia is unknown but probably reflects action of the drug on nerve endings as well as nerve trunks. Normal sensation and skeletal muscle tone return promptly on release of the tourniquet, which allows blood flow to dilute the concentration of local anesthetic.

Ester and amide local anesthetics produce satisfactory effects when used for IV regional anesthesia. Lidocaine is the most frequently selected amide local anesthetic for producing this type of regional anesthesia. Alternatives to lidocaine include prilocaine, mepivacaine, and ropivacaine. The onset, duration, and quality of IV regional anesthesia produced by 50 ml of a 0.5% solution of lidocaine or prilocaine are similar, but plasma concentrations of prilocaine are lower than those of lidocaine after tourniquet deflation (Fig. 7-13) (Bader et al., 1988). The associated degree of methemoglobinemia (3% of hemoglobin as methemoglobin) seen with prilocaine is far below the level needed to produce cyanosis (10% hemoglobin as methemoglobin). The significantly lower plasma prilocaine concentrations after tourniquet deflation may indicate a greater margin of safety for prilocaine compared to lidocaine in terms of potential systemic toxicity. Mepivacaine 5 mg/kg provided superior analgesia to lidocaine 3 mg/kg when utilized for intravenous regional anesthesia (Prieto-Alvarez et al., 2002). Plasma concentrations of lidocaine decreased significantly in the first 60 minutes following

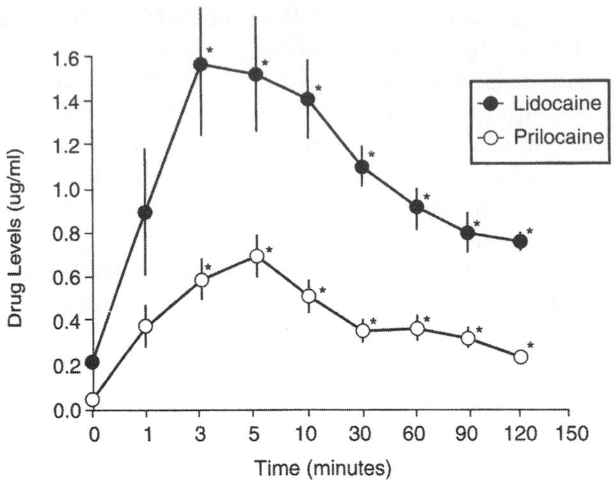

Figure 7-13. After tourniquet deflation, plasma concentrations of lidocaine exceed concentrations of prilocaine. (Mean ± SE; *$P < .05$.) (From Bader AM, Concepcion M, Hurley RJ, et al. Comparison of lidocaine and prilocaine for intravenous regional anesthesia. *Anesthesiology* 1988;69:409–412; with permission.)

tourniquet deflation, whereas blood concentrations of mepivacaine remained below toxic concentrations. Ropivacaine, 1.2 mg/kg and 1.8 mg/kg compared with lidocaine 3 mg/kg produced comparable intravenous regional anesthesia but residual analgesia was longer lasting with ropivacaine (Chan et al., 1999). Chloroprocaine is not selected for IV regional anesthesia because of a high incidence of thrombophlebitis. Bupivacaine is not recommended for IV regional anesthesia considering its greater likelihood than other local anesthetics for producing cardiotoxicity when the tourniquet is deflated at the conclusion of the anesthetic. Ropivacaine, although less likely to produce cardiotoxicity than bupivacaine, is not recommended for IV regional anesthesia.

Epidural Anesthesia

Local anesthetic solutions placed in the epidural or sacral caudal space produce epidural anesthesia by two presumed mechanisms. First, local anesthetic diffuses across the dura to act on nerve roots and the spinal cord as it does when injected directly into the lumbar subarachnoid space to produce spinal anesthesia. Second, local anesthetic also diffuses into the paravertebral area through the intervertebral foramina, producing multiple paravertebral nerve blocks. These slow diffusion processes account for the 15- to 30-minute delay in onset of sensory anesthesia after placement of local anesthetic solutions in the epidural space. Lidocaine is commonly used for epidural anesthesia because of its good diffusion capabilities through tissues. Despite a reasonable safety profile, bupivacaine is being replaced by levobupivacaine and ropivacaine, as these local anesthetics are associated with less risk for cardiac and central nervous system toxicity and are also less likely to result in unwanted postoperative motor blockade.

Bupivacaine and ropivacaine at similar concentrations (0.5% to 0.75%) produce similar prolonged sensory anesthesia (ropivacaine has a greater tendency to block A-delta and C fibers) when used for epidural anesthesia, but the motor anesthesia produced by ropivacaine is less intense and of shorter duration (Brown et al., 1990; Feldman and Covino, 1988). These characteristics of ropivacaine may be advantageous for obstetric patients in labor and for those experiencing acute and chronic pain. The addition of epinephrine 1:200,000 to 0.5% or 0.75% bupivacaine or ropivacaine does not appear to offer an advantage in terms of duration of action (Cederholm et al., 1994). Use of 1% ropivacaine may provide longer sensory anesthesia than 0.75% bupivacaine, whereas the motor block is similar (Niesel et al., 1993; Wood and Rubin, 1993). The lower systemic toxicity of ropivacaine compared with bupivacaine enables ropivacaine to be used for surgical anesthesia in concentrations up to 1% (McClure, 1996). For postoperative analgesia, the infusion of 0.2% ropivacaine at 6 to 10 mL/hour is effective (Erichsen et al., 1996). In children, there is no difference with regard to postoperative analgesia provided by bupivacaine, levobupivacaine, or ropivacaine but unwanted motor blockade was more frequent in patients receiving bupivacaine (Fig. 7-14) (Negri et al., 2004). Epidural analgesia or anesthesia for labor or cesarean delivery is similar with 0.5% bupivacaine or ropivacaine but the duration of motor block is shorter in parturients receiving ropivacaine (Alahuhta et al., 1995). Likewise, 0.25% ropivacaine and 0.25% bupivacaine administered as intermittent doses into the epidural space are equally efficacious in providing relief of labor pain (Muir et al., 1997). The conclusion is that ropivacaine and bupivacaine both provide excellent labor analgesia with no significant differences between the two drugs in the incidence of measured obstetric outcomes (Polley and Columb, 2003b). Increased plasma concentrations of local

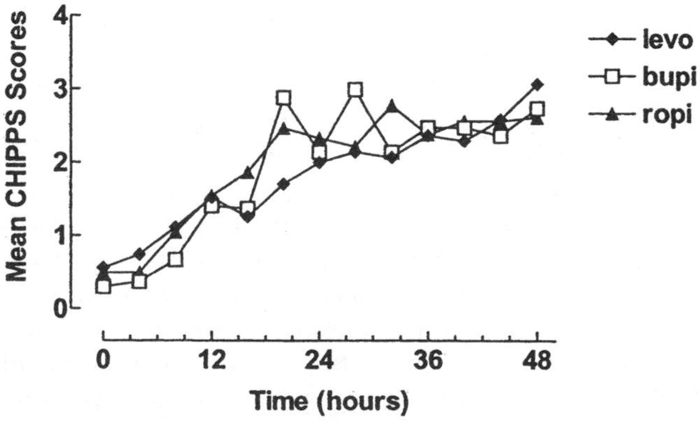

Figure 7-14. Mean postoperative pain scores (Children's and Infant's Postoperative Pain Score, CHIPPS) were similar in patients receiving epidural levobupivacaine (levo), bupivacaine (bupi) and ropivacaine (ropi) infusions. (From Negri PD, Ivani G, Tirri T et al. A comparison of epidural bupivacaine, levobupivacaine, and ropivacaine on postoperative analgesia and motor blockade. *Anesth Analg* 2004;99:45–48; with permission.)

anesthetics after epidural anesthesia are of special importance when this technique is used to provide anesthesia to the parturient. Local anesthetics cross the placenta and may produce detectable, although not necessarily adverse, effects on the fetus for 24 to 48 hours. The fetus and neonate are less able to metabolize mepivacaine, resulting in a prolonged elimination half-time compared with that of adults. Use of a more lipid-soluble and protein-bound local anesthetic such as bupivacaine may limit passage across the placenta to the fetus. Even low doses of lidocaine, such as those used for spinal anesthesia during labor, result in some systemic absorption, as reflected by the presence of lidocaine and its metabolites in neonatal urine for >36 hours (Kuhnert et al., 1986b). Conversely, bupivacaine is undetectable in neonatal plasma 24 hours after cesarean delivery using bupivacaine-induced spinal anesthesia (Kuhnert et al., 1987). Indeed, maternal plasma concentrations of bupivacaine in mothers of those neonates is approximately 5% of that level present after epidural anesthesia, and plasma umbilical vein concentrations are approximately 7% of those present after epidural anesthesia.

In contrast to spinal anesthesia, during epidural anesthesia, there often is not a zone of differential sympathetic nervous system blockade, and the zone of differential motor blockade may average up to four rather than two segments below the sensory level. Another difference from spinal anesthesia is the larger dose required to produce epidural anesthesia, leading to substantial systemic absorption of the local anesthetic. For example, peak plasma concentrations of lidocaine are 3 to 4 μg/mL after placement of 400 mg into the epidural space. Bupivacaine, 70 to 100 mg of 0.5% with 1:200,000 epinephrine placed in the epidural space, results in peak average plasma concentrations of 0.335 μg/mL occurring about 30 minutes after instillation of the local anesthetic (Reynolds, 1971). Peak plasma concentrations of bupivacaine near 1 μg/mL occur when epinephrine is not added to the local anesthetic solution placed in the epidural space. In this regard, addition of epinephrine to the local anesthetic solution may decrease systemic absorption of the local anesthetic by approximately one-third. The peak venous plasma concentration of ropivacaine is 1.3 μg/mL after epidural placement of 200 mg of the local anesthetic. Addition of 1:200,000 epinephrine solution decreases systemic absorption of ropivacaine by approximately one-third. Systemic absorption of epinephrine produces beta-adrenergic stimulation characterized by peripheral vasodilation, with resultant decreases in systemic blood pressure, even though cardiac output is increased by the inotropic and chronotropic effects of epinephrine.

Addition of opioids to local anesthetic solutions placed in the epidural or intrathecal space results in synergistic analgesia (Solomon and Gebhart, 1994). An exception to this analgesic synergy is 2-chloroprocaine, which appears to decrease the effectiveness of epidural opioids when administered with local anesthetic solutions placed into the epidural space (Coda et al., 1997). Combining local anesthetics and opioids for peripheral nerve blocks appears to be ineffective in altering the characteristics or results of the block.

Spinal Anesthesia

Spinal anesthesia is produced by injection of local anesthetic solutions into the lumbar subarachnoid space. Local anesthetic solutions placed into lumbar cerebrospinal fluid act on superficial layers of the spinal cord, but the principal site of action is the preganglionic fibers as they leave the spinal cord in the anterior rami. Because the concentration of local anesthetics in cerebrospinal fluid decreases as a function of distance from the site of injection, and because different types of nerve fibers differ in their sensitivity to the effects of local anesthetics, zones of differential anesthesia develop. Because preganglionic sympathetic nervous system fibers are blocked by concentrations of local anesthetics that are insufficient to affect sensory or motor fibers, the level of sympathetic nervous system denervation during spinal anesthesia extends approximately two spinal segments cephalad to the level of sensory anesthesia. For the same reasons, the level of motor anesthesia averages two segments below sensory anesthesia.

Dosages of local anesthetics used for spinal anesthesia vary according to the (a) height of the patient, which determines the volume of the subarachnoid space, (b) segmental level of anesthesia desired, and (c) duration of anesthesia desired. The total dose of local anesthetic administered for spinal anesthesia is more important than the concentration of drug or the volume of the solution injected. Tetracaine, lidocaine, bupivacaine, ropivacaine, and levobupivacaine are the local anesthetics most likely to be administered for spinal anesthesia.

Spinal anesthesia with lidocaine has been reported to produce a higher incidence of transient neurologic symptoms than spinal anesthesia produced by bupivacaine (see the section on Neurotoxicity). For these reasons, bupivacaine has been proposed as an alternative local anesthetic to lidocaine for spinal anesthesia (Carpenter, 1995; Drasner, 1997). If lidocaine is selected, it may be prudent to limit the dose to 60 mg (Drasner, 1997). Bupivacaine used for spinal anesthesia is more effective than tetracaine in preventing lower-extremity tourniquet pain during orthopedic surgery (Stewart et al., 1988). This effectiveness may reflect the ability of bupivacaine to produce greater frequency-dependent conduction blockade of fibers than does tetracaine. In parturients, the intrathecal placement of bupivacaine, 2.5 mg, plus sufentanil, 10 μg, provided labor analgesia and allowed the patients to continue to ambulate (Campbell et al., 1997). The addition of intrathecal fentanyl 5 μg provides a bupivacaine dose-sparing effect similar to that provided by 15 μg or 25 μg of fentanyl, resulting

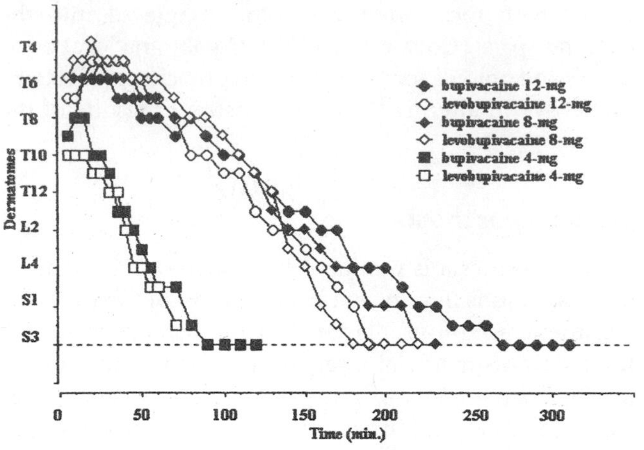

Figure 7-15. Recovery from sensory block occurs at a similar rate following spinal anesthesia produced with equipotent doses of bupivacaine and levobupivacaine. (From Alley EA, Kopacz DJ, McDonald SB et al. Hyperbaric spinal levobupivacaine: A comparison to racemic bupivacaine in volunteers. *Anesth Analg* 2002;94:188–193; with permission.)

in less pruritus but a shortening of the duration of action (Stocks et al., 2001).

Ropivacaine, 3 mL of 0.5% or 0.75%, produces sensory anesthesia, although complete motor blockade was present in only about 50% of patients receiving the lower dose (van Kleef et al., 1994). Ropivacaine is an acceptable local anesthetic to produce spinal anesthesia for cesarean section, and decreased lower extremity blockade compared with bupivacaine may be a desirable feature (Halpern et al., 2003; Khaw et al., 2001). Levobupivacaine has equivalent clinical efficacy to bupivacaine for spinal anesthesia (Fig. 7-15) (Alley et al., 2002). Dibucaine is 1.5 to 2.0 times as potent as tetracaine when used for spinal anesthesia. In the past, chloroprocaine was not recommended for placement in the subarachnoid space because of potential neurotoxicity (Covino et al., 1980; Ravindran et al., 1980; Reisner et al., 1980). However, preservative-free 2-chloroprocaine solutions (2% and 3%) are available for intrathecal injection ("off label use") and have been shown to produce reliable sensory and motor blockade with a short duration and little or no risk of transient neurologic symptoms, making this local anesthetic an attractive selection for outpatient surgical procedures performed under spinal anesthesia (Fig. 7-16) (Drasner, 2005; Kouri and Kopacz, 2004).

The specific gravity of local anesthetic solutions injected into the lumbar cerebrospinal fluid is important in determining spread of the drugs. Addition of glucose to local anesthetic solutions increases the specific gravity of local anesthetic solutions above that of cerebrospinal fluid (hyperbaric). Addition of distilled water lowers the specific gravity of local anesthetic solutions below that of cerebrospinal fluid (hypobaric). Cerebrospinal fluid does not contain significant amounts of cholinesterase enzyme; therefore, the duration of action of ester local anesthetics as well as amides placed in the subarachnoid space depends on systemic absorption of the drug.

Injected intrathecally, tetracaine produces a significant increase in spinal cord blood flow, an effect that can be prevented or reversed by epinephrine (Kozody et al., 1985). Vasodilation is less prominent with lidocaine, and bupivacaine produces vasoconstriction. Predictably, vasoconstrictors appear to be most effective in prolonging tetracaine-induced spinal anesthesia (up to 100%) and less effective at prolonging lidocaine spinal anesthesia, whereas the effect on bupivacaine spinal anesthesia remains controversial and is, at best, minimal.

Physiologic Effects

The goal of spinal anesthesia is to provide sensory anesthesia and skeletal muscle relaxation. It is the accompanying level of sympathetic nervous system blockade, however, that produces physiologic alterations. Plasma concentrations of local anesthetics after subarachnoid injection are too low to produce physiologic changes.

Cardiac Arrest

Cardiac arrest may accompany hypotension and bradycardia associated with spinal anesthesia (Aurory et al., 1997; Lee et al., 2004; Liu and McDonald, 2001; Pollard, 2001). The incidence of hypotension is about 33%, and the incidence of bradycardia approximates 13% in nonobstetric populations. Risk factors for hypotension include sensory anesthesia above T5 and baseline systolic blood pressure of <120 mm Hg. Risk factors for bradycardia include sensory anesthesia above T5, baseline heart rate <60 beats/minute, prolonged P-R interval on the electrocardiogram, and concomitant treatment with beta-blocking drugs. Common features of cardiac arrest in patients receiving spinal anesthesia have included administration of sedation to produce a sleep-like state without spontaneous verbalization and lack of early administration of epinephrine. Even

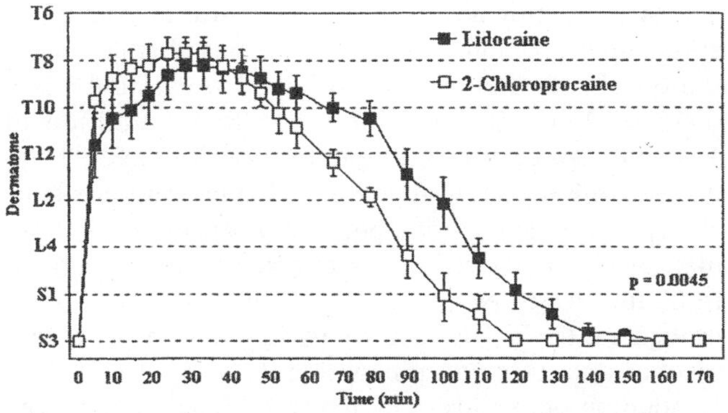

Figure 7-16. Recovery of sensory block is more rapid following spinal anesthesia produced with 2-chlorporocaine than with lidocaine. (From Kouri ME and Kopacz DJ. Spinal 2-chlorporcaine: a comparison with lidocaine in volunteers. *Anesth Analg* 2004;98: 75–80; with permission.)

when therapy is promptly administered, patients may be refractory to treatment, because local anesthetic-induced sympathetic nervous system blockade, which decreases circulating blood volume, may also cause a defective neuroendocrine response to stress. Even early administration of epinephrine in patients being previously monitored with pulse oximetry and capnography may not guarantee a good outcome following neuraxial cardiac arrest (Lee et al., 2004).

Sympathetic nervous system blockade results in arteriolar dilatation, but systemic blood pressure does not decrease proportionally because of compensatory vasoconstriction in areas with intact sympathetic nervous system innervation. Compensatory vasoconstriction occurs principally in the upper extremities and does not involve the cerebral vasculature. Even with total sympathetic nervous system blockade produced by spinal anesthesia, the decrease in systemic vascular resistance is <15%. This change is minimal because smooth muscles of arterioles retain intrinsic tone and do not dilate maximally.

The most important cardiovascular responses produced by spinal anesthesia are those that result from changes in the venous circulation. Unlike arterioles denervated by sympathetic nervous system blockade, venules do not maintain intrinsic tone and thus dilate maximally during spinal anesthesia. The resulting increased vascular capacitance decreases venous return to the heart, leading to decreases in cardiac output and systemic blood pressure. The physiologic effect of spinal anesthesia on venous return emphasizes the risk of extreme systemic hypotension if this technique is instituted in hypovolemic patients. Blockade of preganglionic cardiac accelerator fibers (T1 to T4) results in heart rate slowing, particularly if decreased venous return and central venous pressure decrease the stimulation of intrinsic stretch receptors in the right atrium (Bezold Jarisch reflex). For example, heart rate will increase with a head-down position that increases venous return and central venous pressure so as to stimulate these receptors. During spinal anesthesia, myocardial oxygen requirements are decreased as a result of decreased heart rate, venous return, and systemic blood pressure.

Apnea

Apnea that occurs with an excessive level of spinal anesthesia probably reflects ischemic paralysis of the medullary ventilatory centers due to profound hypotension and associated decreases in cerebral blood flow. Concentrations of local anesthetics in ventricular cerebrospinal fluid are usually too low to produce pharmacologic effects on the ventilatory centers. Rarely is the cause of apnea due to phrenic nerve paralysis.

Analgesia

Lidocaine and procaine have been demonstrated to produce intense analgesia when injected IV. Use of local anesthetics for this purpose, however, is limited by the small margin of safety between IV analgesic doses and those that produce systemic toxicity. Nevertheless, continuous low-dose infusion of lidocaine to maintain a plasma concentration of 1 to 2 μg/mL decreases the severity of postoperative pain and decreases requirements for opioids without producing systemic toxicity (Cassuto et al., 1985). Lidocaine administered IV also decreases anesthetic requirements for volatile drugs (DiFazio et al., 1976). Lidocaine may also be administered IV in the perioperative period as a cough suppressant. In this regard, the cough reflex during intubation of the trachea is suppressed by plasma concentrations of lidocaine >2 μg/mL (Yukioka et al., 1985). Stump pain (neuromas) but not phantom pain (cortical reorganization) following amputation is diminished by intravenous administration of lidocaine (Wu et al., 2002).

Suppression of Ventricular Cardiac Dysrhythmias

In addition to suppressing ventricular cardiac dysrhythmias (see Chapter 17), the IV administration of lidocaine may increase the defibrillation threshold. Failure to recognize this effect could lead to unnecessary revision of the lead system of an implantable cardioverter defibrillator (Peters et al., 1997).

Suppression of Grand Mal Seizures

Grand mal seizures have been suppressed by IV administration of low doses of lidocaine or mepivacaine. Presumably, these and perhaps other local anesthetics, when present at low plasma concentrations, are effective in suppressing seizures through initial depression of hyperexcitable cortical neurons. Nevertheless, inhibitory neurons are usually more sensitive to depressant actions of local anesthetics than are excitatory neurons, and excitatory phenomena predominate.

Antiinflammatory Effects

Local anesthetics modulate inflammatory responses and may be useful in mitigating perioperative inflammatory injury (Hollmann and Durieux, 2000). For example, overreactive inflammatory responses that destroy rather than protect are critical in the development of several perioperative phenomena including postoperative pain, adult respiratory distress syndrome, systemic inflammatory response syndrome, and multiple organ failure. Beneficial effects attributed to epidural anesthesia (pain relief, decreased thrombosis from hypercoagulability) may reflect antiinflammatory effects of local anesthetics. Adverse effects of local anesthetic-induced antiinflammatory effects include retardation of wound healing and increased risk of infection. Nevertheless, there is evidence that local anesthetics also possess significant antibacterial effects (tetracaine > bupivacaine >lidocaine) (Pere et al., 1999).

Mechanism

Antiinflammatory effects of local anesthetics are not dependent on the sodium ion channel blockade that is responsible for the anesthetic effects of these drugs. Local anesthetics may modulate inflammatory responses by inhibiting inflammatory mediator signaling. For example, local anesthetics inhibit platelet-activating factor (an inflammatory mediator), which is an established signaling mechanism in early acute respiratory distress syndrome, a typical postoperative inflammatory disorder (Hollmann et al., 2001b). Many of the mediators (thrombin, thromboxane, platelet activating factor, and interleukins) of the inflammatory and hemostatic systems act through G-protein–coupled receptors. Local anesthetics may inhibit G proteins, resulting in antiinflammatory effects (Hollmann et al., 2002). In addition, local anesthetics inhibit neutrophil accumulation at sites of inflammation and impair free radical and mediator release (Kiefer et al., 2003). Local anesthetics in clinically relevant concentrations inhibit superoxide anion production of platelet-activating factor–primed neutrophils (Hollmann et al., 2001a). Priming is the process whereby the response of neutrophils to a subsequent activating stimulus is potentiated. Levobupivacaine is more effective than bupivacaine and other local anesthetics in suppressing neutrophil priming (Hollmann et al., 2003). Decreased generation of reactive oxygen radicals is associated with decreases in ischemic damage after myocardial infarction.

Bronchodilation

Inhaled lidocaine and ropivacaine attenuate histamine-induced bronchospasm and induce airway anesthesia. This response most likely reflects topical airway anesthesia, as bronchial reactivity is inhibited at plasma concentrations that are lower than those needed to attenuate bronchial reactivity. Nevertheless, dyclonine, a longer lasting and more intense local anesthetic, does not reliably attenuate bronchial hyper-reactivity, suggesting that other properties of local anesthetics may be important (Groeben et al., 2001).

Tumescent Liposuction

Tumescent technique for liposuction characterizes the subcutaneous infiltration of large volumes (5 or more liters) of solution containing highly diluted lidocaine (0.05% to 0.10%) with epinephrine (1:100,000). The taut stretching of overlying blanched skin by the large volume of solution and epinephrine-induced vasoconstriction is the origin of the term, tumescent technique.

The result is sufficient local anesthesia for the liposuction, virtually bloodless aspirates, and prolonged postoperative analgesia. Slow and sustained release of lidocaine into the circulation is associated with plasma concentrations $<1.5\ \mu g/mL$ that peak 12 to 14 hours after injection and then decline gradually over the next 6 to 14 hours (Klein, 1990). Plasma concentrations of epinephrine peak at 3 to 5 times the upper normal limits approximately 3 hours following injection of the solution and return to normal after about 12 hours (Burk et al, 1996).

The recommended adult dose of lidocaine with epinephrine for regional anesthesia is about 7 mg/kg. When highly diluted lidocaine solutions are administered for tumescent liposuction, the dose of lidocaine may range from 35 mg/kg to 55 mg/kg ("mega-dose lidocaine") (Ostad et al., 1996). It is estimated that 1 g of subcutaneous tissue can absorb up to 1 mg of lidocaine ("tissue buffering system"). The injection of additional undiluted lidocaine for concomitant cosmetic procedures must be considered in estimating the likely plasma concentrations of lidocaine that will occur.

Despite the popularity and presumed safety of tumescent liposuction, there are reports of increased mortality associated with this technique (greater than mortality associated with automobile accidents) (Rao et al., 1999). Causes of death may include lidocaine toxicity or local anesthetic-induced depression of cardiac conduction and contractility.

COCAINE TOXICITY

Cocaine produces sympathetic nervous system stimulation by blocking the presynaptic uptake of norepinephrine and dopamine, thus increasing their postsynaptic concentrations. Because of this blocking effect, dopamine remains at high concentrations in the synapse and continues to affect adjacent neurons, producing the characteristic cocaine "high" (Mendelson and Mello, 1996; Leshner, 1996). Chronic exposure to cocaine is postulated to affect adversely dopaminergic function in the brain due to dopamine depletion.

Pharmacokinetics

Once cocaine is absorbed, the pharmacokinetics, regardless of the route of administration, are similar (Hatsukami and Fischman, 1996). Conversely, the route of administration is important in the rate of onset as well as the intensity and duration of cocaine's effects. For example, peak venous plasma concentrations of cocaine are achieved at approximately 30 to 40 minutes after intranasal administration and approximately 5 minutes after IV and smoked cocaine administration. The maximum physiologic effects of intranasal cocaine occur within 15 to 40 minutes, and the maximum subjective effects occur within 10 to 20 minutes. The duration of effects is approximately 60 minutes or longer after peak effects. The subjective effects occur within minutes of IV or smoked cocaine use, and the duration of effect is approximately 30 to 45 minutes. The elimination half-time of cocaine is 60 to 90 minutes, and metabolism is principally by plasma esterases (see the section on Metabolism of Local Anesthetics). Urinary excretion of unchanged cocaine (<1% of the total dose) and metabolites (benzoylecgonine and ecgonine methyl ester representing about 65% of the dose) is similar regardless of the route of administration.

Adverse Physiologic Effects

Acute cocaine administration is known to cause coronary vasospasm, myocardial ischemia, myocardial infarction, and ventricular cardiac dysrhythmias, including ventricular fibrillation (Hollander et al., 1995). Associated hypertension and tachycardia further increase myocardial oxygen requirements at a time when coronary oxygen delivery is decreased by the effects of cocaine on coronary blood flow. Even remote cocaine use can result in myocardial ischemia and hypotension for as long as 6 weeks after discontinuing cocaine use (Weicht and Bernards, 1996; Nademanee et al., 1989). Presumably, delayed episodes of myocardial ischemia are due to cocaine-induced coronary artery vasospasm. In animals, chronic cocaine exposure sensitizes the left anterior descending coronary artery to catecholamines, even in the absence of circulating cocaine. Excessive sensitivity of the coronary vasculature to catecholamines after chronic exposure to cocaine may be due in part to cocaine-induced depletion of dopamine activity. Cocaine-abusing parturients are at higher risk for interim peripartum events such as hypertension, hypotension, and wheezing episodes (Kain et al., 1996). Cocaine produces dose-dependent decreases in uterine blood flow that result in fetal hypoxemia (Woods et al., 1987). Cocaine may produce hyperpyrexia, which could contribute to seizures. Unexpected patient agitation in the perioperative period may reflect the effects of cocaine ingestion (Bernards and Teijeiro, 1996). There is a temporal relationship between the recreational use of cocaine and cerebrovascular accidents (Levine et al., 1989).

Administration of topical cocaine plus epinephrine, or the presence of volatile anesthetics that sensitize the myocardium, may exaggerate the cardiac-stimulating effects of cocaine. Cocaine should be used with caution, if at all, in patients with hypertension or coronary artery disease and in patients receiving drugs that potentiate the effects of catecholamines, such as monoamine oxidase inhibitors.

Treatment

Nitroglycerin has been used to treat cocaine-induced myocardial ischemia (Hollander et al., 1994). Although esmolol has been recommended to treat tachycardia due to cocaine overdose, there is also evidence that beta-adrenergic blockade accentuates coronary artery vasospasm in the setting of acute cocaine overdose (Lange et al., 1990; Pollan and Tadjziechy, 1989). Whether beta-adrenergic blockade is harmful for coronary vasospasm in the setting of chronic cocaine use is not known. Furthermore, administration of beta-blocking drugs in the presence of catecholamine-induced hypertension and tachycardia has been associated with profound cardiovascular collapse and cardiac arrest that is unresponsive to aggressive cardiopulmonary resuscitation (Gourdine et al., 2000). In this situation, administration of a vasodilating drug such as nitroprusside may be the safest intervention. Alpha-adrenergic blockade may be effective in treatment of coronary vasoconstriction due to cocaine, but in the presence of hypotension this intervention is questionable. IV administration of a benzodiazepine such as diazepam is effective for control of seizures associated with cocaine toxicity.

REFERENCES

Adejepon-Yamoah KK, Scott DB, Prescott LF. Impaired absorption and metabolism of oral lignocaine in patients undergoing laparoscopy. *Br J Anaesth* 1973;45:143–147.

Alahuhta S, Rasanen J, Jouppila P, et al. The effects of epidural ropivacaine and bupivacaine for cesarean section on uteroplacental and fetal circulation. *Anesthesiology* 1995;83:23–32.

Albright GA. Cardiac arrest following regional anesthesia with etidocaine or bupivacaine [editorial]. *Anesthesiology* 1979;51: 285–287.

Alley EA, Kopacz DJ, McDonald, et al. Hyperbaric spinal levobupivacaine: a comparison to racemic bupivacaine in volunteers. *Anesth Analg* 2002:94:188–193.

Arevalo MI, Escribano E, Calpena A, et al. Rapid skin anesthesia using a new topical amethocaine formulation: a preclinical study. *Anesth Analg* 2004;98:1407–1412.

Atlee JL, Bosnjak ZJ. Mechanisms for dysrhythmias during anesthesia. *Anesthesiology* 1990;72:347–374.

Bacon GS, Lyons TR, Wood SH. Dyclonine hydrochloride for airway anesthesia: awake endotracheal intubation in a patient with suspected local anesthetic allergy. *Anesthesiology* 1997;86: 1206–1207.

Bader AM, Concepcion M, Hurley RJ, et al. Comparison of lidocaine and prilocaine for intravenous regional anesthesia. *Anesthesiology* 1988; 69:409–412.

Benowitz N, Forsyth RP, Melmon KL, et al. Lidocaine disposition kinetics in monkey and man. I: prediction by a perfusion model. *Clin Pharmacol Ther* 1974;16:87–92.

Bernards CM, Teijeiro A. Illicit cocaine ingestion during anesthesia. *Anesthesiology* 1996;84:218–220.

Biehl D, Shnider SM, Levinson G, et al. Placental transfer of lidocaine: effects of fetal acidosis. *Anesthesiology* 1978;48:409–412.

Bowdle TA, Freund PR, Slattery JT. Propranolol reduces bupivacaine clearance. *Anesthesiology* 1987;66:36–38.

Brown DL, Carpenter RL, Thompson GE. Comparison of 0.5% ropivacaine and 0.5% bupivacaine for epidural anesthesia in patients undergoing lower extremity surgery. *Anesthesiology* 1990;72: 633–636.

Brown DL, Ransom DM, Hall JA, et al. Regional anesthesia, and local anesthetic-induced systemic toxicity: seizure frequency and accompanying cardiovascular changes. *Anesth Analg* 1995;81:321–328.

Brown DT, Beamsih D, Wildsmith JAW. Allergic reaction to an amide local anaesthetic. *Br J Anaesth* 1981;53:435–437.

Burk RW, Guzman-Stein G, Vasconez LO. Lidocaine and epinephrine levels in tumescent technique liposuction. *Plast Reconstr Surg* 1996;97:1379–1384.

Burm AG, van der Meer AD, van Kleef JW, et al. Pharmacokinetics of the enantiomers of bupivacaine following intravenous administration of the racemate. *Br J Clin Pharmacol* 1994;38:125–129.

Burm AGL, Cohen IMC, van Kleef JW, et al. Pharmacokinetics of the enantiomers of mepivacaine after intravenous administration of the racemate in volunteers. *Anesth Analg* 1997;84:85-89.

Butterworth JF, Brownlow RC, Leith JP, et al. Bupivacaine inhibits cyclic-3',5'-adenosine monophosphate production: a possible contributing factor to cardiovascular toxicity. *Anesthesiology* 1993; 79:88–95.

Butterworth JF, James RL, Grimes J. Structure-affinity relationships and stereospecificity of several homologous series of local anesthetics for the B_2-adrenergic receptor. *Anesth Analg* 1997;85: 336–342.

Butterworth JF, Strichartz GR. Molecular mechanisms of local anesthesia: a review. *Anesthesiology* 1990;72:722–734.

Campbell DC, Banner R, Crone LA, et al. Addition of epinephrine to intrathecal bupivacaine and sufentanil for ambulatory labor analgesia. *Anesthesiology* 1997;86:525–531.

Carpenter RL, Smith HS, Bridenbaugh LD. Epinephrine increases the effectiveness of tetracaine spinal anesthesia. *Anesthesiology* 1989; 71:33–36.

Carpenter RL. Hyperbaric lidocaine spinal anesthesia: do we need an alternative? *Anesth Analg* 1995;81:1125–1128.

Cassuto J, Wallin G, Hogstrom S, et al. Inhibition of postoperative pain by continuous low-dose intravenous infusion of lidocaine. *Anesth Analg* 1985;64:971–974.

Cederholm I, Anskar S, Bengtsson M. Sensory, motor, and sympathetic block during epidural analgesia with 0.5% and 0.75% ropivacaine with and without epinephrine. *Reg Anesth* 1994;19:18–33.

Chan V, Weisbrod M, Kaszas Z, et al. Comparison of ropivacaine and lidocaine for intravenous regional anesthesia in volunteers: a preliminary study on anesthetic efficacy and blood level. *Anesthesiology* 1999;90:1602–1608.

Chazalon P, Tourtier JP, Villevielle T, et al. Ropivacaine-induced cardiac arrest after peripheral nerve block: successful resuscitation. *Anesthesiology* 2003;99:1449–1451.

Cheng ACK. Intended epidural anesthesia as possible cause of cauda equina syndrome. *Anesth Analg* 1994;78:157–159.

Chestnut DH, Geiger M, Bates JN, Choi WW. The influence of pH-adjusted 2-chloroprocaine on the quality and duration of subsequent epidural bupivacaine analgesia during labor: a randomized, double blind study. *Anesthesiology* 1989;70:437–441.

Christie JM, Valdes C, Markowsky SJ. Neurotoxicity of lidocaine combined with mexiletine. *Anesth Analg* 1993;77:1291–1294.

Clarkson CW, Hondeghem LM. Mechanism for bupivacaine depression of cardiac conduction: fast block of sodium channels during the action potential with slow recovery from block during diastole. *Anesthesiology* 1985;62:396–405.

Coda B, Bausch S, Haas M, et al. The hypothesis that antagonism of fentanyl analgesia by 2-chloroprocaine is mediated by direct action on opioid receptors. *Reg Anesth* 1997;22:43–48.

Covino BG, Marx GF, Finster M, et al. Prolonged sensory/motor deficits following inadvertent spinal anesthesia [editorial]. *Anesth Analg* 1980;59:399–400.

Covino BG, Wildsmith JAW. Clinical pharmacology of local anesthetic agents. In: Cousins MJ, Bridenbaugh PO (eds). *Neural blockade in clinical anesthesia and management of pain*. Philadelphia. Lippincott-Raven, 1998:97–128.

Crews JC, Rothman TE. Seizure after levobupivacaine for interscalene brachial plexus block. *Anesth Analg* 2003;96:1188–1190.

Curatolo M, Petersen-Felix S, Arendt-Nielsen L, et al. Adding sodium bicarbonate to lidocaine enhances the depth of epidural blockade. *Anesth Analg* 1998;86:341–346.

Datta S, Lambert DH, Gergus J, et al. Differential sensitivities of mammalian nerve fibers during pregnancy. *Anesth Analg* 1983;62: 1070–1072.

Dauphin A, Gupta RN, Young JEM, et al. Serum bupivacaine concentrations during continuous extrapleural infusion. *Can J Anaesth* 1997;44:367–370.

de Jong RH. Last round for a "heavyweight"? *Anesth Analg* 1994; 78:3–4.

Denson DD, Coyle DE, Santos D, et al. Bupivacaine protein binding in the term parturient. Effects of lactic acidosis. *Clin Pharmacol Ther* 1984;35:409–415.

Denson DD. Physiology and pharmacology of local anesthetics. In Sinatra RS, Hord AH, Ginsberg B, Preble LM (eds.): *Acute pain. mechanisms and management*. St Louis, Mosby Year Book, 1992:124

DiFazio CA, Niederlehner JR, Burney RG. The anesthetic potency of lidocaine in the rat. *Anesth Analg* 1976;55:818–821.

Douglas MJ. Neurotoxicity of lidocaine—does it exist? *Can J Anaesth* 1995;42:181–185.

Drasner K. Lidocaine spinal anesthesia: a vanishing therapeutic index? *Anesthesiology* 1997;87:469–472.

Drasner K. Chloroprocaine spinal anesthesia: Back to the future? *Anesth Analg* 2005;100:549–552.

Duncan L, Wildsmith JAW. Liposomal local anesthetics. *Br J Anaesth* 1995;75:260–261.

Ehrlich GE. Racemic mixtures: harmless or potentially toxic? *Am J Hosp Pharm* 1992;49:S15–S18.

Eisenach JC. Regional anesthesia: vintage bordeaux (and Napa valley). *Anesthesiology* 1997;87:467–469.

Erichsen CJ, Sjovall J, Kehlet H, et al. Pharmacokinetics and analgesic effect of ropivacaine during continuous epidural infusion for postoperative pain relief. *Anesthesiology* 1996;84:834–842.

Erichsen CJ, Vibits H, Dahl JB, et al. Wound infiltration with ropivacaine and bupivacaine for pain after inguinal herniotomy. *Acta Anaesthesiol Scand* 1995;39:67–70.

Feldman HS, Covino BG. Comparative motor-blocking effects of bupivacaine and ropivacaine, a new amino amide local anesthetic in the rat and dog. *Anesth Analg* 1988;67:1047–1052.

Fischer LG, Bremer M, Coleman EJ, et al. Local anesthetics attenuate lysophosphatidic acid-induced priming in human neutrophils. *Anesth Analg* 2001;92:1041–1047.

Foster RH, Markham A. Levobupivacaine: a review of its pharmacology and use as a local anesthetic. *Drugs* 2000;59:551–559.

Gajraj NM, Pennant JH, Watcha MF. Eutectic mixture of local anesthetics (EMLA) cream. *Anesth Analg* 1994;78:574–583.

Gerancher JC. Cauda equina syndrome following a single spinal administration of 5% hyperbaric lidocaine through a 25-gauge Whitacre needle. *Anesthesiology* 1997;87:687–689.

Gourdine SB, Hollinger I, Jones J, et al. New York state guidelines on the topical use of phenylephrine in the operating room. *Anesthesiology* 2000;92:859–864.

Groban L, Deal DD, Vernon JC, et al. Cardiac resuscitation after incremental overdosage with lidocaine, bupivacaine, levobupivacaine, and ropivacaine in anesthetized dogs. *Anesth Analg* 2001;92: 37–43.

Groeben H, GroBendts T, Silvanus M-T, et al. Airway anesthesia alone does not explain attenuation of histamine-induced bronchospasm by local anesthetics. A comparison of lidocaine, ropivacaine, and dyclonine. *Anesthesiology* 2001;94:423–428.

Gross JB, Caldwell CB, Shaw LM, et al. The effect of lidocaine infusion on the ventilatory response to hypoxia. *Anesthesiology* 1984;61: 662–665.

Halpern SH, Breen TW, Campbell DC, et al. A multicenter, randomized, controlled trial comparing bupivacaine with ropivacaine for labor analgesia. *Anesthesiology* 2003;98:1431–1435.

Hampl KF, Schneider MC, Pargger H, et al. A similar incidence of transient neurologic symptoms after spinal anesthesia with 2% and 5% lidocaine. *Anesth Analg* 1996;83:1051–1054.

Hatsukami DK, Fischman MW. Crack cocaine and cocaine hydrochloride. Are the differences myth or reality? *JAMA* 1996;276: 1580–1588.

Hickey R, Candido KD, Ramamurthy S, et al. Brachial plexus block with a new local anesthetic: 0.5 percent ropivacaine. *Can J Anaesth* 1990;37:732–738.

Hiller A, Rosenberg PH. Transient neurological symptoms after spinal anaesthesia with 4% mepivacaine and 0.5% bupivacaine. *Br J Anaesth* 1997;79:301–305.

Hodgson PS, Neal JM, Pollock JE et al. The neurotoxicity of drugs given intrathecally (spinal). *Anesth Analg* 1999;88:797–809.

Hollander J, Hoffman R, Gennis P, et al. Nitroglycerine in the treatment of cocaine associated chest pain—clinical safety and efficacy. *Clinical Toxicol* 1994;32:243–256.

Hollander JE, Hoffman RS, Burstein JL, Shih RD, Thode HC Jr. Cocaine-associated myocardial infarction. Mortality and complications. Cocaine-Associated Myocardial Infarction Study Group. *Arch Intern Med* 1995;155:1081–1086.

Hollmann MW, Durieux ME. Local anesthetics and the inflammatory response: a new therapeutic indication? *Anesthesiology* 2000;93: 858–875.

Hollmann MW, Gross G, Jelecin N, et al. Local anesthetic effects on priming and activation of human neutrophils. *Anesthesiology* 2001b;95:113–122.

Hollmann MW, Kurz K, Herroeder S, et al. The effects of S (−)-, R(+)-, and racemic bupivacaine on lysophosphatidate-induced priming of human neutrophils. *Anesth Analg* 2003;97:1053-1058.

Hollmann MW, McIntire WE, Garrison JC, et al. Inhibition of mammalian Gq protein function by local anesthetics. *Anesthesiology* 2002;97:1451–1457.

Hollmann MW, Wieczorek KS, Berger A, et al. Local anesthetic inhibition of G protein-couples receptor signaling by interference with Galpha(q) function. *Mol Pharmacol* 2001a;59:294–299.

Horlocker TT, McGregor DG, Matsushige DK, et al. A retrospective review of 4767 consecutive spinal anesthetics: central nervous system complications. *Anesth Analg* 1997;84:578–584.

Huang YF, Pryor ME, Mather LE, et al. Cardiovascular and central nervous system effects of intravenous levobupivacaine and bupivacaine in sheep. *Anesth Analg* 1998;86:797–802.

Hymes JA, Spraker MK. Racial differences in the effectiveness of a topically applied mixture of local anesthetics. *Reg Anesth* 1986;11: 11–13.

Inoue R, Suganuma T, Echizen H, et al. Plasma concentrations of lidocaine and its principal metabolites during intermittent epidural anesthesia. *Anesthesiology* 1985;63:304–310.

Jakobson B, Nilsson A. Methemoglobinemia associated with a prilocaine-lidocaine cream and trimethoprim-sulphamethoxazole. A case report. *Acta Anaesthesiol Scand* 1985;29:453–455.

Jorfeldt L, Lewis DH, Lofstrom JB, et al. Lung uptake of lidocaine in man. *Reg Anesth* 1980;5:6–7.

Kain ZN, Mayes LC, Ferris CA, et al. Cocaine-abusing parturients undergoing cesarean section. A cohort study. *Anesthesiology* 1996;85:1028–1035.

Kaplan JA, Miller ED, Gallagher EG. Postoperative analgesia for thoracotomy patients. *Anesth Analg* 1975;54:773–777.

Kasten GW, Martin ST. Bupivacaine cardiovascular toxicity: comparison of treatment with bretylium and lidocaine. *Anesth Analg* 1985;64:911–916.

Katz NP, Shapiro DE, Herrmann TE, et al. Rapid onset of cutaneous anesthesia with EMLA cream after pretreatment with a new ultrasound-emitting device. *Anesth Analg* 2004;98:371–376.

Kendig JJ. Clinical implications of the modulated receptor hypothesis: local anesthetics and the heart [editorial]. *Anesthesiology* 1985;62: 382–384.

Khaw KS, Kee WDN, Wong EL, et al. Spinal ropivacaine for cesarean section. A dose-finding study. *Anesthesiology* 2001;95:1346-1350.

Kuboyoma N, Nakoa S, Moriya Y et al. Bupivacaine-included Ca^{2+} release on intracellular Ca^{2+} stores in rat DRG neurons. *Jpn J Pharmacol* 1997;73:98–103.

Kiefer R-T, Ploppa A, Krueger WA, et al. Local anesthetics impair human granulocyte phagocytosis activity, oxidative burst, and CD11b expression in response to *Staphylococcus aureus*. *Anesthesiology* 2003;98:842–848.

Kirkpatrick MB, Sanders RV, Bass JB. Physiologic effects and serum lidocaine concentrations after inhalation of lidocaine from a compressed gas-powered nebulizer. *Am Rev Respir Dis* 1987;136: 447–449.

Klein JA. Tumescent technique for regional anesthesia permits lidocaine doses of 35 mg/kg for liposuction. *J Dermatol Surg Oncol* 1990;16:248–263.

Klein SM, Pierce T, Rubin Y, et al. Successful resuscitation after ropivacaine-induced ventricular fibrillation. *Anesth Analg* 2003;97: 901–903.

Kotelko DM, Shnider SM, Dailey PA, et al. Bupivacaine-induced cardiac arrhythmias in sheep. *Anesthesiology* 1984;60:10–18.

Kouri M, Kopacz DJ. Spinal 2-chloroprocaine: a comparison with lidocaine in volunteers. *Anesth Analg* 2004;98:75–80.

Kozody R, Palahniuk RJ, Cumming MO. Spinal cord blood flow following subarachnoid tetracaine. *Can J Anaesth* 1985;32:23–29.

Kozody R, Palahniuk RJ, Wade JG, et al. The effect of subarachnoid epinephrine and phenylephrine on spinal cord blood flow. *Can Anaesth Soc J* 1984;31:503–507.

Kuhnert BR, Kuhnert PM, Philipson EH, et al. The half-life of 2-chloroprocaine. *Anesth Analg* 1986a;65:273–278.

Kuhnert BR, Philipson EH, Pimental R, et al. Lidocaine disposition in mother, fetus, and neonate after spinal anesthesia. *Anesth Analg* 1986b;65:139–144.

Kuhnert BR, Zuspan KJ, Kuhnert PM, et al. Bupivacaine disposition in mother, fetus, and neonate after spinal anesthesia for caesarean section. *Anesth Analg* 1987;66:407–412.

Kuipers JA, Boer F, de Roode A, et al. Modeling population pharmacokinetics of lidocaine. Should cardiac output be included as a patient factor? *Anesthesiology* 2001;94:566–573.

Lambert DH, Hurley RJ. Cauda equina syndrome and continuous spinal anesthesia. *Anesth Analg* 1991;72:817–819.

Lange R, Cigarroa R, Flores E, et al. Potentiation of cocaine-induced coronary vasoconstriction by beta-adrenergic blockade. *Ann Intern Med* 1990;112:897–903.

Lange RA, Cigarroa RG, Yancy CW, et al. Cocaine-induced coronary artery vasoconstriction. *N Engl J Med* 1989;321:1557–1562.

Lee LA, Posner KL, Domino KB, et al. Injuries associated with regional anesthesia in the 1980s and 1990s: a closed claims analysis. *Anesthesiology* 2004;101:143–152.

Lee-Son S, Wang GK, Concus A, et al. Stereoselective inhibition of neuronal sodium channels by local anesthetics: evidence for two sites of action? *Anesthesiology* 1992;77:324–335.

Leshner AI. Molecular mechanisms of cocaine addiction. *N Engl J Med* 1996;335:128–129.

Levine RA, Brust JCM, Futrell N, et al. Cocaine-induced coronary artery vasoconstriction. *N Engl J Med* 1989;323:699–704.

Liu SS, McDonald SB. Current issues in spinal anesthesia. *Anesthesiology* 2001;94:888–896.

Liu SS, Ware PD, Allen HW, et al. Dose-response characteristics of spinal bupivacaine in volunteers: clinical implications for ambulatory anesthesia. *Anesthesiology* 1996;85:729–736.

Liu SS. Local anesthetics and analgesia. In: Ashburn MA, Rice LJ (eds). *The management of pain*. New York. Churchill Livingstone, 1997;141–170.

Liguori GA, Zayas VM, Chisholm MF. Transient neurologic symptoms after spinal anesthesia with mepivacaine and lidocaine. *Anesthesiology* 1998;88:619–623.

Lynch J, zur Nieden M, Kasper SM, et al. Transient radicular irritation after spinal anesthesia with hyperbaric 4% mepivacaine. *Anesth Analg* 1997;85:872–873.

Marsch SCI, Schaefer H-G, Castelli I. Unusual psychological manifestation of systemic local anesthetic toxicity. *Anesthesiology* 1998;88:531–533.

McAlpine LG, Thomson NC. Lidocaine-induced bronchoconstriction in asthmatic patients: relation of histamine airway responsiveness and effect of preservatives. *Chest* 1989;96:1012–1015.

McClure JH. Ropivacaine. *Br J Anaesth* 1996;76:300–307.

Mendelson JH, Mello NK. Management of cocaine abuse and dependence. *N Engl J Med* 1996;334:965–972.

Moller R, Covino BG. Cardiac electrophysiologic properties of bupivacaine and lidocaine compared with those of ropivacaine, a new amide local anesthetic. *Anesthesiology* 1990;72:322–329.

Moore DC, Crawford RD, Scurlock JE. Severe hypoxia and acidosis following local anesthetic-induced convulsions. *Anesthesiology* 1980;53: 259–260.

Morishima HO, Pederson H, Finster M, et al. Bupivacaine toxicity in pregnant and nonpregnant ewes. *Anesthesiology* 1985;63:134–139.

Mowat JJ, Mok MJ, MacLeod BA, et al. Liposomal bupivacaine: extended duration nerve blockade using large unilamellar vesicles that exhibit a proton gradient. *Anesthesiology* 1996;85: 635–643.

Muir HA, Writer D, Douglas J, et al. Double-blind comparison of epidural ropivacaine 0.25% and bupivacaine 0.25%, for the relief of childbirth pain. *Can J Anaesth* 1997;44:599–604.

Munson ES, Paul WL, Embro WJ. Central-nervous system toxicity of local anesthetic mixtures in monkeys. *Anesthesiology* 1977; 46:179–183.

Nademanee K, Gorelick D, Josephson M, et al. Myocardial ischemia during cocaine withdrawal. *Ann Intern Med* 1989;111:876–880.

Naveira FA, Copeland S, Anderson M, et al. Transient neurologic toxicity after spinal anesthesia, or is it myofascial pain? Two case reports. *Anesthesiology* 1998;88:268–270.

Negri PD, Ivani G, Tirri T et al. A comparison of epidural bupivacaine, levobupivacaine, and ropivacaine on postoperative analgesia and motor blockade. *Anesth Analg* 2004;99:45–48.

Nguyen ST, Cabrtales RE, Bashour CA, et al. Benzocaine-induced methemoglobinemia. *Anesth Analg* 2000;90:369–371.

Niesel HC, Eilingsfeld T, Hornung M, et al. Plain ropivacaine 1% versus bupivacaine 0.75% in epidural anaesthesia. A comparative study in orthopaedic surgery. *Anaesthestist* 1993;42:605–611.

Nolte H, Fruhstorfer H, Edstrom HH. Local anesthetic efficacy of ropivacaine (LEA 103) in ulnar nerve block. *Reg Anesth* 1990; 15:118–124.

Noorily AD, Noorily SH, Otto RA. Cocaine, lidocaine, and tetracaine: Which is best for topical nasal anesthesia? *Anesth Analg* 1995;81:724–727.

Ostad A, Kageyama N, Moy RL. Tumescent anesthesia with a lidocaine dose of 55 mg/kg is safe for liposuction. *Dermatol Surg* 1996;22: 291:921-927.

Pedersen JL, Lilleso J, Hammer N, et al. Bupivacaine in microcapsules prolongs analgesia after subcutaneous infiltration in humans: A dose-finding study. *Anesth Analg* 2004;99:912–918.

Pere P, Lindgren L, Vaara M. Poor antibacterial effect of ropivacaine. Comparison with bupivacaine. *Anesthesiology* 1999;91:884–886.

Pere P, Salonen M, Jokinen M, et al. Pharmacokinetics of ropivacaine in uremic and nonuremic patients after axillary brachial plexus block. *Anesth Analg* 2003;96:563–569

Peters RW, Gilbert TB, Johns-Walton S, et al. Lidocaine-related increase in defibrillation threshold. *Anesth Analg* 1997;85: 299–300.

Pihlajamaki K, Kantro J, Lindberg R, et al. Extradural administration of bupivacaine: pharmacokinetics and metabolism in pregnant and non-pregnant women. *Br J Anaesth* 1990;64:556–562.

Pollan S, Tadjziechy M. Esmolol in the management of epinephrine- and cocaine-induced cardiovascular toxicity. *Anesth Analg* 1989;69:663–664.

Pollard JB. Cardiac arrest during spinal anesthesia: common mechanisms and strategies for prevention. *Anesth Analg* 2001;92: 252–256.

Polley LS, Columb MO. Ropivacaine and bupivacaine: concentrating on dosing. *Anesth Analg* 2003b;96:1251–1253.

Polley LS, Santos AC. Cardiac arrest following regional anesthesia with ropivacaine. Here we go again. *Anesthesiology* 2003a;99: 1253–1254.

Pollock JE, Liu SS, Neal JM, et al. Dilution of spinal lidocaine does not alter the incidence of transient neurologic symptoms. *Anesthesiology* 1999;90:445–450.

Pollock JE, Neal JM, Stephenson CA, et al. Prospective study of the incidence of transient radicular irritation in patients undergoing spinal anesthesia. *Anesthesiology* 1996;84:1361–1367.

Powell DM, Rodeheaver GT, Foresman PA, et al. Damage to tissue defenses by EMLA cream. *J Emerg Med* 1991;9:205–209.

Prierto-Alvarez P, Calas-Guerra A, Fuentes-Bellido J, et al. Comparison of mepivacaine and lidocaine for intravenous regional anaesthesia: pharmacokinetic study and clinical correlation. *Br. J Anaesth* 2002;88:516–519.

Ramanathan J, Bottorff M, Jeter JN, et al. The pharmacokinetics and maternal and neonatal effects of epidural lidocaine in preeclampsia. *Anesth Analg* 1986;65:120–126.

Rao RB, Ely SF, Hoffman RS. Deaths related to liposuction. *N Engl J Med* 1999;340:1471–1475

Ravindran RS, Bond VK, Tasch MD, et al. Prolonged neural blockade following regional analgesia with 2-chloroprocaine. *Anesth Analg* 1980; 59:447–451.

Reisner LS, Hochman BN, Plumer MH. Persistent neurologic deficit and adhesive arachnoiditis following intrathecal 2-chloroprocaine injection. *Anesth Analg* 1980;59:452–454.

Reynolds F. A comparison of the potential toxicity of bupivacaine, lidocaine, and mepivacaine during epidural blockade for surgery. *Br J Anaesth* 1971;43:567–572.

Rigler M, Drasner K, Krejcie T, et al. Cauda equina syndrome after continuous spinal anesthesia. *Anesth Analg* 1991;72:275–281.

Roitman K, Sprung J, Wallace M, et al. Enhancement of bupivacaine cardiotoxicity with cardiac glycosides and β-adrenergic blockers: a case report. *Anesth Analg* 1993;76:658–661.

Rothstein P, Cole J, Pitt BR. Pulmonary extraction of bupivacaine is dose dependent. *Anesthesiology* 1984;61:A236.

Rothstein P, Pitt BR. Pulmonary extraction of bupivacaine and its modification by propranolol. *Anesthesiology* 1983;59:A189.

Sakura S, Sumi M, Sakaguchi Y, et al. The addition of phenylephrine contributes to the development of transient neurologic symptoms after spinal anesthesia with 0.5% tetracaine. *Anesthesiology* 1997;87:771–778.

Schneider M, Ettlin T, Kaufmann M, et al. Transient neurologic toxicity after hyperbaric subarachnoid anesthesia with 5% lidocaine. *Anesth Analg* 1993;76:1154–1157.

Schneider MC, Birnbach DJ. Lidocaine neurotoxicity in the obstetric patient: is the water safe? *Anesth Analg* 2001;92:287–290.

Scott DB, Jebson PJR, Braid B, et al. Factors affecting plasma levels of lignocaine and prilocaine. *Br J Anaesth* 1972;44:1040–1049.

Scott DB, Lee A, Fagan D, et al. Acute toxicity of ropivacaine compared with that of bupivacaine. *Anesth Analg* 1989;69:563–569.

Scott DB. Maximum recommended doses of local anaesthetic drugs. *Br J Anaesth* 1989;63:373–374.

Silvanto M, Tarkkila P, Makela M-L, et al. The influence of ambulation time on the incidence of transient neurologic symptoms after lidocaine spinal anesthesia. *Anesth Analg* 2004;98:642–646

Solomon RE, Gebhart GF. Synergistic antinociceptive interactions among drugs administered to the spinal cord. *Anesth Analg* 1994;78:1164–1169.

Stewart A, Lambert DH, Concepcion MA, et al. Decreased incidence of tourniquet pain during spinal anesthesia with bupivacaine. A possible explanation. *Anesth Analg* 1988;67:833–837.

Stocks GM, Hallworth SP, Ferando R, et al. Minimum local analgesic dose of intrathecal bupivacaine in labor and the effect of intrathecal fentanyl. *Anesthesiology* 2001;94:593–598.

Sugiyama K, Muteik T. Local anesthetics depress the calcium current of rat sensory neurons in culture. *Anesthesiology* 1994;80: 1369–1375.

Sumi M, Sakura S, Kosaka Y. Interthecal hyperbaric 0.5% tetracaine as a possible cause of transient neurologic toxicity. *Anesth Analg* 1996; 82:1076–1077.

Taddio A, Stevens B, Craig K, et al. Efficacy and safety of lidocaine-prilocaine cream for pain during circumcision. *N Engl J Med* 1997;336: 1197–1201.

Tarkkila P, Huhtala J, Tuominen M, et al. Transient radicular irritation after bupivacaine spinal anesthesia. *Reg Anesth* 1996;21: 26–29.

Teillol-Foo WLM, Kassab JY. Topical glyceryl trinitrate and eutectic mixture of local anesthetics in children. A randomized controlled trial on choice of site and ease of venous cannulation. *Anaesthesia* 1991;46:881–884.

Thomas J, Long G, Moore G, Morgan D. Plasma protein binding and placental transfer of bupivacaine. *Clin Pharmacol Ther* 1976;19: 426–434.

Timour Q, Freysz M, Couzon P, et al. Possible role of drug interaction in bupivacaine-induced problems related to intraventricular conduction disorders. *Reg Anesth* 1990;15:180–185.

Tucker GT, Boyes RN, Bridenbaugh PO, et al. Binding of anilide-type local anesthetics in human plasma: I. Relationships between binding, physicochemical properties, and anesthetic activity. *Anesthesiology* 1970;33: 287–293.

Tucker GT, Mather LE. Clinical pharmacokinetics of local anaesthetics. *Clin Pharmacokinet* 1979;4:241–278.

van Kleef JW, Veering BT, Burm AGL. Spinal anesthesia with ropivacaine: a double-blind study on the efficacy and safety of 0.5% and 0.75% solutions in patients undergoing minor lower limb surgery. *Anesth Analg* 1994;78:1125–1130.

Viegas O, Stoelting RK. Lidocaine in arterial blood after laryngotracheal administration. *Anesthesiology* 1975;43:491–493.

Vladimirov M, Nau C, Mok WM, et al. Potency of bupivacaine stereoisomers tested in vitro and in vivo. Biochemical, electrophysiological, and neurobehavioral studies. *Anesthesiology* 2000;93: 744–755.

Weicht GT, Bernards CM. Remote cocaine use as a likely cause of cardiogenic shock after penetrating trauma. *Anesthesiology* 1996;85: 933–935.

Winnie AP, La Vallee DA, De Sosa B, Masud KZ. Clinical pharmacokinetics of local anesthetics. *Can Anaesth Soc J* 1977a;24: 252–262.

Winnie AP, Tay CH, Patel KP, Ramamurthy S, Durrani Z. Pharmacokinetics of local anesthetics during plexus blocks. *Anesth Analg* 1977b;56:852–861.

Wood MB, Rubin AP. A comparison of epidural 1% ropivacaine with 0.75% bupivacaine for lower abdominal gynecologic surgery. *Anesth Analg* 1993;76:1274–1278.

Woods JR, Plessinger MA, Clark KE. Effect of cocaine on uterine blood flow and fetal oxygenation. *JAMA* 1987;257:957–961.

Wu CL, Tell P, Staats PS, et al. Analgesic effects of intravenous lidocaine and morphine on postamputation pain. A randomized double-blind, active placebo-controlled, crossover trial. *Anesthesiology* 2002;96:841–848.

Xuecheng J, Xiaobin W, Bo G, et al. The plasma concentrations of lidocaine after slow versus rapid administration of an initial dose of epidural anesthesia. *Anesth Analg* 1997;84:570–573.

Yokoyama M, Ohashi I, Nakatsuka H, et al. Drug-induced liver disease during continuous epidural block with bupivacaine. *Anesthesiology* 2001;95:259–261.

Yukioka H, Yoshimoto N, Nishimura K, et al. Intravenous lidocaine as a suppressant of coughing during tracheal intubation. *Anesth Analg* 1985;64:1189–1192.

Neuromuscular-Blocking Drugs

8

The principal pharmacologic effect of neuromuscular-blocking drugs is to interrupt transmission of nerve impulses at the neuromuscular junction (NMJ). On the basis of distinct electrophysiologic differences in their mechanisms of action and duration of action, these drugs can be classified as depolarizing neuromuscular-blocking drugs (mimic the actions of acetylcholine) and nondepolarizing neuromuscular-blocking drugs (interfere with the actions of acetylcholine), which are further subdivided into long-, intermediate-, and short-acting drugs (Table 8-1 and Fig. 8-1) (Hunter, 1995). Neuromuscular-blocking drugs are either benzylisoquinolinium compounds or aminosteroid compounds (see Table 8-1) (Hunter, 1995; Moore and Hunter, 2001). Neuromuscular-blocking drugs produce phase I depolarizing neuromuscular blockade, phase II depolarizing neuromuscular blockade, or nondepolarizing neuromuscular blockade.

PHARMACODYNAMICS

The pharmacodynamics of neuromuscular-blocking drugs are determined by measuring the speed of onset and duration of neuromuscular blockade. Clinically, a common method for determining the type, speed of onset, magnitude, and duration of neuromuscular blockade present is to observe or record the skeletal muscle response that is evoked by a supramaximal electrical stimulus delivered from a peripheral nerve stimulator. Most often, contraction of the adductor pollicis muscle (single twitch response to 1 Hz) after electrical stimulation of the ulnar nerves is used to assess the effect of neuromuscular-blocking drugs (Fig. 8-2) (Hunter, 1995). Equal potency between neuromuscular-blocking drugs is determined by measuring the dose needed to produce 95% suppression of the single-twitch response (ED_{95}) (Table 8-2). Unless stated otherwise, the ED_{95} is assumed to represent the potency of the neuromuscular-blocking drug in the presence of nitrous oxide–barbiturate–opioid anesthesia. In the presence of a volatile anesthetic, the ED_{95} is greatly decreased compared with the value in the absence of these anesthetic drugs.

Neuromuscular-blocking drugs affect small, rapidly moving skeletal muscles (eyes, digits) before those of the abdomen (diaphragm). The onset of neuromuscular blockade after administration of a nondepolarizing neuromuscular blocking drug is more rapid but less intense at the laryngeal muscles (vocal cords) than the peripheral muscles (adductor pollicis) (Fig. 8-3) (Meistelman et al., 1992). The sparing effects of nondepolarizing neuromuscular-blocking drugs at the laryngeal muscles may reflect the role of skeletal muscle fiber types (Meistelman et al., 1992). The muscles involved in closure of the glottis (thyroarytenoid muscles) have fast contraction times, whereas the adductor pollicis is composed mainly of slow fibers. The density of acetylcholine receptors is greater in the fast than in the slow contraction fibers. It is likely that more receptors need to be occupied to block a fast muscle than a slow muscle. The more rapid onset of action at the vocal cords than at the adductor pollicis muscle suggests a more rapid equilibration between plasma concentrations and those at the airway muscles when compared with the adductor pollicis. With intermediate- and short-acting nondepolarizing neuromuscular-blocking drugs, the period of laryngeal paralysis is brief and may be dissipating before a maximum effect is reached at the adductor pollicis (see Fig. 8-3) (Meistelman et al., 1992). It is important to recognize that the dose of neuromuscular-blocking drug necessary to produce a given degree of neuromuscular blockade at the diaphragm is about twice the dose required to produce similar blockade of the adductor pollicis muscle (Donati et al., 1986). It is well documented that adductor pollicis monitoring is a poor indicator of laryngeal relaxation (cricothyroid muscle), whereas facial nerve stimulation and monitoring the response of the orbicularis oculi muscle more closely reflects the onset of neuromuscular blockade at the

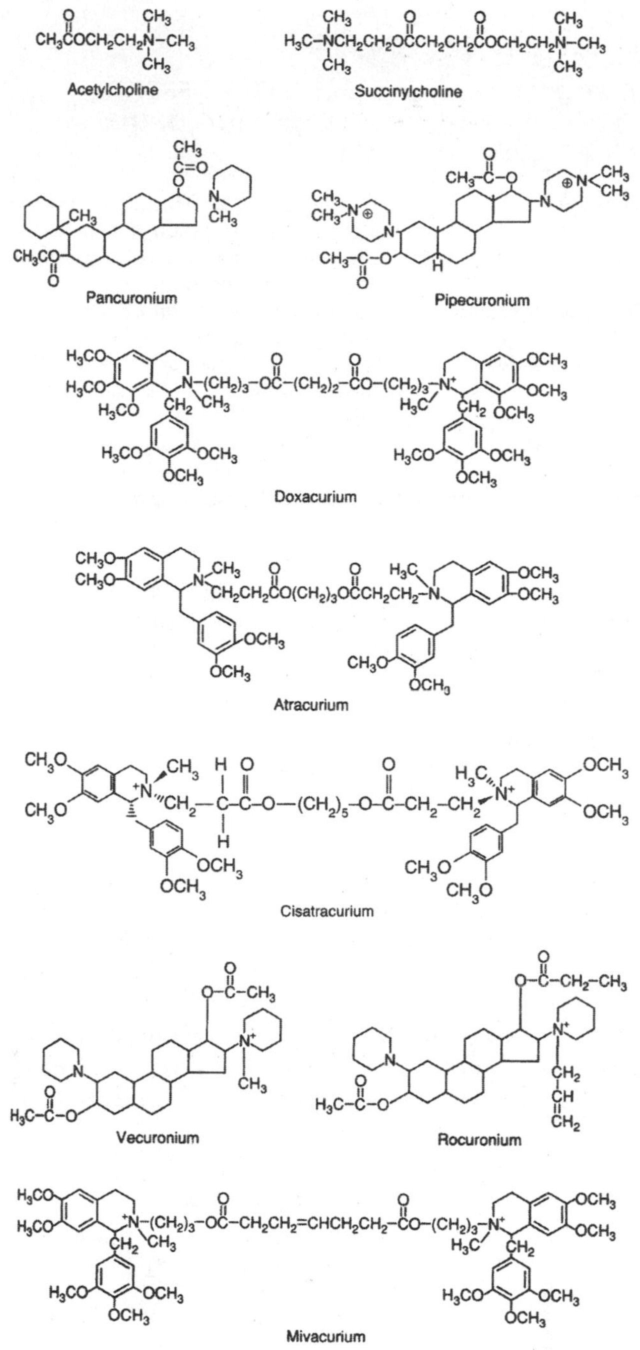

Figure 8-1. Acetylcholine and neuromuscular-blocking drugs.

TABLE 8-1.
CLASSIFICATION OF NEUROMUSCULAR-BLOCKING DRUGS

Clinical Classification	Chemical Classification
Depolarizers	
Succinylcholine	
Nondepolarizers	
Long-acting	
Pancuronium	Aminosteroid
Doxacurium	Aminosteroid
Pipecuronium	Aminosteroid
Intermediate-acting	
Atracurium	Benzylisoquinoline
Vecuronium	Aminosteroid
Rocuronium	Aminosteroid
Cisatracurium	Benzylisoquinoline
Short-acting	
Mivacurium	Benzylisoquinoline

diaphragm (Fig. 8-4) (Moorthy et al., 1996; Meistelman et al., 1992; Ungureanu et al., 1993). Thus, the orbicularis oculi muscle may be preferred to the adductor pollicis as an indicator of laryngeal muscle blockade.

A single-twitch response evoked using a peripheral nerve stimulator reflects events at the postjunctional membrane. Conversely, the response to continuous stimulation (50 to 100 Hz) or train-of-four stimulation (TOF) reflects events at the presynaptic membrane. The differences in effects of nondepolarizing neuromuscular-blocking drugs on responses to single stimulus versus multiple or continuous stimulation most likely reflect differences in the magnitude of presynaptic and postsynaptic effects of these drugs (Bowman, 1980). The electromyogram serves the same purpose as the peripheral nerve stimulator.

PHARMACOKINETICS

Neuromuscular-blocking drugs, because of their quaternary ammonium groups, are highly ionized water-soluble compounds at physiologic pH and possess limited lipid solubility (Table 8-3) (Hunter, 1995; Shanks, 1986). As a result of these two characteristics, the volume of distribution of these drugs is limited, and is similar to the extracellular fluid volume (about 200 mL/kg). In addition, neuromuscular-blocking drugs cannot easily cross lipid membrane barriers such as the blood-brain barrier, renal tubular epithelium, gastrointestinal epithelium, or placenta. Therefore, neuromuscular-blocking drugs do not produce central nervous system (CNS) effects, renal tubular reabsorption is minimal, oral absorption is ineffective, and maternal administration does not affect the fetus. Redistribution of nondepolarizing neuromuscular-blocking drugs also plays a role in the pharmacokinetics of these drugs.

The plasma clearance, volume of distribution, and elimination half-times of neuromuscular-blocking drugs may be influenced by patient age, volatile anesthetics, and the presence of hepatic or renal disease (see Table 8-3) (Hunter, 1995). Renal and hepatic elimination are aided by access to a large fraction of the administered drug due to the high degree of ionization, which maintains high plasma concentrations of drug and also prevents renal reabsorption of excreted drug. Renal disease can greatly alter the pharmacokinetics of long-acting nondepolarizing neuromuscular-blocking drugs. Neuromuscular-blocking drugs are not highly bound to plasma proteins (up to 50%), and it is

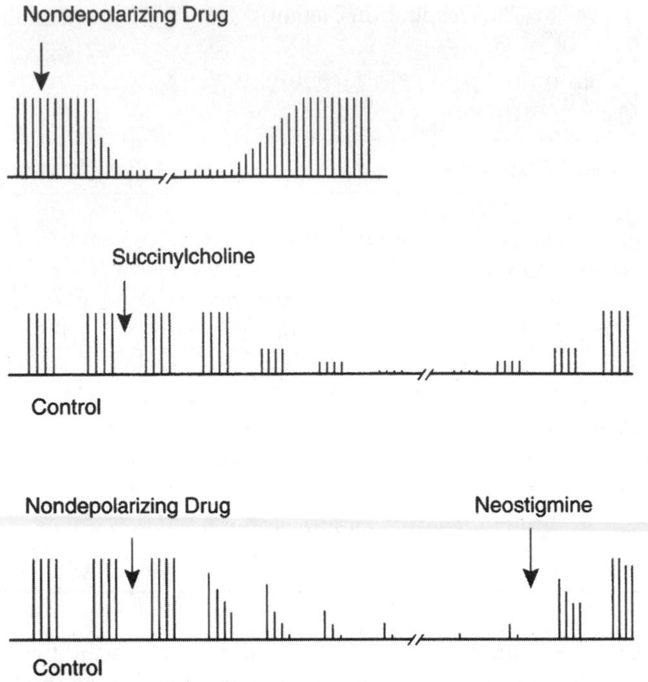

Figure 8-2. Effects of neuromuscular blocking-drugs on the single-twitch and train-of-four responses. The top tracing depicts the effect of a nondepolarizing neuromuscular-blocking drug on the single-twitch response. A depolarizing neuromuscular-blocking drug (succinylcholine) would have the same effect on single-twitch response. The middle tracing depicts the effect of succinylcholine on train-of-four responses characterized by a similar decrease (no fade) in the magnitude of the four twitch responses. The lower tracing depicts the contrasting effects of a nondepolarizing neuromuscular-blocking drug on train-of-four responses characterized by a decrease in the magnitude of the four-twitch responses and the antagonism of the neuromuscular blockade after administration of an anticholinesterase drug, neostigmine. (From Hunter JM. New neuromuscular blocking drugs. *N Engl J Med* 1996;332: 1691–1699; with permission.)

unlikely that plasma protein binding, or any changes in protein binding, will have a significant effect on the renal excretion of neuromuscular-blocking drugs (Pollard, 1992).

Pharmacokinetics of nondepolarizing neuromuscular-blocking drugs are calculated after rapid intravenous (IV) administration of the drug. The rate of disappearance of long-acting nondepolarizing neuromuscular drugs from the plasma is characterized by a rapid initial decline (distribution to tissues) followed by a slower decline (clearance). Despite changes in the distribution of blood flow, inhaled anesthetics have little or no effect on the pharmacokinetics of neuromuscular-blocking drugs. Enhancement of neuromuscular blockade by volatile anesthetics reflects a pharmacodynamic action, as manifested by decreased plasma concentrations of neuromuscular-blocking drugs required to produce a given degree of neuromuscular blockade in the presence of volatile anesthetics. If the volume of distribution is decreased, as by increased protein binding, dehydration, or acute hemorrhage, the same dose of drug produces a higher plasma concentration, and the apparent potency of the drug is augmented. The elimination half-times of neuromuscular-blocking drugs are poorly correlated with the duration of action of these drugs when administered as a rapid IV injection.

TABLE 8-2.
DESCRIPTORS OF THE CLINICAL EFFECTS OF NEUROMUSCULAR BLOCKING DRUGS (SEE FIG. 8-2)

Potency	Effective dose (ED) necessary to depress single-twitch depression 95% (ED_{95})
Onset	Time from injection to onset of maximal single-twitch depression
Duration of Action	Time from injection to return of single-twitch height to 25% or 95%
Recovery Index	Time from 25% return of single-twitch height to 75% return of single-twitch height
Clinical Duration	Time from injection to recovery of the train-of-four ratio to ≥0.7 or ≥0.9

HISTORY

Modern use of neuromuscular-blocking drugs dates from 1932, when purified fractions of *d*-tubocurarine (dTc) were administered to control skeletal muscle spasms in patients with tetanus. In 1940, dTc was administered as an adjuvant to drug-induced electroshock therapy. The first use of dTc to produce surgical skeletal muscle relaxation during general anesthesia was reported in 1942 (Griffith and Johnson, 1942). The use of curarized animals in experiments to determine the parasympathomimetic effects of succinylcholine (SCh) in 1906 masked the neuromuscular-blocking

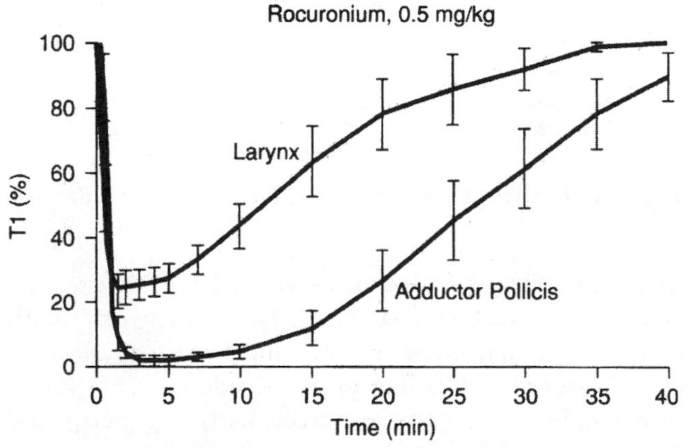

Figure 8-3. The effects of rocuronium (in terms of maximum depression of the single-twitch response) were less intense and the duration of action was less at the adductor muscles of the larynx than at the adductor pollicis. (From Meistelman C, Plaud B, Donati F. Rocuronium (ORG 9426) neuromuscular blockade at the adductor muscles of the larynx and adductor pollicis in humans. *Can J Anaesth* 1992;39:665–669; with permission.)

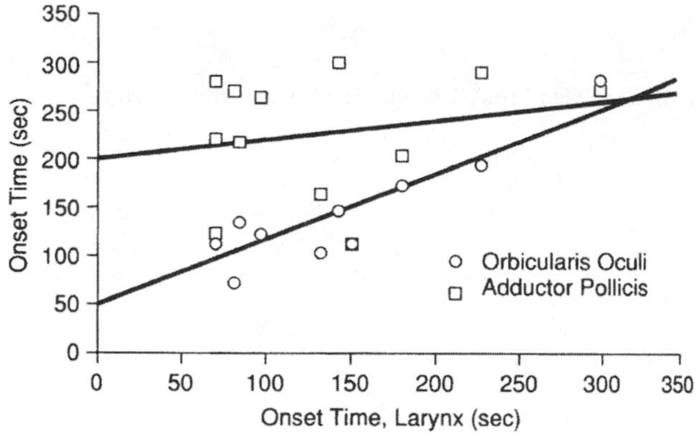

Figure 8-4. Onset time to loss of visible detectable response in the orbicularis oculi and adductor pollicis versus measured onset time to 100% depression of response in laryngeal muscles. No correlation was found between adductor pollicis and laryngeal muscle onset time. Onset time in the orbicularis oculi correlated significantly with that of the laryngeal muscles ($P < .001$). (From Unureanu D, Meistelman C, Frossard J, et al. The orbicularis oculi and the adductor pollicis muscles as monitors of atracurium block of laryngeal muscles. *Anesth Analg* 1993;77:775–779; with permission.)

properties of this drug. It was not until 1949 that the neuromuscular-blocking effects of SCh were recognized. Between 1949 and 1960, dTc and SCh remained the most commonly utilized neuromuscular-blocking drugs. Pancuronium was introduced in 1960 as a long-acting aminosteroid nondepolarizing neuromuscular-blocking drug. In 1980, two new nondepolarizing neuromuscular-blocking drugs, atracurium (benzylisoquinoline) and vecuronium (aminosteroid) were introduced. Cisatracurium followed in 1995, mivacurium in 1997 and most recently, rocuronium was introduced.

CLINICAL USES

Currently, the principal uses of neuromuscular-blocking drugs are to provide skeletal muscle relaxation to facilitate tracheal intubation and to improve surgical working conditions during general anesthesia (Hunter, 1995). A 2 × ED_{95} dose of the nondepolarizing muscle relaxant is often recommended to facilitate tracheal intubation, whereas 90% suppression of single-twitch response is usually considered clinical evidence of adequate drug-induced skeletal muscle relaxation to optimize surgical working conditions. Neuromuscular-blocking drugs lack CNS depressant and analgesic effects. Therefore, these drugs cannot be substituted for anesthetic drugs. Further-more, ventilation of the lungs must be provided mechanically whenever substantial neuromuscular blockade is produced by these drugs. Laryngospasm can be treated effectively with doses of SCh as small as 0.1 mg/kg IV (Chung and Rowbottom, 1993). Uses of neuromuscular-blocking drugs outside the operating room includes management of patients who require mechanical ventilation of the lungs in a critical care environment (adult respiratory distress syndrome, suppression of spontaneous respirations, tetanus) (Hunter, 1995; Miller, 1995).

Clinically, the degree of neuromuscular blockade is typically evaluated by monitoring the evoked skeletal muscle responses produced by an electrical stimulus delivered percutaneously to the ulnar or facial nerves by a peripheral nerve stimulator (Table 8-2). Traditionally, a TOF ratio of >0.7 has been considered to reflect adequate return of skeletal muscle strength to permit spontaneous ventilation after either spontaneous recovery or pharmacologic antagonism of the effects of nondepolarizing neuromuscular blockade. Evidence that pharyngeal dysfunction and a greater likelihood of aspiration is present when the TOF ratio is <0.9 compared to a TOF ratio of >0.9 may require a reassessment of this traditional guideline (Eriksson et al., 1997). Other clinical indicators of residual neuromuscular blockade include grip strength, ability to sustain head lift, vital capacity measurement, and generation of negative inspiratory pressure.

Drug Selection

The choice between depolarizing and nondepolarizing neuromuscular-blocking drugs is influenced by the speed of onset, duration of action, and possibility of drug-induced side effects due to the actions of these drugs at sites other than the NMJ, including those cardiovascular responses due to histamine release evoked by benzylisoquinolinium nondepolarizing neuromuscular-blocking drugs. A rapid onset and brief duration on neuromuscular blockade, as provided by SCh and, to a lesser extent, by mivacurium, is useful when tracheal intubation is the reason for administering a neuromuscular-blocking drug. Rocuronium is the only nondepolarizing neuromuscular-blocking drug that mimics the rapid onset of SCh, but its duration of action is prolonged. When sustained periods of neuromuscular blockade are needed, nondepolarizing neuromuscular-blocking drugs are selected for injection as intermittent doses or as a continuous infusion to provide sustained skeletal muscle paralysis. When a rapid onset of neuromuscular blockade is not considered necessary, skeletal muscle relaxation to facilitate intubation of the trachea can be provided by nondepolarizing neuromuscular-blocking drugs. Certain nondepolarizing neuromuscular-blocking drugs can produce significant decreases in systemic blood pressure (histamine release evoked by atracurium or mivacurium) or increases in heart rate (pancuronium). These drug-induced circulatory effects may be undesirable in the presence of hypovolemia, coronary artery disease, or valvular heart disease. Conversely, bradycardia associated with opioid-based anesthetics, which is masked to some extent by the heart rate–accelerating effects of pancuronium, will not be offset by nondepolarizing neuromuscular-blocking drugs that are devoid of circulatory effects (vecuronium, rocuronium, cisatracurium, doxacurium, pipecuronium).

TABLE 8-3.
COMPARATIVE PHARMACOLOGY OF NONDEPOLARIZING NEUROMUSCULAR-BLOCKING DRUGS

	ED_{95} (mg/kg)	Intubating Dose (mg/kg)	Onset to Maximum Twitch Depression	Duration to Return to ≥25% Control Twitch Height	Duration to Return to Train-of-Four >0.9 (min)	Continuous Infusion (μg/kg/min)
Pancuronium	0.06–0.07	0.1	3–5	60–90	130–220	
Doxacurium	0.03	0.05–0.08	4–6	60–90		
Pipecuronium	0.05–0.06	0.14	3–5	60–90		
Atracurium	0.25	0.4–0.5	3–5	20–35	55–80	4–12
Vecuronium	0.05–0.06	0.08–0.1	3–5	20–35	50–80	1
Rocuronium	0.3	0.6–1.2	1–2	20–35	55–80	3–12
Cisatracurium	0.05	0.1	3–5	20–35	60–90	0.4–4
Mivacurium	0.08	0.25	2–3	12–20	25–40	3–15

	Volume of Distribution (liters/kg)	Clearance (ml/kg/min)	Renal Excretion (% Unchanged)	Biliary Excretion (% Unchanged)	Hepatic Degradation (%)	Hydrolysis in Plasma
Pancuronium	0.26	1.8	80	5–10	10	No
Doxacurium	0.22	2.7	70	30	?	No
Pipecuronium	0.35	3.0	70	20	10	No
Atracurium	0.2	5.5	10	NS	?	Yes*
Vecuronium	0.27	5.2	15–25	40–75	20–30	No
Rocuronium	0.3	4.0	10–25	50–70	10–20	No
Cisatracurium	0.2	4.7–5.3	NS	NS	0	No*
Mivacurium			<10	NS	0	Yes

	Degradation Dependent on Body Temperature	Degradation Dependent on Blood pH	Elimination Dependent on Renal Function	Elimination Dependent on Hepatic Function	Elimination Half-Time (min)		
					Normal	Kidney Failure	Hepatic Failure
Pancuronium	Yes		Yes	Modest	132	240–1050	208–270
Doxacurium	Yes		Yes	No			
Pipecuronium	Yes		Yes	No			
Atracurium	Yes	Yes	No	No	21	18–25	20–25
Vecuronium	Yes	No	Yes	Yes	50–110	80–150	49–198
Rocuronium	Yes	No	Yes	Yes	87	97	97
Cisatracurium	Yes	Yes	No	No	22–30	25–34	21
Mivacurium	Yes	?	?	?	1–3		

NS, not significant.
*Also undergoes chemodegradation (Hofmann elimination).

Sequence of Onset of Neuromuscular Blockade

Neuromuscular-blocking drugs affect small, rapidly moving muscles, such as those of the eyes and digits, before those of the trunk and abdomen. Ultimately, intercostal muscles and finally the diaphragm are paralyzed. Recovery of skeletal muscles usually occurs in the reverse order to that of paralysis, so that the diaphragm is the first to regain normal function. Differences in onset and recovery of varying skeletal muscle groups are probably due to more rapid equilibration of the drug in skeletal muscles with greater blood flow (Hunter, 1995).

IV injection of a nondepolarizing neuromuscular-blocking drug to a person who is awake initially produces difficulty in focusing and weakness in the mandibular muscles followed by ptosis, diplopia, and dysphagia. Relaxation of the small muscles of the middle ear improves acuity of hearing. Consciousness and sensorium remain undisturbed even in the presence of complete neuromuscular blockade.

STRUCTURE–ACTIVITY RELATIONSHIPS

Neuromuscular-blocking drugs are quaternary ammonium compounds that have at least one positively charged nitrogen atom that binds to the alpha subunit of postsynaptic cholinergic receptors (see Fig. 8-1). In addition, these drugs have structural similarities to the endogenous neurotransmitter acetylcholine (see Fig. 8-1). For example, SCh is two molecules of acetylcholine linked through acetate methyl groups. The long, slender, and flexible structure of SCh allows it to bind to and activate cholinergic receptors. Bulky and rigid molecules that are characteristic of nondepolarizing neuromuscular-blocking drugs, although containing portions similar to acetylcholine, cannot activate cholinergic receptors.

Nondepolarizing neuromuscular-blocking drugs are either benzylisoquinolinium compounds or aminosteroid compounds (see Table 8-1) (Hunter, 1995). Pancuronium is the aminosteroid neuromuscular-blocking drug most closely related structurally to acetylcholine. The acetylcholine-like fragments of pancuronium give the steroidal molecule its high degree of neuromuscular-blocking activity and its plasma cholinesterase inhibiting action. Vecuronium and rocuronium are monoquaternary analogues of the bisquaternary nondepolarizing neuromuscular-blocking drug pancuronium. Aminosteroid neuromuscular-blocking drugs lack hormonal activity.

Acetylcholine has a positively charged quaternary ammonium group (four carbon atoms attached to one nitrogen atom) that attaches to negatively charged cholinergic receptors (see Fig. 8-1). The same feature is common to neuromuscular-blocking drugs, which all contain one or more positively charged quaternary ammonium groups. The bisquaternary ammonium structure of most of these drugs suggests that an electrostatic association occurs between two ionized cationic centers of the drug and anionic groups on cholinergic receptors. In view of the monoquaternary structure of some nondepolarizing neuromuscular-blocking drugs, it is not tenable to propose that nondepolarizing neuromuscular-blocking activity depends on an optimal distance between quaternary ammonium groups.

The electrostatic attraction of negatively charged cholinergic receptors for the positively charged quaternary ammonium group occurs at cholinergic sites other than the NMJ, including cardiac muscarinic receptors and autonomic ganglia nicotinic receptors. This lack of specificity for the NMJ means that neuromuscular-blocking drugs could produce cardiovascular effects, particularly as reflected by changes in systemic blood pressure and heart rate.

The specificity of a drug for autonomic ganglia nicotinic receptors versus the NMJ is influenced by the length of the carbon chain separating the two positively charged ammonium groups. Maximal autonomic ganglion blockade occurs when the positive charges are separated by six carbon atoms (hexamethonium), whereas neuromuscular blockade occurs when 10 carbon atoms are present (decamethonium). As a bulky monoquaternary molecule, dTc is more likely to produce autonomic ganglion blockade than is a bisquaternary drug. Indeed, methylation of dTc to the bisquaternary ammonium drug metocurine dramatically decreases the autonomic-blocking properties associated with production of neuromuscular blockade.

Benzylisoquinolinium derivatives are more likely to evoke the release of histamine compared with aminosteroid derivatives, presumably reflecting the presence of a tertiary amine.

NEUROMUSCULAR JUNCTION

The mammalian NMJ is one of the most studied and best understood synapses (Naguib et al., 2002). Immobility, as a component of general anesthesia, is dependent on the function of the NMJ. Neuromuscular-blocking drugs acting directly on the NMJ are a component of most general anesthetics and the function of the NMJ influences responses to anesthetic drugs as well as neuromuscular-blocking drugs. The physiology and pharmacology of the NMJ is critically important to many aspects of anesthesiology including intraoperative care, management in postoperative critical care units, and treatment of chronic pain syndromes.

The NMJ consists of a prejunctional motor nerve ending separated from a highly folded postjunctional membrane of the skeletal muscle fiber by a synaptic cleft that is 20 to 30 nm wide and filled with extracellular fluid (Fig. 8-5) (Drachman, 1978; Standaert, 1994) (see Chapter 55). The nonmyelinated nerve ending contains mitochondria, endoplasmic reticulum, and synaptic vesicles necessary to synthesize the neurotransmitter acetylcholine. The resting transmembrane potential of approximately −90 mv across nerve and skeletal muscle membranes is maintained by the unequal distribution of potassium and sodium ions across the membrane. The NMJ contains three types of nicotinic cholinergic receptors (nAChRs); two are postsynaptic on the skeletal muscle surface—one junctional and the other

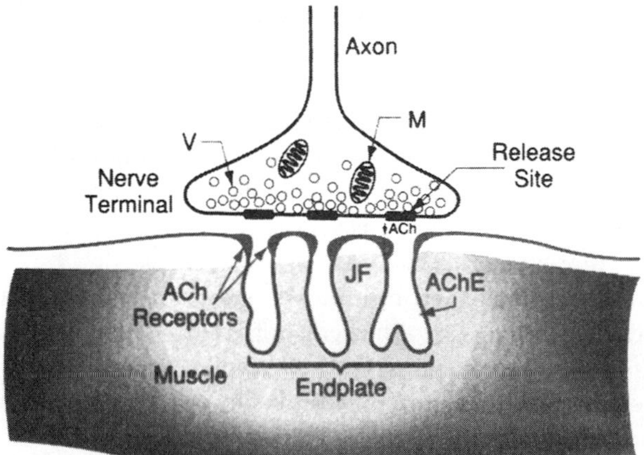

Figure 8-5. Schematic depiction of the neuromuscular junction. Acetylcholine (ACh) is present in vesicles (V) of the axon for release in response to nerve impulses. The neurotransmitter diffuses across the synaptic cleft to attach to receptors that are concentrated on the junctional folds (JF) of the skeletal muscle end-plate. Acetylcholinesterase (AChE) is present in the JF to facilitate rapid hydrolysis of ACh. (From Drachman DA. Myasthenia gravis. *N Engl J Med* 1978;298:136–142; with permission.)

extrajunctional—and one is presynaptic on the nerve ending. The extrajunctional receptors are not involved in normal neuromuscular transmission but may proliferate if the skeletal muscle is diseased, damaged, or denervated, altering the effect of neuromuscular-blocking drugs. The postsynaptic receptors are concentrated on the junctional folds, immediately opposite the sites on the nerve ending where acetylcholine is released.

Acetylcholine

The neurotransmitter at the NMJ is the quaternary ammonium ester acetylcholine. Acetylcholine in motor nerve endings is synthesized by the acetylation of choline under the control of the enzyme choline acetylase. This acetylcholine is stored in synaptic vesicles in motor nerve endings and released into the synaptic cleft as packets (quanta), each of which contains 5,000 to 10,000 molecules of acetylcholine. Arrival of a nerve impulse causes the release of hundreds of quanta of acetylcholine that bind to alpha subunits of nAChRs on postsynaptic membranes, causing a change in membrane permeability to ions. This change in permeability causes a decrease in the transmembrane potential from approximately −90 mv to −45 mv (threshold potential). At this point, a propagated action potential spreads over the surfaces of skeletal muscle fibers leading to their contraction. In the absence of action potentials, quanta of acetylcholine are released randomly, producing miniature endplate potentials of <1 mv that are insufficient to trigger depolarization of the skeletal muscle membrane. Release of acetylcholine is a calcium-dependent process and is triggered by increases in the concentrations of free calcium ions in nerve terminals. It is speculated that a nerve action potential activates adenylate cyclase in membranes of nerve terminals leading to the formation of cyclic adenosine monophosphate (cAMP). cAMP subsequently opens calcium ion channels, causing synaptic vesicles to fuse with the nerve membrane and release acetylcholine (Standaert and Dretchen, 1981). Indeed, drugs such as aminophylline that stimulate formation of cAMP facilitate neuromuscular transmission, and calcium channel-blocking drugs such as verapamil interfere with neuromuscular transmission.

Situated in close proximity to cholinergic receptors is the enzyme acetylcholinesterase. This enzyme is responsible for the rapid hydrolysis (<15 ms) of acetylcholine to acetic acid and choline. Choline can reenter motor nerve endings to again participate in the synthesis of new acetylcholine. The rapid hydrolysis of acetylcholine prevents sustained depolarization of the NMJ.

Postjunctional Nicotinic Acetylcholine Receptors

Postjunctional membranes possess two types of nAChRs that respond to neuromuscular-blocking drugs (Standaert, 1994). nAChRs are present in large numbers on postjunctional membranes. Extrajunctional nAChRs appear throughout skeletal muscles whenever there is deficient stimulation of the skeletal muscle membrane by the nerve.

Fetal Receptors

Fetal nAChRs consist of five subunits designated alpha, beta, gamma, and delta and each subunit is encoded by a different gene (Naguib et al., 2002). In response to acetylcholine, these fetal receptors oscillate between open (acetylcholine attached) and closed (acetylcholine dissociated) states. In the open state, sodium, potassium, and calcium ions flow across the skeletal muscle membrane along electrochemical gradients. The long open period of fetal nAChRs combined with the high electrical resistance of the myotubules allows single acetylcholine quanta to elicit action potentials.

Adult Receptors

Synapse maturation involves the gradual disappearance of fetal nAChRs from junctional and extrajunctional sites and formation of a motor nerve terminal with densely packed synaptic vesicles containing acetylcholine (Naguib et al., 2002). Postsynaptic differentiation is characterized by the formation of a postsynaptic apparatus anchoring nAChRs at a density of 10,000 per μm^2 in the subsynaptic muscle membrane. Subsynaptic myonuclei selectively begin to express a new nAChR subunit, *epsilon*, giving rise to a functionally distinct nAChR subtype known as the adult receptor (Mishina et al., 1986). These mature adult receptors have shorter open periods and higher conductance of sodium, potassium, and calcium ions than fetal nAChRs. Up-regulation and down-regulation of nAChRs occurs in response to physiologic, pathophysiologic, and pharmacologic stimulation (Table 8-4) (Naguib et al., 2002).

TABLE 8-4.
EVENTS ASSOCIATED WITH UP-REGULATION OR DOWN-REGULATION OF NICOTINIC ACETYLCHOLINE RECEPTORS (nAChR)

nAChR Up-Regulation	nAChR Down-Regulation
Spinal cord injury	Myasthenia gravis
Cerebral vascular accident	Anticholinesterase overdose
Thermal injury	Organophosphate poisoning
Prolonged immobility	
Prolonged exposure to neuromuscular-blocking drugs	
Multiple sclerosis	
Guillain-Barre syndrome	

Adapted from Naguib M, Flood P, McArdle, et al. Advances in neurobiology of the neuromuscular junction: Implications for the anesthesiologist. *Anesthesiology* 2002;96:202–231.

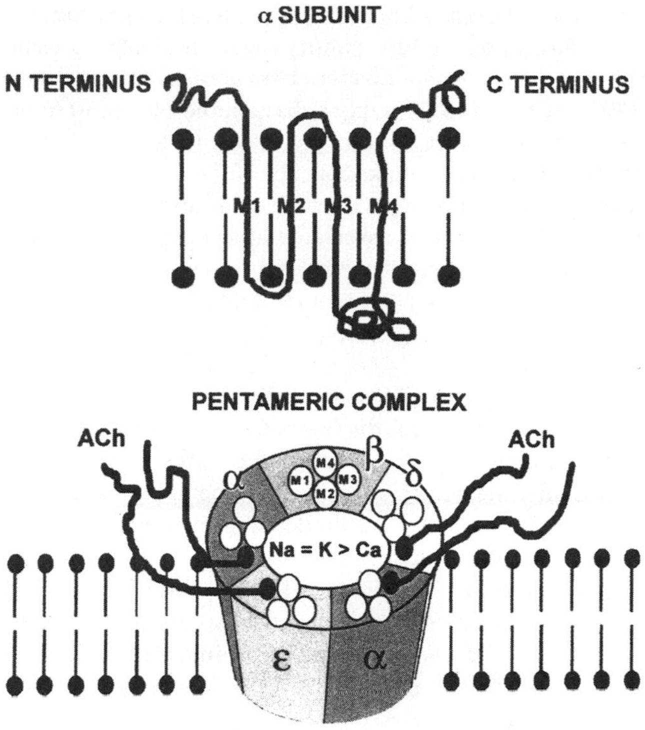

Figure 8-6. Subunit composition of the adult nicotinic acetylcholine receptor (nAChR) consisting of five (two alpha, beta, delta, epsilon) protein subunits. Each subunit contains four helical domains (M1-M4) and the M2 domain forms the channel pore. A single alpha subunit with its N and C termini on the extracellular surface of the membrane lipid bilayer (Top). Between the N and C termini, the alpha subunit forms four helices (M1-M4) that span the membrane bilayer. The pentameric structure of the adult nAChR consists of the N termini of two alpha subunits that form two distinct binding pockets for acetylcholine. (Bottom). The ion channel has equal permeability for sodium and potassium ions, whereas calcium ion permeability contributes about 2.5% of the total permeability. (From Naguib M, Flood P, McArdle, et al. Advances in neurobiology of the neuromuscular junction: Implications for the anesthesiologist. *Anesthesiology* 2002;96:202–231; with permission).

Structure and Function

The function of nAChR endplates depends on five subunit proteins that combine to form the pentameric unit consisting of two alpha subunits in association with single beta, delta, and epsilon subunits (Fig 8-6) (Naguib et al., 2002). These subunits form a transmembrane pore as well as the extracellular binding pockets for acetylcholine and other agonists (depolarizing neuromuscular-blocking drugs) or antagonists (nondepolarizing neuromuscular-blocking drugs). In the absence of acetylcholine or other agonists, the stable closed state of the pore is maintained, which precludes flow of ions along their electrochemical gradients. An important function of the delta and epsilon subunits is to stabilize this closed state. Simultaneous binding of two acetylcholine molecules to nAChRs initiates conformational changes that open the pores and passage of ions occurs. For example, when two molecules bind simultaneously to alpha subunits of a receptor, a channel opens through the center of the receptor, allowing sodium and calcium ions to move into the skeletal muscle and potassium ions to leave. Each NMJ contains several million postjunctional receptors, and a burst of acetylcholine from the nerve ending opens at least 400,000 receptors. As a result, sufficient current flows through these open receptors to depolarize the endplate and create the action potential that triggers contraction of the skeletal muscle. It is the flow of ions that is the basis of normal neuromuscular transmission.

The two alpha subunits, in addition to being the binding sites for acetylcholine, are the sites occupied by neuromuscular-blocking drugs. Nondepolarizing neuromuscular-blocking drugs bind to one or both alpha subunits, but unlike acetylcholine, lack agonist activity (competitive blockade). As a result, conformational changes do not occur, and the receptor channel remains closed. Therefore, ions do not flow through these channels, and depolarization cannot occur at these sites. If enough channels remain closed, there is blockade of neuromuscular transmission. A nondepolarizing neuromuscular-blocking drug may show preference for one of the two alpha subunits. This may result in synergism if two nondepolarizing neuromuscular-blocking drugs with different selective preferences for each alpha subunit are administered simultaneously. The probability of binding is dependent on the concentration of acetylcholine and nondepolarizing neuromuscular-blocking drug at the receptor and the affinity of the receptor for the neurotransmitter or drug. When the neuromuscular-blocking drug diffuses from the nAChRs, the probability of receptor binding of acetylcholine increases, and the effect of the nondepolarizing neuromuscular-blocking drug decreases.

SCh, which is structurally two molecules of acetylcholine bound together, is a partial agonist at nAChRs and depolarizes (opens) the ion channels. This opening requires the binding of only one molecule of SCh to the alpha subunit. The other alpha subunit can be occupied by either acetylcholine or SCh. Because SCh is not hydrolyzed by acetylcholinesterase, the channel remains open for a longer period of time than would be produced by acetylcholine, causing contractions known as *fasciculations* and persistent depolarization of the end-plate and neuromuscular blockade (sustained depolarization prevents propagation of an action potential). Furthermore, SCh can diffuse from nAChRs and repeatedly bind to other nAChRs until it is cleared from the area of the NMJ and is exposed to hydrolysis by plasma cholinesterase.

Large doses of nondepolarizing neuromuscular-blocking drugs may also prevent normal flow of ions by entering the channels formed by nAChRs to produce blockade within the channel. Similar blockade of sodium ion channels is produced by local anesthetics.

Extrajunctional nAChRs

Extrajunctional nAChRs normally are not present in large numbers because their synthesis is suppressed by neural activity. Whenever motor nerves are less active due to trauma or skeletal muscle denervation, these extrajunctional cholinergic receptors proliferate rapidly (Pumplin and Fambrough, 1982). These extrajunctional nAChRs appear over the entire postjunctional membrane rather than being confined to the area of the NMJ.

Extrajunctional nAChRs are highly responsive to agonists such as acetylcholine or SCh. Because extrajunctional nAChRs are formed rapidly after slackening of neural influence on skeletal muscles and are degraded soon after neural influence returns, mixtures of prejunctional nAChRs and extrajunctional nAChRs are present in many clinical situations and may account for differences in responses to neuromuscular-blocking drugs among individuals and various disease states.

Prejunctional nAChRs

Prejunctional nAChRs on motor nerve endings influence the release of neurotransmitters. These prejunctional nAChRs seem to be different from postjunctional nAChRs in (a) their chemical binding characteristics, (b) the nature of the ion channel they control, and (c) their preferential blockade during high-frequency stimulation. Some nondepolarizing neuromuscular-blocking drugs block prejunctional sodium ion channels but not calcium ion channels. As a result, these drugs may interfere with mobilization of acetylcholine from synthesis sites to release sites. Interference with release of acetylcholine, which is calcium dependent, does not occur.

DEPOLARIZING NEUROMUSCULAR-BLOCKING DRUGS

The only depolarizing neuromuscular-blocking drug in clinical use is SCh (see Fig. 8-1). SCh is endowed with two unique and critically important characteristics—it produces intense paralysis rapidly, and its effects are likely to wane before a preoxygenated patient becomes hypoxic (Donati, 2003). SCh, 0.5 to 1 mg/kg IV, has a rapid onset (30 to 60 seconds) and short duration of action (3 to 5 minutes). These characteristics make SCh a useful drug for providing skeletal muscle relaxation to facilitate intubation of the trachea. SCh has several associated adverse effects that can limit or even contraindicate its use.

Dose

The traditional dose of SCh to facilitate tracheal intubation is 1 mg/kg IV although the literature supporting this practice is lacking. In adult patients, the ED_{90} for SCh, as determined after the administration of thiopental while breathing nitrous oxide, is 0.27 mg/kg IV (Smith et al., 1988). Thus, a 1 mg/kg IV dose represents 3.5 to 4 times the ED_{95}. Conceptually, it is anticipated that administration of 1 mg/kg IV to a preoxygenated patient would be associated with return of spontaneous breathing before arterial hypoxemia became significant. Indeed, spontaneous breathing has been observed to occur within about 5 minutes following paralysis produced by SCh. Nevertheless, the average duration to 90% twitch height recovery following 1 mg/kg IV is greater than 10 minutes, reflecting the fact that the diaphragm recovers before the adductor pollicis muscle. In this regard, it has been estimated that a preoxygenated healthy adult can experience 8 minutes of apnea before arterial oxygen saturation decreases to 90% (Benumof et al., 1997).

Decreasing the intubating dose of SCh from 1 mg/kg IV to 0.6 mg/kg IV decreases the duration of twitch depression by >90 seconds and is still associated with acceptable intubating conditions (Fig. 8-7) (Kopman et al., 2003;

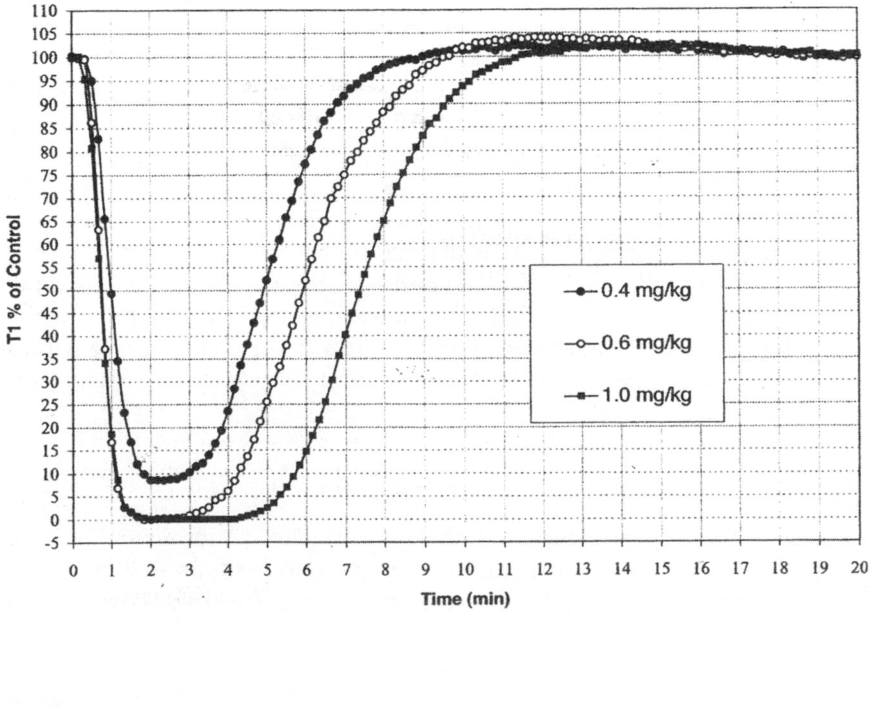

Figure 8-7. Twitch height (T1) as a percent of control at the adductor pollicis versus time from the initial drug bolus for three different doses of succinylcholine. Reducing the dose of succinylcholine from 1.0 mg/kg to 0.60 mg/kg shortens the duration of action at the adductor pollicis by more than 90 seconds. (From Kopman A, Zhaku B, Lai KS, The "intubating dose" of succinylcholine: The effect of decreasing doses on recovery time. *Anesthesiology* 2003;99:1050–1054; with permission.)

Naguib et al., 2003). In this regard, the onset of arterial hypoxemia before the return of spontaneous breathing would seem less likely (but not impossible, considering the variation in responses to SCh) than with the traditional 1 mg/kg IV dose. Nevertheless, decreasing the dose of SCh from 1.0 mg/kg to 0.56 mg/kg does not shorten the time to spontaneous diaphragmatic movement (Naguib et al., 2005). When complete neuromuscular blockage is critical, doses of SCh 1.0 to 1.5 mg/kg IV may still be appropriate. Considering the variability in response to SCh among patients, it is concluded there is no single perfect intubating dose of SCh (Donati, 2003).

Mechanism of Action

SCh attaches to one or both of the alpha subunits of nAChRs and mimics the action of acetylcholine (partial agonist), thus depolarizing the postjunctional membrane. Compared with acetylcholine, the hydrolysis of SCh is slow, resulting in sustained depolarization (opening) of the receptor ion channels. Neuromuscular blockade develops because a depolarized postjunctional membrane cannot respond to subsequent release of acetylcholine (depolarizing neuromuscular blockade). Depolarizing neuromuscular blockade is also referred to as *phase I blockade*. SCh has presynaptic effects, but these are considered minor when compared with postsynaptic effects (Standaert and Adams, 1965). Sustained opening of receptor ion channels and resulting depolarization of postjunctional membranes produced by SCh is associated with leakage of potassium ions from the interior of cells sufficient to produce an average 0.5 mEq/liter increase in serum potassium concentrations.

A single large dose of SCh (>2 mg/kg IV), repeated doses, or a prolonged continuous infusion of SCh may result in postjunctional membranes that do not respond normally to acetylcholine even when the postjunctional membranes have become repolarized (desensitization neuromuscular blockade). The mechanism for the development of desensitization neuromuscular blockade is unknown and, for this reason, designation as *phase II blockade*, which does not imply a mechanism, is the preferred terminology (Hunter and Feldman, 1976). It is likely that combinations of receptor desensitization, ion channel blockade, and entrance of SCh into the cytoplasm of skeletal muscles are responsible for the events that manifest as phase II blockade.

Characteristics of Phase I Blockade

Electrically evoked mechanical responses, using a peripheral nerve stimulator, that are characteristic of phase I blockade are (a) decreased contraction in response to single twitch stimulation, (b) decreased amplitude but sustained response to continuous stimulation, (c) TOF ratio of >0.7, (d) absence of posttetanic facilitation, and (e) augmentation of neuromuscular blockade after administration of an anticholinesterase drug (see Fig. 8-2) (Hunter, 1995). In addition, the onset of phase I blockade is accompanied by skeletal muscle fasciculations that reflect the generalized depolarization of postjunctional membranes produced by SCh.

Characteristics of Phase II Blockade

Electrically evoked mechanical responses, using a peripheral nerve stimulator, that are characteristic of phase II blockade resemble those considered typical of neuromuscular blockade produced by nondepolarizing neuromuscular-blocking drugs (see Fig. 8-2) (Hunter, 1995). Furthermore, phase II blockade can be antagonized with an anticholinesterase drug. Despite the similarities, it is likely that mechanisms of nondepolarizing neuromuscular blockade and SCh-induced phase II blockade differ.

The transition between phase I and phase II blockade is fairly abrupt, occurring with a SCh dose of 2 to 4 mg/kg IV (Fig. 8-8) (Lee, 1975). Clinically, the onset of phase II blockade is often manifested initially as tachyphylaxis and the need to increase the infusion rate of SCh or to administer progressively larger incremental doses. At a single moment, varying degrees of phase I and phase II blockade may be present (Ali and Saverese, 1976). When neuromuscular blockade is predominantly phase I, administering an anticholinesterase drug will enhance existing neuromuscular blockade. Conversely, an anticholinesterase drug will antagonize a predominant phase II blockade. An acceptable approach is to observe the mechanical response evoked by

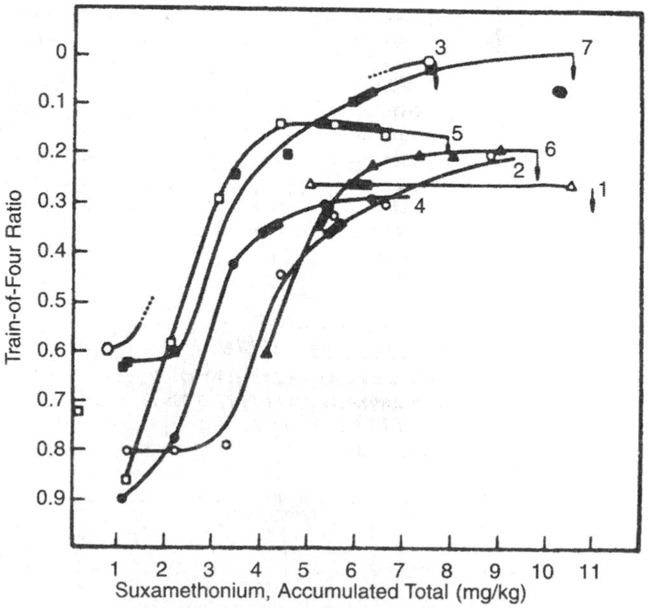

Figure 8-8. The transition between phase I and phase II blockade as depicted by the train-of-four ratio is fairly abrupt, occurring at a total dose of succinylcholine (suxamethonium) of 2 to 4 mg/kg IV. (From Lee C. Dose relationship of phase II, tachyphylaxis and train-of-four fade on suxamethonium-induced dual neuromuscular block in man. *Br J Anaesth* 1975;47:841–845; with permission.)

a peripheral nerve stimulator after administering a small dose of anticholinesterase drug such as edrophonium, 0.1 to 0.2 mg/kg IV. If this small dose of edrophonium improves neuromuscular transmission, it is likely that an additional dose of anticholinesterase drug will antagonize, rather than enhance, neuromuscular blockade produced by SCh.

Duration of Action

The brief duration of action of SCh (3 to 5 minutes) is principally due to its hydrolysis by plasma cholinesterase (pseudocholinesterase) enzyme (Fig. 8-9). Plasma cholinesterase enzyme is synthesized in the liver and is a tetrameric glycoprotein containing four identical subunits, each having one active catalytic site. Despite its importance in the hydrolysis of certain ester-containing drugs such as SCh, the physiologic significance of plasma cholinesterase has not been established (Pantuck, 1993).

The initial metabolite of SCh, succinylmonocholine, is a much weaker neuromuscular blocker (1/20 to 1/80 as potent) than the parent drug. Succinylmonocholine is subsequently hydrolyzed to succinic acid and choline. Rapid hydrolysis makes it difficult to obtain pharmacokinetic data for succinylcholine. Nevertheless, based on isolated tourniquet techniques, it seems likely that significant amounts of SCh are still circulating 3 minutes after injection of the drug (Holst-Larsen, 1976).

Plasma cholinesterase has an enormous capacity to hydrolyze SCh at a rapid rate, so that only a small fraction of the original IV dose of drug actually reaches the NMJ. Because plasma cholinesterase is not present in significant amounts at the NMJ, neuromuscular blockade produced by SCh is terminated by its diffusion away from the NMJ into extracellular fluid. Therefore, plasma cholinesterase influences the duration of action of SCh by controlling the amount of neuromuscular-blocking drug that is hydrolyzed before reaching the NMJ.

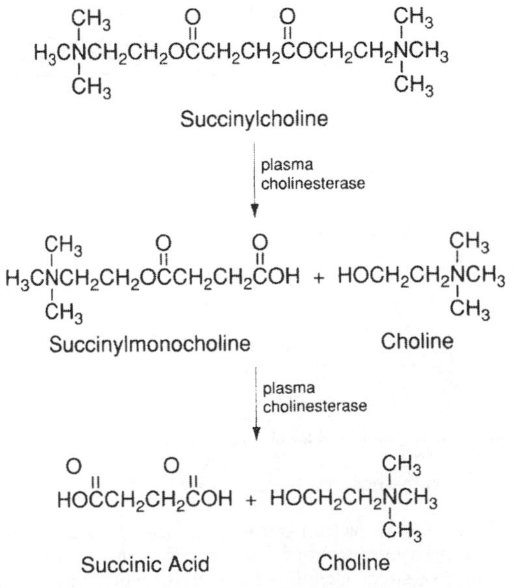

Figure 8-9. The brief duration of action of succinylcholine is due principally to its rapid hydrolysis in plasma by cholinesterase enzyme to inactive metabolites.

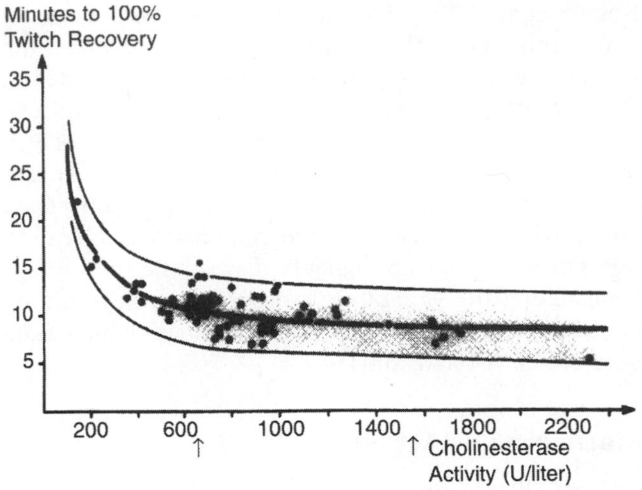

Figure 8-10. The duration of succinylcholine-induced neuromuscular blockade parallels activity of plasma cholinesterase enzyme. (From Viby-Mogensen J. Correlation of succinylcholine duration of action with plasma cholinesterase activity in subjects with the genotypically normal enzyme. *Anesthesiology* 1980;53:517–520; with permission.)

Plasma Cholinesterase Activity

Decreases in the hepatic production of plasma cholinesterase, drug-induced decreases in plasma cholinesterase activity, or the genetically determined presence of atypical plasma cholinesterase result in slowed to absent hydrolysis of SCh and corresponding prolongation of the neuromuscular blockade produced by the drug (Fig. 8-10) (Viby-Mogensen, 1980).

Liver disease must be severe before decreases in plasma cholinesterase production sufficient to prolong SCh-induced neuromuscular blockade occur (Foldes et al., 1956). It is estimated that the incidence of low plasma cholinesterase activity is 6% (Viby-Mogensen, 1980). The elimination half-time of plasma cholinesterase is 8 to 16 hours, and levels of <75% are necessary for prolongation of SCh effect. Neostigmine but not edrophonium causes a profound decrease in plasma cholinesterase activity (Fig. 8-11) (Devcic et al., 1995). Even 30 minutes after administration of neostigmine, the plasma cholinesterase activity remains about 50% of control values. Potent anticholinesterase drugs used in insecticides and occasionally in the treatment of glaucoma and myasthenia gravis, as well as chemotherapeutic drugs (nitrogen mustard and cyclophosphamide), may decrease plasma cholinesterase activity so that prolonged neuromuscular blockade follows administration of SCh. The duration of action of SCh administered after injecting metoclopramide, 10 mg IV, is prolonged, presumably reflecting inhibition of

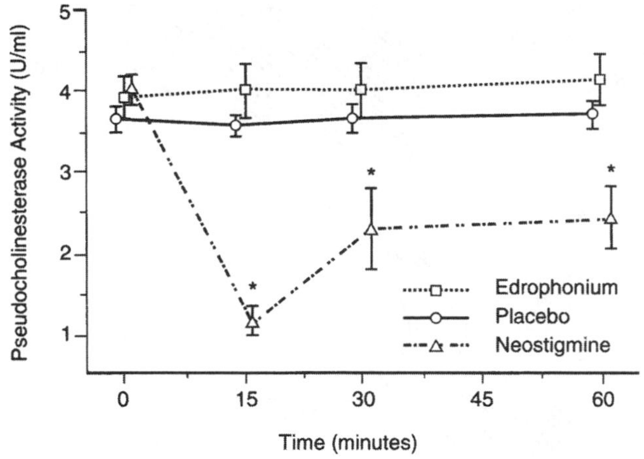

Figure 8-11. Plasma cholinesterase activity before (time 0) and during the first hour after anticholinesterase drug administration. (Values are mean ± SE; *P ≤.01.) (From Devcic A, Munshi CA, Gandhi SK, et al. Antagonism of mivacurium neuromuscular block: neostigmine versus edrophonium. *Anesth Analg* 1995;81:1005–1009; with permission.)

plasma cholinesterase by metoclopramide (Kao and Turner, 1989). High estrogen levels, as observed in parturients at term, are associated with up to 40% decreases in plasma cholinesterase activity. Paradoxically, the duration of action of SCh-induced skeletal muscle paralysis is not prolonged, presumably reflecting an increased volume of distribution of the drug at term (Leighton et al., 1986).

Resistance to the effects of SCh may reflect increased plasma cholinesterase activity (inherited as a C5 isoenzyme variant or acquired), manifesting as an accelerated rate of hydrolysis and a shorter duration of action of SCh (Sugimori, 1986). In obese patients, there is an increase in plasma cholinesterase activity so that SCh requirements may increase (Bentley et al., 1982). Resistance to SCh may also be a result of pharmacodynamic causes, as observed in patients with myasthenia gravis (ED_{95} 2.6 times that in normal patients) (Eisenkraft et al., 1988). In myasthenia gravis, there is a decrease in functional acetylcholine end-plate receptors, with a consequent decrease in the response to the neurotransmitter acetylcholine. Resistance to SCh has been observed in a patient with juvenile hyaline fibromatosis and normal plasma cholinesterase activity (Baraka, 1988).

Atypical Plasma Cholinesterase

The presence of atypical plasma cholinesterase is often recognized only after an otherwise healthy patient experiences prolonged neuromuscular blockade (1 to 3 hours), after a conventional dose of SCh. A single cholinesterase gene is present and nucleotide alterations in this gene are responsible for the numerous variants in the enzyme. The application of techniques of molecular genetics has permitted precise identification of plasma cholinesterase variants (Pantuck, 1993).

Among the several genetically determined variants of plasma cholinesterase, the dibucaine-related variants seem to be the most important (Table 8-5) (Hunter, 1995; Pantuck, 1993). Dibucaine, a local anesthetic with an amide linkage, inhibits the activity of normal plasma cholinesterase enzyme by approximately 80%, compared with only approximately 20% inhibition of the activity of atypical enzyme. A dibucaine number of 80, which reflects 80% inhibition of enzyme activity, confirms the presence of normal plasma cholinesterase enzyme, whereas approximately 1 in every 3,200 patients is homozygous for an atypical plasma cholinesterase enzyme variant and has a dibucaine number of 20. In these patients, neuromuscular blockade after administration of SCh, 1 mg/kg IV, may persist for 3 hours or longer, and 25% recovery of the single-twitch response after a small dose of mivacurium, 0.03 mg/kg IV, takes up to 80 minutes (Ostergaard et al., 1995). Approximately 1 in every 480 patients is heterozygous for atypical plasma cholinesterase enzyme that results in a dibucaine number of 40 to 60. These heterozygous patients may manifest a modestly prolonged duration of neuromuscular blockade (up to 30 minutes) after administration of SCh.

It is important to recognize that the dibucaine number reflects quality of cholinesterase enzyme (ability to hydrolyze SCh) and not the quantity of the enzyme that is circulating in the plasma. For example, decreases in the plasma cholinesterase activity due to liver disease or anticholinesterase drugs are associated with normal (near 80)

TABLE 8-5.
HEREDITARY VARIANTS OF PLASMA CHOLINESTERASE

Genotype	Dibucaine Number	Fluoride Number	Response to Succinylcholine	Frequency
E^uE^u	80	60	Normal	96%
E^aE^a	20	20	Greatly prolonged	1 in 3,200
E^uE^a	60	45	Slightly prolonged	1 in 480
E^uE^f	75	50	Slightly prolonged	1 in 200
E^fE^a	45	35	Greatly prolonged	1 in 20,000

dibucaine numbers. A small number of patients have an isoenzyme of plasma cholinesterase that is associated with an accelerated rate of hydrolysis and a shorter duration of action of SCh (Sugimori, 1986).

Adverse Side Effects

Adverse side effects that may accompany the administration of SCh include (a) cardiac dysrhythmias, (b) hyperkalemia, (c) myalgia, (d) myoglobinuria, (e) increased intragastric pressure, (f) increased intraocular pressure, (g) increased intracranial pressure (ICP), and (h) sustained skeletal muscle contractions. These side effects may limit or even contraindicate the administration of SCh.

Administration of nonparalyzing doses of a nondepolarizing neuromuscular-blocking drug (pretreatment) may attenuate or prevent the occurrence of cardiac dysrhythmias, myalgia, and increases in intragastric and intraocular pressure after IV administration of SCh (Miller and Way, 1971; Miller et al., 1968; Stoelting, 1977; Stoelting and Peterson, 1975). Pretreatment, however, does not influence the magnitude of potassium release evoked by SCh (Stoelting and Peterson, 1975).

Cardiac Dysrhythmias

Sinus bradycardia, junctional rhythm, and even sinus arrest may follow administration of SCh. These cardiac effects reflect the actions of SCh at cardiac muscarinic cholinergic receptors where the drug mimics the physiologic effects of acetylcholine. Cardiac dysrhythmias are most likely to occur when a second dose of SCh is administered approximately 5 minutes after the first dose. This relationship to the second dose suggests a possible role of the metabolites of SCh (succinylmonocholine and choline) in producing bradycardia (Schoenstadt and Whitcher, 1963). Administration of atropine, 6 μg/kg IV, does not prevent heart rate slowing in response to a second dose of SCh (Stoelting, 1977).

In contrast to actions at cardiac muscarinic cholinergic receptors, the effects of SCh at autonomic nervous system ganglia may produce ganglionic stimulation and associated increases in heart rate and systemic blood pressure. The ganglionic stimulation reflects an effect of SCh on autonomic ganglia that resembles the physiologic effect of acetylcholine at these sites.

Hyperkalemia

Hyperkalemia may occur after administration of SCh to patients with (a) clinically unrecognized muscular dystrophy, (b) unhealed third-degree burns, (c) denervation leading to skeletal muscle atrophy, (d) severe skeletal muscle trauma, and (e) upper motor neuron lesions (Cooperman et al., 1970; Gronert and Theye, 1975; Sullivan et al., 1994; Tobey, 1970). Severe abdominal infections have been associated with SCh-induced potassium release (Kohlschutter et al., 1976). The potential for excessive potassium release

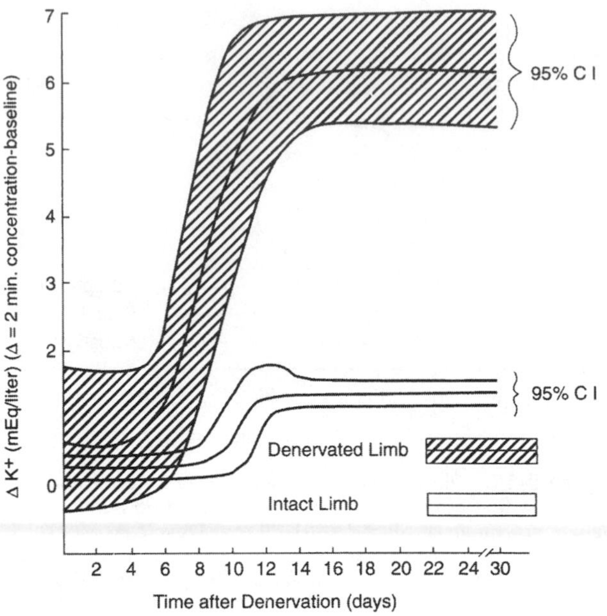

Figure 8-12. Changes in plasma potassium (K+) concentrations begin as early as 4 days after denervation injury in animals, whereas peak increases occur 14 days after injury. (CI, confidence interval.) (From John DA, Tobey RE, Homer LD, et al. Onset of succinylcholine-induced hyperkalemia following denervation. *Anesthesiology* 1976;45:294–299; with permission.)

after denervation may develop within 96 hours and may persist for an indefinite period up to 6 months or longer (Fig. 8-12) (John et al., 1976). There is no evidence of SCh-induced hyperkalemia in patients with Parkinson disease, cerebral palsy, or myelomeningocele, or in those undergoing cerebral aneurysm surgery (Dierdorf et al., 1985; Dierdorf et al., 1986; Manninen et al., 1990; Muzzi et al., 1989). Pretreatment with a subparalyzing dose of a nondepolarizing neuromuscular-blocking drug does not influence the magnitude of potassium release. Preexisting hyperkalemia (>5.5 mEq/L) as associated with renal failure and in the absence of skeletal muscle paralysis is not associated with an increased risk of acute potassium release following intubating doses of SCh (Schow et al., 2002).

SCh-induced rhabdomyolysis, hyperkalemia, and cardiac arrest may occur when SCh is administered to male children with undiagnosed myopathy (Sullivan et al., 1994). Duchenne muscular dystrophy is the most common form of muscular dystrophy, with an incidence of 1 in 3,300 male births. Diagnosis is often not possible until 2 to 6 years of age. Becker muscular dystrophy is also an X-linked muscular dystrophy that is less common (1 in 33,000 male births) and characterized by a more benign clinical course, which may delay clinical diagnosis. Based on these observations, it can be anticipated that a small percentage of the male pediatric population may present for surgery with an occult myopathy. For this reason, some clinicians favor avoiding the use of SCh in pediatric patients when an equally acceptable response can be achieved with a nondepolarizing neuromuscular-blocking drug.

Proliferation of extrajunctional cholinergic receptors providing more sites for potassium to leak outward from cells during depolarization is the presumed explanation for hyperkalemia that follows administration of SCh to patients with denervation injury. This mechanism has not been confirmed in burn injury patients.

Myalgia

Postoperative skeletal muscle myalgia, which is particularly prominent in the skeletal muscles of the neck, back, and abdomen, can occur after administration of SCh, especially to young adults undergoing minor surgical procedures that permit early ambulation. Myalgia localized to neck muscles may be perceived as a pharyngitis ("sore throat") by the patient and attributed to tracheal intubation by the anesthesiologist. It is speculated that unsynchronized contractions of skeletal muscle fibers associated with generalized depolarization produced by SCh lead to myalgia. Indeed, prevention of clinically visible SCh-induced skeletal muscle contractions with prior administration of a nonparalyzing dose of dTc prevents or attenuates the incidence of myalgia after administration of SCh (Stoelting and Peterson, 1975). Surprisingly, use of vecuronium in place of SCh does not decrease the occurrence of myalgia in patients undergoing laparoscopy (Zahl and Apfelbaum, 1989). Inflammation as a cause of SCh-induced myalgia is not supported by data failing to show a protective effect of dexamethasone (Schreiber et al., 2003).

Myoglobinuria

Damage to skeletal muscles is suggested by the occurrence of myoglobinuria after administration of SCh, especially to pediatric patients (Ryan et al., 1971). Presumably, myoglobinuria reflects skeletal muscle damage associated with SCh-induced fasciculations. For reasons that are not clear, myoglobinuria rarely occurs in adults receiving SCh.

Increased Intragastric Pressure

SCh produces inconsistent increases in intragastric pressure (Miller and Way, 1971). When intragastric pressure increases, it seems to be related to the intensity of skeletal muscle fasciculations induced by SCh. Indeed, prevention of clinically visible skeletal muscle fasciculations by prior administration of a nonparalyzing dose of nondepolarizing neuromuscular-blocking drug prevents increases in intragastric pressure produced by the subsequent administration of SCh (Miller and Way, 1971). The risk of increased intragastric pressure (gastroesophageal sphincter may open spontaneously at pressures of >28 cm H_2O) is resulting passage of gastric fluid into the esophagus and pharynx and subsequent inhalation into the lungs. Minimal to absent skeletal muscle fasciculations in children are consistent with the absence of appreciable increases in intragastric pressure that accompany administration of SCh to this age group (Salem et al., 1972).

Increased Intraocular Pressure

SCh causes a maximum increase in intraocular pressure 2 to 4 minutes after its administration (Pandey et al., 1972). This increase in the intraocular pressure is transient, lasting only 5 to 10 minutes. The mechanism by which SCh increases intraocular pressure remains unknown, although contraction of the extraocular muscles with distortion and compression of the globe has long been presumed to be the etiology of these changes (Macri and Grimes, 1957). The fear that such contraction may extrude global contents in a patient with an open eye injury has led clinicians to avoid administration of SCh to these patients (Dillon et al., 1957). This theory has never been substantiated and is challenged by the description of patients with an open eye injury in whom IV administration of SCh did not cause extrusion of global contents (Libonati et al., 1985). Indeed, there is evidence that contraction of extraocular muscles does not contribute to the increase in intraocular pressure that accompanies the administration of SCh (Fig. 8-13) (Kelly et al., 1993). It is likely that the cycloplegic action of SCh, with a deepening of the anterior chamber and increased resistance to outflow of aqueous humor, combined with slight increases in choroidal blood volume and central venous pressure, contributes to the increase in intraocular pressure.

Increased Intracranial Pressure

Increases in ICP after administration of SCh to patients with intracranial tumors or head trauma have not been a consistent observation (Fig. 8-14) (Kovarik et al., 1994).

Sustained Skeletal Muscle Contraction

Incomplete jaw relaxation and masseter jaw rigidity after a halothane-SCh sequence is not uncommon in children (occurs in about 4.4% of patients) and is considered a

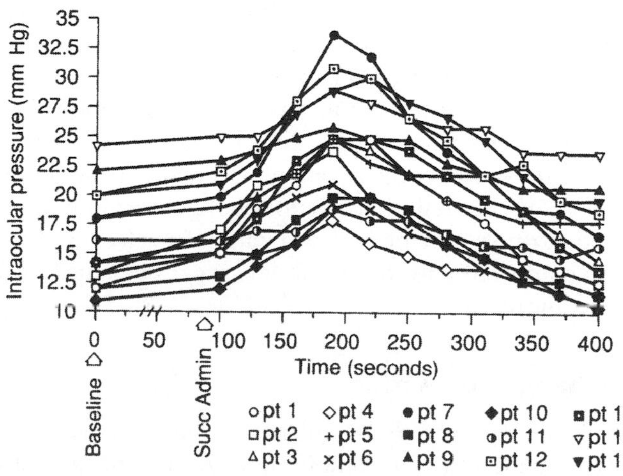

Figure 8-13. Intraocular pressure changes after administration of succinylcholine (Succ Admin), 1.5 mg/kg IV, to patients in whom all extraocular muscles had been previously detached. (From Kelly RE, Dinner M, Turner LS, et al. Succinylcholine increases intraocular pressure in the human eye with the extraocular muscles detached. *Anesthesiology* 1993;79: 948–952; with permission.)

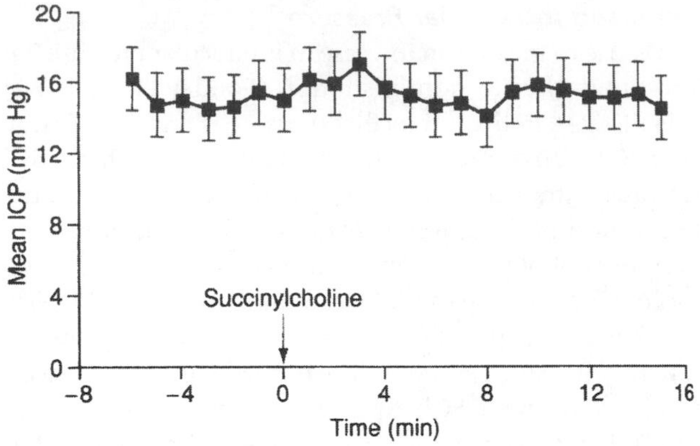

Figure 8-14. Succinylcholine, 1 mg/kg IV, when administered to patients with neurologic injury (median Glasgow coma scale score of 6) did not change mean intracranial pressure (ICP). (From Kovarik WD, Mayberg TS, Lam AM, et al. Succinylcholine does not change intracranial pressure, cerebral blood flow velocity, or the electroencephalogram in patients with neurologic injury. *Anesth Analg* 1994;78:469–473; with permission.)

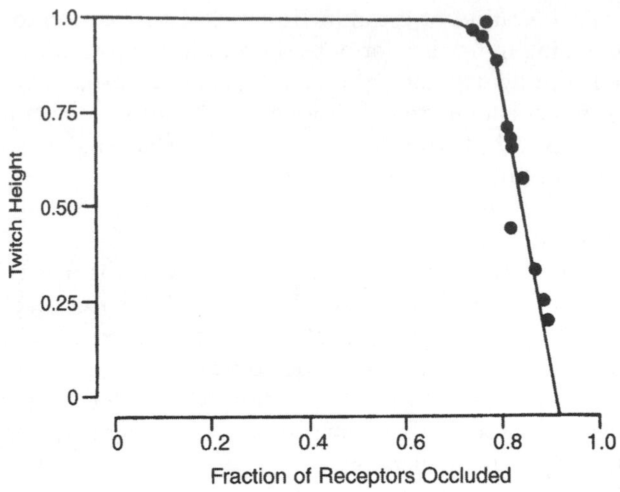

Figure 8-15. Schematic depiction of the number of receptors that must be occupied (receptor occupancy theory) before the existence of neuromuscular blockade is evident as a decrease in twitch height.

normal response (Hannallah and Kaplan, 1994). The difficulty lies in separating the normal response from masseter muscle rigidity that may be associated with the development of malignant hyperthermia (Bevan, 1994).

Sustained skeletal muscle spasm may accompany the administration of SCh to patients with myotonia congenita or myotonia dystrophica (Mitchell et al., 1978). This sustained skeletal muscle contraction may interfere with ventilation of the lungs and become life-threatening.

NONDEPOLARIZING NEUROMUSCULAR-BLOCKING DRUGS

Nondepolarizing neuromuscular-blocking drugs are characterized clinically as long-, intermediate-, and short-acting (see Table 8-1) (Hunter, 1995). Differences in onset, duration of action, rate of recovery, metabolism, and clearance, influence the clinical decision to select one drug over another. Many of the variable patient responses evoked by nondepolarizing neuromuscular-blocking drugs can be explained by differences in pharmacokinetics. In addition, the cost of the newer nondepolarizing neuromuscular-blocking drugs may be a consideration in selecting these drugs compared with older and less expensive drugs such as pancuronium.

Mechanism of Action

Nondepolarizing neuromuscular-blocking drugs are classically thought to act by combining with nicotinic nAChRs without causing any activation of these ion receptor channels. Specifically, these drugs can act competitively with acetylcholine at the alpha subunits of the postjunctional nAChRs without causing a change in the configuration of these receptors. In addition, these drugs, especially at high doses, may act by blocking the ion receptor channels. Nondepolarizing neuromuscular-blocking drugs also act at prejunctional nAChRs, but the actions at postjunctional sites are most important.

Occupation of as many as 70% of the nAChRs by a neuromuscular-blocking drug does not produce evidence of neuromuscular blockade, as reflected by the twitch response to a single electrical stimulus (Fig. 8-15) (Waud and Waud, 1971). Neuromuscular transmission, however, fails when 80% to 90% of the receptors are blocked. This confirms the wide safety margin of neuromuscular transmission and is the basis for the techniques of clinical monitoring of neuromuscular blockade.

Characteristics of Nondepolarizing Neuromuscular Blockade

Characteristic skeletal muscle responses in the presence of nondepolarizing neuromuscular blockade, as evoked by electrical stimulation from a peripheral nerve stimulator, include (a) decreased twitch response to a single stimulus, (b) unsustained response (fade) during continuous stimulation, (c) TOF ratio of <0.7, (d) posttetanic potentiation, (e) potentiation of other nondepolarizing neuromuscular-blocking drugs, and (f) antagonism by anticholinesterase drugs (see Fig. 8-2) (Hunter, 1995). In addition, skeletal muscle fasciculations do not accompany the onset of nondepolarizing neuromuscular blockade.

Skeletal muscle contraction is an all-or-none phenomenon. Each skeletal muscle fiber contracts maximally or does not contract at all. Therefore, when twitch response is decreased, some fibers are contracting normally, whereas others are completely blocked. Fade of skeletal muscle contraction in response to continuous electrical stimulation suggests that some fibers are more susceptible to being

TABLE 8-6.
MECHANISMS OF NEUROMUSCULAR-BLOCKING DRUG–INDUCED CARDIOVASCULAR EFFECTS

	Histamine Release	Cardiac Muscarinic Receptors	Nicotinic Receptors at Autonomic Ganglia
Succinylcholine	Slight	Modest stimulation	Modest stimulation
Pancuronium	None	Modest blockade	None
Doxacurium	None	None	None
Pipecuronium	None	None	None
Atracurium	Slight	None	None
Vecuronium	None	None	None
Rocuronium	None	None	None
Cisatracurium	None	None	None
Mivacurium	Slight	None	None

blocked by neuromuscular-blocking drugs and need a greater sustained release of acetylcholine to trigger their responses.

Cardiovascular Effects

Nondepolarizing neuromuscular-blocking drugs may exert cardiovascular effects through drug-induced release of histamine or other vasoactive substances (prostacyclin release from mast cells), effects at cardiac muscarinic receptors, or effects on nAChRs at autonomic ganglia (Table 8-6). Considerable species difference exists with respect to mechanisms responsible for circulatory effects of neuromuscular-blocking drugs. It is likely that the relative magnitude of circulatory effects varies from patient to patient according to factors such as underlying autonomic nervous system activity, preoperative medication, drugs administered for maintenance of anesthesia, and concurrent drug therapy. Despite the frequent reference to the cardiovascular effects of nondepolarizing neuromuscular-blocking drugs, it is rare that these changes achieve clinical significance.

The difference between the dose of neuromuscular-blocking drug that produces neuromuscular blockade and circulatory effects is defined as the *autonomic margin of safety* (Hughes and Chapple, 1976). An ED_{95} dose of pancuronium that produces neuromuscular blockade is also likely to produce circulatory (heart rate) changes, and the autonomic margin of safety is narrow. Conversely, vecuronium, rocuronium, and cisatracurium have wide autonomic margins of safety because the ED_{95} dose necessary to produce neuromuscular blockade is less than the dose that evokes circulatory changes.

Critical Illness Myopathy

A small fraction of patients with asthma, or acutely injured patients with multiple-organ system failure and who require drug-induced skeletal muscle paralysis to facilitate mechanical ventilation of the lungs for prolonged periods (usually >6 days), manifest skeletal muscular weakness on recovery (Hunter, 1995). These patients exhibit moderate to severe quadriparesis with or without areflexia, but they usually retain normal sensory function. The time course of the weakness is unpredictable, and in some patients the weakness may progress and persist for weeks or months despite discontinuation of the nondepolarizing neuromuscular-blocking drug. Although the mechanism of this myopathy is not known, it is thought to be more common when an aminosteroid nondepolarizing neuromuscular-blocking drug (pharmacologic denervation) such as pancuronium or vecuronium is used to facilitate mechanical ventilation (Hansen-Flaschen et al., 1993; Margolis et al., 1991). Despite this impression, a similar myopathy has been observed in patients treated with atracurium (Meyer et al., 1994; Tousignant et al., 1995). Thus, the steroidal nucleus of aminosteroid nondepolarizing neuromuscular blockers does not seem to be critical to the development of this myopathy. Nevertheless, administration of glucocorticoids before therapy including nondepolarizing neuromuscular-blocking drugs may increase the risk of developing this myopathy. When monitoring of neuromuscular blockade with a peripheral nerve stimulator is combined with clinical guidelines, including adequate sedation and analgesia, smaller doses of nondepolarizing neuromuscular-blocking drugs are used to facilitate mechanical ventilation of the lungs, and prolonged paralysis is less likely (Kheunl-Brady et al., 1994; Lee, 1995). Conversely, others conclude that monitoring the TOF does not prevent the development of a myopathy or polyneuropathy (Prielipp et al., 1994).

The pathophysiology of this myopathy is not well understood. Proposed causes include prolonged neuromuscular blockade resulting from decreased clearance owing to renal and/or hepatic dysfunction or active metabolites of the neuromuscular-blocking drug, as well as metabolic disorders and polypharmacy. Steroid myopathy and polyneuropathy of sepsis have been implicated. The number of steroid receptors in skeletal muscles increases with denervation, and it is possible that increased susceptibility to the myopathic effects of systemically administered steroids occurs. Alternatively, skeletal muscle weakness may not be the result of polyneuropathy but that of dysfunction of the NMJ with some unknown role of the nondepolarizing neuromuscular blockers being present (Tousignant et al., 1995).

Causes of Altered Responses

Drugs administered in the perioperative period may enhance the effects of nondepolarizing neuromuscular-blocking drugs at the NMJ. Examples of drugs that can enhance nondepolarizing neuromuscular blockade include (a) volatile anesthetics, (b) aminoglycoside antibiotics, (c) local anesthetics, (d) cardiac antidysrhythmic drugs, (e) diuretics, and (f) magnesium and lithium. Changes unrelated to concurrent drug therapy, such as (a) hypothermia, (b) acid–base alterations, (c) changes in serum potassium concentrations, (d) adrenocortical dysfunction, (e) thermal (burn) injury, and (f) allergic reactions, may also influence the characteristics of neuromuscular blockade produced by nondepolarizing neuromuscular-blocking drugs. Combinations of nondepolarizing neuromuscular-blocking drugs may produce a degree of neuromuscular blockade that is different from the degree that would be produced by either drug alone. In addition, gender may influence the duration of neuromuscular blockade produced by nondepolarizing neuromuscular-blocking drugs.

Volatile Anesthetics

Volatile anesthetics produce dose-dependent enhancement of the magnitude and duration of neuromuscular blockade due to nondepolarizing neuromuscular-blocking drugs (Fogdall and Miller, 1975; Miller et al., 1971). This enhancement of neuromuscular blockade is greatest with enflurane, isoflurane, desflurane, and sevoflurane and least with nitrous oxide-opioid combinations (Caldwell et al., 1991). Sevoflurane has a marked inhibitory effect on neuromuscular transmission and this, combined with its low blood-gas solubility, results in a rapid onset (within 30 minutes) of sevoflurane-induced potentiation of nondepolarizing neuromuscular-blocking drugs (Suzuki et al., 2000). The potency, infusion requirements and recovery characteristics for rocuronium are similar in the presence of 1.25 MAC isoflurane, desflurane, and sevoflurane (Bock et al., 2000). For unknown reasons, the magnitude of decrease in dose requirements produced by volatile anesthetics seems to be less for intermediate-acting than for long-acting nondepolarizing neuromuscular-blocking drugs (Figs. 8-16 and 8-17) (Rupp et al., 1984; Rupp et al., 1985). Furthermore, changes in the alveolar concentration of volatile anesthetic has less impact on neuromuscular blockade produced by intermediate-acting compared with long-acting neuromuscular-blocking drugs. The advantage of lessened augmentation of intermediate-acting neuromuscular-blocking drugs by volatile anesthetics is a more predictable degree of neuromuscular blockade, without precise knowledge of the alveolar (brain) partial pressure of the anesthetic. Conversely, a disadvantage is that existing neuromuscular blockade is not easily enhanced by increasing the delivered concentration of volatile anesthetic.

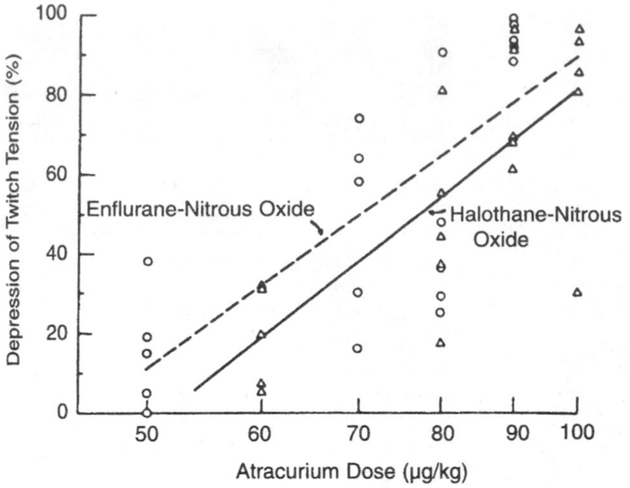

Figure 8-16. Atracurium-induced neuromuscular blockade is enhanced by volatile anesthetics. (From Rupp SM, McChristian JW, Miller RD. Neuromuscular effects of atracurium during halothane–nitrous oxide and enflurane–nitrous oxide anesthesia in humans. *Anesthesiology* 1985;63:16–19; with permission.)

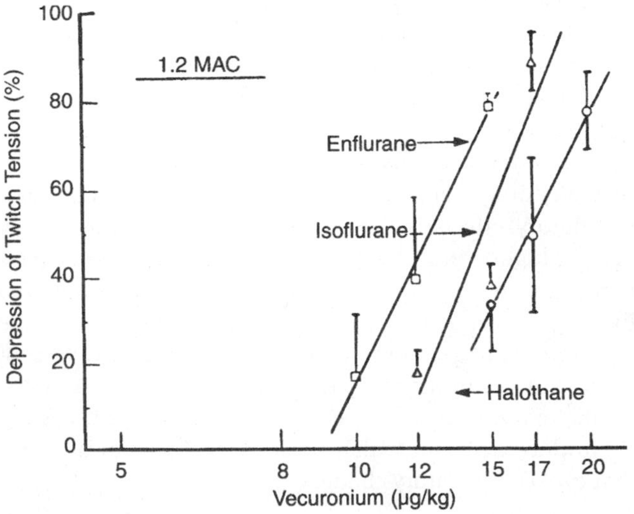

Figure 8-17. Vecuronium-induced neuromuscular blockade is enhanced by volatile anesthetics. (From Rupp SM, Miller RD, Gencarelli P. Vecuronium-induced neuromuscular blockade during enflurane, isoflurane, and halothane anesthesia in humans. *Anesthesiology* 1984;60:102–105; with permission.)

Volatile anesthetics most likely enhance the effects of nondepolarizing neuromuscular-blocking drugs by virtue of anesthetic-induced depression of the CNS, which decreases the tone of skeletal muscles (Waud and Waud, 1975). In addition, volatile anesthetics may decrease the sensitivity of postjunctional membranes to depolarization (Waud and Waud, 1979). Increased skeletal muscle blood flow as a means to deliver more drug to the NMJ is probably important only for the enhanced neuromuscular blockade seen in the presence of isoflurane (Vitez et al., 1975). Inhaled anesthetics do not enhance neuromuscular blockade by decreasing the release of acetylcholine from motor nerve endings or by altering the configuration of cholinergic receptors (Waud and Waud, 1973). Plasma concentrations of nondepolarizing neuromuscular-blocking drugs necessary to depress single-twitch response are less in the presence of volatile anesthetics than in the presence of nitrous oxide-opioid combinations, confirming that potentiation of neuromuscular blockade by volatile anesthetics represents a change in pharmacodynamics rather than a change in pharmacokinetics.

Antibiotics

Several types of antibiotics have been shown to enhance neuromuscular blockade produced by nondepolarizing neuromuscular-blocking drugs. Prominent among the antibiotics that produce this enhancement are the aminoglycoside antibiotics (Chapple et al., 1983; Dotan et al., 2003). Antagonism of antibiotic-potentiated neuromuscular blockade by an anticholinesterase drug or calcium is unpredictable. Antibiotics devoid of neuromuscular-blocking effects are the penicillins and cephalosporins.

Antibiotics may exert effects on the prejunctional membranes similar to those exerted by magnesium, resulting in decreased release of acetylcholine (Sokoll and Gergis, 1981). Likewise, the same antibiotics may stabilize postjunctional membranes; thus, proposing a common mechanism for antibiotic-induced enhancement of neuromuscular blockade probably is impossible.

Inhibition of the presynaptic release of acetylcholine by antibiotics may reflect competition by these drugs with calcium. Indeed, IV injection of calcium may at least transiently antagonize the enhanced neuromuscular blockade associated with the administration of antibiotics. Nevertheless, in addition to facilitating the prejunctional release of acetylcholine, calcium at the same time stabilizes postjunctional membranes to the effects of acetylcholine. These different effects of calcium at the NMJ are consistent with the unpredictable effects of calcium in antagonizing antibiotic-induced enhancement of neuromuscular blockade produced by nondepolarizing neuromuscular-blocking drugs.

Local Anesthetics

Small doses of local anesthetics can enhance neuromuscular blockade produced by nondepolarizing neuromuscular-blocking drugs, whereas large doses of local anesthetics can block neuromuscular transmission. Depending on the dose, local anesthetics interfere with the prejunctional release of acetylcholine, stabilize postjunctional membranes, and directly depress skeletal muscle fibers. In addition, ester local anesthetics compete with other drugs for plasma cholinesterase, thus introducing the possibility of a prolonged drug effect produced by SCh.

Cardiac Antidysrhythmic Drugs

Lidocaine administered IV to treat cardiac dysrhythmias could augment preexisting neuromuscular blockade (Harrah et al., 1970). This potential drug interaction is a consideration when lidocaine is administered IV to patients recovering from general anesthesia that included use of a nondepolarizing neuromuscular-blocking drug.

Quinidine potentiates neuromuscular blockade produced by nondepolarizing and depolarizing neuromuscular-blocking drugs, presumably by interfering with the prejunctional release of acetylcholine (Miller et al., 1967). As with lidocaine, this drug interaction may manifest when quinidine is administered to treat cardiac dysrhythmias in patients who previously have received neuromuscular-blocking drugs during general anesthesia.

Diuretics

Furosemide, 1 mg/kg IV, enhances neuromuscular blockade produced by nondepolarizing neuromuscular-blocking drugs (Miller et al., 1976). This effect most likely reflects furosemide-induced inhibition of cAMP production, leading to decreased prejunctional output of acetylcholine. Conversely, large doses of furosemide may inhibit phosphodiesterase, making more cAMP available and leading to antagonism of nondepolarizing neuromuscular-blocking drugs (Azar et al., 1980). Azathioprine also antagonizes nondepolarizing neuromuscular blockade, presumably by inhibiting phosphodiesterase (Dretchen et al., 1976). This same drug augments neuromuscular blockade produced by SCh.

Mannitol does not influence the degree of neuromuscular blockade produced by nondepolarizing neuromuscular-blocking drugs, even in the presence of diuresis (Matteo et al., 1980). This emphasizes that renal clearance of neuromuscular-blocking drugs depends on glomerular filtration. Osmotic diuretics increase urine output independent of glomerular filtration rate. Chronic hypokalemia due to treatment with diuretics decreases dose requirements for pancuronium and increases the dose of neostigmine necessary to antagonize neuromuscular blockade (Miller and Roderick, 1978a).

Magnesium

Magnesium enhances neuromuscular blockade produced by nondepolarizing neuromuscular-blocking drugs and, to a lesser extent, enhances neuromuscular blockade produced by SCh (Ghoneim and Long, 1970). It has been suggested that the interaction between magnesium and vecuronium is more pronounced than observed with other nondepolarizing neuromuscular-blocking drugs (Sinatra et al., 1985). Speculated mechanisms for this interaction include decreased prejunctional release of acetylcholine and decreased sensitivity (stabilization of postjunctional membranes) to acetylcholine. The effects of magnesium are consistent with the enhancement of neuromuscular blockade produced by nondepolarizing neuromuscular-blocking drugs as administered to patients with pregnancy-induced hypertension (toxemia of pregnancy) who are being treated with magnesium. The mechanism by which these effects of magnesium enhance neuromuscular blockade produced by SCh is not apparent. It is possible that phase II blockade occurs more readily when SCh is administered in the presence of increased plasma concentrations of magnesium.

Lithium

Lithium, as used to treat psychiatric depression, may enhance the neuromuscular-blocking effects of depolarizing and nondepolarizing neuromuscular-blocking drugs (Havdala et al., 1979).

Anticonvulsants

Patients treated chronically with anticonvulsants (phenytoin, carbamazepine) are relatively resistant to some (pancuronium, vecuronium, rocuronium, cisatracurium, pipecuronium, doxacurium) but not all (mivacurium, atracurium) nondepolarizing neuromuscular-blocking drugs (Richard et al., 2005; Spacek et al., 1999a). These patients recover more quickly from neuromuscular blockade, which could put them at risk if movement occurred during delicate neurosurgical procedures. Resistance seems to be related to a pharmacodynamic mechanism, because plasma concentrations of drug needed to produce a given level of neuromuscular blockade are increased compared with the plasma level necessary to produce the same response in untreated patients. Nevertheless, phenytoin and carbamazepine result in resistance to the neuromuscular blocking effects of vecuronium in children reflecting pharmacokinetic (increased hepatic clearance and decreased elimination half-time perhaps reflecting hepatic enzyme induction and/or increased protein binding) rather than pharmacodynamic (plasma concentrations at different degrees of recovery unchanged from controls) changes (Soriano et al., 2001). In contrast to chronic treatment, acute administration of phenytoin has been associated with augmentation of neuromuscular blockade produced by rocuronium (Spacek et al., 1999b).

Cyclosporine

Cyclosporine may prolong the duration of neuromuscular blockade produced by nondepolarizing neuromuscular-blocking drugs (Wood, 1989).

Corticosteroids (see the section, Critical Illness Myopathy)

Cortisol or adrenocorticotrophic hormone can improve neuromuscular function in patients with myasthenia gravis. Conversely, the IV administration of corticosteroids does not alter the characteristics of neuromuscular blockade produced by nondepolarizing neuromuscular-blocking drugs (Schwartz et al., 1986). Enhanced neuromuscular blockade produced when corticosteroids are combined with vecuronium may reflect pharmacologic denervation of nAChRs and contribute to prolonged weakness observed in some critically ill patients (Kindler et al., 2000).

The combination of corticosteroids and neuromuscular blocking-drugs has been utilized in critically ill asthmatic patients in attempts to facilitate mechanical ventilation of the lungs and minimize barotraumas. In patients undergoing this combined treatment regimen for as little as 96 hours, severe skeletal muscle weakness may develop requiring prolonged (weeks or months) of recovery time (critical illness polyneuropathy) (Kindler et al., 2000).

Drugs Acting on the Sympathetic Nervous System

Administration of ephedrine, 0.07 mg/kg IV, prior to injection of rocuronium decreases the onset time by 22%, suggesting that increased cardiac output and skeletal muscle blood flow provides more rapid delivery of rocuronium to the neuromuscular junction (Szmuk et al., 2000). Esmolol, 0.5 mg/kg IV, administered immediately before the induction of anesthesia, delays the onset time of rocuronium by 26%, suggesting that decreased cardiac output and skeletal muscle blood flow slowed delivery of rocuronium to the neuromuscular junction (Szmuk et al., 2000).

Hypothermia

Mild hypothermia doubles the duration of vecuronium-induced neuromuscular blockade. This increased duration of action is due to decreased clearance of vecuronium and a slowed rate of effect site equilibration (Caldwell et al., 2003). Tissue sensitivity to vecuronium is not influenced by core body temperature. Hypothermia prolongs the duration of neuromuscular blockade of pancuronium, presumably reflecting temperature-induced slowing of hepatic enzyme activity and biliary and renal clearance of the drug (Buzello et al., 1985a; Hame et al., 1978). Hypothermia also seems to increase sensitivity of the NMJ to pancuronium. Hypothermia prolongs the duration of action of atracurium and decreases the rate of continuous infusion necessary to maintain a constant degree of neuromuscular blockade (Flynn et al., 1983). Presumably, this enhanced neuromuscular-blocking effect of atracurium reflects decreased degradation of atracurium by Hofmann elimination and decreased metabolism by ester hydrolysis.

Serum Potassium Concentration

An acute decrease in the extracellular concentration of potassium increases the transmembrane potential, causing hyperpolarization of cell membranes. This change manifests as resistance to the effects of depolarizing neuromuscular-blocking drugs and increased sensitivity to nondepolarizing neuromuscular-blocking drugs. Conversely, hyperkalemia decreases the resting transmembrane potential and thus partially depolarizes cell membranes. This change increases the effects of depolarizing neuromuscular-blocking drugs and opposes the action of nondepolarizing neuromuscular-blocking drugs.

Thermal (Burn) Injury

Thermal (burn) injury causes resistance to the effects of nondepolarizing neuromuscular-blocking drugs that manifests approximately 10 days after injury, peaks at approximately 40 days, and declines after approximately 60 days (Fig. 8-18) (Dwersteg et al., 1986; Martyn et al., 1982; Martyn et al., 1983). Despite this typical sequence, at least one report describes resistance lasting 463 days (Martyn et al., 1982). Approximately 30% or more of the body must be burned to produce resistance. The onset time to adequate intubating conditions for rocuronium is prolonged in burned patients compared with nonburned patients and this may be offset by increasing the dose to 1.2 mg/kg IV (Han et al., 2004). A pharmacodynamic explanation as the principal mechanism for this resistance is documented by the need to achieve higher plasma concentrations to produce a given degree of twitch suppression in thermal injury versus nonthermal injury patients (Marathe et al., 1989a; Martyn et al., 1982). In contrast to denervation injury and an associated increase in extrajunctional cholinergic receptors that respond to acetylcholine, resistance to the effects of nondepolarizing neuromuscular-blocking drugs in patients with thermal injury is not associated with changes in the density of these receptors (Marathe et al., 1989b). An altered affinity of nAChRs for nondepolarizing neuromuscular-blocking drugs may be the basis for thermal injury–induced resistance to these drugs.

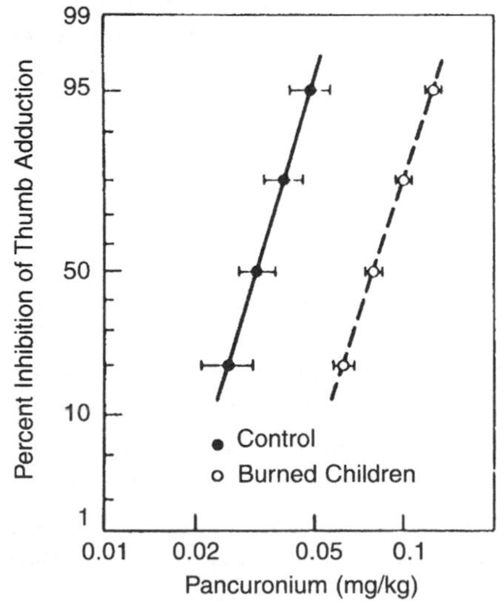

Figure 8-18. Dose response curves for pancuronium are shifted to the right in thermal (burn) injury patients, indicating a resistance to the neuromuscular-blocking effects of the drug (From Martyn JAJ, Liu LMP, Szfelbein SK, et al. The neuromuscular effects of pancuronium in burned children. *Anesthesiology* 1983;59:561–564; with permission.)

Paresis or Hemiplegia

Monitoring neuromuscular blockade with a peripheral nerve stimulator attached to the paretic arm on the side affected by a cerebral vascular accident reveals resistance (decreased sensitivity) to the effects of the neuromuscular-blocking drug compared with the response observed on the unaffected side (Iwasaki et al., 1985; Moorthy and Hilgenberg, 1980). Furthermore, the unaffected arm shows resistance to the effects of neuromuscular-blocking drugs compared with responses observed in normal patients (Shayevitz and Matteo, 1985). As a result, monitoring neuromuscular blockade with a peripheral nerve stimulator after a cerebral vascular accident may underestimate the degree of neuromuscular blockade present at the muscles of ventilation. Resistance to neuromuscular-blocking drugs after a cerebral vascular accident may reflect proliferation of extrajunctional nAChRs that respond to acetylcholine.

Allergic Reactions

Anaphylactic and anaphylactoid reactions occur occasionally after the IV administration of nondepolarizing neuromuscular-blocking drugs and SCh. There may be cross-sensitivity between all the neuromuscular-blocking drugs, reflecting the presence of a common antigenic component, the quaternary ammonium group (Didier et al., 1987). Drugs with single quaternary ammonium groups (pancuronium, vecuronium, rocuronium) are less likely to cause allergic reactions than SCh (Rose and Fisher, 2001). A severe anaphylactic reaction has been reported following administration of cisatracurim to a child, despite the perception that this drug is unlikely to be associated with allergic reactions (Legros et al., 2001). Nevertheless, allergic reactions have been observed after administration of monoquaternary as well as bisquaternary nondepolarizing neuromuscular-blocking drugs. Anaphylactic reactions after the first exposure to a neuromuscular-blocking drug may reflect sensitization from prior contact with cosmetics or soaps that also contain antigenic quaternary ammonium groups. Indeed, females have a greater incidence of allergic reactions to neuromuscular-blocking drugs than do males (2.5:1).

Succinylcholine Followed by a Nondepolarizing Neuromuscular-Blocking Drug

The prior administration of SCh, 1 mg/kg IV, to facilitate tracheal intubation, enhances the magnitude of twitch response suppression produced by the subsequently administered nondepolarizing neuromuscular-blocking drug, even when the evidence of neuromuscular blockade produced by SCh has waned (Ono et al., 1989; Stirt et al., 1983). This is unexpected, because the sequence of SCh followed by a nondepolarizing neuromuscular-blocking drug should be antagonistic. Presumably, postjunctional membranes remain desensitized by SCh, resulting in prolonged effects produced by nondepolarizing neuromuscular-blocking drugs. Despite the initial enhancement, the subsequent duration of action of neuromuscular blockade produced by atracurium or vecuronium is not prolonged by the prior administration of SCh. A smaller prior dose of SCh, 0.5 mg/kg IV, does not enhance the neuromuscular-blocking effects of vecuronium (Fisher and Miller, 1983a).

Gender

The sensitivity of patients to pancuronium, vecuronium, and rocuronium is appreciably different between men and women (Semple et al., 1994; Houghton et al., 1992; Xue et al., 1998). Women are more sensitive to vecuronium than men, as reflected by a 22% decrease in the dose of vecuronium that is necessary to achieve the same degree of neuromuscular blockade. Compared with women, men have lower plasma concentrations of vecuronium after the intravenous administration of the drug and a larger volume of distribution (Xue et al., 1998). The duration of vecuronium-induced neuromuscular blockade is longer in women than men. Women are 30% more sensitive to rocuronium than men (Fig. 8-19) (Xue et al., 1997). This suggests that the routine dose of rocuronium should be decreased in women compared with men. The reason for differences in sensitivity to nondepolarizing muscle relaxants between genders is unclear but may be related to differences in body composition, distribution volume, and plasma protein concentrations. The most likely reason would seem to be a greater percentage of skeletal muscle mass in men, thus increasing the required dose of neuromuscular-blocking drug to produce a response similar to that in women.

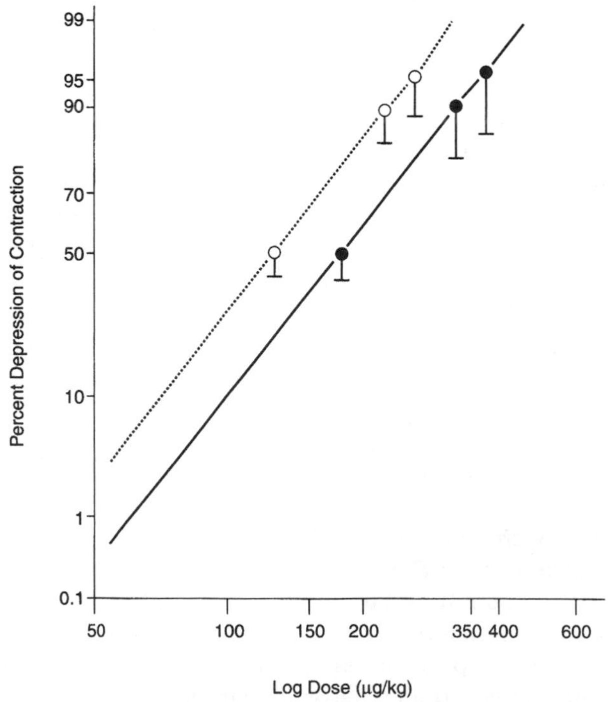

Figure 8-19. Dose response curves of rocuronium in male (*solid circles*) and female (*clear circles*) patients. (From Xue FS, Tong SY, Liao X, et al. Dose-response and time course of effect of rocuronium in male and female anesthetized patients. *Anesth Analg* 1997;85:667–671; with permission.)

LONG-ACTING NONDEPOLARIZING NEUROMUSCULAR-BLOCKING DRUGS

Pancuronium is the most commonly administered long-acting nondepolarizing neuromuscular-blocking drug. Doxacurium and pipecuronium resemble pancuronium but, unlike pancuronium, these drugs are devoid of cardiovascular side effects. The low cost of pancuronium has been cited as an advantage of this drug compared with newer and more expensive nondepolarizing neuromuscular-blocking drugs (Rachel et al., 1993). The benzylisoquinolinium compounds dTc and metocurine (dimethyltubocurarine) and the quaternary amine compound gallamine are examples of long-acting nondepolarizing neuromuscular-blocking drugs that have been replaced in clinical practice with drugs possessing more efficient and predictable clearance mechanisms.

Pancuronium

Pancuronium is a bisquaternary aminosteroid nondepolarizing neuromuscular-blocking drug with an ED_{95} of 70 μg/kg that has an onset of action in 3 to 5 minutes and a duration of neuromuscular blockade lasting 60 to 90 minutes (see Fig. 8-1 and Table 8-3) (Hunter, 1995). Respiratory acidosis enhances pancuronium-induced neuromuscular blockade and opposes its antagonism with neostigmine (Miller and Roderick, 1978b). Changes produced by metabolic acidosis and respiratory and metabolic alkalosis have been inconsistent.

Clearance

An estimated 80% of a single dose of pancuronium is eliminated unchanged in the urine. In the presence of renal failure, the plasma clearance of pancuronium is decreased 33% to 50% (Pollard, 1992). An estimated 10% to 40% of a dose of pancuronium undergoes hepatic deacetylation to 3-desacetylpancuronium, 17-desacetylpancuronium, and 3,17-desacetylpancuronium (Agoston et al., 1973; Hunter, 1995). The 3-desacetylpancuronium metabolite is approximately 50% as potent as pancuronium at the NMJ, whereas the other metabolites have only minimal activity (Miller et al., 1978a).

Patients with total biliary obstruction and hepatic cirrhosis have an increased volume of distribution, decreased plasma clearance, and prolonged elimination half-time of pancuronium (Table 8-7) (Duvaldestin et al., 1978). The large volume of distribution means a large initial dose of

TABLE 8-7.
PHARMACOKINETICS OF PANCURONIUM AND HEPATIC DYSFUNCTION

	Normal Hepatic Function	Cirrhosis
Volume of distribution (mL/kg)	279	416*
Clearance (mL/kg/min)	1.9	1.5*
Elimination half-time (mins)	114	208*

*$P < .05$ compared with normal hepatic function.
Source: Data from Duvaldestin P, Agoston S, Henzel E, et al. Pancuronium pharmacokinetics in patients with liver cirrhosis. *Br J Anaesth* 1978;50:131–136; with permission.

pancuronium is required to produce the same plasma concentration, but the resulting neuromuscular blockade may be prolonged because of decreased clearance.

Aging is associated with decreased clearance of pancuronium from the plasma (Fig. 8-20) (Duvaldestin et al., 1982; Matteo et al., 1985). The resulting prolonged elimination half-time reflects decreasing renal function in the elderly, manifesting as a prolonged duration of neuromuscular blockade. The absence of age-related changes in responsiveness of the NMJ (pharmacodynamics) is confirmed by similar dose–response curves in elderly and young adults (Fig. 8-21) (Duvaldestin et al., 1982).

Cardiovascular Effects

Pancuronium typically produces a modest 10% to 15% increase in heart rate, mean arterial pressure, and cardiac output (Figs. 8-22 and 8-23) (Rathmell et al., 1993;

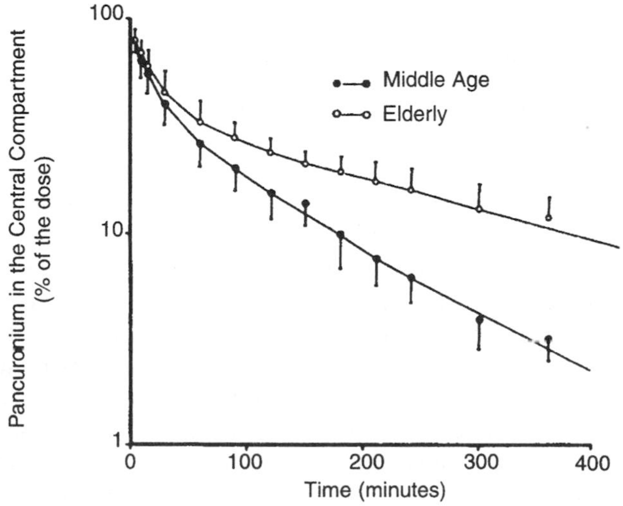

Figure 8-20. Aging is associated with a decreased rate of decline in the plasma concentration of long-acting nondepolarizing neuromuscular-blocking drugs such as pancuronium. (From Duvaldestin P, Saada J, Berger JL, et al. Pharmacokinetics, pharmacodynamics, and dose–response relationship of pancuronium in control and elderly subjects. *Anesthesiology* 1982;56:36–40; with permission.)

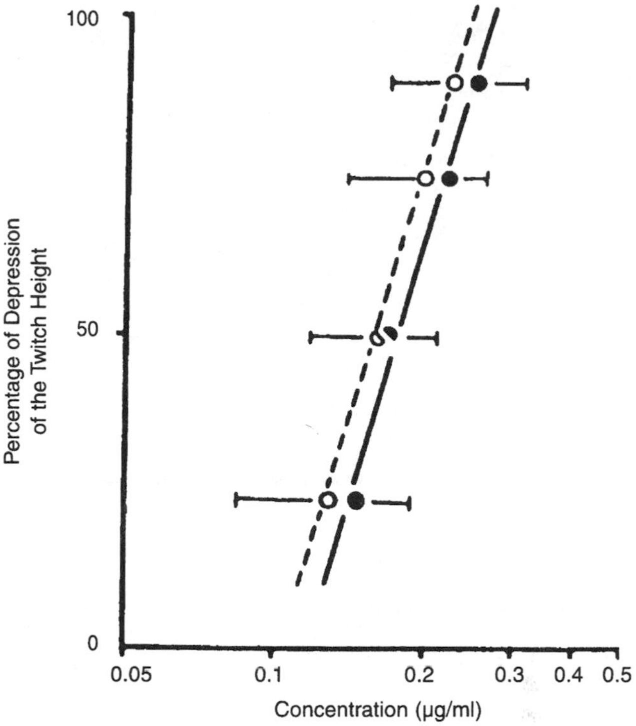

Figure 8-21. The absence of age-related changes in the responsiveness of the neuromuscular junction to long-acting nondepolarizing neuromuscular-blocking drugs such as pancuronium is confirmed by the similarity of plasma concentrations necessary to produce comparable responses in young adults (*solid circles*) and elderly individuals (*clear circles*). (From Duvaldestin P, Saada J, Berger JL, et al. Pharmacokinetics, pharmacodynamics, and dose–response relationship of pancuronium in control and elderly subjects. *Anesthesiology* 1982;56:36–40; with permission.)

Stoelting, 1972). These cardiovascular effects are attributed to selective cardiac vagal blockade (atropine-like effect limited to cardiac muscarinic receptors) and activation of the sympathetic nervous system (Domenech et al., 1976). Both release of norepinephrine from adrenergic nerve endings and blockade of uptake of norepinephrine back into postganglionic nerve endings have been proposed as mechanisms for activation of the sympathetic nervous system by pancuronium (Ivankovich et al., 1975; Vercruyse et al., 1979). Pancuronium may also interfere with the activity of muscarinic receptors that normally inhibit the release of norepinephrine. Likewise, pancuronium may produce blockade at muscarinic receptors that normally release dopamine, thus facilitating transmission through autonomic ganglia by inactivating the inhibitory influence of the dopaminergic cell loop (Scott and Savarese, 1985). The increase in circulating plasma concentrations of catecholamines after IV administration of pancuronium supports a drug-induced activation of the sympathetic nervous system (Domenech et al., 1976).

Pancuronium increases heart rate principally by blocking vagal muscarinic receptors in the sinoatrial node, as evidenced by the ability of prior administration of atropine to block this response. A sympathomimetic effect of pancuronium apparently plays a minor role in heart rate

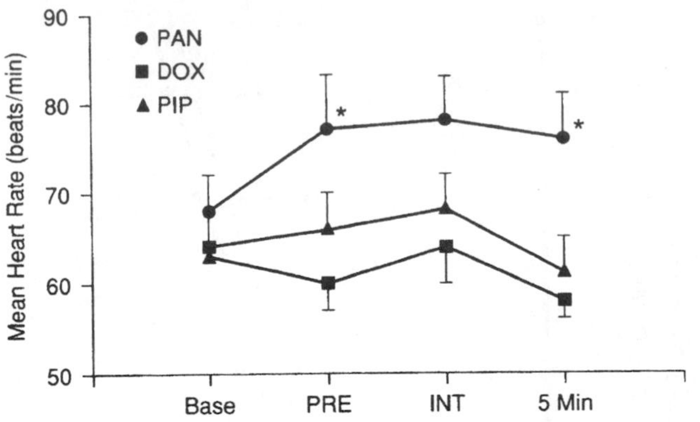

Figure 8-22. Heart rate awake (Base) was measured in awake patients and then 5 minutes after anesthetic induction (PRE) with fentanyl, 50 μg/kg IV, plus 2 × ED_{95} of pancuronium (PAN), doxacurium (DOX), or pipecuronium (PIP); immediately after tracheal intubation (INT); and 5 minutes after tracheal intubation (5 Min). There were no differences between treatment groups at any time. (*$P < .05$ compared with baseline.) (From Rathmel JP, Brooker RF, Prielipp RC, et al. Hemodynamic and pharmacodynamic comparison of doxacurium and pipecuronium during induction of cardiac anesthesia: Does the benefit justify the cost? *Anesth Analg* 1993;76:513–519; with permission.)

responses. Indeed, heart rate responses evoked by pancuronium still occur in patients treated with beta-adrenergic antagonists (Morris et at., 1983). The magnitude of heart rate increase evoked by pancuronium seems more dependent on the preexisting heart rate (an inverse relationship) than the dose or rate of pancuronium administration. Marked increases in heart rate in response to pancuronium seem more likely to occur in patients with altered atrioventricular conduction of cardiac impulses, such as may occur in the presence of atrial fibrillation.

The modest increase in blood pressure after the administration of pancuronium reflects the effect of heart rate on cardiac output in the absence of changes in systemic vascular resistance. Positive inotropic effects of pancuronium have not been demonstrated (Scott and Savarese, 1985).

An increased incidence of cardiac dysrhythmias has been observed after the administration of pancuronium, but not SCh, to patients being treated chronically with digitalis. Cardiac dysrhythmias may reflect sudden changes in the balance of autonomic nervous system activity in favor of the sympathetic nervous system. The cardiac-stimulating effects of pancuronium may also increase the incidence of myocardial ischemia in patients with coronary artery disease (Thomson and Putnins, 1985). Histamine release and autonomic ganglion blockade are not produced by pancuronium.

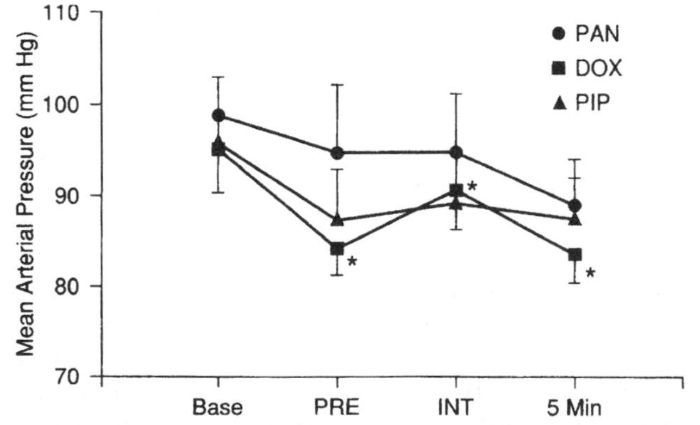

Figure 8-23. Mean arterial pressure at various times after induction of anesthesia and administration of 2 × ED_{95} of pancuronium, doxacurium, and pipecuronium. (*$P < .05$ compared to baseline.) (See the legend for Fig. 8-22 for a description of labels.) (From Rathmel JP, Brooker RF, Prielipp RC, et al. Hemodynamic and pharmacodynamic comparison of doxacurium and pipecuronium with pancuronium during induction of cardiac anesthesia: Does the benefit justify the cost? *Anesth Analg* 1993;76:615–619; with permission.)

Doxacurium

Doxacurium is a benzylisoquinolinium nondepolarizing neuromuscular-blocking drug with an ED_{95} of 30 μg/kg that has an onset of action in 4 to 6 minutes and a duration of neuromuscular blockade lasting 60 to 90 minutes (see Fig. 8-1 and Table 8-3) (Basta et al., 1988; Hunter, 1995). Volatile anesthetics decrease doxacurium dose requirements by 20% to 40% compared with doses required during nitrous oxide-fentanyl anesthesia (Katz et al., 1989). The pharmacokinetics of doxacurium resemble pancuronium with respect to dependence on renal clearance. As with pancuronium, a longer duration of action can be expected when doxacurium is administered to elderly patients, although the intensity of neuromuscular blockade (pharmacodynamics) is not different between young and elderly patients (Koscielniak-Nielsen et al., 1992). Drug-induced histamine release does not occur, and, as a result, cardiovascular changes do not accompany the administration of doxacurium (see Figs. 8-22 and 8-23) (Rathmell et al., 1993).

Pipecuronium

Pipecuronium is a bisquaternary aminosteroid nondepolarizing neuromuscular-blocking drug with an ED_{95} of 50 to 60 μg/kg that has an onset of action in 3 to 5 minutes and a duration of neuromuscular blockade lasting 60 to 90 minutes (see Fig. 8-1 and Table 8-3) (Hunter, 1995; Larijani et al., 1989; Wierda et al., 1989). The potency of pipecuronium is increased, and its duration of action shortened, in infants compared with children and adults (Pittet et al., 1990). The pharmacokinetics of pipecuronium resemble those of pancuronium with respect to dependence on renal clearance (Fig. 8-24) (Caldwell et al., 1989; Wierda et al., 1990). The principal metabolite excreted in the urine is 3-desacetylpipecuronium. Hepatic cirrhosis does not seem to alter the pharmacokinetics or pharmacodynamics of pipecuronium (D'Honneur et al., 1993). The responsiveness of the NMJ to pipecuronium (pharmacodynamics) is not different between young and elderly adults (Ornstein et al., 1992). Drug-induced histamine does not occur, and,

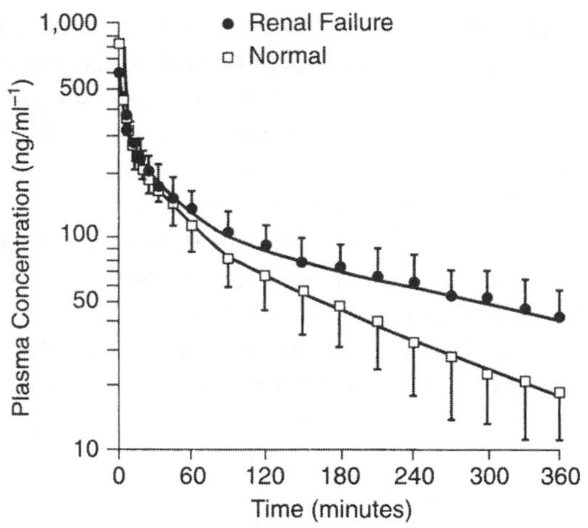

Figure 8-24. Clearance of pipecuronium from the plasma is slowed in patients with renal failure compared with normal patients. (From Caldwell JE, Canfell PC, Castagnoli KP, et al. The influence of renal failure on the pharmacokinetics and duration of action of pipecuronium bromide in patients anesthetized with halothane and nitrous oxide. *Anesthesiology* 1989;70:7–12; with permission.)

as a result, cardiovascular changes do not accompany the administration of pipecuronium (see Figs. 8-22 and 8-23) (Rathmell et al., 1993).

INTERMEDIATE-ACTING NONDEPOLARIZING NEUROMUSCULAR-BLOCKING DRUGS

Atracurium, vecuronium, rocuronium, and cisatracurium are classified as intermediate-acting nondepolarizing neuromuscular-blocking drugs. In contrast to the long-acting nondepolarizing neuromuscular-blocking drugs, these drugs possess efficient clearance mechanisms that minimize the likelihood of significant cumulative effects with repeated injections or continuous infusions. As such, intermediate-acting nondepolarizing neuromuscular-blocking drugs are useful, although they are more expensive alternatives to SCh and pancuronium, especially when tracheal intubation or skeletal muscle relaxation are needed for short operations, such as outpatient procedures.

Compared with long-acting nondepolarizing neuromuscular-blocking drugs, these drugs have (a) a similar onset rate of maximum neuromuscular blockade, with the exception of rocuronium, which is unique because of its rapid onset paralleling that of SCh; (b) approximately one-third the duration of action (hence the designation *intermediate-acting*); (c) a 30% to 50% more rapid rate of recovery; (d) minimal to absent cumulative effects; and (e) minimal to absent cardiovascular effects (Basta et al., 1982; Belmont et al., 1995; Fahey et al., 1981; Hunter, 1995; Hunter, 1996; Konstadt et al., 1995; Lien et al., 1995; Levy et al., 1994). The intermediate duration of action of these drugs is due to their rapid and efficient clearance from the circulation.

The onset of action of rocuronium is more rapid than that of the other intermediate-acting nondepolarizing neuromuscular blockers. This drug may serve as an alternative to SCh when the rapid onset of neuromuscular blockade (within 60 seconds) to facilitate tracheal intubation is desired. The speed of onset of the other intermediate-acting nondepolarizing neuromuscular-blocking drugs may be accelerated by administering an initial small subparalyzing dose (approximately 10% of the drug's ED_{95}) followed in approximately 4 minutes by the larger dose (2 to 3 × ED_{95}) of the drug (Gergis et al., 1983; Mehta et al., 1985; Schwarz et al., 1985; Taboada et al., 1986). This divided dose technique is known as the *priming principle* and is based on the concept that the onset of neuromuscular blockade consists of two steps: (a) initial binding of spare receptors during which no clinical effect is observed, and (b) subsequent deepening of the blockade. Conceptually, the initial subparalyzing dose is presumed to decrease the safety margin of neuromuscular transmission, allowing a more rapid onset of effect after the second larger dose. The priming principle may serve as a useful alternative when administration of SCh is best avoided but a rapid onset of neuromuscular blockade is needed. Nevertheless, the need for the priming principle is questionable when a single large IV dose of rocuronium produces a rapid onset of neuromuscular blockade without the risk of drug-induced weakness in an awake patient (Hunter, 1996).

Neuromuscular blockade produced by intermediate-acting nondepolarizing neuromuscular-blocking drugs is reliably antagonized by anticholinesterase drugs, often within 20 minutes of administering a paralyzing dose of these drugs (Gencarelli and Miller, 1982). Pharmacologic antagonism of neuromuscular blockade is further enhanced by the concomitant spontaneous recovery due to rapid clearance of the drug. Indeed, the incidence of residual neuromuscular blockade present in patients recovering in the postanesthesia care unit is less in patients receiving intermediate-acting compared with long-acting nondepolarizing neuromuscular-blocking drugs, despite the use of pharmacologic antagonism (Bevan et al., 1988).

Atracurium

Atracurium is a bisquaternary benzylisoquinolinium nondepolarizing neuromuscular blocking drug (mixture of ten geometric isomers) with an ED_{95} of 0.2 mg/kg that has an onset of action in 3 to 5 minutes and a duration of neuromuscular blockade lasting 20 to 35 minutes (see Fig. 8-1 and Table 8-3) (Basta et al., 1982; Hunter, 1995). The site of action of atracurium, like that of other nondepolarizing neuromuscular-blocking drugs, is on both presynaptic and postsynaptic cholinergic receptors (Hughes and Payne, 1983). Atracurium may also produce neuromuscular blockade by directly interfering with passage of ions through channels of nicotinic cholinergic receptors. An estimated 82% of atracurium is bound to plasma proteins, presumably albumin (Foldes and Deery, 1983).

Atracurium was designed specifically to undergo spontaneous in vivo degradation (Hofmann elimination) at normal body temperature and pH (Stenlake et al., 1983). The iodide salt besylate provides water solubility, and adjusting the pH of the commercial solution to 3.25 to 3.65 minimizes the likelihood of spontaneous in vitro degradation. In view of its acid pH in vitro, atracurium probably should not be mixed with alkaline drugs such as barbiturates or exposed to solutions with more alkaline pHs, as are present in delivery tubing used for infusion of IV fluids. Exposure of atracurium to an increased pH before its entrance into the circulation could theoretically result in premature breakdown of the drug. The potency of atracurium stored at room temperature decreases approximately 5% every 30 days.

Clearance

Atracurium undergoes spontaneous nonenzymatic degradation at normal body temperature and pH by a base-catalyzed reaction termed *Hofmann elimination* (Fig. 8-25) (Stiller et al., 1985). A second and simultaneously occurring route of metabolism is hydrolysis by nonspecific plasma esterases (see Fig. 8-25) (Stiller et al., 1985). Laudanosine is the major metabolite of both pathways. This metabolite is not active at the NMJ (in contrast to metabolites of many other nondepolarizing neuromuscular-blocking drugs) but may, in very high concentrations, cause CNS stimulation in animals (Shi et al., 1989; Stiller et al., 1985). Electrophilic acrylates are also formed by Hofmann elimination. These acrylates are reactive and, when studied in vitro, are capable of damaging cells by alkylating nucleophiles present in cellular membranes (Nigrovic et al., 1989). The clinical significance, if any, of these acrylates is unknown; however, the concentrations of atracurium used for the in vitro studies were as much as 1,600 times those required to produce neuromuscular blockade in vivo.

Hofmann elimination represents a chemical mechanism of elimination, whereas ester hydrolysis is a biologic mechanism. These two routes of metabolism are independent of hepatic and renal function as well as plasma cholinesterase activity (Merrett et al., 1983). As such, the duration of atracurium-induced neuromuscular blockade is similar in normal patients and those with absent or impaired renal or hepatic function or those with atypical plasma cholinesterase (Hunter et al., 1984; Ward and Neill, 1983). Absence of prolonged neuromuscular blockade after administration of atracurium to patients with atypical cholinesterase emphasizes the dependence of ester hydrolysis of atracurium on nonspecific plasma esterases that are unrelated to plasma cholinesterase (Baraka, 1987). Hofmann elimination and ester hydrolysis also account for the lack of cumulative drug effects with repeated doses or continuous infusions of atracurium. Overall, ester hydrolysis accounts for an estimated two-thirds of degraded atracurium, whereas Hofmann elimination provides a "safety net," especially in patients with impaired hepatic and/or renal function (Stiller et al., 1985).

Laudanosine

Laudanosine is the major metabolite of both pathways of metabolism of atracurium, with Hofmann elimination resulting in two molecules of laudanosine and ester hydrolysis resulting in one molecule of laudanosine for every molecule of atracurium that is metabolized (see Fig. 8-25) (Stiller et al., 1985). Peak plasma concentrations of laudanosine in humans occur 2 minutes after a rapid IV injection of atracurium and remain at approximately 75% of peak levels for nearly 15 minutes (Fahey et al., 1985). Laudanosine depends on the liver for clearance, with approximately 70% excreted in the bile and the remainder in urine (Ward and Weatherley, 1986). Hepatic cirrhosis in humans does not alter clearance of laudanosine, whereas

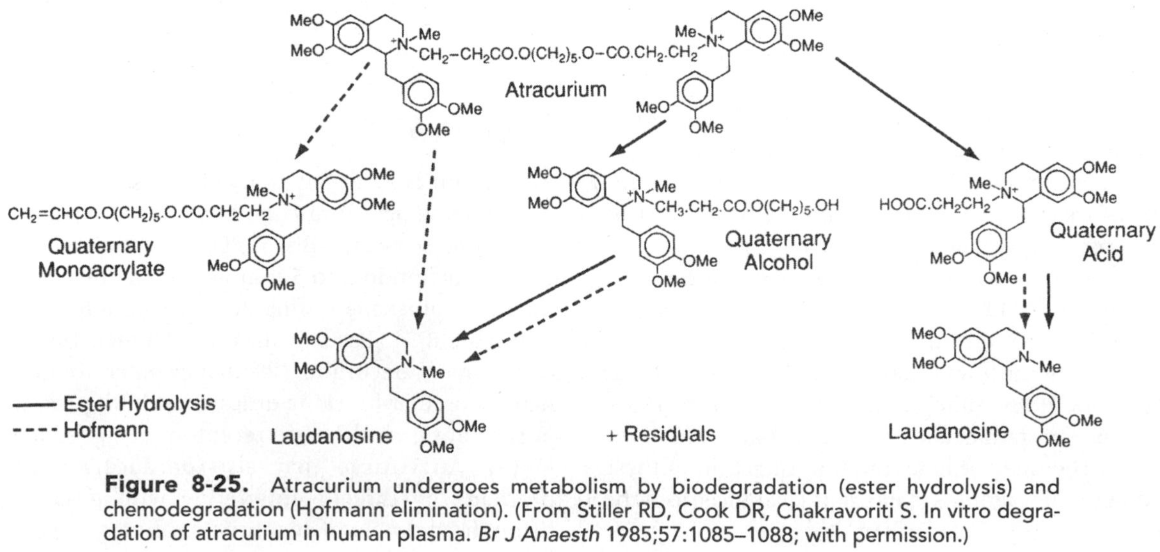

Figure 8-25. Atracurium undergoes metabolism by biodegradation (ester hydrolysis) and chemodegradation (Hofmann elimination). (From Stiller RD, Cook DR, Chakravoriti S. In vitro degradation of atracurium in human plasma. *Br J Anaesth* 1985;57:1085–1088; with permission.)

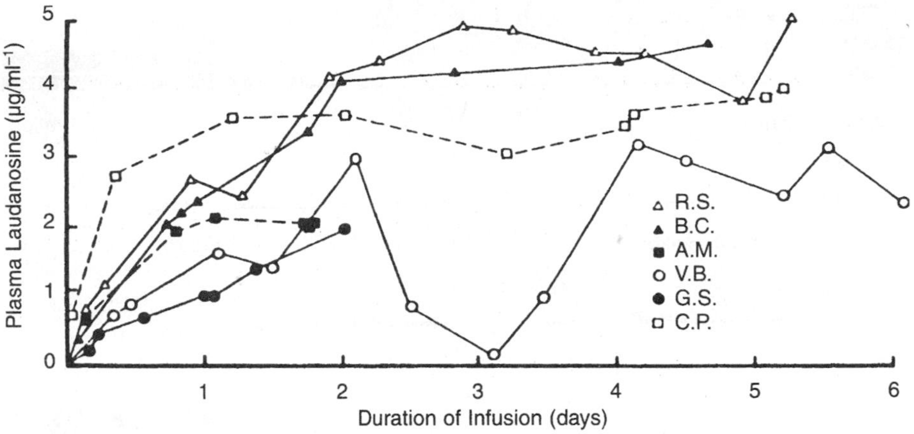

Figure 8-26. Plasma laudanosine concentrations in six patients during atracurium infusion. (From Yate PM, Flynn PJ, Arnold RW, et al. Clinical experience and plasma laudanosine concentrations during infusion of atracurium in the intensive therapy unit. *Br J Anaesth* 1987;59:211–217; with permission.)

excretion of this metabolite is impaired in patients with biliary obstruction (Parker and Hunter, 1989). Despite increases in plasma laudanosine concentrations during each stage of liver transplantation in patients receiving atracurium, these levels are considered to be far below clinically significant concentrations when graft function is satisfactory (Chow et al., 2000; Lawhead et al., 1993). Plasma concentrations of laudanosine after single doses of atracurium, 0.5 mg/kg IV, are higher in patients with renal failure compared with normal patients (Fahey et al., 1985).

Although inactive at the NMJ, animal studies have shown laudanosine to be a CNS stimulant, to increase MAC of volatile anesthetics, and to cause peripheral vasodilation (Fahey et al., 1985; Lanier et al., 1985; Shi et al., 1985). For example, in anesthetized animals receiving a continuous infusion of laudanosine, laudanosine plasma concentrations >6 μg/mL cause hypotension; laudanosine concentrations >10 μg/mL induce epileptic spiking on the electroencephalogram, and plasma concentrations of laudanosine >17 μg/mL produce seizures (Chapple et al., 1987). In this regard, it seems unlikely that administration of atracurium to patients will result in plasma concentrations of laudanosine capable of producing CNS or cardiovascular effects. Indeed, in patients receiving a full paralyzing dose of atracurium (0.5 mg/kg IV), the resulting peak plasma concentrations of laudanosine are approximately 0.3 μg/mL, which is about 20 times less than the plasma concentrations producing cardiovascular effects in animals (Fahey et al., 1985). Anesthetic requirements are not changed in patients receiving as much as 1 mg/kg IV (5 × ED_{95}) of atracurium, suggesting that any CNS-stimulating effect resulting from laudanosine would not be apparent clinically. Clearly, laudanosine resulting from metabolism of atracurium probably will not produce seizure activity in anesthetized patients because skeletal muscle paralysis from atracurium would prevent movement. Furthermore, inhaled anesthetics (with the possible exception of enflurane) or injected drugs such as thiopental would tend to suppress evidence of laudanosine-evoked CNS stimulation. In the absence of CNS depression produced by anesthetics, as in the critical care unit, it is theoretically possible that laudanosine-induced evidence of CNS stimulation could occur. Nevertheless, in patients receiving continuous infusions of atracurium for as long as 6 days, the plasma concentrations of laudanosine remain below those levels in animals associated with cardiovascular or CNS effects (Fig. 8-26) (Chapple et al., 1987; Yate et al., 1987). Furthermore, in an animal model of epilepsy, laudanosine does not alter the incidence of seizure activity (Tateishi et al., 1989).

Acid–Base Changes

Despite pH-dependent Hofmann elimination (accelerated by alkalosis and slowed by acidosis), it is unlikely that the range of pH changes encountered clinically is sufficiently great to alter the rate of Hofmann elimination and thus the duration of atracurium-induced neuromuscular blockade (Payne and Hughes, 1981). Furthermore, pH changes influence the rate of ester hydrolysis in a direction opposite to the change in the rate of Hofmann elimination, such that slowed Hofmann elimination would be offset theoretically by an accelerated rate of ester hydrolysis.

Cumulative Effects

Consistency of onset to recovery intervals after repeated supplemental doses of atracurium is characteristic of this drug and reflects the absence of significant cumulative drug effect (Fig. 8-27) (Ali et al., 1983). The absence of a significant cumulative drug effect is due to rapid clearance of atracurium from the plasma that is independent of renal or hepatic function. Lack of a significant drug cumulative effect minimizes the likelihood of persistent neuromuscular blockade when prolonged surgical procedures require repeated doses or a sustained continuous infusion of atracurium.

Cardiovascular Effects

Systemic blood pressure and heart rate changes do not accompany the rapid IV administration of atracurium in

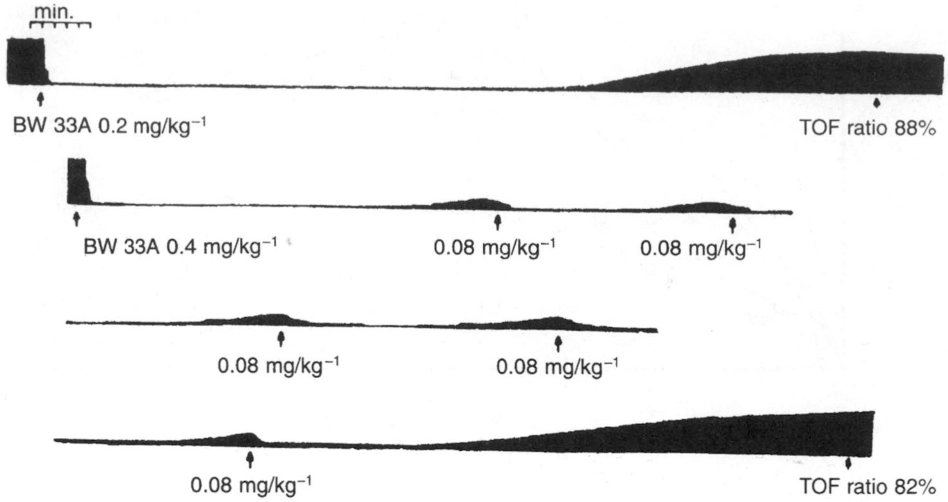

Figure 8-27. Repeated doses of atracurium (BW 33A) do not produce a cumulative drug effect as evidenced by the unchanging time intervals between doses for the same degree of recovery from neuromuscular blockade to occur. (TOF, train-of-four stimulation.) (From Ali HH, Savarese JJ, Basta SJ, et al. Evaluation of cumulative properties of three new nondepolarizing neuromuscular blocking drugs: BW A444U, atracurium, and vecuronium. *Br J Anaesth* 1983;55:107S–111S; with permission.)

doses up to 2 × ED_{95} with background anesthetics including nitrous oxide, fentanyl and isoflurane (Fig. 8-28) (Basta et al., 1982; Hilgenberg et al., 1983; Rupp et al., 1983a; Sokoll et al., 1983). During nitrous oxide-fentanyl anesthesia, the rapid IV administration of 3 × ED_{95} of atracurium increases heart rate by 8.3% and decreases mean arterial pressure by 21.5% (see Fig. 8-28) (Basta et al., 1982). These circulatory changes are transient, occurring 60 to 90 seconds after administration of atracurium and disappearing within 5 minutes. Facial and truncal flushing in some patients suggests release of histamine as the mechanism for the circulatory changes accompanying the rapid administration of high doses of atracurium. Indeed, plasma histamine concentrations increase transiently and parallel heart rate and systemic blood pressure

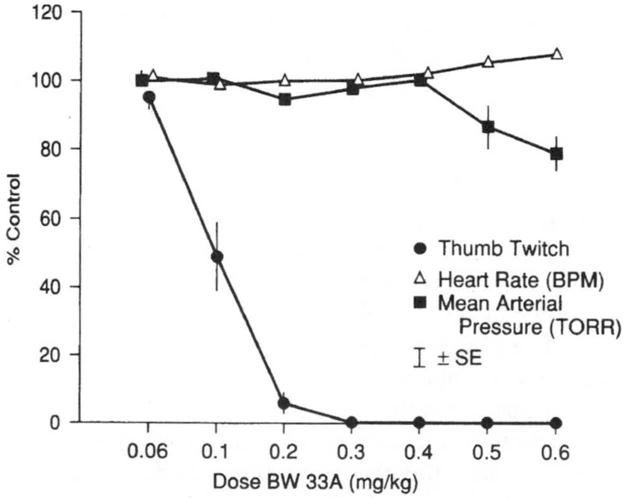

Figure 8-28. Heart rate and systemic blood pressure changes do not occur after the rapid intravenous administration of atracurium (BW 33A) up to doses equivalent to 2 × ED_{95} (0.4 mg/kg IV). Larger doses of atracurium may produce transient increases in heart rate and decreases in systemic blood pressure. (From Basta SJ, Ali HH, Savarese JJ, et al. Clinical pharmacology of atracurium besylate [BW 33A]: a new nondepolarizing muscle relaxant. *Anesth Analg* 1982;61:723–729; with permission.)

changes when atracurium, 0.6 mg/kg IV, is administered rapidly. Conversely, the same dose of atracurium administered over 30 to 75 seconds, or rapidly but in patients pretreated with H_1 and H_2 receptor antagonists, does not evoke circulatory changes despite similar increases in plasma concentrations of histamine as present in those receiving the same dose rapidly but without pretreatment (Scott et al., 1984). It is estimated that the plasma histamine concentration must double before cardiovascular changes manifest clinically. Despite its ability to evoke the release of histamine, the administration of atracurium does not alter ICP in patients with intracranial tumors (Rosa et al., 1986a; Rosa et al., 1986b).

There is evidence that patients treated chronically with H_2 receptor antagonists may experience exaggerated circulatory changes in response to the administration of histamine-releasing drugs (Hosking et al., 1988). In this regard, it is speculated that H_2 receptor antagonists exert a partial antagonist effect on H_3 receptors, thus removing the usual negative feedback role of H_3 receptors in modulating histamine release. As a result, there may be enhanced and sustained release of histamine. Animal evidence also suggests that laudanosine may contribute to transient blood pressure decreases associated with rapid IV administration of large doses of atracurium (Hennis et al., 1986).

Histamine release evoked by atracurium and mivacurium does not occur with short interval repeated injections of these drugs because tissue histamine stores are not replenished for several days. Therefore, a decrease in systemic blood pressure due to drug-induced histamine release is less likely to occur to the same magnitude on repeat dosing. Cardiovascular effects previously attributed to drug-induced histamine release may reflect prostacyclin release and its vasodilating effects on peripheral vasculature mediated by H_1 and H_2 receptors (Fig. 8-29) (Hatano et al., 1990).

Pediatric Patients

Effective doses of atracurium are similar in adults and children (2 to 16 years old), when differences in extracellular

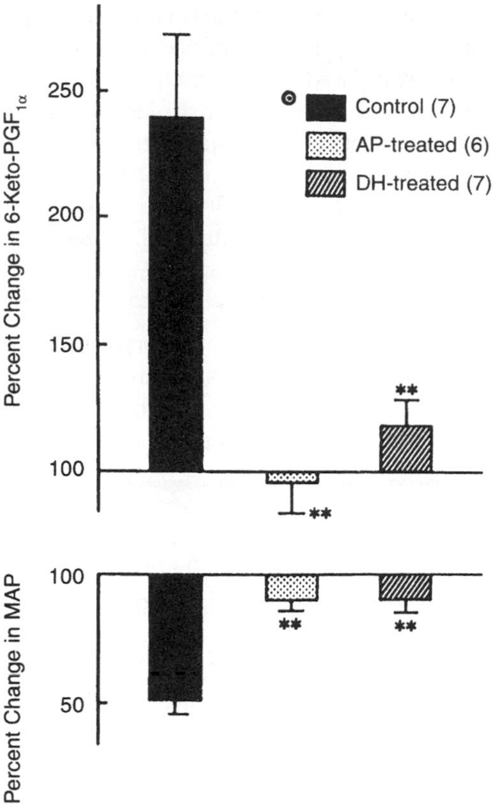

Figure 8-29. Changes (%) in plasma 6-keto-PGF$_{1\alpha}$ concentrations (nonenzymatic metabolite of prostacyclin) and in mean arterial pressure (MAP) 2 minutes after *d*-tubocurarine (dTc) administration to control, aspirin (AP)-treated, and diphenhydramine (DH)-treated patients. The values just before dTc administration are considered 100%. Figures in parentheses indicate the number of patients studied. (*$P < .01$ compared with control.) (From Hatano Y, Arai T, Noda J, et al. Contribution of prostacyclin to *d*-tubocurarine–induced hypotension in humans. *Anesthesiology* 1990;72:28–32; with permission.)

fluid volume are minimized by calculating the dose on a mg/m^2 rather than a mg/kg basis (Brandom et al., 1984). Conversely, infants 1 to 6 months old require approximately one-half the dose of atracurium given to older children to achieve the same degree of neuromuscular blockade (Brandom et al., 1983). Likewise, the continuous infusion rate of atracurium required to maintain a steady-state neuromuscular blockade is 25% less during the first 30 days of life (0.4 mg/kg per hour) compared to patients older than 1 month of age (0.53 mg/kg per hour) (Kalli and Meretoja, 1988). These data imply that infants are more sensitive than children or adults to the neuromuscular-blocking effects of atracurium. Recovery from atracurium-induced neuromuscular blockade, however, is more rapid in infants (23 minutes) than adolescents (29 minutes) (Brandom et al., 1983).

Elderly Patients

Increasing age has no effect on the continuous rate of infusion of atracurium necessary to maintain a constant degree of neuromuscular blockade (d'Hollander et al., 1983). Likewise, the rate of recovery and thus the duration of neuromuscular blockade are similar in young adults and the elderly. This lack of influence of aging on dose requirements of atracurium most likely reflects the independence of clearance mechanisms (Hofmann elimination and ester hydrolysis) from age-related effects on renal and hepatic function. Furthermore, changes in the volume of distribution of atracurium that occur with aging will not influence the clearance of atracurium from the plasma. Failure of aging to alter responsiveness of the NMJ is documented by similar plasma concentrations of atracurium necessary to depress single-twitch response 50% in elderly patients and young adults (Kitts et al., 1990).

Vecuronium

Vecuronium is a monoquaternary aminosteroid nondepolarizing neuromuscular-blocking drug with an ED_{95} of 50 μg/kg that has an onset of action in 3 to 5 minutes and a duration of neuromuscular blockade lasting 20 to 35 minutes (see Fig. 8-1 and Table 8-3) (Hunter, 1995; Fahey et al., 1981; Miller et al., 1984). Structurally, vecuronium is pancuronium without the quaternary methyl group in the A-ring of the steroid nucleus. The absence of this quaternary methyl group decreases the acetylcholine-like character of vecuronium as compared with pancuronium. Indeed, the vagolytic property of vecuronium is decreased approximately 20-fold. The monoquaternary structure of vecuronium increases its lipid solubility compared with pancuronium. Vecuronium is unstable in solution and, for this reason, is supplied as a lyophilized powder that must be dissolved in sterile water before its use.

Clearance

Vecuronium undergoes both hepatic metabolism and renal excretion (Pollard, 1992). The increased lipid solubility of vecuronium compared with that of pancuronium facilitates entrance of vecuronium into hepatocytes, where it undergoes deacetylation to 3-desacetylvecuronium, 17-desacetylvecuronium, and 3,17-desacetylvecuronium (Hunter, 1995; Savage et al., 1980). The 3-desacetylvecuronium metabolite is approximately one-half as potent as the parent compound but it is rapidly converted to the 3,17-desacetylvecuronium derivative. The 3,17-desacetylvecuronium and 17-desacetylvecuronium derivatives have less than one-tenth the neuromuscular blocking properties of vecuronium.

Increased lipid solubility also facilitates biliary excretion of vecuronium. For example, in patients, an estimated 50% of the IV dose of vecuronium may be present in the liver 30 minutes after IV administration, and approximately 40% of the drug is excreted unchanged in the bile in the first 24 hours (Bencini et al., 1986a). Approximately 30% of an administered dose of vecuronium appears in urine as unchanged drug and metabolites in the first 24 hours (Bencini et al., 1986b). The extensive hepatic uptake of vecuronium may account for the rapid decrease in vecuronium plasma concentrations and the drug's short duration of action.

Accidental epidural injection of vecuronium resulted in a prolonged duration of neuromuscular blockade but symptoms of neurologic or cardiovascular toxicity did not occur (Kostopanagiotou et al., 2000). Neuromuscular-blocking drugs may cause excitement and seizures when injected into the central nervous system, but pancuronium and atracurium, are approximately 12 and 28 times, respectively, more potent than vecuronium in eliciting seizures.

Renal Dysfunction

Despite the presumption that the liver is the main organ of elimination, the elimination half-time of vecuronium and 3-desacetylvecuronium is prolonged in patients with renal failure, reflecting a decreased clearance of the drug (Lynam et al., 1988). Increased plasma concentrations of 3-desacetylvecuronium may contribute to persistent skeletal muscle paralysis after prolonged infusion of vecuronium (6 hours to 7 days) to patients in renal failure (Conway, 1992; Segredo et al., 1992). An apparent tolerance to vecuronium in patients with renal failure is suggested by higher plasma concentrations of vecuronium at 25% and 75% recovery compared to patients with normal renal function (Bencini et al., 1986b). This tolerance is consistent with a slower onset of action of vecuronium in patients with renal failure. A similar, but less prominent, degree of tolerance also may occur after administration of atracurium to patients in renal failure (Hunter et al., 1984).

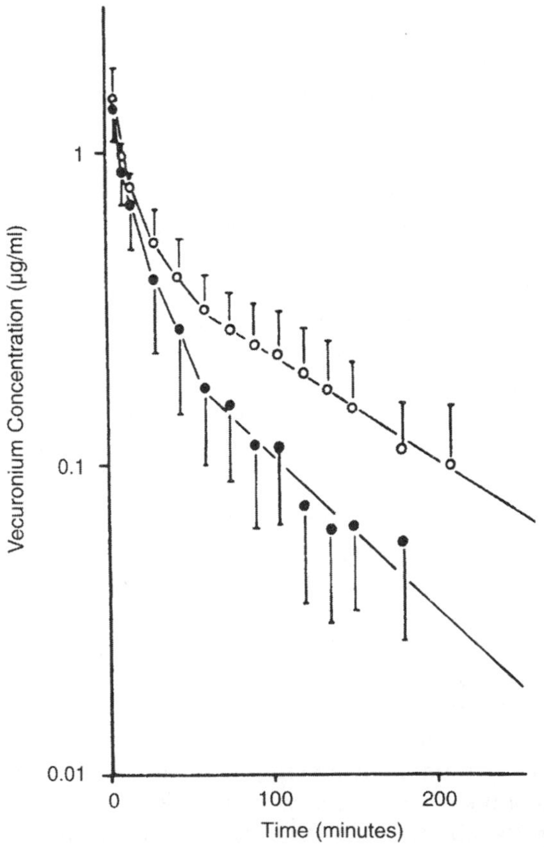

Figure 8-30. Disappearance of vecuronium (0.2 mg/kg IV) from the plasma is slowed in patients with hepatic cirrhosis (*clear circles*) compared with normal patients (*solid circles*). (Mean ± SD.) (From Lebrault C, Berger JL, d'Hollander AA, et al. Pharmacokinetics and pharmacodynamics of vecuronium [ORG NC45] in patients with cirrhosis. *Anesthesiology* 1985;62:601–605; with permission.)

Hepatic Dysfunction

As with atracurium, the elimination half-time of vecuronium, 0.1 mg/kg IV, administered to patients with alcoholic liver disease is not different from that observed in patients without liver disease (Arden et al., 1988). In contrast, vecuronium, 0.2 mg/kg IV, is associated with a prolonged elimination half-time and a corresponding prolonged duration of action in patients with hepatic cirrhosis (Fig. 8-30) (Lebrault et al., 1985). It is possible that other clearance mechanisms, such as renal clearance or diffusion of drug into inactive tissues such as cartilage, offset the effect of impaired hepatic function when smaller doses of vecuronium are administered. In patients with cholestasis who are undergoing biliary surgery, the administration of vecuronium, 0.2 mg/kg IV, results in a prolonged elimination half-time and increased duration of action (Lebrault et al., 1986).

Acid–Base Changes

The impact of acid–base changes on vecuronium-induced neuromuscular blockade depends on whether the changes in blood pH precede or follow the administration of vecuronium (Gencarelli et al., 1983). For example, changes in $PaCO_2$ that precede the administration of vecuronium do not alter the magnitude of neuromuscular blockade. Conversely, hypercarbia introduced after the establishment of vecuronium-induced neuromuscular blockade significantly enhances the effects of vecuronium. For this reason, the onset of hypoventilation, which may occur in the early postoperative period, could enhance neuromuscular blockade.

Cumulative Effects

Vecuronium has a large volume of distribution, reflecting its tissue uptake. After a single dose of vecuronium, the plasma concentration decreases rapidly because of redistribution from central to peripheral compartments. With subsequent doses, any vecuronium present in various peripheral tissue compartments will limit the distribution phase and thus also the rate of decrease in the plasma concentration of vecuronium. As a result, vecuronium can be demonstrated to have a cumulative effect that is less than for pancuronium and greater than for atracurium (Fahey et al., 1981).

Although the effect of renal failure is small, there is a gradual increase in the duration of action with repeated

TABLE 8-8.
COMPARISON OF VECURONIUM-INDUCED NEUROMUSCULAR BLOCKADE IN PEDIATRIC AND ADULT PATIENTS

	Vecuronium (mg/kg)	Onset of Maximum Twitch Suppression (mins)	Duration (mins to 90% Twitch Recovery)	Recovery Index (mins for Twitch Response to Recover From 25% to 75% Control)
Infants	0.07	1.5[a]	73[a]	20[b]
Children	0.07	2.4	35	9
Adults	0.07	2.9	54	13

[a] $P < .05$ compared with adults.
[b] $P < .05$ compared with children.
Source: Data from Fisher DM, Miller RD. Neuromuscular effects of vecuronium (ORG NC45) in infants and children during N_2O, halothane anesthesia. *Anesthesiology* 1983;58:519–523; with permission.

doses, and this cumulative effect is presumed to be a result of gradual saturation of peripheral storage sites (Pollard, 1992). Accumulation of the 3-desacetylvecuronium metabolite of vecuronium may contribute to prolonged effects of this drug, especially with repeated doses of vecuronium administered to patients with renal dysfunction (Segredo et al., 1992).

Cardiovascular Effects

Vecuronium is typically devoid of circulatory effects even with rapid IV administration of doses that exceed 3 × ED_{95} of the drug, emphasizing the lack of vagolytic effects or histamine release associated with the administration of vecuronium (Morris et al., 1983). Nevertheless, occasional increases in the plasma concentrations of histamine without associated systemic blood pressure changes have been observed after administration of vecuronium (Cannon et al., 1988). A modest vagotonic effect of vecuronium is suggested by an increased incidence of bradycardia in patients receiving vecuronium in the absence of prior administration of an anticholinergic drug or in close association with the injection of a potent opioid such as sufentanil (Cozanitis et al., 1987; Inoue et al., 1988; Salmenpera et al., 1983; Starr et al., 1986). In fact, the absence of a neuromuscular-blocking drug-induced vagolytic effect, as produced by pancuronium, may permit direct cardiovascular effects of other drugs (opioid-induced bradycardia) used during anesthesia to manifest. Sinus node exit block and even cardiac arrest has been described in association with vecuronium administration (Milligan and Beers, 1985; Yeaton and Teba, 1988).

Pediatric Patients

The potency of vecuronium in infants (7 to 45 weeks old), children (1 to 8 years old), and adults (18 to 38 years old) is similar during nitrous oxide–halothane anesthesia (Table 8-8) (Fisher and Miller, 1983b). The onset of action is more rapid in infants than in adults, whereas the duration of action is longest in infants and shortest in children (see Table 8-8) (Fisher and Miller, 1983b; Meretoja, 1989). Presumably, a high cardiac output in infants speeds the onset of vecuronium-induced neuromuscular blockade, whereas the longer duration reflects immature enzyme systems in the neonate's liver or an increased volume of distribution. An increased volume of distribution means more drug is sequestered in peripheral compartments and is inaccessible to hepatic and renal clearance mechanisms. Age-related changes in biliary clearance also may contribute to a longer duration of vecuronium-induced neuromuscular blockade in infants.

Elderly Patients

Increasing age is associated with decreases in the continuous rate of infusion of vecuronium necessary to maintain a constant degree of neuromuscular blockade (d'Hollander et al., 1982). Presumably, this reflects decreased plasma clearance of vecuronium due to age-related decreases in hepatic blood flow and renal blood flow and possibly decreased hepatic microsomal enzyme activity. Furthermore, when a continuous infusion of vecuronium is discontinued, the rate of recovery of the single-twitch response is prolonged in the elderly compared with young adults. The delayed rate of recovery could manifest as a prolonged duration of vecuronium-induced neuromuscular blockade in the elderly. In contrast to the detectable impact of aging during and after the continuous infusion of vecuronium, the elimination half-time and dose–response curves as determined from single-twitch responses produced by individual IV doses of vecuronium are not influenced by increasing age (O'Hara et al., 1985; Rupp et al., 1987).

In patients 70 to 80 years old, the volume of distribution and plasma clearance of vecuronium are decreased compared with younger patients (Rupp et al., 1983b). The decrease in volume of distribution is consistent with age-related decreases in skeletal muscle mass and total body water, whereas decreases in plasma clearance most likely reflect decreased hepatic blood flow in the elderly. Evidence of unchanged responsiveness of the NMJ despite increasing age is the similarity of the plasma concentration of vecuronium necessary to depress the single-twitch response 50% in elderly patients and young adult patients (Rupp et al., 1983b).

Obstetric Patients

Insufficient amounts of nondepolarizing neuromuscular-blocking drugs cross the placenta to produce clinically significant effects in the fetus (Dailey et al., 1984; Frank et al., 1983). For example, the maternal-to-fetal ratio of vecuronium after administration of 40–50 μg/kg IV to the mother is 0.11. Concentrations of atracurium in umbilical venous blood are below the sensitivity limits of the assay. The clearance of vecuronium may be accelerated during late pregnancy, possibly reflecting stimulation of hepatic microsomal enzymes by progesterone as well as by cardiovascular changes and fluid shifts that occur during pregnancy. Conversely, the duration of action of vecuronium-induced neuromuscular blockade is prolonged in the immediate postpartum period (Hawkins et al., 1989).

Obesity

The duration of action of vecuronium, but not atracurium, is prolonged in obese (>130% of ideal body weight) compared with nonobese adults (Fig. 8-31) (Weinstein et al., 1988).

Intraocular Pressure

Administration of paralyzing doses of vecuronium or atracurium after induction of anesthesia with thiopental does not change intraocular pressure (Schneider et al., 1986). Furthermore, neuromuscular blockade produced by these drugs does not prevent increases in intraocular pressure in response to tracheal intubation.

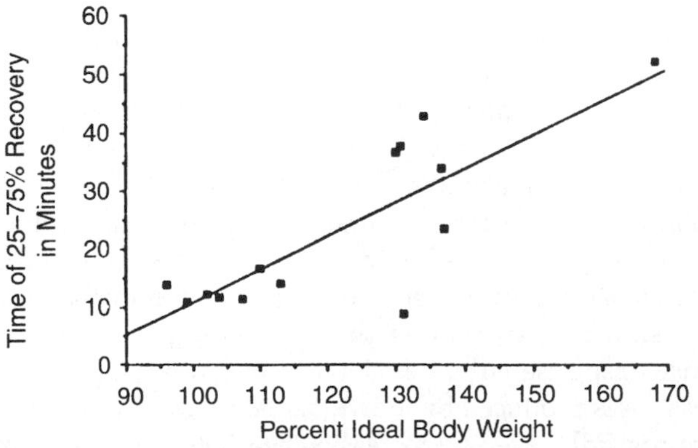

Figure 8-31. The rate of recovery after administration of vecuronium, 0.1 mg/kg IV, is delayed in obese compared with nonobese adults. (From Weinstein JA, Matteo RS, Ornstein E, et al. Pharmacodynamics of vecuronium and atracurium in the obese surgical patient. *Anesth Analg* 1988;67:1149–1153; with permission.)

Malignant Hyperthermia

Malignant hyperthermia does not follow the administration of vecuronium or atracurium to sensitive swine (Buzello et al., 1985b; Ording and Fonsmark, 1988; Rorvik et al., 1988; Skarpa et al., 1983). Prolonged vecuronium-induced neuromuscular blockade has been reported in a patient susceptible to malignant hyperthermia who was pretreated with dantrolene (Driessen et al., 1985). This response could reflect dantrolene-induced decreases in neurotransmitter mobilization at the NMJ due to impaired release of calcium ions from storage sites within cholinergic nerve terminals (Durant et al., 1980). Its seems likely that similar prolongation of neuromuscular blockade could occur with other neuromuscular-blocking drugs administered in the presence of dantrolene.

Rocuronium

Rocuronium is a monoquaternary aminosteroid nondepolarizing neuromuscular-blocking drug with an ED_{95} of 0.3 mg/kg that has an onset of action in 1 to 2 minutes and a duration of neuromuscular blockade lasting 20 to 35 minutes (see Fig. 8-1 and Table 8-3) (Hunter, 1996). Structurally, rocuronium resembles vecuronium except for the presence of a hydroxyl group rather than an acetyl group on the A-ring of the steroid nucleus. The lack of potency of rocuronium compared with vecuronium is thought to be an important factor in determining the rapid onset of neuromuscular blockade produced by this drug. For example, the large number of molecules administered when using a less potent nondepolarizing neuromuscular-blocking drug results in a greater number of molecules being available to diffuse into the NMJ. Thus, a rapid onset of action is more likely to be achieved with a less potent drug such as rocuronium. Indeed, the onset of maximum single-twitch depression after the administration of 3 to $4 \times ED_{95}$ of rocuronium resembles the onset of action of SCh, 1 mg/kg IV (Fig. 8-32) (Magorian et al., 1995). In this regard, rocuronium is the only nondepolarizing neuromuscular-blocking drug that may serve as an alternative to SCh when the rapid onset of neuromuscular blockade is needed to facilitate tracheal intubation and SCh is contraindicated. Nevertheless, the fact that the laryngeal muscles are more resistant to the effects of rocuronium than is the adductor pollicis, means that the onset of large doses of rocuronium will resemble SCh at the adductor pollicis but will be delayed compared with that of SCh at the laryngeal adductors (Wright et al., 1994). Furthermore, unlike SCh, rocuronium produces a duration of neuromuscular blockade that resembles the other intermediate-acting nondepolarizing neuromuscular-blocking drugs. In fact, large doses of rocuronium, as needed to mimic the onset of action of SCh (3 to $4 \times ED_{95}$), produce a duration of action

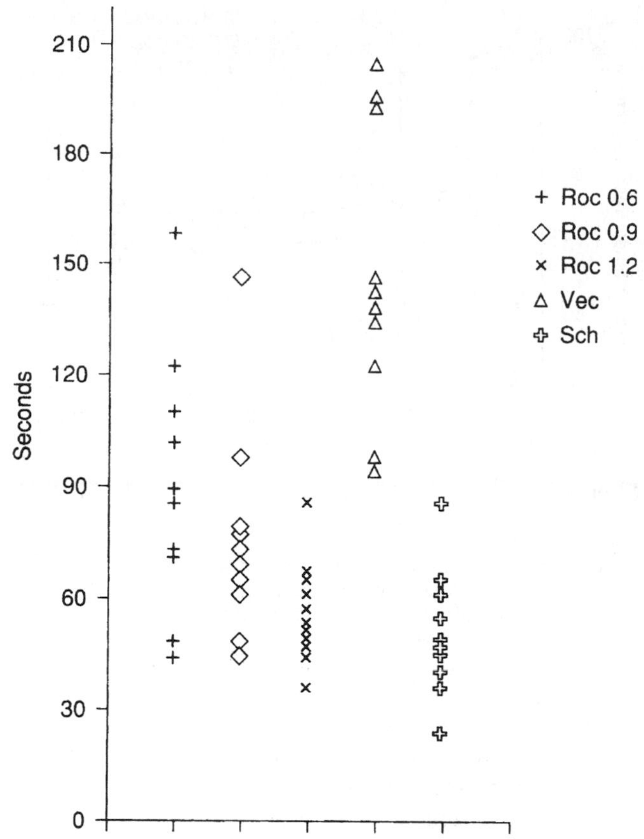

Figure 8-32. Onset to maximum twitch depression is similar after the IV administration of rocuronium (Roc) at doses of 0.9 mg/kg and 1.2 mg/kg and succinylcholine (SCh), 1 mg/kg. (vecuronium.) (From Magorian T, Flannery KB, Miller RD. Vec Comparison of rocuronium, succinylcholine, and vecuronium for rapid sequence induction of anesthesia in adult patients. *Anesthesiology* 1993;79:913–918; with permission.)

that resembles the long-acting nondepolarizing neuromuscular-blocking drug pancuronium.

Similarly, large intramuscular (IM) doses of rocuronium (1 to 8 mg/kg) administered to infants and children permit rapid tracheal intubation, but the duration of these large doses (about 1 hour) may limit clinical usefulness (Reynolds et al., 1996). Conversely, others have reported that IM rocuronium (1 to 1.8 mg/kg) does not consistently produce satisfactory intubating conditions in infants and children and is not an adequate alternative to IM SCh when rapid tracheal intubation is necessary (Kaplan et al., 1999).

As with other nondepolarizing neuromuscular-blocking drugs, the laryngeal adductor muscles and diaphragm are more resistant to rocuronium than the adductor pollicis muscles (see Fig. 8-3) (Meistelman et al., 1992). Complete suppression of the single-twitch response at the adductor pollicis muscle does not confirm that the laryngeal muscles and diaphragm are also paralyzed. Furthermore, the period of maximum laryngeal paralysis may be missed if the onset of complete suppression of single-twitch response at the adductor pollicis is used as the clinical sign of optimal conditions for tracheal intubation (see Fig. 8-3) (Meistelman et al., 1992). Conversely, initiating direct laryngoscopy for tracheal intubation at the time of peak laryngeal muscle paralysis could result in abdominal muscle and diaphragmatic movement when the tracheal tube is placed because these muscles are not yet fully paralyzed. These latter responses are particularly undesirable if the patient is considered to be at risk for pulmonary aspiration of gastric contents. In morbidly obese patients, the duration of action of rocuronium is prolonged when the dose of drug is calculated using real body weight rather than ideal body weight (Leykin et al., 2004a).

Clearance

Animal studies have suggested that rocuronium is largely excreted unchanged (up to 50% in 2 hours) in the bile (Khuenl-Brady et al., 1990; Proost et al., 2000). Deacetylation of rocuronium does not occur, and, unlike vecuronium, 3-hydroxy metabolites with neuromuscular-blocking activity do not occur. Renal excretion of rocuronium may be >30% in 24 hours, and administration of this drug to patients in renal failure may produce a modestly prolonged duration of action (Cooper et al., 1993). Liver disease increases the volume of distribution of rocuronium and could result in a longer duration of action of the drug, especially with repeated doses or prolonged IV administration (Servin et al., 1996). Conversely, a newly transplanted liver seems to eliminate rocuronium normally (Fisher et al., 1997). Compared with young adults, elderly patients (older than 70 years of age) experience a similar speed of onset but a prolonged duration of action after administration of rocuronium, and this latter response is attributed to decreased hepatic clearance mechanisms (Fig. 8-33) (Matteo et al., 1993). The pharmacodynamics of rocuronium are not different in young adults or elderly patients (Fig. 8-34) (Matteo et al., 1993).

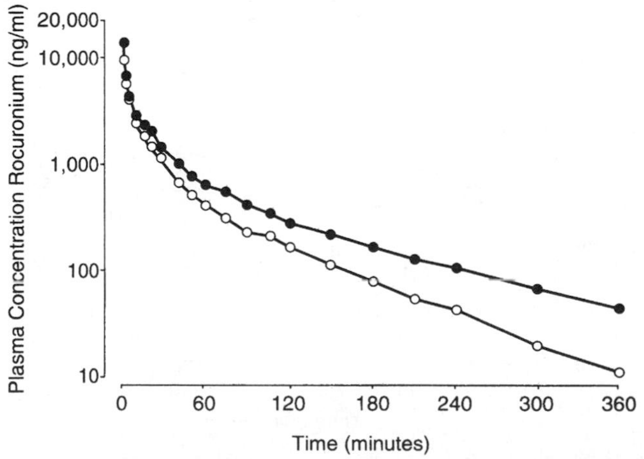

Figure 8-33. Mean plasma concentrations after administration of rocuronium, 600 μg/kg IV, to young adults (*open circles*) or elderly patients (*solid circles*). (From Matteo RS, Ornstein E, Schwartz AE, et al. Pharmacokinetics and pharmacodynamics of rocuronium [ORG 9426] in elderly surgical patients. *Anesth Analg* 1993;77:1193–1197; with permission.)

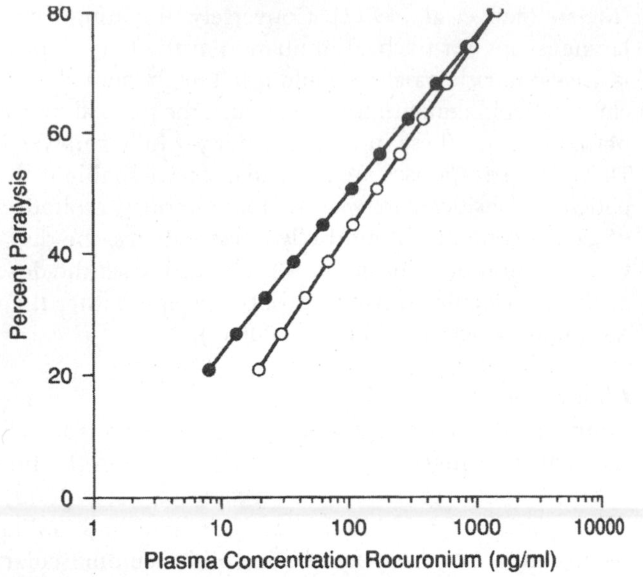

Figure 8-34. The plasma concentration of rocuronium necessary to produce a specific degree of paralysis is not different in elderly (*solid circles*) and young adults (*open circles*). (From Matteo RS, Ornstein E, Schwartz AE, et al. Pharmacokinetics and pharmacodynamics of rocuronium (ORG 9426) in elderly surgical patients. *Anesth Analg* 1993;77:1193–1197; with permission.)

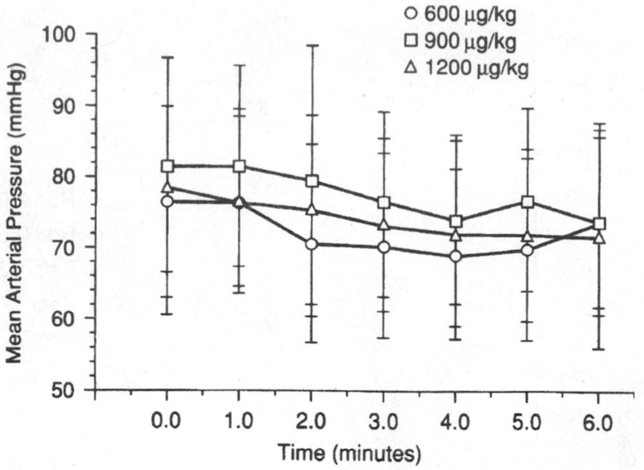

Figure 8-36. Changes in mean arterial pressure (mean ± SD) after intravenous administration of three different doses of rocuronium to adult patients. (From Levy JH, Davis GK, Duggan J, et al. Determination of the hemodynamics and histamine release of rocuronium [ORG 9426] when administered in increased doses under N_2O/O_2-sufentanil anesthesia. *Anesth Analg* 1994;78:318–321; with permission.)

Cardiovascular Effects

Cardiovascular effects or the release of histamine do not follow the rapid IV administration of even large doses of rocuronium (Figs. 8-35, 8-36, and 8-37) (Levy et al., 1994). The absence of histamine release is consistent with other aminosteroid nondepolarizing neuromuscular-blocking drugs. Unlike other aminosteroid neuromuscular-blocking drugs, however, rocuronium may produce a slight vagolytic effect (Hunter, 1996). This feature of rocuronium may be useful in patients undergoing surgical procedures (ophthalmologic, laparoscopic) that may be associated with vagal stimulation. Indeed, reflex bradycardia has been described when atracurium or vecuronium is administered to patients undergoing these types of surgical procedures (Hunter, 1996).

Cisatracurium

Cisatracurium is a benzylisoquinolinium nondepolarizing neuromuscular-blocking drug with an ED_{95} of 50 μg/kg that has an onset of action of 3 to 5 minutes and a dura-

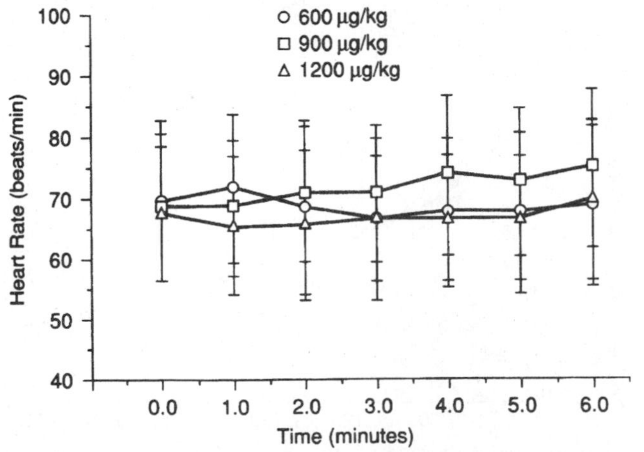

Figure 8-35. Changes in heart rate (mean ± SD) after intravenous administration of three different doses of rocuronium to adult patients. (From Levy JH, Davis GK, Duggan J, et al. Determination of the hemodynamics and histamine release of rocuronium [ORG 9426] when administered in increased doses under N_2O/O_2-sufentanil anesthesia. *Anesth Analg* 1994;78:318–321; with permission.)

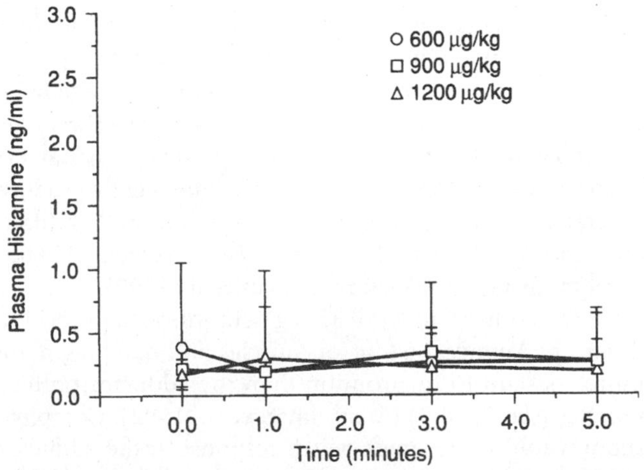

Figure 8-37. Changes in plasma histamine concentrations (mean ± SD) after intravenous administration of three different doses of rocuronium to adult patients. (From Levy JH, Davis GK, Duggan J, et al. Determination of the hemodynamics and histamine release of rocuronium [ORG 9426] when administered in increased doses under N_2O/O_2-sufentanil anesthesia. *Anesth Analg* 1994;78:318–321; with permission.)

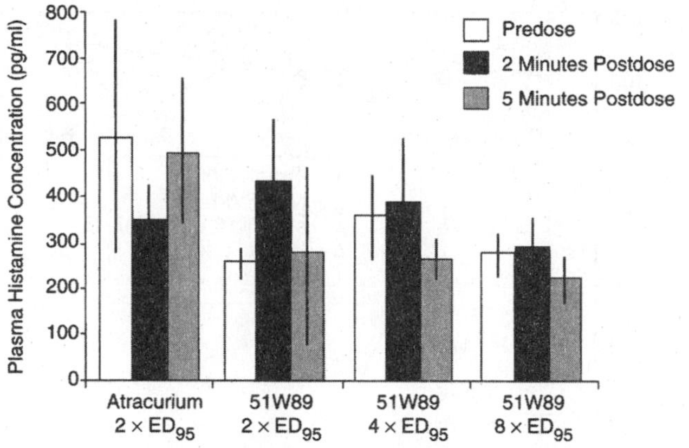

Figure 8-38. Mean plasma histamine concentrations before and after the intravenous administration of atracurium (2 × ED_{95}) and cisatracurium (51W89) (2, 4, and 8 × ED_{95}) to patients anesthetized with nitrous oxide/thiopental/fentanyl. There were no dose-related changes in plasma histamine concentrations in any of the study groups. (From Lien CA, Belmont MR, Abalos A, et al. The cardiovascular effects and histamine-releasing properties of 51W89 in patients receiving nitrous oxide/opioid/barbiturate anesthesia. *Anesthesiology* 1995;82:1131–1138; with permission.)

tion of neuromuscular blockade lasting 20 to 35 minutes (see Fig. 8-1 and Table 8-3) (Belmont et al., 1995; Mellinghoff et al., 1996). Structurally, cisatracurium is the purified form of one of the ten stereoisomers of atracurium, accounting for about 15% of the total mixture. As such, cisatracurium has a similar neuromuscular-blocking profile to atracurium except that the onset of cisatracurium is somewhat slower and its propensity to release histamine is dramatically less (Fig. 8-38) (Doenicke et al., 1997; Lien et al., 1995; Mellinghoff et al., 1996). Neuromuscular blockade is easily maintained at a stable level by infusion at a constant rate and does not diminish over time. In contrast to vecuronium, the rate of spontaneous recovery from cisatracurium-induced neuromuscular blockade is not influenced by the prolonged (average 80 hours) cisatracurium infusion to patients requiring mechanical ventilation of the lungs in a critical care unit (Prielipp et al., 1995). As with the other nondepolarizing neuromuscular-blocking drugs, spontaneous recovery from the neuromuscular blocking effects of cisatracurium is accelerated by administration of an anticholinesterase drug. In morbidly obese patients, the duration of action of cisatracurium is prolonged when the dose of drug is calculated using real body weight rather than ideal body weight (Leykin et al, 2004b).

Clearance

Cisatracurium undergoes degradation principally by Hofmann elimination at physiologic pH and temperature to form laudanosine and a monoquaternary acrylate (Kisor et al., 1996). The monoquaternary acrylate can also undergo Hofmann elimination but at a much slower rate than for cisatracurium. In contrast to atracurium, nonspecific plasma esterases do not seem to be involved in the clearance of cisatracurium. It is estimated that Hofmann elimination accounts for 77% of the clearance of cisatracurium, whereas renal clearance is responsible for another 16%.

The organ-independent clearance of cisatracurium means that this nondepolarizing neuromuscular-blocking drug, like atracurium, can be administered to patients with hepatic or renal dysfunction without a change in its neuromuscular-blocking profile. An efficient clearance mechanism results in the absence of a cumulative effect of cisatracurium, even with prolonged infusion (Prielipp et al., 1995). The pharmacokinetics of cisatracurium are only marginally influenced by advanced age, and these differences are not associated with changes in the recovery profile, although the onset of action is delayed approximately 1 minute in elderly patients due to slower biophase equilibration (Ornstein et al., 1996; Sorooshian et al., 1996). Likewise, minor differences in the pharmacokinetics and pharmacodynamics of cisatracurium in liver transplant and control patients are not associated with clinically significant differences in recovery profiles after a single dose of cisatracurium (Lien et al., 1996).

The metabolites resulting from the degradation of cisatracurium by Hofmann elimination are inactive at the NMJ. In contrast to atracurium, plasma concentrations of laudanosine after administration of a 2 × ED_{95} dose of cisatracurium are fivefold less than that present after a 1.5 × ED_{95} dose of atracurium (Lien et al., 1996). Presumably, the greater potency of cisatracurium compared with atracurium results in fewer molecules being administered and therefore lower plasma concentrations of the metabolite laudanosine.

Cardiovascular Effects

Cisatracurium, in contrast to atracurium, is devoid of histamine-releasing effects, so that cardiovascular changes do not accompany the rapid IV administration of even large doses (8 × ED_{95}) of cisatracurium (see Figs. 8-38 and 8-39) (Lien et al., 1995). In patients with coronary artery disease, the hemodynamic effects of cisatracurium are indistinguishable from those occurring in similar patients receiving vecuronium (Konstadt et al., 1995). Cisatracurium (3 × ED_{95}), administered to adult neurosurgical patients, produces less cerebral hemodynamic changes (intracranial pressure, cerebral perfusion pressure, middle cerebral artery blood flow velocity) compared with equipotent doses of atracurium (Schramm et al., 1998). An anaphylactic reaction has been described after the first exposure to cisatracurium (Clendenen et al., 1997).

SHORT-ACTING NONDEPOLARIZING NEUROMUSCULAR-BLOCKING DRUGS

Mivacurium is the only clinically useful nondepolarizing neuromuscular-blocking drug that is classified as short-acting (see Table 8-1).

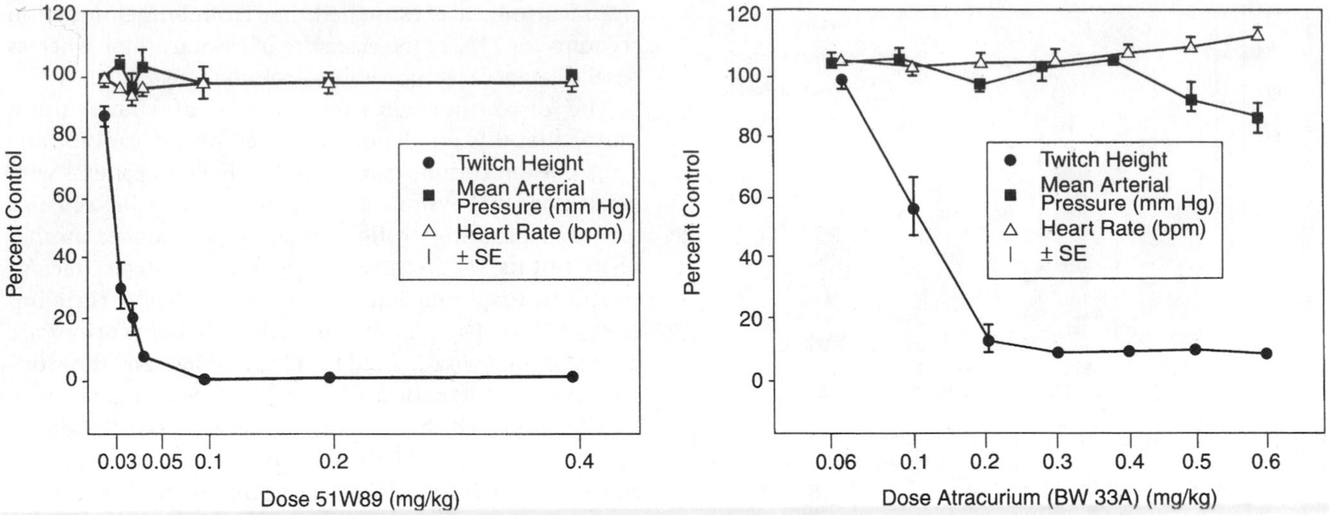

Figure 8-39. Mean twitch height, heart rate, and mean arterial pressure responses to various doses of cisatracurium (51W89) or atracurium. Although significant decreases in mean arterial pressure and increases in heart rate accompanied doses of atracurium of >2 × ED_{95}, no significant changes in heart rate or mean arterial pressure occurred after any dose of cisatracurium. (From Lien CA, Belmont MR, Abalos A, et al. The cardiovascular effects and histamine-releasing properties of 51W89 in patients receiving nitrous oxide/opioid/barbiturate anesthesia. *Anesthesiology* 1995;82:1131–1138; with permission.)

Mivacurium

Mivacurium is a benzylisoquinolinium nondepolarizing neuromuscular-blocking drug with an ED_{95} of 80 μg/kg that has an onset of action in 2 to 3 minutes lasting 12 to 20 minutes (see Fig. 8-1 and Table 8-3) (Hunter, 1995; Savarese et al., 1988). As such, the duration of action of mivacurium is approximately twice that of SCh and 30% to 40% that of the intermediate-acting nondepolarizing neuromuscular-blocking drugs. Mivacurium consists of three stereoisomers. The two most active and equipotent are the trans-trans and cis-trans isomers, whereas the *cis-cis* isomer has only one-tenth the activity of the other isomers (Savarese et al., 1988). Mivacurium does not trigger malignant hyperthermia in susceptible swine (Sufit et al., 1990).

Administration of 2 × ED_{95} of mivacurium produces maximum single-twitch depression at the orbicularis oculi sooner than that observed at the adductor pollicis (Fig. 8-40) (Sayson and Mongan, 1994). This contrasts with SCh, which produces maximum single-twitch depression simultaneously at the orbicularis oculi and adductor pollicis (see Fig. 8-40) (Sayson and Mongan, 1994). With both drugs, recovery of function at the orbicularis oculi occurs sooner than at the adductor pollicis (see Fig. 8-40) (Sayson and Mongan, 1994). It is important to recognize that loss of function of the orbicularis oculi, and not the adductor pollicis, correlates with maximal paralysis of the laryngeal adductor muscles and diaphragm.

Clearance

The *cis-trans* and *trans-trans* isomers of mivacurium are hydrolyzed by plasma cholinesterase at a rate equivalent to 88% that of SCh (Fig. 8-41) (Savarese et al., 1988). Hydrolysis of these two isomers is responsible for the short duration of action of mivacurium, whereas the *cis-cis* isomer, which lacks significant neuromuscular-blocking effects at the NMJ, does not depend on hydrolysis by plasma cholinesterase, and is cleared at a rate closer to that

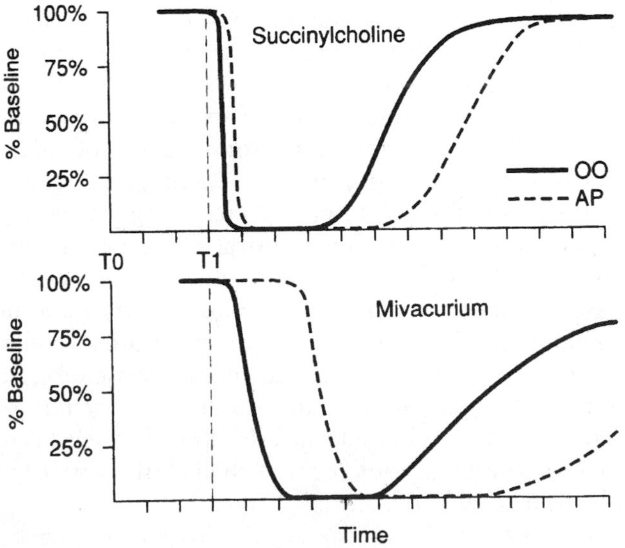

Figure 8-40. The maximum onset of twitch depression after administration of mivacurium, 0.15 mg/kg IV, was more rapid when twitch response was monitored at the orbicularis oculi (OO) muscle than at the adductor pollicis muscle (AP). The onset of maximum twitch depression after administration of succinylcholine, 1 mg/kg IV, was similar at both skeletal muscles. Time is represented as 1 minute per division. (From Sayson SC, Mongan PD. Onset of action of mivacurium chloride: A comparison of neuromuscular blockade monitoring at the adductor pollicis and the orbicularis oculi. *Anesthesiology* 1994;81:35–42; with permission.)

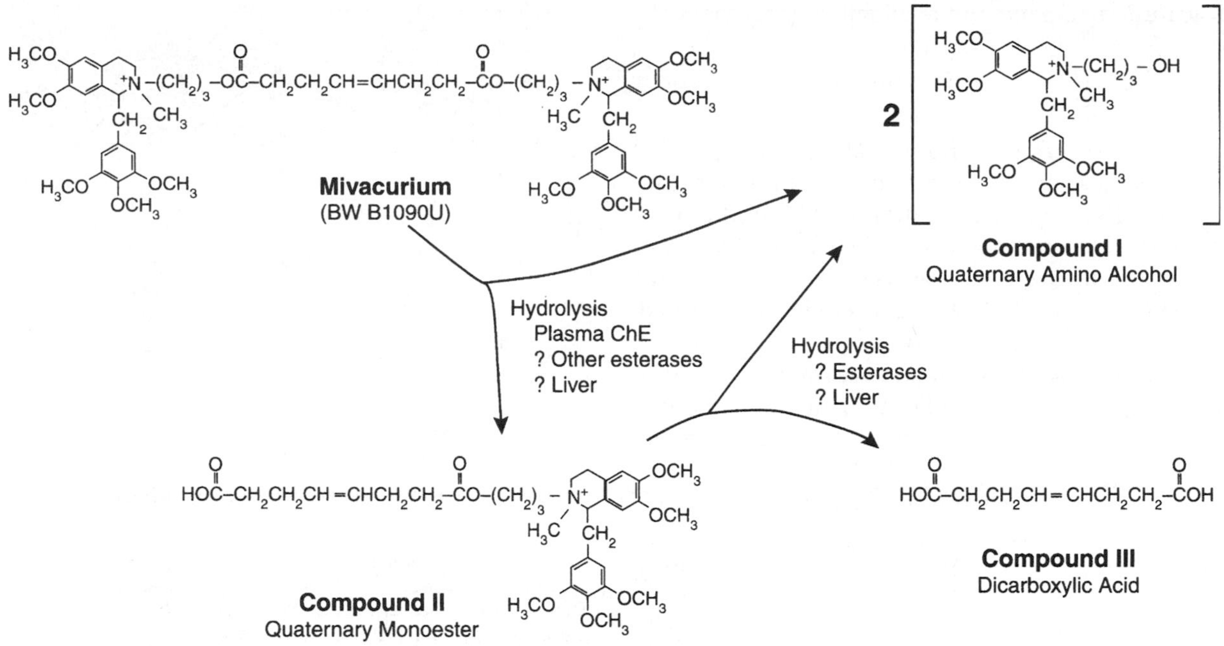

Figure 8-41. Proposed metabolic pathway of mivacurium. (From Savarese JJ, Ali HH, Basta SJ, et al. The clinical neuromuscular pharmacology of mivacurium chloride [BW B1090U]. A short-acting nondepolarizing ester neuromuscular blocking drug. *Anesthesiology* 1988;68:723–732; with permission.)

of the intermediate-acting nondepolarizing neuromuscular-blocking drugs (Lien et al., 1994). The metabolites resulting from hydrolysis of mivacurium include quaternary amino alcohols and quaternary monoesters, which are presumed to be inactive at the NMJ. The rate of hydrolysis of mivacurium by plasma cholinesterase depends on the concentration of mivacurium in the plasma. Thus, the greater the concentration of mivacurium, the more rapid is its breakdown, and unlike the response seen with other neuromuscular-blocking drugs, increasing the dose has only a small impact on the duration of action. Clearance of miviacurium's potent isomers is more rapid in younger patients, which is consistent with the larger mivacurium infusion requirements in children (Markakis et al., 1998).

Atypical Plasma Cholinesterase

The hydrolysis of mivacurium is decreased and its duration of action increased in patients with atypical plasma cholinesterase (Goudsouzin et al., 1993; Maddineni and Mirakhur, 1993; Petersen et al., 1993). In these patients, a normal dose of mivacurium produces an intense neuromuscular blockade. Administration of human plasma cholinesterase has been found to be effective in antagonizing this intense neuromuscular blockade in contrast to the ineffectiveness of anticholinesterase drugs (Ostergaard et al., 1995).

Inhibition of Plasma Cholinesterase Activity

Fluoride is a potent inhibitor of plasma cholinesterase, suggesting that fluoride production, as from the metabolism of fluorinated volatile anesthetics, especially sevoflurane, might impact on the rate of hydrolysis of mivacurium. Nevertheless, fluoride concentrations equivalent to 100 μmol/L do not alter the in vitro half-times of the *cis-trans* and *trans-trans* isomers of mivacurium (Gruber et al., 2002).

Pancuronium potentiates mivacurium more than other nondepolarizing neuromuscular-blocking drugs because it occupies postsynaptic acetylcholine receptors and also slows hydrolysis of mivacurium by inhibiting the activity of plasma cholinesterase. Indeed, the administration of mivacurium following injection of pancuronium results in a prolonged duration of action of mivacurium (Erkola et al., 1996). Even, subparalyzing doses of pancuronium decrease plasma cholinesterase activity and impair the clearance of the two most active isomers of mivacurium (Motamed et al., 2003).

Renal Dysfunction

Renal excretion appears to be a minor pathway for clearance of mivacurium, with an estimated 7% of an administered dose appearing unchanged in urine (Lacroix et al., 1997). A comparison of the neuromuscular-blocking effects of mivacurium in patients with or without renal failure showed a clinically insignificant prolongation of mivacurium in the anephric patients (Phillips and Hunter, 1992). This prolongation was attributed to decreased cholinesterase activity, which is a common finding in the presence of renal failure. In another report, prolonged neuromuscular blockade was observed after administration of mivacurium to a patient in renal failure (Mangar et al., 1993).

Hepatic Dysfunction

The speed of onset of mivacurium-induced neuromuscular blockade is similar in normal patients and those with cirrhosis of the liver, but the duration of action of mivacurium is prolonged in those patients in whom liver disease was associated with decreased plasma cholinesterase activity (Fig. 8-42) (Devlin et al., 1993). Conversely, the increased extracellular fluid volume that occurs in the presence of severe cirrhosis could lead to an increased volume of distribution of mivacurium (similar to pancuronium and atracurium). This increased volume of distribution would result in a less intense neuromuscular blockade that would appear clinically to be resistant to the effects of the nondepolarizing neuromuscular-blocking drug (similar responses have been observed with pancuronium and atracurium) (Devlin et al., 1993).

Pharmacologic Antagonism

Spontaneous recovery from the neuromuscular-blocking effects of mivacurium is rapid, and the need for pharmacologic antagonism has been questioned (Naguib et al., 1996; Pollard, 1992). Furthermore, neostigmine profoundly decreases plasma cholinesterase activity and could thus interfere with the normal rapid spontaneous recovery from mivacurium-induced neuromuscular blockade (see Fig. 8-11) (Devcic et al., 1995). Nevertheless, moderate levels of mivacurium-induced neuromuscular blockade are antagonized readily by anticholinesterases such as neostigmine (Savarese et al., 1988). Edrophonium provides more rapid antagonism of deep mivacurium-induced neuromuscular blockade than does neostigmine (Devcic et al., 1995).

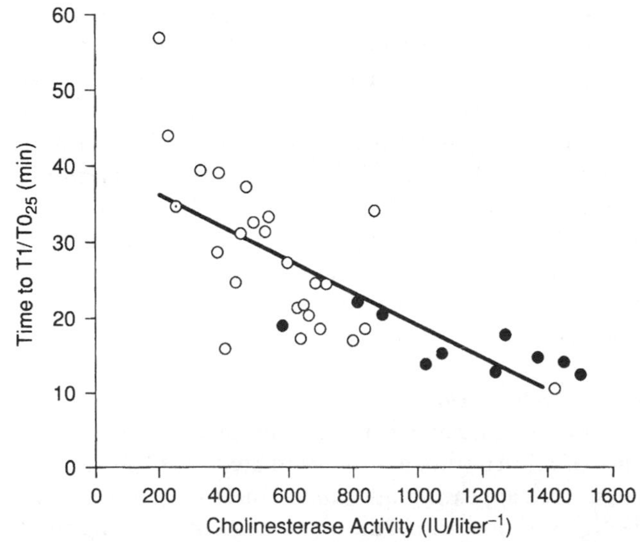

Figure 8-42. Recovery from neuromuscular blockade produced by mivacurium is prolonged in patients with decreased cholinesterase activity, as may be associated with cirrhosis of the liver (*open circles*). Solid circles represents normal patients, whereas the circle with a dot represents a heterozygous patient. (From Devlin JC, Head-Rapson AG, Parker CJR, et al. Pharmacodynamics of mivacurium chloride in patients with hepatic cirrhosis. *Br J Anaesth* 1993;71:227–231; with permission.)

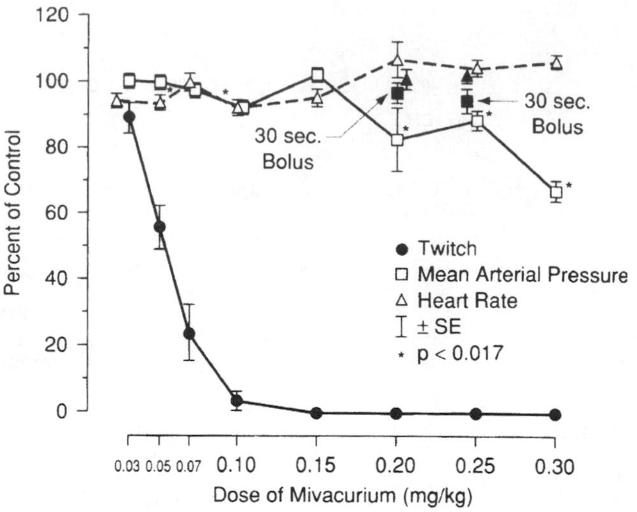

Figure 8-43. Neuromuscular and cardiovascular dose responses to mivacurium after injection over 10 to 15 seconds (except where indicated as 30 seconds). (From Savarese JJ, Ali HH, Basta SJ, et al. The cardiovascular effects of mivacurium chloride [BW 1090U] in patients receiving nitrous oxide–opiate–barbiturate anesthesia. *Anesthesiology* 1989;70:386–394; with permission.)

Cardiovascular Effects

The cardiovascular response to mivacurium is minimal at doses up to $2 \times ED_{95}$ (Fig. 8-43) (Savarese et al., 1989). Administration of $3 \times ED_{95}$ of mivacurium over 10 to 15 seconds evokes sufficient histamine release to transiently decrease the mean arterial pressure 13% to 18% (see Fig. 8-43) (Savarese et al., 1989). Hypotension is more frequent and more pronounced in hypertensive than normotensive patients (Plaud et al., 2002).

Bronchospasm

Although mivacurium is not a potent histamine releaser, the possibility of histamine release and bronchospasm is a consideration, especially in patients with reactive airway disease. Anecdotal experience and analysis of data submitted to the Food and Drug Administration suggests caution in rapid administration of mivacurium to patients with asthma requiring active treatment (Bishop et al., 2003).

Burn Injury

Plasma cholinesterase activity is decreased by burn injury, and it is possible this effect could counter receptor-mediated resistance to the effects of nondepolarizing neuromuscular-blocking drugs, resulting in lack of resistance to mivacurium. Indeed, mivacurium 0.2 mg/kg IV produces similar effects in burned and nonburned patients (Martyn et al.,

2000). In contrast to increased dose requirements for other nondepolarizing neuromuscular blocking drugs, the onset of rapid paralysis can be achieved by normal doses of mivacurium administered to burn injury patients.

GW280430A

GW280430A is a representative of a new class of nondepolarizing neuromuscular-blocking drugs characterized as asymmetric mixed-onium chlorofurmarates (Saverese et al., 2004). This drug undergoes rapid breakdown in plasma by chemical hydrolysis and inactivation by cysteine adduction, resulting in a very short duration of action. In volunteers, the ED_{95} was 0.19 mg/kg, the time to onset of 90% twitch depression ranged from 1.3 to 2.1 minutes, and the duration ranged from 4.7 to 10.1 mintues depending on the dose (Belmont et al., 2004). Transient cardiovascular effects suggestive of histamine release occured when the dose of GW280430A was $3ED_{95s}$ or greater.

REFERENCES

Agoston S, Vermeer GA, Kersten UW, et al. The fate of pancuronium blockade in man. *Acta Anaesthesiol Scand* 1973;17:267–275.

Ali HH, Savarese JJ. Monitoring of neuromuscular function. *Anesthesiology* 1976;45:216–249.

Ali HH, Savarese JJ, Basta SJ, et al. Evaluation of cumulative properties of three new nondepolarizing neuromuscular blocking drugs: BW A444U, atracurium and vecuronium. *Br J Anaesth* 1983;55: S107–S111.

Arden JR, Lynam DP, Castagnoli KP, et al. Vecuronium in alcoholic liver disease: a pharmacokinetic and pharmacodynamic analysis. *Anesthesiology* 1988;68:771–776.

Azar I, Cottrell J, Gupta B, et al. Furosemide facilitates recovery of evoked twitch response after pancuronium. *Anesth Analg* 1980;59:55–57.

Baraka A. Neuromuscular blockade of atracurium versus succinylcholine in a patient with complete absence of plasma cholinesterase activity. *Anesthesiology* 1987;66:80–81.

Baraka AS. Succinylcholine resistance to succinylcholine in myasthenia gravis: a dose-response study. *Anesthesiology* 1988;69:760–763.

Basta SJ, Ali HH, Savarese JJ, et al. Clinical pharmacology of atracurium besylate (BW 33A): a new nondepolarizing muscle relaxant. *Anesth Analg* 1982;61:723–729.

Basta SJ, Savarese JJ, Ali HH, et al. Clinical pharmacology of doxacurium chloride. A new long-acting nondepolarizing muscle relaxant. *Anesthesiology* 1988;69:478–486.

Belmont MR, Lien CA, Quessy S, et al. The clinical neuromuscular pharmacology of 51W89 in patients receiving nitrous oxide/opioid/barbiturate anesthesia. *Anesthesiology* 1995;82:1139–1145.

Bencini AF, Scaf AHJ, Sohn YJ, et al. Disposition and urinary excretion of vecuronium bromide in anesthetized patients with normal renal function or renal failure. *Anesth Analg* 1986a;65: 245–251.

Bencini AF, Scaf AHJ, Sohn YJ, et al. Hepatobiliary disposition of vecuronium bromide in man. *Br J Anaesth* 1986b;58:988–995.

Belmont MR, Lien CA, Tjan J, et al. Clinical pharmacology of GW280430A in humans. *Anesthesiology* 2004;100:768–773.

Bentley JB, Borel JD, Vaughan RW, Gandolfi AJ. Weight, pseudocholinesterase activity, and succinylcholine requirements. *Anesthesiology* 1982;57:48–49.

Benumof JL, Dig R, Benumof R. Critical hemoglobin desideration will occur before return to an unanalyzed state following 1 mg/kg intravenous succinylcholine. *Anesthesiology* 1997;87:979–982.

Bevan DR. Succinylcholine. *Can J Anaesth* 1994;41:465–468.

Bevan DR, Smith CE, Donati F. Postoperative neuromuscular blockade: a comparison between atracurium, vecuronium, and pancuronium. *Anesthesiology* 1988;69:272–276.

Bishop MJ, O'Donnell JT, Salami JR. Mivacurium and bronchospasm. *Anesth Analg* 2003;97:484–485.

Bock M, Klippel K, Nitsche B, et al. Rocuronium potency and recovery characteristics during steady-state desflurane, sevoflurane, isoflurane or propofol anesthesia.. *Anesth Analg* 2000;84:43–47.

Brandom BW, Rudd GD, Cook DR. Clinical pharmacology of atracurium in paediatric patients. *Br J Anaesth* 1983;55:S 117–S121.

Brandom BW, Woelfel SK, Cook DR, et al. Clinical pharmacology of atracurium in infants. *Anesth Analg* 1984;63:309–312.

Buzello W, Schluermann D, Schindler M, et al. Hypothermic cardiopulmonary bypass and neuromuscular blockade by pancuronium and vecuronium. *Anesthesiology* 1985a;62:201–204.

Buzello W, Williams CH, Chandra P, et al. Vecuronium and porcine malignant hyperthermia. *Anesth Analg* 1985b;64:515–519.

Caldwell JE, Canfell PC, Castagnoli RP, et al. The influence of renal failure on the pharmacokinetics and duration of action of pipecuronium bromide in patients anesthetized with halothane and nitrous oxide. *Anesthesiology* 1989;70:7–12.

Caldwell JE, Laster MJ, Magorian T, et al. The neuromuscular effects of desflurane, alone and combined with pancuronium or succinylcholine in humans. *Anesthesiology* 1991;74:412–418.

Caldwell JE, Heier T, Wright PMC, et al. Temperature-dependent pharmacokinetics and pharmacodynamics of vecuronium. *Anesthesiology* 2000;92:84–93.

Cannon JE, Fahey MR, Moss J, et al. Large doses of vecuronium and plasma concentrations. *Can J Anaesth* 1988;35:350–353.

Chapple DJ, Clark JS, Hughes R. Interaction between atracurium and drugs used in anaesthesia. *Br J Anaesth* 1983;55:S17–S22.

Chapple DJ, Miller AA, Ward JB, et al. Cardiovascular and neurological effects of laudanosine. Studies in mice and rats, and in conscious and anaesthetized dogs. *Br J Anaesth* 1987;59:218–225.

Chow B, Bowedn MI, Ho E, et al. Pharmacokinetics and dynamics of atracurium infusions after paediatric orthotopic liver transplantation. *Br J Anaesth* 2000;85:850–855.

Chung DC, Rowbottom SJ. A very small dose of suxamethonium relieves laryngospasm. *Anaesthesia* 1993;48:229–230.

Clendenen SR, Harper JV, Wharen RE Jr, Guarderas JC. Anaphylactic reaction after cisatracurium. *Anesthesiology* 1997;87:690–692.

Conway EE. Persistent paralysis after vecuronium administration. *N Engl J Med* 1992;327:1881–1882.

Cooper RA, Maddineni VR, Mirakhur RK, et al. Time course of neuromuscular effects and pharmacokinetics of rocuronium bromide (ORG 9426) during isoflurane anaesthesia in patients with and without renal failure. *Br J Anaesth* 1993;71:222–226.

Cooperman LH, Strobel GE, Kennell EM. Massive hyperkalemia after administration of succinylcholine. *Anesthesiology* 1970;32: 161–164.

Cozanitis DA, Pouttu J, Rosenberg PH. Bradycardia associated with the use of vecuronium. A comparative study with pancuronium with and without glycopyrronium. *Anaesthesia* 1987;42: 192–194.

Dailey PA, Fisher DM, Shnider SM, et al. Pharmacokinetics, placental transfer, and neonatal effects of vecuronium and pancuronium administered during cesarean section. *Anesthesiology* 1984;60: 569–574.

Devcic A, Munshi CA, Gandhi SK, et al. Antagonism of mivacurium neuromuscular block: neostigmine versus edrophonium. *Anesth Analg* 1995;81:1005–1009.

Devlin JC, Head-Rapson AG, Parker CJR, et al. Pharmacodynamics of mivacurium chloride in patients with hepatic cirrhosis. *Br J Anaesth* 1993;71:27–31.

d'Hollander AA, Luyckx C, Barvais L, De Ville A. Clinical evaluation of atracurium besylate requirement for a stable muscle relaxation during surgery: lack of age-related effects. *Anesthesiology* 1983;59: 237–240.

d'Hollander AA, Massaux F, Nevelsteen M, et al. Age-dependent dose response relationship of ORG NC45 in anaesthetized patients. *Br J Anaesth* 1982;54:563–567.

D'Honneur G, Khalil M, Dominique C, et al. Pharmacokinetics and pharmacodynamics of pipecuronium in patients with cirrhosis. *Anesth Analg* 1993;77:1203–1206.

Didier A, Benzarti M, Senft M, et al. Allergy to suxamethonium: persisting abnormalities in skin tests, specific IgE antibodies and leucocyte histamine release. *Clin Allergy* 1987;17:385–392.

Dierdorf SF, McNiece WL, Rao CC. Effect of succinylcholine on plasma potassium in children with cerebral palsy. *Anesthesiology* 1985;62: 88–90.

Dierdorf SF, McNiece WL, Rao CC, et al. Failure of succinylcholine to alter plasma potassium in children with myelomeningocele. *Anesthesiology* 1986;64:272–273.

Dillon JB, Sabawala P, Taylor DB, et al. Action of succinylcholine on extraocular muscles and intraocular pressure. *Anesthesiology* 1957;18:44–49.

Doenicke A, Soukup J, Hoernecke R, et al. The lack of histamine release with cisatracurium: a double-blind comparison with vecuronium. *Anesth Analg* 1997;84:623–628.

Domenech JS, Garcia RC, Sastain JMR, et al. Pancuronium bromide: an indirect sympathomimetic agent. *Br J Anaesth* 1976;48:1143–1148.

Donati F, Antzaka C, Bevan DR. Potency of pancuronium at the diaphragm and the adductor pollicis muscle in humans. *Anesthesiology* 1986;65:1–5.

Donati F, Meistelman C, Plaud B. Vecuronium neuromuscular blockade at the adductor muscles of the larynx and adductor pollicis. *Anesthesiology* 1991;74:833–837.

Donati F. The right dose of succinylcholine. *Anesthesiology* 2003;99: 1037–1038.

Dotan ZA, Hana R, Simon D, et al. The effect of vecuronium is enhanced by a large rather than a modest dose of gentamicin as compared with no preoperative gentamicin. *Anesth Analg* 2003;96: 750–754.

Drachman DA. Myasthenia gravis. *N Engl J Med* 1978;298:136–142.

Dretchen KL, Morgenroth VH, Standaert FG, et al. Azathioprine: effects on neuromuscular transmission. *Anesthesiology* 1976;45:604–609.

Driessen JJ, Wuis EW, Gielen JM. Prolonged vecuronium neuromuscular blockade in a patient receiving orally administered dantrolene. *Anesthesiology* 1985;62:523–524.

Durant MN, Lee C, Katz RL. The action of dantrolene on transmitter mobilization at the rate NMJ. *Eur J Pharmacol* 1980;68:403–408.

Duvaldestin P, Agoston S, Henzel E, et al. Pancuronium pharmacokinetics in patients with liver cirrhosis. *Br J Anaesth* 1978;50: 1131–1136.

Duvaldestin P, Saada J, Berger JL, et al. Pharmacokinetics, pharmacodynamics, and dose-response relationship of pancuronium in control and elderly subjects. *Anesthesiology* 1982;56:36–40.

Dwersteg JF, Pavlin EG, Heimbach DM. Patients with burns are resistant to atracurium. *Anesthesiology* 1986;65:517–520.

Eisenkraft JB, Book WJ, Mann SM, et al. Resistance to succinylcholine in myasthenia gravis: a dose-response study. *Anesthesiology* 1988; 69:760–763.

Eriksson LI, Sundman E, Olsson R, et al. Functional assessment of the pharynx at rest and during swallowing in partially paralyzed humans: simultaneous videomanometry and mechanomyography of awake human volunteers. *Anesthesiology* 1997;87:1035–1043.

Erkola O, Rautoma P, Meretoja OA. Mivacurium when preceded by pancuronium becomes a long-acting muscle relaxant. *Anesthesiology* 1996;84:562–565.

Fahey MR, Morris RB, Miller RD, et al. Clinical pharmacology of ORG NC45 (Norcuron): a new nondepolarizing muscle relaxant. *Anesthesiology* 1981;55:6–11.

Fahey MR, Rupp SM, Canfell C, et al. Effect of renal function on laudanosine excretion in man. *Br J Anaesth* 1985;57:1049–1051.

Fisher DM, Miller RD. Interaction of succinylcholine and vecuronium during N_2O-halothane anesthesia. *Anesthesiology* 1983a;59:A278.

Fisher DM, Miller RD. Neuromuscular effects of vecuronium (ORG NC45) in infants and children during N_2O, halothane anesthesia. *Anesthesiology* 1983b;58:519–523.

Fisher DM, Ramsay MA, Hein HAT, et al. Pharmacokinetics of rocuronium during the three stages of liver transplantation. *Anesthesiology* 1997;86:1306–1316.

Flynn PJ, Hughes P, Walton B. The use of atracurium in cardiopulmonary bypass with induced hypothermia. *Anesthesiology* 1983;59:A262.

Fogdall RP, Miller RD. Neuromuscular effects of enflurane, alone and combined with *d*-tubocurarine, pancuronium, and succinylcholine, in man. *Anesthesiology* 1975;42:173–177.

Foldes FF, Deery A. Protein binding of atracurium and other short acting neuromuscular blocking agents and their interaction with human cholinesterase. *Br J Anaesth* 1983;55:S31–S34.

Foldes FF, Rendell-Baker L, Birch JH. Causes and prevention of prolonged apnea with succinylcholine. *Anesth Analg* 1956;35:609–613.

Frank M, Flynn PJ, Hughes R. Atracurium in obstetric anaesthesia. *Br J Anaesth* 1983;55:S113–S114.

Gencarelli PJ, Miller RD. Antagonism of ORG NC 45 (vecuronium) and pancuronium neuromuscular blockade by neostigmine. *Br J Anaesth* 1982;54:53–56.

Gencarelli PJ, Siven J, Koot HWJ, et al. The effects of hypercarbia and hypocarbia on pancuronium and vecuronium neuromuscular blockades in anesthetized humans. *Anesthesiology* 1983;59:376–380.

Gergis SD, Sokoll MD, Mehta M, et al. Intubation conditions after atracurium and suxamethonium. *Br J Anaesth* 1983;55:S83.

Ghoneim MM, Long JP. The interaction between magnesium and other neuromuscular blocking agents. *Anesthesiology* 1970;32:23–27.

Goudsouzian NG, d'Hollander AA, Viby-Mogensen J. Prolonged neuromuscular block from mivacurium in two patients with cholinesterase deficiency. *Anesth Analg* 1993;77:183–185.

Griffith HR, Johnson GE. The use of curare in general anesthesia. *Anesthesiology* 1942;3:418–420.

Gronert GA, Theye RA. Pathophysiology of hyperkalemia induced by succinylcholine. *Anesthesiology* 1975;43:89–99.

Gruber M, Lindner R, Prasser C, et al. The effect of fluoride and hypothermia on the in vitro metabolism of mivacurium. *Anesth Analg* 2002;95:397–399.

Hame J, Miller RD, Benet LZ, et al. Pharmacokinetics and pharmacodynamics of *d*-tubocurarine during hypothermia in the cat. *Anesthesiology* 1978;49:324–329.

Han T H, Kim HS, Bae JY, et al. Neuromuscular pharmacodynamics of rocuronium in patients with major burns. *Anesth Analg* 2004;99: 386–92.

Hannallah RS, Kaplan RF. Jaw relaxation after a halothane/succinylcholine sequence in children. *Anesthesiology* 1994;81:99–103.

Hansen-Flaschen J, Cowen J, Raps EC. Neuromuscular blockade in the intensive care unit: more than we bargained for. *Am Rev Respir Dis* 1993;147:234–236.

Harrah MD, Way WL, Katzung BG. The interaction of *d*-tubocurarine with antiarrhythmic drugs. *Anesthesiology* 1970;33:406–410.

Hatano Y, Arai T, Noda J, et al. Contribution of prostacyclin to *d*-tubocurarine-induced hypotension in humans. *Anesthesiology* 1990;72:28–32.

Havdala HS, Borison RL, Diamond BI. Potential hazards and applications of lithium in anesthesiology. *Anesthesiology* 1979;50:534–537.

Hawkins JL, Adenwala J, Camp C, Joyce TH. The effect of H_2-receptor antagonist premedication on the duration of vercuronium-induced neuromuscular blockade in postpartum patients. *Anesthesiology* 1989;71:175–177.

Hennis PJ, Fahey MR, Canfell PC, et al. Pharmacology of laudanosine in dogs. *Anesthesiology* 1986;65:56–60.

Hilgenberg JC, Stoelting RK, Harris WA. Systemic vascular responses to atracurium during enflurane-nitrous oxide anesthesia in humans. *Anesthesiology* 1983;58:242–244.

Holst-Larsen H. The hydrolysis of suxamethonium in human blood. *Br J Anaesth* 1976;48:887–891.

Hosking MP, Lennon RL, Gronert GA. Combined H_1 and H_2 receptor blockade attenuates the cardiovascular effects of high-dose atracurium for rapid sequence endotracheal intubation. *Anesth Analg* 1988;67:1089–1092.

Houghton IT, Aun CST, Oh TE. Vecuronium: an anthropometric comparison. *Anaesthesia* 1992;47:741–746.

Hughes R, Chapple DJ. Effects of non-depolarizing neuromuscular blocking agents on peripheral autonomic mechanisms in cats. *Br J Anaesth* 1976;48:59–67.

Hughes R, Payne JP. Clinical assessment of atracurium using the single twitch and tetanic responses of the adductor pollicis muscles. *Br J Anaesth* 1983;55:S47–S52.

Hunter AR, Feldman SA. Muscle relaxants [editorial]. *Br J Anaesth* 1976;48:277–278.

Hunter JM. New neuromuscular blocking drugs. *N Engl J Med* 1995;332: 1691–1699.

Hunter JM. Rocuronium: the newest aminosteroid neuromuscular blocking drug. *Br J Anaesth* 1996;76:481–483.

Hunter JM, Jones RS, Utting JE. Comparison of vecuronium, atracurium and tubocurarine in normal patients and in patients with no renal function. *Br J Anaesth* 1984;56:941–950.

Inoue K, el-Banayosy A, Stolarski L, Reichelt W. Vecuronium induced bradycardia following induction of anaesthesia with etomidate or thiopentone, with or without fentanyl. *Br J Anaesth* 1988;60:10–17.

Ivankovich AD, Miletich DJ, Albrecht RF, Zahed B. The effect of pancuronium on myocardial contraction and catecholamine metabolism. *J Pharm Pharmacol* 1975;27:837–841.

Iwasaki H, Namiki A, Omote K, et al. Response differences of paretic and healthy extremities to pancuronium and neostigmine in hemiplegic patients. *Anesth Analg* 1985;64:864–866.

John DA, Tobey RE, Homer LD, et al. Onset of succinylcholine-induced hyperkalemia following denervation. *Anesthesiology* 1976;45:294–299.

Kalli I, Meretoja OA. Infusion of atracurium in neonates, infants and children. A study of dose requirements. *Br J Anaesth* 1988;60: 651–654.

Kao YJ, Turner DR. Prolongation of succinylcholine block by metoclopramide. *Anesthesiology* 1989;70:905–908.

Kaplan RF, Uejima T, Lobel G, et al. Intramuscular rocuronium in infants and children: A multicenter study to evaluate tracheal intubating conditions, onset, and duration of action. *Anesthesiology* 1999;91:633–638.

Katz JA, Fragen RJ, Shanks CA, et al. Dose-response relationships of doxacurium chloride in humans during anesthesia with nitrous oxide and fentanyl, enflurane, isoflurane, or halothane. *Anesthesiology* 1989;70:432–436.

Kelly RE, Dinner M, Turner LS, et al. Succinylcholine increases intraocular pressure in the human eye with the extraocular muscles detached. *Anesthesiology* 1993;79:948–952.

Khuenl-Brady KS, Reitstatter B, Schlager A, et al. Long-term administration of pancuronium and pipecuronium in the intensive care unit. *Anesth Analg* 1994;78:1082–1086.

Khuenl-Brady K, Castagnoli KP, Canfell PC, et al. The neuromuscular blocking effects and pharmacokinetics of ORG 9426 and ORG 9616 in the cat. *Anesthesiology* 1990;72:669–674.

Kindler CH, Verotta D, Gray AT, et al. Additive inhibition of nicotinic acetylcholine receptors by corticosteroids and the neuromuscular blocking drug vecuronium. *Anesthesiology* 2000;92:821–832.

Kisor DF, Schmith VD, Wargin WA, et al. Importance of the organ-independent elimination of cisatracurium. *Anesth Analg* 1996;83:1065–1071.

Kitts JB, Fisher DM, Canfell PC, et al. Pharmacokinetics and pharmacodynamics of atracurium in the elderly. *Anesthesiology* 1990;72: 272–275.

Kohlschutter B, Bauer H, Roth F. Suxamethonium-induced hyperkalemia in patients with severe intraabdominal infections. *Br J Anaesth* 1976;48:557–562.

Konstadt SN, Reich DL, Stanley TE, et al. A two-center comparison of the cardiovascular effects of cisatracurium (Nimbex™) and vecuronium in patients with coronary artery disease. *Anesth Analg* 1995;81:1010–1014.

Kopman AF, Zhaku B, Lai KS. The "intubating dose" of succinylcholine: the effect of decreasing doses on recovery time. *Anesthesiology* 2003;99:1050–1054.

Koscielniak-Nielsen ZJ, Law-Min JC, Donati F, et al. Dose-response relations of doxacurium and its reversal with neostigmine in young adults and healthy elderly patients. *Anesth Analg* 1992;74: 845–850.

Kostopanagiotou G, Mylona M, Massoura L, et al. Accidental epidural injection of vecuronium. *Anesth Analg* 2000;91:1550–1551.

Kovarik WD, Mayberg TS, Lam AM, et al. Succinylcholine does not change intracranial pressure, cerebral blood flow velocity, or the electroencephalogram in patients with neurologic injury. *Anesth Analg* 1994;78:469–473.

Lanier WL, Milde JH, Michenfelder JD. The cerebral effects of pancuronium and atracurium in halothane-anesthetized dogs. *Anesthesiology* 1985;63:589–597.

Larijani GE, Bartkowski RR, Azad SS, et al. Clinical pharmacology of pipecuronium bromide. *Anesth Analg* 1989;68:734–739.

Lawhead RG, Matsumi M, Peters KR, et al. Plasma laudanosine levels in patients given atracurium during liver transplantation. *Anesth Analg* 1993;76:569–573.

Lebrault C, Berger JL, d'Hollander AA, et al. Pharmacokinetics and pharmacodynamics of vecuronium (ORG NC45) in patients with cirrhosis. *Anesthesiology* 1985;62:601–605.

Lebrault C, Duvaldestin P, Henzel D, et al. Pharmacokinetics and pharmacodynamics of vecuronium in patients with cholestasis. *Br J Anaesth* 1986;58:983–987.

Lee C. Dose relationship of phase II, tachyphylaxis and train-of-four fade on suxamethonium-induced dual neuromuscular block in man. *Br J Anaesth* 1975;47:841–845.

Lee C. Intensive care unit neuromuscular syndrome? *Anesthesiology* 1995; 83:237–240.

Legros CB, Orliaguet GA, Mayer M-N, et al. Severe anaphylactic reaction to cisatracurium in a child. *Anesth Analg* 2001;92:648–649.

Leighton BL, Cheek TG, Gross JB, et al. Succinylcholine pharmacodynamics in peripartum patients. *Anesthesiology* 1986;64:202–205.

Levy JH, Davis GK, Duggan J, et al. Determination of the hemodynamics and histamine release of rocuronium (ORG 9426) when administered in increased doses under N_2O/O_2-sufentanil anesthesia. *Anesth Analg* 1994;78:318–321.

Leykin Y, Pellis T, Lucca M, et al. The pharmacodynamic effects of rocuronium when dosed according to real body weight and ideal body weight in morbidly obese patients. *Anesth Analg* 2004a;99: 1086–1089.

Leykin Y, Pellis T, Lucca M, et al. The effects of cisatracurium in morbidly obese women. *Anesth Analg* 2004b;99:1090–1094.

Libonati MM, Leahy JJ, Ellison N. The use of succinylcholine in open eye surgery. *Anesthesiology* 1985;62:637–640.

Lien CA, Belmont MR, Abalos A, et al. The cardiovascular effects and histamine-releasing properties of 51W89 in patients receiving nitrous oxide/opioid/barbiturate anesthesia. *Anesthesiology* 1995;82:1131–1138.

Lien CA, Schmith VD, Belmont MR, et al. Pharmacokinetics of cisatracurium in patients receiving nitrous oxide/opioid/barbiturate anesthesia. *Anesthesiology* 1996;84:300–308.

Lien CA, Schmith VD, Embree PB, et al. The pharmacokinetics and pharmacodynamics of the stereoisomers of mivacurium in patients receiving nitrous oxide/opioid/barbiturate anesthesia. *Anesthesiology* 1994;80:1296–1302.

Lynam DP, Cronnelly R, Castagnoli KP, et al. The pharmacodynamics and pharmacokinetics of vecuronium in patients anesthetized with isoflurane with normal renal function or with renal failure. *Anesthesiology* 1988;69:227–231.

Macri FJ, Grimes PA. The effects of succinylcholine on the extraocular striate muscles and on the intraocular pressure. *Am J Ophthalmol* 1957;44:221–229.

Maddineni VR, Mirakhur RK. Prolonged neuromuscular block following mivacurium. *Anesthesiology* 1993;78:1181–1184.

Magorian T, Wood P, Caldwell J, et al. The pharmacokinetics and neuromuscular effects of rocuronium bromide in patients with liver disease. *Anesth Analg* 1995;80:754–759.

Mangar D, Kirchhoff GT, Rose PL, et al. Prolonged neuromuscular block after mivacurium in a patient with end-stage renal disease. *Anesth Analg* 1993;76:866–867.

Manninen PH, Mahendran B, Gelb AW, et al. Succinylcholine does not increase serum potassium levels in patients with acutely ruptured cerebral aneurysm. *Anesth Analg* 1990;70:172–175.

Marathe PH, Dwerstg JF, Pavlin EG, et al. Effect of thermal injury on the pharmacokinetics and pharmacodynamics of atracurium in humans. *Anesthesiology* 1989a;70:752–755.

Marathe PH, Haschke RH, Slattery JT, et al. Acetylcholine receptor density and acetylcholinesterase activity in skeletal muscle of rats following thermal injury. *Anesthesiology* 1989b;70:654–659.

Margolis BD, Khachikian D, Friedman Y, et al. Prolonged reversible quadriparesis in mechanically ventilated patients who received long-term infusion of vecuronium. *Chest* 1991;100:877–878.

Markakis DA, Lau M, Brown R, et al. The pharmacokinetics and steady state pharmacodynamics of mivacurium in children. *Anesthesiology* 1998;88:978–983.

Martyn JAJ, Liu LMP, Szyfelbein SK, et al. The neuromuscular effects of pancuronium in burned children. *Anesthesiology* 1983;59:561–564.

Martyn JAJ, Matteo RS, Szyfelbein SK, et al. Unprecedented resistance to neuromuscular blocking effects of metocurine, with persistence and complete recovery in a burned patient. *Anesth Analg* 1982;61: 614–617.

Martyn JAJ, Goudsouzian NG, Chang YC, et al. Neuromuscular effects of mivacurium in 2- to 12-yr old children with burn injury. *Anesthesiology* 2000;92:31–37.

Matteo RS, Backus WW, McDaniel DD, et al. Pharmacokinetics and pharmacodynamics of *d*-tubocurarine and metocurine in the elderly. *Anesth Analg* 1985;64:23–29.

Matteo RS, Nishitateno K, Pua E, et al. Pharmacokinetics of *d*-tubocurarine in man: effect of an osmotic diuretic on urinary excretion. *Anesthesiology* 1980;52:335–338.

Matteo RS, Ornstein E, Schwartz AE, et al. Pharmacokinetics and pharmacokinetics of rocuronium (ORG 9426) in elderly surgical patients. *Anesth Analg* 1993;77:1193–1197.

Mehta MP, Choi WW, Gergis SD, et al. Facilitation of rapid endotracheal intubations with divided doses of nondepolarizing neuromuscular blocking drugs. *Anesthesiology* 1985;62:392–395.

Mellinghoff H, Radbruch L, Diefenbach C, et al. A comparison of cisatracurium and atracurium: onset of neuromuscular block after bolus injection and recovery after subsequent infusion. *Anesth Analg* 1996;83:1072–1075.

Meretoja AA. Is vecuronium a long-acting neuromuscular blocking agent in neonates and infants? *Br J Anaesth* 1989;62:184–187.

Merrett RA, Thompson CW, Webb FW. In vitro degradation of atracurium in human plasma. *Br J Anaesth* 1983;55:61–66.

Meyer KC, Prielipp RC, Grossman JF, et al. Prolonged weakness after infusion of atracurium in two intensive care unit patients. *Anesth Analg* 1994;78:772–774.

Miller RD. Use of neuromuscular blocking drugs in intensive care unit patients. *Anesth Analg* 1995;81:1–2.

Miller RD, Agoston S, Booij LHDJ, et al. The comparative potency and pharmacokinetics of pancuronium and its metabolites in anesthetized man. *J Pharmacol Exp Ther* 1978;207:539–543.

Miller RD, Roderick L. Diuretic-induced hypokalaemic pancuronium neuromuscular blockade and its antagonism by neostigmine. *Br J Anaesth* 1978a;50:541–544.

Miller RD, Roderick LL. Acid-base balance and neostigmine antagonism of pancuronium neuromuscular blockade. *Br J Anaesth* 1978b;50: 317–324.

Miller RD, Rupp SM, Fisher DM, et al. Clinical pharmacology of vecuronium and atracurium. *Anesthesiology* 1984;61:444–453.

Miller RD, Sohn YJ, Matteo RS. Enhancement of *d*-tubocurarine neuromuscular blockade by diuretics in man. *Anesthesiology* 1976;45: 442–445.

Miller RD, Way WL. Inhibition of succinylcholine-induced increased intragastric pressure by nondepolarizing muscular relaxants and lidocaine. *Anesthesiology* 1971;34:185–188.

Miller RD, Way WL, Dolan WM, et al. Comparative neuromuscular effects of pancuronium, gallamine, and succinylcholine during forane and halothane anesthesia in man. *Anesthesiology* 1971;35: 509–514.

Miller RD, Way WL, Hickey RL. Inhibition of succinylcholine-induced increased intraocular pressure by nondepolarizing muscle relaxants. *Anesthesiology* 1968;29:123–126.

Miller RD, Way WL, Katzung BG. The potentiation of neuromuscular blocking agents by quinidine. *Anesthesiology* 1967;28:1036–1041.

Milligan KR, Beers HT. Vecuronium-associated cardiac arrest. *Anesthesia* 1985;40:385.

Mitchell MM, Ali HH, Savarese JJ. Myotonia and neuromuscular blocking agents. *Anesthesiology* 1978;49:44–48.

Moore EW, Hunter JM. The new neuromuscular blocking agents: Do they offer any advantages? *Br J Anaesth* 2001;87:912–925.

Moorthy SS, Hilgenberg JC. Resistance to nondepolarizing muscle relaxants in paretic upper extremities of patients with residual hemiplegia. *Anesth Analg* 1980;59:624–627.

Moorthy SS, Reddy RV, Dunfield JA, et al. The effect of muscle relaxants on the cricothyroid muscle: a report of three cases. *Anesth Analg* 1996;82:657–660.

Morris RB, Cahalan MK, Miller RD, et al. The cardiovascular effects of vecuronium (ORG NC45) and pancuronium in patients undergoing coronary artery bypass grafting. *Anesthesiology* 1983;58:438–440.

Motamed C, Menad R, Farinotti R, et al. Potentiation of mivacurium blockade by low doses of pancuronium: a pharmacokinetic study. *Anesthesiology* 2003;98:1057–1062.

Muzzi DA, Black S, Cucchiara RF. The lack of effect of succinylcholine on serum potassium in patients with Parkinson's disease. *Anesthesiology* 1989;71:322.

Naguib M, Selim M, Bakhamees HS, et al. Enzymatic versus pharmacologic antagonism of profound mivacurium-induced neuromuscular blockade. *Anesthesiology* 1996;84:1051–1059.

Naguib M, Flood P, McArdle, et al. Advances in neurobiology of the neuromuscular junction: Implications for the anesthesiologist. *Anesthesiology* 2002;96:202–231.

Naguib M, Samarkandi A, Riad W et al. Optimal dose of succinylcholine revisited. *Anesthesiology* 2003;99:1045–1049.

Naguib M, Samarkandi A, Abdullah K, et al. Succinylcholine dosage and apnea-induced hemoglobin desaturation in patients. *Anesthesiology* 2005;102:35–40.

Nigrovic V, Pandya JB, Klaunig JE, et al. Reactivity and toxicity of atracurium and its metabolites in vitro. *Can J Anaesth* 1989;36: 262–268.

O'Hara DA, Fragen RJ, Shanks CA. The effects of age on the dose-response curves for vecuronium in adults. *Anesthesiology* 1985;63:542–544.

Ono K, Manabe N, Ohta Y, et al. Influence of suxamethonium on the action of subsequently administered vecuronium or pancuronium. *Br J Anaesth* 1989;62:324–326.

Ording H, Fonsmark L. Use of vecuronium and doxapram in patients susceptible to malignant hyperthermia. *Br J Anaesth* 1988;60: 445–449.

Ornstein E, Lien CA, Matteo RS, et al. Pharmacodynamics and pharmacokinetics of cisatracurium in geriatric surgical patients. *Anesthesiology* 1996;84:520–525.

Ornstein E, Matteo RS, Schwartz AE, et al. Pharmacokinetics and pharmacodynamics of pipecuronium bromide (Arduan) in elderly surgical patients. *Anesth Analg* 1992;74:841–844.

Ostergaard D, Jensen FS, Viby-Mogensen J. Reversal of intense mivacurium block with human plasma cholinesterase in patients with atypical plasma cholinesterase. *Anesthesiology* 1995;82:1295–1298.

Pandey K, Badola RP, Kumar S. Time course of intraocular hypertension produced by suxamethonium. *Br J Anaesth* 1972;44:191–196.

Pantuck EJ. Plasma cholinesterase: gene and variations. *Anesth Analg* 1993;77:380–386.

Parker CJR, Hunter JM. Pharmacokinetics of atracurium and laudanosine in patients with hepatic cirrhosis. *Br J Anaesth* 1989;62: 177–183.

Payne JP, Hughes R. Evaluation of atracurium in anesthetized man. *Br J Anaesth* 1981;53:45–56.

Petersen RS, Bailey PL, Kalameghan R, et al. Prolonged neuromuscular block after mivacurium. *Anesth Analg* 1993;76:194–196.

Phillips BJ, Hunter JM. Use of mivacurium chloride by constant infusion in the anephric patient. *Br J Anaesth* 1992;68:492–498.

Pittet JF, Tassonju E, Morel DR, et al. Neuromuscular effect of pipecuronium bromide in infants and children during nitrous oxide–alfentanil anesthesia. *Anesthesiology* 1990;72:432–435.

Plaud B, Debaene B, Lequeau F, et al. Mivacurium neuromuscular block at the adductor muscles of the larynx and the adductor pollicis in humans. *Anesthesiology* 1996;85:77–81.

Plaud B, Marty J, Debaene B, et al. The cardiovascular effects of mivacurium in hypertensive patients. *Anesth Analg* 2002;95:379–384.

Pollard BJ. Neuromuscular blocking drugs and renal failure. *Br J Anaesth* 1992;68:545–546.

Prielipp RC, Coursin DB, Scuderi PE, et al. Comparison of the infusion requirements and recovery profile of vecuronium and cisatracurium in intensive care unit patients. *Anesth Analg* 1994;81:3–12.

Prielipp RC, Coursin DB, Scuderi PE, et al. Comparison of the infusion requirements and recovery profiles of vecuronium and cisatracurium 51W89 in intensive care unit patients. *Anesth Analg* 1995;81:3–12.

Proost JH, Eriksson LI, Mirakhur RK, et al. Urinary, biliary and faecal excretion of rocuronium in humans. *Br J Anaesth* 2000;85:717–723.

Pumplin DW, Fambrough DM. Turnover of acetyl-choline receptors in skeletal muscle. *Ann Rev Physiol* 1982;44:319–335.

Rathmell JP, Brooker RF, Prielipp RC, et al. Hemodynamic and pharmacodynamic comparison of doxacurium and pipecuronium with pancuronium during induction of cardiac anesthesia: does the benefit justify the cost? *Anesth Analg* 1993;76:313–319.

Reynolds LM, Lau M, Brown R, et al. Intramuscular rocuronium in infants and children: dose-ranging and tracheal intubating conditions. *Anesthesiology* 1996;85:231–239.

Richard A, Girard F, Girad D, et al. Cisatracurium-induced neuromuscular blockade is affected by chronic phenytoin or carbamazepine treatment in neurosurgical patients. *Anesth Analg* 2005;100; 538–544.

Rorvik K, Husby P, Gramstad L, et al. Comparison of large dose of vecuronium with pancuronium for prolonged neuromuscular blockade. *Br J Anaesth* 1988;61:180–185.

Rosa G, Orfei P, Sanfilippo M, et al. The effects of atracurium besylate (Tracrium) on intracranial pressure and cerebral perfusion pressure. *Anesth Analg* 1986a;65:381–384.

Rosa G, Sanfilippo M, Vilardi V, et al. Effects of vecuronium bromide on intracranial pressure and cerebral perfusion pressure. *Br J Anaesth* 1986b;58:437–440.

Rose M, Fisher M. Rocuronium: high risk for anaphylaxis? *Br J Anaesth* 2001;86:678–682.

Rupp SM, Castagnoli KP, Fisher DM, et al. Pancuronium and vecuronium pharmacokinetics and pharmacodynamics in younger and elderly adults. *Anesthesiology* 1987;67:45–49.

Rupp SM, Fahey MR, Miller RD. Neuromuscular and cardiovascular effects of atracurium during nitrous oxide–isoflurane anaesthesia. *Br J Anaesth* 1983a;55:S67–S70.

Rupp SM, Fisher DM, Miller RD, et al. Pharmacokinetics and pharmacodynamics of vecuronium in the elderly. *Anesthesiology* 1983b;59:A270.

Rupp SM, McChristian JW, Miller RD. Neuromuscular effects of atracurium during halothane–nitrous oxide and enflurane–nitrous oxide anesthesia in humans. *Anesthesiology* 1985;63:16–19.

Rupp SM, Miller RD, Gencarelli P. Vecuronium-induced neuromuscular blockade during enflurane, isoflurane, and halothane anesthesia in humans. *Anesthesiology* 1984;60:102–105.

Ryan JF, Kagen LJ, Hyman AI. Myoglobinemia after a single dose of succinylcholine. *N Engl J Med* 1971;285:824–827.

Salem MR, Wong AY, Lin YH. The effect of suxamethonium in the intragastric pressure in infants and children. *Br J Anaesth* 1972;44:166–170.

Salmenpera M, Peltola K, Takkumen O, et al. Cardiovascular effects of pancuronium and vecuronium during high-dose fentanyl anesthesia. *Anesth Analg* 1983;62:1059–1064.

Savage DS, Sleigh T, Carlyle I. The emergence of ORG NC 45, 1- . . . (2 beta,3 alpha,5 alpha,16 beta,17 beta)-3-17 bis(acetyloxy)-2-(1-piperidinyl)-androstan-16 y1) . . . 1-methylpiperidinium bromide, from the pancuronium series. *Br J Anaesth* 1980;52(suppl 1):S3–S9.

Savarese JJ, Ali HH, Basta SJ, et al. The clinical neuromuscular pharmacology of mivacurium chloride (BW B1090U). A short-acting non-depolarizing ester neuromuscular blocking drug. *Anesthesiology* 1988;68:723–732.

Savarese JJ, Ali HH, Basta SJ, et al. The cardiovascular effects of mivacurium chloride (BW B1090U) in patients receiving nitrous oxide–opiate–barbiturate anesthesia. *Anesthesiology* 1989;70:386–394.

Savarese JJ, Belmont MR, Hashim MA, et al. Preclinical pharmacology of GW280430A (AV430A) in the rhesus monkey and in the cat: a comparison with mivacurium. *Anesthesiology* 2004;100:835–845.

Sayson SC, Mongan PD. Onset of action of mivacurium chloride: a comparison of neuromuscular blockade monitoring at the adductor pollicis and the orbicularis oculi. *Anesthesiology* 1994;81:35–42.

Schneider MJ, Stirt JA, Finholt DA. Atracurium, vecuronium, and intraocular pressure in humans. *Anesth Analg* 1986;65:877–882.

Schoenstadt DA, Whitcher CE. Observations on the mechanism of succinylcholine-induced cardiac arrhythmias. *Anesthesiology* 1963;24:358–362.

Schow AJ, Lubarsky DA, Olson RP, et al. Can succinylcholine be used safely in hyperkalemic patients? *Anesth Analg* 2002;95:119–122.

Schramm WM, Papousek A, Michalek-Sauberer A, et al. The cerebral and cardiovascular effects of cisatracurium and atracurium in neurosurgical patients. *Anesth Analg* 1998;86:123–127.

Schrieber J-W, Mencke T, Biedler A, et al. Postoperative myalgia after succinylcholine: no evidence for an inflammatory origin. *Anesth Analg* 2003;96:1640–1644.

Schwartz AE, Matteo RS, Ornstein E, et al. Acute steroid therapy does not alter nondepolarizing muscle relaxant effects in humans. *Anesthesiology* 1986;65:326–327.

Schwartz S, Ilias W, Lackner F, et al. Rapid tracheal intubation with vecuronium: the priming principle. *Anesthesiology* 1985;62:388–393.

Scott RPF, Savarese JJ. The cardiovascular and autonomic effects of neuromuscular blocking agents. *Semin Anesth* 1985;4:319–334.

Scott RPF, Savarese JJ, Ali HH, et al. Atracurium: clinical strategies for preventing histamine release and attenuating the hemodynamic response. *Anesthesiology* 1984;61:A287.

Segredo V, Caldwell JE, Matthay MA, et al. Persistent paralysis in critically ill patients after long-term administration of vecuronium. *N Engl J Med* 1992;327:524–528.

Semple P, Hope DA, Clyburn P, et al. Relative potency of vecuronium in male and female patients in Britain and Australia. *Br J Anaesth* 1994;72:190–194.

Servin FS, Lavaut E, Kleff U, et al. Repeated doses of rocuronium bromide administered to cirrhotic and control patients receiving isoflurane: a clinical and pharmacokinetic study. *Anesthesiology* 1996;84:1092–1100.

Shanks CA. Pharmacokinetics of the nondepolarizing neuromuscular relaxants applied to calculation of bolus and infusion dosage regiments. *Anesthesiology* 1986;64:72–86.

Shayevitz JR, Matteo RS. Decreased sensitivity to metocurine in patients with upper motor neuron disease. *Anesth Analg* 1985;64:767–772.

Shi WZ, Fahey MR, Fisher DM, et al. Laudanosine (a metabolite of atracurium) increases the minimal alveolar concentration of halothane in rabbits. *Anesthesiology* 1985;63:584–588.

Shi WZ, Fahey MR, Fisher DM, et al. Modification of central nervous system effects of laudanosine by inhalation anaesthetics. *Br J Anaesth* 1989;63:598–600.

Sinatra RS, Philip BK, Naulty JS, et al. Prolonged neuromuscular blockade with vecuronium in a patient treated with magnesium sulfate. *Anesth Analg* 1985;64:1220–1222.

Skarpa M, Dayan AD, Follenfant M, et al. Toxicity testing of atracurium. *Br J Anaesth* 1983;55:S27–S29.

Smith CE, Donati F, Bevan DR. Dose-response curves for succinylcholine: single versus cumulative techniques. *Anesthesiology* 1988;69:338–342.

Sokoll MD, Gergis SD. Antibiotics and neuromuscular function. *Anesthesiology* 1981;55:148–159.

Sokoll MD, Gergis SD, Mehta M, et al. Safety and efficacy of atracurium (BW 33A) in surgical patients receiving balanced or isoflurane anesthesia. *Anesthesiology* 1983;58:450–455.

Soriano SG, Sullivan LJ, Venkatakrishnan K, et al. Pharmacokinetics and pharmacodynamics of vecuronium in children receiving phenytoin or carbamazepine for chronic anticonvulsant therapy. *Br J Anaesth* 2001;86;223–229.

Sorooshian SS, Stafford MA, Eastwood NB, et al. Pharmacokinetics and pharmacodynamics of cisatracurium in young and elderly adult patients. *Anesthesiology* 1996;84:1083–1091.

Spacek A, Neiger FX, Krenn CG, et al. Rocuronium-induced neuromuscular block is affected by chronic carbamazepine therapy. *Anesthesiology* 1999a;90:109–112.

Spacek A, Nickl S, Neiger FX, et al. Augmentation of the rocuronium-induced neuromuscular block by the acutely administered phenytoin. *Anesthesiology* 1999b;90:1551–1555.

Standaert FG. Doughnuts and holes: molecules and muscle relaxants. *Semin Anesth* 1994;13:286–296.

Standaert FG, Adams JE. The actions of succinylcholine on the mammalian motor nerve terminal. *J Pharmacol Exp Ther* 1965;149:113–123.

Standaert FG, Dretchen KL. Cyclic nucleotides in neuromuscular transmission. *Anesth Analg* 1981;60:91–99.

Starr NK, Sethna DH, Estafanous FG. Bradycardia and asystole following the rapid administration of sufentanil with vecuronium. *Anesthesiology* 1986;64:521–523.

Stenlake JB, Waigh RD, Urwin J, et al. Atracurium: conception and inception. *Br J Anaesth* 1983;55:S3–S10.

Stiller RL, Cook DR, Chakravorti S. In vitro degradation of atracurium in human plasma. *Br J Anaesth* 1985;57:1085–1088.

Stirt JA, Katz RL, Murray AL, et al. Modification of atracurium blockade by halothane and by suxamethonium. *Br J Anaesth* 1983;55:S71–S77.

Stoelting RK. The hemodynamic effects of pancuronium and *d*-tubocurarine in anesthetized patients. *Anesthesiology* 1972;36:612–615.

Stoelting RK. Comparison of gallamine and atropine as pretreatment before anesthetic induction and succinylcholine administration. *Anesth Analg* 1977;56:493–495.

Stoelting RK, Peterson C. Adverse effects of increased succinylcholine dose following *d*-tubocurarine pretreatment. *Anesth Analg* 1975;54:282–288.

Sufit RL, Kreul JK, Bellay YM, et al. Doxacurium and mivacurium do not trigger malignant hyperthermia in susceptible value. *Anesth Analg* 1990;71:285–287.

Sugimori T. Shortened action of succinylcholine in individuals with cholinesterase C_5 isozyme. *Can Anaesth Soc J* 1986;33:321–327.

Sullivan M, Thompson WK. Succinylcholine-induced cardiac arrest in children with undiagnosed myopathy. *Can J Anaesth* 1994;41: 497–501.

Suzuki T, Iwasaki K, Fukano N, et al. Duration of exposure to sevoflurane affects does-response relationship of vecuronium. *Br J Anaesth* 2000;85:732–734.

Szmuk P, Ezri T, Jacques E, et al. The onset time of rocuronium is slowed by esmolol and accelerated by ephedrine. *Anesth Analg* 2000;90:1217–1219.

Taboada JA, Rupp SM, Miller RD. Refining the priming principle for vecuronium during rapid-sequence induction of anesthesia. *Anesthesiology* 1986;64:243–247.

Tateishi A, Zornow MH, Scheller MS, et al. Electroencephalographic effects of laudanosine in an animal model of epilepsy. *Br J Anaesth* 1989;62:548–552.

Thomson IR, Putnins CL. Adverse effects of pancuronium during high-dose fentanyl anesthesia for coronary artery bypass grafting. *Anesthesiology* 1985;62:708–713.

Tobey RE. Paraplegia, succinylcholine, and cardiac arrest. *Anesthesiology* 1970;32:359–364.

Tousignant CP, Bevan DR, Eisen AA, et al. Acute quadriparesis in an asthmatic treated with atracurium. *Can J Anaesth* 1995;42:224–227.

Ungureanu D, Meistelman C, Frossard J, et al. The orbicularis oculi and the adductor pollicis muscles as monitors of atracurium block of laryngeal muscles. *Anesth Analg* 1993;77:775–779.

Vercruyse P, Bossuyt P, Hanegreffs G, et al. Gallamine and pancuronium inhibit pre- and post-junctional muscarinic receptors in canine saphenous veins. *J Pharmacol Exp Ther* 1979;209:225–230.

Viby-Mogensen J. Correlation of succinylcholine duration of action with plasma cholinesterase activity in subjects with the genotypically normal enzyme. *Anesthesiology* 1980;53:517–520.

Vitez TS, Miller RD, Eger EI, et al. Comparison in vitro of isoflurane and halothane potentiation of *d*-tubocurarine and succinylcholine neuromuscular blockades. *Anesthesiology* 1974;41:53–56.

Ward S, Neill EAM. Pharmacokinetics of atracurium in acute hepatic failure (with acute renal failure). *Br J Anaesth* 1983;55:1169–1172.

Ward S, Weatherley BC. Pharmacokinetics of atracurium and its metabolites. *Br J Anesth* 1986;58:S6–S10.

Waud BE. Decrease in dose requirements of *d*-tubocurarine by volatile anesthetics. *Anesthesiology* 1979;51:298–302.

Waud BE, Waud DR. The relation between tetanic fade and receptor occlusion in the presence of competitive neuromuscular block. *Anesthesiology* 1971;35:456–464.

Waud BE, Waud DR. Comparison of drug-receptor dissociation constants at the mammalian neuromuscular junction in the presence and absence of halothane. *J Pharmacol Exp Ther* 1973;187:40–46.

Waud BE, Waud DR. The effects of diethyl ether, enflurane and isoflurane at the neuromuscular junction. *Anesthesiology* 1975;42:275–280.

Waud BE, Waud DR. Effects of volatile anesthetics on directly and indirectly stimulated muscle. *Anesthesiology* 1979;50:103–110.

Weinstein JA, Matteo RS, Ornstein E, et al. Pharmacodynamics of vecuronium and atracurium in the obese surgical patient. *Anesth Analg* 1988;67:1149–1153.

Wierda JMKH, Karliczek GF, Vandenbrom RHG, et al. Pharmacokinetics and cardiovascular dynamics of pipecuronium bromide during coronary artery surgery. *Can J Anaesth* 1990;37:183–191.

Wierda JMKH, Richardson FJ, Agoston S. Dose-response relation and time course of action of pipecuronium bromide in humans anesthetized with nitrous oxide isoflurane, halothane, or droperidol and fentanyl. *Anesth Analg* 1989;68:208–213.

Wood GG. Cyclosporine-vecuronium interaction. *Can J Anaesth* 1989; 36:358–366.

Wright PMC, Caldwell JE, Miller RD. Onset and duration of rocuronium and succinylcholine at the adductor pollicis and laryngeal adductor muscles in anesthetized humans. *Anesthesiology* 1994;81:1110–1115.

Xue FS, Tong SY, Liao X, et al. Dose-response and time course of effect of rocuronium in male and female anesthetized patients. *Anesth Analg* 1997;85:667–671.

Xue FS, An G, Liao X, et al. The pharmacokinetics of vecuronium in male and female patients. *Anesth Analg* 1998;86:1322–1327.

Yate PM, Flynn PJ, Arnold RW, et al. Clinical experience and plasma laudanosine concentrations during the infusion of atracurium in the intensive therapy unit. *Br J Anaesth* 1987;59:211–217.

Yeaton P, Teba L. Sinus node exit block following administration of vecuronium. *Anesthesiology* 1988;68:177–178.

Zahl K, Apfelbaum JL. Muscle pain occurs after outpatient laparoscopy despite the substitution of vecuronium for succinylcholine. *Anesthesiology* 1989;70:408–411.

Antícholinesterase Drugs and Cholinergic Agonists

9

Anticholinesterase drugs as represented by edrophonium, neostigmine, and pyridostigmine are most often administered by anesthesiologists to facilitate the speed of recovery from the skeletal muscle effects produced by nondepolarizing neuromuscular-blocking drugs (Fig. 9-1). Another anticholinesterase drug, physostigmine, may be administered to produce nonspecific antagonism of the central nervous system (CNS) effects of certain drugs (see Fig. 9-1). The treatment of patients with myasthenia gravis or glaucoma may include administration of anticholinesterase drugs.

MECHANISM OF ACTION

The mechanism of action of anticholinesterase drugs reflects (a) enzyme inhibition, (b) presynaptic effects, and (c) direct effects on the neuromuscular junction (NMJ) (Bevan et al., 1992).

Enzyme Inhibition

Edrophonium, neostigmine, and pyridostigmine inhibit the enzyme acetylcholinesterase (true cholinesterase), which is normally responsible for the rapid hydrolysis of the neurotransmitter acetylcholine to choline and acetic acid. Acetylcholinesterase is one of the most efficient enzymes known, with a single molecule able to hydrolyze an estimated 300,000 molecules of acetylcholine every minute. Inhibition of the hydrolysis of acetylcholine secondary to administration of an anticholinesterase drug, results in greater availability at its sites of action, which include preganglionic sympathetic and parasympathetic nerve endings and the NMJ (Bevan et al., 1992). This increased availability of acetylcholine at the NMJ is reflected by an increase in the size of the miniature end-plate potentials. Neostigmine and pyridostigmine inhibit the breakdown of acetylcholine by virtue of their being hydrolyzed by acetylcholinesterase. In this process, acetylcholinesterase is carbamylated, and its ability to hydrolyze acetylcholine is decreased. In contrast to neostigmine and pyridostigmine, acetylcholinesterase does not break down edrophonium but rather edrophonium forms a reversible electrostatic attachment to the enzyme. The different mechanisms of action at the molecular level have little impact on the clinical uses of anticholinesterase drugs.

Presynaptic Effects

In the absence of nondepolarizing neuromuscular-blocking drugs, administration of an anticholinesterase drug may produce spontaneous contractions (fasciculations) of skeletal muscles. These presynaptic effects are abolished by a small dose of a nondepolarizing neuromuscular-blocking drug, suggesting that acetylcholine receptors are involved. Likewise, inhibition of acetylcholinesterase could be responsible for these presynaptic effects, reflecting the availability of more neurotransmitters at these sites.

Direct Effects at the Neuromuscular Junction

Anticholinesterase drugs have also been reported to produce some form of neuromuscular blockade, but doses far greater than those ever administered clinically are required to produce this effect (Drury et al., 1987). It is possible that an excess of acetylcholine produced by acetylcholinesterase inhibition at the NMJ causes desensitization (end-plates no longer responsive to acetylcholine).

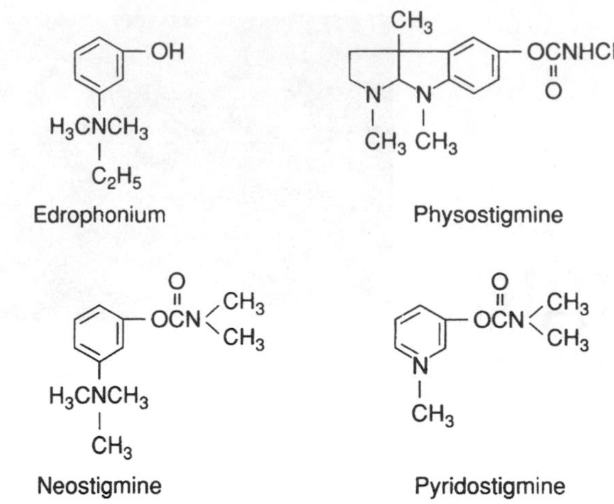

Figure 9-1. Anticholinesterase drugs.

CLASSIFICATION

Anticholinesterase drugs are classified according to the mechanism by which they inhibit the activity of acetylcholinesterase: (a) reversible inhibition, (b) formation of carbamyl esters, and (c) irreversible inactivation by organophosphates.

Reversible Inhibition

Edrophonium is a quaternary ammonium anticholinesterase drug that lacks a carbamyl group, producing reversible inhibition of acetylcholinesterase through its electrostatic attachment to the anionic site on the enzyme (Fig. 9-2). This binding is stabilized further by hydrogen bonding at the esteratic site on the enzyme (see Fig. 9-2). The edrophonium-acetylcholinesterase enzyme complex prevents the natural substrate acetylcholine from approximating correctly with the enzyme. Because a true chemical (covalent) bond is not formed, acetylcholine can easily compete with edrophonium for access to acetylcholinesterase, making the inhibition truly reversible. Indeed, the duration of action of edrophonium is often considered to be brief, reflecting its reversible binding with acetylcholinesterase.

The predominant site of action of edrophonium appears to be presynaptic. This site of action may explain differences in the dose–response relationships compared with longer-acting anticholinesterase drugs that presumably act principally at postsynaptic sites (Cronnelly et al., 1982).

The muscarinic effects of edrophonium are mild compared with longer-acting anticholinesterase drugs. Edrophonium is used to (a) antagonize the effects of nondepolarizing neuromuscular-blocking drugs, (b) diagnose and assess therapy of myasthenia gravis and cholinergic crisis, and (c) evaluate the presence of dual blockade produced by succinylcholine.

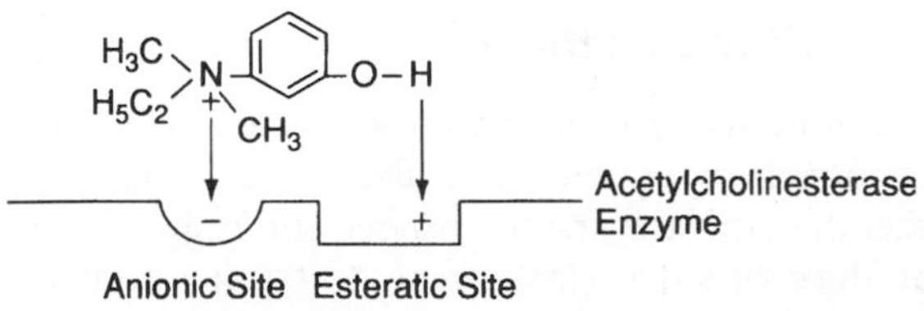

Figure 9-2. Edrophonium produces reversible inhibition of acetylcholinesterase by electrostatic attachment to the anionic site and hydrogen bonding at the esteratic site of the enzyme.

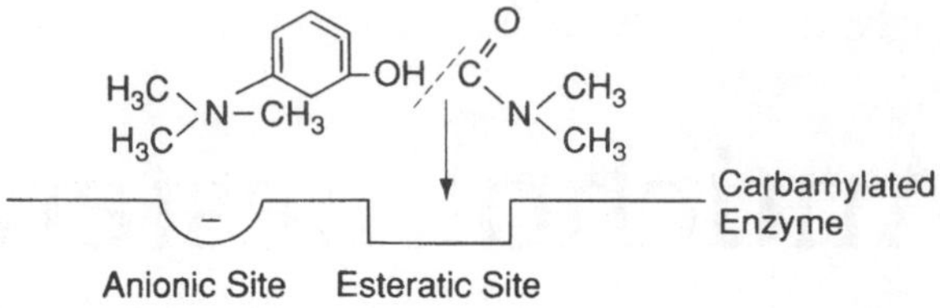

Figure 9-3. Drugs such as physostigmine, neostigmine, and pyridostigmine produce reversible inhibition of acetylcholinesterase by forming a carbamyl ester complex at the esteratic site of the enzyme.

Formation of Carbamyl Esters

Drugs such as physostigmine, neostigmine, and pyridostigmine produce reversible inhibition of acetylcholinesterase by formation of a carbamyl ester complex at the esteratic site of the enzyme (Fig. 9-3). In contrast to edrophonium, these drugs act as competitive substrate substitutes for acetylcholine in the enzyme's normal interaction with acetylcholinesterase. Indeed, the initial formation of the drug–enzyme complex proceeds in the same way as the initial reaction between acetylcholine and acetylcholinesterase. Likewise, the next stage of formation of an intermediate acid–enzyme compound and first split-product proceeds normally. At this stage, there is transfer of a carbamate group to acetylcholinesterase at the esteratic site. This carbamylated acetylcholinesterase cannot hydrolyze acetylcholine until the carbamate-enzyme bond dissociates. Carbamylated acetylcholinesterase has a half-time of 15 to 30 minutes.

Irreversible Inactivation

Organophosphate anticholinesterase drugs combine with acetylcholinesterase at the esteratic site to form a stable

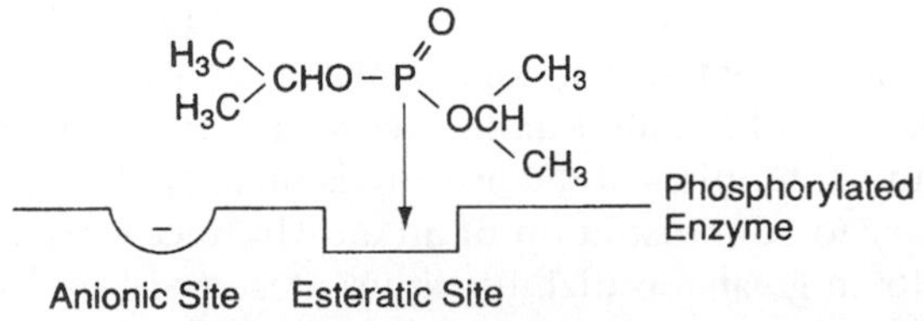

Figure 9-4. Organophosphate anticholinesterase drugs produce irreversible inhibition of acetylcholinesterase by forming a phosphorylate complex at the esteratic site of the enzyme.

inactive complex that does not undergo hydrolysis (Fig. 9-4). Echothiophate interacts with both the esteratic and anionic subsites, thus accounting for its extreme potency. Spontaneous regeneration of acetylcholinesterase either requires several hours or does not occur, thus requiring synthesis of new enzyme.

Echothiophate is the only organophosphate anticholinesterase drug used clinically (see Fig. 9-1). Other organophosphate anticholinesterase drugs, such as parathion and malathion, are used as insecticides. Malathion is a selective insecticide because enzymes necessary for its metabolism are absent in insects. In mammals and birds, malathion undergoes extensive hydrolysis by enzymes known as phosphorylphosphatases before excretion in urine. Nerve gases such as tabum, saran, and soman are extremely lipid-soluble organophosphate inhibitors, and absorption can occur even through intact skin.

STRUCTURE–ACTIVITY RELATIONSHIPS

Acetylcholinesterase consists of an anionic and an esteratic site that are so arranged that they are complementary to the natural substrate acetylcholine (Fig. 9-5). The anionic site of the enzyme binds the quaternary nitrogen of acetylcholine. This binding serves to orient the ester linkage of acetylcholine to the esteratic site of acetylcholinesterase (see Fig. 9-5). The esteratic site is responsible for the hydrolytic process. Thus, acetylcholinesterase has an optimum substrate concentration and is less effective against longer chain substrates. Acetylcholinesterase is highly concentrated at the NMJ but also present in lower concentrations throughout the length of skeletal muscle fibers. In mammals, acetylcholinesterase is encoded by a single gene localized to chromosome 7q22 in humans (Naguib et al., 2002).

At the NMJ, acetylcholinesterase is responsible for rapid hydrolysis of released acetylcholine, thereby controlling the duration of receptor activation (Naguib et al., 2002). Approximately 50% of the released acetylcholine is hydrolyzed during the time of diffusion across the synaptic cleft to reach nicotinic cholinergic receptors (nAChRs). The efficiency of acetylcholinesterase depends on its rapid catalytic activity, and this enzyme ranks as having one of the highest catalytic efficiencies known. It can catalyze acetylcholine hydrolysis (4,000 molecules of acetylcholine hydrolyzed per active site per second) at near diffusion-limited rates. In addition to hydrolysis of acetylcholine, acetylcholinesterase has other functions such as nerve growth-promoting activities and modulation of nAChRs.

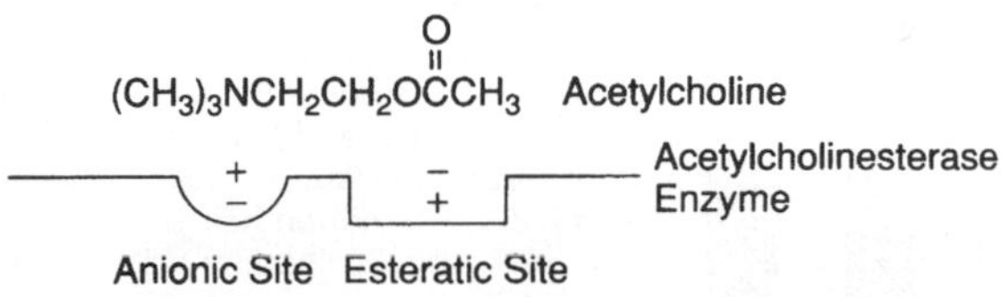

Figure 9-5. The anionic and esteratic sites of acetylcholinesterase are arranged so that they are complementary to the quaternary nitrogen and ester linkage of acetylcholine, respectively.

Neostigmine is a quaternary ammonium derivative of physostigmine, having a greater stability and equal or greater potency (see Fig. 9-1). Pyridostigmine is a closely related congener of neostigmine (see Fig. 9-1). An increase in anticholinesterase potency and duration of action occurs from linking two quaternary ammonium nuclei by a chain of appropriate structure and length. For example, the potent anticholinesterase drug demecarium is two molecules of neostigmine connected at the carbamate nitrogen atoms by a series of ten methylene groups (see Fig. 9-1). Another bisquaternary compound is ambenonium, which binds strongly to acetylcholinesterase and exerts direct effects at both prejunctional and postjunctional membranes (see Fig. 9-1).

PHARMACOKINETICS

In patients with normal renal and hepatic function, there are no significant pharmacokinetic differences among the anticholinesterase drugs (Table 9-1) (Fig. 9-6) (Bevan et al., 1992; Cronnelly, 1985). After a single bolus dose, the plasma concentrations of edrophonium, neostigmine, and pyridostigmine reach a peak and decrease rapidly during the first 5 to 10 minutes. The volume of distribution of these anticholinesterase drugs is in the range of 0.7 to 1.4 liters/kg, and the elimination half-times are 60 to 120 minutes. The clearance of anticholinesterase drugs is in the range of 8 to 16 mL/kg per minute, which is much greater than the glomerular filtration rate.

The similarity in pharmacokinetics among the anticholinesterase drugs means that differences in potency are most likely explained in terms of pharmacodynamics. Affinity for acetylcholinesterase is probably of major importance in determining the relative anticholinesterase potency of these drugs. The fact that edrophonium dose response curves are not parallel to those for neostigmine and pyridostigmine suggests that different mechanisms of action may be involved for the different anticholinesterase drugs (Fig. 9-7) (Cronnelly et al., 1982).

Lipid Solubility

Anticholinesterase drugs containing a quaternary ammonium group (edrophonium, neostigmine, pyridostigmine) are poorly lipid soluble and thus do not easily penetrate lipid cell membrane barriers such as the gastrointestinal tract or blood-brain barrier. Lipid-soluble drugs, such as tertiary amines (physostigmine) and organophosphates, are readily absorbed from the gastrointestinal tract or across mucous membranes and have predictable effects on the CNS.

TABLE 9-1.
COMPARATIVE CHARACTERISTICS OF ANTICHOLINESTERASE DRUGS ADMINISTERED TO ANTAGONIZE NONDEPOLARIZING NEUROMUSCULAR-BLOCKING DRUGS

	Elimination Half-Time (mins)		Volume of Distribution (liters/kg)		Clearance (ml/kg/min)	
	Normal	Anephric	Normal	Anephric	Normal	Anephric
Edrophonium (0.5 kg/kg)	110	206	1.1	0.7	9.6	2.7
Neostigmine (0.043 mg/kg)	77	181	0.7	1.6	9.2	7.8
Pyridostigmine (0.35 mg/kg)	112	379	1.1	1.0	8.6	2.1

	Renal Contribution to Total Clearance (%)	Speed of Onset	Duration (mins)	Principal Site of Action	Anticholinergic Dose (µg/kg)	
					Atropine	Glycopyrrolate
Edrophonium (0.5 mg/kg)	66	Rapid	60	Presynaptic	7*	NR
Neostigmine (0.043 mg/kg)	54	Intermediate	54	Postsynaptic	20	10
Pyridostigmine (0.35 mg/kg)	76	Delayed	76	Postsynaptic	20	10

NR, not recommended.
*10–15 µg/kg if an opioid-based anesthetic.
Source: Data from Bevan DR, Donati F, Kopman AF. Reversal of neuromuscular blockade. *Anesthesiology* 1991;77:785–792; Cronnelly R. Muscle relaxant antagonists. *Semin Anesth* 1985;4:31–40.

Volume of Distribution

The large volume of distribution (0.7 to 1.4 liters/kg) of quaternary ammonium anticholinesterase drugs compared with nondepolarizing neuromuscular-blocking drugs is surprising because these drugs would not be expected to cross lipid membranes easily (see Table 9-1) (Bevan et al., 1992; Cronnelly, 1985). Presumably, this large volume of distribution reflects extensive tissue storage in organs such as the liver and kidneys. The liver, as a site of this tissue uptake, is suggested by the presence of a relatively unchanged volume of distribution in anephric patients compared with normal patients.

Onset of Action

During steady-state infusion of a nondepolarizing muscle relaxant, the onset of action of edrophonium is 1 to 2 minutes, neostigmine 7 to 11 minutes, and pyridostigmine as long as 16 minutes (Fig. 9-8) (Cronnelly et al., 1982). Because the pharmacokinetics of anticholinesterase drugs are similar, it is likely that differences in the onset of action of these drugs reflects a pharmacodynamic mechanism, such as the rate of binding to the enzyme. The reason for the more rapid onset of action of edrophonium is unclear but may reflect a presynaptic effect (acetylcholine release) rather than a postsynaptic (acetylcholinesterase

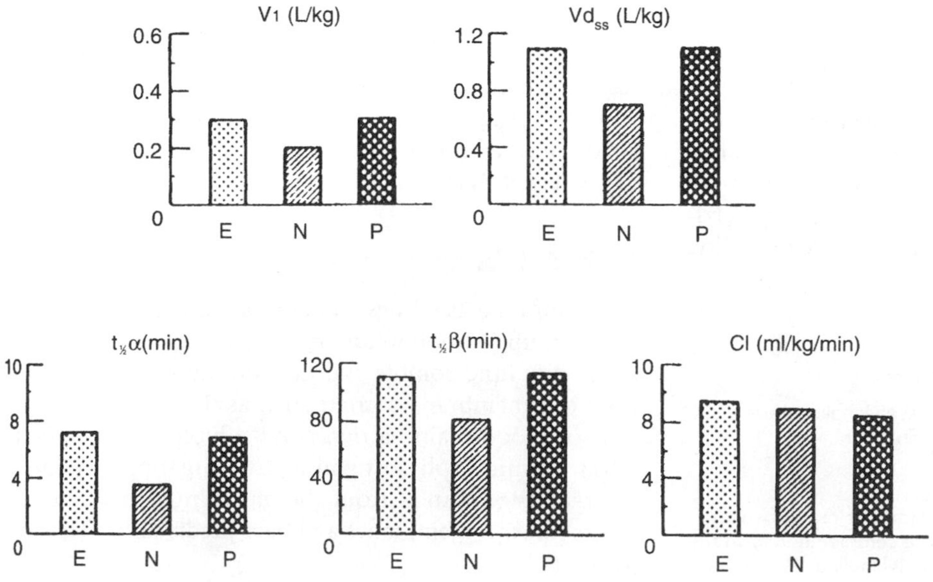

Figure 9-6. Pharmacokinetics of edrophonium (E), pyridostigmine (P), and neostigmine (N) in patients with normal renal and hepatic function. (Cl, clearance; t1/2α, distribution half-time; t1/2β, elimination half time; V_1, initial volume of distribution; Vd_{ss}, volume of distribution at steady state.) (From Cronnelly R. Muscle relaxant antagonists. *Semin Anesth* 1985;4:31–40; with permission.)

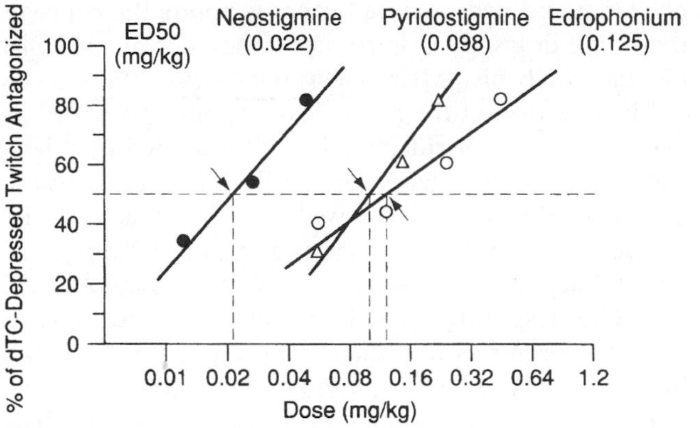

Figure 9-7. The dose response curve for edrophonium is not parallel to the curves for neostigmine and pyridostigmine, suggesting different mechanisms of action among the anticholinesterase drugs. (dTC, *d*-tubocurarine.) (From Cronnelly R, Morris RB, and Miller RD. Edrophonium: Duration of action and atropine requirements in humans during halothane anesthesia. *Anesthesiology* 1982;57:261–266; with permission.)

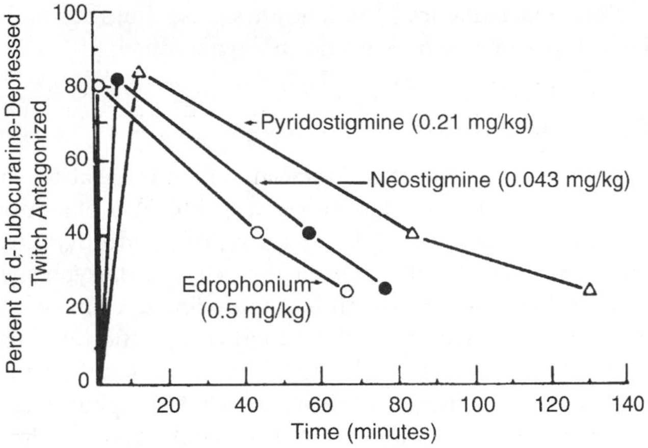

Figure 9-9. Edrophonium produces antagonism of drug-induced neuromuscular blockade that is similar in magnitude to that produced by neostigmine or pyridostigmine. (From Cronnelly R, Morris RB, and Miller RD. Edrophonium: Duration of action and atropine requirement in humans during halothane anesthesia. *Anesthesiology* 1982;57:261–266; with permission.)

inhibition) action, whereas the postsynaptic action is predominant for neostigmine and pyridostigmine. It is also possible that onset times could reflect differences in rate constants at presynaptic and postsynaptic sites of action. The slower onset of action of neostigmine and pyridostigmine compared with edrophonium is not related to the need to form active metabolites (Hennis et al., 1984).

Duration of Action

The duration of action of anticholinesterase drugs is governed largely by the rate of disappearance of these drugs from the plasma (Bevan et al., 1992). For example, the half-time of the carbamylated enzyme (15 to 30 minutes) is much shorter than the elimination half-times of the anticholinesterase drugs (60 to 120 minutes). In clinical practice, anticholinesterase drugs are given when the effect of the nondepolarizing neuromuscular-blocking drug is waning, which makes determination of the actual duration of action of the reversal drug difficult to determine. In this regard, when a constant infusion of a neuromuscular-blocking drug is administered to maintain a constant level of neuromuscular blockade, equivalent durations of action are provided by neostigmine, 0.043 mg/kg IV, pyridostigmine, 0.21 mg/kg IV, and edrophonium, 0.5 mg/kg IV (Fig. 9-9) (Cronnelly et al., 1982; Miller et al., 1974). When twitch height is decreased >90%, the dose of edrophonium may need to be increased to 1 mg/kg IV to produce an onset as rapid as that of neostigmine (Rupp et al., 1986). Although edrophonium in the past has been considered a short-acting drug, controlled studies in anesthetized patients have documented that the duration of action of edrophonium does not differ from that of neostigmine (Cronnelly et al., 1982).

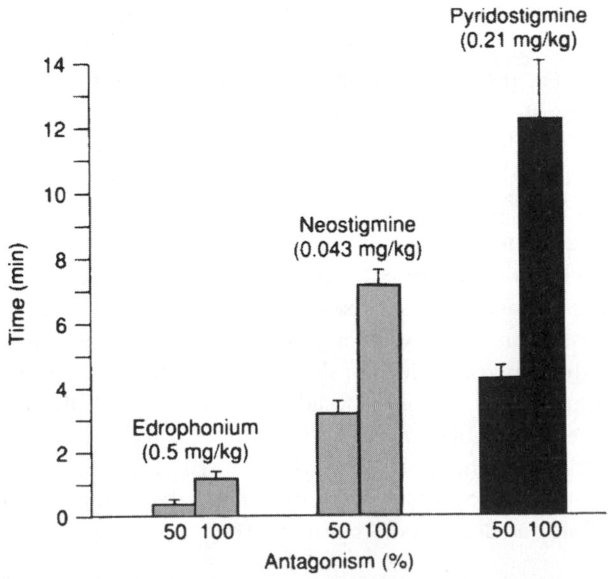

Figure 9-8. Comparison of the onset of action of anticholinesterase drugs as reflected by antagonism of drug-induced neuromuscular blockade. (Mean ± SE.) (From Cronnelly R, Morris RB, Miller RD. Edrophonium: Duration of action and atropine requirement in humans during halothane anesthesia. *Anesthesiology* 1982;57:261–266; with permission.)

Renal Clearance

Anticholinesterase drugs are actively secreted into the lumens of the renal tubules. Renal clearance accounts for approximately 50% of the elimination of neostigmine and approximately 75% of the elimination of edrophonium and pyridostigmine. As a result, the elimination half-times of these drugs are greatly prolonged by renal failure (see Table 9-1) (Bevan et al., 1992; Cronnelly 1985). In fact, the plasma clearance of anticholinesterase drugs in patients in renal failure is prolonged to a greater extent than most of the nondepolarizing neuromuscular-blocking drugs, making the occurrence of recurarization unlikely. In anesthetized patients receiving a functioning renal transplant, the pharmacokinetics of anticholinesterase drugs are similar to those in patients with normal renal function.

Metabolism

In the absence of renal function, hepatic metabolism accounts for 50% of a dose of neostigmine, 30% of a dose of edrophonium, and 25% of a dose of pyridostigmine. The principal metabolite of neostigmine is 3-hydroxyphenyl trimethylammonium, which has approximately one-tenth the antagonist activity of the parent compound (Hennis et al., 1984). The principal metabolite of pyridostigmine is 3-hydroxy-*N*-methylpyridinium, which lacks pharmacologic activity. Edrophonium undergoes conjugation to edrophonium glucuronide, which is presumed to be pharmacologically inactive. Physostigmine is hydrolyzed at its ester linkage, and renal excretion is of minor importance. It can be concluded that metabolites of anticholinesterase drugs do not contribute significantly to the effects of these drugs, including antagonism of neuromuscular blockade produced by nondepolarizing neuromuscular-blocking drugs.

Influence of Patient Age

When neostigmine is administered at a fixed point in recovery from the effects of a nondepolarizing neuromuscular-blocking drug, reversal occurs more rapidly and the dose of neostigmine required to produce equivalent effects is less in infants and children than in adults (Fisher et al., 1983). The difference in dose requirements cannot be explained on the basis of differences in pharmacokinetics, which are similar for neostigmine in pediatric and young adult patients. It is likely that the age-related differences in dose requirements of neostigmine are related to pharmacodynamic mechanisms. In contrast to neostigmine, dose requirements for edrophonium are not different for infants, children, and adults (Fisher et al., 1984). This difference between edrophonium and neostigmine further supports the concepts that these drugs antagonize neuromuscular blockade by different mechanisms (Cronnelly and Morris, 1982).

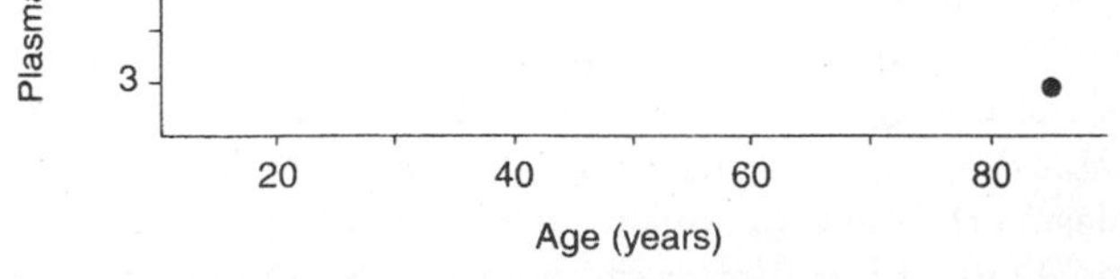

Figure 9-10. Pyridostigmine clearance from the plasma decreases with increasing age of the patient. (From Stone JG, Matteo RS, Ornstein E, et al. Aging alters the pharmacokinetics of pyridostigmine. *Anesth Analg* 1995;81:773–776; with permission.)

The duration of the maximum response produced by neostigmine and pyridostigmine is prolonged in elderly compared with younger patients, reflecting a smaller extracellular fluid volume and slowed rate of plasma clearance in elderly patients (Fig. 9-10) (Stone et al., 1995; Young et al., 1988). Pharmacodynamics are not altered, as emphasized by similar responses evoked by neostigmine at the same plasma concentration in middle-aged and elderly adults. In contrast to neostigmine and pyridostigmine, the duration of action of edrophonium is not prolonged in elderly patients (Matteo et al., 1990). A higher plasma concentration of edrophonium is required to produce the same effects in elderly patients as in younger adults. The observed differences between edrophonium and other anticholinesterase drugs may relate to differences in chemical structure and to the possibility that edrophonium produces antagonism of neuromuscular blockade by a different mechanism than do neostigmine and pyridostigmine.

PHARMACOLOGIC EFFECTS

The pharmacologic effects of anticholinesterase drugs are predictable and reflect the accumulation of acetylcholine at muscarinic and nicotinic cholinergic receptors (nAChRs). Depending on the reason for administration of anticholinesterase drugs, these effects may be considered therapeutic or undesirable.

Muscarinic cholinergic effects, such as bradycardia, salivation, miosis, and hyperperistalsis, are evoked by lower concentrations of acetylcholine than are required for production of nicotinic effects at autonomic ganglia and the NMJ. For this reason, using an anticholinesterase drug to reverse nondepolarizing neuromuscular-blocking drugs also includes administering an anticholinergic drug to prevent adverse muscarinic cholinergic effects that would be associated with the high dose of anticholinesterase drug. The anticholinergic drug selectively blocks the effects of acetylcholine at muscarinic cholinergic receptors and leaves intact the responses to acetylcholine at nAChRs. Neostigmine and pyridostigmine, but not edrophonium, produce marked and prolonged inhibition of plasma cholinesterase activity (Mirakhur, 1986). Indeed, the prolonged effects of succinylcholine administered shortly after reversal of nondepolarizing neuromuscular blockade with neostigmine or pyridostigmine may reflect this enzyme inhibition (Bentz and Stoelting, 1976).

Cardiovascular Effects

The cardiovascular effects of anticholinesterase drugs reflect effects of accumulated acetylcholine at the heart (vagal effects), blood vessels, autonomic ganglia, and postganglionic cholinergic nerve endings. Bradycardia and/or bradydysrhythmia such as nodal and ventricular escape beats and asystole may occur (Bevan et al., 1992). Bradycardia most likely reflects slowing of the conduction of cardiac impulses through the atrioventricular node. These cardiac effects of anticholinesterase drugs can be attenuated by the administration of an anticholinergic drug that blocks muscarinic receptors but not nAChRs. Interestingly, bradycardia and/or sinus arrest may occur when an anticholinesterase drug is administered to a patient with a denervated heart, as accompanies a heart transplant (Backman et al., 1993; Beebe et al., 1994). It is possible that denervation hypersensitivity may have rendered the sinoatrial nodes of these heart transplant patients exquisitely sensitive to neostigmine, despite, the concomitant administration of an anticholinergic drug. Decreases in systemic blood pressure that may accompany accumulation of acetylcholine presumably reflect decreases in systemic vascular resistance, although the coronary and pulmonary circulations may manifest an opposite response.

Gastrointestinal and Genitourinary Tract

Anticholinesterase drugs enhance gastric fluid secretion by parietal cells and increase the motility of the entire gastrointestinal tract, particularly the large intestine. The actions of anticholinesterase drugs on gastrointestinal motility most likely reflect the effects of accumulated acetylcholine on the ganglion cells of Auerbach's plexus and on smooth muscle fibers. There is controversy about the effectiveness of atropine in blocking the increased peristalsis produced by anticholinesterase drugs. Some studies have claimed an increased risk of bowel anastomotic leakage when neostigmine was used to reverse neuromuscular blockade (Aitkenhead, 1984; Bevan et al., 1992). Nevertheless, the incidence of this complication may depend more on surgical technique. The combination of atropine with neostigmine has been found to decrease gastric cardiac sphincter pressure (lower esophageal pressure minus gastric pressure) (Turner and Smith, 1985). Neostigmine and presumably other anticholinesterase drugs may increase the incidence of postoperative nausea and vomiting even when administered with atropine, which has its own antiemetic properties (King et al., 1988). Nausea and gastrointestinal disturbances associated with use of the anticholinesterase drugs to reverse nondepolarizing neuromuscular-blocking drugs is a consideration when patients are to be discharged to home on the day of surgery. In this regard, use of short-acting nondepolarizing neuromuscular-blocking drugs that do not require pharmacologic antagonism is an option.

Neostigmine, 0.5 to 1 mg subcutaneously, may be effective in the treatment of paralytic ileus or atony of the urinary bladder. This treatment, however, should not be used when there is mechanical obstruction of the gastrointestinal tract or urinary bladder. The lower portion of the esophagus is stimulated by neostigmine, resulting in a beneficial increase in tone and peristalsis in patients with achalasia.

Salivary Glands

Anticholinesterase drugs augment production of secretions of glands that are innervated by postganglionic cholinergic fibers. Such glands include the bronchial, lacrimal, sweat, salivary, gastric, intestinal, and acini pancreatic glands. Smooth muscle fibers of bronchioles and ureters are contracted by anticholinesterase drugs. Cholinergic stimulation of the bronchi produces bronchoconstriction, and anticholinesterase drugs have the potential to increase airway resistance.

Eye

Anticholinesterase drugs applied topically to the cornea cause constriction of the sphincter of the iris (miosis) and ciliary muscle. Constriction of the ciliary muscle manifests as inability to focus for near vision. Interference with accommodation is usually shorter in duration than is miosis. Intraocular pressure declines because the outflow of aqueous humor is facilitated.

Myasthenia Gravis

Cholinergic crisis is the risk associated with the administration of anticholinesterase drugs to patients with myasthenia gravis who have also received nondepolarizing neuromuscular-blocking drugs. Indeed, prolonged neuromuscular blockade has been described when neostigmine was administered to a myasthenic patient who had received vecuronium (Kim and Mangold, 1989).

Myotonia

Anticholinesterase drugs share some pharmacologic properties with succinylcholine, including the ability to produce fasciculations and to augment twitch response. For this reason, it has been suggested that these drugs be administered with caution to patients who have absolute contraindications to succinylcholine (Bevan et al., 1992). Examples include myotonia, muscular dystrophies, spinal cord transection, and extensive burns. Nevertheless, problems in such patients are infrequent, with only one report of tonic responses after the administration of neostigmine to two patients with dystrophica myotonica (Buzello et al., 1982).

Beta-Adrenergic Blockade

Theoretically, beta-adrenergic blockade could result in a predominance of parasympathetic nervous system activity at the heart, which might be exaggerated by the subsequent administration of an anticholinesterase drug to reverse nondepolarizing neuromuscular blockade (Sprague, 1975; Prys-Roberts, 1979). Nevertheless, bradycardia does not accompany administration of mixtures of atropine and neostigmine or pyridostigmine to animals with acutely produced beta-adrenergic blockade using propranolol (Wagner et al., 1982).

CLINICAL USES

The principal clinical uses of anticholinesterase drugs are (a) antagonist-assisted reversal of neuromuscular blockade produced by nondepolarizing neuromuscular-blocking drugs, (b) treatment of the CNS effects produced by certain drugs, (c) treatment of myasthenia gravis, (d) treatment of glaucoma, and (e) treatment of paralytic ileus and atony of the urinary bladder. Patients with mild-to-moderate Alzheimers disease may benefit from treatment with anticholinesterase drugs (Cummings, 2004).

Antagonist-Assisted Reversal of Neuromuscular Blockade

Antagonist-assisted reversal of neuromuscular blockade using edrophonium, neostigmine, or pyridostigmine reflects increased availability of acetylcholine at the NMJ due to inhibition of acetylcholinesterase, which is needed to hydrolyze acetylcholine. Physostigmine is not used to reverse neuromuscular blockade because the dose required to achieve this effect is excessive. An increased amount of the neurotransmitter acetylcholine in the region of the NMJ improves the chances that two acetylcholine molecules will bind to the alpha subunits of the nicotinic cholinergic receptor. This binding changes the balance of the competition between acetylcholine and a nondepolarizing neuromuscular-blocking drug in favor the neurotransmitter (acetylcholine) and restores neuromuscular transmission. In addition, anticholinesterase drugs may produce antidromic action potentials and repetitive firing of motor nerve endings (presynaptic effects) (Donati et al., 1983). Postsynaptic and presynaptic mechanisms are dose-related and operate simultaneously to restore neuromuscular transmission in the presence of nondepolarizing neuromuscular-blocking drugs.

Anticholinesterase drugs typically are administered during the time when spontaneous recovery from neuromuscular blockade is occurring, so that the effect of the pharmacologic antagonist adds to the rate of spontaneous recovery from the neuromuscular-blocking drug. For this reason, antagonism of neuromuscular blockade produced by a short- or intermediate-acting drug that undergoes rapid spontaneous recovery by virtue of plasma hydrolysis or Hofmann elimination is much faster than antagonism of a slow recovery long-acting nondepolarizing neuromuscular-blocking drug. This difference is most obvious when reversal is compared at deep levels (>90% twitch depression) of neuromuscular blockade.

At equivalent degrees of spontaneous reversal of twitch height, the train-of-four ratio is greater after the administration of edrophonium than neostigmine or pyridostigmine (Donati et al., 1983). If the train-of-four ratio reflects presynaptic events, then these results would support a presynaptic predominance for edrophonium compared with neostigmine or pyridostigmine. Conceivably, matching the principal site of action of the anticholinesterase drug with that of the nondepolarizing neuromuscular-blocking drug (presynaptic or postsynaptic) would result in more selective antagonism, with a minimal dose of anticholinesterase drug. Despite this logic, there is no evidence that anticholinesterase drugs act by different mechanisms when administered to anesthetized patients to antagonize nondepolarizing neuromuscular blockade. For example, combinations of edrophonium with neostigmine or pyridostigmine result in only additive effects with respect to the degree of antagonism of neuromuscular blockade achieved, suggesting a similar mechanism of action for these anticholinesterase drugs (Donati et al., 1983; Jones et al., 1984). Thus, mixtures of anticholinesterase drugs seem to offer no clinical advantage over the use of adequate doses of the individual drugs alone (Cronnelly and Miller, 1984).

Onset and Duration of Action

Edrophonium has a more rapid onset of action than neostigmine and pyridostigmine, whereas the duration of action of these three anticholinesterase drugs is similar (see Fig. 9-8) (Cronnelly et al., 1982; Miller et al., 1974) (see the section on Pharmacokinetics). Doses of anticholinesterase drugs that produce equivalent degrees of antagonism of neuromuscular blockade are edrophonium, 0.5 mg/kg IV (1 mg/kg IV if >90% twitch depression when reversal is initiated); neostigmine, 0.043 mg/kg IV; and pyridostigmine,

TABLE 9-2.
DOSES OF NEOSTIGMINE OR EDROPHONIUM (μg/kg) REQUIRED FOR 50% (ED_{50}) AND 80% (ED_{80}) RECOVERY OF FIRST TWITCH HEIGHT AFTER INJECTION OF ANTICHOLINESTERASE DRUG WHEN TWITCH HEIGHT IS 10% OF CONTROL

	Pancuronium	Atracurium	Vecuronium
Neostigmine			
ED_{50}	13	10	10
ED_{80}	45	22	24
Edrophonium			
ED_{50}	170	110	180
ED_{80}	680	440	460

Source: Data from Cronnelly R, Morris RB, Miller RD. Edrophonium: Duration of action and atropine requirement in humans during halothane anesthesia. *Anesthesiology* 1982;57: 261–266; Gencarelli PJ, Miller RD. Antagonism of ORG NC45 (vecuronium) and pancuronium neuromuscular blockade by neostigmine. *Br J Anaesth* 1982;54:53–56.

0.21 mg/kg IV (see Fig. 9-9) (Cronnelly et al., 1982; Miller et al., 1974) (see the section on Pharmacokinetics). Nevertheless, the potency ratios of these anticholinesterase drugs varies depending on the nondepolarizing neuromuscular-blocking drug being antagonized and the drug's inherent speed of spontaneous recovery, the depth of the neuromuscular blockade when the reversal is initiated, and the end-point selected (Table 9-2) (Smith et al., 1989). When reversal of intense neuromuscular blockade is attempted (99% twitch depression), the dose response curves for the anticholinesterase drugs are shifted to the right, but the shift is more important for edrophonium and pyridostigmine than for neostigmine (Donati et al., 1989). Thus, neostigmine appears preferable to either edrophonium or pyridostigmine when >90% twitch depression is to be antagonized.

Mixture with Anticholinergic Drugs

Reversal of nondepolarizing neuromuscular blockade requires only the nicotinic cholinergic effects of the anticholinesterase drug. Therefore, muscarinic cholinergic effects of the anticholinesterase drug are attenuated or prevented by the concurrent administration of an anticholinergic drug such as atropine or glycopyrrolate (see Table 9-1) (Bevan et al., 1992; Cronnelly, 1985). It is desirable to administer an anticholinergic drug with a faster onset of action than the anticholinesterase drug to minimize the likelihood of drug-induced bradycardia. Thus, when edrophonium, 0.5 mg/kg IV, is administered, atropine, 7 μg/kg IV, is recommended (see Table 9-1) (Bevan et al., 1992; Cronnelly, 1985). Others have recommended a higher dose of atropine (10 to 15 μg/kg), especially if an opioid-based maintenance anesthetic is being used (Urquhart et al., 1987). Neostigmine has a slower onset of action than edrophonium, and either atropine or glycopyrrolate may be administered as the anticholinergic drug. The dose of atropine is about one-half that of neostigmine (20 μg/kg if the dose of neostigmine is 40 μg/kg), whereas the dose of glycopyrrolate is about one-fourth the dose of neostigmine (see Table 9-1) (Bevan et al., 1992; Cronnelly, 1985). The simultaneous administration of atropine and neostigmine leads to an initial tachycardia because of the more rapid onset of action of atropine (see Fig. 9-10) (Cronnelly et al., 1982). Conversely, the time course of action of glycopyrrolate more closely parallels the onset of action of neostigmine, so that simultaneous administration of these two drugs may result in a more stable heart rate. Late bradycardia is more likely when short-acting atropine rather than long-acting glycopyrrolate is combined with neostigmine. The onset of action of pyridostigmine is very slow, and an initial tachycardia may be expected with either atropine or glycopyrrolate.

Excessive Neuromuscular Blockade

Once acetylcholinesterase is maximally inhibited, administering additional anticholinesterase drug does not further antagonize nondepolarizing neuromuscular blockade. For this reason, persistence of neuromuscular blockade despite large doses of anticholinesterase drugs (neostigmine, 70 μg/kg IV, or equivalent doses of other anticholinesterase drugs) is often an indication to ventilate the patient's lungs mechanically until neuromuscular blockade spontaneously wanes with time. When twitch height has recovered to >10%, the administration of anticholinesterase drugs is more likely to produce predictable effects (Engbaek et al., 1990).

TABLE 9-3.
RECOMMENDED DOSES OF NEOSTIGMINE OR EDROPHONIUM ACCORDING TO RESPONSES TO TRAIN-OF-FOUR (TOF) STIMULATION

TOF Visible Twitches	Fade	Anticholinesterase Drug	Dose (mg/kg)
None*	—	—	—
<2	++++	Neostigmine	0.07
3–4	+++	Neostigmine	0.04
4	++	Edrophonium	0.5
4	+	Edrophonium	0.25

*Postpone administration of anticholinesterase drug until some visible evoked response.
Source: Data from Bevan DR, Donati F, Kopman AF. Reversal of neuromuscular blockade. *Anesthesiology* 1992; 77:785–805.

Events That Influence Reversal of Neuromuscular Blockade

The speed and extent to which neuromuscular blockade is reversed by anticholinesterase drugs are influenced by a number of factors, including the intensity of the neuromuscular blockade at the time pharmacologic reversal is initiated (train-of-four visible twitches) and the nondepolarizing neuromuscular-blocking drug being reversed (Table 9-3 and Fig. 9-11) (Bevan et al., 1992; Katz, 1971). Continued administration of a volatile anesthetic may delay drug-assisted antagonism of nondepolarizing muscle relaxants. Edrophonium is less effective than neostigmine in reversing deep neuromuscular blockade (twitch height <10% of control) produced by continuous infusions of atracurium, vecuronium, and pancuronium (Engbaek et al., 1985; Kopman, 1986).

Edrophonium and neostigmine may not be equally effective for reversal of atracurium (edrophonium is better) and vecuronium (neostigmine is better) (Smith et al., 1989).

Antagonism of neuromuscular blockade by anticholinesterase drugs may be inhibited or even prevented by (a) certain antibiotics, (b) hypothermia, (c) respiratory acidosis associated with a $Paco_2$ of >50 mm Hg, or (d) hypokalemia and metabolic acidosis (Fig. 9-12) (Bevan et al., 1992; Miller et al., 1975). Nevertheless, the clinical effect of drug interactions, hypothermia, and acid–base

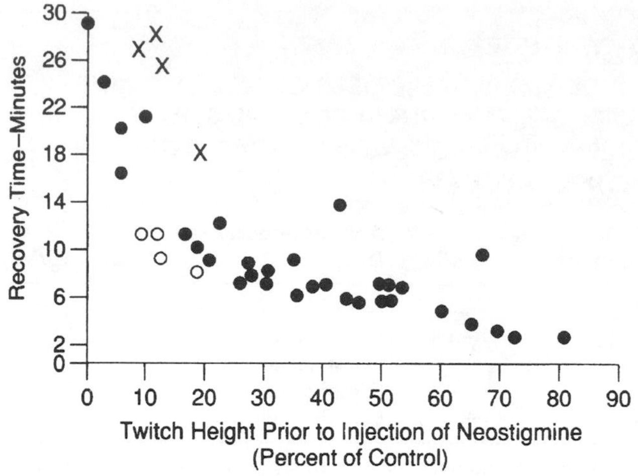

Figure 9-11. The rate of antagonism of drug-induced neuromuscular blockade parallels the magnitude of blockade present just before administration of the anticholinesterase drug. (From Katz RL. Clinical neuromuscular pharmacology of pancuronium. *Anesthesiology* 1971;34:550–556; with permission.)

changes in the ability to reliably reverse nondepolarizing neuromuscular-blocking drugs is difficult to prove (Bevan et al., 1992; Heier et al., 2002). For example, mild hypothermia (<34.5 C) did not change the maximum effect, clearance, or duration of action of neostigmine (Heier et al., 2002). Reversal of phase II block associated with prolonged or repeated use of succinylcholine can be reversed with neostigmine or edrophonium (Futter et al., 1983). In contrast, reversal of phase II block that occurs in patients with atypical plasma cholinesterase with an anticholinesterase drug may not be reliable, and mechanical ventilation of the patient's lungs until the blockade wanes spontaneously may be preferred to attempts at pharmacologic reversal (Bevan and Donati, 1983).

Priming with Anticholinesterases

It has been reported that the time to reach a train-of-four ratio of 0.75 is shorter when edrophonium or neostigmine is administered in divided doses (initial dose when twitch is 10% of control and the remainder of the dose 3 minutes later) (Naguib and Abdultif, 1988). Others have not been able to detect any significant differences in the rate of reversal when the anticholinesterase drug was administered in divided doses (Szalados et al., 1990).

Treatment of Central Nervous System Effects of Certain Drugs

Physostigmine, a lipid-soluble tertiary amine, crosses the blood-brain barrier and thus is effective in antagonizing adverse CNS effects of certain drugs.

Central Anticholinergic Syndrome

Physostigmine, 15 to 60 μg/kg IV, is effective in antagonizing restlessness and confusion (central anticholinergic syndrome) due to atropine or scopolamine (see Chapter 10). Presumably, physostigmine increases concentrations of acetylcholine in the brain, making more neurotransmitters available for interaction with cholinergic receptors. The duration of action of physostigmine is shorter than that of anticholinergic drugs. For this reason, it may be necessary to repeat the dose of physostigmine used in the treatment of central anticholinergic syndrome.

Opioids

Physostigmine abolishes the somnolent effects of opioids and may reverse the depression of the ventilatory response to carbon dioxide, but not analgesia produced by prior administration of morphine (Paaraskeva et al., 2002; Snir-Mor et al., 1983). It is speculated that opioids diminish the

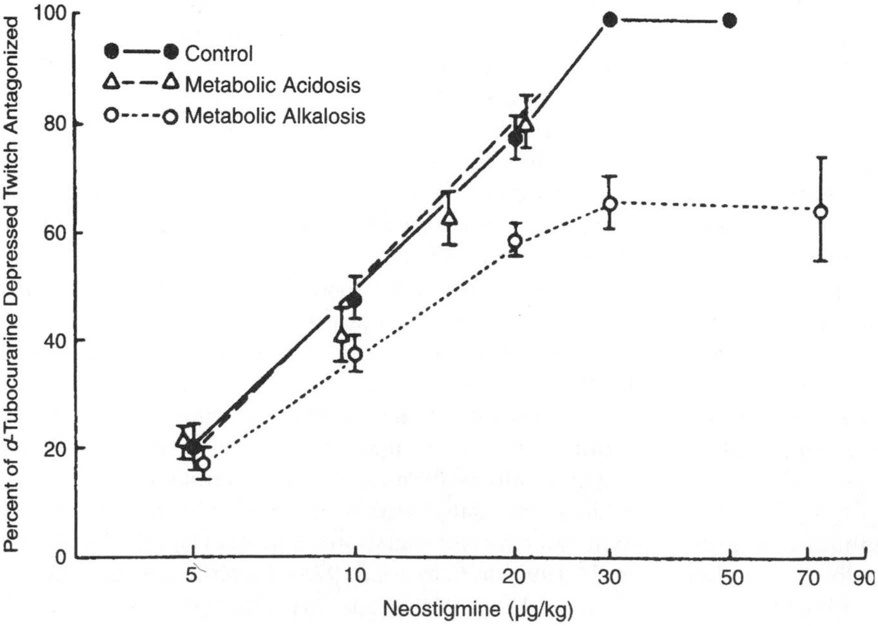

Figure 9-12. Antagonism of drug-induced neuromuscular blockade by anticholinesterase drugs is impaired by metabolic alkalosis. (Mean ± SE.) (From Miller RD, Van Nyhuis LS, Eger EI, et al. The effect of acid-base balance on neostigmine antagonism of *d*-tubocurarine–induced neuromuscular blockade. *Anesthesiology* 1975; 42:377–383; with permission.)

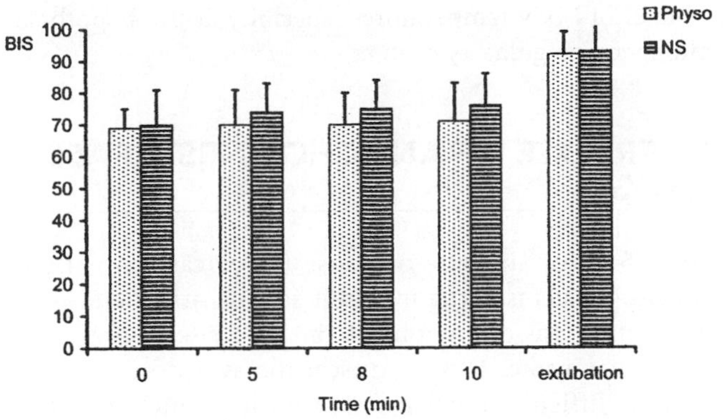

Figure 9-13. Bispectral index (BIS) before and after treatment with physostigmine, 2 mg IV or normal saline (NS), in the presence of 0.6 inspired sevoflurane. Mean ≠ SD. (From Paraskeva A, Konstantinos P, Fassoulaki A, et al. Physostigmine does not antagonize sevoflurane anesthesia assessed by bispectral index or enhance recovery. *Anesth Analg* 2002;54:569–572; with permission.)

ventilatory response to carbon dioxide by decreasing the amount of acetylcholine in the area of the respiratory center that would normally be released in response to hypercarbia. Other data, however, do not support an antagonist effect of physostigmine on opioid-induced depression of ventilation (Bourke et al., 1984). Physostigmine, 2 mg produces analgesia comparable to that produced by meperidine, 50 mg.

Anesthetics

Physostigmine decreases postoperative somnolence after anesthesia with a volatile anesthetic (Hill et al., 1977). Nevertheless, administration of physostigmine, 2 mg IV, during sevoflurane administration does not change the bispectral index or enhance recovery following discontinuation of the volatile anesthetic (Fig. 9-13) (Paraskeva et al., 2002). Reversal of the adverse CNS effects of ketamine by physostigmine while analgesia remains intact has been described (Balmer and Wyte, 1977). Sedative effects of other drugs, including phenothiazines and tricyclic antidepressants, may also be antagonized by physostigmine.

Treatment of Myasthenia Gravis

Neostigmine, pyridostigmine, and ambenonium are the standard anticholinesterase drugs used in the symptomatic treatment of myasthenia gravis. These drugs increase the response of skeletal muscles to repetitive impulses, presumably by increasing the availability of endogenous acetylcholine.

The quaternary ammonium structure of neostigmine and pyridostigmine limits the oral absorption of these drugs. For example, the oral dose of neostigmine is 30 times greater than the IV dose. The interval between oral doses is usually 2 to 4 hours for neostigmine and 3 to 6 hours for pyridostigmine or ambenonium. Muscarinic, cardiovascular, and gastrointestinal side effects are controlled as necessary with anticholinergic drugs.

In assessing the anticholinesterase drug therapy of myasthenia gravis, edrophonium, 1 mg IV, may be administered every 1 to 2 minutes until a change in symptoms is observed. Inadequate anticholinesterase drug therapy is diagnosed if there is a decrease in myasthenic symptoms. Conversely, patients experiencing excessive anticholinesterase drug effects (cholinergic crisis) will manifest increased skeletal muscle weakness with administration of edrophonium. Bromide intoxication has been described in a patient with myasthenia gravis being treated with pyridostigmine bromide (Rothenberg et al., 1990).

Treatment of Glaucoma

Anticholinesterase drugs decrease intraocular pressure in patients with narrow-angle and wide-angle glaucoma, reflecting a decrease in the resistance to outflow of aqueous humor. Treatment of glaucoma with topical administration of long-acting anticholinesterase drugs (echothiophate, demecarium, isoflurophate) for 6 months or longer results in the risk of cataract formation. For this reason, short-acting miotic anticholinesterase drugs are used initially, with introduction of long-acting miotic anticholinesterase drugs only when the therapeutic response to the short-acting drugs is not effective. Topical administration of a beta-adrenergic antagonist, such as timolol, does not produce miosis, but does decrease intraocular pressure by decreasing the secretion of aqueous humor.

Alzheimers Disease

Cholinesterase inhibitors are recommended for treatment of patients with mild to moderate Alzheimer disease (Cummings, 2004). Four centrally active cholinesterase inhibitors (tacrine, donepezil, rivastigmine, galantamine) are available to treat Alzheimer disease, although tacrine is rarely used since it has hepatotoxic effects in nearly 40% of treated patients (Mayeux and Sano, 1999). Liver toxicity produced by tacrine is reversible and easily detected by frequent measurement of plasma concentrations of liver transaminases. Compared with tacrine, the other centrally active anticholinesterase drugs are less toxic, and their duration of action permits more convenient dosage regimens. For example, donepezil is effective with once-a-day dosing and does not produce liver toxicity.

Chronic Fatigue Syndrome

Chronic fatigue syndrome is a complex disorder characterized by long-term disability and no consistently effective treatment. Hypoactivity of the hypothalamic-pituitary-adrenal axis may be present in these patients and those with fibromyalgia. Patients with chronic fatigue syndrome are often intolerant to the anticholinergic effects of tricyclic antidepressants. Galantamine is a selective, reversible, inhibitor of acetylcholinesterase that is active both peripherally and in the central nervous system. The pharmacologic properties of galantamine suggest this drug might be effective in the treatment of patients with chronic fatigue syndrome. Nevertheless, a randomized controlled clinical trial did not demonstrate any benefit of galantamine over placebo in the treatment of these patients (Blacker et al., 2004).

Diagnosis and Management of Cardiac Dysrhythmias

Edrophonium has been administered for the diagnosis and management of cardiac dysrhythmias, especially paroxysmal supraventricular tachycardias including those due to Wolff-Parkinson-White syndrome (Atlee, 1997). Administration of edrophonium, 5 to 10 mg IV (25 to 30 mg over 30 minutes), produces principally muscarinic effects manifesting as slowing of the heart rate with no effect on ventricular conduction, contractility, or peripheral vascular tone. Bradycardia reflects drug-induced muscarinic effects at the sinoatrial node (slowed rate of discharge) and atrioventricular node (increased conduction time). Increased airway secretions and bronchoconstriction (higher risk in patients with asthma or chronic obstructive pulmonary disease) are risks of treatment of cardiac dysrhythmias with edrophonium.

Postoperative Analgesia

Intrathecal (50 to 100 μg) or epidural (1 to 4 μg/kg) injection of neostigmine produces analgesia in the postoperative period and in patients with chronic pain (Lauretti et al. 1998). Epidural combinations of neostigmine 6 to 7 μg/kg (500 μg) with sufentanil 10 μg provides similar duration of analgesia as epidural sufentanil 20 μg and allows effective and selective analgesia devoid of side effects in the first stage of labor (Relents and Lavand'homme, 2004). Neostigmine probably produces analgesia by inhibiting the breakdown of spinally released acetylcholine which is increased in the presence of pain. Disadvantages of intrathecal neostigmine to produce analgesia include a high incidence of nausea and vomiting, pruritus, and prolongation of sensory and motor block produced by spinal anesthesia (Liu et al., 1999). Ventilatory depression characteristic of analgesia produced by opioids does not accompany neostigmine-induced pain relief. Neurotoxicity does not accompany intrathecal injection of commercially available neostigmine preparations containing paraben preservatives (Eisenach et al., 1997).

Postoperative Shivering

Administration of physostigmine, 40 μg/kg IV, at the conclusion of anesthesia decreases the incidence of postoperative shivering similar to meperidine and clonidine (Horn et al., 1998). It is postulated that physostigmine enhances secretion of neurotransmitters that are involved in the control of body temperature, especially at the hypothalamic thermoregulatory centers.

OVERDOSE OF ANTICHOLINESTERASE DRUGS

The effects of an acute overdose (intoxication) with an anticholinesterase drug manifest as muscarinic and nicotinic symptoms on peripheral and CNS sites (Karalliedde and Senanayake, 1989). Muscarinic symptoms include miosis, difficulty focusing, salivation, bronchoconstriction, bradycardia, abdominal cramps, and loss of bladder and rectal control. Nicotinic actions at the NMJ range from skeletal muscle weakness to overt paralysis with resulting apnea. CNS actions include confusion, ataxia, seizures, coma, and depression of ventilation.

The diagnosis of anticholinesterase drug overdose is made by a history of exposure and characteristic signs and symptoms. Organophosphate anticholinesterases are present in insecticides; are absorbed rapidly across alveoli, skin, and the gastrointestinal tract; and may be the cause of toxic symptoms. Accidental poisoning from these drugs most often occurs by inhalation or dermal absorption. The high lipid solubility of organophosphate anticholinesterases ensures that these drugs will cross the blood-brain barrier easily and produce intense effects on the CNS.

Treatment

Treatment of anticholinesterase drug overdose is with atropine, occasionally supplemented by an acetylcholinesterase reactivator, pralidoxime (Fig. 9-14). Atropine, 35 to 70 μg/kg IV administered every 3 to 10 minutes until muscarinic symptoms disappear, is specific for antagonizing the muscarinic effects of acetylcholine, but has no impact on nicotinic actions at the NMJ. The effects of excessive concentrations of acetylcholine at the NMJ and, to a lesser extent, effects at autonomic ganglia, can be reversed by administration of pralidoxime, 15 mg/kg IV, over 2 minutes. This dosage is repeated after 20 minutes if skeletal muscle weakness is not reversed. The CNS effects of excessive concentrations of acetylcholine are not antagonized by pralidoxime. Pralidoxime is more effective in countering the effects of drugs that phosphorylate acetylcholinesterase than against drugs that carbamylate the enzyme. Furthermore, pralidoxime may be ineffective unless it is administered within minutes after exposure to the potent anticholinesterase drug.

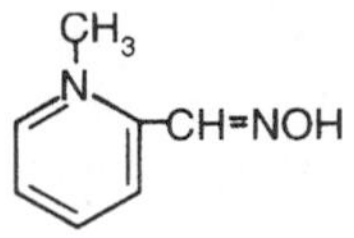

Figure 9-14. Pralidoxime.

In addition to specific pharmacologic antagonism, treatment of anticholinesterase drug overdose includes supportive measures such as intubation of the trachea and mechanical ventilation of the lungs. Seizures may require suppression with drugs such as thiopental or diazepam.

SYNTHETIC CHOLINERGIC AGONISTS

Synthetic cholinergic agonist drugs have as their primary action the activation of cholinergic (muscarinic) receptors that are innervated by postganglionic parasympathetic nerves. Additional actions are exerted on autonomic ganglia and on cells that do not receive extensive parasympathetic innervation but, nevertheless, possess cholinergic (nicotinic) receptors. Acetylcholine has no therapeutic application because of its diffuse sites of action and its rapid hydrolysis by acetylcholinesterase and, to a lesser extent, by plasma cholinesterase.

Derivatives of acetylcholine have been synthesized that have more selective effects and prolonged durations of action. Of the synthetic acetylcholine derivatives, only methacholine, carbachol, and bethanechol have clinical usefulness (Fig. 9-15). These drugs are administered orally, subcutaneously, or topically to the eye. Asthma, coronary artery disease, and peptic ulcer disease are examples of diseases that could be exacerbated by treatment with a cholinergic agonist. For example, bronchoconstriction produced by these drugs could produce an asthmatic attack. Vasodilation and resulting decreases in diastolic blood pressure may decrease coronary blood flow sufficiently to evoke myocardial ischemia in vulnerable patients. Enhanced secretion of acidic gastric fluid in response to treatment with a cholinergic agonist could aggravate the symptoms of peptic ulcer disease. All of the muscarinic effects of cholinergic agonists are blocked selectively by atropine.

Methacholine

Methacholine has a longer duration of action than acetylcholine because its rate of hydrolysis by acetylcholinesterase is slower. Furthermore, methacholine is almost totally resistant to hydrolysis by plasma cholinesterase. Its greater receptor selectivity than acetylcholine is manifested by a lack of significant nicotinic and predominance of muscarinic actions. This drug is rarely used clinically because of the unpredictable nature of its muscarinic effects, especially on the cardiovascular system. Investigation of the role of cholinergic stimulation in reactive airway disease may include a methacholine inhalation challenge (Maclagan and Barners, 1989).

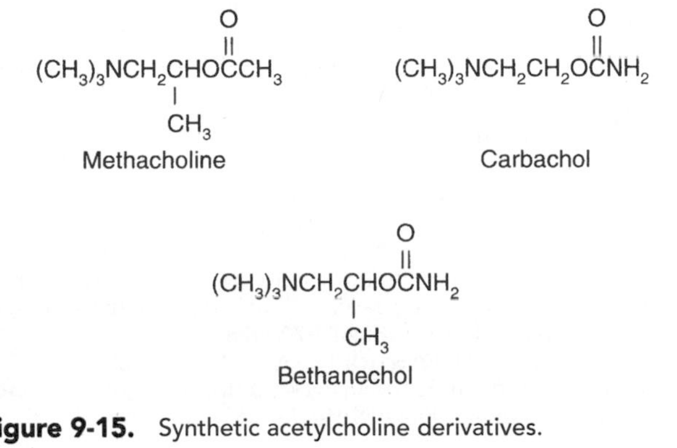

Figure 9-15. Synthetic acetylcholine derivatives.

Carbachol and Bethanechol

Carbachol and bethanechol are totally resistant to hydrolysis by acetylcholinesterase or plasma cholinesterase. Bethanechol has mainly muscarinic actions, but both of these drugs act with some selectivity on smooth muscle of the gastrointestinal tract and urinary bladder. Carbachol retains a high level of nicotinic activity, particularly on autonomic ganglia, which may reflect drug-induced release of endogenous acetylcholine from the terminals of cholinergic fibers.

In contrast to methacholine, the cardiovascular effects of carbachol and bethanechol are less prominent than the effects on the gastrointestinal and urinary tracts. Effects on the gastrointestinal tract include increased lower esophageal sphincter tone, increased peristalsis, and enhanced secretory activity. Nausea, vomiting, and spontaneous defecation are manifestations of increased gastrointestinal motility. Selective effects of carbachol and bethanechol include stimulation of urethral peristalsis and contraction of the detrusor muscle of the urinary bladder. In addition, the trigone and external sphincter are relaxed. These effects evoke evacuation of a neurogenic bladder.

Secretions are increased from all glands that receive parasympathetic nervous system innervation, including the lacrimal, tracheobronchial, salivary, digestive, and exocrine sweat glands. Effects on the respiratory system include, in addition to increased tracheobronchial secretions, bronchoconstriction, and stimulation of the chemoreceptors of the carotid and aortic bodies. When applied topically onto the cornea, these drugs produce miosis.

Bethanechol is used as a stimulant of the smooth muscles of the gastrointestinal tract and the urinary bladder. For example, oral administration of bethanechol may relieve adynamic ileus or gastric atony after bilateral vagotomy. Bethanechol may be useful in combating urinary retention when mechanical obstruction is absent, as in the postoperative and postpartum period and in certain cases of neurogenic bladder, thus avoiding the risk of infection attendant with bladder catheterization. For acute urinary retention, the usual adult dose of bethanechol is 5 mg injected subcutaneously, which can be repeated after 15 to 30 minutes if necessary.

Carbachol is not used for its actions on the gastrointestinal tract and urinary bladder because of its relatively greater nicotinic action at autonomic ganglia. Instead, carbachol is useful as a topical drug in the chronic therapy of

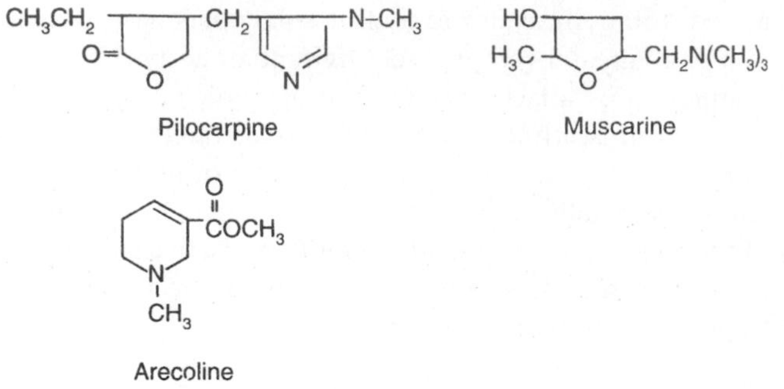

Figure 9-16. Cholinomimetic alkaloids.

narrow-angle glaucoma and to produce miosis during intraocular surgery.

Pilocarpine, Muscarine, and Arecoline

Pilocarpine, muscarine, and arecoline are examples of cholinomimetic alkaloids derived from plants (Fig. 9-16). Pilocarpine has dominant muscarinic actions, and sweat glands are particularly sensitive to this drug, reflecting nicotinic cholinergic effects. Muscarine acts almost exclusively at muscarinic cholinergic receptors and produces cardiac effects that resemble vagal nerve stimulation. Arecoline, like pilocarpine, has effects on muscarinic and nicotinic cholinergic receptors.

The clinical use of these drugs is largely limited to the topical administration of pilocarpine as a miotic in the treatment of glaucoma. Pilocarpine, when applied topically to the cornea, causes miosis, paralysis of accommodation, and a sustained decrease in intraocular pressure. Miosis may persist for several hours, but cycloplegia usually wanes within 2 hours. Pilocarpine is useful for overcoming mydriasis produced by atropine. Atrioventricular heart block has been described following topical corneal pilocarpine (Littmann et al., 1987). Oral doses of pilocarpine may be used to treat xerostomia associated with Sjogren syndrome and radiation therapy involving the salivary glands (Nusair and Rubinow, 1999).

REFERENCES

Aitkenhead AR. Anaesthesia and bowel surgery. *Br J Anaesth* 1984;56:95–102.

Atlee JL. Perioperative cardiac dysrhythmias: diagnosis and management. *Anesthesiology* 1997;86:1397–1424.

Backman SB, Ralley FE, Fox GS. Neostigmine produces bradycardia in a heart transplant patient. *Anesthesiology* 1993;78:777–779.

Balmer HGR, Wyte SR. Antagonism of ketamine or physostigmine [letter]. *Br J Anaesth* 1977;49:510.

Beebe DS, Shumway SJ, Maddock R. Sinus arrest after intravenous neostigmine in two heart transplant patients. *Anesth Analg* 1994;78:779–782.

Bentz WE, Stoelting RK. Prolonged response to succinylcholine following pancuronium reversal with pyridostigmine. *Anesthesiology* 1976;44:258–260.

Bevan DR, Donati F. Succinylcholine apnea: attempted reversal with anticholinesterase. *Can Anaesth Soc J* 1983;30:536–539.

Bevan DR, Donati F, Kopman AF. Reversal of neuromuscular blockade. *Anesthesiology* 1992;77:785–805.

Blacker CVR, Greenwood DT, Wesnes KA, et al. Effect of galantamne hydrobromide in chronic fatigue syndrome: A randomized clinical trial. *JAMA* 2004;292:1195–1204.

Bourke DL, Rosenberg M, Allen PD. Physostigmine: effectiveness as an antagonist of respiratory depression and psychomotor effects caused by morphine or diazepam. *Anesthesiology* 1984;61:523–528.

Buzello W, Krieg N, Schlickewei A. Hazards of neostigmine in patients with neuromuscular disorders. Report of two cases. *Br J Anaesth* 1982;54:529–534.

Cronnelly R. Muscle relaxant antagonists. *Semin Anesth* 1985;4:31–40.

Cronnelly R, Miller RD. Onset and duration of edrophonium-pyridostigmine mixtures. *Anesthesiology* 1984;61:A301.

Cronnelly R, Morris RB. Antagonism of neuromuscular blockade. *Br J Anaesth* 1982;54:183–193.

Cronnelly R, Morris RB, Miller RD. Edrophonium: Duration of action and atropine requirement in humans during halothane anesthesia. *Anesthesiology* 1982;57:261–266.

Cummings JL. Alzheimer's disease. *N Engl J Med* 2004;351:56–67.

Donati F, Ferguson A, Bevan DR. Twitch depression and train-of-four ratio after antagonism of pancuronium with edrophonium, neostigmine, or pyridostigmine. *Anesth Analg* 1983;62:314–316.

Donati F, McCarroll SM, Antzaka C, et al. Dose-response curves for edrophonium, neostigmine, and pyridostigmine after pancuronium and *d*-tubocurarine. *Anesthesiology* 1987;66:471–476.

Donati F, Smith CE, Bevan DR. Dose-response relationships for edrophonium and neostigmine as antagonists of moderate and profound atracurium blockade. *Anesth Analg* 1989;68:13–19.

Drury PJ, Birmingham AT, Healy TEJ. Interaction of adrenaline with neostigmine and tubocurarine at the skeletal neuromuscular junction. *Br J Anaesth* 1987;59:784–790.

Eisenach JC, Hood DD, Curry R. Phase I human safety assessment of intrathecal neostigmine containing methyl- and propylparabens. *Anesth Analg* 1997;85:842–846.

Engbaek J, Ostergaard D, Skovgaard LT, et al. Reversal of intense neuromuscular blockade following infusion of atracurium. *Anesthesiology* 1990;72:803–806.

Fisher DM, Cronnelly R, Miller RD, et al. The neuromuscular pharmacology of neostigmine in infants and children. *Anesthesiology* 1983;59:220–225.

Fisher DM, Cronnelly R, Sharma M, et al. Clinical pharmacology of edrophonium in infants and children. *Anesthesiology* 1984;61:428–433.

Futter ME, Donati F, Sadikot AS, et al. Neostigmine antagonism of succinylcholine phase II block: a comparison with pancuronium. *Can Anaesth Soc J* 1983;30:575–580.

Heier T, Clough D, Wright PMC et al. The influence of mild hypothermia on the pharmacokinetics and time course of action of neostigmine in anesthetized volunteers. *Anesthesiology* 2002;97:90–95.

Hennis PJ, Cronnelly R, Sharma M, et al. Metabolites of neostigmine and pyridostigmine do not contribute to antagonism of neuromuscular blockade in the dog. *Anesthesiology* 1984;62:334–339.

Hill GE, Stanley TH, Sentker CR. Physostigmine reversal of postoperative somnolence. *Can Anaesth Soc J* 1977;24:707–711.

Horn EP, Standl T, Sessler DI, et al. Physostigmine prevents postanesthetic shivering as does meperidine or clonidine. *Anesthesiology* 1998;88:108–113.

Jones RM, Pearce AC, Williams JP. Recovery characteristics following antagonism of atracurium with neostigmine or edrophonium. *Br J Anaesth* 1984;56:453–457.

Karalliedde L, Senanayake N. Organophosphorus insecticide poisoning. *Br J Anaesth* 1989;63:736–750.

Katz RL. Clinical neuromuscular pharmacology of pancuronium. *Anesthesiology* 1971;34:550–556.

Kim JM, Mangold J. Sensitivity to both vecuronium and neostigmine in a seronegative myasthenic patient. *Br J Anaesth* 1989;63:497–500.

King MJ, Milazkiewicz R, Carli F, et al. Influence of neostigmine on postoperative vomiting. *Br J Anaesth* 1988;61:403–406.

Kopman A. Recovery times following edrophonium and neostigmine reversal of pancuronium, atracurium, and vecuronium steady-state infusions. *Anesthesiology* 1986;65:572–578.

Lauretti GR, Hood DD, Eisenach JC, et al. A multi-center study of intrathecal neostigmine for analgesia following vaginal hysterectomy. *Anesthesiology* 1998;89:913–918.

Littmann L, Kempler P, Rohla M et al. Severe symptomatic atrioventricular block induced by pilocarpine eye drops. *Arch Intern Med* 1987;147:586–587.

Liu S, Hodgson PS, Moore JM, et al. Dose-response effects of spinal neostigmine added to bupivacaine spinal anesthesia in volunteers. *Anesthesiology* 1999;90:710–717.

Maclagan J, Barners PJ. Muscarinic pharmacology of the airways. *Trends Pharmacol Sci* 1989;5:88–91.

Matteo RS, Young WL, Orstein E, et al. Pharmacokinetics and pharmacodynamics of edrophonium in elderly surgical patients. *Anesth Analg* 1990;71:334–339.

Mayeux r, Sano M. Treatment of Alzehimer's disease. *N Engl J Med* 1999;341:1671–1677.

Miller RD, Van Nyhuis LS, Eger EI, et al. Comparative times to peak effect and duration of action of neostigmine and pyridostigmine. *Anesthesiology* 1974;41:27–33.

Miller RD, Van Nyhuis LS, Eger EI, et al. The effect of acid-base balance of neostigmine antagonism of *d*-tubocurarine- induced neuromuscular blockade. *Anesthesiology* 1975;42:377–383.

Mirakhur RK. Edrophonium and plasma cholinesterase activity. *Can Anaesth Soc J* 1986;33:588–590.

Naguib M, Abdulatif M. Priming with anticholinesterases: the effect of different priming doses of edrophonium. *Can J Anaesth* 1988;35: 53–57.

Naguib M, Flood P, McArdle, et al. Advances in neurobiology of the neuromuscular junction: Implications for the anesthesiologist. *Anesthesiology* 2002;96:202–231.

Nusair S, Rubinow A. The use of oral pilocarpine in xerostomia and Sjogren's syndrome.*Semin Arthritis Rheum* 1999;28: 360365.

Paraskeva A, Konstantinos P, Fassoulaki A, et al. Physostigmine does not antagonize sevoflurane anesthesia assessed by bispectral index or enhance recovery. *Anesth Analg* 2002;54:569–72.

Prys-Roberts C. Hemodynamic effects of anesthesia and surgery in renal hypertensive patients receiving large doses of beta-receptor antagonists. *Anesthesiology* 1979;51:S22.

Relents F, Lavand'homme PM. Epidural neostigmine combined with sufentanil provides balanced and selective analgesia in early labor. Anesthesiology 2004;101:439–444.

Rothenberg DM, Berns AS, Barkin R, et al. Bromide intoxication secondary to pyridostigmine bromide therapy. *JAMA* 1990;263: 1121–1122.

Rupp SM, McChristian JW, Miller RD, et al. Neostigmine and edrophonium antagonism of varying neuromuscular blockade induced by atracurium, pancuronium, or vecuronium. *Anesthesiology* 1986; 64:711–717.

Smith CE, Donati F, Bevan DR. Dose-response relationships for edrophonium and neostigmine as antagonists of atracurium and vecuronium neuromuscular blockade. *Anesthesiology* 1989;71:37–43.

Snir-Mor I, Weinstock M, Davidson JT, et al. Physostigmine antagonizes morphine-induced respiratory depression in human subjects. *Anesthesiology* 1983;59:6–9.

Sprague DH. Severe bradycardia after neostigmine in a patient taking propranolol to control paroxysmal atrial tachycardia. *Anesthesiology* 1975;42:208–210.

Stone JG, Matteo RS, Ornstein E, et al. Aging alters the pharmacokinetics of pyridostigmine. *Anesth Analg* 1995;81:773–776.

Szalodos JE, Donati F, Bevan DR. Edrophonium priming for antagonism of atracurium neuromuscular blockade. *Can J Anaesth* 1990; 37:197–201.

Turner DAB, Smith G. Evaluation of the combined effects of atropine and neostigmine on the lower oesophageal sphincter. *Br J Anaesth* 1985;57:956–959.

Urquhart ML, Ramsey FM, Royster RL, et al. Heart rate and rhythm following an edrophonium/atropine mixture for antagonism of neuromuscular blockade during fentanyl/N_2O/O_2 anesthesia. *Anesthesiology* 1987;67:561–565.

Wagner DL, Moorthy SS, Stoelting RK. Administration of anticholinesterase drugs in the presence of beta-adrenergic blockade. *Anesth Analg* 1982;61:153–154.

Young WL, Matteo RS, Ornstein E. Duration of action of neostigmine and pyridostigmine in the elderly. *Anesth Analg* 1988;67:775–778

Anticholinergic Drugs

10

Anticholinergic drugs competitively antagonize the effects (parasympatholytic) of the neurotransmitter acetylcholine at cholinergic postganglionic sites designated as muscarinic receptors. Muscarinic cholinergic receptors are present in the heart, salivary glands, and smooth muscles of the gastrointestinal tract and genitourinary tract. Acetylcholine is also the neurotransmitter at postganglionic nicotinic receptors located at the neuromuscular junction (NMJ) and autonomic ganglia. In contrast to effects at muscarinic receptors, usual doses of anticholinergic drugs exert little or no effect at nicotinic cholinergic receptors. As such, anticholinergic drugs may be considered to be selectively antimuscarinic.

Naturally occurring tertiary amine anticholinergic drugs such as atropine and scopolamine are alkaloids of belladonna plants. Semisynthetic congeners of the belladonna alkaloids, represented by glycopyrrolate, are usually quaternary ammonium derivatives. These quaternary ammonium derivatives are often more potent than their parent compounds with respect to peripheral anticholinergic effects, but they lack central nervous system (CNS) activity because of poor penetration into the brain.

STRUCTURE–ACTIVITY RELATIONSHIPS

Naturally occurring anticholinergic drugs (atropine and scopolamine) are esters formed by the combination of tropic or mandelic acid and an organic base (tropine, scopine, or an *N*-methylated derivative of tropine) (Fig. 10-1). Structurally, these drugs resemble cocaine, and atropine, in fact, has weak analgesic actions. Atropine and scopolamine comprise mixtures of equal parts of dextrorotatory and levorotatory isomers, but the anticholinergic effects are due to the levorotatory form. Synthetic anticholinergic drugs such as glycopyrrolate contain mandelic acid rather than tropic acid (see Fig. 10-1). Like acetylcholine, anticholinergic drugs contain a cationic portion that can fit into the muscarinic cholinergic receptor.

MECHANISM OF ACTION

Anticholinergic drugs combine reversibly with muscarinic cholinergic receptors and thus prevent access of the neurotransmitter acetylcholine to these sites. In contrast to acetylcholine, the combination of an anticholinergic drug with the muscarinic receptor does not result in cell membrane changes and associated inhibition of adenylate cyclase or alterations in calcium permeability that would lead to cholinergic responses. Anticholinergic drugs do not prevent the liberation of acetylcholine nor do they react with acetylcholine. As competitive antagonists, the effect of anticholinergic drugs can be overcome by increasing the concentration of acetylcholine in the area of the muscarinic receptors.

Molecular cloning has defined five distinct muscarinic cholinergic receptor subtypes that are designated M_1 through M_5, with each subtype being encoded by distinct cellular genes (Table 10-1) (Lambert and Appadu, 1995). There is a distinct tissue distribution of these subtypes, with M_1 receptors found in the CNS and stomach, M_2 receptors in the lungs and the heart, and M_3 receptors in the CNS, airway smooth muscles, and glandular tissues. The CNS is the principal site for M_4 and M_5 receptors.

Anticholinergic drugs promote airway relaxation by inhibiting M_2 and M_3 muscarinic receptors on airway smooth muscle. The release of acetylcholine from parasympathetic nerves increases during exacerbations of asthma and during endotracheal intubation. Bronchial M_3 receptors mediate muscarinic agonist-induced bronchoconstriction, whereas M_2 receptors antagonize beta-adrenergic receptor–mediated bronchodilation through inhition of adenylyl cylcase activity (Gunst et al., 1989). Vasodilaton of vascular beds by acetylcholine is mediated predominantly by M_3 receptors located on the luminal surfaces of endothelial cells. Stimulation of these receptors is followed by release of nitric oxide and vasodilaton. Cardiac M_3 receptors densely populate cardiac conduction tissues, such as the sinoatrial node and atrioventricular node and the Purkinje fibers, but are sparsely present in the ventricular myocardium. Chronic hypoxia increases the density of M_2 receptors in the cardiac ventricles. There is evidence that edrophonium binds to M_2 and M_3 receptors nonselectively and acts as a competitive antagonist to acetylcholine (Tanito et al., 2001).

Muscarinic cholinergic receptors are examples of G protein-coupled receptors that also depend on second-messenger coupling. The M_1, M_3, and M_5 receptors activate G proteins, leading to phospholipase C stimulation and

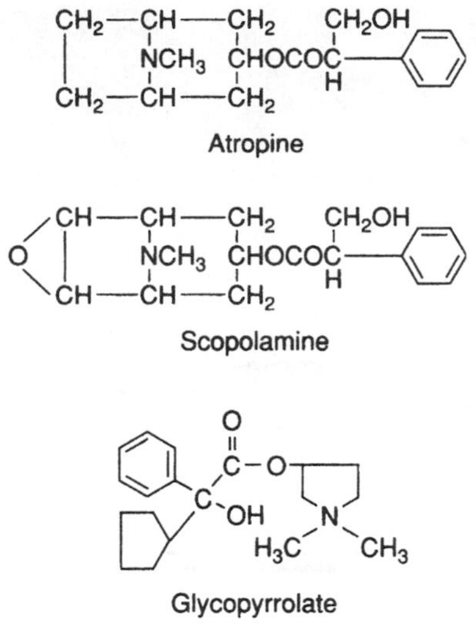

Figure 10-1. Naturally occurring and synthetic anticholinergic drugs.

calcium mobilization. The M_2 and M_4 receptors activate G proteins that mediate inhibition of adenylyl cyclase and inhibition of voltage-sensitive calcium channels (Caulfield, 1993). Evidence for subclasses of muscarinic cholinergic receptors is based upon the variation in sensitivity among different cholinergic receptors as well as differences in potency among the anticholinergic drugs (Goyal, 1989; Lambert and Appadu, 1995). For example, muscarinic cholinergic receptors that control salivary and bronchial secretions (M_3 receptors) are inhibited by lower doses of anticholinergic drugs than are necessary to inhibit receptors that regulate acetylcholine effects on the heart and eyes (M_2 receptors). Even larger doses of anticholinergic drugs inhibit cholinergic control of the gastrointestinal tract and genitourinary tract, thus decreasing the tone and motility of the intestine and inhibiting micturition. Still larger doses of anticholinergic drugs are required to inhibit gastric secretion of hydrogen ions (M_1 receptors). As a result, a dose of anticholinergic drug that inhibits gastric secretion of hydrogen ions invariably affects salivary secretion, heart rate, ocular accommodation, and micturition. The sequence of blockade of effects mediated by activation of muscarinic cholinergic receptors is the same for all anticholinergic drugs.

Examples of differences in anticholinergic potency between drugs are the greater antisialagogue and ocular effects of scopolamine compared with atropine (Table 10-2) (Eger, 1962). The required intramuscular doses for a reliable antisialagogue effect are 10 to 20 μg/kg for atropine, 5 to 8 μg/kg for glycopyrrolate, and about 5 μg/kg for scopolamine (Kirvela et al., 1994). Atropine has greater anticholinergic effects at the heart, bronchial smooth muscles, and gastrointestinal tract than does scopolamine (see Table 10-2) (Eger, 1962). Glycopyrrolate increases metabolic oxygen consumption, whereas atropine has no effect and scopolamine is associated with a decrease (Kirvela et al., 1994).

Atropine, scopolamine, and glycopyrrolate do not discriminate among M_1, M_2, and M_3 receptors; instead they act as highly selective competitive antagonists of acetylcholine at all muscarinic receptors. It is conceivable that an anticholinergic drug could act as a selective antagonist on a specific subclass of muscarinic receptors that mediate unique physiologic responses such as secretion of hydrogen ions by gastric parietal cells. In this regard, pirenzepine seems to be selective in blocking M_1 receptors responsible for gastric hydrogen ion secretion by parietal cells (see Table 10-1) (Lambert and Appadu, 1995). A selective M_2 receptor antagonist, if available, would be useful for prevention and treatment of reflex-induced bradycardia due to parasympathetic nervous system stimulation.

Evidence that anticholinergic drugs are not pure muscarinic cholinergic receptor antagonists is the observation that small doses of atropine, scopolamine, and glycopyrrolate can produce heart rate slowing even when the drug is

TABLE 10-1.
MUSCARINIC RECEPTOR SUBTYPES

	M_1	M_2	M_3	M_4	M_5
Location	CNS Stomach	Heart CNS Airway smooth muscle	CNS Salivary glands Airway smooth Muscle Vascular endothelial cells	CNS Heart	CNS
Clinical effects	Hydrogen ion secretion	Bradycardia	Salivation Bronchodilation Vasodilation	?	?
Clinically selective drugs available	Yes	No	No	No	No

CNS, central nervous system.
Source: Adapted from Lambert DG, Appadu BL. Muscarinic receptor subtypes: Do they have a place in clinical anaesthesia? *Br J Anaesth* 1995;74:497–499.

TABLE 10-2.
COMPARATIVE EFFECTS OF ANTICHOLINERGIC DRUGS

	Sedation	Antisialagogue	Increase Heart Rate	Relax Smooth Muscle	Mydriasis, Cycloplegia	Prevent Motion-Induced Nausea	Decrease Gastric Hydrogen Ion Secretion	Alter Fetal Heart Rate
Atropine	+	+	+++	++	+	+	+	0
Scopolamine	+++	+++	+	+	+++	+++	+	?
Glycopyrrolate	0	++	++	++	0	0	+	0

0, none; +, mild; ++, moderate; +++, marked

administered in the presence of bilateral vagotomy. Previous speculation that heart rate slowing after administration of atropine reflected central vagal action before the peripheral blocking effects could occur is not supported by the occurrence of similar heart rate slowing in response to the administration of glycopyrrolate, which cannot easily cross the blood-brain barrier. Rather, paradoxical slowing of heart rate likely results from blockade of presynaptic inhibitory M_1 receptors on vagus nerve endings, which usually provide negative feedback on further acetylcholine release. This inhibition results in increased acetylcholine release, which initially overcomes the muscarinic blockade on sinoatrial M_2 receptors. Atropine has no heart rate effect on the denervated, acutely transplanted heart.

An additional indirect effect of anticholinergic drugs can result from interference by these drugs with the normal inhibition of the release of endogenous norepinephrine. This indirect action may manifest as a sympathomimetic effect of atropine.

PHARMACOKINETICS

Oral absorption of even the lipid-soluble tertiary amine anticholinergic drugs is not sufficiently predictable for a recommendation of oral administration in the perioperative period. Intramuscular (IM) or intravenous (IV) administration is used most often for delivery of anticholinergic drugs. Administered IV, atropine has an onset of action (as reflected by changes in heart rate) of about 1 minute and a duration of action of 30 to 60 minutes, whereas glycopyrrolate has a slower onset (2 to 3 minutes) and approximately

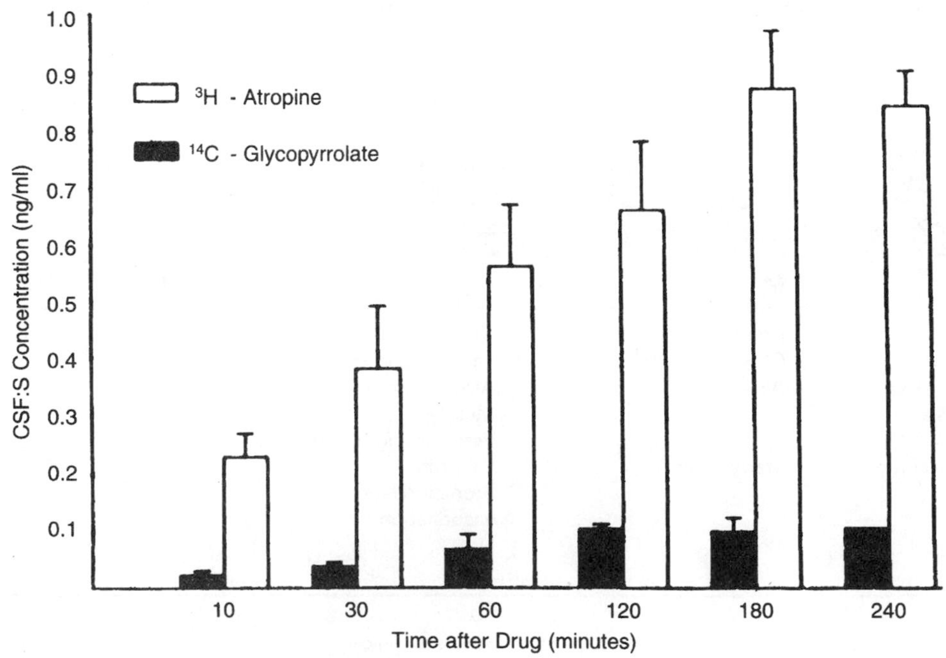

Figure 10-2. Cerebrospinal fluid (CSF)-to-serum (S) concentration ratios (mean ± SE) after intravenous administration of ^{14}C-glycopyrrolate (n = 3) or ^{3}H-atropine (n = 4) to anesthetized dogs. ^{3}H-atropine produced significantly ($P < .05$) higher CSF:S concentration ratios over the 4-hour postdrug period (0.1 mg/kg of each drug) than did ^{14}C-glycopyrrolate. (From Proakis AG, Harris GB. Comparative penetration of glycopyrrolate and atropine across the blood-brain and placental barriers in anesthetized dogs. *Anesthesiology* 1978; 48: 339–344; with permission.)

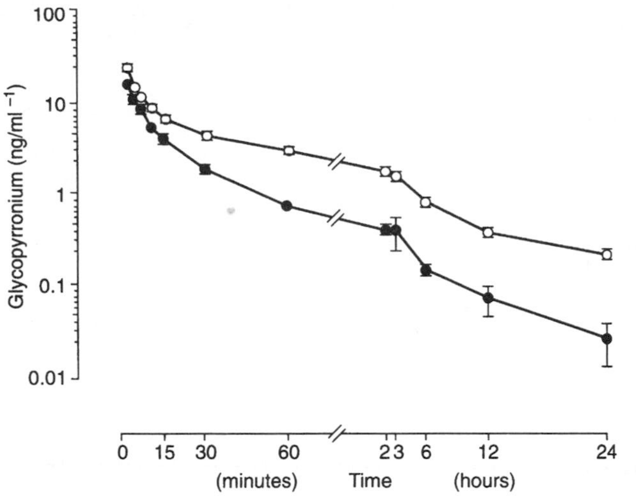

Figure 10-3. Plasma concentrations of glycopyrrolate in 11 uremic (*open circles*) and seven control (*solid circles*) patients. (From Kirvela M, Ali-Melkkila T, Kaila T, et al. Pharmacokinetics of glycopyrronium in uraemic patients. *Br J Anaesth* 1993;71:437–439; with permission.)

the same duration of action as atropine (Bevan et al., 1992).

Atropine and scopolamine are lipid-soluble tertiary amines that easily penetrate the blood-brain barrier (Fig. 10-2) (Proakis and Harris, 1978). In contrast, glycopyrrolate is a poorly lipid-soluble quaternary ammonium compound with minimal ability to cross the blood-brain barrier and produce CNS effects (see Fig. 10-2) (Ali-Melkkila et al., 1990; Proakis and Harris, 1978). Absorption of glycopyrrolate after IM injection is rapid (maximum plasma concentration in about 16 minutes) and comparable with atropine (Ali-Melkkila et al., 1990). Clearance of glycopyrrolate from the plasma is more rapid than atropine (elimination half-time about 1.25 hours versus 2.3 hours), and nearly 80% of glycopyrrolate is excreted unchanged in the urine. The corresponding value for atropine is 18%. Appearance of tropine and tropic acid reflects hydrolysis of atropine to inactive metabolites. Minimal amounts of atropine are destroyed in human plasma, whereas certain animals, such as the rabbit, possess a specific plasma enzyme, atropine esterase, that is capable of hydrolyzing atropine. Conversely, scopolamine is broken down almost entirely in the body, with only approximately 1% appearing unchanged in the urine. The elimination of glycopyrrolate in plasma is significantly prolonged in uremic patients compared with nonuremic patients (Fig. 10-3) (Kirvela et al., 1993).

CLINICAL USES

Anticholinergic drugs are used in a wide variety of clinical conditions and situations (Mirakhur, 1988). However, the lack of selectivity of these drugs makes it difficult to obtain desired therapeutic responses without concomitant side effects (see Table 10-1) (Lambert and Appadu, 1995). The most important uses of anticholinergic drugs in the perioperative period are for (a) preoperative medication, (b) treatment of reflex-mediated bradycardia, and (c) combination with anticholinesterase drugs during pharmacologic antagonism of nondepolarizing neuromuscular-blocking drugs (see Chapter 9). Less common uses of anticholinergic drugs include (a) bronchodilation, (b) biliary and ureteral smooth muscle relaxation, (c) production of mydriasis and cycloplegia, (d) antagonism of gastric hydrogen ion secretion by parietal cells, (e) prevention of motion-induced nausea, and (f) constituents in nonprescription cold remedies.

Preoperative Medication

Historically, atropine was administered IM before the induction of anesthesia to protect the heart from vagal reflexes and to prevent excessive salivary gland secretions. Currently available inhaled or injected anesthetic drugs are not predictably associated with these effects, and it is not mandatory to include an anticholinergic drug in the preoperative medication. When an anticholinergic drug is included in the preoperative medication, the most likely therapeutic goals are to produce sedation or an antisialagogue effect. Anticholinergic drugs in traditional doses used for preoperative medication in adults do not alter gastric fluid pH or volume.

Patients with glaucoma and parturients require special considerations in using anticholinergic drugs for preoperative medication. For example, the mydriatic effects of scopolamine are greater than those of atropine, suggesting caution in the administration of scopolamine to patients with glaucoma (Garde et al., 1978). Atropine, 0.4 mg IM or 1 mg IV, administered with an anticholinesterase drug, seems safe because little or no change in pupil size occurs (Balamoutsos et al., 1980). Glycopyrrolate has the least effect on pupil size of all the anticholinergic drugs used for preoperative medication. Both atropine and scopolamine can cross the placenta, but the fetal heart rate is not significantly changed after IV administration of either atropine or glycopyrrolate (Fig. 10-4) (Abboud et al., 1983; Murad et al., 1981).

Sedation

Scopolamine is selected when sedation is the reason for including an anticholinergic drug in the preoperative medication. Indeed, scopolamine is approximately 100 times more potent than atropine in decreasing the activity of the reticular activating system. Scopolamine, in addition to depressing the cerebral cortex, also affects other areas of the brain, causing amnesia. Typical doses of scopolamine (0.3 to 0.5 mg IM) usually cause sedation, whereas similar doses of atropine produce minimal CNS effects. Nevertheless, atropine has been associated with an increased incidence

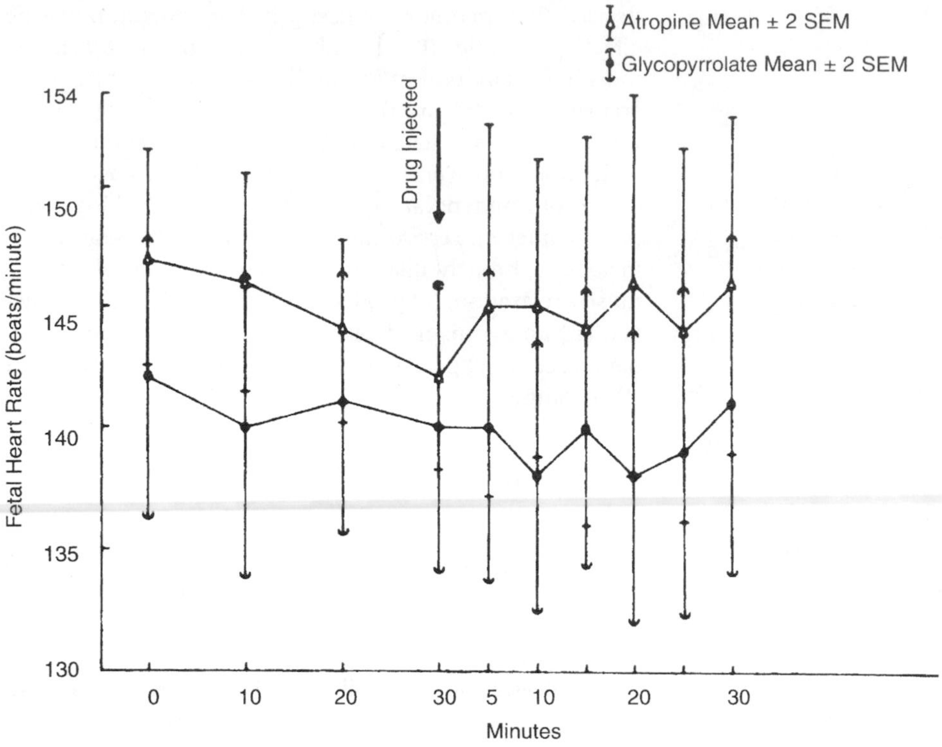

Figure 10-4. Neither atropine nor glycopyrrolate alters fetal heart rate after intravenous administration to the mother. (Mean ± 2 SEM.) (From Abboud T, Raya J, Sadri S, et al. Fetal and maternal cardiovascular effects of atropine and glycopyrrolate. *Anesth Analg* 1983; 62:426–430; with permission.)

of memory deficit after anesthesia compared with glycopyrrolate (Simpson et al., 1987). Furthermore, arousal in the first 30 minutes after cessation of anesthesia is delayed after administration of atropine-neostigmine but not glycopyrrolate-neostigmine mixtures, used to antagonize the effects of nondepolarizing neuromuscular-blocking drugs (Baraka et al., 1980). Scopolamine also greatly enhances the sedative effects of concomitantly administered drugs, especially opioids and benzodiazepines. Indeed, the combination of morphine and scopolamine is favored by many anesthesiologists when a reliable sedative effect from the preoperative medication is desired. Glycopyrrolate, which does not easily cross the blood-brain barrier, is devoid of sedative effects.

Occasionally, CNS effects of anticholinergic drugs, especially scopolamine, cause symptoms ranging from restlessness to somnolence. These symptoms are more likely to occur in elderly patients and should be considered as a possible explanation for delayed awakening from anesthesia or agitation in the early postoperative period. Inhaled anesthetics can potentiate the effects of anticholinergic drugs on the CNS, leading to an increased incidence of postoperative restlessness or somnolence. Physostigmine is effective in reversing restlessness or somnolence due to CNS effects of tertiary amine anticholinergic drugs.

Antisialagogue Effect

Scopolamine is approximately three times more potent as an antisialagogue than atropine. For this reason, scopolamine is often selected when both an antisialagogue effect and sedation are desired results of preoperative medication. In equivalent antisialagogue doses, scopolamine, 0.3 to 0.5 mg IM, is less likely than atropine, 0.4 to 0.6 mg IM, to produce heart rate changes. Glycopyrrolate is selected when an antisialagogue effect, in the absence of sedation, is desired. As an antisialagogue, glycopyrrolate is approximately twice as potent as atropine, and its duration for producing this effect is longer (Murad et al., 1981).

Treatment of Reflex-Mediated Bradycardia

Anticholinergic drugs are the drugs of choice for treating intraoperative bradycardia, particularly that resulting from increased parasympathetic nervous system activity. Administration of atropine, 15 to 70 μg/kg IV, and, to a lesser extent, scopolamine and glycopyrrolate, increase the heart rate by blocking the effects of acetylcholine on the sinoatrial node (Gravenstein et al., 1964; Meyers and Tomeldan, 1979). Indeed, the maximum increase in heart rate produced by atropine indicates the degree of control normally exerted by the vagus nerve on the sinoatrial node. Equivalent doses of glycopyrrolate produce similar increases in heart rate, but the onset of effect is slower than after the administration of atropine (Bevan et al., 1992). On the electrocardiogram, the effect of anticholinergic drugs is to shorten the P-R interval.

In young adults, in whom vagal tone is enhanced, the influence of atropine on heart rate is most evident, whereas in infants or elderly patients, even large doses may fail to increase heart rate. During anesthesia that includes a volatile drug, the dose of atropine needed to increase heart rate may be decreased compared with awake patients, perhaps reflecting depression of vagal centers during anesthesia.

Combination with Anticholinesterase Drugs

Pharmacologic-enhanced antagonism of nondepolarizing neuromuscular-blocking drugs with an anticholinesterase drug requires the concomitant administration of atropine or glycopyrrolate to prevent parasympathomimetic effects that predictably accompany IV administration of edrophonium, neostigmine, or pyridostigmine (see Chapter 9). Depending on the speed of onset of the anticholinesterase drug, atropine (rapid onset) or glycopyrrolate (slower onset) are selected for concomitant administration (see Chapter 9).

Administration of anticholinergic drugs during pharmacologic antagonism of nondepolarizing neuromuscular blockade causes impairment of parasympathetic nervous system control of heart rate that persists into the early postoperative period. These effects are of shorter duration after administration of glycopyrrolate than atropine (van Vlymen and Parlow, 1997; Parlow et al., 1997). In this regard, glycopyrrolate may be preferable in patients at risk for cardiovascular complications. For example, impairment of parasympathetic nervous system activity has been associated with an increased incidence of cardiac dysrhythmias in response to myocardial ischemia and decreased survival after myocardial infarction (Pedretti et al., 1993).

Bronchodilation

The effectiveness of anticholinergic drugs as bronchodilators reflects antagonism of acetylcholine effects on airway smooth muscle via muscarinic receptors, present predominantly in large- and medium-sized airways, that respond to vagal nerve stimulation. The resulting relaxation of bronchial smooth muscle decreases airway resistance and increases dead space, particularly in patients with bronchial asthma or chronic bronchitis. For example, clinical doses of scopolamine decrease airway resistance and increase dead space by about one-third, but this effect depends largely on the degree of preexisting bronchomotor tone. Glycopyrrolate is equally effective as a bronchodilator and is devoid of effects on the CNS, and heart rate effects are minimal to modest (Fig. 10-5) (Gal and Suratt, 1981).

Administration of anticholinergic drugs for preanesthetic medication could result in inspissation of secretions, possibly leading to airway obstruction rather than decreases in airway resistance. Nevertheless, it seems unlikely that a single dose of anticholinergic would predictably produce these adverse effects.

Bronchodilation is more likely to occur when anticholinergic drugs are administered as aerosols. An advantage of aerosol administration is the absence of adverse cardiovascular side effects that are more likely to accompany systemic administration. Atropine, 1 to 2 mg diluted in 3 to 5 mL of normal saline, can be administered via a nebulizer to treat reflex bronchoconstriction due to parasympathetic nervous system stimulation.

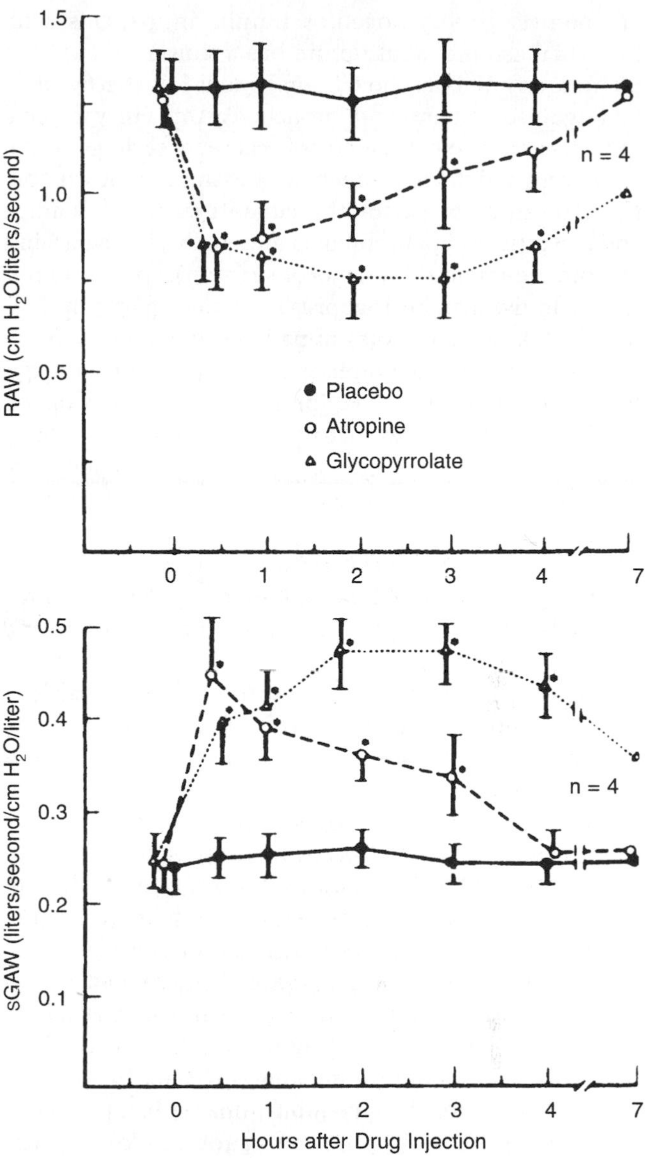

Figure 10-5. Atropine and glycopyrrolate are equally effective in lowering airway resistance (RAW) and increasing airway conductance (sGAW). (From Gal TJ, Suratt PM. Atropine and glycopyrrolate effects on lung mechanics in normal man. *Anesth Analg* 1981;60:85–90; with permission.)

Ipratropium

Ipratropium is a *N*-isopropyl derivative of atropine and is the anticholinergic drug most often selected for aerosol administration to produce bronchodilation in patients with chronic obstructive pulmonary disease (Groeben and Brown, 1996; Gross, 1988). This drug is administered by metered dose inhaler (40 to 80 μg delivered by two to four actuations of the metered-dose inhaler) or by nebulization (0.25 to 0.50 mg). This drug is most effective in preventing and treating bronchospasm that is due to beta-adrenergic antagonists or psychogenic stimuli. In patients with bronchial asthma, ipratropium has a slower onset (30 to 90 minutes and lasts 4 to 6 hours) and is less effective than beta agonists. Patients with bronchial asthma may respond more favorably to beta agonists because these drugs inhibit the release and the subsequent airway smooth muscle contraction caused by chemical mediators such as histamine and leukotrienes (ipratropium is minimally effective against leukotriene-induced bronchoconstriction). Ipratropium is more effective than beta agonists in producing bronchodilation (blocks M_3 receptors) in patients with chronic bronchitis or emphysema, emphasizing the role of cholinergic tone in the latter patients. Ipratropium provides only a modest added bronchodilatory effect when administered with submaximal doses of beta agonists in the treatment of bronchial asthma. No benefit is gained by adding ipratropium to beta-agonists being administered at maximal doses. Paradoxical bronchoconstriction may occur initially following inhalation of ipratropium, reflecting preferential blockade of M_2 receptors by this drug (Groeben and Brown, 1996).

Bronchoconstriction in response to tracheal intubation is thought to be due to an irritant reflex response mediated by acetylcholine from parasympathetic nerves acting on muscarinic receptors of airway smooth muscles. For this reason, it is possible that bronchospasm accompanying placement of a tracheal tube would be responsive to inhaled ipratropium, which blocks muscarinic effects of acetylcholine. Indeed, patients with asthma who develop bronchospasm following tracheal intubation manifest improvement with ipratropium therapy, and prophylactic ipratropium administered before tracheal instrumentation decreases airway resistance following tracheal intubation in patients with a history of chronic cigarette smoking (Kil et al., 1994).

Effects of aerosol ipratropium on the heart rate and intraocular pressure, in contrast to atropine, do not occur, reflecting the minimal systemic absorption (<1% of the inhaled dose) of this quaternary ammonium drug. This limited absorption from the airways also accounts for a prolonged effect at the desired site of action. After inhalation of ipratropium, much of the dose is in fact swallowed, but absorption of unchanged drug from the gastrointestinal tract is insignificant. Effects of this drug on mucociliary activity and mucus secretion in the airways are minimal. Tolerance to the bronchodilator effect of ipratropium has not been observed. This is consistent with the concept that antagonists, in contrast to agonists, do not down-regulate but rather may up-regulate the target receptors.

Biliary and Ureteral Smooth Muscle Relaxation

Atropine decreases the tone of the smooth muscles of the biliary tract and ureter. This modest antispasmodic action, however, is unlikely to overcome opioid-induced spasm of the sphincter of Oddi. Conversely, atropine may prevent spasm of the ureter produced by morphine, supporting the custom of administering atropine with an opioid to manage pain due to a renal stone (renal colic). Therapeutic doses of atropine are thought to diminish the tone of the fundus of the bladder and to increase the tone of the vesicle sphincter, possibly contributing to urinary retention.

Mydriasis and Cycloplegia

Circular muscles of the iris that constrict the pupil are innervated by cholinergic fibers from the third cranial nerve, whereas fibers from the same nerve cause contraction of the ciliary muscles, allowing the lens to become more convex. Anticholinergic drugs placed topically on the cornea block the action of acetylcholine at both these sites, resulting in mydriasis and cycloplegia. Complete recovery from mydriasis and cycloplegia produced by topical atropine requires 7 to 14 days. In patients with glaucoma, relaxation of the ciliary muscles produced by an anticholinergic drug may occlude the angular space, whereas mydriasis obstructs passage of intraocular fluid into the venous circulation, resulting in potentially hazardous increases in intraocular pressure.

Doses of atropine used for preoperative medication are probably inadequate to increase intraocular pressure even in susceptible patients, assuming medications being used to treat glaucoma are continued. Indeed, mydriasis produced by an anticholinergic drug is completely offset by topical placement on the cornea of an anticholinesterase drug such as pilocarpine. Nevertheless, IM administration of scopolamine is a more potent mydriatic than atropine or glycopyrrolate, suggesting the need for caution in using this anticholinergic drug for preoperative medication in patients with glaucoma. IV administration of atropine or glycopyrrolate to prevent or treat reflex- or drug-mediated bradycardia does not produce sufficient tissue levels of the drug in the eye to produce adverse effects in patients with glaucoma.

Antagonism of Gastric Hydrogen Ion Secretion

Anticholinergic drugs have been administered for the control of peptic ulcer disease. Indeed, glycopyrrolate was originally introduced as an anticholinergic drug to control gastric acidity. Nevertheless, none of the anticholinergic drugs is selective for this effect, and the high doses required to inhibit hydrogen ion secretion by gastric parietal cells are often associated with unacceptable secretory, ocular, and cardiac side effects. Furthermore, the efficacy of H_2 receptor antagonists for decreasing hydrogen ion secretion has largely negated the use of anticholinergic drugs for this purpose.

Anticholinergic drugs have predictable effects on the tone and motility of the gastrointestinal tract because the parasympathetic nervous system provides almost exclusive motor innervation of this organ. As with suppression of gastric hydrogen ion secretion, however, large doses of anticholinergic drugs are necessary to alter gastrointestinal motility, often introducing unacceptable side effects. Nevertheless, high doses of anticholinergic drugs do prevent excess peristalsis of the gastrointestinal tract that would otherwise be associated with the administration of an anticholinesterase drug for the antagonism of nondepolarizing neuromuscular-blocking drugs.

Prevention of Motion-Induced Nausea

Transdermal absorption of scopolamine provides sustained therapeutic plasma concentrations that protect against motion-induced nausea without introducing prohibitive side effects such as sedation, cycloplegia, or drying of secretions. For example, a postauricular application of scopolamine delivers the drug at about 5 μg/hour for 72 hours (total absorbed dose is <0.5 mg). Protection against motion-induced nausea is greatest if the transdermal application of scopolamine is initiated at least 4 hours before the noxious stimulus. Administration of transdermal scopolamine after the onset of symptoms is less effective than prophylactic administration. Similar protection against motion-induced nausea by oral or IV administration of scopolamine would require large doses, resulting in undesirable side effects and subsequent poor patient acceptance.

Transdermal application of a scopolamine patch has been shown to exert significant antiemetic effects in patients experiencing motion sickness and in those treated with patient-controlled analgesia or epidural morphine for the management of postoperative pain (Honkavaara et al., 1994). It is well known that motion sickness is caused by stimulation of the vestibular apparatus. It has also been shown that morphine and synthetic opioids increase vestibular sensitivity. It is presumed that scopolamine blocks transmission to the medulla of impulses arising from overstimulation of the vestibular apparatus of the inner ear. Indeed, application of a scopolamine patch before the induction of anesthesia protects against nausea and vomiting after middle ear surgery that is likely to alter function of the vestibular apparatus (Honkavaara et al., 1994). Furthermore, a prophylactic transdermal scopolamine patch applied the evening before surgery decreases but does not abolish the occurrence of nausea and vomiting after outpatient laparoscopy using general anesthesia (Bailey et al., 1990). Conversely, not all reports describe an antiemetic effect in patients treated with transdermal scopolamine who are undergoing general anesthesia (Koski et al., 1990).

Anisocoria has been attributed to contamination of the eye after digital manipulation of the transdermal scopolamine patch (Price, 1985). More than 90% of unilateral dilated pupils occur on the same side as the patch. This diagnosis is confirmed by history and failure of the mydriasis to respond to topical installation of pilocarpine.

Constituents of Nonprescription Cold Remedies

Anticholinergic drugs are common constituents of nonprescription cold remedies. The apparent efficacy of these drugs is most likely due to inhibition of the production of upper airway secretions. With the exception of an allergic mechanism, it is also likely that contributions of antihistamines in cold remedies are primarily due to their anticholinergic effects.

Management of Parkinson Disease

Benzotropine (synthetic anticholinergic containing a tropine base of atropine and the benzohydryl portion of diphenhydramine) and trihexyphenidyl are used in the management of Parkinson disease for their effects on tremor, rigidity, and dystonia (see Chapter 31). These drugs are also useful for treating extrapyramidal side effects of antidopaminergic effects of drugs such as metoclopramide. Disadvantages of using anticholinergics in patients with Parkinson disease include memory impairment, hallucinations, visual blurring, and aggravation of glaucoma, especially in the elderly.

Treatment of Hiccups

Administration of atropine, 0.5 mg IV, has been described to be effective in terminating hiccups that follows placement of a laryngeal mask airway (Kanaya et al., 2001).

CENTRAL ANTICHOLINERGIC SYNDROME

Scopolamine and, to a lesser extent, atropine can enter the CNS and produce symptoms characterized as the central anticholinergic syndrome. Symptoms range from restlessness and hallucinations to somnolence and unconsciousness. Presumably, these responses reflect blockade of muscarinic cholinergic receptors and competitive inhibition of the effects of acetylcholine in the CNS. Glycopyrrolate does not easily cross the blood-brain barrier and thus is not likely to cause central anticholinergic syndrome. Nevertheless, central anticholinergic syndrome has been attributed to the IV administration of glycopyrrolate before the induction of anesthesia (Grum and Osborne, 1991).

Physostigmine, a lipid soluble tertiary amine anticholinesterase drug administered in doses of 15 to 60 μg/kg IV, is a specific treatment for the central anticholinergic syndrome. Treatment may need to be repeated every 1 to 2 hours. Edrophonium, neostigmine, and pyridostigmine are not effective antidotes because the quaternary ammonium structure prevents these drugs from easily entering the CNS. The central anticholinergic syndrome is often mistaken for delayed recovery from anesthesia. Ventilation may be depressed. Differentiation of this syndrome from other causes of perioperative confusion is possible with slow intravenous administration of physostigmine, 0.4 mg/kg.

OVERDOSE

Deliberate or accidental overdose with an anticholinergic drug produces a rapid onset of symptoms characteristic of muscarinic cholinergic receptor blockade. The mouth becomes dry, swallowing and talking is difficult, vision is blurred, photophobia is present, and tachycardia is prominent. The skin is dry and flushed, and a rash may appear especially over the face, neck, and upper chest (blush area). Even therapeutic doses of anticholinergic drugs sometimes may selectively dilate cutaneous vessels in the blush area. Body temperature is likely to be increased by anticholinergic drugs, especially when the environmental temperature is also increased. This increase in body temperature largely reflects inhibition of sweating by anticholinergic drugs, emphasizing that innervation of sweat glands is by sympathetic nervous system nerves that release acetylcholine as the neurotransmitter. Small children are particularly vulnerable to drug-induced increases in body temperature, with "atropine fever" occurring occasionally in this age group after administration of even a therapeutic dose of anticholinergic drug. Minute ventilation may be slightly increased due to CNS stimulation and the impact of an increased physiologic dead space due to bronchodilation. Arterial blood gases are usually unchanged. Skeletal muscle weakness and orthostatic hypotension, when present, reflect nicotinic cholinergic receptor blockade. Fatal events due to an overdose of an anticholinergic drug include seizures, coma, and medullary ventilatory center paralysis.

Small children and infants seem particularly vulnerable to developing life-threatening symptoms after an overdose with an anticholinergic drug. Physostigmine, administered in doses of 15 to 60 μg/kg IV, is the specific treatment for reversal of symptoms. Because physostigmine is metabolized rapidly, repeated doses of this anticholinesterase drug may be necessary to prevent the recurrence of symptoms.

DECREASED BARRIER PRESSURE

Barrier pressure is the difference between gastric pressure and lower esophageal sphincter pressure. Administration of atropine, 0.6 mg IV, or glycopyrrolate, 0.2 to 0.3 mg IV, decreases lower esophageal sphincter pressure, and thus decreases barrier pressure and the inherent resistance to reflux of acidic fluid into the esophagus (Cotton and Smith, 1981). This effect may persist longer with glycopyrrolate (60 minutes) than after administration of atropine (40 minutes). It is presumed, but not documented, that IM administration of anticholinergic drugs produces similar effects on lower esophageal sphincter pressure. The clinical significance, if any, of drug-induced decreases in lower esophageal sphincter pressure remains undocumented.

REFERENCES

Abboud T, Raya J, Sadri S, et al. Fetal and maternal cardiovascular effects of atropine and glycopyrrolate. *Anesth Analg* 1983;62:426–430.

Ali-Melkkila TM, Kaila T, Kanto J, et al. Pharmacokinetics of IM glycopyrronium. *Br J Anaesth* 1990;64:667–669.

Bailey PL, Streisland JB, Pace NL, et al. Transdermal scopolamine reduces nausea and vomiting after outpatient laparoscopy. *Anesthesiology* 1990;72:922–928.

Balamoutsos NG, Drossou FR, Alevizou FR, et al. Pupil size during reversal of muscle relaxants. *Anesth Analg* 1980;59:615–616.

Baraka A, Yared JP, Karam AM, et al. Glycopyrrolate-neostigmine, and atropine-neostigmine mixtures affect postanesthetic times differently. *Anesth Analg* 1980;59:431–434.

Bevan DR, Donati F, Kopman AF. Reversal of neuromuscular blockade. *Anesthesiology* 1992;77:785–805.

Caulfield MP. Muscarinic receptors-characterization, coupling and function. *Pharmacol Ther* 1993;58:319–325.

Cotton BR, Smith G. Comparison of the effects of atropine and glycopyrrolate on lower oesophageal sphincter pressure. *Br J Anaesth* 1981; 53:875–879.

Eger EI. Atropine, scopolamine, and related compounds. *Anesthesiology* 1962;23:365–383.

Gal TJ, Suratt PM. Atropine, and glycopyrrolate effects on lung mechanics in normal man. *Anesth Analg* 1981;60:85–90.

Garde JF, Aston R, Endler GC, et al. Racial mydriatic response to belladonna premedication. *Anesth Analg* 1978;57:572–576.

Goyal RK. Muscarinic receptor subtypes. Physiology and clinical implications. *N Engl J Med* 1989;321:1022–1028.

Gravenstein JS, Andersen TW, DePadua CB. Effects of atropine and scopolamine on the cardiovascular system in man. *Anesthesiology* 1964; 25:123–130.

Groeben H, Brown RH. Ipratropium decreases airway size in dogs by preferential M_2 muscarinic receptor blockade in vivo. *Anesthesiology* 1996;85:867–873.

Gross NJ. Ipratropium bromide. *N Engl J Med* 1988;319:486–494.

Grum DF, Osborne LR. Central anticholinergic syndrome following glycopyrrolate. *Anesthesiology* 1991;74:191–193.

Gunst SJ, Stropp JQ, Flavahan NA. Muscarinic receptor reserve and beta-adrenergic sensitivity in tracheal smooth muscle. *J Appl Physiol* 1989;67:1294–1299.

Honkavaara P, Saarnivaara L, Klemola UM. Prevention of nausea and vomiting with transdermal hyoscine in adults after middle ear surgery during general anaesthesia. *Br J Anaesth* 1994;73:763–766.

Kanaya N, Nakayama M, Kanaya J, et al. Atropine for the treatment of hiccup after laryngeal mask insertion. *Anesth Analg* 2001;93: 791–792.

Kil HK, Rooke GA, Ryan-Dykes MA, et al. Effect of prophylactic bronchodilator treatment on lung resistance after tracheal intubation. *Anesthesiology* 1994;81:43–48.

Kirvela M, Ali-Melkkila T, Kaila T, et al. Pharmacokinetics of glycopyrronium in uraemic patients. *Br J Anaesth* 1993;71:437–439.

Kirvela OA, Kanto JH, Raty HME, et al. Anticholinergic drugs: effects on oxygen consumption and energy expenditure. *Anesth Analg* 1994; 78:995–999.

Koski EMJ, Mattila MAK, Knapik D, et al. Double blind comparison of transdermal hyoscine and placebo for the prevention of postoperative nausea. *Br J Anaesth* 1990;64:16–20.

Lambert DG, Appadu BL. Muscarinic receptor subtypes: Do they have a place in clinical anaesthesia? *Br J Anaesth* 1995;74:497–499.

Meyers EF, Tomeldan SA. Glycopyrrolate compared with atropine in prevention of the oculocardiac reflex during eye muscle surgery. *Anesthesiology* 1979;51:350–352.

Murad SHN, Conklin KA, Tabsh KMA, Brinkman CR, Erkkola R, Nuwayhid B. Atropine and glycopyrrolate: hemodynamic effects and placental transfer in the pregnant ewe. *Anesth Analg* 1981;60: 710–714.

Parlow JL, van Vlymen JM, Odell MJ. The duration of impairment of autonomic control after anticholinergic drug administration in humans. *Anesth Analg* 1997;84:155–159.

Pedretti R, Etro MD, Laporta A, et al. Prediction of late arrhythmic events after acute myocardial infarction from combined use of noninvasive prognostic variables and inducibility of sustained monomorphic ventricular tachycardia. *Am J Cardiol* 1993;71: 1131–1141.

Price BH. Anisocoria from scopolamine patches. *JAMA* 1985;253:1561.

Proakis AG, Harris GB. Comparative penetration of glycopyrrolate and atropine across the blood-brain and placental barriers in anesthetized dogs. *Anesthesiology* 1978;48:339–344.

Simpson KH, Smith RJ, Davies LF. Comparison of the effects of atropine and glycopyrrolate on cognitive function following general anesthesia. *Br J Anaesth* 1987;59:966–969.

Tanito Y, Miwa T, Endou M, et al. Interaction of edrophonium with muscarinic acetylcholine M_2 and M_3 receptors. *Anesthesiology* 2001;94:804–814.

van Vlymen JM, Parlow JL. The effects of reversal of neuromuscular blockade on autonomic control in the perioperative period. *Anesth Analg* 1997;84:148–154.

11

Cyclooxygenase-2 Inhibitors and Nonspecific Nonsteroidal Antiinflammatory Drugs

Cyclooxygenase (COX) is an enzyme that catalyzes the synthesis of prostaglandins from arachidonic acid (Fig. 11-1) (Gajraj, 2003; Gilron et al., 2003). Prostaglandins mediate a large number of bodily processes including inflammation pain secretion of a protective gastric layer, maintenance of renal perfusion, and platelet aggregation. Nonsteroidal antiinflammatory drugs (NSAIDs) block the action of COX enzyme thus reducing the production of prostaglandin mediators. This results in both positive (analgesia, antiinflammatory) and negative (gastric ulceration, decreased renal perfusion, bleeding) effects (Tables 11-1 and 11-2). It is estimated that 30 billion NSAID tablets are ingested annually in the United States (Rajan and Ahlquist, 2003). The elderly consume a disproportionate share of these medications, perhaps reflecting the high prevalence of rheumatic diseases in this age group. Among those aged 65 years and older, it has been estimated that 10% to 15% take prescribed NSAIDs.

CYCLOOXYGENASE ENZYMES

COX activity is associated with two isoenzymes, ubiquitously and constitutively expressed as COX-1 and inflammation-inducible COX-2. COX-1 is found primarily in gastric mucosa, renal parenchyma, and platelets. COX-1 is only slightly up-regulated in response to inflammatory hormones. This enzyme is essesntial in homeostatic processes such as platelet aggregation, gastrointestinal mucosal integrity, and renal function. In contrast, COX-2 is inducible and is expressed mainly at sites of injury (brain and kidneys) and mediates inflammation, fever, pain, and carcinogenesis. COX-2 does not exert a protective role in the tissues in which it is present. Expression of COX-2 may facilitate several oncogenic processes, including tumor invasion, angiogenesis, and metastasis. Transient COX-2 up-regulation in the spinal cord in response to surgical inflammation may be important in central sensitization (Dolan et al., 2003). In response to inflammation, COX-2 expression is significantly up-regulated 10- to 20-fold.

NSAID-mediated suppression of prostaglandins and thromboxanes, which play a homeostatic role in the stomach (prostaglandin E_2 and prostaglandin I_2), kidneys (prostaglandin E_2), and platelets (thromboxane A_2 and prostaglandin I_2) is also thought to be the primary mechanism by which NSAIDs cause some of their adverse effects (see Table 11-1). In addition, inhibition of prostaglandin synthesis by NSAIDs is considered to be the mechanism underlying NSAID-induced bronchospasm and the suppression of new bone formation.

CLASSIFICATION OF NONSTEROIDAL ANTIINFLAMMATORY DRUGS

NSAID is an all-inclusive term denoting a varied group of drugs possessing analgesic, antiinflammatory, and antipyretic effects. These drugs can be categorized into conventional nonspecific inhibitors of both isoforms of COX (ibuprofen, naproxen, aspirin, acetaminophen, ketorolac)

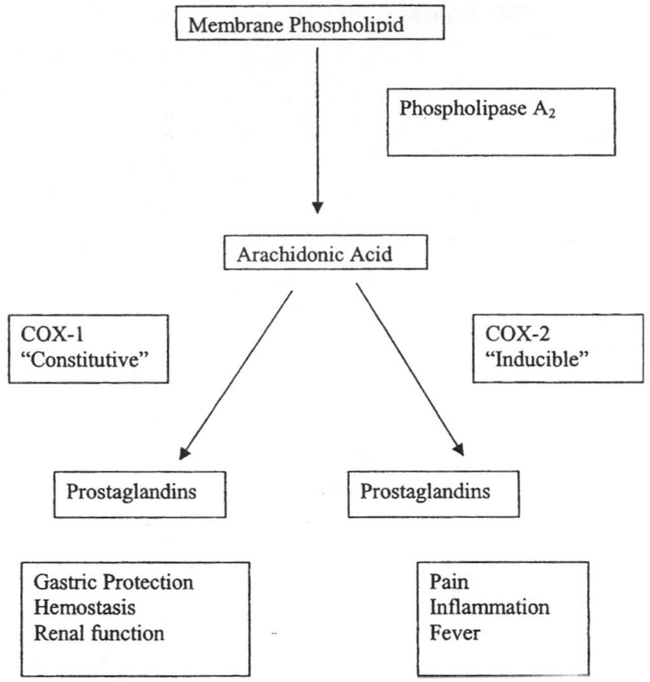

Figure 11-1. Cyclooxygenase (COX) pathways. (From Gilron I, Milne B, Hong M. Cyclooxygenase-2 inhibitors in postoperative pain management: Current evidence and future directions. *Anesthesiology* 2003;99:1198–1208; with permission).

and COX-2 selective inhibitors (celecoxib, rofecoxib, valdecoxib, parecoxib). All NSAIDs and COX-2 inhibitors have ceiling effects and exceeding this dose only increases the risk of drug-induced toxicity. Inhibition of COX-1 is responsible for many of the adverse side effects associated with conventional NSAIDs.

Conventional NSAIDs possess many desirable features (see Table 11-1) (Gajraj, 2003). The hypothesis that COX-1 mediates physiologic functions, whereas COX-2 is important in pathophysiologic processes, led to the development of selective COX-2 enzyme inhibitors (Fig. 11-2)

TABLE 11-1.
CHARACTERISTICS OF NONSTEROIDAL ANTIINFLAMMATORY DRUGS

Decrease activation and sensitization of peripheral nociceptors
Attenuate the inflammatory response
Absence of dependence or addiction potential
Synergistic effects with opioids
Preemptive analgesia (decreased neuronal sensitization)
Absence of depression of breathing
Less nausea and vomiting compared with opioids
Long duration of action
Less dose variability compared with opioids
No pupillary changes
Absence of cognitive effects

Adapted from Gajraj NM. Cyclooxygenase-2 inhibitors. *Anesth Analg* 2003;96:1720–1738.

TABLE 11-2.
POTENTIAL ADVERSE EFFECTS PRODUCED BY NONSTEROIDAL ANTIINFLAMMATORY DRUGS

Inhibition of platelet aggregation
Gastric ulceration
Renal dysfunction
Hepatocellular injury
Asthma exacerbation
Allergic reactions
Tinnitus
Urticaria

(Gajraj, 2003). COX-2 inhibitors represent a significant therapeutic advance because of their improved side-effect profile compared with conventional NSAIDs.

CYCLOOXYGENASE-2 SPECIFIC INHIBITORS

Selective COX-2 specific enzyme inhibitors exhibit analgesic efficacy, comparable with that of conventional antiinflammatory drugs (NSAIDs) (Gajraj, 2003). These drugs lack effects on platelets at therapeutic doses and may be associated with decreased gastrointestinal side effects in patients with arthritis, compared with nonspecific NSAIDs. The risk of acute myocardial infarction and cerebrovascular accident may be increased in patients treated chronically with selective COX-2–specific enzyme inhibitors. Furthermore, the analgesic effects of these drugs may not be superior to that provided by historically older drugs.

Celecoxib

Celecoxib was the first selective COX-2 inhibitor to become clinically available in 1998, and it is recommended

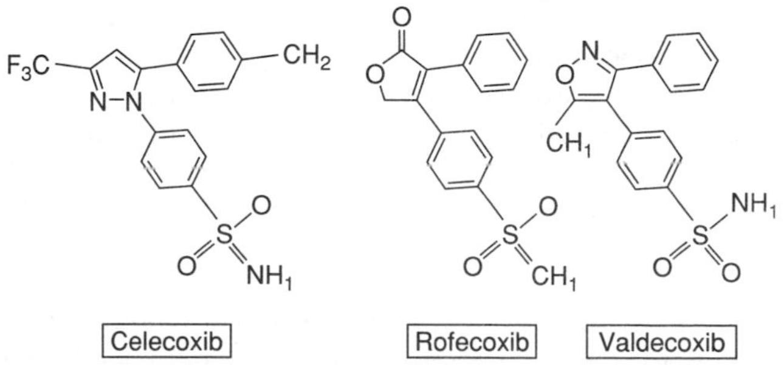

Figure 11-2. Chemical structure of cyclooxygenase-2 inhibitors. Rofecoxib is no longer clinically available. (From Gilron I, Milne B, Hong M. Cyclooxygenase-2 inhibitors in postoperative pain management: Current evidence and future directions. *Anesthesiology* 2003; 99:1198–1208; with permission.)

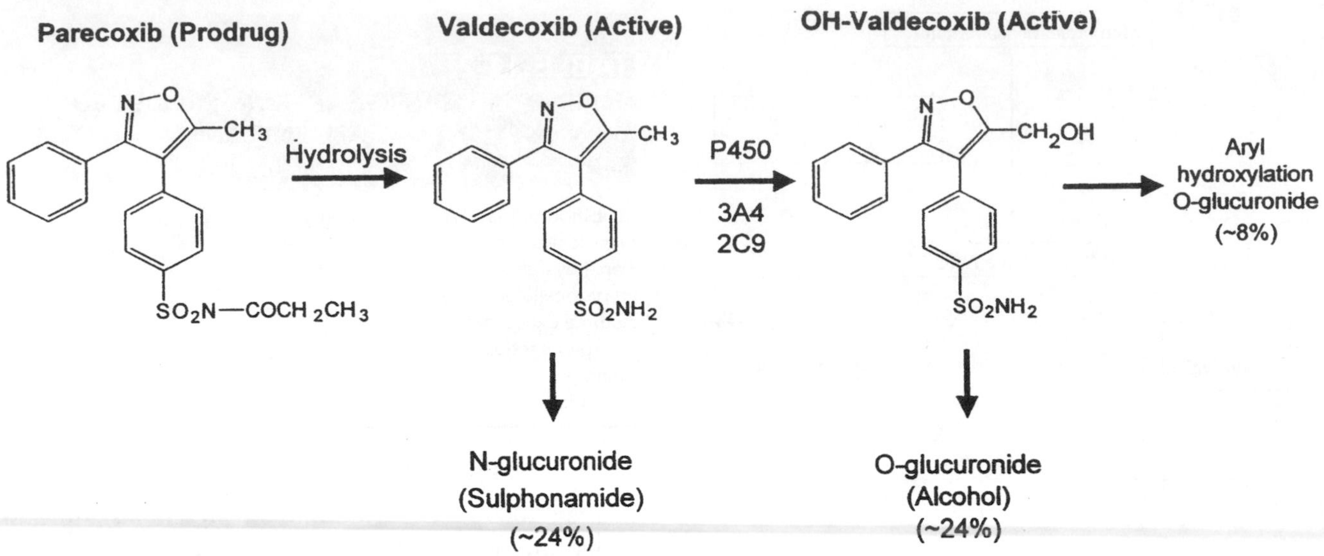

Figure 11-3. Metabolic pathways of parecoxib. (Ibraham A, Park S, Feldman J, et al. Effects of parecoxib, a parenteral COX-2-specific inhibitor, on the pharmacokinetics and pharmacodynamics of propofol. *Anesthesiology* 2002a;96:88-95; with permission).

for the treatment of pain and inflammation associated with osteoarthritis and rheumatoid arthritis. For patients with osteoarthritis, an initial dosage of 200 mg daily is recommended. In patients with rheumatoid arthritis, a dose of 100 to 200 mg twice daily is recommended.

Rofecoxib

Rofecoxib is used for acute pain associated with surgery, beginning with a loading dose of 50 mg followed by 25 mg daily. Treatment of dental pain with rofecoxib 50 mg produces analgesia similar to naproxen and ibuprofen. A single daily dose of 12.5 to 25 mg is recommended for patients with osteoarthritis. A loading dose of 50 mg followed by a further 25 mg daily is recommended for the treatment of menstrual pain associated with primary dysmenorrhea and is equivalent to 550 mg of naproxen. A long-term study to determine the possible protective effect of rofecoxib against the development of cancerous colon polyps revealed a doubling of the risk of myocardial infarction and cerebrovascular accidents in treated patients resulting in the withdrawal of this drug from the market in October 2004.

Valdecoxib

Valdecoxib 40 mg may be administered 1 hour before surgery for relief of postoperative pain and an additional 40 mg after surgery if needed. The recommended dose for treatment of osteoarthritis and rheumatoid arthritis is 10 mg daily. A twice daily dose of 20 mg or a once daily dose of 40 mg is recommended for treatment of menstrual pain associated with primary dysmenorrhea.

Parecoxib

Parecoxib is the only COX-2-specific inhibitor that is available as a parenteral form. For postoperative pain relief, parecoxib 40 mg is administered 1 hour before the surgical procedure and an additional 40 mg after surgery if needed. The dose may be increased to 80 mg in selected patients. Parecoxib is a prodrug that is converted in vivo to valdecoxib (Fig. 11-3) (Iabrahim et al, 2002a).

Pharmacokinetics

As a class of drugs, the NSAIDs are well absorbed from the gastrointestinal tract, have low first-pass hepatic extraction, are highly bound (>95%) to plasma albumin, and exhibit small volumes of distribution. The more lipid-soluble NSAIDs cross the blood-brain barrier more effectively and may have greater central nervous system (CNS) effects (changes in mood and cognition). Most NSAIDs are weakly acidic, with a pK of 3 to 5. The proportion of an NSAID that is not ionized at a particular pH is important because it influences the distribution of these drugs in tissues. For example, acidic NSAIDs become sequestered preferentially in the synovial tissue of inflamed joints, which may be of potential advantage during episodes of arthritis.

Selective COX-2 inhibitors are chemically distinct compounds with differing pharmacokinetics (Table 11-3) (Gajraj, 2003). These drugs differ from nonspecific NSAIDs in that they are all highly lipophilic, neutral, nonacidic molecules with very limited solubility in aqueous media. Celecoxib is a sulfonamide that is extensively distributed into tissues. Metabolism is by cytochrome P-450 enzymes

TABLE 11-3.
PHARMACOKINETICS OF CYCLOOXGYENASE-2 INHIBITORS

	Celecoxib	Rofecoxib*	Valdecoxib
Molecular weight	381.38	314.36	314.36
Elimination half-time (hrs)	12	17	8–11
Volume of distribution (L)	400	86–89	86
Protein binding (%)	98	87	98

*Withdrawn from the market in October 2004 because of an increased incidence of myocardial infarction and cerebrovascular accident in patients treated for longer than 18 months.

to hydroxy, carboxylic acid, and glucuronide derivatives with about 2% of the drug being excreted unchanged by the kidneys. Rofecoxib is a sulfone that is not as well distributed in tissues and is metabolized principally by cytosolic reduction in the liver and <1% appears unchanged in the urine. In this regard, important interactions between rofecoxib and other P450 inhibitors are unlikely. Parecoxib is a parenterally administered inactive prodrug that undergoes rapid amide hydrolysis in vivo to the pharmacologically active COX-2 inhibitor, valdecoxib (Fig. 11-3) (Ibrahim et al., 2002a). Valdecoxib is metabolized primarily to 1-hydroxyvaldecoxib by hepatic cytochrome P450 enzymes. Because both parecoxib and valdecoxib are inhibitors of P-450, there is a potential for these COX-2 inhibitors to inhibit metabolism of other drugs. Propofol is the most commonly used anesthetic drug that undergoes metabolism by P-450 and single dose parecoxib in doses used for postoperative pain management does not alter the disposition or duration of action of propofol (Ibrahim et al., 2002a). Likewise, midazolam is dependent on P450 enzymes for metabolism and parecoxib does not alter the pharmacokinetics or pharmacodynamics of midazolam infusion (Ibrahim et al, 2002b).

Clinical Uses

The perceived beneficial effects of COX-2 inhibitors have resulted in wide-ranging use of these drugs for a variety of indications especially for conditions associated with inflammation and pain (Table 11-4) (Gajraj, 2003).

Analgesic Efficacy

COX-2 inhibitors are useful in the management of patients experiencing pain owing to osteoarthritis, rheumatoid arthritis, acute gout, and dysmenorrhea (Table 11-2) (Gajraj, 2003). Indeed, the majority of adverse effects of

TABLE 11-4.
CLINICAL USES OF CYLCOOXYGENASE-2 INHIBITORS

Drug	Clinical Uses	Dosage
Celecoxib	Osteoarthritis	200 mg every day or 100 mg twice daily
	Rheumatoid arthritis	100–200 mg twice daily
	Familial adenomatous polyposis	400 mg twice daily
	Acute pain and primary dysmenorrhea	400 mg initially, followed by an additional 200 mg if needed, then 200 mg twice daily if needed
Rofecoxib*	Acute pain	50 mg every day
	Osteoarthritis	25 mg every day
	Rheumatoid arthritis	50 mg every day
	Primary dysmenorrhea	50 mg every day
Parecoxid	Acute pain	40 mg every day
Valdecoxib	Acute pain	40 mg every day
	Osteoarthritis	10 mg every day
	Rheumatoid arthritis	10 mg every day
	Primary dysmenorrhea	20 mg twice daily if needed

*Withdrawn from the market in October 2004 because of an increased incidence of myocardial infarction and cerebrovascular accident in patients treated for longer than 18 months
Adapted from Gajraj NM. Cyclooxygenase-2 inhibitors. *Anesth Analg* 2003;96:1720–1738.

NSAIDs are in patients receiving these drugs chronically for the treatment of arthritis. Pain associated with musculoskeletal conditions is effectively treated with COX-2 inhibitors. Acute postoperative pain as associated with major orthopedic surgery and arthroscopy is responsive to COX-2 inhibitors and the lack of antiplatelet effects allows these drugs to be continued throughout the perioperative period. The efficacy of COX-2 inhibitors has been established for dental pain.

Postoperative Pain Management

The administration of NSAIDs is one of the most common nonopioid analgesic techniques used for postoperative pain management (White, 2002). In contrast to the dose-dependent analgesic effects of opioids, NSAIDs appear to exhibit a ceiling effect when used for postoperative analgesia (Fig. 11-2) (O'Hara et al., 1987). NSAIDs are believed to reduce postoperative pain by suppressing COX-mediated production of prostaglandin E_2, which is thought to be the primary inflammatory prostaglandin that directly activates and up-regulates the sensitivity of peripheral nociceptors to cause pain. Prostaglandins have also been shown to cross the blood-brain barrier and exert a role in spinal nociception, thus supporting a spinal analgesic mechanism of NSAIDs. Opioid requirements for postoperative pain management are decreased 20% to 50% by NSAIDs (Kharasch, 2004). COX-2 is constitutively expressed in brain and spinal cord and is up-regulated after persistent noxious inputs such that spinal COX-2 inhibition may be important for decreasing postinjury hyperalgesia.

Postoperative analgesia produced by COX-2 inhibitors is similar to conventional nonselective NSAIDs (Gilron et al., 2003). The primary advantage of COX-2 inhibitors compared with nonselective NSAIDs is the lack of effects on platelet function and bleeding and hence the opportunity for preoperative and postoperative administration (Kharasch, 2004). Furthermore, COX-2 inhibitors may be acceptable (based on data from chronic treatment of patients with arthritis) for administration to patients with a history of gastritis or gastric ulcers who cannot receive conventional NSAIDs. In addition, COX-2 inhibitors may represent a safer alternative to nonselective NSAIDs because they are well tolerated by patients with asthma (McCrory and Lindahl, 2002).

Perioperative inhibition of COX enzyme by NSAIDs may cause serious complications including renal injury, gastric ulceration, and excessive bleeding. Brief perioperative NSAID use in otherwise healthy adults does not seem to cause significant renal dysfunction. Gastrointestinal ulceration or bleeding may occur after even brief use of NSAIDs making this an important risk to consider when selecting these drugs for postoperative pain management. The rare potential for excessive postoperative bleeding owing to NSAIDs is a consideration in selecting NSAIDs to manage postoperative pain. Screening for renal dysfunction, gastritis, gastric ulcers, or bleeding diathesis will minimize these complications.

Protection Against Colorectal Cancer

COX-2 expression increases significantly in most human colorectal cancers. In this regard, chronic use of aspirin and other conventional NSAIDs reduces the risk of colorectal cancer by 40% to 50% (Smalley et al., 1999). The number and size of colon adenomas is decreased by treatment with conventional NSAIDs. COX-2 inhibitors inhibit colon tumor growth in animals and in patients with familial adenomatous polyposis, the administration of celecoxib decreased the number of polyps (Steinbach et al., 2000). Protective effects against esophageal cancer, gastric cancer, and breast cancer may result from treatment with NSAIDs (Half et al., 2002).

Protection Against Dementia

The risk of developing Alzheimer's disease is decreased among those who use NSAIDs (t'Veld et al., 2001). This effect may reflect a decrease in inflammatory processes that result in neuronal destruction

Side Effects

Gastrointestinal Toxicity

NSAID-induced gastrointestinal toxicity is one of the most common drug-related adverse events with upper gastrointestinal endoscopy studies, showing a 15% to 30% incidence of ulcers in the stomach or duodenum of patients taking NSAIDs regularly (Laine, 1996). Concomitant therapy with histamine-2 receptor antagonists, proton pump inhibitors, or misoprostol decreases the incidence of gastrointestinal ulcers associated with NSAIDs (Rostom et al., 2000). Because prostaglandins are involved in the maintenance of gastrointestinal mucosal integrity and because only COX-1 is present in the gastrointestinal tract, it is presumed that gastrointestinal toxicity produced by nonselective NSAIDs is due principally to inhibition of COX-1 activity. Prostaglandins normally protect gastrointestinal mucosa from damage by maintaining mucosal blood flow and increasing mucosal secretion of mucus and bicarbonate. Blockade of COX-1 activity by NSAIDs decreases prostaglandin synthesis and thus lowers gastrointestinal mucosal blood flow and secretion of mucus and bicarbonate. Indeed, the incidence of gastrointestinal side effects (gastric and duodenal ulcers) is decreased about 50% in patients treated with selective COX-2 inhibitors (Bombardier, 2002). Patients with osteoarthritis and rheumatoid arthritis receiving supratherapeutic doses of celecoxib (400 mg twice daily) had a significantly lower incidence of symptomatic ulcers and ulcer complications compared with patients receiving standard therapeutic doses of conventional NSAIDs (Silverstein et al., 2000). However, gastric perforation has been reported in a patient recovering from a gastric ulcer who was treated with celecoxib (Reuben and Steinberg, 1999).

There is no evidence that NSAIDs contribute to gastroesophageal reflux disease. Some NSAID preparations are irritating to the esophageal mucosa, and esophagitis can result if the tablet remains in the esophagus ("pill esophagitis"). Patients with esophageal strictures may be especially susceptible to NSAID-induced esophageal injury.

Corticosteroids, which block COX-2 but not COX-1, are no longer considered ulcerogenic when administered as monotherapy, although they may impair healing of preexisting ulcers. When corticosteroids are administered in combination with nonselective NSAIDs, the risk of ulcer formation is greater than when NSAIDs are used alone.

Coagulation Effects

Platelet aggregation and hemostasis depend on the ability of platelets to generate thromboxane A_2 from prostaglandins. Because platelets do not contain COX-2, all synthesis of thromboxane A_2 in platelets is mediated by COX-1. Conventional nonspecific NSAIDs inhibit COX-1 and impair the ability of platelets to aggregate. Patients receiving anticoagulation therapy should be monitored when receiving nonspecific NSAIDs, especially aspirin which has irreversible effects on platelets. COX-2 inhibitors do not appear to have any significant interactions with anticoagulant drugs (Davies et al., 2000). Preoperative NSAID therapy significantly increases intraoperative and postoperative blood loss in children undergoing tonsillectomy (Marret et al., 2003). COX-2 inhibitors have no effect on platelet aggregation, bleeding time or postoperative blood loss (Leese et al., 2003; Joshi et al., 2003). Thrombotic events may occur more frequently in patients treated with COX-2 inhibitors compared with traditional NSAIDs. Aspirin (75 to 325 mg per day) induces an irreversible inactivation of platelet COX that lasts for the life of the platelet (7 to 10 days) (Schror, 1996).

Cardiac Effects

The risk of experiencing a thrombotic episode or a myocardial infarction may be increased in patients treated with COX-2 inhibitors (Mukherjee et al., 2002). This may reflect COX-2 inhibitor selective suppression of prostaglandin I_2 (vasoprotective) without affecting thromboxane A_2 (procoagulant) (FitzGerald, 2004). An increased risk of myocardial infarction and cerebrovascular accident in patients treated for prolonged periods (18 months or longer) resulted in the withdrawal of rofecoxib from the market in October 2004. There may be an increased incidence of congestive heart failure in patients treated with COX-2 inhibitors. Furthermore, COX-2 inhibitors may serve a protective role by mediating delayed preconditioning against myocardial infarction and stunning (Alcindor et al., 2004). Compared with rofecoxib, naproxen is associated with less of a risk of myocardial infarction, although this drug offers less protection than aspirin.

Hypertensive Effects

Prostaglandins modulate systemic blood pressure by virtue of effects on vascular tone in arteriolar smooth muscle and control of extracellular fluid volume. Prostaglandins counteract the response to vasoconstrictor hormones and can influence sodium balance as a result of their natriuretic effects. It is predictable that NSAIDs may interfere with the pharmacologic control of systemic hypertension, although the average effects of these drugs on blood pressure control is usually quite small (about 5 mm Hg) (Gurwitz et al., 1994; deLeeuw, 1996).

Renal Effects

NSAIDs have no adverse effects on renal function in healthy individuals (Clive and Stoff, 1984). When renal toxicity does manifest, it is likely due to NSAID-induced inhibition of prostaglandin synthesis, leading to renal medullary ischemia. Prostaglandins participate in the autoregulation of renal blood flow and glomerular filtration and also influence the tubular transport of ions and water. Tubulointerstitial nephritis caused by NSAIDs (analgesic nephropathy) was originally shown to be associated with chronic ingestion of phenacetin, which was withdrawn from the market for this reason. Acetaminophen is a phenacetin metabolite that has been associated with an increased incidence of end-stage renal disease (ESRD). It has been estimated that decreased consumption of acetaminophen could lower the incidence of ESRD by 8% to 10% (Perneger et al., 1994). Factors favoring NSAID-induced nephrotoxicity include hypovolemia, preexisting renal disease, congestive heart failure, sepsis, combination with other potentially nephrotoxic drugs or radiographic contrast material, diabetes mellitus, and cirrhosis. There is general agreement that no NSAID other than aspirin can be prescribed with absolute safety with respect to adverse renal effects.

Nonselective NSAIDs interfere with production of vasodilating prostaglandins and may result in decreases in glomerular filtration rate and sodium retention manifesting as systemic hypertension and edema. The nephrotoxic potential of NSAIDs is increased in patients who require prostaglandins for renal vasodilation. Prerenal azotemia reflecting decreased renal perfusion is the most frequent pattern of renal injury related to the use of NSAIDs. Elderly patients are at increased risk for nephrotoxicity in patients treated with NSAIDs. Hyperchloremic metabolic acidosis often in association with hyperkalemia is an effect of NSAIDs particularly in patients with preexisting renal disease. Renal and cardiovascular effects of COX-2 inhibitors are similar to conventional NSAIDs (Harris, 2002). There is evidence that preoperative administration of NSAIDs (ketorolac) to well-hydrated patients anesthetized with sevoflurane does not produce glomerular or tubular dysfunction (Laisalmi et al., 2001). Conversely, postoperative acute renal failure has been observed in an otherwise healthy patient who was taking ibuprofen preoperatively (Sivarajan and Wasse, 1997).

Hepatic Effects

Increases in plasma concentrations of liver transaminases may accompany treatment with NSAIDs. Rare cases of severe hepatic dysfunction with jaundice and hepatic failure may occur during therapy with NSAIDs. If clinical signs and symptoms of liver dysfunction occur, COX-2 therapy should be discontinued.

Allergy

Sulfonamide hypersensitivity is a contraindication to treatment with celecoxib and valdecoxib. COX-2 inhibitors should not be administered to patients who have experienced asthma, urticaria, or allergic-type reactions to aspirin. Patients with respiratory sensitivity to aspirin generally develop dose-dependent reactions to aspirin or COX-1, whereas COX-2 inhibitors are usually well tolerated in these patients.

Asthma

NSAIDs may trigger bronchoconstriction in susceptible asthmatic patients by blocking COX-mediated conversion of arachidonic acid to prostaglandins, especially prostaglandin E_2 which is a potent antiinflammatory substance. This inhibition of prostaglandin production results in shunting of arachidonic acid toward the lipoxygenase pathway and ultimate production of bronchoconstrictor and proinflammatory leukotrienes. A history of asthma exacerbation on exposure to aspirin is a reason to avoid NSAIDs that inhibit COX-1 and COX-2. Nevertheless, the COX-2 inhibitor rofecoxib may be safe in aspirin-sensitive patients. Sodium salicylate, salicylamide, and dextropropoxyphene do not inhibit COX enzymes and can be safely administered to aspirin-sensitive patients.

Aseptic Meningitis

Aseptic meningitis may follow systemic drug administration. Drug-induced meningitis has been observed following administration of NSAIDs (especially ibuprofen) and H_2 receptor antagonists (Burke and Wildsmith, 1997). Signs and symptoms typically appear within a few hours after drug ingestion, but may be delayed for weeks. In addition to the usual features of meningitis, there may be periorbital edema, conjunctivitis, hypotension, parotitis, pancreatitis, fatigue, and seizures. Fever is common. Most patients recover fully when the drug is discontinued. The syndrome is more common in females with underlying autoimmune or collagen vascular disease and is presumed to reflect an acute hypersensitivity reaction. Aseptic meningitis attributed to central nerve block (spinal anesthesia) must be differentiated from drug-induced meningitis.

Bone Healing

NSAIDs may impair bone healing such that these drugs are not recommended for patients undergoing spinal fusion surgery. Earlier suggestions that COX-2 inhibitors did not interfere with bone healing have not been substantiated (Matsumura, 2001).

Drug Interactions

The most common drug interaction is between oral anticoagulants and NSAIDs, resulting in an increased risk of gastrointestinal hemorrhage. Concomitant administration of NSAIDs including COX-2 inhibitors and aspirin increases the risk of gastrointestinal ulceration. COX-2 inhibitors may increase plasma warfarin concentrations, emphasizing the need to monitor anticoagulant therapy. The combination of NSAIDs and potassium-sparing diuretics may increase the risk of hyperkalemia. NSAID-induced decreases in renal function may decrease the clearance of drugs such as digoxin, lithium, and aminoglycoside antibiotics. NSAIDs may interfere with the antihypertensive actions of beta-adrenergic antagonists, diuretics, and angiotensin-converting enzyme inhibitors. Plasma lithium concentrations may increase during treatment with COX-2 inhibitors.

NONSPECIFIC CYCLOOXYGENASE INHIBITORS

NSAIDs that are classified as nonspecific COX inhibitors are represented by a variety of chemical classifications (Table 11-5). These drugs possess analgesic, antiinflammatory, and platelet inhibitory effects. Comparative trials have rarely revealed clinically important differences between these drugs, especially as utilized to treat patients with osteoarthritis or rheumatoid arthritis (Brooks and Day, 1991). Variability between patients in responsiveness and preference for different NSAIDs may reflect fluctuations in the intensity of the inflammatory and noninflammatory rheumatologic diseases that might coincide with exposure to a particular NSAID.

Aspirin (Acetylsalicylic Acid)

Aspirin is an example of a salicylate that produces analgesia through its ability to irreversibly acetylate COX enzyme, leading to a decrease in the synthesis and release of prostaglandins (see Fig. 20-1). Aspirin is a relatively weak inhibitor of renal prostaglandin synthesis and is unlikely to exert any clinically relevant effect at doses below the

TABLE 11-5.
CHEMICAL CLASSIFICATION OF NONSPECIFIC NONSTEROIDAL ANTIINFLAMMATORY DRUGS

Carboxylic acids
Acetylated: aspirin
Nonacetylated: sodium salicylate, salicylamide, diflunisal
Acetic acids
Indomethacin, sulindac, tolmetin
Propionic acids
Ibuprofen, naproxen, fenoprofen, ketoprofen
Enolic acids
Phenylbutazone, piroxicam
Pyrrolopyrrole
Ketorolac

antiinflammatory range (Patrono, 1994). The leukotriene pathway remains intact in the presence of aspirin. Aspirin does not interact with opioid receptors and has little effect on release of histamine or serotonin. Aspirin is rapidly hydrolyzed to salicylic acid (orthohydroxybenzoic acid), which lacks acetylating capacity but inhibits prostaglandin synthesis by a nonacetylation mechanism.

Pharmacokinetics

Aspirin is rapidly absorbed from the small intestine and, to a lesser extent, from the stomach. The rate of absorption is influenced by dissolution rates of the administered tablet and gastric emptying time. If gastric pH is increased, aspirin is more ionized and the rate of absorption is decreased. The presence of food also delays absorption from the gastrointestinal tract. There is no conclusive evidence that sodium bicarbonate given with aspirin (buffered aspirin) has a faster onset of action, greater peak intensity, or longer analgesic effect. In fact, alkalinization of the urine may increase urinary excretion of aspirin, requiring administration of a larger dose to achieve the same plasma concentration. Aspirin that is available in buffered effervescent preparations, however, undergoes more rapid absorption and achieves higher plasma concentrations than the corresponding tablet formulations. These effervescent preparations also cause less gastrointestinal irritation.

Clearance

After absorption into the systemic circulation, aspirin is rapidly hydrolyzed in the liver to salicylic acid. As a result of this rapid hydrolysis, plasma concentrations of aspirin are rarely >20 μg/mL. Nevertheless, aspirin is pharmacologically active and does not require hydrolysis to salicylic acid for its effects. Metabolism of salicylic acid also occurs in the liver, where it is conjugated with glycine to form salicyluric acid. Salicyluric acid is excreted in the urine along with free salicylic acid. Renal excretion of free salicylic acid is highly variable—from up to 85% of the ingested drug when the urine is alkaline to as low as 5% in acidic urine. Plasma concentrations of salicylic acid are increased in the presence of renal dysfunction that is characterized by decreased glomerular filtration rate or decreased secretory activity of proximal renal tubules. The elimination half-time for aspirin is 15 to 20 minutes and for salicylic acid is 2 to 3 hours.

Clinical Uses

Aspirin is most often administered as an (a) analgesic for the symptomatic relief of low-intensity pain associated with headache and with musculoskeletal disorders, such as osteoarthritis and rheumatoid arthritis; (b) antipyretic; and (c) antiplatelet drug for prevention of myocardial infarction and certain forms of ischemic stroke (Patrono, 1994; Schror, 1995). The use of aspirin to treat patients with rheumatoid arthritis has decreased substantially with the availability of COX-1 and COX-2 drugs.

The analgesic action of aspirin is confined to a small dose range, below which there is little effect and above which an increase in dose produces toxic effects with little increase in analgesia. Aspirin is effective as an antipyretic by virtue of its ability to prevent pyrogen-induced release of prostaglandins in the CNS, including the hypothalamus. This is consistent with the known pyrogenic effect of most prostaglandins.

Aspirin is a mainstay therapy for patients experiencing angina and acute myocardial infarction (Collins et al., 1997). It is recommended that aspirin be administered as soon as the diagnosis of myocardial infarction is confirmed. Inhibition of COX-dependent platelet activation may well be responsible for most or all of the protective effects of aspirin. The current recommendation for the dose of aspirin to decrease the incidence of occlusive cardiovascular events in patients at risk for these events is administration of a single loading dose of 200 to 300 mg followed by a daily dose of 75 to 100 mg (Patrono, 1994). In patients with unstable angina, the addition of heparin to aspirin therapy further decreases the risk of myocardial infarction (Oler et al., 1996).

The antiplatelet effect of low-dose aspirin (75 to 325 mg per day) is due to irreversible acetylation of platelet COX-1 by nonhydrolyzed aspirin with the resulting prevention of thromboxane generation. Thromboxane is a potent inducer of platelet release and aggregation. This inhibitory effect is rapid, occurring even before the appearance of aspirin in the systemic circulation, probably as a result of the acetylation of platelet prostaglandin synthase in the portal circulation. Thus, the antiplatelet effect of aspirin is unrelated to its systemic bioavailability. A daily aspirin maintenance dose of 40 mg is sufficient to cause an apparently complete inhibition of platelet COX-1 as evidenced by >95% decrease in serum thromboxane concentrations (Schror, 1995). Ingestion of aspirin 600 mg prolongs the bleeding time by 2 to 3 minutes. Some apparently normal patients manifest marked sensitivity to the effects of aspirin so that their bleeding times are very much prolonged and they have clinically significant bleeding, particularly during or after surgery or trauma. These patients most likely have a mild form of von Willebrand disease. Uremic patients are especially sensitive to bleeding induced by aspirin. A small dose of aspirin that does not prolong the bleeding time of normal patients may prolong bleeding time as much as 15 minutes in uremic patients. Prostaglandins may play a role in the maintenance of patent ductus arteriosus, and drugs that inhibit synthesis of prostaglandins, such as indomethacin, have been used with limited success in neonates to evoke closure of the ductus arteriosus. Excessive production of prostaglandins is present in Bartter's syndrome, and aspirin-like drugs have been used successfully in its treatment.

Side Effects

Major adverse side effects of aspirin therapy are related to gastrointestinal tract dysfunction and inhibition of platelet function. Other side effects include CNS stimulation, hepatic and renal dysfunction, metabolic alterations, uterine effects, and allergic reactions (Schror, 1995; Settipane, 1981; Willard et al., 1992). Epidemiologic evidence has suggested the possibility of an association between the use of aspirin in the treatment of fever in children and the development of Reye syndrome.

Gastric Irritation and Ulceration

Gastrointestinal intolerance is the most common adverse effect of aspirin and is related to the dose administered. However, even low dose aspirin as utilized for cardiovascular prophylaxis may cause gastrointestinal bleeding. Presumably, aspirin-induced decreases in prostaglandin synthesis, which normally inhibits gastric acid secretion, contribute to gastric mucosa ulceration. Resulting hemorrhage manifests as heme test–positive stools and, in severe examples, iron-deficiency anemia. When the aspirin dose is 325 mg administered on alternate days, the incidence of reported gastrointestinal symptoms is only 0.5% greater than in placebo-treated patients (Willard et al., 1992). Gastrointestinal intolerance can be largely prevented by using enteric-coated tablets.

Prolongation of Bleeding Time

Aspirin induces a long-lasting functional defect in platelets that is clinically detectable as a prolongation of the bleeding time (see Table 11-3) (Smith et al., 1996). This platelet dysfunction reflects prevention of the formation of thromboxane, which is a potent stimulant for platelet aggregation. Platelets are exquisitely sensitive to even small doses of aspirin. Aspirin-induced platelet inhibition is irreversible and lasts for the entire life span of the platelet. Furthermore, large doses of aspirin administered chronically decrease production of prothrombin, leading to prolonged prothrombin time. Aspirin should be avoided in patients with severe hepatic dysfunction, vitamin K deficiency, hypoprothrombinemia, or hemophilia because inhibition of platelet aggregation in these patients can result in hemorrhage. Hemorrhagic events, including easy bruising, melena, and epistaxis, are more frequent among patients receiving aspirin.

Aspirin is a ubiquitous ingredient in a variety of over-the-counter preparations such that patients undergoing surgery, even in the absence of medically directed aspirin therapy as for protection against myocardial infarction, may be exposed unknowingly to aspirin. Indeed, preoperative aspirin therapy may increase chest tube drainage and bleeding in patients undergoing coronary artery bypass surgery, but an increased need for blood transfusion in these patients has not been demonstrated (Levy, 1994; Reich et al., 1994; Tuman et al., 1996).

Aspirin ingestion within the previous 7 to 10 days is often considered a relative contraindication to performing invasive surgical procedures. However, aspirin is an important component to the treatment of many patients and withholding therapy for this time may not be prudent. In fact, the practice of withholding aspirin for a prolonged period preoperatively may not be necessary as the aspirin-induced effect as reflected by bleeding time has largely disappeared by 48 hours (Sonksen et al., 1999)

Central Nervous System Stimulation

Excessive doses of aspirin may produce stimulation of the CNS manifesting as hyperventilation and seizures. Hyperventilation is due to direct stimulation of the medullary ventilatory center. Initially, these changes result in respiratory alkalosis, which is promptly compensated for by renal excretion of bicarbonate, sodium, and potassium ions with return of the pH toward normal. Ultimately, however, salicylate overdose is likely to progress to metabolic and respiratory acidosis. Metabolic acidosis reflects depression of renal function with accumulation of strong metabolic acids in addition to derangement of carbohydrate metabolism, leading to an increased formation of pyruvic, lactic, and acetoacetic acids. Adults, in contrast to children, however, rarely develop metabolic acidosis regardless of the severity of the overdose. Hyperthermia and dehydration may be life-threatening results of salicylate overdose.

Tinnitus associated with increased plasma concentrations of salicylates reflects drug-induced increases in labyrinthine pressure or an effect on hair cells of the cochlea. This side effect is the earliest sign of salicylate overdose. Nausea and vomiting are due to irritation of gastric mucosa at low doses and stimulation of the medullary chemoreceptor trigger zone by large doses.

Correction of metabolic acidosis is crucial in the treatment of salicylate overdose because a decrease in pH causes a shift of salicylic acid from plasma into the CNS. Metabolic alkalosis produced by the IV administration of sodium bicarbonate reverses the direction of transfer of salicylic acid and increases renal excretion. Diuretic-induced diuresis combined with IV administration of sodium bicarbonate is effective in speeding renal excretion of salicylic acid.

Hepatic Dysfunction

Salicylates can be associated with increased plasma concentrations of transaminase enzymes, indicating hepatic damage that is usually reversible. Patients with preexisting liver disease are more likely to develop changes in hepatic function in response to salicylates. In severe salicylate intoxication, fatty infiltration of the liver and kidneys may occur.

Renal Dysfunction

In contrast to that of other NSAIDs (especially acetaminophen), the chronic use of aspirin has not been shown to increase the incidence of ESRD (Perneger et al., 1994).

Metabolic Alterations

Large doses of salicylates may cause hyperglycemia and glycosuria and may deplete liver and skeletal muscle glycogen. Salicylates decrease lipogenesis by partially blocking incorporation of free fatty acids.

Uterine Effects

Prolongation of labor by salicylates may reflect loss of the normal uterotropic effects of prostaglandins. Aspirin is likely to be discontinued before the anticipated time of delivery to avoid prolonging labor or increasing postpartum hemorrhage.

Allergic Reactions

Allergic reactions to aspirin, although rare, can be life-threatening. Clinical manifestations may appear within minutes of ingestion and can include vasomotor rhinitis, laryngeal edema, bronchoconstriction, and cardiovascular collapse. Aspirin is more likely than salicylic acid to be associated with an allergic reaction. Patients who are allergic to aspirin cross-react to all inhibitors of prostaglandin synthesis.

Aspirin-Induced Asthma

Aspirin-induced asthma occurs in 8% to 20% of all asthmatic adults (Spector et al., 1979). The incidence of aspirin-induced asthma is even greater in asthmatic patients who also experience rhinosinusitis or have a history of nasal polyps. Aspirin-induced asthma usually occurs within an hour of ingesting aspirin or other NSAIDs (see the section on Ketorolac) and can be accompanied by life-threatening bronchospasm and hypotension. Bronchoconstriction associated with ingestion of aspirin in sensitive patients is likely caused by derangement of arachidonic acid metabolism with increased production of leukotrienes. Cross-sensitivity between aspirin and other NSAIDs must be considered in any patient with asthma. Description of aspirin-induced asthma as aspirin allergy is not accurate as it implies the mechanism for this response is immunologic (Zikowski et al., 1993).

Acetaminophen

Acetaminophen is a widely used analgesic and antipyretic drug that is present in a number of over-the-counter and prescription products. Although acetaminophen is used to treat similar conditions, it is not considered a true NSAID as it lacks significant antiinflammatory effects. In oral doses of 325 to 650 mg every 4 to 6 hours, acetaminophen is a useful alternative to aspirin as an analgesic and antipyretic, especially in pediatric patients and in patients in whom salicylates are not recommended (peptic ulcer disease) or in whom prolongation of bleeding time would be a disadvantage. Unlike salicylates, acetaminophen does not produce gastric irritation, alter aggregation characteristics of platelets, or antagonize the effects of uricosuric drugs. The antiinflammatory effects of acetaminophen are weak (no significant antirheumatic effects), presumably reflecting the modest peripheral inhibiting effects on prostaglandin synthesis produced by this drug. Conversely, strong central inhibition of prostaglandin synthesis confers analgesic and antipyretic effects. Concentrations of acetaminophen between 10 and 20 mg/liter are known to produce an antipyretic effect.

Pharmacokinetics

The systemic absorption of acetaminophen is nearly complete after oral administration, and significant binding to serum proteins does not occur. Acetaminophen is converted by conjugation and hydroxylation in the liver to inactive metabolites with only small amounts of drug being excreted unchanged.

Side Effects

It has been estimated that decreased consumption of acetaminophen could lower the incidence of ESRD by 8% to 10% (Perneger et al., 1994). Indeed, phenacetin, which is metabolized in part to acetaminophen, was withdrawn from clinical use because of its role in analgesic-induced nephropathy (Ronco and Flahault, 1994). After the administration of acetaminophen, its metabolites, especially *p*-aminophenol, are concentrated in the hypertonic renal papillae. This accumulation may explain the occurrence of papillary necrosis as a hallmark of analgesic-induced nephropathy. Apparently *p*-aminophenol is nephrotoxic because its oxidized metabolites bind covalently to sulfhydryl-containing tissue macromolecules and deplete stores of reduced glutathione, leading to cell necrosis. The long-term renal toxicity of NSAIDs may be caused by persistent inhibition of prostaglandin synthesis leading to medullary ischemia.

Hepatic necrosis and death may accompany a single dose of acetaminophen of >15 g. In otherwise healthy adults, hepatic toxicity can occur when daily dosages of acetaminophen exceed 4 g and at even lower daily doses in the presence of alcohol abuse. High doses of acetaminophen result in formation of *N*-acetyl-*p*-benzoquinone, which is believed to be responsible for hepatotoxicity. Normally, this metabolite is scavenged by the intracellular antioxidant, glutathione. In the presence of an overdose there is exhaustion of glutathione stores which allows the toxic reactive metabolite to accumulate and bind to hepatocytes. Alcoholics are at risk for toxicity at lower doses presumably because of increased P-450 activity and decreased glutathione stores. Clinical manifestations of hepatic damage, including jaundice and coagulation defects, occur 2 to 6 days after the overdose. Liver biopsy reveals centrilobular necrosis. Acetylcysteine is an antioxidant that substitutes for glutathione as a scavenger and is highly effective in preventing liver damage from acetaminophen when administered within the first 8 hours after an acetaminophen overdose (Smilkstein et al., 1988).

Genetically determined limitations on metabolism of phenacetin to acetaminophen result in formation of other metabolites with the potential to produce methemoglobinemia and hemolysis. For example, phenacetin may cause methemoglobinemia and hemolytic anemia in patients with a genetic deficiency of glucose-6-phosphate deficiency in erythrocytes. Hemolysis and subsequent jaundice associated with the administration of this drug to patients with a genetic deficiency of this enzyme in erythrocytes are presumed to be due to metabolites that oxidize glutathione and components of erythrocyte membranes, leading to shortened erythrocyte survival. Anuria may accompany severe intravascular hemolysis. Withdrawal of phenacetin from clinical use should eliminate methemoglobinemia due to this cause.

Diflunisal

Diflunisal is a fluorinated salicylic acid derivative that differs chemically from salicylates but possesses analgesic, antipyretic, and antiinflammatory effects. Antiarthritic effects are prominent, but antipyretic actions, although present, are not clinically useful. The most frequent side effects of diflunisal are nausea, vomiting, and gastrointestinal irritation. The effect of diflunisal on platelet function and bleeding time is dose-related but, in contrast to aspirin, is reversible. Acute interstitial nephritis may occur, and transient increases in plasma concentrations of transaminase enzymes may occur.

Indomethacin

Indomethacin is a methylated indole derivative with analgesic, antipyretic, and antiinflammatory effects comparable to those of salicylates. This drug is one of the most potent inhibitors of COX enzyme known. Its antiinflammatory effects are useful in the management of patients with arthritis. Indomethacin is the drug of choice in the treatment of ankylosing spondylitis and may be considered for initial therapy of Reiter's syndrome. Indomethacin provides antiinflammatory effects comparable to those of colchicine in the treatment of acute attacks of gouty arthritis. Conversely, indomethacin does not correct hyperuricemia and therefore is not useful for managing patients with chronic gout. Cardiac failure in neonates caused by patent ductus arteriosus may be controlled with a single dose of indomethacin, emphasizing the ability of this drug to selectively inhibit synthesis of prostaglandins. Indomethacin also appears to be more effective than aspirin in relieving the pain of dysmenorrhea. Patients with Bartter's syndrome have been successfully treated with indomethacin as well as with other inhibitors of prostaglandin synthesis.

Side Effects

Severe adverse side effects limit the usefulness of this drug. Gastrointestinal disturbances and severe frontal headaches are common. Indomethacin inhibits platelet aggregation. Allergic reactions may occur, and cross-sensitivity with salicylates is likely. Liver function tests may become abnormal, and patients with preexisting renal disease may experience an exacerbation. Neutropenia, thrombocytopenia, and aplastic anemia are rare.

Sulindac

Sulindac is a substituted analogue of indomethacin and has similar analgesic, antipyretic, and antiinflammatory effects. The parent drug is inactive (a prodrug) but is reduced in vivo to the sulfide form, which is responsible for pharmacologic effects. The active metabolite is cleared slowly from the plasma, principally into the bile, with an elimination half-time of about 16 hours. Side effects include inhibition of platelet aggregation, gastrointestinal irritation, renal dysfunction, and altered liver function tests. It has been suggested that because sulindac does not seem to affect the renal synthesis of prostaglandins as much as other NSAIDs, it may be the preferred drug in patients with renal disease or impaired renal perfusion, such as those who are hypovolemic (Ciabattoni et al., 1987). Others, however, have failed to demonstrate an advantage for sulindac in these situations (Roberts et al., 1985).

Tolmetin

Tolmetin is an analgesic, antipyretic, and antiinflammatory drug that, like salicylates, causes gastric irritation and prolongs bleeding time. It is more potent than salicylates and less potent than indomethacin or phenylbutazone. After oral administration, absorption is rapid and binding to plasma proteins is extensive (99%). Most of tolmetin is inactivated by decarboxylation.

Propionic Acid Derivatives

Ibuprofen, naproxen, and diclofenac are nonsteroidal propionic acid derivatives with prominent analgesic, antipyretic, and antiinflammatory effects, reflecting inhibition of prostaglandin synthesis. Propionic acid derivatives are as useful as salicylates in treating various forms of arthritis including osteoarthritis, rheumatoid arthritis, and acute gouty arthritis. Naproxen is unique in that its longer elimination half-time makes twice daily administration effective.

Pharmacokinetics

Ibuprofen is primarily eliminated by metabolism to hydroxyl or carboxyl conjugates with $<1\%$ of the drug appearing unchanged in the urine. Naproxen is metabolized by dealkylation by cytochrome P450 and $<10\%$ is excreted unchanged in the urine. Diclofenac is eliminated by metabolism to glucuronide, hydroxy, and sulphate conjugates followed by excretion in the urine and bile. Elimination is rapid with 90% of the clearance occurring within 3 to 4 hours and <1% appearing unchanged in the urine.

Side Effects

Gastrointestinal irritation and mucosal ulceration are usually less severe than the irritation and ulceration that may accompany administration of salicylates. Platelet function is altered but the duration of COX inhibition varies with the specific drug. Inhibition of prostaglandin synthesis may exacerbate renal dysfunction in patients with preexisting renal disease in whom prostaglandins are important for maintaining renal blood flow. It should be assumed that any patient who is hypersensitive to salicylates may also be allergic to propionic acid derivatives.

Drug Interactions

Adverse drug interactions often reflect the extensive plasma protein binding to albumin of propionic acid derivatives. For example, the dose of warfarin must be decreased because of its displacement from protein binding sites as well as alterations in platelet aggregation. Ibuprofen, however, is an exception, presumably because it occupies only a small number of binding sites on albumin. Hematopoietic suppression characterized by agranulocytosis and bone marrow granulocytic aplasia has been associated with chronic administration of ibuprofen (Mamua et al., 1986).

Phenylbutazone

Phenylbutazone is an effective antiinflammatory drug that is useful in the therapy of acute gout and treatment of rheumatoid arthritis. Acute exacerbations of these conditions respond well to this drug, and its use should be reserved for such episodes. Phenylbutazone is an effective alternative to colchicine in acute gout, providing control in 85% of patients within 24 to 36 hours. Because of its toxicity, this drug should be given for short periods not exceeding 7 days. Certainly, phenylbutazone should not be used routinely as an analgesic or antipyretic.

Pharmacokinetics

Phenylbutazone is absorbed rapidly and completely from the gastrointestinal tract. Plasma protein binding approaches 98%. Metabolism of phenylbutazone is extensive, involving glucuronidation and hydroxylation of the phenyl rings on the butyl side chain. Oxyphenbutazone is a metabolite of phenylbutazone with antiinflammatory activity similar to the parent drug. Phenylbutazone and oxyphenbutazone are excreted slowly in urine because extensive plasma protein binding limits glomerular filtration. The elimination half-time of phenylbutazone is 50 to 100 hours, and significant plasma concentrations may persist in the synovial spaces of joints for up to 3 weeks after treatment is discontinued.

Side Effects

Serious side effects of phenylbutazone therapy are frequent and include anemia and agranulocytosis, which limit the usefulness of this drug. Nausea, vomiting, epigastric discomfort, and skin rashes are frequent. Phenylbutazone causes significant sodium retention due to a reversible direct effect on renal tubules. This renal tubular effect is accompanied by decreased urine output. Plasma volume increases as much as 50% and pulmonary edema may occur in patients with poor cardiac function. Weight gain and the appearance of dilutional anemia reflect drug-induced fluid retention.

Phenylbutazone displaces drugs including warfarin, oral hypoglycemics, and sulfonamides from protein-binding sites. Increased bleeding may occur when phenylbutazone and warfarin or aspirin are coadministered. Displacement of thyroid hormone from protein-binding sites complicates interpretation of thyroid function tests. Phenylbutazone decreases uptake of iodine by the thyroid gland, presumably by inhibiting synthesis of organic iodine compounds.

Piroxicam

Piroxicam differs chemically from other NSAIDs but produces similar pharmacologic effects. Like salicylates, this drug inhibits prostaglandin synthesis. Administration of 20 mg in a single dose or in divided doses provides prolonged effects. Extensive protein binding (99%) may displace other drugs such as aspirin or oral anticoagulants from albumin-binding sites.

Ketorolac

Ketorolac is a NSAID that exhibits potent analgesic effects but only moderate antiinflammatory activity when administered IM or IV (Kenny, 1990). This drug is useful for providing postoperative analgesia both as the sole drug (less painful ambulatory procedures) and to supplement opioids. It is likely that ketorolac potentiates the antinociceptive actions of opioids. In contrast to dose-dependent analgesic effects of opioids, ketorolac and other NSAIDs appear to exhibit a ceiling effect with respect to postoperative analgesia (Fig. 11-4) (O'Hara et al., 1987). The use of ketorolac as the sole intraoperative analgesic drug may be associated with an increased incidence of purposeful movement on surgical incision (Ding et al., 1993). Ketorolac, 30 mg IM, produces analgesia that is equivalent to 10 mg of morphine or 100 mg of meperidine. An important benefit of ketorolac-induced analgesia is the absence of ventilatory or cardiovascular depression. Also unlike opioids, ketorolac has little or no effect on biliary tract dynamics, making this

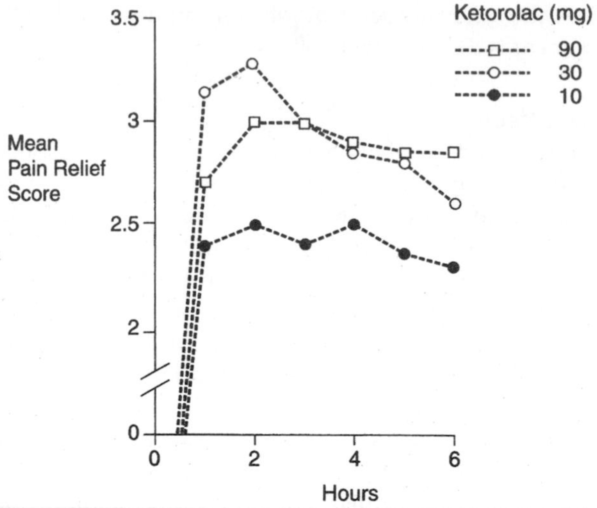

Figure 11-4. Ketorolac as well as other nonsteroidal antiinflammatory drugs exhibit a ceiling effect with respect to dose-dependent analgesic effects. (From O'Hara DA, Fragen RK, Kinzer M, Pemberton D. Ketorolac tromethamine as compared with morphine sulfate for treatment of postoperative pain. *Clin Pharmacol Ther* 1987;41:556–561; with permission.)

drug a useful analgesic when spasm of the biliary tract is undesirable (Krimmer et al., 1992).

Pharmacokinetics

After IM injection, maximum plasma concentrations of ketorolac are achieved within 45 to 60 minutes, and the elimination half-time is about 5 hours (Jung et al., 1987). Protein binding exceeds 99% and clearance of this drug is decreased compared with that of opioids. Clearance is decreased further in elderly individuals, and the dose of ketorolac should be less than that given to younger patients. Ketorolac is metabolized principally by glucuronic acid conjugation.

Side Effects

In common with other NSAIDs, ketorolac inhibits platelet thromboxane production and platelet aggregation by reversible inhibition of prostaglandin synthetase. Bleeding time may be increased by a single IV dose of ketorolac administered to patients with spinal anesthesia (T6 sensory level) but not by general anesthesia (Thwaites et al., 1996). This modest prolongation of bleeding time and marked decrease in platelet aggregation lasts until the drug is eliminated from the body. The difference between platelet responses to ketorolac during general versus spinal anesthesia may reflect a hypercoagulable state produced by the neuroendocrine response to surgical stress that normally occurs during general anesthesia but not spinal anesthesia. Conceptually, this stress response effect on coagulation could offset ketorolac-induced effects on bleeding time, whereas the absence of this effect during spinal anesthesia would permit the effect of ketorolac on platelet aggregation to manifest (Thwaites et al., 1996). Increased postoperative blood loss attributed to administration of ketorolac is a consideration, but the clinical significance remains unproved (Haddow et al., 1993; Rusy et al., 1995).

Life-threatening bronchospasm may follow the administration of ketorolac to patients with nasal polyposis, asthma, and aspirin sensitivity (Haddow et al., 1993; Zikowski et al., 1993). Cross-tolerance between aspirin and other NSAIDs occurs regularly. Although the molecular structures of these drugs may be very different, all share the common mechanism of COX inhibition. Ketorolac appears to have little potential for producing renal toxicity when adequate fluid balance is maintained and renal function does not depend on renal prostaglandins. Patients with congestive heart failure, hypovolemia, or hepatic cirrhosis release vasoactive substances; in these circumstances, prostaglandins are important for preventing renal arteriolar constriction, which may decrease renal blood flow. Modest increases in plasma concentrations of liver transaminase enzymes may occur in some patients treated with ketorolac. Gastrointestinal irritation and perforation, nausea, sedation, and peripheral edema may accompany the administration of this NSAID.

MISCELLANEOUS ANTIARTHRITIS DRUGS

Colchicine

Colchicine decreases inflammation and thus decreases pain in acute gouty arthritis (Fig. 11-5). This drug is unique in that its beneficial antiinflammatory effects are limited to the treatment of acute attacks of gout as well as prophylaxis against such attacks. Relief of pain and inflammation usually occurs within 24 to 48 hours after oral administration. Colchicine is not an analgesic and does not provide relief of other types of pain or inflammation. Colchicine has been reported to prolong survival in patients with cirrhosis of the liver (Kershenobich et al., 1988).

Mechanism of Action

Colchicine does not influence the renal excretion of uric acid but instead alters fibrillar microtubules in granulocytes, resulting in inhibition of the migration of these cells into inflamed areas. This effect decreases the release of lactic acid and other inflammation-producing enzymes. The result is inhibition of the cycle leading to the inflammatory

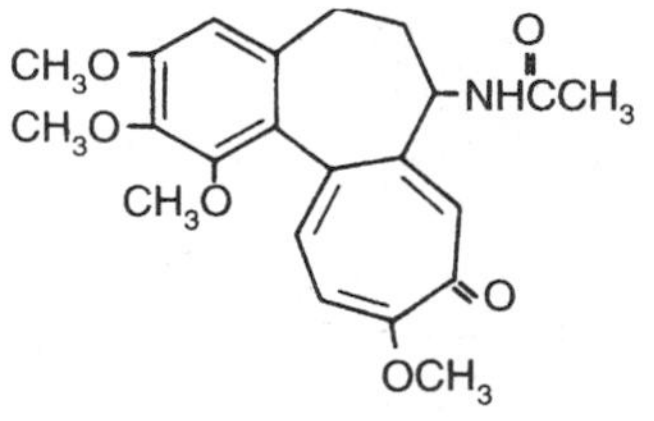

Figure 11-5. Colchicine.

response evoked by crystals of sodium urate that are deposited in joint tissue. Large amounts of colchicine and its metabolites are excreted in the bile; lesser amounts appear in the urine.

Side Effects

Nausea, vomiting, diarrhea, and abdominal pain are the most common side effects of colchicine therapy, occurring in approximately 80% of patients. Gastrointestinal intolerance tends to protect the patient from toxic doses of colchicine. Indeed, oral administration of colchicine must be discontinued as soon as gastrointestinal symptoms appear because hemorrhagic gastroenteritis can result in severe fluid and electrolyte losses. Gastrointestinal side effects may be minimized by administering colchicine IV. Colchicine enhances effects produced by CNS depressants and sympathomimetics. The medullary ventilatory center is depressed. Severe colchicine toxicity may manifest as bone marrow depression with leukopenia and thrombocytopenia.

Allopurinol

Allopurinol is the preferred drug for the therapy of primary hyperuricemia of gout and hyperuricemia that occurs during therapy with chemotherapeutic drugs (Fig. 11-6).

Mechanism of Action

In contrast to uricosuric drugs that facilitate renal excretion of urate, allopurinol interferes with the terminal steps of uric acid synthesis by inhibiting xanthine oxidase, the enzyme that converts xanthine to uric acid. Allopurinol is readily absorbed after oral administration and is rapidly converted to oxypurinol, with <10% of the drug appearing unchanged in the urine. Most of the oxypurinol is excreted unchanged by the kidneys. Oxypurinol is also an inhibitor of xanthine oxidase activity and has an elimination half-time of approximately 21 hours compared with 1.3 hours for allopurinol.

Side Effects

The most common side effect of allopurinol is maculopapular rash, frequently preceded by pruritus. Fever and myalgia may occur. These hypersensitivity-like syndromes may be due to allopurinol acting as a hapten to produce immune complex dermatitis. Pruritus is an indication to discontinue therapy with allopurinol. Allopurinol, acting as a hapten, could also result in nephritis and vasculitis. Hepatic dysfunction, manifesting as increases in plasma concentrations of transaminase enzymes, is common in patients treated with allopurinol.

Allopurinol inhibits the enzymatic inactivation of 6-mercaptopurine and azathioprine such that doses of these drugs must be decreased. Allopurinol also inhibits hepatic drug-metabolizing enzymes, which may result in unexpected prolonged effects produced by drugs that are extensively metabolized, including oral anticoagulants.

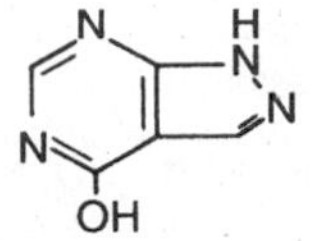

Figure 11-6. Allopurinol.

Uricosuric Drugs

Uricosuric drugs, such as probenecid and sulfinpyrazone, act directly on renal tubules to increase the rate of excretion of uric acid and other organic acids, including penicillin (Fig. 11-7). These drugs are also useful in controlling hyperuricemia resulting from the use of chemotherapeutic drugs or from diseases associated with accelerated destruction of erythrocytes. Salicylates antagonize the uricosuric action of probenecid but not its capacity to inhibit the renal tubular excretion of penicillin. Biliary excretion of rifampin is decreased by probenecid, making it possible to achieve higher plasma concentrations of this antituberculosis drug.

Probenecid

Probenecid is completely absorbed after oral administration, with peak plasma concentrations occurring in 2 to 4 hours. The elimination half-time is approximately 8 hours. Approximately 90% of probenecid is bound to plasma albumin. A total adult daily dose of 1 g of probenecid in four divided doses is necessary to effectively block the renal excretion of penicillin. Plasma concentrations of penicillin achieved in the presence of probenecid are at least twice the level achieved with the antibiotic alone.

Mild allergic reactions characterized as cutaneous rashes occur in 2% to 4% of patients treated with probenecid. This rash is a diagnostic dilemma when probenecid is administered in conjunction with penicillin. Hepatic dysfunction can occur but is rare.

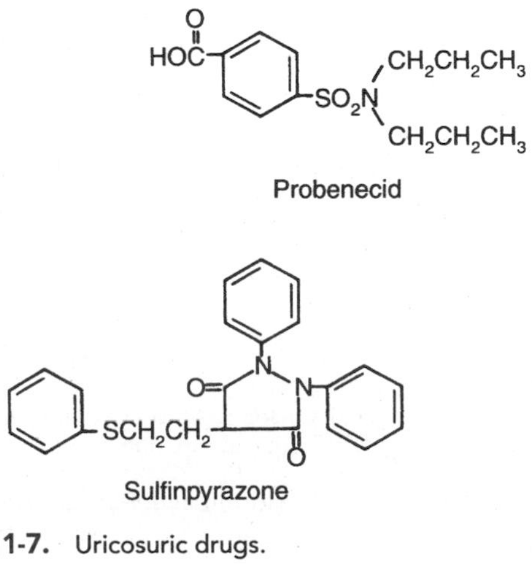

Figure 11-7. Uricosuric drugs.

Sulfinpyrazone

Sulfinpyrazone, an organic congener of phenylbutazone, lacks antiinflammatory effects but instead is a potent inhibitor of renal tubular reabsorption of uric acid. This uricosuric action of sulfinpyrazone is antagonized by salicylates. Renal tubular secretion of many drugs is also decreased. For example, sulfinpyrazone may induce hypoglycemia by decreasing the excretion of oral hypoglycemics.

Sulfinpyrazone is well-absorbed after oral administration. Protein binding approaches 98%. The drug undergoes secretion by proximal renal tubules because protein binding limits its glomerular filtration. Approximately 90% of sulfinpyrazone appears unchanged in urine. The remainder of the drug is metabolized to the parahydroxyl analogue, which also has uricosuric activity.

Gastrointestinal irritation occurs in 10% to 15% of patients treated with sulfinpyrazone, suggesting caution in patients with peptic ulcer disease. Allergic reactions, characterized by rash and fever, occur infrequently. Sulfinpyrazone inhibits platelet function.

REFERENCES

Alcindor D, Krolikowski JG, Pagel PS, et al. Cyclooxygenase-2 mediates ischemic, anesthetic, and pharmacologic preconditioning in vivo. *Anesthesiology* 2004;100:547–554.

Bombardier C. An evidence-based evaluation of the gastrointestinal safety of coxibs. *Am J Cardiol* 2002;89:3–9.

Brooks PM, Day RO. Nonsteroidal antiinflammatory drugs—differences and similarities. *N Engl J Med* 1991;324:1716–1725.

Burke D, Wildsmith JAW. Meningitis after spinal anesthesia. *Br J Anaesth* 1997;78:635–636.

Ching CK, Lam SK. Antacids: indications and limitations. *Drugs* 1994; 47:305–317.

Ciabattoni G, Boss AH, Patrignani P, et al. Effects of sulindac on renal and extrarenal eicosanoid synthesis. *Clin Pharmacol Ther* 1987;41: 380–383.

Collins R, Peto R, Baigent C, Sleight P. Aspirin, heparin, and fibrinolytic therapy in suspected acute myocardial infarction. *N Engl J Med* 1997; 336:847–860.

deLeeuw PW. Nonsteroidal anti-inflammatory drugs and hypertension: the risks in perspective. *Drugs* 1996;51:179–187.

Ding Y, Fredman B, White PF. Use of ketorolac and fentanyl during outpatient gynecologic surgery. *Anesth Analg* 1993;77:205–210.

Dolan S, Kelly JG, Huan M, et al. Transient up-regulation of spinal cyclooxygenase-2 and neuronal nitric oxide synthase following surgical inflammation. *Anesthesiology* 2003;98:170–180.

FitzGerald GA. Coxibs and cardiovascular disease. *N Engl J Med* 2004; 351:1709–1711.

Gajraj NM. Cyclooxygenase-2 inhibitors. *Anesth Analg* 2003;96: 1720–1738.

Gilron I, Milne B, Hong M. Cyclooxygenase-2 inhibitors in postoperative pain management: current evidence and future directions. *Anesthesiology* 2003;99:1198–1208.

Gurwitz ZJH, Avorn J, Bohn RL, et al. Initiation of antihypertensive treatment during nonsteroidal anti-inflammatory drug therapy. *JAMA* 1994;272:781–786.

Haddow GR, Riley E, Isaacs R, et al. Ketorolac, nasal polyposis, and bronchial asthma: a cause for concern. *Anesth Analg* 1993;76: 420–422.

Half E, Tang X, Gwyn K, et al. Cyclooxygenase-2 expression in human breast cancers and adjacent ductal carcinoma in situ. *Cancer Res.* 2002;62:1676–1681.

Harris R. Cyclooxygenase-2 inhibition and renal physiology *Am J Cardiol* 2002;89:10–17.

Ibraham A, Park S, Feldman J, et al. Effects of parecoxib, a parenteral COX-2-specific inhibitor, on the pharmacokinetics and pharmacodynamics of propofol. *Anesthesiology* 2002a;96:88–95.

Ibrahim A, Karikm A, Feldman J, et al. The influence of parecoxib, a parenteral cyclooxygenase-2-specific inhibitor, on the pharmacokinetics and clinical effects of midazolam. *Anesth Analg* 2002b;85: 667–673.

Jung D, Mroszcak E, Bynum L. Pharmacokinetics of ketorolac tromethamine in humans after intravenous, intramuscular and oral administration. *Eur J Clin Pharmacol* 1988;35:423–425.

Kenny GNC. Ketorolac trometamol—a new non-opioid analgesic. *Br J Anaesth* 1990;65:445–447.

Kershenobich D, Vargas F, Garcia-Tsao G, Tamayo RP, Gent M, Rojkind M. Colchicine in the treatment of cirrhosis of the liver. *N Engl J Med* 1988;318:1709–1713.

Kharasch ED. Perioperative COX-2 inhibitors: knowledge and challenges. *Anesth Analg* 2004:98:1–3.

Krimmer H, Bullingham RES, Lloyd J, and Bruch HP. Effects on biliary tract pressure in humans of intravenous ketorolac tromethamine compared with morphine and placebo. *Anesth Analg* 1992;75: 204–207.

Laine L. Nonsteroidal anti-inflammatory drug gastropathy. *Gastrointest Endosc Clin North Am* 1996;6:489–504.

Laisalmi M, Teppo A-M, Koivusalo A-M, et al. The effect of ketorolac and sevoflurane anesthesia on renal glomerular and tubular function. *Anesth Analg* 2001;93:1210–1213.

Levy JH. Aspirin and bleeding after coronary artery bypass grafting. *Anesth Analg* 1994;79:1–3.

Mamua SW, Burton JW, Groat JD, Schulte DA, Lobell M, Zanjani ED. Ibuprofen-associated pure white-cell aplasia. *N Engl J Med* 1986; 314:624–625.

Marret e, Flahault A, Samama C-M, et al. Effects of postoperative, nonsteroidal, antiinflammatory drugs on bleeding risk after tonsillectomy: Meta-analysis of randomized, controlled trials. *Anesthesiology* 2003;98:1497–1502.

McCrory CR, Lindahl SGE. Cyclooxygenase inhibition for postoperative analgesia. *Anesth Analg* 2002;95:169–176.

Mukherjee D, Nissen S, Topol E. Risk of cardiovascular events associated with selective COX-2 inhibitors. *JAMA* 2001;286;954–959.

O'Hara DA, Fragen RJ, Kinzer M, Pemberton D. Ketorolac tromethamine as compared with morphine sulfate for treatment of postoperative pain. *Clin Pharmacol Ther* 1987;41:556–561.

Oler A, Whooley MA, Oler J, et al. Adding heparin to aspirin reduces the incidence of myocardial infarction and death in patients with unstable angina. *JAMA* 1996;276:811–815.

Patrono C. Aspirin as an antiplatelet drug. *N Engl J Med* 1994;330: 1287–1294.

Perneger TV, Whelton PK, Klag MJ. Risk of kidney failure associated with the use of acetaminophen, aspirin, and nonsteroidal antiinflammatory drugs. *N Engl J Med* 1994;331:1675–1679.

Rajan E, Ahlquist DA. Gastrointestinal bleeding. *Sci Am Med* 2003;4:X: 1–15.

Reich DL, Patel GC, Vela-Castos F, et al. Aspirin does not increase homologous blood requirements in elective coronary bypass surgery. *Anesth Analg* 1994;79:4–8.

Reuben SS, Steinberg R. Gastric perforation associated with the use of celecoxib. *Anesthesiology* 1999;91:1548–1549.

Roberts DG, Gerber JG, Barnes JS, et al. Sulindac is not renal sparing in man. *Clin Pharmacol Ther* 1985;38:258–265.

Rostom A, Wells G, Tugwell P et al. The prevention of chronic NSAID-induced upper gastrointestinal toxicity: A Cochrane collaboration metaanalysis of randomized controlled trials. *J Rheumatol* 2000; 27:2203–2214.

Rusy LM, Houck CS, Sullivan LF, et al. A double-blind evaluation of ketorolac tromethamine versus acetaminophen in pediatric tonsillectomy: analgesia and bleeding. *Anesth Analg* 1995;80:226–229.

Schror K. Antiplatelet drugs: a comparative review. *Drugs* 1995;50:7–28.

Settipane GA. Adverse reactions to aspirin and related drugs. *Arch Intern Med* 1981;141:328–332.

Silverstein FE, Faich G, Goldstein JL, et al. Gastrointestinal toxicity with celecoxib vs. nonsteroidal anti-inflammatory drugs for osteoarthritis and rheumatoid arthritis: The CLASS study: A randomized controlled trial. Celecoxib. Long-term Arthritis Safety Study. *JAMA* 2000;248:1247–1257.

Sivarajan M, Wasse L. Perioperative acute renal failure associated with preoperative intake of ibuprofen. *Anesthesiology* 1997;86: 1390–1392.

Smalley W, Ray W. Daugherty J, et al. Use of nonsteroidal anti-inflammatory drugs and incidence of colorectal cancer: a population-based study. *Arch Intern Med* 1999;159:161–166.

Smilkstein MJ, Knapp GL, Kulig KW, Rumack BH. Efficacy of oral *N*-acetylcysteine in the treatment of acetaminophen overdose. *N Engl J Med* 1988;319:1557–1562.

Sonksen JR, Kong KL, Holder R. Magnitude, and time course of impaired primary haemostasis after stopping chronic low and medium dose aspirin in healthy volunteers. *Br J Anaesth* 1999;82: 360–365

Spector SL, Wangaard BS, Farr RS. Aspirin and concomitant idiosyncrasies in adult asthmatic patients. *J Allergy Clin Immunol* 1979;64: 500–506.

Steinbach G, Lynch P, Philips R, et al. The effect of celecoxib, a cyclooxygenase-2 inhibitor, in familial adenomatous polyposis. *N Engl J Med* 2000;342:1946–1952.

Thwaites BK, Nigus DB, Bouska GW, et al. Intravenous ketorolac tromethamine worsens platelet function during knee arthroscopy under spinal anesthesia. *Anaesth Analg* 1996;82:1176–1181.

t'Veld B, Ruitenberg A, Hofman A, et al. Nonsteroidal antiinflammtory drugs and the risk of Alzheimer's disease. *N Engl J Med* 2001;345:1515–1521.

Tuman KJ, McCarthy RJ, O'Connor CJ, et al. Aspirin does not increase allogenic blood transfusion in reoperative coronary artery surgery. *Anesth Analg* 1996;83:1178–1184.

Willard JE, Lange RA, Hills LD. The use of aspirin in ischemic heart disease. *N Engl J Med* 1992;327:175–181.

Zikowski D, Hord AH, Haddox D, et al. Ketorolac-induced bronchospasm. *Anesth Analg* 1993;76:417–419.

Sympathomimetics

12

Sympathomimetics include naturally occurring (endogenous) catecholamines, synthetic catecholamines, and synthetic noncatecholamines. Synthetic noncatecholamines are further subdivided into indirect-acting and direct-acting categories (Table 12-1). These drugs evoke physiologic responses similar to those produced by endogenous activity of the sympathetic nervous system. For example, pharmacologic effects of sympathomimetics, although quantitatively different, may include (a) vasoconstriction, especially in cutaneous and renal circulations; (b) vasodilation in skeletal muscle vasculature; (c) bronchodilation; (d) cardiac stimulation characterized by increased heart rate, increased myocardial contractility, and vulnerability to cardiac dysrhythmias; (e) liberation of free fatty acids from adipose tissues; (f) hepatic glycogenolysis; (g) modulation of insulin, renin, and pituitary hormone secretion; and (h) central nervous system (CNS) stimulation (Lawson and Wallfisch, 1986). The net effect of sympathomimetics on cardiac function is influenced by baroreceptor-mediated reflex responses.

CLINICAL USES

Clinically, sympathomimetics are used most often as positive inotropic agents to increase myocardial contractility, or as vasopressors to increase systemic blood pressure after sympathetic nervous system blockade produced by regional anesthesia. The ability to measure atrial filling pressures and cardiac output via a pulmonary artery catheter as well as calculation of systemic and pulmonary vascular resistances is useful when sympathomimetics are administered as positive inotropes to improve myocardial contractility (Goldberg and Cohn, 1987). Sympathomimetics may also be used as vasopressors to maintain systemic blood pressure during the time needed to eliminate excess inhaled anesthetic or to restore intravascular fluid volume. The prolonged administration of sympathomimetics to support blood pressure in the presence of hypovolemia is not recommended. Indeed, the only time a vasopressor should be administered is when systemic blood pressure must be increased promptly to prevent pressure-dependent decreases in blood flow that could result in tissue ischemia. Disadvantages of using sympathomimetics that lack significant $beta_1$-adrenergic effects to maintain systemic blood pressure include intense vasoconstriction and associated blood pressure increases that evoke reflex-mediated bradycardia, which leads to a decrease in cardiac output.

Other uses of selected sympathomimetics include (a) treatment of bronchospasm in patients with asthma, (b) management of life-threatening allergic reactions, and (c) addition to local anesthetic solutions to retard systemic absorption of the local anesthetic (see Chapter 7).

STRUCTURE ACTIVITY RELATIONSHIPS

All sympathomimetics are derived from beta-phenylethylamine (Fig. 12-1). The presence of hydroxyl groups on the 3 and 4 carbon positions of the benzene ring (dihydroxybenzene) of beta-phenylethylamine, designates it a catechol; drugs with this composition are designated catecholamines. For example, 3,4-dihydroxyphenylethylamine is the endogenous catecholamine dopamine. Hydroxylation of the beta carbon of dopamine results in the endogenous catecholamine and neurotransmitter norepinephrine. The third endogenous catecholamine, epinephrine, results from methylation of the terminal amine of norepinephrine. Addition of an isopropyl group rather than a methyl group to the terminal amine of norepinephrine results in the synthetic catecholamine isoproterenol. The other synthetic catecholamine, dobutamine, possesses a bulky aromatic substituent on the terminal amine. Synthetic noncatecholamines include the beta-phenylethylamine structure but lack hydroxyl groups on the 3 and 4 carbons of the benzene ring (Fig. 12-2).

Receptor Selectivity

The relative selectivity of sympathomimetics for various adrenergic receptors depends on the chemical structure of the drug. Maximal alpha- and beta-adrenergic receptor activity depends on the presence of hydroxyl groups on the 3 and 4 carbons of the benzene ring of beta-phenylethylamine

TABLE 12-1. CLASSIFICATION AND COMPARATIVE PHARMACOLOGY OF SYMPATHOMIMETICS

	Receptors Stimulated			Mechanism of Action	Cardiac Effects			Peripheral Vascular Resistance	Renal Blood Flow	Mean Arterial Pressure	Airway Resistance	Central Nervous System Stimulation	Single Intravenous Dose (70-kg Adult)	Continuous Infusion Dose (70-kg Adult)
	Alpha	$Beta_1$	$Beta_2$		Cardiac Output	Heart Rate	Dysrhythmias							
Natural catecholamines														
Epinephrine	+	++	++	Direct	++	++	+++	±	−−	+	−−	Yes	2–8 μg	1–20 μg/min
Norepinephrine	+++	++	0	Direct	−	−	+	+++	−−−	+++	NC	No	Not used	4–16 μg/min
Dopamine	++	++	+	Direct	+++	+	+	+	+++	+	NC	No	Not used	2–20 μg/kg/min
Synthetic catecholamines														
Isoproterenol	0	+++	+++		+++	+++	+++	−−	−	±	−−−	Yes	1–4 μg	1–5 μg/min
Dobutamine	0	+++	0		+++	+	±	NC	++	+	NC		Not used	2–10 μg/kg/min
Synthetic noncatecholamines														
Indirect-acting														
Ephedrine	++	+	+	Indirect, some direct	++	++	++	+	−−	++	−−	Yes	10–25 mg	Not used
Mephentermine	++	+	+	Indirect	++	++	++	+	−−	++	−	Yes	10–25 mg	Not used
Amphetamines	++	+	+	Indirect	+	+	+	++	−−	+	NC	Yes	Not used	Not used
Metaraminol	++	+	+	Indirect, direct	−	−	+	+++	−−−	+++	NC	No	1.5–5.0 mg	40–500 μg/kg/min
Direct-acting														
Phenylephrine	+++	0	0	Direct	−	−	NC	+++	−−−	+++	NC	No	50–100 μg	20–50 μg/min
Methoxamine	+++	0	0	Direct	−	−	NC	+++	−−−	+++	NC	No	5–10 mg	

0, none; +, minimal increase; ++, moderate increase; +++, marked increase; −, minimal decrease; −−, moderate decrease; −−−, marked decrease; NC, no change.

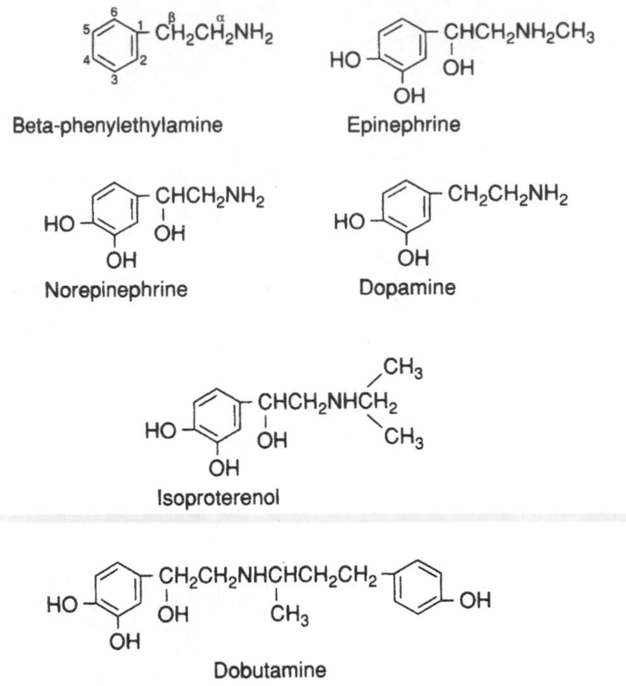

Figure 12-1. Sympathomimetics are derived from beta-phenylethylamine, with a catecholamine being any compound that has hydroxyl groups on the 3 and 4 carbon positions of the benzene ring.

(catecholamine). Epinephrine has the optimal chemical structure for producing alpha- and beta-adrenergic effects (see Fig. 12-1). Any change in chemical structure from epinephrine results in a compound that is less active at alpha- and beta-adrenergic receptors. Indeed, phenylephrine, which lacks the 4-hydroxyl group, is less potent than epinephrine on both alpha- and beta-adrenergic receptors (see Fig. 12-1). Despite decreased potency, the removal of this 4-hydroxyl group increases the alpha$_1$ receptor selectivity of phenylephrine. Substitution on the terminal amine of beta-phenylethylamine increases activity of the drug at beta-adrenergic receptors. For example, norepinephrine possesses minimal beta$_2$-adrenergic agonist activity, whereas this activity is greatly accentuated in epinephrine with the addition of a methyl group to the terminal amine. Beta$_1$ and beta$_2$ receptor activity is maximal in isoproterenol, which contains an isopropyl group on the terminal amine.

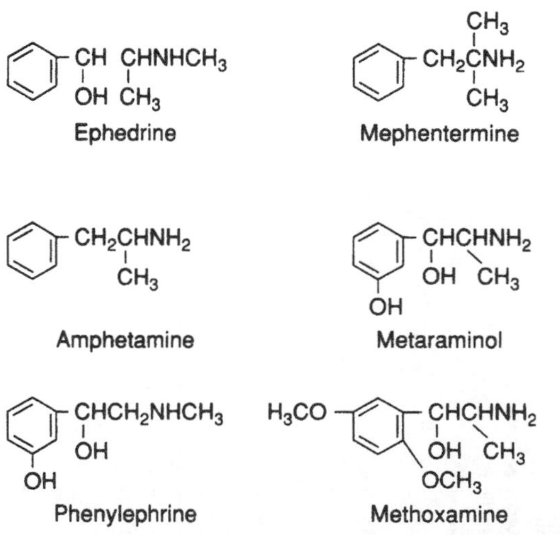

Figure 12-2. Indirect-acting and direct-acting synthetic noncatecholamines.

Hydroxyl groups on the 3 and 5 carbons of the benzene ring of beta-phenylethylamine confer selective beta$_2$ receptor agonist activity on compounds with long-chain substituents (Fig. 12-3). Thus, metaproterenol, terbutaline, and albuterol relax bronchial smooth muscle without evoking significant beta$_1$ receptor-mediated cardiac effects.

The dextrorotatory forms of norepinephrine and epinephrine are approximately one-half as active as the levorotatory isomer. The levorotatory isomer of isoproterenol is more than 1,000 times as active as the dextrorotatory isomer.

Central Nervous System Stimulation

CNS stimulation is prominent with synthetic noncatecholamines that lack substituents on the benzene ring (methamphetamine) (see Fig. 12-2). Substitution of a hydroxyl group on the beta carbon of the ethylamine side chain (ephedrine) decreases CNS stimulant effects, presumably by decreasing lipid solubility. Such a substitution, however, enhances alpha- and beta-adrenergic receptor agonist activity. Thus, ephedrine is less potent than methamphetamine as a CNS stimulant but is more potent as a bronchodilator and cardiac stimulant. Catecholamines have limited lipid solubility and thus are not likely to cross the blood-brain barrier in sufficient amounts to cause CNS stimulation.

MECHANISM OF ACTION

Sympathomimetics exert their pharmacologic effects by activating either directly or indirectly alpha-adrenergic, beta-adrenergic, or dopaminergic receptors which belong to the family of G protein-coupled receptors (Yost, 1993). The first step is binding of the endogenous or exogenous sympathomimetic on the cell surface by a receptor that recognizes the specific ligand. Once bound, this ligand induces a conformational change, enabling the receptor to activate a specific class of G protein. The name *G protein* derives from the fact that these proteins use the binding and hydrolysis of guanosine 5′-triphosphate (GTP) as a timer to limit their duration of action. G proteins are essential intermediaries in cell communication. Once activated, the G protein is free to diffuse in the cell membrane and to encounter the next element of the cycle, an effector protein. Usually, this effector protein will be an intracellular enzyme (adenylate cyclase, phospholipase C) or an ion

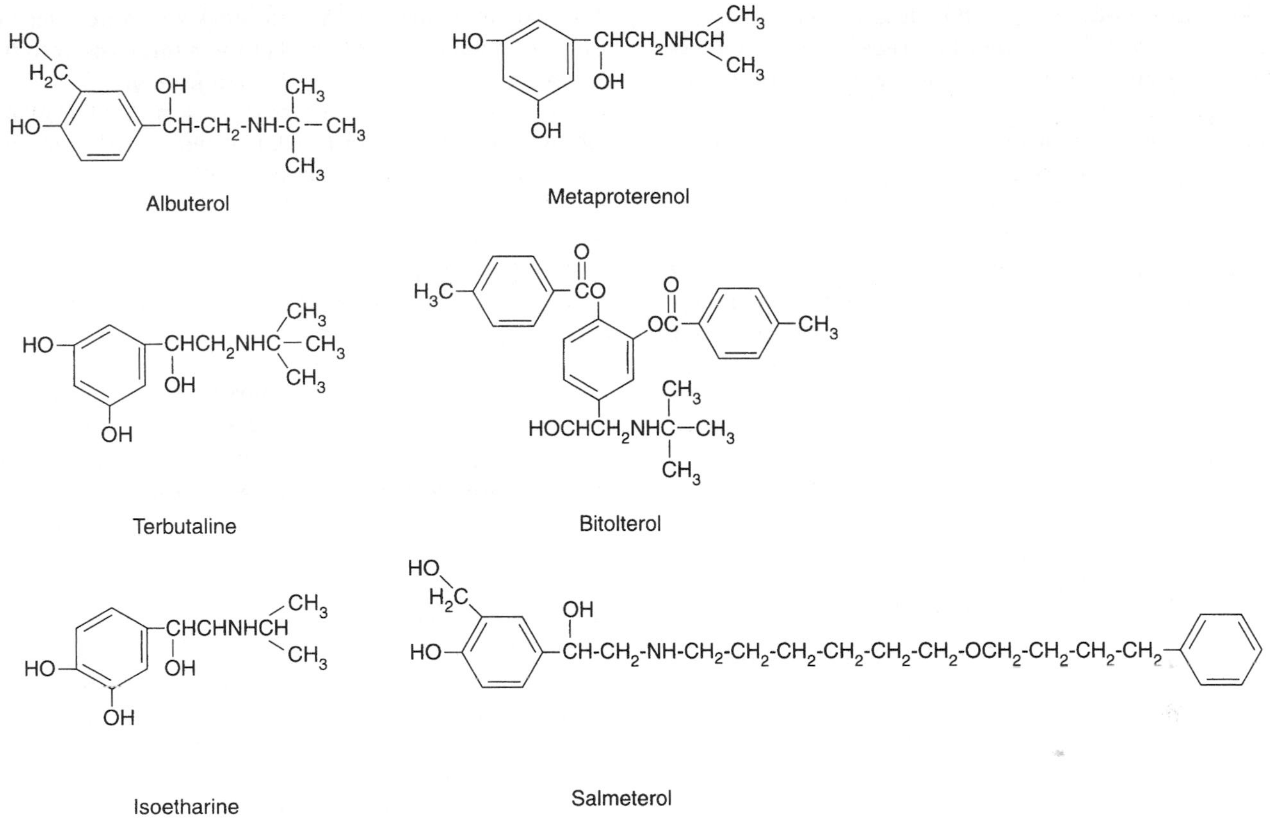

Figure 12-3. Selective $beta_2$-adrenergic agonists.

channel in the cell membrane. This encounter regulates the effector (activation or inhibition of an effector enzyme, opening or closing of an ion channel), changing either the concentration of an intracellular second messenger or the cell membrane potential (Yost, 1993).

Production of cyclic adenosine monophosphate (cAMP) by stimulating the enzyme adenylate cyclase is the speculated mechanism by which sympathomimetics produce pharmacologic effects considered to reflect beta-adrenergic receptor stimulation (Maze, 1981). For example, increased cAMP stimulates protein kinases, which phosphorylate substrates and enhance inward calcium ion flux, which increases cytoplasmic calcium concentrations. This increased availability of calcium enhances the intensity of actin and myosin interaction, manifesting as more forceful myocardial contractility ($beta_1$ effect). Conversely, $beta_2$ receptor activation, characterized by relaxation of bronchial, vascular, and smooth muscles, reflects hyperpolarization of cell membranes and decreased inward calcium ion flux. $Alpha_1$ receptor stimulation increases inward calcium ion flux and also probably facilitates the release of bound intracellular calcium. $Alpha_2$ receptor stimulation inhibits adenylate cyclase activity. Dopamine-mediated activation of adenylate cyclase and subsequent increased intracellular concentrations of cAMP is responsible for renal artery dilation that follows activation of $dopamine_1$ receptors.

It is common to refer to cAMP as the *second messenger*, whereas the water-soluble sympathomimetic that activates adenylate cyclase to catalyze the conversion of adenosine triphosphate to cAMP is referred to as the *first messenger*. The intracellular level of cAMP also is controlled by phosphodiesterase, which hydrolyzes cAMP to an inactive molecule.

An important factor in the pharmacologic response elicited by a sympathomimetic is the density of alpha- and beta-adrenergic receptors in tissues. There is an inverse relationship between the concentration of available sympathomimetic and the number of receptors. For example, increased plasma concentrations of norepinephrine result in a decrease in the density of beta-adrenergic receptors in cell membranes (down-regulation). Likewise, chronic treatment of patients with bronchial asthma using a $beta_2$ agonist results in tachyphylaxis, presumably reflecting decreased receptor density.

The anatomic distribution of alpha- and beta-adrenergic receptors influences the pharmacologic response evoked by sympathomimetics (see Table 12-1). For example, norepinephrine has minimal effects on airway resistance because adrenergic receptors in bronchial smooth muscle are not stimulated by this catecholamine. Conversely, epinephrine and isoproterenol are potent bronchodilators as a result of their ability to activate $beta_2$ receptors. Stimulation of $beta_2$ receptors also inhibits activation of T cells and release of cytokines from airway smooth muscle cells (Halsworth et al., 2001). Cutaneous blood vessels possess alpha-adrenergic receptors, resulting almost exclusively in vasoconstriction when activated by norepinephrine or epinephrine. Smooth muscles of blood vessels supplying skeletal muscles contain both $beta_2$ and $alpha_1$ receptors such that low doses of epinephrine produce beta receptor–mediated vasodilation and high doses produce alpha receptor–mediated vasoconstriction, which overrides evidence of beta stimulation. $Beta_1$ receptors are equally responsive to epinephrine and norepinephrine, whereas $beta_2$ receptors are more sensitive to epinephrine than norepinephrine (Maze, 1981). Skeletal muscle tremors associated with beta-agonist therapy reflects stimulation of $beta_2$ receptors. Lipolysis is mediated by activation of $beta_3$ receptors. The venous circulation contains a high density of $alpha_1$ receptors and venoconstriction as produced by epinephrine enhances venous return.

Indirect-Acting Sympathomimetics

Indirect-acting sympathomimetics are synthetic noncatecholamines that activate adrenergic receptors by evoking the release of the endogenous neurotransmitter norepinephrine from postganglionic sympathetic nerve endings (see Table 12-1 and Fig. 12-2). Presumably, these drugs enter postganglionic sympathetic nerve endings from which they displace norepinephrine outward into the synaptic cleft. Denervation or depletion of neurotransmitter, as with repeated doses of a sympathomimetic, blunts the pharmacologic responses normally evoked by the drug. For some synthetic noncatecholamines, such as ephedrine, pharmacologic effects may reflect combinations of direct and indirect actions.

Indirect-acting sympathomimetics are characterized mostly by alpha- and $beta_1$-adrenergic agonist effects because norepinephrine is a weak $beta_2$-adrenergic agonist (see Table 12-1). The systemic blood pressure response to indirect-acting sympathomimetics is decreased by drugs that decrease sympathetic CNS activity. (Eger and Hamilton, 1959; Miller et al., 1968).

Direct-Acting Sympathomimetics

Direct-acting sympathomimetics include catecholamines and the synthetic noncatecholamines phenylephrine and methoxamine (see Table 12-1 and Fig. 12-2). These sympathomimetics activate adrenergic receptors directly, although the potency of direct-acting synthetic noncatecholamines is less than that of catecholamines. Denervation or depletion of neurotransmitter does not prevent the activity of these drugs. Most direct-acting sympathomimetics activate both alpha- and beta-adrenergic receptors, but the magnitude of alpha and beta activity varies greatly among drugs from almost pure alpha-agonist activity for phenylephrine to almost pure beta-agonist activity for isoproterenol (see Table 12-1).

Sympathetic nervous system blockade, which deprives alpha-adrenergic receptor sites of tonic impulses, results in increased sensitivity of these sites to norepinephrine. As a result, exaggerated systemic blood pressure changes may follow the administration of direct-acting sympathomimetics (Eger and Hamilton, 1959).

METABOLISM

Catecholamines

All drugs containing the 3,4-dihydroxybenzene structure (catecholamines) are rapidly inactivated by the enzymes monoamine oxidase (MAO) or catechol-*O*-methyltransferase (COMT). MAO is an enzyme present in the liver, kidneys, and gastrointestinal tract that catalyzes oxidative deamination. COMT is capable of methylating a hydroxyl group of catecholamines. The resulting inactive methylated metabolites are conjugated with glucuronic acid and appear in urine as 3-methyoxy-4-hydroxymandelic acid, metanephrine (derived from epinephrine), and normetanephrine (derived from norepinephrine).

Despite the importance of enzymatic degradation of catecholamines, the biologic actions of these substances are terminated principally by uptake back into postganglionic sympathetic nerve endings. Inhibition of this uptake mechanism produces a greater potentiation of the effects of epinephrine than does inhibition of either enzyme. The completeness of this uptake mechanism and metabolism is emphasized by the appearance of only minimal amounts of unchanged catecholamines in urine.

The lungs are efficient biochemical filters for central venous blood as reflected by clearance of endogenous catecholamines during pulmonary transit. For example, an estimated 25% of circulating norepinephrine is extracted during a single passage through the lungs in normal resting humans. The lungs clear about 20% of clinical doses of dopamine whereas extraction of dobutamine is minimal (Sumikawa et al., 1991). Because epinephrine traverses the lungs without change, the same concentration exists in arterial and venous blood. In animals, halothane and nitrous oxide decrease removal of norepinephrine from the blood by the lungs (Naito and Gillis, 1973). It is possible that inhaled anesthetics interfere with the amine transport system necessary to deliver norepinephrine into pulmonary cells.

Synthetic Noncatecholamines

Synthetic noncatecholamines lacking a 3-hydroxyl group are not affected by COMT and thus depend on MAO for their metabolism. Metabolism of these sympathomimetics, however, is often slower than that of catecholamines, and inhibition of MAO may even further prolong their duration of action. For this reason, patients treated with

MAO inhibitors may manifest exaggerated responses when treated with synthetic noncatecholamines (see Chapter 19).

The presence of an alpha methyl group, as with ephedrine or amphetamine, inhibits deamination by MAO. Ephedrine may be excreted unchanged in urine. Urinary excretion of unchanged drug is even greater if the urine is acidified, emphasizing the fact that many synthetic noncatecholamines have pK values >9.

ROUTE OF ADMINISTRATION

Oral administration of catecholamines is not effective, presumably reflecting the metabolism of these compounds by enzymes in the gastrointestinal mucosa and liver before they reach the systemic circulation. For this reason, epinephrine is administered subcutaneously (SC) or intravenously (IV). Recommendations to administer epinephrine by the intratracheal route during cardiopulmonary resuscitation have been challenged by data suggesting this route of administration does not result in therapeutic cardiovascular responses (McCrirrick and Monk, 1994). Dopamine, dobutamine, and norepinephrine are administered only IV. Absence of one or both of the 3,4-hydroxyl groups or the presence of an alpha methyl group, as is characteristic of synthetic noncatecholamines, increases oral absorption of these drugs.

NATURALLY OCCURRING CATECHOLAMINES

Naturally occurring catecholamines are epinephrine, norepinephrine, and dopamine (see Table 12-1 and Fig. 12-1).

Epinephrine

Epinephrine is the prototype drug among the sympathomimetics. Its natural functions on release from the adrenal medulla include regulation of (a) myocardial contractility, (b) heart rate, (c) vascular and bronchial smooth muscle tone, (d) glandular secretions, and (e) metabolic processes such as glycogenolysis and lipolysis. It is the most potent activator of alpha-adrenergic receptors, being two to ten times more active than norepinephrine and more than 100 times more potent than isoproterenol. Epinephrine also activates $beta_1$ and $beta_2$ receptors. Oral administration is not effective because epinephrine is rapidly metabolized in the gastrointestinal mucosa and liver. Therefore, epinephrine is administered SC or IV. Absorption after SC injection is slow because of local epinephrine-induced vasoconstriction. Epinephrine is poorly lipid soluble, preventing its ready entrance into the CNS and accounting for the lack of cerebral effects.

Clinical Uses

Clinical uses of epinephrine include (a) addition to local anesthetic solutions to decrease systemic absorption and prolong the duration of action of the anesthetic, (b) treatment of life-threatening allergic reactions, (c) administration during cardiopulmonary resuscitation as the single most important therapeutic drug, and (d) continuous infusion to increase myocardial contractility. The administration of supraphysiologic doses (100 μg/kg) of epinephrine during cardiopulmonary resuscitation has not been shown to be more effective than standard doses (10 μg/kg) of this catecholamine (Beatriz et al., 2004).

Side Effects

Cardiovascular Effects

The cardiovascular effects of epinephrine result from epinephrine-induced stimulation of alpha- and beta-adrenergic receptors (see Table 12-1). Small doses of epinephrine (1 to 2 μg/minute IV) administered to adults stimulate principally $beta_2$ receptors in peripheral vasculature. Stimulation of $beta_1$ receptors occurs at somewhat larger doses (4 μg/minute IV), whereas large doses of epinephrine (10 to 20 μg/minute IV) stimulate both alpha- and beta-adrenergic receptors with the effects of alpha stimulation predominating in most vascular beds, including the cutaneous and renal circulations. A single rapid injection of epinephrine, 2 to 8 μg IV, produces transient cardiac stimulation lasting 1 to 5 minutes, usually without an overshoot of systemic blood pressure or heart rate. During continuous infusion, the concomitant administration of a vasodilator can offset epinephrine-induced vasoconstriction, especially in the splanchnic and renal circulations.

Epinephrine stimulates $beta_1$ receptors to cause an increase in systolic blood pressure, heart rate, and cardiac output. There is a modest decrease in diastolic blood pressure, reflecting vasodilation in skeletal muscle vasculature due to stimulation of $beta_2$ receptors. The net effect of these systemic blood pressure changes is an increase in pulse pressure and minimal change in mean arterial pressure. Because mean arterial pressure does not change greatly, there is little likelihood that baroreceptor activation will occur to produce reflex bradycardia. Epinephrine increases heart rate by accelerating the rate of spontaneous phase 4 depolarization, which also increases the likelihood of cardiac dysrhythmias. Increased cardiac output reflects epinephrine-induced increases in heart rate, myocardial contractility, and venous return. Repeated doses of epinephrine produce similar cardiovascular effects in contrast to tachyphylaxis that accompanies administration of synthetic noncatecholamines that evoke the release of norepinephrine.

Epinephrine predominantly stimulates $alpha_1$ receptors in the skin, mucosa, and hepatorenal vasculature, producing intense vasoconstriction. In skeletal muscle vasculature, epinephrine principally stimulates $beta_2$ receptors, producing vasodilation. The net effect of these peripheral vascular changes is preferential distribution of cardiac output to skeletal muscles and decreased systemic vascular resistance. Renal blood flow is substantially decreased by epinephrine, even in the absence of changes in systemic blood pressure. Indeed, epinephrine is estimated to be two to ten times more potent than norepinephrine for increasing renal vascular resistance. The secretion of renin is increased due to epinephrine-induced stimulation of beta receptors in the kidneys. In usual therapeutic doses, epinephrine has no significant vasoconstrictive effect on cerebral arterioles. Coronary blood flow is enhanced by epinephrine, even at doses that do not alter systemic blood pressure.

Chronic increases in the plasma concentrations of epinephrine, as in patients with pheochromocytoma, result in a decrease of plasma volume because of a loss of protein-free fluid into the extracellular space. Arterial wall damage and local areas of myocardial necrosis may also accompany chronic circulating excesses of epinephrine. Conventional doses of epinephrine, however, do not produce these effects.

Airway Smooth Muscle

Smooth muscles of the bronchi are relaxed by virtue of epinephrine-induced activation of $beta_2$ receptors. This bronchodilator effect of epinephrine is converted to bronchoconstriction in the presence of beta-adrenergic blockade, reflecting epinephrine-induced stimulation of alpha receptors. $Beta_2$ stimulation, by increasing intracellular concentrations of cAMP, decreases release of vasoactive mediators associated with symptoms of bronchial asthma.

Metabolic Effects

Epinephrine has the most significant effects of all the catecholamines on metabolism. $Beta_1$ receptor stimulation due to epinephrine increases liver glycogenolysis and adipose tissue lipolysis, whereas $alpha_1$ receptor stimulation inhibits release of insulin. Liver glycogenolysis results from epinephrine-induced activation of hepatic phosphorylase enzyme. Lipolysis is due to epinephrine-induced activation of triglyceride lipase, which accelerates the breakdown of triglycerides to form free fatty acids and glycerol. Infusions of epinephrine usually increase plasma concentrations of cholesterol, phospholipids, and low-density lipoproteins.

Release of epinephrine and resulting glycogenolysis and inhibition of insulin secretion is the most likely explanation for the hyperglycemia that commonly occurs during the perioperative period. In addition, epinephrine can produce inhibition of glucose uptake by peripheral tissues, which is also due, in part, to inhibition of insulin secretion. Increased plasma concentrations of lactate presumably reflect epinephrine-induced glycogenolysis in skeletal muscles.

Electrolytes

Selective $beta_2$-adrenergic agonist effects of low-dose infusion of epinephrine (0.05 μg/kg/minute IV) are speculated to reflect activation of the sodium-potassium pump in skeletal muscles, leading to a transfer of potassium ions into cells (Fig. 12-4) (Brown et al., 1983). The observation that serum potassium measurements in blood samples obtained immediately before induction of anesthesia are lower than measurements 1 to 3 days preoperatively is presumed to reflect stress-induced release of epinephrine (Fig. 12-5) (Kharasch and Bowdle, 1991). The ability of a nonselective $beta_1$ and $beta_2$ antagonist (propranolol) but not a cardioselective $beta_1$ antagonist (atenolol) to prevent "preoperative hypokalemia" is consistent for a $beta_2$-adrenergic agonist effect as the explanation for potassium transfer (Fig. 12-6) (Kharasch and Bowdle, 1991). In making therapeutic decisions based on a preinduction serum potassium measurement, especially in patients without a reason to experience hypokalemia, one should consider the possible role of preoperative anxiety and the release of epinephrine.

Epinephrine-induced hypokalemia could contribute to cardiac dysrhythmias that occasionally accompany stimulation of the sympathetic nervous system. Conversely, epinephrine may stimulate the release of potassium from the liver, tending to offset the decrease in extracellular concentration of this ion produced by entrance into skeletal muscles. Among the endocrine glands, only the salivary glands respond significantly to epinephrine, producing thick, sparse secretions.

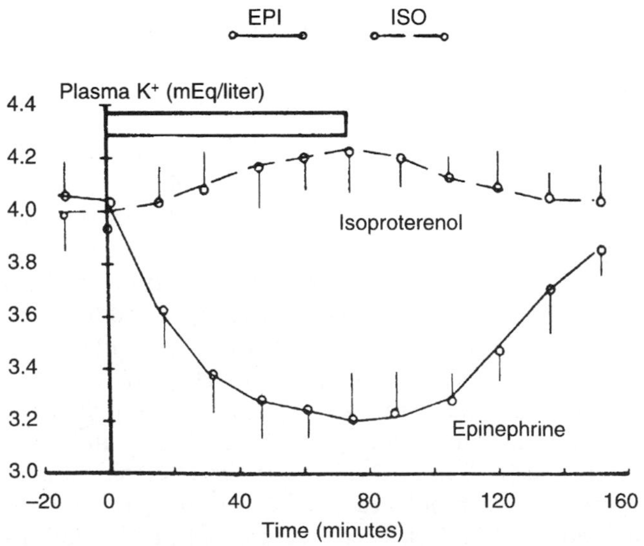

Figure 12-4. Selective $beta_2$-adrenergic agonist effects of epinephrine are responsible for stimulating the movement of potassium ions (K^+) into cells, with a resulting decrease in the serum potassium concentration. (From Brown MJ, Brown DC, Murphy MB. Hypokalemia from beta-2 receptor stimulation by circulating norepinephrine. *N Engl J Med* 1983;309:1414–1419; with permission.)

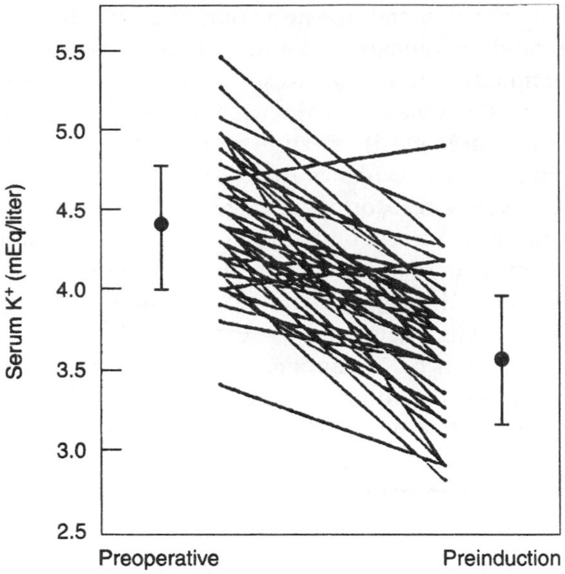

Figure 12-5. Individual and mean (± SD) plasma potassium (K^+) concentrations determined 1 to 3 days preoperatively and immediately before the induction (preinduction) of anesthesia. (From Kharasch ED, Bowdle TA. Hypokalemia before induction of anesthesia and prevention by beta-2 adrenoceptor antagonism. *Anesth Analg* 1991;72:216–220; with permission.)

Ocular Effects

Epinephrine causes contraction of the radial muscles of the iris, producing mydriasis. Contraction of the orbital muscles produces an appearance of exophthalmus considered characteristic of hyperthyroidism. Adrenergic receptors responsible for these ocular effects are probably alpha receptors because norepinephrine is less potent than epinephrine and isoproterenol has practically no ocular effects.

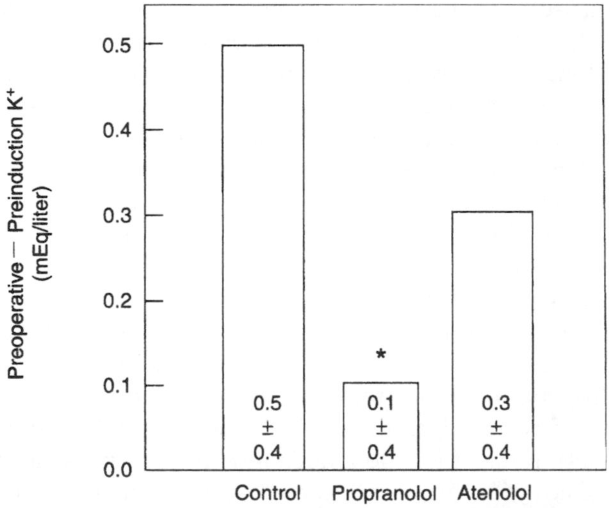

Figure 12-6. Propranolol, but not atenolol, was effective in blunting the difference between preoperative and preinduction serum potassium (K^+) concentrations compared with patients (controls) not receiving a beta antagonist. Data are mean ± SD. The asterisk denotes a significant difference ($P < .02$) between controls and patients treated with propranolol. (From Kharasch ED, Bowdle TA. Hypokalemia before induction of anesthesia and prevention by beta-2 adrenoceptor antagonism. *Anesth Analg* 1991;72:216–220; with permission.)

Gastrointestinal and Genitourinary Effects

Epinephrine, norepinephrine, and isoproterenol produce relaxation of gastrointestinal smooth muscle. Activation of beta-adrenergic receptors relaxes the detrusor muscle of the bladder, whereas activation of alpha-adrenergic receptors contracts the trigone and sphincter muscles.

Coagulation

Blood coagulation is accelerated by epinephrine, presumably due to increased activity of factor V. A hypercoagulable state present during the intraoperative and postoperative period may reflect stress-associated release of epinephrine. Epinephrine increases the total leukocyte count but at the same time causes eosinopenia.

Treatment of Overdose (see Phenylephrine, Treatment of Overdose)

Norepinephrine

Norepinephrine is the endogenous neurotransmitter released from postganglionic sympathetic nerve endings. It is approximately equal in potency to epinephrine for stimulation of $beta_1$ receptors, but unlike epinephrine, norepinephrine has little agonist effect at $beta_2$ receptors (see Table 12-1). Norepinephrine is a potent alpha-agonist that produces intense arterial and venous vasoconstriction in all vascular beds and lacks bronchodilating effects on airway smooth muscle. Hyperglycemia is unlikely to occur as a result of norepinephrine.

Cardiovascular Effects

A continuous infusion of norepinephrine, 4 to 16 μg/minute, may be used to treat refractory hypotension such as may occur in the early period after ligation of the vascular supply to a pheochromocytoma. Placement of norepinephrine in a 5% glucose solution provides sufficient acidity to prevent oxidation of the catecholamine. Extravasation during infusion can produce severe local vasoconstriction and possible necrosis.

IV administration of norepinephrine results in intense vasoconstriction in the vasculature of skeletal muscles, liver, kidneys, and skin. The resulting increase in systemic vascular resistance decreases venous return to the heart and increases systolic, diastolic, and mean arterial pressure (see Table 12-1). Decreased venous return to the heart combined with baroreceptor-mediated reflex decreases in heart rate due to the marked increase in mean arterial pressure tend to decrease cardiac output despite $beta_1$ effects of norepinephrine. Peripheral vasoconstriction may decrease tissue blood flow so much that metabolic acidosis occurs. Chronic infusion of norepinephrine or increased circulating concentrations of this catecholamine, as may be associated with pheochromocytoma, cause precapillary vasoconstriction, and loss of protein-free fluid into the extracellular space.

Dopamine

Dopamine is an endogenous catecholamine that is the immediate precursor of norepinephrine. Dopamine regulates cardiac, vascular, and endocrine function and is an important neurotransmitter in the CNS and peripheral nervous system. The pharmacology of dopamine is complex as this catecholamine differentially stimulates a variety of dopaminergic and adrenergic receptors. For example, dopamine is a relatively nonspecific agonist at both $dopamine_1$ and $dopamine_2$ receptors and the alpha and beta-adrenergic receptors. $Dopamine_1$ receptors are located postsynaptically and when activated elicit vasodilation (renal, mesenteric, coronary, cerebral vessels) and inhibition of sodium-potassium adenosine triphosphate (Goldberg and Rajfer, 1985). Activation of these receptors is mediated by adenylate cyclase. $Dopamine_2$ receptors are principally presynaptic and inhibit adenylate cyclase activity and release of norepinephrine. Nausea and vomiting produced by dopamine probably reflect stimulation of $dopamine_2$ receptors. Dopamine receptors may be associated with the neural mechanism for "reward" that is associated with cocaine and alcohol dependence.

Rapid metabolism of dopamine mandates its use as a continuous infusion (1 to 2 μg/kg/minute) to maintain therapeutic plasma concentrations. Dopamine should be dissolved in 5% glucose in water for IV administration to avoid inactivation of the catecholamine that may occur in alkaline solutions. Depending on the dose, dopamine stimulates principally $dopamine_1$ receptors (0.5 to 3 μg/kg/minute IV) in the renal vasculature to produce renal vasodilation, $beta_1$ receptors (3 to 10 μg/kg/minute IV) in the heart, and alpha receptors (>10 μg/kg/minute IV) in the peripheral vasculature. Despite identical IV infusion rates, there may be a 10 to 75 fold variability in plasma dopamine concentrations that are produced (MacGregor et al, 2000). Extravasation of dopamine, like norepinephrine, produces intense local vasoconstriction, which may be treated with local infiltration of phentolamine. Dopamine is not effective orally and does not cross the blood-brain barrier in sufficient amounts to cause CNS effects. The immediate precursor of dopamine, L-dopa, is absorbed from the gastrointestinal tract and readily crosses the blood-brain barrier. Hyperglycemia that is commonly present in patients receiving a continuous infusion of dopamine is likely to reflect drug-induced inhibition of insulin secretion.

Clinical Uses

Dopamine is used clinically to increase cardiac output in patients with low systemic blood pressure, increased atrial filling pressures, and low urine output as may be present after cardiopulmonary bypass. It is unique among the catecholamines in being able to simultaneously increase (a) myocardial contractility, (b) renal blood flow, (c) glomerular filtration rate, (d) excretion of sodium, and (e) urine output. There is evidence that dopamine inhibits renal tubular solute reabsorption, suggesting that diuresis and natriuresis that frequently accompanies dopamine administration may occur independently of the effect on renal blood flow (Hilberman et al., 1984). Inhibition of aldosterone secretion may contribute to increased sodium excretion produced by dopamine. In adults, dopamine produces a greater diuresis and natriuresis than does dobutamine (Sweny, 1991).

Renal Dose Dopamine

The term *renal dose dopamine* refers to continuous infusion of small doses (1 to 3 μg/kg/minute) of dopamine to patients at risk for development of acute renal failure. This description is misleading as dopamine has many effects at sites other than the kidneys even at these low doses, and it also implies an unproved beneficial effect on renal function (Cottee and Saul, 1996). In fact, no randomized controlled studies have demonstrated a decrease in the incidence of acute renal failure when dopamine is administered to patients considered to be at risk for developing acute renal failure (abdominal aortic cross-clamping, cardiopulmonary bypass) (Baldwin et al., 1994; Byrick and Rose, 1990).

In patients receiving dopamine before a "renal insult," there is a clear diuretic effect but no evidence that the creatinine clearance or need for hemodialysis is altered (Cottee and Saul, 1996). Despite drug-induced diuresis, there is no evidence that urine output in the presence of low cardiac output and/or hypovolemia protects renal function. The use of dopamine after the renal insult has occurred has not been shown to improve glomerular filtration rate. There is evidence that the beneficial effect of low-dose dopamine on renal blood flow and glomerular filtration rate observed in healthy individuals is due to drug-induced increases in cardiac output, and this benefit is lost in early renal failure (Girbes et al., 1996; ter Wee et al., 1986). There is also evidence that arterial hypoxemia attenuates the renal effects of dopamine, and dopamine antagonists (droperidol, metoclopramide) are known to antagonize the effects of dopamine on the kidneys (Blumberg et al., 1988). Risks of low-dose dopamine include tachycardia, cardiac dysrhythmias, myocardial ischemia, attenuation of the ventilatory response to hypoxia, increased intrapulmonary shunting, and development of mesenteric ischemia (Thompson and Cockrill, 1994). Gastrointestinal mucosal ischemia and subsequent translocation of bacteria or bacterial toxins play a role in the development of multiple organ dysfunction syndrome, and it is possible that low-dose dopamine could be exacerbating this process. In the absence of data confirming the efficacy of dopamine in preventing acute renal failure (also true for mannitol and furosemide), it is concluded by many that renal dose dopamine cannot be recommended (Baldwin et al., 1994; Cottee and Saul, 1996; Thompson and Cockrill, 1994).

Side Effects

Cardiovascular Effects

Dopamine increases cardiac output by stimulation of $beta_1$ receptors. This increase in cardiac output is usually accompanied by only modest increases in heart rate, systemic blood pressure, and systemic vascular resistance. A portion of the positive inotropic effect of dopamine is due to stimulation of release of endogenous norepinephrine, which may predispose to the development of cardiac dysrhythmias. Nevertheless, dopamine is less dysrhythmogenic than epinephrine. The release of norepinephrine caused by dopamine may be an unreliable mechanism for increasing cardiac output when cardiac catecholamine stores are depleted, as in patients in chronic cardiac failure. In septic patients, dopamine but not norepinephrine, as administered to maintain an acceptable mean arterial pressure, may result in an uncompensated increase in splanchnic oxygen requirements (Marik and Mohedin, 1994). Decreases in hepatic blood flow associated with epidural anesthesia are reversed by dopamine (5 μg/kg/minute IV) (Tanaka et al., 1997).

The divergent pharmacologic effects of dopamine and dobutamine make their use in combination potentially useful. For example, infusions of the combination of dopamine and dobutamine have been noted to produce a greater improvement in cardiac output, at lower doses, than can be achieved by either drug alone. Each drug dilates different vascular beds such that the summation of afterload reduction by both drugs could produce a greater improvement in cardiac output than could be achieved by either drug alone, even at the same level of inotropism. Dopamine could distribute the cardiac output to the renal and mesenteric vascular beds while dobutamine could provide additional afterload reduction by dilating the vascular beds of skin and skeletal muscles. The objective of combination therapy is to increase coronary perfusion and cardiac output while decreasing afterload, a goal that mimics the effect achieved by the intraaortic balloon pump. In an animal model, both dopamine and dobutamine produce similar increases in pulmonary vascular resistance, whereas the response to hypoxic pulmonary vasoconstriction is not altered (Lejeune et al., 1987).

Ventilation Effects

Infusion of dopamine interferes with the ventilatory response to arterial hypoxemia, reflecting the role of dopamine as an inhibitory neurotransmitter at the carotid bodies (Ward and Belville, 1982). The result is unexpected depression of ventilation in patients who are being treated with dopamine to increase myocardial contractility. Indeed, arterial blood gases have been observed to deteriorate during infusion of dopamine (Lemaire, 1983).

Intraocular Pressure

Continuous infusions of dopamine to critically ill patients are associated with increases in intraocular pressure (Brath et al, 2001). This may create a risk in patients with preexisting glaucoma especially if they are sedated and mechanically ventilated.

SYNTHETIC CATECHOLAMINES

The two clinically useful synthetic catecholamines are isoproterenol and dobutamine (see Table 12-1 and Fig. 12-1). Dopexamine is an analogue of dopamine that predominantly stimulates $beta_2$ and $dopamine_1$ receptors.

Isoproterenol

Isoproterenol is the most potent activator of all the sympathomimetics at $beta_1$ and $beta_2$ receptors, being two to three times more potent than epinephrine and at least 100 times more active than norepinephrine. In clinical doses, isoproterenol is devoid of alpha-agonist effects. Metabolism of isoproterenol in the liver by COMT is rapid, necessitating a continuous infusion to maintain therapeutic plasma concentrations. Uptake of isoproterenol into postganglionic sympathetic nerve endings is minimal.

Clinical Uses

A continuous infusion of isoproterenol, 1 to 5 μg/minute, is effective in increasing the heart rate in adults in the presence of heart block. Isoproterenol is used to provide sustained increases in heart rate before insertion of a temporary or permanent cardiac pacemaker in the treatment of bradydysrhythmias. The use of isoproterenol as an inotropic drug has decreased with the availability of dobutamine and phosphodiesterase inhibitors. Likewise, the use of isoproterenol as a bronchodilator has been supplanted by availability of specific $beta_2$ agonists.

Cardiovascular Effects

The cardiovascular effects of isoproterenol reflect activation of $beta_1$ receptors in the heart and $beta_2$ receptors in the vasculature of skeletal muscles. For example, in an adult, continuous infusion of isoproterenol, 1 to 5 μg/minute, greatly increases heart rate, myocardial contractility, and cardiac automaticity, whereas vasodilation in skeletal muscles decreases systemic vascular resistance. The net effect of these changes is an increase in cardiac output that is usually sufficient to increase systolic blood pressure. The mean arterial pressure, however, may decrease due to decreases in systemic vascular resistance and associated decreases in diastolic blood pressure. Decreased diastolic blood pressure and cardiac dysrhythmias induced by isoproterenol may decrease coronary blood flow at the same time that myocardial oxygen requirements are increased by tachycardia and increased myocardial contractility. This combination of events may be undesirable in patients with coronary artery disease. Compensatory baroreceptor-mediated reflex slowing of the heart rate does not occur during infusion of isoproterenol because mean arterial pressure is not increased.

Dobutamine

Dobutamine is a synthetic catecholamine that acts as a selective $beta_1$-adrenergic agonist. Both of the isomers of dobutamine are beta-agonists whereas at $alpha_1$ receptors these isomers exert opposing agonist and antagonist effects. Rapid metabolism of dobutamine dictates its administration as a continuous infusion at 2 to 10 μg/kg/minute to maintain therapeutic plasma concentrations. Like dopamine, dobutamine should be dissolved in 5% glucose in water for infusion to avoid inactivation of the catecholamine that may occur in an alkaline solution.

Clinical Uses

Dobutamine produces potent beta-adrenergic agonist effects at does <5 μg/kg/minute IV. As a result, dobutamine increases myocardial contractility ($beta_1$ receptors) and causes a modest degree of peripheral vasodilation ($beta_2$ receptors). The levorotatory isomer of dobutamine stimulates $alpha_1$ receptors at doses >5 μg/kg/min and prevents further vasodilation from occurring. Dobutamine is used to improve cardiac output in patients with congestive heart failure, particularly if heart rate and systemic vascular resistance are increased. Combinations of drugs may be useful to increase the spectrum of activity and improve the distribution of cardiac output. For example, dobutamine may be used to increase output, and a low dose of dopamine may be added to favor renal perfusion. Vasodilators may be combined with dobutamine or dopamine to decrease afterload to optimize cardiac output in the presence of increased systemic vascular resistance.

Cardiovascular Effects

Dobutamine produces dose-dependent increases in cardiac output and decreases in atrial filling pressures without associated significant increases in systemic blood pressure and heart rate. The small increase in heart rate compared with isoproterenol reflects a lesser effect of dobutamine on the sinoatrial node. In contrast to dopamine, dobutamine does not have any clinically important vasoconstrictor activity and calculated systemic vascular resistance is usually not greatly altered. Indeed, dobutamine may be ineffective in patients who require increased systemic vascular resistance rather than augmentation of cardiac output to increase systemic blood pressure. In patients with increased pulmonary artery pressure after mitral valve replacement, the infusion of dobutamine (up to 10 μg/kg/minute) increases cardiac output and decreases systemic and pulmonary vascular resistance (Schwenzer and Miller, 1989). These changes were associated with increased intrapulmonary shunt flow. Minimal effects of dobutamine on heart rate and blood pressure reduce the likelihood of adverse increases in myocardial oxygen requirements during infusion of this drug. Unlike dopamine, dobutamine does not act indirectly by stimulating the release of endogenous norepinephrine from the heart, nor does this catecholamine activate dopaminergic receptors to increase renal blood flow. Renal flow, however, improves as a result of drug-induced increases in cardiac output. Dobutamine but not dopamine is a coronary artery vasodilator. Redistribution of cardiac output in the presence of dobutamine may contribute to increased cutaneous heat loss manifesting as an additional decrease in body temperature (Shitara et al., 1996).

High doses of dobutamine (>10 μg/kg/minute IV) may predispose the patient to tachycardia and cardiac dysrhythmias. Nevertheless, cardiac dysrhythmias are unlikely, presumably because of the absence of endogenous catecholamine release. Conduction velocity through the atrioventricular node, however, is increased by dobutamine, raising the possibility that excessive increases in heart rate could occur in patients with atrial fibrillation.

Dopexamine

Dopexamine is a synthetic catecholamine that activates dopaminergic and $beta_2$ receptors. Dopexamne is structurally related to dopamine but is devoid of alpha receptor effects and has a greater affinity for beta receptors. Mild positive inotropic effects reflect principally $beta_2$-adrenergic agonist actions and potentiation of endogenous norepinephrine due to blockade of reuptake. Dopexamine improves creatinine clearance and decreases systemic inflammation without altering splanchnic oxygenation in patients undergoing cardiopulmonary bypass (Berendes et al., 1997).

SYNTHETIC NONCATECHOLAMINES

Synthetic noncatecholamines that possess potential clinical usefulness include, but are not limited to, ephedrine, mephentermine, amphetamine, metaraminol, phenylephrine, and methoxamine (see Table 12-1 and Fig. 12-2) (Smith and Corbascio, 1970).

Ephedrine

Ephedrine is an indirect-acting synthetic noncatecholamine that stimulates alpha- and beta-adrenergic receptors. The pharmacologic effects of this drug are due in part to endogenous release of norepinephrine (indirect-acting), but the drug also has direct stimulant effects on adrenergic receptors (direct-acting). Ephedrine is resistant to metabolism by MAO in the gastrointestinal tract, thus permitting unchanged drug to be absorbed into the circulation after oral administration. IM injection of ephedrine is also acceptable because drug-induced local vasoconstriction is insufficient to greatly delay systemic absorption. Up to 40% of a single dose of ephedrine is excreted unchanged in urine. Some ephedrine is deaminated by MAO in the liver, and conjugation also occurs. The slow inactivation and excretion of ephedrine are responsible for the prolonged duration of action of this sympathomimetic.

Ephedrine, unlike epinephrine, does not produce marked hyperglycemia. Mydriasis accompanies the administration of ephedrine, and CNS stimulation does occur, although less than that produced by amphetamine.

Clinical Uses

Ephedrine, 10 to 25 mg IV administered to adults, is a commonly selected sympathomimetic when drug therapy is used to increase systemic blood pressure in the presence of sympathetic nervous system blockade produced by regional anesthesia or hypotension due to inhaled or injected anesthetics. In an animal model, ephedrine more specifically corrected the noncardiac circulatory changes produced by spinal anesthesia than did a selective alpha- or beta-agonist drug (Butterworth et al., 1986). Until recently, ephedrine was considered the preferred sympathomimetic for administration to parturients experiencing decreased systemic blood pressure owing to spinal or epidural anesthesia. Support for this practice was the observation in pregnant ewes that uterine blood flow was not greatly altered when ephedrine was administered to restore maternal blood pressure to normal after production of sympathetic nervous system blockade (Ralston et al., 1974; McGrath et al., 1994). Recent reviews of trials of ephedrine versus phenylephrine have concluded that systemic blood pressure control is similar with both drugs but phenylephrine is associated with a higher umbilical artery pH at delivery than ephedrine (Lee et al., 2002). Administration of phenylephrine by infusion during cesarean section to maintain maternal systolic blood pressure at baseline is associated with a lower incidence of fetal acidosis than is ephedrine (Cooper et al., 2002). Based on these data it seems that alpha-agonists such as phenylephrine may be a safe alternative to ephedrine for treatment of maternal hypotension.

Ephedrine can be used as chronic oral medication to treat bronchial asthma because of its bronchodilating effects by activation of beta$_2$-adrenergic receptors. Compared with epinephrine, the onset of action of ephedrine is slow, becoming complete only 1 hour or more after administration. A decongestant effect accompanying oral administration of ephedrine produces symptomatic relief from acute coryza. Ephedrine, 0.5 mg/kg IM, has an antiemetic effect similar to that of droperidol but with less sedation when administered to patients undergoing outpatient laparoscopy using general anesthesia (Rothenberg et al., 1991).

Cardiovascular Effects

The cardiovascular effects of ephedrine resemble those of epinephrine, but its systemic blood pressure–elevating response is less intense and lasts approximately ten times longer. It requires approximately 250 times more ephedrine than epinephrine to produce equivalent systemic blood pressure responses. IV administration of ephedrine results in increases in systolic and diastolic blood pressure, heart rate, and cardiac output. Renal and splanchnic blood flows are decreased, whereas coronary and skeletal muscle blood flows are increased. Systemic vascular resistance may be altered minimally because vasoconstriction in some vascular beds is offset by vasodilation (beta$_2$ stimulation) in other areas. These cardiovascular effects are due, in part, to alpha receptor–mediated peripheral arterial and venous vasoconstriction. The principal mechanism, however, for cardiovascular effects produced by ephedrine is increased myocardial contractility due to activation of beta$_1$ receptors. In the presence of preexisting beta-adrenergic blockade, the cardiovascular effects of ephedrine may resemble responses more typical of alpha-adrenergic receptor stimulation.

A second dose of ephedrine produces a less intense systemic blood pressure response than the first dose. This phenomenon, known as tachyphylaxis, occurs with many sympathomimetics and is related to the duration of action of these drugs. Tachyphylaxis probably represents a persistent blockade of adrenergic receptors. For example, ephedrine-induced activation of adrenergic receptors persists even after systemic blood pressure has returned to near predrug levels by virtue of compensatory cardiovascular changes. When ephedrine is administered at this time, the receptor sites still occupied by ephedrine limit available sites and the blood pressure response is less. Alternatively, tachyphylaxis may be due to depletion of norepinephrine stores.

Mephentermine

Mephentermine is an indirect-acting synthetic noncatecholamine that stimulates alpha- and beta-adrenergic receptors. Structurally, it is closely related to methylamphetamine but has only modest CNS-stimulating qualities. Administered IV, mephentermine produces cardiovascular effects that resemble those of ephedrine. Despite its positive inotropic effect, however, mephentermine exerts a modest antidysrhythmic effect.

Amphetamine

Amphetamine and related sympathomimetics (dextroamphetamine and methamphetamine) resemble ephedrine in evoking alpha- and beta-adrenergic receptor stimulation but differ from ephedrine in producing significant CNS stimulation. The CNS stimulant effects, as well as appetite-suppressant actions, reflect release of norepinephrine from storage sites in the CNS. Tachyphylaxis is prominent, and drug dependence is predictable, considering the ability of these drugs to stimulate the CNS.

Acute IV administration of dextroamphetamine to dogs increases anesthetic requirements, presumably reflecting the release of norepinephrine into the CNS (Johnston et al., 1974). Conversely, chronic administration of dextroamphetamine decreases CNS stores of catecholamines, and anesthetic requirements may be decreased (Johnston et al., 1974). Excretion of amphetamine is negligible in alkaline urine (2% to 3%) because the drug exists predominantly in the nonionized fraction that is readily reabsorbed by renal tubules. For this reason, treatment of amphetamine overdose includes acidification of the urine.

Modafinil

Modafinil is a wakefulness-promoting drug that is effective for treatment of patients with excessive daytime sleepiness associated with narcolepsy. The mechanism of action of modafinil is not known. This drug is chemically unrelated to amphetamine. A feeling of fatigue and sedation following recovery from general anesthesia may be countered by administration of modafinil (Larijani et al., 2004).

Metaraminol

Metaraminol is a synthetic noncatecholamine that stimulates alpha- and beta-adrenergic receptors by indirect and direct effects. This sympathomimetic undergoes uptake into postganglionic sympathetic nerve endings, where it substitutes for norepinephrine and acts as a weak false neurotransmitter. Indeed, chronically administered metaraminol (2 to 3 hours by continuous infusion) decreases systemic blood pressure in hypertensive patients, presumably reflecting the lesser vasoconstrictor potency (estimated to be one-tenth) of this sympathomimetic compared with that of norepinephrine. Sudden withdrawal of a metaraminol infusion can lead to profound hypotension until the nerve ending stores of norepinephrine are replenished. Metaraminol is not a substrate for MAO or COMT.

Cardiovascular Effects

Metaraminol produces more intense peripheral vasoconstriction and less increase in myocardial contractility than ephedrine. Administration of metaraminol, 1.5 to 5.0 mg IV to adults, produces a sustained increase in systolic and diastolic blood pressure that is due almost entirely to peripheral vasoconstriction, emphasizing the predominant alpha-agonist effect of this sympathomimetic. Vasoconstriction decreases renal and cerebral blood flow. Reflex bradycardia often accompanies drug-induced increases in systemic blood pressure, resulting in a decrease in cardiac output. If heart rate slowing is prevented by atropine, then metaraminol can increase cardiac output similar to that of ephedrine. Like phenylephrine, infusion of metaraminol to maintain maternal blood pressure during cesarean section is associated with less fetal acidosis than ephedrine (Kee et al, 2001).

Phenylephrine

Phenylephrine is a synthetic noncatecholamine that stimulates principally $alpha_1$-adrenergic receptors by a direct effect, with only a small part of the pharmacologic response being due to its ability to evoke the release of norepinephrine (indirect-acting). There is a minimal effect on beta-adrenergic receptors. The dose of phenylephrine necessary to stimulate $alpha_1$ receptors is far less than the dose that stimulates $alpha_2$ receptors. Resulting venoconstriction is greater than arterial constriction. Structurally, phenylephrine is 3-hydroxyphenylethylamine; it differs from epinephrine only in lacking a 4-hydroxyl group on the benzene ring. Clinically, phenylephrine mimics the effects of norepinephrine but is less potent and longer lasting. CNS stimulation is minimal.

Clinical Uses

Phenylephrine, 50 to 200 μg IV, is often administered to adults to treat systemic blood pressure decreases that accompany sympathetic nervous system blockade produced by a regional anesthetic or peripheral vasodilation, which accompanies administration of injected or inhaled anesthetics. Treatment of tetracaine-induced hypotension with phenylephrine restores systolic, diastolic, and mean arterial pressure, whereas heart rate and cardiac output decrease (Brooker et al., 1997). Phenylephrine is believed to be particularly useful in patients with coronary artery disease and in patients with aortic stenosis because this drug, in contrast to other sympathomimetics, increases coronary perfusion pressure without chronotropic side effects.

Phenylephrine has been used as a continuous infusion (20 to 50 μg/minute) in adults to sustain systemic blood pressure at normal levels during carotid endarterectomy. The reflex vagal effects produced by phenylephrine can be used to slow heart rate in the presence of hemodynamically significant supraventricular tachydysrhythmias. Phenylephrine sufficient to increase systemic blood pressure in combination with inhaled nitric oxide results in a greater improvement in arterial oxygenation than with either drug alone (Pearl, 1997). Topically applied, phenylephrine is a nasal decongestant and produces mydriasis without cycloplegia. The initial dose of topical phenylephrine should not exceed 0.5 mg (four drops of 0.25% solution) (Gourdine et al., 2000). Phenylephrine, like epinephrine, is effective in prolonging spinal anesthesia when added to local anesthetic solutions that are placed in the subarachnoid space (see Chapter 7).

Obstetrical Anesthesia

Recent reviews of trials of ephedrine versus phenylephrine have concluded that systemic blood pressure control is similar with both drugs but phenylephrine is associated with a higher umbilical artery pH at delivery than ephedrine (Lee et al., 2002). Administration of phenylephrine by infusion during cesarean section to maintain maternal systolic blood pressure at baseline is associated with a lower incidence of fetal acidosis than is ephedrine (Cooper et al., 2002). Based on these data it seems that alpha-agonists such as phenylephrine may be a safe alternative to ephedrine for treatment of maternal hypotension.

IV administration of phenylephrine, but not ephedrine, to prevent maternal hypotension during combined spinal-epidural anesthesia for cesarean section decreases the rostral spread of spinal anesthesia (Fig. 12-7) (Cooper et al., 2004). A possible explanation is greater epidural vein constriction with phenylephrine than ephedrine, thereby decreasing epidural vein engorgement. As a result, phenylephrine would be associated with a decrease in epidural space pressure compared with ephedrine.

Side Effects

Cardiovascular Effects

Rapid IV injection of phenylephrine to patients with coronary artery disease produces dose-dependent peripheral vasoconstriction and increases in systemic blood pressure that are accompanied by decreases in cardiac output (Fig. 12-8) (Schwinn and Reves, 1989). Decreases in cardiac output may reflect increased afterload but more likely are due to baroreceptor-mediated reflex bradycardia in response to drug-induced increases in diastolic blood pressure. It is possible that decreases in cardiac output could limit the associated increases in systemic blood pressure. Rapid administration of phenylephrine, 1 μg/kg IV, to anesthetized patients with coronary artery disease causes a transient impairment of left ventricular global function (Goertz et al., 1993). Oral clonidine premedication augments the pressor response to phenylephrine, presumably due to clonidine-induced potentiation of $alpha_1$-mediated vasoconstriction (Inomata et al., 1995). Renal, splanchnic, and cutaneous blood flows are decreased but coronary blood flow is increased. Pulmonary artery pressure is increased by phenylephrine.

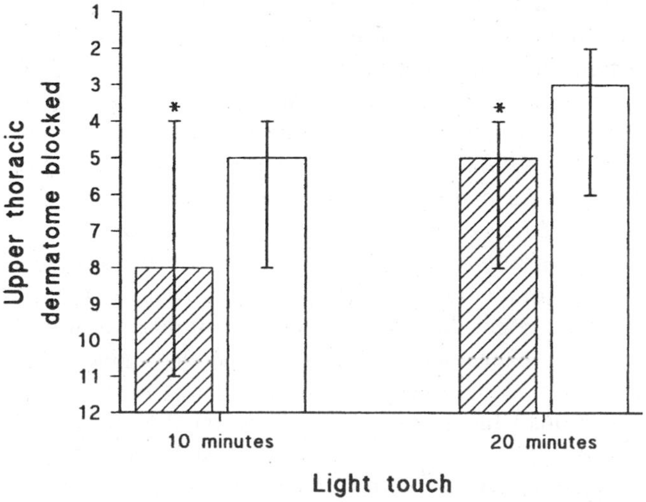

Figure 12-7. Upper dermatome blockade to light touch 10 minutes and 20 minutes postspinal in the presence of phenylephrine (hatched bars) or ephedrine (open bars). *P < 0.026 at 10 minutes and P < 0.009 at 20 minutes. (From Cooper DW, Jeyaraj L, Hynd R, et al. Evidence that intravenous vasopressors can affect rostral spread of spinal anesthesia in pregnancy. *Anesthesiology* 2004; 101:28–33; with permission.)

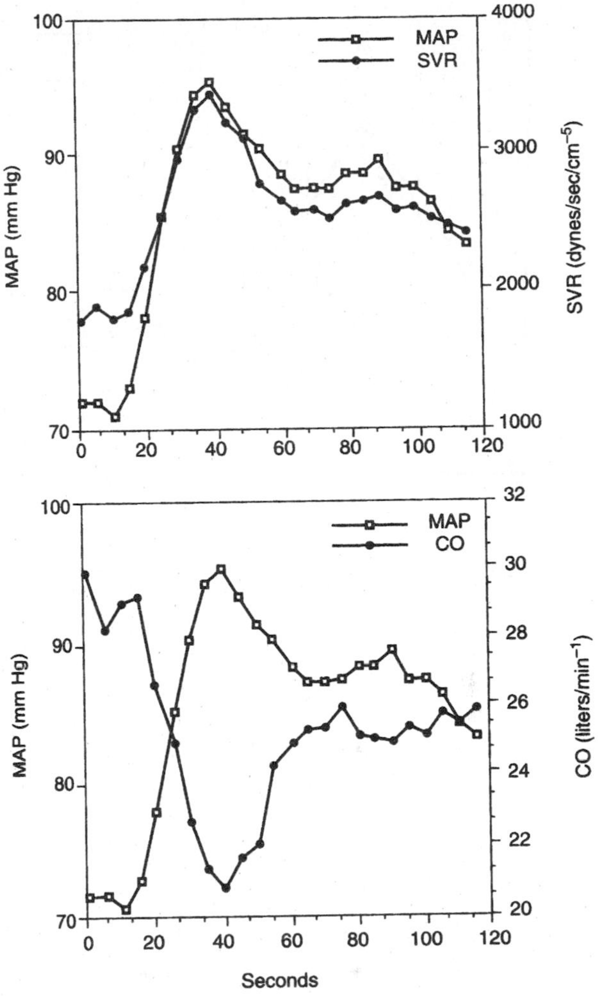

Figure 12-8. Hemodynamic response to rapid intravenous injection of phenylephrine in a single patient. Mean arterial pressure (MAP) and systemic vascular resistance (SVR) increase and cardiac output (CO) decreases in response to phenylephrine, with peak effects occurring 42 seconds after drug administration. (From Schwinn DA, Reves JG. Time course and hemodynamic effects of alpha-1 adrenergic bolus administration in anesthetized patients with myocardial disease. *Anesth Analg* 1989;68:571–578; with permission.)

Metabolic Effects

Stimulation of alpha receptors by a continuous infusion of phenylephrine during acute potassium loading interferes with the movement of potassium ions across cell membranes into cells (Fig. 12-9) (Williams et al., 1984).

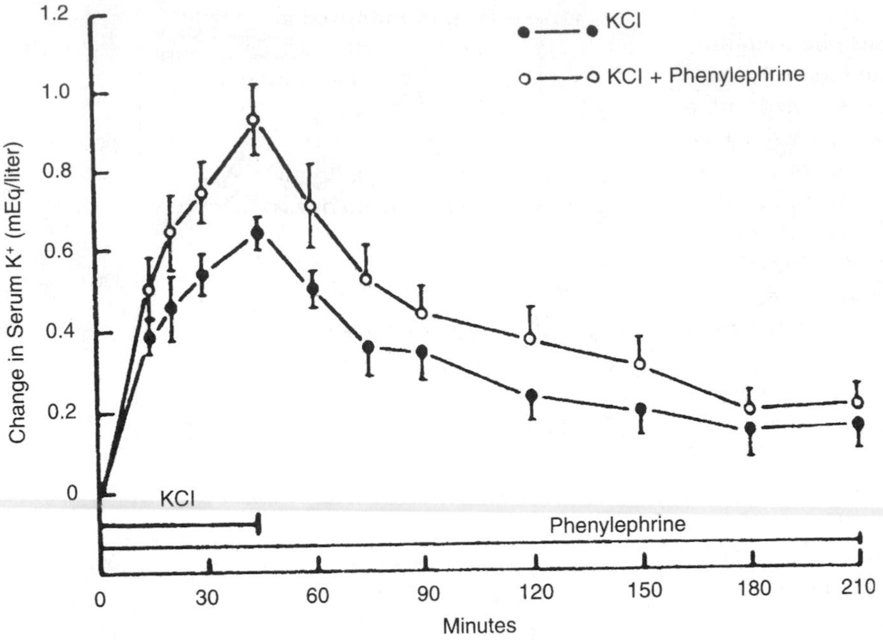

Figure 12-9. Plasma potassium (K^+) concentrations during the infusion of potassium chloride (KCl) increase more in patients also receiving phenylephrine. (From Williams ME, Rosa RM, Silva P, et al. Impairment of extrarenal potassium disposal by alpha-adrenergic stimulation. *N Engl J Med* 1984; 311:145–149; with permission.)

Administration of phenylephrine in the absence of an acute potassium load does not change the plasma potassium concentration. This effect of alpha-adrenergic stimulation on movement of potassium ions across cell membranes is opposite to that produced by beta$_2$-receptor stimulation (see Fig. 12-6) (Brown et al., 1983).

Treatment of Overdose

Systemic manifestations of sympathetic nervous system activation (systemic hypertension, tachycardia, baroreceptor-mediated bradycardia) may accompany vascular absorption of alpha-agonists (phenylephrine, epinephrine) when utilized as topical or injected vasoconstrictors in the surgical field. Treatment of these systemic effects with beta-adrenergic blocking drugs may be followed by pulmonary edema and irreversible cardiovascular collapse (Gourdine et al., 2000).

Systemic hypertension secondary to alpha stimulation increases systemic vascular resistance. This shifts blood from the peripheral circulation into the pulmonary vasculature, which is less sensitive to the effects of vasoconstrictors, increasing left ventricular filling pressure. The increased systemic vascular resistance increases impedance to left ventricular ejection and increases end-diastolic volumes and pressures. The ability of the heart to increase heart rate and contractility are important compensatory mechanisms to preserve cardiac output under these circumstances. Beta-blockers interfere with these compensatory mechanisms and their administration in the presence of phenylephrine or epinephrine overdose may be followed by cardiovascular collapse.

Systemic hypertension induced by topically applied or injected alpha-agonists may not require treatment. The duration of action of phenylephrine and epinephrine is brief and hypertension may resolve spontaneously without pharmacologic interventions. Severe hypertension may require pharmacologic interventions but treatment must not decrease the ability of the stressed myocardium to increase contractility and heart rate. In this circumstance, vasodilating drugs such as nitroprusside or nitroglycerin is recommended. Should cardiovascular collapse occur in relation to administration of a beta-blocker, glucagon (5 to 10 mg IV) may be a consideration.

Methoxamine

Methoxamine is a synthetic noncatecholamine that acts directly and selectively on alpha-adrenergic receptors. This drug resembles phenylephrine but has a longer duration of action, and large doses of methoxamine have an inhibitory effect on beta-receptors and may produce bradycardia. Methoxamine, 5 to 10 mg IV administered to adults, causes intense arterial vasoconstriction that manifests as increased systolic and diastolic blood pressure and baroreceptor-mediated reflex bradycardia that contributes to a decrease in cardiac output. Venoconstriction is minimal after administration of methoxamine. Renal blood flow is decreased to a greater extent than after equally potent doses of norepinephrine. Conversely, coronary blood flow may increase as a result of increased perfusion pressure and increased time for coronary blood flow to occur due to reflex bradycardia. Atropine prevents reflex bradycardia and the associated decrease in cardiac output. Methoxamine exerts a modest antidysrhythmic effect by an unknown mechanism.

Midodrine

Midodrine is an alpha$_1$-adrenergic agonist that activates receptors on arterioles and veins to increase systemic vascular resistance. After oral administration, the drug is extensively absorbed and undergoes enzymatic hydrolysis to its active metabolite, desylymidodrine. Neurogenic orthostatic hypotension as may accompany autonomic neuropathies (diabetes mellitus, amyloidosis) may be responsive to treatment with midodrine (Low et al., 1997).

SELECTIVE BETA$_2$-ADRENERGIC AGONISTS

Selective beta$_2$-adrenergic agonists specifically relax bronchiole and uterine smooth muscle, but in contrast to isoproterenol, generally lack stimulating (beta$_1$) effects on the heart. Nevertheless, high concentrations of these drugs are likely to cause stimulation of beta$_1$ receptors. The chemical structure of selective beta$_2$-adrenergic agonists (placement of hydroxyl groups on the benzene ring at sites different than the catecholamines) renders them resistant to methylation by COMT, thus contributing to their sustained duration of action (see Figs. 12-1 and 12-3).

Clinical Uses

Beta$_2$-adrenergic agonists are the preferred treatment for acute episodes of asthma and the prevention of exercise-induced asthma (Nelson, 1995). Currently used beta$_2$-adrenergic agonists may be divided into those with an intermediate duration of action (3 to 6 hours) and those that are long-acting (>12 hours) (Table 12-2) (Nelson, 1995). Among the intermediate-acting drugs, there is little reason to choose one over the other. Metaproterenol is less beta$_2$-specific than other agonists and hence more likely to cause cardiac stimulation. This is usually not a problem with the customary dose used (two inhalations at intervals of 4 hours). Beta$_2$-adrenergic agonists are also used regularly in patients with chronic obstructive pulmonary disease, resulting in improved air flow and exercise tolerance. The long-acting beta$_2$-adrenergic agonist salmeterol is highly lipophilic and has a high affinity for the beta$_2$ receptor, resulting in prolonged activation at this site. In addition to the treatment of bronchospasm, beta$_2$-adrenergic agonists may also be administered as continuous infusions to stop premature uterine contractions (tocolytics).

Route of Administration

Beta$_2$-adrenergic bronchodilators can be administered orally, by inhalation, or subcutaneously (SC) or via IV injection. The inhaled route is preferred because the side effects are fewer for any given degree of bronchodilation. Inhalation is as effective as parenteral administration for treating acute, severe attacks of asthma in most patients, although some who have severe bronchial obstruction may benefit initially from parenteral therapy.

Inhaled beta$_2$-adrenergic agonists can be administered as an aerosol from a jet or ultrasonic nebulizer, or they can be administered from a metered-dose inhaler either as a propellant-generated aerosol or as a breath-propelled dry powder. With optimal inhalation technique (discharge the inhaler while taking a slow deep breath over 5 to 6 seconds, and then hold the breath at full inspiration for 10 seconds) approximately 12% of the drug is delivered from the metered-dose inhaler to the lungs; the remainder is deposited in the mouth, pharynx, and larynx (Nelson, 1995). The presence of a tracheal tube decreases by approximately 50% to 70% the amount of drug delivered by a metered-dose inhaler that reaches the trachea (Crogan and Bishop, 1989). Actuation of the metered-dose inhaler during a mechanically delivered inspiration increases the amount of drug that passes beyond the distal end of the tracheal tube. In general, the dose required in a nebulizer is six to ten times that used in a metered-dose inhaler to produce the same degree of bronchodilation.

TABLE 12-2.
COMPARATIVE PHARMACOLOGY OF SELECTIVE BETA$_2$-ADRENERGIC AGONIST BRONCHODILATORS

	Beta$_2$ Selectivity	Peak Effect (mins)	Duration of Action (hrs)	Concentration (μg per puff)	Method of Administration
Intermediate-acting (3–6 hrs)					
Albuterol	++++	30–60	4	90	MDI, oral
Metaproterenol	+++	30–60	3–4	200	Oral, subcutaneous
Terbutaline	++++	60	4	200	MDI, oral, subcutaneous
Isoetharine	++	15–60	2–3	340	MDI, solution
Bitolterol	++++	30–60	5	370	MDI
Long-acting (>12 hrs)					
Salmeterol	++++		>12	21	MDI

++, minimal stimulation; +++, moderate stimulation; ++++, marked stimulation; MDI, metered-dose inhaler; solution, solution of nebulization.

Side Effects

The widespread distribution of beta$_2$-adrenergic receptors makes it likely that undesired responses may result when beta$_2$-adrenergic agonists undergo systemic absorption. The ability to minimize these systemic side effects by decreasing plasma drug concentrations is an advantage of administering beta$_2$-adrenergic bronchodilators by inhalation.

The principal side effect of beta$_2$-adrenergic agonists treatment is tremor, which is caused by direct stimulation of beta$_2$ receptors in skeletal muscles. Increased heart rate is less common with the selective beta$_2$-adrenergic agonists, but even stimulation of beta$_2$ receptors may result in vasodilation and reflex tachycardia. Furthermore, some of the beta-adrenergic receptors in the heart are beta$_2$; thus, direct stimulation of the heart results from the use of selective beta$_2$-adrenergic agonists. In patients with acute, severe asthma, beta$_2$-adrenergic agonists may cause a transient decrease in arterial oxygenation presumed to reflect relaxation of compensatory vasoconstriction in areas of decreased ventilation. This is not a serious problem if supplemental oxygen is administered. Increased mortality in patients with severe asthma and treated with beta$_2$-adrenergic agonists is most likely a reflection of the severity of the asthma rather than a toxic effect of the drug therapy (Mullen et al., 1993; Suissa et al., 1994).

Acute metabolic responses to beta$_2$-adrenergic agonists include hyperglycemia, hypokalemia, and hypomagnesemia. Because these responses diminish with chronic administration, such changes are not important in patients receiving long-term therapy. Lactic acidosis may occur in association with beta$_2$ agonist therapy perhaps reflecting excess glycogenolysis and lipolysis from beta$_2$ receptor activation (Liem et al., 2003).

Albuterol

Albuterol is the preferred selective beta$_2$-adrenergic agonist for the treatment of acute bronchospasm due to asthma. Administration is most often by metered-dose inhaler, producing about 100 μg per puff; the usual dose is two puffs delivered during deep inhalations 1 to 5 minutes apart. This dose may be repeated every 4 to 6 hours, not to exceed 16 to 20 puffs daily. Alternatively, 2.5 to 5 mg of albuterol (0.5 to 1 ml of 0.5% solution in 5 ml of normal saline) may be administered by nebulization every 15 minutes for three to four doses, followed by treatments hourly during the initial hours of therapy. The duration of action of an inhaled dose is about 4 hours, but significant relief of symptoms may persist up to 8 hours. The effects of albuterol and volatile anesthetics on bronchomotor tone are additive (Tobias and Hirshman, 1990).

Continuous nebulization of albuterol using a large reservoir system to deliver up to 15 mg/hour for 2 hours may be appropriate and necessary in the presence of life-threatening asthma. Tachycardia and hypokalemia may accompany these large doses of albuterol. Nevertheless, larger doses and more frequent dosing intervals for inhaled beta-adrenergic agonist therapy are needed in acute severe asthma due to decreased deposition at the site of action (low tidal volumes and narrowed airways), alteration in the dose-response curve, and altered duration of activity. Inhaled albuterol (four puffs) blunts airway responses to tracheal intubation in asthmatic patients (Maslow et al., 2000).

Metaproterenol

Metaproterenol is a selective beta$_2$-adrenergic agonist used to treat asthma. Administered by metered-dose inhaler, the daily dosage should not exceed 16 puffs, with each metered-aerosol actuation delivering approximately 650 μg. Oral administration is followed by excretion as conjugates of glucuronic acid.

Terbutaline

Terbutaline is a predominantly beta$_2$-adrenergic agonist that may be administered orally, SC, or by inhalation to treat asthma. The SC administration of terbutaline (0.25 mg) produces responses that resemble those of epinephrine, but the duration of action is longer. The SC dose of terbutaline for children is 0.01 mg/kg. Administered by metered-dose inhaler, the daily dose should not exceed 16 to 20 puffs, with each metered-dose actuation delivering about 200 μg.

Bitolterol

Bitolterol is a selective beta$_2$-adrenergic agonist that resembles albuterol but is more potent and lasts longer. When inhaled, bitolterol is a prodrug that is converted primarily by pulmonary esterases to the active catecholamine colterol. Cardiovascular side effects are rare. The daily dosage should not exceed 16 to 20 puffs, with each metered-aerosol actuation delivering approximately 270 μg.

Isoetharine

Isoetharine resembles isoproterenol structurally but has less beta$_1$ activity and produces fewer adverse effects. Used by hand nebulizer, the drug is delivered by one to two inhalations. If the therapeutic response is inadequate after 1 minute, this dose may be repeated once and every 2 to 4 hours thereafter. The metered-dose inhaler delivers approximately 340 μg with each actuation. Overall, this drug is less selective than other beta$_2$-adrenergic agonists, and its duration of action is brief.

Ritodrine

Ritodrine is the beta$_2$-adrenergic agonist most often used to stop uterine contractions of premature labor (Fig. 12-10).

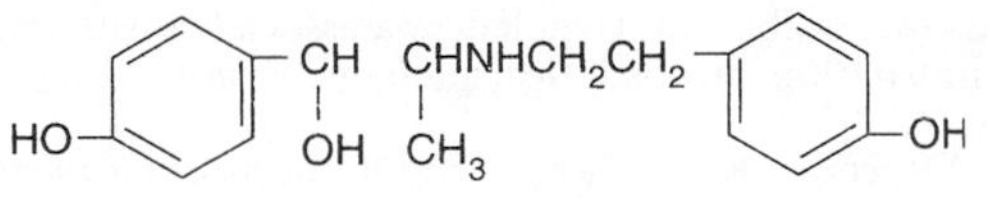

Figure 12-10. Ritodrine.

The inhibitory action of ritodrine on uterine activity reflects stimulation of $beta_2$ receptors through activation of adenylate cyclase. Although ritodrine predominantly stimulates $beta_2$ receptors, it also has some $beta_1$ effects manifesting as tachycardia. Ritodrine is administered as a continuous infusion at doses up to 350 μg/kg/minute until uterine contractions are inhibited for at least 12 hours. Metabolism to inactive conjugates occurs in the liver and about half the drug is excreted unchanged in the urine. Teratogenic effects have not been shown to accompany the prenatal use of ritodrine after 20 weeks of gestation. Although ritodrine therapy decreases the incidence of delivery within 48 hours of the start of treatment, this immediate effect has not led to a decrease in the overall rate of preterm delivery (Moutquin et al., 1992).

Side Effects

Ritodrine readily crosses the placenta such that cardiovascular and metabolic side effects may occur in the mother and fetus (Benedetti, 1983). Although mean arterial pressure changes little, there is a dose-related tachycardia and increase in cardiac output that most likely results from a reflex response to decreases in diastolic blood pressure combined with direct actions on cardiac $beta_1$ receptors. Secretion of renin is increased, leading to decreased excretion of sodium, potassium, and water. Pulmonary edema may occur if hydration is aggressive during infusion of the drug, leading to the recommendation that total fluid intake be restricted to <2 liters in 24 hours and that the electrocardiogram be monitored continuously (Benedetti, 1983). Evidence of cardiac disease limits the use of ritodrine as a tocolytic. Exaggerated systemic blood pressure decreases are possible when ritodrine is given with other drugs that can cause hypotension, such as volatile anesthetics.

Maternal hypokalemia may be associated with infusion of ritodrine (Hurlbert et al., 1981; Moravec and Hurlbert, 1980). Hypokalemia presumably reflects $beta_2$-adrenergic agonist effects that favor translocation of potassium ions into the cells. Because total body potassium stores are unaltered, treatment is not indicated. The possibility of an additive hypokalemic effect with potassium-depleting diuretics should be considered.

Ritodrine, like other $beta_2$-adrenergic agonists, can cause marked hyperglycemia. Persistent maternal hyperglycemia may evoke sufficient insulin release to cause reactive hypoglycemia in the fetus. Administration of ritodrine to insulin-dependent diabetics has been followed by ketoacidosis despite prior SC doses of insulin (Mordes et al., 1982). Concomitant administration of glucocorticoids to promote fetal lung maturation could aggravate the diabetic state in these patients and contribute to the beta-agonist actions of ritodrine in promoting glycogenolysis and lipolysis. Nevertheless, abrupt metabolic deterioration is not common in diabetics who receive glucocorticoids without ritodrine. Continuous infusion of insulin may be indicated in the diabetic parturient receiving IV ritodrine. Maximum rates of ritodrine infusion may result in at least doubling of previous insulin requirements. Certainly, plasma glucose and potassium concentrations should be monitored during IV administration of ritodrine.

REFERENCES

Baldwin L, Henderson A, Hickman P. Effect of postoperative low-dose dopamine on renal function after elective major vascular surgery. *Ann Intern Med* 1994;120:744–747.

Beatriz M, Perondi M, Reis AG, et al. A comparison of high-dose and standard-dose epinephrine in children with cardiac arrest. *N Engl J Med* 2004;350:1722–30.

Benedetti TJ. Maternal complications of parenteral -sympathomimetic therapy for premature labor. *Am J Obstet Gynecol* 1983;1:145–146.

Berendes E, Mollhoff T, Van Aken H, et al. Effects of dopexamine on creatine clearance, systemic inflammation, and splanchnic oxygenation in patients undergoing coronary artery bypass grafting. *Anesth Analg* 1997;84:950–957.

Blumberg AL, Dubb JW, Allison NL, et al. Selectivity of metoclopramide for endocrine versus renal effects of dopamine in normal humans. *J Cardiovasc Pharmacol* 1988;11:181–186.

Brath PC, MacGregor DA, Ford JG, et al. Dopamine, and intraocular pressure in critically ill patients. *Anesthesiology* 2000;93:1398–1400.

Brooker FR, Butterworth JF, Kitzman DW, et al. Treatment of hypotension after hyperbaric tetracaine spinal anesthesia: a randomized, double-blind, cross-over comparison of phenylephrine and epinephrine. *Anesthesiology* 1997;86:797–805.

Brown MJ, Brown DC, Murphy MB. Hypokalemia from beta-2 receptor stimulation by circulating epinephrine. *N Engl J Med* 1983; 309:1414–1419.

Butterworth JF, Piccione W, Berribeitia LD, et al. Augmentation of venous return by adrenergic agonists during spinal anesthesia. *Anesth Analg* 1986;65:612–616.

Byrick RJ, Rose DK. Pathophysiology and prevention of acute renal failure: the role of the anaesthetist. *Can J Anaesth* 1990;37: 457–467.

Cooper DW, Carpenter M, Mowbray P, et al. Fetal, and maternal effects of phenylephrine and ephedrine during spinal anesthesia for cesarean delivery. *Anesthesiology* 2002;97:1582–1590.

Cooper DW, Jeyaraj L, Hynd R, et al. Evidence that intravenous vasopressors can affect rostral spread of spinal anesthesia in pregnancy. *Anesthesiology* 2004;101:28–33.

Cottee DBF, Saul WP. Is renal dose dopamine protective or therapeutic? No. *Controv Crit Care Med* 1996;12:687–695.

Crogan SJ, Bishop MJ. Delivery efficiency of metered dose aerosols given via endotracheal tubes. *Anesthesiology* 1989;70:1008–1010.

Eger EI, Hamilton WK. The effect of reserpine on the action of various vasopressors. *Anesthesiology* 1959;20:641–645.

Girbes ARJ, Lieverse AG, Smith AJ, et al. Lack of specific renal haemodynamic effects on different doses of dopamine after infrarenal aortic surgery. *Br J Anaesth* 1996;77:753–757.

Goertz AW, Lindner KH, Seefelder C, et al. Effect of phenylephrine bolus administration on global left ventricular function in patients with coronary artery disease and patients with valvular aortic stenosis. *Anesthesiology* 1993;78:834–841.

Goldberg IF, Cohn JN. New inotropic drugs for heart failure. *JAMA* 1987; 258:493–497.

Goldberg LI, Rajfer SI. Dopamine receptors: applications in clinical cardiology. *Circulation* 1985;72:246–252.

Gourdine SB, Hollinbger I, Jones J et al. New York State Guidelines on the topical use of phenylephrine in the operating room. *Anesthesiology* 2000;92:859–870.

Halsworth CH, Lee TH, Hirst SJ. $Beta_2$-adrenoceptor agonists inhibit release of eosinophil-activating cytokines from human airway smooth muscle cells. *Br J Pharmacol* 2001;132:729–733.

Hilberman M, Maseda J, Stinson EB, et al. The diuretic properties of dopamine in patients after open-heart operation. *Anesthesiology* 1984;61:489–494.

Hurlbert BJ, Edelman JD, David K. Serum potassium levels during and after terbutaline. *Anesth Analg* 1981;60:723–725.

Inomata S, Nishikawa T, Kihara S, Akiyoshi Y. Enhancement of pressor response to intravenous phenylephrine following oral clonidine medication in awake and anaesthetized patients. *Can J Anaesth* 1995;42:119–125.

Johnston PR, Way WL, Miller RD. The effect of central nervous system catecholamine-depleting drugs on dextroamphetamine-induced elevation of halothane MAC. *Anesthesiology* 1974;41:57–61.

Kee WDN, Lau TK, Khaw KS et al. Comparison of metaraminol and ephedrine infusions for maintaining arterial pressure during spinal anesthesia for elective cesarean section. *Anesthesiology* 2001;95:317–313.

Kharasch ED, Bowdle TA. Hypokalemia before induction of anesthesia and prevention by beta-2 adrenoceptor antagonism. *Anesth Analg* 1991;72:216–220.

Larijani GE, Goldberg ME, Hojat M, et al. Modafinil improves recovery after general anesthesia. *Anesth Analg* 2004;98:976–981.

Lawson NW, Wallfisch HK. Cardiovascular pharmacology: a new look at the pressors. In: Stoelting RK, Barash PG, Gallagher TJ, eds. *Advances in anesthesia*. Chicago: Year Book, 1986:195–270.

Lee A, Ngan KWD, Gin T. A quantitative, systematic review of randomized controlled trials of ephedrine versus phenylephrine for the management of hypotension during spinal anesthesia for cesarean delivery. *Anesth Analg* 2002;94:920–926.

Lejeune P, Leeman M, Deloff T, Naeije R. Pulmonary hemodynamic response to dopamine and dobutamine in hyperoxic and in hypoxic dogs. *Anesthesiology* 1987;66:49–54.

Lemaire F. Effects of catecholamines on pulmonary right-to-left shunt. *Int Anesthesiol Clin* 1983;21:43–58.

Liem EB, Mnolokin SC, Mahla ME. Albuterol-induced lactic acidosis. *Anesthesiology* 2003;99:505–506.

Low PA, Gilden JL, Freeman R, et al. Efficacy of midodrine vs. placebo in neurogenic orthostatic hypotension: a randomized, double-blind multicenter study. *JAMA* 1997;277:1046–1051.

MacGregor DA, Smith TE, Prielipp RC et al. Pharmacokinetics of dopamine in healthy male subjects. *Anesthesiology* 2000;92: 338–346.

Marik PE, Mohedin M. The contrasting effects of dopamine and norepinephrine on systemic and splanchnic oxygen utilization in hyperdynamic sepsis. *JAMA* 1994;272:1354–1357.

Maslow AD, Regan MM, Israel E, et al. Inhaled albuterol, but not intravenous lidocaine, protects against intubation-induced bronchoconstriction in asthma. *Anesthesiology* 2000;95: 1198–1204.

Maze M. Clinical implications of membrane receptor function in anesthesia. *Anesthesiology* 1981;55:160–171.

McCrirrick A, Monk CR. Comparison of i.v. and intra-tracheal administration of adrenaline. *Br J Anaesth* 1994;72:529–532.

McGrath JM, Chestnut DH, Vincent RD, et al. Ephedrine remains the vasopressor of choice for treatment of hypotension during ritodrine infusion and epidural anesthesia. *Anesthesiology* 1994;80: 1073–1081.

Miller RD, Way WL, Eger EI. The effects of alpha-methyldopa, reserpine, guanethidine, and iproniazid on minimum alveolar anesthetic requirements (MAC). *Anesthesiology* 1968;29:1153–1158.

Moravec MA, Hurlbert BJ. Hypokalemia associated with terbutaline administration in obstetrical patients. *Anesth Analg* 1980;59: 917–920.

Mordes D, Kreutner K, Metzger W, et al. Dangers of intravenous ritodrine in diabetic patients. *JAMA* 1982;248:973–975.

Moutquin JM, Milner RA, Mohide PT, et al. Treatment of preterm labor with the beta-adrenergic agonist ritodrine. *N Engl J Med* 1992;327:308–313.

Mullen M, Mullen B, Carey M. The association between beta-agonist use and death from asthma: a meta-analytic integration of case-control studies. *JAMA* 1993;270:1842–1845.

Naito H, Gillis CN. Effects of halothane and nitrous oxide on removal of norepinephrine from the pulmonary circulation. *Anesthesiology* 1973;39:575–580.

Nelson HS. Beta-adrenergic bronchodilators. *N Engl J Med* 1995;333: 499–506.

Pearl RG. Phenylephrine and inhaled nitric oxide in adult respiratory distress syndrome: when are two better than one? *Anesthesiology* 1997;87:1–3.

Ralston DH, Shnider SM, deLorimier AA. Effects of equipotent ephedrine, metaraminol, mephentermine, and methoxamine on uterine blood flow in the pregnant ewe. *Anesthesiology* 1974;40: 354–370.

Rothenberg DM, Parnass SM, Litwack K, et al. Efficacy of ephedrine in the prevention of postoperative nausea and vomiting. *Anesth Analg* 1991;72:58–61.

Schwenzer KJ, Miller ED. Hemodynamic effects of dobutamine in patients following mitral valve replacement. *Anesth Analg* 1989;68:467–472.

Schwinn DA, Reves JG. Time course and hemodynamic effects of alpha-1 adrenergic bolus administration in anesthetized patients with myocardial disease. *Anesth Analg* 1989;68:571–578.

Shitara T, Wajima Z, Ogawa R. Dobutamine infusion modifies thermoregulation during general anesthesia. *Anesth Analg* 1996;83: 1154–1159.

Smith NT, Corbascio AN. The use and misuse of pressor agents. *Anesthesiology* 1970;33:58–101.

Suissa S, Blais L, Ernst P. Patterns of increasing beta-agonist use and the risk of fatal or near-fatal asthma. *Eur Respir J* 1994;7:1602–1609.

Sumikawa K, Hayashi Y, Yamatodani A, et al. Contribution of the lungs to the clearance of exogenous dopamine in humans. *Anesth Analg* 1991; 72:622–626.

Sweny P. Haemofiltration and haemodiafiltration—theoretical and practical aspects. *Curr Anaesth Crit Care* 1991;2:37–43.

Tanaka N, Nagata N, Hamakawa T, et al. The effect of dopamine on hepatic blood flow in patients undergoing epidural anesthesia. *Anesth Analg* 1997;85:286–290.

ter Wee PM, Smit AJ, Rosman JB, et al. Effect of intravenous infusion of low-dose dopamine on renal function in normal individuals and in patients with renal disease. *Am J Nephrol* 1986;6:42–46.

Thompson BT, Cockrill BA. Renal-dose dopamine: a siren song? *Lancet* 1994;344:7–8.

Tobias JD, Hirshman CA. Attenuation of histamine-induced airway constriction by albuterol during halothane anesthesia. *Anesthesiology* 1990;72:105–110.

Ward DS, Belville JW. Reduction of hypoxic ventilatory drive by dopamine. *Anesth Analg* 1982;61:333–337.

Williams ME, Rosa RM, Silva P, et al. Impairment of extrarenal potassium disposal by alpha-adrenergic stimulation. *N Engl J Med* 1984;311:145–149.

Yost CS. G proteins: basic characteristics and clinical potential for the practice of anesthesia. *Anesth Analg* 1993;77:822–834.

Digitalis and Related Drugs

13

Digitalis is the term used for cardiac glycosides that occur naturally in many plants, including the foxglove plant. Digoxin, digitoxin, and ouabain are examples of clinically useful cardiac glycosides (Fig. 13-1). Nonglycoside and noncatecholamine drugs that may be administered for similar clinical purposes as cardiac glycosides include specific phosphodiesterase (PDE) III inhibitors, calcium, and glucagon (Fig. 13-2) (Skoyles and Sherry, 1992).

CLINICAL USES

Cardiac glycosides are used most often during the perioperative period for the management of supraventricular tachydysrhythmias (paroxysmal atrial tachycardia, atrial fibrillation, atrial flutter) associated with a rapid ventricular response rate based on the ability of these drugs to slow conduction of cardiac impulses through the atrioventricular node. The use of cardiac glycosides to treat acute decreases in left ventricular contractility is uncommon because of the availability of more potent and less toxic drugs. For example, patients treated with digoxin have a decreased risk of death from heart failure but an increased incidence of sudden death, presumably due to cardiac dysrhythmias (similar to increased risk of sudden death described for other positive inotropic drugs) (Packer, 1997; Digitalis Investigation Group, 1997). Based on this observation, cardiac glycosides may be selected only for treatment of symptoms that persist after administration of drugs (angiotensin-converting enzyme inhibitors, beta-adrenergic antagonists) that do decrease overall mortality (Packer, 1997). Nevertheless, cardiac glycosides continue to have an important therapeutic role in the treatment of chronic congestive heart failure. Digitalis preparations may not be of benefit in high-output cardiac failure, such as that caused by hyperthyroidism or thiamine deficiency. Before administering a cardiac glycoside to treat a supraventricular dysrhythmia, it is important to confirm that the cardiac dysrhythmia is not due to digitalis toxicity.

Intravenous (IV) administration of propranolol or esmolol combined with digoxin may provide more rapid control of supraventricular tachydysrhythmias and minimize the likelihood of toxicity by permitting decreases in the dose of both classes of drugs. Direct current cardioversion in the presence of digitalis may be hazardous because of an alleged risk for developing cardiac dysrhythmias, including ventricular fibrillation. In approximately 30% of patients with Wolff-Parkinson-White syndrome, digitalis decreases refractoriness in the accessory conduction pathway to the point that rapid atrial impulses can cause ventricular fibrillation. Digitalis may be harmful in patients with hypertrophic subaortic stenosis because increased myocardial contractility intensifies the resistance to ventricular ejection.

STRUCTURE ACTIVITY RELATIONSHIPS

The basic structure of cardiac glycosides is that of a steroid cyclopentenophenanthrene nucleus that consists of a glycone and an aglycone portion (see Fig. 13-1). As such, cardiac glycosides are related chemically to bile acids and sex hormones. The glycone portion is sugar—often glucose, but closely related sugars such as digitoxose may also be present. Glycones are pharmacologically inactive but are necessary to ensure fixation of cardiac glycosides to cardiac muscle. It is the aglycone portion of cardiac glycosides that produces the pharmacologic activity on the heart characterized as "digitalis-like."

MECHANISM OF ACTION

The complex mechanisms of the positive inotropic effect evoked by cardiac glycosides includes direct effects on the heart that modify its electrical and mechanical activity and indirect effects evoked by reflex alterations in autonomic nervous system activity.

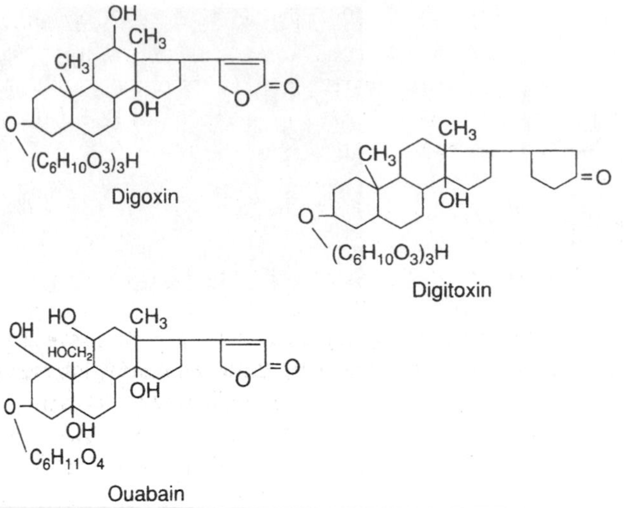

Figure 13-1. Cardiac glycosides.

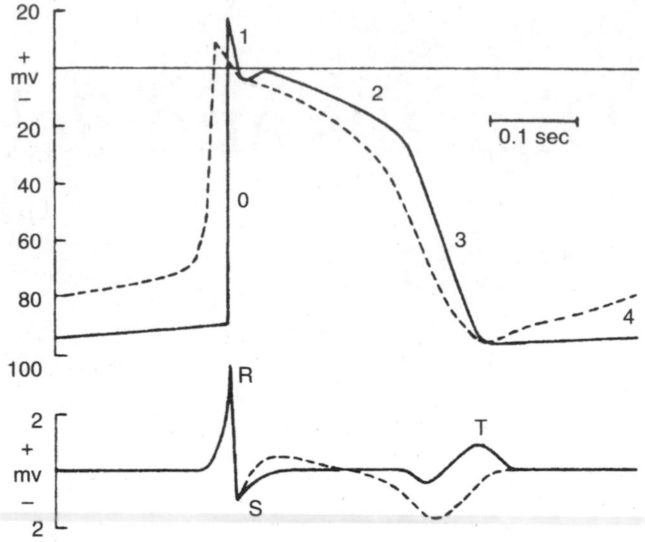

Figure 13-3. Schematic depiction of the effects of digitalis (*dashed line*) on the transmembrane potential and electrocardiogram (ECG) compared with records in the absence of digitalis. In the presence of digitalis, the resting transmembrane potential becomes less negative and the slope of phase 4 spontaneous depolarization is increased (automaticity is enhanced). The change in the slope and duration of phases 2 and 3 of the cardiac action potential change the S-T segment and T wave and shorten the R-T interval on the ECG. (From Hoffman BF, Bigger JT. Digitalis and allied cardiac glycosides. In: Gilman AG, Goodman LS, Rall TW, Murad F, eds. *The pharmacological basis of therapeutics*, 7th ed. New York: Macmillan, 1985:716; with permission.)

Direct Effects on the Heart

Cardiac glycosides selectively and reversibly inhibit the sodium-potassium adenosine triphosphatase (ATP) ion transport system (sodium pump) located in the sarcolemma of cardiac cell membranes. Cardiac glycosides bind to the alpha subunit on the extracellular surface of the ATPase enzyme, inducing a conformational change that interferes with outward transport of sodium ions across cardiac cell membranes. The resulting increase in sodium ion concentration in cardiac cells leads to decreased extrusion of calcium ions by the sodium pump mechanism. It is presumed that this increased intracellular concentration of calcium ions is responsible for the positive inotropic effects of cardiac glycosides. Conceptually, increased amounts of calcium ions become available to react with contractile proteins to generate a greater force of myocardial contraction. The positive inotropic effects produced by cardiac glycosides occur without changes in heart rate and are associated with decreases in left ventricular preload, afterload, wall tension, and oxygen consumption in the failing heart (Kulick and Rahimtoola, 1991).

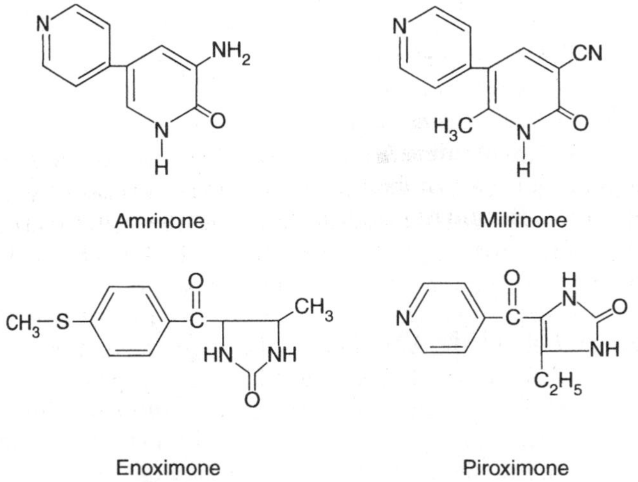

Figure 13-2. Selective phosphodiesterase III inhibitors that function as noncatecholamine, nonglycoside cardiac inotropic agents.

Many of the known effects of cardiac glycosides on the cardiac action potential can be explained on the basis of drug-induced inhibition of the sodium-potassium ATPase ion transport system. Indeed, this ion transport system is essential for maintaining normal gradients for sodium and potassium ions that determine depolarization and excitability characteristics of cardiac cell membranes. For example, cardiac glycosides decrease resting transmembrane potentials and thus increase automaticity (excitability) of cardiac cells by virtue of alterations in potassium ion gradients (Fig. 13-3) (Hoffman and Bigger, 1985). Automaticity is also accentuated by drug-induced increases in the slope of phase 4 depolarization. Inhibition of outward transport of sodium ions decreases the slope of phase 0 of the cardiac action potential. The decrease in the duration of the cardiac action potential results largely from shortening of the duration of phase 2. Excessive digitalis-induced increases in intracellular calcium ion concentrations decrease the spread of excitatory current from one myocardial cell to another, manifesting as impaired conduction of cardiac impulses.

Alterations in Autonomic Nervous System Activity

Autonomic nervous system effects of cardiac glycosides include increased parasympathetic nervous system activity due to sensitization of arterial baroreceptors (carotid sinus) and activation of vagal nuclei and the nodose ganglion in the central nervous system (CNS). Enhanced parasympathetic nervous system activity produced by therapeutic concentrations of digitalis decreases activity of the sinoatrial node and prolongs the effective refractory period, and thus the time for conduction of cardiac impulses through the atrioventricular node. The manifestation of these effects is a slowed heart rate, especially in the presence of atrial fibrillation. Furthermore, the relative predominance of parasympathetic to sympathetic nervous system activity produced by digitalis is consistent with suppression of ectopic cardiac pacemakers. Indirect neurally mediated effects of therapeutic concentrations of digitalis on the specialized ventricular conduction system are less important than effects on the sinoatrial and atrioventricular node.

PHARMACOKINETICS

The assay of plasma concentrations of cardiac glycosides has greatly improved the understanding of the pharmacokinetics of these drugs. At equilibrium, the concentration of cardiac glycosides in the heart is 15 to 30 times greater than those in the plasma. The concentration of cardiac glycosides in skeletal muscles is approximately one-half that in the heart.

Digoxin

Absorption of digoxin after oral administration is approximately 75% in the first hour, with peak plasma concentrations occurring in 1 to 2 hours (Table 13-1) (Hoffman and Bigger, 1985). Intramuscular (IM) administration of digoxin is painful and absorption is often unpredictable. Therapeutic plasma concentrations of digoxin can be achieved rapidly with IV administration of the drug (up to 10 μg/kg over approximately 30 minutes), producing an appreciable effect in 5 to 30 minutes. After achievement of therapeutic plasma concentrations of digoxin by either the oral or IV route, the maintenance oral dose is adjusted according to the individual patient's response, the electrocardiogram (ECG), and the plasma concentration of digoxin. The maintenance dose must be equal to the daily loss (clearance) of the drug.

Clearance of digoxin from the plasma is primarily by the kidneys, with approximately 35% of the drug excreted daily. In the presence of renal dysfunction, the elimination half-time of digoxin is depressed in proportion to the decrease in creatinine clearance. For example, the elimination half-time of digoxin is 31 to 33 hours in the presence of normal renal function and up to 4.4 days in the absence of renal function. A practical rule is that the dose of digoxin should be decreased by 50% when the serum creatinine concentration is 3 to 5 mg/dL and by 75% in the absence of renal function.

TABLE 13-1.
COMPARISON OF DIGOXIN AND DIGITOXIN

	Digoxin	Digitoxin
Average digitalizing dose		
Oral	0.75–1.50 mg	0.8–1.2 mg
Intravenous	0.5–1.0 mg	0.8–1.2 mg
Average daily maintenance dose		
Oral	0.125–0.500 mg	0.05–0.20 mg
Intravenous	0.25 mg	0.1 mg
Onset of effect		
Oral	1.5–6.0 hrs	3–6 hrs
Intravenous	5–30 mins	30–120 mins
Absorption from the gastrointestinal tract	75%	90–100%
Plasma protein binding	25%	95%
Route of elimination	Renal	Hepatic
Enterohepatic circulation	Minimal	Marked
Elimination half-time	31–33 hrs	5–7 days
Therapeutic plasma concentration	0.5–2.0 ng/mL	10–35 ng/mL

Source: Data from Hoffman BF, Bigger JT. Digitalis and allied cardiac glycosides. In: Gilman AG, Goodman LS, Rall TW, Murad F, eds. *The pharmacological basis of therapeutics*, 7th ed. New York. Macmillan, 1985:716; with permission.

The principal inactive tissue reservoir site for digoxin is the skeletal muscles. A decrease in the size of this reservoir, as in elderly patients, results in increased plasma and myocardial levels of digoxin. Minimal amounts of digoxin accumulate in fat. Approximately 25% of digoxin is bound to protein. Occasionally, patients form antibodies to digoxin, which prevents a therapeutic effect. Metabolism of digoxin is minimal, with a few patients forming the inactive metabolite dihydrodigoxin.

Digitoxin

Absorption of digitoxin after oral administration is 90% to 100%, reflecting the greater lipid solubility of this cardiac glycoside compared with digoxin (see Table 13-1) (Hoffman and Bigger, 1985). Digitoxin is actively metabolized by hepatic microsomal enzymes; one of these metabolites is digoxin. Approximately 10% of the digoxin appears unchanged in the urine. The elimination half-time of digitoxin and its metabolites is 5 to 7 days. Hepatic disease does not appreciably alter the elimination half-time of digitoxin, emphasizing the large reserve capacity of the liver for metabolic degradation of digitoxin. Likewise, impaired renal function does not alter plasma concentrations of digitoxin. The long elimination half-time of digitoxin is an advantage for maintaining therapeutic plasma concentrations should a patient fail to receive several doses.

Ouabain

Ouabain is administered in doses of 1.5 to 3.0 μg/kg IV to provide rapid increases in myocardial contractility or to decrease the heart rate in rapid ventricular response atrial fibrillation. It is unlikely, however, that ouabain offers any advantages over digoxin administered IV for the same reasons. The total adult IV dose of ouabain should not exceed 1 mg in 24 hours. Ouabain is rapidly excreted in urine, with approximately 50% of the unchanged drug being recovered in 8 hours. A longer-acting digitalis preparation should be substituted for ouabain when maintenance therapy is indicated. Ouabain is not effective when administered orally, reflecting destruction of its glycoside portion in the gastrointestinal tract.

CARDIOVASCULAR EFFECTS

The principal cardiovascular effect of digitalis glycosides administered to patients with cardiac failure is a dose-dependent increase in myocardial contractility that becomes significant with less than full digitalizing doses. The positive inotropic effect manifests as increased stroke volume, decreased heart size, and decreased left ventricular end-diastolic pressure. Indeed, cardiac glycosides can double stroke volume from a failing and dilated left ventricle. The ventricular function curve (Frank-Starling curve) is shifted to the left (Fig. 13-4). Improved renal perfusion due to an overall increase in cardiac output favors mobilization and excretion of edema fluid, accounting for the diuresis that often accompanies the administration of cardiac glycosides to patients in cardiac failure. Excessive sympathetic nervous system activity that occurs as a compensatory response to cardiac failure is decreased with the improved circulation that accompanies administration of cardiac glycosides. The resulting decrease in systemic vascular resistance further enhances forward left ventricular stroke volume.

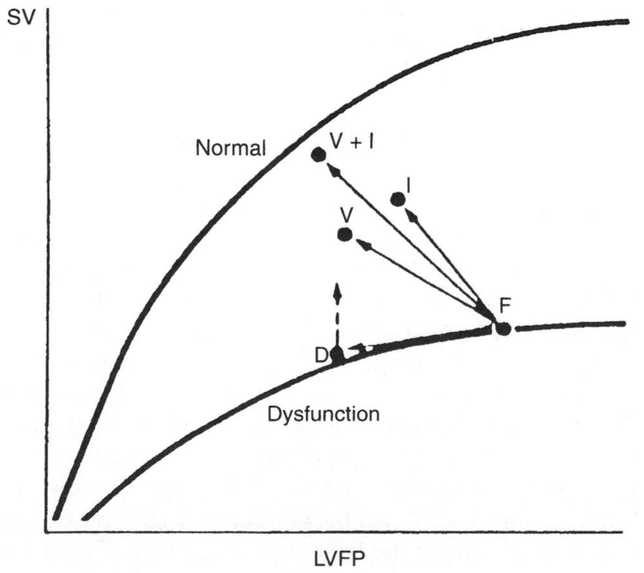

Figure 13-4. Cardiac glycosides shift the ventricular function curve of the failing myocardium to the left. (LVFP, left ventricular filling pressure; SV, stroke volume.)

In addition to positive inotropic effects, cardiac glycosides enhance parasympathetic nervous system activity, leading to delayed conduction of cardiac impulses through the atrioventricular node and decreases in heart rate. The magnitude of this negative dromotropic and chronotropic effect depends on the preexisting activity of the autonomic nervous system. Increased parasympathetic nervous system activity decreases contractility in the atria, but direct positive inotropic effects of cardiac glycosides more than offset these nervous system–induced negative inotropic effects on the ventricles.

Cardiac glycosides also increase myocardial contractility in the absence of cardiac failure. Nevertheless, the resulting tendency for cardiac output to increase may be offset by decreases in heart rate and direct vasoconstricting effects of cardiac glycosides on arterial, and to a lesser extent, venous smooth muscle. Indeed, cardiac output is often unchanged or even decreased when cardiac glycosides are administered to patients with normal hearts.

ELECTROCARDIOGRAPHIC EFFECTS

The electrophysiologic effects of therapeutic plasma concentrations of cardiac glycosides manifest on the ECG as (a) prolonged P-R intervals due to delayed conduction of cardiac impulses through the atrioventricular node, (b) shortened QTc intervals because of more rapid ventricular repolarization, (c) ST segment depression (scaphoid or scooped-out) due to a decreased slope of phase 3 depolarization of cardiac action potentials, and (d) diminished amplitude or inversion of T waves. The P-R interval is rarely prolonged to >0.25 second, and the effect on the QTc interval is independent of parasympathetic nervous system activity. Changes in the ST segment and T wave do not correlate with therapeutic plasma concentrations of cardiac glycosides. Furthermore, ST segment and T wave changes on the ECG may suggest myocardial ischemia. When digitalis is discontinued, the changes on the ECG disappear in approximately 20 days.

DIGITALIS TOXICITY

Cardiac glycosides have a narrow therapeutic range. Indeed, it is estimated that approximately 20% of patients who are being treated with cardiac glycosides experience some form of digitalis toxicity. The therapeutic effects of cardiac glycosides develop at approximately 35% of the fatal dose, and cardiac dysrhythmias typically manifest at approximately 60% of the fatal dose. The only difference between various cardiac glycosides when toxicity develops is the duration of adverse effects.

There is general agreement that the toxic effects of cardiac glycosides result from inhibition of the sodium-potassium ATPase ion transport system, which leads to an accumulation of intracellular sodium and calcium ions and a corresponding decrease in intracellular potassium ions. It is presumed that increased intracellular calcium ion concentrations that accompany digitalis toxicity are responsible for associated ectopic cardiac dysrhythmias. The slope of phase 4 depolarization of the cardiac action potential is enhanced by digitalis, especially in the ventricles.

Causes

The most frequent cause of digitalis toxicity in the absence of renal dysfunction is the concurrent administration of diuretics that cause potassium depletion. During anesthesia, hyperventilation of the patient's lungs can decrease the serum potassium concentration an average of 0.5 mEq/liter for every 10 mm Hg decrease in $PaCO_2$ (Edwards and Winnie, 1977). Hypokalemia probably increases myocardial binding of cardiac glycosides, resulting in an excess drug effect. Indeed, binding of cardiac glycosides to the sodium-potassium ATPase enzyme complex is inhibited by increases in the plasma concentration of potassium. Other electrolyte abnormalities that contribute to digitalis toxicity include hypercalcemia and hypomagnesemia. An increase in sympathetic nervous system activity as produced by arterial hypoxemia increases the likelihood of digitalis toxicity. Elderly patients with decreased skeletal muscle mass and decreased renal function are vulnerable to the development of digitalis toxicity if the usual doses of digoxin are administered. Impaired renal function and electrolyte changes (hypokalemia, hypomagnesemia) that may accompany cardiopulmonary bypass could predispose the patient to the development of digitalis toxicity.

Diagnosis

Digitalis is often administered in situations in which the toxic effects of the drug are difficult to distinguish from the effects of the cardiac disease. For this reason, determination of the plasma concentration of the cardiac glycoside may be used to indicate the likely presence of digitalis toxicity. For example, a plasma digoxin concentration of <0.5 ng/mL eliminates the possibility of digitalis toxicity. Plasma concentrations between 0.5 and 2.5 ng/mL are usually considered therapeutic, and levels >3 ng/mL are definitely in a toxic range. Infants and children have an increased tolerance to cardiac glycosides, and their range of therapeutic concentrations for digoxin is 2.5 to 3.5 ng/mL.

It must be appreciated that the relationship between plasma concentrations and observed pharmacologic effects is not always consistent. For example, therapeutic plasma concentrations of digoxin, despite clinical symptoms of digitalis toxicity, are frequently observed in the presence of electrolyte disturbances and recent myocardial infarction. Conversely, high therapeutic plasma concentrations of digoxin, without symptoms of digitalis toxicity, are frequently observed in the treatment of patients with supraventricular tachydysrhythmias, which require large doses to decrease the ventricular response rate.

Anorexia, nausea, and vomiting are early manifestations of digitalis toxicity. These symptoms, when present preoperatively in patients receiving cardiac glycosides, should arouse suspicion of digitalis toxicity. Excitation of the chemoreceptor trigger zone is the principal mechanism responsible for vomiting. Transitory amblyopia and scotomata have been observed. Pain simulating trigeminal neuralgia may be an early sign of digitalis toxicity. The extremities may also be a site of discomfort.

Electrocardiogram

There are no unequivocal features on the ECG that confirm the presence of digitalis toxicity (Atlee, 1997). Nevertheless, toxic plasma concentrations of digitalis typically cause atrial or ventricular cardiac dysrhythmias (increased automaticity) and delayed conduction of cardiac impulses through the atrioventricular node (prolonged P-R interval on the ECG), culminating in incomplete to complete heart block. Atrial tachycardia with block is the most common cardiac dysrhythmia attributed to digitalis toxicity. Activity of the sinoatrial node may also be directly inhibited by high doses of cardiac glycosides. Conduction of cardiac impulses through specialized conducting tissues of the ventricles is not altered, as evidenced by the failure of even toxic plasma concentrations of digoxin to alter the duration of the QRS complex on the ECG. Ventricular fibrillation is the most frequent cause of death from digitalis toxicity.

Treatment

Treatment of digitalis toxicity includes (a) correction of predisposing causes (hypokalemia, hypomagnesemia, arterial hypoxemia), (b) administration of drugs (phenytoin, lidocaine, atropine) to treat cardiac dysrhythmias, and (c) insertion of a temporary artificial transvenous cardiac pacemaker if complete heart block is present. Supplemental potassium decreases the binding of digitalis to cardiac muscle and thus directly antagonizes the cardiotoxic effects of cardiac glycosides. Serum potassium concentrations should be determined before treatment because supplemental potassium in the presence of a high preexisting plasma level of potassium will intensify atrioventricular block and depress the automaticity of ectopic pacemakers in the ventricles, leading to complete heart block. If renal function is normal and atrioventricular conduction block is not present, it is acceptable to rapidly administer potassium, 0.025 to 0.050 mEq/kg IV, to treat life-threatening cardiac dysrhythmias associated with digitalis toxicity. Phenytoin (0.5 to 1.5 mg/kg IV over 5 minutes) or lidocaine (1 to 2 mg/kg IV) is effective in suppressing ventricular cardiac dysrhythmias caused by digitalis; phenytoin is also effective in suppressing atrial dysrhythmias. Atropine, 35 to 70 μg/kg IV, can be administered to increase heart rate by offsetting excessive parasympathetic nervous system activity produced by toxic plasma concentrations of digitalis. Propranolol is effective in suppressing increased automaticity produced by digitalis toxicity, but its tendency to increase atrioventricular node refractoriness limits its usefulness when conduction blockade is present.

Life-threatening digitalis toxicity can be treated by administering antibodies (Fab fragments) to the drug, thus decreasing the plasma concentration of cardiac glycosides available to attach to cell membranes. The Fab-digitalis complex is eliminated by the kidneys.

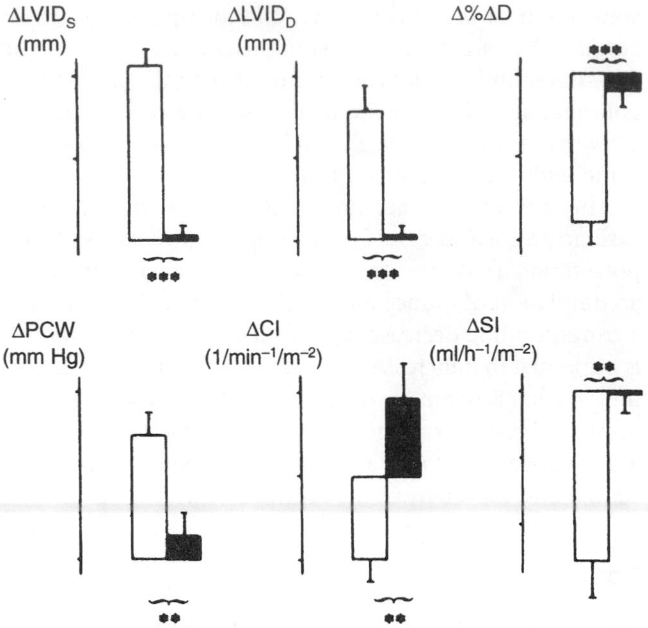

Figure 13-5. Preoperative and postoperative measurements (mean ± SE) of cardiac function in patients with coronary artery disease receiving digitalis (*black bars*) or not receiving digitalis (*clear bars*). (Δ%ΔD, shortening fraction; ΔCI, change in cardiac index; $\Delta LVID_D$, end-diastolic left ventricular internal dimension; $\Delta LVID_S$, end-systolic left ventricular internal dimension; ΔPCW, pulmonary capillary occlusion pressure; ΔSI, change in stroke index; $^{**}P < .01$; $^{***}P < .001$.) (From Pinaud MLJ, Blanloeil YAG, Souron RJ. Preoperative prophylactic digitalization of patients with coronary artery disease: a randomized echocardiographic and hemodynamic study. *Anesth Analg* 1983;62:865–869; with permission.)

PREOPERATIVE PROPHYLACTIC DIGITALIS

Preoperative prophylactic administration of digitalis to patients without signs of cardiac failure is controversial. The obvious disadvantage of prophylactic use of digitalis is the administration of a drug with a narrow therapeutic-to-toxic dose difference to patients with no obvious need for the drug. Furthermore, there may be difficulty in differentiating anesthetic-induced cardiac dysrhythmias from those due to digitalis toxicity (Chung, 1981). Indeed, events such as alterations in renal function, decreases in serum potassium concentration due to hyperventilation of the patient's lungs, and increases in sympathetic nervous system activity are likely to occur intraoperatively and thus increase the likelihood of an increased pharmacologic effect from circulating digitalis.

Despite these theoretical disadvantages, there is evidence that patients with limited cardiac reserve may benefit from prophylactic administration of digitalis. For example, the preoperative administration of digoxin orally (0.75 mg in divided doses the day before surgery and 0.25 mg before induction of anesthesia) decreases the occurrence of postoperative supraventricular cardiac dysrhythmias in elderly patients undergoing thoracic or abdominal surgery (Chee et al., 1982). Prophylactic administration of digoxin also decreases evidence of impaired cardiac function in patients with coronary artery disease recovering from anesthesia (Fig. 13-5) (Pinaud et al., 1983). Based on these observations, it may be reasonable to conclude that beneficial effects of prophylactic digitalis administered to appropriately selected patients in the preoperative period outweigh the potential hazards of digitalis toxicity. Certainly, there are no data to support discontinuing digitalis in any patient preoperatively, including those undergoing cardiopulmonary bypass. It is particularly important to continue digitalis therapy throughout the perioperative period in patients who are receiving the drug for heart rate control.

DRUG INTERACTIONS

Quinidine produces a dose-dependent increase in the plasma concentration of digoxin that becomes apparent within 24 hours after the first dose of the antidysrhythmic drug. This effect of quinidine may be due to displacement of digoxin from binding sites in tissues.

Succinylcholine, or any other drug that can abruptly increase parasympathetic nervous system activity, could theoretically have an additive effect with cardiac glycosides. Cardiac dysrhythmias also could reflect succinylcholine-induced catecholamine release and resulting cardiac irritability. Despite these theoretical concerns, clinical experience does not support the occurrence of an increased incidence of cardiac dysrhythmias in patients being treated with cardiac glycosides and receiving succinylcholine (Bartolone and Rao, 1983).

Sympathomimetics with beta-adrenergic agonist effects as well as pancuronium may increase the likelihood of cardiac dysrhythmias in the presence of cardiac glycosides (Bartolone and Rao, 1983). IV administration of calcium may precipitate cardiac dysrhythmias in patients receiving cardiac glycosides. Any drug that facilitates renal loss of potassium ions increases the likelihood of hypokalemia and associated digitalis toxicity. The simultaneous administration of an oral antacid and digitalis decreases the gastrointestinal absorption of cardiac glycosides. Fentanyl, enflurane, and, to a lesser extent, isoflurane protect against digitalis-enhanced cardiac automaticity (Ivankovich et al., 1976).

SELECTIVE PHOSPHODIESTERASE INHIBITORS (NONCATECHOLAMINE, NONGLYCOSIDE CARDIAC INOTROPIC AGENTS)

Selective phosphodiesterase inhibitors are a heterogenous group of noncatecholamine and nonglycoside compounds that exert a competitive inhibitory action on an isoenzyme fraction of PDE (PDE III) (see Fig. 13-2) (Skoyles and Sherry, 1992). This inhibition decreases the hydrolysis of cyclic adenosine monophosphate (cAMP) and cyclic guanosine monophosphate (cGMP), leading to increased intracellular concentrations of cAMP and cGMP in the myocardium and vascular smooth muscle. Increased intracellular concentrations of cAMP result in stimulation of protein kinases that phosphorylate substances responsible for inward movement of calcium ions. The effects of catecholamines, which also increase cAMP concentrations through beta-adrenergic stimulation, are potentially enhanced by PDE III inhibition. Although PDE III isoenzymes exist in airway smooth muscle, bronchodilation is not a predominant clinical effect of the current cardiac-selective PDE III inhibitors.

The overall effect of selective PDE III inhibitors is to combine positive inotropic effects with vascular and airway smooth muscle relaxation. The positive inotropic effects of these selective PDE inhibitors result principally from inhibition of cardiac PDE III, leading to an increase in myocardial cAMP content. Selective PDE inhibitors act independently of beta-adrenergic receptors and will increase myocardial contractility in patients with myocardial depression from beta receptor blockade and those who have become refractory to catecholamine therapy. Selective PDE III inhibitors not only exert positive inotropic effects by increasing availability of calcium for contractile activation but also facilitate diastolic relaxation by enhancing calcium removal from the myoplasm.

The hemodynamic response to selective PDE inhibitors exceeds cardiac glycosides and is complementary and synergistic to the actions of catecholamines. These drugs can be used in conjunction with digitalis without provoking digitalis toxicity. The PDE III inhibitors have their greatest clinical usefulness in the management of acute cardiac failure (as after a myocardial infarction) in patients who would benefit from combined inotropic and vasodilator therapy.

Amrinone

Amrinone is a bipyridine derivative that acts as a selective PDE III inhibitor and produces dose-dependent positive inotropic and vasodilator effects manifesting as increased cardiac output and decreased left ventricular end-diastolic pressure (LeJemtel et al., 1980). Heart rate may increase and systemic blood pressure may decrease. Controversy exists as to whether the predominant action of amrinone is inotropic or vasodilating. Amrinone possesses neither antidysrhythmic nor dysrhythmogenic properties. The elimination half-time of amrinone is approximately 6 hours, with the principal route of excretion being that of unchanged drug in the urine.

Route of Administration

Amrinone is effective when administered orally as well as IV. Administration of a single dose, 0.5 to 1.5 mg/kg IV, increases cardiac output within 5 minutes, with detectable positive inotropic effects persisting for approximately 2 hours. After the initial injection, continuous infusion of 2 to 10 μg/kg/minute produces positive inotropic effects that are maintained during the infusion (tachyphylaxis does not occur) and for several hours after discontinuation of the infusion. The recommended maximum daily dose of amrinone is 10 mg/kg including the initial loading dose, which may be repeated 30 minutes after the first injection. In view of the dependence of amrinone on renal excretion, it is presumed that the dose should be decreased in patients with severe renal dysfunction. Patients who have failed to respond to catecholamines may respond to amrinone. The vasodilating effects of amrinone can accelerate the cooling rate of core temperature during deliberate mild hypothermia for neurosurgical procedures (Inoue et al., 2001).

Side Effects

An adverse effect of amrinone is occasional hypotension due to vasodilation. Thrombocytopenia may occur with chronic therapy. In animals, chronic administration of amrinone has been associated with hepatic dysfunction. Overall, the therapeutic index of amrinone is approximately 100:1 compared with 1.2:1 for cardiac glycosides.

Milrinone

Milrinone is a bypyridine derivative that, like amrinone, produces positive inotropic and vasodilating effects. It has minimal effects on heart rate and myocardial oxygen consumption. Administration of 50 μg/kg IV followed by a continuous infusion, 0.5 μg/kg/minute, maintains plasma milrinone concentrations at or above therapeutic levels (Bailey et al., 1994). The elimination half-time of milrinone is 2.7 hours, and approximately 80% of the drug is excreted unchanged by the kidneys (Skoyles and Sherry, 1992). The dose of milrinone should be decreased in patients with severe renal dysfunction (glomerular filtration rate of <50 mL/minute). Nevertheless, both milrinone and amrinone have a wide therapeutic ratio and the risk of overdose, even in the presence of renal dysfunction, is low.

Milrinone may be useful in the management of acute left ventricular dysfunction as may follow cardiac surgery. Successful weaning of high-risk patients from cardiopulmonary bypass may be enhanced by administration of milrinone (Rathmell et al., 1998). The inotropic effects of milrinone are attenuated by acidosis presumably reflecting decreased cAMP formation in acidotic muscle (Tanaka et al., 1998). Despite its beneficial hemodynamic actions, chronic oral therapy with milrinone may increase morbidity and mortality in patients with severe chronic heart failure (Packer et al., 1991). Similar disappointing results have been obtained with other specific PDE inhibitors, although improved survival may be seen when lower doses of the drugs are used (Packer, 1993).

Enoximone and Piroximone

Enoximone and piroximone are imidazole derivatives that act as highly selective PDE III inhibitors to increase myocardial contractility (see Fig. 13-2). Enoximone has an elimination half-time of 4.3 hours and is metabolized mainly by the liver. In this regard, the pharmacokinetics of enoximone are influenced by renal function. The dose of enoximone is 0.5 mg/kg IV followed by a continuous infusion of 5 to 20 μg/kg/minute.

NONSELECTIVE PHOSPHODIESTERASE INHIBITORS

Theophylline

Theophylline (aminophylline is theophylline in complex with ethylenediamine to increase its solubility) is a PDE inhibitor that, in contrast to selective PDE III inhibitors, is capable of inhibiting all fractions of PDE isoenzymes (I–V) (Skoyles and Sherry, 1992). Although inhibition of PDE is often proposed as the explanation for all the actions of theophylline, this is probably not the sole mechanism at therapeutic concentrations. The intracellular accumulation of cGMP may be partly responsible for mediating smooth muscle relaxation produced by theophylline. Methylxanthines also act as competitive antagonists of adenosine receptors, which could explain some of the effects of theophylline on the CNS and cardiac conduction system and may underlie the efficacy of theophylline in antagonizing bronchoconstriction. Theophylline has complex effects on circulation through a combination of brainstem vasomotor stimulation, smooth muscle relaxation, and diuresis.

Pharmacokinetics

Theophylline is metabolized by the liver and excreted by the kidneys. Frequent monitoring of plasma concentrations is indicated because there is significant individual variation in the response to theophyllene reflecting differences in liver dysfunction due to cardiac failure or alcoholism, treatment with cimetidine, or extremes of age. Conversely, cigarette smoking speeds metabolism of theophylline. The elimination half-time of theophylline is approximately 8.7 hours in nonsmoking adults and 5.5 hours in adults who smoke.

Side Effects

Theophylline, unlike selective PDE III inhibitors, has a very narrow therapeutic margin. For example, therapeutic plasma concentrations of theophylline are between 10 and 20 μg/mL, with toxic responses, including cardiac dysrhythmias, becoming more prevalent at plasma concentrations of >20 μg/mL. In the presence of toxic plasma concentrations of aminophylline, the subsequent administration of volatile anesthetics may be associated with the development of cardiac dysrhythmias. Aminophylline readily crosses the placenta and may produce toxicity in infants of mothers receiving this drug during labor. Theophylline may relax the gastroesophageal sphincter, leading to gastroesophageal reflux.

Clinical Uses

Administration of aminophylline (loading dose 5 mg/kg IV followed by 0.5 to 1.0 mg/kg/hour IV) has been recommended in the past for the treatment of bronchospasm due to an acute exacerbation of asthma. Nevertheless, the degree of bronchodilation obtained with aminophylline is not different than that produced by selective beta$_2$-adrenergic agonists. This has led to a recommendation that IV administration of aminophylline be considered only when beta$_2$-adrenergic agonists and corticosteroids produce an inadequate response (Rees, 1984). Any protective effect of aminophylline on histamine reactivity most likely results from release of endogenous catecholamines.

Pentoxifylline

Pentoxifylline is a methylxanthine derivative that increases flexibility of erythrocytes and decreases viscosity of blood, thereby improving capillary blood flow and associated tissue oxygenation. Patients with intermittent claudication due to chronic occlusive arterial disease of the limbs begin to experience improvement within 2 to 4 hours after initiation of oral administration of pentoxifylline, 400 mg every 8 hours. This drug is neither a vasodilator nor an anticoagulant and is unrelated to aspirin or dipyridamole.

Side effects are rare but may include hypotension, angina pectoris, and cardiac dysrhythmias. Bleeding or prolonged prothrombin time may occur in the presence of anticoagulants or platelet aggregation inhibitors. Pentoxifylline is compatible with digitalis and beta-adrenergic antagonists.

CALCIUM

Calcium, when injected IV, produces an intense positive inotropic effect lasting 10 to 20 minutes and manifesting as increases in stroke volume and decreases in left ventricular end-diastolic pressure (Denlinger et al., 1975). Heart rate and systemic vascular resistance decrease. The inotropic effects of calcium are enhanced in the presence of preexisting hypocalcemia. The risk of cardiac dysrhythmias when calcium is administered intravenously to patients receiving digitalis should be considered, especially if hypokalemia is also present.

Calcium chloride, 5 to 10 mg/kg IV to adults, may be administered to improve myocardial contractility and stroke volume at the conclusion of cardiopulmonary bypass. Indeed, myocardial contractility at the conclusion of cardiopulmonary bypass may be decreased by hypocalcemia because of (a) use of potassium-containing cardioplegia solutions, (b) administration of citrated stored whole blood, and (c) treatment of metabolic acidosis with sodium bicarbonate. A 10% solution of calcium chloride contains more calcium than a 10% calcium gluconate solution, although the availability of ionized calcium is prompt regardless of the intravenous preparation administered (see Chapter 35).

GLUCAGON

Glucagon is a polypeptide hormone produced by the alpha cells of the pancreas. Like catecholamines, glucagon enhances formation of cAMP, but unlike catecholamines, it does not act via beta-adrenergic receptors. Inhibition of PDE enzyme does not occur. Glucagon also evokes the release of catecholamines, but this is not the predominant mechanism of its cardiovascular effects. The principal cardiac indication for glucagon is to increase myocardial contractility and heart rate in the presence of beta-adrenergic blockade. Because glucagon is a peptide, it must be administered IV or IM.

Cardiovascular Effects

Glucagon, as a rapid injection (1 to 5 mg IV to adults) or as a continuous infusion (20 mg/hour), reliably increases stroke volume and heart rate independent of adrenergic receptor stimulation. Tachycardia, however, may be sufficiently great to interfere with the augmented cardiac output. Abrupt increases in heart rate can occur when glucagon is administered to patients in atrial fibrillation. Mean arterial pressure may increase modestly, whereas systemic vascular resistance is unchanged or decreased. In contrast to other sympathomimetics, glucagon enhances automaticity in the sinoatrial and atrioventricular nodes without increasing automaticity in the ventricles. The renal effect is similar to that of dopamine, but glucagon is less potent. In contrast to these acute cardiovascular effects, the chronic administration of glucagon is not effective in evoking sustained positive inotropic and chronotropic effects.

Side Effects

In awake patients, IV administration of glucagon often evokes nausea and vomiting. Hyperglycemia is a predictable effect after IV administration of glucagon. Paradoxical hypoglycemia may occur in patients lacking sufficient hepatic glycogen stores to offset the increased insulin release caused by glucagon. Hypokalemia reflects increased secretion of insulin and subsequent intracellular transfer of glucose and potassium. Glucagon stimulates release of catecholamines and could evoke systemic hypertension in patients with unrecognized pheochromocytomas. In this regard, glucagon, 1 to 2 mg IV, has been used as a provocative test in the differential diagnosis of pheochromocytoma. This dose of glucagon will evoke a threefold or greater increase in the plasma concentration of catecholamines 1 to 3 minutes after administration to a patient with a pheochromocytoma. A simultaneous increase in systemic blood pressure of at least 20/15 mm Hg is also likely.

MYOFILAMENT CALCIUM SENSITIZERS

Myofilament calcium sensitizers (pimobendan, sulmazole, levosimendan) are positive inotropic drugs that improve myocardial contractility independent of increases in intracellular cAMP or calcium concentrations. These drugs enhance the response of myofilament contractile elements to calcium without altering the availability of this ion. As a result, interaction between actin and myosin filaments is prolonged, and increased myocardial contractility occurs. Desensitization of myofilaments to activating effects of calcium may occur during myocardial ischemia and stunning and these drugs may be particularly useful in these circumstances (Jamali et al., 1997). The PDE III inhibiting properties of myofilament calcium sensitizers produces arterial and venous dilation that likely also contributes to the positive inotropic effects of these drugs.

REFERENCES

Atlee JL. Perioperative cardiac dysrhythmias: diagnosis and management. *Anesthesiology* 1997;86:1397–1424.

Bailey JM, Levy JH, Kikura M, et al. Pharmacokinetics of intravenous milrinone in patients undergoing cardiac surgery. *Anesthesiology* 1994;81:616–622.

Bartolone RS, Rao TLK. Dysrhythmias following muscle relaxant administration in patients receiving digitalis. *Anesthesiology* 1983;58: 567–569.

Chee TP, Prakash NS, Desser KB, Benchimol A. Postoperative supraventricular arrhythmias and the role of prophylactic digoxin in cardiac surgery. *Am Heart J* 1982;104:974–977.

Chung DC. Anesthetic problems associated with the treatment of cardiovascular disease: I. Digitalis toxicity. *Can Anaesth Soc J* 1981;28: 6–16.

Denlinger JP, Kaplan JA, Lecky JH, Wollman H. Cardiovascular responses to calcium administered intravenously to man during halothane anesthesia. *Anesthesiology* 1975;42:390–397.

Digitalis Investigation Group. The effect of digoxin on mortality and morbidity in patients with heart failure. *N Engl J Med* 1997;336: 525–533.

Edwards R, Winnie AP, Ramamurphy S. Acute hypocapnic hypokalemia: an iatrogenic complication. *Anesth Analg* 1977;56:786–792.

Hoffman BF, Bigger JT. Digitalis and allied cardiac glycosides. In: Gilman AG, Goodman LS, Rall TW, Murad F, eds. *The pharmacological basis of therapeutics*, 7th ed. New York: Macmillan, 1985: 716–747.

Inoue S, Kawaguchi M, Sakamoto T, et al. Amrinone can accelerate the cooling rate of core temperature during deliberate mild hypothermia for neurosurgical procedures. *Br J Anaesth* 2001;86:633–668.

Ivankovich AD, Miletich DJ, Grossman RK, Albrecht RF, el-Etr AA, Cairoli VJ. The effect of enflurane, isoflurane, fluroxene, methoxyflurane and diethyl ether anesthesia on ouabain tolerance in the dog. *Anesth Analg* 1976;55:360–365.

Jamali IN, Kersten JR, Pagel PS, et al. Intracoronary levosimendan enhances contractile function of stunned myocardium. *Anesth Analg*1997;85:23–29.

Kulick DL, Rahimtoola SH. Current role of digitalis therapy in patients with congestive heart failure. *JAMA* 1991;265:2995–2997.

LeJemtel TH, Keung E, Ribner HS, et al. Sustained beneficial effects of oral amrinone on cardiac and renal function in patients with severe congestive heart failure. *Am J Cardiol* 1980;45:123–129.

Packer M. The search for the ideal positive inotropic agent. *N Engl J Med* 1993;329:201–202.

Packer M. End of the oldest controversy in medicine: are we ready to conclude the debate on digitalis? *N Engl J Med* 1997;336: 575–576.

Packer M, Carver JR, Rodeheffer RJ, et al. Effect of oral milrinone on mortality in severe chronic heart failure. *N Engl J Med* 1991;325: 1468–1475.

Pinaud MLJ, Blanloeil YAG, Souron RJ. Preoperative prophylactic digitalization of patients with coronary artery disease—a randomized echocardiographic and hemodynamic study. *Anesth Analg* 1983;62:865–869.

Rathmell JP, Prielipp RC, Butterworth JF, et al. A multicenter, randomized, blind comparison of amrinone and milrinone after elective cardiac surgery. *Anesth Analg* 1998;86:683–690.

Rees J. Drug treatment in acute asthma. *BMJ* 1984;288:1819–1821.

Skoyles JR, Sherry KM. Pharmacology, mechanisms of action and uses of selective phosphodiesterase inhibitors. *Br J Anaesth* 1992;68: 293–302.

Tanaka M, Ishikawa T, Nishikawa T, et al. Influence of acidosis on cardiotonic effects of milrinone. *Anesthesiology* 1998;88:725–734.

Alpha- and Beta-Adrenergic Receptor Antagonists

14

Alpha- and beta-adrenergic receptor antagonists prevent the interaction of the endogenous neurotransmitter norepinephrine or sympathomimetics with the corresponding adrenergic receptors (Foex, 1984). Interference with normal adrenergic receptor function attenuates sympathetic nervous system homeostatic mechanisms and evokes predictable pharmacologic responses.

ALPHA-ADRENERGIC RECEPTOR ANTAGONISTS

Alpha-adrenergic receptor antagonists bind selectively to alpha-adrenergic receptors and interfere with the ability of catecholamines or other sympathomimetics to provoke alpha responses. Drug-induced alpha-adrenergic blockade prevents the effects of catecholamines and sympathomimetics on the heart and peripheral vasculature. The inhibitory action of epinephrine on insulin secretion is prevented. Orthostatic hypotension, baroreceptor-mediated reflex tachycardia, and impotence are invariable side effects of alpha-adrenergic blockade. Furthermore, absence of beta-adrenergic blockade permits maximum expression of cardiac stimulation from norepinephrine. These side effects prevent the use of nonselective alpha-adrenergic antagonists in the management of ambulatory essential hypertension.

Mechanism of Action

Phentolamine, prazosin, and yohimbine are competitive (reversible binding with receptors) alpha-adrenergic antagonists. In contrast, phenoxybenzamine binds covalently to alpha-adrenergic receptors to produce an irreversible and insurmountable type of alpha-receptor blockade. Once alpha blockade has been established with phenoxybenzamine, even massive doses of sympathomimetics are ineffective until the effect of phenoxybenzamine is terminated by metabolism.

Phentolamine and phenoxybenzamine are nonselective alpha-antagonists acting at postsynaptic $alpha_1$ receptors as well as presynaptic $alpha_2$ receptors. Prazosin is selective for $alpha_1$ receptors, whereas yohimbine is selective for $alpha_2$ receptors.

Phentolamine

Phentolamine is a substituted imidazoline derivative that produces transient nonselective alpha-adrenergic blockade (Fig. 14-1). Administered intravenously (IV), phentolamine produces peripheral vasodilation and a decrease in systemic blood pressure that manifests within 2 minutes and lasts 10 to 15 minutes. This vasodilation reflects $alpha_1$ receptor blockade and a direct action of phentolamine on vascular smooth muscle. Decreases in blood pressure elicit baroreceptor-mediated increases in sympathetic nervous system activity manifesting as cardiac stimulation. In addition to reflex stimulation, phentolamine-induced $alpha_2$ receptor blockade permits enhanced neural release of norepinephrine manifesting as increased heart rate and cardiac output. Indeed, cardiac dysrhythmias and angina pectoris may accompany the administration of phentolamine. Hyperperistalsis, abdominal pain, and diarrhea may be caused by a predominance of parasympathetic nervous system activity. Phentolamine undergoes principally hepatic metabolism and only about 10% of the drug is excreted unchanged in the urine.

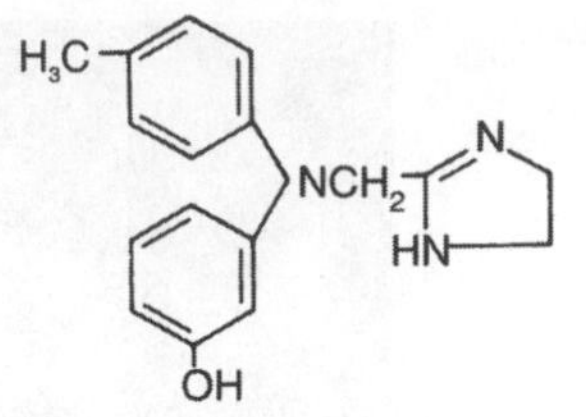

Figure 14-1. Phentolamine.

Clinical Uses

The principal use of phentolamine is the treatment of acute hypertensive emergencies, as may accompany intraoperative manipulation of a pheochromocytoma or autonomic nervous system hyperreflexia. Administration of phentolamine, 30 to 70 μg/kg IV, produces a prompt but transient decrease in systemic blood pressure. A continuous infusion of phentolamine may be used to maintain normal blood pressure during the intraoperative resection of a pheochromocytoma. Local infiltration with a phentolamine-containing solution (2.5 to 5.0 mg in 10 mL) is appropriate when a sympathomimetic is accidentally administered extravascularly.

Phenoxybenzamine

Phenoxybenzamine is a haloalkylamine derivative that acts as a nonselective alpha-adrenergic antagonist by combining covalently with alpha-adrenergic receptors (Fig. 14-2). Blockade at postsynaptic $alpha_1$ receptors is more intense than at $alpha_2$ receptors.

Pharmacokinetics

Absorption of phenoxybenzamine from the gastrointestinal tract is incomplete. Onset of alpha-adrenergic blockade is slow, taking up to 60 minutes to reach peak effect even after IV administration. This delay in onset is due to the time required for structural modification of the phenoxybenzamine molecule, which is necessary to render the drug pharmacologically active. The elimination half-time of phenoxybenzamine is about 24 hours, emphasizing the likelihood of cumulative effects with repeated doses.

Cardiovascular Effects

Phenoxybenzamine administered to a supine, normovolemic patient in the absence of increased sympathetic nervous system activity produces little change in systemic blood pressure. Orthostatic hypotension, however, is prominent, especially in the presence of preexisting hypertension or hypovolemia. In addition, impairment of compensatory vasoconstriction results in exaggerated blood pressure decreases in response to blood loss or vasodilating drugs such as volatile anesthetics. Despite decreases in blood pressure, cardiac output is often increased and renal blood flow is not greatly altered unless preexisting renal vasoconstriction is present. Cerebral and coronary vascular resistances are not changed. Alpha-adrenergic blockade produced by maternal treatment may result in neonatal hypotension and respiratory distress in the first 72 hours of life (Aplin et al., 2004).

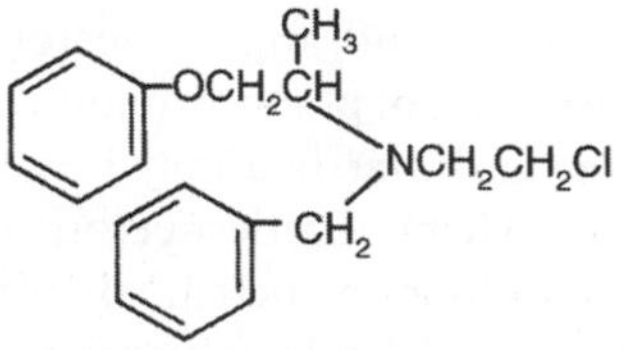

Figure 14-2. Phenoxybenzamine.

Noncardiac Effects

Phenoxybenzamine prevents the inhibitory action of epinephrine on the secretion of insulin. Catecholamine-induced glycogenolysis in skeletal muscles or lipolysis is not altered. Stimulation of the radial fibers of the iris is prevented, and miosis is a prominent component of the response to phenoxybenzamine. Sedation may accompany chronic phenoxybenzamine therapy. Nasal stuffiness is due to unopposed vasodilation in mucous membranes in the presence of alpha-adrenergic blockade.

Clinical Uses

Phenoxybenzamine, 0.5 to 1.0 mg/kg orally (prazosin is a alternative) is administered preoperatively to control blood pressure in patients with pheochromocytoma. Chronic alpha-adrenergic blockade, by relieving intense peripheral vasoconstriction, permits expansion of intravascular fluid volume as reflected by a decrease in the hematocrit. Excessive vasoconstriction with associated tissue ischemia, as accompanies hemorrhagic shock, may be reversed by phenoxybenzamine, but only after intravascular fluid volume has been replenished.

Treatment of peripheral vascular disease characterized by intermittent claudication is not favorably influenced by alpha-adrenergic blockade because cutaneous rather than skeletal muscle blood flow is increased. The most beneficial clinical responses to alpha-adrenergic blockade are in diseases with a large component of cutaneous vasoconstriction, such as Raynaud syndrome.

Yohimbine

Yohimbine is a selective antagonist at presynaptic $alpha_2$ receptors, leading to enhanced release of norepinephrine from nerve endings. As a result, this drug may be useful in the treatment of the rare patient suffering from idiopathic orthostatic hypotension. In the past, impotence had been successfully treated with yohimbine in male patients with vascular, diabetic, and psychogenic origins. Yohimbine readily crosses the blood-brain barrier and may be associated with increased skeletal muscle activity and tremor. Excessive doses of yohimbine may produce tachycardia, hypertension, rhinorrhea, paresthesias, and dissociative states.

Observations that $alpha_2$ adrenergic agonists can decrease anesthetic requirements by actions on presynaptic $alpha_2$ receptors in the central nervous system (CNS) suggests a possible interaction of yohimbine with volatile anesthetics.

Prazosin

Prazosin is a selective postsynaptic $alpha_1$ receptor antagonist that leaves intact the inhibiting effect of $alpha_2$ receptor activity on norepinephrine release from nerve endings (see Chapter 15). As a result, prazosin is less likely than nonselective alpha-adrenergic antagonists to evoke reflex tachycardia. Prazosin dilates both arterioles and veins. Following oral administration the onset of action is approximately 30 minutes and the duration of action is about 4 to 6 hours. Elimination of prazosin is principally by hepatic metabolism.

Terazosin

Alpha-blocker therapy of benign prostatic hypertrophy is based on $alpha_1$-mediated innervation of prostatic smooth muscle that controls contraction of the prostate and obstruction of the bladder outlet. Terazosin is a long-acting orally effective $alpha_1$-adrenergic antagonist that may be useful in the treatment of benign prostatic hyperplasia by virtue of its ability to relax prostatic smooth muscle.

Tamulosin

Tamulosin is an orally effective $alpha_{1a}$-adrenergic antagonist that is indicated for the treatment of the signs and symptoms of benign prostatic hyperplasia. Side effects may include orthostatic hypotension, vertigo, and syncope. The clearance of tamulosin is decreased in the presence of cimetidine.

Tolazoline

Tolazoline is a competitive nonselective alpha-adrenergic receptor antagonist. This drug has been used to treat persistent pulmonary hypertension of the newborn but its use for this purpose has been largely replaced by nitric oxide. Side effects of tolazoline include systemic hypotension with reflex tachycardia, cardiac dysrhythmias, and pulmonary and gastrointestinal hemorrhages. Tolazoline is excreted mainly unchanged by the kidneys.

BETA-ADRENERGIC RECEPTOR ANTAGONISTS

Beta-adrenergic receptor antagonists bind selectively to beta-adrenergic receptors and interfere with the ability of catecholamines or other sympathomimetics to provoke beta responses. Drug-induced beta-adrenergic blockade prevents the effects of catecholamines and sympathomimetics on the heart and smooth muscles of the airways and blood vessels. Beta-antagonist therapy should be continued throughout the perioperative period to maintain desirable drug effects and to avoid the risk of sympathetic nervous system hyperactivity associated with abrupt discontinuation of these drugs. Propranolol is the standard beta-adrenergic antagonist drug to which all other beta-adrenergic antagonists are compared.

Mechanism of Action

Beta-adrenergic receptor antagonists exhibit selective affinity for beta-adrenergic receptors, where they act by competitive inhibition. Binding of antagonist drugs to beta-adrenergic receptors is reversible such that the drug can be displaced from the occupied receptors if sufficiently large amounts of agonist become available. Competitive antagonism causes a rightward displacement of the dose-response curve for the agonist, but the slope of the curve remains unchanged, emphasizing that sufficiently large doses of the agonist may still exert a full pharmacologic effect. Chronic administration of beta-adrenergic antagonists is associated with an increase in the number of beta-adrenergic receptors.

Beta-adrenergic receptors are G-protein coupled receptors and their occupancy by agonists (norepinephrine, epinephrine) stimulates G proteins that in turn activates adenylate cyclase to produce cyclic adenosine monophosphate (cAMP). cAMP activates protein kinases which phosphorylates proteins including L-type voltage-dependent calcium channels and troponin C in a variety of tissues (especially myocardium). The net effect of beta-adrenergic stimulation in the heart is to produce positive chronotropic, inotropic, and dromotropic effects and these are the responses that are blunted by beta-adrenergic receptor antagonists. It is estimated that about 75% of beta receptors in the myocardium are $beta_1$ whereas $beta_2$ receptors account for about 20% of beta receptors.

Structure Activity Relationships

Beta-adrenergic antagonists are derivatives of the beta-agonist drug isoproterenol (Fig. 14-3). Substituents on the benzene ring determine whether the drug acts on beta-adrenergic receptors as an antagonist or agonist. The levorotatory forms of beta-antagonists and agonists are more potent than the dextrorotatory forms. For example, the dextrorotatory isomer of propranolol has $<1\%$ of the potency of the levorotatory isomer for blocking beta-adrenergic receptors.

Classification

Beta-adrenergic receptor antagonists are classified as nonselective for $beta_1$ and $beta_2$ receptors (propranolol, nadalol, timolol, pindolol) and cardioselective (metoprolol, atenolol, acebutolol, betaxolol, esmolol, bisoprolol) for

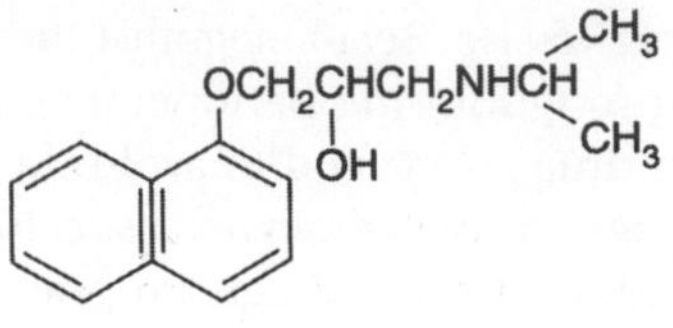
Propranolol

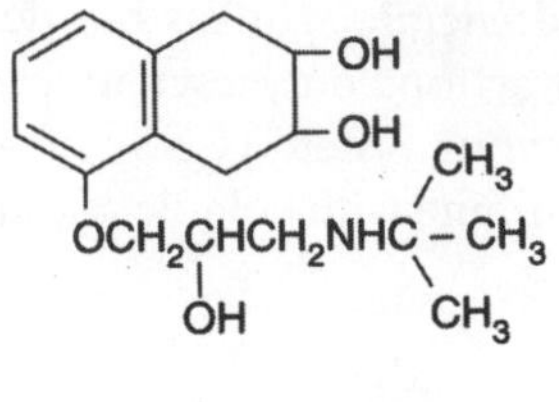
Nadolol

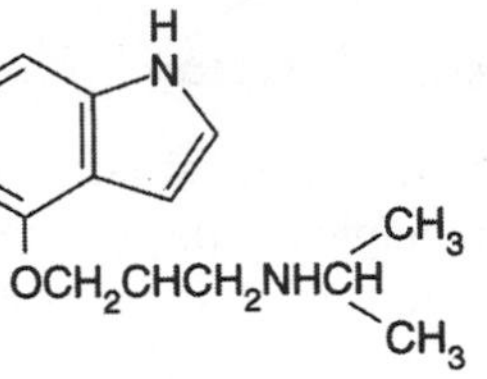
Pindolol

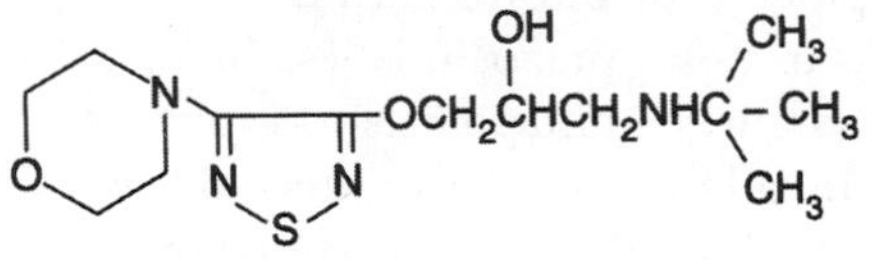
Timolol

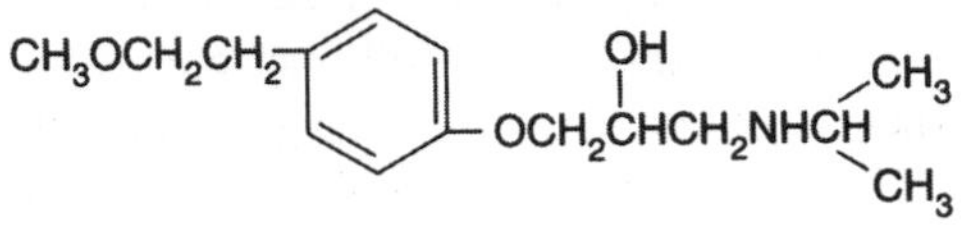
Metoprolol

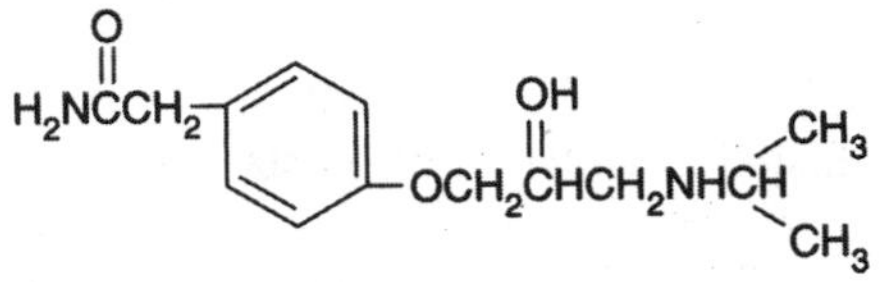
Atenolol

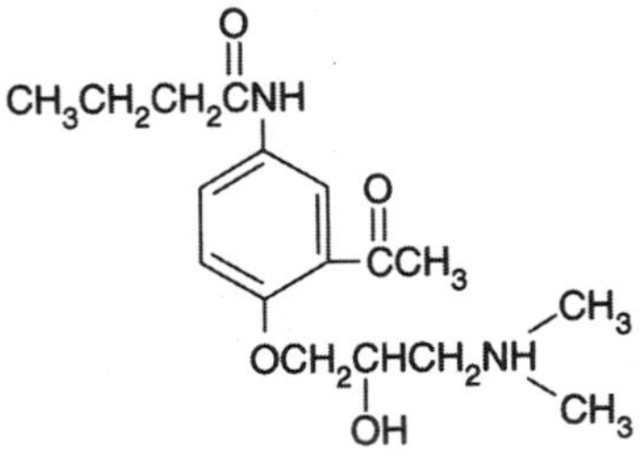
Acebutolol

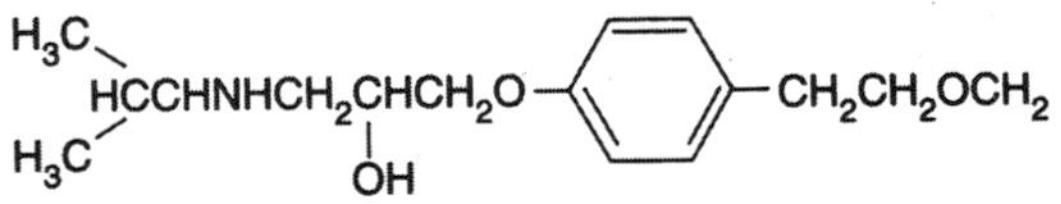
Betaxolol

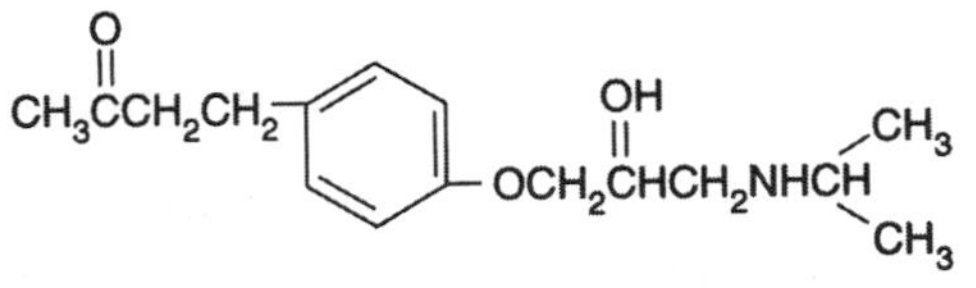
Esmolol

Figure 14-3. Beta-adrenergic antagonists.

$beta_1$ receptors (Tables 14-1 and 14-2). It is important to recognize that beta-receptor selectivity is dose dependent and is lost when large doses of the antagonist are administered. This emphasizes that selectivity should not be interpreted as specificity for a specific type of beta-adrenergic receptor. Beta-adrenergic antagonists are further classified as partial or pure antagonists on the basis of the presence or absence of intrinsic sympathomimetic activity (see Tables 14-1 and 14-2). Drugs that exhibit cardiac selectivity for $beta_1$ receptors (cardioselective) are better suited for administration to patients with asthma and reactive airway disease. Theoretically, cardioselective drugs are better suited for treatment of patients with essential hypertension as these drugs lack inhibition of peripheral $beta_2$ receptors that produce vasodilation.

$Beta_1$-receptor blockade is associated with slowing of the sinus rate, slowing of conduction of cardiac impulses through the atrioventricular node, and a decrease in inotropy. These effects are relatively greater during activity than during rest. The result is a decrease in myocardial

TABLE 14-1.
COMPARATIVE CHARACTERISTICS OF BETA-ADRENERGIC RECEPTOR ANTAGONISTS

	Propranolol	Nadolol	Pindolol	Timolol	Metoprolol	Aternolol	Acebutolol	Betaxolol	Esmolol
Cardiac selectivity	No	No	No	No	Yes	Yes	Yes	Yes	Yes
Partial agonist activity	No	No	Yes	No	No	No	Yes	No	No
Protein binding (%)	90–95	30	40–60	10	10	5	25		55
Clearance	Hepatic	Renal	Hepatic Renal	Hepatic	Hepatic	Renal	Hepatic Renal	Hepatic Renal	Plasma hydrolysis
Active metabolites	Yes	No	No	No	No	No	Yes		No
Elimination half-time (hrs)	2–3	20–24	3–4	3–4	3–4	6–7	3–4	11–22	0.15
First-pass hepatic metabolism (estimate) (%)	75	Minimal	10–15	50	60	10	60		
Blood level variability	++++	+	++	+++	++++	+	++		
Adult oral dose (mg)	40–360	40–320	5–20	10–30	50–400	50–200	200–800	10–20	
Adult intravenous dose (mg)	1–10		0.4–2	0.4–1	1–15	5–10	12.5–50		10–80 IV 50–300 μg/kg/min

+, minimal; ++, modest; +++, moderate; ++++, marked.

TABLE 14-2.
COMPARATIVE CHARACTERISTICS OF BETA-ADRENERGIC RECEPTOR ANTAGONISTS EFFECTIVE IN THE TREATMENT OF CONGESTIVE HEART FAILURE

	Metoprolol (Extended Release)	Carvedilol	Bisoprolol
Cardiac selectivity	Yes	No	Yes
Partial agonist activity	No	No	No
Initial oral dose*	6.25 mg twice daily	3.125 mg twice daily	1.25 mg daily
Desired dosage range*	50–150 mg daily	25–50 mg twice daily	5 mg daily

*Recommended doses for treatment of patients with mild to moderate congestive heart failure.

oxygen demand, with a subsequent decrease in the occurrence of myocardial ischemia during exercise. The decrease in heart rate also increases diastolic perfusion time, which may enhance myocardial perfusion. Beta$_2$-receptor blockade increases the risk of bronchospasm in patients with reactive airway disease and may worsen the clinical symptoms of peripheral vascular disease.

Beta-adrenergic antagonists may produce some degree of membrane stabilization in the heart and thus resemble quinidine. This membrane stabilization effect, however, is detectable only at plasma concentrations that are far higher than needed to produce clinically adequate beta-adrenergic blockade.

Pharmacokinetics

The principal difference in pharmacokinetics between all the beta-adrenergic receptor antagonists is the elimination half-time ranging from brief for esmolol (about 10 minutes) to hours for the other drugs (see Table 14-1). Elimination half-time is considered in the perioperative period when redosing intervals are being developed or when conversion to another beta-adrenergic receptor drug is planned. Among the beta-adrenergic receptor antagonists only propranolol is highly protein bound. The volume of distribution of these drugs is high and they are rapidly distributed following intravenous administration.

Beta-adrenergic receptor antagonists are eliminated by several different pathways and this must be considered in the presence of renal and/or hepatic dysfunction (see Table 14-1). The therapeutic plasma concentration varies greatly among these drugs and between patients (interpatient variability). Explanations for interpatient variability include (a) differences in basal sympathetic nervous system tone, (b) flat dose response curves for the drug so changes in plasma concentrations evoke minimal changes in pharmacologic effects, (c) impact of active metabolites, and (d) genetic differences in beta-adrenergic receptors that influence how an individual patient responds to a given drug and plasma concentration.

Propranolol

Propranolol is a nonselective beta-adrenergic receptor antagonist that lacks intrinsic sympathomimetic activity and thus is a pure antagonist (see Table 14-1). Antagonism of beta$_1$ and beta$_2$ receptors produced by propranolol is about equal. As the first beta-adrenergic antagonist introduced clinically, propranolol is the standard drug to which all beta-adrenergic antagonists are compared. Typically, propranolol is administered in stepwise increments until physiologic plasma concentrations have been attained, as indicated by a resting heart rate of 55 to 60 beats per minute.

Cardiac Effects

The most important pharmacologic effects of propranolol are on the heart. Because of beta$_1$-receptor blockade, propranolol decreases heart rate and myocardial contractility, resulting in decreased cardiac output. These effects on heart rate and cardiac output are especially prominent during exercise or in the presence of increased sympathetic nervous system activity. Heart rate slowing induced by propranolol lasts longer than the negative inotropic effects, suggesting a possible subdivision of beta$_1$ receptors. Concomitant blockade of beta$_2$ receptors by propranolol increases peripheral vascular resistance, including coronary vascular resistance. Although prolongation of systolic ejection and dilatation of the cardiac ventricles caused by propranolol increases myocardial oxygen requirements, the oxygen-sparing effects of decreased heart rate and myocardial contractility predominate. As a result, propranolol may relieve myocardial ischemia, even though drug-induced increases in coronary vascular resistance oppose coronary blood flow. Sodium retention associated with propranolol therapy most likely results from intrarenal hemodynamic changes that accompany drug-induced decreases in cardiac output.

Pharmacokinetics

Propranolol is rapidly and almost completely absorbed from the gastrointestinal tract, but systemic availability of the drug is limited by extensive hepatic first-pass metabolism, which may account for 90% to 95% of the absorbed dose. There is considerable individual variation in the magnitude of hepatic first-pass metabolism, accounting for up to 20-fold differences in plasma concentrations of propranolol in patients after oral administration of comparable doses (Shand, 1975). Hepatic first-pass metabolism is the reason the oral dose of propranolol (40 to 800

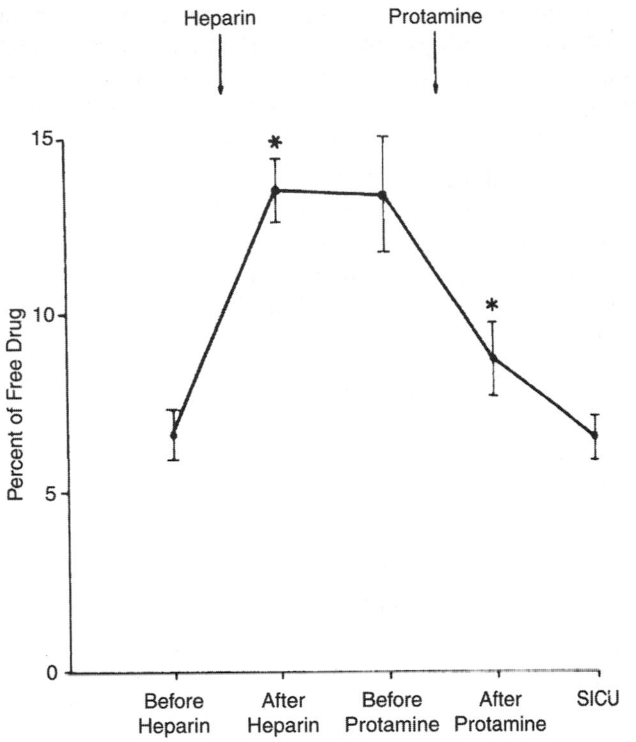

Figure 14-4. Heparin administration is associated with decreased plasma protein binding of propranolol manifesting as an increased plasma concentration of free (unbound) drug. (Mean ± SE; *P <.05.) (SICU, surgical intensive care unit.) (From Wood M, Shand DG, Wood AJJ. Propranolol binding in plasma during cardiopulmonary bypass. *Anesthesiology* 1979;51:512–516; with permission.)

mg/day) must be substantially greater than the IV dose (0.05 mg/kg given in increments of 0.5 to 1.0 mg every 5 minutes). Propranolol is not effective when administered intramuscularly.

Protein Binding

Propranolol is extensively bound (90% to 95%) to plasma proteins. Heparin-induced increases in plasma concentrations of free fatty acids due to increased lipoprotein lipase activity result in decreased plasma protein-binding of propranolol (Fig. 14-4) (Wood et al., 1979). In addition, hemodilution that occurs when cardiopulmonary bypass is initiated may alter protein binding of drugs because of the nonphysiologic protein concentration in the pump prime.

Metabolism

Clearance of propranolol from the plasma is by hepatic metabolism. An active metabolite, 4-hydroxypropranolol, is detectable in the plasma after oral administration of propranolol. Indeed, cardiac beta-blocking activity after equivalent doses of propranolol is greater after oral than after IV administration, presumably reflecting the effects of this metabolite, which is equivalent in activity to the parent compound. The elimination half-time of propranolol is 2 to 3 hours, whereas that of 4-hydroxypropranolol is even briefer. The plasma concentration of propranolol or the total dose does not correlate with its therapeutic effects. Furthermore, the assay for propranolol may not detect 4-hydroxypropranolol.

Elimination of propranolol is greatly decreased when hepatic blood flow decreases. In this regard, propranolol may decrease its own clearance rate by decreasing cardiac output and hepatic blood flow. Alterations in hepatic enzyme activity may also influence the rate of hepatic metabolism. Renal failure does not alter the elimination half-time of propranolol, but accumulation of metabolites may occur.

Clearance of Local Anesthetics

Propranolol decreases clearance of amide local anesthetics by decreasing hepatic blood flow and inhibiting metabolism in the liver (Bowdle et al., 1987). For example, in humans, propranolol causes clearance to be decreased to a much greater extent (46%) than would be predicted from a maximum 25% decrease in hepatic blood flow, implying that drug metabolism in the liver has also been affected (Conrad et al., 1983). Bupivacaine clearance is relatively insensitive to changes in hepatic blood flow (low extraction drug), suggesting that the 35% decrease in clearance of this local anesthetic reflects propranolol-induced decreases in metabolism (Fig. 14-5) (Bowdle et al., 1987). Because clearance of drugs with low extraction ratios is inversely related to plasma protein

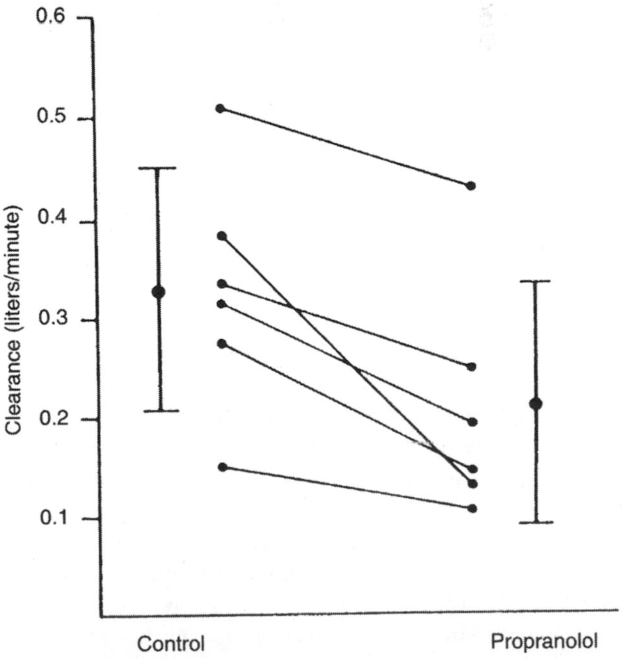

Figure 14-5. Bupivacaine clearance is decreased 35% in subjects treated with propranolol compared with control measurements. (From Bowdle TA, Freund PR, Slattery JT. Propranolol reduces bupivacaine clearance. *Anesthesiology* 1987;66:36–38; with permission.)

binding, an increase in bupivacaine binding to $alpha_1$-acid glycoprotein (responsible for 90% binding of bupivacaine) caused by propranolol could explain a decrease in clearance. Nevertheless, propranolol does not alter $alpha_1$-acid glycoprotein concentrations (Conrad et al., 1983). It is conceivable that systemic toxicity of bupivacaine could be increased by propranolol and presumably other beta antagonists that interfere with the clearance of this and other amide local anesthetics.

Clearance of Opioids

Pulmonary first-pass uptake of fentanyl is substantially decreased in patients being treated chronically with propranolol (Roerig et al., 1989). As a result, two to four times as much injected fentanyl enters the systemic circulation in the time period immediately after injection. This response most likely reflects the ability of one basic lipophilic amine (propranolol) to inhibit the pulmonary uptake of a second basic lipophilic amine (fentanyl).

Nadolol

Nadolol is a nonselective beta-adrenergic receptor antagonist that is unique in that its long duration of action permits once-daily administration.

Pharmacokinetics

Nadolol is slowly and incompletely absorbed (an estimated 30%) from the gastrointestinal tract. Metabolism does not occur, with about 75% of the drug being excreted unchanged in urine and the remainder in bile. Therefore, wide individual variations in plasma concentrations that occur with nadolol cannot be attributed to differences in metabolism, as occur with propranolol. The elimination half-time is 20 to 40 hours, accounting for the need to administer this drug only once a day. The elimination half-time of pindolol is 3 to 4 hours, and this is increased to >11 hours in patients with renal failure.

Timolol

Timolol is a nonselective beta-adrenergic receptor antagonist that is as effective as propranolol for various therapeutic indications. In addition, timolol is effective in the treatment of glaucoma because of its ability to decrease intraocular pressure, presumably by decreasing the production of aqueous humor. Timolol is administered as eyedrops in the treatment of glaucoma, but systemic absorption may be sufficient to cause resting bradycardia and increased airway resistance. Indeed, bradycardia and hypotension that are refractory to treatment with atropine have been observed during anesthesia in pediatric and adult patients receiving topical timolol with or without pilocarpine (Mishra et al., 1983). Timolol may be associated with impaired control of ventilation in neonates, resulting in unexpected postoperative apnea (Bailey, 1984). Immaturity of the neonate's blood-brain barrier may facilitate access of this drug to the CNS.

Pharmacokinetics

Timolol is rapidly and almost completely absorbed after oral administration. Nevertheless, extensive first-pass hepatic metabolism limits the amount of drug reaching the systemic circulation to about 50% of that absorbed from the gastrointestinal tract. Protein binding of timolol is not extensive. The elimination half-time is about 4 hours.

Metoprolol

Metoprolol is a selective $beta_1$-adrenergic receptor antagonist that prevents inotropic and chronotropic responses to beta-adrenergic stimulation. Conversely, bronchodilator, vasodilator, and metabolic effects of $beta_2$ receptors remain intact such that metoprolol is less likely to cause adverse effects in patients with chronic obstructive airway disease or peripheral vascular disease, and in patients vulnerable to hypoglycemia. It is important to recognize, however, that selectivity is dose related, and large doses of metoprolol are likely to become nonselective, exerting antagonist effects at $beta_2$ receptors as well as $beta_1$ receptors. Indeed, airway resistance may increase in asthmatic patients treated with metoprolol, although the magnitude of increase will be less than that evoked by propranolol. Furthermore, metoprolol-induced increases in airway resistance are more readily reversed with $beta_2$-adrenergic agonists such as terbutaline.

Pharmacokinetics

Metoprolol is readily absorbed from the gastrointestinal tract, but this is offset by substantial hepatic first-pass metabolism such that only about 40% of the drug reaches the systemic circulation. Protein binding is low; it is estimated to account for about 10% of the drug. None of the hepatic metabolites have been identified as active. A small amount (<10%) of the drug appears unchanged in urine. The elimination half-time of metoprolol is 3 to 4 hours. Plasma concentrations of metoprolol do not correlate with therapeutic effects of the drug.

Atenolol

Atenolol is the most selective $beta_1$-adrenergic antagonist that may have specific value in patients in whom the continued presence of $beta_2$ receptor activity is desirable. In patients at risk for coronary artery disease who must undergo noncardiac surgery, treatment with IV atenolol before and immediately after surgery, followed by oral therapy during the remainder of the hospitalization, decreases mortality and the incidence of cardiovascular complications for as long as 2 years (Mangano et al., 1996). Perioperative administration of atenolol to patients at high risk for coronary artery disease significantly decreases the incidence of postoperative myocardial ischemia (Wallace et al., 1998).

The antihypertensive effect of atenolol is prolonged, permitting this drug to be administered once daily for the treatment of hypertension. Like nadolol, atenolol does not enter the CNS in large amounts, but fatigue and mental depression still occur. Unlike nonselective beta-adrenergic antagonists, atenolol does not appear to potentiate insulin-induced hypoglycemia and can thus be administered with caution to patients with diabetes mellitus whose hypertension is not controlled by other antihypertensives.

Pharmacokinetics

About 50% of an orally administered dose of atenolol is absorbed from the gastrointestinal tract, with peak concentrations occurring 1 to 2 hours after oral administration. Atenolol undergoes little or no hepatic metabolism and is eliminated principally by renal excretion. The elimination half-time is 6 to 7 hours; this may increase to more than 24 hours in patients with renal failure. Therapeutic plasma concentrations of atenolol are 200 to 500 ng/mL.

Betaxolol

Betaxolol is a cardioselective $beta_1$-adrenergic antagonist with no intrinsic sympathomimetic activity and weak membrane-stabilizing activity. High doses can be expected to produce some $beta_2$-adrenergic antagonist effects on bronchial and vascular smooth muscle. Absorption after an oral dose is nearly complete. Its elimination half-time is 11 to 22 hours, making it one of the longest-acting beta-adrenergic antagonists. Clearance is primarily by metabolism, with renal elimination contributing less to overall removal of the drug from the plasma. A single oral dose daily is useful for the treatment of hypertension. A topical preparation is used as an alternative to timolol for treatment of chronic open-angle glaucoma. The risk of bronchoconstriction in patients with airway hyperreactivity may be less with betaxolol than with timolol.

Bisoprolol

Bisoprolol is a $beta_1$-selective antagonist drug without significant intrinsic agonist activity. The elimination half-time is 9 to 12 hours. Bisoprolol is eliminated equally by renal and nonrenal mechanisms. Metabolites are pharmacologically inactive. The most prominent pharmacologic effect of bisoprolol is a negative chronotropic effect. Bisoprolol is useful in the treatment of essential hypertension and has been shown to improve survival in patients with mild to moderate congestive heart failure (see Table 14-2).

Esmolol

Esmolol is a rapid-onset and short-acting selective $beta_1$-adrenergic receptor antagonist that is administered only IV (see Fig. 14-3). After a typical initial dose of 0.5 mg/kg IV over about 60 seconds, the full therapeutic effect is evident within 5 minutes, and its action ceases within 10 to 30 minutes after administration is discontinued. These characteristics make esmolol a useful drug for preventing or treating adverse systemic blood pressure and heart rate increases that occur intraoperatively in response to noxious stimulation, as during tracheal intubation. For example, esmolol, 150 mg IV, administered about 2 minutes before direct laryngoscopy and tracheal intubation provides reliable protection against increases in both heart rate and systolic blood pressure, which predictably accompanies tracheal intubation (Fig. 14-6) (Helfman et al., 1991).

Lidocaine or fentanyl is effective in blunting the increase in systolic blood pressure associated with laryngoscopy and tracheal intubation, but heart rate is not influenced (see Fig. 14-6) (Helfman et al., 1991). Other reports describe prevention of perioperative tachycardia and hypertension with esmolol, 100 to 200 mg IV, administered over 15 seconds before the induction of anesthesia (Oxorn et al., 1990; Sheppard et al., 1990). Prior administration of esmolol, 500 μg/kg/minute IV, to patients undergoing electroconvulsive therapy with anesthesia induced by methohexital plus succinylcholine results in attenuation of the heart rate increase and a decrease in the length of the electrically-induced seizures (Howie et al., 1990). Esmolol has been used during resection of pheochromocytoma and may be useful in the perioperative management of thyrotoxicosis, pregnancy-induced hypertension, and epinephrine- or cocaine-induced cardiovascular toxicity

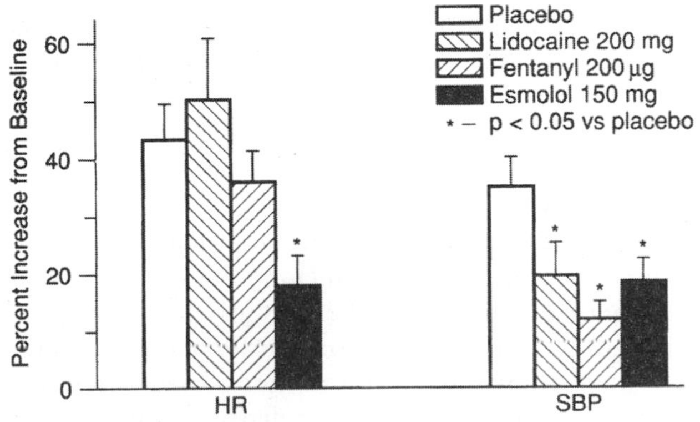

Figure 14-6. Maximum percent increases in heart rate (HR) and systolic blood pressure (SBP) after induction of anesthesia and direct laryngoscopy with tracheal intubation in patients pretreated with saline, lidocaine, fentanyl, or esmolol. All three drugs blunt the increase in SBP, but only esmolol is also effective in attenuating the increase in HR. (From Helfman SM, Gold MI, DeLisser EA, et al. Which drug prevents tachycardia and hypertension associated with tracheal intubation: lidocaine, fentanyl, or esmolol? *Anesth Analg* 1991;72:482–486; with permission.)

(Nicholas et al., 1988; Ostman et al., 1988; Pollan and Tadjziechy, 1989; Thorne and Bedford, 1989; Zakowski et al., 1989). Conversely, treatment of excessive sympathetic nervous system activity produced by cocaine or systemic absorption of topical or subcutaneous epinephrine with beta-adrenergic receptor antagonists has been associated with fulminant pulmonary edema and irreversible cardiovascular collapse (Gourdine et al., 2000). It is possible that acute drug-induced beta-receptor antagonism removes the ability of the heart to increase heart rate and myocardial contractility to compensate for catecholamine-induced increases in left ventricular afterload. In this regard, persistent symptomatic systemic hypertension owing to catecholamine-induced sympathetic nervous system stimulation is more safely treated with a peripheral vasodilator drug such as sodium nitroprusside or nitroglycerin. Detrimental effects of catecholamine release during anesthesia in patients with hypertrophic obstructive cardiomyopathy and in patients experiencing hypercyanotic spells associated with tetralogy of Fallot may be blunted by administration of esmolol (Ooi et al., 1993).

The $beta_1$ selectivity of esmolol may unmask $beta_2$-mediated vasodilation by epinephrine-secreting tumors. Administration of esmolol to patients chronically treated with beta-adrenergic antagonists has not been observed to produce additional negative inotropic effects (de Bruijn et al., 1987). The presumed reason for this observation is that esmolol, in the dose used, does not occupy sufficient additional beta receptors to produce detectable increases in beta blockade. Likewise, esmolol infused during cardiopulmonary bypass is not associated with adverse effects after discontinuation of cardiopulmonary bypass (Cork et al., 1995).

Esmolol (1 mg/kg IV followed by 250 μg/kg/minute IV) significantly decreases the plasma concentration of propofol required to prevent patient movement in response to a surgical skin incision (Johansen et al., 1997). This effect does not seem to be explained by a pharmacokinetic interaction between the two drugs.

Pharmacokinetics

Esmolol is available for IV administration only. The only other beta-adrenergic antagonists that may be administered IV are propranolol and metoprolol. The commercial preparation of esmolol is buffered to pH 4.5 to 5.5, which may be one of the factors responsible for pain on injection. The drug is compatible with commonly used IV solutions and nondepolarizing neuromuscular-blocking drugs. The elimination half-time of esmolol is about 9 minutes, reflecting its rapid hydrolysis in the blood by plasma esterases that is independent of renal and hepatic function (Hall, 1992). Less than 1% of the drug is excreted unchanged in urine, and about 75% is recovered as an inactive acid metabolite. Clinically insignificant amounts of methanol also occur from the hydrolysis of esmolol. Plasma esterases responsible for the hydrolysis of esmolol are distinct from plasma cholinesterase, and the duration of action of succinylcholine is not predictably prolonged in patients treated with esmolol (McCammon et al., 1985). Evidence of the short duration of action of esmolol is return of the heart rate to predrug levels within 15 minutes after discontinuing the drug. Indeed, plasma concentrations of esmolol are usually not detectable 15 minutes after discontinuing the drug. Poor lipid solubility limits transfer of esmolol into the CNS or across the placenta (Ostman et al., 1988).

Side Effects

The side effects of beta-adrenergic antagonists are similar for all available drugs, although the magnitude may differ depending on their selectivity and the presence or absence of intrinsic sympathomimetic activity. Beta-adrenergic antagonists exert their most prominent pharmacologic effects as well as side effects on the cardiovascular system. These drugs may also alter airway resistance, carbohydrate and lipid metabolism, and the distribution of extracellular ions. Beta-adrenergic antagonists may cause hypoglycemia (Brown and Brown, 2004). Additive effects between drugs used for anesthesia and beta-adrenergic antagonists may occur. Beta-adrenergic antagonists penetrate the blood-brain barrier and cross the placenta. Gastrointestinal side effects include nausea, vomiting, and diarrhea. Fever, rash, myopathy, alopecia, and thrombocytopenia have been associated with chronic beta-adrenergic antagonist treatment. Beta-adrenergic antagonists have been reported to decrease plasma concentrations of high-density lipoproteins and to increase triglyceride and uric acid levels.

The principal contraindication to administration of beta-adrenergic antagonists is preexisting atrioventricular heart block or cardiac failure not caused by tachycardia. Administration of beta-adrenergic antagonists to hypovolemic patients with compensatory tachycardia may produce profound hypotension (Ramsey, 1991). Nonselective beta-adrenergic antagonists or high doses of selective beta-adrenergic antagonists are not recommended for administration to patients with chronic obstructive airway disease. In patients with diabetes mellitus, there is the risk that beta-adrenergic blockade may mask the signs of hyperglycemia and thus delay its clinical recognition.

Cardiovascular System

Beta-adrenergic antagonists produce negative inotropic and chronotropic effects. In addition, the conduction speed of cardiac impulses through the atrioventricular node is slowed and the rate of spontaneous phase 4 depolarization is decreased. Preexisting atrioventricular heart block due to any cause may be accentuated by beta-adrenergic antagonists.

The cardiovascular effects of beta-adrenergic blockade reflect removal of sympathetic nervous system innervation to the heart (beta$_1$ blockade) and not membrane stabilization, which occurs only at high plasma concentrations of the antagonist drug. In addition, nonselective beta-adrenergic blockade resulting in beta$_2$-adrenergic receptor antagonism may impede left ventricular ejection due to unopposed alpha-adrenergic receptor-mediated peripheral vasoconstriction. The magnitude of cardiovascular effects produced by beta-adrenergic antagonists is greatest when preexisting sympathetic nervous system activity is increased, as during exercise or in patients in cardiac failure. Indeed, the tachycardia of exercise is consistently attenuated by beta-adrenergic antagonists. Furthermore, administration of a beta-antagonist may precipitate cardiac failure in a patient who was previously compensated. Resting bradycardia is minimized and cardiac failure is less likely to occur when a partial beta-adrenergic antagonist with intrinsic sympathomimetic activity is administered. Acute cardiac failure is rare with oral administration of beta-adrenergic antagonists.

Classically, beta-adrenergic antagonists prevent inotropic and chronotropic effects of isoproterenol as well as baroreceptor-mediated increases in heart rate evoked by decreases in systemic blood pressure in response to peripheral vasodilator drugs. Conversely, the influence of beta-adrenergic antagonists on the cardiac-stimulating effects of calcium, glucagon, and digitalis preparations is not detectable. Likewise, beta-adrenergic antagonists do not alter the response to alpha-adrenergic agonists such as epinephrine or phenylephrine. Indeed, the pressor effect of epinephrine is enhanced because the nonselective beta antagonists prevent the beta$_2$-vasodilating effect of epinephrine and leave unopposed its alpha-adrenergic effect. The presence of unopposed alpha-adrenergic–induced vasoconstriction may provoke paradoxical hypertension and may even precipitate cardiac failure in the presence of diseased myocardium that cannot respond to sympathetic nervous system stimulation because of beta-adrenergic blockade. Unexpected hypertension has occurred in patients receiving clonidine who subsequently receive a nonselective beta-adrenergic antagonist (Nies and Shand, 1973). Presumably, blockade of the vasodilating effect normally produced by activity of beta$_2$ receptors leaves unopposed alpha-adrenergic effects to provoke peripheral vasoconstriction with resulting hypertension.

Patients with peripheral vascular disease do not tolerate well the peripheral vasoconstriction associated with beta$_2$ receptor blockade produced by nonselective beta-adrenergic antagonists. Indeed, the development of cold hands and feet is a common side effect of beta blockade. Vasospasm associated with Raynaud's disease is accentuated by propranolol.

The principal antidysrhythmic effect of beta-adrenergic blockade is to prevent the dysrhythmogenic effect of endogenous or exogenous catecholamines or sympathomimetics. This reflects a decrease in sympathetic nervous system activity. Membrane stabilization is probably of little importance in the antidysrhythmic effects produced by usual doses of beta-adrenergic antagonists.

Treatment of Excess Myocardial Depression

The usual clinical manifestations of excessive myocardial depression produced by beta-adrenergic blockade include bradycardia, low cardiac output, hypotension, and cardiogenic shock (DeLima et al., 1995). Bronchospasm and depression of ventilation may also be associated with an overdose of beta-adrenergic antagonist drugs. Seizures and prolonged intraventricular conduction of cardiac impulses are thought to be the result of local anesthetic properties of certain beta-adrenergic antagonists (see Table 14-1). Hypoglycemia is a rare manifestation of beta-adrenergic antagonist overdose.

Excessive bradycardia and/or decreases in cardiac output due to drug-induced beta blockade should be treated initially with atropine in incremental doses of 7 μg/kg IV. Atropine is likely to be effective by blocking vagal effects on the heart and thus unmasking any residual sympathetic nervous system innervation. If atropine is ineffective, drugs to produce direct positive chronotropic and inotropic effects are indicated. For example, continuous infusion of the nonselective beta-adrenergic agonist isoproterenol, in doses sufficient to overcome competitive beta blockade, is appropriate. The necessary dose of isoproterenol may be 2 to 25 μg/minute IV (60 μg/minute IV was not effective in one report), which is five to 20 times the necessary dose in the absence of beta blockade (DeLima et al., 1995). When a pure beta-adrenergic antagonist is responsible for excessive cardiovascular depression, a pure beta$_1$-adrenergic agonist such as dobutamine is recommended because isoproterenol, with beta$_1$- and beta$_2$-adrenergic agonist effects, could produce vasodilation before its inotropic effect develops. Dopamine is not recommended because alpha-adrenergic-induced vasoconstriction is likely to occur with the high doses required to overcome beta blockade.

Glucagon administered to adults, 1 to 10 mg IV followed by 5 mg/hour IV, effectively reverses myocardial depression produced by beta-adrenergic antagonists at normal doses because these drugs do not exert their effects by means of beta-adrenergic receptors. For example, glucagon stimulates adenylate cyclase and increases intracellular cAMP concentrations independent of beta-adrenergic receptors (DeLima et al., 1995). Calcium chloride, 250 to 1,000 mg IV, may also act independent of beta-adrenergic receptors to offset excessive cardiovascular depression produced by beta-adrenergic antagonists. Glucagon appears to be particularly effective in the presence of life-threatening bradycardia and has been described as the drug of choice to treat massive beta-adrenergic antagonist overdose (DeLima et al., 1995).

In the presence of bradycardia that is unresponsive to pharmacologic therapy, it may be necessary to place a transvenous artificial cardiac pacemaker. Hemodialysis should be reserved to remove minimally protein-bound, renally excreted beta-adrenergic antagonists in patients refractory to pharmacologic therapy.

Airway Resistance

Nonselective beta-adrenergic antagonists such as propranolol consistently increase airway resistance as a manifestation of bronchoconstriction due to blockade of $beta_2$ receptors. These airway resistance effects are exaggerated in patients with preexisting obstructive airway disease. Because bronchodilation is a $beta_2$-adrenergic agonist response, selective $beta_1$-adrenergic antagonists such as metoprolol and esmolol are less likely than propranolol to increase airway resistance.

Metabolism

Beta-adrenergic antagonists alter carbohydrate and fat metabolism. For example, nonselective beta-adrenergic antagonists such as propranolol interfere with glycogenolysis that ordinarily occurs in response to release of epinephrine during hypoglycemia. This emphasizes the need for $beta_2$-receptor activity in glycogenolysis. Furthermore, tachycardia, which is an important warning sign of hypoglycemia in insulin-treated diabetics, is blunted by beta-adrenergic antagonists. For this reason, nonselective beta-adrenergic antagonists are not recommended for administration to patients with diabetes mellitus who may be at risk for developing hypoglycemia because of treatment with insulin or oral hypoglycemics. Altered fat metabolism is evidenced by failure of sympathomimetics or sympathetic nervous system stimulation to increase plasma concentrations of fatty-free acids in the presence of beta-adrenergic blockade.

Distribution of Extracellular Potassium

Distribution of potassium across cell membranes is influenced by sympathetic nervous system activity as well as insulin. Specifically, stimulation of $beta_2$-adrenergic receptors seems to facilitate movement of potassium intracellularly. As a result, beta-adrenergic blockade inhibits uptake of potassium into skeletal muscles, and the plasma concentration of potassium may be increased. Indeed, increases in the plasma concentration of potassium associated with infusion of this ion are greater in the presence of beta-adrenergic blockade produced by propranolol (Fig. 14-7) (Rosa et al., 1980). In animals, increases in the plasma concentration of potassium after administration of succinylcholine last longer when beta-adrenergic blockade is present (McCammon and Stoelting, 1984). In view of the speculated role of $beta_2$ receptors in regulating plasma concentrations of potassium, it is likely that selective $beta_1$-adrenergic antagonists would impair skeletal muscle uptake of potassium less than nonselective beta-adrenergic antagonists.

Interaction with Anesthetics

Myocardial depression produced by inhaled or injected anesthetics could be additive with depression produced by beta-adrenergic antagonists. Nevertheless, clinical experience and controlled studies in patients and animals have confirmed that additive myocardial depression with beta-adrenergic antagonists and anesthetics is not excessive, and treatment with beta-adrenergic antagonists may therefore be safely maintained throughout the perioperative period (Foex, 1984). An exception may be patients treated with timolol in whom profound bradycardia has been observed in the presence of inhaled anesthetics.

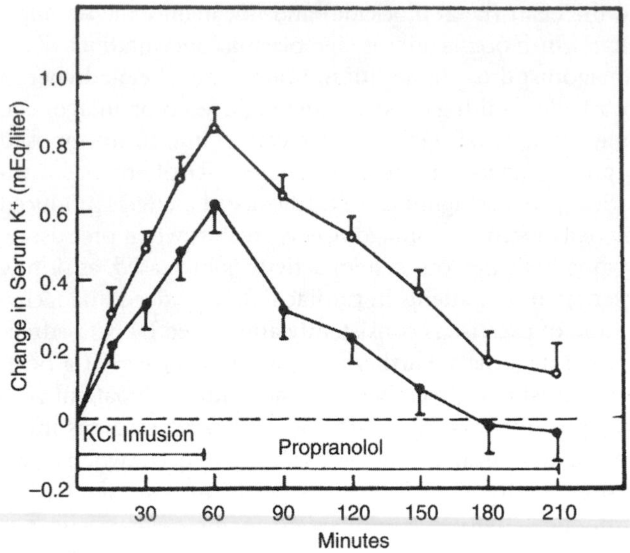

Figure 14-7. Increases in plasma (serum) potassium concentration (K^+) in response to infusion of potassium chloride (KCl) are greater in the presence of propranolol (*clear circles*) than in its absence (*solid circles*). Mean ± SE. (From Rosa RM, Silva P, Young JB, et al. Adrenergic modulation of extrarenal potassium disposal. *N Engl J Med* 1980;302:431–434; with permission.)

Additive cardiovascular effects with inhaled anesthetics and beta-adrenergic antagonists seem to be greatest with enflurane and least with isoflurane (Foex, 1984). Sevoflurane and desflurane, like isoflurane, do not seem to be associated with significant additive cardiovascular effects when administered to patients being treated with beta-adrenergic antagonists. Cardiac output and systemic blood pressure are similar with or without beta-adrenergic blockade in the presence of 1 or 2 MAC isoflurane (Philbin and Lowenstein, 1976). Even acute hemorrhage does not alter the interaction between isoflurane and beta-adrenergic antagonists (Horan et al., 1977a; Roberts et al., 1976). In contrast, cardiac depression is more likely to occur in the presence of beta blockade when acute hemorrhage occurs in animals anesthetized with enflurane (Horan et al., 1977b). Cardiovascular responses to even high doses of opioids such as fentanyl are not altered by preexisting beta-adrenergic blockade. In the presence of anesthetic drugs that increase sympathetic nervous system activity (ketamine), or when excessive sympathetic nervous system activity is present because of hypercarbia, the acute administration of a beta-adrenergic antagonist may unmask direct negative inotropic effects of concomitantly administered anesthetics, with resulting decreases in systemic blood pressure and cardiac output (Foex and Ryder, 1981).

Nervous System

Beta-adrenergic antagonists may cross the blood-brain barrier to produce side effects. For example, fatigue and lethargy are commonly associated with chronic propranolol therapy. Vivid dreams are frequent, but psychotic reactions are rare. Memory loss and mental depression have been alleged to occur, although beta-adrenergic antagonist therapy has not been shown to produce these effects (Bright and Everitt, 1992). Peripheral paresthesias have been described. Atenolol and nadolol are less lipid soluble than other beta-adrenergic antagonists and thus may be associated with a lower incidence of CNS effects.

Fetus

Beta-adrenergic antagonists can cross the placenta and cause bradycardia, hypotension, and hypoglycemia in newborn infants of mothers who are receiving the drug. Breast milk is also likely to contain beta-adrenergic antagonists administered to the mother.

Withdrawal Hypersensitivity

Acute discontinuation of beta-adrenergic antagonist therapy can result in excess sympathetic nervous system activity that manifests in 24 to 48 hours. Presumably, this enhanced activity reflects an increase in the number of beta-adrenergic receptors (up-regulation) during chronic therapy with beta-adrenergic antagonists. Continuous infusion of propranolol, 3 mg/hour IV, is effective in maintaining therapeutic plasma concentrations in adult patients who cannot take drugs orally during the perioperative period (Smulyan et al., 1982).

Clinical Uses

Clinical uses of beta-adrenergic antagonists are multiple and in equivalent doses, all beta-adrenergic antagonists seem to be equally effective in producing desired therapeutic effects (Table 14-3). It is accepted that patients being treated with beta-adrenergic receptor antagonists should have their medication continued uninterrupted through the perioperative period. It is also recommended that patients at high risk for myocardial ischemia and presenting for major surgery should be treated with beta-adrenergic receptor antagonists beginning preoperatively and continuing into the postoperative period.

TABLE 14-3.
CLINICAL USES OF BETA-ADRENERGIC BLOCKERS

Treatment of essential hypertension
Management of angina pectoris
Treatment of acute coronary syndrome
Perioperative beta-adrenergic receptor blockade
Treatment of intraoperative myocardial ischemia
Suppression of cardiac dysrhythmias
Management of congestive heart failure
Prevention of excessive sympathetic nervous system activity
Preoperative preparation of hyperthyroid patients
Treatment of migraine headache

Treatment of Essential Hypertension

Chronic therapy with beta-adrenergic antagonists results in gradual decreases in systemic blood pressure. The antihypertensive effect of beta-adrenergic blockade is largely dependent on decreases in cardiac output due to decreased heart rate. Large doses of beta-adrenergic antagonists may decrease myocardial contractility as well. In many patients, systemic vascular resistance remains unchanged. An important advantage in the use of beta-adrenergic antagonists for the treatment of essential hypertension is the absence of orthostatic hypotension. Often a beta-adrenergic antagonist is used in combination with a vasodilator to minimize reflex baroreceptor–mediated increases in heart rate and cardiac output produced by the vasodilator. All orally administered beta-adrenergic antagonists appear to be equally effective antihypertensive drugs. Release of renin from the juxtaglomerular apparatus that occurs in response to stimulation of $beta_2$ receptors is prevented by nonselective beta-adrenergic antagonists such as propranolol. This may account for a portion of the antihypertensive effect of propranolol, especially in patients with high circulating plasma concentrations of renin. Because drug-induced decreases in secretion of renin will lead to decreased release of aldosterone, beta-adrenergic antagonists will also prevent the compensatory sodium and water retention that accompanies treatment with a vasodilator.

Management of Angina Pectoris

Orally administered beta-adrenergic antagonists are equally effective in decreasing the likelihood of myocardial ischemia manifesting as angina pectoris. This desirable response reflects drug-induced decreases in myocardial oxygen requirements secondary to decreased heart rate and myocardial contractility. The effective dose usually decreases resting heart rate to <60 beats per minute. A more important measure is the heart rate during exercise, which should not exceed 75% of the heart rate at which myocardial ischemia occurs.

The concept that beta-adrenergic antagonists and calcium-channel blockers act on different determinants of the myocardial oxygen supply-to-demand ratio suggests combined uses of these drugs would be beneficial in the management of patients with coronary artery disease. Nevertheless, the evidence from clinical studies suggests that patients managed with combined therapy do not experience greater beneficial therapeutic effects but may experience more adverse effects than if they had received optimal treatment with a single drug (Packer, 1989).

Treatment of Acute Coronary Syndrome

It is recommended that all patients who experience an acute myocardial infarction receive IV beta-adrenergic antagonists (assuming no contraindications are present) as early as possible, whether or not they receive reperfusion therapy. Treatment with beta-adrenergic antagonists is contraindicated in the presence of severe bradycardia, unstable left ventricular failure, atrioventricular heart block). Relative contraindications to treatment with beta-adrenergic antagonists includes asthma or reactive airway disease, mental depression, and peripheral vascular disease. Diabetes mellitus is not a contraindication to treatment with beta-adrenergic antagonists recognizing that signs of hypoglycemia may be masked. The incidence of nonfatal reinfarction and recurrent myocardial ischemia is decreased compared with patients in whom oral metoprorol was initiated 6 days following myocardial infarction (TIMI Study Group, 1988). Beta-adrenergic antagonist prophylaxis after acute myocardial infarction is considered to be one of the most scientifically substantiated, cost-effective preventive medical treatments. Whether beta-adrenergic antagonists can decrease mortality in patients with angina pectoris who have not yet experienced a myocardial infarction is unknown.

The cardioprotective effect of beta-adrenergic antagonists is present with both cardioselective and nonselective drugs (see Tables 14-1 and 14-2). The mechanism of the cardioprotective effect is uncertain, but antidysrhythmic actions may be important. A nonselective beta-adrenergic antagonist that prevents epinephrine-induced decreases in plasma potassium concentrations (a $beta_2$-mediated response) may be useful in decreasing the incidence of ventricular dysrhythmias.

Perioperative Beta-Adrenergic Receptor Blockade

Perioperative beta-adrenergic receptor blockade is recommended for patients considered at risk for myocardial ischemia (known coronary artery disease, positive preoperative stress tests, diabetes mellitus treated with insulin, left ventricular hypertrophy) during high-risk surgery (vascular surgery, thoracic surgery, intraperitoneal surgery, anticipated large blood loss) (London et al., 2002; Shojania et al., 2002). The goal of preoperative therapy is a resting heart rate between 65 and 80 beats per minute (Auerbach and Goldman, 2002). All beta-adrenergic receptor antagonists except those with intrinsic sympathetic nervous system activity decrease mortality. Perioperative myocardial ischemia is the single most important potentially reversible risk factor for mortality and cardiovascular complications after noncardiac surgery. Administration of atenolol for 7 days before and after noncardiac surgery in patients at risk for coronary artery disease may decrease mortality and the incidence of cardiovascular complications for as long as 2 years after surgery (Mangano et al., 1996). In another report, administration of atenolol intravenously before induction of anesthesia and every 12 hours after noncardiac surgery for 7 days to patients at high risk for coronary artery disease reduced the incidence of postoperative myocardial ischemia by 30% to 50% (Wallace et al., 1998). Decreases in perioperative myocardial ischemia are associated with reductions in the risk for death at 24 months. The incidence of bronchospasm, hypotension, bradycardia, and cardiac dysrhythmias was not increased in treated patients. The mechanism for the beneficial effects of perioperative beta-adrenergic receptor blockade is not known but is most likely multifactorial (Table 14-4). It is not known if patients with cardiac risk factors but no signs of underlying coronary artery disease will benefit from perioperative administration of a beta-adrenergic antagonist (Eagle and Froehlich, 1996).

TABLE 14-4.
POSSIBLE EXPLANATIONS FOR CARDIOPROTECTIVE EFFECTS PRODUCED BY PERIOPERATIVE BETA-ADRENERGIC RECEPTOR BLOCKADE

Decreased myocardial oxygen consumption and demand
Less stress on potentially ischemic myocardium owing to decreased heart rate and myocardial contractility
Attenuation of effects of endogenous catecholamines
Redistribution of coronary blood flow to ischemic areas
Increased coronary blood flow owing to increased diastolic time
Plaque stabilization owing to decrease in shear forces
Cardiac antidysrhythmic effects
Antiinflammatory effects (?)

Preoperatively, oral therapy can be initiated with atenolol 50 mg or bisoprolol 5 to 10 mg daily or metoprolol 25 to 50 mg twice daily. If the patient is seen the morning of surgery, atenolol 5 to 10 mg IV or metoprolol 5 to10 IV can be titrated. Esmolol is an acceptable drug to achieve beta-adrenergic receptor blockade during surgery and postoperatively in the intensive care unit where continuous IV infusions can be monitored. Alternatively, IV atenolol or metoprolol can be administered until the patient can take oral atenolol or bisoprolol. Beta-adrenergic receptor antagonists with sypmathomimetic actions are not likely selections to produce perioperative beta-blockade.

Treatment of Intraoperative Myocardial Ischemia

Appearance of evidence of myocardial ischemia on the electrocardiogram or as wall motion abnormalities on the transesophageal echocardiogram may benefit from treatment with a beta-adrenergic receptor-blocking drug, assuming the absence of contraindications (severe reactive airway disease, shock, left ventricular failure) and the presence of an adequate concentration of inhaled anesthetic drugs. The drug selected should be titrated IV to the desired heart rate (about 60 beats/minute) to attenuate myocardial ischemia. Treatment options include esmolol (1–1.5 mg/kg IV followed by a continuous infusion of 50–300 μg/kg/minute), metoprolol (5 mg IV), atenolol (5 to 10 mg IV), or propranolol (1 to 10 mg IV). The advantage of esmolol is the ability to titrate its effects to the desired heart rate. Nitroglycerin is often added to this treatment regimen.

Suppression of Cardiac Dysrhythmias

Beta-adrenergic receptor-blocking drugs are effective in the treatment of cardiac dysrhythmias as a result of enhanced sympathetic nervous system stimulation (thryotoxicosis, phenochromocytoma, perioperative stress). Esmolol and propranolol are effective for controlling the ventricular response rate to atrial fibrillation and atrial flutter. These drugs are also effective for controlling atrial dysrhythmias following cardiac surgery. Propranolol may be effective for controlling torsades de pointes in patients with prolonged QTc intervals on the electrocardiogram. Acebutolol, emtoprolol, atenolol, propranolol, and timolol are approved for prevention of sudden death following acute myocardial infarction.

Management of Congestive Heart Failure

Controlled studies have demonstrated that metoprolol, carvedilol, and bisoprolol improve ejection fraction and increase survival in patients in chronic heart failure (see Table 14-2). Sustained-release metoprolol is associated with improved survival (Hjalmarson et al., 2000). Carvedilol, a nonselective beta blocker with vasodilator and antioxidant properties, has been shown to decrease mortality associated with congestive heart failure. (Colucci et al., 1996). When beta-blocking drugs are used to treat congestive heart failure, the initial doses of beta blockers should be minimal and gradually increased.

Prevention of Excessive Sympathetic Nervous System Activity

Beta-adrenergic blockade is associated with attenuated heart rate and blood pressure changes in response to direct laryngoscopy and tracheal intubation (Foex, 1984; Prys-Roberts et al., 1973). Hypertrophic obstructive cardiomyopathies are often treated with beta-adrenergic antagonists. Tachycardia and cardiac dysrhythmias associated with pheochromocytoma and hyperthyroidism are effectively suppressed by propranolol. The likelihood of cyanotic episodes in patients with tetralogy of Fallot is minimized by beta blockade. Propranolol has been used intraoperatively to prevent reflex baroreceptor–mediated increases in heart rate evoked by vasodilators administered to produce controlled hypotension. Even anxiety states as caused by public speaking have been treated with propranolol.

Preoperative Preparation of Hyperthyroid Patients

Thyrotoxic patients can be prepared for surgery in an emergency by IV administration of propranolol or esmolol or electively by oral administration of propranolol (40 to 320 mg daily) (Lee et al., 1982; Lennquits et al., 1985). Advantages of beta-adrenergic antagonists include rapid suppression of excessive sympathetic nervous system activity and elimination of the need to administer iodine or antithyroid drugs.

COMBINED ALPHA- AND BETA-ADRENERGIC RECEPTOR ANTAGONISTS

Labetalol

Labetalol is a unique parenteral and oral antihypertensive drug that exhibits selective $alpha_1$- and nonselective $beta_1$- and $beta_2$-adrenergic antagonist effects (Fig. 14-8) (MacCarthy and Bloomfield, 1983; Wallin and O'Neill, 1983). Presynaptic $alpha_2$ receptors are spared by labetalol such that released norepinephrine can continue to inhibit further release of catecholamines via the negative feedback mechanism resulting from stimulation of $alpha_2$ receptors. Labetalol is one-fifth to one-tenth as potent as phentolamine in its ability to block alpha receptors and is approximately one-fourth to one-third as potent as propranolol in blocking beta receptors. In humans, the beta- to alpha-blocking potency ratio is 3:1 for oral labetalol and 7:1 for IV labetalol.

Pharmacokinetics

Metabolism of labetalol is by conjugation of glucuronic acid, with 5% of the drug recovered unchanged in urine. The elimination half-time is 5 to 8 hours and is prolonged in the presence of liver disease and unchanged by renal dysfunction.

Cardiovascular Effects

Administration of labetalol lowers systemic blood pressure by decreasing systemic vascular resistance ($alpha_1$ blockade), whereas reflex tachycardia triggered by vasodilation is attenuated by simultaneous beta blockade. Cardiac output remains unchanged. In addition to producing vasodilation by $alpha_1$ blockade, labetalol may cause vasodilation that is mediated by $beta_2$-adrenergic agonist activity (Baum et al., 1981). The maximum systemic blood pressure–lowering effect of an IV dose of labetalol (0.1 to 0.5 mg/kg) is present in 5 to 10 minutes.

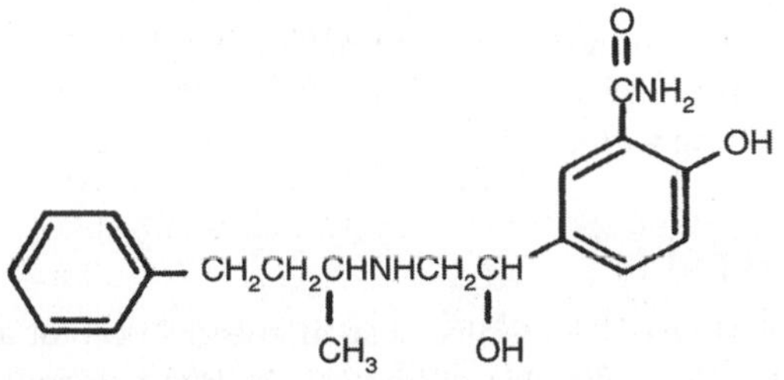

Figure 14-8. Labetalol.

Clinical Uses

Labetalol is a safe and effective treatment for hypertensive emergencies. For example, labetalol has been administered IV to control severe hypertension that may be associated with an epinephrine overdose as may occur during submucosal injection to produce surgical hemostasis (Larsen, 1990). Conversely, caution has been urged in using beta-adrenergic blockers to treat phenylephrine and epinephrine overdose resulting from systemic absorption following topical application (Gourdine et al., 2000). Large bolus doses of labetalol (2 mg/kg IV) administered to treat hypertensive emergencies may result in excessive decreases in blood pressure, whereas smaller doses (20 to 80 mg IV) are less likely to produce undesirable decreases in blood pressure (Lebel et al., 1985; Wilson et al., 1983). Repeated doses of labetalol, 20 to 80 mg IV, may be administered about every 10 minutes until the desired therapeutic response is achieved (Wilson et al., 1983). Rebound hypertension after withdrawal of clonidine therapy and hypertensive responses in patients with pheochromocytoma can be effectively treated with labetalol. Labetalol is also effective in the treatment of angina pectoris. Availability of both an oral (100 to 600 mg twice a day) and IV preparation is useful for converting a patient with a hypertensive crisis to oral therapy after initial control with IV therapy.

Labetalol, 0.1 to 0.5 mg/kg IV, can be administered to anesthetized patients to attenuate increases in heart rate and blood pressure that are presumed to result from abrupt increases in the level of surgical stimulation. It is possible that existing depressant effects of the anesthetic drugs could accentuate the blood pressure–lowering properties of labetalol. In contrast to the results with nitroprusside, controlled hypotension produced with intermittent injections of labetalol, 10 mg IV, is not associated with increases in heart rate, intrapulmonary shunt, or cardiac output (Goldberg et al., 1990).

Side Effects

Orthostatic hypotension is the most common side effect of labetalol therapy. Bronchospasm is possible in susceptible patients, reflecting the beta-adrenergic antagonist effects of labetalol. Other adverse effects associated with beta-adrenergic antagonists (congestive heart failure, bradycardia, heart block) are a potential risk of labetalol therapy, but the likely incidence and severity is substantially decreased. Incomplete alpha-adrenergic blockade in the presence of more complete beta blockade could result in excessive alpha stimulation (Larsen, 1990). Fluid retention in patients treated chronically with labetalol is the reason for combining this drug with a diuretic during prolonged therapy.

Carvedilol

Carvedilol is a nonselective beta-adrenergic receptor antagonist with $alpha_1$-blocking activity. This drug has no intrinsic beta-adrenergic agonist effect. Following oral administration carvedilol is extensively metabolized to products with pharmacologic activity possessing weak vasodilator actions. The elimination half-time is 7 to 10 hours and protein binding is extensive. Carvedilol is indicated for the treatment of mild to moderate congestive heart failure owing to ischemia or cardiomyopathy (see Table 14-2). This drug is also useful for the treatment of essential hypertension.

REFERENCES

Aplin Sc, Yee KF, Cole MJ. Neonatal effects of long-term maternal phenoxybenzamine therapy. *Anesthesiology* 2004;100:1608–1610.

Auerbach AD, Goldman L. Beta-blockers and reduction of cardiac events in noncardiac surgery. *JAMA* 2002;287:1435–1444.

Bailey PL. Timolol and postoperative apnea in neonates and young infants. *Anesthesiology* 1984;61:622.

Baum T, Watkins RW, Sybertz EJ, et al. Antihypertensive and hemodynamic actions of Sch 19927, the R,R-isomer of labetalol. *J Pharmacol Exp Ther* 1981;218:441–452.

Bowdle TA, Freund PR, Slattery JT. Propranolol reduces bupivacaine clearance. *Anesthesiology* 1987;66:36–38.

Bright RA, Everitt DE. Beta-blockers and depression: evidence against an association. *JAMA* 1992;267:1783–1787.

Brown DR, Brown MJ. Hypoglycemia associated with preoperative metoprolol administration. *Anesth Analg* 2004;99:1427–1428.

Colucci WS, Packer M, Bristow MR, et al. Carvedilol inhibits clinical progression in patients with mild symptoms of heart failure. *Circulation* 1996;94:1199–1205.

Conrad KA, Beyers JM, Finley PR, et al. Lidocaine elimination: effects of metoprolol and propranolol. *Clin Pharmacol Ther* 1983;33:133–138.

Cork RC, Kramer TH, Dreischmeier B, et al. The effect of esmolol given during cardiopulmonary bypass. *Anesth Analg* 1995;80:28–40.

de Bruijn NP, Croughwell N, Reves JG. Hemodynamic effects of esmolol in chronically beta-blocked patients undergoing aortocoronary bypass surgery. *Anesth Analg* 1987;66:137–141.

DeLima LGR, Kharasch ED, Butler S. Successful pharmacologic treatment of massive atenolol overdose: sequential hemodynamics and plasma atenolol concentrations. *Anesthesiology* 1995;83:204–207.

Eagle KA, Froehlich JB. Reducing cardiovascular risk in patients undergoing noncardiac surgery. *N Engl J Med* 1996;335:1761–1763.

Foex P. Alpha- and beta-adrenoceptor antagonists. *Br J Anaesth* 1984;56:751–765.

Foex P, Ryder WA. Interactions of adrenergic beta-receptor blockade (oxprenolol) and P_{CO_2} in the anesthetized dog: influence of intrinsic sympathomimetic activity. *Br J Anaesth* 1981;53:19–26.

Goldberg ME, McNulty SE, Azad SS, et al. A comparison of labetalol and nitroprusside for inducing hypotension during major surgery. *Anesth Analg* 1990;70:537–542.

Gourdine SB, Hollinger I, Jones J, et al. New York state guidelines on the topical use of phenylephrine in the operating room. *Anesthesiology* 2000;92:859–864.

Hall RI. Esmolol—just another beta blocker? *Can J Anaesth* 1992;39:757–764.

Helfman SM, Gold MI, DeLisser EA, et al. Which drug prevents tachycardia and hypertension associated with tracheal intubation: lidocaine, fentanyl, or esmolol? *Anesth Analg* 1991;72:482–486.

Hjalmarson A, Goldstein S, Gagerberg B, et al. Effects of controlled-release metoprolol on total mortality, hospitalizations, and well-being in patients with heart failure: The Metoprolol CR/XL Randomized Intervention Trial in Congestive Heart Failure (MERIT-HF). MERIT-HF Study Group. *JAMA* 2000;283:1295–1302.

Horan BF, Prys-Roberts C, Hamilton WK, et al. Haemodynamic responses to enflurane anaesthesia and hypovolaemia in the dog, and their modification by propranolol. *Br J Anaesth* 1977a;49:1189–1197.

Horan BF, Prys-Roberts C, Roberts JG, et al. Haemodynamic responses to isoflurane anaesthesia and hypovolaemia in the dog, and their modification by propranolol. *Br J Anaesth* 1977b;49:1179–1187.

Howie MB, Black HA, Zvara D, et al. Esmolol reduces autonomic hypersensitivity and length of seizures induced by electroconvulsive therapy. *Anesth Analg* 1990;71:384–388.

Johansen JW, Flaishon R, Sebel PS. Esmolol reduces anesthetic requirement for skin incision during propofol/nitrous oxide/morphine anesthesia. *Anesthesiology* 1997;86:364–371.

Larsen LS. Labetalol in the treatment of epinephrine overdose. *Ann Emerg Med* 1990;19:680–682.

Lebel M, Langlois S, Belleau LJ, et al. Labetalol infusion in hypertensive emergencies. *Clin Pharmacol Ther* 1985;37:615–618.

Lee TC, Coffey RJ, Currier BM, et al. Propranolol and thyroidectomy in the treatment of thyrotoxicosis. *Ann Surg* 1982;195:766–772.

Lennquits S, Jortso E, Anderberg B, et al. Beta blockers compared with antithyroid drug as preoperative treatment in hyperthyroidism: drug tolerance, complications, and postoperative thyroid function. *Surgery* 1985;98:1141–1146.

MacCarthy EP, Bloomfield SS. Labetalol: a review of its pharmacology, pharmacokinetics, clinical uses and adverse effects. *Pharmacotherapy* 1983;3:193–219.

Mangano DT, Layug EL, Wallace A, et al. Effect of atenolol on mortality and cardiovascular morbidity after noncardiac surgery. *N Engl J Med* 1996;335:1713–1720.

McCammon RL, Hilgenberg JC, Sandage BW, Stoelting RK. The effect of esmolol on the onset and duration of succinylcholine-induced neuromuscular blockade. *Anesthesiology* 1985;63:A317.

McCammon RL, Stoelting RK. Exaggerated increase in serum potassium following succinylcholine in dogs with beta blockade. *Anesthesiology* 1984;61:723–725.

Mishra P, Calvey TN, Williams NE, et al. Intraoperative bradycardia and hypotension associated with timolol and pilocarpine eye drops. *Br J Anaesth* 1983;55:897–899.

Nicholas E, Deutschman CS, Allo M, et al. Use of esmolol in the intraoperative management of pheochromocytoma. *Anesth Analg* 1988;67:1114–1117.

Nies AS, Shand DG. Clinical pharmacology of propranolol. *Circulation* 1975;52:6–15.

Ooi LG, O'Shea PJ, Wood AJ. Use of esmolol in the postbypass management of hypertrophic obstructive cardiomyopathy. *Br J Anaesth* 1993;70:104–106.

Ostman PL, Chestnut DH, Robillard JE, et al. Transplacental passage and hemodynamic effects of esmolol in the gravid ewe. *Anesthesiology* 1988;69:738–741.

Oxorn D, Knox JWD, Hill J. Bolus doses of esmolol for the prevention of perioperative hypertension and tachycardia. *Can J Anaesth* 1990;37:206–209.

Packer M. Combined beta-adrenergic and calcium-entry blockade in angina pectoris. *N Engl J Med* 1989;320:709–717.

Philbin DM, Lowenstein E. Lack of beta-adrenergic activity of isoflurane in the dog: a comparison of circulatory effects of halothane and isoflurane after propranolol administration. *Br J Anaesth* 1976;48:1165–1170.

Pollan S, Tadjziechy M. Esmolol in the management of epinephrine and cocaine-induced cardiovascular toxicity. *Anesth Analg* 1989; 69:663–664.

Prys-Roberts C, Foex P, Biro GP, et al. Studies of anaesthesia in relation to hypertension. V. Adrenergic beta-receptor blockade. *Br J Anaesth* 1973;45:671–681.

Ramsey JG. Esmolol. *Can J Anaesth* 1991;38:155–158.

Roberts JG, Foex P, Clarke TNS, et al. Haemodynamic interactions of high-dose propranolol pretreatment and anaesthesia in the dog. III. The effects of haemorrhage during halothane and trichloroethylene anaesthesia. *Br J Anaesth* 1976;48:411–418.

Roerig DL, Kotryl KJ, Ahlf SB, Dawson CA, Kampine JP. Effect of propranolol on the first pass uptake of fentanyl in the human and rat lung. *Anesthesiology* 1989;71:62–68.

Rosa RM, Silva P, Young JB, et al. Adrenergic modulation of extrarenal potassium disposal. *N Engl J Med* 1980;302:431–434.

Shand DG. Drug therapy—propranolol. *N Engl J Med* 1975;293: 280–285.

Sheppard S, Eagle CJ, Strunin L. A bolus dose of esmolol attenuates tachycardia and hypertension after tracheal intubation. *Can J Anaesth* 1990;37:202–205.

Shjojania KG, Duncan BW, McDonald KM, et al. Safe but sound: patient safety meets evidence-based medicine. *JAMA* 2002;288: 508–513.

Smulyan H, Weinberg SE, Howanitz PJ. Continuous propranolol infusion following abdominal surgery. *JAMA* 1982;247:2539–2542.

Thorne AC, Bedford RF. Esmolol for perioperative management of thyrotoxic goiter. *Anesthesiology* 1989;71:291–294.

The TIMI Study Group. Immediate versus delayed catheterization and angioplasty following thrombolytic therapy for acute myocardial infarction. *JAMA* 1988;260:2849–2856.

Wallace A, Layug B, Tateo I, et al. Prophylactic atenolol reduces postoperative myocardial ischemia. *Anesthesiology* 1998;88:7–17.

Wallin JD, O'Neill WM. Labetalol: current research and therapeutic status. *Arch Intern Med* 1983;143:485–490.

Wilson DJ, Wallin JD, Vlachakis ND, et al. Intravenous labetalol in the treatment of severe hypertensive and hypertensive emergencies. *Am J Med* 1983;75:95–102.

Wood M, Shand DG, Wood AJJ. Propranolol binding in plasma during cardiopulmonary bypass. *Anesthesiology* 1979;51:512–516.

Zakowski M, Kaufman B, Berguson P, et al. Esmolol use during resection of pheochromocytoma: report of three cases. *Anesthesiology* 1989;20: 875–877.

Antihypertensive Drugs

15

Drugs used to treat systemic hypertension include sympatholytics, angiotensin-converting enzyme (ACE) inhibitors, angiotensin receptor blockers, calcium channel blockers, vasodilators, and diuretics (Table 15-1) (Oparil and Calhoun, 2000). To some extent, these drugs all act by interfering with normal homeostatic mechanisms. Efficacy, toxicity, and suitable combinations of antihypertensive drugs can often be predicted by considering both the sites and mechanisms of action of these drugs. The effectiveness of a given drug, however, cannot be taken as evidence that its mechanism of action relates to the pathogenesis of systemic hypertension.

The potential interaction between antihypertensive drugs and anesthetics has been exaggerated. When interactions are likely, they are usually predictable and can thus be avoided or their significance minimized. Specific concerns during the administration of anesthesia to patients being treated with antihypertensive drugs include (a) attenuation of sympathetic nervous system activity, (b) modification of the response to sympathomimetic drugs, and (c) sedation. Attenuation of sympathetic nervous system activity is reflected by orthostatic hypotension and exaggerated systemic blood pressure decreases during anesthesia in response to (a) acute blood loss, (b) body position change, or (c) decreased venous return due to positive-pressure ventilation of the lungs. Antihypertensive drugs that result in depletion of norepinephrine from nerve endings or that act on peripheral vascular smooth muscle decrease the sensitivity to predominantly indirect-acting sympathomimetic drugs. Conversely, sympathetic nervous system blockade, which deprives the alpha-adrenergic receptors of tonic impulses, may result in exaggerated responses to catecholamines and direct-acting sympathomimetic drugs.

Maintenance of antihypertensive drug therapy during the perioperative period is associated with fewer fluctuations in systemic blood pressure and heart rate during anesthesia. Patients who receive antihypertensive drug therapy during the perioperative period are also less likely to exhibit cardiac dysrhythmias (Prys-Roberts et al., 1971). It is an inescapable conclusion that previously effective antihypertensive drug therapy should be continued without interruption during the perioperative period. In this regard, the usual dose and unique pharmacology of each antihypertensive drug as well as the physiologic reflexes that occur in response to drug-induced blood pressure changes must be considered when planning the management of anesthesia. The incidence of sleep apnea is increased in hypertensive patients perhaps reflecting the impact of recurrent arterial hypoxemia induced by sleep apnea on systemic blood pressure (Fletcher, 1995).

SYMPATHOLYTICS

Beta-Adrenergic Blockers

Beta-adrenergic blockers used as single-drug therapy for systemic hypertension seem to be most effective in young and middle-aged patients, as well as those with coronary artery disease. Use of a beta blocker as antihypertensive therapy is different, in terms of dosage intervals, from its use as an antianginal therapy. In patients with angina, inadequate serum drug levels may result in increased risk for myocardial ischemia. In contrast, increasing dosage intervals in patients with mild to moderate hypertension often improves compliance and is relatively safe. Propranolol is the beta blocker that has been in use the longest, but a number of other available beta-blocking drugs have a more acceptable pharmacologic profile (see Chapter 14).

Mechanism of Action

Beta blockers can be classified according to whether they exhibit selective or nonselective properties and whether they possess intrinsic sympathomimetic activity. A beta blocker with selective properties binds primarily to $beta_1$ (cardiac) receptors, whereas a beta blocker with nonselective properties has equal affinity for $beta_1$ and $beta_2$ (vascular and bronchial smooth muscle, metabolic) receptors. The beta blockers with intrinsic sympathomimetic activity tend to produce less bradycardia and thus are less likely to unmask left ventricular dysfunction. These drugs are also less likely to produce vasospasm and thus to exacerbate symptoms of peripheral vascular disease. The antihypertensive effect of

TABLE 15-1.
DRUGS USED TO TREAT SYSTEMIC HYPERTENSION

Sympatholytics
- ***Beta-adrenergic blockers*** (acebutolol, atenolol, betaxolol, bisoprolol, carteolol, metoprolol, nadolol, penbutolol, pindolol, propranolol, timolol)
- ***Combined alpha-adrenergic blockers*** (labetalol)
- ***Alpha-adrenergic blockers*** (prazosin, terazosin, doxazosin)
- ***Centrally acting blockers*** (clonidine, dexmedetomidine)

Angiotensin-converting enzyme inhibitors (captopril, enalapril, benazepril, fosinopril, lisinopril, quinapril, ramipril, spiropril, moxeipril, perindopril, trandolapril)
Angiotensin II receptor inhibitors (losartan, valsartan, candesartan, eprosartan, irbeasartan, telmisartan)
Calcium channel blockers (verapamil, diltiazem, nifedipine, nicardipine, isradipine, amlodipine, felodipine))
Vasodilating drugs (hydrazaline, minoxidil)
Diuretics
- ***Thiazides*** (chlorothiazinde, hydrochlorothiazide, bendroflumethiazide, hydroflumethiazide, methyclothiazide, polythiazide, trimethiazide, indapamide)
- ***Loop diuretics*** (bumetanide, ethacrynic acid, furosemide, torsemide)
- ***Potassium-sparing diuretics*** (amiloride, spironolactone, triamterene)

beta blockers may be attenuated by nonsteroidal antiinflammatory drugs.

In contrast to nonselective beta blockers, selective $beta_1$ blockers (acebutolol, atenolol, metoprolol) administered in low doses are unlikely to produce bronchospasm, decrease peripheral blood flow, or mask hypoglycemia. For these reasons, $beta_1$ blockers are preferred drugs for patients with pulmonary disease, insulin-dependent diabetes mellitus, or symptomatic peripheral vascular disease. The intrinsic sympathomimetic effect of acebutolol and pindolol is advantageous for patients with bradycardia and possibly for those with congestive heart failure. Metoprolol, propranolol, and timolol are considered to be cardioprotective.

Side Effects

Treatment of hypertension with beta blockers involves certain risks, including bradycardia, congestive heart failure, bronchospasm, claudication, masking of hypoglycemia, sedation, impotence, and possibly precipitation of angina pectoris with abrupt discontinuation of the drug. Patients with any degree of congestive heart failure or preexisting heart block cannot tolerate more than modest doses of beta blockers. Patients with asthma should probably not be treated with beta blockers. Long-term antihypertensive therapy with beta blockers may result in development or worsening of glucose intolerance. Beta blockers potentially increase the risk of serious hypoglycemia in diabetic patients because they blunt autonomic nervous system responses that would warn of hypoglycemia. Nevertheless, the incidence of hypoglycemia has not been shown to be increased in diabetic patients being treated with beta-adrenergic antagonists to control hypertension (Shorr et al., 1997).

Labetalol

Labetalol combines $alpha_1$-adrenergic and beta-adrenergic blocking properties and appears to also produce a direct vasodilating effect. The presence of alpha-adrenergic blocking properties results in less bradycardia and negative inotropic effects compared with beta blockers. These alpha properties, however, may result in orthostatic hypotension. The incidence of bronchospasm is similar to that seen with atenolol or metoprolol. Treatment with labetalol may result in plasma aminotransferase elevations. Withdrawal complications are less likely with this drug than with beta blockers. Metabolites of labetalol in the plasma may lead to the false diagnosis of pheochromocytoma (Bouloux et al., 1985). Paresthesias (scalp tingling) and urinary retention may accompany treatment of hypertension with this drug.

Prazosin

Prazosin is a selective postsynaptic $alpha_1$-adrenergic receptor antagonist resulting in vasodilating effects on both arterial and venous vasculature (Fig. 15-1). Absence of presynaptic $alpha_2$ receptor antagonism leaves intact the normal inhibitory effect on norepinephrine release from nerve endings. This drug is unlikely to elicit reflex increases in cardiac output and renin release. When prazosin is used as the sole antihypertensive drug to treat mild to moderate hypertension, it appears to be less effective than a thiazide diuretic. However, when used as a secondary drug in combination with a diuretic, prazosin has proved to be quite effective for the treatment of young patients with moderately severe hypertension. Patient acceptance of prazosin has been relatively high.

In addition to treating essential hypertension, prazosin may be of value for decreasing afterload in patients with congestive heart failure. Prazosin may also be a useful drug for the preoperative preparation of patients with pheochromocytoma. This drug has been used to relieve the vasospasm of Raynaud phenomenon. Another useful indication for prazosin in the treatment of essential hypertension is the presence of benign prostatic hypertrophy in older males, as this drug decreases the size of the gland (Foglar et al., 1995).

Pharmacokinetics

Prazosin is nearly completely metabolized, and <60% bioavailability after oral administration suggests the

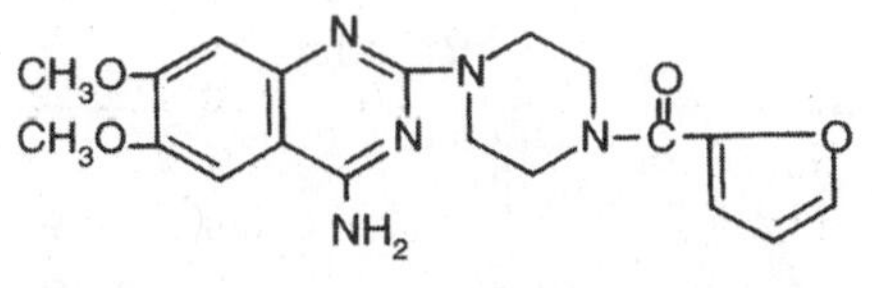

Figure 15-1. Prazosin.

occurrence of substantial first-pass hepatic metabolism. The elimination half-time is about 3 hours and is prolonged by congestive heart failure but not renal dysfunction. The fact that this drug is metabolized in the liver permits its use in patients with renal failure without altering the dose.

Cardiovascular Effects

Prazosin decreases systemic vascular resistance without causing reflex-induced tachycardia or increases in renin activity as occurs during treatment with hydralazine or minoxidil. Failure to alter plasma renin activity reflects continued activity of $alpha_2$ receptors that normally inhibit the release of renin. Vascular tone in both resistance and capacitance vessels is decreased, resulting in decreased venous return and cardiac output. Because of its greater affinity for alpha receptors in veins than in arteries, prazosin produces hemodynamic changes (orthostatic hypotension) that resemble those of nitroglycerin more than those of hydralazine.

Side Effects

The side effects of prazosin include vertigo, fluid retention, and orthostatic hypotension. Fluid retention requires the concomitant administration of a diuretic. On rare occasions, after the first dose of prazosin, a patient may experience sudden syncope that is usually postural and often dose related. Presumably, acute peripheral vasodilation is responsible for this rare syncopal response. Nonsteroidal antiinflammatory drugs may interfere with the antihypertensive effect of prazosin. Dryness of the mouth, nasal congestion, nightmares, urinary frequency, lethargy, and sexual dysfunction may accompany treatment with this drug.

Hypotension during epidural anesthesia may be exaggerated in the presence of prazosin, reflecting drug-induced $alpha_1$ blockade that prevents compensatory vasoconstriction in the unblocked portions of the body (Lydiatt et al., 1993). The resulting decrease in systemic vascular resistance results in hypotension that may not be responsive to the usual clinical doses of an $alpha_1$-adrenergic agonist such as phenylephrine. In this situation, administration of epinephrine may be necessary to increase systemic vascular resistance and systemic blood pressure. Conceivably, the combination of prazosin and a beta blocker could result in particularly refractory hypotension during regional anesthesia due to potentially blunted responses to $beta_1$ as well as $alpha_1$ agonists.

Terazosin and Doxazosin

Terazosin and doxazosin resemble prazosin, acting as $alpha_1$ receptor antagonists. Likewise, their side effects are similar to those of prazosin. An advantage of these drugs is their efficacy when taken once a day.

Clonidine

Clonidine is a centrally acting selective partial $alpha_2$-adrenergic agonist (220:1 $alpha_2$ to $alpha_1$) that acts as an antihypertensive drug by virtue of its ability to decrease sympathetic nervous system output from the central nervous system (CNS) (Fig. 15-2). This drug has proved to be particularly effective in the treatment of patients with severe hypertension or renin-dependent disease. The usual daily adult dose is 0.2 to 0.3 mg orally. The availability of a transdermal clonidine patch designed for weekly administration is useful for surgical patients who are unable to take oral medications.

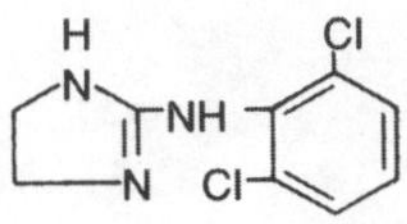

Figure 15-2. Clonidine.

Other Clinical Uses

Alpha-adrenergic agonists (clonidine and dexmedetomidine) induce sedation, decrease anesthetic requirements and improve perioperative hemodynamic (attenuate blood pressure and heart rate responses to surgical stimulation) and sympathoadrenal stability (Fig. 15-3) (Kimibayashi and Maze, 2000). In addition, $alpha_2$ receptors within the spinal cord modulate pain pathways resulting in analgesia. Routine use of clonidine as an anesthetic adjuvant and provision of postoperative sedation without depression of ventilation have been limited by its relatively long half-time of 6 to 10 hours. Dexmedetomidine has a half-time of only 2 to 3 hours and is more potent than clonidine at $alpha_2$ receptors.

Analgesia

Preservative-free clonidine administered into the epidural or subarachnoid space (150 to 450 μg) produces dose-dependent analgesia and, unlike opioids, does not produce depression of ventilation, pruritus, nausea and vomiting, or delayed gastric emptying (Asai et al., 1997; Eisenach et al., 1996; Filos et al., 1994). Urinary retention, which is a common complication of epidural opioids, is uncommon when epidural clonidine is administered to produce postoperative analgesia. Activation of postsynaptic $alpha_2$ receptors in the substantia gelatinosa of the spinal cord is the presumed mechanism by which clonidine produces analgesia. As such, clonidine and morphine, when used concomitantly as neuraxial analgesics, do not exhibit cross-tolerance (Milne et al., 1985). Hypotension, sedation, and dryness of the mouth may accompany use of neuraxial clonidine to produce analgesia. The addition of clonidine, 1 μg/kg, to lidocaine as used for total intravenous regional anesthesia enhances postoperative analgesia (Reuben et al., 1999). Intravenous regional administration of clonidine, 1 μg/kg is effective in relieving sympathetically mediated pain (Reuben et al., 1998).

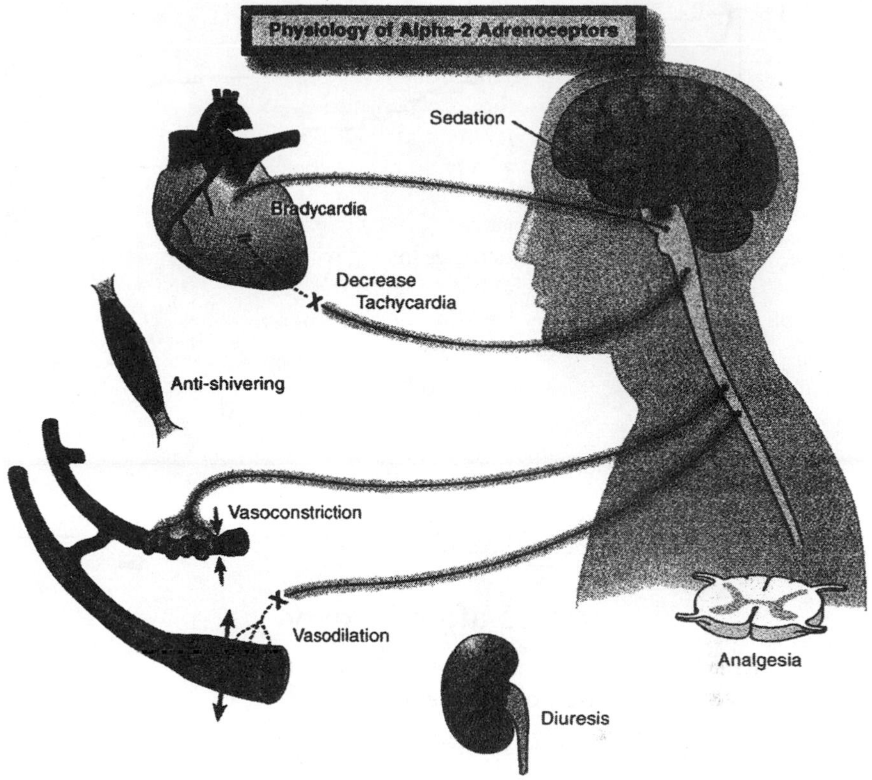

Figure 15-3. Schematic depiction of effects that are mediated by $alpha_2$ adrenergic receptors. The site for sedation is the locus ceruleus of the brain stem whereas the principal site of analgesia is most likely the spinal cord. In the heart, the dominant effect of $alpha_2$ stimulation is attenuation of tachycardia through block of the cardioaccelerator nerves and bradycardia through vagal stimulation. In the peripheral vasculature, there are vasodilatory effects reflecting sympatholysis and vasoconstriction mediated by $alpha_2$ receptors in smooth muscle cells. (From Kamibayashi T, Maze M. Clinical uses of $alpha_2$-adrenergic agonists. *Anesthesiology* 2000;93:1345–1349; with permission.)

Preanesthetic Medication

Oral clonidine preanesthetic medication (5 μg/kg) (a) blunts reflex tachycardia associated with direct laryngoscopy for intubation of the trachea, (b) decreases intraoperative lability of blood pressure and heart rate, (c) decreases plasma catecholamine concentrations, and (d) dramatically decreases anesthetic requirements for inhaled (MAC) and injected drugs (Aantaa et al., 1997; Ghignone et al., 1987; Quintin et al., 1996). This same preanesthetic medication dose of clonidine enhances the postoperative analgesia provided by intrathecal morphine plus tetracaine without increasing the intensity of the side effects from morphine (Fig. 15-4) (Goyagi and Nishikawa, 1996).

Sympathetic nervous system activation owing to administration of desflurane and ketamine is blunted by clonidine (Taittonen et al., 1998). For example, oral clonidine premedication, 5 μg/kg administered 90 minutes before induction of anesthesia, attenuates the blood pressure and heart rate increases that normally follow the administration of ketamine, 1 mg/kg IV (Doak and Duke, 1993). It has been observed that oral clonidine preanesthetic medication augments rather than attenuates the pressor responses to intravenous (IV) ephedrine (Goyagi et al., 1998). This augmented response is a consideration in selecting the dose of ephedrine should it be necessary to treat hypotension associated with clonidine administration during the perioperative period. The fact that the most pronounced effect of clonidine seems to be a decrease in sympathetic nervous system activity introduces the possibility that cardiovascular responses to hypotension could be attenuated. Nevertheless, there is evidence that plasma concentrations of catecholamines can increase in response to hypotension despite the prior administration of clonidine (Dodd et al., 1997).

Prolonging the Effects of Regional Anesthesia

Addition of clonidine, 75 to 150 μg, to a solution containing tetracaine or bupivacaine and placed in the subarachnoid

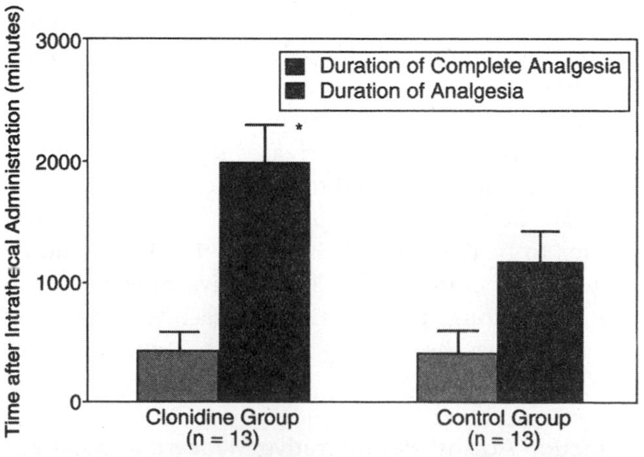

Figure 15-4. Clonidine, 5 μg/kg orally as preoperative medication, enhances the postoperative analgesia of intrathecal morphine plus tetracaine. (*$P < .05$ versus the control group. Values are mean ± SEM.) (From Goyagi T, Nishikawa T. Oral clonidine premedication enhances the quality of postoperative analgesia by intrathecal morphine. *Anesth Analg* 1996;82:1192–1196; with permission.)

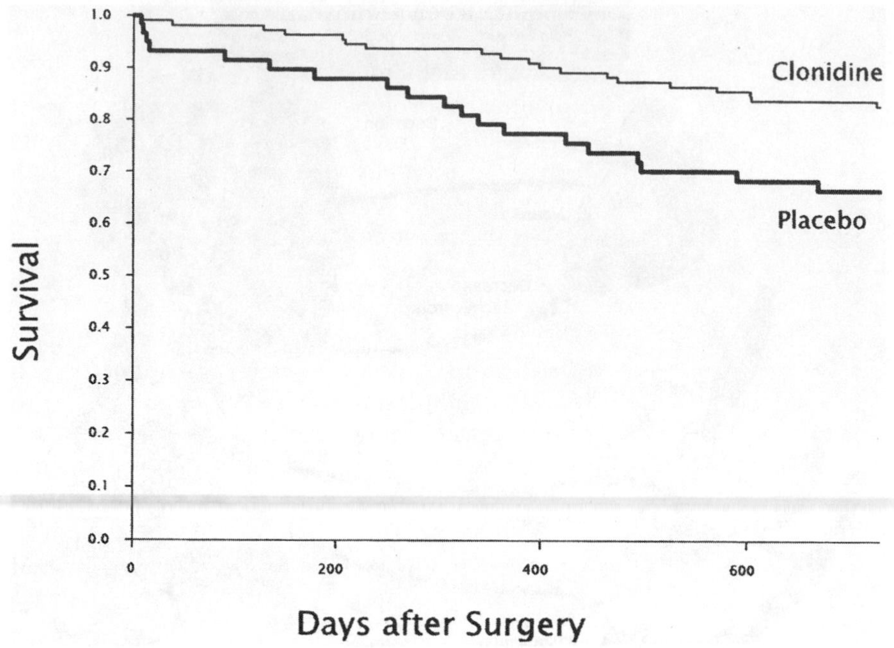

Figure 15-5. Survival for clonidine-treated versus placebo treated patients. Clonidine significantly decreased the incidence of death. (From Wallace AW, Galindez D, Salahieh A, et al. Effect of clonidine on cardiovascular morbidity and mortality after noncardiac surgery. *Anesthesiology* 2004; 101:284–293, with permission.)

space prolongs the duration of sensory and motor blockade produced by the local anesthetic (Bonnet et al., 1989; Goyagi and Nishikawa, 1996). Clonidine, 150 µg added to intrathecal bupivacaine, seems to be the preferred dose in terms of prolonging the anesthetic and analgesic effects without introducing unwanted side effects (Strebel et al., 2004). The need for infusion of fluids and the decrease in diastolic blood pressure may be greater in patients receiving clonidine-containing local anesthetic solutions. Fetal bradycardia may limit the usefulness of subarachnoid clonidine in obstetrics (Eisenach and Dewan, 1990). Oral clonidine, 150 to 200 µg, administered 1.0 to 1.5 hours before institution of spinal anesthesia with tetracaine or lidocaine results in a significant prolongation of sensory anesthesia (Liu et al., 1995; Ota et al., 1994). In another report, oral clonidine, 200 µg, shortened the onset time of tetracaine's sensory block and prolonged the duration of sensory and motor block (Singh et al., 1994). However, clonidine premedication increases the risk of clinically significant bradycardia and hypotension. The mechanism whereby oral clonidine prolongs spinal anesthesia remains to be determined (Liu et al., 1995). Addition of 0.5 µg/kg of clonidine to 1% mepivacaine-containing solution prolongs the duration of brachial plexus block performed via the axillary approach (Singelyn et al., 1996).

Protection Against Perioperative Myocardial Ischemia

Clonidine decreases myocardial ischemia, infarction, and mortality following cardiovascular surgery. The decrease in overall mortality associated with clonidine is superior to that observed in patients treated with beta blockers (Goldman, 2003; Nishina et al., 2002). Clonidine 0.2 mg orally or as a transdermal patch administered the evening before surgery or on the morning of surgery to patients at risk for coronary artery disease and continued for 4 days postoperatively decreased the incidence of perioperative myocardial ischemia with minimal hemodynamic effects (Wallace et al., 2004). Clonidine reduced the incidence of postoperative mortality for up to 2 years (Fig. 15-5) (Wallace et al, 2004).

Diagnosis of Pheochromocytoma

Clonidine, 0.3 mg orally, will decrease the plasma concentration of catecholamines in normal patients but not in the presence of pheochromocytoma (Bravo et al., 1981). This reflects the ability of clonidine to suppress the endogenous release of catecholamines from nerve endings but not diffusion of excess catecholamines into the circulation from a pheochromocytoma.

Treatment of Opioid and Alcohol Withdrawal Syndrome

Administration of large doses of naloxone to patients addicted to opioids markedly increases efferent sympathetic neural outflow and catecholamine plasma concentrations, and evokes cardiovascular stimulation despite general anesthesia, apparently unmasking dampening effects of chronic opioid agonist administration on the sympathetic nervous system. Clonidine, 10 µg/kg IV decreases sympathetic nervous system activity that is associated with cardiovascular stimulation and attenuates increases in plasma catecholamine concentrations when naloxone is administered during general anesthesia to patients addicted to opioids (Kienbaum et al., 2002).

Adrenergic agonists are effective in the treatment of alcohol withdrawal syndrome in patients who may not respond to high doses of benzodiazepines or opioids. Preoperative administration of clonidine 150 μg, intrathecally or orally, prevents significant postoperative alcohol withdrawal syndrome in ethanol-dependent patients (Dobrydnjov et al., 2004).

Treatment of Shivering

Administration of clonidine, 75 μg IV, stops shivering (Kamibayashi and Maze, 2000). This desirable effect may reflect the ability of clonidine, like volatile anesthetics, opioids, and propofol, to inhibit central thermoregulatory control. Indeed, drugs that inhibit thermoregulatory vasoconstriction may cause core hypothermia and inhibit shivering. There is evidence that clonidine produces little or no increase in the sweating threshold (triggering core temperature) (see Chapter 41). As evidence of its ability to inhibit thermoregulatory control, clonidine decreases the vasoconstriction and shivering thresholds.

Mechanism of Action

$Alpha_2$-adrenergic agonists produce clinical effects by binding to $alpha_2$ receptors of which there are three subtypes ($alpha_{2A}$, $alpha_{2B}$, $alpha_{2C}$) that are distributed ubiquitously, and each may be uniquely responsible for some, but not all, of the actions of $alpha_2$ agonists (Kamibayashi and Maze, 2000). $Alpha_{2A}$ receptors mediate sedation, analgesia, and sympatholysis whereas $alpha_{2B}$ receptors mediate vasoconstriction and possibly antishivering effects. The startle response may reflect activation of $alpha_{2C}$ receptors.

One of the highest densities of $alpha_2$ receptors is present in the pontine locus ceruleus, an important source of sympathetic nervous system innervation of the forebrain and a vital modulator of vigilance. Sedative effects evoked by $alpha\text{-}_2$-agonists most likely reflect inhibition of this nucleus (Nelson et al., 2003). Clonidine stimulates $alpha_2$-adrenergic inhibitory neurons in the medullary vasomotor center. As a result, there is a decrease in sympathetic nervous system outflow from central nervous system (CNS) to peripheral tissues. Decreased sympathetic nervous system activity is manifested as peripheral vasodilation and decreases in systemic blood pressure, heart rate, and cardiac output. The ability of clonidine to modify the function of potassium channels in the CNS (cell membranes become hyperpolarized) may be the mechanism for profound decreases in anesthetic requirements produced by clonidine and other even more selective $alpha_2$-adrenergic agonists such as dexmedetomidine. $Alpha_2$ receptors on blood vessels mediate vasoconstriction and on peripheral sympathetic nervous system nerve endings inhibit release of norepinephrine. Neuraxial placement of clonidine inhibits spinal substance P release and nociceptive neuron firing produced by noxious stimulation.

The quality of sedation produced by $alpha_2$ agonists differs from sedation produced by drugs (midazolam, propofol) that act on gamma-aminobutyric acid receptors (GABA) (Shelly, 2001). For example, dexmedetomidine, acting on $alpha_2$ receptors produces sedation by decreasing sympathetic nervous system activity and the level of arousal. The result is a calm patient who can be easily aroused to full consciousness. Drugs that activate GABA receptors produce a clouding of consciousness and can cause paradoxical agitation as well as tolerance and dependence.

Pharmacokinetics

Clonidine is rapidly absorbed after oral administration and reaches peak plasma concentrations within 60 to 90 minutes. The elimination half-time of clonidine is between 9 and 12 hours, with approximately 50% metabolized in the liver whereas the rest is excreted unchanged in urine. The duration of hypotensive effect after a single oral dose is about 8 hours. The transdermal route requires about 48 hours to produce therapeutic plasma concentrations.

Cardiovascular Effects

The decrease in systolic blood pressure produced by clonidine is more prominent than the decrease in diastolic blood pressure. In patients treated chronically, systemic vascular resistance is little affected, and cardiac output, which is initially decreased, returns toward predrug levels. Homeostatic cardiovascular reflexes are maintained, thus avoiding the problems of orthostatic hypotension or hypotension during exercise. The ability of clonidine to decrease systemic blood pressure without paralysis of compensatory homeostatic reflexes is highly desirable. Renal blood flow and glomerular filtration rate are maintained in the presence of clonidine therapy.

Respiratory Effects

$Alpha_2$ agonists have minimal depressant effects on ventilation and these agonists do not potentiate ventilatory depressant effects of opioids. For example, clonidine does not significantly potentiate morphine-induced depression of ventilation (Bailey et al., 1991). However, the simultaneous IV administration of clonidine and fentanyl may lead to accumulation of fentanyl, which may increase the risk for depression of ventilation (Bernard et al., 1994). Clonidine does not significantly potentiate morphine-induced depression of ventilation (Bailey et al., 1991).

Side Effects

The most common side effects produced by clonidine are sedation and xerostomia. Consistent with sedation and, perhaps more specifically, an agonist effect on postsynaptic $alpha_2$ receptors in the CNS are nearly 50% decreases in anesthetic requirements for inhaled anesthetics (MAC) and injected drugs in patients pretreated with clonidine administered in the preanesthetic medication (Ghignone et al., 1987). Patients pretreated with clonidine often manifest lower plasma concentrations of catecholamines in response to surgical stimulation and occasionally require treatment of bradycardia with an IV anticholinergic. As with other antihypertensive drugs, retention of sodium and water often occurs such that combination of clonidine with a diuretic is often necessary. Conversely, a diuretic effect during general anesthesia has been described after administration of oral clonidine, 2.5 to 5.0 μg/kg, as preanesthetic medication (Hamaya et al., 1994). Skin rashes are frequent, impotence occurs occasionally, and orthostatic hypotension is rare. Despite the fact that clonidine prevents opioid-induced skeletal muscle rigidity and produces skeletal muscle flaccidity, $alpha_2$ agonists have no effect on the responses evoked by neuromuscular blocking drugs (Talke et al., 1999).

Rebound Hypertension

Abrupt discontinuation of clonidine therapy can result in rebound hypertension as soon as 8 hours and as late as 36 hours after the last dose (Husserl and Messerli, 1981). Rebound hypertension is most likely to occur in patients who were receiving >1.2 mg of clonidine daily. The increase in systemic blood pressure may be associated with a >100% increase in circulating concentrations of catecholamines and intense peripheral vasoconstriction. Symptoms of nervousness, diaphoresis, headache, abdominal pain, and tachycardia often precede the actual increase in systemic blood pressure. Beta-adrenergic blockade may exaggerate the magnitude of rebound hypertension by blocking the $beta_2$-vasodilating effects of catecholamines and leaving unopposed their alpha-vasoconstricting actions. Likewise, tricyclic antidepressant therapy may exaggerate rebound hypertension associated with abrupt discontinuation of clonidine therapy (Stiff and Harris, 1983). Indeed, tricyclic antidepressants can potentiate the pressor effects of norepinephrine.

Rebound hypertension can usually be controlled by reinstituting clonidine therapy or by administering a vasodilating drug such as hydralazine or nitroprusside. Beta-adrenergic blocking drugs are useful but probably should be administered only in the presence of alpha-adrenergic blockade to avoid unopposed alpha-vasoconstricting actions. In this regard, labetalol with alpha- and beta-antagonist effects may be useful in the management of patients experiencing rebound hypertension. If oral clonidine therapy is interrupted because of surgery, use of transdermal clonidine provides a sustained therapeutic level of drug for as long as 7 days (White and Gilbert, 1985). For a planned withdrawal, the clonidine dosage should be gradually decreased over 7 days or longer.

Rebound hypertension after abrupt discontinuation of chronic treatment with antihypertensive drugs is not unique to clonidine (Husserl and Messerli, 1981). For example, abrupt discontinuation of beta-blocker therapy has been associated with clinical evidence of excessive sympathetic nervous system activity. Antihypertensive drugs that act independently of central and peripheral sympathetic nervous system mechanisms (direct vasodilators, ACE inhibitors) do not seem to be associated with rebound hypertension after sudden discontinuation of therapy.

Dexmedetomidine

Dexmedetomidine is a highly selective, specific, and potent $alpha_2$-adrenergic agonist (1,620:1 $alpha_2$ to $alpha_1$) (Bloor et al., 1992; Sandler, 1996). This drug is the dextroisomer and pharmacologically active component of medetomidine, which has been used for many years in veterinary practice for its hypnotic, sedative, and analgesic effects. Compared with clonidine, dexmedetomidine is seven to ten times more selective for $alpha_2$ receptors and has a shorter duration of action than clonidine. In this regard, dexmedetomidine is considered a full agonist at the $alpha_2$ receptor, whereas clonidine is a partial agonist (ratio of $alpha_2$ to $alpha_1$ activity for clonidine is 220:1) (Sandler, 1996). Atipamezole is a specific and selective $alpha_2$ receptor antagonist that rapidly and effectively reverses the sedative and cardiovascular effects of IV dexmedetomidine (Scheinin et al., 1998).

Pharmacokinetics

The elimination half-time of dexmedetomidine is 2 to 3 hours compared with 6 to 10 hours for clonidine. Dexmedetomidine is highly protein bound (>90%) and undergoes extensive hepatic metabolism. The resulting methyl and glucuronide conjugates are excreted by the kidneys. Dexmedetomidine has weak inhibiting effects on cytochrome P450 enzyme systems that might manifest as increased plasma concentrations of opioids as administered during anesthesia (Buhrer et al., 1994).

Clinical Uses

As with clonidine, pretreatment with dexmedetomidine attenuates hemodynamic responses to tracheal intubation, decreases plasma catecholamine concentrations during anesthesia, decreases perioperative requirements for inhaled anesthetics and opioids, and increases the likelihood of hypotension (see Fig. 15-3) (Jalonen et al., 1997; Kamibayashi and Maze, 2000). Dexmedetomidine decreases MAC for volatile anesthetics in animals by >90% compared with a plateau effect between 25% to 40% for clonidine (Fig. 15-6) (Segal et al., 1988). In patients, isoflurane MAC was decreased 35% and 48% by dexmedetomidine plasma concentrations of 0.3 ng/mL and 0.6 ng/mL, respectively (Aantaa et al., 1997). Despite marked dose-dependent analgesia and sedation produced by this drug, there is only mild depression of ventilation. Dexmedetomidine in high doses (loading dose of 1 μg/kg

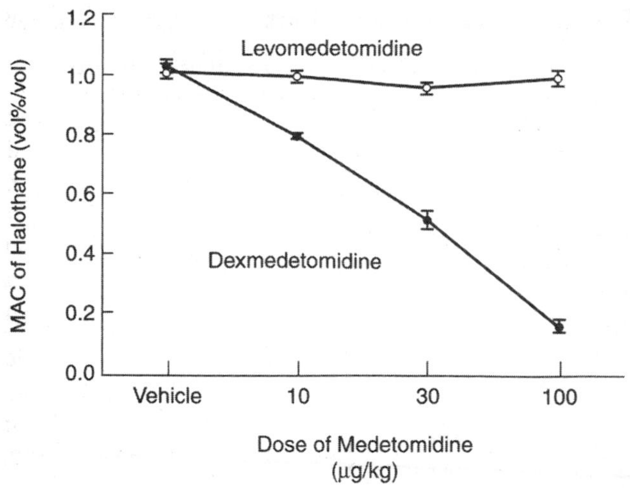

Figure 15-6. Dexmedetomidine produces dose-dependent decreases in halothane MAC in rats. Levomedetomidine did not produce any changes in MAC. Data are mean ± SEM. (From Segal IS, Vickery RG, Walton JK, et al. Dexmedetomidine diminishes halothane anesthetic requirements in rats through a postsynaptic alpha-2 adrenergic receptor. *Anesthesiology* 1988; 69:818–823; with permission.)

IV followed by 5 to 10 µg/kg/hour IV) produces total IV anesthesia without associated depression of ventilation (Ramsay and Luterman, 2004). The preservation of breathing provides a potential anesthetic technique for patients with a difficult upper airway. As with clonidine, dexmedetomidine has been reported to be effective in attenuating the cardiostimulatory and postanesthetic delirium effects of ketamine (Levanen et al., 1995). Addition of 0.5 µg/kg dexmedetomidine to lidocaine being administered to produce IV regional anesthesia improves the quality of anesthesia and postoperative analgesia without causing side effects (Memis et al. 2004). Dexmedetomidine markedly increases the range of temperatures not triggering thermoregulatory defenses. For this reason, dexmedetomidine, like clonidine, is likely to promote perioperative hypothermia and also prove to be an effective treatment for shivering (Talke et al., 1997). Severe bradycardia may follow the administration of dexmedetomidine and cardiac arrest has been reported in a patient receiving a dexmedetomidine infusion as a supplement to general anesthesia (Ingersoll-Weng, et al., 2004).

Postoperative Sedation

Dexmedetomidine (200 to 700 µg/kg/hour IV) is useful for sedation of postoperative critical care patients in an intensive care unit environment, particularly when mechanical ventilation via a tracheal tube is necessary. In comparison with remifentanil, dexmedetomidine infusions do not result in clinically significant depression of ventilation and sedation exhibits some similarity with natural sleep (Hsu et al., 2004). Following tracheal extubation, dexmedetomidine-sedated patients breathe spontaneously and appear calm and relaxed (Venn et al., 1999). Both clonidine and dexmedetomidine are useful in the intensive care unit to prevent drug withdrawal symptoms following long-term sedation with benzodiazepines. Because of its sympatholytic and vagomimetic actions, dexmedetomidine may be accompanied by systemic hypotension, and bradycardia. The ability to specifically antagonize the sedative effects of dexmedetomidine with atipamezole may be useful (Scheinin et al., 1998).

ANGIOTENSIN-CONVERTING ENZYME INHIBITORS

Angiotensin-converting enzyme (ACE) inhibitors represent a major advance in the treatment of all forms of hypertension because of their potency and minimal side effects, resulting in improved patient compliance (Croog et al., 1986). These drugs are free of many of the CNS side effects associated with other antihypertensive drugs, including depression, insomnia, and sexual dysfunction. Other adverse effects, such as congestive heart failure, bronchospasm, bradycardia, and exacerbation of peripheral vascular disease, are not seen with ACE inhibitors. Similarly, metabolic changes induced by diuretic therapy, such as hypokalemia, hyponatremia, and hyperglycemia, are not observed. Rebound hypertension, as seen with clonidine, has not been observed with ACE inhibitors.

ACE inhibitors are most effective in treating systemic hypertension secondary to increased renin production. These drugs have been established as first-line therapy in patients with systemic hypertension, congestive heart failure, and mitral regurgitation. ACE inhibitors are more effective and possibly safer than other antihypertensive drugs in the treatment of hypertension in diabetics (Hummel et al., 1986). There is also evidence that ACE inhibitors delay the progression of diabetic renal disease (Remiss and Regiment, 1993). These compounds may cause left ventricular hypertrophy to regress (remodeling of the myocardium), which could make ACE inhibitors useful for patients who are at risk for development of congestive heart failure.

Mechanism of Action

ACE inhibitors block the conversion of angiotensin I to angiotensin II, a potent vasoconstrictor responsible for arterial smooth muscle constriction, increased aldosterone secretion, and sympathetic nervous system stimulation. Angiotensin II normally binds to a specific cell membrane receptor (AT_1) that ultimately leads to increased release of calcium from sarcoplasmic reticulum to produce vasoconstriction. Decreased generation of angiotensin II results in decreased vasoconstrictive effects. In addition, plasma concentrations of aldosterone are decreased resulting in reduced sodium and water retention. ACE inhibitors also block the breakdown of bradykinin, an endogenous vasodilator substance, which contributes to the antihypertensive effects of these drugs. ACE inhibitors, like statins, reduce activation of LDL receptors and thus decrease plasma concentrations of LDL cholesterol. If the concentration of LDL cholesterol is already sufficiently low, ACE inhibitors may no longer be effective in reducing the rate of cardiovascular events (Pitt, 2004).

ACE inhibitors can be classified according to the structural element that interacts with the zinc ion of the enzyme as well as the form in which the drug is administered (prodrug or active form). Administration of ACE inhibitors as prodrugs increases oral bioavailability prior to their hepatic metabolism to the active drug. Enalapril is the prodrug of the active ACE inhibitor, enalaprilat, and conversion may be altered in patients with hepatic dysfunction. Captopril and lisinopril are not prodrugs. The major difference among clinically used ACE inhibitors is in duration of action (Table 15-2) (Mirenda and Grissom, 1991).

Side Effects

Cough, upper respiratory congestion, rhinorrhea, and allergic-like symptoms seem to be the most common side effects of ACE inhibitors (Israili et al., 1992). It is speculated that these airway responses reflect potentiation of the effects of kinins due to drug-induced inhibition of peptidyl-dipeptidase activity and subsequent breakdown of bradykinin. If respiratory distress develops, prompt injection of epinephrine (0.3 to 0.5 mL of a 1:1,000 dilution subcutaneously) is advised. Angioedema is a potentially life-threatening complication of treatment with ACE inhibitors (Brown et al., 1997). Decreases in glomerular filtration rate may occur in patients treated with ACE inhibitors. For this reason, ACE inhibitors are used with caution in patients with preexisting renal dysfunction and are not recommended for patients with renal artery stenosis. Hyperkalemia is possible due to decreased production of aldosterone. The risk of hyperkalemia is greatest in patients with recognized risk factors (congestive heart failure with renal insufficiency) (Palmer, 2004). Measurement of plasma concentrations of potassium may be indicated in treated patients.

Preoperative Management

Adverse circulatory effects during anesthesia are recognized in patients chronically treated with ACE inhibitors leading some to recommend that these drugs be discontinued 12 to 24 hours before anesthesia and surgery (Bertrand et al., 2001). Prolonged hypotension has been observed in patients undergoing general anesthesia for minor surgery in whom ACE inhibitor therapy was maintained until the morning of surgery. Indeed, the incidence of hypotension during induction of anesthesia in hypertensive patients chronically treated with ACE inhibitors was greater when ACE inhibitor therapy was continued until the morning of surgery compared with patients in whom therapy was discontinued at least 12 hours (captopril) or 24 hours (enalapril) preoperatively (Coriat et al., 1994). Surgical procedures involving major body fluid shifts have also been associated with hypotension in patients treated with ACE inhibitors. In patients about to undergo extensive surgical procedures involving large blood or fluid shifts, it may be an acceptable option to discontinue ACE inhibitor therapy and substitute shorter-acting IV antihypertensive drugs should the need arise (Mirenda and Grissom, 1991). Nevertheless, treatment with ACE inhibitors does not increase the incidence of hypotension after induction of anesthesia in patients with infarction-induced myocardial dysfunction (Ryckwaert and Colson, 1997). Exaggerated hypotension attributed to continued ACE inhibitor therapy has been responsive to crystalloid fluid infusion and/or administration of a sympathomimetic such as ephedrine or phenylephrine. If hypotension is refractory to treatment with ephedrine, treatment with a vasopressin analogue, terlipressin (1 mg IV), may be effective (Boccara et al., 2003. Morelli et al., 2005). Terlipressin is a long-acting (half-time 6 hours) analog of vasopressin with a higher vascular selectivity for vascular receptors compared with vasopressin. ACE inhibitors may increase insulin sensitivity and hypoglycemia, which is a concern when these drugs are administered to patients with diabetes mellitus. Nevertheless, there is no evidence that the incidence of hypoglycemia is greater in diabetics being treated with ACE inhibitors for control of hypertension (Shorr et al., 1997).

TABLE 15-2.
PHARMACOLOGIC EFFECTS OF SINGLE DOSES OF ANGIOTENSIN-CONVERTING ENZYME INHIBITORS

Drug	Dose (mg)	Prodrug	Time of Onset of Effect (min)	Time of Peak (hrs)	Duration of Effect (hrs)	Effect on Venous System	Effect on Arterial System
Captopril	100	No	15–30	1–2	6–10	++	+++
Enalapril	20	Yes	60–120	4–8	18–30	++	+++
Lisinopril	10	No	60	2–4	18–30	++	+++
Ramipril	20	Yes	30–60	3–8	24–60		

Captopril

Captopril is an orally effective (12.5 to 25.0 mg every 8 to 12 hours) antihypertensive drug that acts by competitive inhibition of angiotensin I–converting enzyme (peptidyl-dipeptidase) (Fig. 15-7). This is the enzyme that converts inactive angiotensin I to active angiotensin II. Angiotensin II is responsible for stimulating secretion of aldosterone by the adrenal cortex. As a result of inhibition of this enzyme by captopril, there is a predictable decrease in circulating plasma concentrations of angiotensin II and aldosterone accompanied by compensatory increases in angiotensin I and renin levels. The increase in plasma concentrations of renin reflects the loss of negative feedback control normally provided by angiotensin II. The decrease in aldosterone secretion results in a slight increase in serum potassium levels.

Pharmacokinetics

Captopril is well absorbed after oral administration, with 25% to 30% of the drug reversibly bound to protein in the circulation. Inhibition of converting enzyme occurs within 15 minutes after oral administration. Excretion of unchanged drug in the urine accounts for about 50% of captopril. The short elimination half-time of captopril (approximately 2 hours) appears to be due in part to its oxidation to the dimer and mixed sulfides, all of which are excreted by the kidneys.

Cardiovascular Effects

The antihypertensive effects of captopril are due to a decrease in systemic vascular resistance as a result of decreased sodium and water retention. Decreased systemic vascular resistance is particularly prominent in the kidneys, whereas cerebral blood flow and coronary blood flow appear to remain autoregulated. Typically, captopril decreases systemic blood pressure without concomitant alterations in cardiac output or heart rate. Orthostatic hypotension is unlikely because this drug does not interfere with sympathetic nervous system activity. The absence of a compensatory reflex-mediated increase in heart rate when blood pressure is decreased suggests that captopril may cause changes in baroreceptor sensitivity (Williams, 1988). Captopril may improve the efficacy of vasodilators in treating congestive heart failure, presumably by blocking vasodilator-induced increases in renin output. Dramatic reversal of vascular and renal effects of scleroderma may follow the administration of captopril.

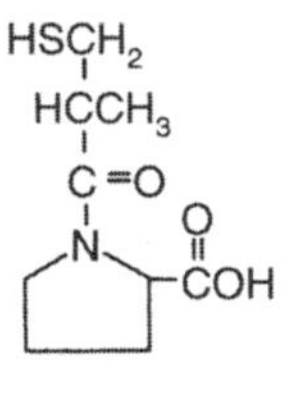

Figure 15-7. Captopril.

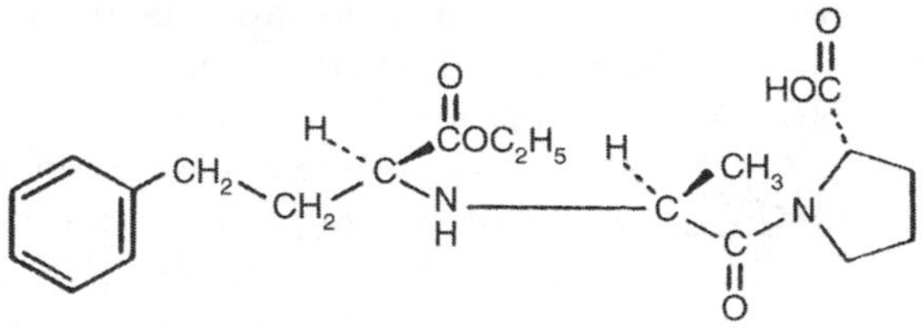

Figure 15-8. Enalapril.

Side Effects

Rash or pruritus occurs in about 10% of patients, and alteration or loss of taste (dysgeusia) occurs in 2% to 4%. Nonsteroidal antiinflammatory drugs may antagonize the antihypertensive effects of captopril, suggesting the possible role of prostaglandin synthesis in the blood pressure–lowering effects of this drug. Captopril may increase the serum potassium concentration and cause hyperkalemia, especially in patients with impaired renal function or when a potassium-sparing diuretic is administered simultaneously (Williams, 1988). This effect on the serum potassium concentration reflects drug-induced interference with the major stimulus for release of aldosterone. Granulocytopenia has occurred in about 0.3% of patients, being most frequent in patients with severe renal disease. The gravest but rarest side effect of captopril is angioedema, which may be due to a drug-induced inhibition of the metabolism of bradykinin.

Enalapril

Enalapril is an ACE inhibitor that resembles captopril with respect to pharmacologic effects (Fig. 15-8). This drug binds tightly to the enzyme such that a single daily oral dose may be effective. Enalapril is a prodrug that is metabolized in the liver to its active form, enalaprilat. This active form lacks the sulfhydryl group thought to be responsible for some of the adverse effects of captopril. Indeed, rash, granulocytopenia, and renal insufficiency have occurred less often with enalapril than with captopril. Patients chronically treated with ACE inhibitors who are unable to tolerate oral medication can continue their antihypertensive therapy without interruption with IV administration of enalapril. The value of this IV preparation in the management of perioperative hypertension as compared with other drugs is undetermined.

ANGIOTENSIN II RECEPTOR INHIBITORS

Angiotensin II receptor inhibitors produce antihypertensive effects by blocking the vasoconstrictive actions of angiotensin II without affecting ACE activity.

Losartan

Losartan is an orally effective antihypertensive drug that acts as an antagonist at angiotensin II receptors (AT_1).

Angiotensin II is formed from angiotensin I by the action of ACE and functions as the primary vasoactive hormone of the renin-angiotensin system. Substantial first-pass hepatic metabolism through cytochrome P450 occurs after oral administration of this drug. Losartan and its active carboxylic acid metabolite block the vasoconstrictor and aldosterone-secretion effects of angiotensin II by selectively inhibiting the binding of angiotensin II to the AT_1 receptors found principally in vascular smooth muscles. The active metabolite of losartan is 10 to 40 times more potent than the parent drug in inhibiting the pressor effects of angiotensin II. Once daily dosing (25 to 50 mg) is sufficient.

Side Effects

Compared with ACE inhibitors, cough related to bradykinin accumulation is significantly less with losartan therapy. Hyperkalemia is a potential side effect, especially with concomitant use of potassium-sparing diuretics. Both the parent drug and active metabolite undergo biliary excretion and dose requirements are decreased in the presence of hepatic, but not renal dysfunction. As with ACE inhibitors, losartan is not recommended for treatment of patients with renal artery stenosis. Lithium reabsorption is increased in treated patients introducing the risk of lithium toxicity.

Removal of the negative feedback of angiotensin II causes a two- to threefold increase in plasma renin activity and consequent increase in angiotensin II plasma concentrations. Drugs that act directly on the renin-angiotensin system can cause fetal and neonatal morbidity and death when administered during pregnancy, emphasizing the need to discontinue these drugs when pregnancy is detected.

As with ACE inhibitors, hypotension following induction of anesthesia has been observed in patients being treated with angiotensin II receptor blockers causing some to recommend these drugs be discontinued on the day before surgery (Bertrand et al., 2001).

CALCIUM CHANNEL BLOCKERS

Although calcium channel blockers were introduced initially as second-line drugs for the treatment of angina pectoris, and in the case of verapamil, for supraventricular tachydysrhythmias, their hypotensive effects inevitably resulted in their clinical use as antihypertensive drugs (see Chapter 18). For treatment of essential hypertension, these drugs may be considered as vasodilators. Calcium channel blockers have been particularly successful in treating hypertension in the elderly, African Americans, and salt-sensitive patients. The incidence of myocardial ischemia may be increased in patients being treated with high doses of short-acting nifedipine, verapamil, and diltiazem (Furberg et al., 1995; Psaty et al., 1995). A similar risk has not been found with longer-acting forms of calcium channel blockers. The use of calcium channel blockers does not require concurrent sodium restriction, which makes these drugs unique antihypertensive drugs and perhaps the drugs of choice for patients who find sodium restriction unacceptable.

VASODILATING DRUGS

Hydralazine

Hydralazine is a phthalazine derivative that activates guanylate cyclase to produce vascular relaxation (Fig. 15-9) (see Chapter 16). Decreases in systemic blood pressure reflect these direct relaxant effects on vascular smooth muscle, the dilatation effect on arterioles being greater than on veins. Vasodilatory effects are more pronounced on the coronary, cerebral, renal, and splanchnic circulations. When used in the treatment of chronic systemic hypertension, hydralazine is most often administered in combination with a beta blocker and a diuretic. Concomitant administration of a beta blocker limits the reflex increase in sympathetic nervous system activity induced by hydralazine. Beta blockers effectively prevent tachycardia and increased secretion of renin. Side effects are minimal when administered as part of combination therapy.

Treatment of a hypertensive crisis can be accomplished with hydralazine, 2.5 to 10.0 mg IV. The antihypertensive effect begins within 10 to 20 minutes after IV administration and lasts 3 to 6 hours. Nevertheless, the systemic blood pressure response to hydralazine is unpredictable and prolonged hypotension is not unusual (Abe, 1993).

Pharmacokinetics

Extensive hepatic first-pass metabolism limits the availability of hydralazine after oral administration. Acetylation seems to be the major route of metabolism of hydralazine. Rapid acetylators have lower bioavailability (about 30%) than do slow acetylators (about 50%) after oral administration of hydralazine. During chronic oral dosing, slow acetylators attain higher concentrations of hydralazine in plasma than do those who acetylate the drug rapidly. The elimination half-time averages 3 hours. After IV administration, <15% of the drug appears unchanged in urine.

Cardiovascular Effects

Hydralazine often decreases diastolic blood pressure more than systolic blood pressure. Systemic vascular resistance is decreased. Heart rate, stroke volume, and cardiac output increase, reflecting reflex baroreceptor-mediated increases

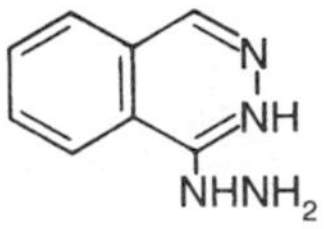

Figure 15-9. Hydralazine

in sympathetic nervous system activity due to decreases in systemic blood pressure. Nevertheless, tachycardia induced by hydralazine is greater than would be expected solely on a reflex basis and is poorly correlated with changes in blood pressure. This exaggerated heart rate increase may reflect a direct effect of hydralazine on the heart and in the CNS in addition to baroreceptor-mediated responses.

The preferential dilation of arterioles over veins minimizes the incidence of orthostatic hypotension and promotes an increase in cardiac output. The effect of hydralazine develops gradually over about 15 minutes, even after IV administration. Splanchnic, coronary, cerebral, and renal blood flow usually increase. Glomerular filtration rate, renal tubular function, and urine volume are not consistently affected. Renin activity is often increased, presumably reflecting hydralazine-induced reflex increases in sympathetic nervous system activity leading to increased secretion of renin by renal juxtaglomerular cells.

Side Effects

Like other vasodilators, hydralazine causes sodium and water retention if a diuretic is not given concomitantly. Other common side effects of hydralazine include vertigo, diaphoresis, nausea, and tachycardia. Myocardial stimulation associated with hydralazine therapy can evoke angina pectoris and produces changes on the electrocardiogram characteristic of myocardial ischemia. Side effects are less frequent and less severe when the dose of hydralazine is increased slowly, and tolerance may develop with continued administration. Drug fever, urticaria, polyneuritis, anemia, and pancytopenia are rare but require termination of hydralazine therapy. Peripheral neuropathies have been successfully treated with pyridoxine. Hydrazine-containing compounds, such as hydralazine, may lead to enhanced defluorination of enflurane (Mazze et al., 1982).

A systemic lupus erythematosus–like syndrome occurs in 10% to 20% of patients treated chronically (>6 months) with hydralazine, especially if the daily dose is >200 mg. The syndrome occurs predominantly in patients who are slow acetylators. Symptoms disappear when the drug is discontinued, differentiating it from the true disease.

Minoxidil

Minoxidil is an orally active antihypertensive drug that decreases systemic blood pressure by direct relaxation of arteriolar smooth muscle (Fig. 15-10). It has little effect on venous capacitance vessels. Like hydralazine, minoxidil increases the influx of potassium into vascular smooth muscle, resulting in hyperpolarization and vasodilation. Used with a diuretic and either a beta blocker or another potent sympatholytic, minoxidil is effective in treating the severest forms of hypertension (renal failure, transplant rejection, renovascular disease). Use of this drug is decreasing because ACE inhibitors and calcium-blocking drugs may be as effective with fewer side effects.

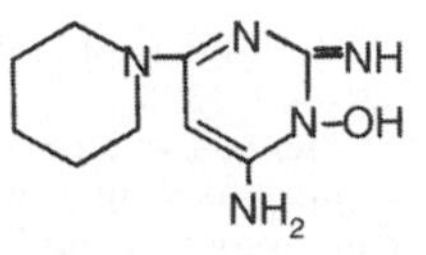

Figure 15-10. Minoxidil.

Pharmacokinetics

About 90% of an oral dose of minoxidil is absorbed from the gastrointestinal tract, and peak plasma levels are attained within 1 hour. Metabolism to inactive minoxidil glucuronide is extensive, and only 10% of the drug is recovered unchanged in urine. The elimination half-time is about 4 hours.

Cardiovascular Effects

The hypotensive effect of minoxidil is accompanied by marked increases in heart rate and cardiac output. This reflex stimulation of the sympathetic nervous system is also accompanied by increases in the plasma concentrations of norepinephrine and renin, with associated sodium and water retention. Orthostatic hypotension is not prominent in patients treated with minoxidil.

Side Effects

Fluid retention, manifesting as weight gain and edema, is a common side effect of minoxidil therapy. Furosemide or even dialysis may be necessary if fluid retention is unresponsive to less potent diuretics. Pulmonary hypertension associated with minoxidil is more likely due to fluid retention than a unique effect of this drug on pulmonary vasculature. A potentially serious side effect of minoxidil therapy that presumably reflects accumulation of fluid in a serous cavity is the development of pericardial effusion and cardiac tamponade, especially if severe renal dysfunction is present (Husserl and Messerli, 1981). Echocardiographic studies are helpful if pericardial effusion is suspected.

Abnormalities on the electrocardiogram are characterized by flattening or inversion of the T-wave and increased voltage of the QRS complex. During long-term therapy, T-wave abnormalities usually disappear and the QRS voltage is decreased.

Hypertrichosis, most notable around the face and arms, is an unpleasant but harmless side effect that appears, to some degree, in nearly all patients treated for >1 month. This side effect cannot be attributed to any definite endocrine abnormality.

DIURETICS

Diuretics are now less commonly used to initiate and maintain antihypertensive therapy than they were in the past (see Chapter 25). To augment patient compliance, relatively inexpensive diuretics and those that need to be taken only once daily are preferred. Because of their greater cost, their shorter duration of action, and the limited evidence that they are effective antihypertensive drugs, the potent diuretics (furosemide, ethacrynic acid, bumetanide) are usually reserved for patients with evidence of renal insufficiency in whom thiazide diuretics are ineffective. For patients with documented allergy to thiazides, ethacrynic acid is the diuretic of choice.

Diuretic-induced hypokalemia is a fairly frequent side effect. The diuretic's duration of action is apparently a major determinant of its tendency to cause hypokalemia, with the longer-acting drugs producing a more continuous kaliuresis. Prolonged hypokalemia will impair glucose metabolism and increase the incidence of ventricular irritability. Drug-induced hypokalemia is particularly important to avoid in patients with coronary artery disease and those being treated with digitalis.

Potassium-sparing diuretics are less potent than the other diuretics. These drugs are of special value for treatment of patients at increased risk if hypokalemia occurs. Conversely, because there is a risk of drug-induced hyperkalemia, these drugs should be used with caution in patients with impaired renal function and in those being treated with an ACE inhibitor.

REFERENCES

Aantaa R, Maakola ML, Kallio A, et al. Reduction of the minimum alveolar concentration of isoflurane by dexmedetomidine. *Anesthesiology* 1997;86:1055–1060.

Abe K. Vasodilators during cerebral aneurysm surgery. *Can J Anaesth* 1993;40:775–790.

Asai T, McBeth C, Stewart JIM. Effect of clonidine on gastric emptying of liquids. *Br J Anaesth* 1997;78:28–33.

Bailey PL, Sperry RJ, Johnson GK, et al. Respiratory effects of clonidine alone and combined with morphine in humans. *Anesthesiology* 1991;74:43–48.

Bernard JM, Lagarde D, Souron R. Balanced postoperative analgesia: effect of intravenous clonidine on blood gases and pharmacokinetics of intravenous fentanyl. *Anesth Analg* 1994;79:1126–1131.

Bertrand M, Godet G, Meersschaert K, et al. Should the angiotensin II antagonists be discontinued before surgery? *Anesth Analg* 2001;92; 26–30.

Boccara G, Ouattara A, Godet G, et al. Terlipressin versus norepinephrine to correct refractory arterial hypotension after general anesthesia in patients chronically treated with rennin-angiotensin system inhibitors. *Anesthesiology* 2003;98:1338–1344.

Bloor BC, Ward DS, Belleville JP, et al. Effects of intravenous dexmedetomidine in humans. II. Hemodynamic changes. *Anesthesiology* 1992;77:1134–1142.

Bonnet F, Brun-Buisson V, Saada M, et al. Dose-related prolongation of hyperbaric tetracaine spinal anesthesia by clonidine in humans. *Anesth Analg* 1989;68:619–622

Bouloux PM, Feathersonte RM, Clement-Jones V, Rees LH, Goligher JE. Erroneous diagnosis of phaeochromocytoma in hypertensive patient on labetalol. *J R Soc Med* 1985;78:588–589.

Bravo EL, Taraji RC, Fouad FM, Vidt DG, Gifford RW. Clonidine suppression: a useful aid in the diagnosis of pheochromocytoma. *N Engl J Med* 1981;305:623–626.

Brown NJ, Snowden M, Griffin MR. Recurrent angiotensin-converting enzyme inhibitor-associated angioedema. *JAMA* 1997;278: 232–233.

Buhrer M, Mappes A, Lauber R, et al. Dexmedetomidine decreases thiopental dose requirement and alters distribution pharmacokinetics. *Anesthesiology* 1994;80:1216–1221.

Coriat P, Richer C, Douraki T, et al. Influence of chronic angiotensin-converting enzyme inhibition on anesthetic induction. *Anesthesiology* 1994;81:299–307.

Croog SH, Levine S, Testa MA, et al. The effects of antihypertensive therapy on the quality of life. *N Engl J Med* 1986;314:1657–1661.

Doak GJ, Duke PC. Oral clonidine premedication attenuates the haemodynamic effects associated with ketamine anaesthetic induction in humans. *Can J Anaesth* 1993;40:612–618.

Dobrydnjov I, Axelsson K, Berggren L, et al. Intrathecal and oral clonidine as prophylaxis for postoperative alcohol withdrawal syndrome: a randomized double-blinded study. *Anesth Analg* 2004;98:738–744.

Dodd JM, Breslow MJ, Dorman T, Rosenfeld BA. Preserved sympathetic response to hypotension despite perioperative alpha$_2$ agonist administration. *Anesth Analg* 1997;84:1208–1210.

Eisenach JC, DeKock M, Klimscha W. Alpha$_2$-adrenergic agonists for regional anesthesia: a clinical review of clonidine (1984–1995). *Anesthesiology* 1996;85:655–674.

Eisenach JC, Dewan DM. Intrathecal clonidine in obstetrics: sheep studies. *Anesthesiology* 1990;72:663–668.

Filos KS, Goudas LC, Patroni O, et al. Hemodynamic and analgesic profile after intrathecal clonidine in humans. A dose response study. *Anesthesiology* 1994;81:591–601.

Fletcher EC. The relationship between systemic hypertension and obstructive sleep apnea: facts and theory. *Am J Med* 1995;98: 118–123

Foglar R, Shibta K, Horie K, et al. Use of recombinant alpha-1 adrenoceptors to characterize subtype selectivity of drugs for the treatment of prostatic hypertrophy. *Eur J Pharmacol* 1995;288: 201–206.

Furberg CD, Psaty BM, Meyer JV. Nifedipine: dose-related increase in mortality in patients with coronary heart disease. *Circulation* 1995; 92:1326–1331.

Ghignone M, Calvillo O, Quintin L. Anesthesia and hypertension: the effect of clonidine on perioperative hemodynamics and isoflurane requirements. *Anesthesiology* 1987;67:3–10.

Glassman AH, Stetner F, Walsh T, et al. Heavy smokers, smoking cessation, and clonidine: results of double-blind, randomized trial. *JAMA* 1988; 259:2863–2867.

Goyagi T, Makoto T, Nishikawa T. Oral clonidine enhances the pressor response to ephedrine during spinal anesthesia. *Anesth Analg* 1998;87:1336–1339.

Gold MS, Pottash AC, Sweeney DR, et al. Opiate withdrawal using clonidine: a safe, effective and rapid nonopiate treatment. *JAMA* 1980;242: 343–346.

Goldman L. Evidence-based perioperative risk reduction. *Am J Med* 2003;114:763–764.

Goyagi T, Nishikawa T. Oral clonidine premedication enhances the quality of postoperative analgesia by intrathecal morphine. *Anesth Analg* 1996;82:1192–1196.

Hamaya Y, Nishikawa T, Dohi S. Diuretic effect of clonidine during isoflurane, nitrous oxide, and oxygen anesthesia. *Anesthesiology* 1994;81:811–819.

Hsu Y-W, Cortinez LI, Robertson KM, et al. Dexmedetomidine pharmacodynamics: Part I. Crossover comparison of the respiratory effects of dexmedetomidine and remifentanil in healthy volunteers. *Anesthesiology* 2004;101:1066–1076.

Husserl FE, Messerli FH. Adverse effects of antihypertensive drugs. *Drugs* 1981;22:188–210.

Ingersoll-Weng E, Manecke GR, Thistlethwaite PA. Dexmedetomidine and cardiac arrest. *Anesthesiology* 2004;100:738–739.

Israili ZH, Hall WD. Cough and angioneurotic edema associated with angiotensin-converting enzyme inhibitor therapy: a review of the literature and pathophysiology. *Ann Intern Med* 1992;117: 234–239.

Jalonen J, Hynynen M, Kuitunen A, et al. Dexmedetomidine as an anesthetic adjunct in coronary artery bypass grafting. *Anesthesiology* 1997;86:331–345.

Kamibayashi T, Maze M. Clinical uses of alpha$_2$-adrenergic agonists. *Anesthesiology* 2000;93:1345–1349.

Kienbaum P, Heuter T, Michel MC, et al. Sympathetic neural activation evoked by μ-receptor blockade in patients addicted to opioids is abolished by intravenous clonidine. *Anesthesiology* 2002; 96:346–351.

Levanen J, Makela ML, Scheinin H. Dexmedetomidine premedication attenuates ketamine-induced cardiostimulatory effects and postanesthetic delirium. *Anesthesiology* 1995;82:1117–1125.

Liu S, Chiu AA, Neal JM, et al. Oral clonidine prolongs lidocaine spinal anesthesia in human volunteers. *Anesthesiology* 1995;82: 1353–1359.

Lydiatt CA, Fee MP, Hill GE. Severe hypotension during epidural anesthesia in a prazosin-treated patient. *Anesth Analg* 1993;76: 1152–1153.

Mazze RI, Woodruff RE, Heerdt ME. Isoniazid-induced enflurane defluorination in humans. *Anesthesiology* 1982;57:5–8.

Memis D, Turan A, Karamanhoglu B, et al. Adding dexmedetomidine to lidocaine for intravenous regional anesthesia. *Anesth Analg* 2004;98:835–840.

Milne B, Cervenko FW, Jhamandas K, et al. Local clonidine: analgesia and effect on opiate withdrawal in the rat. *Anesthesiology* 1985;62: 34–38.

Mirenda JV, Grissom TE. Anesthetic implications of the renin-angiotensin system and angiotensin-converting enzyme inhibitors. *Anesth Analg* 1991;72:667–683.

Morelli A, Tritapepe L, Rocco M, et al. Terlipressin versus norepinephrine to counteract anesthesia-induced hypotension in patients treated with renin-angiotensin inhibitors: Effects on systemic and regional hemodynamics. *Anesthesiology* 2005;102:12–19.

Nelson LE, Lu J, Guo T, et al. The alpha$_2$ adrenoreceptor agonist dexmedetomidine converges on an endogenous sleep-promoting pathway to exert its sedative effects. *Anesthesiology* 2003;98: 428–436.

Nishina K, Mikawa K, Useugi T, et al. Efficacy of clonidine for prevention of perioperative myocardial ischemia: A critical appraisal and meta-analysis of the literature. *Anesthesiology* 2002;96:323–329.

Oparil S, Calhoun DA. High blood pressure. *Sci Am Med* 2000;1: III:1–16.

Ota K, Namidi A, Iwasaki H, et al. Dosing interval for prolongation of tetracaine spinal anesthesia by oral clonidine in humans. *Anesth Analg* 1994;79:1117–1120.

Palmer BF. Managing hyperkalemia caused by inhibitors of the rennin-angiotensin-aldosterone system. *N Engl J Med* 2004;351:585–592.

Pitt B. ACE inhibitors for patients with vascular disease without left ventricular dysfunction—may they rest in PEACE? *N Engl J Med* 2004;351:2115–2117.

Prys-Roberts C, Meloche R, Foex P. Studies of anaesthesia in relation to hypertension. I: Cardiovascular responses to treated and untreated patients. *Br J Anaesth* 1971;43:122–137.

Psaty BM, Heckbert SR, Koepsell TD, et al. The risk of myocardial infarction associated with antihypertensive drug therapies. *JAMA* 1995; 274:620–624.

Quintin L, Bouilloc X, Butin E, et al. Clonidine for major vascular surgery in hypertensive patients: a double-blind, controlled, randomized study. *Anesth Analg* 1996;83:687–695.

Ramsay MAE, Luterman DL. Dexmedetomidine as a total intravenous anesthetic agent. *Anesthesiology* 2004;101:787–790.

Remuzzi G, Ruggenenti P. Slowing the progression of diabetic nephropathy *N Engl J Med* 1993;329:1496–1497.

Reuben SS, Steinberg RB, Klatt JL, et al. Intravenous regional anesthesia using lidocaine and clonidine. *Anesthesiology* 1999;91:654–658.

Reuben SS, Steinberg RB, Madabhushi L, et al. Intravenous regional clonidine in the management of sympathetically maintained pain. *Anesthesiology* 1998;89:527–530.

Ryckwaert R, Colson P. Hemodynamic effects of anesthesia in patients with ischemic heart failure chronically treated with angiotensin-converting enzyme inhibitors. *Anesth Analg* 1997;84:945–949.

Sandler AN. The role of clonidine and alpha$_2$-agonists for postoperative analgesia. *Can J Anaesth* 1996;43:1191–1194.

Scheinin H, Aantaa R, Anttila M, et al. Reversal of the sedative and sympatholytic effects of dexmedetomidine with a specific alpha$_2$ adrenoceptor antagonist atipamezole. A pharmacodynamic and kinetic study in healthy volunteers. *Anesthesiology* 1998;89:574–584.

Segal IS, Vickery RG, Walton JK, Doze VA, Maze M. Dexmedetomidine diminishes halothane anesthetic requirements in rats through a postsynaptic alpha 2 adrenergic receptor. *Anesthesiology* 1988;69: 818–823.

Shelly MP. Dexmedetomidine: a real innovation or more of the same? *Br J Anaesth* 2001;87:677–678.

Shorr RI, Ray WA, Daugherty JR, et al. Antihypertensives and the risk of serious hypoglycemia in older persons using insulin or sulfonylureas. *JAMA* 1997;278:40–43.

Singelyn FJ, Gouverneur JM, Robert A. A minimum dose of clonidine added to mepivacaine prolongs the duration of anesthesia and analgesia after axillary brachial plexus block. *Anesth Analg* 1996; 83:1046–1050.

Singh H, Liu J, Gaines GY, White PF. Effect of oral clonidine and intrathecal fentanyl on tetracaine spinal block. *Anesth Analg* 1994;79:1113–1116.

Stiff JL, Harris DB. Clonidine withdrawal complicated by amitriptyline therapy. *Anesthesiology* 1983;59:73–74.

Strebel S, Gurzeler JA, Schneider MC, et al. Small-dose intrathecal clonidine and isobaric bupivacaine for orthopedic surgery: a dose-response study. *Anesth Analg* 2004;99:1231–1238.

Stuhmeier KD, Mainzer B, Ciepka J, et al. Small, oral dose of clonidine reduces the incidence of intraoperative myocardial ischemia in patients having vascular surgery. *Anesthesiology* 1996;85:706–712.

Taittonen MT, Kirvela OA, Aantaa R, et al. The effect of clonidine or midazolam premedication on perioperative responses during ketamine anesthesia. *Anesth Analg* 1998;87:161–166.

Talke P, Tayefeh F, Sessler DI, et al. Dexmedetomidine does not alter the sweating threshold, but comparably and linearly decreases the vasoconstriction and shivering thresholds. *Anesthesiology* 1997;87: 835–841.

Talke PO, Caldwell JE, Richardson CA, et al. The effects of dexmedetomidine on neuromuscular blockade in human volunteers. *Anesth Analg* 1999;88:633–639.

Venn RM, Bradshaw CJ, Spencer R, et al. Preliminary UK experience of dexmedetomidine, a novel agent for postoperative sedation in the intensive care unit. *Anaesthesia* 1999;54:1136–1142.

Wallace AW, Galindez D, Salahieh A, et al. Effect of clonidine on cardiovascular morbidity and mortality after noncardiac surgery. *Anesthesiology* 2004;101:284–293.

White WB, Gilbert JC. Transdermal clonidine in a patient with resistant hypertension and malabsorption. *N Engl J Med* 1985;313: 1418.

Williams GH. Converting-enzyme inhibitors in the treatment of hypertension. *N Engl J Med* 1988;319:1517–1525.

Peripheral Vasodilators, Nitric Oxide, and Nitrovasodilators

16

Peripheral vasodilators that act on the systemic circulation are most frequently used clinically to (a) treat hypertensive crises, (b) produce controlled hypotension, and (c) facilitate left ventricular forward stroke volume, as in patients with regurgitant valvular heart lesions or acute cardiac failure (Abe, 1993). Nitrovasodilators that are administered intravenously (IV) as a continuous infusion include sodium nitroprusside (SNP) and nitroglycerin. Conceptually, vasodilators decrease systemic blood pressure by decreasing systemic vascular resistance (arterial vasodilators) or by decreasing venous return and cardiac output (venous vasodilators). Vasodilator therapy is the standard initial treatment in symptomatic patients with left ventricular dysfunction. Preload reducing vasodilators (nitroglycerin) alleviate pulmonary and systemic congestive symptoms, whereas arterial vaosodilators (SNP) reverse deleterious effects of peripheral vasoconstriction.

Nitrovasodilators produce systemic and pulmonary vasodilation through generation of nitric oxide (NO) intracellularly, leading to stimulation of guanylate cyclase and increases in the intracellular concentrations of cyclic guanosine 3′5′-monophosphate (cGMP) manifesting as vascular smooth muscle relaxation. cGMP activates protein kinases that phosphorylate various peptides leading to decreased intracellular concentrations of calcium ions similar to the effects of cyclic adenosine monophosphate. NO is an endogenous gas that may be administered by inhalation to produce selective relaxation of the pulmonary vasculature.

NITRIC OXIDE

NO is recognized as a chemical messenger in a multitude of biologic systems, with homeostatic activity in the modulation of cardiovascular tone (vasorelaxant effect), platelet regulation, and a neurotransmitter function in the central nervous system (CNS). In addition, NO has a role in gastrointestinal smooth muscle relaxation, in immune regulation, and as an effector molecule for the volatile anesthetics (Schroeder and Kuo, 1995). NO is administered by inhalation to produce selective relaxation of the pulmonary vasculature.

Synthesis and Transport

NO is synthesized in endothelial cells from the amino acid L-arginine by a family of calcium-activated enzymes known as NO synthases. As a gas, NO diffuses from the producing cells into target cells, where it activates guanylate cyclase to increase the cGMP concentration, which in turn results in vasodilation. NO has a half-time of <5 seconds under normal physiologic conditions, which ensures a relatively localized action. NO binds to the iron of heme-based proteins and thus is avidly bound and inactivated by hemoglobin. A major metabolic transformation of NO, at least when it is given by inhalation, is by means of hemoglobin into nitrate.

Physiologic Effects

The physiologic effects of endogenous NO reflect the distribution of NO synthase and the functional effects of inhibiting or stimulating the pathway (Moncada and Higgs, 1993; Quinn et al., 1995; Schroeder and Kuo, 1995).

Cardiovascular System

In the systemic circulation, flow-induced shear stress and pulsatile arterial flow result in the continual release of NO so that NO regulates systemic vascular resistance and pulmonary vascular resistance under baseline conditions. Indeed, normal production of NO is an important indicator of normal endothelial function. Endothelial production of NO also appears to determine the distribution of cardiac output, particularly with respect to the pulmonary and cerebral circulations. NO is a major factor in autoregulation because endothelial cells increase NO production in response to decreased oxygenation. NO release is important for opposing the pulmonary hypertensive response to multiple stimuli, including arterial hypoxemia. NO has negative inotropic and chronotropic effects. The fact that arteries generate more NO than veins is consistent with the observation that internal mammary artery bypass grafts remain patent more often than do venous grafts.

Inhaled NO causes vasodilation that is proportional to the pulmonary vascular resistance in the presence of pulmonary vasoconstriction. Inhaled NO has very little effect on pulmonary vascular resistance if pulmonary vascular tone is not increased or if pulmonary hypertension is secondary to fixed or fibrotic disease similarly if the pulmonary artery pressure is elevated secondary to increased cardiac output or if left atrial pressure is increased, inhaled NO is unlikely to produce a significant effect.

Inhibition of NO production in animals results in sustained systemic hypertension suggesting the cardiovascular system is exposed to a continuous NO-dependent vasodilator tone. NO-related vascular relaxation is decreased in patients with essential hypertension but it is unclear if this is a cause or consequence of hypertension.

Pulmonary System

NO may contribute to bronchodilation. Formation of NO in the upper airways could result in selective dilatation of blood vessels supplying ventilated segments, and NO has been proposed as an important mediator of ventilation-to-perfusion matching.

Platelets

NO inhibits platelet activation, aggregation, and adhesion by activation of platelet guanylate cyclase, which results in decreased intracellular calcium. The effects of NO are synergistic with prostacyclin, allowing the endothelium to maintain its antithrombotic properties.

Nervous System

Endogenous NO is a neurotransmitter in the brain, spinal cord, and peripheral nervous system. NO is released in response to stimulation of the excitatory *N*-methyl-D-aspartate (NMDA) glutamate receptor. There is evidence that NO may be important in the formation of memory. As a neurotransmitter, NO may be involved in antinociception and in modulating anesthetic effects. In the peripheral nervous system, nerves previously characterized as nonadrenergic and noncholinergic are now known to synthesize and release NO as a neurotransmitter. These peripheral nerves may innervate the myenteric plexus and produce relaxation of the smooth muscle of the gastrointestinal tract. These same peripheral nerves innervate the corpora cavernosa of the penis, resulting in penile erection. Sildenafil is a phosphodiesterase-5 inhibitor that acts by increasing the local availability of endogenous NO. In this regard, sidenafil may be administered to increase the response to inhaled NO (Bigatello et al., 2000).

Immune Function

NO appears to modulate inflammation and is involved in host defenses and immunologic function. For example, activation of macrophages by cytokines results in induction of NO synthase with the production of large amounts of NO. These high concentrations of NO damage bacteria, fungi, and protozoa. Activated macrophages can also kill tumor cells.

Pathophysiology

Essential hypertension may reflect decreased NO release, whereas the hypotension associated with septic shock may reflect excess release of NO. Arginine decreases blood pressure in patients with essential hypertension, and the effects of angiotensin-converting enzyme inhibitors may be due to their ability to prolong the half-time of bradykinin, which stimulates the release of NO from endothelial cells. Defective NO production may play a primary role in atherosclerosis by producing platelet aggregation, platelet-induced vasoconstriction, and leukocyte adhesion. NO is rapidly inactivated by hemoglobin, suggesting that vasospasm after subarachnoid hemorrhage may be a result of decreased NO activity. Defective NO production may cause or contribute to pulmonary hypertension. The hyperdynamic state of cirrhosis may result from excessive production of NO because of induction of NO synthetase. Myocardial ischemia and reperfusion impair NO production. NO may increase pulmonary artery occlusion pressure and produce pulmonary edema in patients with left ventricular dysfunction.

In the gastrointestinal tract, diminished activity of neuronal NO has been demonstrated in pyloric stenosis and achalasia. NO modulates morphine-induced constipation. In the CNS, excess NO has been implicated in the pathogenesis of epilepsy. In the immune system, absence of NO may predispose to infection, whereas excessive production of NO might be a mechanism of inflammation.

Mechanism of Anesthesia

NO appears to be involved in excitatory neurotransmission in the CNS, and NO synthase inhibition suppresses excitatory transmission mediated by NMDA (Quinn et al., 1995). A role for NO in central nociceptive pathways and in maintaining wakefulness has been reported (Dzoljic and DeVries, 1994; Meller et al., 1992). Suppression of formation of NO by anesthetics could decrease excitatory neurotransmission (block glutamatergic and muscarinic excitatory function) and increase inhibitory neurotransmission (enhance gamma-aminobutyric acid inhibitory function), leading to an overall enhancement of the anesthetic state (Johns, 1996; Nakamura and Mori, 1993). Administration of NO synthase inhibitors causes a dose-dependent decrease in minimum alveolar concentration (MAC) in animals (Johns, 1996).

Clinical Uses

Inhaled NO has multiple clinical uses and potential benefits (Table 16-1) (Troncy et al., 1997; Haddad et al., 2000). The "I-NO vent delivery system" is intended to add NO to a ventilator breathing system so that the inspired NO concentration remains constant despite changes in minute ventilation (Young et al., 1997). The use of inhaled NO for therapy of pulmonary disease is based on the finding that NO rapidly binds and is inactivated by hemoglobin. Inhaled NO can diffuse from alveoli to pulmonary vascular muscle (alveolocapillary diffusion coefficient is three to five times more rapid than for carbon monoxide) and produces pulmonary vasodilation but will not produce systemic effects because NO that diffuses into blood is immediately inactivated. Thus, inhaled NO functions as a selective pulmonary vasodilator for the management of diseases associated with pulmonary hypertension. Pulmonary hypertension, which may follow cardiopulmonary bypass, may reflect endothelial dysfunction because of cardiopulmonary bypass. In this situation, inhaled NO, 20 ppm, may be efficacious (Fig. 16-1) (Rich et al., 1993).

Inhaled NO, 10 to 20 ppm, has been used for therapy of persistent pulmonary hypertension of the newborn (Kinsella et al., 1992; Roberts et al., 1997). Such therapy decreases the need for extracorporeal membrane oxygen therapy, although mortality has not been shown to be decreased (Neonatal Inhaled Nitric Oxide Study Group, 1997). Inhalation of NO in premature infants with respiratory distress syndrome decreases the incidence of chronic lung disease and death (Schreiber et al., 2003). The outcome benefit of inhaled NO has been limited to the decreased need for extracorporeal membrane oxygenation in newborns with pulmonary hypertension.

TABLE 16-1.
POTENTIAL BENEFICIAL EFFECTS OF INHALED NITRIC OXIDE

Bronchodilation
Improved ventilation/perfusion matching
Decreased right ventricular pressures
Decreased intracardiac shunt
Increased right ventricular ejection fraction
Decreased pulmonary artery pressures
Decreased pulmonary vascular resistance
Increased cardiac output
Increased arterial oxygenation

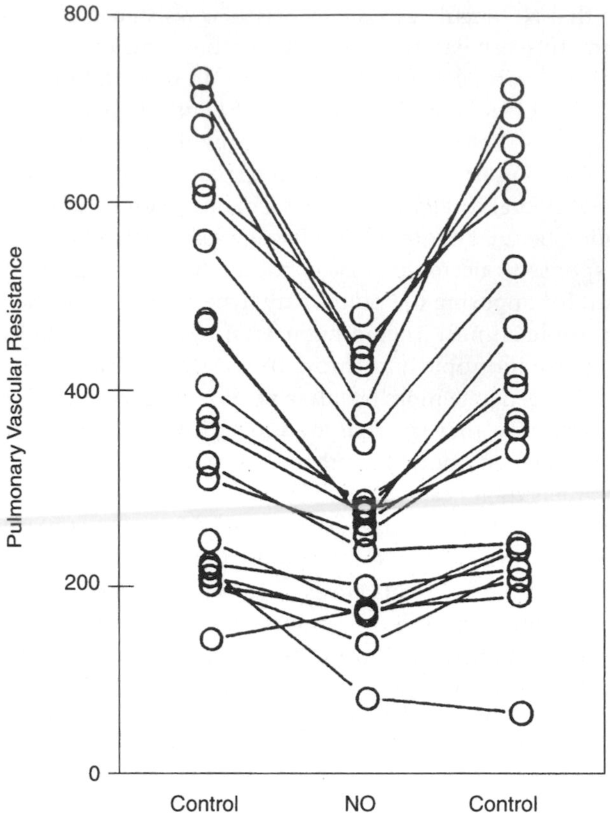

Figure 16-1. Pulmonary vascular resistance (dyne/cm/s^{-5}) before, during, and after inhalation of nitric oxide (NO) for each patient before cardiopulmonary bypass. (From Rich GF, Murphy GD, Roos CM, et al. Inhaled nitric oxide: selective pulmonary vasodilation in cardiac surgical patients. *Anesthesiology* 1993;78:1028–1035; with permission.)

Acute Lung Injury and Adult Respiratory Distress Syndrome

Current cumulative evidence from clinical trials suggests that NO is not indicated in the routine therapy of patients with acute lung injury or adult respiratory distress syndrome (ARDS) (Adhikari and Granton, 2004). Inhaled NO (5 ppm) administered to patients with acute lung injury not due to sepsis results in short-term oxygenation improvements but has no impact on the duration of mechanical ventilatory support or mortality (Taylor et al, 2004). Thus, this expensive therapy is not recommended as standard care for these patients. In severe cases of ARDS for which refractory arterial hypoxemia or pulmonary hypertension are major clinical problems, short-term physiologic improvements may be crucial for patient survival and in these instances, NO may have a role as "salvage" therapy along with other strategies such as high-frequency oscillatory ventilation. The degree of improvement in arterial oxygenation is likely to be related to pulmonary vascular resistance before treatment (Young et al., 1994). The improvement in arterial oxygenation occurs because inhaled NO (in contrast to IV vasodilators) is distributed according to ventilation so that the associated vasodilation increases blood flow to well-ventilated alveoli (improved matching of ventilation to perfusion). The beneficial effects of inhaled NO on arterial oxygenation and the pulmonary circulation are associated with a significant inhibition of platelet aggregation, although the bleeding time remains unchanged (Samama et al., 1995). Absence of systemic effects in the presence of inhaled NO reflects its rapid inactivation by hemoglobin. By decreasing pulmonary hypertension and improving arterial oxygenation, inhaled NO may provide time for the lungs to heal.

Cardiac Transplantation

Inhaled NO may be used for preoperative assessment of the reversibility of pulmonary hypertension in establishing the need for either heart or heart and lung transplantation. Inhaled NO may be a useful intervention following cardiac transplantation, as the donor heart has not been previously exposed to increased pulmonary vascular resistance as may be present in the recipient. In this situation, inhaled NO produces pulmonary vasodilation and may improve right ventricular function and increase cardiac output. The benefit from decreased right ventricular afterload caused by NO may be particularly apparent in patients who require a left ventricular assist device.

Toxicity

Inhaled NO increases methemoglobin levels as NO combines with hemoglobin. The increases in methemoglobin concentrations are usually modest. Life-threatening rebound arterial hypoxemia and pulmonary hypertension may accompany discontinuation of inhaled NO therapy (Haddad et al., 2000). Because of the variability in rebound pulmonary hypertension, it is important to wean patients from inhaled NO slowly. NO is oxidized to nitrogen dioxide (NO_2) especially in the presence of high concentrations of oxygen. NO_2 is a known pulmonary toxin ("silo filler's disease") and is a possible product of the interaction of NO with oxygen. It is conceivable that NO_2 concentrations could produce pulmonary toxicity during treatment with NO. Continuous monitoring of inspired NO and NO_2 concentrations is important to provide an early warning of possible pulmonary toxicity.

SODIUM NITROPRUSSIDE

SNP is a direct-acting, nonselective peripheral vasodilator that causes relaxation of arterial and venous vascular smooth muscle (Friederich and Butterworth, 1995). It is comprised of a ferrous ion center complexed with five cyanide (CN^-) moieties and a nitrosyl group (Fig. 16-2). The molecule is 44% cyanide by weight and is soluble in water. SNP lacks significant effects on nonvascular smooth muscle and on cardiac muscle. Its onset of action is almost immediate, and its duration is transient, requiring continuous IV administration to maintain a therapeutic effect. The extreme potency of SNP necessitates careful titration of dosage as provided by continuous infusion devices and frequent monitoring of systemic blood pressure, often by an intraarterial catheter attached to a transducer.

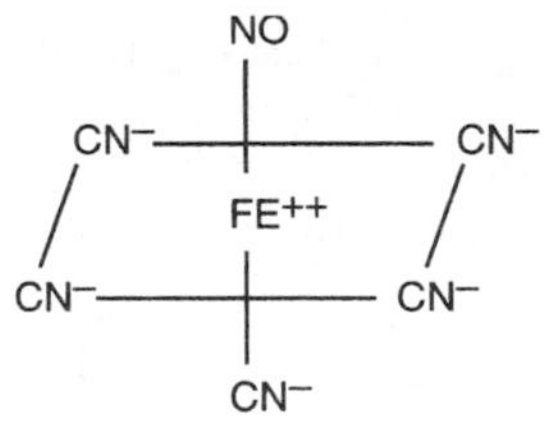

Figure 16-2. Nitroprusside.

Mechanism of Action

When infused IV, SNP interacts with oxyhemoglobin, dissociating immediately and forming methemoglobin while releasing cyanide and NO (Fig. 16-3) (Friederich and Butterworth, 1995). Once released, NO activates the enzyme guanylate cyclase present in vascular smooth muscle, resulting in increased intracellular concentrations of cGMP (Fig. 16-4) (Friederich and Butterworth, 1995). cGMP inhibits calcium entry into vascular smooth muscle cells and may increase calcium uptake by the smooth endoplasmic reticulum to produce vasodilation (Moncada and Higgs, 1993). As such, NO is the active mediator responsible for the direct vasodilating effect of SNP. In contrast to the organic nitrates (nitroglycerin), which require the presence of thio-containing compounds to generate NO, SPN spontaneously generates this product, thus functioning as a prodrug.

Metabolism

Metabolism of SNP begins with the transfer of an electron from the iron of oxyhemoglobin to SNP, yielding methemoglobin and an unstable SNP radical (see Fig. 16-3) (Friederich and Butterworth, 1995). This electron transfer is independent of electron activity. The unstable SNP radical promptly breaks down, releasing all five cyanide ions, one of which reacts with methemoglobin to form cyanomethemoglobin. The remaining free cyanide ions are available to rhodanese enzyme in the liver and kidneys for conversion to thiocyanate. Rhodanese uses thiosulfate ions as sulfur donors, and most adults can detoxify approximately 50 mg of SNP using existing sulfur stores. Normal adult methemoglobin concentrations (about 0.5% of all hemoglobin) are capable of binding the cyanide released from 18 mg of SNP. Cyanomethemoglobin remains in dynamic equilibrium with free cyanide and is considered nontoxic. The nonenzymatic release of cyanide from SNP is not inhibited by hypothermia as may be present during cardiopulmonary bypass, whereas enzymatic conversion of cyanide to thiocyanate may be delayed (Moore et al., 1985).

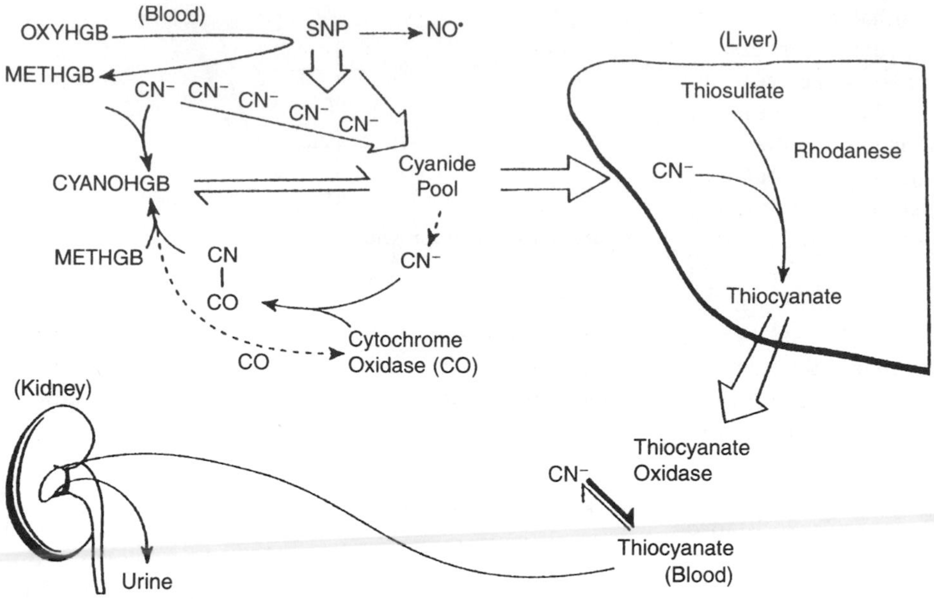

Figure 16-3. Metabolism of nitroprusside (SNP) to cyanide (CN), nitric oxide (NO), and thiocyanate. (CYANOHGB, cyanohemoglobin; METHGB, methemoglobin; OXYHGB, oxyhemoglobin.) (From Friederich JA, Butterworth JF. Sodium nitroprusside: twenty years and counting. *Anesth Analg* 1995;81:152–162; with permission.)

Toxicity

Cyanide toxicity, methemoglobinemia, and effects due to high plasma concentrations of thiocyanate represent the potential toxic effects of treatment with SNP.

Cyanide Toxicity

A healthy adult can eliminate cyanide via the liver at a rate equivalent to cyanide production during SNP infusion equivalent to approximately 2 μg/kg per minute (Curry and Arnold-Capell, 1991; Zerbe and Wagner, 1993). Clinical evidence of cyanide toxicity may occur when the rate of IV SNP infusion is >2 μg/kg per minute or when sulfur donors and methemoglobin are exhausted, thus allowing cyanide radicals to accumulate. Because any free cyanide radical may bind inactive tissue cytochrome oxidase and prevent oxidative phosphorylation, increased cyanide concentrations may precipitate tissue anoxia, anaerobic metabolism, and lactic acidosis. Children may be less able to mobilize thiosulfate stores despite increasing cyanide concentrations, leading to accelerated toxicity.

Regardless of the SNP infusion rate or total administered dose, cyanide toxicity should be suspected in any patient who is resistant to the hypotensive effects of the drug despite maximum infusion rates (>2 μg/kg per minute or 10 μg/kg per minute for no longer than 10 minutes) or in a previously responsive patient who becomes unresponsive to the systemic blood pressure-lowering effects of SNP (tachyphylaxis). Mixed venous PO_2 is increased in the presence of cyanide toxicity, indicating paralysis of cytochrome oxidase and inability of tissues to use oxygen. At the same time, metabolic acidosis (plasma lactate concentrations of >10 mM, which correlates with blood cyanide concentrations of >40 μM) develops as a reflection of anaerobic metabolism in the tissues. Decreased cerebral oxygen use is evidenced by the increased cerebral venous oxygen content. In awake patients, CNS dysfunction (mental status changes, seizures) may occur.

Blood cyanide concentrations required for clinical toxicity appear to exceed 40 μM, and deaths have been reported with cyanide concentrations of >77 μM (Curry and Arnold-Capell, 1991). There is controversy about the definitive method for assaying blood cyanide concentrations and the importance of photodecomposition during the assay or the infusion. The clinical value of blood cyanide concentration measurements is further limited due to the delay (ranging from several hours to days) before the results are available. Conversely, the base deficit, which is a readily available clinical determination, correlates well with the blood lactate concentration. For example, plasma lactate concentrations exceeding 10 mM

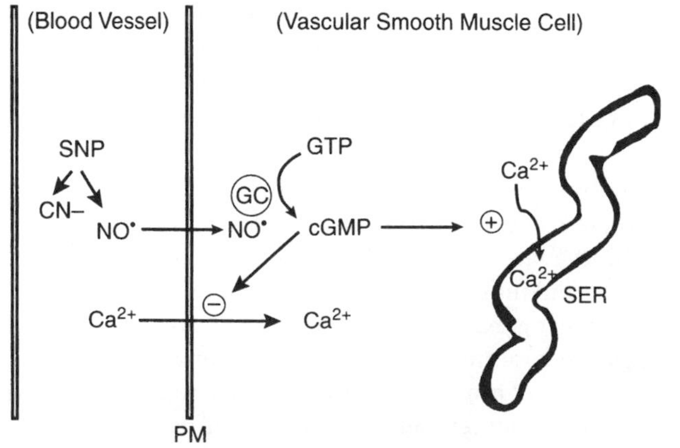

Figure 16-4. Mechanism of action of sodium nitroprusside (SNP). (cGMP, cyclic guanosine 3′5′-monophosphate; CN^-, cyanide; GC, guanylate cyclase; GTP, guanosine triphosphate; NO•, nitric oxide; PM, plasma membrane; SER, smooth endoplasmic reticulum.) (From Friederich JA, Butterworth JF. Sodium nitroprusside: twenty years and counting. *Anesth Analg* 1995;81:152–162; with permission.)

correlate well with blood cyanide concentrations exceeding 40 μM.

The phenomenon of resistance to the therapeutic effects of SNP may be related to an abnormality in the cyanide-thiocyanate pathway that allows cyanide to accumulate (Davies et al., 1975). For example, patients with Leber optic atrophy or tobacco amblyopia manifest increased blood concentrations of cyanide. Although there are no documented cases of adverse effects due to SNP administration to patients with these abnormalities, there is likewise no evidence that the drug would be safe (Friederich and Butterworth, 1995). The mechanism by which cyanide results in resistance or tachyphylaxis to the blood pressure-lowering effects of SNP is not confirmed but could reflect cyanide-induced stimulation of cardiac output, which would tend to offset the hypotensive effects of the vasodilator. Furthermore, most patients who are resistant or develop tachyphylaxis to the hypotensive effects of SNP are children or young adults. It is speculated that active baroreceptor reflexes in this age group evoke increases in sympathetic nervous system activity in response to drug-induced decreases in systemic blood pressure. As a result, a larger initial dose or a subsequent increase in the dose of SNP is required to decrease the blood pressure, leading to the likelihood of dose-dependent cyanide toxicity. A beta antagonist such as propranolol can be administered to blunt these baroreceptor-mediated responses and thus decrease the total dose of SNP required to produce the desired blood pressure effect. Likewise, volatile anesthetics blunt baroreceptor reflex activity, thus contributing to decreased dose requirements for SNP.

There is no evidence that preexisting hepatic or renal disease increases the likelihood of cyanide toxicity. In fact, renal failure may prevent sulfate excretion, which allows production of more thiosulfate to act as a sulfur donor and thus convert cyanide to thiocyanate (Fig. 16-5) (Tinker and Michenfelder, 1980).

SNP should be used cautiously in pregnant patients due to the potential for fetal cyanide toxicity. However, this is not a major concern when modest SNP doses (<3 μg/kg per minute IV) are administered for short durations. In this regard, SNP is acceptable for producing acute afterload reduction in parturients.

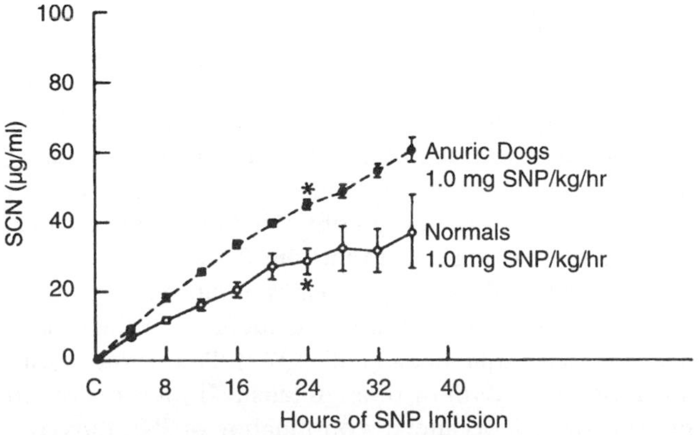

Figure 16-5. Plasma thiocyanate (SCN) concentrations in anuric and normal dogs receiving nitroprusside (SNP). (From Tinker JH, Michenfelder JD. Increased resistance to nitroprusside–induced cyanide toxicity in anuric dogs. *Anesthesiology* 1980;52:40–47; with permission.)

Treatment of Cyanide Toxicity

Appearance of tachyphylaxis in a previously sensitive patient in association with metabolic acidosis and increased mixed venous PO_2 mandates immediate discontinuation of SNP and administration of 100% oxygen despite normal oxygen saturation. Sodium bicarbonate is administered to correct metabolic acidosis. Sodium thiosulfate, 150 mg/kg IV administered over 15 minutes, is a recommended treatment for cyanide toxicity (Friederich and Butterworth, 1995). Thiosulfate acts as a sulfur donor to convert cyanide to thiocyanate. If cyanide toxicity is severe, with deteriorating hemodynamics and metabolic acidosis, the recommended treatment is slow IV administration of sodium nitrate, 5 mg/kg. Sodium nitrate converts hemoglobin to methemoglobin, which acts as an antidote by converting cyanide to cyanomethemoglobin. Alternatively, hydroxocobalamin (vitamin B_{12a}), which binds cyanide to form cyanocobalamin (vitamin B_{12}) can be administered (25 mg per hour IV to a maximum of 100 mg) to treat cyanide toxicity. In addition to being expensive, hydroxocobalamin may produce a reddish discoloration of the skin and mucous membranes (Hall and Rumack, 1987).

Thiocyanate Toxicity

Thiocyanate is cleared slowly by the kidneys, with an elimination half-time of 3 to 7 days (Friederich and Butterworth, 1995). Clinical thiocyanate toxicity is rare, as thiocyanate is 100-fold less toxic than cyanide. In patients with normal renal function, 7 to 14 days of SNP infusion in the 2 to 5 μg/kg per minute range may be required to produce potentially toxic thiocyanate blood concentrations. SNP infusions for 3 to 6 days may result in thiocyanate toxicity in patients with chronic renal failure who are not undergoing periodic hemodialysis.

Nonspecific symptoms of thiocyanate toxicity include fatigue, tinnitus, nausea, and vomiting. Clinical evidence of neurotoxicity produced by thiocyanate includes hyperreflexia, confusion, psychosis, and miosis. Toxicity may progress to seizures and coma. Increased thiocyanate concentrations competitively inhibit uptake and binding of iodine in the thyroid gland, sometimes producing clinical hypothyroidism. Thiocyanate clearance can be facilitated by dialysis. Oxyhemoglobin can slowly oxidize thiocyanate back to sulfate and cyanide, but this is insufficient to cause cyanide toxicity.

Methemoglobinemia

Adverse effects from methemoglobinemia produced by SNP breakdown are unlikely even in patients with a congenital inability to convert methemoglobin to hemoglobin (methemoglobin reductase deficiency) (Friederich and Butterworth,

1995). The total SNP dose required to produce 10% methemoglobinemia exceeds 10 mg/kg. Patients receiving such high doses of SNP who present with evidence of impaired oxygenation despite an adequate cardiac output and arterial oxygenation should have methemoglobinemia included in the differential diagnosis. Measurement of methemoglobin via co-oximetry may be helpful in these patients.

Isosulfan Blue Dye

Isosulfan blue as injected for detection of an axillary sentinel node in breast cancer may cause discoloration of the plasma, resulting in the pulse oximeter readings to be falsely low in the presence of normal arterial oxygen partial pressures (Rizzi et al., 2000). Co-oximetry does not reveal methemoglobin in the presence of systemic absorption of isosulfan blue dye. The presence of any substance in blood that absorbs light in the red or infrared spectrum can alter oxygen saturation readings. Other dyes known to interfere with the accuracy of pulse oximeter readings include indigo carmine, indocyanine green, and methylene blue. Isosulfan blue dye has also been associated with anaphylactoid reactions (Sprung et al., 2003).

Phototoxicity

It is recommended that SNP be mixed only in 5% glucose in water and that this solution be protected continuously from exposure to light by wrapping the container and delivery tubing with aluminum foil. This recommendation reflects the potential rapid conversion of SNP to aquapentacyanoferrate in the presence of light with the subsequent release of hydrogen cyanide (Friederich and Butterworth, 1995). Nevertheless, differences in cyanide concentrations do not occur in light-exposed compared with light-protected solutions during the first 8 hours (Ikeda et al., 1987). When protected from light, in vitro breakdown to cyanide is not excessive in the first 24 hours after the solution of SNP is prepared.

Dose and Administration

The recommended initial dose of SNP is 0.3 μg/kg per minute IV titrated to a maximum rate of 10 μg/kg per minute IV, with the maximum rate not to be infused longer than 10 minutes (Food and Drug Administration, 1991). This drug has an immediate onset and short duration of action, requiring continuous infusion to produce a sustained pharmacologic effect. An indwelling arterial catheter for continuous monitoring of systemic blood pressure is recommended. Delivery of the SNP infusion as protected from light by aluminum foil is most often via an infusion pump.

SNP infusion rates of >2 μg/kg per minute IV result in dose-dependent accumulation of cyanide and the risk of cyanide toxicity must be considered. Potentially useful approaches to decreasing the risk of cyanide toxicity include combining SNP with another drug (volatile anesthetic, beta-adrenergic antagonist) to decrease the dose of SNP needed to achieve the desired pharmacologic effect on systemic blood pressure. Alternatively, SNP can be administered concurrently with thiosulfate or hydroxocobalamin when an infusion rate of SNP >2 μg/kg per minute IV is needed.

Effects on Organ Systems

The principal pharmacologic effects of SNP are manifest on the (a) cardiovascular system, (b) cerebral blood flow, (c) hypoxic pulmonary vasoconstriction, and (d) platelet aggregation. SNP lacks direct effects on the CNS and autonomic nervous system. In animals, SNP-induced decreases in systemic blood pressure do not result in hepatic hypoxia or changes in hepatic blood flow (Sivarajan et al., 1985). Furthermore, hepatic blood flow does not change when cardiac output is maintained in anesthetized patients, despite 20% to 60% decreases in systemic blood pressure produced by SNP (Chauvin et al., 1985).

Cardiovascular System

SNP produces direct venous and arterial vasodilation, resulting in prompt decreases in systemic blood pressure. Systemic vascular resistance is decreased as evidence of arterial vasodilation, whereas venous return is decreased because of vasodilation of venous capacitance vessels. It is likely that decreases in right atrial pressure reflect pooling of blood in the veins. Baroreceptor-mediated reflex responses to SNP-induced decreases in systemic blood pressure manifest as tachycardia and increased myocardial contractility. These reflex-mediated responses may oppose the blood pressure-lowering effects of SNP. Although decreased venous return would tend to decrease cardiac output, the net effect is often an increase in cardiac output due to reflex-mediated increases in peripheral sympathetic nervous system activity combined with decreased impedance to left ventricular ejection. In the setting of left ventricular failure, SNP decreases systemic vascular resistance, pulmonary vascular resistance, and right atrial pressure, whereas the effect on cardiac output depends on the initial left ventricular end-diastolic pressure. There is no evidence that SNP exerts direct inotropic or chronotropic effects on the heart.

SNP-induced decreases in systemic blood pressure may result in decreases in renal function. Release of renin may accompany blood pressure decreases produced by SNP and contribute to blood pressure overshoots when the drug is discontinued (Khambatta et al., 1979). Pretreatment with a competitive inhibitor of angiotensin II prevents blood pressure overshoots after discontinuation of SNP, thus confirming the participation of the renin-angiotensin system in this response (Delaney and Miller, 1980). Increased plasma concentrations of catecholamines also accompany

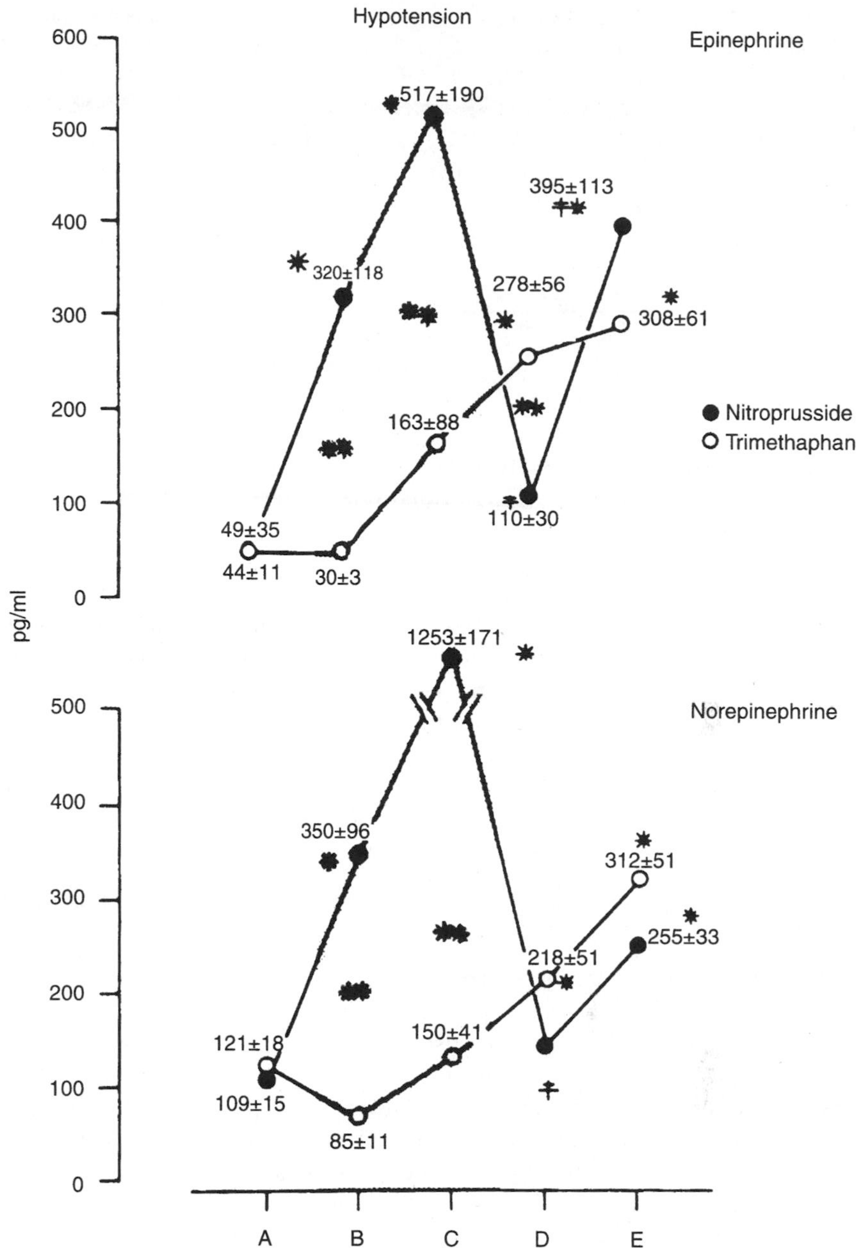

Figure 16-6. Increased plasma concentrations of epinephrine and norepinephrine accompany hypotension induced by nitroprusside but not by trimethaphan. (From Knight PR, Lane GA, Hensinger RN, et al. Catecholamine and renin-angiotensin response during hypotensive anesthesia induced by sodium nitroprusside or trimethaphan camsylate. *Anesthesiology* 1983; 59:248–253; with permission.)

hypotension produced by SNP but not that produced by trimethaphan (Fig. 16-6) (Knight et al., 1983).

SNP may increase the area of damage associated with a myocardial infarction. It is speculated that SNP causes an intracoronary steal of blood flow away from ischemic areas by arteriolar vasodilation (Becker, 1978). Coronary steal occurs because SNP dilates resistance vessels in nonischemic myocardium, resulting in diversion of blood flow away from ischemic areas where blood vessels are already maximally dilated. Clinical evidence of coronary steal phenomenon is the appearance of ischemic changes on the electrocardiogram (ECG). Decreases in diastolic blood pressure produced by SNP may also contribute to myocardial ischemia by decreasing coronary perfusion pressure and associated coronary blood flow (Sivarajan et al., 1985).

Cerebral Blood Flow

SNP is a direct vasodilator, leading to increased cerebral blood flow and cerebral blood volume. These changes, when they occur in patients with decreased intracranial compliance, may cause undesirable increases in intracranial pressure (greater than the increase produced by nitro glycerin). It is likely that the rapidity of systemic blood pressure decrease produced by SNP exceeds the capacity of the cerebral circulation to autoregulate its blood flow such that intracranial pressure and cerebral blood flow change simultaneously but in opposite directions (Rogers et al., 1979). Nevertheless, increases in intracranial pressure produced by SNP are maximal during modest decreases (<30%) in mean arterial pressure. When SNP-induced decreases in mean arterial pressure are >30% of the awake

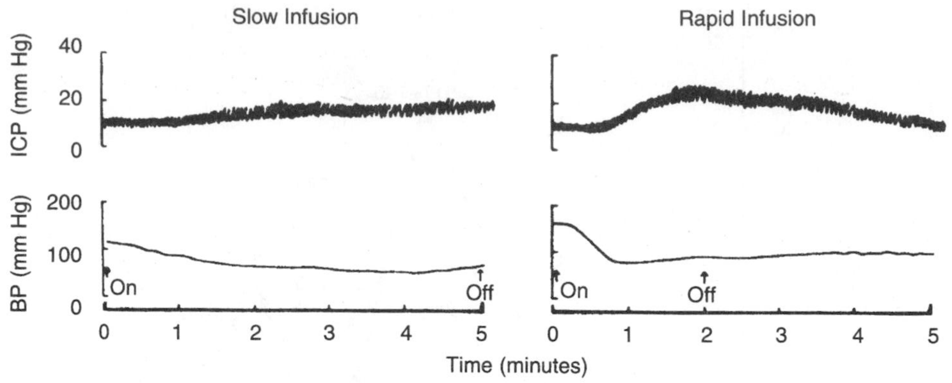

Figure 16-7. Compared with rapid infusion, the slow intravenous administration of nitroprusside does not increase the intracranial pressure (ICP). (BP, blood pressure.) (From Marsh ML, Aidinis SJ, Naughton KVH, et al. The technique of nitroprusside administration modifies the intracranial pressure response. *Anesthesiology* 1979;51:538–541; with permission.)

level, the intracranial pressure decreases to below the awake level (Turner et al., 1977). Furthermore, decreasing blood pressure slowly over 5 minutes with SNP in the presence of hypocarbia and hyperoxia negates the increase in intracranial pressure that accompanies the rapid infusion of nitroprusside (Fig. 16-7) (Marsh et al., 1979). Patients with known inadequate cerebral blood flow as associated with dangerously increased intracranial pressure or carotid artery stenosis should probably not be treated with SNP. During cardiopulmonary bypass, SNP has been shown to have no direct effect on cerebral vasculature and autoregulation is preserved (Rogers et al., 1991). Clearly, the potential adverse effects of SNP on intracranial pressure are not present if the drug is administered after the dura has been surgically opened.

Hypoxic Pulmonary Vasoconstriction

Decreases in the PaO_2 may accompany the infusion of SNP and other peripheral vasodilators used to produce controlled hypotension. Attenuation of hypoxic pulmonary vasoconstriction by peripheral vasodilators is the presumed mechanism for this effect on arterial oxygenation (Colley et al., 1979). Addition of propranolol to the vasodilator regimen does not alter the magnitude of decrease in PaO_2 (Miller et al., 1982). Furthermore, peripheral vasodilator-induced decreases in blood pressure may be more likely to increase the shunt fraction in patients with normal lungs than in those with chronic obstructive pulmonary disease (Casthely et al., 1982). It is speculated that hypotension in normal patients leads to decreased pulmonary artery pressure such that preferential perfusion of dependent but poorly ventilated alveoli occurs. In contrast, patients with chronic obstructive pulmonary disease may develop destructive vascular changes that prevent alterations in the distribution of pulmonary blood flow in response to vasodilation. The addition of positive end-expiratory pressure may reverse vasodilator-induced decreases in the PaO_2 (Berthelsen et al., 1986).

Platelet Aggregation

Increased intracellular concentrations of cGMP, as produced by SNP and nitroglycerin, have been shown to inhibit platelet aggregation (Brodde et al., 1982). Infusion rates of SNP of >3 μg/kg per minute may result in decreases in platelet aggregation and increased bleeding time (Fig. 16-8) (Hines and Barash, 1989). Even the postoperative stress-induced increase in platelet aggregation is absent in SNP-treated patients (Dietrich et al., 1996). Increased bleeding time could also be the result of vasodilation secondary to a direct effect of SNP on vascular tone. Intraoperative bleeding is not increased in SNP-treated patients, suggesting that decreased ability of platelets to aggregate during and after controlled hypotension does not have an adverse clinical effect (Dietrich et al., 1996).

Clinical Uses

Despite the risk of cyanide toxicity, SNP remains the drug most likely to be selected for production of controlled hypotension during anesthesia and surgery and for treatment of hypertensive emergencies (Friederich and Butterworth, 1995). SNP may also be selected for an additional wide range of medical (acute and chronic heart failure) and surgical indications (aortic surgery, cardiac surgery requiring cardiopulmonary bypass, pheochromocytoma resection).

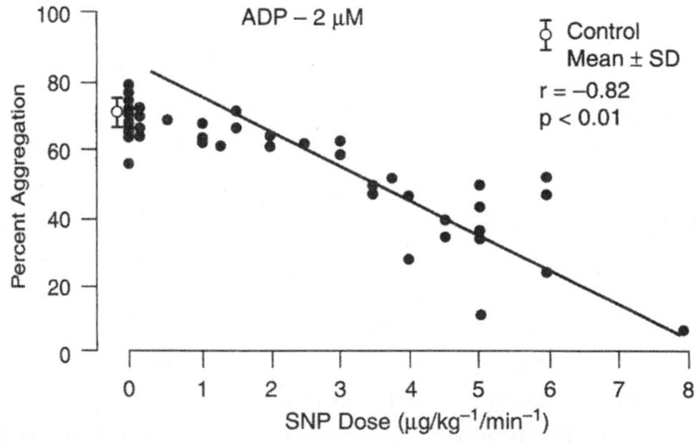

Figure 16-8. Platelet aggregation (%) at varying infusion rates of nitroprusside (SNP). (ADP, adenosine diphosphate.) (From Hines R, Barash PG. Infusion of sodium nitroprusside induces platelet dysfunction in vitro. *Anesthesiology* 1989;70: 611–615; with permission.)

Controlled Hypotension

The ability of SNP to rapidly and predictably decrease mean arterial pressure to desired levels makes this vasodilator a useful drug, especially during operations requiring nearly a bloodless field (spine surgery, neurosurgery), as well as decreasing transfusion requirements. Among those drugs used to produce controlled hypotension, SNP is most likely to maintain cerebral perfusion. Mean arterial pressures of 50 to 60 mm Hg can be maintained in healthy patients without apparent complications. The initial recommended infusion rate is 0.3 to 0.5 μg/kg per minute. The infusion rate may be increased as necessary to produce the desired mean arterial pressure but should not exceed 2 μg/kg per minute. A maximum rate of 10 μg/kg per minute IV not to exceed 10 minutes may be considered. Other cardiovascular depressant drugs (volatile anesthetics, beta-adrenergic antagonists, calcium channel blockers) may be administered simultaneously to decrease the dose requirements for SNP and thus decrease the risk of cyanide toxicity. Beta-adrenergic antagonists are effective in decreasing dose requirements for SNP but also contribute to a decreased cardiac output, which may be undesirable in patients with impaired left ventricular function.

Hypertensive Emergencies

Rapid onset, ease of titration, rapid dissipation of its effects after discontinuation, and efficacy regardless of the etiology of the hypertension contribute to the popularity of SNP in managing hypertensive crises. Typically, SNP is administered as a temporary initial treatment with replacement by longer-lasting medications as soon as feasible.

SNP, 1 to 2 μg/kg IV as a rapid injection, is useful to offset systemic blood pressure increases produced by direct laryngoscopy for intubation of the trachea (Stoelting, 1979). SNP effectively controls systemic hypertension without increasing intraocular pressure.

Cardiac Disease

SNP infusion, by virtue of decreasing left ventricular afterload, may be of benefit in the management of patients with mitral or aortic regurgitation or congestive heart failure and after acute myocardial infarction complicated by left ventricular failure. The clinical significance of SNP-induced coronary steal is unclear. Nevertheless, it is common to use nitroglycerin in preference to SNP after an acute myocardial infarction. However, in those patients with continuing left ventricular dysfunction, particularly in association with regurgitant valvular lesions, SNP can rapidly improve cardiac function and clinical stability, provided adequate ventricular filling pressures are maintained (Francis, 1991).

In the presence of chronic congestive heart failure, SNP enhances ventricular function by decreasing impedance to ventricular ejection, permitting the ventricles to eject to lower end-diastolic volumes (Cohn, 1996). Preload is decreased by blood pooling in venous capacitance vessels, further contributing to decreased ventricular end-diastolic volume. When filling pressures are increased, SNP will improve cardiac output with only minimum increases in heart rate. If, despite adequate filling pressures, cardiac output fails to increase during SNP therapy, then addition of an inotrope (dopamine, dobutamine, and epinephrine) is indicated.

Aortic Surgery

Surgical repair of thoracic aortic aneurysms, dissections, and coarctations may include SNP to attenuate proximal hypertension associated with cross-clamping the aorta. When used to control proximal hypertension, SNP may aggravate hypotension distal to the clamp. A possible contribution of SNP to spinal cord ischemia, a devastating complication of aortic surgery, has prompted an assessment of the effects of SNP on spinal cord blood flow (Friederich and Butterworth, 1995).

Cardiac Surgery

Systemic hypertension during cardiac surgery may reflect activation of the renin-angiotensin system and increased plasma concentrations of catecholamines. Regardless of the etiology of the hypertension, SNP is often chosen to decrease the blood pressure. Administration of SNP during the rewarming phase of cardiopulmonary bypass results in vasodilation that permits increased flow rates and, thus, improved heat delivery to peripheral tissues. As a result, the decrease in nasopharyngeal temperature after cessation of cardiopulmonary bypass is minimized (Fig. 16-9) (Noback and Tinker, 1980). SNP is an effective pulmonary vasodilator and may be useful for the treatment of pulmonary hypertension after heart valve replacement, especially in the presence of systemic hypertension and increased filling pressures. NO is an alternative to SNP when a drug is needed to decrease pulmonary vascular resistance.

NITROGLYCERIN

Nitroglycerin is an organic nitrate that acts principally on venous capacitance vessels and large coronary arteries to produce peripheral pooling of blood and decreased cardiac ventricular wall tension (Fig. 16-10) (Kaplan et al., 1980; Parker, 1987). As the dose of nitroglycerin is increased, there is also relaxation of arterial vascular smooth muscle. Nitroglycerin can produce pulmonary vasodilation equivalent to the degree of systemic arterial vasodilation. The most common clinical use of nitroglycerin is sublingual or IV administration for the treatment of angina pectoris as a result of either atherosclerosis of the coronary arteries or intermittent vasospasm of these vessels. Production of controlled hypotension has also been achieved with the continuous infusion of nitroglycerin.

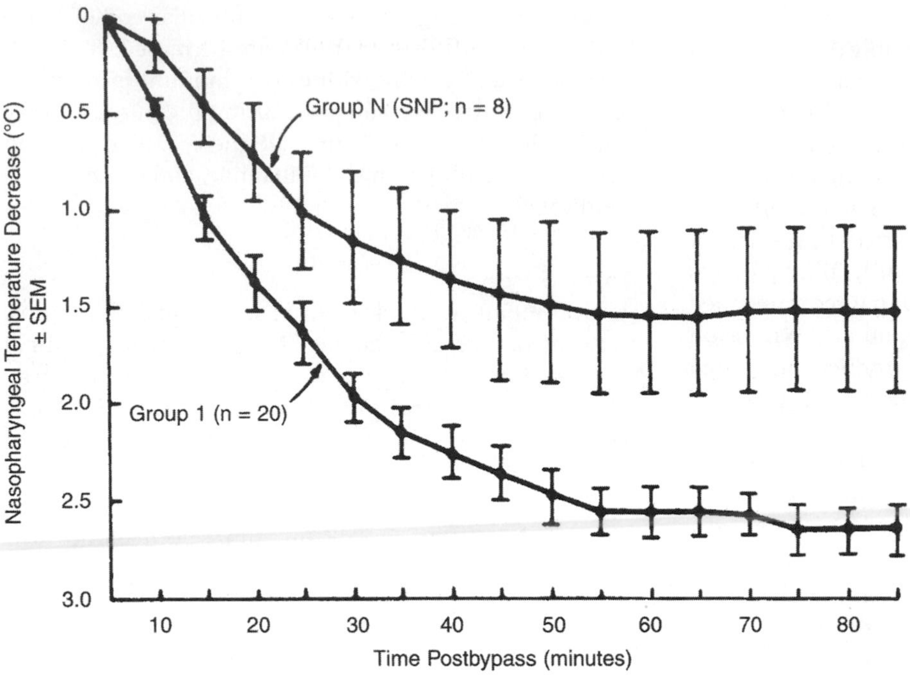

Figure 16-9. Nitroprusside (SNP)-induced vasodilation during the rewarming phase of cardiopulmonary bypass minimizes the subsequent decrease in nasopharyngeal temperature (group II) compared with untreated patients (group 1). (From Noback CR, Tinker JR. Hypothermia after cardiopulmonary bypass in man: amelioration by nitroprusside-induced vasodilation during rewarming. *Anesthesiology* 1980;53:277–280; with permission.)

Route of Administration

Nitroglycerin is most frequently administered by the sublingual route, but it is also available as an oral tablet, a buccal or transmucosal tablet, a lingual spray, and a transdermal ointment or patch. Sublingual administration of nitroglycerin results in peak plasma concentrations within 4 minutes. Only about 15% of the blood flow from the sublingual area passes through the liver, which limits the initial first-pass hepatic metabolism of nitroglycerin. In contrast, nitroglycerin is well absorbed after oral administration but it is largely inactive because of first-pass hepatic metabolism.

Transdermal absorption of nitroglycerin, 5 to 10 mg over 24 hours, provides sustained protection against myocardial ischemia. The plasma concentration resulting from transdermal absorption of nitroglycerin is low, but tolerance to the drug effect occurs when the patches are left in place >24 hours. It is possible that removing the patches after 14 to 16 hours will prevent the development of tolerance.

Continuous infusion of nitroglycerin, via special delivery tubing to decrease absorption of the drug into plastic, is a useful approach to maintain a constant delivered concentration of nitroglycerin.

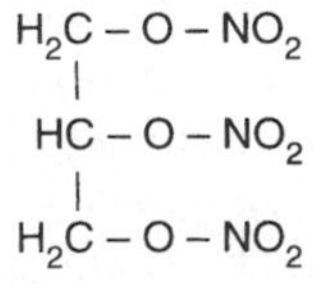

Figure 16-10. Nitroglycerin.

Mechanism of Action

Nitroglycerin, like SNP, generates NO, which stimulates production of cGMP to cause peripheral vasodilation (see the section on Sodium Nitroprusside, Mechanism of Action) (Friederich and Butterworth, 1995). In contrast to SNP, which spontaneously produces NO, nitroglycerin requires the presence of thio-containing compounds. In this regard, the nitrate group of nitroglycerin is biotransformed to NO through a glutathione-dependent pathway involving both glutathione and glutathione-S-transferase. Nitroglycerin is not recommended in patients with hypertrophic obstructive cardiomyopathy or in the presence of severe aortic stenosis, and venous pooling may be followed by syncope.

Pharmacokinetics

Nitroglycerin has an elimination half-time of about 1.5 minutes (Parker, 1987). There is a large volume of distribution, reflecting tissue uptake, and it has been estimated that only 1% of total body nitroglycerin is present in the plasma. For this reason, plasma nitroglycerin concentrations may vary widely because of minor changes in tissue binding.

Methemoglobinemia

The nitrite metabolite of nitroglycerin is capable of oxidizing the ferrous ion in hemoglobin to the ferric state with the production of methemoglobin (Fibuch et al., 1979; Zurick et al., 1984). Treatment of methemoglobinemia is with methylene blue, 1 to 2 mg/kg IV, administered over 5 minutes, to facilitate the conversion of methemoglobin to hemoglobin.

High doses of nitroglycerin may produce methemoglobinemia in patients with hepatic dysfunction.

Tolerance

A limitation to the use of all nitrates is the development of tolerance to their vasodilating effects. Tolerance is dose-dependent and duration-dependent, usually manifesting within 24 hours of sustained treatment. If ischemia occurs during continuous administration of nitroglycerin, responsiveness to the antiischemic effects of the nitrate can usually be restored by increasing the dose. The mechanism of tolerance is not well understood but may reflect a change in the vasculature that limits the vasodilating effects of the nitrates. A drug-free interval of 12 to 14 hours is recommended to reverse tolerance to nitroglycerin and other nitrates. Rebound myocardial ischemia may occur during the drug-free interval.

Effects on Organ Systems

The principal pharmacologic actions of nitroglycerin manifest as cardiovascular effects. Nitroglycerin also acts on smooth muscles in the airways and gastrointestinal tract. For example, bronchial smooth muscle is relaxed regardless of the preexisting tone (Byrick et al., 1983). Smooth muscle of the biliary tract, including the sphincter of Oddi, is relaxed (see the section, Sphincter of Oddi Spasm). Esophageal muscle tone is decreased, as is ureteral and uterine smooth muscle tone, although these later effects are somewhat unpredictable. Like SNP, nitroglycerin is a cerebral vasodilator and may increase intracranial pressure in patients with decreased intracranial compliance (Gagnon et al., 1979).

Cardiovascular Effects

Nitroglycerin doses up to 2 μg/kg per minute IV produce dilatation of veins that predominates over that produced in arterioles (Gerson et al., 1982). Venodilation results in decreased venous return as well as decreased left and right ventricular end-diastolic pressures. In normal individuals and patients with coronary artery disease, but in the absence of cardiac failure, nitroglycerin decreases cardiac output. This decreased cardiac output reflects decreased venous return as nitroglycerin is devoid of any direct inotropic effect on the heart. Heart rate is often not changed or only slightly increased during administration of nitroglycerin.

Nitroglycerin-induced decreases in systemic blood pressure depend more on blood volume than do blood pressure changes produced by SNP. Indeed, marked hypotension may occasionally follow sublingual administration of nitroglycerin, especially if the patient is standing, as this position augments venous pooling and further decreases cardiac output. Excessive decreases in diastolic blood pressure may decrease coronary blood flow. These decreases in diastolic blood pressure may also evoke baroreceptor-mediated reflex increases in sympathetic nervous system activity manifesting as tachycardia and increased myocardial contractility. The combination of decreased coronary blood flow and changes that increase myocardial oxygen requirements may provoke angina pectoris in susceptible patients.

Calculated systemic vascular resistance is usually relatively unaffected by nitroglycerin. Pulmonary vascular resistance is, however, consistently decreased, presumably reflecting a direct relaxant of nitroglycerin on pulmonary vasculature (Tinker and Michenfelder, 1976). The principal limitation for using nitroglycerin to treat pulmonary hypertension is the rapid development of tolerance. Similar to other vasodilators, nitroglycerin will inhibit hypoxic pulmonary vasoconstriction and worsen gas exchange in patients with ARDS.

Nitroglycerin primarily dilates larger conductance vessels of the coronary circulation, often leading to an increase in coronary blood flow to ischemic subendocardial areas. In contrast, SNP may produce a coronary steal phenomenon. Indeed, the frequency of S-T segment elevation on the ECG during acute coronary artery occlusion in dogs is decreased by nitroglycerin but increased by SNP (Chiariello et al., 1976). Therefore, nitroglycerin has been recommended for the treatment of hypertension in patients with coronary artery disease (Kaplan et al., 1976).

Nitroglycerin produces a dose-related prolongation of bleeding time that parallels the decrease in systemic blood pressure (Fig. 16-11) (Lichtenthal et al., 1985). As with SNP, increased intracellular concentrations of cGMP produced by nitroglycerin have been shown to inhibit platelet aggregation (Brodde et al., 1982). Increased bleeding time could also be the result of vasodilation secondary to a direct effect of nitroglycerin on vascular tone.

Clinical Uses

Angina Pectoris

Sublingual nitroglycerin, 0.3 mg, is the most useful of the organic nitrates for the acute and chronic treatment and prevention of angina pectoris because of atherosclerotic coronary artery disease or coronary artery vasospasm (Parker and Parker, 1998). Failure of three sublingual tablets in a 15-minute period to relieve angina pectoris may reflect myocardial infarction. Other, more expensive, sublingual nitrates do not appear to be more effective than nitroglycerin (see the section on Isosorbide Dinitrate). Application of 2% nitroglycerin ointment produces sustained protection from angina pectoris for up to 4 hours. Nitroglycerin, 0.5 to 1.0 μg/kg per minute IV, has not been documented to prevent changes of myocardial ischemia on the ECG of patients anesthetized with nitrous oxide-fentanyl and paralyzed with pancuronium (Gallagher et al., 1986; Thomson et al., 1984). Nitroglycerin does, however, decrease the incidence of hypertension as may occur during direct laryngoscopy and intubation of the trachea.

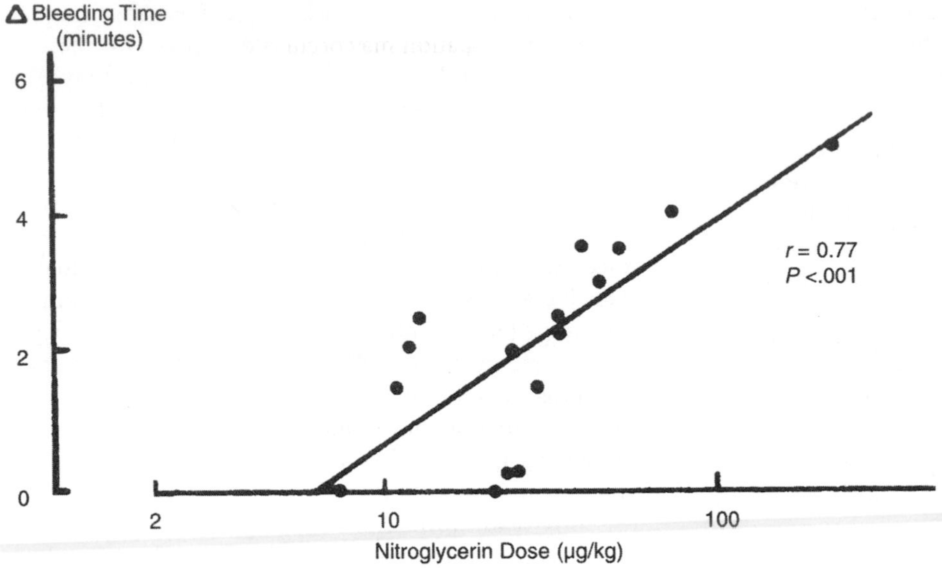

Figure 16-11. Nitroglycerin produces dose-related increases in bleeding time. (From Lichtenthal PR, Rossi EC, Louis G, et al. Dose-related prolongation of the bleeding time by intravenous nitroglycerin. *Anesth Analg* 1985;64:30–33; with permission.)

Mechanism of Action

The ability of nitroglycerin to decrease myocardial oxygen requirements is the most likely mechanism by which this drug relieves angina pectoris in patients with atherosclerotic disease of the coronary arteries. For example, nitroglycerin-induced venodilation and increased venous capacitance decreases venous return (preload) to the heart, resulting in decreased ventricular end-diastolic pressure and volume and, therefore, decreased myocardial oxygen requirements. In addition, any drug-induced decrease in systemic vascular resistance decreases afterload and myocardial oxygen requirements. Nitroglycerin does not increase total coronary blood flow in patients with angina pectoris due to atherosclerosis.

The ability of nitroglycerin to dilate selectively large conductive coronary arteries may be an important mechanism in the relief of angina pectoris due to vasospasm. Specifically, nitroglycerin appears to cause redistribution of coronary blood flow to ischemic areas of subendocardium by selective dilation of large epicardial vessels. Indeed, nitroglycerin increases the washout rate of radioactive xenon from ischemic areas of the ventricle, indicating that blood flow to this region has increased. Nitroglycerin, in contrast to SNP, may decrease the area of damage associated with a myocardial infarction, presumably by preferentially diverting blood flow to the ischemic area.

Side Effects

Headache is common and may be severe after administration of sublingual nitroglycerin. Presumably, headache reflects dilation of meningeal vessels. Vascular dilatation in the face and neck manifests as facial flushing. Tolerance, which occurs with frequent exposure to high doses of organic nitrates, does not develop with the intermittent sublingual administration of nitroglycerin as used to treat angina pectoris. Nitroglycerin may decrease sensitivity to heparin by interfering with the binding of heparin to antithrombin III. It is possible that achievement of a desired anticoagulant endpoint will require an increased dose of heparin in the presence of nitroglycerin, whereas excessive heparin-induced effects could accompany discontinuation of nitroglycerin.

Acute Coronary Syndrome

Routine administration of intravenous nitroglycerin to patients receiving early thrombolytic therapy is probably not beneficial. Intravenous administration of nitroglycerin is most likely to be beneficial in patients with persistent or recurrent angina pectoris after reperfusion therapy and in patients in whom reperfusion therapy is not administered. In these patients, nitroglycerin may improve regional myocardial function and decrease infarct size. Nitroglycerin should be administered cautiously in patients with suspected right ventricular infarction as these patients are highly dependent on preload and may become acutely hypotensive when vasodilation from nitroglycerin occurs. Inhibition of platelet adherence and aggregation by nitroglycerin should be beneficial in decreasing thrombosis within coronary arteries.

Cardiac Failure

Nitroglycerin primarily decreases preload and relieves pulmonary edema. Infusion of nitroglycerin to patients with acute myocardial infarction can improve cardiac output, relieve pulmonary congestion, and decrease myocardial oxygen requirements, thus potentially limiting the size of the myocardial infarction.

Acute Hypertension

Nitroglycerin may be effective in controlling acute increases in systemic blood pressure that may accompany noxious stimulation in the parturient, as during cesarean section (Snyder et al., 1979). This drug crosses the placenta because of its low molecular weight (227) and nonionized state but should not produce adverse metabolic or CNS effects in the fetus. Conversely, a theoretical concern exists about the possible adverse effects of cyanide that is detectable in fetal blood after administration of SNP to the mother.

Controlled Hypotension

Nitroglycerin can be used to produce controlled hypotension, but it is less potent than SNP. For example, equivalent decreases in systemic blood pressure are achieved by the continuous infusion of nitroglycerin, 4.7 μg/kg per minute, and SNP, 2.5 μg/kg per minute (Fahmy, 1978). At comparable systolic blood pressures, the mean and diastolic blood pressures are higher with nitroglycerin than with SNP. Evidence of myocardial ischemia may appear on the ECG during infusion of SNP, presumably reflecting the impact of decreased diastolic blood pressure on coronary blood flow (Fahmy, 1978). Because nitroglycerin acts predominantly on venous capacitance vessels, the production of controlled hypotension using this drug may be more dependent on intravascular fluid volume compared with SNP. Low intracranial compliance restricts the use of nitroglycerin before opening the dura.

Sphincter of Oddi Spasm

Nitroglycerin can relax vascular smooth muscles, including those in the gastrointestinal tract, and may have a dilating effect on the sphincter of Oddi. In this regard, spasm of the sphincter of Oddi, as may occur during laparoscopic cholecystectomy, is effectively treated with intravenous nitroglycerin (Toyoyama et al., 2001). Pain that mimics angina pectoris but is due to opioid-induced biliary tract spasm may be relieved by nitroglycerin. Relief of this pain by nitroglycerin may lead to the incorrect conclusion that myocardial ischemia had been present.

ERECTILE DYSFUNCTION DRUGS

Erectile dysfunction drugs act as selective inhibitors of cGMP-specific phosphodiesterase type 5, which is the predominant enzyme metabolizing cGMG in the corpus cavernosum (Goldstein et al., 1998). By selectively inhibiting cGMP catabolism in cavernosal smooth muscle cells, erectile dysfunction drugs may restore the natural erectile response to sexual stimulation. Consistent with their known effects on cGMP, erectile dysfunction drugs can potentiate the hypotensive effects of nitrates. For this reason, concurrent administration of nitroglycerin and erectile dysfunction drugs within 24 hours is not recommended as life-threatening hypotension from exaggerated systemic vasodilation may occur (Cheitlin et al., 1999).

ISOSORBIDE DINITRATE

Isosorbide dinitrate is a commonly administered oral nitrate for the prophylaxis of angina pectoris. Given orally, isosorbide dinitrate is well absorbed from the gastrointestinal tract. It exerts a physiologic effect lasting up to 6 hours when taken in large doses of 60 to 120 mg. The longer-acting sustained release form provides a prolonged antianginal effect and improves exercise tolerance for up to 6 hours. Isosorbide dinitrate may also be administered sublingually, producing an effect lasting up to 2 hours.

Isosorbide dinitrate has predominant effects on the venous circulation and improves regional distribution of myocardial blood flow in patients with coronary artery disease. The metabolite of isosorbide dinitrate, isosorbide-5-mononitrate, is more active than the parent compound. Orthostatic hypotension accompanies acute administration of isosorbide dinitrate, but tolerance to this and other pharmacologic effects seems to develop with chronic therapy.

HYDRALAZINE

Hydralazine is a direct systemic arterial vasodilator that activates guanylate cyclase to produce vasorelaxation (see Chapter 16). Arterial vasodilation may produce reflex sympathetic nervous system stimulation with resulting increases in heart rate and myocardial contractility. The accompanying increase in cardiac output may increase pulmonary artery pressure if pulmonary vasodilation does not occur. The use of hydralazine to treat pulmonary hypertension is not recommended since accompanying systemic vasodilation may result in severe systemic hypotension.

DIPYRIDAMOLE

Dipyridamole is most often administered in combination with warfarin to patients with prosthetic heart valves as prophylaxis against thromboembolism (Fig. 16-12). This

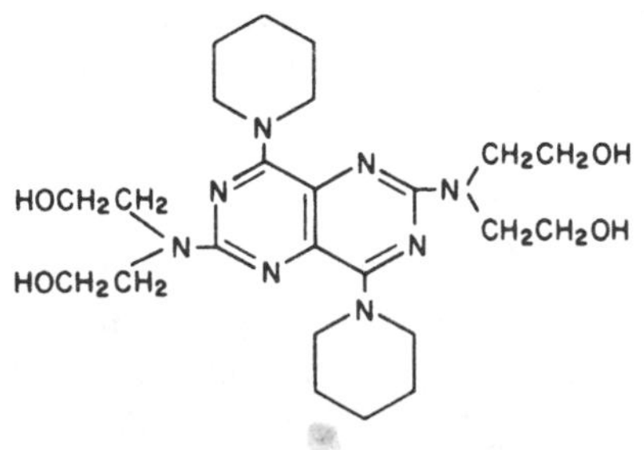

Figure 16-12. Dipyridamole.

clinical use reflects the ability of dipyridamole, like aspirin, to inhibit platelet aggregation. Dipyridamole may interfere with platelet function by potentiating the effect of prostacyclin or by inhibiting phosphodiesterase enzyme activity, thus increasing intracellular concentrations of cyclic adenosine monophosphate (cAMP).

Dipyridamole may also be administered orally as prophylaxis against angina pectoris. In this regard, dipyridamole decreases coronary vascular resistance by acting principally on small resistance vessels in the coronary circulation, with little effect on resistance to flow in ischemic areas of the myocardium where blood vessels are already maximally dilated. These actions of dipyridamole are linked to the metabolism and transport of adenosine and adenine nucleotides. Adenosine is released from ischemic myocardium, acting as a vasodilator and an important signal for the autoregulation of coronary artery blood flow. Indeed, dipyridamole inhibits cellular uptake of adenosine.

PAPAVERINE

Papaverine is a nonspecific smooth muscle relaxant present in opium but unrelated chemically or pharmacologically to the opioid alkaloids (Fig. 16-13). It is possible that papaverine-induced vasodilation is related to its ability to inhibit phosphodiesterase, leading to increased intracellular concentrations of cAMP. Papaverine has not been demonstrated to be efficacious in any condition.

TRIMETHAPHAN

Trimethaphan is a peripheral vasodilator and ganglionic blocker that enjoyed some initial popularity for production of controlled hypotension but its use has been abandoned in favor of drugs such as SNP and nitroglycerin. Trimethaphan acts rapidly but so briefly that it must be administered as a continuous infusion. Because trimethaphan directly relaxes capacitance vessels and blocks autonomic nervous system reflexes, it lowers systemic blood pressure by decreasing cardiac output and systemic vascular resistance (Harioka et al., 1984). Histamine release does not contribute to decreases in blood pressure produced by trimethaphan (Fahmy and Soter, 1985). In contrast to SNP, trimethaphan-induced decreases in blood pressure are not associated with increases in plasma concentrations of catecholamines and renin, reflecting the effects of ganglionic blockade (see Fig. 16-6) (Knight et al., 1983). Increases in heart rate secondary to the administration of trimethaphan most likely reflect parasympathetic nervous system ganglionic blockade.

Ganglionic blockade produced by trimethaphan reflects occupation of receptors normally responsive to acetylcholine as well as stabilization of postsynaptic membranes against the actions of acetylcholine liberated from presynaptic nerve endings. The route of metabolism of trimethaphan is unclear, although hydrolysis by plasma cholinesterase has been suggested. As a quaternary ammonium drug, trimethaphan has a limited ability to cross the blood-brain barrier, and CNS effects are unlikely.

Mydriasis, decreased gastrointestinal activity including ileus, and urinary retention reflecting ganglionic blockade accompany administration of trimethaphan. Drug-induced mydriasis interferes with neurologic evaluation of patients after intracranial surgery.

DIAZOXIDE

Diazoxide, a benzothiadiazine derivative, is related chemically to the thiazide diuretics (Fig. 16-14). This drug is used to treat acute systemic blood pressure increases, as in patients with accelerated and severe hypertension associated with glomerulonephritis. For example, diazoxide, 1 to 3 mg/kg IV (30 mg miniboluses up to 150 mg in a single injection), administered to a hypertensive patient produces a decrease in systolic and diastolic blood pressure within 1 to 2 minutes that lasts 6 to 7 hours. The drug can be repeated at intervals of 5 to 15 minutes. Diazoxide is highly protein bound, and it was previously thought that the drug had to be given as a bolus to exceed the binding capacity of albumin. Subsequent experience has shown that an adequate therapeutic response can be obtained with a slower infusion (Garrett and Kaplan, 1982). Diazoxide is eliminated principally as unchanged drug by the kidneys, with an elimination half-time of 28 hours. Although excessive systemic blood pressure decreases are unlikely, a disadvantage of diazoxide, compared with SNP, is the inability to titrate the dose of this drug in accordance with the patient's response.

Cardiovascular Effects

Diazoxide-induced decreases in systemic blood pressure are associated with significant increases in cardiac output

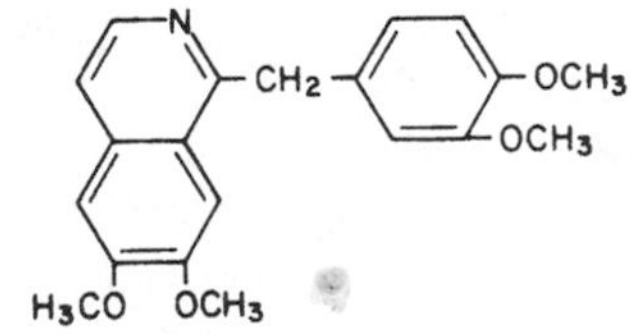

Figure 16-13. Papaverine.

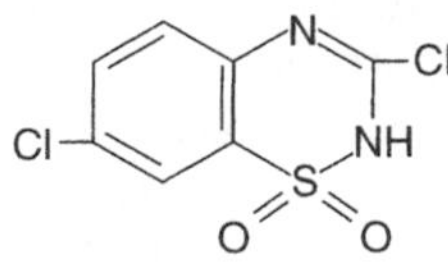

Figure 16-14. Diazoxide.

and often an increase in heart rate. Systemic vascular resistance is decreased. Because diazoxide increases cardiac output and left ventricular ejection velocity, this drug is not likely to be recommended for the treatment of hypertension associated with a dissecting aortic aneurysm. Excessive hypotension that evokes reflex sympathetic nervous system stimulation resulting in myocardial ischemia could occur in these patients. The hypotensive effect of diazoxide may be accentuated in patients receiving beta-adrenergic antagonists because baroreceptor-mediated reflex increases in sympathetic nervous system activity (increased heart rate and cardiac output) are attenuated or prevented. The principal site of action of diazoxide is on the arteriolar resistance rather than venous capacitance vessels.

Side Effects

Unlike thiazide diuretics, diazoxide causes sodium and water retention, which may result in congestive heart failure in susceptible patients. This effect may necessitate concomitant administration of a thiazide diuretic. Retention of sodium occurs independently of decreases in glomerular filtration rate and renal blood flow that predictably accompany diazoxide-induced decreases in systemic blood pressure. Diazoxide is a powerful uterine relaxant and is capable of stopping labor. Hyperglycemia can occur 4 to 5 hours after a single IV injection, reflecting a drug-induced alpha-adrenergic agonist-like inhibition of insulin release from the pancreas. Thiazide diuretics may enhance the hyperglycemic effects of diazoxide. Blood glucose concentrations should be monitored daily during chronic use of diazoxide, as hyperglycemic, hyperosmolar, nonketoacidotic coma has occurred. Stimulation of catecholamine release prohibits the use of diazoxide in patients with pheochromocytoma.

PURINES

Adenosine

Adenosine is an endogenous nucleoside present in all cells of the body. It is formed as a product of enzymatic breakdown of either adenosine triphosphate or S-adenosylhomocysteine (Fig. 16-15). The precise function of endogenous adenosine is unknown, but its actions tend to maintain the balance between oxygen delivery and oxygen demand in the heart and other organs (Camm and Garratt, 1991).

Adenosine is a potent dilator of coronary arteries and is capable of decreasing myocardial oxygen consumption by its antiadrenergic and negative chronotropic actions. Consequently, adenosine can be viewed as a locally acting metabolite that has a homeostatic role in protecting the heart against hypoxia. The half-time of endogenously released adenosine is very brief (0.6 to 1.5 seconds) because of its deamination to inosine in the plasma and its uptake by erythrocytes. The principal electrophysiologic actions of adenosine on supraventricular tissues (sinoatrial node and atrium) are mediated by stimulation of potassium channels (identical to those stimulated by acetylcholine), resulting in hyperpolarization of atrial myocytes and a decrease in the diastolic depolarization (phase 4) of the pacemaker cells of the sinoatrial node. Ventricular myocytes do not possess these adenosine-sensitive potassium channels.

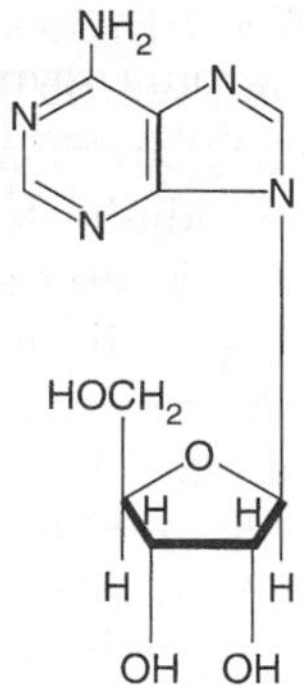

Figure 16-15. Adenosine.

Clinical Uses

Adenosine is administered clinically as an alternative to verapamil to treat paroxysmal supraventricular tachycardia as well as to aid in the diagnosis of tachydysrhythmias (Camm and Garratt, 1991). In addition, its vasodilatory effects make it a potentially useful drug for inducing controlled hypotension and as an alternative to dipyridamole for pharmacologic stress testing (O'Keefe et al., 1992; Owall et al., 1987).

Supraventricular Tachycardia

Adenosine is administered as an alternative to verapamil to terminate paroxysmal supraventricular tachycardia and narrow complex regular tachycardia when the diagnosis (atrial or junctional) is in doubt (Camm and Garratt, 1991). For adult patients, the initial dose is 6 mg IV, followed by 12 mg IV if the first dose is ineffective. A further dose of 18 mg IV may be given if the 12-mg dose is ineffective but well tolerated by the patient. Lower initial doses should be given to patients receiving concomitant dipyridamole therapy (blocks nucleoside transport) or who have undergone cardiac transplantation, because of supersensitivity to adenosine. Because of its very brief elimination half-time, intervals between doses can be as short as 60 seconds without risking a cumulative effect. In a child, adenosine, 0.2 mg/kg IV, has been reported to be effective for terminating supraventricular tachycardia during anesthesia (Litman et al., 1991). Continuous ECG monitoring and the availability of equipment for cardioversion are necessary in patients being treated with adenosine.

Adenosine is not effective in the treatment of atrial flutter, atrial fibrillation, and ventricular tachycardia. In the absence of a functioning artificial cardiac pacemaker, adenosine should not be administered in the presence of second- or third-degree atrioventricular heart block or in the presence of sick sinus syndrome. Adenosine administered rapidly to an awake patient may be associated with dyspnea, flushing, and chest pain. Bronchospasm may accompany IV administration of adenosine, particularly to patients with pre-existing airway hypersensitivity (Bennett-Guerrero and Young, 1994).

Controlled Hypotension

Adenosine-induced controlled hypotension is characterized by the rapid onset and stable level of hypotension that is promptly reversed when the infusion is discontinued (Sollevi et al., 1984). Rapid recovery of systemic blood pressure reflects the brief elimination half-time of adenosine. During controlled hypotension produced by adenosine, there is a large decrease in systemic vascular resistance and a modest increase in heart rate. Cardiac output is enhanced, coronary sinus blood flow is increased, and cardiac filling pressures are maintained, suggesting the absence of negative inotropic effects and minimal changes in venous capacitance and venous return to the heart (Bloor et al., 1985). The rate of adenosine infusion required to produce controlled hypotension (approximately 220 μg/kg per minute) is unlikely to result in plasma concentrations that alter cardiac automaticity or conduction of cardiac impulses (Owall et al., 1987). Furthermore, the necessary infusion rate of adenosine can be decreased by about one third when patients are pretreated with an adenosine uptake inhibitor, such as dipyridamole (Sollevi et al., 1984).

The unchanged adenosine infusion requirements to maintain sustained decreases in blood pressure for as long as 2 hours confirm the absence of tachyphylaxis. Likewise, plasma concentrations of renin and catecholamines do not increase, which is again consistent with unchanging adenosine dose requirements and the absence of rebound hypertension when the infusion is discontinued (Bloor et al., 1985; Owall et al., 1987). Acid-base disturbances do not accompany adenosine-induced hypotension. Uric acid levels may increase 10% to 20% when adenosine is used for controlled hypotension, suggesting caution in selecting this drug for patients with a purine metabolic disturbance such as gout (Owall et al., 1987).

Acadesine

Acadesine is a purine nucleoside analogue that may decrease myocardial ischemic injury by selectively increasing the availability of adenosine in ischemic tissues. In this regard, acadesine limits the severity of postbypass myocardial ischemia (Leung et al., 1994). Uric acid is a metabolite of acadesine, and plasma uric acid concentrations may increase slightly in treated patients.

REFERENCES

Abe K. Vasodilators during cerebral aneurysm surgery. *Can J Anaesth* 1993;40:775–790.

Adhikari N, Granton JT. Inhaled nitric oxide for acute lung injury. No place for NO? *JAMA* 2004;291:1629–1631.

Becker LC. Conditions for vasodilator-induced coronary steal in experimental myocardial ischemia. *Circulation* 1978;57:1103–1110.

Bennett-Guerrero E, Young CC. Bronchospasm after intravenous adenosine administration. *Anesth Analg* 1994;79:386–388.

Berthelsen P, St. Haxholdt O, Husum R, et al. PEEP reverses nitroglycerin-induced hypoxemia following coronary artery bypass surgery. *Acta Anaesthesiol Scand* 1986;30:243–246.

Bigatello LM, Hess D, Dennehy KC, et al. Sildenafil can increase the response to inhaled nitric oxide. *Anesthesiology* 2000;92:1827–1829.

Bloor BC, Fukunaga AF, Ma C, et al. Myocardial hemodynamics during induced hypotension: a comparison between sodium nitroprusside and adenosine triphosphate. *Anesthesiology* 1985;63:517–525.

Brodde OE, Anlauf M, Graben N, et al. In vitro and in vivo down-regulation of human platelet $alpha_2$-adrenoreceptors by clonidine. *Eur J Clin Pharmacol* 1982;23:403–409.

Byrick RJ, Hobbs EG, Martineau R, et al. Nitroglycerin relaxes large airways. *Anesth Analg* 1983;62:421–425.

Camm AJ, Garratt CJ. Adenosine and supraventricular tachycardia. *N Engl J Med* 1991;325:1621–1629.

Casthely PA, Lear S, Cottrell JE, et al. Intrapulmonary shunting during induced hypotension. *Anesth Analg* 1982;61:231–235.

Chauvin M, Bonnet F, Montembault C, et al. Hepatic plasma flow during sodium nitroprusside-induced hypotension in humans. *Anesthesiology* 1985;63:287–293.

Cheitlin MD, Hutter AM, Brindis RG, et al. ACC/AHA expert consensus document: use of sildenafil (Viagra) in patients with cardiovascular disease. *J Am Coll Cardiol* 1999;33:273–281.

Chiariello M, Gold HK, Leinbach RC, et al. Comparison between the effects of nitroprusside and nitroglycerin on ischemic injury during acute myocardial infarction. *Circulation* 1976;54:766–773.

Cohn JN. The management of chronic heart failure. *N Engl J Med* 1996; 335:490–498.

Colley PS, Cheney FW Jr, Hlastala MP. Ventilation-perfusion and gas exchange effects of sodium nitroprusside in dogs with normal and edematous lungs. *Anesthesiology* 1979;50:489–495.

Curry SC, Arnold-Capell P. Toxic effects of drugs used in the ICU. Nitroprusside, nitroglycerin, and angiotensin-converting enzyme inhibitors. *Crit Care Clin* 1991;7:555–581.

Davies DW, Greiss L, Steward DJ. Sodium nitroprusside in children: observations on metabolism during normal and abnormal responses. *Can Anaesth Soc J* 1975;22:553–560.

Delaney TJ, Miller ED. Rebound hypertension after sodium nitroprusside prevented by saralism in rats. *Anesthesiology* 1980;52:154–156.

Dietrich GV, Hessen M, Boldt J, et al. Platelet function, and adrenoceptors during and after induced hypotension using nitroprusside. *Anesthesiology* 1996;85:1334–1340.

Dzoljic MR, DeVries R. Nitric oxide synthase inhibition reduces wakefulness. *Neuropharmacology* 1994;33:1505–1509.

Fahmy NR. Nitroglycerin as a hypotensive drug during general anesthesia. *Anesthesiology* 1978;49:17–20.

Fibuch EE, Cecil WT, Reed WA. Methemoglobinemia associated with organic nitrate therapy. *Anesth Analg* 1979;58:521–523.

Food and Drug Administration. New labeling for sodium nitroprusside emphasized risk of cyanide toxicity. *JAMA* 1991;265:487.

Francis GS. Vasodilators in the intensive care unit. *Am Heart J* 1991;121:1875–1878.

Friederich JA, Butterworth JF. Sodium nitroprusside: twenty years and counting. *Anesth Analg* 1995;81:152–162.

Gagnon RL, Marsh ML, Smith RW, et al. Intracranial hypertension caused by nitroglycerin. *Anesthesiology* 1979;51:86–87.

Gallagher JD, Moore RA, Jose AB, et al. Prophylactic nitroglycerin infusions during coronary artery bypass surgery. *Anesthesiology* 1986;64:785–789.

Garrett BN, Kaplan NM. Efficacy of slow infusion of diazoxide in treatment of severe hypertension without organ hypoperfusion. *Am Heart J* 1982;103:390–394.

Gerson JI, Allen FB, Seltzer JL, et al. Arterial and venous dilation by nitroprusside and nitroglycerin—is there a difference? *Anesth Analg* 1982;61:256–260.

Goldstein I, Lue TF, Padma-Nathan H, et al. Oral sildenafil in the treatment of erectile dysfunction. *N Engl J Med* 1998;338:1397–1404.
Haddad E, Lowson SM, Johns RA, et al. Use of inhaled nitric oxide perioperatively and in intensive care patients. *Anesthesiology* 2000;92:1821–1825.
Hall AH, Rumack BH. Hydroxocobalamin/sodium thiosulfate as a cyanide antidote. *J Emerg Med* 1987;5:115–121.
Hines R, Barash PG. Infusion of sodium nitroprusside induces platelet dysfunction in vitro. *Anesthesiology* 1989;70:611–615.
Ikeda S, Schweiss JF, Frank PA, et al. In vitro cyanide release from sodium nitroprusside. *Anesthesiology* 1987;66:381–385.
Johns RA. Nitric oxide, cyclic guanosine monophosphate, and the anesthetic state. *Anesthesiology* 1996;85:457–459.
Kaplan JA, Dunbar RW, Jones EL. Nitroglycerin infusion during coronary artery surgery. *Anesthesiology* 1976;45:14–21.
Kaplan JA, Finlayson DC, Woodward S. Vasodilator therapy after cardiac surgery: a review of the efficacy and toxicity of nitroglycerin and nitroprusside. *Can Anaesth Soc J* 1980;27:154–158.
Khambatta HJ, Stone G, Khan E. Hypertension during anesthesia on discontinuation of sodium nitroprusside-induced hypotension. *Anesthesiology* 1979;51:127–130.
Kinsella JP, Neish SR, Sheffer E, et al. Low-dose inhalational nitric oxide in persistent pulmonary hypertension of the newborn. *Lancet* 1992;340:819–820.
Knight PR, Lane GA, Hensinger RN, et al. Catecholamine and renin-angiotensin response during hypotensive anesthesia induced by sodium nitroprusside or trimethaphan camsylate. *Anesthesiology* 1983;59:248–253.
Leung JM, Stanley T, Mathew J, et al. An initial multicenter, randomized controlled trial on the safety and efficacy of acadesine in patients undergoing coronary artery bypass graft surgery. *Anesth Analg* 1994;78:420–434.
Lichtenthal PR, Rossi EC, Louis G, et al. Dose-related prolongation of the bleeding time by intravenous nitroglycerin. *Anesth Analg* 1985;64:30–33.
Litman RS, Keon TP, Campbell FW. Termination of supraventricular tachycardia with adenosine in a healthy child undergoing anesthesia. *Anesth Analg* 1991;73:665–667.
Marsh ML, Aidinis SJ, Naughton KVH, et al. The technique of nitroprusside administration modifies the intracranial pressure response. *Anesthesiology* 1979;51:538–541.
Meller ST, Pechman PS, Gebhart GF, et al. Nitric oxide mediates the thermal hyperalgesia produced in a model of neuropathic pain in the rat. *Neuroscience* 1992;50:7–10.
Michenfelder JD, Theye RA. Canine systemic and cerebral effects of hypotension induced by hemorrhage, trimethaphan, halothane, or nitroprusside. *Anesthesiology* 1977;46:188–195.
Miller JR, Benumof JL, Trousdale FR. Combined effects of sodium nitroprusside and propranolol on hypoxic pulmonary vasoconstriction. *Anesthesiology* 1982;57:267–271.
Moncada S, Higgs A. The L-arginine-nitric oxide pathway. *N Engl J Med* 1993;329:2002–2012.
Moore RA, Geller EA, Gallagher JD, et al. Effect of hypothermic cardiopulmonary bypass on nitroprusside metabolism. *Clin Pharmacol Ther* 1985;37:680–683.
Nakamura K, Mori K. Nitric oxide and anesthesia. *Anesth Analg* 1993;77:877–879.
Neonatal Inhaled Nitric Oxide Study Group. Inhaled nitric oxide in full-term and nearly full-term infants with hypoxic respiratory failure. *N Engl J Med* 1997;336:597–604.
Noback CR, Tinker JR. Hypothermia after cardiopulmonary bypass in man: amelioration by nitroprusside-induced vasodilation during rewarming. *Anesthesiology* 1980;53:277–280.
O'Keefe JH, Bateman TM, Silvestri RT, et al. Safety and diagnostic accuracy of adenosine thallium-201 scintigraphy in patients unable to exercise and those with left bundle branch block. *Am Heart J* 1992;124:614–621.
Owall A, Gordon E, Lagerkranser M, et al. Clinical experience with adenosine for controlled hypotension during cerebral aneurysm surgery. *Anesth Analg* 1987;66:229–234.
Parker JD, Parker JO. Nitrate therapy for stable angina pectoris. *N Engl J Med* 1998;338:520–526.
Quinn AC, Petros DL, Valance P. Nitric oxide: an endogenous gas. *Br J Anaesth* 1995;74:443–451.
Rich GF, Murphy GD, Roos CM, et al. Inhaled nitric oxide: selective pulmonary vasodilation in cardiac surgical patients. *Anesthesiology* 1993;78:1028–1035.
Rizzi RR, Thomas K, Pilnik S. Factious desaturation due to isosulfan dye injection. *Anesthesiology* 2000;93:1146–1147.
Roberts JD, Fineman JR, Morin CF, et al. Inhaled nitric oxide and persistent pulmonary hypertension of the newborn. *N Engl J Med* 1997;336:605–610.
Rogers AT, Prough DS, Gravlee GP, et al. Sodium nitroprusside infusion does not dilate cerebral resistance vessels during hypothermic cardiopulmonary bypass. *Anesthesiology* 1991;74:820–826.
Rogers MC, Hamburger C, Owen K, et al. Intracranial pressure in the cat during nitroglycerin induced hypotension. *Anesthesiology* 1979;51:227–229.
Samama CM, Diaby M, Fellahi JL, et al. Inhibition of platelet aggregation by inhaled nitric oxide in patients with acute respiratory distress syndrome. *Anesthesiology* 1995;83:56–65.
Schreiber MD, Gin-Mestan, Marks JD, et al. Inhaled nitric oxide in premature infants with respiratory distress syndrome. *N Engl J Med* 2003;349:2099–2107.
Schroeder RA, Kuo PC. Nitric oxide: physiology and pharmacology. *Anesth Analg* 1995;81:1052–1059.
Sivarajan M, Amory DW, McKenzie SM. Regional blood flows during induced hypotension produced by nitroprusside or trimethaphan in the rhesus monkey. *Anesth Analg* 1985;64:759–766.
Sprung J, Tully M, Ziser A. Anaphylactic reactions to isosulfan blue dye during sentinel node lymphadenectomy for breast cancer. *Anesth Analg* 2003;96;1051–1053.
Snyder SW, Wheeler AS, James FM. The use of nitroglycerin to control severe hypertension of pregnancy during cesarean section. *Anesthesiology* 1979;51:563–564.
Sollevi A, Lagerkranser M, Irestedt L, et al. Controlled hypotension with adenosine in cerebral aneurysm surgery. *Anesthesiology* 1984;61:400–405.
Stoelting RK. Attenuation of blood pressure response to laryngoscopy and tracheal intubation with sodium nitroprusside. *Anesth Analg* 1979;58:116–119.
Taylor RW, Zimmerman JL, Dellinger RP, et al. Low-dose inhaled nitric oxide in patients with acute lung injury: a randomized controlled trial. *JAMA* 2004;291:1603–1609.
Thomson IR, Mutch WAC, Culligan JD. Failure of intravenous nitroglycerin to prevent intraoperative myocardial ischemia during fentanyl-pancuronium anesthesia. *Anesthesiology* 1984;61:385–393.
Tinker JH, Michenfelder JD. Sodium nitroprusside: pharmacology, toxicity and therapeutics. *Anesthesiology* 1976;45:340–354.
Tinker JH, Michenfelder JD. Increased resistance to nitroprusside-induced cyanide toxicity in anuric dogs. *Anesthesiology* 1980;52:40–47.
Toyoyama H, Kariya N, Hase I et al. The use of intravenous nitroglycerin in a case of spasm of the sphincter of Oddi during laparoscopic cholecystectomy. *Anesthesiology* 2001;94:708–709.
Troncy E, Francoeur M, Blaise G. Inhaled nitric oxide: clinical applications, indications, and toxicology. *Can J Anaesth* 1997;44:973–988.
Turner JM, Powell D, Gibson RM. Intracranial pressure changes in neurosurgical patients during hypotension induced with sodium nitroprusside or trimethaphan. *Br J Anaesth* 1977;49:419–424.
Wang HH, Liu LMP, Katz RI. A comparison of the cardiovascular effects of sodium nitroprusside and trimethaphan. *Anesthesiology* 1977;46:40–48.
Young JD, Brampton WJ, Knighton JD, et al. Inhaled nitric oxide in acute respiratory failure in adults. *Br J Anaesth* 1994;73:499–502.
Young JD, Roberts M, Gale LB. Laboratory evaluation of the 1-NOvent nitric oxide delivery device. *Br J Anaesth* 1997;79:398–401.
Zerbe NF, Wagner BK. Use of vitamin B_{12} in the treatment and prevention of nitroprusside-induced cyanide toxicity. *Crit Care Med* 1993;21:465–467.
Zurick AM, Wagner RH, Starr NJ, et al. Intravenous nitroglycerin, methemoglobinemia, and respiratory distress in a postoperative cardiac surgical patient. *Anesthesiology* 1984;61:464–466.

Cardiac Antidysrhythmic Drugs

17

Cardiac dysrhythmias occur in the perioperative period, manifesting most often as atrial fibrillation following cardiac surgery and less often as ventricular dysrhythmias (Atlee, 1997; Creswell et al., 1993). The use of antidysrhythmic drugs for treatment and prevention of cardiac dysrhythmias is limited by the potential for these drugs to depress left ventricular contractility and the triggering of new dysrhythmias (Ben-David and Zipes, 1993) (see the section, Prodysrhythmic Effects). Improved survival for patients receiving implantable cardioverter defibrillator devices compared with antidysrhythmic drugs has altered the treatment paradigms for patients with ventricular dysrhythmias (Zipes, 2001). Likewise, catheter ablation techniques are preferred treatments for many supraventricular dysrhythmias including atrial and certain types of atrial fibrillation (Morady, 1999). For these reasons, pharmacologic treatment of cardiac dysrhythmias is principally used to treat atrial fibrillation and atrial flutter that is not responsive to catheter ablation treatment and for patients with implantable cardioverter-defibrillator devices who are receiving frequent but needed electrical shocks.

Pharmacologic treatment of cardiac dysrhythmias and disturbances in conduction of cardiac impulses with antidysrhythmic drugs is based on an understanding of the electrophysiologic basis of the abnormality and the mechanism of action of the therapeutic drug to be administered (Atlee and Bosnjak, 1990; Atlee, 1997). The two major physiologic mechanisms that cause ectopic cardiac dysrhythmias are reentry and enhanced automaticity. Factors underlying cardiac dysrhythmias associated with either mechanism include arterial hypoxemia, electrolyte and acid-base abnormalities, myocardial ischemia, altered sympathetic nervous system activity, bradycardia, and the administration of certain drugs. It is not commonly appreciated that alkalosis is even more likely than acidosis to trigger cardiac dysrhythmias. Hypokalemia and hypomagnesemia predispose to ventricular dysrhythmias and must be suspected in patients who are being treated with diuretics. Increased sympathetic nervous system activity lowers the threshold for ventricular fibrillation, a phenomenon that is attenuated by beta blockers and vagal stimulation. Bradycardia can lead to ventricular dysrhythmias by causing a temporal dispersion of refractory periods among Purkinje fibers, creating an electrical gradient between adjacent cells. Enlargement of a failing left ventricle stretches individual myocardial cells and can thereby induce cardiac dysrhythmias. A decrease in left ventricular volume by the administration of digitalis, diuretics, or vasodilators helps to control cardiac dysrhythmias that are precipitated by this mechanism.

In many patients, correction of identifiable precipitating events is not sufficient to suppress cardiac ectopic dysrhythmias, and therefore specific cardiac antidysrhythmic drugs may be administered. Drugs administered for the chronic suppression of cardiac dysrhythmias pose little threat to the uneventful course of anesthesia and should be continued up to the time of induction of anesthesia (Atlee, 1997; Lucas et al., 1990). The majority of cardiac dysrhythmias that occur during anesthesia do not require therapy. Cardiac dysrhythmias, however, do require treatment when (a) they cannot be corrected by removing the precipitating cause, (b) hemodynamic function is compromised, and (c) the disturbance predisposes to more serious cardiac dysrhythmias. During the perioperative period, cardiac antidysrhythmic drugs are most often administered by the intravenous (IV) route.

The mechanism of cardiac dysrhythmias may be different with or without anesthesia. For example, anesthetic-related cardiac dysrhythmias have been ascribed to abnormal pacemaker activity characterized by suppression of the sinoatrial node, with the emergence of latent pacemakers within or below the atrioventricular tissues (Atlee and Bosnjak, 1990). Furthermore, development of reentry circuits is likely to be important in the mechanism of cardiac dysrhythmias that occur during anesthesia. Certainly, anesthetics, particularly volatile drugs, may have effects on the specialized conduction system for cardiac impulses.

MECHANISM OF ACTION

Cardiac antidysrhythmic drugs produce pharmacologic effects by blocking passage of ions across sodium, potassium, and calcium ion channels present in the heart (see Fig. 47-1). The cardiac action potential is the result of multiple inward and outward ion currents with specific ion channels responsible for each of the five phases. The duration of each phase of the action potential differs in atrial compared with ventricular myocardium and the specialized systems for conduction of cardiac impulses differ in ion channel density. Ion channels are large membrane-bound glycoproteins that provide a pathway across cell membranes for the passage of ions. Ion channels exist in different states (open, inactivated, closed). In the inactivated state, the ion channel is unresponsive to a continued or new stimulus. The resting state is more prevalent during diastole, the active state occurs during the upstroke of the action potential, and the inactivated state occurs during the plateau phase of repolarization.

The effects of cardiac antidysrhythmic drugs on the action potential and effective refractory period of the cardiac action potential determine the clinical effect of these drugs. Drugs that primarily block inward sodium ion flow will slow conduction and result in suppression of the maximum upstroke velocity (V_{max}) of the cardiac action potential. Potassium-channel blocking drugs prolong repolarization by prolonging the duration of the cardiac action potential and the effective refractory resulting in prolongation of the QTc interval on the ECG. Calcium channels are present in cardiac cells, and the alpha subunit of L and T calcium ion channels is the site of cardiac antidysrhythmic drug action.

CLASSIFICATION

Cardiac antidysrhythmic drugs are most commonly classified into four groups based primarily on the ability of the drug to control dysrhythmias by blocking specific ion channels and currents during the cardiac action potential (Tables 17-1 and 17-2) (Langberg and DeLugrio, 1999; Williams, 1970). Few cardiac antidysrhythmic drugs demonstrate pure effects on cardiac ion channels and other characteristics including the impact of the drug on autonomic nervous system activity and myocardial contractility may be more important clinically. Antidysrhythmic drugs differ in their pharmacokinetics and efficacy in treating specific types of cardiac dysrhythmias (Tables 17-3 and 17-4) (Lucas et al., 1990).

Class I Drugs

Class I drugs inhibit fast sodium channels during depolarization (phase 0) of the cardiac action potential with resultant decreases in depolarization rate and conduction velocity (Fig. 17-1) (Langberg and DeLugrio, 1999).

TABLE 17-1.
CLASSIFICATION OF CARDIAC ANTIDYSRHYTHMIC DRUGS

Class I (Inhibit Fast Sodium Ion Channels)
Class IA
Quinidine
Procainamide
Disopyramide
Moricizine
Class IB
Lidocaine
Tocainide
Mexiletine
Class IC
Flecainide
Propafenone
Class II (Decrease Rate of Depolarization)
Esmolol
Propranolol
Acebutolol
Class III (Inhibit Potassium Ion Channels)
Amiodarone
Sotalol
Ibutilide
Dofetilide
Bretylium
Class IV (Inhibit Slow Calcium Channels)
Verapamil
Diltiazem

Class IA Drugs

Class IA drugs (quinidine, procainamide, disopyramide, moricizine) lengthen both the action potential duration and the effective refractory period reflecting sodium channel inhibition and lengthening of repolarization owing to potassium channel blockade.

Class IB Drugs

Class IB drugs (lidocaine, mexiletine, tocainide, phenytoin) are less powerful sodium channel blockers and unlike Class IA drugs, shorten the action potential duration and refractory period in normal cardiac ventricular muscle. In ischemic tissue, lidocaine may also block adenosine triphosphate (ATP)-dependent channels, thus preventing ischemic-mediated shortening of ventricular depolarization.

Class IC Drugs

Class IC drugs (flecainide, propafenone) are potent sodium-channel blockers and markedly decrease the rate of phase 0 depolarization and speed of conduction of cardiac impulses. These drugs have little effect on the duration of the cardiac action potential and the effective refractory period in ventricular myocardial cells but do shorten the duration of the action potential in Purkinje fibers. This

TABLE 17-2.
ELECTROPHYSIOLOGIC AND ELECTROCARDIOGRAPHIC EFFECTS OF CARDIAC ANTIDYSRHYTHMIC DRUGS

	Class IA	Class IB	Class IC	Class II	Class III	Class IV
Depolarization rate (phase 0)	Decreased	No effect	Greatly decreased	No effect	No effect	No effect
Conduction velocity	Decreased	No effect	Greatly decreased	Decreased	Decreased	No effect
Effective refractory period	Greatly increased	Decreased	Increased	Decreased	Greatly increased	No effect
Action potential duration	Increased	Decreased	Increased	Increased	Greatly increased	Decreased
Automaticity	Decreased	Decreased	Decreased	Decreased	Decreased	No effect
P-R duration	No effect	No effect	Increased	No effect or increased	Increased	No effect or increased
QRS duration	Increased	No effect	Greatly increased	No effect	Increased	No effect
QTc duration	Greatly increased	No effect or decreased	Increased	Decreased	Greatly increased	No effect

inhomogeneity of effects on the rate of cardiac depolarization plus the slowing of cardiac conduction may contribute to the prodysrhythmic effects of these drugs.

Class II Drugs

Class II drugs are represented by beta-adrenergic antagonists. Beta-adrenergic antagonists decrease the rate of spontaneous phase 4 depolarization resulting in decreased autonomic nervous system activity, which may be important in suppression of ventricular dysrhythmias during myocardial ischemia and reperfusion. Drug-induced slowing of heart rate with resulting decreases in myocardial oxygen requirements is desirable in patients with coronary artery disease. Beta-adrenergic antagonists slow the speed of conduction of cardiac impulses through atrial tissues resulting in prolongation of the P-R interval on the electrocardiogram (ECG), whereas the duration of action of the cardiac action potential in ventricular myocardium is not altered. These drugs are effective in decreasing the incidence of dysrhythmia-related morbidity and mortality although the exact mechanism for this beneficial effect remains unclear.

Class III Drugs

Class III drugs (amiodarone, sotalol, bretylium) block potassium ion channels resulting in prolongation of cardiac

TABLE 17-3.
PHARMACOKINETICS OF CARDIAC ANTIDYSRHYTHMIC DRUGS

	Principal Clearance Mechanism	Protein Binding (%)	Elimination Half-Time (hrs)	Therapeutic Plasma Concentration
Quinidine	Hepatic	80–90	5–12	1.2–4.0 μg/mL
Procainamide	Renal/hepatic	15	2.5–5.0	4–8 μg/mL
Disopyramide	Renal/hepatic	15	8–12	2–4 μg/mL
Lidocaine	Hepatic	55	1.4–8.0	1–5 μg/mL
Tocainide	Hepatic/renal	10–30	12–15	4–10 μg/mL
Mexiletine	Hepatic	60–75	6–12	0.75–2.00 μg/mL
Flecainide	Hepatic	30–45	13–30	0.3–1.5 μg/mL
Propafenone	Hepatic	>95	5–8	
Propranolol	Hepatic	90–95	2–4	10–30 ng/mL
Amiodarone	Hepatic	96	8–107 days	1.5–2.0 μg/mL
Sotalol	Renal			
Verapamil	Hepatic	90	4.5–12.0	100–300 ng/mL

TABLE 17-4.
EFFICACY OF CARDIAC ANTIDYSRHYTHMIC DRUGS

	Conversion of Atrial Fibrillation	Paroxysmal Supraventricular Tachycardia	Premature Ventricular Contractions	Ventricular Tachycardia
Quinidine	+	++	++	+
Procainamide	+	++	++	++
Disopyramide	+	++	++	++
Lidocaine	+	0	++	++
Tocainide	0	0	++	++
Mexiletine	0	0	++	++
Moricizine	0	0	++	++
Flecainide	0	+	++	++
Propafenone	0	+	++	++
Propranolol	+	++	+	+
Amiodarone	+	++	++	++
Sotalol	++	+	+	+
Verapamil	+	++	0	0
Diltiazem	+	++	0	0
Digitalis	++	++	0	0
Adenosine	0	++	0	0

0, no effect; +, effective; ++, highly effective

depolarization, action potential duration, and the effective refractory period. These effects are beneficial in preventing cardiac dysrhythmias by decreasing the proportion of the cardiac cycle during which myocardial cells are excitable and thus susceptible to a triggering event. Reentrant tachycardias may be suppressed if the action potential duration becomes longer than the cycle length of the tachycardia circuit.

In addition to class III effects, amiodarone exhibits sodium channel blockade (class I), beta-blockade (class II), and calcium channel blockade (class IV). Sotalol is a racemic mixture of levorotatory (L) and dextrorotatory (D) isomers that possess similar class III effects. In addition, the L isomer of sotalol acts as a beta-adrenergic antagonist whereas the D isomer may increase mortality in patients with ventricular dysfunction and recent myocardial infarction. The lower incidence of prodysrhythmia effects seen with amiodarone or racemic sotalol treatment may be related to beneficial class II effects.

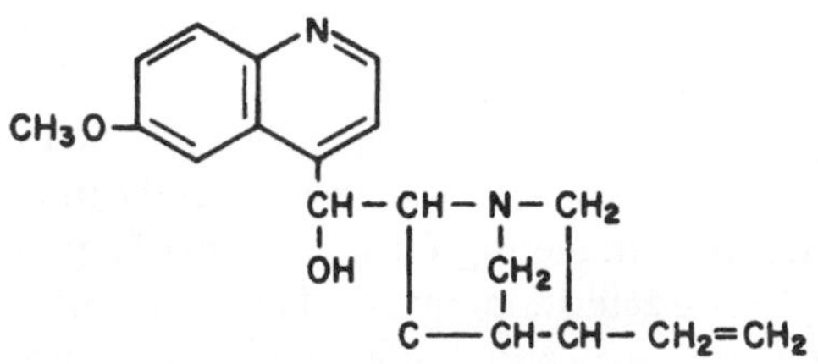

Figure 17-1. Quinidine.

Class IV Drugs

Class IV drugs (verapamil, diltiazem) act by inhibiting inward slow calcium ion currents that may contribute to the development of ventricular tachycardia. As such, these drugs are useful in the treatment of idiopathic ventricular tachycardia.

PRODYSRHYTHMIA EFFECTS

Prodysrhythmia effects describe bradydysrhythmias or tachydysrhythmias that represent new cardiac dysrhythmias associated with chronic antidysrhythmic drug treatment (Ben-David and Zipes, 1993). Types of prodysrhythmias include torsades de pointes, incessant ventricular tachycardia, and wide complex ventricular rhythm (Langberg and DeLugrio, 1999).

Torsades de Pointes

Torsades de pointes (polymorphic ventricular tachycardia and ventricular fibrillation) is the most common prodysrhythmia and is triggered by early-after depolarizations in a setting of delayed repolarization and increased duration of refractoriness manifesting as prolongation of the QTc interval on the ECG. Class IA (quinidine and disopyramide) and class III drugs (amiodarone) prolong the QTc interval by potassium channel blockade provide the setting for torsades de pointes. Drug-induced torsades de pointe is often associated with bradycardia because the QTc interval is longer at slower heart rates. Exacerbating factors such as hypokalemia, hypomagnesemia, poor left ventricular function, and concomitant administration of other QT-prolonging drugs, are important predisposing factors in the development of this prodysrhythmia.

Incessant Ventricular Tachycardia

Incessant ventricular tachycardia may be precipitated by cardiac antidysrhythmic drugs that slow conduction of cardiac impulses (class IA and class IC drugs) sufficiently to create a continuous ventricular tachycardia circuit (reentry). Incessant ventricular tachycardia is more likely to occur with high doses of class IC drugs and in patients with a prior history of sustained ventricular tachycardia and poor left ventricular function. Ventricular tachycardia due to this mechanism is generally slower because of the drug effect but may be resistant to drugs or electrical therapy. This prodysrhythmia is rarely associated with class IB drugs, which have a weaker blocking effect on sodium channels.

Wide Complex Ventricular Rhythm

Wide complex ventricular rhythm is usually associated with class IC cardiac antidysrhythmic drugs in the setting of structural heart disease. Excessive plasma concentrations of the antidysrhythmic drug or an abrupt change in the dose may result in this prodysrhythmia. Wide complex ventricular rhythm is thought to reflect a reentrant tachycardia and easily degenerates to ventricular fibrillation.

EFFICACY AND RESULTS OF TREATMENT WITH CARDIAC ANTIDYSRHYTHMIC DRUGS

Suppression of ventricular ectopy with a cardiac antidysrhythmic drug does not prevent future life-threatening dysrhythmias and may increase mortality (Langberg and DeLugrio, 1999). In fact, patients treated with class IC cardiac antidysrhythmic drugs experienced a higher incidence of sudden cardiac arrest reflecting the prodysrhythmic effects of these drugs. Conversely, beta-adrenergic antagonists that do not typically suppress ventricular dysrhythmias appear to decrease mortality and the risk of life-threatening ventricular dysrhythmias. In patients with a history of myocardial infarction and ventricular dysrhythmias, mortality was increased in those who received class IA and class IC drugs whereas mortality was decreased with amiodarone and beta-adrenergic antagonists (Kennedy et al., 1994). Survivors of cardiac arrest have a high risk of subsequent ventricular fibrillation and treatment of these patients with amiodarone results in fewer life-threatening cardiac events. The prodysrhythmic and negative inotropic effects of class IA and class IC cardiac antidysrhythmic drugs precludes their administration to patients with congestive heart failure. In these patients, administration of amiodarone appears to be safe and may suppress prodysrhythmias.

PROPHYLACTIC ANTIDYSRHYTHMIC THERAPY

Lidocaine is not recommended as prophylactic treatment for patients in the early stages of acute myocardial infarction and without malignant ventricular ectopy (Teo et al., 1993). In fact, lidocaine does not decrease and may increase mortality because of an increase in the occurrence of fatal bradydysrhythmias and asystole.

Calcium-channel antagonists are not recommended as routine treatment of patients with acute myocardial infarction because mortality is not decreased by these drugs. Calcium-channel blockers may be administered to patients in whom myocardial ischemia persists despite treatment with aspirin, heparin, nitroglycerin, and beta-adrenergic antagonists.

Magnesium is involved in many enzymatic reactions and produces systemic and coronary vasodilation, inhibits platelet aggregation, and decreases myocardial reperfusion injury. Data on the ability of magnesium to decrease mortality following myocardial infarction are conflicting (Schechter et al., 1995). Treatment with magnesium is indicated in patients following an acute myocardial infarction who develop torsades de pointes ventricular tachycardia (Ryan et al., 1999).

DECISION TO TREAT CARDIAC DYSRHYTHMIAS

Drug treatment of cardiac dysrhythmias is not uniformly effective and frequently causes side effects (see the section on Prodysrhythmic Effects) (Atlee, 1997; Roden, 1994). The benefit of antidysrhythmic drugs is clearest when it results in the immediate termination of a sustained tachycardia. There is no doubt that the termination of ventricular tachycardia by lidocaine or supraventricular tachycardia by adenosine or verapamil is a true benefit of antidysrhythmic therapy. Furthermore, in this limited period, side effects are less likely. Conversely, it has been difficult to demonstrate that antidysrhythmic drugs alleviate symptoms related to chronic cardiac dysrhythmias, a situation in which the risk of side-effects is greater. The increase in long-term mortality associated with certain cardiac antidysrhythmic drugs (Cardiac Arrhythmia Suppression Trial [CAST] and other trials) raises the possibility that some antidysrhythmics result in sensitization of the myocardium to intercurrent triggering factors (myocardial ischemia, neurohumoral activation, myocardial stretch, slow healing process after a myocardial infarction) that then elicit cardiac dysrhythmias (Roden, 1994). The mechanism by which beta-adrenergic antagonists decrease mortality after an acute myocardial infarction is not known.

The value of monitoring plasma drug concentrations in minimizing the risks associated with antidysrhythmic therapy is not established. In fact, many side-effects appear to depend as much on the nature and extent of the underlying heart disease as on increased plasma drug concentrations (Roden, 1994).

QUINIDINE

Quinidine is a class IA drug that is effective in the treatment of acute and chronic supraventricular dysrhythmias (Fig. 17-1) (Grace and Camm, 1998). A frequent indication for quinidine is to prevent recurrence of supraventricular tachydysrhythmias or to suppress premature ventricular contractions. For example, quinidine is often administered to slow the atrial rate in the presence of atrial fibrillation. Indeed, about 25% of patients with atrial fibrillation will convert to normal sinus rhythm when treated with quinidine. Supraventricular tachydysrhythmias associated with Wolff-Parkinson-White syndrome are effectively suppressed by quinidine.

It is common to administer prior digitalis when treating atrial fibrillation with quinidine because an occasional patient will manifest a paradoxical increase in the rate of ventricular response when quinidine is administered. Of interest is an occasional patient in whom a previously stable plasma concentration of digoxin increases dramatically when quinidine is acutely added to the treatment regimen (Leahey et al., 1980). Apparently, quinidine causes displacement of digoxin from myocardial and peripheral tissue stores. An associated decrease in renal excretion of digoxin is due to a decrease in the renal tubular secretion of digoxin.

Quinidine is most often administered orally in a dose of 200 to 400 mg four times daily. Oral absorption of quinidine is rapid, with peak concentrations in the plasma attained in 60 to 90 minutes and an elimination half-time of 5 to 12 hours. The therapeutic blood level of quinidine is 1.2 to 4.0 μg/mL. Intramuscular (IM) injection is not recommended because of associated pain at the injection site. Quinidine can be administered IV (50 to 75 mg per hour) when administration by the oral route is unsatisfactory. The IV administration of quinidine is limited because peripheral vasodilation and myocardial depression can occur.

Mechanism of Action

Quinidine is the dextroisomer of quinine and, like quinine, has antimalarial and antipyretic effects. Unlike quinine, however, quinidine has intense effects on the heart. For example, quinidine decreases the slope of phase 4 depolarization, which explains its effectiveness in suppressing cardiac dysrhythmias caused by enhanced automaticity. Quinidine increases the fibrillation threshold in the atria and ventricles. Quinidine-induced slowing of the conduction of cardiac impulses through normal and abnormal fibers may be responsible for the ability of quinidine to occasionally convert atrial flutter or fibrillation to normal sinus rhythm. This drug can abolish reentry dysrhythmias by prolonging conduction of cardiac impulses in an area of injury, thus converting one-way conduction blockade to two-way conduction blockade. A decrease in the atrial rate during atrial flutter or fibrillation may reflect slowed conduction velocity, a prolonged effective refractory period in the atria, or both.

Metabolism and Excretion

Quinidine is hydroxylated in the liver to inactive metabolites, which are excreted in the urine. About 20% of quinidine is excreted unchanged in the urine. Enzyme induction significantly shortens the duration of action of quinidine. The concurrent administration of phenytoin, phenobarbital, or rifampin may lower blood levels of quinidine by enhancing liver clearance. Because of its dependence on renal excretion and hepatic metabolism for clearance from the body, accumulation of quinidine or its metabolites may occur in the presence of impaired function of these organs. About 80% to 90% of quinidine in plasma is bound to albumin. Quinidine accumulates rapidly in most tissues except the brain.

Side Effects

Quinidine has a low therapeutic ratio, and side effects are predictable if the plasma concentration becomes excessive. As the plasma concentration increases to more than 2 μg/mL, the P-R interval, QRS complex, and QTc interval on the ECG are prolonged; thus, ECG monitoring of patients being treated with quinidine is useful. A 50% increase in the duration of the QRS complex requires a decrease in the dosage of quinidine or heart block will likely ensue. Occasionally, uniquely susceptible patients being treated with quinidine experience syncope or sudden death despite low plasma concentrations of the drug (Morganroth and Goin, 1991). Quinidine syncope may reflect the occurrence of ventricular dysrhythmias due to delayed intraventricular conduction of cardiac impulses. Persons with preexisting prolongation of the QTc interval or evidence of atrioventricular heart block on the ECG should not be treated with quinidine. Paradoxical ventricular tachycardia can occur occasionally and is often preceded by prolongation of the QTc interval.

Quinidine can cause significant hypotension, particularly if administered IV. This response most likely reflects peripheral vasodilation from alpha-adrenergic blockade. In some patients, combined therapy with quinidine and verapamil has caused hypotension, which is probably the result of an additive blockade of alpha-adrenergic receptors by the two drugs (Maisel et al., 1985). High plasma concentrations depress myocardial contractility, which is further accentuated by hyperkalemia.

Patients in normal sinus rhythm treated with quinidine may show an increase in heart rate that is a result of presumably either an anticholinergic action and/or a reflex increase in sympathetic nervous system activity. This atropine-like action of quinidine opposes its direct depressant actions on the sinoatrial and atrioventricular nodes.

Allergic reactions may include drug rash or a drug fever that is occasionally associated with leukocytosis. Thrombocytopenia is a rare occurrence that is caused by drug–platelet complexes that evoke production of antibodies. Discontinuation of quinidine results in return of the platelet count to normal in 2 to 7 days. Nausea, vomiting, and diarrhea occur in about one-third of treated patients.

Like other cinchona alkaloids and salicylates, quinidine can cause cinchonism. Symptoms of cinchonism include tinnitus, decreased hearing acuity, blurring of vision, and gastrointestinal upset. In severe cases, there may be abdominal pain and mental confusion.

Because quinidine is an alpha-adrenergic-blocking drug, it can interact in an additive manner with drugs that cause vasodilation. For example, nitroglycerin can cause exaggerated orthostatic hypotension in patients being treated with quinidine.

Quinidine interferes with normal neuromuscular transmission and may accentuate the effect of neuromuscular-blockings drugs. Recurrence of skeletal muscle paralysis in the immediate postoperative period has been observed in association with the administration of quinidine (Way et al., 1967).

PROCAINAMIDE

Procainamide is as effective as quinidine for the treatment of ventricular tachydysrhythmias but is not as effective in abolishing atrial tachydysrhythmias (Fig. 17-2). Premature ventricular contractions and paroxysmal ventricular tachycardia are suppressed in most patients within a few minutes after IV administration. In urgent situations (ventricular tachydysrhythmias, atrial tachycardias in the presence of accessory pathways) in which a therapeutic blood level must be achieved rapidly, procainamide can be administered IV at a rate not exceeding 100 mg every 5 minutes until the cardiac dysrhythmia is controlled or the total dose reaches about 15 mg/kg. When the cardiac dysrhythmia is controlled, a constant rate of infusion (2 to 6 mg per minute) is used to maintain a therapeutic concentration of procainamide. The systemic blood pressure and ECG (QRS complex) are monitored continuously during infusion of this drug. The therapeutic blood level of procainamide is 4 to 8 μg/mL. Although procainamide and quinidine have a broader spectrum of antidysrhythmic effects than lidocaine (useful in the treatment of supraventricular and ventricular cardiac dysrhythmias), they are rarely used during anesthesia because of their propensity to produce hypotension.

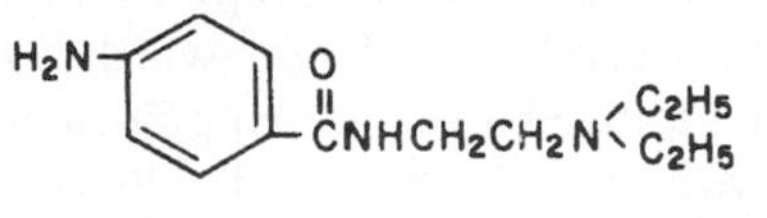

Figure 17-2. Procainamide.

Mechanism of Action

Procainamide is an analogue of the local anesthetic procaine. Procainamide possesses an electrophysiologic action similar to that of quinidine but produces less prolongation of the QTc interval on the ECG. As a result, paradoxical ventricular tachycardia is a rare feature of procainamide therapy. Procainamide has no vagolytic effect and can be used in patients with atrial fibrillation to suppress ventricular irritability without increasing the ventricular rate. Like quinidine, procainamide may prolong the QRS complex and cause ST-T wave changes on the ECG.

Metabolism and Excretion

Procainamide is eliminated by renal excretion and hepatic metabolism. In humans, 40% to 60% of procainamide is excreted unchanged by the kidneys. The dose of procainamide must be decreased when renal function is abnormal. In the liver, procainamide that has not been excreted unchanged by the kidneys is acetylated to *N*-acetyl procainamide (NAPA), which is also eliminated by the kidneys. This metabolite is cardioactive and probably contributes to the antidysrhythmic effects of procainamide. In the presence of renal failure, plasma concentrations of NAPA may reach dangerous levels. Eventually, 90% of an administered dose of procainamide is recovered as unchanged drug or its metabolites.

The activity of the *N*-acetyltransferase enzyme response for the acetylation of procainamide is genetically determined. In patients who are rapid acetylators, the elimination half-time of procainamide is 2.5 hours compared with 5 hours in slow acetylators. The blood level of NAPA exceeds that of procainamide in rapid but not slow acetylators.

Unlike its analogue, procaine, procainamide is highly resistant to hydrolysis by plasma cholinesterase. Evidence of this resistance is the fact that only 2% to 10% of an administered dose of procainamide is recovered unchanged in the urine as paraaminobenzoic acid.

Only about 15% of procainamide is bound to plasma proteins. Despite this limited binding in plasma, procainamide is avidly bound to tissue proteins with the exception of the brain.

Side Effects

The incidence of side effects is high when procainamide is used as an antidysrhythmic drug. Hypotension that results from procainamide is more likely to be caused by direct myocardial depression than peripheral vasodilation. Indeed, rapid IV injection of procainamide is associated with hypotension, whereas higher plasma concentrations slow conduction of cardiac impulses through the atrioventricular node and intraventricular conduction system. Ventricular asystole or fibrillation may occur when procainamide is administered in the presence of heart block, as associated with digitalis toxicity. Direct myocardial depression that occurs at high plasma concentrations of procainamide is exaggerated by hyperkalemia. As with quinidine, ventricular dysrhythmias may accompany excessive plasma concentrations of procainamide..

Chronic administration of procainamide may be associated with a syndrome that resembles systemic lupus erythematosus. Serositis, arthritis, pleurisy, or pericarditis may develop, but unlike systemic lupus erythematosus, vasculitis is not usually present. Patients with this lupus-like syndrome often develop antinuclear antibodies (positive antinuclear antibody test). Slow acetylators are more likely than rapid acetylators to develop antinuclear antibodies. Symptoms disappear when procainamide is discontinued.

As with many drugs, procainamide may cause drug fever or an allergic rash. Although agranulocytosis is rare, leukopenia and thrombocytopenia may be seen after chronic use of procainamide, often in association with the lupus-like syndrome. The most common early, noncardiac complications of procainamide are gastrointestinal disturbances, including nausea and vomiting.

DISOPYRAMIDE

Disopyramide is comparable to quinidine in effectively suppressing atrial and ventricular tachydysrhythmias (Fig. 17-3). Absorption of oral disopyramide is almost complete, resulting in peak blood levels within 2 hours of administration. Therapeutic plasma concentrations of disopyramide are 2 to 4 μg/mL. About 50% of the drug is excreted unchanged by the kidneys. As a result, the typical elimination half-time of 8 to 12 hours is prolonged in the presence of renal dysfunction. A dealkylated metabolite with less antidysrhythmic and atropine-like activity than the parent drug accounts for about 20% of the drug's elimination.

Side Effects

The most common side-effects of disopyramide are dry mouth and urinary hesitancy, both of which are caused by the drug's anticholinergic activity. Some patients taking disopyramide also experience blurred vision or nausea.

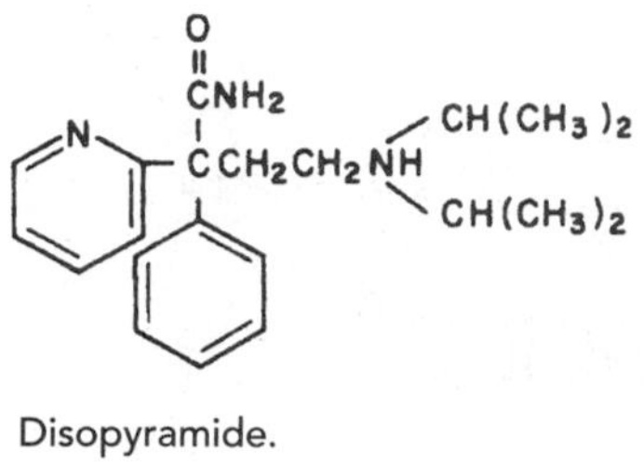

Figure 17-3. Disopyramide.

Prolongation of the QTc interval on the ECG and paradoxical ventricular tachycardia (similar to quinidine) may occur. For this reason, disopyramide should be administered cautiously if patients have known cardiac conduction effects. Disopyramide has significant myocardial depressant effects and can precipitate congestive heart failure and hypotension. The potential for direct myocardial depression, especially in patients with preexisting left ventricular dysfunction, seems to be greater with this drug than with quinidine and procainamide.

MORICIZINE

Moricizine is a phenothiazine derivative with modest efficacy in the treatment of sustained ventricular dysrhythmias. In view of its prodysrhythmic effects, this drug is reserved for the treatment of life-threatening ventricular dysrhythmias. It is not effective in the treatment of atrial dysrhythmias. Moricizine decreases the fast inward sodium ion current and also decreases automaticity.

Side Effects

Prodysrhythmic effects occur in 3% to 15% of patients treated chronically with moricizine. Patients with poor left ventricular function tolerate moricizine and small increases in systemic blood pressure and heart rate may accompany therapy. Plasma concentrations of theophylline may increase in patients treated with moricizine.

LIDOCAINE

Lidocaine is used principally for suppression of ventricular dysrhythmias, having minimal effects on supraventricular tachydysrhythmias (see Chapter 7). This drug is particularly effective in suppressing reentry cardiac dysrhythmias, such as premature ventricular contractions and ventricular tachycardia. The efficacy of prophylactic lidocaine therapy for preventing early ventricular fibrillation after acute myocardial infarction has not been documented and is no longer recommended. In fact, lidocaine does not decrease and may increase mortality because of an increase in the occurrence of fatal bradydysrhythmias and asystole.

In adult patients with a normal cardiac output, hepatic function, and hepatic blood flow, an initial administration of lidocaine, 2 mg/kg IV, followed by a continuous infusion of 1 to 4 mg per minute should provide therapeutic plasma lidocaine concentrations of 1 to 5 μg/mL. Decreased cardiac output and/or hepatic blood flow, as produced by anesthesia, acute myocardial infarction, or congestive heart failure, may decrease by 50% or more the initial dose and the rate of lidocaine infusion necessary to maintain therapeutic plasma levels. Concomitant administration of drugs such as propranolol and cimetidine can result in decreased hepatic clearance of lidocaine. An advantage of lidocaine compared with quinidine or procainamide is the more rapid onset and prompt disappearance of effects when the continuous infusion is terminated. This permits moment-to-moment titration of the infusion rate, which is necessary to produce a sustained antidysrhythmic effect. Lidocaine for IV administration differs from that used for local anesthesia because it does not contain a preservative. Lidocaine is also well absorbed after oral administration but is subject to extensive hepatic first-pass metabolism. As a result, only about one-third of an oral dose of lidocaine reaches the circulation. IM absorption of lidocaine is nearly complete. In an emergency situation, lidocaine, 4 to 5 mg/kg IM, will produce a therapeutic plasma concentration in about 15 minutes. This level is maintained for about 90 minutes.

Mechanism of Action

Lidocaine delays the rate of spontaneous phase 4 depolarization by preventing or diminishing the gradual decrease in potassium ion permeability that normally occurs during this phase. The effectiveness of lidocaine in suppressing premature ventricular contractions reflects its ability to decrease the rate of spontaneous phase 4 depolarization. The ineffectiveness of lidocaine against supraventricular tachydysrhythmias presumably reflects its inability to alter the rate of spontaneous phase 4 depolarization in atrial cardiac cells.

In usual therapeutic doses, lidocaine administered as an antidysrhythmic drug has no significant effect on either the QRS or QTc interval on the ECG or on atrioventricular conduction. In high doses, however, lidocaine can decrease conduction in the atrioventricular node as well as in the His-Purkinje system.

Metabolism and Excretion

Lidocaine is metabolized in the liver, and resulting metabolites may possess cardiac antidysrhythmic activity (see Chapter 7).

Side Effects

Lidocaine is essentially devoid of effects on the ECG or cardiovascular system when the plasma concentration remains <5 μg/mL. In contrast to quinidine and procainamide, lidocaine does not alter the duration of the QRS complex on the ECG, and activity of the sympathetic nervous system is not changed. Lidocaine depresses cardiac contractility less than any other antidysrhythmic drug used to suppress ventricular dysrhythmias. Toxic plasma concentrations of lidocaine (>5 to 10 μg/mL) produce peripheral vasodilation and direct myocardial depression, resulting in hypotension. In addition, slowing of conduction of cardiac impulses may manifest as bradycardia, a prolonged P-R interval, and widened QRS complex on the ECG.

The principal side effects of lidocaine used to treat cardiac dysrhythmias are neurologic. Stimulation of the central nervous system (CNS) occurs in a dose-related manner, with symptoms appearing when plasma concentrations of lidocaine are >5 μg/mL. Seizures are possible at plasma concentrations of 5 to 10 μg/mL. CNS depression, apnea, and cardiac arrest are possible when plasma lidocaine concentrations are >10 μg/mL. The convulsive threshold for lidocaine is decreased during arterial hypoxemia, hyperkalemia, or acidosis, emphasizing the importance of monitoring these parameters during continuous infusion of lidocaine to patients for suppression of ventricular dysrhythmias.

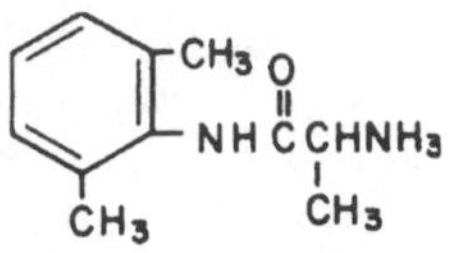

Figure 17-4. Tocainide.

TOCAINIDE

Tocainide, like mexiletine, is an orally effective amine analogue of lidocaine that is used for the chronic suppression of ventricular cardiac tachydysrhythmias (Fig. 17-4). Its side-effects resemble those of mexiletine, but in rare patients this drug has caused severe bone marrow depression (leukopenia, anemia, thrombocytopenia) and pulmonary fibrosis (Chabal et al., 1992). The usual adult dose is 400 to 800 mg administered every 8 hours. As with mexiletine, the combination of tocainide with a beta-adrenergic blocker or another antidysrhythmic drug has a synergistic effect.

MEXILETINE

Mexiletine is an orally effective amine analogue of lidocaine that is used for the chronic suppression of ventricular cardiac tachydysrhythmias (Fig. 17-5). Combination with a beta blocker or another antidysrhythmic drug such as quinidine or procainamide results in a synergistic effect that permits a decrease in the dose of mexiletine and an associated decrease in the incidence of side effects. Electrophysiologically, mexiletine is similar to lidocaine. The addition of the amine side group enables mexiletine to avoid significant hepatic first-pass metabolism that limits

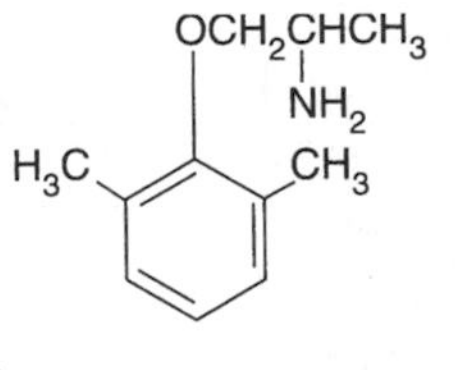

Figure 17-5. Mexiletine.

the effectiveness of orally administered lidocaine. The usual adult dose is 150 to 200 mg every 8 hours. Mexiletine may be effective in decreasing neuropathic pain for patients in whom alternative pain medications have been unsatisfactory (Chabal et al., 1992).

Side Effects

Epigastric burning may occur and is often relieved by taking the drug with meals. Neurologic side effects include tremulousness, diplopia, vertigo, and occasionally slurred speech.

Cardiovascular side effects resemble lidocaine. Increases in liver enzymes may occur especially in patients manifesting congestive heart failure. Blood dyscrasias occur rarely. Prodysrhythmic effects may manifest in occasional treated patients. Toxic effects may develop at plasma concentrations only slightly above therapeutic levels.

PHENYTOIN

Phenytoin is particularly effective in suppression of ventricular dysrhythmias associated with digitalis toxicity (see Chapter 30). This drug is effective, although to a lesser extent than quinidine, procainamide, and lidocaine, in the treatment of ventricular dysrhythmias due to other causes. Phenytoin may be useful in the treatment of paradoxical ventricular tachycardia or torsades de pointes that is associated with a prolonged QTc interval on the ECG. Treatment of atrial tachydysrhythmias with phenytoin is not very effective.

Phenytoin can be administered orally or IV IM administration is too unreliable to treat cardiac dysrhythmias. The IV dose is 100 mg (1.5 mg/kg) every 5 minutes until the cardiac dysrhythmia is controlled or 10 to 15 mg/kg (maximum 1,000 mg) has been administered. Because phenytoin can precipitate in 5% dextrose in water, it is preferable to give the drug via a delivery tubing containing normal saline. Slow IV injection into a large peripheral or central vein is recommended to minimize the likelihood of discomfort or thrombosis at the injection site. Therapeutic blood levels range from 10 to 18 μg/mL.

Mechanism of Action

The effects of phenytoin on automaticity and velocity of conduction of cardiac impulses resemble those of lidocaine. Phenytoin exerts a greater effect on the electrocardiographic QTc interval than does lidocaine, and shortens the QTc interval more than any of the other antidysrhythmic drugs. Phenytoin has no significant effect on the ST-T waves or the QRS complex. It does not significantly depress the myocardium in usual doses but can cause hypotension when administered in high doses rapidly. Conduction of cardiac impulses through the atrioventricular node is improved, but activity of the sinus node may be depressed. The ability of some volatile anesthetics to depress the sinoatrial node is a consideration if administration of phenytoin during general anesthesia is planned.

Metabolism and Excretion

Phenytoin is hydroxylated and then conjugated with glucuronic acid for excretion in the urine. The elimination half-time is about 24 hours. Because phenytoin is metabolized by the liver, impaired hepatic function may result in higher than normal blood levels of the drug. Blood levels of phenytoin can be lowered by drugs, such as barbiturates, that enhance its rate of metabolism. Warfarin, phenylbutazone, and isoniazid may inhibit metabolism and increase phenytoin blood levels. Uremia increases the unbound fraction of phenytoin relative to the plasma-bound portion.

Side Effects

Phenytoin toxicity most commonly manifests as CNS disturbances, especially cerebellar disturbances. Symptoms include ataxia, nystagmus, vertigo, slurred speech, sedation, and mental confusion. Cerebellar symptoms correlate with phenytoin blood levels of >18 μg/mL. Cardiac dysrhythmias that have not been suppressed at this concentration are unlikely to respond favorably to further increases in the dosage of phenytoin. Phenytoin partially inhibits insulin secretion and may lead to increased blood glucose levels in patients who are hyperglycemic. Leukopenia, granulocytopenia, and thrombocytopenia may occur as a manifestation of drug-induced bone marrow depression. Nausea, skin rash, and megaloblastic anemia may occur.

FLECAINIDE

Flecainide is a fluorinated local anesthetic analogue of procainamide that is more effective in suppressing ventricular premature beats and ventricular tachycardia than quinidine and disopyramide (Fig. 17-6). Flecainide is also effective for the treatment of atrial tachydysrhythmias. Because it delays conduction in the bypass tracts, flecainide can be effective for the treatment of tachydysrhythmias due to reentry mechanisms as associated with the Wolff-Parkinson-White syndrome. Chronic treatment of ventricular dysrhythmias with flecainide after myocardial infarction is not recommended due to an increased incidence of sudden

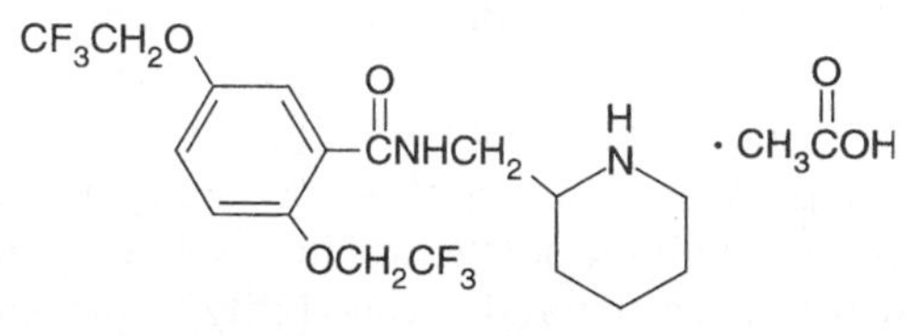

Figure 17-6. Flecainide.

death in treated patients (Echt et al., 1991). Thus, flecainide should be reserved for the treatment of life-threatening dysrhythmias.

Oral absorption of flecainide is excellent, and a prolonged elimination half-time (about 20 hours) makes a twice daily dose of 100 to 200 mg acceptable. About 25% of flecainide is excreted unchanged by the kidneys, and the remainder appears as weakly active metabolites. Elimination of flecainide is decreased in patients with congestive heart failure or renal failure. Flecainide competes with metabolic pathways utilized by other drugs and as a result may increase the plasma concentrations of digoxin and propranolol. Coadministration of amiodarone and flecainide can double plasma flecainide concentrations. Phenytoin and other drugs that stimulate hepatic P-450 enzymes may speed the elimination of flecainide. The therapeutic plasma concentration of flecainide ranges from 0.2 to 1.0 μg/mL. Flecainide has a moderate negative inotropic effect and a prodysrhythmic effect, especially in patients with preexisting decreased left ventricular function. Vertigo and difficulty in visual accommodation are common dose-related side-effects of flecainide therapy.

Side Effects

Prodysrhythmic effects occur in a significant number of treated patients especially in the presence of left ventricular dysfunction. Flecainide prolongs the QRS complex by 25% or more and, to a lesser extent, prolongs the P-R interval on the ECG. These changes suggest the possibility of atrioventricular or infranodal conduction block of cardiac impulses. Flecainide may depress sinoatrial node function as do beta-adrenergic antagonists and calcium-channel blockers. For these reasons, flecainide is not administered to patients with second- and third-degree atrioventricular heart block. Pacing threshold is increased, emphasizing caution in the use of this drug in patients with artificial cardiac pacemakers.

PROPAFENONE

Propafenone, like flecainide, is an effective antidysrhythmic drug for suppression of ventricular and atrial tachydysrhythmias. This drug possesses weak beta-adrenergic-blocking and calcium-blocking effects. Propafenone may be prodysrhythmic, especially in patients with poor left ventricular function and sustained ventricular tachycardia.

Absorption after oral administration is excellent, and peak plasma levels occur in about 3 hours. The rate of metabolism is genetically determined with about 90% of patients able to metabolize propafenone efficiently in the liver. The principal metabolites in those who metabolize the drug rapidly are pharmacologically active and equivalent in antidysrhythmic potency to the parent drug. Because of extensive metabolism, the availability of propafenone increases significantly in the presence of liver disease.

Side Effects

Prodysrhythmic effects are more likely to occur in patients with preexisting ventricular dysrhythmias. Propafenone depresses the myocardium and may cause conduction abnormalities such as sinoatrial node slowing, atrioventricular block, and bundle-branch block. Small doses of quinidine inhibit the metabolism of propafenone, whereas propafenone interferes with the metabolism of propranolol and metoprolol resulting in increased plasma concentrations of these beta-blockers. This drug also increases the plasma concentration of warfarin and may prolong the prothrombin time. Vertigo, disturbances in taste, and blurred vision are the common side-effects. Nausea and vomiting may occur, and, rarely, cholestatic hepatitis or worsening of asthma manifests.

BETA-ADRENERGIC ANTAGONISTS

Beta-adrenergic antagonists are effective for treatment of cardiac dysrhythmias related to enhanced activity of the sympathetic nervous system (perioperative stress, thyrotoxicosis, pheochromocytoma). Propranolol and esmolol are effective for controlling the rate of ventricular response in patients with atrial fibrillation and atrial flutter (see Chapter 14). Multifocal atrial tachycardia may respond to esmolol or metoprolol but is best treated with amiodarone. Comparable doses of metoprolol (5 to 15 mg IV over 20 minutes, which lasts 5 to 7 hours) produces antidysrhythmic effects similar to those of propranolol, as well as the same potential side effects. Acebutolol is effective in the treatment of frequent premature ventricular contractions. Beta-adrenergic antagonists, especially propranolol, may be effective in controlling torsades de pointes for patients with prolonged QTc intervals. Acebutolol, propranolol, and metoprolol are approved for prevention of sudden death following myocardial infarction. For example, in contrast to class I antidysrhythmic drugs, propranolol decreases sudden death as well as reinfarction rates in the first year after acute myocardial infarction (Teo et al., 1993).

Mechanism of Action

The antidysrhythmic effects of beta-adrenergic antagonists most likely reflect blockade of the responses of beta receptors in the heart to sympathetic nervous system stimulation, as well as the effects of circulating catecholamines. As a result, the rate of spontaneous phase 4 depolarization is decreased and the rate of sinoatrial node discharge is decreased. The rate of conduction of cardiac impulses through the atrioventricular node is slowed as reflected by a prolonged P-R interval on the ECG. This drug has little effect on the ST-T wave, although it may shorten the overall QTc interval. Beta-adrenergic antagonists can depress the myocardium not only by beta blockade but also by direct depressant effects on cardiac muscle. In addition to beta-adrenergic blockade, these drugs cause alterations in the electrical activity of myocardial cells. This cell membrane effect is probably responsible for some of the antidysrhythmic effects of beta-adrenergic antagonists. Indeed, dextropropranolol, which lacks beta-adrenergic antagonist activity, is an effective cardiac antidysrhythmic.

The usual oral dose of propranolol for chronic suppression of ventricular dysrhythmias is 10 to 80 mg every 6 to 8 hours. The total daily dose is determined by the physiologic effects of propranolol on the heart rate and systemic blood pressure. Effective beta blockade is usually achieved in an otherwise normal person when the resting heart rate is 55 to 60 beats/minute. For emergency suppression of cardiac dysrhythmias in an adult, propranolol may be administered IV in a dose of 1 mg per minute (3 to 6 mg). The onset of action after IV administration is within 2 to 5 minutes, the peak effect at the atrioventricular node is within 10 to 15 minutes, and the duration of action is 3 to 4 hours. Administration at 1-minute intervals is intended to minimize the likelihood of excessive pharmacologic effects on the conduction of cardiac impulses. In patients with marginal systemic blood pressure or left ventricular dysfunction, the rate of administration may need to be slowed and the total dose limited to <3 mg.

Metabolism and Excretion

Orally administered propranolol is extensively metabolized in the liver, and a hepatic first-pass effect is responsible for the variation in plasma concentration; the therapeutic plasma concentration of propranolol may vary from 10 to 30 ng/mL. Propranolol readily crosses the blood-brain barrier. The principal metabolite of propranolol is 4-hydroxypropranolol, which possesses weak beta-adrenergic antagonist activity. This active metabolite most likely contributes to the antidysrhythmic activity after the oral administration of propranolol. The elimination half-time of propranolol is 2 to 4 hours, although the antidysrhythmic activity usually persists for 6 to 8 hours.

Side Effects

Bradycardia, hypotension, myocardial depression, and bronchospasm are side effects of beta-adrenergic antagonists that reflect the ability of these drugs to inhibit sympathetic nervous system activity. Patients with any degree of congestive heart failure are highly dependent on increased sympathetic nervous system activity as a compensatory mechanism. Attenuation of this compensatory response may accentuate congestive heart failure. In addition, the direct depressant effects of propranolol on myocardial contractility may further accentuate congestive heart failure. The use of propranolol in patients with preexisting atrioventricular heart block is not recommended. Propranolol may cause drug fever, an allergic rash, or nausea and may increase esophageal reflux. Cold extremities and worsening of Raynaud disease may occur. Interference with glucose metabolism may manifest as hypoglycemia in patients being treated for diabetes mellitus. The most common central nervous system (CNS) side effects are mental depression and fatigue. Reversible alopecia may occur. Up-regulation of beta-adrenergic receptors occurs with chronic administration of beta-adrenergic antagonists such that abrupt discontinuation of treatment may lead to supraventricular tachycardia that is particularly undesirable in patients with coronary artery disease. Slowly tapering the dose of beta-adrenergic antagonist will prevent withdrawal responses.

AMIODARONE

Amiodarone is a potent antidysrhythmic drug with a wide spectrum of activity against refractory supraventricular and ventricular tachydysrhythmias. In the presence of ventricular tachycardia or fibrillation that is resistant to electrical defibrillation, amiodarone 300 mg IV is recommended. Lidocaine or procainamide are recommended during cardiopulmonary resuscitation only when amiodarone has been ineffective. Preoperative oral administration of amiodarone decreases the incidence of atrial fibrillation after cardiac surgery (Daoud et al., 1997). It is also effective for suppression of tachydysrhythmias associated with Wolff-Parkinson-White syndrome because it depresses conduction in the atrioventricular node and the accessory bypass tracts. Similar to beta blockers and unlike class I drugs, amiodarone decreases mortality after myocardial infarction (Nademanee et al., 1993).

After initiation of oral therapy, a decrease in ventricular tachydysrhythmias occurs within 72 hours. The maintenance dose can usually be gradually decreased to about 400 mg daily for suppression of ventricular tachydysrhythmias and 200 mg daily for suppression of supraventricular tachydysrhythmias. Administered IV over 2 to 5 minutes, a dose of 5 mg/kg produces a prompt antidysrhythmic effect that lasts up to 4 hours. Therapeutic blood concentrations of amiodarone are 1.0 to 3.5 μg/mL. After discontinuation of chronic oral therapy, the pharmacologic effect of amiodarone lasts for a prolonged period (up to 60 days), reflecting the prolonged elimination half-time of this drug.

Mechanism of Action

Amiodarone, a benzofurane derivative, is 37% iodine by weight and structurally resembles thyroxine (Fig. 17-7). It prolongs the effective refractory period in all cardiac tissues, including the sinoatrial node, atrium, atrioventricular node, His-Purkinje system, ventricle, and, in the case of Wolff-Parkinson-White syndrome, accessory bypass tracts. Amiodarone has an antiadrenergic effect (noncompetitive blockade of alpha and beta receptors) and a minor negative inotropic effect, which may be offset by the drug's

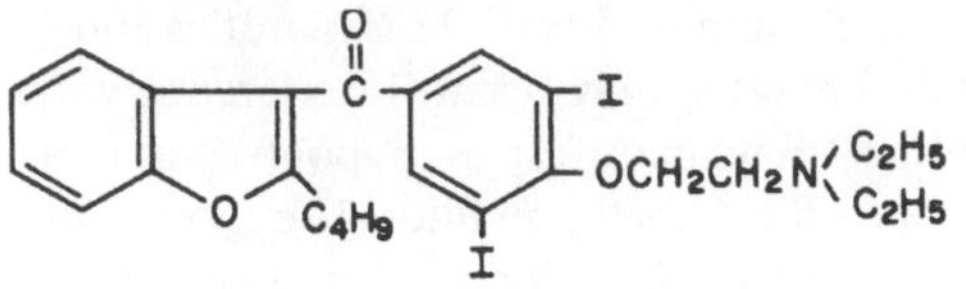

Figure 17-7. Amiodarone.

potent vasodilating properties (Gottlieb et al., 1994). Amiodarone acts as an antianginal drug by dilating coronary arteries and increasing coronary blood flow.

Metabolism and Excretion

Amiodarone has a prolonged elimination half-time (29 days) and large volume of distribution (Fig. 17-8) (Kannan et al., 1982). This drug is minimally dependent on renal excretion as evidenced by an unchanged elimination half-time in the absence of renal function (Kannan et al., 1982). The principal metabolite, desethylamiodarone, is pharmacologically active and has a longer elimination half-time than the parent drug, resulting in accumulation of this metabolite with chronic therapy. Protein binding of amiodarone is extensive, and the drug is not easily removed by hemodialysis. There is an inconsistent relationship between the plasma concentration of amiodarone and its pharmacologic effects. Indeed, the ultimate concentration of drug in the myocardium is 10 to 50 times that present in the plasma.

Side Effects

Side effects in patients treated chronically with amiodarone are common, especially when the daily maintenance dose exceeds 400 mg (Mason, 1987).

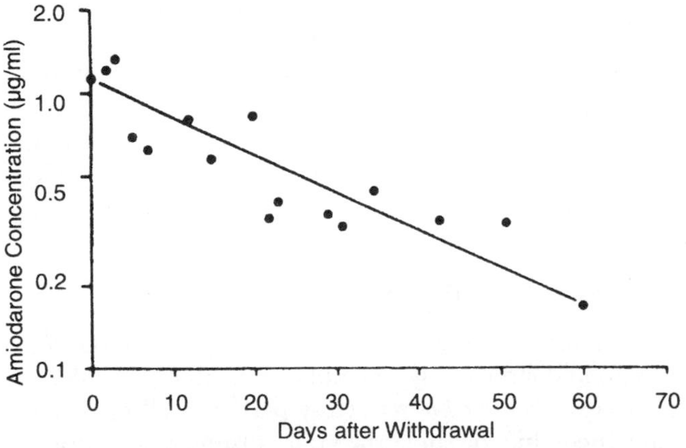

Figure 17-8. After discontinuation of amiodarone, the plasma concentration decreases slowly, resulting in a prolonged elimination half-time. (From Kannan R, Nademannee K, Hendrickson JA, et al. Amiodarone kinetics after oral doses. *Clin Pharmacol Ther* 1982;31:438–444; with permission.)

Pulmonary Toxicity

The most serious side effect of amiodarone is pulmonary alveolitis (pneumonitis) (Dusman et al., 1990; Martin and Rosenow, 1988). The overall incidence of amiodarone-induced pulmonary toxicity is estimated at 5% to 15% of treated patients, with a reported mortality of 5% to 10%. The cause of this drug-induced pulmonary toxicity is not known but may reflect the ability of amiodarone to enhance production of free oxygen radicals in the lungs that in turn oxidize cellular proteins, membrane lipids, and nucleic acids. It is suggested that high-inspired oxygen concentrations may accelerate these reactions (Kay et al., 1988). For this reason, it may be prudent to restrict the inspired concentration of oxygen in patients receiving amiodarone and undergoing general anesthesia to the lowest level capable of maintaining adequate systemic oxygenation (Herndon et al., 1992). Indeed, postoperative pulmonary edema has been reported in patients being treated chronically with amiodarone (Herndon et al., 1992). Furthermore, there is evidence that patients with preexisting evidence of amiodarone-induced pulmonary toxicity are at increased risk for developing adult respiratory distress syndrome after surgery that requires cardiopulmonary bypass (Kupferschmid et al., 1989; Nalos et al., 1987). It must be recognized, however, that no animal model has established a cause-and-effect relationship between oral amiodarone administration and secondary oxygen-enhanced pulmonary toxicity.

There are two distinct types of presentation of patients with amiodarone-induced pulmonary toxicity (Martin and Rosenow, 1988). The more common form of pulmonary toxicity consists of a slow insidious onset of progressive dyspnea, cough, weight loss, and pulmonary infiltrates on the chest x-ray. The second form of pulmonary toxicity has a much more acute onset of dyspnea, cough, arterial hypoxemia, and occasionally fever that may mimic an infectious pneumonia. Postoperative pulmonary edema attributed to amiodarone-induced pulmonary toxicity reflects this acute form of onset.

Cardiovascular

Like quinidine and disopyramide, amiodarone may prolong the QTc interval on the ECG, which may lead to an increased incidence of ventricular tachydysrhythmias, including torsades de pointes (prodysrhythmia effect). Heart rate often slows and is resistant to treatment with atropine. Responsiveness to catecholamines and sympathetic nervous system stimulation is decreased as a result of drug-induced inhibition of alpha- and beta-adrenergic receptors. Direct myocardial depressant effects are presumed to be minimal (MacKinnon et al., 1983). IV administration of amiodarone may result in hypotension, most likely reflecting the peripheral vasodilating effects of this drug. Atrioventricular heart block may also occur when the drug is administered IV. The negative inotropic effects of amiodarone may be enhanced in the presence of general anesthesia, beta-adrenergic blockers, and calcium-channel blockers (Teasdale and Downar, 1990). Drugs that inhibit automaticity of the sinoatrial node (lidocaine) could accentuate the effects of amiodarone and increase the likelihood of sinus arrest. The potential need for a temporary artificial cardiac (ventricular) pacemaker and administration of a sympathomimetic such as isoproterenol may be a consideration in patients being treated with this drug and scheduled to undergo surgery (Navalgund et al., 1986).

Ocular, Dermatologic, Neurologic, and Hepatic

Corneal microdeposits occur in most patients during amiodarone therapy, but visual impairment is unlikely. Photosensitivity and rash develop in up to 10% of patients. Rarely, there may be a cyanotic discoloration (slate-gray pigmentation) of the face that persists even after the drug is discontinued. Neurologic toxicity may manifest as peripheral neuropathy, tremors, sleep disturbance, headache, or proximal skeletal muscle weakness (Heger et al., 1981). Transient, mild increases in plasma transaminase concentrations may occur, and fatty liver infiltration has been observed (Heger et al., 1981).

Pharmacokinetic

Amiodarone inhibits hepatic P-450 enzymes resulting in increased plasma concentrations of digoxin, procainamide, quinidine, warfarin, and cyclosporine. Amiodarone also displaces digoxin from protein-binding sites. The digoxin dose may be decreased as much as 50% when administered in the presence of amiodarone. Amiodarone also increases the plasma concentrations of quinidine, procainamide, and phenytoin. The anticoagulant effects of warfarin are potentiated because amiodarone may directly depress vitamin K-dependent clotting factors.

Endocrine

Amiodarone contains iodine and has effects on thyroid metabolism, causing either hypothyroidism or hyperthyroidism in 2% to 4% of patients (see Fig. 17-7). Thyroid dysfunction may develop insidiously in these patients. Hyperthyroidism has occurred up to 5 months after discontinuation of amiodarone. Patients with preexisting thyroid dysfunction seem more likely to develop amiodarone-related alterations in thyroid function. Hyperthyroidism is best detected by finding an increased plasma concentration of triiodothyronine. Hypothyroidism is best detected by finding an increased plasma concentration of thyroid-stimulating hormone.

Amiodarone-induced hyperthyroidism reflecting the release of iodine from the parent drug is often refractory to conventional therapy. These patients may be intolerant of beta-adrenergic blockade because of their underlying cardiomyopathies. When medical management fails, the performance of surgical thyroidectomy provides prompt metabolic control. Bilateral superficial cervical plexus blocks have been described for anesthetic management of subtotal thyroidectomy in these patients (Klein et al., 1997).

SOTALOL

Sotalol is administered for the treatment of sustained ventricular tachycardia or ventricular fibrillation (Hohnloser and Woosley, 1994). This drug is also approved for the treatment of atrial tachydysrhythmia including atrial fibrillation as may follow cardiac surgery. Sotalol is a nonselective beta-adrenergic antagonist drug at low doses, and at higher doses, it prolongs the cardiac action potential in the atria, ventricles, and accessory bypass tracts. Sotalol is not recommended in patients with asthma, left ventricular dysfunction, and cardiac conduction abnormalities including prolonged QTc intervals on the ECG. Because of its prodysrhythmic effects, this drug is usually restricted for use in patients with life-threatening ventricular dysrhythmias.

The daily oral dose of sotalol is 240 to 320 mg administered twice daily. Because sotalol is excreted mainly by the kidneys, the dosing intervals should be lengthened in patients with renal dysfunction. Sotalol does not bind to plasma proteins, is not metabolized, and it does not cross the blood-brain barrier to any extent. Beta-adrenergic blocking effects of this drug primarily reflect activity of the levorotatory isomer.

Side Effects

The most dangerous side effect of sotalol is torsades de pointes, reflecting prolongation of the QTc interval on the ECG. Torsades de pointes is dose related, occurring in 0.5% of patients receiving 80 mg of sotalol daily and in 5.8% of patients receiving more than 320 mg daily. The beta-blocking effects of sotalol result in decreased myocardial contractility, bradycardia, and delayed conduction of cardiac impulses through the atrioventricular node. Other side-effects of sotalol include fatigue, dyspnea, vertigo, and nausea.

IBUTILIDE

Ibutilide is effective for the conversion of recent onset atrial fibrillation or atrial flutter to normal sinus rhythm. Hepatic metabolism is extensive with production of inactive metabolites with the exception of hydroxy metabolites that possess weak antidysrhythmic effects. Polymorphic ventricular tachycardia with or without prolongation of the QTc interval on the ECG may occur during ibutilide treatment, especially in patient with predisposing factors (impaired left ventricular function, preexisting prolonged QTc intervals, hypokalemia, hypomagnesemia).

DOFETILIDE

Dofetilide is effective for the conversion of recent onset atrial fibrillation or atrial flutter to normal sinus rhythm, as well as the maintenance of normal sinus rhythm in patients who have been successfully cardioverted. Oral absorption is greater than 90%, and 80% of the drug is excreted unchanged in the urine. Dosage adjustments are indicated based on renal function. Trimethoprim, cimetidine, and prochlorperazine can inhibit renal clearance of dofetilide. Prodysrhythmic effects of dofetilide may occur when it is coadministered with calcium-channel blocking drugs. Dofetilide does not depress myocardial contractility. Torsades de pointes occurs in a dose-related manner, especially in patients with preexisting left ventricular dysfunction.

BRETYLIUM

Bretylium is no longer recommended for treatment of ventricular fibrillation during cardiopulmonary resuscitation as it is less effective than amiodarone and has more side-effects. This drug causes a direct early release of norepinephrine from adrenergic nerve endings, which can result in transient hypertension. Ultimately, the presence of bretylium in adrenergic nerve endings prevents the release of norepinephrine and may lead to orthostatic hypotension and bradycardia. Bretylium also potentiates the action of norepinephrine and epinephrine on adrenergic receptors by inhibiting the uptake of catecholamines.

Bretylium is not easily obtained for clinical use and if available can only be administered IM or IV. The usual dose is 5 to 10 mg/kg IV administered every 10 to 30 minutes to a maximum dose of 30 mg/kg (Atlee, 1997). Nausea and hypotension (because of peripheral vasodilation) are common after rapid IV administration of bretylium. Conversely, because of the initial release of norepinephrine, transient hypertension and increased ventricular irritability may occur after the first few doses, especially in patients also receiving digitalis. The elimination half-time of bretylium is 8 to 12 hours, which is directly related to renal clearance. In this regard, the dose of bretylium should be decreased when administered to patients with renal dysfunction to avoid cumulative drug effects. About 70% of the drug is excreted unchanged in urine in the first 24 hours, and by 48 hours, 98% of the initially injected drug can be recovered unchanged in urine. Hepatic metabolism has not been demonstrated for bretylium.

VERAPAMIL AND DILTIAZEM

Among the calcium-channel blockers, verapamil and diltiazem have the greatest efficacy for the treatment of cardiac dysrhythmias (Atlee, 1997) (see Chapter 18). Verapamil is highly effective in terminating paroxysmal supraventricular tachycardia, a reentrant tachycardia whose pathway usually includes the atrioventricular node. This drug also effectively controls the ventricular rate in most patients who develop atrial fibrillation or flutter. Verapamil, however, does not have a depressant effect on accessory tracts and thus will not slow the ventricular response rate in patients with Wolff-Parkinson-White syndrome. In fact, verapamil may cause reflex sympathetic nervous system activity that enhances conduction of cardiac impulses over accessory tracts and thus increases the ventricular response rate similar to digitalis. Verapamil has little efficacy in the therapy for ventricular ectopic beats.

The usual dose of verapamil for suppression of paroxysmal supraventricular tachycardia is 5 to 10 mg IV (75 to 150 μg/kg) over 1 to 3 minutes followed by a continuous infusion of about 5 μg/kg per minute to maintain a sustained effect. The administration of calcium gluconate, 1 g IV, approximately 5 minutes before administration of verapamil may decrease verapamil-induced hypotension without altering the drug's antidysrhythmic effects (Salerno et al., 1987). Chronic treatment with oral verapamil, 80 to 120 mg every 6 to 8 hours, may be useful for prevention of paroxysmal supraventricular tachycardia and for control of the ventricular response rate in atrial fibrillation or atrial flutter. Diltiazem, 20 mg IV, produces antidysrhythmic effects similar to those of diazepam, and the potential side effects are similar.

Mechanism of Action

Verapamil and the other calcium channel blockers inhibit the flux of calcium ions across the slow channels of vascular smooth muscle and cardiac cells. This effect on calcium ion flux manifests as a decreased rate of spontaneous phase 4 depolarization. Verapamil has a substantial depressant effect on the atrioventricular node and a negative chronotropic effect on the sinoatrial node. This drug exerts a negative inotropic effect on cardiac muscle and produces a moderate degree of vasodilation of the coronary arteries and systemic arteries.

Metabolism and Excretion

An estimated 70% of an injected dose of verapamil is eliminated by the kidneys, whereas up to 15% may be present in the bile. A metabolite, norverapamil, may contribute to the parent drug's antidysrhythmic effects. The need for a large oral dose is related to the extensive hepatic first-pass effect that occurs with the oral route of administration.

Side Effects

The side effects of verapamil used to treat cardiac dysrhythmias reflect its effects on calcium ion flux into cardiac cells. Atrioventricular heart block is more likely in patients with preexisting defects in the conduction of cardiac impulses.

Direct myocardial depression and decreased cardiac output are likely to be exaggerated in patients with poor left ventricular function. Peripheral vasodilation may contribute to hypotension. There may be potentiation of anesthetic-produced myocardial depression, and the effects of neuromuscular-blocking drugs may be exaggerated.

By decreasing hepatic blood flow, cimetidine may increase the plasma concentration of verapamil. Verapamil, like quinidine, may increase the plasma concentration of digoxin by 50% to 75%. Excessive bradycardia has been observed when verapamil and propranolol are administered simultaneously.

OTHER CARDIAC ANTIDYSRHYTHMIC DRUGS

Digitalis

Digitalis preparations such as digoxin are effective cardiac antidysrhythmics for stabilization of atrial electrical activity and the treatment and prevention of atrial tachydysrhythmias (see Chapter 13). Because of their vagolytic effects, these drugs can also slow conduction of cardiac impulses through the atrioventricular node and thus slow the ventricular response rate in patients with atrial fibrillation. Conversely, digitalis preparations enhance conduction of cardiac impulses through accessory bypass tracts and can dangerously increase the ventricular response rate in patients with Wolff-Parkinson-White syndrome. The usual oral dose of digoxin is 0.5 to 1.0 mg in divided doses over 12 to 24 hours. Digitalis toxicity is a risk and may manifest as virtually any cardiac dysrhythmia (most commonly atrial tachycardia with block).

Adenosine

Adenosine is an endogenous nucleoside that slows conduction of cardiac impulses through the atrioventricular node, making it an effective alternative to calcium-channel blockers (verapamil) for the treatment of paroxysmal supraventricular tachycardia, including that due to conduction through accessory pathways in patients with Wolff-Parkinson-White syndrome (Lerman and Belardinelli, 1991). This drug is not effective in the treatment of atrial fibrillation, atrial flutter, or ventricular tachycardia. The usual dose of adenosine is 6 mg IV followed, if necessary, by a repeat injection of 6 to 12 mg IV about 3 minutes later.

Adenosine receptors represent a logical target for treatment of pain. Adenosine agonists result in blockade of acute nociception and reduce hypersensitivity to thermal or mechanical stimuli in the presence of sensitization after peripheral inflammation or nerve injury. This response most likely reflects actions on extracellular G protein-coupled receptors present in the periphery and CNS, primarily in the spinal cord. Intrathecal administration of adenosine produces selective inhibition of hypersensitivity presumed to be due to central sensitization (Eisenach et al., 2002).

Mechanism of Action

Adenosine has cardiac electrophysiologic effects similar to those of the calcium-channel blockers verapamil and diltiazem (Atlee, 1997). It stimulates cardiac adenosine$_1$ receptors to increase potassium ion currents, shorten the action potential duration, and hyperpolarize cardiac cell membranes. In addition, adenosine decreases cyclic adenosine monophosphate concentrations. Its short-lived cardiac effects (elimination half-time 10 seconds) are due to carrier-mediated cellular uptake and metabolism to inosine by adenosine deaminase. Methylxanthines inhibit the actions of adenosine by binding to adenosine$_1$ receptors. Conversely, dipyridamole (adenosine uptake inhibitor) and cardiac transplantation (denervation hypersensitivity) potentiate the effects of adenosine.

Side Effects

The side effects associated with the rapid IV administration of adenosine include facial flushing, headache, dyspnea, chest discomfort, and nausea. Adenosine may produce transient atrioventricular heart block. Bronchospasm, although an uncommon complication, has been observed after the IV administration of adenosine, even in the absence of preexisting wheezing (Aggarwal et al., 1993; Bennett-Guerrero and Young, 1994). It is recommended that adenosine be used with caution, if at all, in patients known to have active wheezing. Several theories have been proposed to account for adenosine's bronchoconstrictor effect, including activation of adenosine receptors on the bronchial smooth muscle, mast cell degranulation, and stimulation of bronchoconstrictor prostaglandin formation (Crimi et al., 1989). The pharmacologic effects of adenosine are antagonized by methylxanthines (theophylline, caffeine) and potentiated by dipyridamole.

REFERENCES

Aggarwal A, Farber NE, Warltier DC. Intraoperative bronchospasm caused by adenosine. *Anesthesiology* 1993;79:1132–1135.

Atlee JL. Perioperative cardiac dysrhythmias: diagnosis and management. *Anesthesiology* 1997;86:1397–1424.

Atlee JL, Bosnjak ZJ. Mechanisms of cardiac dysrhythmias during anesthesia. *Anesthesiology* 1990;72:347–374.

Ben-David J, Zipes DP. Torsades de pointes and proarrhythmia. *Lancet* 1993;341:1578–1583.

Bennett-Guerrero E, Young CC. Bronchospasm after intravenous adenosine administration. *Anesth Analg* 1994;79:386–388.

Chabal C, Jacobson L, Mariano A, et al. The use of oral mexiletine for the treatment of pain after peripheral nerve injury. *Anesthesiology* 1992;76:513–517.

Creswell LL, Schuessler RB, Rosenbloom M, et al. Hazards of postoperative atrial arrhythmias. *Ann Thorac Surg* 1993;56:539–545.

Crimi N, Palermo F, Polosa R, et al. Effect of indomethacin on adenosine-induced bronchoconstriction. *J Allergy Clin Immunol* 1989; 83:921–925.

Daoud EG, Strickberger SA, Man KC, et al. Preoperative amiodarone as prophylaxis against atrial fibrillation after heart surgery. *N Engl J Med* 1997;337:1785–1791.

Dusman RE, Marshall SS, Miles WM, et al. Clinical features of amiodarone-induced pulmonary toxicity. *Circulation* 1990;82:51–59.

Echt DS, Liebson PR, Mitchell LB, et al. Mortality in patients receiving encainide, flecainide, or placebo: the Cardiac Arrhythmia Suppression Trial. *N Engl J Med* 1991;324:781–788.

Eisenach JC, Hood DD, Curry R. Preliminary efficacy assessment of intrathecal injection of an American formulation of adenosine in humans. *Anesthesiology* 2002;96:29–34.

Gottlieb SS, Riggio DW, Lauria S, et al. High dose oral amiodarone loading exerts important hemodynamic actions in patients with congestive heart failure. *J Am Coll Cardiol* 1994;23:560–566.

Grace AA, Camm AJ. Quinidine. *N Engl J Med* 1998;338:35–45.

Heger JJ, Prystowsky EN, Jackman WM, et al. Amiodarone: clinical efficacy and electrophysiology during long-term therapy for recurrent ventricular tachycardia or ventricular fibrillation. *N Engl J Med* 1981;305:539–545.

Herndon JC, Cook AO, Ramsay AE, et al. Postoperative unilateral pulmonary edema: possible amiodarone pulmonary toxicity. *Anesthesiology* 1992;76:308–312.

Hohnloser SH, Woosley RL. Sotalol. *N Engl J Med* 1994;331:31–37.

Kannan R, Nademannee K, Hendrickson JA, et al. Amiodarone kinetics after oral doses. *Clin Pharmacol Ther* 1982;31:438–444.

Kay GN, Epstein AE, Kirklin JK, et al. Fatal postoperative amiodarone pulmonary toxicity. *Am J Cardiol* 1988;62:490–492.

Kennedy HL, Brooks MM, Barker AH, et al. Beta blocker therapy in the Cardiac Arrhythmia Suppression Trial. CAST Investigators. *Am J Cardiol* 1994;74:674–680.

Klein SM, Greengrass RA, Knudsen N, et al. Regional anesthesia for thyroidectomy in two patients with amiodarone-induced hyperthyroidism. *Anesth Analg* 1997;85:22–24.

Kupferschmid JP, Rosengart TK, McIntosh CL, et al. Amiodarone-induced complications after cardiac operation for obstructive hypertrophic cardiomyopathy. *Ann Thorac Surg* 1989;48:359–364.

Langberg JJ, DeLurgio DB. Ventricular arrhythmias. *Sci Am Med* 1999; 1:VI:1–12.

Leahey EB, Reiffel JA, Giardina EV, et al. The effect of quinidine and other oral antiarrhythmic drugs on serum digoxin. *Ann Intern Med* 1980;92:605–611.

Lerman BB, Belardinelli L. Cardiac electrophysiology of adenosine: basic and clinical concepts. *Circulation* 1991;83:1449–1455.

Lucas WJ, Maccioli GA, Mueller RA. Advances in oral antiarrhythmic therapy: implications for the anaesthetist. *Can J Anaesth* 1990;37: 94–101.

MacKinnon G, Landymore R, et al. Should oral amiodarone be used for sustained ventricular tachycardia in patients requiring open-heart surgery? *Can J Surg* 1983;26:355–357.

Maisel AS, Motulskyl HJ, Insel PA. Hypotension after quinidine plus verapamil: possible additive competition at alpha-adrenergic receptors. *N Engl J Med* 1985;312:1267–1274.

Martin WJ, Rosenow EC. Amiodarone pulmonary toxicity: recognition and pathogenesis (part 1). *Chest* 1988;93:1067–1075.

Mason JW. Amiodarone. *N Engl J Med* 1987;316:455–463.

Morady F. Radio-frequency ablation as treatment for cardiac arrhythmias. *N Engl J Med* 1999;340:534–539.

Morganroth J, Goin JE. Quinidine-related mortality in the short- to medium-term treatment of ventricular arrhythmias: a meta-analysis. *Circulation* 1991;84:1977–1983.

Nadeemanee K, Singh BN, Stevenson WG, et al. Amiodarone and post-MI patients. *Circulation* 1993;88:764–769.

Nalos PC, Kass RM, Gang ES, et al. Life-threatening postoperative pulmonary complications in patients with previous amiodarone pulmonary toxicity undergoing cardiothoracic operations. *J Thorac Cardiovasc Surg* 1987;93:904–912.

Navalgund AA, Alifimoff JK, Jakymec AJ, Bleyaert AL. Amiodarone-induced sinus arrest successfully treated with ephedrine and isoproterenol. *Anesth Analg* 1986;65:414–416.

Roden DM. Risks and benefits of antiarrhythmic therapy. *N Engl J Med* 1994;331:785–791.

Ryan TJ, Antman EM, Brooks NH, et al. 1999 Update: ACC/AHA guidelines for the management of patients with acute myocardial infarction. *J Am Coll Cardiol* 1999;34:890–899.

Salerno DM, Anderson B, Sharkey PJ, et al. Intravenous verapamil for treatment of multifocal atrial tachycardia with and without calcium pretreatment. *Ann Intern Med* 1987;107:623–628.

Schechter M, Hod H, Chouraqui P, et al. Magnesium therapy in acute myocardial infarction when patients are not candidates for thrombolytic therapy. *Am J Cardiol* 1995;75:321–328.

Teasdale S, Downar E. Amiodarone and anaesthesia. *Can J Anaesth* 1990;37:151–155.

Teo KK, Yusuf S, Furberg CD. Effects of prophylactic antiarrhythmic drug therapy in acute myocardial infarction: an overview of results from randomized controlled trials. *JAMA* 1993;270: 1589–1594.

Way WL, Katzung BG, Larson CP. Recurarization with quinidine. *JAMA* 1967;200:163–164.

Williams VEM. Cardiac arrhythmias. In: Sandoe E, Fiensted-Jensen E, Olson KH, eds. Astra, Sodertalje, Sweden, 1970:449.

Zipes DP. Implantable cardioverter-defibrillator: a Volkswagen or Rolls Royce. *Circulation* 2001;103:1372–1377.

Calcium-Channel Blockers

18

Calcium-channel blockers (also known as *calcium-entry blockers* and *calcium antagonists*) are a diverse group of structurally unrelated compounds that selectively interfere with inward calcium ion movement across myocardial and vascular smooth muscle cells (Durand et al., 1991; Kaplan, 1989). Calcium ions play a key role in the electrical excitation of cardiac cells and vascular smooth muscle cells.

Commercially available calcium-channel blockers are classified, based on chemical structure, as (a) phenylalkylamines, (b) dihydropyridines, and (c) benzothiazepines (Table 18-1 and Fig. 18-1). The phenylalkylamines and benzothiazepines are selective for the atrioventricular node, whereas the dihydropyrimidines are selective for the arteriolar beds (Kanneganti and Halpern, 1996). Common side effects of calcium-channel blockers include systemic hypotension, peripheral edema, flushing, and headache. The various calcium-channel blockers differ in terms of side effects, usual doses, metabolism, and duration of action (Tables 18-2 and 18-3).

MECHANISM OF ACTION

Calcium-channel blockers bind to receptors on voltage-gated calcium ion channels (L, N, and T subtypes) resulting in maintenance of these channels in an inactive (closed) state. As a result, calcium influx is decreased and there is a reduction in intracellular calcium. The L-type channel (slow channel) has five subunits: alpha$_1$, alpha$_2$, beta, gamma, and delta. The alpha$_1$ subunit forms the central part of the channel and provides the main pathway for calcium ion entry into cells. All clinically utilized calcium-channel blockers bind to a unique site on the alpha$_1$ subunit of the L-type calcium channels and thus diminish entry of calcium ions into cells. These structurally diverse drugs differ in their tissue selectivity, their binding-site location on the alpha$_1$ subunit, and their mechanism of calcium blockade.

Voltage-gated calcium ion channels are present in the cell membranes of skeletal muscle, vascular smooth muscle, cardiac muscle, mesenteric muscle, glandular cells, and neurons (Fig. 18-2) (Kanneganti and Halpern, 1996). Calcium ion influx through L-type calcium channels is responsible for phase 2 of the cardiac action potential, which is important in excitation/contraction coupling in cardiac and vascular smooth muscle and depolarization in sinoatrial and atrioventricular nodal tissue. Thus blockade of slow calcium channels by calcium-channel blockers predictably results in slowing of the heart rate, reduction in myocardial contractility, decreased speed of conduction of cardiac impulses through the atrioventricular node, and vascular smooth muscle relaxation (Reeves, 1984).

Direct activation of the vascular smooth muscle cell voltage-gated channels by neural impulses initiates an action potential, calcium ion influx, and myofilament contraction (see Fig. 18-2) (Kanneganti and Halpern, 1996). This process is known as *excitation-contraction coupling*. The intracellular calcium combines with calmodulin, the calcium-binding protein, to form the calcium-calmodulin complex. This complex activates myosin and causes the formation of cross-bridges with actin. These cross-bridges begin the process of muscular contraction.

PHARMACOLOGIC EFFECTS

The pharmacologic effects of calcium-channel blockers may be predicted by considering the normal role of calcium ions in the production of action potentials, especially in cardiac cells. It is predictable that calcium-channel blockers will produce (a) decreased myocardial contractility, (b) decreased heart rate, (c) decreased activity of the sinoatrial node, (d) decreased rate of conduction of cardiac impulses through the atrioventricular node, and (e) vascular smooth muscle relaxation with associated vasodilation

TABLE 18-1.
CLASSIFICATION OF CALCIUM-CHANNEL BLOCKERS

Phenylalkylamines
Verapamil
Dihydropyrimidines
Nifedipine
Nicardipine
Nimodipine
Isradipine
Felodipine
Amlodipine
Benzothiazepines
Diltiazem

and decreases in systemic blood pressure (Reves et al., 1982, Reves, 1984). Calcium-channel blockers produce these effects to varying degrees (Table 18-2).

All of the calcium-channel blockers are effective for the treatment of coronary artery spasm. Calcium-channel blockers decrease vascular smooth muscle contractility, thereby increasing coronary blood flow and causing peripheral vasodilation with reductions in systemic vascular resistance and systemic blood pressure. These drug-induced responses contribute to the anti-ischemic effects characteristic of calcium-channel blockers. Because calcium-channel blockers dilate the coronary arteries via a mechanism that is different from that of nitrates, the two classes of drugs complement each other in the treatment of coronary artery spasm. Calcium-channel blockers are also effective for the treatment of chronic stable angina pectoris caused by fixed obstructive coronary artery lesions and for the treatment of unstable angina pectoris.

All calcium-channel blockers exert negative inotropic effects that are most significant with verapamil and diltiazem.

PHENYLALKYLAMINES

The phenylalkylamines bind to the intracellular portion of the L-type channel alpha$_1$ subunit when the channel is in an open state and conceptually occlude the channel (Fig. 18-3) (Kanneganti and Halpern, 1996).

Verapamil

Verapamil is a synthetic derivative of papaverine that is supplied as a racemic mixture. The dextroisomer of verapamil is devoid of activity at slow calcium channels and

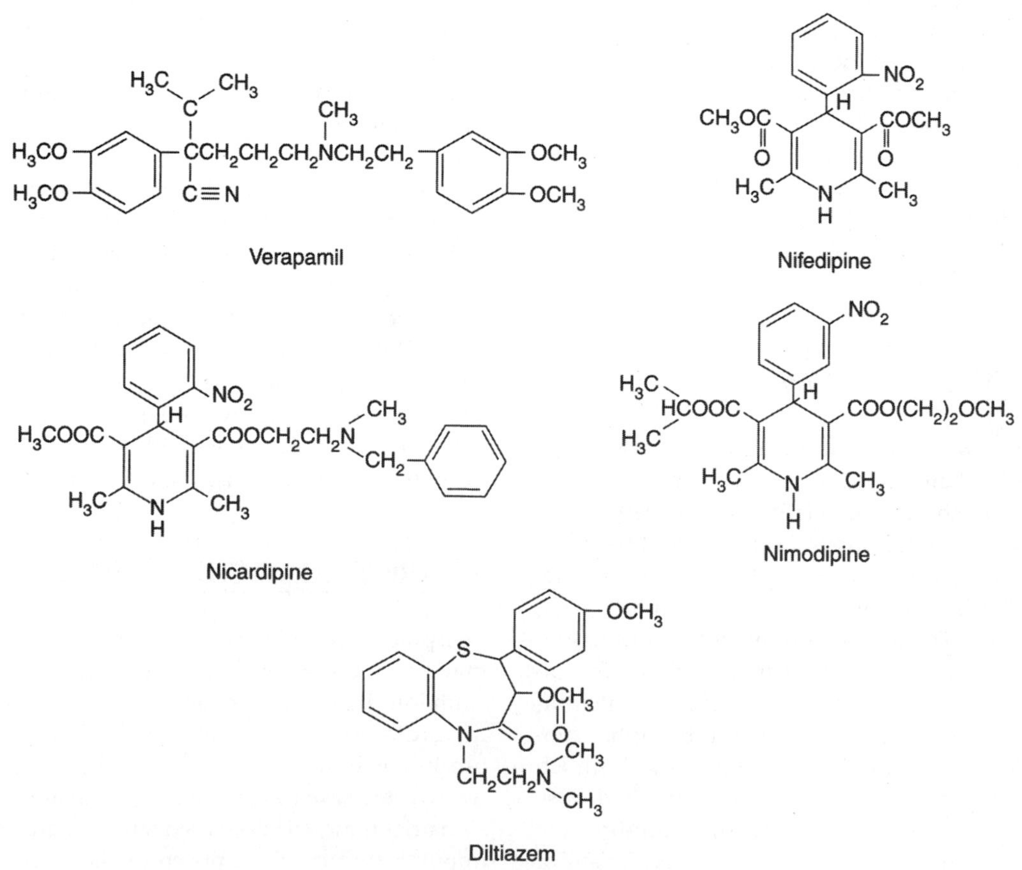

Figure 18-1. Calcium-channel blockers.

TABLE 18-2.
COMPARATIVE PHARMACOLOGIC EFFECTS OF CALCIUM-CHANNEL BLOCKERS

	Verapamil	Nifedipine	Nicardipine	Diltiazem
Systemic blood pressure	Decrease	Decrease	Decrease	Decrease
Heart rate	Decrease	Increase to no change	Increase to no change	Decrease
Myocardial depression	Moderate	Moderate	Slight	Moderate
Sinoatrial node depression	Moderate	None	None	Slight
Atrioventricular node conduction	Marked	None	None	Moderate depression
Coronary artery dilation	Moderate	Marked	Greatest	Moderate
Peripheral artery dilation	Moderate	Marked	Marked	Moderate

instead acts on fast sodium channels, accounting for the local anesthetic effects of verapamil (1.6 times as potent as procaine) (Kraynack et al., 1982). The levoisomer of verapamil is specific for slow calcium channels, and the predominance of this action accounts for the classification of verapamil as a calcium-blocking drug.

Side Effects

Verapamil has a major depressant effect on the atrioventricular node, a negative chronotropic effect on the sinoatrial node, a negative inotropic effect on cardiac muscle, and a moderate vasodilating effect on coronary and systemic arteries. The negative inotropic effects of verapamil seem to be exaggerated in patients with preexisting left ventricular dysfunction. For these reasons, verapamil should not be administered to patients in heart failure or patients with severe bradycardia, sinus node dysfunction, or atriventricular nodal block. Likewise, this drug's negative inotropic and chronotropic effects may be enhanced in the presence of concomitant treatment with beta-adrenergic antagonists. Isoproterenol may be useful to increase heart rate in the presence of drug-induced heart block. Verapamil may precipitate ventricular dysrhythmias in patients with Wolff-Parkinson-White syndrome.

TABLE 18-3.
PHARMACOKINETICS OF CALCIUM-CHANNEL BLOCKERS

	Verapamil	Nifedipine	Nicardipine	Nimodipine	Diltiazem
Dosage					
Oral	80–160 mg every 8 hrs	10–30 mg every 8 hrs	20 mg every 8 hrs	30–60 mg every 4–6 hrs	60–90 mg every 8 hrs
Intravenous	75–150 μg/kg	5–15 μg/kg		10 μg/kg	75–150 μg/kg
Absorption (%)					
Oral	>90	>90		>90	
Bioavailability (%)	10–20	65–70	30	5–10	40
Onset of effect (mins)					
Oral	<30	<20	20–60	30–90	30
Sublingual		3			
Intravenous	1–3	1–3	1–3	1–3	
First-pass hepatic extraction after oral administration (%)	75–90	40–60	20–40	90	70–80
Protein binding (%)	83–93	92–98	95	99	98
Clearance					
Renal (%)	70	80	55	20	35
Hepatic (%)	15	<15	45	80	60
Active metabolites	Yes	No		Yes	
Therapeutic plasma concentration (ng/mL)	50–250	10–100	5–100	10–30	100–250
Elimination half-time (hrs)	3–7	3–7	3–5	2	4–6

Source: Data from Reves JG, Kissin I, Lell WA, Tosone S. Calcium entry blockers: uses and implications for anesthesiologists. *Anesthesiology* 1982;57:504–518; Durand PG, Lehot JJ, Foex P. Calcium-channel blockers and anaesthesia. *Can J Anaesth* 1991;38:75–89.

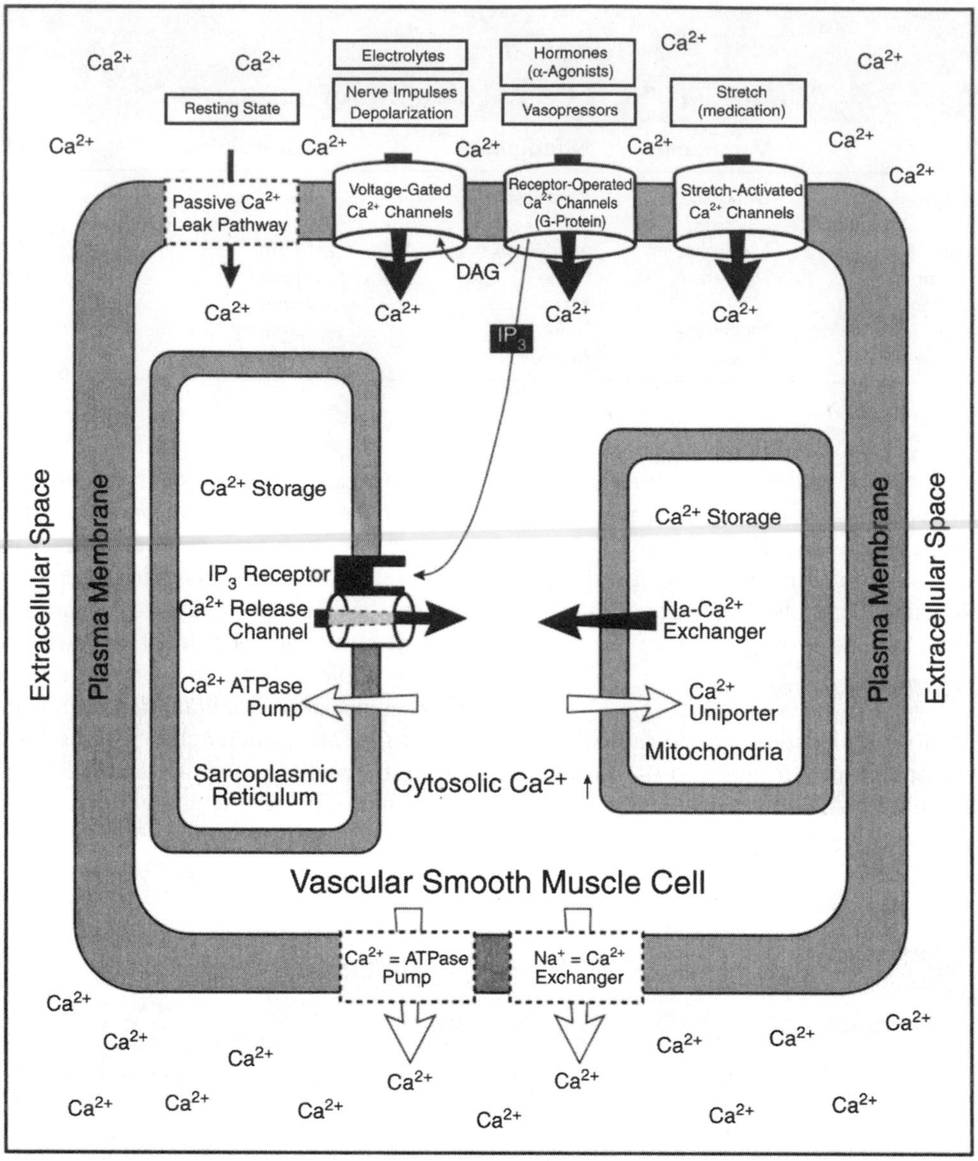

Figure 18-2. Calcium ion entry and exit from a vascular smooth muscle cell. Calcium enters the cytosol (*black arrows*) of the vascular smooth muscle cell either from the extracellular space through the plasma membrane (*top of diagram*) or from the intracellular storage areas. The primary entry sites for calcium ions are the voltage-gated channels. (From Kanneganti M, Halpern NA. Acute hypertension and calcium-channel blockers. *New Horizons* 1996;4:19–25; with permission.)

Clinical Uses

Verapamil is effective in the treatment of supraventricular tachydysrhythmias, reflecting its primary site of action on the atrioventricular node (see Chapter 17). The mild vasodilating effects produced by verapamil make this drug useful in the treatment of vasospastic angina pectoris and essential hypertension. Indeed, calcium-channels blockers are as effective as beta-blockers in relieving angina pectoris. Verapamil is not as active as nifedipine in its effects on vascular smooth muscle and therefore causes a less pronounced decrease in systemic blood pressure and less reflex peripheral sympathetic nervous system activity. Verapamil is effective in the treatment of symptomatic hypertrophic cardiomyopathy with or without left ventricular outflow obstruction (Spirito et al., 1997). Calcium-channel antagonists should not be routinely administered for acute myocardial infarction as postinfarction mortality is not decreased (Opie, 2000).

Verapamil may be useful in the treatment of maternal and fetal tachydysrhythmias as well as premature labor (Murad et al., 1985a). Administered intravenously (IV) to parturients, verapamil prolongs atrioventricular conduction of the fetus despite limited placental transport of the drug. Fetal hepatic extraction of verapamil is substantial, as evidenced by a plasma concentration in the fetal carotid artery that is less than that in the umbilical vein. Verapamil may decrease uterine blood flow, suggesting caution in the

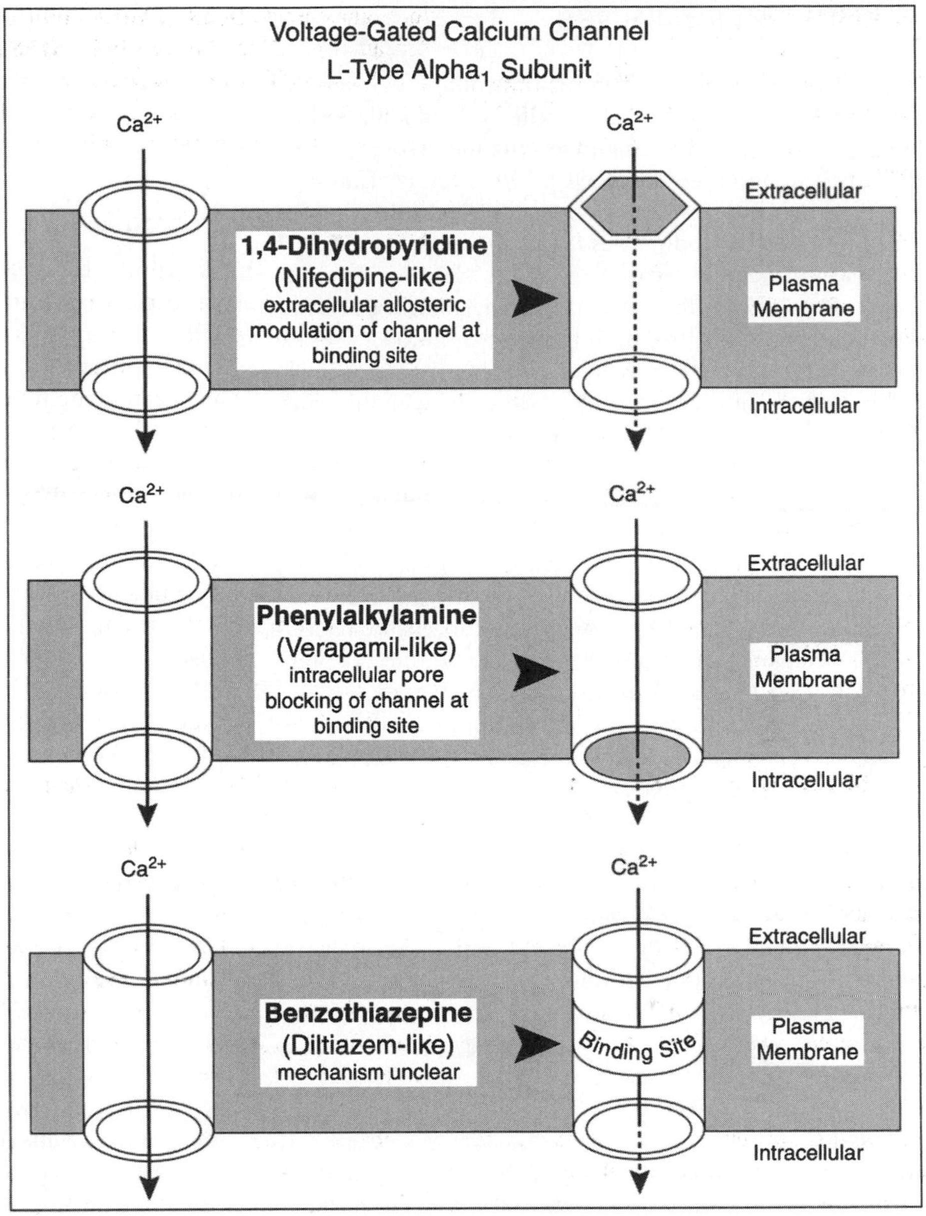

Figure 18-3. Mechanism of action of the three classes of calcium-channel blockers. (From Kanneganti M, Halpern NA. Acute hypertension and calcium-channel blockers. *New Horizons* 1996; 4:19–25; with permission.)

administration of this drug to parturients with impaired uteroplacental perfusion (Murad et al., 1985b).

Pharmacokinetics

Oral verapamil is almost completely absorbed, but extensive hepatic first-pass metabolism limits bioavailability to 10% to 20% (Table 18-3). As a result, the oral dose (80 to 160 mg three times daily) is about 10 times the IV dose. The therapeutic plasma concentration of verapamil is 100 to 300 ng/mL. The activity of oral verapamil peaks in 30 to 45 minutes compared with about 15 minutes following IV administration. Pharmacologic effects following IV administration of verapamil appear within 2 to 3 minutes and may last 6 hours.

Demethylated metabolites of verapamil predominate, with norverapamil possessing sufficient activity to contribute to the antidysrhythmic properties of the parent drug. In view of the nearly complete hepatic metabolism of verapamil, almost none of the drug appears unchanged in the urine. Conversely, an estimated 70% of an injected dose of verapamil is recovered in urine as metabolites and about 15% is excreted via bile. Chronic oral administration of verapamil or the presence of renal dysfunction leads to the accumulation of norverapamil.

The elimination half-time of verapamil is 6 to 12 hours, and this may be prolonged in patients with liver disease. In this regard, chronic treatment with verapamil has rarely been associated with increased plasma concentrations of transaminase enzymes. Like nifedipine, verapamil is highly protein bound (90%), and the presence of other drugs (lidocaine, diazepam, propranolol) can increase the pharmacologically active, unbound portion of the drug.

DIHYDROPYRIMIDINES

The dihydropyridines prevent calcium entry into the vascular smooth cells by extracellular allosteric modulation of the L-type voltage-gated calcium ion channels (see Fig. 18-3) (Kanneganti and Halpern, 1996). The primary affinity of the dihydropyridines nifedipine, nicardipine, isradipine, felodipine, and amlodipine is for the peripheral arterioles, whereas nimodipine favors cerebral vessels. The vasodilating effects of these drugs on venous capacitance vessels are minimal. As with other peripheral vasodilators, a reflex tachycardia attributed to sympathetic nervous system activity or baroreceptor reflexes may be observed with the acute administration of dihydropyridines.

Nifedipine

Nifedipine is a dihydropyridine derivative with greater coronary and peripheral arterial vasodilator properties than verapamil. There is minimal effect on venous capacitance vessels. Unlike verapamil, nifedipine has little or no direct depressant effect on sinoatrial or atrioventricular node activity. Peripheral vasodilation and the resulting decrease in systemic blood pressure produced by nifedipine activate baroreceptors, leading to increased peripheral sympathetic nervous system activity most often manifesting as an increased heart rate. This increased sympathetic nervous system activity counters the direct negative inotropic, chronotropic, and dromotropic effects of nifedipine. Nevertheless, nifedipine may produce excessive myocardial depression, especially in patients with preexisting left ventricular dysfunction or concomitant therapy with a beta-adrenergic antagonist drug. The presence of aortic stenosis may also exaggerate the cardiac depressant effects of nifedipine.

Clinical Uses

Nifedipine is administered orally with a 10 to 30 mg dose producing an effect in about 20 minutes with a peak effect between 60 and 90 minutes. Nifedipine is used to treat patients with angina pectoris, especially that due to coronary artery vasospasm.

Pharmacokinetics

Absorption of an oral or sublingual dose of nifedipine is about 90%, with onset of an effect being detectable within about 20 minutes after administration (see Table 18-3). It is likely that most of the absorption of sublingual nifedipine is via the gastrointestinal tract from swallowed saliva. Protein binding approaches 90%. Hepatic metabolism is nearly complete, with elimination of inactive metabolites principally in urine (about 80%) and, to a lesser extent, in bile. The elimination half-time is 3 to 7 hours.

Side Effects

The side effects of nifedipine include flushing, vertigo, and headache. Less common side effects include peripheral edema (venodilation), hypotension, paresthesias, and skeletal muscle weakness. Glucose intolerance and hepatic dysfunction occur rarely. Nifedipine may induce renal dysfunction. Abrupt discontinuation of nifedipine has been associated with coronary artery vasospasm.

Nicardipine

Nicardipine lacks effects on the sinoatrial node and atrioventricular node and has minimal myocardial depressant effects. This drug has the greatest vasodilating effects of all the calcium entry blockers, with vasodilation being particularly prominent in the coronary arteries. Combination with a beta-adrenergic antagonist for the treatment of angina is a consideration, as dihydropyridine calcium-channel blockers do not significantly depress the sinoatrial node. Of all the antianginal drugs, the dihydropyridine calcium-channel blockers produce the greatest dilatation of the peripheral arterioles. Therefore, either nifedipine or nicardipine may be particularly useful in patients who have residual hypertension despite beta-adrenergic blockade.

Nicardipine is available in IV and oral preparations (other dihydropyridine calcium-channel blockers are available only as oral preparations). A long elimination half-time is the basis for the recommendation that about 72 hours should elapse before increasing the oral dose. Nicardipine is metabolized in the liver and is highly protein bound (about 95%). The side effects of nicardipine are similar to nifedipine.

Clinical Uses

Nicardipine is used as a tocolytic drug having a similar tocolytic effect as salbutamol but with fewer side effects. When nicardipine is administered as a tocolytic it binds to the inside of myometrial L-type voltage-dependent calcium ion channels, causing them to remain closed, and thus inhibits uterine contractility. Pulmonary edema associated with salbutamol used as a tocolytic has also been reported in a parturient treated with nicardipine (Bal et al., 2004). Nicardipine, 40 μg/kg IV administered immediately before performing electroconvulsive therapy is effective in blunting acute hemodynamic responses to the treatment (Zhanag et al., 2005).

Nimodipine

Nimodipine is a highly lipid-soluble analogue of nifedipine. Lipid solubility facilitates its entrance into the central nervous system, where it blocks the influx of extracellular calcium ions necessary for contraction of large cerebral arteries.

Clinical Uses

The lipid solubility of nimodipine and its ability to cross the blood-brain barrier is responsible for the potential value of this drug in treating patients with subarachnoid hemorrhage.

Cerebral Vasospasm

The vasodilating effect of nimodipine on cerebral arteries is uniquely valuable in preventing or attenuating cerebral vasospasm that often accompanies subarachnoid hemorrhage (Verma, 2000). The initial event in the development of vasospasm may be an intracellular influx of calcium ions that cause contraction of smooth muscle cells in large cerebral arteries. Administration of nimodipine, 0.7 mg/kg orally as an initial dose followed by 0.35 mg/kg every 4 hours for 21 days, is associated with a decreased incidence of neurologic deficits due to cerebral vasospasm in patients who had experienced subarachnoid hemorrhage (Allen et al., 1983). Blood and cerebrospinal fluid levels of nimodipine with this dosing regimen were 6.9 ng/mL and 0.77 ng/mL, respectively. In comatose patients who cannot take oral medications, the recommendation is to extract the contents of the nimodipine capsule into a syringe and administer the drug into a nasogastric tube. To ensure delivery of the drug into the stomach via a nasogastric tube, it is necessary to add up to 30 mL of saline to the nimodipine-containing solution (Gelmers et al., 1988). Side effects have not been observed with the oral administration of nimodipine. Symptoms of excessive nimodipine effect would be expected to be related to cardiovascular effects such as peripheral vasodilation with associated systemic hypotension. Theoretically, drug-induced cerebral vasodilation could evoke increases in intracranial pressure, particularly in patients with preexisting decreases in intracranial compliance.

Cerebral Protection

Nimodipine has also been evaluated for cerebral protection after global ischemia as associated with cardiac arrest. The theoretical basis for considering calcium-channel blockers for this purpose is the observation that lack of oxygen interferes with maintenance of the normal calcium ion gradient across cell membranes, leading to a massive increase (at least 200-fold) in the intraneuronal concentrations of this ion. In this regard, nimodipine is associated with improved neurologic outcome when administered to primates within 5 minutes after experiencing 17 minutes of cerebral ischemia (Steen et al., 1985). The dose of nimodipine used (10 μg/kg IV followed by 1 μg/kg per minute IV) was associated with decreases in blood pressure that responded to infusion of fluids and/or dopamine.

Amlodipine

Amlodipine is a dihydropyridine derivative that is available for only oral administration (5 to 10 mg) resulting in a peak plasma concentration in 6 to 12 hours. Elimination half-time is 30 to 40 hours and about 90% of the drug undergoes hepatic metabolism to inactive products. Amlodipine appears to have minimal detrimental effects on myocardial contractility and provides anti-ischemic effects comparable to beta-blockers in patients with acute coronary syndrome (Opie, 2000). The combination of amlodipine and beta-blockers may be more effective in the treatment of myocardial ischemia than either drug alone.

BENZOTHIAZEPINES

Benzodiazepines act at the L-type channel alpha$_1$ subunit, although the mechanism of action is not well understood (see Fig. 18-3) (Kanneganti and Halpern, 1996). The benzodiazepine diltiazem may have two additional effects: It may act on the sodium-potassium pump, decreasing the amount of intracellular sodium available for exchange with extracellular calcium, and it may inhibit calcium-calmodulin binding.

Diltiazem

Diltiazem, like verapamil, blocks predominantly the calcium channels of the atrioventricular node and is therefore a first-line medication for the treatment of supraventricular tachydysrhythmias (see Chapter 17). It may also be used for the chronic control of essential hypertension. The effects of diltiazem on the sinoatrial and atrioventricular nodes and its vasodilating properties appear to be intermediate between those of verapamil and the dihydropyridines. Diltiazem exerts minimal cardiodepressant effects and is unlikely to interact with beta-adrenergic-blocking drugs to decrease myocardial contractility (Packer, 1989).

Clinical Uses

The clinical use and drug interactions for diltiazem are similar to those of verapamil. Diltiazem is available as an oral capsule and can also be administered IV, especially for the management of angina pectoris. The recommended IV dose is 0.25 to 0.35 mg/kg over 2 minutes and is repeated in 15 minutes, if needed. After the initial IV dose, diltiazem can be given by continuous infusion of about 10 mg/hour for up to 24 hours.

Pharmacokinetics

Oral absorption of diltiazem is excellent with an onset of action in 15 minutes and a peak effect in about 30 minutes (see Table 18-3). The drug is 70% to 80% bound to proteins and is excreted as inactive metabolites principally in bile (about 60%) and, to a lesser extent, in urine (about 35%). Active metabolites of diltiazem include desacetyldiltiazem and desmethyldiltiazem. The elimination half-time for the parent drug is 4 to 6 hours and about 20 hours for metabolites. As with verapamil, liver disease may necessitate a decrease in the dosage of diltiazem.

DRUG INTERACTIONS

The known pharmacologic effects of calcium-channel blockers on cardiac, skeletal, and vascular smooth muscle, as well as on the conduction velocity of cardiac impulses, make drug interactions possible (Durand et al., 1991). Verapamil and diltiazem have depressant effects on the generation of cardiac action potentials at the sinoatrial node and slow the movement of cardiac impulses through the atrioventricular node. Therefore, patients with preexisting cardiac conduction abnormalities may experience greater degrees of atrioventricular heart block with concurent administration of beta-blockers or digoxin. Myocardial depression and peripheral vasodilation produced by volatile anesthetics could be exaggerated by similar actions of calcium-channel blockers. Vasodilating effects of calcium-channel blockers could result in exaggerated systemic hypotension should these drugs be administered to hypovolemic patients.

The likelihood of adverse circulatory changes due to interactions between calcium-channel blockers and anesthetic drugs would seem to be greater in patients with preexisting atrioventricular heart block or left ventricular dysfunction. Nevertheless, treatment with calcium-channel blockers can be continued until the time of surgery without risk of significant drug interactions, especially with respect to conduction of cardiac impulses (Henling et al., 1984). Toxicity reflecting an overdose of calcium-channel blockers may be partially reversed with intravenous administration of calcium or dopamine.

Anesthetic Drugs

Calcium-channel blockers are vasodilators and myocardial depressants. In fact, the negative inotropic effects, depressant effects on sinoatrial node function, and peripheral vasodilating effects of these drugs and those of volatile anesthetics are similar, and there is evidence that volatile anesthetics have blocking effects on calcium channels (Merin, 1987). For these reasons, calcium-channel blockers must be administered with caution to patients with impaired left ventricular function or hypovolemia. Patients treated with a combination of beta-adrenergic blockers and nifedipine tolerate high-dose fentanyl anesthesia and do not show evidence of additive depression of cardiac function when verapamil is infused (Kapur et al., 1986). Conversely, in anesthetized patients with preexisting left ventricular dysfunction, administration of verapamil is associated with myocardial depression and decreased cardiac output (Chew et al., 1981). Furthermore, IV administration of verapamil or diltiazem during open-chest surgery in patients with depressed ventricular function and anesthetized with a volatile anesthetic may be associated with further decreases in ventricular function (Merin, 1987).

Treatment of cardiac dysrhythmias with calcium-channel blockers in anesthetized patients produces only transient decreases in systemic blood pressure and infrequent prolongation of the P-R interval on the ECG. Because of the tendency to produce atrioventricular heart block, verapamil should be used cautiously in patients being treated with digitalis or beta-adrenergic blocking drugs. Nevertheless, in patients with preoperative evidence of cardiac conduction abnormalities, the chronic combined administration of calcium-channel blockers and beta-adrenergic antagonists is not associated with cardiac conduction abnormalities in the perioperative period (Table 18-4) (Henling et al., 1984). Beta-adrenergic agonists increase the number of functioning slow calcium

TABLE 18-4.
EFFECT OF CHRONIC ANTIANGINAL THERAPY ON PERIOPERATIVE HEART RATE (beats/min) AND P-R INTERVAL (ms)

	Before Induction	After Induction	10 mins after Cardiopulmonary Bypass
Control			
Heart rate	72	71	87
P-R interval	160	156	164
Calcium-channel blockers			
Heart rate	69	70	86
P-R interval	168	169	175
Beta-adrenergic antagonists			
Heart rate	59	65	78
P-R interval	168	171	183
Nifedipine plus beta-adrenergic antagonists			
Heart rate	67	69	86
P-R interval	175	177	186

Source: Data from Henling CE, Slogoff S, Kodali SV, Arlund C. Heart block after coronary artery bypass—effect of chronic administration of calcium-entry blockers and beta-blockers. *Anesth Analg* 1984;63:515–520.

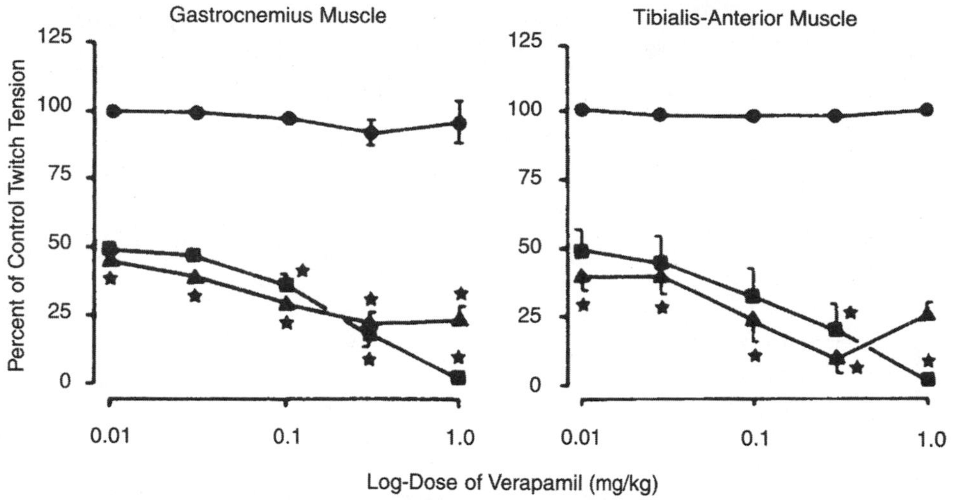

Figure 18-4. Infusion of verapamil in the absence of neuromuscular-blocking drugs (*solid circles*) does not alter twitch height response (twitch tension) of indirectly stimulated rabbit skeletal muscle. When twitch tension is decreased to about 50% of control by the continuous infusion of pancuronium (*solid squares*) or succinylcholine (*solid triangles*), the addition of verapamil further decreases twitch tension. (*$P < .05$ compared with the twitch tension before verapamil; mean ± SE.) (From Durant NN, Nguyen N, Katz RL. Potentiation of neuromuscular blockade by verapamil. *Anesthesiology* 1984;60:298–303; with permission.)

channels in myocardial cell membranes through a cyclic adenosine monophosphate mechanism and readily counter the effects of calcium-channel blockers. Nevertheless, there is no evidence that patients being treated chronically with calcium-channel blockers are at increased risk for anesthesia.

Neuromuscular-Blocking Drugs

Calcium-channel blockers alone do not produce a skeletal muscle relaxant effect (Fig. 18-4) (Durant et al., 1984). Conversely, these drugs potentiate the effects of depolarizing and nondepolarizing neuromuscular-blocking drugs (see Fig. 18-4) (Durant et al., 1984; van Poorten et al., 1984). This potentiation resembles that produced by mycin antibiotics in the presence of neuromuscular-blocking drugs (see Chapter 28). The local anesthetic effects of verapamil and diltiazem, reflecting inhibition of sodium ion flux via fast sodium channels, may also contribute to the potentiation of neuromuscular-blocking drugs. Observations of skeletal muscle weakness after administration of verapamil to a patient with muscular dystrophy are inconsistent with diminished release of neurotransmitter (Zalman et al., 1983). Therefore, the neuromuscular effects of verapamil may be more likely to manifest in patients with a compromised margin of safety of neuromuscular transmission.

Antagonism of neuromuscular blockade may be impaired because of diminished presynaptic release of acetylcholine in the presence of a calcium-channel blocker (Lawson et al., 1983). Indeed, calcium ions are necessary for the release of acetylcholine at the neuromuscular junction. In one report, edrophonium but not neostigmine was effective in antagonizing nondepolarizing neuromuscular blockade that was potentiated by verapamil (Jones et al., 1985).

Local Anesthetics

Verapamil and diltiazem have potent local anesthetic activity, which may increase the risk of local anesthetic toxicity when regional anesthesia is administered to patients being treated with this drug (Rosenblatt et al., 1984).

Potassium-Containing Solutions

Calcium-channel blockers slow the inward movement of potassium ions. For this reason, hyperkalemia in patients being treated with verapamil may occur after much smaller amounts of exogenous potassium infusion as associated with the use of potassium chloride to treat hypokalemia or administration of stored whole blood (Nugent et al., 1984). In animals, however, pretreatment with verapamil does not alter the increases in plasma potassium concentrations that follow the administration of succinylcholine (Roth et al., 1985).

Dantrolene

The ability of both verapamil and dantrolene to inhibit intracellular calcium ion flux and excitation-contraction coupling would suggest this combination might be useful in the treatment of malignant hyperthermia. In swine, however, the administration of dantrolene in the presence of verapamil or diltiazem results in hyperkalemia and cardiovascular collapse (Fig. 18-5) (Saltzman et al., 1984). A

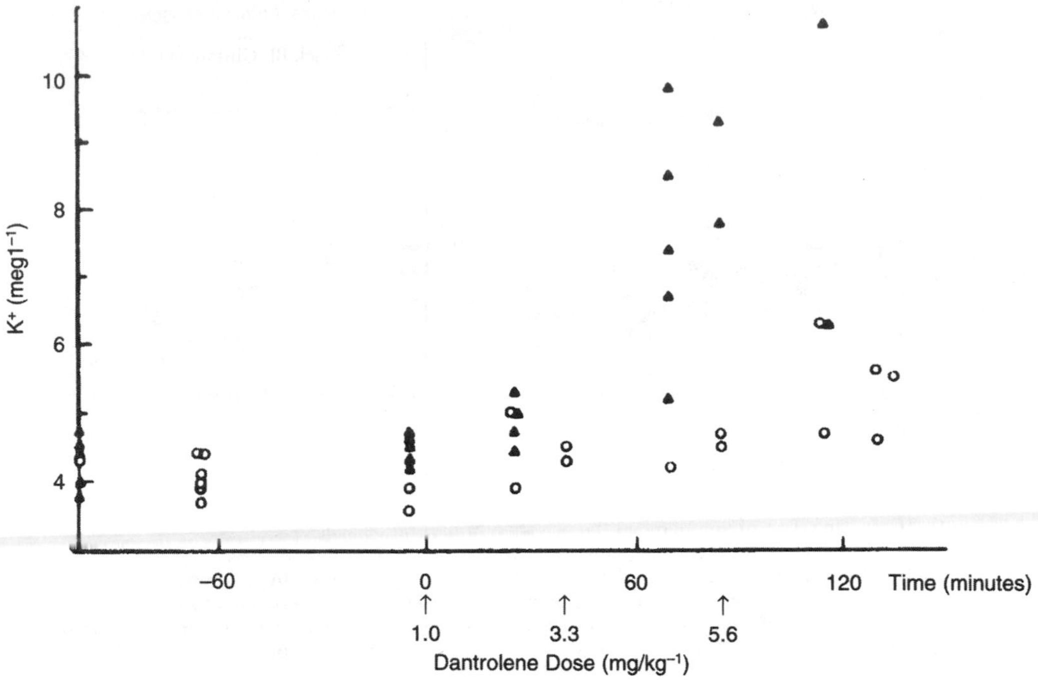

Figure 18-5. Administration of dantrolene to swine pretreated with verapamil (*solid triangles*) results in hyperkalemia compared with animals receiving only dantrolene (*open circles*). (From Saltzman LS, Kates RA, Corke BC, et al. Hyperkalemia and cardiovascular collapse after verapamil and dantrolene administration in swine. *Anesth Analg* 1984;63:473–478; with permission.)

patient receiving verapamil developed hyperkalemia and myocardial depression within 1.5 hours of being treated with dantrolene administered IV (Rubin and Zablocki, 1987). This same patient did not experience hyperkalemia when nifedipine was substituted for verapamil before pretreatment with dantrolene.

Whenever calcium-channel blockers, especially verapamil or diltiazem, and dantrolene must be administered concurrently, invasive hemodynamic monitoring and frequent measurement of the plasma potassium concentration are recommended. It is speculated that verapamil alters normal homeostatic mechanisms for regulation of plasma potassium concentrations and may result in hyperkalemia from dantrolene-induced potassium release. Furthermore, there is evidence that verapamil does not influence the ability of known triggering drugs to evoke malignant hyperthermia in susceptible animals (Gallant et al., 1985).

Platelet Function

Calcium-channel blockers may interfere with calcium-mediated platelet functions.

Digoxin

Calcium-channel blockers may increase the plasma concentration of digoxin, presumably by decreasing its plasma clearance.

H-2 Antagonists

Cimetidine and ranitidine by altering hepatic enzyme activity and/or hepatic blood flow may increase the plasma concentrations of calcium-channel blockers.

RISKS OF CHRONIC TREATMENT

Despite the popularity of calcium-channel blockers in the treatment of cardiovascular diseases (essential hypertension, angina pectoris), there is increasing concern about the long-term safety of these drugs, especially the short-acting dihydropyrimidine derivatives (Chobanian, 1996). For example, the risk of developing cardiovascular complications has been described as being greater in patients treated with nifedipine compared with those receiving placebo or conventional therapy (Furberg et al., 1995). Increased perioperative bleeding and an increased incidence of gastrointestinal hemorrhage have been reported in patients receiving a dihydropyrimidine derivative (Pahor et al., 1996a; Wagenknecht et al., 1995). The risk of developing cancer may be increased in those treated with calcium-channel blockers compared with beta-adrenergic antagonists or angiotensin-converting enzyme inhibitors (Pahor et al., 1996b). For these reasons, treatment with calcium-channel blockers, especially short-acting dihydropyrimidine derivatives, should generally be reserved for second-step rather than initial therapy (Chobanian, 1996).

CYTOPROTECTION

Drug-induced calcium-channel blockade may provide cytoprotection against ischemic reperfusion injury. By decreasing calcium ion entry into cells and the conversion of xanthine dehydrogenase to xanthine oxidase (dependent on the calcium/calmodulin complex), calcium-channel blockers may limit the accumulation of oxygen free radicals. Calcium-channel blockers may attenuate renal injury from nephrotoxic drugs such as cisplatinum and radiocontrast dyes. The vasodilator effects of calcium-channel blockers and resultant control of systemic hypertension may result in increases in renal blood flow and glomerular filtration rate, thus favoring natriuresis.

REFERENCES

Allen GS, Ahn HS, Preziosi TJ, et al. Cerebral arterial spasm: a controlled trial of nimodipine in patients with subarachnoid hemorrhage. *N Engl J Med* 1983;308:619–624.

Bal L, Thierry S, Brocas E, et al. Pulmonary edema induced by calcium-channel blockade for tocolysis. *Anesth Analg* 2004;99:910–911.

Chew CYC, Hecht HS, Collett JT, et al. Influence of severity of ventricular dysfunction on hemodynamic responses to intravenously administered verapamil in ischemic heart disease. *Am J Cardiol* 1981;47:917–922.

Chobanian AV. Calcium-channel blockers: lessons learned from MIDAS and other clinical trials. *JAMA* 1996;276:829–830.

Durand PG, Lehot JJ, Foex P. Calcium-channel blockers and anaesthesia. *Can J Anaesth* 1991;38:75–89.

Durant NN, Nguyen N, Katz RL. Potentiation of neuromuscular blockade by verapamil. *Anesthesiology* 1984;60:298–303.

Furberg CD, Posaty BM, Meyer JV. Nifedipine: dose-related increase in mortality in patients with coronary heart disease. *Circulation* 1995;92:1326–1331.

Gallant EM, Foldes FF, Rempel WE, Gronert GA. Verapamil is not a therapeutic adjunct to dantrolene in porcine malignant hyperthermia. *Anesth Analg* 1985;64:601–606.

Gelmers HJ, Gorter K, deWeerdt CJ, et al. A controlled trial of nimodipine in acute ischemic stroke. *N Engl J Med* 1988;318:303–307.

Henling CE, Slogoff S, Kodali SV, Arlund C. Heart block after coronary artery bypass—effect of chronic administration of calcium-entry blockers and beta-blockers. *Anesth Analg* 1984;63:515–520.

Jones RM, Cashman JN, Casson WR, et al. Verapamil potentiation of neuromuscular blockade: failure of reversal with neostigmine but prompt reversal with edrophonium. *Anesth Analg* 1985;64:1021–1025.

Kanneganti M, Halpern NA. Acute hypertension and calcium-channel blockers. *New Horizons* 1996;4:19–25.

Kaplan NM. Calcium entry blockers in the treatment of hypertension: current status and future prospects. *N Engl J Med* 1989;262:817–823.

Kapur PA, Norel EJ, Dajee H, et al. Hemodynamic effects of verapamil administration after large doses of fentanyl in man. *Can Anaesth Soc J* 1986;33:138–144.

Kraynack BJ, Lawson NW, Gintautas J. Local anesthetic effect of verapamil in vitro. *Reg Anesth* 1982;7:114–117.

Lawson NW, Kraynack BJ, Gintautas J. Neuromuscular and electrocardiographic responses to verapamil in dogs. *Anesth Analg* 1983;62:50–54.

Merin RG. Calcium channel blocking drugs and anesthetics: is the drug interaction beneficial or detrimental? *Anesthesiology* 1987;66:111–113.

Murad SHN, Tabsh KMA, Conklin KA, et al. Verapamil: placental transfer and effects on maternal and fetal hemodynamics and atrioventricular conduction in the pregnant ewe. *Anesthesiology* 1985a;62:49–53.

Murad SHN, Tabsh KMA, Shilyanski G, et al. Effects of verapamil on uterine blood flow and maternal cardiovascular function in the awake pregnant ewe. *Anesth Analg* 1985b;64:7–10.

Nugent M, Tinker JH, Moyer TP. Verapamil worsens rate of development and hemodynamic effects of acute hyperkalemia in halothane-anesthetized dogs. Effects of calcium therapy. *Anesthesiology* 1984;60:435–439.

Opie LH. First line drugs in chronic stable effort angina: the case for newer, longer-acting calcium channel blocking drugs. *J Am Coll Cardiol* 2000;36:1967–1971.

Packer M. Combined beta-adrenergic and calcium-entry blockade in angina pectoris. *N Engl J Med* 1989;320:709–717.

Pahor M, Guralnik JM, Furberg CD, et al. Risk of gastrointestinal hemorrhage with calcium antagonists in hypertensive patients over 67. *Lancet* 1996a;347:1061–1066.

Pahor M, Guralnik JM, Salive ME, et al. Do calcium-channel blockers increase the risk of cancer? *Am J Hypertens* 1996b;9:695–699.

Reves JG, Kissin I, Lell WA, Tosone S. Calcium entry blockers: uses and implications for anesthesiologists. *Anesthesiology* 1982;57:504–518.

Reves JG. The relative hemodynamic effects of calcium entry blockers. *Anesthesiology* 1984;61:3–5.

Rosenblatt RM, Weaver JM, Want Y, Tallman RD. Verapamil potentiates the toxicity of local anesthetics. *Anesth Analg* 1984;63:269.

Roth JL, Nugent M, Gronert GA. Verapamil does not alter succinylcholine-induced increases in serum potassium during halothane anesthesia in normal dogs. *Anesth Analg* 1985;64:1202–1204.

Rubin AS, Zablocki AD. Hyperkalemia, verapamil, and dantrolene. *Anesthesiology* 1987;66:246–249.

Saltzman LS, Kates RA, Corke BC, et al. Hyperkalemia and cardiovascular collapse after verapamil and dantrolene administration in swine. *Anesth Analg* 1984;63:473–478.

Spirito P, Seidman CE, McKenna WJ, et al. The management of hypertrophic cardiomyopathy. *N Engl J Med* 1997;336:775–780.

Steen PA, Gisvold SE, Milde JH, et al. Nimodipine improves outcome when given after complete cerebral ischemia in primates. *Anesthesiology* 1985;62:406–414.

van Poorten JE, Chasmana KM, Kuypers SM, et al. Verapamil and reversal of vecuronium neuromuscular blockade. *Anesth Analg* 1984;63:155–157.

Verma A. Opportunities for neuroprotection in traumatic brain injury. *J Head Trauma Rehabil* 2000;15:1149–1156.

Wagenknecht LE, Furberg CD, Hammon JW, et al. Surgical bleeding: unexpected effect of a calcium antagonist. *BMJ* 1995;310:776–777.

Zalman F, Perloff JK, Durant NW, et al. Acute respiratory failure following intravenous verapamil in Duchenne's muscular dystrophy. *Am Heart J* 1983;105:510–511.

Drugs Used for Psychopharmacologic Therapy

19

Drugs used for psychopharmacologic therapy include antidepressants, anxiolytics, lithium, and antipsychotics. The development of relatively safe and effective psychotherapeutic drugs has made it possible to effectively treat as ambulatory patients many individuals with depression and anxiety disorders. Antidepressants and anxiolytics are the drugs most likely to be prescribed by primary care physicians for the treatment of depression in adults. Lithium and antipsychotic drugs are useful for treatment of bipolar disorders and psychotic disorders including schizophrenia. It is estimated that between 2% and 4% of the population is treated for a depressive illness at some time in life, and mood disorders requiring antidepressant therapy are an increasingly frequent occurrence in the elderly population.

It is now accepted that anesthesia can be safely administered to patients being treated with drugs used to treat mental illness (El-Ganzouri et al., 1985; Michaels et al., 1984). There appears to be growing acceptance that the problem of drug interactions between psychopharmacologic drugs and drugs administered in the perioperative period is less than previously perceived and that past recommendations for discontinuation of antidepressant therapy are not justified. Nevertheless, it remains important to remain alert for potential drug interactions (Wells and Bjorksten, 1989). This is particularly true in elderly patients, who constitute the majority of patients on antidepressant drugs.

ANTIDEPRESSANTS

Considering the wide range of disorders for which antidepressant drugs are effective, the term *antidepressant* has become a misnomer (Table 19-1). The broad spectrum of effectiveness of antidepressants does not imply a common pathophysiology but rather reflects the diverse roles of monoamine neurotransmitters in the human nervous system.

Antidepressants are logically classified based on their chemical structures and their acute neuropharmacologic effects (Table 19-2). The precise mechanism by which antidepressants work is unknown, but they appear to act by altering noradrenergic neurotransmission and/or serotoninergic neurotransmission (see Table 19-2). This suggests that antidepressants work by increasing the amount of norepinephrine and serotonin in synapses. Nevertheless, the most important observation not explained by this hypothesis is the time course of clinical improvement. Neurobiologically, reuptake blockade or monoamine oxidase (MAO) inhibition (necessary for breakdown of free norepinephrine and serotonin) occurs promptly after initiation of antidepressant therapy, but clinical improvement typically does not occur for 2 to 4 weeks. Perhaps adaptive changes including downregulation of neurotransmitter receptors are necessary before evidence of clinical improvement appears.

Selective Serotonin Reuptake Inhibitors

The selective serotonin reuptake inhibitors (SSRIs) are the most broadly prescribed class of antidepressants and are the drugs of choice for the treatment of mild to moderate depression (Richelson, 2001). SSRIs are the first line pharmacotherapy for panic disorder and obsessive-compulsive syndrome. These drugs are also effective in treatment of social phobia and post-traumatic stress disorder. SSRIs that share the ability to block the reuptake of serotonin (and thus enhance serotonergic activity) include fluoxetine, paroxetine, sertraline, fluvoxamine, citalopram, and escitalopram. Other newer SSRIs are believed to act on

TABLE 19-1. CLINICAL USES OF ANTIDEPRESSANT DRUGS

Unipolar and bipolar depression
Panic disorder
Social phobia
Posttraumatic stress syndrome
Neuropathic pain
Migraine prophylaxis
Obsessive-compulsive disorder
Bulimia
Childhood attention-deficit hyperactivity disorder

serotonin and norepinephrine pathways in the brain by a variety of mechanisms, including dual serotonin and norepinephrine reuptake blockade (venlafaxine) and $alpha_2$ receptor blockade (mirtazapine) (Harvey et al., 2000). Different SSRIs have different side-effect profiles, so patients who do not respond to one drug or who fail to tolerate the drug may do well on a different SSRI. Standard practice dictates trying several SSRIs before moving to another class of medication.

There is abundant evidence that serotonin receptors are involved in the etiology of anxiety. Potent inhibition of serotonin reuptake appears to be necessary for effectiveness in the treatment of obsessive-compulsive disorders. Compared with tricyclic antidepressants, SSRIs lack anticholinergic properties, do not cause postural hypotension or delayed conduction of cardiac impulses, and do not appear to have a major effect on the seizure threshold. Perhaps the most important advantage of SSRIs compared with tricyclic antidepressants is the safety of SSRIs when taken in overdose (Buckley and McManus, 2002). The exception may be venlafaxine that may be similar to tricyclic antidepressants with respect to overdose-associated risks and in having proconvulsant and cardiac side effects (Whyte, 2003). Common side effects of SSRIs include insomnia, agitation, headache, nausea, and diarrhea. A prominent cause of noncompliance with SSRI therapy is

TABLE 19-2. COMPARATIVE PHARMACOLOGY OF ANTIDEPRESSANT DRUGS

	Sedative Potency	Anticholinergic Potency	Orthostatic Hypotension
Selective serotonin-uptake inhibitors			
Fluoxetine	+	+	+
Sertraline	+	+	+
Paroxetine	+	+	+
Fluvoxamine	+	+	+
Citalopram	+	+	+
Escitalopram	+	+	+
Bupropion	+	+	+
Venlafaxine	+	+	May cause hypertension in some individuals
Trazodone	+++	+	+++; associated with cardiac dysrhythmias
Nefazodone	++	+	++
Tricyclic and related cyclic compounds*			
Amitriptyline	+++	++++	+++
Amoxapine	+	+	++
Clomipramine	+++	+++	+++
Desipramine	+	+	++
Doxepin	+++	++	++
Imipramine	++	++	+++
Nortriptyline	+	+	0
Protriptyline	+	+++	+
Trimipramine	+++	++	++
Mirtazapine			
Monoamine oxidase inhibitors			
Phenelzine	+	+	+++
Tranylcypromine	+	+	+++
Isocarboxazid	+	+	+++

0, none; +, mild; ++, moderate; +++, marked; ++++, greatest.
*All tricyclic and related cyclic compounds may produce cardiac dysrhythmias.

drug-induced sexual dysfunction (delayed ejaculation, anorgasmia, decreased libido) (Hirschfeld, 1999).

Abrupt discontinuation of SSRIs with short elimination half-times (paroxetine, venlafaxine) may be associated with dizziness, paresthesias, myalgias, irritability, insomnia, and visual disturbances. Tapering all SSRIs before discontinuance is recommended especially for drugs with short elimination half-times (Coupland et al., 1996).

In September 2004, the Food and Drug Administration recommended a "black box" warning for newer antidepressant drugs, primarily SSRIs (Newman, 2004). This warning is based on evidence that suicidal tendencies in children and adolescents may be increased in those age groups when they are treated with SSRIs. Nevertheless, the risk is small and many patients benefit from treatment with SSRIs emphasizing the need to individualize therapy.

Fluoxetine

Fluoxetine was the first SSRI introduced in the United States in 1988 (Gram, 1994). The drug is commonly administered once daily in the morning to decrease the risk of insomnia. Because fluoxetine has a prolonged elimination half-time (1 to 3 days for acute administration and 4 to 6 days for chronic administration), the drug can be taken every other day. An active metabolite, norfluoxetine, has an elimination half-time of 4 to 16 days. A therapeutic effect produced by fluoxetine is usually evident in 2 to 4 weeks. Because of this drug's prolonged elimination half-time, increases in dosage are often limited to no more often than once every 4 weeks.

Side Effects

The most common side effects of fluoxetine are nausea, anorexia, insomnia, sexual dysfunction, agitation, and neuromuscular restlessness, which may mimic akathisia. Appetite suppression associated with fluoxetine therapy may help patients achieve weight loss (Goldstein et al., 1994). Like tricyclic antidepressants, fluoxetine may be an effective analgesic for treatment of chronic pain as may be associated with rheumatoid arthritis (Rani et al., 1996). Fluoxetine does not cause hypotension, and changes in conduction of cardiac impulses seem infrequent. Bradycardia causing syncope has been reported in occasional elderly patients (Gram, 1994). Because of its long elimination half-time, fluoxetine should be discontinued for about 5 weeks before initiating treatment with an MAO inhibitor. The long elimination half-time of fluoxetine appears to prevent withdrawal symptoms induced by abrupt discontinuance of the drug. An overdose with fluoxetine alone is not associated with the risk of cardiovascular and central nervous system (CNS) toxicity.

Drug Interactions

Among the SSRIs, fluoxetine is the most potent inhibitor of certain hepatic cytochrome P-450 enzymes. As a result, this drug may increase the plasma concentrations of drugs that depend on hepatic metabolism for clearance. For example, the addition of fluoxetine to treatment with a tricyclic antidepressant drug may result in a two- to fivefold increase in the plasma concentration of the tricyclic drug. Neuroleptic drugs may inhibit the metabolism of fluoxetine or vice versa. Several cardiac antidysrhythmic drugs as well as some beta-adrenergic antagonists may be metabolized by the same enzyme system that is inhibited by fluoxetine, resulting in potentiation of these drug effects. MAO inhibitors combined with fluoxetine may cause the development of a serotonin syndrome characterized by anxiety, restlessness, chills, ataxia, and insomnia (Gram, 1994). The combination of fluoxetine and lithium or carbamazepine may also provoke this potentially fatal syndrome.

Sertraline

Sertraline was the second SSRI introduced in the United States and has a spectrum of efficacy similar to fluoxetine. This drug has a shorter elimination half-time (25 hours) than fluoxetine and is a less potent inhibitor of hepatic microsomal enzymes. A potentially active metabolite has an elimination half-time of 60 to 70 hours.

Compared with fluoxetine, sertraline may cause more gastrointestinal symptoms (nausea, diarrhea) but may be less likely to cause insomnia and agitation. The recommended washout period before starting an MAO inhibitor is 14 days.

Paroxetine

Paroxetine was the third SSRI introduced in the United States and has an efficacy similar to that of fluoxetine. This drug has a relatively short elimination half-time (24 hours), and there are no active metabolites. Side effects resemble those of other SSRIs with the exception of a possibly increased incidence of sedation. The levels of paroxetine in breast milk are greater than levels in patients receiving fluoxetine or sertraline. Paroxetine produces less inhibition of hepatic cytoplasmic P-450 enzymes than is fluoxetine. Enhancement of the anticoagulant effect of warfarin reflects competition for common protein-binding sites. The recommended washout period before starting an MAO inhibitor is 14 days.

Fluvoxamine

Fluvoxamine is effective in the management of obsessive-compulsive disorders. In addition, this drug probably has a spectrum of therapeutic efficacy similar to that of other SSRIs. The most common side effects associated with this drug are nausea, vomiting (possibly a greater frequency than with other SSRIs), headache, sedation, insomnia, and sexual dysfunction. Although it produces less inhibition of hepatic cytoplasmic P-450 enzymes than the other SSRIs, fluvoxamine may still cause clinically significant drug interactions.

Bupropion

Bupropion, which is structurally related to amphetamine, is effective in the treatment of major depression, producing improvement in 2 to 4 weeks. In addition, bupropion is effective for smoking cessation. The mechanism of action of bupropion is obscure but may include inhibition of dopamine and norepinephrine reuptake. This drug does not inhibit MAO. Bupropion is associated with a greater incidence of seizures (about 0.4%) than other antidepressants (Johnston et al., 1991). Some patients experience stimulant-like effects early in therapy. Like the SSRIs, bupropion has no anticholinergic effects, does not cause postural hypotension, and lacks significant effects on conduction of cardiac impulses. Unlike the SSRIs, bupropion is not associated with significant drug interactions and is not commonly associated with sexual dysfunction. Ataxia and myoclonus have occurred rarely. Bupropion should not be administered in combination with an MAO inhibitor.

Venlafaxine

Venlafaxine is perceived to have a profile of efficacy similar to that of the tricyclic antidepressants but has a more favorable side effect profile. Like the tricyclic antidepressants, this drug inhibits the reuptake of norepinephrine and serotonin and may potentiate the action of dopamine in the central nervous system (CNS). Unlike tricyclic antidepressants, venlafaxine does not produce anticholinergic effects or postural hypotension. Side effects include insomnia, sedation, and nausea. At high doses, a modest but persistent increase in diastolic blood pressure occurs in 5% to 7% of patients. Venlafaxine is metabolized by cytochrome P-450 enzymes and also acts as a weak inhibitor of these enzymes. The elimination half-time is 5 hours and that of its active metabolite is 11 hours. Venlafaxine should not be used in combination with an MAO inhibitor, and the recommended washout period is 14 days.

Trazodone

Trazodone inhibits serotonin reuptake and may also act as a serotonin agonist via an active metabolite. Although effective in the management of depression, its greatest efficacy may be treatment of insomnia induced by SSRIs or bupropion. Common side effects of trazodone include sedation, orthostatic hypotension, nausea, and vomiting. Priapism may occur in males. This drug lacks effects on conduction of cardiac impulses but on rare occasions has been associated with cardiac dysrhythmias. The elimination half-time of this drug is brief (3 to 9 hours), and toxicity associated with an overdose is less than what accompanies an overdose of tricyclic antidepressants and MAO inhibitors. Combination therapy with an MAO inhibitor is not recommended.

Nefazodone

Nefazodone is chemically related to trazodone but with fewer $alpha_1$-adrenergic-blocking properties. Like trazodone, this drug inhibits reuptake of serotonin and norepinephrine. The risk of sedation and priapism may be less than in patients treated with trazodone. The principal side effects are nausea, dry mouth, and sedation. Orthostatic hypotension may occur. Nefazodone-induced inhibition of cytochrome P-450 results in elevated plasma concentrations of benzodiazepines, antihistamines, and of protease inhibitors used in the treatment of HIV infection. Combination therapy with an MAO inhibitor is not recommended.

Tricyclic and Related Antidepressants

Before the availability of SSRIs, tricyclic antidepressants and related cyclic antidepressants were the most commonly used drugs to treat depression (see Table 19-2). Although tricyclic antidepressants are highly effective, they have been supplanted as first-line drugs in many clinical situations because of their unfavorable side-effect profile (largely resulting from their anticholinergic, antiadrenergic, and antihistaminic properties). Tricyclic antidepressants also have a narrow therapeutic index and are potentially lethal in overdose (resulting in part from inhibition of sodium ion channels) reflecting a slowing of conduction of cardiac impulses and appearance of life threatening cardiac dysrhythmias.

Measurement of plasma drug levels for the tricyclics imipramine, desipramine, and nortriptyline can be useful in guiding therapeutic decisions. Generally, plasma levels should not exceed 225 ng/mL when imipramine is administered. Plasma levels should not exceed 125 ng/mL when desipramine is administered, and the therapeutic range for nortriptyline is 50 to 150 ng/mL. It is preferable to taper tricyclic and tetracyclic antidepressants during a 4-week period to avoid the risk of withdrawal symptoms (chills, coryza, muscle aches). These symptoms have been attributed to supersensitivity of the cholinergic nervous system.

Chronic Pain Syndromes

The tricyclic antidepressants (especially amitriptyline and imipramine), in doses lower than those used to treat depression, may be useful in the treatment of chronic neuropathic pain. Because of their structural similarities to local anesthetics, it is possible that tricyclic antidepressants produce antiinflammatory effects similar to local anesthetics. Since many chronic pain syndromes include an inflammatory component, it is possible that the clinical efficacy of tricyclic antidepressants in chronic pain patients is due to inhibition of an overactive inflammatory system (Strumper et al., 2003).

Structure–Activity Relationships

The structure of tricyclic antidepressants resembles that of local anesthetics and phenothiazines (Fig. 19-1). Similar to local anesthetics, tricyclic antidepressants include a hydrophobic portion linked to an amide via a linear intermediate moiety. Tricyclic denotes the three-ring chemical structure of the central portion of the molecule

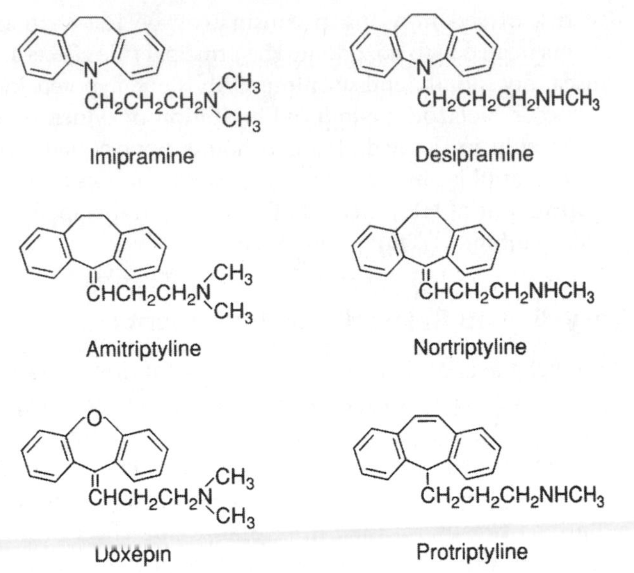

Figure 19-1. Tricyclic antidepressants.

(see Fig. 19-1). Imipramine, which is the prototype of the tricyclic antidepressants, differs from phenothiazine only in the replacement of the sulfur atom with an ethylene linkage to produce a seven-membered central ring. Desipramine is the principal metabolite of imipramine, and nortriptyline is the demethylated metabolite of amitriptyline. Maprotiline is a tetracyclic antidepressant with a clinical profile that resembles imipramine. Mirtazapine is a tetracyclic antidepressant that may enhance central norepinephrine and serotonin activity in the CNS. Maprotiline and mirtazapine should not be administered to patients being treated with MAO inhibitors.

Mechanism of Action

Tricyclic antidepressants act at several transporters and receptors, but their antidepressant effect is likely produced by blocking the reuptake (uptake) of serotonin and/or norepinephrine at presynaptic terminals, thereby increasing the availability of these neurotransmitters. These drugs can be categorized into tertiary amines, which inhibit reuptake of both serotonin and norepinephrine (amitriptyline, imipramine, clomipramine) and secondary amines, which are primarily norepinephrine reuptake inhibitors (desipramine, nortriptyline). Despite the prompt onset of this effect, the development of a therapeutic antidepressant effect is inexplicably delayed for 2 to 3 weeks. For this reason, there is doubt that antidepressant effects are totally due to an accumulation of biogenic amines in the brain. Furthermore, some drugs without effects on uptake of biogenic amines are effective antidepressants. It seems likely that potentiation of monoaminergic neurotransmission in the brain is only an early event in a complex cascade of events that eventually results in an antidepressant effect. Indeed, chronic administration of these drugs is associated with (a) decreased sensitivity of postsynaptic $beta_1$ and $serotonin_2$ receptors and of presynaptic $alpha_2$ receptors, and (b) increased sensitivity of postsynaptic $alpha_1$ receptors.

Pharmacokinetics

Tricyclic antidepressants are efficiently absorbed from the gastrointestinal tract after oral administration, reflecting high lipid solubility. Peak plasma concentrations occur within 2 to 8 hours after oral administration. Therapeutic plasma concentrations (parent drug plus the pharmacologically active demethylated metabolites) are 100 to 300 ng/mL, whereas toxicity is likely at levels >500 ng/mL. Tricyclic antidepressants are strongly bound to plasma and tissue proteins, which, in combination with high lipid solubility, results in a large volume of distribution (up to 50 liters/kg) for these drugs. The long elimination half-time (17 to 30 hours) and wide range of therapeutic plasma concentrations make once-daily dosing intervals effective.

Metabolism

Tricyclic antidepressants are oxidized by microsomal enzymes in the liver with subsequent conjugation with glucuronic acid. The individual variation in rate of metabolism between patients is 10- to 30-fold. Metabolism is likely to be slowed in elderly patients. The elimination of tricyclic antidepressants occurs over several days, with 1 week or longer required for excretion.

Imipramine is metabolized to the active compound desipramine. Both these active compounds are inactivated by oxidation of hydroxy metabolites and by conjugation with glucuronic acid. Nortriptyline, which is the pharmacologically active demethylated metabolite of imipramine and amitriptyline, can accumulate to levels that exceed the precursors. Doxepin also appears to be converted to an active metabolite, nordoxepin, by demethylation.

Side Effects

The side effects of tricyclic antidepressants occur frequently, most commonly manifesting as (a) anticholinergic effects, (b) cardiovascular effects, and (c) CNS effects (see Table 19-2). Marked individual variation in the incidence and type of side effects that may be related to the plasma concentrations of the tricyclic antidepressant and its active metabolites.

Anticholinergic Effects

The anticholinergic effects of tricyclic antidepressants are prominent, especially at high doses. Amitriptyline causes the highest incidence of anticholinergic effects (dry mouth, blurred vision, tachycardia, urinary retention, slowed gastric emptying, ileus), whereas desipramine produces the fewest such effects (see Table 19-2). Anticholinergic delirium may occur in elderly patients even at therapeutic doses of these drugs. Serious anticholinergic toxicity may reflect the results of polypharmacy with more than one anticholinergic drug (over-the-counter preparations to treat diarrhea or insomnia). Elderly patients have greater sensitivity to anticholinergic and other receptor effects compared with younger patients being treated with tricyclic antidepressants.

Cardiovascular Effects

Orthostatic hypotension and modest increases in heart rate are the most common cardiovascular side effects of tricyclic antidepressants, presumably reflecting drug-induced inhibition of norepinephrine reuptake into presynaptic nerve terminals. Orthostatic hypotension may be particularly hazardous in elderly patients, who are at increased risk of fractures when they fall. The risk of hypotension during general anesthesia in patients treated with tricyclic antidepressants is low but has been reported (Malan et al., 2001). Previous suggestions that tricyclic antidepressants increase the risks of cardiac dysrhythmias and sudden death have not been substantiated in the absence of drug overdose (Thompson et al., 1983). Furthermore, in the absence of severe preexisting cardiac dysfunction, tricyclic antidepressants lack adverse effects on left ventricular function and may even possess cardiac antidysrhythmic properties (Veith et al., 1982). Reports that doxepin is less cardiotoxic than other tricyclic antidepressants have not been confirmed.

Tricyclic antidepressants produce depression of conduction of cardiac impulses through the atria and ventricles, manifesting on the electrocardiogram (ECG) as prolongation of the P-R interval, widening of the QRS complex, and flattening or inversion of the T wave. Nevertheless, these changes on the ECG are probably benign and gradually disappear with continued therapy (Thompson et al., 1983). Atropine is a useful treatment when tricyclic antidepressants dangerously slow atrioventricular or intraventricular conduction of cardiac impulses.

Direct cardiac depressant effects may reflect quinidine-like actions of tricyclic antidepressants on the heart. Conceivably, there could also be enhancement of depressant cardiac effects of anesthetics by tricyclic antidepressants. Quinidine-like properties of tricyclic antidepressants are thought to reflect slowing of sodium ion flux into cells, resulting in altered repolarization and conduction of cardiac impulses.

Central Nervous System Effects

Sedation associated with tricyclic antidepressant therapy may be desirable for management of agitated patients. Amitriptyline and doxepin produce the greatest degree of sedation (see Table 19-2). Tricyclic antidepressants, especially maprotiline and clomipramine, lower the seizure threshold, raising the question of the advisability of administering these drugs to patients with seizure disorders or to those receiving drugs that may produce seizures. Children seem to be especially vulnerable to the seizure-inducing effects of tricyclic antidepressants. Treatment with tricyclic antidepressants may enhance the CNS-stimulating effects of enflurane. Weakness and fatigue are attributable to CNS effects and may resemble those seen in patients treated with phenothiazines. Extrapyramidal reactions are rare, although a fine tremor develops in about 10% of patients, especially the elderly. Because of their cardiac toxicity, tendency to cause seizures, and depressant properties on the CNS, the tricyclic antidepressants may be fatal if taken in an overdose. The combination of a tricyclic antidepressant and an MAO inhibitor may result in CNS toxicity manifesting as hyperthermia, seizures, and coma.

Drug Interactions

The anticholinergic effects and catecholamine uptake-blocking properties of tricyclic antidepressants are most likely to be responsible for drug interactions. Drug interactions may be prominent with (a) sympathomimetics, (b) inhaled anesthetics, (c) anticholinergics, (d) antihypertensives, and (e) opioids. Binding of tricyclic antidepressants to plasma albumin can be decreased by competition from other drugs, including phenytoin, aspirin, and scopolamine.

Sympathomimetics

The systemic blood pressure response to the administration of sympathomimetics to patients treated with tricyclic antidepressants is complex and unpredictable. Even inclusion of epinephrine in the local anesthetic solutions used to produce epidural anesthesia and, to a lesser extent, spinal anesthesia has been questioned (Boakes et al., 1973). It has been suggested that indirect-acting sympathomimetics may produce exaggerated pressor responses due to an increased amount of norepinephrine available to stimulate postsynaptic adrenergic receptors. Although acute administration of tricyclic antidepressants increases sympathetic nervous system synaptic activity due to norepinephrine reuptake blockade, chronic administration of these drugs may result in decreased sympathetic nervous system transmission due to down regulation of beta-adrenergic receptors (Spiss et al., 1984; Braverman et al., 1987). It would appear that for patients recently started on tricyclic antidepressants, exaggerated pressor responses should be anticipated whether or not direct-acting or indirect-acting sympathomimetics are administered, although pressor responses may be more pronounced with an indirect-acting drug such as ephedrine. Smaller than usual doses of direct-acting sympathomimetics that are titrated to a specific hemodynamic response are recommended. For individuals chronically treated with tricyclic antidepressants (>6 weeks), administration of either a direct-acting or indirect-acting sympathomimetic is acceptable, although a prudent approach may be to decrease the initial dose of drug to about one-third the usual dose. Conversely, conventional sympathomimetics may not be effective in restoring systemic blood pressure in patients chronically treated with tricyclic antidepressants because adrenergic receptors are either desensitized or catecholamine stores are depleted. In these patients, a potent direct-acting sympathomimetic such as norepinephrine may be the only effective management for hypotension (Sprung et al., 1997).

Induction of anesthesia may be associated with an increased incidence of cardiac dysrhythmias in patients treated with tricyclic antidepressants. Likewise, the dose of exogenous epinephrine necessary to produce cardiac dysrhythmias during anesthesia with a volatile anesthetic is decreased by tricyclic antidepressants (Wong et al., 1980). Theoretically, increased availability of norepinephrine in the CNS could result in increased anesthetic requirements for inhaled anesthetics.

Anticholinergics

Because the anticholinergic side effects of drugs may be additive, the use of centrally active anticholinergic drugs for preoperative medication of patients treated with tricyclic antidepressants could increase the likelihood of postoperative delirium and confusion (central anticholinergic syndrome) (see Chapter 10). Glycopyrrolate would theoretically be less likely to evoke this type of drug interaction in patients being treated with tricyclic antidepressants.

Antihypertensives

Rebound hypertension after abrupt discontinuation of clonidine may be accentuated and prolonged by concomitant tricyclic antidepressant therapy (Stiff and Harris, 1983). Conceivably, increased plasma concentrations of catecholamines can persist for longer periods in the presence of tricyclic antidepressants that prevent uptake of norepinephrine back into sympathetic nerve endings.

Opioids

In animals, tricyclic antidepressants augment the analgesic and ventilatory depressant effects of opioids. Likewise, the sedative and depressant effects of barbiturates are increased in animals. If these responses also occur in patients, it is predictable that doses of these drugs should be decreased to avoid exaggerated or prolonged depressant effects.

Tolerance

Tolerance to anticholinergic effects (dry mouth, blurred vision, tachycardia) and orthostatic hypotension develops during chronic therapy with tricyclic antidepressants. Conversely, tolerance to desirable effects often fails to develop. Abrupt discontinuation of high doses of tricyclic antidepressants may be associated with a mild withdrawal syndrome characterized by malaise, chills, coryza, and skeletal muscle aching.

Overdose

Tricyclic antidepressant overdose is life-threatening, as the progression from an alert state to unresponsiveness may be rapid (Frommer et al., 1987). Intractable myocardial depression or ventricular cardiac dysrhythmias are the most frequent terminal events.

Presenting features of tricyclic antidepressant overdose include agitation and seizures followed by coma, depression of ventilation, hypotension, hypothermia, and striking evidence of anticholinergic effects including mydriasis, flushed dry skin, urinary retention, and tachycardia. The QRS complex on the ECG may be prolonged to >100 ms. Indeed, the likelihood of seizures and ventricular dysrhythmias is increased when the duration of the QRS complex is >100 ms (Boehnert and Lovejoy, 1985). Conversely, plasma concentrations of tricyclic antidepressants do not allow prediction of the likely occurrence of seizures or cardiac dysrhythmias (Boehnert and Lovejoy, 1985).

The comatose phase of tricyclic antidepressant overdose lasts 24 to 72 hours. Even after this phase passes, the risk of life-threatening cardiac dysrhythmias persists for up to 10 days, necessitating continued monitoring of the ECG in these patients.

Treatment of a life-threatening overdose of a tricyclic antidepressant is directed toward management of CNS and cardiac toxicity (Table 19-3) (Frommer et al., 1987). Coma usually resolves in 24 hours but is frequently severe enough to require invasive airway support. Extrapyramidal effects and organic brain syndrome usually require supportive care only, although judicious use of physostigmine, 0.5 to 2 mg given intravenously (IV), for treatment of anticholinergic psychosis may be indicated.

Seizures may precede cardiac arrest and should be treated aggressively with diazepam. After initial suppression of seizure activity with diazepam, it may be necessary to provide sustained effects with a longer-acting drug such as phenytoin. Acidosis associated with seizure activity may

TABLE 19-3.
PHARMACOLOGIC TREATMENT OF TRICYCLIC ANTIDEPRESSANT OVERDOSE

Symptom	Treatment
Seizures	Diazepam Sodium bicarbonate Phenytoin
Ventricular cardiac dysrhythmias	Sodium bicarbonate Lidocaine Phenytoin
Heart block	Isoproterenol
Hypotension	Crystalloid or colloid solutions Sodium bicarbonate Sympathomimetics Inotropics

Source: Data from Frommer DA, Kulig KW, Marx JA, et al. Tricyclic antidepressant overdose. *JAMA* 1987;257:521–526; with permission.

abruptly increase the unbound fraction of tricyclic antidepressants in the circulation and predispose to cardiac dysrhythmias. In this regard, alkalization of the plasma (pH >7.45) either by IV administration of sodium bicarbonate or deliberate hyperventilation of the patient's lungs can temporarily reverse drug-induced cardiotoxicity. Lidocaine and phenytoin may be used subsequently to provide sustained suppression of cardiac ventricular dysrhythmias.

Hypotension may be the result of direct tricyclic antidepressant-induced vasodilation, alpha-adrenergic blockade, or myocardial depression. Patients remaining hypotensive despite intravascular fluid replacement and alkalinization of the plasma, may require systemic blood pressure support with sympathomimetics, inotropics, or both.

Gastric lavage may be useful in the early treatment, but this is most safely performed with a cuffed tracheal tube already in place. Activated charcoal significantly absorbs drugs throughout the gastrointestinal tract ("intestinal dialysis"). Conversely, avid protein binding of tricyclic antidepressants negates any therapeutic value of hemodialysis or drug-induced diuresis.

Monoamine Oxidase Inhibitors

MAO inhibitors constitute a heterogenous group of drugs that block the enzyme that metabolizes biogenic amines, increasing the availability of these neurotransmitters in the CNS and peripheral autonomic nervous system. MAO inhibitors are rarely used because their administration is complicated by side effects (hypotension), lethality in overdose, and lack of simplicity in dosing. Patients treated with MAO inhibitors must follow a specific tyramine-free diet because of the potential for pharmacodynamic interactions with tyramine that can result in systemic hypertension (Table 19-4). Many patients with major depression who do not respond to cyclic antidepressants improve with MAO

TABLE 19-4.
DIETARY RESTRICTIONS IN PATIENTS TREATED WITH MONOAMINE OXIDASE INHIBITORS

Prohibited foods
Cheese
Liver
Fava beans
Avocados
Chianti wine
Prohibited drugs
Cyclic antidepressants
Fluoxetine
Cold or allergy medications
Nasal decongestants
Sympathomimetic drugs
Opioids (especially meperidine)

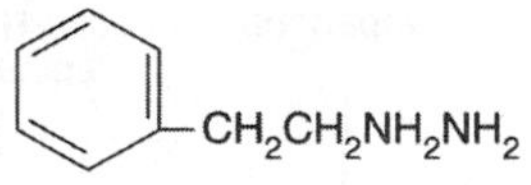

Phenelzine

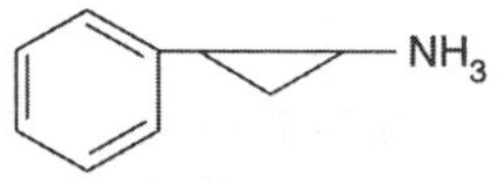

Tranylcypromin

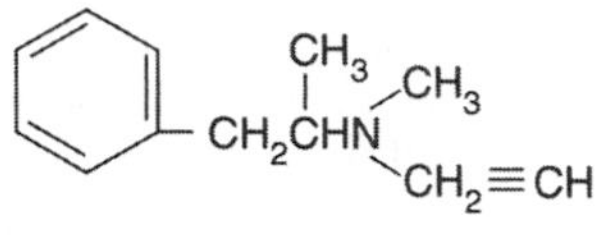

Selegiline

Figure 19-2. Monoamine oxidase inhibitors.

inhibitors. MAO inhibitors are also effective in the treatment of panic disorder. The dosage of MAO inhibitors is the same in the elderly as in younger adults because elderly persons often have higher levels of MAO and because the metabolism of these drugs does not seem to be affected by age.

The only MAO inhibitors approved in the United States for the treatment of depression or panic disorder are phenelzine, tranylcypromine, and isocarboxazid (see Fig. 19-2). Another MAO inhibitor, selegiline (formerly termed *deprenyl*) has been shown to be effective in the treatment of early Parkinson's disease. These drugs are administered orally, being readily absorbed from the gastrointestinal tract.

Monoamine Oxidase Enzyme System

MAO is a flavin-containing enzyme found principally on outer mitochondrial membranes. The enzyme functions via oxidative deamination to inactivate several monoamines including dopamine, serotonin (5-hydroxytryptamine), norepinephrine, and epinephrine. MAO is divided into two subtypes (MAO-A and MAO-B) based on different substrate specificities (Fig. 19-3) (Michaels et al., 1984; Wells and Bjorksten, 1989). MAO-A preferentially deaminates serotonin, norepinephrine, and epinephrine, whereas MAO-B preferentially deaminates phenylethylamine. Platelets contain exclusively MAO-A and the placenta exclusively MAO-B. About 60% of human brain MAO activity is of the A subtype.

Mechanism of Action

MAO inhibitors act by forming a stable, irreversible complex with MAO enzyme, especially with cerebral neuronal MAO (Stack et al., 1988). As a result, the amount of neurotransmitter (norepinephrine) available for release from CNS neurons increases. These effects, however, are not limited to the brain, and the concentration of norepinephrine also increases in the sympathetic nervous system. Because

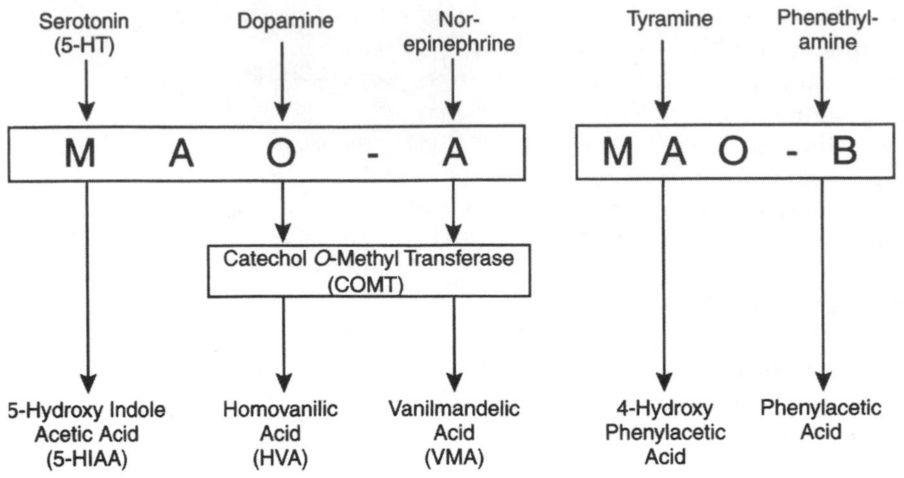

Figure 19-3. The two forms of monoamine oxidase enzyme (MAO-A and MAO-B) exhibit substrate selectivity. (From Michaels I, Serrins M, Shier NQ, et al. Anesthesia for cardiac surgery in patients receiving monoamine oxidase inhibitors. *Anesth Analg* 1984;63: 1041–1044; with permission.)

MAO inhibitors cause irreversible enzyme inhibition, their effects are prolonged as the synthesis of new enzyme is a slow process.

Due to its location in the outer mitochondrial membrane, MAO in neurons is only capable of deaminating substrates that are free within the cytoplasm and are unable to gain access to substrates once they are bound in the storage vesicles. As a result, cytoplasmic concentrations of monoamines are maintained at a low level.

Side Effects

The most common serious side effect of MAO inhibitors is orthostatic hypotension, which may be especially prominent in elderly patients. Orthostatic hypotension may reflect accumulation of the false neurotransmitter octopamine in the cytoplasm of postganglionic sympathetic nerve endings. Release of this less potent vasoconstrictor in response to neural impulses is the most likely explanation for orthostatic hypotension as well as the antihypertensive effect that has been associated with chronic MAO inhibitor therapy.

Phenelzine has anticholinergic-like side effects and may produce sedation in some patients. Tranylcypromine has no anticholinergic side effects but has mild stimulant effects that may cause insomnia. Impotence and anorgasmy are side effects of MAO inhibitors. Some patients complain of paresthesias that may respond to pyridoxine therapy. Weight gain is a common side effect of treatment with MAO inhibitors. Hepatitis is a rare complication of MAO inhibitor therapy. Effects of MAO inhibitors on the electroencephalogram (EEG) are minimal and not seizure-like, which contrasts with tricyclic antidepressants. Also in contrast with tricyclic antidepressants is the failure of MAO inhibitors to produce cardiac dysrhythmias (Wong et al., 1980).

Dietary Restrictions

MAO enzyme present in the liver, gastrointestinal tract, kidneys, and lungs seems to perform a protective function in deactivating circulating monoamines. In particular, this enzyme appears to form the initial defense against monoamines absorbed from foods, such as tyramine and beta-phenylethanolamine, which would otherwise produce an indirect sympathomimetic response and precipitous hypertension. MAO-A is found in the gastrointestinal tract and liver, where it acts to metabolize bioactive amines such as tyramine. The MAO inhibitors used in the United States as antidepressants inhibit MAO-A and MAO-B nonselectively. Selegiline, when used to treat Parkinson's disease, selectively inhibits MAO-B and patients do not need to follow a tyramine-free diet. At high doses (30 mg per day), however, even selegiline becomes a nonselective MAO inhibitor, making dietary precautions necessary (see Table 19-4).

Because patients treated with MAO inhibitors cannot metabolize dietary tyramine and other monoamines, these compounds can enter the systemic circulation and be taken up by sympathetic nervous system nerve endings. This uptake can elicit massive release of endogenous catecholamines and result in a hyperadrenergic crisis characterized by hypertension, hyperpyrexia, and cerebral vascular accident. Therefore, patients taking MAO inhibitors should be instructed to report promptly the onset of serious headache, nausea, vomiting, or chest pain. The precipitous hypertension resembles that which occurs with the release of catecholamines from a pheochromocytoma. Treatment of hypertension is with a peripheral vasodilator such as nitroprusside (see Chapter 16). Cardiac dysrhythmias that persist after control of systemic blood pressure are treated with lidocaine or a beta-adrenergic antagonist.

Drug Interactions

In addition to interacting with foods, MAO inhibitors can interact adversely with opioids, sympathomimetic drugs, tricyclic antidepressants, and SSRIs. These interactions can result in hypertension, CNS excitation, delirium, seizures, and death. In animals, anesthetic requirements for volatile anesthetics are increased, presumably reflecting accumulation of norepinephrine in the CNS.

Opioids and Monoamine Oxidase Inhibitors

Administration of meperidine to a patient treated with MAO inhibitors may result in an excitatory (type I) response (agitation, headache, skeletal muscle rigidity, hyperpyrexia) or a depressive (type II) response characterized by hypotension, depression of ventilation, and coma (Pavy et al., 1995). Enhanced serotonin activity in the brain is presumed to be responsible for excitatory reactions evoked by meperidine. Meperidine is capable of inhibiting neuronal serotonin uptake. Slowed breakdown of meperidine due to *N*-demethylase inhibition by MAO inhibitors is the presumed explanation for hypotension and depression of ventilation. About 20% of MAO inhibitor-treated patients have experienced excitatory reactions in response to meperidine. There is evidence that meperidine toxicity is increased only when both MAO-A and MAO-B are inhibited (Wells and Bjorksten, 1994). Derivatives of meperidine (fentanyl, sufentanil, alfentanil) have been associated with adverse reactions in patients treated with MAO inhibitors, although the incidence seems to be less than with meperidine (Insler et al., 1994). Morphine does not inhibit uptake of serotonin, but its opioid effects may be potentiated in the presence of MAO inhibitors.

Sympathomimetics and Monoamine Oxidase Inhibitors

There is no experimental evidence to support the recommendation that all sympathomimetic drugs be avoided in patients treated with MAO inhibitors. The most consistent observation has been an occasional patient who experienced an exaggerated systemic blood pressure response after the administration of an indirect-acting vasopressor such as ephedrine. The hypertensive response is presumed to reflect an exaggerated release of norepinephrine from neuronal nerve endings. If needed, the use of a direct-acting sympathomimetic (phenylephrine) is preferable to an indirect-acting drug, keeping in mind that receptor hypersensitivity may enhance the systemic blood pressure response to these drugs as well. Regardless of the drug selected, the recommendation is to decrease the dose to about one third of normal, with additional titration of doses based on cardiovascular responses (Wells and Bjorksten, 1994).

Overdose

Overdose with an MAO inhibitor is reflected by signs of excessive sympathetic nervous system activity (tachycardia, hyperthermia, mydriasis), seizures, and coma. Treatment is supportive in addition to gastric lavage. Dantrolene has been suggested as a treatment for skeletal muscle rigidity and associated symptoms of hypermetabolism after an overdose with MAO inhibitors (Kaplan et al., 1986).

Management of Anesthesia

In the past, it was a common recommendation to discontinue MAO inhibitors 2 to 3 weeks before elective surgery based on the concern that life-threatening cardiovascular and CNS instability could occur during anesthesia and surgery when these drugs were present. This policy of drug withdrawal seems to be based more on anecdotes and isolated responses than on controlled scientific studies. Furthermore, discontinuation of effective therapy potentially places patients at risk from their psychiatric disturbances. There is growing appreciation that anesthesia can be safely administered in most patients being chronically treated with MAO inhibitors (Wells and Bjorksten, 1989). When anesthesia is administered to patients treated with MAO inhibitors, it remains prudent to consider certain drug interactions and to avoid certain drugs, if possible (Stack et al., 1988; Wells and Bjorksten, 1989).

Selection of Drugs Used during Anesthesia

The anesthetic technique selected should minimize the possibility of sympathetic nervous system stimulation or drug-induced hypotension. Regional anesthesia as in parturients is acceptable, recognizing the disadvantage of these techniques should hypotension require administration of a sympathomimetic (Pavy et al., 1995). If regional anesthesia is performed, a cautious approach is not to add epinephrine to the local anesthetic solution, although problems have not been reported with a 1:200,000 dilution. An advantage of regional anesthesia is postoperative analgesia such that the need for opioids is negated or minimized. Etomidate and thiopental have been administered to MAO inhibitor-treated patients undergoing electroconvulsive therapy without adverse effects. Responses to nondepolarizing neuromuscular-blocking drugs are not altered by MAO inhibitors.

ANXIOLYTICS

Benzodiazepines

Benzodiazepines (see Chapter 5) are used clinically as anxiolytics, sedatives, anticonvulsants, and muscle relaxants. They appear to produce all these effects by facilitating the actions of gamma-aminobutyric acid (GABA), the major inhibitory neurotransmitter in the nervous system.

The effectiveness of benzodiazepines, combined with the high frequency of anxiety and insomnia in the adult population, has led to these drugs being widely prescribed. Few patients who receive benzodiazepines for valid indications abuse them or become addicted. Benzodiazepines have less of a tendency to produce tolerance, less potential for abuse, and a large margin of safety if taken in an overdose. A history of alcohol abuse or substance abuse is a relative contraindication to use of benzodiazepines for treatment of anxiety.

When benzodiazepines are used to treat situational anxiety or generalized anxiety disorder, low doses (diazepam, 2 to 5 mg three times daily) are typically selected to minimize sedation. Sedation associated with administration of benzodiazepines to treat anxiety usually subsides within 2 weeks. For short-term treatment of situational anxiety or longer-term treatment of generalized anxiety disorders, a total daily dose of >30 mg of diazepam or its equivalent is almost never needed. For the treatment of panic disorder, the high-potency, short-acting benzodiazepine alprazolam has the longest record of efficacy, although the long-acting benzodiazepine clonazepam is gaining increasing acceptance. Problems with benzodiazepine rebound and withdrawal symptoms can be minimized if low-potency, long-acting drugs are used for the treatment of generalized anxiety disorders. Elderly patients manifest greater sedation and greater impairment of psychomotor performance than younger persons receiving the same dose.

Buspirone

Buspirone is a nonbenzodiazepine that is effective in the treatment of generalized anxiety disorders (onset of anxiolytic effects over several days) but not panic disorder. This drug is a partial agonist at serotonin receptors, resulting in decreased serotonin turnover and anxiolytic effects. Buspirone has no direct effects on GABA receptors and thus no pharmacologic cross-reactivity with benzodiazepines, barbiturates, or alcohol. Buspirone lacks sedative, anticonvulsant, and skeletal muscle-relaxing effects characteristic of benzodiazepines. Absorption from the gastrointestinal tract is 100%, but extensive hepatic first-pass metabolism decreases bioavailability to 4%. The elimination half-time is 2 to 11 hours. Buspirone does not produce dependence and does not appear to be highly toxic if taken in overdose. The principal disadvantage seems to be a slow onset of effect (1 to 2 weeks), which may be interpreted as ineffectiveness by patients experiencing acute anxiety.

LITHIUM

Lithium is considered the drug of choice for the treatment of bipolar disorders. It has many neurobiologic effects, but it is not known which components are necessary for its efficacy in the treatment of bipolar disorders (Price and Heninger, 1994). One possible mechanism is the ability of lithium to inhibit a second-messenger system that transduces signals from many neurotransmitter receptors that ultimately lead to release of calcium ions from intracellular storage sites. With repeated firing, a neuron that has been exposed to lithium would become relatively depleted of second messengers and signal transmission would be dampened, especially in hyperactive neurons. Full therapeutic effects of lithium may take several weeks. The goal for treatment of acute mania is to maintain plasma lithium concentrations between 1.0 and 1.2 mEq/liter. Plasma lithium concentrations should be measured 10 to 12 hours after the last oral dose, and levels should not be drawn sooner than 4 to 5 days after the latest change in dosage.

Pharmacokinetics

Lithium is distributed throughout the total body water and is excreted almost entirely by the kidneys. Lithium, like sodium, is filtered by the glomerulus and reabsorbed by the proximal, but not distal, renal tubules. Thus, its renal excretion is not enhanced by thiazide diuretics, which act selectively on the distal renal tubules. In fact, because proximal reabsorption of lithium and sodium is competitive, depletion of sodium as produced by dehydration, decreased sodium intake, and thiazide and loop diuretics may increase reabsorption of lithium by proximal renal tubules, resulting in as much as a 50% increase in the plasma concentration of lithium. Potassium-sparing diuretics (triamterene, spironolactone) do not facilitate reabsorption of lithium and, in fact, may increase excretion. Nonsteroidal antiinflammatory drugs, by altering renal blood flow, may produce marked increases in the plasma concentration of lithium.

Safe and effective use of lithium can be monitored only by measuring plasma concentrations. The therapeutic range for acute mania is 1.0 to 1.2 mEq/liter, with oral doses averaging 900 to 1,800 mg per day. Plasma lithium concentrations should be measured about 12 hours after the last oral dose. Because the elimination half-time is about 24 hours and the time to reach steady state is four to five elimination half-times, plasma concentrations should be measured no sooner than 5 days after a change in dosage, unless toxicity is suspected. In elderly patients and in patients with renal disease, the elimination half-time for lithium is prolonged; the time to equilibration can be delayed to 7 days or longer. If toxicity is suspected, lithium should be withheld and the plasma concentration determined immediately, taking into account the time that has elapsed since the last dose.

Side Effects

The most common serious side effects of lithium occur at the kidneys, manifesting as polydipsia and polyuria. An estimated 20% of treated patients excrete >3 liters of urine daily, reflecting an impaired renal-concentrating ability due to the inhibitory effect of lithium on intracellular adenosine monophosphate formation in the renal tubules. The potassium-sparing diuretic amiloride is effective in decreasing urine volume without affecting the plasma concentrations of either lithium or potassium. It is recommended that renal function be evaluated by measuring blood urea nitrogen or plasma creatinine every 6 months.

TABLE 19-5.
DRUG INTERACTIONS WITH LITHIUM

Drug	Interaction
Thiazide diuretics	Increased plasma lithium concentration as a result of decreased renal clearance
Furosemide	Usually no change in the plasma lithium concentration
Nonsteroidal antiinflammatory drugs	Increased plasma lithium concentration as a result of decreased renal clearance (exceptions are aspirin and sulindac)
Aminophylline	Decreased plasma lithium concentration as result of increased renal clearance
Angiotensin-converting enzyme inhibitors	May increase plasma lithium concentration
Neuroleptic drugs	Lithium may exacerbate extrapyramidal symptoms or increase the risk of the neuroleptic malignant syndrome
Anticonvulsant drugs (carbamazepine)	Concurrent use with lithium may result in additive neurotoxicity
Beta-adrenergic antagonists	Decrease lithium-induced tremor
Neuromuscular blocking drugs	Lithium may prolong the duration of action

Source: Adapted from Price LH, Heninger GR. Lithium in the treatment of mood disorders. *N Engl J Med* 1994;331:591–598.

Changes on the ECG characterized by T wave flattening or inversion occur in some patients being treated with lithium, but there seem to be no related clinical effects. These changes are reversible within 2 weeks when lithium is discontinued. Clinically significant lithium-induced cardiac conduction disturbances are rare, although sinoatrial node dysfunction and sinoatrial node block have been described. Patients with preexisting sinoatrial node dysfunction (sick sinus syndrome) should probably be treated with lithium only if they have an artificial cardiac pacemaker in place.

Hypothyroidism develops in about 5% of patients treated with lithium and is more common in women than men. For this reason, it is recommended that TSH levels be measured every 6 months. If necessary, levothyroxine therapy may be initiated without discontinuing lithium.

Clinically important dermatologic toxicities of lithium include acne and exacerbations of psoriasis or a new onset of psoriasis. Patients may complain of memory disturbance and cognitive slowing. Hand tremor occurs in 25% to 50% of treated patients and diminishes with time and in response to a decrease in the dose of lithium or treatment with a beta-adrenergic antagonist. Rarely, lithium may cause extrapyramidal effects.

The association of sedation with lithium therapy suggests that anesthetic requirements for injected and inhaled drugs could be decreased. High plasma concentrations of lithium may delay recovery from the CNS depressant effects of barbiturates (Mannisto and Saarnivaara, 1976). Responses to depolarizing and nondepolarizing neuromuscular-blocking drugs may be prolonged in the presence of lithium (Hill et al., 1977).

Drug Interactions (see Table 19-5)

Toxicity

Diuretic therapy, sodium restriction, and sodium wasting increase reabsorption of lithium and thus increase plasma lithium concentrations. Patients being treated with lithium should avoid nonsteroidal antiinflammatory drugs and diuretics.

Many symptoms and signs of toxicity are closely correlated with the plasma lithium concentration (Table 19-6) (Price and Heninger, 1994). Mild lithium toxicity is reflected by sedation, nausea, skeletal muscle weakness, and changes on the ECG characterized by widening of the QRS complex. Atrioventricular heart block, hypotension, cardiac dysrhythmias, and seizures may occur when plasma concentrations of lithium are >2 mEq per liter. It is not uncommon for elderly patients who excrete lithium slowly to become confused, even in the presence of therapeutic plasma concentrations of this ion. Significant lithium toxicity is a medical emergency that may require aggressive treatment, including hemodialysis. If renal function is adequate, excretion of lithium ions can be modestly accelerated by osmotic diuresis and IV administration of sodium bicarbonate.

Treatment-Resistant Bipolar Disorder

An estimated 30% of patients with bipolar disorder cannot tolerate or do not respond to lithium. In these individuals, the anticonvulsants carbamazepine and valproic acid may be efficacious. Side effects of carbamazepine, although rare, include leukopenia, aplastic anemia, and hepatitis. It

TABLE 19-6.
SIGNS AND SYMPTOMS OF LITHIUM TOXICITY

Toxic Effects	Plasma Lithium Concentration (mEq/liter)	Signs and Symptoms
Mild	1.0–1.5	Lethargy Irritability Skeletal muscle weakness Tremor Slurred speech Nausea
Moderate	1.6–2.5	Confusion Drowsiness Restlessness Unsteady gait Coarse tremor Dysarthria Skeletal muscle fasciculations Vomiting
Severe	>2.5	Impaired consciousness (coma) Delirium Ataxia Extrapyramidal symptoms Seizures Impaired renal function

Source: Adapted from Price LH, Heninger GR. Lithium in the treatment of mood disorders. *N Engl J Med* 1994;331:591–598.

is recommended that liver function tests and complete blood counts be followed in patients being treated with carbamazepine.

ANTIPSYCHOTIC (NEUROLEPTIC) DRUGS

The antipsychotic drugs are a chemically diverse group of compounds (phenothiazines, thioxanthenes, butyrophenones) that are useful in the treatment of schizophrenia, mania, depression with psychotic features, and certain organic psychoses (Table 19-7). Schizophrenic patients who have not responded to standard antipsychotics may respond to clozapine. In addition, antipsychotic drugs are used to treat Tourette syndrome and certain movement disorders. Some of these drugs may also be used as antiemetics.

Phenothiazines and thioxanthenes have a high therapeutic index and relatively flat dose-response curve, accounting for the remarkable safety of these drugs over a wide dose range. Even large overdoses are unlikely to cause life-threatening depression of ventilation. These drugs do not produce physical dependence, although abrupt discontinuation may be accompanied by skeletal muscle discomfort.

Structure–Activity Relationships

Phenothiazines have a three-ring structure in which two benzene rings are linked by a sulfur and a nitrogen atom (see Fig. 19-4). If the nitrogen atom at position 10 is replaced by a carbon atom with a double bond to the side-chain, the compound becomes a thioxanthene. Phenothiazines and thioxanthenes used to treat psychiatric disease have three carbon atoms interposed between position 10 of the central ring and the first amino nitrogen atom of the side-chain at this position. In addition, the amine is always tertiary. This structure contrasts with that of phenothiazines

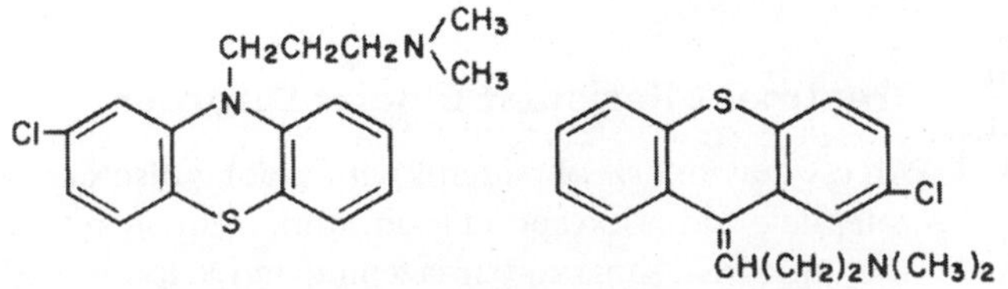

A,B Chlorpromazine Chlorprothixene

Figure 19-4. Phenothiazines (**A**) and thioxanthenes (**B**).

TABLE 19-7.
COMPARATIVE PHARMACOLOGY OF ANTIPSYCHOTIC (NEUROLEPTIC) DRUGS

Category and Drug	Sedative Potency	Anticholinergic Potency	Orthostatic Hypotension Potency	Extrapyramidal Potency
Phenothiazines				
Chlorpromazine	+++	++	+++	+
Triflupromazine	+++	++	+++	++
Thioridazine	+++	+++	+++	+
Fluphenazine	++	+	+	+++
Perphenazine	+	+	+	+++
Trifluoperazine	++	+	+	+++
Thioxanthenes				
Chlorprothixene	+++	+++	+++	+
Thiothixene	+	+	+	+++
Dibenzodiazepines				
Clozapine	+++	+++	+++	0
Loxapine	++	++	++	+++
Butyrophenones				
Haloperidol	+	+	+	+++
Droperidol	+	+	+	+++
Diphenylbutylpiperidines				
Primozide	+	+	+	+++
Benzisoxazole				
Risperidone	+	+	++	+

0, none; +, mild; ++, moderate; +++, marked.

with significant antihistamine activity (promethazine) or phenothiazines with significant anticholinergic activity (ethopropazine, diethazine), which have only two carbon atoms separating the amino group from position 10 of the central ring. Loss of a methyl group or other substituents on the tertiary amino group, as can occur during metabolism, results in a loss of pharmacologic activity.

Mechanism of Action

The mechanism of action of antipsychotic drugs is thought to be due to blockade of dopamine receptors (especially dopamine$_2$ receptors) in the basal ganglia and limbic portions of the forebrain (Baldessarini and Frankenburg, 1991; Richter, 1981). All antipsychotic drugs achieve maximum clinical efficacy over a period of weeks, emphasizing the importance of distinguishing the acute receptor-antagonist effects of antipsychotic drugs from their chronic effects. Interference with the neurotransmitter functions of dopamine by these drugs is suggested by extrapyramidal side effects. Blockade of dopamine receptors in the chemoreceptor trigger zone of the medulla is responsible for the antiemetic effect of these drugs.

Pharmacokinetics

Phenothiazines and thioxanthenes often display erratic and unpredictable patterns of absorption after oral administration. These drugs are highly lipid soluble and accumulate in well-perfused tissues such as the brain. Passage across the placenta and accumulation of drug in the fetus is possible. Avid binding to protein in plasma and tissues limits the effectiveness of hemodialysis in removing these drugs.

Metabolism

Metabolism of phenothiazines and thioxanthenes is principally by oxidation in the liver followed by conjugation. Most oxidative metabolites are pharmacologically inactive, with a notable exception being 7-hydroxychlorpromazine. Metabolites appear primarily in urine and to a lesser extent in bile. Typical elimination half-times of these drugs are 10 to 20 hours, permitting once-daily dosing intervals. The elimination half-time may be prolonged in the fetus and in the elderly, who have decreased capacity to metabolize these drugs.

Side Effects

With the exception of clozapine, the chronic use of phenothiazines and thioxanthenes may be complicated by serious side effects, most likely reflecting drug-induced blockade of dopamine receptors, especially in the forebrain (Baldessarini and Frankenburg, 1991). Despite the common occurrence of side effects, these drugs have a large margin of safety and overdoses are rarely fatal.

Extrapyramidal Effects

Tardive dyskinesia may occur in 20% of patients who receive antipsychotic drugs for >1 year. Only clozapine has not been implicated as a cause of this potentially permanent side effect. Elderly patients and women of all ages seem to be more susceptible to the development of tardive dyskinesia. Manifestations of tardive dyskinesia include abnormal involuntary movements that may affect the tongue, facial and neck muscles, upper and lower extremities, truncal musculature, and, occasionally, skeletal muscle groups involved in breathing and swallowing. Tardive dyskinesia only rarely remits, and there is no treatment. Compensatory increases in the function of dopamine activity in the basal ganglia may be responsible for the development of tardive dyskinesia.

Acute dystonic reactions occur in approximately 2% of treated patients and are most likely to occur within the first 72 hours of therapy. Dystonic reactions are most common in young men and in patients taking high-potency antipsychotics. Acute skeletal muscle rigidity and cramping may develop, usually in the musculature of the neck, tongue, face, and back. Opisthotonos and oculogyric crises may occur. The sudden onset of respiratory distress in a patient on neuroleptics may reflect laryngeal dyskinesia (laryngospasm) (Koek and Pi, 1989). Acute dystonia responds dramatically to diphenhydramine, 25 to 50 mg IV. Extrapyramidal side effects including tremor, masked facies, and skeletal muscle rigidity may occur, especially in elderly patients. Patients with antipsychotic-induced akathisia often appear restless (inability to tolerate inactivity), which may be confused with the underlying psychotic disorder.

Cardiovascular Effects

IV administration of chlorpromazine causes a decrease in systemic blood pressure resulting from (a) depression of vasomotor reflexes mediated by the hypothalamus or brainstem, (b) peripheral alpha-adrenergic blockade, (c) direct relaxant effects on vascular smooth muscle, and (d) direct cardiac depression. Risperidone is an antipsychotic drug that has been associated with exaggerated systemic hypotension during a spinal anesthetic, perhaps reflecting risperidone-induced alpha-blockade (Williams and Hepner, 2004). Alpha-adrenergic blockade produced by chlorpromazine is sufficient to blunt or prevent the pressor effects of epinephrine. Miosis that occurs predictably may also be due to alpha-adrenergic blockade. A cardiac antidysrhythmic effect of chlorpromazine may reflect the potent local anesthetic activity of this drug. These drugs usually do not cause cardiac dysrhythmias. Rarely, antipsychotic drugs prolong the QTc interval on the ECG and therefore predispose to the development of ventricular tachycardia (Kriwisky et al., 1990). Thioridazine and pimozide are potent calcium-channel blockers, which may contribute to their cardiac toxicity, including prolongation of the QTc interval on the ECG.

Oral administration of these drugs is associated with less pronounced systemic blood pressure-lowering effects. Indeed, tolerance to the hypotensive effect develops so that after several weeks of therapy, the blood pressure returns toward normal. Nevertheless, some element of orthostatic hypotension may persist for the duration of therapy.

Neuroleptic Malignant Syndrome

Neuroleptic malignant syndrome occurs in 0.5% to 1.0% of all patients treated with antipsychotic drugs. Risk factors for the development of this syndrome may include dehydration and intercurrent illness. The syndrome typically develops over 24 to 72 hours in young men and is characterized by (a) hyperthermia; (b) generalized hypertonicity of skeletal muscles; (c) instability of the autonomic nervous system manifesting as alterations in systemic blood pressure, tachycardia, and cardiac dysrhythmias; and (d) fluctuating levels of consciousness (Guze and Baxter, 1985). Autonomic nervous system dysfunction may precede the onset of other symptoms. Increased skeletal muscle tone may so decrease chest wall expansion that it becomes necessary to provide mechanical support of ventilation. Skeletal muscle rigidity may be severe enough to cause myonecrosis leading to increased creatine phosphokinase levels, myoglobinuria, and renal failure. Liver transaminase enzymes are likely to be increased. Mortality is 20% to 30%, with common causes of death being ventilatory failure, cardiac failure and/or dysrhythmias, renal failure, and thromboembolism.

The cause of neuroleptic malignant syndrome is not known and, as a result, treatment is empirical and includes supportive measures and the administration of the direct-acting muscle relaxant dantrolene and the dopamine agonists bromocriptine or amantadine (Rosenberg and Green, 1989). The reported efficacy of dopamine agonists in the treatment of skeletal muscle rigidity as well as the prevention of the onset of the syndrome with abrupt withdrawal of levodopa therapy suggests a role of dopamine receptor blockade in the development of this syndrome (Granato et al., 1983).

Malignant hyperthermia associated with anesthesia as well as the central anticholinergic syndrome may mimic the neuroleptic malignant syndrome (Guze and Baxter, 1985). A distinguishing feature is the ability of nondepolarizing muscle relaxants to produce flaccid paralysis in patients experiencing the neuroleptic malignant syndrome but not in those experiencing malignant hyperthermia (Sangal and Dimitrijevic, 1985).

Endocrine Effects

Prolactin levels are increased as a result of blockade of dopamine receptors and loss of the normal inhibition of prolactin secretion. Galactorrhea and gynecomastia may accompany excess prolactin secretion. Amenorrhea is a possible but rare complication of therapy. Decreased secretion of corticosteroids may be due to diminished corticotropin release from the anterior pituitary. Chlorpromazine may impair glucose tolerance and the release of insulin in some patients. Hypothalamic effects may manifest as weight gain and occasionally abnormalities of thermoregulation.

Sedation

Sedation produced by antipsychotic drugs appears to be due to antagonism of alpha$_1$-adrenergic, muscarinic, and histamine (H_1) receptors. With chronic therapy, tolerance develops to the sedative effects produced by these drugs.

Antiemetic Effects

The antiemetic effects of antipsychotic drugs reflect their interaction with dopaminergic receptors in the chemoreceptor trigger zone of the medulla (see Chapter 26). These drugs seem most effective in preventing opioid-induced nausea and vomiting. Perphenazine, 5 mg IV, has been shown to be as effective as ondansetron, 4 mg IV, and droperidol, 1.25 mg IV, for prevention of postoperative vomiting after gynecologic surgery (Desilva et al., 1995). Unlike these other antiemetics, perphenazine was not associated with side effects such as sedation or hypotension, making this phenothiazine derivative useful as an inexpensive prophylactic antiemetic. Perphenazine, 70 μg/kg IV, decreases the incidence of vomiting in children during the first 24 hours after tonsillectomy (Splinter and Roberts, 1997). The CNS dopaminergic activity of phenothiazines, which results in their antiemetic effects, may also produce extrapyramidal symptoms. These symptoms, which are easily treated with benztropine, appear to be rare.

Obstructive Jaundice

Obstructive jaundice that is considered to be an allergic reaction occurs rarely 2 to 4 weeks after administration of phenothiazines or thioxanthenes. Indeed, there is prompt recurrence of jaundice if the offending drug, usually chlorpromazine, is again administered. If jaundice is not observed in the first month of therapy, it is unlikely to occur at a later date.

Hypothermia

An effect of chlorpromazine on the hypothalamus is most likely responsible for the poikilothermic effect of this drug. In the past, this effect was used to facilitate the production of surgical hypothermia.

Seizure Threshold

Many antipsychotic drugs decrease the seizure threshold and produce a pattern on the EEG similar to that associated with seizure disorders. Chlorpromazine causes slowing of the EEG pattern, with some increase in burst activity and spiking. Sensory evoked potentials are often decreased in amplitude, and there is an increase in latency.

Skeletal Muscle Relaxation

Chlorpromazine causes skeletal muscle relaxation in some types of spastic conditions, presumably by actions on the CNS because the drug is devoid of actions at the neuromuscular junction.

Drug Interactions

The ventilatory depressant effects of opioids are likely to be exaggerated by antipsychotic drugs. Likewise, the miotic and sedative effects of opioids are increased, and the analgesic actions are likely to be potentiated. These drugs may interfere with the actions of exogenously administered dopamine, and the effects of alcohol are enhanced.

Clozapine

Clozapine is the only antipsychotic that does not seem to cause tardive dyskinesia or extrapyramidal side effects (Baldessarini and Frankenburg, 1991). Among the most common side effects are sedation, nausea and vomiting, and orthostatic hypotension. Excessive salivation, especially during sleep, is a common but paradoxical and poorly explained effect of this strongly anticholinergic drug. Another presumed manifestation of a parasympatholytic effect is sustained mild sinus tachycardia. Caution is advised in the use of such an anticholinergic drug in patients at risk for glaucoma, ileus, or urinary retention. Low-grade fever sometimes occurs early in the use of clozapine. Clozapine has been combined safely with lithium and antidepressant drugs, but there may be a risk of excessive sedation if this drug is combined with a benzodiazepine.

Agranulocytosis is a particularly serious side effect of clozapine, occurring in <1% of patients (Baldessarini and Frankenburg, 1991). For this reason, weekly monitoring of the white blood cell count is recommended in treated patients.

The incidence of seizures is 2% to 4% in those treated with high doses of clozapine. Some clinicians prescribe an anticonvulsant when high doses of clozapine (>500 mg per day) are administered or in patients with a history of epilepsy. Valproic acid may be selected as the anticonvulsant as this drug does not alter the metabolism of clozapine.

Butyrophenones

Butyrophenones, such as droperidol and haloperidol, structurally resemble and evoke pharmacologic effects similar to those of phenothiazines and thioxanthenes (Fig. 19-5). Butyrophenones can decrease anxiety that accompanies psychoses. Conversely, butyrophenones are less effective against anxiety such as that present in the preoperative period.

Droperidol is the butyrophenone most often administered in the preoperative period. Haloperidol has a longer

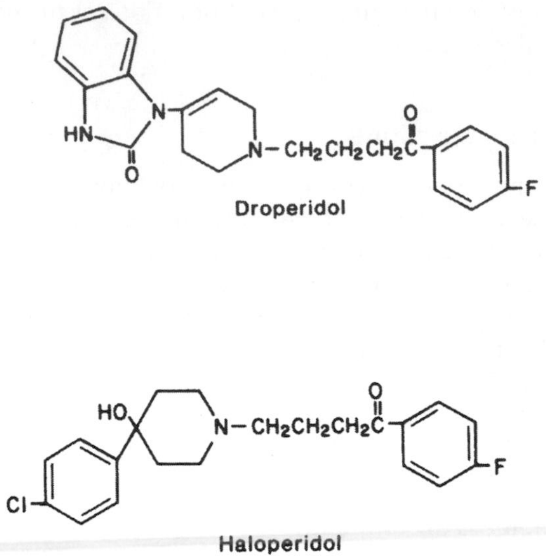

Figure 19-5. Butyrophenones.

duration of action than droperidol and lacks significant alpha-adrenergic antagonist effects such that decreases in systemic blood pressure are unlikely. The principal use of haloperidol is as a long-acting antipsychotic drug and for treatment of agitation and delirium in the intensive care unit.

Ziprasidone is a atypical antipsychotic drug that may be a useful alternative to haloperidol for the treatment of delirium (Young and Lujan, 2004). Like haloperidol, ziprasidone is associated with antidopaminergic side effects (extrapyramidal effects, tardive dyskinesia) and can cause prolongation of the QTc interval on the ECG (not recommended in patients with QTc >500 msec, recent myocardial infarction, uncompensated congestive heart failure).

Pharmacokinetics

In patients anesthetized with nitrous oxide-fentanyl, the elimination half-time of droperidol is 104 minutes, clearance is 14.1 mL/kg per minute, and the volume of distribution 2.04 liters/kg (Fischler et al., 1986). The total body clearance of droperidol is similar to hepatic blood flow (perfusion dependent), emphasizing the importance of hepatic metabolism rather than hepatic enzyme activity (capacity dependent) in elimination of this drug. In this regard, potential accumulation of droperidol is more likely to occur when the hepatic blood flow is decreased rather than with an alteration in hepatic enzyme activity. The short elimination half-time is not consistent with the prolonged CNS effects of droperidol, which may reflect slow dissociation of the drug from receptors or retention of droperidol in the brain. Droperidol is metabolized in the liver, with maximal excretion of metabolites occurring during the first 24 hours.

Side Effects

The side effects of butyrophenones resemble those described for phenothiazines and thioxanthenes.

Central Nervous System

The outwardly calming effect of droperidol may mask an overwhelming fear of surgery. This dysphoric response detracts from the use of droperidol in the preoperative period, especially as preoperative medication (Lee and Yeakel, 1975). Akathisia (most often a feeling of restlessness in the legs) may accompany administration of droperidol as preoperative medication (Ward, 1989). As a dopamine antagonist, droperidol evokes extrapyramidal reactions in about 1% of patients (Rivera et al., 1975; Wiklund and Ngai, 1971). For this reason, droperidol should not be administered to patients who are concurrently being treated for Parkinson disease. Acute laryngeal dystonia (laryngospasm) is a rare extrapyramidal reaction to the butyrophenones (Koek and Pi, 1989). Diphenhydramine administered IV is an effective treatment for droperidol-induced extrapyramidal reactions.

Droperidol is a cerebral vasoconstrictor that causes a decrease in cerebral blood flow, but cerebral metabolic rate for oxygen is not greatly altered. Failure to decrease the metabolic rate despite decreased cerebral blood flow could be undesirable in patients with cerebral vascular disease. The reticular activating system is not depressed, and alpha rhythm persists on the EEG. Droperidol does not produce amnesia, nor does it have an anticonvulsant action.

Cardiovascular Effects

Droperidol can decrease systemic blood pressure as a result of actions in the CNS and by peripheral alpha-adrenergic blockade (Whitwam and Russell, 1971). The decrease in blood pressure is usually minimal, although occasionally a patient may experience marked hypotension. Systemic and pulmonary vascular resistance is only modestly and transiently decreased. Myocardial contractility is not altered by droperidol.

Hypertension has been reported after administration of droperidol to patients with pheochromocytoma (Bittar, 1979; Sumikawa and Amakata, 1977). This systemic blood pressure response reflects droperidol-induced release of catecholamines from the adrenal medulla as well as inhibition of catecholamine uptake into chromaffin granules (Fig. 19-6) (Sumikawa et al., 1985).

Droperidol is a cardiac antidysrhythmic and protects against epinephrine-induced dysrhythmias (Bertolo et al., 1972). The mechanism for the cardiac antidysrhythmic effect has not been established but may reflect blockade of alpha-adrenergic receptors in the myocardium, stabilization of excitable membranes of cardiac cells by local anesthetic effects of droperidol, and decreases in systemic blood pressure that decrease the likelihood of pressure-dependent cardiac dysrhythmias. Large doses of droperidol,

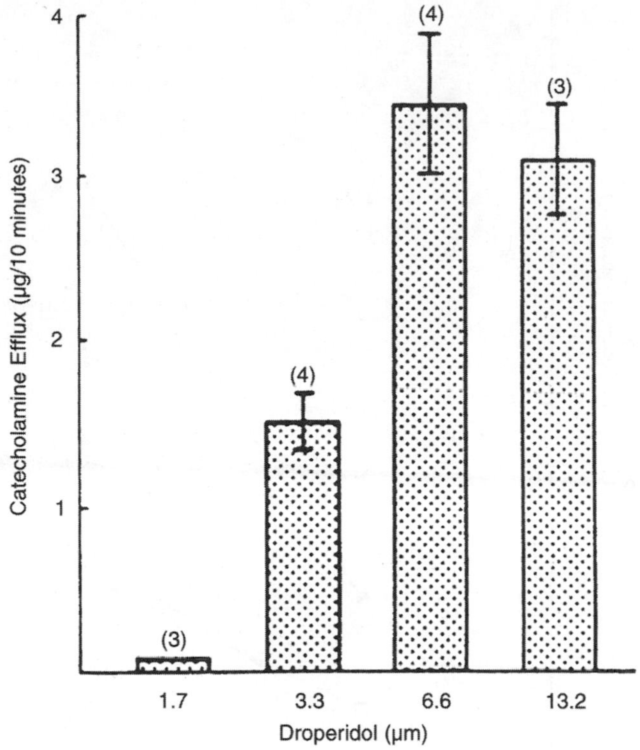

Figure 19-6. Catecholamine efflux (mean ± SE) from the perfused dog adrenal medulla is increased by droperidol. The number of experiments is indicated by the figure in parentheses. (From Sumikawa K, Hirano H, Amakata Y, et al. Mechanism of the effect of droperidol to induce catecholamine efflux from the adrenal medulla. *Anesthesiology* 1985;62:17–22; with permission.)

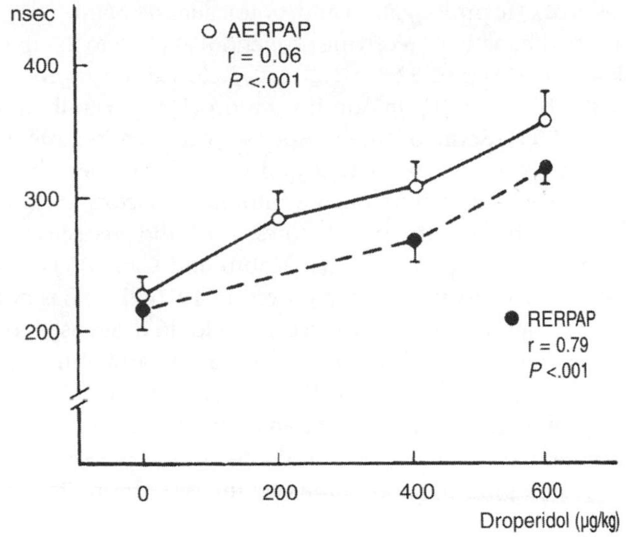

Figure 19-7. Droperidol produces dose-dependent prolongation of the antegrade and retrograde effective refractory period of accessory pathways. (AERPAP, antegrade effective refractory period of accessory pathways; RERPAP, retrograde effective refractory period of accessory pathways.) (From Gomez-Arnau J, Marquez-Montes J, Avello F. Fentanyl and droperidol effects on the refractoriness of the accessory pathway in the Wolff-Parkinson-White syndrome. *Anesthesiology* 1983;58:307–313; with permission.)

0.2 to 0.6 mg/kg IV, decrease conduction of cardiac impulses along accessory pathways responsible for tachydysrhythmias that occur in patients with Wolff-Parkinson-White syndrome (Fig. 19-7) (Gomez-Arnau et al., 1983).

Prolonged QTc Interval

Prolonged QTc syndrome is a malfunction of cardiac ion channels resulting in impaired ventricular repolarization that can lead to a characteristic polymorphic ventricular tachycardia known as torsades de pointes (Kies et al., 2005). The single most common cause of the withdrawal or restriction of the use of drugs that are already in clinical use is the prolongation of the QTc interval on the ECG associated with torsades de pointes (polymorphic ventricular tachycardia) (Liu and Juurlink, 2004; Roden, 2004). This prolongation most often results from delayed ventricular repolarization, a process that is mediated by the efflux of intracellular potassium. The channels responsible for the current are susceptible to blockade by many drugs, producing a suitable environment for the development of torsades de pointes, which may lead to sudden death. Nondrug factors associated with prolongation of the QTc interval include female gender, advanced age, electrolyte disturbances (hypokalemia, hypomagnesemia), congestive heart failure, bradycardia, myocardial ischemia, and congential long Q-T syndromes.

Several classes of noncardiac drugs (droperidol, thiopental, propofol, isoflurane, sevoflurane, succinylcholine, neostigmine, atropine, glycopyrrolate, metoclopramide, macrolide and quinolone antibiotics, SSRIs, $5HT_3$ receptor antagonists) produce dose-dependent prolongation of the QTc interval on the ECG in some patients (Liu and Juurlink, 2004). Although these drugs can provoke torsades de pointes in susceptible patients, the risk of this response in patients with no other risk factors is minimal. Nevertheless, even in low-risk patients, drug interactions can lead to life-threatening torsades de pointes. These drug interactions are characterized by (a) additive or synergistic effects when two drugs capable of prolonging the QTc are administered (haloperidol and amitriptyline) or (b) the simultaneous administration of a drug that interferes with the metabolism of a second drug capable of prolonging the QTc interval (resulting increased plasma concentration of the second drug increases the risk of torsades de pointes). Drugs capable of inhibiting P-450 enzyme and thus delaying the metabolism of second drugs capable of prolonging the QTc interval include calcium channel blockers, antifungal drugs, SSRIs, macrolide and quinolone antibiotics, antiretroviral drugs, and amiodarone.

Droperidol is capable of prolonging the QTc interval on the ECG (Drolet et al., 1999; Habib and Gan, 2003; Reilly et al., 2000, Scuderi, 2003). Although the QTc prolongation effect peaks 2 to 3 minutes following IV administration of droperidol, the effects may persist for several hours.

Cases of QTc prolongation and/or torsades de pointes have occurred in patients receiving droperidol at (1.25 to 2.5 mg) as well as doses (0.625 to 1.25 mg) below those approved by the Food and Drug Administration (FDA) (Habib and Gan, 2003). Some of these responses occurred in patients without known risk factors and some have been fatal. Nevertheless there were many confounding factors in these cases that make it impossible to establish the precise cause of the adverse cardiac events (Habib and Gan 2003). Of note, since droperidol was approved in 1970, there has not been a single case report where droperidol in doses used for the management of postoperative nausea and vomiting has been associated with QTc prolongation, cardiac dysrhythmias, or cardiac arrest (Gan et al., 2002, Gan 2004). Although even small doses of droperidol (<1.25 mg IV) may cause prolongation of the QTc interval, this prolongation is considered clinically insignificant (Zhang et al., 2004; White, 2004).

Based on these reports a "black box warning" has been added to the package insert for droperidol. This warning includes the requirement that all patients should undergo a 12-lead ECG prior to the administration of droperidol to determine if a prolonged QTc interval is present (>440 msec for males and >450 msec for females). When treatment with droperidol is selected, ECG monitoring should be performed before administration of droperidol and continued for 2 to 3 hours. Furthermore, droperidol should be administered with caution to patients who may be at risk for development of prolonged QTc syndrome (congestive heart failure, bradycardia, hypokalemia, elderly, concomitant administration of other drugs known to prolong the QTc interval). Sudden death during treatment with haloperidol has been attributed to drug-induced prolongation of the QTc interval on the ECG (Kriwisky et al., 1990).

When considering the effects of drugs on the QTc interval it is important to recognize that it is difficult to measure this interval with precision (Gan, 2004). There is inherent imprecision in identifying the end of the T wave and variation in the onset of the QRS complex on some ECG leads providing different QT values, depending on the leads selected for the measurement. Even paper speed and sensitivity can influence QT measurements. Automatic QTc measurement techniques have been found to be less accurate in cardiac patients than in healthy controls. Indeed, calculation of the QTc interval is ambiguous as there are numerous different formulae and each produces different results.

Ventilation

Resting ventilation and the ventilatory response to carbon dioxide are not altered by droperidol (Soroker et al., 1978). Furthermore, droperidol administered IV augments the ventilatory response evoked by arterial hypoxemia, presumably by blocking the action of the inhibitory neurotransmitter dopamine at the carotid body (Fig. 19-8) (Ward, 1984). For this reason, droperidol may be an acceptable preoperative medication in patients with chronic obstructive airway disease who depend on carotid body drive to prevent hypoventilation.

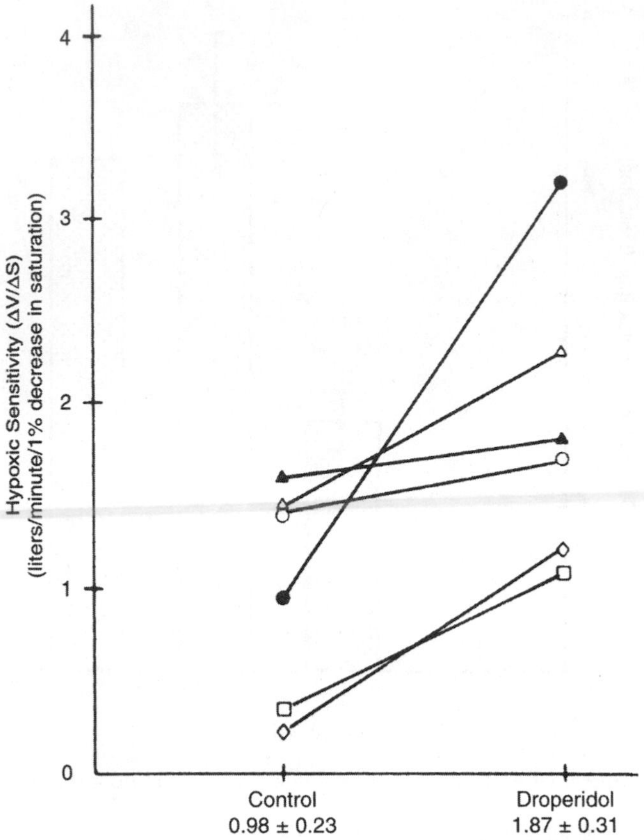

Figure 19-8. The ventilatory response to arterial hypoxemia (hypoxic sensitivity) is enhanced by droperidol. Solid symbols represent repeated experiments on the same subjects as those represented by the open symbols. (From Ward DS. Stimulation of hypoxic ventilatory drive by droperidol. *Anesth Analg* 1984;63: 106–110; with permission.)

Clinical Uses

Clinical uses of droperidol are principally limited to production of neuroleptanalgesia and as an antiemetic.

Neuroleptanalgesia

Droperidol combined with fentanyl is administered for the production of neuroleptanalgesia. A commercially available 50:1 combination of droperidol with fentanyl is known as *Innovar*. This fixed combination of drugs is not associated with enhanced depression of ventilation as compared with either drug alone (Harper et al., 1976). Droperidol does not enhance analgesia produced by fentanyl but rather prolongs its duration of action. Orthostatic hypotension and dysphoria are more likely to occur after the administration of Innovar compared with fentanyl alone.

Neuroleptanalgesia is characterized by trance-like (cataleptic) immobility in an outwardly tranquil patient who is dissociated and indifferent to the external surroundings. Analgesia is intense, allowing performance of a variety of diagnostic and minor surgical procedures such as bronchoscopy and cystoscopy. The disadvantages of neuroleptanalgesia are prolonged CNS depression and failure to depress sympathetic nervous system responses predictably to painful stimulation.

The mechanism by which droperidol produces anesthesia is not known but likely involves inhibition of synaptic transmission by ligand-gated ion channels. Gamma-aminobutyric acid ($GABA_A$) and neuronal nicotinic acetylcholine receptors (nAChRs) are important in the mechanism of action of injected and inhaled anesthetics. There is evidence that droperidol inhibits activation of $GABA_A$ and nAChRs receptors within a concentration range that might result in anxiety, dysphoria, and restlessness that limit the clinical usefulness of high-dose droperidol anesthesia (Flood and Coates, 2002).

Antiemetic

Droperidol is a powerful antiemetic agent as a result of inhibition of $dopamine_2$ receptors in the chemoreceptor trigger zone of the medulla (see Chapter 26). Despite the black box warning there is a question whether small antiemetic doses (1.25 mg or less) introduce the risk of prolonged QTc interval on the ECG (Habib and Gan, 2003). Over nearly three decades, droperidol, 0.625 to 1.25 mg IV, has become widely accepted as a safe, cost-effective first-line therapy for the management of postoperative nausea and vomiting (Henzi et al., 2000; White, 2002). The use of droperidol, 1.25 mg IV is associated with greater effectiveness, lower cost and similar patient satisfaction compared with 0.625 mg droperidol IV or ondansetron 4 mg IV (Hill et al., 2000). Droperidol (1.25 mg) was as effective as dexamethasone (4 mg) and ondansetron (4 mg) in decreasing the incidence of postoperative nausea and vomiting by about 26% when administered as preoperative prophylaxis (Apfel et al., 2004). Labyrinthine-induced vomiting (motion sickness) is not influenced by droperidol.

CANNABIS

Cannabis is an alkaloid mixture of more than 400 compounds derived from the *Cannabis sativa* plant. Cannabis has been used for thousands of years and is presently the most commonly used illicit drug in the world. The most abundant cannabinoids are delta-9-tetrahydrocannabinol (D9THC), cannabidiol, and cannabinol (Smith, 2000). D9THC is the main psychotropically active cannabinoid. Two principal endogenous cannabis receptors (CB1 and CB2) have been identified. CB1 receptors are present in the CNS (especially spinal cord) and CB2 receptors are located peripherally and linked with cells in the immune system. Both receptors are members of the G protein family and like opioid receptors exert their actions by modulating second-messenger activity (adenylate cyclase activity) and calcium ion function. Endogenous cannabinoid agonists (anandamide, 2-arachidonylglycerol) have been identified and produce effects similar to D9THC.

Pharmacokinetics

Cannabinoids undergo substantial hepatic first pass metabolism following oral administration such that only 10% to 20% of the ingested dose reaches the systemic circulation. This metabolism produces large amounts of active metabolite, 11-hydroxy-delta-9-tetrahydrocannabinol that is as active as the parent compound (D9THC) and has a prolonged half-time. The peak clinical effect after oral administration occurs after 1 to 2 hours and duration of action is 4 to 6 hours. In contrast, inhalation administration results in onset of action within seconds.

Toxicity

Euphoria and feeling of relaxation occurs at plasma cannabinoid concentrations of about 3 ng/mL and this can be produced by 2 to 3 mg of D9THC. Acute intoxication may cause perceptual alterations, distortion of time, intensification of normal sensory experiences, decreased reaction times, poor motor skills, increased appetite, impairment of skilled activities, tachycardia, and hypotension. The greatest concern is the creation of long-term toxicity and development of physical dependence. Cannabis is often mixed with tobacco to make it burn more efficiently. Materials that are present in cannabis smoke are carcinogenic. Chronic inhalation of cannabis smoke is associated with an increased incidence of chronic obstructive lung disease and carcinoma of the lung and larynx. Persistent use of cannabis may be associated with decreased reproductive potential and reduced production of testosterone.

Clinical Uses

D9THC is increasingly used for the long-term treatment of nausea, vomiting, cachexia, and management of chronic pain (Deusch et al., 2004). Scientific studies to confirm the efficacy of cannabis are lacking and anecdotal evidence is often cited to support clinical uses. The role of the endogenous cannabinoid system is not fully understood but evidence suggests it is involved with analgesia, cognition, appetite, vomiting, bronchodilation, inflammation, and immune control (Smith, 2000). Cannabinoids are highly lipid soluble and the presence of CB1 receptors in the spinal cord suggests potential analgesic efficacy if placed in the epidural or intrathecal space. Although use of cannabis for analgesia introduces the potential for psychic and physical dependence, there is considerably less risk than the undesirable side effects associated with opioids. Pure

D9THC may be effective in the treatment of chemotherapy-induced nausea and vomiting and is a recognized appetite stimulant in patients with terminal disease. Relief of skeletal muscle spasms in patients with multiple sclerosis has been described. The use of D9THC may be associated with an increased risk of myocardial infarction and thromboangiitis obliterans, perhaps reflecting D9THC-induced platelet activation (Deusch et al., 2004).

REFERENCES

Apfel CC, Korttila K, Abdalla M, et al. A factorial trial of six interventions for the prevention of postoperative nausea and vomiting. *N Engl J Med* 2004;350:2441–2451.

Baldessarini RJ, Frankenburg FR. Clozapine: a novel antipsychotic agent. *N Engl J Med* 1991;324:746–754.

Bertolo L, Novakovic L, Penna M. Antiarrhythmic effects of droperidol. *Anesthesiology* 1972;37:529–535.

Bittar DA. Innovar-induced hypertensive crisis in patients with pheochromocytoma. *Anesthesiology* 1979;50:366–369.

Boakes AJ, Laurence DR, Teoh PC, et al. Interactions between sympathomimetic amines and antidepressant agents in man. *BMJ* 1973;1:311–315.

Boehnert MT, Lovejoy FH. Value of the QRS duration versus the serum drug level in predicting seizures and ventricular arrhythmias after an acute overdose of tricyclic antidepressants. *N Engl J Med* 1985;313:474–479.

Braverman B, McCarthy RJ, Ivankovich AD. Vasopressor challenges during chronic MAOI or TCA treatment in anesthetized dogs. *Life Sci* 1987;40:2587–2595.

Buckley NA, McManus PR. Fatal toxicity of serotonergic and other antidepressant drugs: analysis of United Kingdom mortality data. *Br Med J* 2002;325:1332–1336.

Coupland NJ, Bell CJ, Potokar JP. Serotonin reuptake inhibitor withdrawal. *J Clin Psychopharmacol* 1996;16:356–360.

Desilva PHDP, Darvish AH, McDonald SM, et al. The efficacy of prophylactic ondansetron, droperidol, perphenazine, and metoclopramide in the prevention of nausea and vomiting after major gynecologic surgery. *Anesth Analg* 1995;81:139–143.

Deusch E, Kress HG, Kraft B, et al. The procoagulatory effects of delta-9-tetrahydrocannabinol in human platelets. *Anesth Analg* 2004; 99:1127–1130.

Drolet B, Zhang S, Deschenes D et al. Droperidol lengthens cardiac repolarization due to block of the rapid component of the delayed rectifier potassium current. *J Cardiovas Electrophysiol* 1999; 10:1597–1604.

El-Ganzouri AR, Ivankovich AD, Braverman B, et al. Monoamine oxidase inhibitors: should they be discontinued preoperatively? *Anesth Analg* 1985;64:592–596.

Fischler M, Bonnet F, Trang H, et al. The pharmacokinetics of droperidol in anesthetized patients. *Anesthesiology* 1986;64:486–489.

Flood P, Coates KM. Droperidol inhibits $GABA_A$ and neuronal nicotinic receptor activation. *Anesthesiology* 2002;96:987–993.

Frommer DA, Kulig KW, Marx JA, et al. Tricyclic antidepressant overdose. *JAMA* 1987;257:521–526.

Gan TJ, White PF, Scuderi PE, et al. FDA "black box" warning regarding use of droperidol for postoperative nausea and vomiting: is it justified? *Anesthesiology* 2002;97:287–290.

Gan TJ. "Black box" warning on droperidol: A report of the FDA convened expert panel. *Anesth Analg* 2004;98:1809.

Goldstein DJ, Rampey AH, Enas GG, et al. Fluoxetine: a randomized clinical trial in the treatment of obesity. *Int J Obes Relat Metab Disord* 1994;18:129–135.

Gomez-Arnau J, Marquez-Montes J, Avello F. Fentanyl and droperidol effects on the refractoriness of the accessory pathway in the Wolff-Parkinson-White syndrome. *Anesthesiology* 1983;58:307–313.

Gram LF. Fluoxetine. *N Engl J Med* 1994;331:1354–1361.

Granato JE, Stern BJ, Ringel A, et al. Neuroleptic malignant syndrome: successful treatment with dantrolene and bromocriptine. *Ann Neurol* 1983;14:89–90.

Guze BH, Baxter LR. Neuroleptic malignant syndrome. *New Engl J Med* 1985;313:163–166.

Habib AS, Gan TJ. Food and Drug Administration black box warning on the perioperative use of droperidol: a review of the cases. *Anesth Analg* 2003;96:1377–1379.

Harper MH, Hickey RF, Cromwell TH, et al. The magnitude and duration of respiratory depression produced by fentanyl plus droperidol in man. *J Pharmacol Exp Ther* 1976;199:464–468.

Harvey AT, Rudolph RL, Preskorn SH. Evidence of the dual mechanism of action of venlafaxine. *Arch Gen Psychiatry* 2000;57: 503–508.

Henzi I, Sondergegger J, Tarmer MR. Systematic review. Efficacy, dose-response, and adverse effects of droperidol for prevention of postoperative nausea and vomiting. *Can J Anesth* 2000;47: 537–551.

Hill GE, Wong KC, Hodges MR. Lithium carbonate and neuromuscular blocking agents. *Anesthesiology* 1977;46:122–126.

Hill RP, Lubarsky DA, Phillips-Bute B, et al. Cost-effectiveness of prophylactic antiemetic therapy with ondansetron, droperidol, or placebo. *Anesthesiology* 2000;92:958–967.

Insler SR, Kraenzler EJ, Licina MR, et al. Cardiac surgery in a patient taking monoamine oxidase inhibitors: an adverse fentanyl reaction. *Anesth Analg* 1994;78:593–597.

Johnston AJ, Lineberry CG, Ascher JAA. 102-Center prospective study of seizure in association with bupropion. *J Clin Psychiatry* 1991; 52:450–456.

Kaplan RF, Feinglass NG, Webster W, et al. Phenelzine overdose treated with dantrolene sodium. *JAMA* 1986;255:642–644.

Kies SJ, Pabelick CM, Hurley HA, et al. Anesthesia for patients with congenital long QT syndrome. *Anesthesiology* 2005;102: 204–210.

Koek RJ, Pi EH. Acute laryngeal dystonic reactions to neuroleptics. *Psychosomatics* 1989;30:359–364.

Kriwisky M, Perry GY, Tarchitsky D, et al. Haloperidol-induced torsades de pointes. *Chest* 1990;98;482–484.

Lee CM, Yeakel AE. Patients refusal of surgery following Innovar premedication. *Anesth Analg* 1975;54:224–226.

Liu BA, Juurlink DN. Drugs and the QT interval—caveat doctor. *N Engl J Med* 2004;351:1053–1056.

Malan TP, Nolan PE, Lichtenthal PR, et al. Severe, refractory hypotension during anesthesia in a patient on chronic clomipramine therapy. *Anesthesiology* 2001;95:264–266.

Mannisto PT, Saarnivaara L. Effect of lithium and rubidium on the sleeping time caused by various anaesthetics in the mouse. *Br J Anaesth* 1976;48:185–189.

Michaels I, Serrins M, Shier NQ, et al. Anesthesia for cardiac surgery in patients receiving monoamine oxidase inhibitors. *Anesth Analg* 1984;63:1041–1044.

Newman TB. A black-box warning for antidepressants in children? *N Engl J Med* 2004;351:1595–1597.

Pavy TJG, Kliffer AP, Douglas MJ. Anaesthetic management of labour and delivery in a woman taking long-term MAOI. *Can J Anaesth* 1995;42:618–620.

Price LH, Heninger GR. Lithium in the treatment of mood disorders. *N Engl J Med* 1994;331:591–598.

Rani PU, Naidu MUR, Prasad VB, et al. An evaluation of antidepressants in rheumatic pain conditions. *Anesth Analg* 1996;83:371–375.

Reilly JG, Ayis SA, Ferrier IN, et al. QTc-interval abnormalities and psychotropic drug therapy in psychiatric patients. *Lancet* 2000;355: 1048–1052.

Richelsoln E. Pharmacology of antidepressants. *Mayo Clin Proc* 2001; 76:511–516.

Richter JJ. Current theories about the mechanisms of benzodiazepines and neuroleptic drugs. *Anesthesiology* 1981;54:66–72.

Rivera VM, Keichian AH, Oliver RE. Persistent parkinsonism following neuroleptanalgesia. *Anesthesiology* 1975;42:635–637.

Roden DM. Drug-induced prolongation of the QT interval. *N Engl J Med* 2004;350:1013–1022.

Rosenberg MR, Green M. Neuroleptic malignant syndrome: review of response to therapy. *Arch Intern Med* 1989;149:1927–1931.

Rozen RC, Lane RM, Menza M. Effects of SSRIs on sexual function: a critical review. *J Clin Psychopharmacol* 1999;19:67–73.

Sangal R, Dimitrijevic R. Neuroleptic malignant syndrome: successful treatment with pancuronium. *JAMA* 1985;254:2795–2796.

Scuderi PE. Droperidol: many questions, few answers. *Anesthesiology* 2003;98:289–290.
Smith G. Cannabis: Time for scientific evaluation of this ancient remedy? *Anesth Analg* 2000;90:237–240.
Soroker D, Barjilay E, Konichezky S. Respiratory function following premedication with droperidol or diazepam. *Anesth Analg* 1978; 57:695–699.
Spiss CK, Smith CM, Maze M. Halothane-epinephrine arrhythmias and adrenergic responsiveness after chronic imipramine administration in dogs. *Anesth Analg* 1984;63:825–828.
Splinter WM, Roberts DJ. Perphenazine decreases vomiting by children after tonsillectomy. *Can J Anaesth* 1997;44:1308–1310.
Sprung J, Schoenwald PK, Levy P, et al. Treating intraoperative hypotension in a patient on long-term tricyclic antidepres-sants: a case of aborted aortic surgery. *Anesthesiology* 1997;86:990–992.
Stack CG, Rogers P, Linter PSK. Monoamine oxidase inhibitors and anaesthesia. *Br J Anaesth* 1988;60:222–227.
Stiff JL, Harris DB. Clonidine withdrawal complicated by amitriptyline therapy. *Anesthesiology* 1983;59:73–74.
Strumper D, Durieux ME, Hollmann MW et al. Effects of antidepressants on function and viability of human neutrophils. *Anesthesiology* 2003;98:1356–1362.
Sumikawa K, Amakata Y. The pressor effect of droperidol on a patient with pheochromocytoma. *Anesthesiology* 1977;46:359–361.
Sumikawa K, Hirano H, Amakata Y, et al. Mechanism of the effect of droperidol to induce catecholamine efflux from the adrenal medulla. *Anesthesiology* 1985;62:17–22.
Thompson TL, Moran MG, Nies AS. Psychotropic drug use in the elderly. *N Engl J Med* 1983;308:194–198.
Veith RC, Raskind MA, Caldwell JH, et al. Cardiovascular effects of tricyclic antidepressants in depressed patients with chronic heart disease. *N Engl J Med* 1982;306:954–959.
Ward DS. Stimulation of hypoxic ventilatory drive by droperidol. *Anesth Analg* 1984;63:106–110.
Ward NG. Akathisia associated with droperidol during epidural anesthesia. *Anesthesiology* 1989;71:786–787.
Wells DG, Bjorksten AR. Monoamine oxidase inhibitors revisited. *Can J Anaesth* 1989;36:64–74.
White PF. Droperidol: A cost-effective antiemetic for over thirty years. *Anesth Analg* 2002;95:789–790.
White PF. Prevention of postoperative nausea and vomiting–a multimodal solution to a persistent problem. *N Engl J Med* 2004;350: 2511–2512.
Whitwam JG, Russell WJ. The acute cardiovascular changes and adrenergic blockade by droperidol in man. *Br J Anaesth* 1971;43:581–591.
Wiklund RA, Ngai SH. Rigidity and pulmonary edema after Innovar in a patient on levodopa therapy: report of a case. *Anesthesiology* 1971;35:545–547.
Williams JH, Hepner DL. Risperidone and exaggerated hypotension during a spinal anesthetic. *Anesth Analg* 2004;98:240–241.
Wong KC, Puerto AX, Puerto BA, et al. Influence of imipramine and pargyline on the arrhythmogenicity of epinephrine during halothane, enflurane, or methoxyflurane anesthesia in dogs. *Anesthesiology* 1980;53:S25.
Young CC, Lujan E. Intravenous ziprasidone for treatment of delirium in the intensive care unit. *Anesthesiology* 2004;101:794–795.
Zhang Y, Luo Z, White PF. A model for evaluating droperidol's effect on the median QTc interval. *Anesth Analg* 2004;98:1330–1335.

Prostaglandins

20

Prostaglandins are among the most prevalent of the naturally occurring, physiologically active endogenous substances (autacoids). They have been detected in almost every tissue and body fluid. Indeed, the cellular mechanisms responsible for the formation of prostaglandins are present in all organs of the body. No other autacoids (histamine, serotonin, angiotensin II, plasma kinins) show more numerous and diverse effects than do the prostaglandins. Because prostaglandins act as local hormones, it is difficult to assess their activity in the intact organism.

NOMENCLATURE AND STRUCTURE–ACTIVITY RELATIONSHIPS

The designation of a substance as a prostaglandin reflects the initial belief that the biologically active substance (a lipid-soluble acid) present in human semen resulting in relaxation of the uterus was a secretion of the prostate gland. The generic term *eicosanoids* refers to the 20-carbon, hairpin-shaped fatty acid chain that includes a cyclopentane ring, characteristic of prostaglandins (Fig. 20-1).

The letters PG denote the word prostaglandin. A third letter indicates the structure of the cyclopentane ring, such that PGE has a different ring structure than PGF. A subscript that follows the third letter denotes the number of double bonds in the structure as well as the fatty acid precursor of the prostaglandin. For example, PGE_1 has one double bond, whereas PGE_2 has two double bonds. The subscript 2 also designates arachidonic acid as the fatty acid precursor. Prostaglandins with two double bonds are referred to as *dienoic prostaglandins*. Monoenoic and trienoic prostaglandins have one and three double bonds, respectively. These prostaglandins tend to have less biologic activity. Alpha or beta after the subscript indicates the orientation of the hydroxyl group at the number 9 carbon atom to the plane of the cyclopentane ring.

SYNTHESIS

The principal precursor of dienoic prostaglandins in mammalian cells is the polyunsaturated 20-carbon essential fatty acid, arachidonic acid (Harris, 1992). Monoenoic and trienoic prostaglandins are derived from dihydrolinoleic and eicospentanoic acid. Arachidonic acid is a ubiquitous component of cell membranes and is released by the action of phospholipase C and phospholipase A_2. Phospholipase enzymes are activated by various physical and chemical stimuli and inhibited by corticosteroids. Histamine is known to activate phospholipase enzymes, leading to the formation of prostaglandins, including prostacyclin. Inhaled anesthetics, as a result of their solubility in lipid cell membranes, may increase the availability of arachidonic acid as a substrate (Shayevitz et al., 1985). Once cleaved from the cell membranes, arachidonic acid becomes available to serve as a substrate for production of prostaglandins via either the cyclooxygenase (COX) or the lipoxygenase pathway (Fig. 20-2).

Cyclooxygenase

COX is a widely distributed complex of microsomal enzymes necessary for the initial synthesis (oxidation) of prostaglandins (PGE_2 and PGH_2) known as *endoperoxides* (see Fig. 20-2). Subsequent conversion of PGH_2 to thromboxane (TXA_2) and prostacyclin (PGI_2) requires the activity of tissue-specific enzymes, thromboxane synthetase and prostacyclin synthetase (see Fig. 20-2). There are two distinct isoforms of COX (COX-1 and COX-2), which are encoded by two different genes and differentially expressed in a variety of tissues. In particular, COX-1 is expressed in platelets and gastric mucosa. COX-2 is expressed in inflamed tissues (response to mitogenic stimuli and inflammatory cytokines such as interleukin-1 and tumor necrosis factor) and the brain and spinal cord. Involvement of COX-2 in pain perception thus involves the localized production of prostaglandins at sites of tissue damage and inflammation and centrally in the spinal cord. In contrast to the wide tissue distribution of cox, thromboxane synthetase

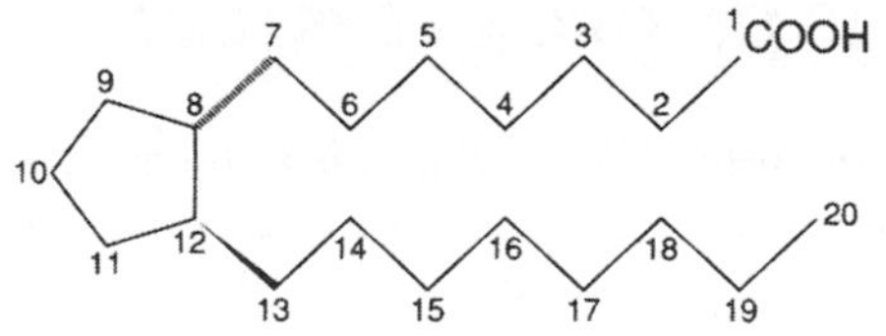

Figure 20-1. A 20-carbon hairpin-shaped fatty acid chain is characteristic of prostaglandins.

is principally present in platelets and the lungs, whereas prostacyclin synthetase is principally present in vascular endothelium.

Lipoxygenase

Lipoxygenase enzymes are localized principally in platelets, vascular endothelium, the lungs, and leukocytes. Compounds formed by enzyme-induced lipoxygenation of arachidonic acid are termed *leukotrienes*. Compounds formed by these enzymes from arachidonic acid include 5-hydroperoxyeicosatetraenoic acid (HPETE) and its degradation product, 12-hydroxyeicosatetraenoic acid (HETE) (see Fig. 20-2). The term *leukotriene* denotes the initial discovery of these substances in leukocytes. Increased concentrations of leukotrienes have been measured in several disease states, including bronchial asthma, neonatal arterial hypoxemia with pulmonary hypertension, and the adult respiratory distress syndrome (Matthay et al., 1984). Leukotriene D (formerly designated as *slow-reacting substance of anaphylaxis*) has preferential effects on peripheral airways and is a more potent bronchoconstrictor than histamine. Furthermore, leukotriene-induced increases in vascular permeability occur at lower concentrations than when histamine is present. Leukotriene B released from alveolar macrophages and other leukocytes stimulates neutrophil adhesion to endothelial cells, with subsequent degranulation, enzyme release, and superoxide generation (Samuelsson, 1983).

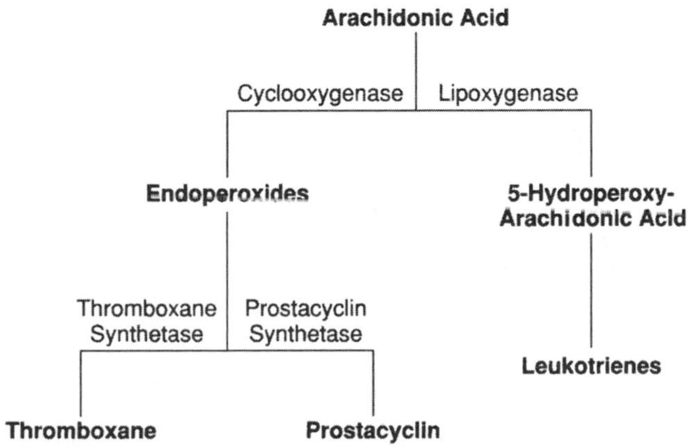

Figure 20-2. Synthesis of prostaglandins from arachidonic acid occurs via a cyclooxygenase pathway and a lipoxygenase pathway.

MECHANISM OF ACTION

In many tissues, prostaglandins act on specific cell membrane receptors to activate adenylate cyclase with the resulting increase in intracellular concentrations of cyclic 3′,5′-adenosine monophosphate (cAMP) (Kerins et al., 1991). cAMP activates protein kinase A to express its effects, including decreased free intracellular calcium in vascular smooth muscle, resulting in vascular relaxation. The acidic lipid nature of prostaglandins is unique among autacoids and other substances that react with specific cell membrane receptors. Prostacyclin also stimulates release of nitric oxide from endothelial cells.

Prostaglandins are produced during inflammation by the action of COX. These prostaglandins increase the sensitivity of nociceptors and nociceptive neurons to other pain-producing stimuli such as histamine, bradykinin, and thermal changes. Excessive production of prostaglandins in the periphery (peripheral sensitization) leads to modifications in gene expression in the central nervous system (CNS) that result in hyperalgesia and allodynia (central sensitization).

METABOLISM

Initial metabolism of prostaglandins to inactive substances is rapid and catalyzed by specific enzymes that are widely distributed in the body in such organs as the lungs, kidneys, and liver and in the gastrointestinal tract. For example, 95% of infused PGE_2 is inactivated during one passage through the lungs. The unique position of the pulmonary circulation between the venous and arterial circulations allows the lungs to act as a filter for many of the prostaglandins, thus protecting the cardiovascular system and other organs from prolonged effects due to recirculation of these substances. Thromboxane is hydrolyzed rapidly (elimination half-time 30 seconds) to an inactive product, thus largely limiting its actions to the microenvironment of its release. Prostacyclin, with an elimination half-time of about 3 minutes, is nonenzymatically converted to 6-keto-$PGF_{1\alpha}$ (Kerins et al., 1991). Measurement of plasma concentrations of 6-keto-$PGF_{1\alpha}$ serves as an indicator of prostacyclin release or lack of release as in the presence of known inhibitors (aspirin, ibuprofen) or H_1 receptor antagonists (diphenhydramine).

The initial rapid metabolism of prostaglandins is followed by slower breakdown, during which the existing inactive metabolites are oxidized by enzymes responsible for oxidation of most fatty acids. The liver is the major site for this oxidation; the resulting metabolites appear in urine, often as dicarboxylic acid.

PROSTACYCLIN (PGI_2, EPOPROSTENIL)

Prostacyclin is derived from arachadonic acid and is synthesized predominantly by endothelial cells. Prostacyclin is a vasodilator and the most potent known inhibitor of platelet aggregation. Endothelial release of nitric oxide is stimulated by prostacyclin. Prostacyclin has an elimination half-time of about 6 minutes and is spontaneously hydrolyzed at a plasma pH 7.4 to inactive metabolizes. Prostacyclin is supplied as a powder that must be dissolved in a glycine buffer and protected from photodegradation. Intravenous (IV) administration of prostacyclin has the significant disadvantage of not being a selective pulmonary vasodilator thus producing parallel decreases in pulmonary and systemic vascular resistance and increasing intrapulmonary shunting. Conversely, inhaled prostacyclin and inhaled nitric oxide seem comparable in terms of their ability to selectively decrease pulmonary artery pressure and improve arterial oxygenation (Lowson, 2002). Inhaled prostacyclin is not metabolized within the lung to any significant extent, and systemic absorption of prostacyclin is determined by measuring the plasma concentrations of its major inactive metabolite, 6-keto-$PGF_{1\alpha}$

ILOPROST

Iloprost is a stable and long-acting (elimination half-time 20 to 30 minutes) carbacyclin derivative of prostacyclin that is a potent inhibitor of platelet aggregation. This drug produces its platelet effect immediately and platelet activity returns usually within 3 hours after cessation of its administration. It has no effect on the activity of coagulation factors other than platelets. Iloprost causes vasodilation, but it is associated with less hypotension than prostacyclin. Nevertheless, iloprost may produce hypotension that is resistant to relatively large doses of phenylephrine (Kraenzler and Starr, 1988).

EFFECTS ON ORGAN SYSTEMS

The possible role of prostaglandins as mediators of effects on organ systems depends on the system under consideration (Table 20-1) (Oates et al., 1988). For example, inhibitors of prostaglandin synthesis usually have little effect on the cardiovascular system or the lungs, suggesting a negligible role of prostaglandins in the basal regulation of these systems. Conversely, normal platelet function and hemostasis are likely to be under strict regulation of prostaglandins, as emphasized by the ability of nonsteroidal antiinflammatory drugs to interfere with normal platelet aggregation. Renal blood flow may be influenced by the presence or absence of prostaglandins in the kidneys. The finding of low basal levels of prostaglandins in hypertensive patients suggests that a deficiency of vasodilator prostaglandins may be associated with essential hypertension (Gurwitz et al., 1994).

Hematologic System

Thromboxane, the principal COX product of arachidonic acid in platelets, acts as an intense stimulus for platelet aggregation, presumably reflecting inhibition of adenylate cyclase and subsequent decreased cAMP synthesis in platelets. Conversely, prostacyclin is the most potent endogenous inhibitor of platelet aggregation, and its release from vascular endothelium opposes platelet aggregation. Prostacyclin binds to receptors on platelets that activate adenylate cyclase and increase intracellular concentrations of cAMP, leading to decreased platelet adhesiveness and prolonged platelet survival.

A normal thromboxane-to-prostacyclin ratio is important in maintaining platelet activity and coagulation. An increase in this ratio, as may occur when atherosclerotic plaques release substances that inhibit synthesis of prostacyclin, results in a predominance of thromboxane activity, manifesting as platelet aggregation and vasoconstriction.

TABLE 20-1.
COMPARATIVE EFFECTS OF PROSTAGLANDINS

	Platelet Aggregation	Systemic Vascular Resistance	Airway Resistance	Uterine Muscle Tone	Gastric Acid Secretion
Thromboxane (TXA_2)	I	I	I		
Prostacyclin (PGI_2)	D	D	?I		
Iloprost	D	D	D		
Alprostadil (PGE_1)	D	D	I	I	
Misoprostol		NC		I	D
Carboprost				I	
Dinoprost ($PGF_2\alpha$)		I,D	I	I	
Dinoprostone (PGE_2)				I	

I, increased; D, decreased; NC, no change.

This sequence of events could lead to decreased blood flow in the area of an atherosclerotic plaque, manifesting as ischemia or infarction in organs such as the heart, brain, and kidneys. A similar imbalance in the thromboxane-to-prostacyclin ratio in the venous circulation could lead to venous thromboembolism.

Bleeding disorders are likely in the presence of thromboxane depletion or excess prostacyclin. The speculated role of platelet aggregation in myocardial ischemia suggests a potentially useful role for prostacyclin in both dilating coronary arteries and preventing aggregation of platelets. These same effects of prostacyclin could be useful in treating acute ischemic pain in extremities and in promoting healing of ischemic extremities.

Prostacyclin present in low concentrations in the plasma may be responsible for preventing aggregation of normal platelets. A break in the vascular endothelium releases thromboxane, causing intense local vasoconstriction and platelet aggregation, leading to formation of a hemostatic plug. It seems likely that COX enzyme in the platelets that synthesize thromboxane is more sensitive to inhibition by aspirin than is the same enzyme in vascular endothelium that synthesizes prostacyclin. As a result, thromboxane production in platelets is inhibited by small doses of aspirin, whereas large doses of aspirin inhibit both thromboxane and prostacyclin production. If a patient is being treated with low doses of aspirin, thromboxane is no longer present to oppose prostacyclin, and platelet aggregation does not occur. Prostacyclin use is limited by its intense vasodilating activity, which may result in hypotension. Epoprostenol (PGI_2) can be administered to inhibit platelet aggregation during hemodialysis with or without heparin. The use of epoprostenol as an antithrombotic drug is limited by its chemical instability and systemic vasodilation effects resulting in hypotension.

Iloprost added to the cardiopulmonary bypass circuit preserves circulating platelet counts and prevents platelet granule release during simulated extracorporeal circulation (Addonizio et al., 1985). This drug may be useful during cardiac surgery to prevent interaction of platelets with antigens such as heparin in patients with heparin-induced thrombocytopenia.

Cardiovascular System

Prostaglandins play an important role in cardiovascular homeostasis by promoting vasodilation and enhancing sodium excretion (de Leeuw, 1996). The effects of prostaglandins on cardiac function are complex and depend on direct inotropic effects, the activity of the sympathetic nervous system relative to the parasympathetic nervous system, and the metabolic status of the heart. For example, PGE_2 produces an increase in heart rate and myocardial contractility by direct inotropic effects as well as by increasing reflex sympathetic nervous system activity. The IV administration of prostacyclin causes a decrease in systemic blood pressure resulting from a decrease in systemic vascular resistance, reflecting vasodilation in several vascular beds, including coronary, renal, mesenteric, and skeletal muscle circulations. Blockade of the arachidonic acid pathway will not only decrease the formation of antihypertensive prostaglandins such as PGE_2 and prostacyclin but also the prohypertensive prostaglandins such as thromboxane A_2 and PHG_2. Local generation of PGE_2 and prostacyclin may participate in the transition of the fetal circulation to that of a normal neonate. Indeed, prostaglandin synthesis inhibitors may contribute to the closure of the ductus arteriosus. The activity of vascular smooth muscle in various vascular beds may be modulated by the relative magnitude of vasoconstriction and vasodilation produced by thromboxane and prostacyclin, respectively. For example, events leading to coronary artery spasm and thrombosis may arise from a deficiency of prostacyclin-induced vasodilation relative to thromboxane-induced vasoconstriction.

Mesenteric traction during aortic surgery may produce facial flushing, decreased systemic blood pressure, and systemic vascular resistance, and increased heart rate and cardiac output (Hudson et al., 1990). These changes are associated with increased plasma concentrations of 6-keto-$PGF_{1\alpha}$, suggesting that prostacyclin is a mediator. Indeed, ibuprofen, a cox inhibitor, prevents facial flushing and cardiovascular changes associated with mesenteric traction (Hudson et al., 1990).

Alprostadil (PGE1, Prostin VR Pediatric)

Alprostadil (PGE_1) is a vasodilator prostaglandin that binds to cell surface prostaglandin receptors that are part of the G-protein superfamily causing activation of adenylate cyclase (Fig. 20-3) (Lowson, 2002). Alprostadil has a variety of pharmacologic effects, the most important of which are vasodilation, inhibition of platelet aggregation, and stimulation of gastrointestinal and uterine smooth muscle. Alprostadil is normally present within the lungs where it produces pulmonary smooth muscle relaxation Alprostadil is a stable compound at pH 7.4 and is rapidly metabolized by 15-hydrogyprostaglandin dehydrogenase to inactive products.

Clinical Uses

Alprostadil is a potent relaxant of vascular smooth muscles and when administered IV maintians the patency of

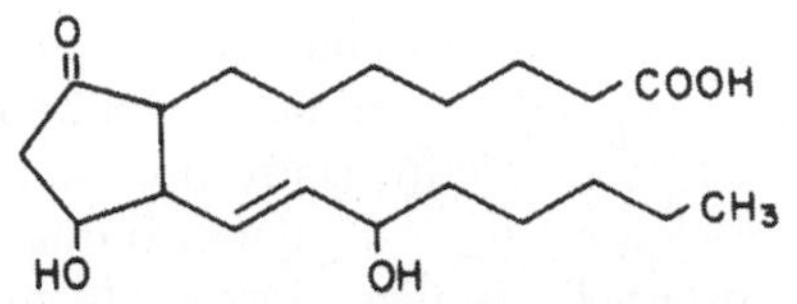

Figure 20-3. Alprostadil [prostaglandin E_1 (PGE_1)].

the ductus arteriosus in infants with congenital heart disease (pulmonary atresia, tetralogy of Fallot) until a surgical shunt can be performed (Lowson, 2002). This prostaglandin has also been administered for treatment of pulmonary hypertension in patients with mitral valve disease, acute respiratory distress syndrome, and following heart transplantation. Alprostadil is metabolized so rapidly that it must be administered as a continuous infusion. Nearly 70% of circulating alprostadil is metabolized in one passage through the lungs, and the metabolites are excreted by the kidneys. Depression of ventilation, bronchoconstriction, flushing, bradycardia, and hyperthermia may be evoked by continuous infusion of this drug (Lewis et al., 1981). Despite the fact that the lungs remove nearly 70% of alprostadil during a single passage, it has not been confirmed that pulmonary selectivity for alprostadil is present.

Pulmonary Circulation

Pulmonary vasoconstriction may be related to increased circulating concentrations of thromboxane, PGE_2, and $PGE_{2\alpha}$. Pulmonary vasoconstriction, pulmonary hypertension, and bronchoconstriction that, on rare occasions, are associated with the administration of protamine may reflect protamine-induced production of the prostaglandin vasoconstrictor thromboxane (Nuttall et al., 1991). Prostacyclin is a ubiquitous, potent vasodilator released primarily from endothelial cells but also from other cell types. It is critical for maintaining low pulmonary vascular resistance and plays a major role in the transitional circulation.

As a potent pulmonary vasoconstrictor, $PGF_{2\alpha}$ has been shown to enhance vasoconstriction in an atelectatic lung, diverting pulmonary blood flow to ventilated alveoli and increasing the Pao_2 (Scherer et al., 1985). In essence, $PGF_{2\alpha}$ is capable of potentiating hypoxic pulmonary vasoconstriction and thus improving arterial oxygenation. Because 70% to 98% of this prostaglandin is inactivated in one passage across the lung, it is possible, with the proper infusion rate, to selectively produce effects on the pulmonary vasculature to the exclusion of the systemic circulation.

Prostacyclin

Prostacyclin has a brief half-time (about 3 mintues) necessitating its administration by the IV route. IV prostacyclin has an established role in the long-term management of primary pulmonary hypertension.

Inhaled (aerosolized) prostacyclin has been shown to produce greater descreases in pulmonary vascular resistance than nitric oxide (Lowson, 2002). Inhaled prostacyclin, in common with nitric oxide has no effect on pulmonary vascular resistance in patients with normal pulmonary vasculature. Inhaled prostacyclin has some potential advantages over inhaled nitric oxide. For example, the lack of toxicity of prostacyclin (unlike nitric oxide, methemoglobin formation is not a risk of prostacyclin therapy) or its metabolites suggests that accurate measurement of the concentrations of delivered drug and its metabolites in inspiratory and expiratory gases is not necessary. Furthermore, in contrast to inhaled nitric oxide, the apparatus for delivery of prostacyclin is inexpensive and readily available. The daily cost of prostacyclin is only a fraction of that of inhaled nitric oxide.

Inhaled prostacyclin is useful for treatment of patients with pulmonary hypertension and acute right ventricular failure after cardiac surgery. Selective pulmonary vasodilation decreases right ventricular afterload thus improving right ventricular ejection and cardiac output without descreasing systemic blood pressure. Impaired platelet function is a poterntial but unsubstantiated undesirable effect of prostacyclin therapy in patients following cardiac surgery.

Inhaled prostacyclin administered to patients with acute respiratory distress syndrome produces selective pulmonary vasodilation and increase in Pao_2 comparable to that produced by inhaled nitric oxide (Fig. 20-4) (Zwissler

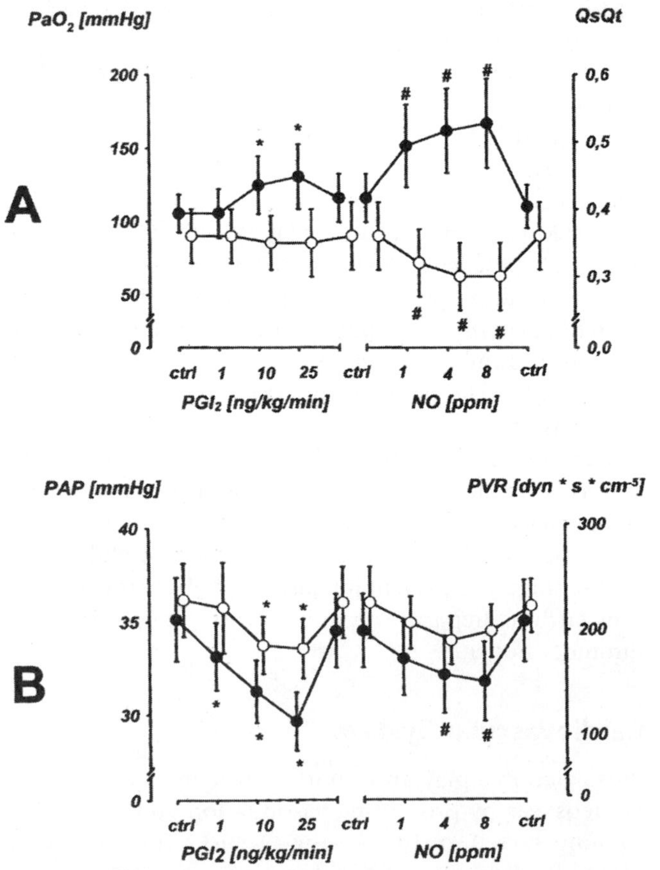

Figure 20-4. The effects of three doses of inhaled prostacyclin (PGI_2) (1, 10, and 25 μg/kg/min) and inhaled nitric oxide (NO) (1,4, and 8 ppm) on mean pulmonary artery pressure (PAP, closed circles) and pulmonary vascular resistance (PVR) (open circles). All data are mean ± SE. (From Zwissler B, Kemming, G Habler, O, et al. Inhaled prostacyclin versus inhaled nitric oxide in adult respiratory distress syndrome. *Am J Respir Crit Care Med* 1996;154: 1671–1677; with permission.)

et al., 1996). Conversely, prostacyclin administered IV to these patients is limited by systemic hypotension and increased pulmonary venous admixture.

Inhaled prostacyclin can selectively decrease pulmonary artery pressure and improve Pao_2 in pediatric patients with hypoxic respiratory failure associated with pulmonary hypertension although its relative efficacy compared with nitric oxide is not determined. Inhibition of platelet aggregation may explain the therapeutic benefit of prostacyclin in patients with pulmonary hypertension secondary to thromboembolic diseases. Prostacyclin has been used as long-term therapy in patients with pulmonary hypertension or as a bridge to transplantation (Conte et al., 1998).

Side Effects

Prostacyclin is a potent vasodilator and side effects to inhaled prostacyclin include anxiety, flushing, digginess, nausea and vomiting, chest and abdominal pain, tachycardia and bradycardia. As described with sudden cessation of inhaled nitric oxide, abrupt withdrawal of infusions of prostacyclin infusions including accidental interruptions in drug delivery systems and sudden large decreases in the dosage, may result in severe rebound pulmonary hypertension and cardiogenic shock (Fig. 20-5) (Augoustides, et al., 2004).

Iloprost

Inhaled iloprost has comparable pulmonary hemodynamic effects to inhaled nitric oxide and prostacyclin (Lowson, 2002). Compared with prostacyclin, iloprost is soluble in saline obviating the need for an alkaline buffer; is less viscous, which aids in nebulization; and significantly longer-acting, permitting intermittent rather than continuous nebulization. The plasma half-time of iloprost is 20 to 30 minutes and the hemodynamic effects of a single

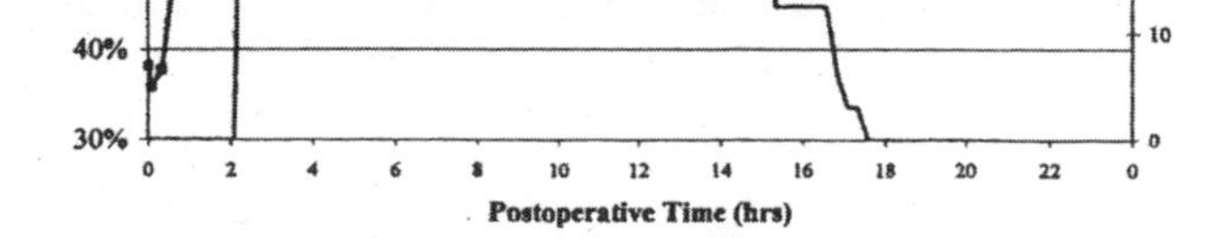

Figure 20-5. Relationship of pulmonary hypertension to cesssation of inhaled prostacyclin administration. PASP, pulmonary artery systolic pressure; SSP, systemic systolic pressure; PGI_2, inhaled prostacyclin. (From Augoustides JG, Culp K, Smith S. Rebound pulmonary hypertension and cardiogenic shock after withdrawal of inhaled prostacyclin. *Anesthesiology* 2004;100:1023–1025; with permission.)

inhaled dose lasts approximatley 1 hour. In patients with primary pulmonary hypertension, inhaled iloprost lowers pulmonary vascular resistance up to 30% within 2 to 5 mintues and lasts up to 75 mintues. The need for a permanent central venous catheter is negated by the effectiveness of inhaled iloprost. Inhaled iloprost appears to have comparable hemodynamic effects to inhaled nitric oxide.

Uniprost

Uniprost is an analogue of prostacyclin that is administered subcutaneously by a portable pump similar to that used for infusion of insulin. Improved pulmonary hemodynamics and exercise tolerance may accompany the administraton of uniprost (McLaughlin et al., 2000).

Beraprost

Beraprost is a chemically stable analog of prostacyclin that is effective when administered orally. Improved pulmonary hemodynamics and improved survival rates in patients with primary pulmonary hypertension may parallel the administration of beraprost (Vissa et al., 2001).

Lungs

The lungs are a major site of prostaglandin synthesis. Prostaglandins may produce bronchoconstriction or bronchodilation. Indeed, an imbalance between production of thromboxane and prostacyclin in the lungs might contribute to symptoms of bronchial asthma. Asthmatic patients experience increased airway resistance with far lower inhaled amounts of PGF_2 than do normal patients. Both PGE_1 and PGE_2 produce bronchodilation when given by aerosol, but the associated irritant effect of this inhalation offsets their clinical usefulness. There is conflicting evidence about whether prostacyclin is a bronchoconstrictor (Wetzel, 1995).

Leukotrienes are several thousand times more potent as constrictors of bronchial smooth muscle than is histamine. A predominant role of leukotrienes in asthma-induced bronchoconstriction in individual patients is suggested by the ineffectiveness of antihistamines. Furthermore, the relatively slow metabolism of leukotrienes in the lungs contributes to long-lasting bronchoconstriction. Aspirin-induced asthma may reflect inhibition of the COX pathway by the drug, leading to increased availability of arachidonic acid to the lipoxygenase pathway to form leukotrienes (see Fig. 20-2).

Kidneys

Intrarenal release of prostaglandins may be an important mechanism for modulating renal blood flow and glomerular filtration rate. Indeed, the kidneys are a major site of prostaglandin synthesis. Prostaglandins influence vascular tone directly in renal afferent arterioles and indirectly in renal efferent arterioles, via the modulation of the renin-angiotensin system. Other effects of prostaglandins include augmentation of the effects of the kallikrein-kinin system, mediation of renin release in response to a decrease in renal blood flow or renal perfusion pressure, and moderation of adrenergic vasoconstriction (de Leeuw et al., 1996). Inhibition of the COX system with nonsteroidal antiinflammatory drugs and aspirin does not have clinically significant effects on renal hemodynamics in patients with normal kidneys. Conversely, when renal vasoconstrictor systems have been activated, inhibition of the production of vasodilator prostaglandins (PGE_2 or prostacyclin) by nonsteroidal antiinflammatory drugs may interfere with normal renal prostaglandin protective mechanisms and accentuate catecholamine-induced renal vasoconstriction (Harris, 1992).

Misoprostol

Misoprostol is a PGE_1 analogue with oral bioavailability that improves renal function and decreases the incidence of acute rejection in renal transplant patients treated concurrently with cyclosporine and prednisone (Moran et al., 1990). Indeed, cyclosporine-induced nephrotoxicity may reflect inhibition of the synthesis of renal prostaglandins.

Misoprostol inhibits the secretion of gastric acid by a direct action on parietal cells, which may reflect intracellular interference with histamine-induced activation of adenylate cyclase (Walt, 1992). This prostaglandin maintains or increases mucosal blood flow in response to gastric irritants and may increase secretion of mucus and bicarbonate by the gastric and duodenal mucosa. For these reasons, misoprostol is recommended for the prevention of nonsteroidal antiinflammatory drug-induced gastric ulcers in patients at high risk. It is rapidly absorbed after oral administration (peak plasma concentrations in about 30 minutes) and then promptly metabolized. Renal excretion is minimal, and the dose does not need adjustment in patients with renal dysfunction. An important side effect of misoprostol is increased uterine contraction, which can provoke abortion. In this regard, misoprostol is an option to PGE_2 for the termination of pregnancy (Jain and Mishell, 1994). Nausea, vomiting, and diarrhea associated with the use of prostaglandins to induce abortion reflect stimulation of smooth muscle of the gastrointestinal tract as well as the uterus. Misoprostol has no major CNS or cardiovascular side effects.

Gastrointestinal Tract

Certain prostaglandins inhibit gastric acid secretion (Penston and Wormsley, 1989). Indeed, comparison of high-dose misoprostol with cimetidine has shown similar rates of healing of duodenal ulcers. Likewise, enprostil was as effective as cimetidine in the treatment of duodenal ulcers. Nevertheless, prostaglandin therapy is not considered a preferred alternative to H_2 receptor antagonists in the management of patients with peptic ulcer disease.

Uterus

The nongravid and gravid uterus is predictably contracted by PGE_2 and $PGF_{2\alpha}$, leading to the speculation that these prostaglandins are important in the initiation and maintenance of labor. Infusion of these prostaglandins results in prompt and dose-dependent increases in uterine muscle tone. In contrast to oxytocin, this effect of prostaglandins is observed at all stages of pregnancy, accounting for the usefulness of certain prostaglandins for inducing labor as well as abortion. Prompt depression of progesterone output and reabsorption of the corpus luteum follow parenteral injection of $PGF_{2\alpha}$ to animals. This effect interrupts early pregnancy, which is dependent on luteal rather than placental progesterone.

Increased synthesis of prostaglandins in the endometrium is speculated to be a cause of dysmenorrhea. Indeed, inhibitors of prostaglandin synthesis such as aspirin or indomethacin decrease pain associated with dysmenorrhea. Chronic use of aspirin increases the average length of gestation and the duration of spontaneous labor. Likewise, these inhibitors of prostaglandin synthesis decrease contractions of the uterus in premature labor and could increase the likelihood of postpartum uterine atony.

Prostaglandins may be important in the control of the uteroplacental circulation. Changes in the production of prostaglandins have been implicated in the pathophysiology of pregnancy-induced hypertension.

Carboprost

Carboprost is a synthetic analogue of naturally occurring $PGF_{2\alpha}$ (Fig. 20-6). The addition of a methyl group at carbon 15 results in a longer duration of action. Drug-induced uterine contractions are similar to those that accompany labor. Induction of elective abortion with carboprost is successful in >90% of patients between 12 and 20 weeks of gestation. Mean time to abortion is 16 hours after intramuscular injection of carboprost. Adverse effects are common but usually are not serious. Vomiting and diarrhea occur in >60% of patients. Body temperature increases of 1° to 2°C occur in nearly 10% of patients and must be differentiated from fever due to endometritis. Delivery of a live fetus with carboprost-induced abortion is possible.

Dinoprost

Dinoprost is $PGF_{2\alpha}$ that is administered intraamniotically to induce uterine contractions (Fig. 20-7). The mean time

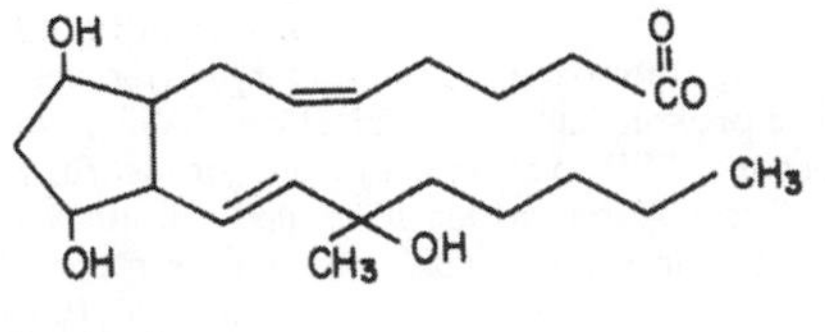

Figure 20-6. Carboprost.

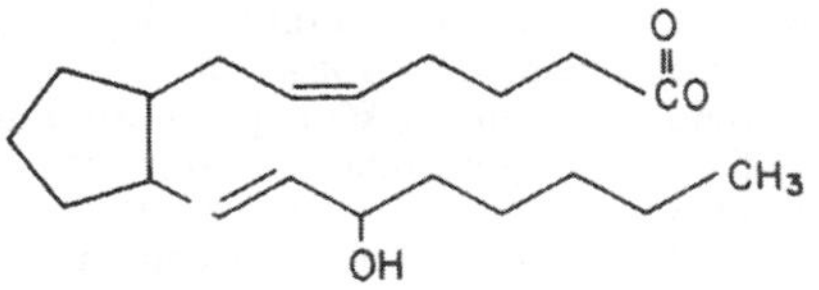

Figure 20-7. Dinoprost.

to abortion is about 20 hours. Nausea and vomiting occur in most patients and can often be ameliorated by antiemetics. Bronchospasm may occur in asthmatic patients. Grand mal seizures are possible in patients prone to epilepsy. Inadvertent IV administration produces bronchospasm and hypotension or hypertension.

Dinoprostone

Dinoprostone is PGE_2 and produces physiologic-like uterine contractions by activating adenylate cyclase and thus increasing intracellular concentrations of calcium ions (Fig. 20-8).

Therapeutically, this prostaglandin is most often administered as a vaginal suppository to induce elective abortion. Side effects of PGE_2 include increases in heart rate and cardiac output as well as tachypnea and hyperthermia that may mimic the onset of sepsis (Hughes and Hughes, 1989). Diuresis is speculated to reflect increased renal blood flow secondary to renal artery dilation. In addition, PGE_2 stimulates steroid formation in the adrenal cortex by activating adenylate cyclase while suppressing epinephrine-induced lipolysis.

Immune System

Prostaglandins such as prostacyclin contribute to the signs and symptoms of inflammation, accentuating the pain and edema produced by bradykinin. Conversely, other prostaglandins suppress the release of chemical mediators from mast cells of patients experiencing allergic reactions.

Antibody responses may be decreased by PGE_1, possibly allowing greater acceptance of tissue transplants. Indeed, immunosuppressant effects of certain tumors may reflect their ability to produce prostaglandins. Hypercalcemia associated with a tumor may reflect osteolytic activity of certain prostaglandins. Overproduction of PGD_2 is principally responsible for the systemic (flushing, tachycardia, hypotension) and pulmonary (bronchoconstriction) manifestations of mastocytosis (Oates et al., 1988).

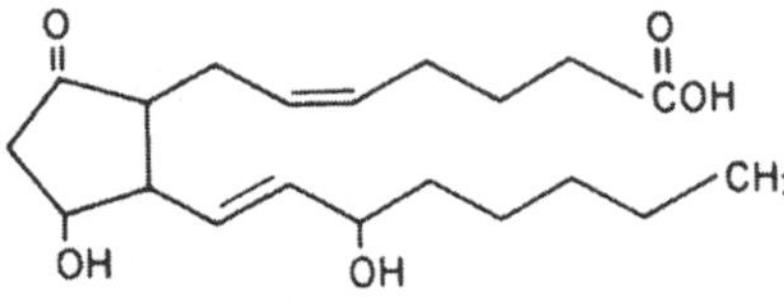

Figure 20-8. Dinoprostone.

LEUKOTRIENE ANTAGONISTS

Inhibitors of the leukotriene pathway are useful drugs in the management of patients with bronchial asthma. Leukotrienes are synthesized from arachidonic acid and are released from membrane phospholipids when inflammatory cells are activated.

Zileuton

Zileuton is a 5-lipoxygenase inhibitor that impairs the conversion of arachidonic acid to leukotriene A_4 thus inhibiting the generation of leukotrienes involved in asthma and inflammation. Oral absorption is rapid, protein binding exceeds 90%, and the elimination half-time is 2.5 hours. Metabolism involves cytochrome P-450 enzymes and metabolites appear in the bile and urine. Side effects of zileuton include dyspepsia, arthralgia, chest pain, fever, and somnolence. This drug is not recommended for administration to patients with hepatic dysfunction.

Montelukast and Zafirlukast

Montelukast and zafirlukast are cysteinyl-leukotriene$_1$ antagonists that competitively block the ability of leukotrienes to bind to cysteinyl-leukotriene$_1$ receptors. Bronchospasm, vasoconstriction, and eosinophil recruitment are in part mediated by leukotriene binding to these receptors. Oral absorption is rapid, protein binding approaches 99%, and elimination half-time is 2.5 to 5 hours. Cytochrome P-450 enzymes are responsible for hepatic metabolism and metabolites are excreted in the bile. Renal dysfunction does not influence the dose of these drugs. Coadministration of montelukast and warfarin may result in decreased clearance of warfarin and prolongation of the prothrombin time. Side effects may include elevation of the plasma concentrations of liver transaminase enzymes.

REFERENCES

Augoustides JG, Culp K, Smith S. Rebound pulmonary hypertension and cardiogenic shock after withdrawal of inhaled prostacyclin. *Anesthesiology* 2004;100:1023–1025.

Cole RB, Abman S, Azis KU, et al. Prolonged prostaglandin E infusion: histologic effects on patent ductus arteriosus. *Pediatrics* 1981;67:816–819.

Conte JV, Gaine SP, Orens JB, et al. The influence of continuous intravenous prostacyclin therapy for primary pulmonary hypertension on the timing and outcome of transplantation. *J Heart Lung Transplant* 1998;17:679–684.

de Leeuw PW. Nonsteroidal anti-inflammatory drugs and hypertension: the risks in perspective. *Drugs* 1996;51:179–187.

Gurwitz JH, Avorn J, Bohn RL, et al. Initiation of antihypertensive treatment during nonsteroidal anti-inflammatory drug therapy. *JAMA* 1994;272:781–786.

Harris K. The role of prostaglandins in the control of renal function. *Br J Anaesth* 1992;69:233–235.

Hudson JC, Wurm WH, O'Donnell TF, et al. Ibuprofen pretreatment inhibits prostacyclin release during abdominal exploration in aortic surgery. *Anesthesiology* 1990;72:443–449.

Hughes WA, Hughes SC. Hemodynamic effects of prostaglandin E_2. *Anesthesiology* 1989;70:713–716.

Jain JJ, Mishell DR. A comparison of intravaginal misoprostol with prostaglandin E_2 for termination of second-trimester pregnancy. *N Engl J Med* 1994;331:290–293.

Kerins DM, Murray R, Fitzgerald GA. Prostacyclin and prostaglandin E_1: molecular mechanisms and therapeutic utility. *Prog Hemost Thromb* 1991;10:307–337.

Kraenzler EJ, Starr NJ. Heparin-associated thrombocytopenia: management of patients for open heart surgery. Case reports describing the use of Hoprost. *Anesthesiology* 1988;69:964–967.

Lewis AB, Scheinman MM, Gonzalez R, et al. Side-effects of therapy with prostaglandin E in infants with critical congenital heart disease. *Circulation* 1981;64:893–898.

Lowson SM. Inhaled alternatives to nitric oxide. *Anesthesiology* 2002;96:1504–1513.

Matthay M, Ischenbacher W, Goetzl E. Elevated concentrations of leukotriene D_4 in pulmonary edema fluid of patients with adult respiratory distress syndrome. *J Clin Immunol* 1984;4:479–483.

McLaughlin VV, Hess DM, Sigman J, et al. Long term effects of UT-15 on hemodynamics and exercise tolerance in primary pulmonary hypertension. *Eur Respir J* 2000;16:394S–399S.

Moran M, Mozes MF, Maddux MS, et al. Prevention of acute graft rejection by the prostaglandin E_1 analogue of misoprostol in renal-transplant recipients treated with cyclosporin and prednisone. *N Engl J Med* 1990;322:1183–1188.

Nuttall GA, Murray MJ, Bowie EJW. Protamine-heparin-induced pulmonary hypertension in pigs: effects of treatment with a thromboxane receptor antagonist on hemodynamics and coagulation. *Anesthesiology* 1991;74:138–145.

Oates JA, Fitzgerald GA, Branch RA, et al. Clinical implications of prostaglandin and thromboxane A_2 formation. *N Engl J Med* 1988;319:689–698.

Penston JG, Wormsley KG. Histamine H_2-receptor antagonists versus prostaglandins in the treatment of peptic ulcer. *Drugs* 1989;37:391–401.

Samuelsson B. Leukotrienes: mediators of immediate hypersensitivity reactions and inflammation. *Science* 1983;220:568–575.

Scherer RW, Vigfusson G, Hultsch E, et al. Prostaglandin F_2 alpha improves oxygen tension and reduces ventilation admixture during one-lung ventilation in anesthetized paralyzed dogs. *Anesthesiology* 1985;62:23–28.

Shayevitz JR, Traystman RJ, Adkinson NF, et al. Inhalation anesthetics augment oxidant-induced pulmonary vasoconstriction: evidence for a membrane effect. *Anesthesiology* 1985;63:624–632.

Vizza CD, Sciomer S, Morelli S, et al. Long-term treatment of pulmonary arterial hypertension with beraprost, an oral prostacyclin analogue. *Heart* 2001;86:661–666.

Walt RP. Misoprostol for the treatment of peptic ulcer and antiinflammatory drug-induced gastroduodenal ulceration. *N Engl J Med* 1992;327:1575–1580.

Zwissler B, Kemming G, Habler O, et al. Inhaled prostacyclin versus inhaled nitric oxide in adult respiratory distress syndrome. *Am J Respir Crit Care Med* 1996;155:991–996.

Histamine and Histamine Receptor-Antagonists

21

HISTAMINE

Histamine is a low-molecular-weight, naturally occurring hydrophilic endogenous amine (autacoid) that produces a variety of physiologic and pathologic responses in different tissues and cells through G-protein coupled membrane receptors (Fig. 21-1). Histamine is also an important chemical mediator of inflammation in allergic disease. Mast cells located in the skin, lungs, and gastrointestinal tract as well as circulating basophils contain large amounts of histamine. Histamine does not easily cross the blood-brain barrier, and central nervous system (CNS) effects are usually not evident.

Synthesis

Synthesis of histamine in tissues is by decarboxylation of histidine. Histamine is stored in vesicles in a complex with heparin. Stored histamine is subsequently released in response to antigen–antibody reactions or in response to certain drugs. Histamine ingested with food is largely destroyed in the liver or lungs or excreted in urine.

Metabolism

There are two pathways of histamine metabolism in humans. The most important pathway involves methylation catalyzed by histamine-*N*-methyltransferase, which is further degraded by monoamine oxidase. In the other pathway, histamine undergoes oxidative deamination catalyzed by diamine oxidase (histaminase), which is a nonspecific enzyme widely distributed in body tissues. Resulting metabolites from both pathways are pharmacologically inactive and excreted in urine.

Receptors

The effects of histamine are mediated via histamine receptors and at least three histamine receptors subtypes have been identified and classified as H_1, H_2, and H_3 (Table 21-1) (Maze, 1981; Simons and Simons, 1994). All three receptor subtypes are found to varying degrees in the heart.

H_1 Receptors

H_1 receptors have been defined pharmacologically by the actions of their respective agonists and antagonists. The gene encoding the H_1 receptor has been cloned. Histamine acting through H_1 receptors and inositol phospholipid hydrolysis evokes smooth muscle contraction in the respiratory and gastrointestinal tracts and is a factor in causing pruritus and sneezing by sensory nerve stimulation (Simons and Simons, 1994). Histamine induces vascular endothelium to release nitric oxide, which stimulates guanylate cyclase to increase levels of cyclic guanosine monophosphate in vascular smooth muscles, causing vasodilation. Acting through H_1 and H_2 receptors, histamine causes increased capillary permeability, hypotension, tachycardia, flushing, and headache. The release of prostacyclin from vascular endothelium is mediated via H_1 receptors. Indeed, histamine activates the enzyme phospholipase, which leads to the release of prostacyclin. Histamine-induced effects mediated by activation of H_1 receptors are suppressed by specific H_1 receptor antagonists (Table 21-2).

H_1 receptors are found in conductive tissue of the atrioventricular node and slow heart rate by decreasing atrioventricular nodal conduction. Cardiac H_1 receptors are also found in epicardial coronary vessels, where they mediate vasoconstriction.

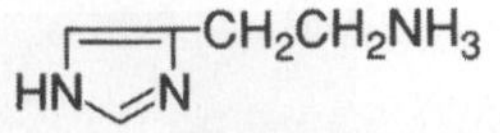

Figure 21-1. Histamine.

H_2 Receptors

Activation of H_2 receptors by histamine results in stimulation of gastric hydrogen ion secretion. Increased myocardial contractility and heart rate reflect histamine activation of these receptors in the heart. H_2 receptors are also present in the CNS. Increased capillary permeability and relaxation of vascular smooth muscles reflects histamine activation of both H_1 and H_2 receptors. Occupation of H_2 receptors by histamine activates adenylate cyclase, thus increasing intracellular concentration of cyclic adenosine monophosphate (cAMP). The increased levels of cAMP activate the proton pump of the gastric parietal cells to secrete hydrogen ions.

Histamine-induced effects mediated by activation of H_2 receptors are suppressed by specific H_2-receptor antagonists (see Table 21-2). H_2 receptors in the CNS are blocked by lysergic acid diethylamide. Similar CNS actions of cimetidine, an H_2-receptor antagonist, would be consistent with confusional states noted occasionally in patients with renal dysfunction and in those receiving high doses of cimetidine.

H_2 receptors are widely distributed through the myocardium and nodal tissues where they exert positive inotropic and chronotropic effects. The vasodilating effects of H_2 receptors in the coronary vasculature opposes the vasoconstricting effects of H_1 receptors.

H_3 Receptors

H_3 receptors found in the heart are localized to presynaptic postganglionic sympathetic nervous system fibers where they act as autoinhibitory to presynaptic norepinephrine release.

H_3 receptors, when stimulated, cause the inhibition of the synthesis and release of histamine. Activity of these receptors may be impaired by H_2 antagonists. This inhibition of H_3 activity could result in enhancement of histamine release when histamine-releasing drugs are administered to patients who have been pretreated with H_2 antagonists. For this reason, it may be prudent to avoid rapid intravenous (IV) injection of drugs known to be capable of evoking the release of histamine in patients receiving concomitant treatment with H_2 antagonists. Indeed, atracurium-induced systemic blood pressure decreases are greater in patients pretreated only with an H_2 antagonist compared with an H_1 antagonist or a combination of an H_1 and an H_2 antagonist (Hosking et al., 1988).

Effects on Organ Systems

Histamine exerts profound effects on the cardiovascular system, airways, and gastric hydrogen ion secretion. Histamine in large doses stimulates ganglion cells and chromaffin cells in the adrenal medulla, evoking the release of catecholamines. CNS effects do not accompany the peripheral release of histamine because this compound cannot easily cross the blood-brain barrier.

Cardiovascular System

The predominant cardiovascular effects of histamine are due to dilatation of arterioles and capillaries, leading to (a) flushing, (b) decreased peripheral vascular resistance, (c) decreases in systemic blood pressure, and (d) increased capillary permeability. Vascular dilatation results from a direct effect of histamine on the blood vessels, mediated by

TABLE 21-1.
EFFECTS MEDIATED BY ACTIVATION OF HISTAMINE RECEPTORS

	Receptor Subtype Activated
Increased intracellular cyclic guanosine monophosphate	H_1
Mediate release of prostacyclin	H_1
Slowed conduction of cardiac impulses through the atrioventricular node	H_1
Coronary artery vasoconstriction	H_1
Bronchoconstriction	H_1
Increased intracellular cyclic adenosine monophosphate	H_2
Central nervous system stimulation	H_2
Cardiac dysrhythmias	H_2
Increased myocardial contractility	H_2
Increased heart rate	H_2
Coronary artery vasodilation	H_2
Bronchodilation	H_2
Increased secretion of hydrogen ions by gastric parietal cells	H_2
Increased capillary permeability	H_1, H_2
Peripheral vascular vasodilation	H_1, H_2
Inhibit synthesis and release of histamine	H_3

TABLE 21-2.
CLASSIFICATION OF HISTAMINE RECEPTOR ANTAGONISTS

	Sedative Effects	Anticholinergic Activity	Antiemetic Effects	Duration of Action (hrs)	Adult Dose (mg)
H_1 antagonists (first generation)					
Diphenhydramine	Marked	Marked	Moderate	3–6	50
Pyrilamine	Mild	None	None	3–6	25–50
Chlorpheniramine	Mild	Mild	None	4–12	2–4
Promethazine	Moderate	Marked	Marked	4–24	25–50
Hydroxyzine	—	—	—	—	—
H_1 antagonists (second generation)					
Fexofenadine	Absent	None	None	12	20–40
Loratadine	Absent	None	None	24	10
Levocabastine	Absent	None	None	—	—
H_2 antagonists					
Cimetidine	Mild*	None	None	5–7	300
Ranitidine	None	None	None	8–12	150
Famotidine	None	None	None	12	20–40
Nizatidine	None	None	None	8–12	15

*Manifests as confusion and agitation.

both H_1 and H_2 receptors independent of autonomic nervous system innervation. Activation of either type of receptor can evoke maximal vasodilation, but H_1 receptors are activated at lower concentrations of histamine, producing a rapid onset and transient vasodilatation compared with a slower onset and more sustained vasodilation in response to H_2-receptor activation. Although peripheral vasodilation is generalized, flushing is most obvious in the skin of the face and upper part of the body (blush area). Increased capillary permeability is characterized as outward passage of plasma proteins and fluid into the extracellular fluid space, manifesting as edema. This increased capillary permeability is due to histamine-induced contraction of capillary endothelial cells, thus exposing the freely permeable basement membranes of capillaries to protein-containing intravascular fluid.

In addition to peripheral vasodilatation, histamine can produce inotropic, chronotropic, and antidromic effects. Positive inotropic effects are due to histamine-mediated stimulation of H_2 receptors as well as the ability of histamine to evoke the release of catecholamines from the adrenal medulla. Positive chronotropic effects and the development of cardiac dysrhythmias reflect direct activation of H_2 receptors by histamine as well as an indirect effect due to histamine-induced catecholamine release. Slowed conduction of cardiac impulses through the atrioventricular node is due to histamine activation of H_1 receptors. Changes in the threshold for ventricular fibrillation may be caused by the liberation of small amounts of histamine that are not detectable as changes in the plasma concentration. It is conceivable that regional tissue release of histamine could contribute to cardiac dysrhythmias. Coronary artery vasoconstriction is mediated by H_1 receptors, whereas coronary artery vasodilation is mediated by H_2 receptors (Simons and Simons, 1994).

The triple response elicited by histamine in the skin consists of (a) dilatation of capillaries in the injured area, (b) edema due to increased permeability of the capillaries, and (c) a flare consisting of dilated arteries surrounding the edema. The flare component of the triple response is an example of the ability of histamine to stimulate nerve endings. Histamine also causes pruritus when injected into superficial layers of the skin.

Decreases in systemic blood pressure induced by histamine are prevented by the prior administration of the combination of H_1 and H_2 receptor antagonists (Philbin et al., 1981). Blockade of either receptor alone does not completely prevent the subsequent blood pressure-lowering effects of histamine.

Airways

Histamine activates H_1 receptors to constrict bronchial smooth muscles, whereas stimulation of H_2 receptors relaxes bronchial smooth muscles. In normal patients, the bronchoconstrictor action of histamine is negligible. Conversely, patients with obstructive airway disease, such as asthma or bronchitis, are more likely to develop increases in airway resistance in response to histamine.

Gastric Hydrogen Ion Secretion

Histamine evokes copious secretion of gastric fluid containing high concentrations of hydrogen ions. This response occurs in the presence of plasma concentrations of histamine that do not alter systemic blood pressure. A doubling of the plasma histamine concentration is usually considered necessary to evoke changes in blood pressure (Rosow et al., 1980).

Increased gastric hydrogen ion secretion is believed to result from a direct stimulant effect of histamine on gastric parietal cells where, acting on H_2 receptors that are linked to adenylate cyclase, histamine activates a membrane enzyme pump (hydrogen-potassium-ATPase) that extrudes protons. The presence of vagal activity results in even a higher rate of hydrogen ion secretion. For example, after vagotomy in humans, the maximal secretory response to histamine decreases to about one-third of its usual value. Cholinergic blockade, as is produced by high doses of atropine, also decreases the gastric secretory response to histamine.

Allergic Reactions

During allergic reactions, histamine is only one of several chemical mediators released, and its relative importance in producing symptoms is greatly dependent on the species studied. Likewise, protection afforded by histamine receptor antagonists is highly variable and species dependent. In humans, histamine receptor antagonists (antihistamines) are effective in preventing edema formation and pruritus. Hypotension is attenuated but not totally blocked, whereas bronchoconstriction is often not prevented, emphasizing the predominant role of leukotrienes in this response in humans.

Responses to histamine-releasing drugs are better controlled by histamine receptor antagonists than are allergic responses (Moss and Rosow, 1983). Fewer chemical mediators are presumably involved in drug-induced responses, and histamine and possibly prostacyclin are relatively more important.

Clinical Uses

Histamine has been used to assess the ability of the gastric parietal cells to secrete hydrogen ions and to determine parietal cell mass. Anacidity or hyposecretion of hydrogen ions in response to histamine may reflect pernicious anemia, atrophic gastritis, or gastric carcinoma. Hypersecretion of hydrogen ions in response to histamine is present in Zollinger-Ellison syndrome and may be found in the presence of duodenal ulcer. Distressing side effects produced by histamine alone can be decreased by prior administration of an H_1-receptor antagonist that does not oppose histamine-induced gastric secretion. An alternative to histamine for gastric function tests is pentagastrin, a synthetic pentapeptide derivative of gastrin. Side effects from pentagastrin are minimal.

The fact that intradermal histamine causes a flare that is mediated by axon reflexes allows a test for the integrity of sensory nerves that may be of value in the diagnosis of certain neurologic conditions. The stimulant effect of histamine on chromaffin cells has been used in the past as a provocative test in patients with pheochromocytoma.

HISTAMINE-RECEPTOR ANTAGONISTS

Depending on what responses to histamine are inhibited, drugs are classified as H_1- or H_2-receptor antagonists (see Table 21-2). This classification is similar to terminology applied to drugs that act as antagonists at alpha or beta receptors. H_1- and H_2-receptor antagonists are presumed to act by occupying receptors on effector cell membranes, to the exclusion of agonist molecules, without themselves initiating a response. For histamine receptor antagonists, this is a competitive and reversible interaction. It is important to recognize that H_1- and H_2-receptor antagonists do not inhibit release of histamine but rather attach to receptors and prevent responses mediated by histamine.

H_1-Receptor Antagonists

H_1-receptor antagonists are characterized as first-generation and second-generation receptor antagonists (Fig. 21-2) (Simons, 2004; Simons and Simons, 1994). First-generation drugs tend to produce sedation, whereas second-generation drugs are relatively nonsedating (see Table 21-2). H_1-receptor antagonists are highly selective for H_1 receptors, having little effect on H_2 or H_3 receptors. First-generation H_1-receptor antagonists may also activate muscarinic cholinergic, 5-hydroxytryptamine (serotonin), or alpha-adrenergic receptors, whereas few of the second-generation antagonists have any of these properties. The selectivity of the second-generation antagonists for H_1 receptors decreases CNS toxicity. An increased understanding of the molecular pharmacologic features of these drugs has resulted in their reclassification as inverse agonists rather than as H_1-receptor antagonists (Simons, 2004). H_1-receptor antagonists act as inverse agonists that combine with and stabilize the inactive form of the H_1 receptor, shifting the equilibrium toward the inactive state.

Pharmacokinetics

H_1-receptor antagonists are well absorbed after oral administration, often reaching peak plasma concentrations within 2 hours (Table 21-3) (Simons, 2004; Simons and Simons, 1994). Protein binding ranges from 78% to 99%. Most H_1-receptor antagonists are metabolized by the hepatic microsomal mixed-function oxidase system. Plasma concentrations are relatively low after single oral doses, which indicates first-pass hepatic extraction. Values for the elimination half-times of these drugs are variable. For example, the elimination half-time of chlorpheniramine is >24 hours and that of acrivastine is about 2 hours (see Table 21-3) (Simons, 2004; Simons and Simons, 1994). Acrivastine is excreted mostly unchanged in urine, as is cetirizine, the active carboxylic metabolite of hydroxyzine.

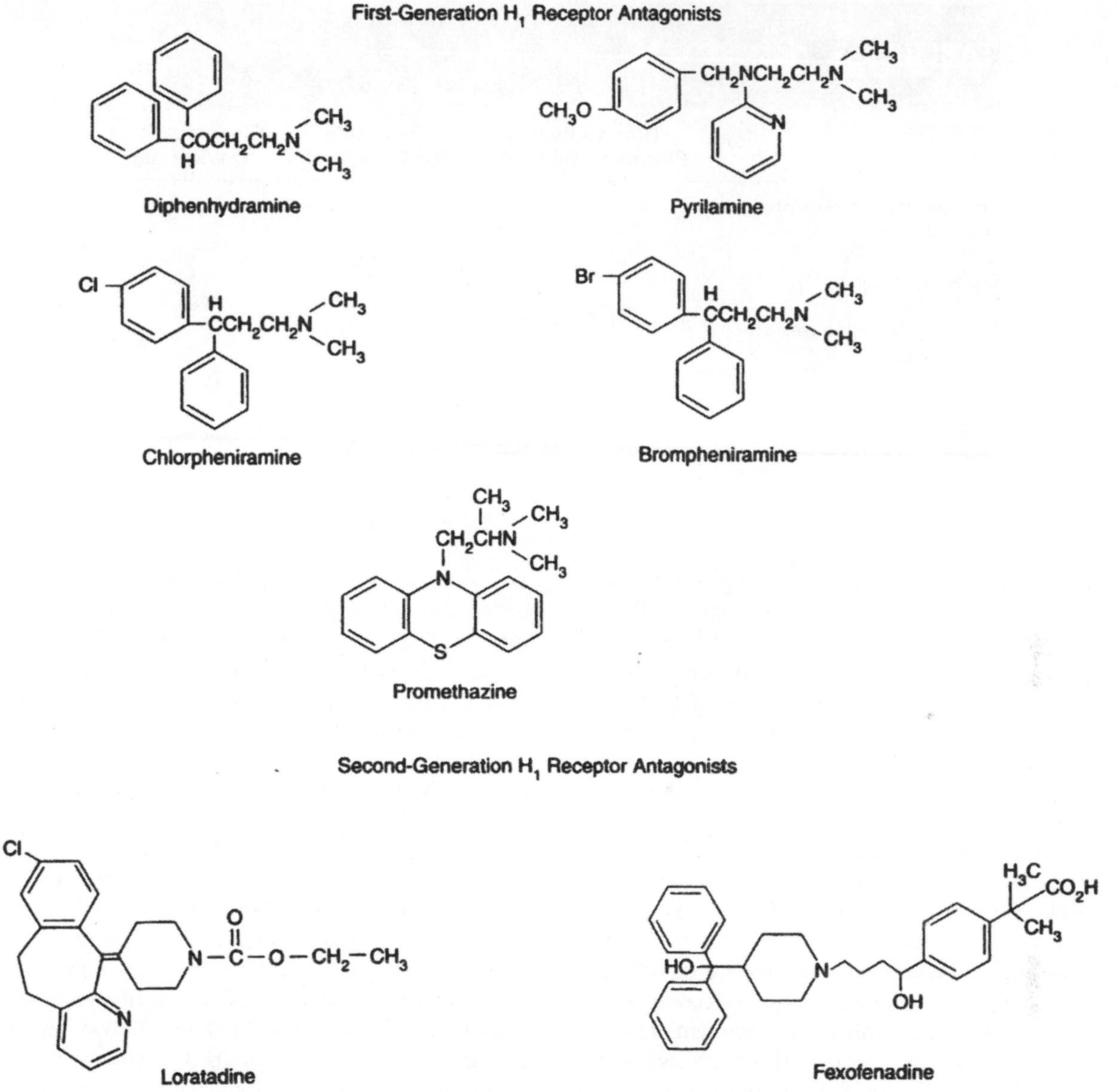

Figure 21-2. First-generation and second-generation H_1-receptor antagonists.

Side Effects

First-generation H_1 antagonists often have adverse effects on the CNS, including somnolence, diminished alertness, slowed reaction time, and impairment of cognitive function. Anticholinergic effects such as dry mouth, blurred vision, urinary retention, and impotence may be noted. Tachycardia is common, and prolongation of the QTc interval on the electrocardiogram (ECG), heart block, and cardiac dysrhythmias have occurred. First-generation H_1-receptor antagonists are still prescribed because they are effective and inexpensive. Administration of these drugs at bedtime is sometimes recommended because drug-related somnolence is of no concern during the night. Indeed, H_1-receptor antagonists may be sold as nonprescription sleeping aids.

Second-generation H_1 antagonists are unlikely to produce CNS side effects such as somnolence unless the recommended doses are exceeded. Enhancement of the effects of diazepam or alcohol are unlikely by second-generation drugs. Fexofenadine, a metabolite of terfenadine, does not prolong the QTc interval on the ECG, even in large doses. Patients with hepatic dysfunction, cardiac disorders associated with prolongation of the QTc interval, or metabolic disorders such as hypokalemia or hypomagnesemia may be especially prone to adverse cardiovascular effects of H_1 receptor antagonists. Most second-generation H_1-receptor antagonists are not removed by hemodialysis.

Antihistamine intoxication is similar to anticholinergic poisoning and may be associated with seizures and cardiac conduction abnormalities resembling tricyclic

TABLE 21-3.
PHARMACOKINETICS OF H_1 RECEPTOR ANTAGONISTS

	Time to Peak Plasma Level (hrs)	Elimination Half-Time (hrs)	Clearance Rate (ml/kg/min)
First-generation receptor antagonists			
Chlorpheniramine	2.8	27.9	1.8
Diphenhydramine	1.7	9.2	23.3
Hydroxyzine	2.1	20.0	98
Second-generation receptor antagonists			
Loratadine	1.0	11.0	202
Acrivastine	0.85–1.4	1.4–2.1	4.56
Azelastine	5.3	22	8.5

Source: Data from Simons FE, Simons KJ. The pharmacology and use of H1-receptor antagonist drugs. *N Engl J Med* 1994;330:1663–1670.

antidepressant overdose. Older nonsedating antihistamine drugs (terfenadine, astemizole) were associated with prolongation of the QTc interval and atypical (torsades de pointes) ventricular tachycardia both after overdose and after coadministration of macrolide antibiotics, or other drugs that interfere with their elimination. These drugs were removed from the market in 1999.

Clinical Uses

H_1 receptor antagonists are among the most widely used of all medications (Simons, 2004). H_1 receptor antagonists prevent and relieve the symptoms of allergic rhinoconjunctivitis (sneezing, nasal and ocular itching, rhinorrhea, tearing, and conjunctival erythema) but they are less effective for the nasal congestion characteristic of a delayed allergic reaction. In contrast to their role in the treatment of allergic rhinitis, H_1-receptor antagonists provide little benefit in the treatment of upper respiratory tract infections and are of no benefit in the management of otitis media. Depending on the H_1-receptor antagonist selected and its dose, pretreatment may provide some protection against bronchospasm induced by various stimuli (histamine, exercise, cold dry air). Earlier concerns about drying of secretions in patients with asthma have not been substantiated. In patients with chronic urticaria, H_1-receptor antagonists relieve pruritus and decrease the number, size, and duration of urticarial lesions. In some patients with refractory urticaria, concurrent treatment with an H_2-receptor antagonist (cimetidine, ranitidine) may enhance relief of pruritus. In addition to a direct effect on H_2 receptors, which account for 10% to 15% of all histamine receptors on the vasculature, this effect may be due in part to the ability of some H_2-receptor antagonists to inhibit the metabolism of H_1-receptor antagonists by the hepatic cytochrome P-450 system, leading to an increased plasma and tissue concentration of H_1-receptor antagonists. The second-generation H_1-receptor antagonists (cetirizine, fexofenadine, loratadine, desloratadine, azelastine) are supplanting first-generation drugs (diphenhydramine, chlorpheniramine, cyproheptadine) in the treatment of allergic rhinoconjunctivitis and chronic urticaria (Simons and Simons, 1994). Their greater cost can be justified because of a more favorable risk-benefit ratio, and because they are less toxic to the CNS. For example, effects of first generation H_1-receptor antagonists last beyond the sedative effects resulting in delayed reaction times.

Diphenhydramine is prescribed as a sedative, an antipruritic, and as an antiemetic. When administered alone, it modestly stimulates ventilation by augmenting the interaction of hypoxic and hypercarbic ventilatory drives. When diphenhydramine is administered in combination with systemic or neuraxial opioids to control nausea and pruritus, there is the conceptual risk of additive depression of ventilation. However, diphenhydramine counteracts opioid-induced decreases in the slope of the ventilatory response to carbon dioxide and does not exacerbate the opioid-induced depression of the hypoxic ventilatory response during moderate hypercarbia (Babenco et al., 1998).

The rich distribution of histamine receptors in the myocardium and coronary vasculature predisposes the heart to cardioregulatory changes during massive histamine release that characterizes type 1 immune-mediated hypersensitivity (anaphylactic) reactions. Use of antihistamines in the acute treatment of anaphylactic reactions is directed at blocking further histamine-mediated vasodilation and resulting homodynamic instability, as well as decreasing respiratory and other systemic complications. As such, the administration of H_1-receptor antagonists plus the administration of epinephrine is indicated in the treatment of acute anaphylaxis. H_1-receptor antagonists are also useful in the ancillary treatment of pruritus, urticaria, and angioedema. These drugs may also be administered prophylactically for anaphylactoid reactions to radiocontrast dyes. Second-generation H_1 receptor antagonists such as terfenadine, fexofenadine, and astemizole have low water solubility, and, unlike first-generation drugs, are not available for parenteral use. The addition of H_2 receptor antagonists to H_1 receptor antagonists in the treatment of anaphylaxis speeds the resolution of symptoms. Concerns of possible attenuation of H_2-mediated increases in inotropy and chronotropy, thereby limiting potential cardioexcitatory compensatory mechanisms, does not seem to be significant clinically (Nault et al., 2002). Dimenhydrinate is a H_1 receptor antagonist that is the theoclate salt of diphenhydramine.

Dimenhydrinate has been used to treat motion sickness as well as postoperative nausea and vomiting. It is speculated that the efficacy of dimenhydrinate in motion sickness and inner ear diseases may be due to inhibition of the integrative functioning of the vestibular nuclei by decreasing vestibular and visual input. Manipulation of the extraocular muscles as in strabismus surgery may trigger an "oculo-emetic" reflex similar to the well-described oculocardiac reflex. If the afferent arc of this reflex is also dependent on the integrity of the vestibular nuclei apparatus, then dimenhydrinate may attenuate or block this reflex and decrease the incidence of postoperative nausea and vomiting. Administration of dimenhydrinate, 20 mg IV, to adults decreases vomiting after outpatient surgery (Bidwai et al., 1989). In children, dimenhydrinate, 0.5 mg/kg IV, significantly decreases the incidence of vomiting after strabismus surgery and is not associated with prolonged sedation (Vener et al., 1996). Compared with serotonin antagonists, dimenhydrinate is an inexpensive antiemetic.

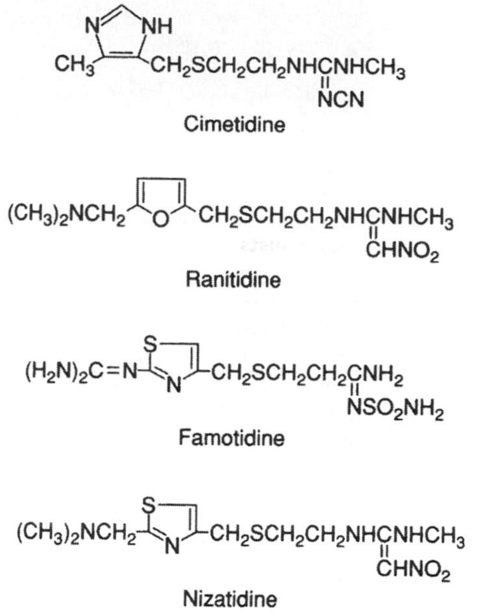

Figure 21-3. H_2-receptor antagonists.

H_2-Receptor Antagonists

Cimetidine, ranitidine, famotidine, and nizatidine are H_2-receptor antagonists that produce selective and reversible inhibition of H_2-receptor-mediated secretion of acidic gastric fluid (Fig. 21-3) (Feldman and Burton, 1990). The relationship between gastric hypersecretion of fluid containing high concentrations of hydrogen ions and peptic ulcer disease emphasizes the potential value of a drug that selectively blocks this response. Despite the presence of H_2 receptors throughout the body, inhibition of histamine binding to the receptors on gastric parietal cells is the major beneficial effect of H_2 receptor antagonists.

Mechanism of Action

The histamine receptors on the basolateral membranes of acid-secreting gastric parietal cells are of the H_2 type and thus are not blocked by conventional H_1 antagonists. The occupation of H_2 receptors by histamine released from mast cells and possibly other cells activates adenylate cyclase, increasing the intracellular concentrations of cAMP. The increased concentrations of cAMP activates the proton pump of gastric parietal cells (an enzyme designated as hydrogen-potassium-ATPase) to secrete hydrogen ions against a large concentration gradient in exchange for potassium ions (Feldman and Burton, 1990). H_2 receptor antagonists competitively and selectively inhibit the binding of histamine to H_2 receptors, thereby decreasing the intracellular concentrations of cAMP and the subsequent secretion of hydrogen ions by the parietal cells.

The relative potencies of the four H_2 receptor antagonists for inhibition of secretion of gastric hydrogen ions varies from 20- to 50-fold, with cimetidine as the least potent and famotidine the most potent (Table 21-4) (Feldman and Burton, 1990). The duration of inhibition ranges from approximately 6 hours for cimetidine to 10 hours for ranitidine, famotidine, and nizatidine. None of the four H_2-receptor antagonists have produced any consistent effects on lower esophageal sphincter function or the rate of gastric emptying. Discontinuation of chronic H_2-receptor antagonist therapy is followed by rebound hypersecretion of gastric acid.

Pharmacokinetics

The absorption of cimetidine, ranitidine, and famotidine is rapid after oral administration. Because of extensive first-pass hepatic metabolism, however, the bioavailability of these drugs is approximately 50% (see Table 21-4) (Feldman and Burton, 1990). Nizatidine does not undergo significant hepatic first-pass metabolism, and its bioavailability after oral administration approaches 100%. The average time to peak plasma concentrations of the four H_2-receptor antagonists ranges from 1 to 3 hours after oral administration. Because the volume of distribution for all four drugs exceeds the body's total body water content, some binding (13% to 35%) to proteins must occur (see Table 21-4) (Feldman and Burton, 1990).

Cimetidine is widely distributed in most organs but not fat. Approximately 70% of the total body content of

TABLE 21-4.
PHARMACOKINETICS OF H_2 RECEPTOR ANTAGONISTS

	Cimetidine	Ranitidine	Famotidine	Nizatidine
Potency	1	4–10	20–50	4–10
EC_{50} (μg/mL)*	250–500	60–165	10–13	154–180
Bioavailability (%)	60	50	43	98
Time to peak plasma concentration (hrs)	1–2	1–3	1.0–3.5	1–3
Volume of distribution (liters/kg)	0.8–1.2	1.2–1.9	1.1–1.4	1.2–1.6
Plasma protein binding (%)	13–26	15	16	26–35
Cerebrospinal fluid: plasma	0.18	0.06–0.17	0.05–0.09	Unknown
Clearance (mL/min)	450–650	568–709	417–483	667–850
Hepatic clearance (%)				
Oral	60	73	50–80	22
Intravenous	25–40	30	25–30	25
Renal clearance (%)				
Oral	40	27	25–30	57–65
Intravenous	50–80	50	65–80	75
Elimination half-time (hrs)	1.5–2.3	1.6–2.4	2.5–4	1.1–1.6
Decrease dose in presence of renal dysfunction	Yes	Yes	Yes	Yes
Hepatic dysfunction	No	No	No	No
Interfere with drug metabolism by cytochrome P-450 enzymes	Yes	Minimal	No	No

*EC_{50} denotes the plasma concentration of the drug necessary to inhibit the pentagastrin-stimulated secretion of hydrogen ions by 50%.
Source: Data from Feldman M, Burton ME. Histamine-2-receptor antagonists. *N Engl J Med* 1990;323:1672–1680.

cimetidine is found in skeletal muscles. The volume of distribution is not altered by renal disease but is increased by severe hepatic disease and can be altered by changes in systemic blood pressure and cardiac output. All four drugs are present in breast milk and can cross the placenta and blood-brain barrier. The presence of cimetidine in cerebrospinal fluid is increased in patients with severe hepatic disease. The dose of cimetidine may need to be decreased to avoid mental confusion in patients with severe liver disease. The volume of distribution of cimetidine is also decreased about 40% in elderly patients, presumably reflecting the decrease in skeletal muscle mass associated with aging.

Although there is considerable variation in the clearance and elimination half-times of H_2-receptor antagonists, their plasma elimination half-times range from 1.5 to 4 hours (see Table 21-4) (Feldman and Burton, 1990). The elimination of all four drugs occurs by a combination of hepatic metabolism, glomerular filtration, and renal tubular secretion. Hepatic metabolism is the principal mechanism for clearance from the plasma of oral doses of cimetidine, ranitidine, and famotidine, and renal excretion is the principal pathway for clearance from the plasma of an oral dose of nizatidine. The liver may metabolize 25% to 40% of an IV dose of nizatidine. Only nizatidine appears to have an active metabolite (*N*-2-monodesmethyl-nizatidine), possessing about 60% of the activity of the parent drug. Hepatic metabolism of cimetidine occurs primarily by conversion of its side-chain to a thioether or sulfoxide, and these inactive products appear in the urine as 5-hydroxymethyl and/or sulfoxide metabolites. The renal clearance of all four H_2-receptor antagonists is typically two to three times greater than creatinine clearance, reflecting extensive renal tubular secretion. Renal failure increases the elimination half-time of all four drugs, with the greatest effect on nizatidine and famotidine. Decreases in the doses of all four drugs are recommended for patients with renal dysfunction. Doses of H_2-receptor antagonists may also need to be decreased in patients with acute burns. Only 10% to 20% of total body cimetidine or ranitidine is cleared by hemodialysis.

Hepatic dysfunction does not seem to significantly alter the pharmacokinetics of H_2-receptor antagonists. Increasing age must be considered when determining the dose of H_2-receptor antagonists. For example, cimetidine clearance decreases 75% between the ages of 20 years and 70 years (Feldman and Burton, 1990). There is also a 40% decrease in the volume of distribution of cimetidine in elderly patients. The elimination half-time of ranitidine and famotidine may be increased up to twofold in elderly patients.

Clinical Uses

H_2 receptor antagonists are most commonly administered for the treatment of duodenal ulcer disease associated with hypersecretion of gastric hydrogen ions. In the preoperative period, H_2-receptor antagonists have been administered as chemoprophylaxis to increase the pH of gastric fluid before induction of anesthesia (Coombs et al., 1979; Stoelting, 1978; Weber and Hirschman, 1979). For this reason, H_2 antagonists have been advocated as useful drugs in the preoperative medication to decrease the risk of acid pneumonitis if inhalation of acidic gastric fluid occurs in the perioperative period. One approach is to administer cimetidine, 300 mg orally (3 to 4 mg/kg), 1.5 to 2.0 hours before the induction of anesthesia, with or without a similar dose the preceding evening (Stoelting, 1978). Famotidine given the evening before and the morning of surgery or on the morning of surgery was equally effective in decreasing gastric fluid pH in outpatients and inpatients, and there was no difference between famotidine doses of 20 mg or 40 mg (Fig. 21-4) (Talke and Solanki, 1993). The ability of H_2-receptor antagonists to decrease gastric fluid volume is unpredictable. Furthermore, H_2-receptor antagonists, in contrast to antacids, have no influence on the pH of the gastric fluid that is already present in the stomach. Cimetidine crosses the placenta but does not adversely affect the fetus when administered before cesarean section (Hodgkinson et al., 1983; Johnston et al., 1983).

Preoperative preparation of patients with allergic histories or patients undergoing procedures associated with an increased likelihood of allergic reactions (radiographic contrast dye administration) may include prophylactic oral administration of an H_1-receptor antagonist (diphenhydramine, 0.5 to 1.0 mg/kg) and an H_2 receptor antagonist (cimetidine, 4 mg/kg) every 6 hours in the 12 to 24 hours preceding the possible triggering event. A corticosteroid administered at least 24 hours earlier is commonly added to this regimen. Dramatic reversals of life-threatening allergic reactions after the IV administration of cimetidine may reflect the cumulative effect of prior epinephrine administration in the presence of a prolonged circulation time (DeSoto and Turk, 1989; Kelly and Prielipp, 1990). In fact, such treatment could exacerbate bronchospasm due to sudden unmasking of unopposed histamine effects of H_1 receptors on bronchial smooth muscle. The risk of further hypotension is also a consideration with IV administration of cimetidine. Furthermore, H_2 receptor activity could have desirable effects during allergic reactions including increased myocardial contractility and coronary artery vasodilation.

Drug-induced histamine release that may follow the rapid IV administration of certain drugs (morphine, atracurium, mivacurium, protamine) is not prevented by pretreatment with an H_1-receptor antagonist in combination with an H_2-receptor antagonist (Moss et al., 1981).

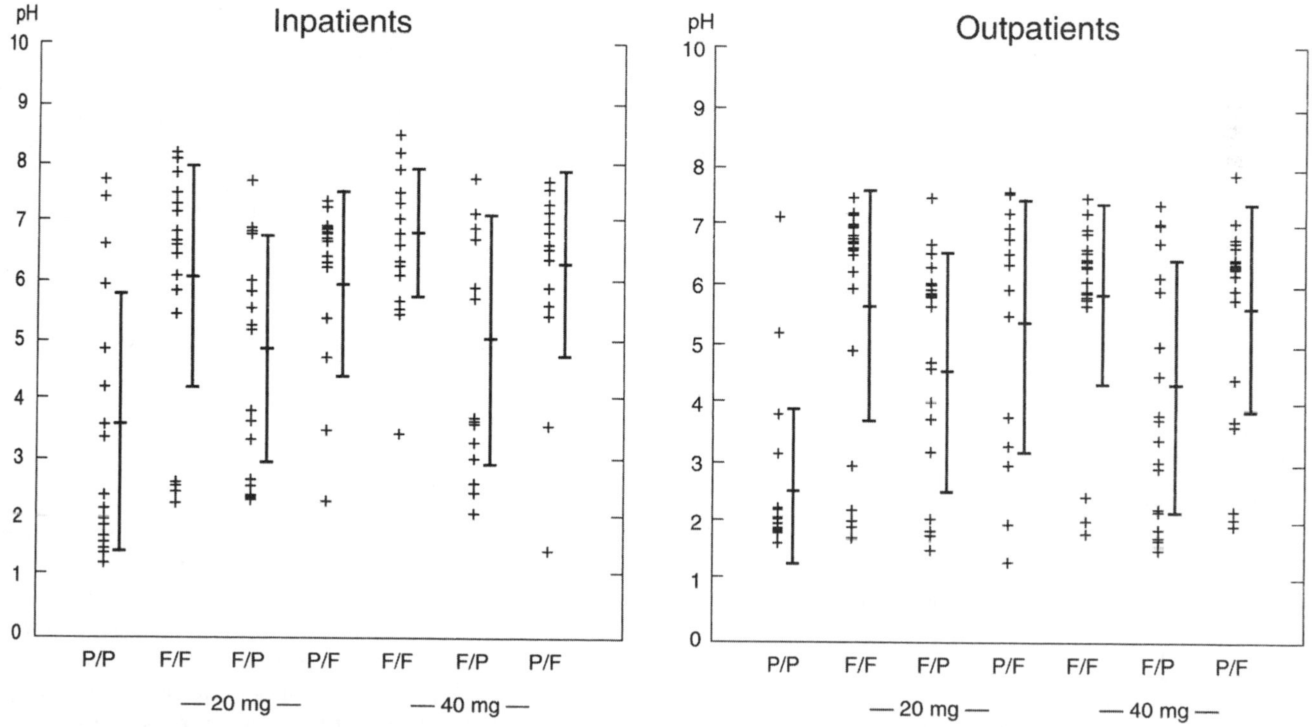

Figure 21-4. Gastric fluid pH values in inpatients and outpatients displayed as individual data points and the mean ± SD for each group. (F, famotidine 20 mg or 40 mg; P, placebo; groups, night before surgery/morning of surgery.) (From Talke PO, Solanki DR. Dose-response study of oral famotidine for reduction of gastric acidity and volume in outpatients and inpatients. *Anesth Analg* 1993;77:1143–1148; with permission.)

The magnitude of the systemic blood pressure decrease that occurs in response to drug-induced histamine release is less, confirming that prior occupation of histamine receptors with a specific antagonist drug attenuates the cardiovascular effects of subsequently released histamine (Philbin, 1981). Pretreatment with an H_1-receptor antagonist (diphenhydramine) or H_2-receptor antagonist (cimetidine) alone is not effective in preventing the cardiovascular effects of histamine that is released in response to drug administration, emphasizing the role of both H_1 and H_2 receptors in these responses. In fact, drug-induced histamine release may be exaggerated in patients pretreated with only H_2-receptor antagonists (see the section on H_3 Receptors).

Side Effects

The frequency of severe side effects is low with all four H_2-receptor antagonists (Table 21-5). The risk for experiencing adverse side effects during treatment with an H_2-receptor antagonist is increased by the presence of multiple medical illnesses, hepatic or renal dysfunction, and advanced age. The most common adverse side effects are diarrhea, headache, fatigue, and skeletal muscle pain. Side effects that occur with a prevalence of $<1\%$ include mental confusion, dizziness, somnolence, gynecomastia, galactorrhea, thrombocytopenia, increased plasma levels of liver enzymes, drug fever, bradycardia, tachycardia, and cardiac dysrhythmias. Cardiac reactions are most likely related to blockade of cardiac H_2 receptors. Mental confusion in patients being treated with cimetidine may be more likely in the presence of hepatic or renal dysfunction. Changes in mental status usually occur in the elderly and tend to be associated with high doses of cimetidine administered IV, often to patients in an intensive care unit. Delayed awakening from anesthesia has been attributed to lingering CNS effects of cimetidine (Viegas et al., 1982). Most patients have an improvement in mental status 24 to 48 hours after discontinuing cimetidine. Ranitidine and famotidine also cross the blood-brain barrier and have been anecdotally reported to produce mental confusion. Mental confusion has rarely been observed in ambulatory patients being treated chronically with H_2 receptor antagonists.

Cimetidine and, to a lesser extent, ranitidine increase the plasma concentrations of prolactin, which may result in galactorrhea in females and gynecomastia in males. Famotidine, and nizatidine do not appear to increase plasma prolactin levels. Cimetidine, but not the other H_2-receptor antagonists, inhibits the binding of dihydrotestosterone to androgen receptors. Indeed, impotence and loss of libido may occur in males receiving chronic high-dose treatment with cimetidine.

The adverse effects of H_2-receptor antagonists on hepatic function are typically reflected by reversible increases in the plasma level of aminotransaminase enzymes, mostly in patients receiving large IV doses of H_2-receptor antagonists. H_2-receptor antagonists probably do not markedly alter hepatic blood flow.

Cardiac dysrhythmias (sinus bradycardia, sinus arrest, sinus arrest with idioventricular escape rhythm, complete atrioventricular heart block) have been described after either oral or IV administration of H_2-receptor antagonists (Schoenwald et al., 1999). Most of the described dysrhythmias have occurred after chronic and uncomplicated administration. Rare descriptions of fatal cardiac arrest with the first IV administration of famotidine have been reported (Schonewald et al., 1999). Cardiac effects of H_2-receptor stimulation are similar to $beta_1$ stimulation mediated by cyclic AMP. This would explain why blockade of H_2 receptors might evoke bradycardia. Furthermore, blockade of H_2 receptors could increase H_1 receptor effects including negative dromotropic effects. Bradycardia and hypotension are generally associated with rapid IV administration of these drugs, most often to critically ill or elderly patients (Iberti et al., 1986). The mechanism for hypotension appears to be peripheral vasodilation. A prudent approach is to administer these drugs over 15 to 30 minutes when IV administration is needed.

Prolonged H_2-receptor blockade and associated gastric achlorhydria may weaken the gastric barrier to bacteria and predispose to systemic infections (Cristiano and Paradisi, 1982). Likewise, pulmonary infections from inhaled secretions may be more likely if the acid-killing effect on bacteria in the stomach is altered. Nevertheless, if acid suppression increases the risk of pneumonia, that risk is small and usually amenable to therapy (Gregor, 2004). Sustained increases of gastric fluid pH may lead to an overgrowth of other organisms such as *Candida albicans*. This may account for the occasional case of *Candida* peritonitis observed after peptic ulcer perforation in patients treated with cimetidine. Prolonged increases of gastric fluid pH also result in the production of nitroso-compounds because of an increase in nitrate-reducing bacteria (Milton-Thompson et al., 1982). Nitroso-derivatives are potent mutagens in vitro, but there is no

TABLE 21-5.
SIDE EFFECTS OF H_2-RECEPTOR ANTAGONISTS

Interaction with cerebral H_2 receptors (headache, somnolence, confusion)
Interaction with cardiac H_2 receptors (bradycardia, hypotension, heart block)
Hyperprolactinemia
Acute pancreatitis
Increased hepatic transaminases
Alcohol dehydrogenase dehydration
Thrombocytopenia
Agranulocytosis
Interstitial nephritis
Interfere with drug metabolism by cytochrome P-450

evidence that this occurs in vivo in association with chronic cimetidine therapy.

Cimetidine, but not ranitidine or famotidine, has been shown to augment cell-mediated immunity through its blockade of H_2 receptors on T lymphocytes (Feldman and Burton, 1990).

Drug Interactions

Numerous drug interactions have been described between H_2-receptor antagonists, most commonly cimetidine, and other drugs (Table 21-6) (Feldman and Burton, 1990). Drug interactions generally occur when a new drug is either started or discontinued. In this regard, measurement of plasma drug concentrations or laboratory measurements of an effect (prothrombin time) may be useful.

The principal type of drug interaction reported with cimetidine is impairment of the hepatic metabolism of another drug because of the binding of cimetidine to the heme portion of the cytochrome P-450 oxidase system. Cimetidine retards metabolism of drugs such as propranolol and diazepam that normally undergo high hepatic extraction (Donovan et al., 1981; Klotz and Reimann, 1980). Slowed metabolism and prolonged elimination half-time with associated exaggerated pharmacologic effects of propranolol and diazepam have been documented with only 24 hours of treatment with cimetidine (Figs. 21-5 and 21-6) (Feely et al., 1981; Klotz and Reimann, 1980). In contrast, benzodiazepines, such as oxazepam and lorazepam, that are eliminated almost entirely by glucuronidation are not altered by cimetidine-induced effects on P-450 enzyme activity. Cimetidine may slow metabolism of lidocaine and thus increase the possibility of systemic toxicity (Feely et al., 1982). In contrast, plasma concentrations of bupivacaine after epidural anesthesia for cesarean section are not influenced by a single dose of cimetidine administered before

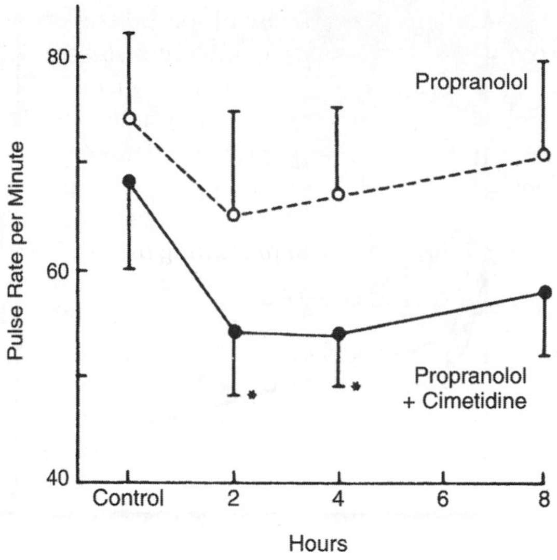

Figure 21-5. The effect of propranolol on resting heart rate is accentuated by the concomitant administration of cimetidine. (Mean ± SD; n = 5; *$P < .05$.) (From Feely J, Wilkinson GR, Wood AJJ. Reduction of liver blood flow and propranolol metabolism by cimetidine. *N Engl J Med* 1981;304:692–696; with permission.)

TABLE 21-6.
DRUG INTERACTIONS WITH CIMETIDINE

Drug	Effect of Cimetidine on Plasma Concentration	Clearance of Drug (% Decrease)	Mechanism
Ketoconazole	Decreased	No change	Decreased absorption due to increased gastric fluid pH that slows dissolution
Warfarin*	Increased	23–36	Decreased hydroxylation of dextrorotatory isomer
Theophylline*	Increased	12–34	Decreased methylation
Phenytoin*	Increased	21–24	Decreased hydroxylation (?)
Propranolol	Increased	20–27	Decreased hydroxylation
Nifedipine	Increased	38	Unknown
Lidocaine	Increased	14–30	Decreased *N*-dealkylation
Quinidine	Increased	25–37	Decreased 3-hydroxylation (?)
Imipramine	Increased	40	Decreased *N*-demethylation
Desipramine	Increased	36	Decreased hydroxyltion in rapid metabolizers
Triazolam	Increased	27	Decreased hydroxylation
Meperidine	Increased	22	Decreased oxidation
Procainamide*	Increased	28	Competition for renal tubular secretion

*Lesser drug interactions also occur with ranitidine.
Source: Data from Feldman M, Burton ME. Histamine-2-receptor antagonists. *N Engl J Med* 1990;323:1672–1680.

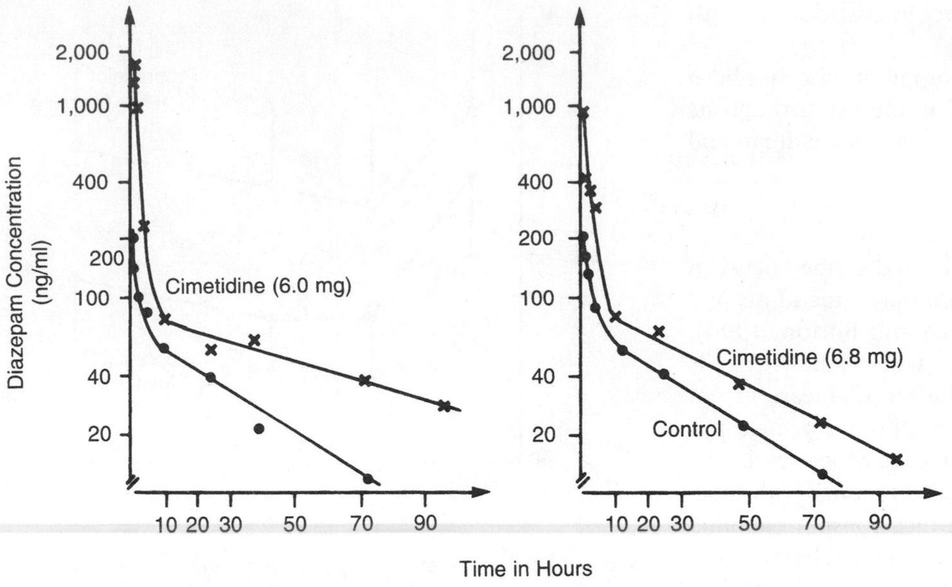

Figure 21-6. The rate of decline in the plasma concentration of diazepam, 0.1 mg/kg IV, is slowed by the prior administration of cimetidine, 6.0 to 6.8 mg/kg. (From Klotz U, Reimann I. Delayed clearance of diazepam due to cimetidine. *N Engl J Med* 1980;302: 1012–1014; redrawn with permission.)

induction of anesthesia (Fig. 21-7) (Flynn et al., 1989; Kuhnert et al., 1987). This is important because bupivacaine has a narrow therapeutic range due to its cardiotoxicity, and cimetidine is likely to be used for aspiration pneumonitis prophylaxis before cesarean section performed under epidural anesthesia with this local anesthetic. A previous suggestion that the duration of action of succinylcholine is significantly prolonged in patients receiving cimetidine has not been confirmed (Woodworth et al., 1989). Indeed, plasma cholinesterase activity is not altered by cimetidine (Kambam and Franks, 1988). Ranitidine, although more potent than cimetidine, binds less avidly to the cytochrome P-450 enzyme system and has less potential than cimetidine to alter the oxidative metabolism of other drugs. Famotidine and nizatidine do not bind notably to the cytochrome P-450 enzyme system and thus have very limited potential for inhibiting the metabolism of other drugs.

H_2-receptor antagonists compete with cationic compounds for renal tubular secretion. Because of the competition of cimetidine and ranitidine with creatinine for renal tubular secretion, serum creatinine levels are increased about 15%. Cimetidine and ranitidine, but not famotidine, impair renal tubular secretion of procainamide and theophylline. Impairment of renal theophylline clearance with cimetidine is probably negligible compared with impairment of the hepatic metabolism of theophylline.

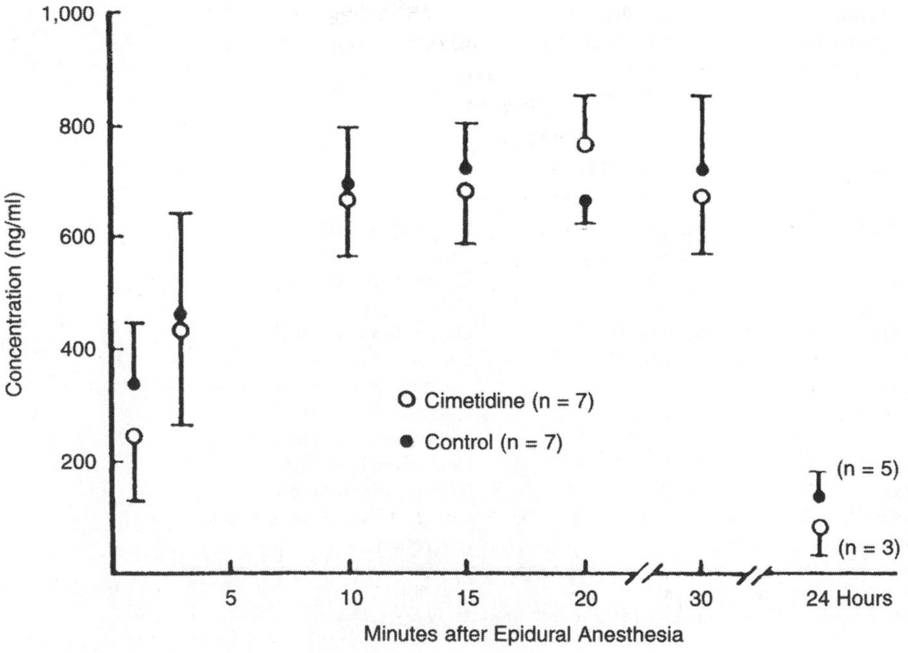

Figure 21-7. Maternal plasma levels of bupivacaine after epidural anesthesia. (From Kuhnert BR, Zuspan KJ, Kuhnert PM, et al. Lack of influence of cimetidine on bupivacaine levels during parturition. *Anesth Analg* 1987;66:986–990; with permission.)

All four H_2-receptor antagonists have the potential to alter the absorption of some drugs by increasing the gastric fluid pH. Cimetidine has been reported to enhance the absorption of ethanol from the stomach as a result of inhibition of gastric alcohol dehydrogenase.

In addition to drug interactions produced by H_2-receptor antagonists, several drugs alter the disposition of the antagonists. Magnesium and aluminum hydroxide antacids decrease by 30% to 40% respectively the bioavailability of cimetidine, ranitidine, and famotidine. Despite this impaired absorption, therapeutic blood levels of the H_2 antagonist can still be achieved, and rigorous separation of dosage schedules during combined drug therapy is probably unnecessary (Russell et al., 1984). Hepatic metabolism of cimetidine may be enhanced if phenobarbital is administered concurrently.

PROTON PUMP INHIBITORS

Proton pump inhibitors (omeprazole, esomeprazole, lansoprazole, pantoprazole, rabeprazole) are the most effective antisecretory drugs available for controlling gastric acid acidity and volume (Table 21-7). The final step in gastric acid secretion is the membrane enzyme proton pump (hydrogen-potassium-ATPase) that moves hydrogen ions across the gastric parietal cell membranes in exchange for potassium ions. The secretion of hydrochloric acid by gastric parietal cells ultimately depends on the function of the proton (hydrogen ion) pump. Proton pump inhibitors are the drugs of choice in the treatment of moderate to severe gastroesophageal reflux disease, hypersecretory disorders, and peptic ulcer disease.

Omeprazole

Omeprazole is a substituted benzimidazole that acts as a prodrug that becomes a proton pump inhibitor (Fig. 21-8) (Klinkenberg-Knol et al., 1995; Maton, 1991). As a weak base, omeprazole is concentrated in the secretory canaliculi of the gastric parietal cells. It is at this site that omeprazole is

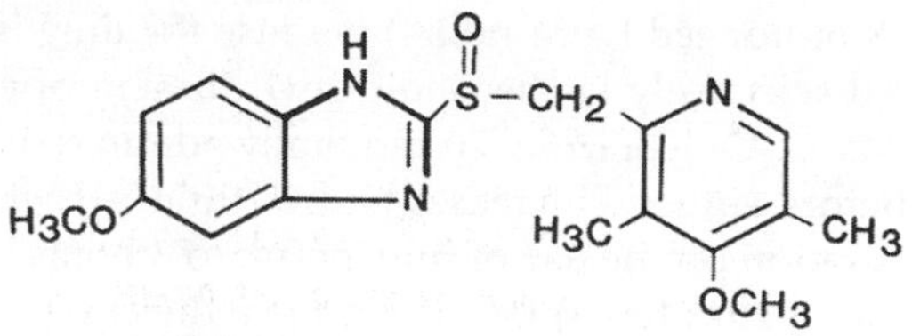

Figure 21-8. Omeprazole.

pronated to its active form, which inhibits the enzyme pump. The initial dose of omeprazole will only inhibit those proton pumps present and working on the luminal surface. As pumps are generated and inserted into the luminal surfaces, further doses are required to inhibit these new pumps. Therefore, omeprazole takes several days to exert its maximal inhibitory effect on gastric acid secretion. Daily administration results in about 66% inhibition of gastric acid secretion after 5 days. Likewise, discontinuation of omeprazole is not followed immediately by return of gastric acid secretion (Sachs, 1997).

Omeprazole provides prolonged inhibition of gastric acid secretion, regardless of the stimulus, and it inhibits daytime and nocturnal acid secretion and meal-stimulated acid secretion to a significantly greater degree than do the H_2-receptor antagonists. This drug heals duodenal and possibly gastric ulcers more rapidly than do the H_2-receptor antagonists. In patients with bleeding peptic ulcers and signs of recent bleeding, treatment with omeprazole decreases the rate of bleeding and the need for surgery (Khuroo et al., 1997). Omeprazole is superior to H_2-receptor antagonists for the treatment of reflux esophagitis and is the best pharmacologic treatment of Zollinger-Ellison syndrome (Maton, 1991).

Preoperative Medication

As preoperative medication, omeprazole effectively increases gastric fluid pH and decreases gastric fluid volume (Nishina et al., 1994). In this regard, the onset of the gastric antisecretory effect of omeprazole after a single oral dose (20 mg) occurs within 2 to 6 hours. The duration of

TABLE 21-7.
PHARMACOKINETICS OF PROTON PUMP INHIBITORS

	Bioavailability	Time to Peak Plasma Concentration (hrs)	Protein Binding	Elimination Half-Time (hrs)	Hepatic Metabolism	Interfere with Cytochrome P-450
Omeprazole	60%	2–4	>90%	0.5–1.0	Yes	Minimal
Esomeprazole	60%	2–4	>90%	0.5–1.0	Yes	Minimal
Lasoprazole	85%	1.5–3.0	97%	1.5	Yes	Minimal
Pantoprazole	77%	2.5	98%	1.9	Yes	No
Rabeprazole	85%	2.9–3.8	96%	1	Yes	No

action is prolonged (>24 hours) because the drug is concentrated selectively in the acidic environment of gastric parietal cells. Omeprazole, 20 mg orally administered the night before surgery, increases gastric fluid pH whereas administration on the day of surgery (up to 3 hours before induction of anesthesia) fails to improve the environment of the gastric fluid (Nishina et al., 1994). This suggests that omeprazole should be administered >3 hours before anticipated induction of anesthesia to ensure adequate chemoprophylaxis.

Side Effects

Omeprazole crosses the blood-brain barrier and may cause headache, agitation, and confusion. Gastrointestinal side effects include abdominal pain, flatulence, nausea, and vomiting. Small bowel bacterial overgrowth may occur owing to acid suppression. The loss of the inhibitory effect of gastric acid results in increased plasma concentrations of gastrin. There is no need to decrease the dose of proton pump inhibitors in the presence of renal or hepatic dysfunction.

Esomeprazole

Esomeprazole is the levorotatory isomer of omeprazole. This levo isomer is metabolized differently in the liver resulting in greater plasma concentrations of the drug compared with the racemic drug, omeprazole.

Pantoprazole

Pantoprazole is a potent and fast-acting proton pump inhibitor. Administration of IV pantoprazole (40 mg) and ranitidine (50 mg) 1 hour before the induction of anesthesia is effective in decreasing gastric fluid volume and pH (Memis et al., 2003).

CROMOLYN

Cromolyn inhibits antigen-induced release of histamine and other autocoids, including leukotrienes, from pulmonary mast cells as well as from mast cells at other sites during antibody-mediated allergic responses (Fig. 21-9). Cromolyn does not prevent the interaction between cell-bound immunoglobulin E and specific antigens but rather suppresses the secretory response elicited by the reaction. Release of histamine from basophils is not altered by cromolyn. Cromolyn does not relax bronchial or vascular smooth muscle.

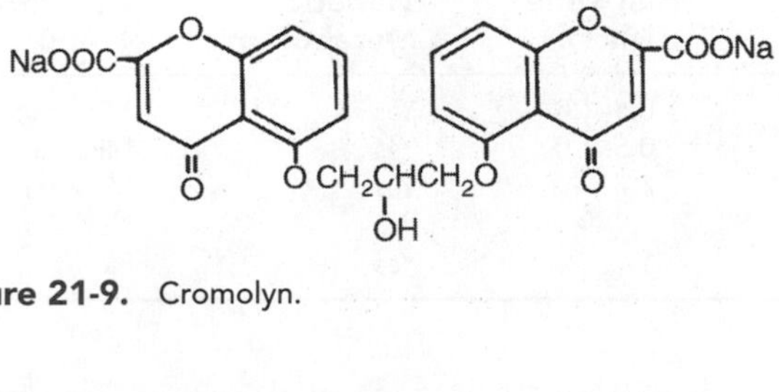

Figure 21-9. Cromolyn.

Cromolyn acts as an inhibitor of inflammation apparently by preventing the release of chemical mediators from mast cells. Antigen activation of mast cells results in intracellular influx of chloride ions through chloride channels, which in turn maintains activation of calcium channels, allowing intracellular entry of calcium ions leading to degranulation. Oral absorption of cromolyn is poor, and the drug is therefore administered by inhalation. After inhalation, 8% to 10% of the drug enters the systemic circulation, where its elimination half-time is about 80 minutes. Cromolyn is not metabolized, being excreted unchanged in the urine and bile in approximately equal amounts.

Side effects of cromolyn are rare and usually insignificant. Infrequent but serious side effects, probably attributable to allergic reactions to the drug, include laryngeal edema, angioedema, urticaria, and anaphylaxis.

The principal use of cromolyn is in the prophylactic treatment of bronchial asthma. Given before an antigenic challenge, cromolyn inhibits bronchoconstriction and prevents signs of an acute asthmatic attack. This protective effect can last for several hours. Evidence that cromolyn has no role in the treatment of established bronchoconstriction is the observation that its administration as early as 1 minute after an antigen challenge is ineffective in altering the response.

REFERENCES

Babenco HD, Blouin RT, Conard PF, et al. Diphenhydramine increases ventilatory drive during alfentanil infusion. *Anesthesiology* 1998; 89:642–647.

Bidwai AW, Meuleman T, Thatte WP. Prevention of postoperative nausea with dimenhydrinate (Dramamine) and droperidol (Inapsine). *Anesth Analg* 1989;68:S25.

Coombs DW, Hooper D, Colton T. Acid aspiration prophylaxis by use of preoperative oral administration of cimetidine. *Anesthesiology* 1979;51:352–356.

Cristiano P, Paradisi F. Can cimetidine facilitate infections by the oral route? *Lancet* 1982;2:45.

DeSoto H, Turk P. Cimetidine in anaphylactic shock refractory to standard therapy. *Anesth Analg* 1989;69:264–265.

Donovan M, Hagerty A, Pael L, et al. Cimetidine and bioavailability of propranolol. *Lancet* 1981;1:164.

Feely J, Wilkinson GR, McAllister CB, Wood AJ. Increased toxicity and reduced clearance of lidocaine by cimetidine. *Ann Intern Med* 1982;96:592–594.

Feely J, Wilkinson GR, Wood AJJ. Reduction of liver blood flow and propranolol metabolism by cimetidine. *N Engl J Med* 1981;304: 692–695.

Feldman M, Burton ME. Histamine-2-receptor antagonists. *N Engl J Med* 1990;323:1672–1680.

Flynn RJ, Moore J, Collier PS, et al. Does pretreatment with cimetidine and ranitidine affect the disposition of bupivacaine? *Br J Anaesth* 1989;62:87–91.

Gregor JC. Acid suppression and pneumonia. A clinical indication for rational prescribing. *JAMA* 2004;292:2012–2013.

Hodgkinson R, Glassenberg R, Joyce TH, et al. Comparison of cimetidine (Tagamet) with antacid for safety and effectiveness in reducing gastric acidity before elective cesarean section. *Anesthesiology* 1983;59:86–90.

Hosking MP, Lennon RL, Gronert GA. Combined H_1 and H_2 receptor blockade attenuates the cardiovascular effects of high-dose atracurium for rapid sequence endotracheal intubation. *Anesth Analg* 1988;67:1089–1092.

Iberti TJ, Paluch TA, Helmer L, et al. The hemodynamic effects of intravenous cimetidine in intensive care unit patients: a double-blind, prospective study. *Anesthesiology* 1986;64:87–89.

Johnston JR, Moore J, McCaughey W, et al. Use of cimetidine as an oral antacid in obstetric anesthesia. *Anesth Analg* 1983;62:720–726.

Kambam JR, Franks JJ. Cimetidine does not affect plasma cholinesterase activity. *Anesth Analg* 1988;67:69–70.

Kelly JS, Prielipp RC. Is cimetidine indicated in the treatment of acute anaphylactic shock? *Anesth Analg* 1990;71:104–105.

Khuroo MS, Yattoo GN, Javid G, et al. A comparison of omeprazole and placebo for bleeding peptic ulcer. *N Engl J Med* 1997;336: 1054–1058.

Klinkenberg-Knol EC, Festen HPM, Meuwissen SGM. Pharmacological management of gastroesophageal reflux disease. *Drug* 1995;49: 695–710.

Klotz U, Reimann I. Delayed clearance of diazepam due to cimetidine. *N Engl J Med* 1980;302:1012–1014.

Kuhnert BR, Zuspan KJ, Kuhnert PM, et al. Lack of influence of cimetidine on bupivacaine levels during parturition. *Anesth Analg* 1987; 66:986–990.

Maton PN. Omeprazole. *N Engl J Med* 1991;324:965–975.

Maze M. Clinical implications of membrane receptor function in anesthesia. *Anesthesiology* 1981;55:160–171.

Memis D, Turan A, Karamanlioglu B, et al. The effect of intravenous pantoprazole and ranitidine for improving preoperative gastric fluid properties in adults undergoing elective surgery. *Anesth Analg* 2003;97:1360–1363.

Milton-Thompson GJ, Lightfoot NF, Ahmet Z, et al. Intragastric acidity, bacteria, nitrite, and N-nitroso compounds before, during and after cimetidine treatment. *Lancet* 1982;1:1091–1095.

Moss J, Rosow CE. Histamine release by narcotics and muscle relaxants in humans. *Anesthesiology* 1983;59:330–339.

Moss J, Rosow CE, Savarese JJ, et al. Role of histamine in the hypotensive action of *d*-tubocurarine in humans. *Anesthesiology* 1981;55:19–25.

Nault MA, Milne B, Parlow JL. Effects of the selective H_1 and H_2 histamine receptor antagonists loratadine and ranitidine on autonomic control of the heart. *Anesthesiology* 2002;96:336–341.

Nishina K, Mikawa K, Maekawa N, et al. Omeprazole reduces preoperative gastric fluid acidity and volume in children. *Can J Anaesth* 1994;41:925–929.

Philbin DM, Moss J, Akins CW, et al. The use of H_1 and H_2 histamine blockers with high dose morphine anesthesia: a double-blind study. *Anesthesiology* 1981;55:292–296.

Rosow CE, Basta SJ, Savarese JJ, et al. Correlation of cardiovascular effects with increases in plasma histamine. *Anesthesiology* 1980;53:S270.

Russell WL, Lopez LM, Normann SA, et al. Effect of antacids on predicted steady-state cimetidine concentrations. *Dig Dis Sci* 1984; 29:385–389.

Sachs G. Proton pump inhibitors and acid related diseases. *Pharmacotherapy* 1997;17:22–37.

Simons FE, Simons KJ. The pharmacology and use of H_1-receptor antagonist drugs. *N Engl J Med* 1994;330:1663–1670.

Simons FE. Advances in H_1-antihistamines. *N Engl J Med* 2004;351: 2203–2217.

Stoelting RK. Gastric fluid pH in patients receiving cimetidine. *Anesth Analg* 1978;57:675–677.

Talke PO, Solanki DR. Dose-response study of oral famotidine for reduction of gastric acidity and volume in outpatients and inpatients. *Anesth Analg* 1993;77:1143–1148.

Vener DF, Carr AS, Sikich N, et al. Dimenhydrinate decreases vomiting after strabismus surgery in children. *Anesth Analg* 1996;82: 728–731.

Viegas OJ, Stoops CA, Ravindran RS. Reversal of cimetidine-induced postoperative somnolence. *Anesthesiol Rev* 1982;9:30–31.

Weber L, Hirshman CA. Cimetidine for prophylaxis of aspiration pneumonitis: comparison of intramuscular and oral dose schedules. *Anesth Analg* 1979;58:426–427.

Woodworth GE, Sears DH, Grove TM, et al. The effect of cimetidine and ranitidine on the duration of action of succinylcholine. *Anesth Analg* 1989;68:295–297.

Serotonin, Plasma Kinins, and Renin

22

SEROTONIN

Serotonin [5-hydroxytryptamine (5-HT)] is a widely distributed endogenous vasoactive substance (autacoid) that evokes complex changes in the cardiovascular system (cerebral, coronary, and pulmonary vascular vasoconstriction) and functions as an important neurotransmitter in emesis and pain transmission (Hindle, 1994). About 90% of the body's stores of serotonin are present in the enterochromaffin cells of the gastrointestinal tract, with the remainder present in the central nervous system (CNS) and platelets. The function of serotonin in platelets is not known but may reflect an inactive storage site for serotonin that escapes from cells, particularly in the gastrointestinal tract. Indeed, the potentiating effect of serotonin on platelet aggregation is small, and platelets depleted of serotonin function normally.

Mechanism of Action

Receptors specific for serotonin are confirmed by the effectiveness of serotonin antagonist drugs. Serotonin receptors are classified as 5-HT_1 through 5-HT_4 (Gyermek, 1995; Hindle, 1994). Genetic studies have shown that DNA sequences of 5-HT_{1A} receptors match part of the DNA sequences of the beta-adrenergic receptor, which may account for the fact that these receptors share some common agonists and antagonists. Cerebral vasoconstriction is mediated by 5-HT_1 receptors, whereas vasoconstriction in the coronary arteries and pulmonary vessels seems to be mediated by 5-HT_2 receptors. Treatment of migraine headache with the 5-HT_1-receptor agonist sumatriptan is based on the presumption that vasodilation causes a shunting of blood away from capillary beds, leading to cerebral hypoxia.

The discovery and use of 5-HT_3-receptor antagonists have revolutionized the management of drug-induced nausea and vomiting. The 5-HT_3 receptors are unique among the 5-HT receptors. In contrast to the other 5-HT receptors, which are linked functionally to G protein-mediated neural, muscular, or glandular mechanisms, the 5-HT_3 receptors are directly coupled to fast sodium and potassium ion channels (Gyermek, 1995). These channels transmit and modulate neural responses in the peripheral and CNS. The 5-HT_3 receptors are presumed to have roles in peripheral neuronal pathways that are involved in visceral pain mechanisms and central neuronal pathways that are involved in emesis, appetite, addiction, pain, and anxiety.

The gastrokinetic effects of metoclopramide may reflect stimulation of 5-HT_4 receptors (see Chapter 26). Serotonin may exert its analgesic effects by causing the release of gamma-aminobutyric acid, which inhibits nociceptive impulses. Physiologically, serotonin acts as a cerebral stimulant ("waking neurotransmitter"), and it is likely that all 5-HT receptors are involved in the etiology of anxiety.

Synthesis and Metabolism

Serotonin is synthesized in cells from the amino acid precursor tryptophan, which is derived from dietary sources (Fig. 22-1). An estimated 1% of dietary tryptophan is converted to serotonin. The conversion of tryptophan to serotonin is mediated by tryptophan hydroxylase, an enzyme that is present in the enterochromaffin cells of the small intestine but not present in platelets. Carcinoid tumors that synthesize serotonin may divert so much tryptophan from protein synthesis to produce serotonin that hypoalbuminemia and pellagra result.

Metabolism of serotonin occurs mainly by oxidative deamination mechanisms (monoamine oxidase enzymes) and is similar to the breakdown of other amines, such as catecholamines. The principal metabolite of serotonin is 5-hydroxyindoleacetic acid, and its urinary excretion is used clinically as an indicator of the level of endogenous metabolism of serotonin (see Fig. 22-1). Patients with

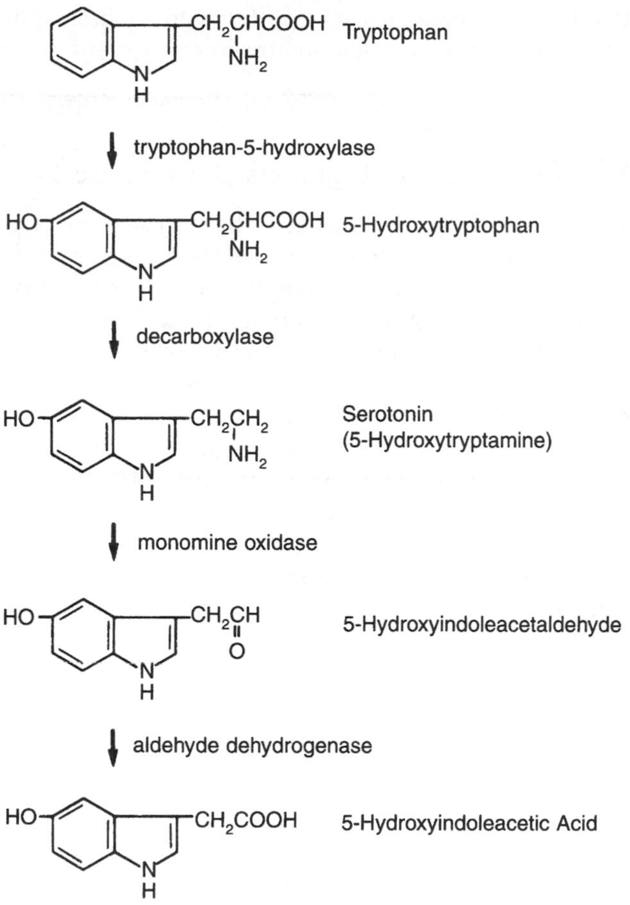

Figure 22-1. Synthesis and metabolism of serotonin.

carcinoid tumors or those who have recently ingested certain foods, such as bananas, manifest an increased urinary excretion of this metabolite.

Serotonin Agonists

Clinically useful serotonin agonists include sumatriptan, fenfluramine, and dexfenfluramine.

Sumatriptan

Sumatriptan is a 5-HT_1-receptor agonist that is useful in the treatment of migraine headache and cluster headache. Doppler ultrasound studies in patients with migraine headache show reversal of middle cerebral artery vasodilation and relief of headache after administration of sumatriptan (Friberg et al., 1991). Subcutaneous injection of sumatriptan, 6 mg, has been reported to be effective in the treatment of postdural puncture headache (Carp et al., 1994). The elimination half-time of sumatriptan is about 2 hours, and it is likely that a repeated injection will be necessary in many patients. In view of the cerebral vasoconstrictive properties of sumatriptan, it is possible that it could have similar effects on the coronary circulation. For this reason, it may not be prudent to administer this drug to patients with known coronary artery disease.

Fenfluramine and Dexfenfluramine

Fenfluramine is a sympathomimetic amine that is structurally similar to amphetamine and epinephrine. Dexfenfluramine is the chemical isomer of fenfluramine. The CNS effects of the drug combination of fenfluramine and dexfenfluramine ("Fen/Phen") tend to cancel each other so that most patients primarily experience weight loss without mood alteration. The satiated feeling and appetite suppression associated with fenfluramine and dexfenfluramine reflect the ability of these drugs to stimulate the release of serotonin from nerve endings and platelets and to inhibit the cellular uptake and metabolism of serotonin. It is the relatively select ability of these drugs to activate serotonergic pathways in the brain that is presumed to be responsible for the anorectic action. Side effects (especially valvular heart disease) attributed to treatment with fenfluramine or dexfenfluramine led to voluntary withdrawal of these drugs by the manufacturer in September 1997.

Serotonin Antagonists

Tricyclic antidepressants inhibit the uptake of serotonin back into tryptaminergic nerve endings similar to the effect exerted on catecholamines. Lysergic acid derivatives are specific competitive antagonists at receptors normally responsive to serotonin. Other drugs that act as serotonin antagonists include H_1-receptor blockers of the ethylenediamine type; phenothiazines, especially chlorpromazine; and beta-haloalkylamines such as phenoxybenzamine.

Methysergide

Methysergide is a congener of lysergic acid but lacks significant CNS effects (Fig. 22-2). It inhibits peripheral vasoconstriction evoked by serotonin. Clinical uses include prophylaxis against development of migraine and other vascular headaches. This drug is not effective after a headache has developed. Methysergide is useful in treating malabsorption and diarrhea in patients with carcinoid syndrome. It may also alleviate similar symptoms in patients with postgastrectomy dumping syndrome. Methysergide depresses prolactin secretion, perhaps by dopamine-like actions. An infrequent but serious side effect of treatment

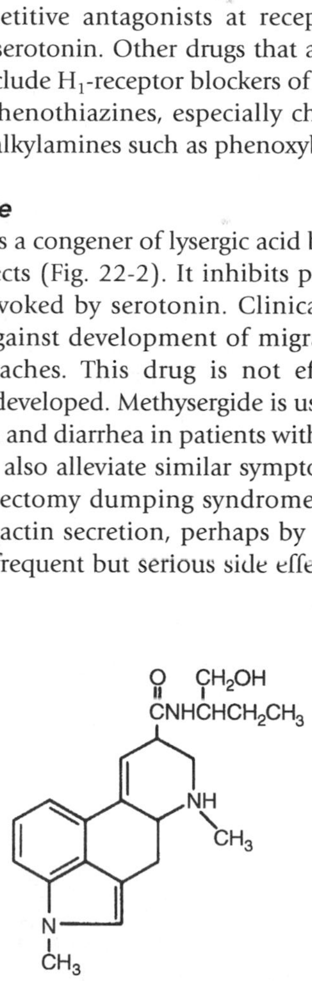

Figure 22-2. Methysergide.

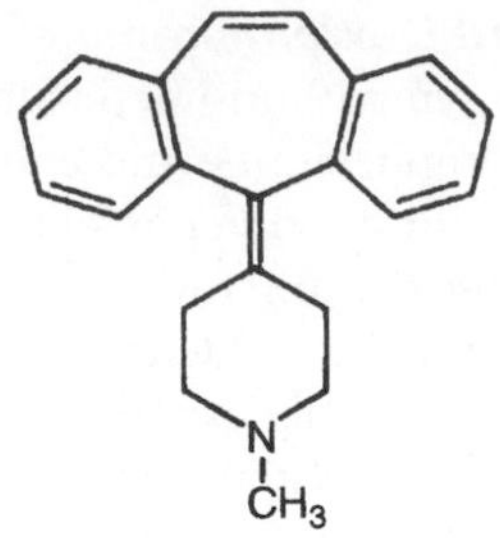

Figure 22-3. Cyproheptadine.

with methysergide is an inflammatory reaction that may manifest as retroperitoneal, pleuropulmonary, coronary, or endocardial fibrosis.

Cyproheptadine

Cyproheptadine resembles the structure of H_1-receptor antagonists and is able to block receptors for both histamine and serotonin (Fig. 22-3). In addition, this drug possesses weak anticholinergic activity and mild CNS depressant properties. The actions of cyproheptadine as an antagonist drug during allergic reactions are not relevant, because serotonin is not involved in human allergic responses. Uses of this drug are principally for the treatment of intestinal hypermotility associated with carcinoid syndrome and in the postgastrectomy dumping syndrome. Side effects of cyproheptadine include sedation and dry mouth, as a reflection of H_1-receptor antagonism. Increased growth in children has been observed, perhaps as a result of altered secretion of insulin and growth hormone.

Ketanserin

Ketanserin is a quinazoline derivative that selectively antagonizes the effects of serotonin at peripheral 5-HT_2 receptors, thus attenuating serotonin-induced vasoconstriction, bronchoconstriction, and platelet aggregation (Fig. 22-4) (Marwood and Stokes, 1984). This drug, however, is nonspecific in that it has substantial affinity for alpha$_1$ receptors, H_1 receptors, and, to a lesser degree, dopamine receptors. In addition, ketanserin appears to inhibit sympathetic nervous system outflow from the CNS.

Uses of ketanserin include treatment of patients with carcinoid syndrome (5 to 30 mg infused over 3 minutes) and management of systemic hypertension. It is possible that the antihypertensive effects of this drug reflect alpha$_1$ antagonist effects unrelated to actions of serotonin receptors.

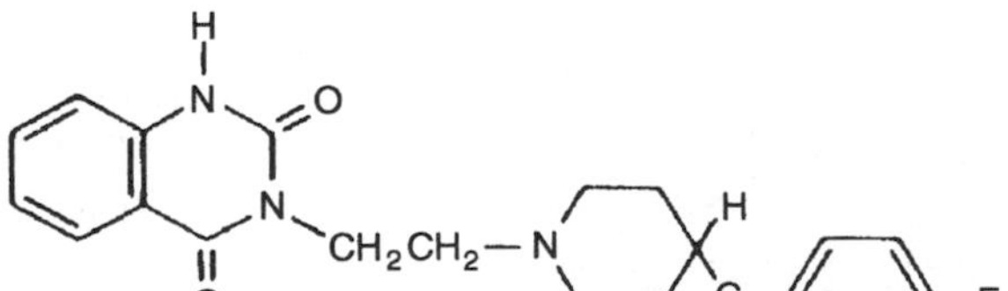

Figure 22-4. Ketanserin.

5-HT_3-Receptor Antagonists (Antiemetics)

The 5-HT_3 receptors are excitatory ligand-gated nonselective cation channels belonging to the gamma aminobutryic acid (GABA) receptor superfamily. The ion channel is a pentamer consisting of five monomers that form a central pore that can be readily permeated by small cations. The 5-HT_3 receptors are extensively distributed on enteric neurones in the gastrointestinal tract and brain. Serotonin is released from the enterochromaffin cells of the small intestine, stimulates the vagal afferents through 5-HT_3 receptors and initiaties the vomiting reflex. Antagonism of the effect of serotonin at 5-HT_3 receptors results in an antiemetic effect. 5-HT_3 receptor antagonists are selective for these receptors with almost no significant binding with other 5-HT receptor subtypes.

Clinical Uses

The 5-HT_3-receptor antagonists represent (ondansetron, tropisetron, graniestron, dolasetron) a significant advance in the prophylaxis and treatment of nausea and vomiting because they are highly specific and evoke minimal side effects. Drugs that act as competitive antagonists at 5-HT_3 receptors are useful antiemetics in the prophylaxis and treatment of chemotherapy and radiation therapy-induced nausea and vomiting (Fig. 22-5) (Gyermek, 1995, Wolf, 2000). Furthermore, these 5-HT_3-receptor antagonists have proved to be highly effective in the prevention and treatment of postoperative nausea and vomiting. It is estimated that one-third of patients undergoing surgery and anesthesia will experience postoperative nausea and vomiting that may be more distressing to the patient than the operative pain. These serotonin-receptor antagonists are not effective in the treatment of motion-induced nausea and vomiting and treatment of postoperative nausea and vomiting owing to vestibular stimulation because the vestibular apparatus and the nucleus of the tractus solitarius are rich in muscarinic and histamine receptors.

The convenience of use is the reason for the popularity of 5-HT_3-receptor antagonists and corticosteroids (used most often in combination) for management of postoperative nausea and vomiting. Unlike prevention and treatment of chemotherapy-induced emesis that are guided by evidence-based consensus guidelines, recommendations regarding the timing of prophylactic antiemetic therapy (with the preanesthetic medication versus, near the conclusion of surgery) cannot be made on the basis of scientific data (Fauser et al., 1999). However, if patients experience breakthrough postoperative nausea and vomiting despite prophylaxis, they should be treated with an antiemetic

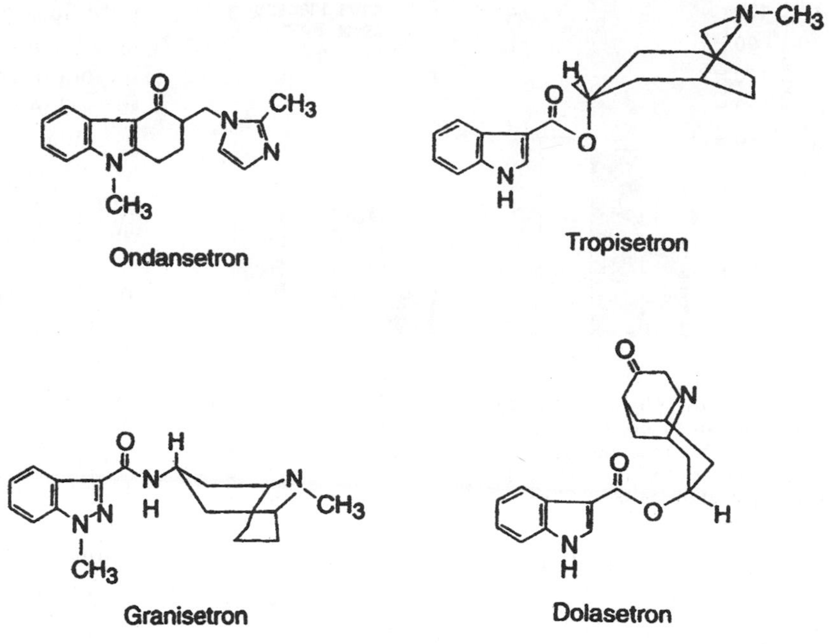

Figure 22-5. Structure of 5-HT_3 receptor antagonists (antiemetics) compared with serotonin.

from a different class than used for prophylaxis (Rose and Watcha, 1999).

Comparison with Other Antiemetics

Ondansetron (4 mg), dexamethasone (4 mg), and droperidol (1.25 mg) administered intravenously (IV) as prophylactic therapy before induction of general anesthesia are equally effective in decreasing the incidence of postoperative nausea and vomiting by about 26% (Apfel et al., 2004). The cost-benefit ratio does not support the use of 5-HT_3-receptor antagonists for routine antiememtic prophylaxis (White, 2004).

Pharmacokinetics

The 5-HT_3-receptor antagonists are readily absorbed after oral administration and readily cross the blood–brain barrier. Following IV administration, the maximum brain concentration is achieved within a few minutes. These antagonists are moderatly bound to protein (60% to 75%). Metabolism is by different subtypes of cytochrome P-450 enzymes and metabolites undergo principally renal excretion.

Ondansetron

Ondansetron is a carbazalone derivative that is structurally related to serotonin and possesses specific 5-HT_3 subtype receptor antagonist properties, without altering dopamine, histamine, adrenergic, or cholinergic receptor activity (Bodner and White, 1991). As a result, ondansetron is free of neurologic effects in contrast to droperidol and metoclopramide (Sprung et al., 2003). Ondansetron is effective when administered orally or IV and has an oral bioavailability of about 60% with therapeutic blood concentrations appearing 30 to 60 minutes after administration. Metabolism to inactive metabolites occurs predominantly in the liver and the elimination half-time is 3 to 4 hours.

The most commonly reported side effects from treatment with ondansetron are headache and diarrhea. Transient increases in the plasma concentrations of liver transaminase enzymes have been observed only in patients receiving chemotherapy and may be due to these drugs rather than ondansetron. Cardiac dysrhythmias and conduction disturbances (atrioventricular block) have been reported after the IV administration of ondansetron and metoclopramide (Baguley et al., 1997; Wolf, 2000). A severe episode of acute myocardial ischemia has been described following IV administration of ondansetron to a patient with no history of cardiac abnormalities (Bosek et al., 2000). Ondansetron and other 5-HT_3 receptor antagonists can cause slight prolongation of the QTc interval on the electrocardiogram (ECG) of treated patients but this has not created the same level of concern as that ascribed to droperidol.

It is estimated that for every 100 patients who receive ondansetron for the prevention of postoperative nausea and vomiting, 20 patients will not vomit who would have vomited without treatment ("number needed to treat"), and three of those 100 patients will develop a headache who would have not had this adverse effect without the drug ("number needed to harm") (Tramer et al., 1997). Sedation, hypotension, dysphoria, and extrapyramidal symptoms that may accompany administration of alternative antiemetic drugs (promethazine, droperidol, metoclopramide) do not accompany administration of ondansetron. Ondansetron, 4 to 8 mg IV (administered over 2 to 5 minutes immediately before the induction of anesthesia), is highly effective in decreasing the incidence of

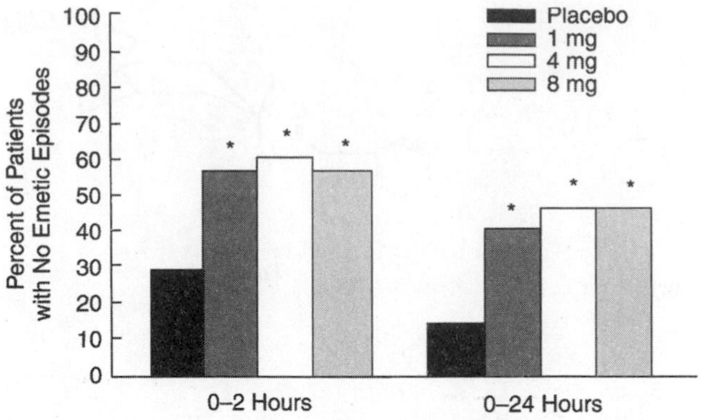

Figure 22-6. The percentage of patients in each study group having no emetic episodes during the initial period (0 to 2 hours) and during the follow-up period (0 to 24 hours). (**P* <.001 compared to placebo.) (From Scuderi P, Wetchler B, Sung YF, et al. Treatment of postoperative nausea and vomiting after outpatient surgery with the 5-HT_3 antagonist ondansetron. *Anesthesiology* 1993;78:15–20; with permission.)

postoperative nausea and vomiting in a susceptible patient population (ambulatory gynecologic surgery, middle ear surgery) (Honkavaara, 1996; McKenzie et al., 1993). Oral (0.15 mg/kg) or IV (0.05 to 0.15 mg/ kg) administration of ondansetron is effective in decreasing the incidence of postoperative vomiting in preadolescent children undergoing ambulatory surgery, including tonsillectomy and strabismus surgery (Furst and Rodarte, 1994; Rose et al., 1994, 1996; Watcha et al., 1995). In addition to prophylaxis, ondansetron, 1 to 8 mg IV (0.1 mg/kg up to 4 mg in children), is highly effective in the treatment of postoperative nausea and vomiting (Fig. 22-6) (Khalil et al., 1996; Scuderi et al., 1993).

Overall, it can be concluded that ondansetron, although highly effective in decreasing the incidence and intensity of postoperative nausea and vomiting, does not totally eliminate this complication. The most significant feature of ondansetron prophylaxis and treatment is the relative freedom from side effects as compared with previously used classes of antiemetic drugs. The cost of ondansetron is greater than that of other antiemetics such as the phenothiazines, antihistamines, and butyrophenones. There is some evidence that prophylactic droperidol (0.625 to 1.25 mg IV) and ondansetron are similarly effective in decreasing the incidence of postoperative nausea and vomiting in high-risk patients (Pan and Moore, 1996; Steinbrook et al., 1996; Sniadach and Alberts, 1997; Tang et al., 1998). Nevertheless, the remote risk of a prolonged QTc interval on the ECG of patients receiving droperidol (usually doses higher than those utilized for prophylaxis or treatment of nausea and vomiting) is a consideration when selecting droperidol based on its lower cost. Use of propofol for induction and maintenance of anesthesia may be as effective as ondansetron in preventing postoperative nausea and vomiting (Gan et al., 1996). The addition of ondansetron (4 mg IV) or dolasetron (12.5 mg IV) does not improve the antiemetic efficacy of droperidol (0.625 mg IV) and dexamethasone (4 mg IV) when they were used for routine prophylaxis in patients undergoing office-based surgical procedures (Tang, et al., 2003).

Ondansetron 8 mg IV is an effective treatment for pruritus associated with neuraxial morphine (Borgeat and Stirnermann, 1999). The intensity of pruritus linked with cholestatic liver disease is decreased by ondansetron.

Tropisetron

Tropisetron is an indoleacetic acid ester of tropine that possesses highly selective 5-HT_3-receptor-blocking effects. Compared with ondansetron, tropisetron has a longer elimination half-time (7.3 hours versus 3.5 hours). Overall, the beneficial effects and side effects of tropisetron resemble ondansetron (Scholz et al., 1998). This drug is effective in the treatment of symptoms related to carcinoid syndrome and may also possess gastrokinetic properties. As an antiemetic, tropisetron is effective in prevention of chemotherapy and radiotherapy-induced emesis and in the prevention of postoperative nausea and vomiting when administered (2 to 5 mg IV) before the induction of general anesthesia (Alon et al., 1996 Boogaerts et al., 2000). Rescue treatment using a single dose of tropisetron is often effective in decreasing further nausea and vomiting (Alon et al., 1998). Tropisetron did not prevent postoperative nausea and vomiting associated with epidural morphine whereas dexamethasone (5 mg IV) was effective (Wang et al., 2002).

Granisetron

Granisetron is a more selective 5-HT_3-receptor antagonist than ondansetron. Like ondansetron, granisetron is effective orally and IV. Doses as low as 0.02 to 0.04 mg/kg IV have been described as effective in prevention of chemotherapy-induced emesis and prevention of postoperative nausea and vomiting (Cieslak et al., 1996; Fujii et al., 1994; Wolf, 2000). Concomitant administration of dexamethasone significantly improved the acute antiemetic efficacy of granisetron (Fujii et al., 2000). Metabolism to inactive metabolites occurs in the liver with only about 10% of the drug excreted unchanged by the kidneys. The elimination half-time of granisetron (9 hours) is 2.5 times longer than that of ondansetron and thus may require less frequent dosing. For example, a single dose of granisetron may be effective for 24 hours. Side effects are mild and include headache, sedation, and diarrhea. The high cost of granisetron may limit its clinical application (Cieslak et al., 1996).

Dolasetron

Dolasetron is a highly potent and selective 5-HT_3-receptor antagonist that is effective in the prevention of chemotherapy-induced nausea and vomiting and postoperative nausea and vomiting following either oral or IV administration. After its administration, dolasetron is rapidly metabolized to hydrodolasetron, which is responsible for the antiemetic effect. Hydrodolasetron has an elimination half-time of approximately 8 hours and is approximately 100 times more potent as a serotonin antagonist than the parent compound.

A single IV dose of dolasetron, 1.8 mg, is equivalent to ondansetron, 32 mg IV, and granisetron, 3 mg IV, in preventing chemotherapy-induced nausea and vomiting. Established postoperative nausea and vomiting is effectively blunted by dolasetron, 12.5 mg IV (Diemunsch et al., 1997; Kovac et al., 1997). Oral dolasetron, 25 to 50 mg, is effective as prophylaxis for decreasing postoperative nausea and vomiting. Although serotonergic pathways are involved in the development of postoperative shivering, dolestron was not effective in preventing this complication (Piper et al., 2002). Side effects include headache, dizziness, and increased appetite. It is unclear if an increased heart rate attributed to dolestron is different from the incidence observed in placebo treated patients (Wolf, 2000).

PLASMA KININS

Plasma kinins are polypeptides that include kallidin and bradykinin. These two kinins are the result of enzyme-induced cleavage of kininogens that exist in the plasma as alpha$_2$ globulins. These alpha$_2$ globulin enzymes are collectively referred to as *kininogenases* and include kallikreins, trypsin, and plasmin.

Plasma kinins are the most potent known endogenous vasodilators. Furthermore, in low plasma concentrations, kinins (a) increase capillary permeability, (b) produce edema, and (c) evoke intense burning pain by acting on nerve endings. Plasma kinins are about ten times more potent than histamine in causing vasodilation. Injected IV, plasma kinins cause flushing in the blush area and dilation in renal, coronary, and cerebral arterioles. Vasodilation results in marked decreases in systolic and diastolic blood pressure. In contrast to their effects on arterioles, plasma kinins tend to constrict large veins, leading to increased venous return. Increased venous return combined with reflexively increased baroreceptor reflex activity due to diastolic hypotension results in increased cardiac output and heart rate. Increased capillary permeability produced by plasma kinins resembles that occurring in response to histamine and serotonin. Indeed, intradermal injections of plasma kinins produce a "wheal and flare" response. Plasma kinins may increase airway resistance in patients with reactive airway disease, such as bronchial asthma.

Mechanism of Action

Specific plasma kinin receptors are postulated, whereas some responses to kinins may be mediated by the production of prostaglandins. Certain of the direct effects on blood vessels may reflect the ability of kinins to evoke the release of histamine from mast cells.

Pharmacokinetics

The elimination half-time of plasma kinins is <15 s, with >90% metabolized during a single passage through the lungs. Other tissues are also capable of rapidly metabolizing plasma kinins. The enzyme responsible for this rapid metabolism is known as *converting enzyme* (peptidyl dipeptidase) and is identical to the enzyme necessary for the conversion of angiotensin I to angiotensin II.

Bradykinin

Bradykinin (so named because it produces slow contraction of the gastrointestinal tract) is formed from a high-molecular-weight kininogen by the action of the enzyme kallikrein. Typically, minimal amounts of bradykinin are present because plasma kallikrein circulates in an inactive form known as *prekallikrein*. Changes that activate prekallikrein and lead to the formation of bradykinin include alterations in pH or temperature and contact with negatively charged surfaces such as collagen when exposed by tissue damage. Indeed, many of the factors that activate prekallikrein are involved in factor XII-initiated coagulation and fibrinolysis.

Hereditary angioedema is associated with the absence of the C1 esterase inhibitor of the complement system, which is also an inhibitor of kallikrein. For this reason, it is speculated that episodes of edema that are characteristic of this disease may be in part due to excess formation of bradykinin. Other diseases that may be associated with excess formation of plasma kinins such as bradykinin include (a) septic shock, (b) allergic reactions, and (c) carcinoid syndrome. Conversely, inadequate amounts of bradykinin may be associated with essential hypertension. Indeed, accumulation of plasma kinins resulting from inhibition of the converting enzyme by captopril may contribute to the systemic blood pressure-lowering effects of this drug.

Aprotinin

Aprotinin is a naturally occurring serine protease inhibitor that decreases activation of plasminogen and the activity of plasmin. Decreased bleeding is thought to reflect inhibition of fibrinolysis, reduction of thrombin generation, and preservation of platelet function. The current opinion is that aprotinin inhibits bleeding mainly through plasmin inhibition. Antiinflammatory properties of aprotinin are reflected by decreases in interleukins and nitric oxide production with subsequent reductions in membrane injury associated with oxidant stress (Freedman et al., 2000) Aprotinin is classified as an antifibrinolytic, anticoagulant, platelet protective, and antiinflammatory drug. The enzymatic activity of aprotinin is generally expressed in kallikrein inactivator units (KIU), with 1 KIU defined as the amount of aprotinin that decreases the activity of 2 biologic kallikrein units by 50%. One mg of aprotinin is equivalent to 7,143 KIU. Effective inhibition of plasmin requires a plasma concentration of >50 KIU/mL (Levy et al., 1994). A 2,000,000-KIU dose is needed to achieve the higher plasma concentration necessary to inhibit kallikrein.

Side Effects

The epithelial cells of the proximal renal tubules have a great avidity for aprotinin, which accumulates in these cells during the first 12 to 24 hours to be later metabolized and eliminated during the next 4 to 5 days (Feindt et al., 1995). This accumulation in renal tubular cells can result in spilling of normally filtered proteins in to the urine (*tubular overloading*). Mild increases in serum creatinine concentrations may occur but are usually well tolerated (D'Ambra and Risk, 1990; Feindt et al., 1995). Although the use of high doses of aprotinin and hypothermia during cardiopulmonary bypass could theoretically lead to renal toxicity (renal vasoconstriction due to inhibition of kallikrein and prostaglandins), clinical experience has not shown untoward renal effects to occur in this setting. Nevertheless, since aprotinin may occasionally cause afferent renovasoconstriction, concomitant therapy with known afferent renovasoconstrictors such as radiocontrast dye or nonsteroidal antiinflammatory drugs is not recommended (Horl, 2000). As a protein derived from bovine lungs, aprotinin possesses antigenic properties in humans (Dietrich et al., 2001). Following administration of aprotinin, formation of antiaprotinin immunoglobulins (IgG and IgE) antibodies may occur. Anaphylactic and analphylactoid reactions may manifest even for patients receiving topical applications of aprotinin. The incidence of allergic reactions evoked by aprotinin is estimated to be 2.8%. Patients who receive aprotinin during an initial cardiac operation may develop antiaprotinin antibodies and thus be at risk for experiencing antigen-antibody dependent anaphylactic reactions. Pretesting for IgG and IgE levels is not a useful screening tool as results are nonspecific. Administration of a test dose of 10,000 KIU is recommended before IV administration of aprotonin.

The use of antifibrinolytic drugs introduces the theoretical concern of thrombotic events. Nevertheless, studies in cardiac surgical patients do not show an increased risk for graft thrombosis in the early postoperative period. Despite the potential risk for thrombosis, the incidence of stroke appears to be decreased in patients treated with aprotinin (Smith, 1996).

Pharmacokinetics

Plasma aprotinin concentrations decrease rapidly after IV administration because of redistribution to peripheral tissues (Levy et al., 1994). During the elimination phase, which is primarily renal, accumulation of aprotinin takes place in proximal tubular epithelial cells of the kidneys, where the drug may be gradually broken down over several days. Approximately 80% of an injected dose of aprotinin can be localized in the kidneys 4 hours after injection. Clearance of aprotinin is 35.5 mL per minute, and the volume of distribution at steady state is 26.5 liters (Levy et al., 1994). The elimination half-time of aprotinin after administration of a single IV dose is 7 to 10 hours. It is possible that the pharmacokinetics of this drug could be altered by anesthesia, intraoperative hemodynamic changes, and the effects of cardiopulmonary bypass, including hypothermia, hemodilution, nonpulsatile flow, and the exclusion of the heart and lungs from the circulation.

Clinical Uses

Therapeutic uses of aprotinin, including use in cases of acute pancreatitis, shock syndromes, and hyperfibrinolytic hemorrhage, are based on its ability to inhibit proteases such as trypsin, plasmin, and plasma and tissue kallikrein (see Chapter 36). Aprotinin is commonly used for the prevention and treatment of surgical hemorrhage.

Cardiac Surgery

Aprotinin can decrease perioperative blood loss and transfusion requirements by 40% to 80% in cardiac surgical patients undergoing cardiopulmonary bypass especially in patients treated with aspirin and those undergoing repeated cardiac surgery (Royston et al., 1987). The mechanism of this beneficial effect is incompletely understood but appears to reflect aprotinin's ability to inhibit plasmin as well as kallikrein, resulting in inhibition of fibrinolytic activity. A protective effect of aprotinin on platelet function may also occur. These mechanisms for the protective effect of aprotinin are consistent with the concept that an acquired platelet defect is most likely responsible when increased bleeding occurs after conclusion of cardiopulmonary bypass. Nevertheless, a consistent beneficial effect of aprotinin on bleeding time has not been demonstrated (Hardy and Desroches, 1992).

Aprotinin inhibits cardiopulmonary bypass related inflammatory responses in part by preventing transmigration of leukocytes through vascular endothelium Intraoperative and postoperative infusion of aprotinin has resulted in more successful weaning from intra-aortic balloon counterpulsation and has been shown to decrease troponin T release (Randomized trial, 2001). Aprotinin does not alter the incidence of graft occlusion or myocardial infarction following cardiopulmonary bypass.

The activated coagulation time (ACT) is prolonged in the presence of heparin plus aprotinin when celite is used as the surface activator. Prolongation of the ACT in the presence of heparin plus aprotinin does not occur when kaolin is used as the surface activator. It is therefore erroneous to conclude that the anticoagulant effect of aprotinin as determined by the celite-ACT is heparin-like, and the dose of heparin should not be altered in the presence of aprotinin. For cardiac surgery, a plasma aprotinin concentration of

TABLE 22-1.
INFUSION PROTOCOL DESIGNED TO MAINTAIN THE PLASMA APROTININ CONCENTRATION AT APPROXIMATELY 250 KIU/mL

	Infusion Rate
Induction to skin incision (0 to 30 mins)	52,000 KIU/min
Skin incision to 60 mins	26,000 KIU/min
60 mins to end of surgery	10,400 KIU/min
Add to prime of cardiopulmonary bypass circuit	500,000 KIU

KIU, kallikrein inhibitor units.
Source: Data from Levy JH, Bailey JM, Salmenpera M. Pharmacokinetics of aprotinin in preoperative cardiac surgical patients. *Anesthesiology* 1994;80:1013–1018.

250 KIU/mL (at least 200 KIU/mL needed to inhibit kallikrein) is recommended as a target to be achieved by the infusion protocol (Table 22-1) (Levy et al., 1994). In patients receiving aprotinin and heparin anticoagulation for cardiopulmonary bypass, celite ACT values should exceed 750 seconds and kaolin ACT should be more than 450 seconds (Hunt et al., 1992). The thromboelastograph trace is altered in the presence of aprotinin when celite and kaolin are used as activators but not when tissue factor is the activator (Avidan et al., 2001).

Total Hip Replacement

The use of high-dose aprotinin (2,000,000 KIU IV followed by 500,000 KIU per hour until the conclusion of surgery) during total hip replacement surgery or major lower extremity surgery for sepsis or malignant tumors results in decreases in total blood loss and the amount of blood transfused (Capdevila et al., 1998). The incidence of deep-vein thrombosis is not increased in aprotinin-treated patients.

RENIN

Renin is a proteolytic enzyme that is synthesized and stored by the juxtaglomerular cells present in the walls of renal afferent arterioles as they enter the glomeruli. The most important stimulus for the release of renin is a decrease in renal perfusion pressure associated with hemorrhage, dehydration, chronic sodium ion depletion, or renal artery stenosis. The secretion of renin is also increased by sympathetic nervous system stimulation caused by activation of beta-adrenergic receptors.

Formation of Angiotensins

Release of renin initiates the formation of active hormones known as *angiotensins*. The first step is the reaction of renin

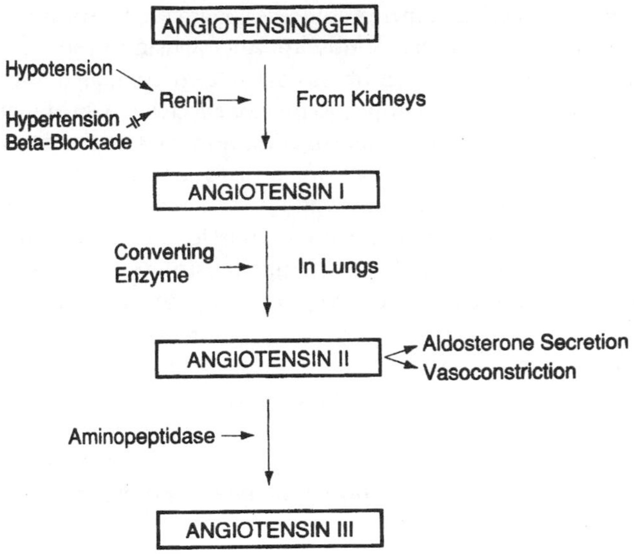

Figure 22-7. Schematic diagram of the renin-angiotensin-aldosterone system.

with circulating angiotensinogen, a substrate synthesized in the liver, to form a decapeptide prohormone known as *angiotensin I* (Fig. 22-7). This prohormone is promptly hydrolyzed to the octapeptide angiotensin II by converting enzyme (peptidyl dipeptidase) that is present in the highest concentrations in the lungs. Indeed, the lungs convert 20% to 40% of angiotensin I to angiotensin II in a single circulation. The same converting enzyme is also responsible for the breakdown of plasma kinins, creating the situation in which the most potent endogenous vasoconstrictor (angiotensin II) and vasodilator (bradykinin) are cleared by the same enzyme. Angiotensin II is metabolized to the pentapeptide angiotensin II by aminopeptidase enzyme (see Fig. 22-7).

The renin-angiotensin-aldosterone system does not play an active role in the sodium-repleted patient but is of major importance in maintaining systemic blood pressure and intravascular fluid volume during sodium depletion or in the presence of hypovolemia. Furthermore, plasma renin activity is increased in only about 15% of patients with essential hypertension. Nevertheless, the frequent efficacy of renin-angiotensin antagonists in treating essential hypertension suggests a much broader involvement than would be indicated solely by increases in plasma renin activity.

Effects on Organ Systems

Vasoconstriction and stimulation of the synthesis and secretion of aldosterone by the adrenal cortex are the principal physiologic effects of angiotensin II. Aldosterone causes renal conservation of sodium with retention of water and loss of potassium and hydrogen ions. Other less intense effects include stimulation of the heart and sympathetic nervous system and increased release of arginine vasopressin hormone (antidiuretic hormone). Angiotensin III produces similar but less marked physiologic effects compared with angiotensin II. For example, its pressor effect is <50% of that of angiotensin II. Angiotensin III, however, is as potent or more so for evoking release of aldosterone when compared with angiotensin II. Angiotensin I has <1% of the activity of angiotensin II on vascular smooth muscles, the heart, or the adrenal cortex. The effects of angiotensin are most likely mediated through specific receptors on cell membranes.

Cardiovascular Effects

Angiotensin II produces vasoconstriction of precapillary arterioles and, to a lesser extent, postcapillary venules. Angiotensin II is the most powerful endogenous vasoconstrictor, being 40 times more potent than norepinephrine. This intense vasoconstriction reflects a direct action of angiotensin II on vascular smooth muscles and indirect activation of the sympathetic nervous system. The vasoconstrictive effect is greatest in skin, splanchnic vasculature, and kidneys, with blood flow being greatly decreased to these sites. Coronary artery vasoconstriction may jeopardize the adequacy of coronary blood flow. Vasoconstriction is less in cerebral vessels and even weaker in vessels to skeletal muscles. In fact, total blood flow in these two regions may increase as the increased perfusion pressure more than offsets a modest increase in systemic vascular resistance. Likewise, changes in pulmonary vascular resistance are usually modest.

Angiotensin II acts directly on cardiac cells to prolong the plateau phase of the cardiac action potential, which increases inward calcium ion movement that activates the contractile elements. Central and peripheral stimulant effects on the sympathetic nervous system may increase heart rate and myocardial contractility. Nevertheless, increased systemic blood pressure may activate baroreceptors, which reflexively slows heart rate and decreases myocardial contractility. Changes in central venous pressure are modest, because angiotensin II has weak vasoconstrictor effects on large veins and thus decreases venous capacitance less than norepinephrine. The net result of all these changes is often a decrease in cardiac output.

Angiotensin II decreases intravascular fluid volume through loss of extracellular fluid in response to constriction of postcapillary venules, which increases capillary filtration pressure. In addition, angiotensin II increases vascular permeability in large arterioles by causing separation of the endothelial cells.

Central Nervous System

CNS effects of angiotensin II occur despite the fact that peptides are generally regarded as being incapable of crossing the blood–brain barrier. Sustained hypertension reflects enhanced central outflow of sympathetic nervous system impulses caused by effects of angiotensin II on the medullary vasomotor center. Angiotensin II can also enhance release of adrenocorticotrophic hormone, presumably via a CNS action.

Peripheral Autonomic Nervous System

The peripheral autonomic nervous system effects of angiotensin II include stimulation of sympathetic nervous system ganglion cells and facilitation of ganglionic transmission. This may result in increased responsiveness of the innervated organ to norepinephrine as well as increased output of norepinephrine from postganglionic sympathetic nerve endings. Angiotensin-induced prolongation of the nerve action potential with the influx of calcium ions contributes to the facilitation of norepinephrine release in response to each nerve impulse.

Angiotensin II stimulates release of catecholamines from the adrenal medulla by directly depolarizing the chromaffin cells. Resulting hypertension may be particularly marked in patients with pheochromocytoma.

Adrenal Cortex

Angiotensin II directly stimulates the synthesis and secretion of aldosterone from the adrenal cortex by facilitating the calcium-dependent mechanism necessary for the conversion of cholesterol to pregnenolone. This effect occurs with low concentrations of angiotensin II that lack effects on systemic blood pressure. Aldosterone subsequently acts on the kidneys to cause retention of sodium and excretion of potassium and hydrogen ions. The stimulant effects of angiotensin II on aldosterone secretion are increased when the plasma sodium concentration is decreased or when the plasma potassium concentration is increased. These changes in responsiveness presumably reflect alterations in the number of receptors for angiotensin II on the zona glomerulosa cells.

In addition to angiotensin II, hyponatremia, hyperkalemia, and adrenocorticotrophic hormone can stimulate the zona glomerulosa of the adrenal cortex to release aldosterone. Indeed, control of aldosterone secretion is not lost after bilateral nephrectomies, although responsiveness is blunted.

Factors That Alter Plasma Renin Activity

Institution of positive end-expiratory pressure results in significant increases in plasma renin activity, plasma aldosterone concentration, and circulating levels of arginine vasopressin hormone (Annat et al., 1983). Nitroprusside-induced hypotension is associated with modest increases in plasma renin activity and marked increases in the plasma concentrations of arginine vasopressin hormone (Fig. 22-8) (Knight et al., 1983). Propranolol administered during nitroprusside-induced hypotension prevents the usual increase in plasma renin activity (Marshall et al., 1981). Plasma renin activity increases may contribute to tachyphylaxis during infusion of nitroprusside as well as overshoot of systemic blood pressure above predrug levels when nitroprusside is discontinued. In contrast to

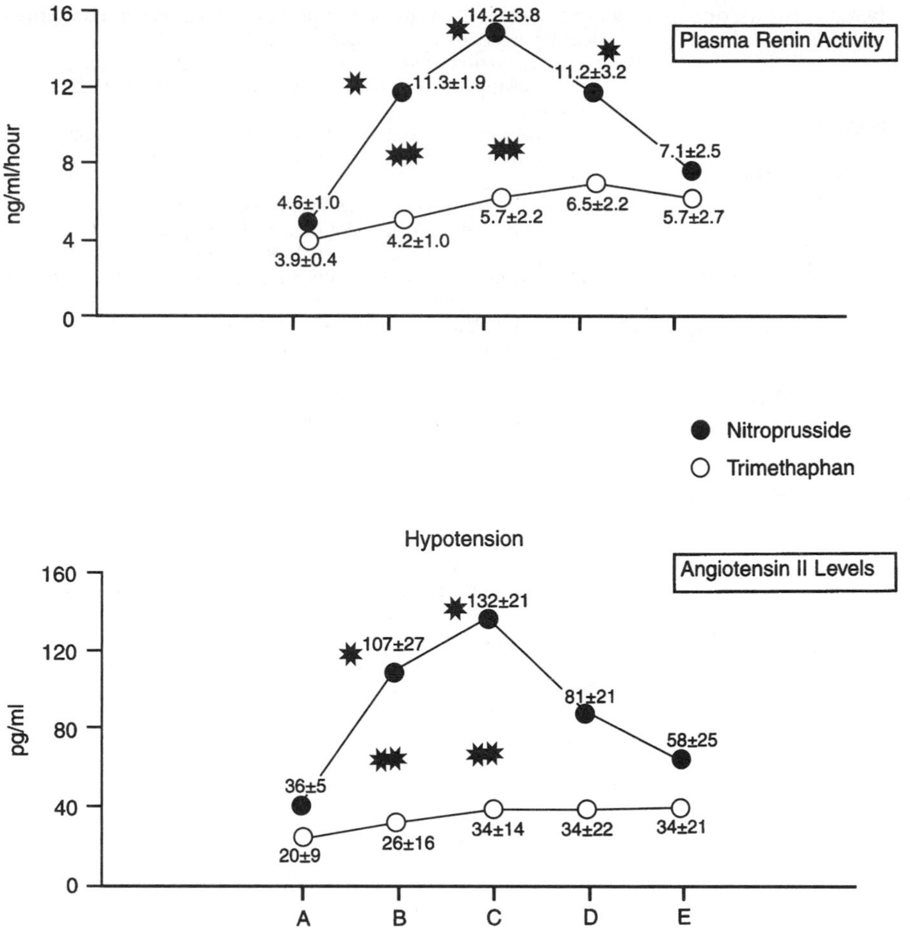

Figure 22-8. Plasma renin activity and angiotensin II concentrations are increased during nitroprusside-induced hypotension (*open circles*) but not during decreases in systemic blood pressure produced by trimethaphan (*solid circles*). (From Knight PR, Lane GA, Hensinger RN, et al. Catecholamine and renin-angiotensin response during hypotensive anesthesia induced by sodium nitroprusside or trimethaphan camsylate. *Anesthesiology* 1983;59:248–253; with permission.)

nitroprusside, systemic blood pressure decreases produced by trimethaphan do not cause an increase in plasma renin activity, presumably because blockade of sympathetic nervous system ganglia by this vasodilator inhibits the release of renin (see Fig. 22-8) (Knight et al., 1983). There is no evidence that anesthetics influence the rate of conversion of angiotensin I to angiotensin II (Miller et al., 1979).

Activation of the sympathetic nervous system may contribute to the release of renin via stimulation of beta-adrenergic receptors in the kidneys. Indeed, plasma renin activity and plasma concentrations of aldosterone increase dramatically during cardiopulmonary bypass (Fig. 22-9) (Bailey et al., 1975). Therefore, the renin-angiotensin-aldosterone system may play a role in systemic blood pressure regulation during cardiopulmonary bypass, which

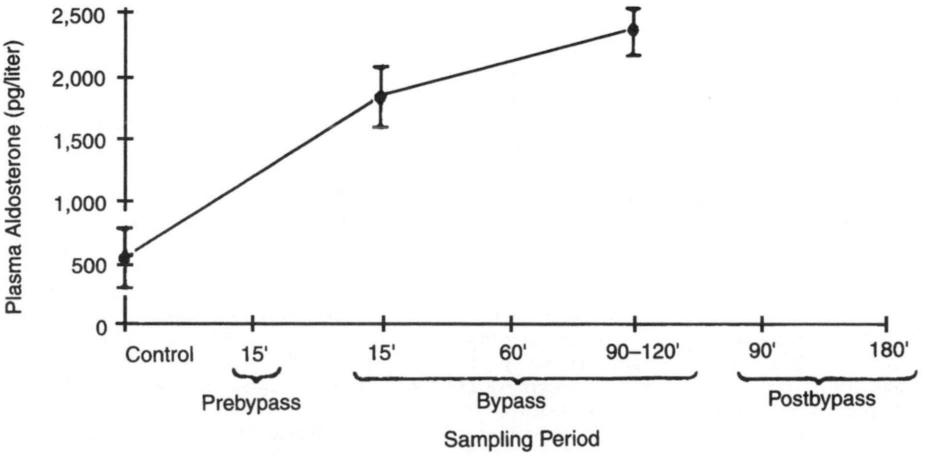

Figure 22-9. Plasma aldosterone concentrations increase dramatically during cardiopulmonary bypass. (From Bailey DR, Miller ED, Kaplan JA, et al. The renin-angiotensin-aldosterone system during cardiac surgery with morphine-nitrous oxide anesthesia. *Anesthesiology* 1975;42:538–544; with permission.)

could manifest as urinary excretion of potassium associated with hypokalemia.

Exogenous Infusion of Angiotensin II

Infusion of commercially available angiotensin II produces intense vasoconstriction and increases in systemic blood pressure. Too rapid an infusion can increase blood pressure to dangerous levels and produce myocardial ischemia. Compared with norepinephrine, angiotensin (a) is a more potent vasoconstrictor, (b) produces a more sustained effect, (c) infrequently causes cardiac dysrhythmias, and (d) is less likely to be associated with hypotension when a chronic infusion is abruptly discontinued. Spasm of the vein used for infusion does not occur, and tissue necrosis has not manifested, even with extravasation of angiotensin II. Like norepinephrine, angiotensin II diminishes intravascular fluid volume by promoting the translocation of fluid from the circulation to tissues. As a constrictor of capacitance vessels, angiotensin II is less potent than norepinephrine. The lack of a positive inotropic effect on the heart may be a disadvantage of angiotensin II compared with norepinephrine.

Antagonists of the Renin-Angiotensin-Aldosterone System

Antagonists of the renin-angiotensin-aldosterone system act by blocking receptors responsive to angiotensin II (losartan) and by inhibiting activity of the converting enzyme necessary for conversion of angiotensin I to angiotensin II (captopril) (see Chapter 15). In addition, beta-adrenergic blockade impairs secretion of renin by sympathetic nervous system stimulation of juxtaglomerular cells. Furthermore, clonidine may decrease renin secretion by an action within the CNS.

REFERENCES

Alon E, Kocian R, Nett PC, et al. Tropisetron for the prevention of postoperative nausea and vomiting in women undergoing gynecologic surgery. *Anesth Analg* 1996;82:338–341.

Alon E, Buchser E, Herrera E, et al. Tropisetron for treating established postoperative nausea and vomiting. A randomized double-blind, placebo-controlled study. *Anesth Analg* 1998;86:617–623.

Annat G, Viale JP, Xuan BB, et al. Effect of PEEP ventilation on renal function, plasma renin, aldosterone, neurophysins and urinary ADH, and prostaglandins. *Anesthesiology* 1983;58:136–141.

Apfel CC, Korttila K, Abdalla M, et al. A factorial trial of six interventions for the prevention of postoperative nausea and vomiting. *N Engl J Med* 2004;350:2441–2551.

Avidan MS, DaFonseca J, Parmar K, et al. The effects of aprotinin on thromboelastography with three different activators. *Anesthesiology* 2001;95:1169–1174.

Baguley WA, Hay WT, Mackie KP, et al. Cardiac dysrhythmias associated with the intravenous administration of ondansetron and metoclopramide. *Anesth Analg* 1997;84:1380–1381.

Bailey DR, Miller ED, Kaplan JA, et al. The renin-angiotensin-aldosterone system during cardiac surgery with morphine-nitrous oxide anesthesia. *Anesthesiology* 1975;42:538–544.

Bodner M, White PF. Antiemetic efficacy of ondansetron after outpatient laparoscopy. *Anesth Analg* 1991;73:250–254.

Boogaerts JG, Bardiau FM, Seidel L, et al. Tropisetron in the prevention of postoperative nausea and vomiting. *J Clin Anesth* 2000;12: 402–408.

Borgeat A, Stirnermann H-R. Ondansetron is effective to treat spinal or epidural morphine induced pruritus. *Anesthesiology* 1999;90: 432–436.

Bosek V, Hu P, Robinson LA. Acute myocardial ischemia after administration of ondansetron hydrochloride. *Anesthesiology* 2000;92: 885–887.

Capdevila X, Calvet Y, Biboulet P, et al. Aprotinin decreases blood loss and homologous transfusions in patients undergoing major orthopedic surgery. *Anesthesiology* 1998;88:50–57.

Carp H, Singh PJ, Vadhera R, Jayaram A. Effects of the serotonin-receptor agonist sumatriptan on postdural puncture headache: report of six cases. *Anesth Analg* 1994;79:180–182.

Cieslak GD, Watcha MF, Phillips MB, et al. The dose-response relation and cost-effectiveness of granisetron for the prophylaxis of pediatric postoperative emesis. *Anesthesiology* 1996;85:1076–1085.

D'Ambra MN, Risk SC. Aprotinin, erythropoietin and blood substitutes. *Int Anesthesiol Clin* 1990;28:237–240.

Diemunsch P, Leeser J, Feiss P, et al. Intravenous dolasetron mesilate ameliorates postoperative nausea and vomiting. *Can J Anaesth* 1997;44:173–181.

Dietrich W, Spath P, Zuhlsdorf M, et al. Anaphylactic reactions to aprotinin reexposure in cardiac surgery. Relation to antiaprotinin immunoglobulin G and E antibodies. *Anesthesiology* 2001;95: 64–71.

Fauser AA, Felhauer M, Hoffmann M, et al. Guidelines for antiemetic therapy. Acute emesis. *Eur J Cancer* 1999;35:361–370.

Feindt PR, Walcher S, Volkmer I, et al. Effects of high-dose aprotinin on renal function in aortocoronary bypass grafting. *Ann Thorac Surg* 1995;60:1076–1080.

Friberg L, Oleson J, Iversen HK, et al. Migraine pain associated with middle cerebral artery dilation: reversal by sumatriptan and dihydroergotamine. *Cephalalgia* 1991;11:165–168.

Fujii Y, Tanaka H, Toyooka H. Optimal anti-emetic dose of granisetron for preventing postoperative nausea and vomiting. *Can J Anaesth* 1994;41:794–797.

Fujii Y, Saitoh Y, Tanaka H, et al. Granisetron/dexamethasone combination for the prevention of postoperative nausea and vomiting after laparoscopic cholecystectomy. *Eur J Anesthesiol* 2000;17:64–68.

Furst SR, Rodarte A. Prophylactic antiemetic treatment with ondansetron in children undergoing tonsillectomy. *Anesthesiology* 1994;81:799–803.

Gan TJ, Ginsberg B, Grant AP, et al. Double-blind, randomized comparison of ondansetron and intraoperative propofol to prevent postoperative nausea and vomiting. *Anesthesiology* 1996;85:1036–1042.

Gyermek L. 5-HT_3 receptors: pharmacologic and therapeutic aspects. *J Clin Pharmacol* 1995;35:845–855.

Hardy JF, Desroches J. Natural and synthetic antifibrinolytics in cardiac surgery. *Can J Anaesth* 1992;39:353–365.

Hindle AT. Recent developments in the physiology and pharmacology of 5-hydroxytryptamine. *Br J Anaesth* 1994;73:395–407.

Honkavaara P. Effect of ondansetron on nausea and vomiting after middle ear surgery during general anaesthesia. *Br J Anaesth* 1996; 76:316–318.

Horl WH. Aprotinin and renal function in patients undergoing cardiac surgery. *Br J Anaesth* 2000;84:3–5.

Hunt BJ, Segal H, Yahoub M. Aprotinin and heparin monitoring during cardiopulmonary bypass. *Circulation* 1992;86:410–412.

Khalil S, Rodarte A, Weldon BC, et al. Intravenous ondansetron in established postoperative emesis in children. *Anesthesiology* 1996; 85:270–276.

Knight PR, Lane GA, Hensinger RN, et al. Catecholamine and renin-angiotensin response during hypotensive anesthesia induced by sodium nitroprusside or trimethaphan camsylate. *Anesthesiology* 1983;59:248–253.

Kovac AL, Scuderi P, Boerner TF, et al. Treatment of postoperative nausea and vomiting with single intravenous doses of dolasetron mesylate: a multicenter trial. *Anesth Analg* 1997;85:546–552.

Levy JH, Bailey JM, Salmenpera M. Pharmacokinetics of aprotinin in preoperative cardiac surgical patients. *Anesthesiology* 1994;80: 1013–1018.

Marshall WK, Bedford RF, Arnold WP, et al. Effects of propranolol on the cardiovascular and renin-angiotensin systems during hypotension

produced by sodium nitroprusside in humans. *Anesthesiology* 1981; 55:277–280.
Marwood JF, Stokes GS. Serotonin (5HT) and its antagonists: involvement in cardiovascular system. *Clin Exp Pharmacol Physiol* 1984; 11:439–456.
McKenzie R, Kovac A, O'Connor, et al. Comparison of ondansetron versus placebo to prevent postoperative nausea and vomiting in women undergoing ambulatory gynecologic surgery. *Anesthesiology* 1993;78:21–28.
Miller ED, Gianfagna W, Ackerly JA, Peach MJ. Converting-enzyme activity and pressure responses to angiotensin I and II in the rat awake and during anesthesia. *Anesthesiology* 1979;50:88–92.
Pan PH, Moore CH. Intraoperative antiemetic efficacy of prophylactic ondansetron versus droperidol for cesarean section patients under epidural anesthesia. *Anesth Analg* 1996;83:982–986.
Piper SN, Rohn KD, Maleck WM et al. Dolestron for preventing postanesthetic shivering. *Anesth Analg* 2002;94:106–111.
Randomized trial of aspirin, sibrafiban, or both for secondary prevention after acute coronary syndromes. *Circulation* 2001;103: 1727- 1733.
Rose JB, Brenn BR, Corddry DH, et al. Preoperative oral ondansetron for pediatric tonsillectomy. *Anesth Analg* 1996;82:558–562.
Rose JB, Martin TM, Corddry DH, et al. Ondansetron reduces the incidence and severity of poststrabismus repair vomiting in children. *Anesth Analg* 1994;79:486–489.
Rose JB, Watcha MF. Postoperative nausea and vomiting. In: Benumof JL, Saidman LJ, eds: Anesthesia and *p*erioperative *c*omplications, 2nd edition. Mosby, St Louis, 1999;425–440.
Royston D, Bidstrup BP, Taylor KM, et al. Effect of aprotinin on need for blood transfusion after repeat open-heart surgery. *Lancet* 1987; 2:1289–1291.
Scholz J, Hennes HJ, Steinfath M, et al. Tropiestron or ondansetron compared with placebo for prevention of postoperative nausea and vomiting. *Eur J Anesthesiol* 1998;15:676–685.
Scuderi P, Wetchler B, Sung YF, et al. Treatment of postoperative nausea and vomiting after outpatient surgery with the 5-HT_3 antagonist ondansetron. *Anesthesiology* 1993;78:15–20.
Smith PK. Aprotinin: Safe and effective only with the full-dose regimen. *Ann Thorac Surg* 1996;62:1575–1577.
Sniadach MS, Alberts MS. A comparison of the prophylactic antiemetic effect of ondansetron and droperidol on patients undergoing gynecologic laparoscopy. *Anesth Analg* 1997;85:797–783.
Sprung J, Choudhry FM, Hall BA. Extrapyramidal reactions to ondansetron: Cross-reactivity between ondansetron and prochlorperazine? *Anesth Analg* 2003;96:1376–1376
Steinbrook RA, Freiberger D, Gosnell JL, et al. Prophylactic antiemetics for laparoscopic cholecystectomy: ondansetron versus droperidol plus metoclopramide. *Anesth Analg* 1996;83:1081–1083.
Tang J, Watcha MF, White PF, et al. The effect of timing of ondansetron administration on its efficacy, cost-effectiveness, and cost-benefit as a prophylactic anti-emetic in the ambulatory setting. *Anesth Analg* 1998;86:274–282.
Tang J, Chen X, White PF, et al. Antiemetic prophylaxis for office-based surgery. Are the 5HT_3 receptor antagonists beneficial? *Anesthesiology* 2003;98:293–298.
Tramer MR, Reynolds JM, Moore RA, et al. Efficacy, dose-response, and safety of ondansetron in prevention of postoperative nausea and vomiting: a quantitative systematic review of randomized placebo-controlled trials. *Anesthesiology* 1997;87:1277–1289.
Wang J-J, Tzeng J-I, Ho, S-T, et al. The propyhylactic effect of tropisetron on epidural morphine-related nausea and vomiting: A comparison of dexamethasone with saline. *Anesth Analg* 2002;94:749–753.
Watcha MF, Bras PJ, Cieslak GD, et al. The dose-response relationship of ondansetron in preventing postoperative emesis in pediatric patients undergoing ambulatory surgery. *Anesthesiology* 1995;82: 47–52.
White PF. Prevention of postoperative nausea and vomiting-a multimodal solution to a persistent problem. *N Engl J Med* 2004;350: 2511–2512.
Wolf H. Preclinical and clinical pharmacology of the 5-HT3 receptor antagonists. *Scand J Rheumatol* 2000;29:37–45.

Hormones as Drugs

23

Preparations that contain synthetic hormones identical to those secreted endogenously by endocrine glands may be administered as drugs. These synthetic hormones resemble the endogenous substances in structure and activity. Typically, the clinical application of these drugs is for hormone replacement to provide a physiologic effect. In certain patients, however, large doses of synthetic hormones are used to exert a pharmacologic effect. Recombinant deoxyribonucleic acid (DNA) technology permits the incorporation of synthetic genes that code for the synthesis of specific human hormones by bacteria, thus permitting production of pure hormones devoid of allergic properties.

ANTERIOR PITUITARY HORMONES

Anterior pituitary hormones include (a) growth hormone; (b) prolactin; (c) gonadotropins, including luteinizing hormone and follicle-stimulating hormone; (d) adrenocorticotrophic hormone (ACTH); and (e) thyroid-stimulating hormone (TSH). Growth hormone, gonadotropins, and ACTH can be administered in the form of synthetic drugs.

Perioperative replacement of anterior pituitary hormones may be necessary for patients receiving exogenous hormones because of a prior hypophysectomy. For example, cortisol must be provided continuously. Conversely, thyroid hormones have such a long elimination half-time that they can be omitted for several days without adverse effects. Likewise, the loss of other anterior pituitary hormones has no immediate physiologic implications.

Growth Hormone

Growth hormone is used to treat hypopituitary dwarfism, based on documentation that the plasma concentration of the hormone is inadequate. In this regard, radioimmunoassays for growth hormone are used to measure plasma concentrations of the hormone. Treatment must be maintained for several months to years, corresponding to childhood secretion patterns of this hormone. Injection of hormone at weekly intervals is usually adequate for treatment despite an elimination half-time of about 20 minutes.

Octreotide

Octreotide is a somatostatin analogue that inhibits the release of growth hormone, making it an effective treatment for patients with acromegaly (Lamberts et al., 1996). Long-term treatment with octreotide (>1 month) is associated with an increased incidence of cholesterol gallstones (occurring in 20% to 30% of treated patients). Because somatostatin analogues inhibit the secretion of insulin, decreased glucose tolerance and even overt hyperglycemia might be expected during treatment with octreotide. Octreotide may be a life-saving treatment in patients experiencing an acute carcinoid crisis although bolus injection of this somatostatin analog may be accompanied by bradycardia and second- and third-degree heart block (Dilger et al., 2004).

Gonadotropins

Gonadotropins are used most often for the treatment of infertility and cryptorchism. Induction of ovulation can be stimulated in females who are infertile because of pituitary insufficiency. Excessive ovarian enlargement and maturation of many follicles, leading to multiple births, is a possibility. Gonadotropins are effective only by parenteral injection. Radioimmunoassays are useful in measuring plasma and urine concentrations of gonadotropins.

Adrenocorticotrophic Hormone

The physiologic and pharmacologic effects of ACTH result from this hormone's stimulation of secretion of corticosteroids from the adrenal cortex, principally cortisol. An important clinical use of ACTH is as a diagnostic aid in patients with suspected adrenal insufficiency. For example, a normal increase in the plasma concentration of cortisol in response to the administration of ACTH rules out primary adrenocortical insufficiency. Furthermore, ACTH may be administered therapeutically to evoke the release of cortisol. Treatment of disease states with ACTH is not physiologically equivalent to administration of a specific hormone because ACTH exposes the tissues to a mixture of glucocorticoids, mineralocorticoids, and androgens. Indeed, there may be associated retention of sodium, development of hypokalemic metabolic alkalosis, and appearance of acne, which are unlikely to accompany selective-acting corticosteroids.

Absorption of ACTH after intramuscular (IM) injection is prompt. After intravenous (IV) injection, ACTH disappears rapidly from the plasma, with an elimination half-time of about 15 minutes. Maximal stimulation of the adrenal cortex is produced by ACTH. Allergic reactions ranging from mild fever to life-threatening anaphylaxis may be associated with administration of ACTH.

THYROID GLAND HORMONES

The thyroid gland is the source of triiodothyronine (T_3), thyroxine (T_4), and calcitonin (Fig. 23-1). Commercial preparations of T_3 and T_4 are available for the treatment of hypothyroidism, as may be encountered in patients with a simple goiter. The effectiveness of treatment is judged by the return of the plasma concentration of TSH to normal and a decrease in the size of the goiter. Certain carcinomas of thyroid gland, particularly papillary tumors, may remain sensitive to TSH. Indeed, administration of thyroid hormones may suppress the responsiveness and cause regression of the malignant lesion. Thyroid hormones enhance the effects of coumarin anticoagulants by increasing catabolism of vitamin K-dependent clotting factors. Cholestyramine binds to orally administered thyroid hormone in the gastrointestinal tract.

Levothyroxine

Levothyroxine is the most frequently administered drug for the treatment of diseases requiring thyroid hormone replacement. Oral administration is preferred, but IV injection is acceptable in emergency situations. Most patients can be maintained in a euthyroid state with 100 to 200 mg daily.

Liothyronine

Liothyronine is the levorotatory isomer of T_3 and is 2.5 to 3.0 times as potent as levothyroxine. Its rapid onset and short duration of action preclude use of liothyronine for long-term thyroid replacement.

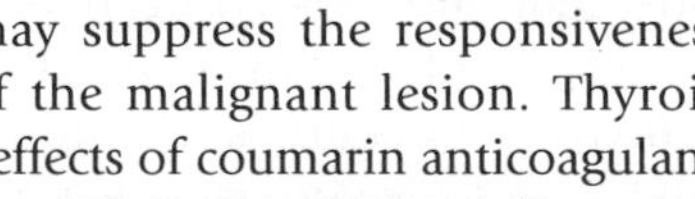

Triiodothyronine (T_3)

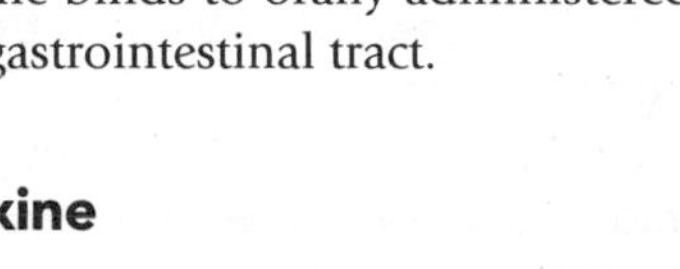

Thyroxine (tetraiodothyronine, T_4)

Figure 23-1. Thyroid gland hormones.

Calcitonin

Calcitonin is a 32-amino acid hormone secreted by the thyroid gland. Endogenous release of this hormone decreases plasma calcium concentrations as a reflection of decreased osteoclast activity and bone resorption. Pharmacologic doses of calcitonin are effective in relieving pain and decreasing the complications of Paget disease.

DRUGS THAT INHIBIT THYROID HORMONE SYNTHESIS

A large number of substances are capable of interfering with the synthesis of thyroid hormones. These compounds include (a) antithyroid drugs, (b) inhibitors of the iodide transport mechanism, (c) iodide, and (d) radioactive iodine.

Antithyroid Drugs

Propylthiouracil and methimazole are antithyroid drugs that inhibit the formation of thyroid hormone by interfering with the incorporation of iodine into tyrosine residues of thyroglobulin (Fig. 23-2) (Cooper, 1984). In addition to blocking hormone synthesis, these drugs also inhibit the peripheral deiodination of T_4 and T_3. These drug-induced effects on thyroid hormone synthesis render antithyroid drugs useful in the treatment of hyperthyroidism before elective thyroidectomy.

Antithyroid drugs are not available as parenteral preparations, necessitating their administration by way of a gastric tube if drugs cannot be administered orally, such as during thyroid storm. Drug-induced decreases in excessive thyroid activity usually require several days, because preformed hormone must be depleted before symptoms begin to wane. In a few patients, especially those with severe hyperthyroidism, definite improvement is evident in 1 to 2 days.

Side Effects

The side effects produced by propylthiouracil and methimazole are similar. The most common reaction is a urticarial or

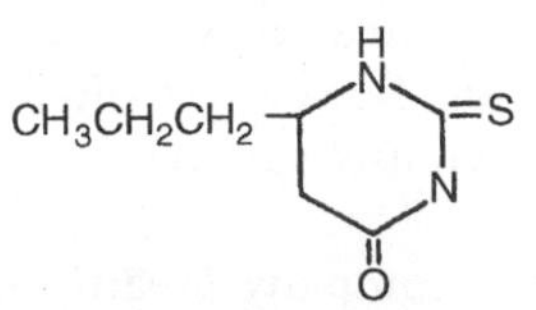

Propylthiouracil

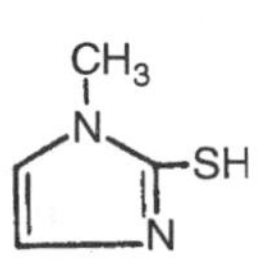

Methimazole

Figure 23-2. Antithyroid drugs.

papular skin rash often associated with pruritus, which occurs in about 3% of patients. This rash may disappear spontaneously without interrupting treatment. In others, this side effect necessitates changing to the other drug, because cross-sensitivity is not likely.

Granulocytopenia and agranulocytosis are serious but rare side effects that are most likely to occur in the first 2 months of therapy with an antithyroid drug. Periodic white blood cell counts, although helpful for detecting gradual decreases in the leukocyte count, should not be relied on to detect agranulocytosis because of the rapidity with which this complication can develop. Fever or pharyngitis may be the earliest manifestation of the development of agranulocytosis. Recovery is likely if the antithyroid drug is discontinued at the first sign of this side effect.

Antithyroid drugs cross the placenta and appear in breast milk. Placental passage, however, is limited for propylthiouracil, making it the preferred drug for use in the parturient.

Inhibitors of Iodide Transport Mechanisms

Inhibitors of iodide transport mechanisms are thiocyanate and perchlorate. These ions are similar in size to iodide and, in some way, interfere with the uptake of iodide ions by the thyroid gland. Thiocyanate can result from the metabolism of sodium nitroprusside (see Chapter 16) or ingestion of cabbage, neither of which is likely to be clinically significant. Perchlorate is capable of producing aplastic anemia and is thus rarely used.

Iodide

Iodide is the oldest available therapy for hyperthyroidism, providing a paradoxical treatment that is effective for reasons that are not fully understood. The response of the patient with hyperthyroidism to iodide is often discernible within 24 hours, emphasizing that release of hormone into the circulation is quickly interrupted. Indeed, the most important clinical effect of high doses of iodide is inhibition of the release of thyroid hormone. This may reflect the ability of iodide to antagonize the ability of TSH and cyclic adenosine monophosphate (cAMP) to stimulate hormone release.

Iodide is particularly useful in the treatment of hyperthyroidism before elective thyroidectomy. Indeed, the combination of oral potassium iodide and propranolol is a recommended approach (Feek et al., 1980). The vascularity of the thyroid gland is also decreased by iodide therapy. Chronic treatment with iodide, however, is often associated with a recurrence of previously suppressed excessive thyroid gland activity.

Allergic reactions may accompany treatment with iodide or administration of organic preparations that contain iodide. Angioedema and laryngeal edema may become life-threatening.

Radioactive Iodine

Among the radioactive isotopes of iodine, ^{131}I is the most frequently administered. This isotope is rapidly and efficiently trapped by thyroid gland cells, and the subsequent emission of destructive beta rays acts almost exclusively on these cells, with little or no damage to surrounding tissue. It is possible to completely destroy the thyroid gland with ^{131}I. Indeed, hypothyroidism occurs in about 10% of treated patients in the first year after ^{131}I administration and increases about 2% to 3% each year thereafter. For this reason, iatrogenic hypothyroidism must be considered preoperatively in any patient who has previously been treated with ^{131}I.

Hyperthyroidism is treated with orally administered ^{131}I, with symptoms of excessive thyroid gland activity gradually abating over a period of 2 to 3 months. One-half to two-thirds of patients are cured by a single dose of isotope, and the remainder require an additional one to two doses. Despite the safety and effectiveness of ^{131}I, surgery is often selected for patients $<$30 years of age because of the concern about potential carcinogenic effects of radiation. Nevertheless, there is no evidence that ^{131}I has ever caused cancer in adults.

The principal indication for ^{131}I treatment is hyperthyroidism in elderly patients and in those with heart disease. Indeed, hypothyroidism is not a common sequela after treatment with ^{131}I for toxic nodular goiter, the usual cause of hyperthyroidism in elderly patients. The use of ^{131}I is contraindicated during pregnancy because the fetal thyroid gland would concentrate the isotope.

Most thyroid cancers except for follicular cancer accumulate little radioactive iodine. As a result, the therapeutic effectiveness of ^{131}I for treatment of thyroid cancer is limited.

OVARIAN HORMONES

An understanding of the synthesis and action of ovarian hormones, including estrogens and progesterone, permits therapeutic interventions in certain disease states. Equally important is the therapeutic use of drugs that can mimic effects of these hormones and act as contraceptives.

Estrogens

Estrogens are effective in treating unpleasant side effects of menopause (Fig. 23-3). Senile or atrophic vaginitis responds to topical estrogen. There is no evidence that administration of estrogens delays the progression of atherosclerosis in postmenopausal women. There is abundant evidence that administration of estrogen to postmenopausal women prevents bone loss (protects against osteoporosis) and also prevents vertebral and femoral bone fractures (Belchetz, 1994). Estrogens are administered to decrease milk production in

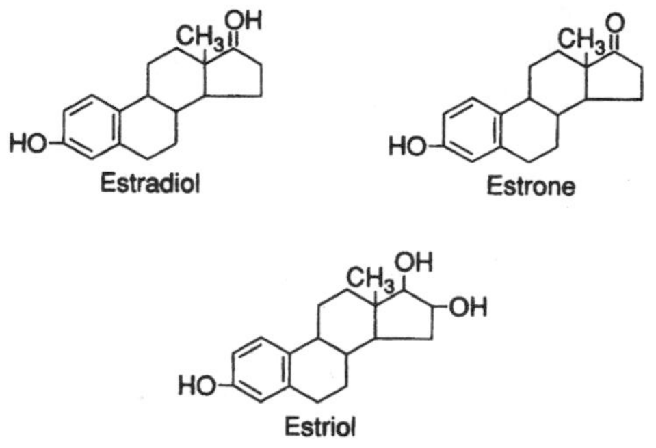

Figure 23-3. Estrogens.

the postpartum period. The presence of receptors for estrogen increases the likelihood of a palliative response to estrogen therapy in women with metastatic breast cancer. An important use of estrogens is in combination with progestins as oral contraceptives.

Route of Administration

The absorption of most estrogens and their derivatives from the gastrointestinal tract is prompt and nearly complete. Metabolism in the liver, however, limits the effectiveness of orally administered estrogens. Topical and IM administration of estrogens is also effective. Radioimmunoassay methods are highly specific and sensitive for measuring the plasma concentrations of estrogens.

Side Effects

The most frequent unpleasant symptom associated with the use of estrogens is nausea. Large doses of estrogens may cause retention of sodium and water, which is particularly undesirable in patients with cardiac or renal disease. There is an increased incidence of vaginal and cervical adenocarcinoma in daughters of mothers treated with diethylstilbestrol or other synthetic estrogens during the first trimester of pregnancy. Most of the affected women have been 20 to 25 years old when diagnosed. Use of estrogen by postmenopausal women increases the risk of developing endometrial cancer.

Antiestrogens

Clomiphene and tamoxifen act as antiestrogens by binding to estrogen receptors (Fig. 23-4) (see Chapter 29). Tamoxifen is administered for a period of 5 years to postmenopausal women with breast cancer that was characterized by estrogen-responsive receptors. It is of interest that tamoxifen has estrogenic activity in some tissues, including bone. The loss of normal feedback inhibition of estrogen synthesis causes an increased secretion of gonadotropins. The most prominent effect on increased plasma concentrations of gonadotropins is the enlargement of the ovaries and enhancement of fertility in otherwise infertile women. Endometrial stimulation and an increased incidence of temperature disturbances ("hot flashes") may accompany treatment with tamoxifen.

Tissue-Specific Estrogens

Raloxifene is a nonsteroidal benzothiophene that acts as a selective estrogen-receptor modulator (Delmas et al., 1997). In this regard, raloxifene preserves the beneficial effects of estrogens (prevention of bone loss and lowering of plasma cholesterol concentrations) without any associated effects on reproductive organs. For example, endometrial stimulation does not accompany treatment with raloxifene. Tissue-specific estrogen agonist or antagonist actions of raloxifene may be related to estrogen receptor-mediated gene activation.

Progesterone

Orally active derivatives of progesterone are designated *progestins* (Fig. 23-5). Progestins are often combined with estrogens as oral contraceptives. Dysfunctional uterine bleeding can be treated with small doses of a progestin for a few days, with the goal being induction of progesterone-withdrawal bleeding. Progestins, like estrogens, are effective in suppressing lactation in the immediate postpartum period. Palliative treatment of metastatic endometrial carcinoma is achieved with progestins. Absorption of progestins from the gastrointestinal tract is rapid, but hepatic first-pass metabolism is extensive.

Antiprogestins

Antiprogestins inhibit the hormonal effects of progesterone and are the most effective and safest means of medical abortion (Spitz and Bardin, 1993). In this regard, mifepristone (RU 486) can be administered in a single oral dose to produce termination of pregnancy (Fig. 23-6). The combination of mifepristone with a prostaglandin administered

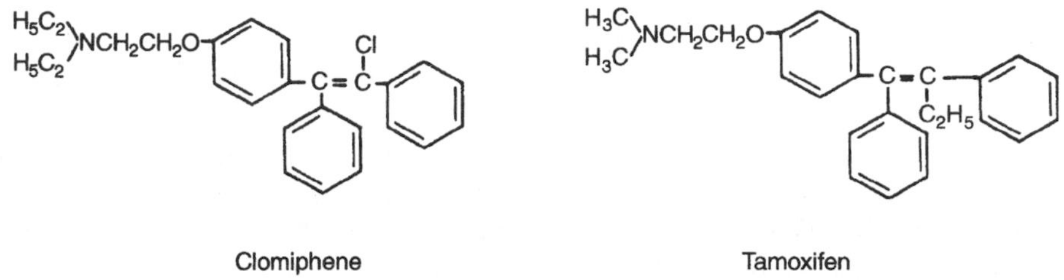

Figure 23-4. Antiestrogens.

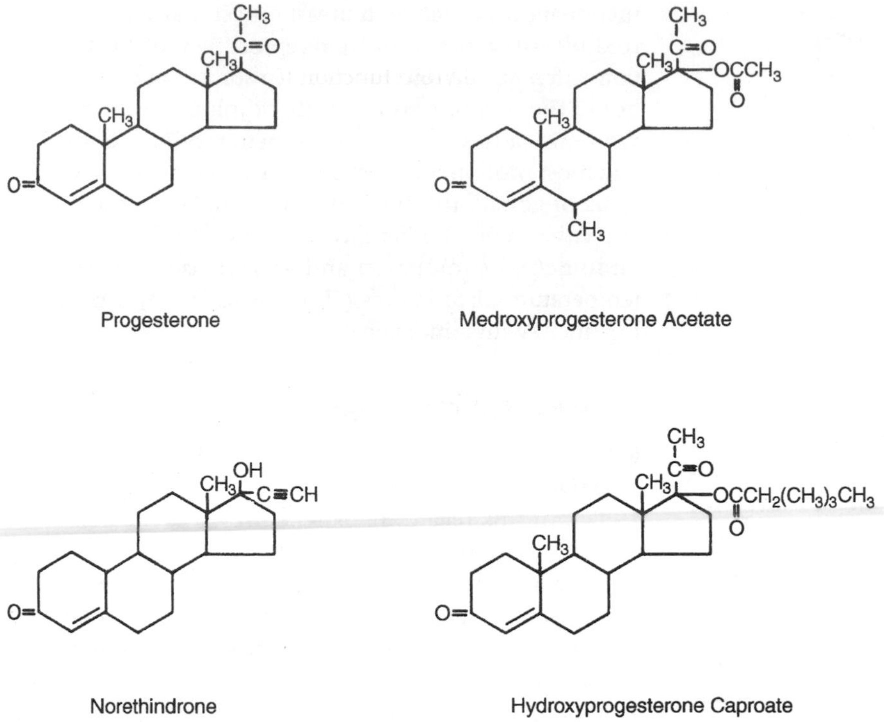

Figure 23-5. Progestins.

48 hours later by IM injection (sulprostone), by vaginal suppository (gemeprost), or orally (misoprostol) has resulted in a rate of complete abortion approaching 100%. Mifepristone has been used as a postcoital contraceptive within 72 hours of unprotected intercourse. In addition to its antiprogesterone properties, mifepristone has antiglucocorticoid activity and is useful in the treatment of patients with hypercortisolism. Side effects of mifepristone include vaginal bleeding, nausea, vomiting, abdominal pain, and fatigue.

Oral Contraceptives

Oral contraceptives are most often a combination of an estrogen and a progestin. This combination inhibits ovulation, presumably by preventing release of follicle-stimulating hormone by estrogen and luteinizing hormone by progesterone.

Side Effects

Estrogens in combined preparations are believed to be responsible for most, if not all of the side effects of oral contraceptives. For example, estrogens seem to be responsible for the increased incidence of thromboembolism. Indeed, patients taking estrogens manifest increased blood concentrations of some clotting factors as well as increased platelet aggregation. Nausea, vomiting, weight gain, and breast discomfort resembling early pregnancy are attributed to the estrogen component of oral contraceptives. The incidence of myocardial infarction and stroke is increased in patients who chronically take oral contraceptives (Kaplan, 1978). Hypertension occurs in about 5% of women taking oral contraceptives chronically (Laragh, 1976). This response probably reflects estrogen-induced increases in circulating plasma concentrations of renin and angiotensin, with associated retention of sodium and water.

Oral contraceptives containing high doses of estrogen may produce alterations in the glucose tolerance curves of patients with preclinical diabetes mellitus. These drugs increase the concentration of cholesterol in bile, which is consistent with an increased incidence of cholelithiasis. Benign hepatomas have been associated with the use of oral contraceptives. An increased incidence of breast cancer in patients taking oral contraceptives has not been documented. Depression of mood and fatigue have been attributed to the progestin component of oral contraceptives.

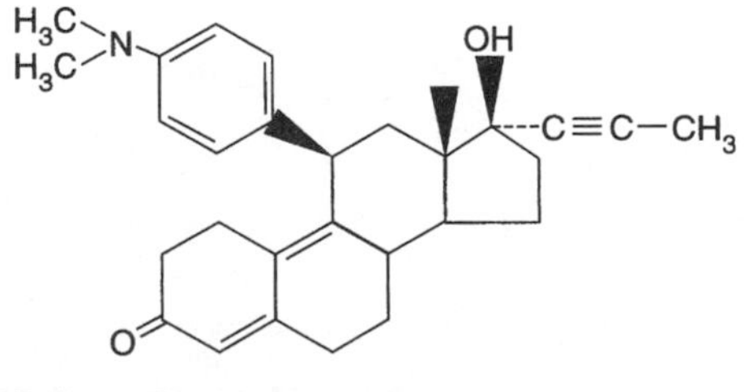

Figure 23-6. Mifepristone (RU 486).

ANDROGENS

Androgens are most often administered to males to stimulate the development and maintenance of secondary sexual characteristics (Fig. 23-7). The most common indication of androgen therapy in females is palliative management of

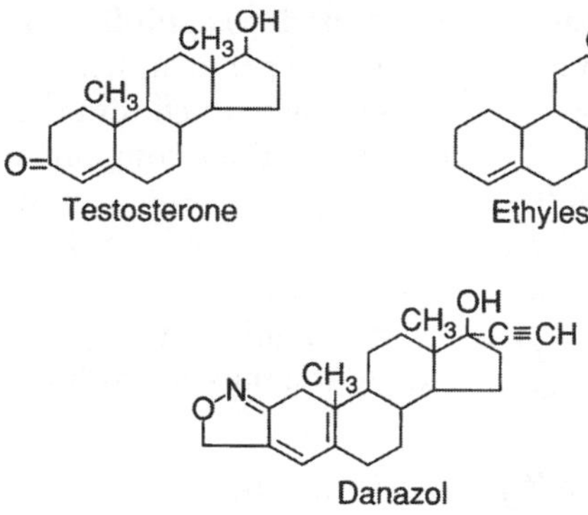

Figure 23-7. Androgens.

metastatic breast cancer. Androgens enhance erythropoiesis by stimulation of renal production of erythropoietin as well as by direct dose-related stimulation of erythropoietin-sensitive elements in bone marrow. In addition, there is a drug-induced increase in 2,3-diphosphoglycerate levels, which decreases hemoglobin affinity for oxygen, thus enhancing the availability of oxygen to tissues. For these reasons, androgen therapy is often instituted in patients with aplastic anemia or hemolytic anemia. Androgen-anabolic steroids have been used in the treatment of chronic debilitating diseases. These drugs promote a feeling of well-being and may improve appetite when administered to patients with terminal illnesses. The efficacy of anabolic steroids to improve athletic performance is not documented and is condemned on ethical grounds. Certain androgens may be useful in the treatment of hereditary angioedema.

Route of Administration

Testosterone administered orally is readily absorbed but is metabolized so extensively by the liver that therapeutic effects do not occur. Alkylation of androgens at the 17 position retards their hepatic metabolism and permits such derivatives to be effective (see Fig. 23-7). About 99% of testosterone circulating in the plasma is bound to sex hormone-binding globulin. As a result, this globulin determines the concentration of free testosterone in the plasma and thus its elimination half-time, which is 10 to 20 minutes.

Side Effects

Dose-related cholestatic hepatitis and jaundice are particularly likely to accompany androgen therapy for palliation in neoplastic disease. Increases in the plasma alkaline phosphatase and transaminase enzymes are also likely. Prolonged therapy (>1 year) with androgens, as for management of anemia, is associated with an increased incidence of hepatic cancer. Retention of sodium and water is also likely to accompany palliative treatment of cancer with high doses of androgens. Androgens increase the potency of coumarin anticoagulants and the likelihood of spontaneous hemorrhage. Androgens can decrease the concentration of thyroid-binding globulin in plasma and thus influence thyroid function tests.

Danazol

The low androgenic activity of danazol makes it the preferred androgen for treatment of hereditary angioedema (see Fig. 23-7). In treated patients, there is a remission of symptoms as well as increased production of previously deficient plasma protein factors. As with other androgens, danazol therapy has been associated with abnormal liver function tests and jaundice. Danazol also decreases breast pain and nodularity in many women with fibrocystic breast disease. Symptoms of endometriosis are decreased, and fertility may be restored in danazol-treated women. In patients with hemophilia A, danazol increases factor VIII activity and decreases the incidence of hemorrhage (Gralnick et al., 1985).

Finasteride

Finasteride is a competitive 5-alpha-reductase inhibitor that does not bind to the androgen receptor (Fig. 23-8) (Rittmaster, 1994). As a result of this drug-induced enzyme inhibition, dihydrotestosterone production from testosterone does not occur. In the absence of dihydrotestosterone, the androgen effects on the prostate and skin do not occur. Finasteride is administered orally (5 mg once daily) for the treatment of benign prostatic hyperplasia. Treatment of male pattern baldness, hirsutism, and acne may represent other potentially useful applications for finasteride. There is no evidence that finasteride is beneficial in men with established prostate cancer. The elimination half-time after oral administration is 6 to 8 hours. The only important side effects of finasteride are related to decreased sexual function. Finasteride has no effect on serum lipids or bone density. Prostate-specific antigen concentrations are decreased by treatment with finasteride, introducing the concern that detection of prostate cancer could be masked in patients treated with this drug.

CORTICOSTEROIDS

The actions of corticosteroids are classified according to the potencies of these compounds to (a) evoke distal renal

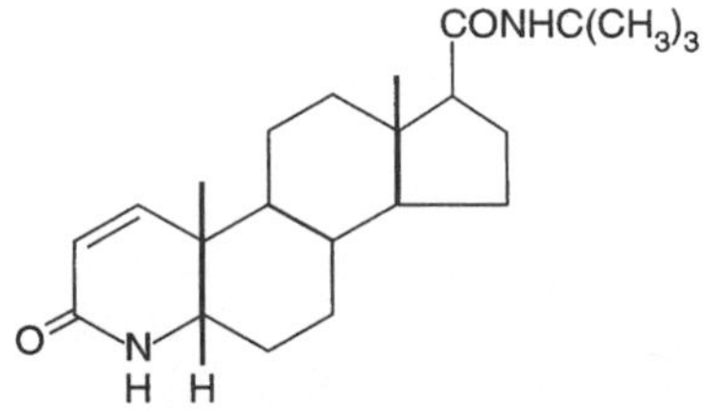

Figure 23-8. Finasteride.

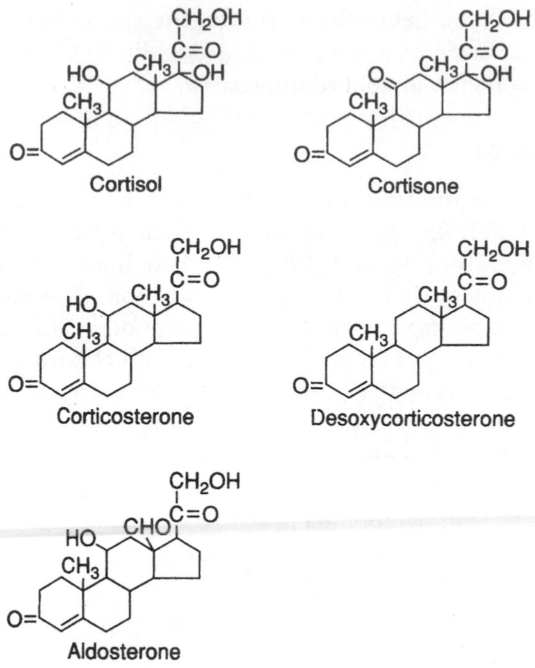

Figure 23-9. Endogenous corticosteroids.

tubular reabsorption of sodium in exchange for potassium ions (mineralocorticoid effect), or (b) produce an antiinflammatory response (glucocorticoid effect). Naturally occurring corticosteroids are cortisol (hydrocortisone), cortisone, corticosterone, desoxycorticosterone, and aldosterone (Fig. 23-9). Several synthetic corticosteroids are available, principally for use to produce antiinflammatory effects. Although it is possible to separate mineralocorticoid and glucocorticoid effects using synthetic drugs, it has not been possible to separate the various components of glucocorticoid effects. Consequently, all synthetic corticosteroids, when used in pharmacologic doses for their antiinflammatory effects, also produce less desirable effects, such as suppression of the hypothalamic-pituitary-adrenal (HPA) axis, weight gain, and skeletal muscle wasting.

Structure–Activity Relationships

All corticosteroids are constructed on the same primary molecular framework, designated as the steroid nucleus (see Fig. 23-9). Changes in molecular structure may result in altered biologic responses due to changes in absorption, protein binding, rate of metabolism, and intrinsic effectiveness of the drug at receptors. Modifications of structure, such as introduction of a double bond in prednisolone and prednisone, have resulted in synthetic corticosteroids with more potent glucocorticoid effects than the two closely related natural hormones, cortisol and cortisone, respectively (Table 23-1). At the same time, mineralocorticoid effects and the rate of hepatic metabolism of these synthetic drugs are less than those of the natural hormones. Despite increased antiinflammatory effects, it has not been possible to separate this response from alterations in carbohydrate and protein metabolism. This suggests that the multiple manifestations of drug-induced glucocorticoid effects are mediated by the same receptor.

TABLE 23-1.
COMPARATIVE PHARMACOLOGY OF ENDOGENOUS AND SYNTHETIC CORTICOSTEROIDS

	Antiinflammatory Potency	Sodium Retaining Potency	Equivalent Dose (mg)	Elimination Half-Time (hrs)	Duration of Action (hrs)	Route of Administration
Cortisol	1	1	20	1.5–3.0	8–12	Oral, Topical, IV, IM, IA
Cortisone	0.8	0.8	25	0.5	8–36	Oral, Topical, IV, IM, IA
Prednisolone	4	0.8	5	2–4	12–36	Oral, Topical, IV, IM, IA
Prednisone	4	0.8	5	2–4	12–36	Oral
Methylprednisolone	5	0.5	4	2–4	12–36	Oral, Topical, IV, IM, IA, Epidural
Betamethasone	25	0	0.75	5	36–54	Oral, Topical, IV, IM, IA
Dexamethasone	25	0	0.75	3.5–5.0	36–54	Oral, Topical, IV, IM, IA
Triamcinolone	5	0	4	3.5	12–36	Oral, Topical, IV, IM, Epidural
Fludrocortisone	10	250	2	—	24	Oral, Topical, IV, IM
Aldosterone	0	3,000				

IV, intravenous; IM, intramuscular; IA, intraarticular

Mechanism of Action

Glucocorticoids attach to cytoplasmic receptors to stimulate changes in the transcription of defined on 456 DNA and thus the synthesis of proteins. Two distinct types of corticosteroid receptors have been identified (mineralocorticoid and glucocorticoid). Mineralocorticoid receptors are present in high concentrations in distal renal tubules and the hippocampus. In contrast, glucocorticoids receptors are more widely distributed and do not bind aldosterone making these receptors glucocorticoid-selective. Local mechanisms that result in release of steroids from their carrier proteins serve to facilitate steroid entry into cells. Target cells also contain an enzyme, 11-beta hydroxysteroid dehydrogenase that controls the interconversion of cortisol (active) and cortisone (inert). The concentration of glucocorticoids receptors may fluctuate and thus influence responsiveness to glucocorticoids.

Maintenance of Homeostasis

Permissive and protective effects of glucocorticoids are critical for the maintenance of homeostasis during severe stress. The permissive and protective actions of glucocorticoids are complementary and permit the individual to effect an appropriate stress response and to maintain homeostasis.

Permissive Actions

Permissive actions of glucocorticoids occur at low physiologic steroid concentrations and serve to prepare the individual for responding to stress. These permissive actions of glucocorticoids maintain basal activity of the HPA by providing negative feedback and by setting the threshold for a response to stress.

Protective Actions

The protective mode of glucocorticoids occurs when high plasma concentrations of steroids exert antiinflammatory and immunosuppressive effects. This protective response prevents the host-defense mechanisms that are activated during stress from overshooting and damaging the organism. Other important protective actions of glucocorticoids include redirection of metabolism to meet energy needs during stress.

Pharmacokinetics

Synthetic cortisol and its derivatives are effective orally (see Table 23-1). Antacids, but not food, interfere with the oral absorption of corticosteroids. Water-soluble cortisol succinate can be administered IV to achieve prompt increases in plasma concentrations. More prolonged effects are possible with IM injection. Cortisone acetate may be given orally or IM but cannot be administered IV. The acetate preparation is a slow-release preparation lasting 8 to 12 hours. After release, cortisone is converted to cortisol in the liver. Corticosteroids are also promptly absorbed after topical application or aerosol administration.

Cortisol is highly bound (90% or more) in the plasma to corticosteroid-binding globulin. Nevertheless, cortisol and related compounds readily cross the placenta. Small amounts of cortisol appear unchanged in the urine, but at least 70% is conjugated in the liver to inactive or poorly active metabolites. These water-soluble conjugated metabolites appear in the urine and bile. The elimination half-time of cortisol is 1.5 to 3.0 hours but its biologic effects persist for several hours.

Cortisol is released from the adrenal glands in an episodic manner and the frequency of pulses follows a circadian rhythm that is linked to the sleep-wake cycle. Maximal plasma concentrations of cortisol occur just before awakening and the lowest levels occur 8 to 10 hours later. Stress-induced changes in the plasma concentrations of cortisol are superimposed on the background baseline release of cortisol. Synthesis of cortisol is governed by ACTH that is controlled by the hypothalamic hormones, corticotropin-releasing hormone and arginine vasopressin.

Synthetic Corticosteroids

Synthetic corticosteroids administered for their glucocorticoid effects include prednisolone, prednisone, methylprednisolone, betamethasone, dexamethasone, and triamcinolone (see Table 23-1) (Fig. 23-10). Fludrocortisone is a synthetic halogenated derivative of cortisol that is administered for its mineralocorticoid effect (see Table 23-1 and

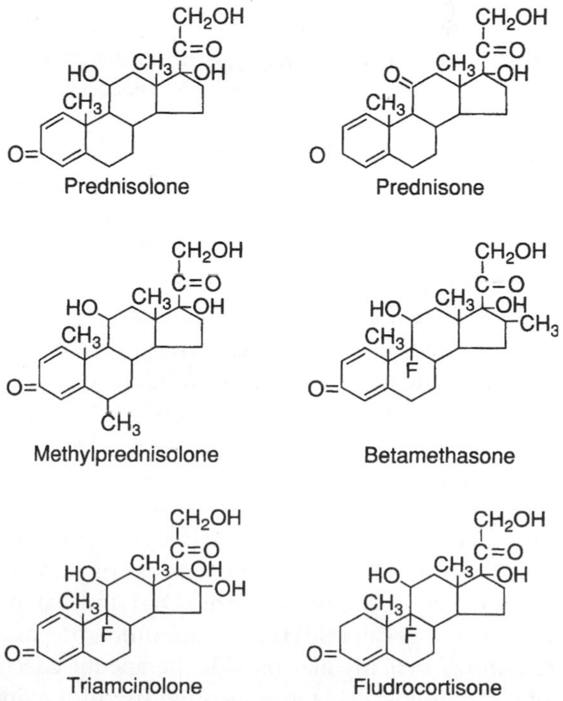

Figure 23-10. Synthetic corticosteroids.

Fig. 23-10). Naturally occurring corticosteroids, such as cortisol and cortisone, are also available as synthetic drugs (see Table 23-1 and Fig. 23-9).

Prednisolone

Prednisolone is an analogue of cortisol that is available as an oral or parenteral preparation. The antiinflammatory effect of 5 mg of prednisolone is equivalent to that of 20 mg of cortisol. This drug and prednisone are suitable for sole replacement therapy in adrenocortical insufficiency because of the presence of glucocorticoid and mineralocorticoid effects.

Prednisone

Prednisone is an analogue of cortisone that is available as an oral or parenteral preparation. It is rapidly converted to prednisolone after its absorption from the gastrointestinal tract. Its antiinflammatory effect and clinical uses are similar to those of prednisolone.

Methylprednisolone

Methylprednisolone is the methyl derivative of prednisolone. The antiinflammatory effect of 4 mg of methylprednisolone is equivalent to that of 20 mg of cortisol. The acetate preparation administered intraarticularly has a prolonged effect. Methylprednisolone succinate is highly soluble in water and is used IV to produce an intense glucocorticoid effect.

Betamethasone

Betamethasone is a fluorinated derivative of prednisolone. The antiinflammatory effect of 0.75 mg is equivalent to that of 20 mg of cortisol. Betamethasone lacks the mineralocorticoid properties of cortisol and thus is not acceptable for sole replacement therapy in adrenocortical insufficiency. Oral or parenteral administration is acceptable.

Dexamethasone

Dexamethasone is a fluorinated derivative of prednisolone and an isomer of betamethasone. The antiinflammatory effect of 0.75 mg is equivalent to that of 20 mg of cortisol. Oral and parenteral preparations are available. The acetate preparation is used as a long-acting repository suspension. Dexamethasone sodium phosphate is water soluble, rendering it appropriate for parenteral use. This corticosteroid is commonly chosen to treat certain types of cerebral edema.

Triamcinolone

Triamcinolone is a fluorinated derivative of prednisolone. The antiinflammatory effect of 4 mg is equivalent to that of 20 mg of cortisol. Triamcinolone has less mineralocorticoid effect than does prednisolone. Oral and parenteral preparations are available. The hexacetonide preparation injected intraarticularly may provide therapeutic effects for 3 months or longer. This drug is often used for epidural injections in the treatment of lumbar disc disease.

During the first days of treatment with triamcinolone, mild diuresis with sodium loss may occur. Conversely, edema may occur in patients with decreased glomerular filtration rates. Triamcinolone does not increase urinary potassium loss except when administered in large doses.

An unusual adverse side effect of triamcinolone is an increased incidence of skeletal muscle weakness. Likewise, anorexia rather than appetite stimulation, and sedation rather than euphoria may accompany administration of triamcinolone.

Clinical Uses

The only universally accepted clinical use of corticosteroids and their synthetic derivatives is as replacement therapy for deficiency states. With this exception, the use of corticosteroids in disease states is empirical and not curative, although antiinflammatory responses exert an intense palliative effect. The safety of corticosteroids is such that it is acceptable to administer a single large dose in a life-threatening situation on the presumption that unrecognized adrenal or pituitary insufficiency may be present.

Prednisolone or prednisone are recommended when an antiinflammatory effect is desired. The low mineralocorticoid potency of these drugs limits sodium and water retention when large doses are administered to produce the desired glucocorticoid effect. It must be recognized, however, that the antiinflammatory effect of corticosteroids is palliative, because the underlying cause of the response remains. Nevertheless, suppression of the inflammatory response may be life-saving in some situations. Conversely, masking of the symptoms of inflammation may delay diagnosis of life-threatening illness, such as peritonitis due to perforation of a peptic ulcer.

Deficiency States

Acute adrenal insufficiency requires electrolyte and fluid replacement as well as supplemental corticosteroids. Cortisol is administered at a rate of 100 mg IV every 8 hours after an initial injection of 100 mg. Management of chronic adrenal insufficiency in adults is with the daily oral administration of cortisone, 25.0 to 37.5 mg. A typical regimen is 25.0 mg in the morning and 12.5 mg in the late afternoon. This schedule mimics the normal diurnal cycle of adrenal secretion. An orally effective mineralocorticoid such as fludrocortisone, 0.1 to 0.3 mg daily, is required by most patients.

Allergic Therapy

Topical corticosteroids are capable of potent antiinflammatory effects and are the mainstay of allergic therapy. These medications interfere with the inflammatory response and multiple aspects of the allergic cascade. Unlike, antihistamines that provide pharmacologic effects within 1 to 2 hours, topical corticosteroids may require 3 to 5 days of treatment to produce a therapeutic effect. Corticosteroids work by inhibiting the production of inflammatory cytokines and chemokines, thus decreasing inflammation, cellular edema, and cellular recruitment to sites of disease. Oral administration of steroids is effective but the risk of unacceptable side effects with chronic treatment limits use by this route. Side effects, although possible with topical administration of corticosteroids, are usually not significant.

Asthma

Asthma is an inflammatory disease of the lungs and inhaled glucocorticoids (beclomethasone, triamcinolone, flunisolide) are often recommended as first-line therapy for controlling the symptoms of asthma and in preventing exacerbations (Barnes, 1995). Inhaled glucocorticoids are highly lipophilic and rapidly enter airway cells, where they have direct inhibitory effects on many of the cells involved in airway inflammation. One possible antiinflammatory mechanism is the modulation of the release of cytokines from inflammatory cells. For patients with mild asthma, one dose a day using a metered-dose inhaled may be sufficient, whereas four daily doses may be required in patients with severe asthma. It is estimated that 80% to 90% of the dose inhaled from the metered-dose inhaler is deposited in the oropharynx and swallowed. Inhaled glucocorticoids have oropharyngeal side effects that include dysphonia and candidiasis. Dysphonia occurs in approximately one-third of treated patients and may reflect myopathy of the laryngeal muscles that is reversible when treatment is stopped. Inhaled glucocorticoids, in doses of 1,500 μg per day or less in adults and 400 μg per day or less in children, have little if any effect on pituitary adrenal function.

Parenteral corticosteroids are important in the preoperative preparation of patients with reactive airway disease and in the treatment of intraoperative bronchospasm. Doses equivalent to 1 to 2 mg/kg of cortisol (or the equivalent dose of prednisolone) are commonly recommended. Preoperative corticosteroid administration 1 to 2 hours before induction of anesthesia is important because the beneficial effects of corticosteroids may not be fully manifest for several hours. Corticosteroids also enhance and prolong the responses to beta-adrenergic agonists. Some enhancement of beta-agonist effect may be present within 1 hour, but 4 to 6 hours are required for an antiinflammatory effect. In patients with bronchial hyperactivity, preoperative treatment with combined corticosteroids (40 mg orally for 5 days) and salbutamol (0.2 mg puffs for 5 days) but not salbutamol alone minimizes intubation-evoked bronchoconstriction (Silvanus et al., 2004).

Manifestations of allergic diseases that are of limited duration, such as hay fever, contact dermatitis, drug reactions, angioneurotic edema, and anaphylaxis, can be suppressed by adequate doses of corticosteroids. Life-threatening allergic reactions, however, must be treated with epinephrine, because the onset of the antiinflammatory effect produced by corticosteroids is delayed. Indeed, any beneficial effect of corticosteroids in the management of severe allergic reactions is probably related to suppression of the antiinflammatory response rather than to inhibition of production of immunoglobulins.

Antiemetic Effect

Dexamethasone prevents postoperative nausea and vomiting only when administered near the beginning of surgery, probably by reducing surgery-induced inflammation due to inhibition of prostaglandin synthesis (Wang et al., 2000). In addition, dexamethasone may exert antiemetic effects by increasing the release of endorphins resulting in mood elevation and appetite stimulation. Prophylactic administration of dexamethasone 4 mg, ondansetron 4 mg, or droperidol 1.25 mg produced similar decreases (about 26%) in the incidence of postoperative nausea and vomiting (Apfel et al., 2004). Because antiemetic interventions are similarly effective and act independently, it is recommended that the safest and least expensive antiemetic should be selected for prophylaxis. Prophylaxis is rarely warranted in low-risk patients, moderate-risk patients may benefit from a single intervention, and multiple interventions should be reserved for high-risk patients (Apfel et al., 2004). Rescue treatments are ineffective when the same drug has already been administered for prophylaxis. A suggested treatment strategy is to administer dexamethasone in conjunction with total intravenous anesthesia as first-line and second-line methods of prophylaxis against postoperative nausea and vomiting and to reserve serotonin antagonists as a rescue treatment (Apfel et al., 2004). Dexamethasone is also effective in suppressing chemotherapy-induced nausea and vomiting. The elimination half-time of dexamethasone is about 3 hours, but antiemetic effects, unlike other classes of antiemetics, often persist as long as 24 hours

Postoperative Analgesia

Glucocorticoids inhibit phospholipase enzyme that is necessary for the inflammatory chain reaction along both the cyclooxygenase and lipoxygenase pathways. As a result, glucocorticoids may be effective in decreasing postoperative pain but with a different side-effect profile than nonsteroidal antiinflammatory drugs. For example, administration of betamethasone 12 mg IM 30 minutes before induction of anesthesia for outpatient foot or hemorrhoid surgery, resulted in reductions in postoperative pain and the incidence of postoperative nausea and vomiting (Aasboe et al., 1998). Dexamethasone, 4 mg IV administered before the induction of anesthesia for anorectal surgery was associated with a shortened time to discharge from the ambulatory surgery unit (Coloma et al., 2001).

Cerebral Edema

Corticosteroids in large doses are of value in the reduction or prevention of cerebral edema and the resulting increases in intracranial pressure that may accompany intracranial tumors and metastatic lesions. There is no doubt about the benefit of corticosteroids in the treatment of cerebral edema resulting from global ischemic injury. Conversely, cerebral edema due to closed head injury is not predictably responsive to corticosteroids. Dexamethasone, with minimal mineralocorticoid activity, is frequently selected to decrease cerebral edema and associated increases in intracranial pressure.

Aspiration Pneumonitis

The use of corticosteroids in the treatment of aspiration pneumonitis is controversial. There is evidence in animals that corticosteroids administered immediately after the inhalation of acidic gastric fluid may be effective in decreasing pulmonary damage (Dudley and Marshall, 1974). Conversely, other data show no beneficial effect or suggest that the use of corticosteroids may enhance the likelihood of Gram-negative pneumonia (Downs et al., 1974; Wynne et al., 1981). Despite the absence of confirming evidence that corticosteroids are beneficial, it is not uncommon for the treatment of aspiration pneumonitis to include the empiric use of pharmacologic doses of these drugs.

Lumbar Disc Disease

An alternative to surgical treatment of lumbar disc disease is the epidural placement of corticosteroids (Haddox, 1992). Corticosteroids may decrease inflammation and edema of the nerve root that has resulted from compression. A common regimen is epidural injection of 25 to 50 mg of triamcinolone, or 40 to 80 mg of methylprednisolone, in a solution containing lidocaine at or near the interspace corresponding to the distribution of pain. In animals, the epidural injection of triamcinolone, 2 mg/kg, interferes with the ability of the adrenal cortex to release cortisol in response to hypoglycemia for 4 weeks. Injection of triamcinolone, 80 mg, into the lumbar epidural space of patients with lumbar disc disease results in acute suppression of plasma concentrations of ACTH and cortisol between 15 minutes (midazolam sedation) and 45 minutes (midazolam not administered) of corticosteroid injection (Kay et al., 1994). Median suppression of the HPA axis was <1 month and all patients had recovered by 3 months. Exogenous corticosteroid coverage during this potentially vulnerable period should be considered in patients undergoing major stress, especially if the adrenocortical response to ACTH is subnormal. Although epidural injections of methylprednisolone may result in short-term improvement of symptoms (pain, sensory loss) due to sciatic nerve compression from a herniated nucleus pulposus, this treatment offers no significant functional benefit nor does it decrease the need for surgery (Carette et al., 1997).

Immunosuppression

In organ transplantation, high doses of corticosteroids are often administered at the time of surgery to produce immunosuppression and decrease the risk of rejection of the newly transplanted organ. Smaller maintenance doses of corticosteroids are continued indefinitely, and the dosage is increased if rejection of the transplanted organ is threatened. Azathioprine is an antimetabolite that is used to suppress the immune system in recipients of organ transplants. Side effects associated with azathioprine include fever, rash, and acute idiosyncratic reactions characterized by life-threatening upper airway edema and cardiovascular collapse (Jungling and Shangraw, 2000).

Arthritis

The criterion for initiating corticosteroid therapy in patients with rheumatoid arthritis is progressive disability despite maximal medical therapy. Corticosteroids are administered in the smallest dose possible that provides significant but not complete symptomatic relief. The usual initial dose is prednisolone, 10 mg or its equivalent, in divided doses. Intraarticular injection of corticosteroids is recommended for treatment of episodic manifestations of acute joint inflammation associated with osteoarthritis. However, painless destruction of the joint is a risk of this treatment.

Collagen Diseases

Manifestations of collagen diseases, such as polymyositis, polyarteritis nodosa, and Wegener granulomatosis, but not scleroderma, are decreased and longevity is improved by corticosteroid therapy. Fulminating systemic lupus erythematosus is a life-threatening illness that is aggressively treated initially with large doses of prednisone, 1 mg/kg, or its equivalent. Large doses of corticosteroids are effective for inducing a remission of sarcoidosis. In temporal arteritis, corticosteroid therapy is necessary to prevent blindness, which occurs in about 20% of untreated patients. Some forms of nephrotic syndrome respond favorably to corticosteroids. Rheumatic carditis may be suppressed by large doses of corticosteroids.

Ocular Inflammation

Corticosteroids are used to suppress ocular inflammation (uveitis and iritis) and thus preserve sight. Instillation of corticosteroids into the conjunctival sac results in therapeutic concentrations in the aqueous humor. Topical corticosteroid therapy often increases intraocular pressure. For this reason, it is recommended that intraocular pressure be monitored when topical corticosteroids are used for >2 weeks. Corticosteroids are not recommended in herpes simplex infections (dendritic keratitis) of the eye. Topical corticosteroids should not be used for treatment of ocular abrasions, because delayed healing and infections may occur.

Cutaneous Disorders

Topical administration of corticosteroids is frequently effective in the treatment of skin diseases. Effectiveness is increased by application of the corticosteroid as an ointment under an occlusive dressing. Systemic absorption is also occasionally enhanced to the degree that suppression of the HPA axis occurs or manifestations of Cushing syndrome appear. Corticosteroids may also be administered systemically for treatment of severe episodes of acute skin disorders and exacerbations of chronic disorders.

Postintubation Laryngeal Edema

Treatment of postintubation laryngeal edema may include administration of corticosteroids, such as dexamethasone, 0.1 to 0.2 mg/kg IV. Nevertheless, the efficacy of corticosteroids for treatment of this condition has not been confirmed. Dexamethasone, 0.6 mg/kg orally is an effective treatment for children with mild croup (Bjornson et al., 2004).

Ulcerative Colitis

Corticosteroid therapy is indicated in selected patients with chronic ulcerative colitis. A disadvantage of this therapy is that signs and symptoms of intestinal perforation and peritonitis may be masked.

Myasthenia Gravis

Corticosteroids are usually reserved for patients with myasthenia gravis who are unresponsive to medical or surgical therapy. These drugs seem to be most effective after thymectomy. The mechanism of beneficial effects produced by corticosteroids is not known but may reflect drug-induced suppression of the production of an immunoglobulin that normally binds to the neuromuscular junction.

Respiratory Distress Syndrome

Administration of corticosteroids at least 24 hours before delivery decreases the incidence and severity of respiratory distress syndrome in neonates born between 24 and 36 weeks' gestation. Dexamethasone administered for prolonged periods (42 days) improves pulmonary and neurodevelopmental outcome of low-birth-weight infants at risk for bronchopulmonary dysplasia (Cummings et al., 1989).

Leukemia

The antilymphocytic effects of glucocorticoids are used to advantage in combination chemotherapy of acute lymphocytic leukemia and lymphomas, including Hodgkin disease and multiple myeloma. For example, prednisone and vincristine produce remissions in about 90% of children with lymphoblastic leukemia.

Cardiac Arrest

Glucocorticoids have been given to patients after global brain ischemia. This practice is based on the well-established benefit of these drugs in the treatment of perifocal vasogenic edema around an intrinsic mass. Nevertheless, the value of glucocorticoids in the treatment of intracellular cytotoxic edema, as is thought to occur after global ischemia, is unproved. Indeed, glucocorticoids have not been shown to improve survival or neurologic recovery rate after cardiac arrest, and their administration to these patients is not recommended (Jastremski et al., 1989).

Side Effects

The side effects of chronic corticosteroid therapy include (a) suppression of the HPA axis, (b) electrolyte and metabolic changes, (c) osteoporosis, (d) peptic ulcer disease, (e) skeletal muscle myopathy, (f) central nervous system dysfunction, (g) peripheral blood changes, and (h) inhibition of normal growth. Increased susceptibility to bacterial or fungal infection accompanies treatment with corticosteroids. Corticosteroid administration is associated with greater clearance of salicylates and decreased effectiveness of anticoagulants. Systemic corticosteroids used for short periods of time (<7 days) even at high doses are unlikely to cause adverse side effects. Inhaled corticosteroids are unlikely to evoke adverse systemic effects.

Suppression of the Hypothalamic-Pituitary-Adrenal Axis

The HPA is a hormonal circuit consisting of the hypothalamus in the brain, the pituitary gland and adrenal glands. This circuit is responsible for production of glucocorticoids (principally cortisol) that are critical to maintenance of homeostasis during physical and emotional stress. Corticosteroid therapy, including epidural administration used to treat lumbar disc disease, may result in suppression of the HPA axis, with the result that release of cortisol in response to stress, such as that produced by surgery, is blunted or does not occur. It is not possible to define the precise dose of corticosteroid or duration of therapy that will produce suppression of the HPA axis in a given patient, because there is marked variation among patients. Typically, however, the larger the dose and the more prolonged the therapy, the greater the likelihood of suppression. When appropriate, a dose of corticosteroid administered every other day is less likely to suppress the anterior pituitary release of ACTH than is the daily administration. Inhaled glucocorticoids used to treat asthma are not likely to suppress the HPA axis.

Corticosteroid Supplementation

Corticosteroid supplementation should be increased whenever the patient being treated for chronic hypoadrenocorticism undergoes a surgical procedure. This recommendation is based on the concern that these patients are susceptible to cardiovascular collapse because they cannot release additional endogenous cortisol in response to the stress of surgery. More controversial is the management of patients who may manifest suppression of the HAP axis because of current or previous administration of corticosteroids for treatment of a disease unrelated to pituitary or adrenal function. Recommendations that prescribe supraphysiologic doses have been advocated despite the absence of supporting scientific data (Salem et al., 1994). In adrenalectomized primates undergoing general anesthesia and surgery, the animals receiving physiologic replacement doses of cortisol were indistinguishable from those receiving supraphysiologic doses (10 times the normal production rate) of cortisol (Udelsman et al., 1986). Subphysiologically treated animals (one-tenth the normal production rate) were hemodynamically unstable during surgery and had a significantly higher mortality rate. Based on these animal data, it was concluded that there is no advantage in supraphysiologic glucocorticoid prophylaxis during surgical stress, and replacement doses of cortisol equivalent to the daily unstressed cortisol production rate are sufficient to allow homeostatic mechanisms to function during surgery (Udelsman et al., 1986).

A rational regimen for corticosteroid supplementation in the perioperative period is the administration of cortisol, 25 mg IV, at the induction of anesthesia followed by a continuous infusion of cortisol, 100 mg, during the following 24 hours (Symreng et al., 1981). This approach maintains the plasma concentration of cortisol above normal during major surgery in patients receiving chronic treatment with corticosteroids and manifesting a subnormal response to the preoperative infusion of ACTH (Fig. 23-11) (Symreng et al., 1981). In those instances in which events such as burns or sepsis could exaggerate the need for exogenous corticosteroid supplementation, the continuous infusion of cortisol, 100 mg every 12 hours, should be sufficient. Indeed, endogenous cortisol production during stress introduced by major surgery or extensive burns is not >150 mg daily (Hardy and Turner, 1957; Hume et al., 1962). It is likely that patients undergoing minor operations will need minimal to no additional corticosteroid coverage during the perioperative period.

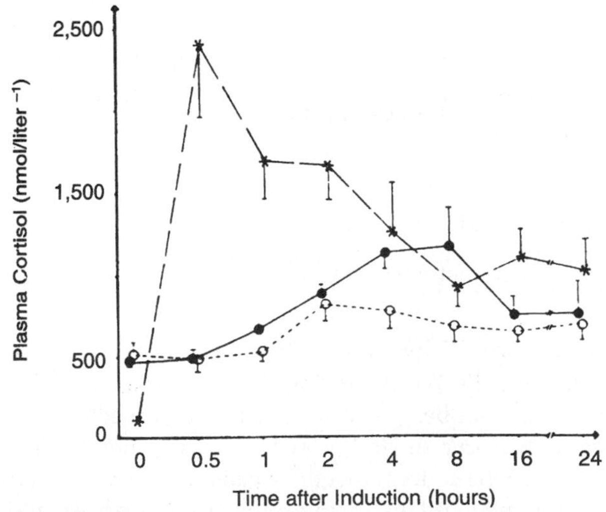

Figure 23-11. Administration of cortisol, 25 mg IV, plus a continuous infusion of 100 mg over 24 hours, maintains the plasma cortisol concentration above normal in patients (*) receiving chronic treatment with corticosteroids and manifesting a subnormal response to the preoperative infusion of adrenocorticotropic hormone. (From Symreng T, Karlberg BE, Kagedal B, et al. Physiological cortisol substitution of long-term steroid-treated patients undergoing major surgery. *Br J Anesth* 1981;53:949–953; with permission.)

An alternative glucocorticoid supplementation regimen is based on the magnitude of the planned surgical procedure (Salem et al., 1994). For minor surgical stress (inguinal hernia repair), the daily cortisol secretion rate and static plasma cortisol measurements suggest that the glucocorticoid requirement is about 25 mg of cortisol. If the postoperative course is uncomplicated, the patient can be returned the next day to the prior glucocorticoid maintenance dose. For moderate surgical stress (nonlaparoscopic cholecystectomy, colon resection, total hip replacement), cortisol production rates suggest the glucocorticoid requirement is about 50 to 75 mg daily of cortisol for 1 to 2 days. For major surgical stress (pancreatoduodenectomy, esophagectomy, cardiopulmonary bypass), the glucocorticoid dose should be 100 to 150 mg of cortisol daily for 2 to 3 days. Even with this coverage, vascular collapse has been described in a patient experiencing massive hemorrhage during surgery (Ratner et al., 1996). It is known that after uncomplicated major surgery, the plasma cortisol concentrations decrease rapidly. The circulating plasma cortisol concentrations are normal by 24 to 48 hours after surgical stress in most patients.

In addition to IV supplementation with cortisol, patients receiving daily maintenance doses of a corticosteroid should also receive this dose with the preoperative medication on the day of surgery. There is no objective evidence to support increasing the maintenance dose of corticosteroid preoperatively.

Electrolyte and Metabolic Changes

Hypokalemic metabolic alkalosis reflects mineralocorticoid effects of corticosteroids on distal renal tubules, leading to enhanced absorption of sodium and loss of potassium. Edema and weight gain accompany this corticosteroid effect.

Corticosteroids inhibit the use of glucose in peripheral tissues and promote hepatic gluconeogenesis. The resulting corticosteroid-induced hyperglycemia can usually be managed with diet, insulin, or both. The dose requirement for oral hypoglycemics may be increased by corticosteroids.

There is a redistribution of body fat characterized by deposition of fat in the back of the neck (buffalo hump), supraclavicular area, and face (moon facies) and loss of fat from the extremities. The mechanism by which corticosteroids elicit this redistribution of fat is not known.

Peripherally, corticosteroids mobilize amino acids from tissues. This catabolic effect manifests as decreased skeletal muscle mass, osteoporosis, thinning of the skin, and a negative nitrogen balance.

Osteoporosis

Osteoporosis, vertebral compression fractures, and rib fractures are common and serious complications of corticosteroid therapy that can be found in patients of all ages.

Corticosteroids appear to inhibit the activities of osteoblasts and stimulate osteoclasts by inhibition of calcium absorption from the gastrointestinal tract, which causes an increased secretion of parathyroid hormone. Osteoporosis is an indication for withdrawal of corticosteroid therapy. Evidence of osteoporosis should be sought on radiographs of the spines of patients being treated chronically with corticosteroids. The presence of osteoporosis could predispose patients to fractures during positioning in the operating room. Bisphosphonates are effective in decreasing vertebral fractures in patients taking corticosteroids (O'Dell, 2004).

Peptic Ulcer Disease

Although a cause-and-effect relationship has not been proved, the incidence of peptic ulcer disease seems to be increased by chronic corticosteroid therapy. Indeed, corticosteroids may decrease the normal protective barrier provided by gastric mucus.

Skeletal Muscle Myopathy

Skeletal muscle myopathy characterized by weakness of the proximal musculature is occasionally observed in patients taking large doses of corticosteroids. In some patients, this skeletal muscle weakness is so severe that ambulation is not possible and corticosteroid therapy must be discontinued.

Central Nervous System Dysfunction

Corticosteroid therapy is associated with an increased incidence of neuroses and psychoses. Behavioral changes include manic depression and suicidal tendencies. Cataracts develop in almost all patients who receive prednisone, 20 mg daily, or its equivalent for 4 years.

Peripheral Blood Changes

Corticosteroids tend to increase the hematocrit and number of circulating leukocytes. Conversely, a single dose of cortisol decreases by almost 70%—the number of circulating lymphocytes, and by more than 90%—the number of circulating monocytes in 4 to 6 hours. This acute lymphocytopenia most likely reflects sequestration from the blood rather than destruction of cells.

Inhibition of Normal Growth

Inhibition or arrest of growth can result from the administration of relatively small doses of glucocorticoids to children. The mechanism of this effect is presumed to be the generalized inhibitory effect of glucocorticoids on DNA synthesis and cell division.

Inhibitors of Corticosteroid Synthesis

Metyrapone

Metyrapone decreases cortisol secretion by inhibition of the 11-beta-hydroxylation reaction, resulting in accumulation of 11-deoxycortisol. Metyrapone may induce acute adrenal insufficiency in patients with decreased adrenocortical function. A deficiency of mineralocorticoids does not occur, because metyrapone-induced inhibition of 11-beta-hydroxylation results in increased production of the mineralocorticoid 11-desoxycorticosterone.

Metyrapone has been used to treat excessive adrenocortical function that results from adrenal neoplasms that function autonomously or as a result of ectopic production of ACTH by tumors.

Aminoglutethimide

Aminoglutethimide inhibits the conversion of cholesterol to 20-alpha-hydroxycholesterol, which interrupts production of both cortisol and aldosterone. Thus, this drug is effective in decreasing the excessive secretion of cortisol in autonomously functioning adrenal tumors and in hypersecretion resulting from ectopic production of ACTH.

NONSTEROID DRUGS THAT PRODUCE IMMUNOSUPPRESSION

Nonsteroid drugs are commonly administered to decrease the immune response and associated rejection of newly transplanted organs. Treatment of rheumatoid arthritis may include drugs that interfere with the inflammatory response at the site of injury.

Cyclosporine

Cyclosporine is a metabolite produced by the fungus *Tolpolcadium inflatum gams*. The drug selectively inhibits helper T lymphocyte-mediated immune responses by blocking the transcription of cytokine genes while not affecting B lymphocytes. Cyclosporine binds and inhibits calmodulin, an intracytoplasmic protein, that is involved in calcium-mediated activities and is required for activation of T cells. Use of this immunosuppressant drug in combination with corticosteroids has greatly increased the success of organ transplantation. Cyclosporine must be administered before T lymphocytes undergo proliferation as a result of exposure to specific antigens presented by organ transplantation. Cyclosporine is primarily eliminated by metabolism by cytochrome P-450 enzymes in the liver and wall of the gastrointestinal tract with $<1\%$ excreted unchanged in the urine.

Pharmacokinetics

Cyclosporine has a narrow therapeutic range with adverse clinical consequences accompanying either underdosing or overdosing. A correlation exists between cyclosporine blood levels and acute rejection. Monitoring of cyclosporine blood concentrations is important to determine the optimum therapeutic doses in each patient (Kahan et al., 1996). Drugs inhibiting or inducing P-450 activity may alter cyclosporine blood concentrations. For example, ketoconazole and diltiazem allow decreases in the dose of cyclosporine whereas P-450 inhibitors such as rifampicin and anticonvulsants can significantly decrease cyclosporine blood concentrations.

Side Effects

Nephrotoxicity is the most important adverse effect, occurring in 25% to 38% of patients treated with cyclosporine. For this reason, it is recommended that renal function tests be performed regularly during therapy. In renal transplant patients, it may be difficult to differentiate cyclosporine nephrotoxicity from acute rejection reactions. Nonsteroidal antiinflammatory drugs are avoided in cyclosporine-treated patients because the combination could precipitate renal failure. Cyclosporine-induced hypertension associated with activation of the sympathetic nervous system and resulting renal and systemic vasoconstriction often requires medical therapy, especially in heart transplant patients (Scherrer et al., 1990). Limb paresthesias occur in about 50% of patients. Although cyclosporine is not believed to cross the blood–brain barrier, there is significant incidence of headache, confusion, and somnolence. Seizures of new onset may be triggered by cyclosporine therapy. The use of cyclosporine almost doubles the incidence of cholestasis with hyperbilirubinemia and elevation of liver transaminase in renal transplant recipients. Rarely, patients have experienced allergic reactions to cyclosporine. Other side effects include gingival hyperplasia, hirsutism, and hyperglycemia. To avoid interactions with plasticizers in infusion bags, cyclosporine is dispensed from glass bottles.

Tacrolimus

Tacrolimus is a potent immunosuppressant with a 10- to 100-fold greater activity compared with cyclosporine. The clinical efficacy of tacrolimus is similar to cyclosporine and both drugs are equally nephrotoxic. Compared with cyclosporine, tacrolimus induces less systemic hypertension.

Disease-Modifying Antirheumatic Drugs

Rheumatoid arthritis is an autoimmune disease that affects approximately 1% of the population. Production of cytokines are central to the damaging cascade that ultimately damages synovial joints. Drugs that act as immunomodulators are available for the treatment of rheumatoid arthritis. Methotrexate remains the most commonly used disease-modifying antirheumatic drug but newer drugs may serve as useful alternatives (Table 23-2) (Olsen and Stein, 2004) (see Chapter 29).

Leflunomide

Leflunomide inhibits pyrimidine synthesis by acting as a competitive inhibitor of intracellular enzyme, dihydroorotate dehydrogenase. Pyrimidines are responsible for proliferative effects associated with rheumatoid arthritis. Leflunomide is a prodrug that undergoes conversion following oral absorption to its active metabolite, A77 1726 which is highly protein bound and has an elimination half-time of about 14 days.

Side Effects

This drug inhibits cytochrome P-450 and may increase the anticoagulant effect of warfarin, whereas rifampin increases the plasma concentration of leflunomide. The most significant side effect of treatment with leflunomide is hepatic dysfunction associated with increases in plasma concentrations of transaminase enzymes in 2% to 4% of the patients. The risk of severe liver injury is small and considering the benefits of the treatment are considered acceptable. Nevertheless,

TABLE 23-2.
DISEASE-MODIFYING ANTIRHEUMATIC DRUGS

Drug	Mechanism of Action	Route of Administration	Elimination Half-Time	Monitoring Recommendation
Leflunomide	Inhibits pyrimidine synthesis	Oral	14 days	Baseline blood count and enzymes and then monthly until stable and then every 2 to 3 months
Etanercept	Binds tumor necrosis factor	Subcutaneous	96 hours	Be alert for infections (tuberculosis, histoplasmosis)
Adalimumab	Human anti-tumor necrosis factor antibody	Subcutaneous	14 days	As for etanercept
Infliximab	Chimeric anti-tumor necrosis factor antibody	Intravenous	9 days	As for etanercept
Anakinra	Interleukin-1 receptor antagonist	Subcutaneous	6 hours	Baseline blood count and then monthly for 3 months and every 3 months thereafter

Adapted from Olsen NJ, Stein CM. New drugs for rheumatoid arthritis. *N Engl J Med* 2004;350:2167–2169.

this drug is not recommended for administration to patients with known liver disease. Monitoring of systemic blood pressure is indicated as new hypertension may be associated with initiation of leflunomide treatment. Reversible alopecia, peripheral neuropathy, pancytopenia, and interstitial pneumonitis may also occur. Leflunomide is teratogenic in animals and given the long elimination half-time of this drug it is necessary to discontinue leflunomide in advance of considering conception.

Tumor Necrosis Factor Antagonists (Etanercept, Adalimumab, Infliximab)

Tumor necrosis factor (TNF) antagonists are among the most effective treatments available for patients with rheumatoid arthritis (Table 23-2) (Olsen and Stein, 2004). The response is typically rapid occurring within a few weeks of initiating therapy. TNF antagonists should not be initiated in the presence of active infection and must be discontinued if an acute infection develops.

Adverse events that accompany TNF-antagonists include infections (tuberculosis, histoplasmosis, *Pneumocystitis carinii* pneumonia), cancer (lymphoma), multiple sclerosis-like demyelinating diseases, lupus-like autoimmune disease, liver dysfunction, aplastic anemia, aseptic meningitis, and allergic reactions.

Adalimumab is a recombinant human immunoglobulin monoclonal antibody that binds to TNF-alpha resulting in impaired cytokine binding to its receptors and lysis of cells that express TNF-alpha.

Anakinra

Anakinra is a recombinant form of human interleukin-1-receptor antagonist that targets type-1 interleukin receptors that are expressed in many tissues. Interleukin-1 concentrations are increased in inflamed joints associated with rheumatoid arthritis. Elimination of anakinra is by the kidneys and the dose must be decreased in patients with renal dysfunction. The most common side effect is skin irritation at the injection site. The risk of bacterial infections may be increased but opportunistic infections do not seem to occur.

MELATONIN

Melatonin (*N*-acetyl-5-methoxytryptamine) is the principal substance secreted by the pineal gland (Fig. 23-12) (Brzezinski, 1997). The mammalian pineal gland is a neuroendocrine transducer. Photic information from the retina is transmitted to the pineal gland through the suprachiasmatic nucleus of the hypothalamus and the sympathetic nervous system. The neural input to the gland is norepinephrine and the output is melatonin. The synthesis and release of melatonin are stimulated by darkness and inhibited by light. As the synthesis of melatonin increases, the hormone enters the bloodstream through passive diffusion.

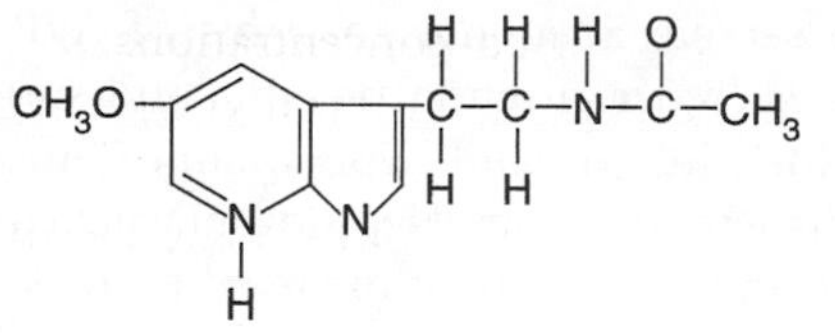

Figure 23-12. Melatonin.

Melatonin is rapidly metabolized, chiefly in the liver, by hydroxylation to 6-hydroxymelatonin, and, after conjugation with sulfuric or glucuronic acid, is excreted in the urine. IV melatonin is rapidly distributed, and the elimination half-time is 0.5 to 5.6 minutes. The bioavailability of orally administered melatonin varies widely.

Dose-dependent physiologic effects of melatonin include biologic regulation of circadian rhythms, sleep, mood, and perhaps reproduction, tumor growth, and aging (Brzezinski, 1997). In humans, the circadian rhythm for the release of melatonin from the pineal gland is closely synchronized with the habitual hours of sleep. Alterations in synchronization due to phase shifts (acute change in time zones or working hours) are correlated with sleep disturbances. Ingestion of melatonin affects the speed of falling asleep as well as the duration and quality of sleep and has hypnotic effects. The circadian cycle of body temperature is linked to the 24-hour cycle of subjective sleepiness and inversely related to serum melatonin concentrations. Nevertheless, sleep-promoting doses of melatonin do not have any effect on body temperature. It is unclear whether the beneficial effect of exogenous melatonin on symptoms of jet lag are due to a hypnotic effect or resynchronization of the circadian rhythm.

POSTERIOR PITUITARY HORMONES

Arginine vasopressin (AVP) (formerly known as antidiureitc hormone, ADH) and oxytocin are the two principal hormones secreted by the posterior pituitary. The target sites for AVP are the renal-collecting ducts, where this hormone acts to increase permeability of cell membranes to water. As a result, water is passively reabsorbed from renal-collecting ducts into extracellular fluid. Nonrenal actions of AVP include intense arterial vasoconstriction (stimulates vascular V1a receptors), accounting for its alternative designation as vasopressin. Oxytocin elicits contractions of the uterus, which are indistinguishable from those that occur in spontaneous labor.

Arginine Vasopressin

AVP and its congeners (desmopressin, lypressin) are useful in the treatment of diabetes insipidus that results from inadequate secretion of the hormone by the posterior pituitary.

Failure to secrete adequate amounts of AVP results in polyuria and hypernatremia. Trauma and surgery in the region of the pituitary and hypothalamus are recognized causes of diabetes insipidus. Nephrogenic diabetes insipidus resulting from an inability of the renal tubules to respond to adequate amounts of centrally produced AVP does not respond to exogenous administration of the hormone or its congeners.

The oral hypoglycemic chlorpropamide sensitizes renal tubules to the effects of low circulating concentrations of AVP, accounting for its beneficial effects in patients with diabetes insipidus. Inhibition of prostaglandin production produced by chlorpropamide may be responsible for increased sensitivity of the renal tubules to AVP. This drug is not effective in the treatment of nephrogenic diabetes insipidus. A high incidence of hypoglycemic reactions detracts from the therapeutic value of chlorpropamide in the treatment of diabetes insipidus. Acetaminophen and indomethacin probably enhance the effects of AVP by a similar inhibitory effect on the synthesis of prostaglandins. Clofibrate may directly stimulate secretion of AVP by the posterior pituitary, leading to a significant antidiuretic action in patients with diabetes insipidus. The combination of clofibrate with chlorpropamide may produce an additive effect, emphasizing the speculated differences in mechanism of action of these drugs. Thiazide diuretics exert a paradoxical antidiuretic action in patients with nephrogenic diabetes insipidus and serve as the only drugs effective in the treatment of this disorder.

Inappropriate and excessive secretion of AVP with subsequent retention of water and dilutional hyponatremia may occur in patients with head injuries, intracranial tumors, meningitis, and pulmonary infections. Aberrant production of AVP is observed most commonly in patients with cancer, especially oat cell carcinoma, in which the tumor itself produces AVP. In these patients, the antibiotic demeclocycline promotes diuresis by antagonizing the effects of AVP on renal tubules.

Vasopressin

Vasopressin is the exogenous preparation of AVP used for (a) treatment of AVP-sensitive diabetes insipidus, (b) evaluation of the urine-concentrating abilities of the kidneys after administration of fluorinated volatile anesthetics, (c) management of uncontrolled hemorrhage from esophageal varices, (d) hemodynamic stabilization in the presence of hemorrhagic and septic shock, and (e) management of refractory cardiac arrest. This drug is not effective in the management of patients with nephrogenic diabetes insipidus.

Diabetes Insipidus

Vasopressin administered IV is used for the initial evaluation of patients with suspected diabetes insipidus, which may follow head trauma or hypophysectomy. Under these circumstances, polyuria may be transient, and a longer antidiuretic effect (1 to 3 days) as produced by IM vasopressin tannate in oil could produce water intoxication. Oral administration of vasopressin is followed by rapid inactivation by trypsin, which cleaves a peptide linkage. Likewise, IV administration of vasopressin results in a brief effect because of rapid enzymatic breakdown of peptides in the tissues, especially the kidneys.

Esophageal Varicies

Vasopressin may serve as an adjunct in the control of bleeding esophageal varices and during abdominal surgery in patients with cirrhosis and portal hypertension. Infusion of 20 units over 5 minutes results in marked decreases in hepatic blood flow lasting about 30 minutes. Only a moderate increase in systemic blood pressure occurs. This effect on the portal circulation is attributable to marked splanchnic vasoconstriction. An alternative to systemic administration is the infusion of vasopressin directly into the superior mesenteric artery. It has not been established whether selective arterial administration is safer than systemic administration with respect to cardiac and vascular side effects.

Refractory Cardiac Arrest

Vasopressin is an alternative to epinephrine for vasopressor therapy during cardiopulmonary resuscitation. Vasopressin 40 units IV was similar to epinephrine 1 mg IV for managment of ventricular fibrillation and pulseless electrical activity. Vasopressin was more effective than epinephrine for management of asystole and the treatment of refractory cardiac arrest (Wenzel et al., 2004). The American Heart Association recommends that vasopressin, at a one-time only dose of 40 units IV be considered instead of epinephrine 1 mg IV every 3 to 5 minutes for patients who are being treated for cardiac arrest. Vasopressin functions as a vasoconstrictor when it is administered in supraphysiologic doses which serves to displace peripheral blood volume to the central circulation without some of the adverse effects produced by epinephrine. This drug needs to only be administered once during cardiopulmonary resuscitation because of its 10 to 20 minute elimination half-time.

Hemorrhagic and Septic Shock

Catecholamine-resistant hypotension is a complication of septic shock and severe multiple-organ dysfunction syndrome. Excess generation of nitric oxide and vasodilatory prostaglandins may contribute to progressive loss of vascular tone. Vasopressin infusion is effective in reversing systemic hypotension in catecholamine-resistant septic shock (Dunser et al., 2001). Vasopressin has been effective in treating hypotension owing to anaphylaxis and to severe catecholamine deficiency owing to resection of a pheochromocytoma (Augoustides et al., 2004; Schummer et al., 2004).

Vasopressin administered during cardiac arrest and hemorrhagic shock may improve vital organ blood flow during cardiopulmonary resuscitation and stabilize cardiocirculatory function after successful resuscitation (Voelckel et al., 2000).

Side Effects

Vasoconstriction and increased systemic blood pressure occur only with doses of vasopressin that are much larger than those administered for the treatment of diabetes insipidus. This response is because of a direct and generalized effect on vascular smooth muscles that is not antagonized by denervation or adrenergic-blocking drugs. Facial pallor due to cutaneous vasoconstriction may also accompany large doses of vasopressin. The magnitude of increase in systemic blood pressure caused by vasopressin depends, to some extent, on the reactivity of the baroreceptor reflexes. For example, when baroreceptor reflexes are depressed by anesthesia, smaller amounts of vasopressin are capable of evoking a pressor response. Pulmonary artery pressures are also increased by vasopressin.

Vasopressin, even in small doses, may produce selective vasoconstriction of the coronary arteries, with decreases in coronary blood flow manifesting as angina pectoris, electrocardiographic evidence of myocardial ischemia, and, in some instances, myocardial infarction. Ventricular cardiac dysrhythmias may accompany these cardiac effects.

Large doses of vasopressin stimulate gastrointestinal smooth muscle, and the resulting increased peristalsis may manifest as abdominal pain, nausea, and vomiting. Smooth muscle of the uterus is also stimulated by large doses of vasopressin.

A decrease in platelet count has been attributed to AVP-mediated platelet aggregation via V_1 receptors (Dunser et al., 2004). AVP infusion in advanced vasodilatory shock does not increase plasma concentrations of Factor VIII, von Willebrand factor antigen and ristocetin co-factor. Allergic reactions ranging from urticaria to anaphylaxis may occasionally follow the administration of vasopressin. Prolonged use of vasopressin may result in antibody formation and a shortened duration of action of the drug.

Desmopressin

Desmopressin (DDAVP) is a synthetic analogue of AVP with an intense antidiuretic (V_2) effect and decreased pressor (V_1) effect. Through its V_2 effects, DDAVP also causes endothelial cells to release von Willebrand factor, tissue-type plasminogen activator, and prostaglandins. The elimination half-time of DDAVP is 2.5 to 4.4 hours (Horrow, 1990). There are fewer side effects produced by DDAVP than are associated with vasopressin, although nausea and increases in systemic blood pressure can occur.

Administered intranasally twice daily, using a calibrated catheter (Rhinyle), DDAVP is the drug of choice in the treatment of diabetes insipidus due to inadequate production of AVP by the posterior pituitary. DDAVP, like all the AVP analogues, is not effective in the treatment of nephrogenic diabetes insipidus. Increased release of von Willebrand factor accounts for the hemostatic activity of DDAVP in patients with uremia, chronic liver disease, and certain types of hemophilia by promoting platelet adhesiveness to the vascular endothelium. DDAVP has also been reported to minimize intraoperative blood loss in patients undergoing cardiac surgery with cardiopulmonary bypass, whereas other reports find no effect on blood loss in patients undergoing cardiac surgery or spinal fusion surgery (Frankville et al., 1991; Guay et al., 1992; Mongan and Hosking, 1992). Desmopressin does not decrease bleeding following cardiopulmonary bypass in patients who were maintained on aspirin therapy until the day before surgery (Pleym et al., 2004). DDAVP administered IV may decrease systemic vascular resistance leading to hypotension (Frankville et al., 1991).

Lypressin

Lypressin is a synthetic analogue of AVP that produces antidiuresis for about 4 hours after intranasal administration. Its short duration of action limits its usefulness in the treatment of diabetes insipidus.

Oxytocin

Oxytocin, along with ergot derivatives and certain prostaglandins, is sufficiently selective in its stimulation of uterine smooth muscle to be clinically useful.

Clinical Uses

The principal clinical uses of oxytocin are to induce labor at term and to counter uterine hypotonicity and decrease hemorrhage in the postpartum or postabortion period.

For induction of labor, a continuous infusion is preferred, because the low dose of oxytocin needed can be precisely controlled. Indeed, the sensitivity of the uterus to oxytocin increases as pregnancy progresses. To induce labor, a dilute solution (10 mU/mL) is administered by a constant infusion pump beginning at 1 to 2 mU per minute. This infusion rate is increased 1 to 2 mU per minute every 15 to 30 minutes until an optimal response (uterine contraction every 2 to 3 minutes) is obtained. The average dose of oxytocin to induce labor is 8 to 10 mU per minute. Infusion rates up to 40 mU per minute of oxytocin may be necessary to treat uterine atony initially after delivery. IM injections of oxytocin are commonly used to provide sustained uterine contractions in the postpartum period.

All preparations of oxytocin used clinically are synthetic, and their potency is described in units. These synthetic preparations are identical to the hormone normally released from the posterior pituitary, but devoid of contamination by other polypeptide hormones and proteins found in natural proteins.

Side Effects

High doses of oxytocin produce a direct relaxant effect on vascular smooth muscles that manifests as a decrease in systolic and diastolic blood pressure and the appearance of flushing. Reflex tachycardia and increased cardiac output accompany the transient decrease in systemic blood pressure. The amounts of oxytocin administered for most obstetric purposes are inadequate to produce marked alterations in systemic blood pressure. A marked decrease in blood pressure, however, may occur if oxytocin is administered to patients with blunted compensatory reflex responses, as may be produced by anesthesia. Likewise, hypovolemic patients may be particularly susceptible to oxytocin-induced hypotension.

In the past, oxytocin preparations were often contaminated with ergot alkaloids, resulting in exaggerated systemic blood pressure increases when administered to patients previously treated with a sympathomimetic. Modern synthetic commercial preparations are pure oxytocin and do not introduce the risk of exaggerated vasoconstriction when administered in the presence of a sympathomimetic drug.

Oxytocin exhibits a slight AVP-like activity when administered in high doses, introducing the possibility of water intoxication if an excessive volume of fluid is administered. The risk of this complication can be minimized by infusion of oxytocin in an electrolyte-containing solution rather than glucose in water.

Ergot Derivatives

Ergot is the product of a fungus that grows on grain. Ingestion of contaminated grain results in generalized and intense vasoconstriction, reflecting the peripheral vascular effects of ergot alkaloids. The ergot alkaloids, ergotamine and ergonovine, are derivatives of 6-methylergoline. Hydrolysis of ergonine yields lysergic acid diethylamide and methylergonovine. Methysergide is formed by the addition of a methyl group to the indole nitrogen of methylergonovine.

Clinical Uses

All the natural alkaloids of ergot produce dose-related increases in the motor activity of the uterus. The sustained increase of resting uterine tone produced by high doses of ergot precludes its use for induction of labor but increases its value in the postpartum or postabortion period to control bleeding and maintain uterine contraction. Ergonovine is less toxic and produces a more rapid uterine response than ergotamine. For these reasons, ergonovine and its semisynthetic derivative methylergonovine have replaced other ergot derivatives. Ergonovine and methylergonovine are rapidly absorbed after oral or IM (0.2 mg) administration, producing a uterotonic action within about 10 minutes that lasts 3 to 6 hours. Administered IV (0.2 mg), uterine contraction occurs within 30 to 45 seconds. The uterine-stimulating effects of these drugs most likely reflect interactions with specific receptors.

Ergotamine may be effective in relieving migraine headaches. This beneficial effect may be due to ergotamine-induced constriction of dilated cerebral blood vessels, particularly in the meningeal branches of the external carotid artery. In addition to decreasing cerebral blood flow, ergotamine decreases hyperperfusion of regions supplied by the basilar artery and decreases shunting of blood via arteriovenous anastomoses. Caffeine increases approximately twofold the absorption of ergotamine after oral administration. Metabolism is almost complete, as emphasized by minimal recovery of unchanged drug in the urine. Storage in the tissues probably accounts for prolonged therapeutic and toxic effects, despite an elimination half-time of about 2 hours. Other types of headache are not improved and may even be aggravated by ergotamine.

Ergoloid is the combination of three ergot alkaloids (dihydroergocristine, dihydroergocomine, and dihydroergocryptine [as the mesylates]) that may provide symptomatic relief in some elderly patients manifesting changes of idiopathic mental decline (Alzheimer's disease). Improvement in cognitive and emotional symptoms is presumed to reflect a drug-induced effect on cerebral metabolism and not a direct cerebrovascular action. After oral administration, the elimination half-time of ergoloid is about 4 hours. Side effects of treatment with ergoloid include nausea, vomiting, and gastric irritation. Sinus bradycardia occasionally occurs. A sublingual preparation of ergoloid may produce local tissue irritation.

Side Effects

Ergonovine and methylergonovine are weak peripheral vasoconstrictors but produce additive effects with sympathomimetics, such as ephedrine and phenylephrine (Munson, 1965). IV injection of these drugs has been associated with intense vasoconstriction leading to acute hypertension, seizures, cerebrovascular accidents, and retinal detachment (Abouleish, 1976). For this reason, these drugs should be used cautiously, if at all, in patients with pregnancy-induced hypertension and essential hypertension. Both drugs should be avoided in patients with atherosclerotic peripheral vascular disease. Nausea and vomiting most likely reflect a direct central nervous system effect.

CHYMOPAPAIN

Chymopapain is a proteolytic enzyme used in the treatment of herniated lumbar intervertebral disc disease that has not responded to conservative therapy. Injected into the intervertebral disc, chymopapain dissolves the proteoglycan portion of the nucleus pulposus but does not affect collagenous components. Evidence of dissolution of the nucleus pulposus is the appearance in the urine of glycosaminoglycans of the type known to occur in the human intervertebral disc. Dissolution of the nucleus pulposus of the herniated intervertebral disc by chymopapain is known as *chemonucleolysis*. The recommended dose is 2,000 to 5,000 units per disc in a volume of 1 to 2 mL. The maximal dose in a patient with multiple disc herniations is 10,000 units.

Side Effects

Injection of chymopapain into the intervertebral disc space has been associated with allergic reactions of varying severity, including cardiovascular collapse and death (Rajagopalan et al., 1974). Almost all allergic reactions occur immediately but occasionally the symptoms do not appear for up to 2 hours, emphasizing the need for close observation after the injection. The allergic potential of chymopapain appears to be greatest in females and those with known preexisting allergies. Known allergy to papaya is a contraindication to injection of chymopapain, because this enzyme is derived from the crude latex of Carica papaya. Preoperative oral administration of a corticosteroid (prednisone, 50 mg) plus H_1 (diphenhydramine, 50 to 100 mg) and H_2 (cimetidine, 300 to 600 mg) receptor antagonists as a single dose with the preoperative medication or up to four doses every 6 hours in the 24 hours preceding the induction of anesthesia for injection of chymopapain may decrease the incidence and severity of allergic reactions (Bruno et al., 1984). Using preoperative histamine-receptor antagonists and avoiding chemonucleolysis in patients with known allergies have decreased the incidence of allergic reactions after the injection of chymopapain to 0.44% (Moss et al., 1985). Chymopapain should not be injected into the subarachnoid space because it is highly toxic to the neural contents.

REFERENCES

Aasboe V, Raeder JC. Groegaard B. Betamethasone reduces postoperative pain and nausea after ambulatory surgery. *Anesth Analg* 1998; 87:319–323.

Abouleish E. Postpartum hypertension and convulsion after oxytoxic drugs. *Anesth Analg* 1976;55:813–815.

Apfel CC, Korttila K, Abdalla M, et al. A factorial trial of six interventions for the prevention of postoperative nausea and vomiting. *N Engl J Med* 2004;350:2441–2451.

Augoustides JC, Abrams M, Berkowitz D, et al. Vasopressin for hemodynamic rescue in catecholamine-resistant vasoplegic shock after resection of massive pheochromocytoma. *Anesthesiology* 2004;101: 1022–1024.

Barnes PJ. Inhaled glucocorticoids for asthma. *N Engl J Med* 1995;332: 868–875.

Belchetz PE. Hormonal treatment of postmenopausal women. *N Engl J Med* 1994;330:1062–1072.

Bjornson CL, Klassen TP, Williamson J, et al. A randomized trial of a single dose of oral dexamethasone for mild croup. *N Engl J Med* 2004;351:1306–1313.

Brzezinski A. Melatonin in humans. *N Engl J Med* 1997;336:186–195.

Bruno LA, Smith DS, Bloom MJ, et al. Sudden hypotension with a test dose of chymopapain. *Anesth Analg* 1984;63:533–535.

Carette S, Leclaire R, Marcoux S, et al. Epidural corticosteroid injections for sciatica due to herniated nucleus pulposus. *N Engl J Med* 1997;336:1634–1640.

Coloma M, Duffy LL, White PF et al. Dexamethasone facilitates discharge after outpatient anorectal surgery. *Anesth Analg* 2001;92: 85–88.

Cooper DS. Antithyroid drugs. *N Engl J Med* 1984;311:1353–1362.

Cummings JJ, D'Eugenio DB, Gross SJ. A controlled trial of dexamethasone in preterm infants at high risk for bronchopulmonary dysplasia. *N Engl J Med* 1989;320:1505–1510.

Delmas PD, Bjarnason NH, Mitlak BH, et al. Effects of raloxifene on bone mineral density, serum cholesterol concentrations, and uterine endometrium in postmenopausal women. *N Engl J Med* 1997; 337:1641–1647.

Dilger JA, Rho EH, Que FG, et al. Octreotide-induced bradycardia and heart block during surgical resection of a carcinoid tumor. *Anesth Analg* 2004;98:318–320.

Downs JB, Chapman RL, Modell JH, et al. An evaluation of steroid therapy in aspiration pneumonitis. *Anesthesiology* 1974;40:129–135.

Dudley WR, Marshall BE. Steroid treatment for acid-aspiration pneumonia. *Anesthesiology* 1974;40:136–141.

Dunser MW, Mayr AJ, Ulmer H, et al. The effects of vasopressin on systemic hemodynamics in catecholamine-resistant septic shock and postcardiotomy shock: A retrospective analysis. *Anesth Analg* 2001;93:7–13.

Feek CM, Stewart J, Sawers A, et al. Combination of potassium iodide and propranolol in preparation of patients with Grave's disease for thyroid surgery. *N Engl J Med* 1980;302:883–885.

Frankville DD, Harper GB, Lake CL, et al. Hemodynamic consequences of desmopressin administration after cardiopulmonary bypass. *Anesthesiology* 1991;74:988–996.

Gralnick HR, Maisonneuve P, Sultan Y, et al. Benefits of danazol treatment in patients with hemophilia A (classic hemophilia). *JAMA* 1985;253: 1151–1153.

Guay J, Reinberg C, Poitras B, et al. A trial of desmopressin to reduce blood loss in patients undergoing spinal fusion for idiopathic scoliosis. *Anesth Analg* 1992;75:405–410.

Haddox JD. Lumbar and cervical epidural steroid therapy. *Anesth Clin North Am* 1992;10:179–203.

Hardy JD, Turner MD. Hydrocortisone secretion in man: studies of adrenal vein blood. *Surgery* 1957;42:194–201.

Horrow JC. Desmopressin and antifibrinolytics. *Int Anesthesiol Clin* 1990;28:230–236.

Hume DM, Bell C, Bartter FC. Direct measurement of adrenal secretion during operative trauma and convalescence. *Surgery* 1962;52: 174–187.

Jastremski M, Sutton-Tyrrell K, PerVaagenes PH, et al. Glucocorticoid treatment does not improve neurologic recovery following cardiac arrest. *JAMA* 1989;262:3427–3430.

Jungling AS, Shangraw RE. Massive airway edema after azathioprine. *Anesthesiology* 2000;92:888–890.

Kahan BD, Welsh M, Schoenberg L et al. Variable oral absorption of cyclosporine. A biopharmaceutical risk factor for chronic renal allograft rejection. *Transplantation* 1996;62:599–606.

Kaplan NM. Cardiovascular complications of oral contraceptives. *Annu Rev Med* 1978;29:31–40.

Kay J, Findling JW, Raff H. Epidural triamcinolone suppresses the pituitary-adrenal axis in human subjects. *Anesth Analg* 1994;79: 501–505.

Lamberts SWJ, van der Lely AJ, de Herder WW, et al. Octreotide. *N Engl J Med* 1996;334:246–254.

Laragh JH. Oral contraceptive-induced hypertension: nine years later. *Am J Obstet Gynecol* 1976;126:141–147.

Mongan PD, Hosking MP. The role of desmopressin acetate in patients undergoing coronary artery bypass surgery: a controlled clinical trial with thromboelastographic risk stratification. *Anesthesiology* 1992; 77:38–46.

Moss J, Roizen MF, Norbdy ET, et al. Decreased incidence and mortality of anaphylaxis to chymopapain. *Anesth Analg* 1985;64:1197–1201.

Munson WM. The pressor effect of various vasopressor-oxytoxic combinations: a laboratory study and review. *Anesth Analg* 1965;44: 114–119.

O'Dell JR. Therapeutic strategies for rheumatoid arthritis. *N Engl J Med* 2004;350:2591–2602.

Olsen NJ, Stein CM. New drugs for rheumatoid arthritis. *N Engl J Med* 2004;350:2167–2179.
Pleym H, Stenseth R, Waqhba A, et al. Prophylactic treatment with desmopressin does not reduce postoperative bleeding after coronary surgery in patients treated with aspirin before surgery. *Anesth Analg* 2004;98:578–584.
Rajagopalan R, Tindal S, MacNab LT, et al. Anaphylactic reactions to chymopapain during general anesthesia: a case report. *Anesth Analg* 1974;53:191–193.
Ratner EF, Allen R, Mihm F, et al. Failure of steroid supplementation to prevent operative hypotension in a patient receiving chronic steroid therapy. *Anesth Analg* 1996;82:1294–1296.
Rittmaster RS. Finasteride. *N Engl J Med* 1994;330:120–126.
Salem M, Tainsh RE Jr, Bromberg J, et al. Perioperative glucocorticoid coverage. A reassessment 42 years after emergence of a problem. *Ann Surg* 1994;219:416–425.
Scherrer U, Vissing SF, Morgan BJ, et al. Cyclosporine-induced sympathetic activation and hypertension after heart transplantation. *N Engl J Med* 1990;323:693–699.
Schummer W, Schummer C, Wippermann J, et al. Anaphylactic shock: Is vasopressin the drug of choice? *Anesthesiology* 2004;101:1025–1027.
Silvanus M-T, Groeben H, Peters J. Corticosteroids and inhaled salbutamol in patients with reversible airway obstruction markedly decrease the incidence of bronchoconstriction after tracheal intubation. *Anesthesiology* 2004;100:1052–1057.
Spitz IM, Bardin CW. Mifepristone (RU 486)—a modulator of progestin and glucocorticoid action. *N Engl J Med* 1993;329:404–412.
Symreng T, Karlberg BE, Kagedal B, et al. Physiological cortisol substitution of long-term steroid-treated patients undergoing major surgery. *Br J Anaesth* 1981;53:949–953.
Udelsman R, Ramp J, Gallucci WT, et al. Adaptation during surgical stress: a reevaluation of the role of glucocorticoids. *J Clin Invest* 1986; 77:1377–1381.
Voelckel WG, Lurie KG, Lindner KH et al. Vasopressin improves survival after cardiac arrest in hypovolemic shock. *Anesth Analg* 2000; 91:627–634.
Wang JJ, Ho ST, Tzeng JI, et al. The effect of timing of dexamethasone administration on its efficacy as a prophylactic antiemetic for postoperative nausea and vomiting. *Anesth Analg* 2000;91:136–139.
Wenzel V, Krismer AC, Arntz HR, et al. A comparison of vasopressin and epinephrine for out-of-hospital cardiopulmonary resuscitation. *N Engl J Med* 2004;350:105–113.
Wynne JW, DeMarco FJ, Hood CI. Physiological effects of corticosteroids in foodstuff aspiration. *Arch Surg* 1981;116:46–49.

Insulin and Oral Hypoglycemics

24

Insulin administered exogenously is the only effective treatment for type 1 diabetes (formerly known as insulin-dependent diabetes mellitus). Oral hypoglycemic drugs may serve as alternatives to exogenous administration of insulin to patients with type 2 diabetes (formerly known as noninsulin-dependent diabetes mellitus). The vast majority of cases of diabetes are either type 1 or type 2 in an approximate ratio of 1:9. There are an estimated 10.2 million diagnosed and 5.4 million undiagnosed cases of diabetes mellitus in the United States.

INSULIN

Insulin is synthesized in the beta cells of the islets of Langerhans as a single polypeptide proinsulin, which is the precursor molecule to insulin (Fig 24-1) (Genuth, 2001; Larner, 1985). The peptide that connects the amino terminus of the A chain to the carboxyl termins of the B chain is designated the connecting (C) peptide. Proinsulin is converted to insulin and C-peptide and these two molecules are stored together in secretory granules. Stimulation of pancreatic beta cells results in the release of equimolar amounts of insulin C-peptide. Thus, plasma concentrations of insulin C-peptide reflect functional activity of pancreatic beta cells.

Mechanism of Action

The cellular actions of insulin begin with its binding to plasma membrane insulin receptors. As a result, tyrosine molecules in the intracelluar portions of the transmembrane receptors are autophosphorylated, creating tyrosine kinase activity in the receptors. Intracellular insulin receptor substrates are then tyrosine phosphorylated by the receptors. Phosphorylated insulin receptor substrates then activate or inactivate numerous enzymes (phosphatidylinositol-3-kinase) and other mediating molecules. An important effect of these insulin-stimulated cascades is translocation of glucose (Glut-4) transporters to plasma membranes, where they (a) facilitate glucose diffusion into cells, (b) shift intracellular glucose metabolism toward storage as glycogen by activating glycogen synthetase, (c) stimulate cellular uptake of amino acids, phosphate, potassium and magnesium, (d) stimulate protein synthesis and inhibition of proteolysis, and (e) regulate gene expression via insulin regulatory elements in target deoxyribonucleic acid (DNA) molecules. In addition to insulin regulation and synthesis of target enzymes, sensitivity of target tissues to enzymes is the other major determinant of insulin action. Insulin resistance occurs when there is an impaired intracellular insulin signal that results in decreased recruitment of glucose transport proteins to the plasma membrane and subsequent decreased glucose uptake. Compensatory hyperinsulinemia is necessary to overcome this resistance of peripheral tissues to the effects of insulin. A feedback loop exsits between insulin responsiveness in target tissues and insulin secretion by pancreatic beta cells.

Insulin receptors become fully saturated with low circulating concentrations of insulin. For example, continuous infusion of insulin, 1 to 2 U per hour, has the same or even greater pharmacologic effect than a single larger intravenous (IV) dose that is cleared rapidly from the circulation. Large doses of insulin, however, will last longer and exert a greater net effect than small doses.

The number of insulin receptors seems to be inversely related to the plasma concentration of insulin. This relationship may reflect the ability of insulin to regulate the population of its receptors. Obesity and insulin-dependent diabetes mellitus appear to be associated with a decrease in the number of insulin receptors.

Pharmacokinetics

The elimination half-time of insulin injected IV is 5 to 10 minutes in normal patients or in the presence of diabetes

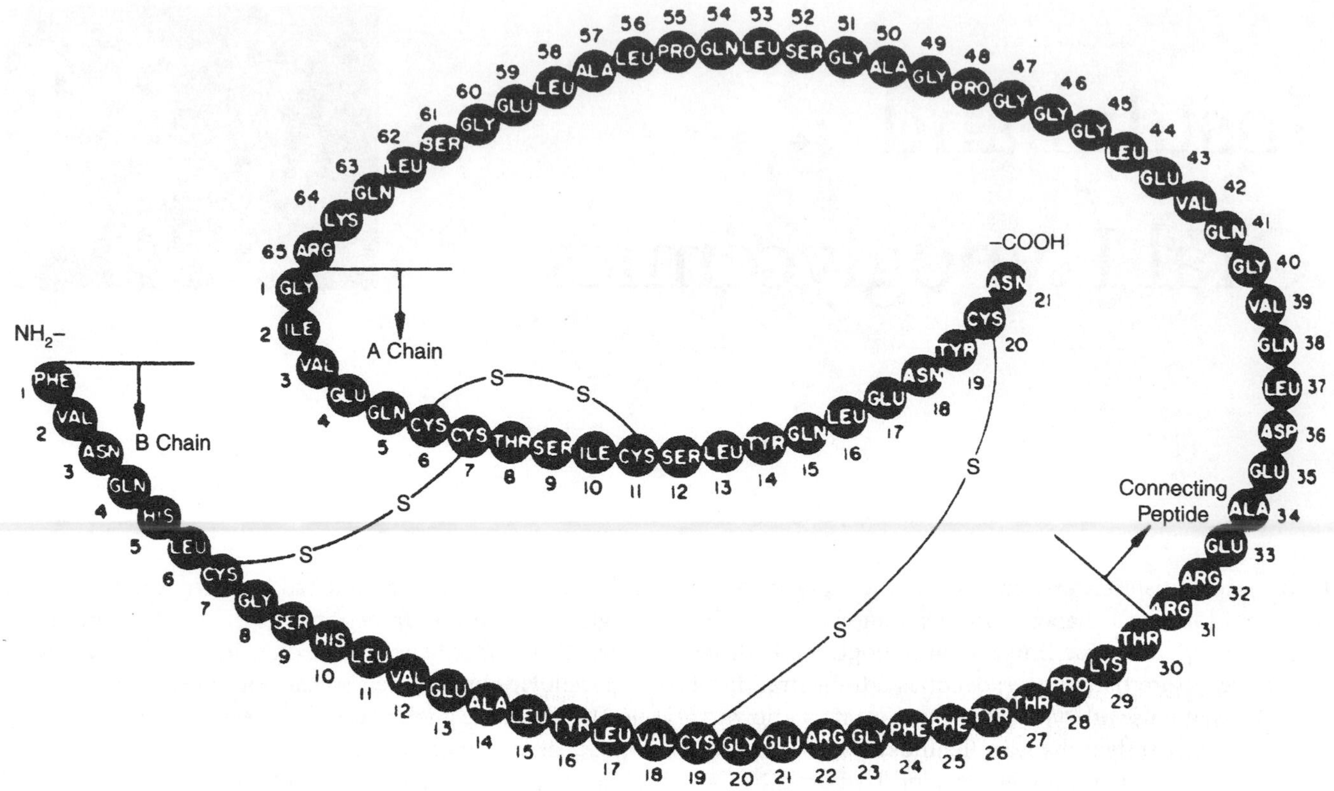

Figure 24-1. Proinsulin, which is converted to insulin by proteolytic cleavage of amino acids 31, 32, 64, 65, and the connecting peptide. (From Larner J. Insulin and oral hypoglycemic drugs: glucagon. In: Gilman AG, Goodman LS, Rall TW, Murad F, eds. *The pharmacological basis of therapeutics*, 7th ed. New York: Macmillan, 1985; with permission.)

mellitus. Insulin is metabolized in the kidneys and liver by a proteolytic enzyme. Approximately 50% of the insulin that reaches the liver by way of the portal vein is metabolized in a single passage through the liver. Nevertheless, renal dysfunction alters the disappearance rate of circulating insulin to a greater extent than does hepatic disease. Indeed, unexpected prolonged effects of insulin may occur in patients with renal disease, reflecting impairment of both metabolism and excretion of this hormone by the kidneys. Peripheral tissues such as skeletal muscles and fat can bind and inactivate insulin, but this is of minor quantitative significance.

Despite rapid clearance from the plasma after IV injection of insulin, there is a sustained pharmacologic effect for 30 to 60 minutes because insulin is tightly bound to tissue receptors. Insulin administered subcutaneously is released slowly into the circulation to produce a sustained biologic effect.

Insulin is secreted into the portal venous system in the basal state at a rate of approximately 1 U per hour. Food intake results in a prompt five- to tenfold increase in the rate of insulin secretion. The total daily secretion of insulin is approximately 40 U. The sympathetic and parasympathetic nervous systems innervate the insulin-producing islet cells and thus influence the basal rate of hormone secretion as well as the response to stress. For example, alpha-adrenergic stimulation decreases and beta-adrenergic or parasympathetic nervous system stimulation increases the basal secretion of insulin. The insulin response to glucose is greater for oral ingestion than for IV infusion. This reflects the release of glucose-dependent insulinotropic polypeptide in response to oral ingestion of glucose and an augmented pancreatic beta cell response.

Insulin Preparations and Delivery

Human insulin manufactured using recombinant DNA technology has replaced insulin extracted from beef and pork pancreas. Allergy or immunoresistance that could accompany administration of animal insulins is no longer a significant problem. In rare instances of local allergy to human insulin, pure porcine insulin or lispro insulin can be substituted. The basic principle of insulin replacement is to provide a slow, long-acting, continuous supply of insulin that mimics the nocturnal and interprandial basal secretion of normal pancreatic beta cells (Hirsch, 1999). In addition, a rapid and relatively short-acting form of insulin delivered before meals mimics the normal meal-stimulated (prandial) release of insulin. Insulin analogues permit more accurate replication of the basal and prandial components of insulin replacement therapy with an attendant decrease in the risk of hypoglycemia (Hirsch, 2005).

TABLE 24-1.
CLASSIFICATION OF INSULIN PREPARATIONS

[NPE1]

	Hours after Subcutaneous Administration		
Insulin Preparation	**Onset**	**Peak**	**Duration**
Rapid acting			
Regular crystalline zinc (CZI)	0.5–1.0	2–3	6–8
Very rapid acting			
Lispro	0.25–0.5	0.5–1.5	4–6
Insulin aspart	0.25–0.5	0.5–1.5	4–6
Intermediate acting			
Lente (NPH)	1	4–8	10–14
Long acting			
Ultralente	1	10–14	18–24
Glargine	1.5	none	30

A number of insulin preparations for subcutaneous administration are available (Table 24-1) (Genuth, 2001). There is variability in the pharmacokinetic characteristics of these insulins from individual to individual and even within the same individual from day to day. Rates of insulin absorption from subcutaneous sites differ with the injection site (absorption from abdominal sites least variable), depth and angle of injection, ambient temperature, and exercise of an injected extremity.

Commercially prepared insulin is bioassayed, and its physiologic activity (potency), based on the ability to decrease the blood glucose concentration, is expressed in units. The potency of insulin is 22 to 26 U per mg. Insulin U-100 (100 U per ml) is the most commonly used commercial preparation. A total daily exogenous dose of insulin for treatment of diabetes mellitus is usually in the range of 20 to 60 U. This insulin requirement, however, may be acutely increased by stress associated with sepsis or trauma.

Continuous subcutaneous insulin infusion (CSII) utilizing an external pump provides basal delivery of insulin (0.5 to 1.0 U per hour) and more predictable acute increases in plasma insulin before meals by delivering bolus doses of insulin. Crystalline zinc insulin (regular insulin) and lispro insulin are the only preparations used for CSII delivery pumps. There is no advantage to giving insulin by IV bolus rather than as a continuous IV infusion.

It is now accepted that intensive insulin treatment regimens to maintain near normoglycemia are the preferred therapy of patients with diabetes mellitus. Different combinations of insulin preparations can be used to approximate normal plasma insulin profiles. Type 1 diabetes is almost never controlled on less than two subcutaneous injections daily of intermediate- or long-acting insulin combined with rapid-acting insulin. Concern that insulin might be atherogenic and increase the incidence of acute myocardial infarction is not sufficiently documented to justify withholding doses of insulin necessary to achieve optimal blood glucose control (Shorr et al., 1997). Long-term metabolic control of diabetes is best monitored by measurement of glycosylated hemoglobin (HbA_{1c}) which reflects glycemia over the previous 8 weeks. A HbA_{1c} value $<7.5\%$ best decreases the risk for microvascular complications.

Lispro

Lispro is an insulin analogue designed to provide a pharmacokinetic profile that more closely parallels physiologic insulin secretion and needs. A feature of natural or synthetic human insulin is that six molecules associate with a zinc molecule to form hexamers. Insulin heaxamers must dissociate to monomers before they can be absorbed from subcutaneous injection sites. This feature is the reason that crystalline zinc insulin (regular insulin) has a peak action 2 to 4 hours after its subcutaneous injection and must be administered 30 to 60 minutes before eating to effectively limit postprandial hyperglycemia. By exchanging lysine and proline at positions 28 and 29 of the insulin B chain, hexamer formation is prevented and the monomer is rapidly absorbed from the injection site. Therefore, lispro insulin injected subcutaneously begins to act within 15 minutes, the peak effect is reached in 0.5–1.5 hours, and the duration of action is only 4 to 6 hours. Lispro injected just before eating provides a postprandial plasma insulin concentration profile similar to that of normal insulin secretion. An important benefit of lispro is a decrease in postprandial hyperglycemia and less risk of hypoglycemia that may follow injection of regular insulin. However, loss of the late action of regular insulin may result in recurrent hyperglycemia before the next meal. In this regard, patients being treated with lispro may not show a decrease in HbA_{1c} unless their doses of basal insulin (neutral protamine Hagedorn [NPH], Lente, or Ultralente) are increased.

Insulin Aspart

Insulin Aspart is a synthetic rapid-acting analogue with a profile of action and therapeutic benefits similar to lispro.

Glargine

Glargine is a long-acting insulin analogue that is used as a basal insulin replacement. This insulin preparation has no discernible peak and manifests a longer duration of action than Ultralente insulin. Glargine may be administered as a single bedtime injection to provide basal insulin for 24 hours with less nocturnal hypoglycemia (Ratner et al., 2000).

Regular Insulin (Crystalline Zinc Insulin)

Regular insulin is a fast-acting preparation and is the only form of insulin that can be administered IV as well as subcutaneously. This form of insulin can be mixed in the same syringe with other insulin preparations, assuming that the pH of the solutions is similar.

Administration of regular insulin is preferred for treating the abrupt onset of hyperglycemia or the appearance of ketoacidosis. In the perioperative period, regular insulin is administered as a single IV injection (1 to 5 U) or as a continuous infusion (0.5 to 2.0 U per hour) to treat metabolic derangements associated with diabetes mellitus.

Isophane Protamine Insulin

Isophane protamine insulin (NPH) is an intermediate-acting preparation whose absorption from its subcutaneous injection site is delayed because the insulin is conjugated with protamine. The acronym NPH designates a neutral solution (N), protamine (P), and origin in Hagedorn's (H) laboratory (Hagedorn et al., 1936). This insulin preparation contains 0.005 mg/U of protamine.

Ultralente Insulin

Ultralente insulin is long-acting, reflecting the large particle size and crystalline form of this insulin preparation. This insulin preparation lacks protamine but has limited clinical usefulness because of its slow onset and prolonged duration of action.

Side Effects

Side effects of treatment with insulin may manifest as (a) hypoglycemia, (b) allergic reactions, (c) lipodystrophy, (d) insulin resistance, and (e) drug interactions.

Hypoglycemia

The most serious side effect of insulin therapy is hypoglycemia. Patients vulnerable to hypoglycemia are those who continue to receive exogenous insulin in the absence of carbohydrate intake, as may occur in the perioperative period, especially before surgery. Initial symptoms of hypoglycemia reflect the compensatory effects of increased epinephrine secretion, manifesting as diaphoresis, tachycardia, and hypertension. Rebound hyperglycemia caused by sympathetic nervous system activity in response to hypoglycemia (Somogyi effect) may mask the correct diagnosis. Symptoms of hypoglycemia involving the central nervous system (CNS) include mental confusion progressing to seizures and coma. The intensity of CNS effects reflects the dependence of the brain on glucose as a selective substrate for oxidative metabolism. A prolonged period of hypoglycemia may result in irreversible brain damage.

The diagnosis of hypoglycemia during general anesthesia is difficult because classic signs of sympathetic nervous system stimulation are likely to be masked by the anesthetic drugs. If signs of sympathetic nervous system stimulation due to hypoglycemia occur, they are likely to be confused with responses evoked by painful surgical stimulation in an anesthetized patient, leading to the erroneous decision to increase the dose of anesthetic drugs. Furthermore, autonomic nervous system neuropathy associated with diabetes mellitus could alter the usual heart rate and systemic blood pressure changes caused by hypoglycemia (Burgos et al., 1989). Nonselective beta-adrenergic antagonists may also mask signs and symptoms of hypoglycemia.

Severe hypoglycemia is treated with 50 to 100 mL of 50% glucose solution administered IV. Alternatively, glucagon, 0.5 to 1.0 mg IV or administered subcutaneously, may be used. Nausea and vomiting are frequent side effects of glucagon treatment. In the absence of CNS depression, carbohydrates may be administered orally.

Allergic Reactions

Use of human insulin preparations has eliminated the problem of systemic allergic reactions that could result from administration of animal-derived insulins. Local allergic reactions to insulin are approximately 10 times more frequent than systemic allergic reactions. These local allergic reactions are characterized by an erythematous indurated area that develops at the site of insulin injection. The cause of local allergic reactions is likely to be noninsulin materials in the insulin preparations. Chronic exposure to low doses of protamine in NPH insulin may serve as an antigenic stimulus for the production of antibodies against protamine. These patients remain asymptomatic until a relatively large dose of protamine is administered IV to antagonize the anticoagulant effects of heparin. Indeed, patients with diabetes and treated with NPH insulin have been described as having an increased incidence of allergic reactions to protamine (Steward et al., 1984). There are also data suggesting that the incidence of allergic reactions to protamine is not increased in patients treated with NPH insulin compared with nondiabetics (Levy et al., 1989).

Lipodystrophy

Lipodystrophy reflects atrophy of fat at the sites of subcutaneous injection of insulin. This side effect is minimized by frequently changing the site used for injection of insulin.

TABLE 24-2.
ORAL DRUGS FOR TREATMENT OF TYPE 2 DIABETES MELLITUS

Sulfonylureas (stimulate insulin secretion; hypoglycemia a risk)
Glyburide
Glipizide
Glimepiride
Tolbutamide
Chlorpropamide
Acetohexamide
Meglitinides (stimulate insulin secretion; hypoglycemia a risk)
Repaglinide
Nateglinide
Biguanides (inhibit glucose production by the liver; hypoglycemia not a risk)
Metformin
Thiazolidinediones (increase sensitivity to insulin for glucose uptake by skeletal muscles and adipose tissues; hypoglycemia not a risk)
Rosiglitazone
Pioglitazone
Alpha-Glucosidase inhibitors (slow digestion and absorption of carbohydrates from the diet; hypoglycemia not a risk)
Acarbose
Miglitol

Insulin Resistance

Patients requiring >100 units of exogenous insulin daily are considered to be manifesting insulin resistance. Even this value is high, because insulin requirements for pancreatectomized adults are often as low as 30 U. The use of human insulins has eliminated the problem of immunoresistance that could accompany administration of animal insulins. Acute insulin resistance is associated with trauma, as produced by surgery and infection.

Drug Interactions

Hormones administered as drugs that counter the hypoglycemic effect of insulin include adrenocorticotrophic hormone, estrogens, and glucagon. Epinephrine inhibits the secretion of insulin and stimulates glycogenolysis. Certain antibiotics (tetracycline or chloramphenicol), salicylates, and phenylbutazone increase the duration of action of insulin and may have a direct hypoglycemic effect. The hypoglycemic effect of insulin may be potentiated by monoamine oxidase inhibitors.

ORAL HYPOGLYCEMICS

Oral drugs representing different mechanisms of action are available for controlling plasma glucose concentrations in patients with type 2 diabetes mellitus (Table 24-2). None of these drugs will adequately control hyperglycemia indefinitely. Therefore, use of combinations of oral drugs from the onset of treatment may be indicated (Riddle, 2000). Even insulin may be administered with sulfonylureas and meglitinides. The effect on HbA_{1c} is similar for these drugs.

Sulfonylureas

Sulfonylurea compounds are orally effective drugs capable of lowering blood glucose concentrations even to hypoglycemic levels (Fig. 24-2) (Gerich, 1989; Mooradian,

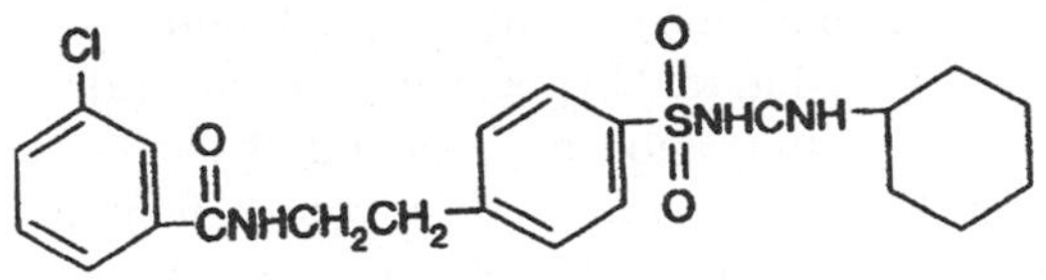

Glyburide

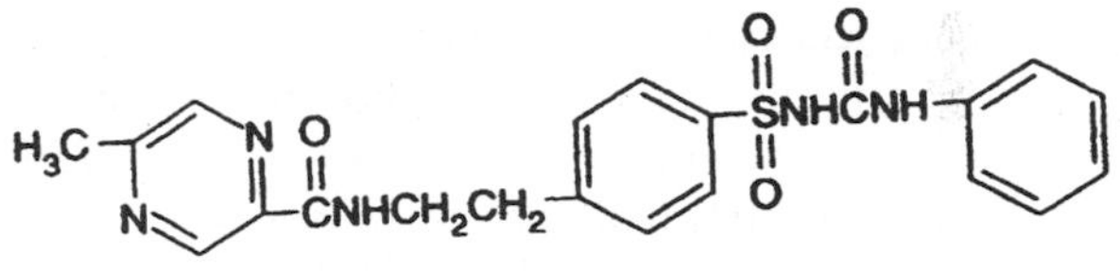

Glipizide

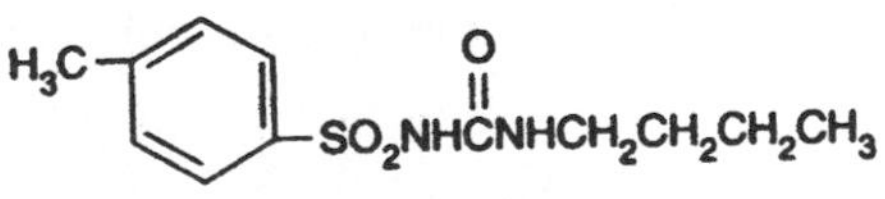

Tolbutamide

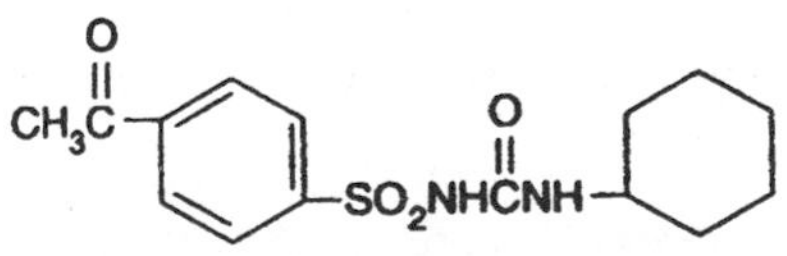

Acetohexamide

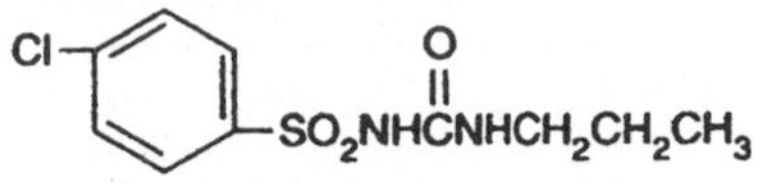

Chlorpropamide

Figure 24–2. Oral hypoglycemics derived from sulfonylurea.

TABLE 24-3.
CLASSIFICATION AND PHARMACOKINETICS OF SULFONYLUREA ORAL HYPOGLYCEMICS

	Relative Potency	Daily Dose Range (mg)	Doses/Day	Duration of Action (hrs)	Elimination Half-Time (hrs)*
Glyburide	150	2.5–20	1–2	18–24	4.6–12
Glipizide	100	5–40	1–2	12–24	4–7
Tolbutamide	1	500–1,000	2–3	6–12	4–8
Acetohexamide	2.5	250–1,500	2	12–18	1.3–6
Chlorpropamide	6	100–750	1	36	30–36

*Approximate

1996). The drug-induced improvement in blood glucose control is associated with decreased hepatic production of very low-density lipoproteins as well as amelioration of hypertriglyceridemia. However, as many as 20% of patients with type 2 diabetes mellitus who begin sulfonylurea therapy do not have an adequate hypoglycemic response to maximal doses (termed *primary failures*), and each year, an additional 10% to 15% of patients who responded initially fail to respond to sulfonylurea therapy (termed *secondary failure*). The sulfonylureas have no effect on and no role in the treatment of patients with type 1 diabetes mellitus. Although sulfonylureas are derivatives of sulfonamides, they have no antibacterial actions. These drugs should not be administered to patients with known allergy to sulfa drugs.

Mechanism of Action

The principal site of action of sulfonylurea drugs is the pancreatic islet (beta) cells, where these drugs act on specific receptors to inhibit adenosine triphosphate-sensitive potassium ion channels in beta cells. As a result, there is an influx of calcium and stimulation of exocytosis (release) of insulin storage granules. Although sulfonylureas decrease insulin resistance, this effect probably plays a minor role, if any, in decreasing blood glucose concentrations.

Pharmacokinetics

Oral hypoglycemics are readily absorbed from the gastrointestinal tract, with the most important distinguishing features being differences in duration of action and elimination half-time (Table 24-3) (Gerich, 1989). These drugs are weakly acidic and circulate bound to protein (90% to 98%), principally to albumin. Metabolism in the liver is extensive, and resulting active and inactive metabolites are eliminated by renal tubular secretion. Approximately 50% of glyburide is excreted in feces.

Side Effects

Sulfonylureas are generally well tolerated, with the most common severe complication of these drugs being hypoglycemia (Table 24-4). The greatest risk of hypoglycemia occurs with drugs with the longest elimination half-times, glyburide and chlorpropamide, Sulfonylureas may have durations of action for up to 7 days. Although hypoglycemia secondary to sulfonylureas may be infrequent, it is often more prolonged and more dangerous than hypoglycemia secondary to insulin (Table 24-5).

Hypoglycemia caused by sulfonylureas may require prolonged infusion of glucose-containing solutions. Risk factors for sulfonylurea-induced hypoglycemia include (a) impaired nutrition, as in the perioperative period, (b) age >60 years, (c) impaired renal function, and (d) concomitant drug therapy than can potentiate sulfonylureas (phenylbutazone, sulfonamide antibiotics, warfarin) or in itself produce hypoglycemia (alcohol or salicylates). Renal disease decreases elimination of sulfonylureas and their active metabolites, thus increasing the likelihood of hypoglycemia. In this regard, only small amounts of tolbutamide and glipizide are

TABLE 24-4.
SIDE EFFECTS OF SULFONYLUREA ORAL HYPOGLYCEMICS

	Overall Incidence of Side Effects (%)	Incidence of Hypoglycemia (%)	Antidiuretic	Diuretic
Glyburide	7	4–6	No	Yes
Glipizide	6	2–4	No	Yes
Tolbutamide	3	<1	Yes	Yes
Acetohexamide	4	1	No`	Yes
Chlorpropamide	9	4–6	Yes	No

TABLE 24-5.
COMPARISON OF SULFONYLUREA THERAPY WITH INSULIN THERAPY

Sulfonylurea	Insulin
Failed initial response in 10% to 15% of patients	No maximum dose
Secondary failure rate each year among treated patients is about 10%	
Hypoglycemia may be more severe	Hypoglycemia may be more frequent
Associated cardiac complications	Lipid levels lowered
Patients may prefer oral medication	Patients may resist injections

excreted unchanged in urine, making these drugs preferable for patients with renal disease. Sulfonylureas cross the placenta and may produce fetal hypoglycemia.

Increased cardiovascular mortality may be associated with sulfonylureas, especially tolbutamide. In this regard, sulfonylureas have a less beneficial effect on plasma lipid levels than does insulin (Nathan et al., 1988). Sulfonylureas close K_{ATP} channels and inhibit ischemic preconditioning, a cardioprotective mechanism (Brady and Terzic, 1998). For this reason, it may be recommended that sulfonylureas be discontinued 24 to 48 hours prior to elective surgery in high-risk patients. Hyperglycemia also prevents ischemic preconditioning and institution of insulin therapy may be indicated when sulfonylureas are discontinued preoperatively. Approximately 1% to 3% of patients treated with oral hypoglycemics experience gastrointestinal disturbances including nausea, vomiting, abnormal liver function tests, and cholestasis. Sulfonylureas are not recommended for patients with hepatic dysfunction as liver disease may prolong the elimination half-time and enhance the hypoglycemic action of all the sulfonylureas except acetohexamide. Disulfiram-like reactions and inappropriate secretion of arginine vasopressin hormone with resulting hyponatremia are unique side effects of chlorpropamide.

Clinically Useful Sulfonylureas

Glyburide

Glyburide stimulates insulin secretion over a 24-hour period after a morning oral dose (Feldman, 1985). Peak plasma levels occur approximately 3 hours after oral administration. Peripheral effects include increased sensitivity to insulin and inhibition of hepatic glucose production. Metabolism is in the liver, with metabolites excreted equally in urine and feces. One of the hepatic metabolites of glyburide has approximately 15% of the activity of the parent compound. A mild diuretic effect accompanies use of this drug. When administration is discontinued, the drug is cleared from the plasma in about 36 hours.

Glipizide

Glipizide stimulates insulin secretion over a 12-hour period after a morning oral dose. Peak plasma levels occur approximately 1 hour after oral administration. Peripheral effects include increased glucose uptake and suppression of hepatic glucose output (Lebovitz, 1985). These effects on insulin secretion persist for prolonged periods (at least 3 years) without evidence of tolerance. Metabolism in the liver produces inactive substances (in contrast to glyburide), which are excreted in the urine. A mild diuretic effect accompanies use of this drug. Relatively rapid clearance from the plasma should minimize the potential for glipizide to produce long-lasting hypoglycemia.

Glimepiride

Glimepiride decreases blood glucose concentrations by stimulating release of insulin from the pancreas and may decrease hepatic glucose production. Combination therapy with insulin is appropriate for secondary failure to oral sulfonylureas.

Tolbutamide

Tolbutamide is the shortest-acting and least potent sulfonylurea (see Table 24-2) (Gerich, 1989). It is extensively metabolized in the liver to much less potent compounds that are excreted in urine. Of all the sulfonylureas, tolbutamide probably causes the fewest side effects, although it can produce hypoglycemia and hyponatremia.

Acetohexamide

Acetohexamide differs from other sulfonylureas in that most of its hypoglycemic action is due to its principal metabolite hydroxyhexamide, which is 2.5 times as potent as the parent compound. After oral ingestion, peak plasma concentrations of acetohexamide and its active metabolite occur after 1.5 hours and 3.5 hours, respectively. This drug is not recommended for patients with renal disease because the kidneys excrete the active metabolite. This is the only sulfonylurea with uricosuric properties, making it an appropriate drug for the diabetic patient with gout.

Chlorpropamide

Chlorpropamide is the longest-acting sulfonylurea, with a duration of action that may approach 72 hours (see Table 24-3) (Gerich, 1989). The maximal effect of chlorpropamide may not be apparent for 7 to 14 days, and several weeks may be required for complete elimination of the drug. Because 20% of a dose is excreted, unchanged, impaired renal function can lead to chlorpropamide accumulation and an enhanced hypoglycemic effect. Chlorpropamide is unique in being associated with reactions similar to those produced by disulfiram (facial flushing after ingestion of alcohol) and can cause severe hyponatremia. Approximately 5% of patients treated with chlorpropamide have serum sodium concentrations of <129 mEq per liter, but they are usually asymptomatic. Risk factors for the development of hyponatremia include age >60 years, female gender, and the concomitant administration of thiazide diuretics. If all these risk factors are present, the frequency of hyponatremia increases threefold.

Meglitinides

Repaglinide and the phenylalanine derivative, nateglinide differ in structure and timing of action from sulfonylurea drugs. Although these drugs may exert effects on beta cells similar to sulfonylurea drugs, they have a more prompt peak effect (about 1 hour) and a shorter duration of action (about 4 hours). Beta cell stimulants lower HbA_{1c} about 1%. Repaglinide and nateglinide must be administered 15 to 30 minutes before a meal and should never be ingested while fasting. The short duration of action and the fact these drugs are only active in the presence of glucose should decrease the risk of prolonged hypoglycemic episodes (Lebovitz, 1999).

Alpha-Glucosidase Inhibitors

Acarbose and miglitol are alpha-glucosidase inhibitors that decrease carbohydrate digestion and absorption of disaccharides by interfering with intestinal glucosidase activity (Gerich, 1989). This action results in slow release of glucose from food and therefore slow absorption from the gastrointestinal tract. HbA_{1c} generally decreases 0.5% to 0.8%. These drugs are useful only as monotherapy when postprandial hyperglycemia is the main problem. Flatulence, abdominal cramping, and diarrhea are frequent side effects that result from indigested carbohydrates reaching bacteria in the lower colon. With the exception of infrequent increases in liver transaminases, these drugs are considered nontoxic (Mooradian, 1996). Although hypoglycemia does not occur with monotherapy, it can occur when alpha-glucosidase inhibitors are added to sulfonylureas or insulin.

Biguanides

Biguanides are recognized to be effective in the treatment of non-insulin-dependent diabetes. The advantage of biguanides is their ability to decrease blood glucose concentrations with only a very low risk for hypoglycemia. In addition, they have a positive effect on blood lipid concentrations and lead to a mild weight reduction in obese patients. Nevertheless, after the introduction of sulfonylureas, biguanides were largely abandoned because of the risk of severe lactic acidosis. In fact, the use of biguanides in the United States was stopped in 1975 for this reason (Gan et al., 1992).

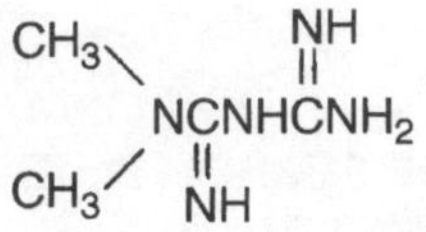

Figure 24-3. Metformin.

Metformin

In 1995, the biguanide metformin was approved for use in the United States (Fig. 24-3) (Bailey, 1993; Gerich, 1989; Mooradian, 1996). Metformin produces satisfactory results in approximately 50% of cases in which sulfonylureas have failed. In contrast to sulfonylureas, metformin does not cause hypoglycemia and is thus considered an antihyperglycemic drug rather than a hypoglycemic drug. Although the risk of metformin-induced lactic acidosis is remote (estimated to be 10 to 20 times less likely than with phenformin), it is still a possible side effect that has been described during the intraoperative period (Mercker et al., 1997; Mooradian, 1996; Stumvoll et al., 1995). For this reason, some have recommended discontinuing metformin 48 hours or longer before elective operations (Mercker et al., 1997). If metformin cannot be omitted before surgery, it is prudent to monitor for the development of lactic acidosis (arterial blood gases and pH, serum lactate concentrations, renal function) in the perioperative period.

Pharmacokinetics

In contrast to sulfonylureas, metformin is not bound to plasma proteins and does not undergo metabolism. It is eliminated by the kidneys, with 90% of an oral dose excreted in approximately 12 hours. Peak plasma concentrations of metformin occur approximately 2 hours after oral administration. The drug has an elimination half-time of 2 to 4 hours, requiring its administration up to three times a day (500 to 1,000 mg with meals). In view of its dependence on renal clearance, metformin should be administered with caution, if at all, to patients with renal dysfunction.

Mechanism of Action

Metformin acts primarily by decreasing excessive hepatic and renal glucose production most likely through inhibiting gluconeogenesis. Because insulin also inhibits gluconeogenesis and metformin requires the presence of insulin to be effective, metformin may be considered a hepatic insulin sensitizer. The blood glucose-lowering effect of metformin is not mediated through stimulation of endogenous insulin secretion (Mooradian, 1996). Hypoglycemia almost never occurs because of metformin monotherapy. Metformin also decreases plasma concentrations of triglycerides and cholesterol.

Side Effects

The most common side effects of metformin are anorexia, nausea, and diarrhea, which occur initially in 5% to 20% of patients. Fewer than 5% of patients experience side effects sufficient to warrant withdrawal of the drug. In contrast to sulfonylureas, metformin does not cause hypoglycemia. The most serious, although rare, side effect of metformin therapy is lactic acidosis.

Lactic Acidosis

Metformin binds to mitochondrial membranes, leading to decreased intracellular adenosine triphosphate and increased adenosine monophosphate concentrations. Glucose is metabolized anaerobically. The resulting pyruvate is reduced to lactate, which is usually metabolized quickly in the liver. For this reason, metformin should be administered with caution, if at all, to patients with hepatic dysfunction. Dehydration, renal dysfunction manifesting as increased plasma concentrations of creatinine, IV administration of radiographic iodinated contrast media, acute myocardial infarction, congestive heart failure and arterial hypoxemia and sepsis could accentuate metformin-induced lactic acidosis. Hemodialysis along with bicarbonate administration can be effective therapy for metformin-induced lactic acidosis. Management of biguanide-induced lactic acidosis is symptomatic because the underlying pathologic change (blockade of the mitochondrial respiratory chain) cannot be treated.

Thiazolidinediones

Thiazolidinediones (TZDs) act principally at skeletal muscles and adipose tissue to decrease insulin resistance that is present in nearly all type 2 diabetics (Henry, 1997). Like metformin, TZDs require the presence of insulin and are especially effective in obese patients. As monotherapy these drugs decrease HbA_{1c} 1% to 1.5%. The clinical effect takes 4 to 12 weeks to become evident. TZDs can cause weight gain, which is partly extracellular fluid. The accumulation of extracellular fluid presents as edema fluid that is undesirable when concurrent congestive heart failure exists. The possibility of drug-induced liver dysfunction is the reason to periodically measure plasma concentrations of hepatic transaminases. TZDs tend to decrease plasma concentrations of triglycerides and increase HDL and LDL cholesterol levels.

Combination Therapy

In patients with persistent hyperglycemia, none of the oral hypoglycemic drugs reliably normalize HbA_{1c} when used as monotherapy presumably because they act principally by correcting single abnormalities. Combination therapies support the logic of targeting two or more different causes of hyperglycemia simultaneously. For example, one approach is to decrease insulin resistance in the liver with metformin while increasing insulin secretion with sulfonylureas or meglitinide. Alpha-glucosidase inhibitors complement the different actions of these two classes of drugs. Exogenous insulin may also be part of combination therapy.

The primary aim of combination therapy is to decrease HbA_{ic}, whereas reductions in the daily insulin dose are a secondary benefit.

REFERENCES

Bailey CJ. Metformin—an update. *Gen Pharmacol* 1993;24:1299–1309.

Brady PA, Terzic A. The sulfonylurea controversy: More questions from the heart. *J Am Coll Cardiol* 1998;31:950–956.

Burgos LG, Ebert TJ, Asiddao C, et al. Increased intraoperative cardiovascular morbidity in diabetics with autonomic neuropathy. *Anesthesiology* 1989;70:591–597.

Feldman JM. Glyburide: Second-generation sulfonylurea hypoglycemic agent; history, chemistry, metabolism, pharmacokinetics, clinical use and adverse effects. *Pharmacotherapy* 1985;5:43–62.

Gan SC, Barr J, Arieff AI, et al. Biguanide-associated lactic acidosis. Case report and review of the literature. *Arch Intern Med* 1992;152: 2333–2336.

Genuth S. Exogenous insulin administration and cardiovascular risk in non-insulin-dependent and insulin-dependent diabetes mellitus. *Ann Intern Med* 1996;124:104–112.

Genuth S. Diabetes mellitus. *Sci Am Med* 2001;9:VI:1–34.

Gerich JE. Oral hypoglycemic agents. *N Engl J Med* 1989;321:1231–1243.

Hagedorn HC, Jensen BN, Krarup NB, et al. Protamine insulinate. *JAMA* 1936;106:179–180.

Henry RR. Thiazolidinediones. *Curr Ther Diabetes* 1997;26:553–559.

Hirsch IB. Type 1 diabetes mellitus and the use of flexible insulin regimens. *Am Fam Physician* 1999;60:2343–2349.

Hirsch IB. Insulin analogues. *N Engl J Med* 2005;352:174–183.

Larner J. Insulin and oral hypoglycemic drugs: glucagon. In: Gilman AG, Goodman LS, Rall TW,

Lebovitz HE. Glipzide: second-generation sulfonylurea hypoglycemic agent. Pharmacology, pharmacokinetics, and clinical use. *Pharmacotherapy* 1985;5:63–77.

Lebovitz HE. Insulin secretagogues: old and new. *Diabetes Rev* 1999;7:139–146.

Levy JH, Schwieger IM, Zaidan JR, et al. Evaluation of patients at risk for protamine reactions. *J Thorac Cardiovasc Surg* 1989;98:200–204.

Mercker SK, Maier C, Doz P, et al. Lactic acidosis as a serious perioperative complication of antidiabetic biguanide medication with metformin. *Anesthesiology* 1997;87:1003–1005.

Mooradian AD. Drug therapy of non–insulin-dependent diabetes mellitus in the elderly. *Drugs* 1996;51.931–941.

Murad F, eds. *The pharmacological basis of therapeutics*, 7th ed. New York: Macmillan, 1985:1490–1516.

Nathan DM, Roussell A, Godine JE. Glyburide or insulin for metabolic control in non–insulin-dependent diabetes mellitus. A randomized double-blind study. *Ann Intern Med* 1988;108:334–340.

Ratner RE, Hirsch IB, Neifing JL, et al. Less hypoglycemia with insulin glargine in intensive insulin therapy for type 1 diabetes. *Diabetes Care* 2000;23:639–645.

Riddle M. The 2 defects of type 2 diabetes: combining drugs to treat both insulin deficiency and insulin resistance. *Am J Med* 2000; 108:S1–S6.

Steward WJ, McSweeney SM, Kellett MA, et al. Increased risk of severe protamine reactions in NPH insulin-dependent diabetics undergoing cardiac catheterization. *Circulation* 1984;70:788–792.

Stumvoll M, Nurjhan N, Perriello G, et al. Metabolic effects of metformin in non–insulin-dependent diabetes mellitus. *N Engl J Med* 1995;333: 550–554.

Diuretics

25

Diuretics are among the most frequently prescribed drugs, with the classic pharmacologic response being diuresis. These drugs may be classified according to their site of action on renal tubules and the mechanism by which they alter the excretion of solute (Tables 25-1 and 25-2 and Fig. 25-1) (Merin and Bastron, 1986).

All diuretics may cause hypovolemia and azotemia but these side effects are most likely to occur with loop diuretics (Table 25-3). Hypokalemic alkalosis, hyperglycemia, and hyperuricemia ("clinical gout") are common dose-dependent complications of both thiazide and loop diuretics. Thiazides decrease calcium excretion and may cause hypercalcemia in patients with underlying conditions (sarcoidosis) that facilitate calcium absorption from the gastrointestinal tract. Thiazides are more likely to cause hyponatremia especially in patients who habitually drink large amounts of fluids. Patients at the greatest risk for developing hyperkalemia in the presence of potassium-sparing diuretics are those receiving angiotensin-converting enzyme (ACE) inhibitors or angiotensin II blocking drugs and patients with acute renal failure.

THIAZIDE DIURETICS

Thiazide diuretics are most often administered for maintenance treatment of essential hypertension in which the combination of diuresis, natriuresis, and vasodilation are synergistic (Fig. 25-2) (see Chapter 15). In combination with thiazide diuretics, the dose of more potent antihypertensive drugs can often be decreased 25% to 50%, thus minimizing drug-induced side effects. A thiazide diuretic may be utilized to mobilize edema fluid associated with renal, hepatic, or cardiac dysfunction. Less common uses of thiazide diuretics include management of diabetes insipidus and treatment of hypercalcemia. Thiazide diuretics are readily absorbed from the gastrointestinal tract and excreted principally by the kidneys.

Mechanism of Action

Thiazide diuretics produce diuresis by inhibiting reabsorption of sodium and chloride ions, principally in the cortical portions of the ascending loops of Henle and, to a lesser extent, in the proximal renal tubules and distal renal tubules (see Table 25-2) (Merin and Bastron, 1986). The result is a marked increase in the urinary excretion of sodium, chloride, and bicarbonate ions (Table 25-4) (Tonnesen, 1983). An associated increased excretion of potassium ions into the renal tubules occurs whenever there is enhanced distal delivery of sodium and water. This emphasizes that the normal driving force for potassium excretion by distal renal tubules is the transtubular electrical potential difference created by sodium reabsorption. Thiazide diuretics, by inhibiting sodium reabsorption, lead to the delivery of higher concentrations of sodium to the distal renal tubules and the subsequent enhancement of secretion of potassium into the renal tubules. The diuretic effect of thiazide diuretics is independent of acid-base balance.

Antihypertensive Effect

The antihypertensive effect of thiazide diuretics is due initially to a decrease in extracellular fluid volume, often with a decrease in cardiac output. The sustained antihypertensive effect of thiazide diuretics, however, is due to peripheral vasodilation, which requires several weeks to develop. This peripheral vasodilation may reflect a diminished effect of sympathetic nervous system activity at peripheral vascular smooth muscle, which correlates with the decrease in total body stores of sodium. This diuretic-induced decrease in systemic vascular resistance is accompanied by at least a partial correction of the decreased extracellular fluid volume. The importance of diuretic-induced sodium excretion is suggested by the absence of an antihypertensive effect when thiazide diuretics are administered to anephric animals.

Side Effects

Thiazide diuretic–induced hypokalemic, hypochloremic, metabolic alkalosis is a common side effect when these drugs are administered chronically for maintenance treatment of essential hypertension (see Table 25-3). Depletion

TABLE 25-1.
CLASSIFICATION OF DIURETIC

	Clinical Uses
Thiazide diuretics	
Chlorothiazide	Essential hypertension, edema due to congestive heart failure, renal failure, hepatic failure
Hydrochlorothiazide	Same as chlorothiazide
Bendroflumethiazide	Same as chlorothiazide
Hydroflumethiazide	Same as chlorothiazide
Methylclothiazide	Same as chlorothiazide
Polythiazide	Same as chlorothiazide
Trichlormethiazide	Same as chlorothiazide
Indapamide	Same as chlorothiazide
Loop diuretics	
Furosemide	Severe essential hypertension, edema due to congestive heart failure, renal failure, hepatic failure
Ethacrynic acid	
Bumetanide	Same as furosemide
Torsemide	Same as furosemide
Osmotic diuretics	
Mannitol	Intracranial hypertension, prophylaxis against or treatment of the oliguric phase of acute renal failure
Urea	
Potassium-sparing diuretics	
Triamterene	Edema associated with congestive heart failure, renal failure, hepatic failure
Amiloride	Essential hypertension, or edema due to congestive heart failure, often in combination with thiazide or loop diuretics
Aldosterone antagonists (potassium-sparing)	
Spironolactone	Edema associated with congestive heart failure, renal failure, hepatic failure
Carbonic anhydrase inhibitors	
Acetazolamide	Glaucoma, altitude sickness, persistent metabolic alkalosis
Dopamine-receptor agonists	
Dopamine	Not recommended as prophylaxis against oliguric phase of acute renal failure
Fenoldopam	

of sodium and magnesium ions may accompany kaliuresis. Cardiac dysrhythmias may occur as the result of diuretic-induced hypokalemia or hypomagnesemia. Other important side effects of hypokalemia that may occur include (a) skeletal muscle weakness, (b) gastrointestinal ileus, (c) nephropathy characterized by polyuria and azotemia, (d) increased likelihood of developing digitalis toxicity, and (e) potentiation of nondepolarizing neuromuscular-blocking drugs.

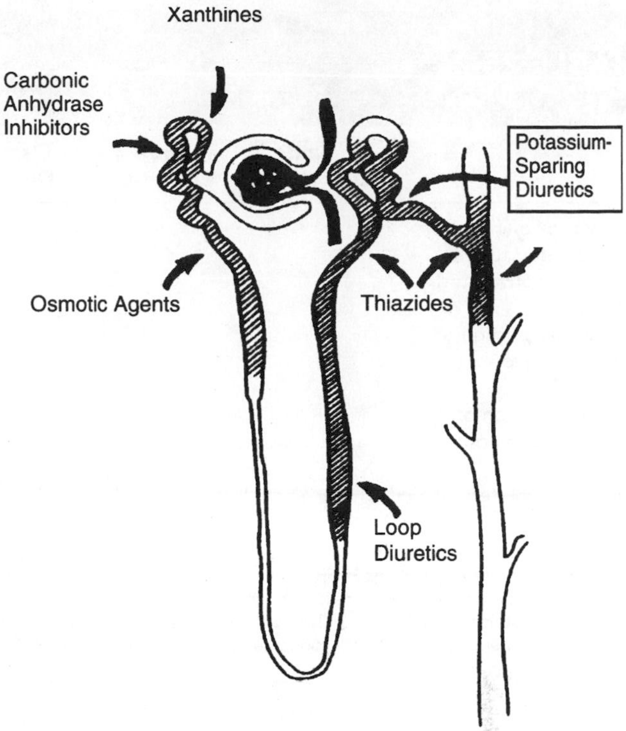

Figure 25-1. Sites of action of diuretics.

Intravascular fluid volume status should be considered in all patients treated with thiazide diuretics and scheduled for surgery. The presence of orthostatic hypotension in such patients should arouse suspicion that intravascular fluid volume is decreased. Laboratory evidence of hemoconcentration (increased hematocrit and increased blood urea nitrogen concentration) and decreased right or left atrial filling pressures are further evidence of hypovolemia.

Thiazide diuretics may cause hyperglycemia and aggravate diabetes mellitus. The mechanism of hyperglycemia is unknown but may reflect drug-induced inhibition of insulin release from the pancreas and blockade of peripheral glucose use.

Inhibition of renal tubular secretion of urate by thiazide diuretics can result in hyperuricemia. This thiazide-induced retention of uric acid can exacerbate gouty arthritis, even in patients treated with probenecid.

Borderline renal or hepatic function may deteriorate further during treatment with thiazide diuretics, presumably

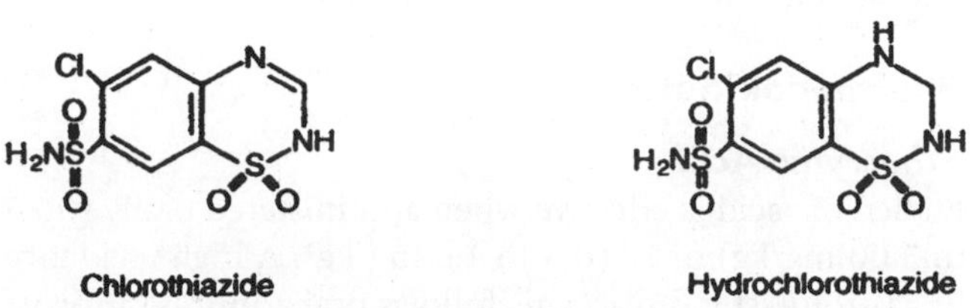

Figure 25-2. Thiazide diuretics.

TABLE 25-2.
SITES OF ACTION OF DIURETICS

	Thiazide Diuretics	Loop Diuretics	Osmotic Diuretics	Potassium Sparing Diuretics	Aldosterone Antagonists	Carbonic Anhydrase
Early proximal convoluted tubule		+	+			
Proximal convoluted tubule	+	+				+++
Medullary portion of ascending loop of Henle		+++	+++			
Cortical portion of ascending loop of Henle	+++	+	+			
Distal convoluted tubule	+	+	+	+++		+
Collecting duct					+++	

+, minor site of action; +++, major site of action.
Source: Adapted from Merin RG, Bastron RD. Diuretics. In: Smith NT, Miller RD, Corbascio AN, eds. *Drug interactions in anesthesia.* Philadelphia: Lea & Febiger, 1986:206–224; with permission.

reflecting drug-induced decreases in blood flow to these organs. A maculopapular rash occurs in 1% or more of patients treated with chlorothiazide.

LOOP DIURETICS

Ethacrynic acid, bumetanide and furosemide are diuretics that inhibit reabsorption of sodium (most potent saliuretic drugs available) and chloride primarily in the medullary portions of the ascending limbs of the loops of Henle (Fig. 25-3; see Table 25-2) (Merin and Bastron, 1986). This site of action accounts for the designation of these drugs as loop diuretics. Intravenous (IV) administration of either ethacrynic acid or furosemide produces within 2 to 10 minutes a diuretic response that is independent of acid–base changes (see Table 25-3) (Tonnesen, 1983). Indeed, responsiveness to furosemide is directly related to the glomerular filtration rate over a wide range. Furosemide also evokes renal production of prostaglandins resulting in renal vasodilation and increased renal blood flow. These renovascular effects of furosemide produce redistribution of renal blood flow from the inner to the outer renal cortex and contribute to the diuretic effects of this drug. Furosemide-induced increases in renal blood flow are inhibited by nonsteroidal antiinflammatory drugs manifesting as an attenuated diuretic effect.

Pharmacokinetics

Ethacrynic Acid

Ethacrynic acid is effective when administered orally (0.75 to 3.00 mg/kg) or IV (0.5 to 1.0 mg/kg). A high incidence of gastrointestinal reactions follows oral administration of this diuretic. Protein binding is extensive. Ethacrynic acid is excreted by the kidneys as unchanged drug and an unstable metabolite.

Furosemide

Furosemide is effective when administered orally (0.75 to 3.00 mg/kg) or IV (0.1 to 1.0 mg/kg). Protein binding to albumin is extensive, accounting for approximately 90% of the drug. Glomerular filtration and renal tubular secretion account for approximately 50% of furosemide excretion. Approximately one-third of a dose of furosemide is metabolized or excreted unchanged in the bile. The elimination half-time is <1 hour, accounting for the short duration of action of furosemide.

Clinical Uses

Clinically, furosemide is used far more often than ethacrynic acid. Loop diuretics should be administered only to patients with a normal or increased intravascular fluid volume. Acute hypovolemia may result from administration of loop diuretics to hypovolemic patients and the resulting hypotension may further exacerbate renal ischemic injury and concentrate nephrotoxins in the renal tubules.

Common clinical uses of furosemide include (a) mobilization of edema fluid due to renal, hepatic, or cardiac

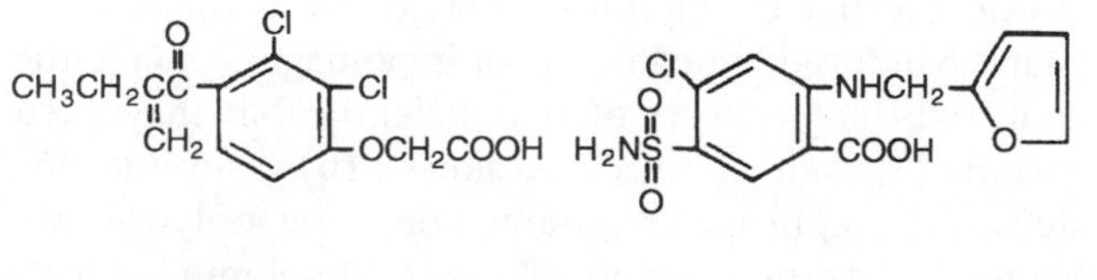

Ethacrynic Acid Furosemide

Figure 25-3. Loop diuretics.

TABLE 25-3.
SIDE EFFECTS OF DIURETICS

	Hypokalemic, Hyperchloremic, Metabolic Alkalosis	Hyperkalemia	Hyperglycemia	Hyperuricemia	Hyponatremia
Thiazide diuretics	Yes	No	Yes	Yes	Yes
Loop diuretics	Yes	No	Minimal	Minimal	Yes
Potassium-sparing	No	Yes	Minimal	—	Minimal
Aldosterone	No	Yes	No	No	Yes

dysfunction; (b) treatment of increased intracranial pressure; and (c) inhibition of cellular uptake of calcium for treatment of hypercalcemia, and (d) differential diagnosis of acute oliguria. Loop diuretics have little use in the chronic treatment of essential hypertension. Indeed, the antihypertensive effect of furosemide is due entirely to its ability to decrease intravascular fluid volume, which, if it occurs rapidly, may evoke baroreceptor reflex-mediated increases in sympathetic nervous system activity. Acceleration of the excretion of other drugs, such as long-acting nondepolarizing neuromuscular-blocking drugs, by furosemide-induced diuresis is limited because this diuretic does not increase glomerular filtration rate or renal tubular secretion.

Mobilization of Edema Fluid

Furosemide, 0.1 to 1 mg/kg IV, produces a prompt diuresis of edema fluid that has accumulated due to renal, hepatic, or cardiac dysfunction. Peripheral vasodilation precedes the onset of diuresis, and the associated decrease in venous return is consistent with the prompt and efficacious effects of furosemide in the management of acute pulmonary edema. Furosemide may also increase lymph flow through the thoracic duct.

Treatment of Increased Intracranial Pressure

Furosemide decreases intracranial pressure by inducing systemic diuresis, decreasing cerebrospinal fluid production by interfering with sodium ion transport in glial tissue, and by resolving cerebral edema by improving cellular water transport. This diuretic-induced decrease in intracranial pressure is not accompanied by changes in cerebral blood flow or plasma osmolarity. Furosemide can be administered as single-drug therapy (0.5 to 1.0 mg/kg IV) or as a lower dose (0.1 to 0.3 mg/kg IV) in combination with mannitol. Furosemide is not as effective as mannitol for decreasing intracranial pressure. Alterations in the blood-brain barrier do not influence the immediate or subsequent effects of furosemide on intracranial pressure. This characteristic contrasts with that of mannitol, which may produce rebound intracranial hypertension if a disrupted blood-brain barrier allows mannitol to enter the central nervous system (CNS). A combination of furosemide and mannitol is more effective in decreasing intracranial pressure than either drug alone, but severe dehydration and electrolyte imbalance are also more likely.

Differential Diagnosis of Acute Oliguria

Furosemide administered in small doses (0.1 mg/kg IV) will stimulate diuresis in the presence of excessive arginine vasopressin hormone (antidiuretic hormone) effect. This drug must not be used, however, to treat acute oliguria due to decreased intravascular fluid volume because furosemide-induced diuresis could further exaggerate hypovolemia and

TABLE 25-4.
EFFECTS OF DIURETICS ON URINE COMPOSITION

	Volume (ml/min)	pH	Sodium (mEq/L)	Potassium (mEq/L)	Chloride (mEq/L)	Bicarbonate
No drug	1	6.4	50	15	60	1
Thiazide diuretics	13	7.4	150	25	150	25
Loop diuretics	8	6.0	140	25	155	1
Osmotic diuretics	10	6.5	90	15	110	4
Potassium-sparing diuretics	3	7.2	130	10	120	15
Carbonic anhydrase Inhibitors	3	8.2	70	60	15	120

Source: Adapted from Tonnesen AS. Clinical pharmacology and use of diuretics. In: Hershey SG, Bamforth BJ, Zauder H, eds. *Review courses in anesthesiology*. Philadelphia: Lippincott, 1983;217–226; with permission.

aggravate renal ischemic changes that result from poor renal blood flow. Furthermore, continued urine output in the presence of furosemide can no longer be considered evidence of adequate intravascular fluid volume, cardiac output, and renal blood flow.

The use of furosemide to treat acute renal failure is controversial. Attempts to convert oliguric renal failure into the nonoliguric form, which is associated with a lower mortality, have not proved beneficial when compared with untreated controls (Byrick and Rose, 1990). Indeed, conversion of oliguric to nonoliguric renal failure does not appear to alter the outcome once dialysis becomes necessary (Brown et al., 1981). Nevertheless, in these patients increased urine flow does facilitate fluid management and nutritional support and tends to slow the development of hyperkalemia and metabolic acidosis.

Side Effects

Side effects of loop diuretics most often manifest as abnormalities of fluid and electrolyte balance. Loss of potassium and chloride is prominent, and hypokalemia is a constant threat in patients treated with furosemide (see Table 25-3). Preoperative evaluation of patients treated chronically with furosemide may include laboratory testing to rule out hypokalemic, hyponatremic, and hypomagnesemic metabolic alkalosis.

Acute or chronic treatment of patients with diuretics, including loop diuretics, may result in acute tolerance ("braking phenomenon"). Acute tolerance is presumed to reflect sodium and water retention (activation of the renin-angiotensin system) in the presence of contracted extracellular fluid volume (Brater, 1994). Treatment of this acute tolerance is extracellular volume repletion. With chronic use of diuretics, there is evidence of a compensatory hypertrophy of those portions of the renal tubule (especially distal convoluted tubules) responsible for sodium retention. When this occurs in a patient treated chronically with furosemide, it may be possible to reestablish a diuretic effect with the administration of a thiazide diuretic.

In animals, loop diuretics deplete myocardial potassium stores and increase the likelihood of digitalis toxicity. Hypokalemia has been associated with enhancement of the effects of nondepolarizing neuromuscular-blocking drugs. As with thiazide diuretics, loop diuretics may cause hyperuricemia, but this is rarely clinically significant. Likewise, hyperglycemia, although possible, is less likely to occur than with thiazide diuretics.

Furosemide increases renal tissue concentrations of aminoglycosides and enhances the possible nephrotoxic effects of these antibiotics. Cephalosporin nephrotoxicity may also be increased by furosemide. Furosemide has been associated with allergic interstitial nephritis similar to that occasionally produced by penicillin. Cross-sensitivity may exist when a patient allergic to other sulfonamides is given furosemide. The renal clearance of lithium is decreased in the presence of diuretic-induced decreases in sodium reabsorption. Consequently, plasma concentrations of lithium may be acutely increased by the IV administration of furosemide in the perioperative period (Havdala et al., 1979). In the presence of symptomatic hypercalcemia, furosemide may lower the plasma concentration of calcium by stimulating urine output.

Development of deafness, either transient or permanent, is a rare dose-dependent complication produced by furosemide and ethacrynic acid. This side effect is most likely to occur with prolonged increases in the plasma concentration of these drugs in the presence of other ototoxic drugs. Drug-induced changes in the electrolyte composition of the endolymph is a possible mechanism. Patients who are allergic to drugs containing a sulfonamide nucleus (certain antibiotics, thiazide diuretics) may be at increased risk for developing allergic reactions when treated with furosemide (Hansbrough et al., 1987). A similar cross-sensitivity with ethacrynic acid is less likely because this diuretic lacks a sulfonamide nucleus (see Figs. 25-2 and 25-3).

OSMOTIC DIURETICS

Osmotic diuretics such as mannitol and urea (a) are freely filterable at the glomerulus, (b) undergo limited reabsorption from renal tubules, (c) resist metabolism, and (d) are pharmacologically inert. These characteristics permit administration of osmotic diuretics in sufficiently large quantities to alter the osmolarity of the plasma, glomerular filtrate, and renal tubular fluid, resulting in osmotic diuresis. Portions of the renal tubules (proximal renal tubules, loops of Henle) that are highly permeable to water represent the principal site of action of osmotic diuretics.

Mannitol

Mannitol is the most frequently used osmotic diuretic. Structurally, mannitol is a six-carbon sugar that does not undergo metabolism (Fig. 25-4). It is not absorbed from the gastrointestinal tract, which necessitates its exclusive use by IV injection to achieve a diuretic effect. Mannitol does not enter cells, and its only means of clearance from the plasma is by glomerular filtration.

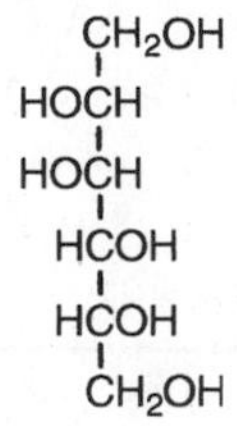

Figure 25-4. Mannitol.

Mechanism of Action

After administration, mannitol is completely filtered at the glomeruli, and none of the filtered drug is subsequently reabsorbed from the renal tubules (see Table 25-2) (Merin and Bastron, 1986). As a result, mannitol increases the osmolarity of renal tubular fluid and prevents reabsorption of water. Sodium is diluted in this retained water in the renal tubules, leading to less reabsorption of this ion. As a result of this osmotic effect in the renal tubular fluid, there is an osmotic diuretic effect with urinary excretion of water, sodium, chloride, and bicarbonate ions (see Table 25-4) (Tonnesen, 1983). Urinary pH is not altered by mannitol-induced osmotic diuresis (see Table 25-4) (Tonnesen, 1983).

In addition to causing renal tubular effects, IV administration of mannitol also increases plasma osmolarity, thus drawing fluid from intracellular to extracellular spaces. This increased plasma osmolarity may result in an acute expansion of the intravascular fluid volume. Redistribution of fluid from intracellular sites decreases brain bulk and may preferentially increase renal blood flow to the medulla. Likewise, the acute increase in intravascular fluid volume may have detrimental effects in patients with poor myocardial function. Mannitol is a scavenger of oxygen-free radicals, which may prevent cellular swelling and reduce renal tubular obstruction.

Clinical Uses

Mannitol is administered for (a) prophylaxis against acute renal failure, (b) differential diagnosis of acute oliguria, (c) treatment of increases in intracranial pressure, and (d) decreasing intraocular pressure.

Prophylaxis Against Acute Renal Failure

Mannitol is used as prophylaxis ("renal protection protocols") against acute renal failure, which may occur after (a) cardiovascular surgery, (b) transplantation surgery, (c) extensive trauma, (d) surgery in the presence of jaundice, and (e) in nephrotoxic conditions (hemolytic transfusion reactions). Despite experimental data that administration of mannitol before an ischemic insult will decrease the likelihood of renal damage there is often the absence of data in patients to confirm these impressions (Byrick and Rose, 1990).

Prophylactic administration of mannitol and low-dose dopamine during and after infrarenal cross-clamping of the abdominal aorta has not been shown to prevent transient deteriorations in renal function in patients whose hemodynamic stability is maintained (Byrick and Rose, 1990). Despite the clinical perception that diuresis is an indication of renal function preservation, there is data demonstrating that urine output alone is not an accurate predictor of renal function in the postoperative period (Alpert et al., 1984). Furthermore, serum creatinine concentrations and creatinine clearance are not improved after mannitol administration to patients undergoing surgery on the abdominal aorta (Nicholson et al., 1996; Paul et al., 1986). Perhaps the principal advantage of mannitol-induced diuresis is easier patient management with respect to fluid and blood administration. There is no question that mannitol reliably produces diuresis in patients undergoing cardiac surgery but, as with abdominal aortic surgery, there is no evidence of a renal protective effect. Furthermore, patients receiving large doses of mannitol in the cardiopulmonary bypass priming solution are at risk for devlopment of hypovolemia and hypokalemia in the postoperative period.

The protective effect of mannitol as used for the prevention of acute renal failure after a transfusion reaction is unproven. The rationale for its use, which is relief of renal tubular obstruction by precipitated hemoglobin, has been largely discounted. Mannitol is not superior to saline for preventing radiocontrast dye-induced renal dysfunction (Solomon et al., 1994). Renal transplant surgery is an example of a renal protective effect of mannitol. The incidence of acute renal failure is less in patients receiving mannitol before revascularization of the transplanted kidney (VanValenberg et al., 1984).

Differential Diagnosis of Acute Oliguria

Mannitol, 0.25 g/kg IV, is useful in the differential diagnosis of acute oliguria. For example, urine output is increased by mannitol when the cause of acute oliguria is decreased intravascular fluid volume. Conversely, when glomerular or renal tubular function is severely compromised, mannitol will not increase urine flow.

Treatment of Increased Intracranial Pressure

Mannitol, 0.25 to 1.00 g/kg IV, decreases intracranial pressure by increasing plasma osmolarity, which draws water from tissues, including the brain, along an osmotic gradient. In addition, mannitol may facilitate decreases in intracranial pressure by decreasing cerebrospinal fluid volume by virtue of decreasing the rate of formation of this fluid (Fig. 25-5) (Donato et al., 1994).

Mannitol begins to exert an effect within 10 to 15 minutes and is effective for about 2 hours. There is little difference in the effect of this dose range on intracranial pressure, but the larger dose may last longer (Marsh et al., 1977). Furthermore, larger doses and repeated administration can result in metabolic derangements. Importantly, mannitol is not associated with a high incidence of rebound increases in intracranial pressure. An intact blood-brain barrier is necessary to prevent entrance of mannitol into the CNS. If the blood-brain barrier is not intact, mannitol may enter the brain, drawing fluid with it and producing rebound cerebral edema. Regardless, the brain eventually adapts to sustained increases in plasma osmolarity such that chronic use of mannitol is likely to become less effective for lowering intracranial pressure.

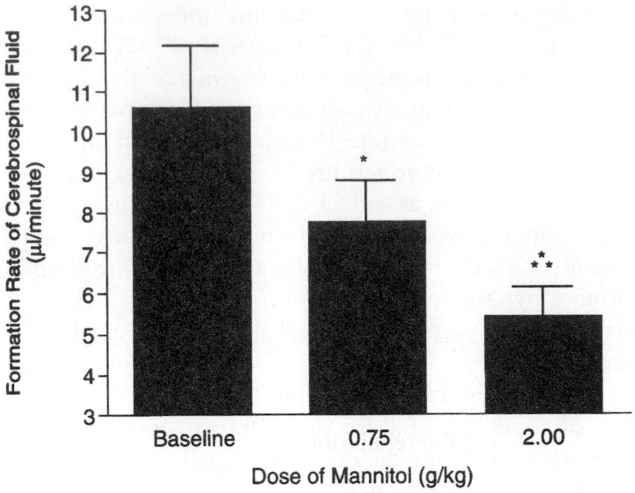

Figure 25-5. The formation rate of cerebrospinal fluid as measured in animals was decreased in a dose-dependent manner by mannitol. (*, significant difference from baseline; **, significant difference from the low-dose condition.) (From Donato T, Shapiro Y, Artru A, et al. Effect of mannitol on cerebrospinal fluid dynamics and brain tissue edema. *Anesth Analg* 1994;78:58–66; with permission.)

Mannitol has been shown to cause vasodilation of vascular smooth muscle, which is dependent on the dose and rate of administration (Ravussin et al., 1988). Mannitol-induced vasodilation affects intracranial and extracranial vessels and can transiently increase cerebral blood volume and intracranial pressure while simultaneously decreasing systemic blood pressure (Cottrell et al., 1977; Domaingue and Nye, 1985). Because mannitol may initially increase intracranial pressure, it is a common recommendation to infuse the selected dose over about 10 minutes and in conjunction with treatments that decrease intracranial volume (corticosteroids, hyperventilation of the lungs).

Reduction of Intraocular Pressure

Mannitol, glycerin, and isosorbide are occasionally used for the short-term reduction of intraocular pressure in patients undergoing ophthalmologic surgery. By increasing plasma osmolarity, fluid leaves the intraocular space along an osmotic gradient. Glycerin and isosorbide are administered orally and may contribute to an increased gastric fluid volume at the time of anesthetic induction. A maximal reduction in intraocular pressure and vitreous volume occurs approximately 1 hour after oral administration of glycerin, with a return to pretreatment levels in approximately 5 hours. Metabolism of glycerin to glucose can cause hyperglycemia and glycosuria, emphasizing the need for caution in administering this substance to patients with diabetes mellitus. Because it is rapidly metabolized, glycerin produces minimal diuresis, and routine urinary bladder catheterization for surgery is not required. Isosorbide does not adversely affect blood glucose levels and is preferred in patients with diabetes mellitus.

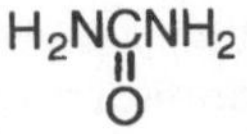

Figure 25-6. Urea.

Side Effects

In patients with oliguria secondary to cardiac failure, acute mannitol-induced increases in intravascular fluid volume may precipitate pulmonary edema. For this reason, furosemide may be a preferred drug for treatment of increased intracranial pressure in patients with left ventricular dysfunction. Prolonged use of mannitol may cause hypovolemia, electrolyte disturbances, and plasma hyperosmolarity due to excessive excretion of water and sodium. Nephrotoxins and prolonged renal ischemia may damage the renal tubular epithelium so that renal tubules are no longer impermeable to mannitol and the osmotic effect of the diuretic is lost.

Diuresis secondary to mannitol does not alter the elimination rate of long-acting nondepolarizing neuromuscular-blocking drugs. This is predictable because these neuromuscular-blocking drugs depend on glomerular filtration, which is not altered by mannitol. Venous thrombosis is not likely to occur after the IV administration of mannitol, and tissue necrosis is unlikely if extravasation occurs.

Urea

Urea, 1.0 to 1.5 g/kg IV, is an effective osmotic diuretic, but unlike mannitol, its small molecular size results in reabsorption of more than 60% of urea filtered by the glomerulus (Fig. 25-6). This drug eventually penetrates cells and crosses the blood-brain barrier, resulting in a greater degree of rebound increase in intracranial pressure than occurs after administration of mannitol. Another disadvantage of urea is the associated high incidence of venous thrombosis and the possibility of tissue necrosis if extravasation of urea-containing solutions occurs. Increased blood urea nitrogen concentrations after administration of urea should not be confused with acute renal failure.

POTASSIUM-SPARING DIURETICS

Potassium-sparing diuretics such as triamterene and amiloride act directly on renal tubular transport mechanisms in the distal convoluted tubules independent of aldosterone to produce diuresis (Fig. 25-7; see Table 25-2)

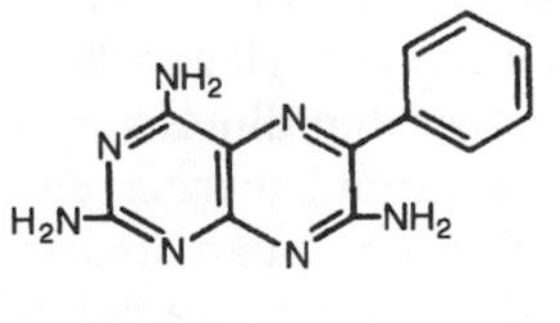

Triamterene

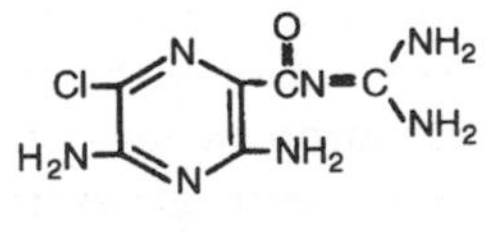

Amiloride

Figure 25-7. Potassium-sparing diuretics.

(Merin and Bastron, 1986). This diuresis is characterized by an increase in the urinary excretion of sodium, chloride, and bicarbonate ions, and an increase in the urine pH (see Table 25-4) (Tonnesen, 1983). Diuresis is accompanied by no increase or a decrease in potassium excretion in the urine (see Table 25-4) (Tonnesen, 1983). The lack of diuretic-induced potassium excretion results from inhibition of potassium secretion into distal renal tubules.

Pharmacokinetics

Triamterene is readily absorbed from the gastrointestinal tract whereas amiloride is only incompletely absorbed. Amiloride is more potent than triamterene and is not metabolized (Saggar-Malik and Cappuccio, 1993). Triamterene is a pteridine with a structural resemblance to folic acid (see Fig. 25-7). The metabolism of triamterene is extensive, and some of its metabolites have diuretic activity. The elimination half-time for triamterene is 3 to 5 hours and for amiloride is about 18 hours. Alterations in the pharmacokinetics of triamterene occur in patients with renal disease; thus, this drug should be used with caution in such patients.

Clinical Uses

Potassium-sparing diuretics are most often used in combination with loop diuretics or thiazide diuretics to augment diuresis and limit renal loss of potassium. These drugs are not available as parenteral formulations and are unlikely to be administered to patients in the perioperative period or to critically ill patients. Because amiloride and triamterene act at sites more distal in the nephron than thiazides, these drugs are inherently less effective. The combination of a thiazide and potassium-sparing diuretic maximizes diuretic efficiency of both types of drugs while offsetting their opposite effects on urinary excretion of potassium. Aerosolized amiloride administered to patients with cystic fibrosis improves sputum viscosity, presumably by inhibiting excessive absorption of sodium across the airway epithelium (Knowles et al., 1990).

Side Effects

Hyperkalemia is the principal side effect of therapy with potassium-sparing diuretics (see Table 25-4). Unlike other diuretics, these drugs do not produce hyperuricemia. Patients at risk for developing acute renal failure may be at risk for developing hyperkalemia if treatment with potassium-sparing diuretics are continued. Hyperkalemia is also a risk in patients receving these diuretics in the presence of other durgs that are also associated with increased plasma postassium concentrations (nonsteroidal antiinflammatory, angiotensin-converting enzyme inhibitors, beta-blockers).

ALDOSTERONE ANTAGONISTS

Spironolactone is a synthetic steroid analog that acts as a potassium-sparing diuretic. This drug bears a close structural resemblance to aldosterone (Fig. 25-8; see Table 25-2) (Merin and Bastron, 1986).

Mechanism of Action

Spironolactone binds to cytoplasmic mineralocorticoid receptors on collecting ducts and acts as a competitive antagonist to aldosterone. Indeend, spironolactone is effective only when aldosterone is present. Normally, aldosterone augments the renal tubular reabsorption of sodium and chloride ions and increases the excretion of potassium ions. Spironolactone blocks these renal tubular effects of aldosterone, as reflected by inhibition of the reabsorption of sodium and chloride. Binding of spironolactone to the receptor complex prevents the aldosterone-receptor complex from translocating to the cell's nucleus (inhibits gene expression). This is consistent with the observation that the drug's onset of action takes 2 to 4 days for full pharmacologic effects to be reached. Furthermore, the effects of spironolactone on aldosterone transport last for 48 to 72 hours after spironolactone is discontinued emphasizing the risk of hyperkalemic, hyperchloremic acidosis in patients receiving this drug and who develop acute renal failure.

Pharmacokinetics

Oral absorption of spironolactone approaches 70% of the administered dose. Spironolactone undergoes extensive hepatic first-pass metabolism. Binding to plasma proteins is extensive, and virtually no unchanged drug appears in urine. Canrenone is a major metabolite of spironolactone, which can, in turn, be metabolized to canrenoate. Canrenone is an active aldosterone antagonist, whereas canrenoate has no pharmacologic activity (Saggar-Malik and Cappuccio, 1993).

Clinical Uses

Spironolactone is often prescribed for treatment of refractory edematous states due to congestive heart failure and cirrhosis of the liver on the assumption that decreased

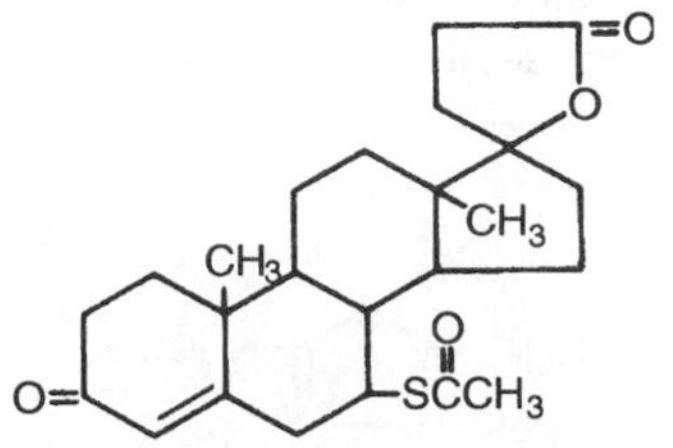

Figure 25-8. Spironolactone.

hepatic function and metabolism lead to increased plasma concentrations of aldosterone. The antihypertensive effect of this diuretic is similar to that of the thiazide diuretics, but side effects are different. The combination of spironolactone and a thiazide diuretic is an attempt to maximize diuretic efficiency of both drugs while offsetting their opposite effects on potassium secretion.

Side Effects

Hyperkalemia, especially in the presence of renal dysfunction, is the most serious side effect of treatment with spironolactone (see Table 25-3). In contrast to thiazide diuretics, spironolactone does not cause hypokalemia, hyperglycemia, or hyperuricemia (see Table 25-3).

CARBONIC ANHYDRASE INHIBITORS

Acetazolamide is the prototype of a class of sulfonamide drugs that bind avidly to carbonic anhydrase enzyme, producing noncompetitive inhibition of enzyme activity, principally in the proximal renal tubules (Fig. 25-9; see Table 25-2) (Merin and Bastron, 1986). As a result of this enzyme inhibition, the excretion of hydrogen ions is diminished and loss of bicarbonate ions is increased (see Table 25-3) (Tonnesen, 1983). Chloride is retained by the kidneys to offset the loss of bicarbonate and thus maintain the ionic balance. Decreased availability of hydrogen ions in the distal renal tubules results in excretion of potassium in exchange for sodium. The net effect of all these changes is excretion of an alkaline urine in the presence of hyperchloremic metabolic acidosis. The diuretic action of acetazolamide is not altered by metabolic or respiratory acidosis. After oral administration, acetazolamide is excreted unchanged by the kidneys in about 24 hours.

Clinical Uses

Acetazolamide, 250 to 500 mg orally, is adminstered to treat altitude sickness and to decrease intraocular pressure in the treatment of glaucoma. Decreased intraocular pressure reflects the presence of high concentrations of carbonic anhydrase enzyme in the ocular structures and a resulting decrease in the formation of aqueous humor when enzyme activity is inhibited by acetazolamide. Formation of cerebrospinal fluid is also inhibited by acetazolamide. Acetazolamide inhibits seizure activity, presumably by producing metabolic acidosis.

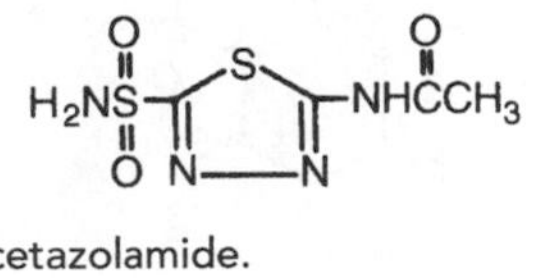

Figure 25-9. Acetazolamide.

Beneficial effects of acetazolamide in the management of familial periodic paralysis may reflect drug-induced metabolic acidosis, which increases the local concentration of potassium in skeletal muscles. Acetazolamide, by producing metabolic acidosis, may stimulate ventilation in patients who are hypoventilating as a compensatory response to metabolic alkalosis. Conversely, the loss of bicarbonate ions necessary to buffer carbon dioxide may result in the exacerbation of respiratory acidosis in patients with chronic obstructive airway disease, leading to CNS depression.

DOPAMINE RECEPTOR AGONISTS

Examples of drugs that augment renal function and exert diuretic effects via actions at dopamine receptors include dopamine and fenoldopam (see Table 25-1). In addition to actions at dopamine receptors, these drugs also exert effects at alpha and beta receptors (see Table 25-5) (Garwood and Hines, 1998).

Dopamine receptors are classified as dopamine-1 and dopamine-2 subtypes. Dopamine-1 receptors, but not dopamine-2 receptors, stimulate adenylate cyclase and phospholipase and the formation of cyclic adenosine monophosphate. In the renal vasculature, dopamine-1 receptors mediate vasodilation and increase renal blood flow and glomerular filtration rate. In renal tubules, stimulation of dopamine-1 receptors inhibits sodium reabsorption and promotes natriuresis. Dopamine-2 receptors in the renal vasculature inhibit norepinephrine release from postganglioninc sympathetic nerve endings but renal blood flow and glomerular filtration rate do not increase.

Dopamine

Dopamine is a mixed dopamine-1 and dopamine-2 agonist at low doses (1 to 3 μg/kg per minute) and at higher doses $beta_1$ agonist effects evoked by dopamine increase cardiac output, renal perfusion pressure and renal blood flow. Stimulation of dopamine-1 receptors in the renal tubules stimulates natriuresis. Dopamine could provide renoprotective effects by inhibiting the sodium pump and decreasing renal tubule oxygen consumption. Indeed, dopamine is often included as part of protocols to preserve renal function. Nevertheless, data confirming a prophylactic renal protective effect of low-dose dopamine are lacking and routine use of dopamine for this purpose cannot be recommended (Perdue et al., 1998; Galley, 2000; O'Hara, 2000). When patients with preexisting renal dysfunction undergoing angiography received prophylactic dopamine the serum creatinine concentrations increased more than in patients receiving saline (Gare et al., 1999). Furthermore, the pharmacodynamic effect of dopamine is unpredictable because of interindividual variability in its pharmacokinetics such that low-dose dopamine may result in plasma concentrations considered to be in the alpha-agonist range in some patients (MacGregor et al., 2000). Undesirable tachycardia and progressive renal vasoconstriction may accompany dopamine alpha and beta agonist-induced effects.

Dopamine is also synthesized endogenously in renal tubular cells from L-dopa resulting in inhibition of the sodium/potassium ATPase pump (Holtback et al., 2000).

Fenoldopam

Fendoldopam is a relatively selective postsynaptic dopamine-1 agonist with weak 5-hydroxytryptamine-2 receptor agonist activity and no significant dopamine-2, alpha and beta agonist effects. Infusion of fendoldopam (0.1 to 0.5 μg/kg/minute) produces renal vasodilation and increased renal blood flow without changes in systemic blood pressure. Higher doses of fenoldopam may decrease systemic blood pressure, but unlike sodium nitroprusside, these fenolopam-induced decreases in blood pressure do not decrease renal blood flow. The principal use of fenoldopam is as an IV antihypertensive drug. A renoprotective effect of fenoldopam has not been established.

Short-term fenoldopam infusion (0.1 μg/kg/minute) in combination with norepinephrine and dobutamine increased gastric mucosal perfusion in patients with septic shock (Morelli et al., 2004). Intestinal mucosa has been identified as an import target for injury during septic shock. Alterations in blood flow within the intestinal wall (ischemia) may be a contributing factor to mucosal injury and multiple organ dysfunction.

REFERENCES

Alpert RA, Roizen MF, Hamilton WK, et al. Intraoperative urinary output does not predict postoperative renal function in patients undergoing abdominal aortic revascularization. *Surgery* 1984;95:707–711.

Brater DC. Diuretic resistance: Mechanisms and therapeutic strategies. *Cardiology* 1994;84:57–67.

Brown C, Ogg C, Cameron J. High dose furosemide in acute renal failure: A controlled trial. *Clin Nephrol* 1981.15:90–96.

Byrick RJ, Rose DK. Pathophysiology and prevention of acute renal failure: the role of the anaesthetist. *Can J Anaesth* 1990;37:457–467.

Cottrell JE, Robustelli A, Post K, et al. Furosemide and mannitol-induced changes in intracranial pressure and serum osmolarity and electrolytes. *Anesthesiology* 1977;47:28–30.

Domaingue CM, Nye DH. Hypotensive effect of mannitol administered rapidly. *Anaesth Intensive Care* 1985;13:134–136.

Donato T, Shapira Y, Artru A, et al. Effect of mannitol on cerebrospinal fluid dynamics and brain tissue edema. *Anesth Analg* 1994;78. 58–66.

Galley HR. Renal-dose dopamine: Will the message now get through? *Lancet* 2000;256:2112–2113.

Gare M, Haviv YS, Ben-Yehuda A et al. The renal effect of low-dose dopamine in high-risk patients undergoing coronary angiography. *J Am Coll Cardiol* 1999;34:1682–1688.

Garwood S, Hines R. Perioperative renal preservation: Dopexamine and fenoldopam-new agents to augment renal performance. *Semin Anes Periop Med Pain* 1998;17:311–316.

Hansbrough JR, Wedner J, Chaplin DD. Anaphylaxis to intravenous furosemide. *J Allergy Clin Immunol* 1987;80:538–541.

Havdala HS, Borison RL, Diamond BI. Potential hazards and applications of lithium in anesthesiology. *Anesthesiology* 1979;50: 534–537.

Holtback U, Kruse MS, Brismar H, et al. Intrarenal dopamine coordinates the effect of antinatriuretic and natriuretic factors. *Acta Physiol Scand* 2000:168:215–218.

Knowles MR, Church NL, Waltner WE, et al. A pilot study of aerosolized amiloride for the treatment of lung disease in cystic fibrosis. *N Engl J Med* 1990;322:1189–1194.

MacGregor DA, Smith TE, Prielipp RC, et al. Pharmacokinetics of dopamine in healthy male subjects. *Anesthesiology* 2000;92: 338–346.

Marsh ML, Marshall LF, Shapiro HM. Neurosurgical intensive care. *Anesthesiology* 1977;47:149–163.

Merin RG, Bastron RD. Diuretics. In: Smith NT, Miller RD, Corbascio AN, eds. *Drug interactions in anesthesia*. Philadelphia: Lea & Febiger, 1986:206–224.

Morelli A, Rocco M, Conti G, et al. Effects of short-term fenoldopam infusion on gastric mucosal blood flow in septic shock. *Anesthesiology* 2004:101:576–582.

Nicholson ML, Baker DM, Hopkinson BR, et al. Randomized controlled trial of the effect of mannitol on renal reperfusion injury during aortic surgery. *Br J Surg* 1996;83:1230–1233.

O'Hara JF. Low-dose "renal" dopamine. *Anesthesiol Clin North America* 2000:18:835–851.

Paul MD, Mazer D, Byrick RJ, et al. Influence of mannitol and dopamine on renal function during elective infrarenal aortic clamping in man. *Am J Nehprol* 1986;6:427–434.

Perdue PW, Balser JR, Lipsett PA et al. "Renal dose" dopamine in surgical patients: Dogma or science? *Ann Surg* 1998;227:470.

Ravussin P, Abou-Madi M, Archer D, et al. Changes in CSF pressure after mannitol in patients with and without elevated CSF pressure. *J Neurosurg* 1988;69:869–876.

Saggar-Malik AK, Cappuccio FP. Potassium supplements, and potassium-sparing diuretics. A review and guide to appropriate use. *Drugs* 1993;46:986–1008.

Solomon R. Werner C, Mann D et al. Effects of saline, mannitol, and furosemide to prevent acute decreases n renal function induced by radiocontrast agents. *N Engl J Med* 1994;331:1416–1420.

Tonnesen AS. Clinical pharmacology and use of diuretics. In: Hershey SG, Bamforth BJ, Zauder H, eds. *Review courses in anesthesiology*. Philadelphia: Lippincott, 1983:217–226.

Van Valenberg PLJ, Hoitsma AJ, Tiggeler RGWAL, et al. Mannitol as an indispensable constituent of an intraoperative hydration protocol for the prevention of acute renal failure after renal cadaveric transplantation. *Transplantation* 1987;44:784–788.

Antacids and Gastrointestinal Prokinetics

26

ANTACIDS

Antacids are drugs that neutralize or remove acid from gastric contents. Clinically useful antacids are aluminum, calcium, and magnesium salts that react with hydrochloric acid to form neutral, less acidic, or poorly soluble salts. In addition, drug-induced increases in gastric fluid pH to >5 result in inactivation of pepsin and produce bile-chelating effects. Neutralization of gastric fluid pH increases gastric motility via the action of gastrin (aluminum hydroxide is an exception) and increases lower esophageal sphincter tone by a mechanism that is independent of gastrin.

Antacids produce a beneficial effect on the rate of duodenal ulcer healing that is similar to H_2-receptor antagonists (Ching and Lam, 1994). Furthermore, antacids provide prompt symptomatic relief of duodenal ulcer pain and are inexpensive compared with H_2-receptor antagonists or proton pump inhibitors. The efficacy of antacids in promoting gastric ulcer healing is controversial. Antacids provide symptomatic relief from symptoms produced by reflux esophagitis, but there is no evidence that antacids are better than placebo in healing reflux esophagitis (Klinkenberg-Knol et al., 1995). Although antacids are commonly prescribed with nonsteroidal antiinflammatory drugs for prophylaxis against drug-induced gastroduodenal mucosa injury, there is little evidence to support the efficacy of this practice (Ching and Lam, 1994).

Commercial Antacid Preparations

Each kind of antacid has advantages and disadvantages. For example, sodium bicarbonate is potent and well absorbed, but its sodium content can be hazardous to patients with heart disease or hypertension. Nonabsorbable antacids that contain magnesium hydroxide as the sole active ingredient almost invariably produce osmotic diarrhea. Calcium carbonate is a potent acid neutralizer but it may induce an increase in gastric acid secretion hours after its ingestion. Aluminum hydroxide is not a potent neutralizer, and because it interferes with phosphate absorption, it can cause hypophosphatemia. Conversely, aluminum hydroxide may decrease plasma phosphate concentrations in patients with renal insufficiency. Because the various antacids have different potencies and side effects, they are commonly combined in commercial preparations (Table 26-1). Liquid preparations are generally more effective than tablets for neutralizing gastric acid in vivo.

Sodium Bicarbonate

The high solubility of bicarbonate results in a prompt and rapid antacid action in the stomach. This effect, however, is brief, and systemic alkalosis is possible. Sodium bicarbonate is useful if the goal is to alkalinize the urine. Patients with hypertension or heart disease may not tolerate the increased sodium load associated with chronic use of this antacid.

Magnesium Hydroxide

Magnesium hydroxide (milk of magnesia) produces prompt neutralization of gastric acid and is not associated with significant acid rebound. In contrast to aluminum hydroxide, a prominent laxative effect (osmotic diarrhea) is characteristic of magnesium hydroxide. Systemic absorption of magnesium may be sufficient to cause neurologic, neuromuscular, and cardiovascular impairment in patients with renal dysfunction. In normal patients, absorption of magnesium is associated with little risk of systemic alkalosis. Magnesium is often combined with aluminum hydroxide.

TABLE 26-1.
CONTENTS (mg per 5 mL) OF PARTICULATE ANTACIDS

	Aluminum Hydroxide	Magnesium Hydroxide	Calcium Carbonate	Sodium
Aludrox	307	103		1.1
Amphojel	320			6.9
Di-Gel	282	85		10.6
Gelusil	200	200		0.7
Maalox	225	200		1.35
Mylanta	200	200		0.68
Riopan	480			0.3
Tums			500	<3
Win Gel	180	160		<2.5

Calcium Carbonate

Calcium carbonate produces prompt and effective neutralization of gastric acid. Although systemic absorption is slight, sufficient absorption occurs with chronic therapy to produce a detectable metabolic alkalosis. The plasma concentration of calcium is increased transiently. Clinically, dangerous hypercalcemia may occur in patients with renal disease. The administration of calcium carbonate-containing antacids may be accompanied by hypophosphatemia. Even small amounts of calcium carbonate-containing antacids evoke hypersecretion of hydrogen ions (acid rebound) (Clayman, 1980). The chalky taste of calcium carbonate is a disadvantage. The release of carbon dioxide in the stomach may cause eructation and flatulence. Constipation is minimized by including magnesium oxide with calcium carbonate. Acute appendicitis has been produced by impacted calcium carbonate fecaliths.

Aluminum Hydroxide

Aluminum hydroxide is actually a mixture of aluminum hydroxide, aluminum oxide, and some fixed carbon dioxide as carbonate. Systemic absorption of aluminum is minimal, but in patients with renal disease, the plasma and tissue concentrations of aluminum may become excessive (Berlyne et al., 1970). Encephalopathy in patients undergoing hemodialysis has been attributed to intoxication with aluminum (Alfrey et al., 1976). Among the compounds formed in the intestine from aluminum hydroxide are insoluble aluminum phosphates, which pass through the gastrointestinal tract unabsorbed. Hypophosphatemia can occur and is the basis for the occasional therapeutic use of aluminum hydroxide in the treatment of phosphate nephrolithiasis. Decreased phosphate absorption is accompanied by increased calcium ion absorption, which sometimes causes hypercalcuria and nephrolithiasis. Hypomagnesemia can also occur. Aluminum compounds, in contrast to other antacids, cause slowing of gastric emptying and marked constipation. These effects, in addition to an unpleasant taste, contribute to poor patient acceptance.

Complications of Antacid Therapy

The only adverse effects shared by all antacids are those resulting from changes in gastric fluid and urine pH and alterations in acid–base status. Chronic alkalinization of gastric fluid has been suggested as a cause of increased susceptibility to various acid-sensitive bacilli. Alkalinization of the urine may predispose to urinary tract infections; if it is chronic, urolithiasis is possible. Increased urine pH may persist >24 hours after administration of an antacid, leading to changes in the renal elimination of drugs. Other potential complications of antacid therapy include (a) acid rebound, (b) milk-alkali syndrome, and (c) phosphorus depletion.

Acid Rebound

Acid rebound is a side effect that is unique to calcium-containing antacids. This response is characterized by a marked increase in gastric acid secretion that takes place several hours after neutralization of gastric acid. It is not known if acid rebound persists as a problem if chronic treatment with calcium carbonate is used. Acid rebound may be related to transient hypercalcemia that develops in some patients who ingest calcium carbonate.

Milk-Alkali Syndrome

The milk-alkali syndrome is characterized by hypercalcemia, increased blood urea nitrogen and plasma creatinine concentrations, and systemic alkalosis as reflected by a high plasma concentration of bicarbonate ions. The plasma calcium phosphate concentration is usually increased. There may be a marked decrease in renal function with calcification of the renal parenchyma. This syndrome is most commonly associated with ingestion of large amounts of calcium carbonate plus >1,000 mL of milk daily. Magnesium and aluminum-containing antacids have not been implicated in this syndrome.

Phosphorus Depletion

Phosphorus depletion can occur in patients who ingest large doses of aluminum salts because these antacids bind phosphate ions in the gastrointestinal tract, thus preventing their absorption. This effect may actually be beneficial in patients with renal disease because it can decrease the plasma phosphate concentration. Individuals with phosphorus depletion may experience anorexia, skeletal muscle weakness, and malaise. Osteomalacia, osteoporosis, and fractures may occur. If it is necessary to administer aluminum-containing antacids on a chronic basis to patients with osteomalacia or osteoporosis, phosphate supplements should be considered.

Drug Interactions

Because gastric alkalinization hastens gastric emptying, antacids other than aluminum compounds will hasten delivery of drugs into the small intestine. This may facilitate absorption of drugs that are poorly absorbed or it may shorten the time available for absorption. The rate of absorption of salicylates, indomethacin, and naproxen is increased when gastric fluid pH is increased. Aluminum hydroxide accelerates absorption and increases bioavailability of diazepam by an unknown mechanism. Conversely, bioavailability of certain drugs may be decreased because of their capacity to form complexes with antacids. For example, antacids decrease bioavailability of orally administered cimetidine by approximately 15% (Gugler et al., 1981). For this reason, it may be recommended that at least 1 hour elapse between ingestion of an antacid and oral administration of cimetidine. Antacids containing aluminum, and to a lesser extent, calcium or magnesium, interfere with the absorption of tetracyclines and possibly digoxin from the gastrointestinal tract.

Antacid Selection

There is considerable variation in the acid-neutralizing effects of different antacids (see Table 26-1). Poorly absorbed antacids are preferred in the treatment of peptic ulcer disease. Mixtures of aluminum hydroxide and magnesium hydroxide are used most frequently. Calcium carbonate has a greater neutralizing capacity, but it is infrequently administered because of concern about systemic absorption of calcium and calcium-induced acid rebound. Whether mixtures of antacids have greater beneficial effects than those produced by the individual antacid remains controversial.

Preoperative Administration of Antacids

The potential value of preoperative administration of antacids is based on the unproved presumption that drug-induced increases in the gastric fluid pH would decrease the likelihood of the development of severe acid pneumonitis should inhalation (aspiration) of gastric fluid occur (Warner et al., 1993). Despite the predictable ability of antacids to increase gastric fluid pH, it has not been documented that prophylactic administration of antacids to a high-risk patient population (parturients) decreases mortality (Tompkinson et al., 1982). Furthermore, antacids or other prophylactic drugs administered to alter gastric fluid pH or volume (H_2 antagonists, metoclopramide) do not influence the incidence of regurgitation and aspiration.

The duration of antacid action is highly dependent on gastric emptying time. For example, opioid-induced slowing of gastric motility prolongs the pH-elevating effects of antacids in these patients compared with the effects of antacids in patients not receiving opioids (O'Sullivan and Bullingham, 1985). Repeated administration of antacids, such as to the parturient who has also received opioids, can result in greatly increased gastric fluid volume at the time general anesthesia is induced. In this regard, it seems more logical to administer an antacid as a single dose approximately 30 minutes before the anticipated induction of general anesthesia.

Even a single dose of antacid may increase the gastric fluid volume, and it has been speculated that this effect could offset desirable effects on pH if aspiration should occur. Nevertheless, in an animal model, mortality was 90% after inhalation of 0.3 mL/kg gastric fluid with a pH of 1.0 compared with 20% mortality after inhalation of 1 mL/kg of gastric fluid with a pH of 2.0 (Table 26-2) (James et al., 1984). These animal data suggest that an increased gastric fluid volume will not increase mortality from aspiration as long as the gastric fluid pH is increased.

Particulate Antacids

Occasional failure of particulate antacids to increase gastric fluid pH may reflect inadequate mixing with stomach contents or an unusually large volume of gastric fluid such that the standard dose of antacid is inadequate to neutralize gastric hydrogen ions. Layering is also common with particulate antacids (Holdsworth et al., 1980). Pneumonitis associated with functional and histologic changes in the

TABLE 26-2.
MORTALITY RATE (%) FOR RATS AFTER ASPIRATION OF SOLUTIONS OF VARIOUS pHs AND VOLUMES

	Fluid pH					
Volume (ml/kg)	1.0	1.4	1.8	2.5	3.5	5.8
0.2	20	0				
0.3	90	0	9			
0.4	90	40	9	0		
1.0	100	90	20	0	0	0
2.0	100	100	27	30	20	10
4.0	100	100	38	20	40	30

Source: Data from James CF, Modell JH, Gibbs CP, et al. Pulmonary aspiration effects of volume and pH in the rat. *Anesth Analg* 1984;63;665–668; with permission.

lungs may reflect a foreign body reaction to inhaled particulate antacid particles. Indeed, aspiration of particulate antacids in a dog model produced changes comparable to those induced by acid (Gibbs et al., 1979). Clinical reports suggest that particulate antacids have caused or aggravated aspiration pneumonitis in humans (Bond et al., 1979; Heaney and Jones, 1979).

Nonparticulate Antacids

Nonparticulate (clear) antacids such as sodium citrate are less likely to cause a foreign body reaction if aspirated, and their mixing with gastric fluid is more complete than is that of particulate antacids (Gibbs et al., 1979; Holdsworth et al., 1980). Furthermore, the onset of effect is more rapid with sodium citrate than with particulate antacids that require a longer time for adequate mixing with gastric fluid. Sodium citrate, 15 to 30 mL of a 0.3-mol solution administered 15 to 30 minutes before the induction of anesthesia, is effective in reliably increasing gastric fluid pH in pregnant and nonpregnant patients (Gibbs et al., 1979). The pH of 0.3 mol sodium citrate is approximately 8.4, accounting for its unpleasant taste and frequent need to add a flavoring material to improve its palatability.

Bicitra is a nonparticulate antacid-containing sodium citrate and citric acid that provides effective buffering of gastric fluid pH (Eyler et al., 1982). Polycitra is a nonparticulate antacid containing sodium citrate, potassium citrate, and citric acid that has greater buffering capacity than Bicitra. Bicitra and Polycitra are more palatable than sodium citrate, possibly due to their lower pHs of 4.5 and 5.2, respectively.

SUCRALFATE

Sucralfate is a complex salt of sucrose sulfate and aluminum hydroxide (Fig. 26-1) (McCarthy, 1991). Administered orally (1 g 1 hour before meals and at bedtime), the tablet disintegrates in the stomach and in the presence of acid forms a viscous suspension that binds with high affinity to both normal and defective mucosa. Aluminum released from the dissolution of sucralfate binds with proteins, peptides, drugs, metals, and large molecules such as mucins. Aluminum absorption during sucralfate therapy is comparable to that during treatment with aluminum hydroxide, and aluminum intoxication may occur. For this reason, sucralfate should be used with caution in patients with renal disease. The poor water solubility of sucralfate results in very little systemic absorption of the intact compound. Sucralfate interferes with the absorption and bioavailability of several drugs including tetracycline and quinolone antibiotics, phenytoin, digoxin, and amitriptyline. Delayed absorption of H_2-receptor antagonists does not seem to be clinically significant. Nosocomial pneumonia appears to be associated less frequently with sucralfate than with antacid therapy.

Clinically, sucralfate appears to be safe and effective in the treatment of patients with duodenal or gastric ulcers. This compound lacks antacid action but instead adheres to the ulcer to form a cytoprotective barrier against pepsin penetration. Simultaneous administration of antacids may interfere with the efficacy of sucralfate. Sucralfate is effective in preventing stress bleeding in patients receiving long-term mechanical ventilation, but it has no demonstrated advantage over H_2-antagonist drugs.

GASTROINTESTINAL PROKINETICS

Motility-modulating drugs exert their therapeutic effects by increasing lower esophageal sphincter tone, enhancing peristaltic contractions, and accelerating the rate of gastric emptying.

Metoclopramide

Metoclopramide (methoxychloroprocainamide) is a dopamine antagonist that is structurally similar to procainamide but lacks local anesthetic activity (Fig. 26-2). Metoclopramide acts as a gastrointestinal prokinetic drug

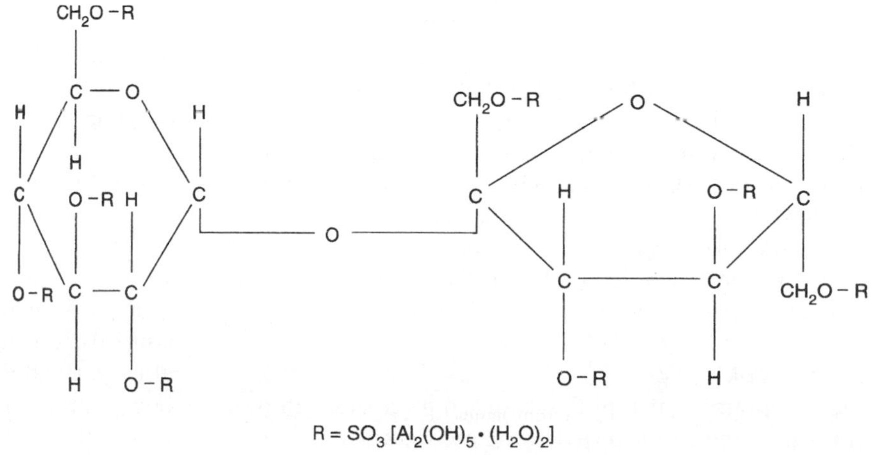

Figure 26-1. Sucralfate.

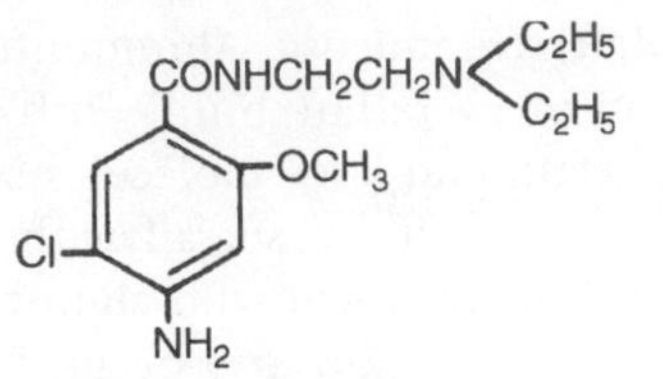

Figure 26-2. Metoclopramide.

that increases lower esophageal sphincter tone and stimulates motility of the upper gastrointestinal tract in normal persons and parturients (Brock-Utne et al., 1978). Gastric hydrogen ion secretion is not altered. The net effect is accelerated gastric clearance of liquids and solids (decreased gastric emptying time) and a shortened transit time through the small intestine.

Mechanism of Action

Metoclopramide produces selective cholinergic stimulation of the gastrointestinal tract (gastrokinetic effect) consisting of (a) increased smooth muscle tension in the lower esophageal sphincter and gastric fundus, (b) increased gastric and small intestinal motility, and (c) relaxation of the pylorus and duodenum during contraction of the stomach (Schulze-Delrieu, 1981). The cholinergic stimulating effects of metoclopramide are largely restricted to smooth muscles of the proximal gastrointestinal tract and require some background cholinergic activity. There is evidence that metoclopramide sensitizes gastrointestinal smooth muscles to the effects of acetylcholine, which explains the observation that metoclopramide, unlike conventional cholinergic drugs, requires background cholinergic activity to be effective. Postsynaptic activity results from the ability of metoclopramide to cause the release of acetylcholine from cholinergic nerve endings. Indeed, atropine opposes metoclopramide-induced increases in lower esophageal sphincter tone and gastrointestinal hypermotility, indicating that metoclopramide acts on postganglionic cholinergic nerves intrinsic to the wall of the gastrointestinal tract.

Metoclopramide acts as a dopamine-receptor antagonist, but any effects on dopamine-induced inhibition of gastrointestinal motility are not considered to be clinically significant (Klinkenberg-Knol et al., 1995). In the central nervous system (CNS), metoclopramide blocks dopamine receptors. As a result, metoclopramide may produce extrapyramidal side effects. Stimulation of prolactin secretion also reflects inhibition of the CNS effects of dopamine. Metoclopramide-induced antagonism of dopamine-agonist effects on the chemoreceptor trigger zone (located outside the blood-brain barrier) would theoretically contribute to an antiemetic effect.

Pharmacokinetics

Metoclopramide is rapidly absorbed after oral administration, reaching peak plasma concentrations in 40 to 120 minutes (Schulze-Delrieu, 1981). Extensive first-pass hepatic metabolism limits bioavailability to about 75%. Most patients achieve therapeutic plasma concentrations of 40 to 80 ng/mL after 10 mg of metoclopramide administered orally. The elimination half-time is 2 to 4 hours. Metoclopramide readily crosses the blood-brain barrier and the placenta. The concentration of metoclopramide in breast milk may exceed the plasma concentration. Approximately 85% of an oral dose of metoclopramide appears in the urine, equally divided between unchanged drug and sulfate and glucuronide conjugates. Impairment of renal function prolongs the elimination half-time and necessitates a decrease in metoclopramide dosage.

Clinical Uses

Clinical uses of metoclopramide include (a) preoperative decrease of gastric fluid volume, (b) production of an antiemetic effect, (c) treatment of gastroparesis, and (d) symptomatic treatment of gastroesophageal reflux. Administration of metoclopramide, 10 to 20 mg intravenously (IV), may be useful to speed gastric emptying before the induction of anesthesia, to facilitate small-bowel intubation, or to speed gastric emptying to improve radiographic examination of the small intestine. Metoclopramide has been used to improve the effectiveness of oral medication if other drugs or the patient's underlying condition slows gastric emptying. Increased prolactin secretion evoked by metoclopramide has been proposed as a means to test the function of the anterior pituitary or to improve lactation in the postpartum period (Schulze-Delrieu, 1981).

Preoperative Decrease in Gastric Fluid Volume

Metoclopramide, 10 to 20 mg IV over 3 to 5 minutes administered 15 to 30 minutes before induction of anesthesia, results in increased lower esophageal sphincter tone and decreased gastric fluid volume (Wyner and Cohen, 1982). More rapid IV administration may produce abdominal cramping. This gastric emptying effect of metoclopramide may be of potential benefit before the induction of anesthesia in (a) patients who have recently ingested solid food, (b) trauma patients, (c) obese patients, (d) patients with diabetes mellitus and symptoms of gastroparesis, and (e) parturients, especially those with a history of esophagitis ("heartburn"), suggesting lower esophageal sphincter dysfunction and gastric hypomotility. Nevertheless, beneficial effects of metoclopramide on gastric fluid volume may be difficult to document in otherwise normal patients with low gastric fluid volumes who are awaiting elective surgery (Table 26-3) (Cohen et al., 1984).

Regardless of the effects of gastric fluid volume, the administration of metoclopramide does not reliably alter gastric fluid pH. Furthermore, it is important to recognize that opioid-induced inhibition of gastric motility may not be reversible with metoclopramide. Likewise,

TABLE 26-3.
VOLUME OF GASTRIC CONTENTS AND pH IN STUDY GROUPS (MEAN ± SE)

	Metoclopramide (n = 30)	Placebo (n = 28)
Gastric volume (range)	24 ± 2 mL (3–600)	30 ± 5 mL (4–155)
Volume <25 mL	16* (53%)	15* (54%)
Gastric pH (range)	2.86 ± 0.27 (1–6)	2.55 ± 5 mL (1–5.5)
pH <2.5	12* (40%)	16* (57%)

*Number of patients
Source: Data from Cohen SE, Jasson J, Talafre ML, et al. Does metoclopramide decrease the volume of gastric contents in patients undergoing cesarean section? *Anesthesiology* 1984;61:604–607; with permission.)

the beneficial cholinergic stimulant effects of metoclopramide on the gastrointestinal tract may be offset by concomitant administration of atropine in the preoperative medication. Under no circumstances do metoclopramide or other prophylactic drugs (antacids or H_2 antagonists) replace the need for proper airway management, including placement of a cuffed endotracheal tube in the awake patient or after induction of general anesthesia.

Production of an Antiemetic Effect

The antiemetic effect of metoclopramide in preventing postoperative nausea and vomiting is equivocal and in some reports no clinically relevant effect on the incidence of postoperative nausea and vomiting can be demonstrated (Henzi et al., 1999). The antiemetic property of metoclopramide probably results from antagonism of dopamine's effects in the chemoreceptor trigger zone. Additional antiemetic effects are provided by metoclopramide-induced increases in lower esophageal sphincter tone and facilitation of gastric emptying in the small intestine. These latter effects reverse the gastric immobility and cephalad peristalsis that accompany the vomiting reflex. Gastric stasis induced by morphine is reversed by metoclopramide, and opioid-induced nausea and vomiting, which can accompany preoperative medication or postoperative pain management, are blunted by this drug.

Treatment of Gastroparesis

Treatment of gastroparesis, as associated with diabetes mellitus, is often managed with orally administered metoclopramide, 10 to 20 mg. Both the prokinetic and antiemetic effects of metoclopramide contribute to its efficacy in treating gastroparesis and associated symptoms. There is evidence that metoclopramide, 10 mg IV, speeds the rate of gastric emptying of solids in patients with diabetic gastroparesis (Fig. 26-3) (Wright et al., 1985).

Symptomatic Treatment of Gastroesophageal Reflux

A possible benefit of metoclopramide in the management of patients with gastroesophageal reflux and associated symptoms of esophagitis ("heartburn") is suggested by the ability of this drug to increase lower esophageal sphincter tone. Metoclopramide has been useful in decreasing the symptoms of esophagitis, but there is no evidence that treatment with this drug facilitates healing of the esophagus (Klinkenberg-Knol et al., 1995).

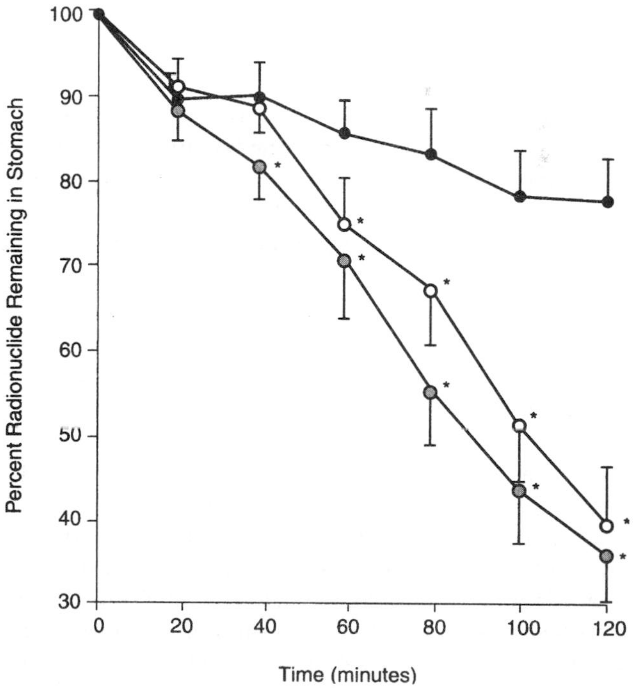

Figure 26-3. Gastric emptying time (mean ± SD) after ingestion of a test meal (radioactive-labeled chicken, liver, and beef stew) in patients with diabetes mellitus (*solid circles*), patients with diabetes mellitus and the test meal followed by metoclopramide, 10 mg IV (*open circles*), and patients without diabetes mellitus (*gray circles*). (From Wright RA, Clemente R, Wathen R. Diabetic gastroparesis: an abnormality of gastric emptying of solids. *Am J Med Sci* 1985;289:240–243; with permission.)

Side Effects

Abdominal cramping may follow rapid IV administration (<3 minutes) of metoclopramide. Intravenous administration of metoclopramide may also be associated with hypotension, tachycardia, bradycardia, and cardiac dysrhythmias. Sedation, dysphoria, agitation, dry mouth, glossal or periorbital edema, hirsutism, and urticarial or maculopapular rash are rare side effects that have not been observed after single doses of metoclopramide (Cohen et al.,1984). Breast enlargement, galactorrhea, or menstrual irregularities that occur rarely are presumed to reflect metoclopramide-induced increases in plasma prolactin concentrations. For this reason, patients with a history of breast cancer probably should not be treated chronically with metoclopramide.

Dystonic extrapyramidal reactions (oculogyric crises, opisthotonus, trismus, torticollis) occur in <1% of patients treated chronically with metoclopramide. Although usually developing if large oral doses (40 to 80 mg daily) are administered chronically, there are reports of neurologic dysfunction related to the preoperative administration of metoclopramide (Scheller and Sears, 1987). These extrapyramidal reactions are identical to the Parkinson syndrome evoked by antipsychotic drugs that antagonize the CNS actions of dopamine (Grimes et al., 1982). Akathisia, a feeling of unease and restlessness in the lower extremities, may follow the IV administration of metoclopramide, resulting in cancellation of scheduled surgery (LaGorio et al., 1998).

Placental transfer of metoclopramide occurs rapidly, but adverse fetal effects with single doses have not been observed (Cohen et al., 1984). The usual dopamine-induced inhibition of aldosterone secretion is prevented by metoclopramide. As a result, the possibility of sodium retention and hypokalemia should be considered, especially in patients who develop peripheral edema during chronic therapy.

Metoclopramide may increase the sedative actions of CNS depressants and the incidence of extrapyramidal reactions caused by certain drugs. For this reason, metoclopramide should probably not be administered in combination with phenothiazine or butyrophenone drugs or to patients with preexisting extrapyramidal symptoms or seizure disorders. Patients being treated with monoamine oxidase inhibitors or tricyclic antidepressants should likewise probably not receive metoclopramide. Metoclopramide decreases bioavailability of orally administered cimetidine by 25% to 50% (Gugler et al., 1981). It would seem prudent not to administer metoclopramide to a patient with a suspected or known mechanical obstruction to gastric emptying. Likewise, metoclopramide is not administered after gastrointestinal surgery such as pyloroplasty or intestinal anastomosis because it stimulates gastric motility and may delay healing.

Metoclopramide has an inhibitory effect on plasma cholinesterase activity when tested in vivo, which may explain occasional observations of prolonged responses to succinylcholine and mivacurium in patients receiving these drugs (Kao et al., 1990; Skinner et al., 1999). Parturients may be at increased risk for this response considering the already decreased plasma cholinesterase activity associated with pregnancy. Likewise, the metabolism of ester local anesthetics could be slowed by metoclopramide-induced decreases in plasma cholinesterase activity.

Cisapride

Cisapride is a gastrointestinal prokinetic drug that stimulates gastric emptying, increases lower esophageal sphincter tone, and enhances motility in the small and large intestine (shortens mouth to cecum transit time) by enhancing the release of acetylcholine from nerve endings in the myenteric plexus of the gastrointestinal mucosa (Klinkenberg-Knol et al., 1995; Rowbotham, 1989). In contrast to metoclopramide, cisapride lacks dopamine-antagonist effects. Like metoclopramide, cisapride has no effect on gastric hydrogen ion secretion or gastric fluid volume.

Opioid-induced gastric stasis, which may be an important cause of postoperative nausea and vomiting, is reversed by cisapride, 10 mg intramuscularly administered 2 hours before the opioid (Rowbotham and Nimmo, 1987). Administration of cisapride before antagonism of neuromuscular blockade with atropine and neostigmine does not prevent the ability of atropine to decrease lower esophageal sphincter tone (Jones et al., 1989). Cisapride is effective in relieving the symptoms of gastroesophageal reflux and is effective in facilitating healing of mild esophagitis.

Domperidone

Domperidone is a benzimidazole derivative that, like metoclopramide, acts as a specific dopamine antagonist that stimulates peristalsis in the gastrointestinal tract, speeds gastric emptying, and increases lower esophageal sphincter tone (Fig. 26-4) (Brock-Utne et al., 1980). Unlike metoclopramide, domperidone does not easily cross the blood-brain barrier and does not appear to have any anticholinergic activity. Its gastrokinetic actions have therefore been attributed to its peripheral dopaminergic activity. Because it lacks dopaminergic effects in the CNS, this drug is not associated with extrapyramidal

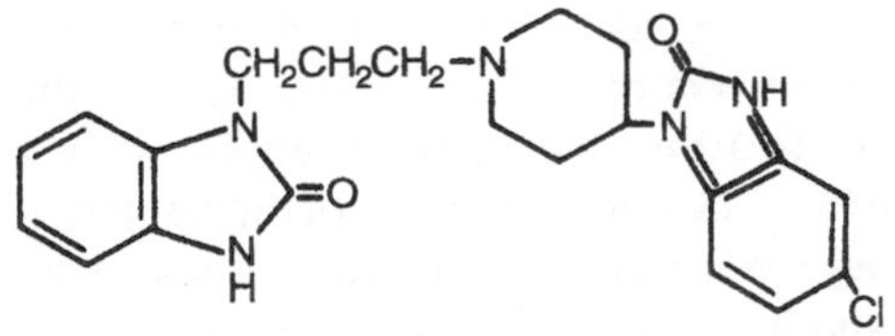

Figure 26-4. Domperidone.

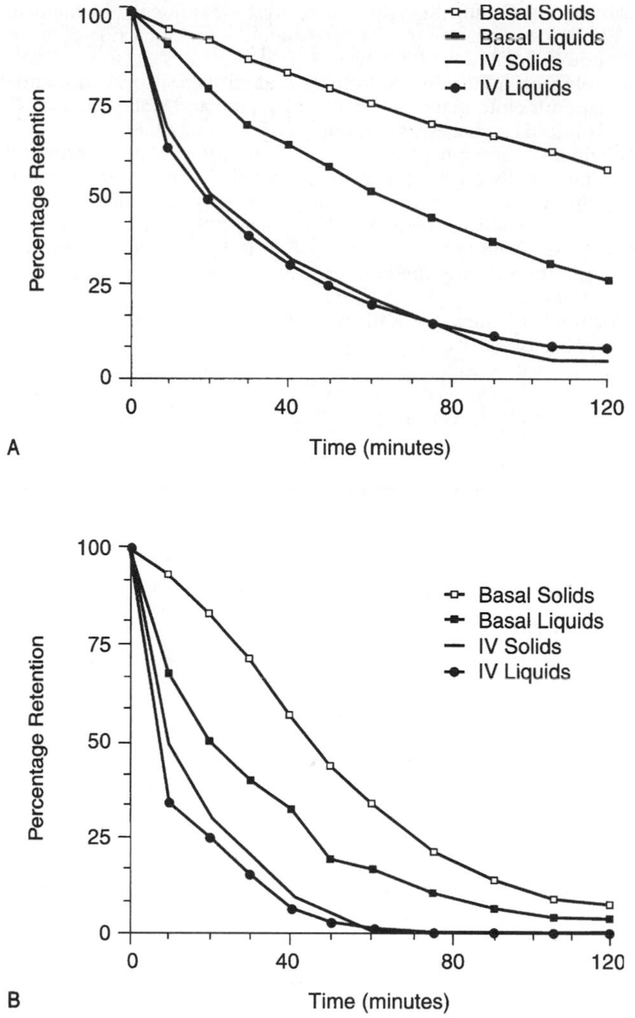

Figure 26-5. Erythromycin, 200 mg intravenously over 15 minutes, followed by ingestion of a radioactive-labeled meal (scrambled egg, toast, and water) resulted in more rapid emptying of solids and liquids (IV solids and IV liquids) in patients with diabetic gastroparesis (**A**) and patients without diabetes (**B**) compared with gastric emptying times in the absence of erythromycin (basal solids and basal liquids). (From Urbain JLC, Vantrappen G, Janssens J, et al. Intravenous erythromycin dramatically accelerates gastric emptying in gastroparesis diabeticorum and normals and abolishes the emptying discrimination between solids and liquids. *J Nucl Med* 1990;31:1490–1493; with permission.)

symptoms. Restriction of its dopamine antagonist effects to the periphery allows domperidone to influence the chemoreceptor trigger zone, which is outside the blood-brain barrier, without affecting the basal ganglia. The value of domperidone as prophylaxis against or treatment of postoperative nausea and vomiting is unclear (Fragen and Caldwell, 1979).

Domperidone is rapidly absorbed after oral or intramuscular administration. Extensive metabolism occurs in the liver, and biliary excretion of inactive metabolites is the main route of elimination. The elimination half-time is approximately 7 hours.

Erythromycin

The antibiotic erythromycin increases lower esophageal sphincter tone, enhances intraduodenal coordination, and promotes emptying of gastric liquids and solids in patients with diabetic gastroparesis, in patients awaiting emergency surgery, and in normal patients (Fig. 26-5) (see Chapter 28) (Kopp et al., 1997; Urbain et al., 1990). These gastric prokinetic properties are attributed to the erythromycin's cholinergic stimulatory properties (Chaussade et al., 1994).

REFERENCES

Alfrey AC, LeGendre GR, Kaehny WS. The dialysis encephalopathy syndrome. Possible aluminum intoxication. *N Engl J Med* 1976; 294:184–188.

Berlyne GM, Ben-Ari J, Pest D, et al. Hyperalbuminemia from aluminum resins in renal failure. *Lancet* 1970;2:494–496.

Bond VK, Stoelting RK, Gupta CD. Pulmonary aspiration syndrome after inhalation of gastric fluid-containing antacids. *Anesthesiology* 1979;51:452–453.

Brock-Utne JG, Dow TGB, Welman S, et al. The effect of metoclopramide on lower oesophageal sphincter tone in late pregnancy. *Anaesth Intensive Care* 1978;6:26–29.

Brock-Utne JG, Downing JW, Dimopoulos GE, et al. Effect of domperidone on lower esophageal sphincter tone in late pregnancy. *Anesthesiology* 1980;52:321–323.

Chaussade S, Michpopoulos S, Sogni P, et al. Motilin agonist erythromycin increases human lower esophageal sphincter pressure by stimulation of cholinergic nerves. *Dig Dis Sci* 1994;39:381–384.

Ching CK, Lam SK. Antacids: indications and limitations. *Drugs* 1994;47:305–317.

Clayman CB. The carbonate affair: chalk one up [editorial]. *JAMA* 1980;244:2554.

Cohen SE, Jasson J, Talafre ML, et al. Does metoclopramide decrease the volume of gastric contents in patients undergoing cesarean section? *Anesthesiology* 1984;61:604–607.

Eyler SW, Cullen BF, Murphy ME, et al. Antacid aspiration in rabbits: a comparison of Mylanta and Bicitra. *Anesth Analg* 1982;61:288–292.

Fragen RJ, Caldwell N. Antiemetic effectiveness of intramuscularly administered domperidone. *Anesthesiology* 1979;51:460–461.

Gibbs CP, Schwartz DJ, Wynne JW, et al. Antacid pulmonary aspiration in the dog. *Anesthesiology* 1979;51:380–385.

Gibbs CP, Spohr L, Schmidt D. The effectiveness of sodium citrate as an antacid. *Anesthesiology* 1982;57:44–46.

Grimes JD, Hassan MN, Preston DN. Adverse neurologic effects of metoclopramide. *Can Med Assoc J* 1982;126:23–25.

Gugler R, Brand M, Somogyi A. Impaired cimetidine absorption due to antacids and metoclopramide. *Eur J Clin Pharmacol* 1981;20: 225–228.

Heaney GAH, Jones HD. Aspiration syndrome in pregnancy [letter]. *Br J Anaesth* 1979;51:266–267.

Henszi I, Walder B, Tramer MR. Metoclopramide in the prevention of postoperative nausea and vomiting:: A quantitative systematic review of randomized, placebo-controlled studies. *Br J Anaesth* 1999,83.761-771.

Holdsworth JD, Johnson K, Mascall G, et al. Mixing of antacids with stomach contents. *Anaesthesia* 1980;35:641–650.

James CF, Modell JH, Gibbs CP, et al. Pulmonary aspiration effects of volume and pH in the rat. *Anesth Analg* 1984;63:665–668.

Jones MJ, Mitchell WD, Hindocha N. Effects on the lower oesophageal sphincter of cisapride given before the combined administration of atropine and neostigmine. *Br J Anaesth* 1989;62:124–128.

Kao YJ, Teliez J, Turner DR. Dose-dependent effect of metoclopramide on cholinesterases and suxamethonium metabolism. *Br J Anaesth* 1990;65:220–224.

Klinkenberg-Knol EC, Festen HPM, Meuwissen SGM. Pharmacological management of gastro-oesophageal reflux disease. *Drugs* 1995;49: 695–710.

Kopp VJ, Mayer DC, Shaheen NJ. Intravenous erythromycin promotes gastric emptying prior to emergency anesthesia. *Anesthesiology* 1997;87:703–705.

La Gorio J, Thompson VA, Sternberg D, et al. Akathisia and anesthesia: refusal of surgery after the administration of metoclopramide. *Anesth Analg* 1998;87:224–227.

McCarthy DM. Sucralfate. *N Engl J Med* 1991;325:1017–1025.

O'Sullivan GM, Bullingham RE. Noninvasive assessment by radiotelemetry of antacid effect during labor. *Anesth Analg* 1985;64:95–100.

Rowbotham DJ. Cisapride and anaesthesia. *Br J Anaesth* 1989;62: 121–123.

Rowbotham DJ, Nimmo WS. Effect of cisapride on morphine-induced delay in gastric emptying. *Br J Anaesth* 1987;59:536–539.

Scheller MS, Sears KL. Postoperative neurologic dysfunction associated with preoperative administration of metoclopramide. *Anesth Analg* 1987;66:274–276.

Schulze-Delrieu K. Drug therapy: metoclopramide. *N Engl J Med* 1981; 305:28–33.

Skinner HJ, Girling KJ, Whitehurst A, et al. Influence of metoclopramide on plasma cholinesterase and duration of action of mivacurium. *Br J Anaesth* 1999;82:542–545.

Tompkinson J, Turnbull A, Robson R, et al. Report on confidential enquiries into maternal deaths in England and Wales 1976–1978. London: Her Majesty's Stationery Office 1982:79–80.

Urbain JLC, Vantrappen G, Janssens J, et al. Intravenous erythromycin dramatically accelerates gastric emptying in gastroparesis diabeticorum and normals and abolishes the emptying discrimination between solids and liquids. *J Nucl Med* 1990;31:1490–1493.

Warner MA, Warner ME, Weber JG. Clinical significance of pulmonary aspiration during the perioperative period. *Anesthesiology* 1993; 78:56–62.

Wright RA, Clemente R, Wathen R. Diabetic gastroparesis: an abnormality of gastric emptying of solids. *Am J Med Sci* 1985;289: 240–243.

Wyner J, Cohen SE. Gastric volume in early pregnancy: effect of metoclopramide. *Anesthesiology* 1982;57:209–212.

Anticoagulants

27

Anticoagulants are drugs that delay or prevent the clotting of blood by direct or indirect actions on the coagulation system. The anticoagulants in clinical use are heparin and enoxaparin (low-molecular-weight heparin), which are administered subcutaneously (SC) or intravenously (IV), and coumarin compounds, which are administered orally. These drugs have no effect on the thrombus (clot) after it is formed. Antithrombotic drugs such as aspirin usually influence the formation of thrombus by interfering with the normal adhesive and aggregation activity of platelets. Thrombolytic drugs are those that possess inherent fibrinolytic effects or enhance the body's fibrinolytic system.

HEPARIN

Unfractionated heparin is composed of a mixture of highly sulfated glycosaminoglycans that produce their anticoagulant effects by binding to antithrombin (previously known as *antithrombin III*), which is normally present as a naturally circulating anticoagulant. This binding with heparin, however, enhances by about 1,000 times the ability of antithrombin to inactivate a number of coagulation enzymes, including thrombin and activated factors X, XII, XI, and IX. There is evidence that heparin's principal inhibitory effect on coagulation is through inhibition of thrombin-induced activation of factor V and factor VII (Hirsh, 1991a). As such, heparin functions as an anticoagulant by accelerating the normally occurring antithrombin-induced neutralization of activated clotting factors. In addition to its anticoagulant effects, heparin inhibits platelet function (Hirsh, 1991a).

Commercial Preparations

Commercial preparations of heparin are heterogenous, their components having molecular weights ranging from 3,000 to 30,000 daltons. Only about one-third of heparin binds to antithrombin, and this fraction is responsible for most of its anticoagulant effect. Heparin for clinical uses is most commonly prepared from bovine lung and bovine or porcine gastrointestinal mucosa. Heparin is also present endogenously in basophils, mast cells, and the liver and the biologic activities of commercial preparations of heparin parallel endogenous heparin. The designation *heparin* emphasizes, is the abundance of this substance in the liver.

Standardization of heparin potency is based on in vitro comparison with a known standard. A unit of heparin is defined as the volume of heparin-containing solution that will prevent 1 mL of citrated sheep blood from clotting for 1 hour after the addition of 0.2 mL of 1:100 calcium chloride. Heparin must contain at least 120 *United States Pharmacopeia* (USP) units per mL. Because the potency of different commercial preparations of heparin may vary greatly, the heparin dose should always be prescribed in units.

Pharmacokinetics

Heparin is a poorly lipid-soluble, high-molecular-weight substance that cannot cross lipid barriers in significant amounts. As a result, heparin is poorly absorbed from the gastrointestinal tract and is usually administered by intravenous (IV) or subcutaneous (SC) injection. Intramuscular (IM) administration of heparin is avoided due to the risk of hematoma formation. Heparin does not cross the placenta and can be administered to the mother without producing anticoagulation in the fetus.

After injection, heparin circulates bound to many plasma proteins. The pharmacokinetics of heparin are complicated and incompletely understood (Hirsh, 1991a). There is no suitable chemical assay for heparin, so the investigation of its kinetics has depended on measurements of its biologic activity. Over the range of heparin concentrations used clinically, the dose-response relationship is not linear; instead, the anticoagulant response increases disproportionately in intensity and duration as the dose increases (deSwart et al., 1982). For example, the elimination half-time after a heparin dose of 100 U/kg IV was 56 minutes and increased to 152 minutes after a dose of 400 U/kg IV. Decreases in body temperature below 37°C greatly prolong the elimination half-time for heparin (Bull et al., 1975). Hepatic and renal dysfunction may also increase the elimination half-time of heparin.

After IV doses of heparin, a fraction of the drug is eliminated in the urine as a depolymerized and less sulfated molecule that retains about 50% of its original activity (Hirsh, 1991a). The precise pathway of heparin elimination is uncertain, and reports of the influence of renal and hepatic disease on its pharmacokinetics have been inconsistent. There is no evidence that the pharmacokinetics or anticoagulant properties of the forms of heparin derived from porcine or bovine sources are different. Among drugs that may influence the anticoagulant effect of heparin is nitroglycerin, which may increase the required dose of heparin (Becker et al., 1990). A lower dose of nitroglycerin did not show this effect (Bode et al., 1990). Heparin binds to many different proteins, which may neutralize the anticoagulant activity of this drug. Indeed, increased plasma concentrations of these proteins may contribute to heparin resistance in patients with inflammatory disorders and cancer (Anderson and Saenko, 2002).

Laboratory Evaluation of Coagulation

The anticoagulant response to heparin varies widely among patients with thromboembolic disease, possibly because of variations in the plasma concentrations of heparin-binding proteins. There is evidence that the clinical efficacy of heparin is optimized if the anticoagulant effect is maintained above a defined minimal level and the risk of spontaneous bleeding is increased as the dose of heparin increases.

Activated Plasma Thromboplastin Time

Heparin treatment is usually monitored to maintain the ratio of the activated plasma thromboplastin time (APTT) within a defined range of approximately 1.5 to 2.5 times the predrug value, which is typically 30 to 35 seconds. An excessively prolonged APPT (>120 seconds) is readily shortened by omitting a dose because heparin has a brief elimination half-time. When low-dose heparin is used, laboratory tests may not be required to monitor treatment because the dosage and schedule are well known.

Activated Coagulation Time

Heparin effect and its antagonism by protamine are commonly monitored in patients undergoing surgical procedures by measuring the activated coagulation time (ACT). Because the ACT is easy to use and reliable for high heparin concentrations, it has become the mainstay of heparin anticoagulation monitoring. In addition to the presence of a heparin effect, the ACT may be influenced by hypothermia, thrombocytopenia, presence of contact activation inhibitors (aprotinin), and preexisting coagulation deficiencies (fibrinogen, factor XII, factor VII). When aprotinin is present, the recommendation is to use kaolin-ACT rather than celite-ACT determinations.

A baseline value for the ACT is determined (a) before the IV administration of heparin, (b) approximately 3 minutes after administration, and (c) at 30-minute intervals thereafter. A dose-response curve for heparin can be constructed with the dose of heparin in mg/kg on the vertical axis and the ACT in seconds on the horizontal axis (Fig. 27-1) (Bull et al., 1975). A line connecting the points before and 3 minutes after heparin is used to calculate the additional dose of heparin necessary to achieve an acceptable ACT. The control ACT is usually 90 to 120 seconds. During cardiopulmonary bypass, the anticoagulant effect of heparin is often considered adequate if the ACT is >300 seconds, questionable with ACT between 180 and 300 seconds, and inadequate at <180 seconds. In animals, however, fibrin monomers may appear during cardiopulmonary bypass at an ACT of >400 seconds (Young et al., 1978). The need to measure ACT repeatedly is emphasized by the fourfold variation in heparin sensitivity between patients and the threefold variation in the rate at which heparin is metabolized. Furthermore, ACT values can be misleading during cardiopulmonary bypass with respect to heparin-induced anticoagulation because of the effects of hypothermia and hemodilution on the measurement system (Despotis et al., 1994).

The ACT is performed by mixing whole blood with an activation substance that has a large surface area, such as celite (diatomaceous earth, silicon dioxide) or kaolin (aluminum silicate). Contact of the activator with the blood initiates activation of the clotting cascade. Commercially available timing systems are used clinically to measure the ACT. These devices detect the onset of clot formation. Nevertheless, results between different commercial devices to measure the ACT are not interchangeable, especially if the type of activator (celite or kaolin) is different.

Clinical Uses

Heparin is effective in the prevention and treatment of venous thrombosis and pulmonary embolism, in the prevention of mural thrombosis after myocardial infarction (MI), in the treatment of patients with unstable angina and acute MI, and in the prevention of coronary artery rethrombosis after thrombolysis (Hirsh, 1991a). Heparin is also used to prevent thrombosis in extracorporeal devices during cardiovascular surgery and hemodialysis, to treat selected cases of disseminated intravascular coagulation, and to treat fetal growth retardation in pregnant women. Heparin is administered IV (bolus or infusion) or by deep SC injection. When administered intravenously, heparin has an immediate onset of action, whereas subcutaneous administration results in variable bioavailability with an onset of action in 1 to 2 hours.

Prophylaxis Against Venous Thromboembolism

General surgical patients and medical patients may be treated with SC heparin or low-molecular-weight heparin (enoxaparin) in an attempt to decrease the likelihood of

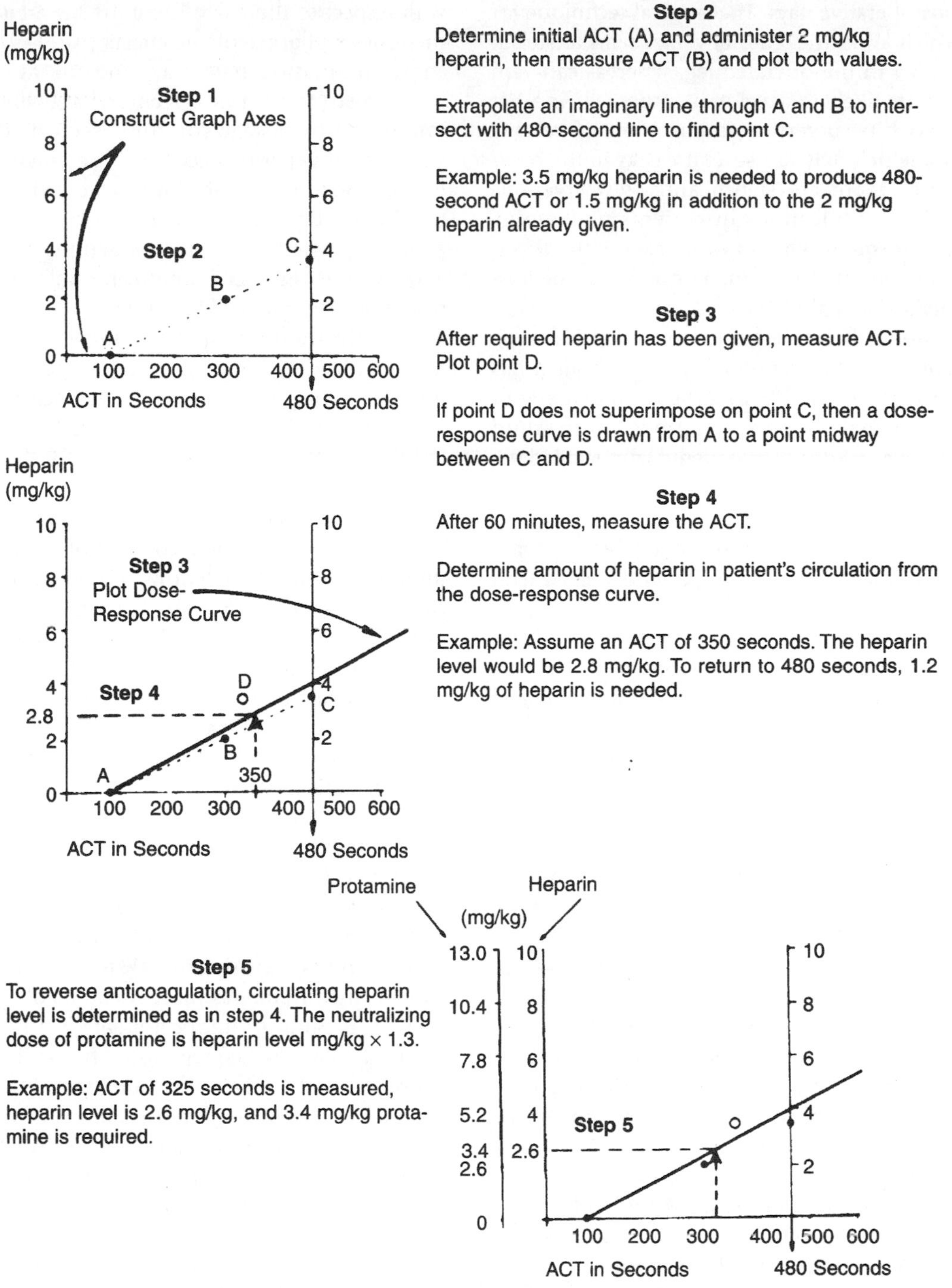

Figure 27-1. Calculation of heparin and protamine doses based on measurement of the activated coagulation time (ACT). (From Bull BS, Huse WM, Brauer FS, et al. Heparin therapy during extracorporeal circulation. II. The use of a dose-response curve to individualize heparin in protamine dosage. *J Thorac Cardiovasc Surg* 1975;69:785–789; with permission.)

venous thromboembolism (Bergqvist et al., 1996). Before the availability of enoxaparin, low-dose heparin, 5,000 U SC every 8 to 12 hours, was a common recommendation (Hirsh, 1991a). The use of low-dose heparin is associated with an increased incidence of wound hematoma but with no increase in the incidence of major bleeding. Low-dose heparin has been shown to decrease the incidence of venous thrombosis after acute MI.

Among surgical patients, those undergoing total hip replacement are at unique risk for developing deep-vein thrombosis (DVT). Currently, the best option for decreasing the risk of DVT, which occurs in an estimated 50% to 60% of patients without prophylaxis, is administration of enoxaparin, which is also cost effective (Bergqvist et al., 1996). The risk of DVT is more protracted after hip surgery than after general surgery, when it usually develops during the first few postoperative days. The surgical technique for hip surgery, which kinks the femoral vein, seems to stimulate proximal DVT in the operated leg, whereas calf-vein thrombosis is more likely to develop in either leg. Another effect unique to hip surgery is impairment of venous hemodynamics, which may last several weeks in the operated leg. Indeed, there are significantly fewer venous thromboembolic complications in patients undergoing elective hip replacement when prophylaxis with enoxaparin is given for 1 month rather than only during the hospitalization (Bergqvist et al., 1996).

Venous thromboembolism is a common, life-threatening complication of major trauma. Pulmonary embolism has been observed to occur in 2% to 22% of patients with major trauma, and fatal pulmonary embolism is the third most common cause of death in patients who survive the first 24 hours. In this regard, enoxaparin is also more efficacious than low-dose heparin in preventing DVT in patients recovering from major trauma (Geerts et al., 1996). The risk of major bleeding in patients treated with enoxaparin or low-dose heparin is low.

Treatment of Venous Thromboembolism

Patients with venous thromboembolism should be treated with 5,000 U IV of heparin followed by a continuous infusion of 30,000 U every 24 hours (Hirsh, 1991a). The goal is to maintain the APPT at 1.5 to 2.5 times the laboratory control value.

Heparin is the anticoagulant of choice in pregnant patients for treatment of venous thromboembolism or in parturients with prosthetic heart valves because it does not cross the placenta and it does not produce untoward effects in the fetus or newborn. Use of high doses of heparin for prolonged periods (>5 months) is problematic, because it may cause osteoporosis (Ginsberg et al., 1990). Anticoagulation is maintained for 3 to 6 months as shortening the time to 4 to 6 weeks doubles the frequency of recurrence of venous thromboembolism during the next 12 to 24 months.

Treatment of Unstable Angina and Acute MI

Patients with unstable angina or acute MI should receive 5,000 U IV of heparin followed by a continuous infusion of 24,000 U every 24 hours (Hirsh, 1991a). A similar heparin regimen may be instituted in conjunction with thrombolytic therapy for acute MI.

Side Effects

Hemorrhage

Hemorrhage is the most common serious side effect of heparin therapy. This risk increases with the intensity of anticoagulation required, preexisting coagulation defects, and concurrent use of other drugs that impact on coagulation, and the need for instrumentation (surgical procedures, performance of regional anesthesia). Advantages of heparin with respect to the risk of hemorrhage are the easy assessment of its pharmacologic effects (APTT, thrombin time), short elimination half-time, and the availability of an antagonist (protamine). Hemorrhage due to heparin is minimized by dosage control based on laboratory measurement of heparin effect. The concomitant use of aspirin is a risk factor for heparin-induced bleeding. Nevertheless, the risk of adding aspirin to a short course of regular therapeutic doses of heparin is low. Serious concurrent illness and chronic heavy consumption of alcohol increase the risk of heparin-induced bleeding.

Heparin should not be administered to patients with known bleeding tendencies or to persons undergoing intraocular or intracranial surgery. Placement of a needle or catheter in the lumbar subarachnoid or epidural space to inject a drug has been questioned for the patient who is receiving, or will receive, heparin. The concern is related to the possible occurrence of an epidural hematoma and compression of the spinal cord if a blood vessel was punctured during these injections. Likewise, hematomas and compression of peripheral nerves may be more likely to occur in association with the performance of peripheral nerve blocks with heparin. Despite these concerns, a large retrospective study has not confirmed an increased incidence of epidural hematoma formation in patients receiving a spinal or epidural anesthetic followed by heparin anticoagulation (Rao and El-Etr, 1981).

Thrombocytopenia

Thrombocytopenia due to heparin administration can be divided into two syndromes (Slaughter and Greenberg, 1997; Stow and Burrows, 1987). The most common syndrome is mild, occurring in 30% to 40% of heparin-treated patients manifesting as platelet counts of <100,000 cells/mm^3. This mild thrombocytopenia is attributed to drug-induced platelet aggregation. It typically manifests between 3 and 15 days after initiation of therapy (median 10 days) but has been reported to begin within hours in patients previously exposed to heparin (Warkentin and Kelton, 1989). Even a trivial intraoperative exposure to heparin flush has been associated with acute heparin-induced thrombocytopenia (Ling and Warkentin, 1998). The platelet count usually returns to baseline within 4 days after heparin is discontinued.

A second, more severe and even life-threatening syndrome develops in 0.5% to 6.0% of patients, manifesting as severe thrombocytopenia (<50,000 cells/mm^3), often with associated resistance to the effects of heparin and the occurrence of thrombotic events (heparin-induced thrombocytopenia and thrombosis [HITT] syndrome). This severe response typically develops after 6 to 10 days of heparin therapy and is probably due to formation of heparin-dependent antiplatelet antibodies that trigger platelet aggregation and resulting thrombocytopenia. Indeed, platelet-associated immunoglobulin G (IgG) antibodies have been demonstrated in these patients. The diagnosis is confirmed by in vitro platelet aggregation studies. Heparin therapy must be immediately discontinued in these patients. All patients treated chronically with heparin (regardless of the route of administration) should be monitored with periodic platelet counts.

Patients with a history of life-threatening heparin-induced thrombocytopenia who subsequently require surgical procedures involving cardiopulmonary bypass present a therapeutic dilemma. In these patients, anticoagulation for cardiopulmonary bypass has been produced by use of antithrombotic drugs that do not produce immune-mediated thrombocytopenia (see the section, Antithrombotic Drugs).

Allergic Reactions

Heparin is obtained from animal tissues; thus, caution should be used in its administration to a patient with a preexisting history of allergy. Indeed, fever, urticaria, and even cardiopulmonary changes occasionally occur after administration of heparin.

Cardiovascular Changes

Rapid IV infusion of large doses of heparin (300 U/kg) as administered before cardiopulmonary bypass may cause modest decreases in mean arterial pressure and pulmonary artery pressure (Konchigeri, 1984). These changes principally reflect decreases in systemic vascular resistance, perhaps due to a direct heparin-induced relaxant effect on vascular smooth muscles. Ionized calcium concentrations are decreased in a dose-dependent manner by in vitro, but not in vivo, administration of heparin (Goto et al., 1985). These results indicate that systemic blood pressure decreases that are occasionally observed after administration of heparin are not related to changes in the plasma concentrations of ionized calcium.

Altered Protein Binding

Acute IV administration of heparin, as before cardiac catheterization or initiation of cardiopulmonary bypass, displaces alkaline drugs from protein-binding sites. Evidence of this displacement is increased circulating concentrations of unbound fractions of propranolol and diazepam after the administration of heparin (Fig. 27-2) (Wood et al., 1980). It is conceivable that increased pharmacologic effects of propranolol and diazepam would accompany this heparin-induced decrease in protein binding. Certainly, measurement of plasma concentrations of drugs in heparinized blood must be interpreted differently than in the absence of heparin.

Altered Cell Morphology

Heparin added to whole blood distorts the morphology of leukocytes and erythrocytes. For this reason, heparinized blood is not acceptable for tests that involve complement, isoagglutinins, or erythrocyte fragility. The hematocrit, white blood cell count, and erythrocyte sedimentation rate are not altered by the presence of heparin.

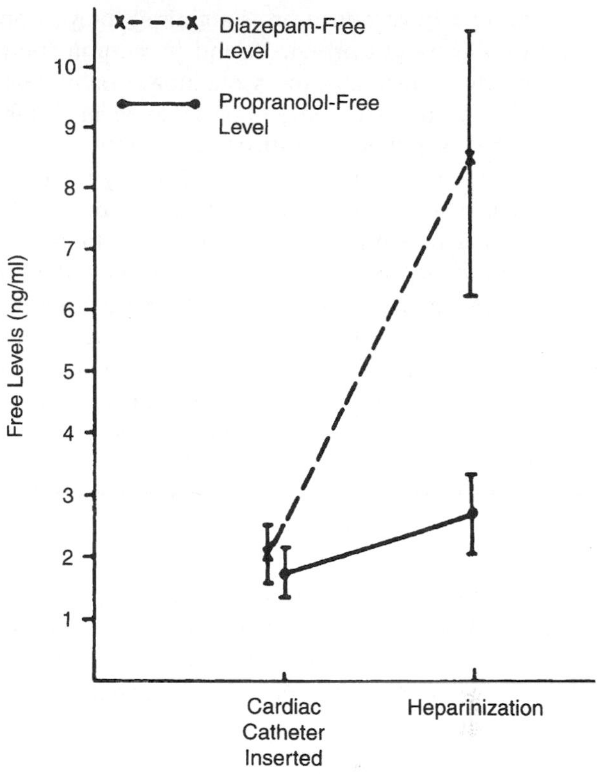

Figure 27-2. Administration of heparin displaces diazepam and propranolol from protein-binding sites, leading to an increase in the unbound (free) concentration of these drugs in the plasma. (From Wood AJJ, Robertson D, Robertson RM, et al. Elevated plasma free drug concentrations of propranolol and diazepam during cardiac catheterization. *Circulation* 1980;62:1119–1122; with permission.)

Decreased Antithrombin Concentrations

Paradoxically, patients who receive intermittent or continuous therapy with heparin manifest a progressive reduction of antithrombin activity to values that are approximately one-third of normal (Marciniak and Gockerman, 1977). Thus, a heparin-induced decrease in the activity of antithrombin may paradoxically increase the thrombotic tendency in humans. Estrogen-containing contraceptives also decrease concentrations of antithrombin; this is consistent with the clinical impression that the incidence of thromboembolic episodes is increased in patients who take these drugs. Patients with genetically determined low levels of antithrombin have a tendency to develop thromboembolism and may manifest increased dose requirements for heparin (Anderson, 1986). When heparin resistance is secondary to a deficiency in antithrombin, administration of fresh frozen plasma restores the levels to normal and promotes the anticoagulant effects of heparin.

Reversal of Heparin-Induced Anticoagulation

Protamine

Protamine is the specific antagonist of heparin's anticoagulant effect. Protamine is strongly alkaline (nearly two-thirds of the amino acid composition is arginine), polycationic low-molecular weight protein found in salmon sperm. The positively charged alkaline protamine combines with the negatively charged acidic heparin to form a stable complex that is devoid of anticoagulant activity. These heparin-protamine complexes are removed by the reticuloendothelial system. Clearance of protamine by the reticuloendothelial system (within 20 minutes) is more rapid than heparin clearance that may explain, in part, the phenomenon of heparin rebound. The dose of protamine required to antagonize heparin is typically 1 mg for every 100 U of heparin predicted to still be circulating. A more specific dose of protamine is calculated by in vitro titration of the patient's blood with protamine (see Fig. 27-1) (Bull et al., 1975). A guideline is administration of 1.3 mg/kg of protamine for each 100 U of heparin present as calculated from the ACT.

Protamine administered IV in the absence of heparin interacts with platelets and proteins, including fibrinogen. These interactions may manifest as an anticoagulant effect of protamine. Adverse cardiovascular responses to protamine include hypotension, pulmonary hypertension, and allergic reactions.

Hypotension

Rapid IV injection of protamine may be associated with histamine release, causing facial flushing, tachycardia, and hypotension. Indeed, the alkaline characteristic of protamine makes it predictable that histamine release could occur, especially after rapid IV injection. Nevertheless, injection of protamine over at least 5 minutes is not associated with changes in circulating plasma concentrations of histamine, and systemic blood pressure is not altered (Stoelting et al., 1984). Furthermore, there is no compelling evidence that protamine has direct negative inotropic effects (Conahan et al., 1981; Hines and Barash, 1986). Patients with poor left ventricular function, however, may be more susceptible to protamine-induced decreases in systemic blood pressure because compensatory increases in cardiac output to offset peripheral vasodilation are limited (Michaels and Barash, 1983).

The site of IV administration may influence the subsequent circulatory changes evoked by protamine. For example, administration of protamine into the right atrium of anesthetized dogs is followed by (a) increases in the plasma concentration of histamine, (b) increases in cardiac output, and (c) decreases in systemic blood pressure and systemic vascular resistance (Casthely et al., 1986). These changes do not occur if protamine is injected into a peripheral vein or into the left atrium. It is speculated that the heparin-protamine complex that evokes the release of histamine in the lungs is diluted before reaching the lungs if protamine is injected into a peripheral vein or left atrium. Despite these animal data, IV or intraatrial injection of protamine to patients has not been documented to produce different circulatory effects (Milne et al., 1983; Kronenfeld et al., 1987).

Pulmonary Hypertension

In rare cases, protamine neutralization of heparin can result in secretion of thromboxane and 5-hydroxy tryptamine (serotonin) manifesting as pulmonary vasoconstriction, pulmonary hypertension, and bronchoconstriction (Blaise, 1998). Arterial hypoxemia reflects ventilation-perfusion mismatching due to pulmonary edema secondary to pulmonary hypertension. These responses do not occur in patients manifesting systemic blood pressure changes traditionally attributed to protamine-induced histamine release. Pretreatment with cyclooxygenase inhibitors such as indomethacin or aspirin blunts the increase in pulmonary vascular resistance (Conzen et al., 1989). Inhibition of nitric oxide release does not play a role in the pulmonary hypertension response to protamine (Hakim et al., 1995).

Allergic Reactions

Allergic reactions to protamine have been described most often in patients receiving protamine-containing insulin preparations (Doolan et al., 1981; Moorthy et al., 1980). For example, there are approximately 2.8 mg of protamine per 100 U of protamine zinc insulin and 0.5 mg per 100 U of isophane (NPH) insulin. Presumably, chronic exposure to low doses of protamine in patients treated with protamine-containing insulin preparations evokes the production of antibodies against protamine. In this situation, the subsequent administration of large doses of protamine, as required to antagonize heparin-induced anticoagulation, may result in life-threatening allergic reactions. The occurrence of an allergic reaction evoked by protamine may be confirmed by increased plasma tryptase concentrations (Takenoshita et al., 1996). Patients who are allergic to fish may also be at increased risk for development of allergic reactions to protamine (Knape et al., 1981). The presence of circulating antisperm antibodies in vasectomized or infertile males has not been associated with allergic reactions to protamine (Horrow, 1985).

Patients known to be allergic to protamine and requiring heparin anticoagulation, as for cardiopulmonary bypass, present a unique problem (Campbell et al., 1984). Proposed options include (a) pretreatment with histamine-receptor antagonists followed by a slow trial of protamine infusion; (b) complete avoidance of protamine, which allows the heparin effect to dissipate spontaneously; and (c) administration of an alternate heparin antagonist, hexadimethrine. Spontaneous dissipation of heparin effect may take several hours and is likely to be associated with substantial bleeding, requiring the administration of multiple blood transfusions.

Platelet Factor 4

Platelet factor 4 (PF4) is a heparin-binding protein stored in the alpha granules of platelets that is released during platelet aggregation. In an animal model, PF4 reverses heparin anticoagulation without the adverse effects of protamine on complement activation or on the cardiovascular system (Cook et al., 1992). Because PF4 is a naturally occurring polypeptide in humans, it would also have the advantage of being less antigenic. Recombinant PF4 reverses heparin-induced anticoagulation after cardiopulmonary bypass and may be an alternative to protamine in the protamine-allergic patient (Levy et al., 1995).

Heparinase-I

Heparinase-I is a specific heparin degrading enzyme that may represent an alternative to protamine. This drug lyses heparin at its alpha-glycoside linkages. Heparinase-I has been effective in restoring the activated clotting time following cardiopulmonary bypass (Heres et al., 2001).

LOW-MOLECULAR-WEIGHT HEPARINS

Enoxaparin and dalteparin are low-molecular-weight heparins derived from standard commercial-grade unfractionated heparin by chemical depolymerization to yield fragments approximately one-third the size of heparin (Weitz, 1997). These fragments are heterogenous in size, with a mean molecular weight of 4,000 to 5,000 daltons. Depolymerization of heparin results in a change in its anticoagulant profile, pharmacokinetics, and effects on platelet function. Compared with heparin, which has an antiactivated factor X to antiactivated factor II activity of about 1:1, enoxaparin has a corresponding ratio that varies between 4:1 and 2:1. The pharmacokinetics of enoxaparin and dalteparin between patients are more consistent than heparin because these drugs bind less avidly to proteins than does heparin. This contributes to superior bioavailability at low doses and more predictable anticoagulant responses. Indeed, the protection against venous thromboembolism in high-risk medical and surgical patients is better with enoxaparin than with heparin (see the section on Heparin, Prophylaxis against Venous Thromboembolism) (Bergqvist et al., 1996; Geerts et al., 1996). Anticoagulation during carotid endarterectomy in patients with heparin-induced thrombocytopenia has been safely produced by enoxaparin (Gottlieb et al., 1997). Enoxaparin and dalteparin exhibits less binding to endothelial cells than does heparin, a property that accounts for their longer elimination half-time (4 to 5 hours) that permits once daily dosing without laboratory monitoring. Therapeutic doses do not usually affect the prothrombin time and APTT. Pentasaccharide consists of very low-molecular-weight heparin fragments and has an elimination half-time of about 24 hours.

The risk of bleeding from therapeutic doses of low-molecular-weight heparin approaches that of unfractionated heparin. Therefore, care should be taken to delay surgery for 12 hours after the last dose. If emergency reversal of anticoagulation is needed, protamine neutralizes about 65% of anti-Xa activity of low-molecular-weight heparin (Roberts et al., 2004).

Spinal and Epidural Hematomas

The risk of spontaneous hematoma formation may be increased in the presence of low-molecular-weight heparin and indwelling epidural catheters for administration of postoperative analgesia and by concomitant use of other drugs that affect hemostasis (nonsteroidal antiinflammatory drugs, platelet inhibitors) and by traumatic or repeated attempts to accomplish entry into the epidural or subarachnoid space (Wysowski et al., 1998). This increased risk of hematoma formation is a consideration when selecting regional anesthesia in patients being treated with low-molecular-weight heparin preparations.

DANAPAROID

Danaparoid is a glycosaminoglycuronan that is derived from porcine intestinal mucosa and consists of a mixture of heparin sulfate, dermatan sulfate, and chondroitin sulfate. This low-molecular-weight heparinoid compound attenuates fibrin formation principally by binding of antithrombin. Elimination of danaparoid is predominately through the kidneys. Danaparoid is effective in decreasing the incidence of DVT following total hip arthroplasty. The risk of immune-induced thrombocytopenia should be minimal.

FONDAPARINUX

Fondaparinux is a synthetic anticoagulant composed of the five saccharide units that make up the active site of heparin that binds antithrombin. The fondaparinum-antithrombin complex inhibits factor Xa but has no direct activity against thrombin. Administered SC, fondaparinux is rapidly absorbed and has an elimination half-tine of 15 hours, making it acceptable for once daily dosing. Metabolism does not occur and the drug is eliminated by the kidneys. Clinical uses of fondaparinux include prevention of DVT and pulmonary embolism.

ORAL ANTICOAGULANTS

Oral anticoagulants are derivatives of 4-hydroxycoumarin (coumarin) (Fig. 27-3) (Hirsch, 1991b). The essential chemical characteristics of coumarin derivatives for anticoagulant activity are an intact D-hydroxycoumarin residue with a

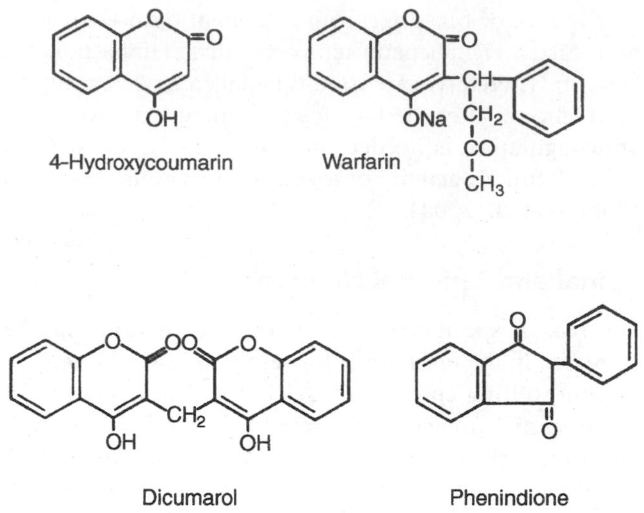

Figure 27-3. Oral anticoagulants are derivatives of 4-hydroxycoumarin.

carbon substitution at the number three position. Warfarin is the most frequently used anticoagulant because of its predictable onset and duration of action and its excellent bioavailability after oral administration (Table 27-1). Treatment usually begins with an oral warfarin dose of 5 to 10 mg, and the average maintenance dose is 5 mg; however, the dose varies widely among individuals. Disadvantages of oral anticoagulants include a delayed onset of action, the need for regular laboratory monitoring, difficulty in reversal should a surgical procedure create concern about bleeding, and the need to be administered orally should gastrointestinal dysfunction be present.

Mechanism of Action

Warfarin inhibits vitamin K epoxide reductase and thus blocks the conversion of vitamin K epoxide to vitamin K (Fig. 27-4) (Furie and Furie, 1990). Subsequent depletion of vitamin K results in the production of hemostatically defective vitamin K–dependent coagulation proteins (prothrombin; factors VII, IX, and X). Platelet activity is not altered by oral anticoagulants.

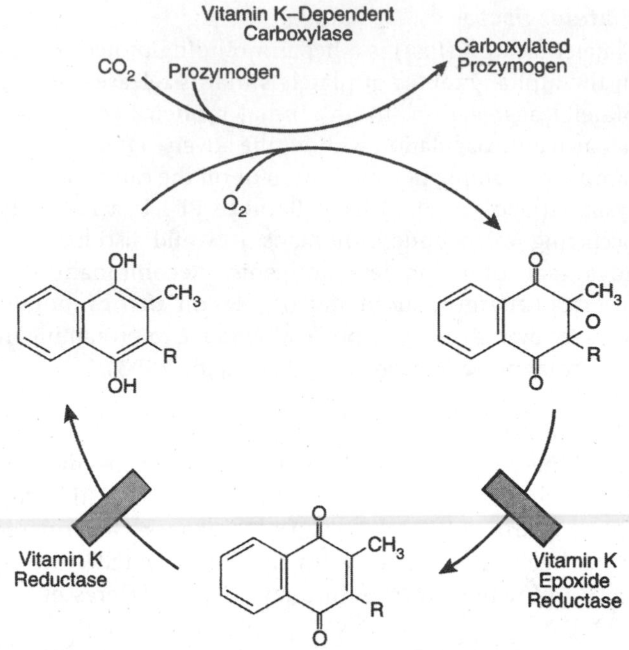

Figure 27-4. Warfarin inhibits vitamin K epoxide reductase and vitamin K reductase (*hatched box*) and thus prevents the conversion of vitamin K epoxide to vitamin KH2. Vitamin KH2 is a cofactor for the carboxylation of inactive proenzymes (factors II, VII, IX, and X) to the carboxylated proenzyme in a reaction that is catalyzed by vitamin K–dependent carboxylase and requires carbon dioxide and oxygen. (From Furie B, Furie BC. Molecular basis of vitamin K-dependent gamma-carboxylation. *Blood* 1990;75:1753–1762, with permission.)

The anticoagulant effect of oral or IV warfarin is delayed for 8 to 12 hours, reflecting the onset of inhibition of clotting factor synthesis and the elimination half-time of previously formed clotting factors that are not altered by the oral anticoagulant. Peak effects of warfarin do not occur for 36 to 72 hours.

Pharmacokinetics

Warfarin is rapidly and completely absorbed, with peak concentrations occurring within 1 hour after ingestion. It is 97% bound to albumin, and this contributes to its negligible

TABLE 27-1.
COMPARATIVE PHARMACOLOGY OF ORAL ANTICOAGULANTS

	Time to Peak Effect (hrs)	Duration after Discontinuation (days)	Initial Adult Dose (mg)	Maintenance Adult Dose (mg)
Warfarin	36–72	2–5	15 first day 10 second day 10 third day	2.5–10
Dicumarol	36–48	2–6	200–300 first day	25–200
Phenindione	18–24	1–2	300 first day 200 second day	25–200

renal excretion and long elimination half-time of 24 to 36 hours after oral administration. The elimination half-time may be prolonged by exposure to trace concentrations of anesthetic vapors, presumably reflecting inhibition of warfarin metabolism (Ghoneim et al., 1975). Extensive protein binding prevents diffusion into erythrocytes, cerebrospinal fluid, and breast milk. Warfarin, however, does cross the placenta and produces exaggerated effects in the fetus, who has limited ability to synthesize clotting factors. Warfarin is metabolized to inactive metabolites that are conjugated with glucuronic acid and ultimately excreted in bile (enterohepatic circulation) and urine.

Laboratory Evaluation

Treatment with oral anticoagulants is best guided by measurement of the prothrombin time. The prothrombin time is particularly sensitive to three of the four vitamin K-dependent clotting factors (prothrombin and factors VII and X). Commercial prothrombin time reagents vary markedly in their responsiveness to warfarin-induced decreases in clotting factors. Therefore, prothrombin time results obtained with different reagents are not interchangeable between laboratories. This problem of variability in the responsiveness of prothrombin time reagents has been overcome by the introduction of a standardized system of reporting known as the *international normalized ratio* (INR). For most indications, a moderate anticoagulant effect with a targeted INR of 2.0 to 3.0 is appropriate.

An excessively prolonged prothrombin time is not readily shortened by omitting a dose because of the long elimination half-time of oral anticoagulants. Likewise, an inadequate therapeutic effect is not readily corrected by increasing the dose because of the delayed onset of therapeutic effect. This slow response of oral anticoagulants contrasts with the rapid and predictable changes made possible by altering the dose of heparin.

Unexpected fluctuations in the dose response to warfarin may reflect changes in diet, undisclosed drug use, poor patient compliance, surreptitious self-medication, or intermittent alcohol consumption. Concomitant medication with over-the-counter and prescription drugs can augment or inhibit the anticoagulant effect of coumarin drugs on hemostasis or interfere with platelet function. Patients receiving coumarin drugs are sensitive to fluctuating levels of dietary vitamin K, which is obtained predominantly from leafy green vegetables. The effect of coumarin can be potentiated in sick patients with poor vitamin K intake, particularly if they are treated with antibiotics and IV fluids without vitamin K supplementation. Preexisting liver disease and advanced age are associated with enhanced effects of oral anticoagulants.

Clinical Uses

Oral anticoagulants are effective in the prevention of venous thromboembolism, the prevention of systemic embolization in patients with prosthetic heart valves or atrial fibrillation, and the prevention of stroke, recurrent MI, and death in patients with acute MI (Hirsh, 1991b). Oral anticoagulants are effective in preventing venous thrombosis after hip surgery and major gynecologic surgery at a targeted INR of 2.0 to 3.0 (Clagett et al., 1995). These drugs are effective both when the treatment begins before surgery and when it begins on the first postoperative day. The risk of clinically important bleeding is small, but because warfarin prophylaxis is more complicated to use than fixed low-dose heparin therapy, warfarin is generally reserved for patients at very high risk, such as those with a history of previous venous thrombosis or those having major orthopedic procedures (Hirsh, 1991b). It is probably necessary to continue anticoagulant therapy for up to 3 months after an initial course of heparin in patients with proximal DVT (Hull et al., 1982).

Management before Elective Surgery

It is prudent to check the prothrombin time and INR before anesthesia and surgery (Roberts et al., 2004). Relatively minor surgical procedures can be safely performed in patients receiving oral anticoagulants. For major surgery, discontinuation of oral anticoagulants 1 to 3 days preoperatively is recommended to permit the prothrombin time to return to within 20% of its normal range (Tinker and Tarhan, 1978). This approach, followed by reinstitution of the oral anticoagulant regimen 1 to 7 days postoperatively, is not accompanied by an increased incidence of thromboembolic complications in vulnerable patients, such as those with prosthetic heart valves. In emergency situations, oral or IV administration of 1 to 2 mg of vitamin K is utilized to reverse the anticoagulant effect. If immediate reversal is needed, for performance of high-risk surgical procedures such as craniotomy, administration of recombinant factor VIIa, 1 to 2 units of fresh frozen plasma, or a prothrombin complex concentrate is effective (Roberts et al., 2004).

Drug Interactions

Drug interactions that increase plasma warfarin levels and potentiate its anticoagulant effect may do so by inhibiting metabolic clearance of the drug. The metabolic clearance of warfarin is inhibited by phenylbutazone and amiodarone. Cimetidine and omeprazole inhibit the metabolic clearance of the less active dextroisomer of warfarin and therefore have a small effect on the prothrombin time. Plasma warfarin concentrations are decreased and the drug's anticoagulant effect decreased by drugs that impair its absorption from the gastrointestinal tract (cholestyramine) and those drugs that increase the metabolic clearance of both isomers by inducing activity of mixed-function oxidases (barbiturates, rifampin, carbamazepine). The second- and third-generation cephalosporins augment the anticoagulant effect of warfarin by inhibiting the cyclic interconversion of vitamin K. Heparin has the potential to increase warfarin's anticoagulant effect, but even if heparin is administered in therapeutic doses, its effect on the prothrombin time is limited. Aspirin and nonsteroidal antiinflammatory drugs inhibit platelet function and have the potential to increase the risk of warfarin-associated bleeding. Serious gastrointestinal bleeding may occur if large doses of aspirin (1 g per day) and high-intensity warfarin therapy are used in combination (Chesebro et al., 1983; Dale et al., 1980). It has not been determined if low doses of aspirin (160 mg per day), which have minimal gastric side effects but antithrombotic efficacy, can be used safely in combination with warfarin (Hirsh, 1991b).

Side Effects

Bleeding is the main complication of oral anticoagulant therapy. The risk of bleeding is influenced by the intensity of the anticoagulant therapy, the patient's underlying disorder, and the concomitant use of aspirin. Bleeding that occurs when the INR is <3.0 is frequently associated with an obvious underlying cause (neoplasm, peptic ulcer). These drugs may increase the incidence of intracranial hemorrhage after a cerebrovascular accident. Compression neuropathy has been observed in treated patients after brachial artery puncture to obtain a sample for blood gas analysis. Treatment of mild hemorrhage is with administration of vitamin K, 10 to 20 mg orally or 1 to 5 mg IV at a rate of 1 mg per minute, which will usually return the prothrombin time to a normal range within 4 to 24 hours.

The most important nonhemorrhagic side effect of warfarin therapy is skin necrosis. This uncommon complication usually occurs between 3 and 8 days of therapy and is caused by extensive thrombosis of the venules and capillaries within the subcutaneous fat. Skin necrosis at the site of SC heparin administration has also been described (Christiaens and Nieuwenhuis, 1996).

Oral anticoagulants cross the placenta and can produce a characteristic embryopathy, central nervous system damage, or fetal bleeding. Embryopathic changes (nasal hypoplasia, stippled epiphyses) have been observed only if warfarin is administered during the first trimester. Conversely, central nervous system abnormalities (blindness, agenesis of the corpus callosum) have been observed with exposure to warfarin during any trimester of pregnancy. Heparin is the preferred anticoagulant if anticoagulants are indicated during pregnancy. Warfarin does not induce an anticoagulant effect in the breast-fed infant if the drug is administered to a nursing mother.

THROMBOLYTIC DRUGS

Pharmacologic thrombolysis is produced by drugs that act as plasminogen activators to convert the endogenous proenzyme plasminogen to the fibrinolytic enzyme plasmin (fibrinolysin) (Table 27-2). The goal of thrombolytic therapy is to restore circulation through a previously occluded artery or vein, most often a coronary artery (Bates, 1992). Fibrinolytic therapy has revolutionized the treatment of acute coronary syndrome as it has been established that these drugs significantly improve survival. In this regard, fibrinolytic therapy should be instituted in patients who present with S-T segment elevation or heart

TABLE 27-2.
COMPARISON OF THROMBOLYTIC DRUGS

	Streptokinase	Alteplase	Antistreplase
Dose (intravenous)	1.5 million units 1 hour	100 mg (1.25 mg/kg infused over 3 hours	30 units over 2–5 minutes
Clinical uses	ACS, PE	ACS, PE	ACS, PE
Site of action	Plasminogen	Plasminogen	Plasminogen
Elimination half-time	23 minutes	<5 minutes	<5 minutes
Clearance	Hepatic	Hepatic	Hepatic
Reperfusion success rate	50% to 70%	60% to 80%	60% to 80%
Antidote	Antifibrinolytics	Antifibrinolytics	Antifibrinolytics
Hypotensive effect	Moderate	Minimal	Minimal
Allergic reactions	Yes	No	No
Stop before surgery	3 hours	1 hour	1 hour
Prolongation of PT/PTT	Yes/Yes	Yes/Yes	Yes/Yes
Cost	Expensive	Very expensive	Very expensive

ACS, acute coronary syndrome; PE, pulmonary embolism
PT, prothrombin time; PTT, activated plasma thromboplastin time

Chapter 27: Anticoagulants 515

TABLE 27-3.
SELECTION OF PATIENTS TO RECEIVE THROMBOLYTIC DRUGS

Relative contraindications
Trauma or surgery more than 14 days previously
Chronic and severe hypertension
Active peptic ulcer disease
Treatment with anticoagulants
Known bleeding diathesis
Significant liver dysfunction
Prior exposure to streptokinase or anistreplase (not a problem with urokinase or alteplase)
Absolute contraindications
Active internal bleeding
Trauma or surgery in the last 14 days
Recent head trauma or known intracranial aneurysm
History of hemorrhagic cerebrovascular accident
Systemic blood pressure >200/120 mm Hg
Previous allergic reaction (applicable only for streptokinase and anistreplase)
Traumatic cardiopulmonary resuscitation
Suspected aortic dissection
Diabetic hemorrhagic retinopathy
Pregnancy

block on the electrocardiogram up to at least 12 hours after the onset of symptoms (Collins et al., 1997). Indeed, thrombolytic therapy is usually considered appropriate in patients who are seen in the early stages of MI and who do not have specific contraindications to this form of therapy (Table 27-3) (Becker et al., 1991). Plasminogen activators are more capable of dissolving newly formed clot (platelet-rich and formed by weaker fibrinogen bonds) than older clot that is more tightly bound with fibrin. Because the incidence of reocclusion after the institution of thrombolytic therapy is relatively frequent (about 20%), antithrombotic therapy with heparin for the first 24 hours is commonly used. Aspirin should also be started promptly in all patients with suspected acute coronary syndrome (acute MI or unstable angina) (Collins et al., 1997).

Spontaneous bleeding (especially intracranial hemorrhage) is the principal risk of thrombolytic drug therapy (Levine et al., 1992; Tiefenbrunn and Ludbrook, 1989). Bleeding is particularly likely in patients who have recently experienced trauma or undergone surgery or invasive diagnostic procedures, emphasizing that these drugs do not distinguish between the fibrin of a thrombus and the fibrin of a hemostatic plug. Other patient characteristics that increase the risk of bleeding include generalized hemostatic defect, a history of gastrointestinal hemorrhage or recent stroke, and serious comorbid conditions. Bleeding including intracranial hemorrhage is more common and more serious with thrombolytic drugs than with anticoagulants. The risk of bleeding is not different among the various thrombolytic drugs. Severe bleeding can be treated with transfusions of fresh frozen plasma, cryoprecipitate, or platelets and drugs that have antifibrinolytic effects (epsilon aminocaproic acid, aprotinin).

Streptokinase

Streptokinase is a protein produced by beta-hemolytic streptococci. In contrast to other plasminogen activators, streptokinase is not an enzyme and does not convert plasminogen directly to plasmin by proteolytic cleavage. Instead, streptokinase binds noncovalently to plasminogen, converting it to a plasminogen-activator complex that acts on other plasminogen molecules to generate plasmin. The elimination half-time is about 23 minutes and infusion may decrease systemic vascular resistance with resulting hypotension. Streptokinase is the least expensive of the thrombolytic drugs.

Streptokinase is not fibrin specific and can produce a systemic thrombolytic state. As a bacterial product, streptokinase may stimulate antibody production and subsequent allergic reactions and fever. Antistreptococcal antibodies, present in variable titers in most patients before streptokinase treatment, induce an amnestic response that makes repeated treatment difficult or impossible for a period of months or years after an initial course of treatment. Allergic reactions (fever, shivering, rarely anaphylaxis) in patients being treated with streptokinase reflect the presence of antistreptococcal antibodies from prior bacterial infections. Laboratory monitoring of streptokinase can be limited to a thrombin time, which is used as a marker for an effective lytic state. If the thrombin time is not prolonged within the first few hours of commencing treatment, resistance to streptokinase due to a high titer of antistreptococcal antibodies should be suspected.

Alteplase (Recombinant Tissue Plasminogen Activator)

Alteplase is a fibrin-specific thrombolytic drug that is synthesized by endothelial cells as a single-chain polypeptide. This drug is at least ten times more expensive than streptokinase but does seem to be somewhat more effective in opening an infarct-related artery, especially if therapy cannot be initiated in the first 3 hours. Clearance from the plasma is primarily by the liver with an elimination half-time of <5 minutes. The difference in cost between streptokinase and alteplase presents a difficult ethical and economic dilemma as differences in mortality in patients treated with streptokinase or alteplase seem small to nonexistent (Becker et al., 1991). Alteplase is recommended for treatment of acute ischemic stroke if the patient's symptoms have a definitive onset of less than 3 hours.

Anistreplase (Anisoylated Plasminogen Streptokinase Activator Complex)

Anistreplase was synthesized in an effort to produce a thrombolytic drug that had a longer duration of action than either streptokinase or alteplase. Indeed, an advantage of anistreplase therapy is ease of administration because it can be administered as a single IV injection (AIMS Trial Study Group, 1990).

DIRECT THROMBIN INHIBITORS

Direct thrombin inhibitors (antithrombotic drugs) suppress platelet function and are used for treatment of arterial and venous thrombotic disease (Table 27-4) (Roberts et al., 2004). Platelet thrombi commonly occur in arterial walls, emphasizing the logic of using drugs that inhibit platelet aggregation in treating arterial thromboembolic diseases, especially those that lead to MI or cerebrovascular accident. Oral anticoagulants have no effect on platelet function; thus, they are unlikely to be useful in the treatment of thrombotic disease in the arterial system. Examples of antithrombotic drugs are hirudin, aspirin, dipyridamole, and dextran.

Recombinant Hirudin

Recombinant hirudin (desirudin, lepirudin) is a 65-amino acid peptide antithrombotic drug that produces drugs that produce anticoagulation by direct inhibition of thrombin. Bivalirudin is a synthetic peptide based on hirudin. Unlike heparin, hirudin does not depend on antithrombin for its anticoagulant activity. Unlike heparin, hirudin inhibits clot-bound and free thrombin and is not associated with immune thrombocytopenia (White et al., 1998). The risk of spontaneous bleeding is not increased in patients treated with hirudin compared with heparin. The ability of drugs in this class to penetrate the network of fibrin filaments and neutralize fibrin-bound thrombin may be beneficial in the treatment of platelet-rich arterial thrombi as well as the prevention of venous thromboembolic disease (Ewenstein, 1997). Desirudin is a safe and more efficacious intervention than low-molecular-weight heparin in the prevention of DVT in patients undergoing total hip replacement (Eriksson et al., 1997). Hirudin is an alternative to heparin in patients who require anticoagulation for surgery but who have developed heparin resistance or heparin-induced thrombocytopenia (Koster et al., 1998; Latham et al., 2000; Sun et al., 2001). Administered IV the onset of action is rapid and the peak effect occurs in about 4 hours.

Ximelagatran

Ximelagatran is an orally effective direct thrombin inhibitor that may be effective in prophylaxis against and treatment of thromboembolism. It is rapidly absorbed and converted to its active component (melagatran) that acts as a reversible inhibitor of free and clot-bound thrombin. Monitoring of coagulation or dose adjustments is not necessary. Elimination haft-time is about 3 hours and the drug is cleared by the kidneys. There are no known food or drug interactions with ximelagatran.

Oral ximelagatran administered the morning after total knee replacement was superior to warfarin for prevention of venous thromboembolism (Francis et al., 2003). Patients treated with ximelagatran do not experience an increased incidence of bleeding but transient increases in the plasma concentrations of transaminase enzymes may occur (Schulman et al., 2003).

Argatroban

Argatroban is an arginine derivative that is a highly specific thrombin inhibitor. In addition to its antithrombin activity, argatroban promotes nitric oxide release contributing to improved perfusion in patients with peripheral vascular disease. Argatroban is an alternative to heparin for anticoagulation in patients requiring cardiopulmonary bypass especially in the presence of heparin-induced thrombocytopenia (Lewis et al., 2001).

TABLE 27-4.
PROPERTIES OF DIRECT THROMBIN INHIBITORS

Drug	Route of Administration	Excretion	Clinical Uses	Stop before Surgery (hrs)	Prolong PT/PTT	Antidote
Hirudin	Intravenous	Renal	Heparin-induced thrombocytopenia	8	Yes/Yes	Hemodialysis
Ximelagatran	Oral	Renal	Thromboprophylaxis Treatment of DVT	24	Yes/Yes	None
Argatroban	Intravenous	Hepatic	Heparin-induced thrombocytopenia	4–6	Yes/Yes	None
Bivalirudin	Intravenous	Hepatic	Coronary Interventions	2–3	Yes/Yes	None

DVT, deep vein thrombosis.
Adapted from Roberts HR, Monroe DM, Escobar MA. Current concepts of hemostasis: implications for therapy. *Anesthesiology* 2004;100:722–730.

TABLE 27-5.
PROPERTIES OF ADENOSINE DIPHOSPHATE INHIBITORS

	Site of Action	Route of Adminis-tration	Elimination Half-Time	Clearance	Antidote	Stop before Surgery	Prolong PT/PTT	Clinical Uses
Aspirin	COX 1–2	Oral	20 mins	Hepatic	None	7 days	No/No	ACS Stroke
Dipyridamole	Adenosine	Oral	40 mins	Hepatic	None	24 hrs	No/No	PVD
Clopidogrel	ADP	Oral	7 hrs	Hepatic	None	5 days	No/No	CAD PVD
Ticlopidine	ADP	Oral	4 days		None	10 days	No/No	CAD PVD

ACS, acute coronary syndrome; PVD, peripheral vascular disease; CAD, coronary artery disease.

ADENOSINE DIPHOSPHATE INHIBITORS

Adenosine diphosphate (ADP) inhibitors are used principally for prevention of arterial thrombosis and act by inhibiting platelet aggregation by different mechanisms (Table 27-5) (Roberts et al., 2004).

Aspirin

Aspirin inhibits thromboxane synthesis by interfering with the activity of cyclooxygenase 1 and 2 enzymes and the subsequent release of adenosine diphosphate by platelets and their aggregation (see Chapter 11). Because platelet aggregation is presumed to play an important role in reocclusion after thrombolytic therapy, it is common to administer aspirin (325 mg daily) before instituting thrombolytic therapy. Despite rapid clearance from the body, the effects of aspirin on platelets are irreversible and last for the life of the platelet.

Clopidogrel and Ticlopidine

Clopidogrel and ticlopidine are prodrugs that are converted to active metabolites in the liver that block ADP receptors on surfaces of platelets. Blocking the action of ADP on platelets inhibits platelet activation, aggregation, and degranulation. Clopidogrel and ticlopidine irreversibly modify ADP receptors resulting in inhibition for the life of the platelet (7 to 10 days). Both drugs act in concert with aspirin and have been used with aspirin to prevent clotting of coronary stents (Cadroy et al., 2000). The combination of aspirin and clopidogrel may be complicated by postoperative bleeding (Moore and Power, 2004). The current recommendation is to discontinue clopidogrel 7 days and ticlopidine about 4 days before elective surgery and to avoid regional anesthesia until the effects of these drugs have dissipated (Roberts et al., 2004). Platelet transfusion may be useful for restoring hemostasis. Side effects of these ADP-receptor antagonists include neutropenia, thrombotic thrombocytopenic purpura, and hepatic dysfunction. Intracranial and gastrointestinal hemorrhage are potential adverse responses.

Dipyridamole

Dipyridamole is most often administered in combination with warfarin to patients with prosthetic heart valves as prophylaxis against thromboembolism reflecting its ability, like aspirin, to inhibit platelet aggregation (see Chapter 16).

Dextran

Dextran-70 prolongs bleeding time, and polymerization of fibrin and platelet function may be impaired (see Chapter 36). For these reasons, dextran may have some value in the prevention of postoperative thromboembolic disease.

PLATELET GLYCOPROTEIN IIb/IIIa ANTAGONISTS

Platelet glycoprotein IIb/IIIa antagonists act at the corresponding fibrinogen receptor that is important for platelet aggregation. These drugs block fibrinogen binding to platelet glycoprotein IIb/IIIa receptors that is the final common pathway of platelet aggregation (Table 27-6) (Fig. 27-5) (Kam and Egan, 2002).

Clinical Uses

Thrombus formation initiated by platelets is important in the pathogenesis of acute coronary syndrome (unstable angina, myocardial infarction), angioplasty failure and stent thrombosis. Glycoprotein IIb/IIIa antagonists are indicated for the acute coronary syndrome and in patients undergoing interventional cardiology procedures (Anderson et al., 2001). For example, abciximab reduces the incidence of MI after percutaneous coronary interventional procedures. Although aspirin lowers the risk associated with

TABLE 27-6.
PROPERTIES OF GLYCOPROTEIN IIb/IIIa ANTAGONISTS

Drug	Structure	Route of Administration	Elimination Half-Time (hrs)	Excretion	Clinical Uses	Stop Before Surgery (hrs)	Prolong PT/PTT	Antidote
Abciximab	Monoclonal antibodies	Intravenous	12–24	Plasma proteases	ACS PCI	72	No/No	None
Eptifibatide	Peptide	Intravenous	2–4	Renal	ACS PCI	24	No/No	None
Tirofiban	Nonpeptide	Intravenous	2–4	Renal (30%–60%) Biliary (40%–70%)	ACS	24	No/No	Hemodialysis

ACS, acute coronary syndrome; PCI, percutaneous coronary interventions.
Adapted from Kam PCA and Egan MK. Platelet glycoprotein IIb/IIIa antagonists. Pharmacology and clinical developments. *Anesthesiology* 2002;96:1237–1249 and Roberts HR, Monroe DM, Escobar MA. Current concepts of hemostasis: Implications for therapy. *Anesthesiology* 2004;100:722–730.

thrombus formation, the IV administration of glycoprotein IIb/IIIa antagonists further decreases the incidence of cardiac and cerebral ischemic events, coronary angioplasty complications, and coronary stenting occlusion.

Monitoring

It is recommended to maintain the ACT between 200 and 400 seconds in patients being treated with glycoprotein IIb/IIIa antagonists. Platelet counts should be monitored and therapy discontinued if thrombocytopenia (platelet count <100,000 cells/mm^3) develops. The effects of these drugs can be reversed with platelet transfusions.

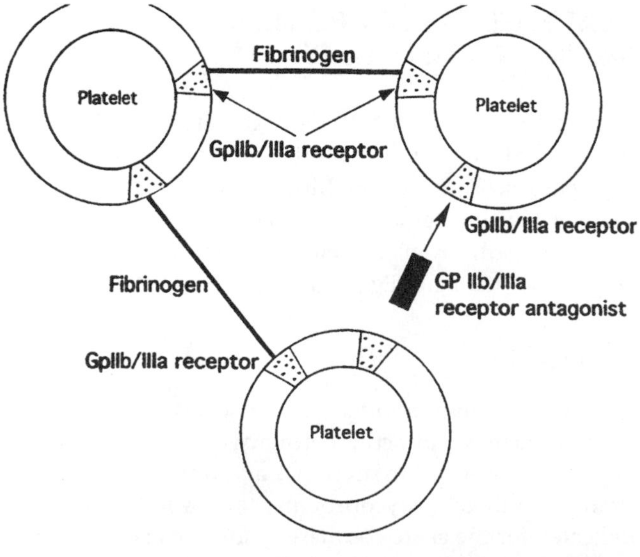

Figure 27-5. Schematic depiction of glycoprotein IIb/IIIa antagonist action on platelets. (From Kam PCA and Egan MK. Platelet glycoprotein IIb/IIIa antagonists. Pharmacology and clinical developments. *Anesthesiology* 2002;96:1237–1249; with permission.)

Anesthetic Considerations

Increasing numbers of patients presenting for surgery are receiving glycoprotein IIb/IIIa antagonists. Avoiding regional anesthesia in patients recently treated with glycoprotein IIb/IIIa antagonists would seem prudent. If possible, it is reasonable to delay surgery for a few hours after administration of these drugs (see Table 27-6). Nevertheless, there is evidence that increased bleeding does not accompany surgery performed in the presence of these drugs (Lincoff et al., 2000). It is possible that the heparin dose should be decreased in patients receiving glycoprotein IIb/IIIa antagonists and undergoing cardiopulmonary bypass (Gammie et al., 1998).

REFERENCES

AIMS Trial Study Group. Long-term effects of intravenous anistreplase in acute MI: final report of the AIMS study. *Lancet* 1990;335:427.

Anderson JAM, Saenko EL. Heparin resistance. *Br J Anaesth* 2002;88:467–469.

Anderson KM, Califf RM, Stone GW, et al. Long-term mortality benefit with abciximab in patients undergoing percutaneous coronary intervention. *J Am Coll Cardiol* 2001;87:537–541.

Bates ER. Is survival in acute MI related to thrombolytic efficacy or the open-artery hypothesis? A controversy to be investigated with gusto. *Chest* 1992;101:S140.

Becker RC, Corrao JM, Bovill EG, et al. Intravenous nitroglycerin-induced heparin resistance: a qualitative antithrombin III abnormality. *Am Heart J* 1990;119:1254–1261.

Becker RC, Corraro JM, Harrington R, et al. Recombinant tissue-type plasminogen activator: current guidelines for clinical use in acute MI. *Am Heart J* 1991;121:220.

Bergqvist D, Benoni G, Bjorgell O, et al. Low-molecular-weight heparin (enoxaparin) as prophylaxis against venous thromboembolism after total hip replacement. *N Engl J Med* 1996;335:696–700.

Blaise G. Heparin and protamine interaction. *Can J Anaesth* 1998;45:1144–1147.

Bode V, Welzel D, Franz G, et al. Absence of drug interaction between heparin and nitroglycerin: randomized placebo-controlled cross-over study. *Arch Intern Med* 1990;150:2117–2119.

Bull BS, Huse WM, Brauer FS, et al. Heparin therapy during extracorporeal circulation. II. The use of a dose-response curve to individualize heparin and protamine dosage. *J Thorac Cardiovasc Surg* 1975;69:785–789.

Cadroy Y, Bossavy JP, Thalamas C, et al. Early potent antithrombotic effect with combined aspirin and a loading dose of clopidogrel on experimental arterial thrombogenesis in humans. *Circulation* 2000;101:2823–2828.

Campbell FW, Goldstein MF, Atkins PC. Management of the patient with protamine hypersensitivity for cardiac surgery. *Anesthesiology* 1984;61:761–764.

Casthely PA, Goodman K, Fyman PN, et al. Hemodynamic changes after the administration of protamine. *Anesth Analg* 1986;65:78–80.

Chesebro JH, Fuster V, Elveback LR, et al. Trial of combined warfarin plus dipyridamole or aspirin therapy in prosthetic heart valve replacement: danger of aspirin compared with dipyridamole. *Am J Cardiol* 1983;51:1537–1541.

Christiaens GCML, Nieuwenhuis HK. Heparin-induced skin necrosis. *N Engl J Med* 1996;335:715.

Clagett GP, Anderson FA, Heit J, et al. Prevention of venous thromboembolism. *Chest* 1995;108:S312–S34.

Collins R, Peto R, Baigent C, et al. Aspirin, heparin, and fibrinolytic therapy in suspected acute MI. *N Engl J Med* 1997;336:847–860.

Conahan TJ, Andrews RW, MacVaugh H. Cardiovascular effects of protamine sulfate in man. *Anesth Analg* 1981;60:33–36.

Conzen PF, Habazettl H, Gutmann R, et al. Thromboxane mediation of pulmonary hemodynamic responses after neutralization of heparin by protamine in pigs. *Anesth Analg* 1989;68:25–31.

Cook JJ, Niewiarowski S, Yan Z, et al. Platelet factor 4 reverses heparin anticoagulation in the rat without adverse effects of heparin-protamine complexes. *Circulation* 1992;85:1102–1109.

Dale J, Myhre E, Lowe D. Bleeding during acetylsalicylic acid and anticoagulant therapy in patients with reduced platelet reactivity after aortic valve replacement. *Am Heart J* 1980;99:746–752.

Despotis GJ, Summerfield AL, Joist JH, et al. Comparison of activated coagulation time and whole blood heparin measurements with laboratory plasma anti-Xa heparin concentration in patients having cardiac operations. *J Thorac Cardiovasc Surg* 1994;108:1076–1082.

deSwart CAM, Nijmeyer B, Roelofs JMM, et al. Kinetics of intravenously administered heparin in normal humans. *Blood* 1982; 60:1251–1258.

Doolan L, McKenzie L, Krafcheck J, et al. Protamine sulfate hypersensitivity. *Anaesth Intensive Care* 1981;9:147–149.

Eriksson BI, Wille-Jorgensen P, Kalebo P, et al. A comparison of recombinant hirudin with a low molecular-weight heparin to prevent thromboembolic complications after total hip replacement. *N Engl J Med* 1997;337:329–335.

Ewenstein B. Antithrombotic agents and thromboembolic disease. *N Engl J Med* 1997;337:1383–1384.

Francis CW, Berkowitz SD, Comp PC, et al. Comparison of ximelagatran with warfarin for the prevention of venous thromboembolism after total knee replacement. *N Engl J Med* 2003;349:1703–1712.

Furie B, Furie BC. Molecular basis of vitamin K-dependent gamma-carboxylation. *Blood* 1990;75:1753–1762.

Gammie JS, Zenati M, Kormos RL, et al. Abciximab and excessive bleeding in patients undergoing emergency cardiac operations. *Ann Thorac Surg* 1998;65:465–469.

Geerts WH, Jay RM, Code KI, et al. A comparison of low-dose heparin with low-molecular weight heparin as prophylaxis against venous thromboembolism after major trauma. *N Engl J Med* 1996;335: 701–707.

Ghoneim MM, Delle M, Wilson WR, et al. Alteration of warfarin kinetics in man associated with exposure to an operating room environment. *Anesthesiology* 1975;43:333–336.

Ginsberg JS, Kowalchuk G, Hirsch J, et al. Heparin effect on bone density. *Thromb Haemost* 1990;64:286–289.

Goto H, Kushihashi T, Benson KT, et al. Heparin, protamine, and ionized calcium in vitro and in vivo. *Anesth Analg* 1985;64:1081–1084.

Gottlieb A, Tabares AH, Levy P, et al. Use of low molecular weight heparin in patients with heparin-induced thrombocytopenia undergoing carotid endarterectomy. *Anesthesiology* 1996;85:678–681.

Hakim TS, Picone A, Oleary CE, et al. Protamine-induced pulmonary vasoconstriction in heparinized pigs. *Anesth Analg* 1995;81:38–43.

Heres EK, Horrow JC, Gravlee GP et al. A dose-determining trial of heparinase-I (Neutralise®) for heparin neutralization in coronary artery surgery. *Anesth Analg* 2001;93:1446–1452.

Hines RL, Barash PG. Protamine: does it alter right ventricular function? *Anesth Analg* 1986;65:1271–1274.

Hirsch J. Heparin. *N Engl J Med* 1991a;324:1565–1573.

Hirsch J. Oral anticoagulant drugs. *N Engl J Med* 1991b;324:1865–1875.

Horrow JC. Protamine: a review of its toxicity. *Anesth Analg* 1985;64: 348–361.

Hull R, Delmore T, Carter C, et al. Adjusted subcutaneous heparin versus warfarin sodium in the long-term treatment of venous thrombosis. *N Engl J Med* 1982;306:189–194.

Kam PCA, Egan MK. Platelet glycoprotein IIb/IIIa antagonists. Pharmacology and clinical developments. *Anesthesiology* 2002;96: 1237–1249.

Knape JA, Schuller JL, DeHaan P, et al. An anaphylactic reaction to protamine in a patient allergic to fish. *Anesthesiology* 1981;55: 324–325.

Konchigeri HN. Hemodynamic effects of heparin in patients undergoing cardiac surgery. *Anesth Analg* 1984;63:235.

Koster A, Kuppe H, Hetzer R, et al. Emergent cardiopulmonary bypass in five patients with heparin-induced thrombocytopenia type II employing recombinant hirudin. *Anesthesiology* 1998;89: 777–780.

Kronenfeld MA, Garguilo R, Weinberg P, et al. Left atrial injection of protamine does not reliably prevent pulmonary hypertension. *Anesthesiology* 1987;67:578–580.

Latham P, Revelis AF, Joshi GP, et al. Use of recombinant hirudin in patients with heparin-induced thrombocytopenia with thrombosis requiring cardiopulmonary bypass. *Anesthesiology* 2000;92: 263–266.

Levine MN, Goldhaber SZ, Califf RM, et al. Hemorrhagic complications of thrombolytic therapy in the treatment of MI and venous thromboembolism. *Chest* 1992;102:S364.

Levy JH, Cormack JG, Morales A. Heparin neutralization by recombinant platelet factor 4 and protamine. *Anesth Analg* 1995;81: 35–37.

Lewis BE, Wallis DE, Berkowitz SD, et al. Argatroban anticoagulant therapy in patients with heparin-induced thrombocytopenia. *Circulation* 2001;103:1838–1843

Lincoff AM, LeNarz LA, Despotis GJ, et al. Abciximab and bleeding during coronary surgery: results from the EPILOG and EPISTENT trials. Improve Long-Term Outcome with Abciximab GP IIb/IIIa blockade. Evaluation of Platelet IIb/IIIa Inhibition in STENTING. *Ann Thorac Surg* 2000;70:516–526.

Ling E, Warkentin TE. Intraoperative heparin flushes and subsequent acute heparin-induced thrombocytopenia. *Anesthesiology* 1998;89: 1567–1569.

Marciniak E, Gockerman JP. Heparin-induced decrease in circulating antithrombin-III. *Lancet* 1977;2:581–584.

Michaels IAL, Barash PG. Hemodynamic changes during protamine administration. *Anaesth Analg* 1983;62:831–835.

Milne B, Rogers K, Cervenko F, et al. Haemodynamic effects of intra-aortic versus intravenous administration of protamine for reversal of heparin in man. *Can Anaesth Soc J* 1983;30:347–351.

Moore M, Power M. Perioperative hemorrhage and combined clopidogrel and aspirin therapy. *Anesthesiology* 2004;101:792–794.

Moorthy SS, Pond W, Rowland RG. Severe circulatory shock following protamine (an anaphylactic reaction). *Anesth Analg* 1980;59: 77–78.

Rao TLK, El-Etr AA. Anticoagulation following placement of epidural and subarachnoid catheters: an evaluation of neurologic sequelae. *Anesthesiology* 1981;55:618–620.

Roberts HR, Monroe DM, Escobar MA. Current concepts of hemostasis; Implications for therapy. *Anesthesiology* 2004;100:722–730.

Schulman S, Wahlander K, Lundstrom T, et al. Secondary prevention of venous thromboembolism with the oral direct thrombin inhibitor ximelagatran. *N Engl J Med* 2003;349:1713–1721.

Slaughter TF, Greenberg CS. Heparin-associated thrombocytopenia and thrombosis: implications for perioperative management. *Anesthesiology* 1997;87:667–675.

Stoelting RK, Henry DP, Verburg KM, et al. Haemodynamic changes and circulating histamine concentrations following protamine administration to patients and dogs. *Can Anaesth Soc J* 1984;31: 534–540.

Stow PJ, Burrows FA. Anticoagulants in anaesthesia. *Can J Anaesth* 1987;34:632–649.

Sun Y, Greilich PE, Wilson SIO, et al. The use of lepirudin for anticoagulation in patients with heparin-induced thrombocytopenia during major vascular surgery. *Anesth Analg* 2001;92:344–346.

Takenoshita M, Sugiyama M, Okuno Y, et al. Anaphylactoid reaction to protamine confirmed by plasma tryptase in a diabetic patient during open heart surgery. *Anesthesiology* 1996;84: 233–235.

Tiefenbrunn AJ, Ludbrook PA. Coronary thrombolysis—it's worth the risk. *JAMA* 1989;261:2107–2108.

Tinker JH, Tarhan S. Discontinuing anticoagulant therapy in surgical patients with cardiac valve prosthesis. Observations in 180 operations. *JAMA* 1978;239:738–740.

Warkentin TE, Kelton JG. Heparin-induced thrombocytopenia. *Annu Rev Med* 1989;40:31–44.

Weitz JI. Low-molecular-weight heparins. *N Engl J Med* 1997;337: 688–698.

White HD, Ellis CJ, French JK et al. Hirudin (desirudin) and Hirulog (bivalirudin) in acute ischaemic syndromes and the rationale for the Hirulog/Early Reperfusion Occlusion (HERO-2) Study. *Aust N Z J M* 1998;28:551–554.

Wood AJJ, Robertson D, Robertson RM, Wilkinson GR, Wood M. Elevated plasma free drug concentrations of propranolol and diazepam during cardiac catheterization. *Circulation* 1980;62: 1119–1122.

Wysowski DK, Talarico L, Bacsanyi J, et al. Spinal and epidural hematoma and low-molecular-weight heparin. *N Engl J Med* 1998; 338:1774–1775.

Young JA, Kisker CT, Doty DB. Adequate anticoagulation during cardiopulmonary bypass determined by activated clotting time and the appearance of fibrin monomer. *Ann Thorac Surg* 1978;26: 231–240.

Antimicrobials

28

The excessive use of antimicrobials (antibiotics) for the treatment of conditions for which these drugs provide little or no benefit (upper respiratory tract infections, bronchitis) has contributed to the emergence of bacterial resistance. It is estimated that 21% of all prescriptions written for antimicrobials are for ambulatory patients seen in physicians' offices with the diagnosis of upper respiratory tract infections or bronchitis (Gonzales et al., 1997).

The therapeutic value and associated dangers of antimicrobials are particularly relevant to the care of patients in the perioperative period and intensive care unit who are at risk for hospital-acquired infections (Table 28-1). The essential feature of effective chemotherapeutic drugs for treatment of microbial diseases is the ability to inhibit microorganisms at concentrations that are tolerated by the host. The most successful antimicrobials are those that target anatomic structures or biosynthetic functions unique to specific microorganisms (Table 28-2). The choice of an antimicrobial is determined by both the properties of the individual drug and the nature of the infecting organism as confirmed by bacteriologic investigation (Tables 28-3 and 28-4). In seriously ill or immunocompromised patients, selection of bactericidal rather than bacteriostatic antimicrobials is often recommended (Table 28-5). Narrow-spectrum antimicrobials should be considered before broad-spectrum antimicrobials or combination therapy is prescribed to preserve normal flora of the patient (Table 28-6). These normal bacterial floras help prevent colonization by pathogens, because they compete for nutrients and produce their own antimicrobial substances. Normal bacterial floras assume special importance in hospitalized patients because the hospital may serve as a reservoir of resistant bacteria from previously treated patients. It is inadvisable to use less than the recommended dose of antimicrobials except in the presence of renal and occasionally hepatic dysfunction.

ANTIMICROBIAL PROPHYLAXIS FOR SURGICAL PROCEDURES

The use of antimicrobial prophylaxis in surgery involves a risk-to-benefit evaluation that varies depending on the nature of the operative procedure (Table 28-7). It is generally believed that prophylactic antimicrobials should be administered intravenously (IV) shortly before the surgical incision (no more than 2 hours before the incision) with the infusion completed before induction of anesthesia (Classen et al., 1992). Nevertheless, the size of the bacterial inoculum may be more important than the precise timing of the prophylactic antimicrobial administration. Data to support administration of prophylactic antibiotics before certain operations are often lacking. For clean elective surgical procedures such as mastectomy and thyroidectomy in which no tissue (other than the skin) carrying an indigenous flora is penetrated, the risks of routine antimicrobial prophylaxis outweigh the possible benefits. Because of their broad antimicrobial spectrum and low incidence of associated allergic reactions, cephalosporins (most often a cost-effective first-generation cephalosporin such as cefazolin or cephapirin) are the antimicrobials of choice for surgical procedures in which skin flora and normal flora of the gastrointestinal and genitourinary tracts are the most likely pathogens. A possible exception is in colorectal and abdominal operations, for which the prominence of anaerobes makes cefoxitin, cefotetan, or cefmetazole a more appropriate choice. However, even in these cases bowel preparation with oral antimicrobials may provide a less costly alternative. In general, adequate surgical prophylaxis can be achieved with treatment regimens ranging from a single dose to 48 hours of cephalosporin administration. Vancomycin is a useful prophylactic antimicrobial for patients undergoing placement of cardiovascular or joint prostheses. The emergence of resistant bacterial strains related to the use of prophylactic antimicrobials is a concern, although there is no proof that a brief course of treatment results in the emergence of resistant microorganisms (Kaiser, 1986). Pseudomembranous colitis is the most frequent complication of prophylactic antimicrobials, including the cephalosporins.

ANTIMICROBIAL SELECTION

Prompt identification of the causative organism is essential for the selection of appropriate antimicrobial drugs. The

TABLE 28-1.
CLASSIFICATION OF ANTIMICROBIALS

Class of Drug	Specific Drugs
Penicillinase-susceptible	Penicillin G Penicillin V
Penicillinase-resistant	Methicillin Oxacillin Nafcillin Cloxacillin Dicloxacillin
Penicillinase-susceptible with activity against Gram-negative bacilli	Ampicillin Amoxicillin Carbenicillin Mezlocillin Piperacillin Azlocillin
Penicillins with beta-lactamase inhibitors	Amoxicillin-clavulanic acid Ampicillin-sulbactam
Cephalosporins	See Table 28-10
Carbapenems	Imipenem
Monobactams	Aztreonam
Aminoglycosides	Streptomycin Kanamycin Gentamicin Tobramycin Amikacin Neomycin
Tetracyclines	Tetracycline Doxycycline
Macrolides	Erythromycin Clarithromycin Azithromycin
Lincomycins	Clindamycin
Dichloroacetic acid derivative	Chloramphenicol
Glycopeptide derivative	Vancomycin
Streptogramins	Quinupristin-dalfopristin
Oxazolidinones	Linezolid
Polymyxins	Polymyxin B Colistimethate
Polypeptide derivative	Bacitracin
Sulfonamides	Sulfisoxazole Sulfamethoxazole Sulfasalazine Sulfacetamide
Pyrimidine derivative	Trimethoprim
Miscellaneous	Metronidazole
Fluoroquinolones	Norfloxacin Ciprofloxacin Ofloxacin Lomefloxacin
Urinary tract disinfectants	Nitrofurantoin Fosfomycin
Antifungal drugs	Amphotericin B Nystatin Miconazole

TABLE 28-2.
MECHANISM OF ACTION OF ANTIMICROBIAL DRUGS

Drug	Anatomic Site of Biosynthetic Function Targeted by Antimicrobial Drug
Penicillins Cephalosporins Vancomycin	Interfere with synthesis of the mucopeptide layer of the bacterial cell wall, which is absent in host cells
Polymyxins	Alter permeability of bacterial cell membrane, allowing leakage of cell contents
Aminoglycosides Tetracyclines	Act on the 30S subunit of the bacterial ribosome so as to inhibit bacterial protein synthesis at the translational level
Chloramphenicol Erythromycin Clindamycin	Act on the 50S subunit of the bacterial ribosome so as to inhibit bacterial protein synthesis at the translational level
Sulfonamides	Inhibit microbial synthesis of folic acid
Quinolones	Inhibit bacterial DNA gyrase, which is the enzyme responsible for maintaining the helical structure of DNA
Rifampin	Selectively inhibits the bacterial DNA-dependent RNA polymerase but does not affect this enzyme in host cells

TABLE 28-3.
CONSIDERATIONS IN THE SELECTION OF AN ANTIMICROBIAL DRUG

Identification of the infecting organism (Gram stain, culture)
Determination of the antimicrobial susceptibility of the offending microorganism
Need for a bactericidal or bacteriostatic drug
Site of infection (need to cross the blood-brain barrier)
Host factors (immunosuppression, allergy, renal or hepatic dysfunction)
Need for combinations of antimicrobials
Route of administration
Duration of treatment
Risk of development of resistant strains in certain environments (hospital)
Cost (efficacy and toxicity may influence selection of more expensive drug)

TABLE 28-4.
ANTIMICROBIAL DRUGS OF CHOICE FOR TREATMENT OF VARIOUS INFECTIONS

Infection	Drug of Choice
Gram-positive cocci	
Staphylococcus aureus	
Methicillin-resistant	Vancomycin
Non–penicillinase-producing	Penicillin G
Penicillinase-producing	Methicillin
Staphylococcus epidermidis	Vancomycin or a cephalosporin
Streptococcus	Penicillin G, penicillin V, or ampicillin
Pneumococcus	Penicillin G or penicillin V
Gram-negative cocci	
Neisseria gonorrhoeae	Ceftriaxone
Bacterial meningitis	Penicillin G
Enteric Gram-negative bacilli	
Respiratory tract strains	Penicillin G
Escherichia coli	Ampicillin or a cephalosporin
Klebsiella	Cephalosporin
Proteus mirabilis	Ampicillin
Other Gram-negative bacilli	
Haemophilus influenzae	
Bronchitis	Trimethoprim with sulfamethoxazole
Meningitis or epiglottitis	Cefotaxime or ceftriaxone
Legionnaires disease	Erythromycin
Pseudomonas aeruginosa	
Urinary tract infections	Quinolone antimicrobial
Other infections	Gentamicin or tobramycin
Acid-fast bacilli	
Mycobacterium tuberculosis	Isoniazid plus rifampin plus pyrazinamide
Fungi	Amphotericin B
Mycoplasma	Erythromycin
Viruses	
Herpes simplex	Acyclovir
Cytomegalovirus	Ganciclovir
Influenza	Amantadine or rimantadine
Respiratory syncytial virus	Ribavirin
Varicella-zoster	Acyclovir
Human immunodeficiency virus	Combinations of antiretroviral drugs

TABLE 28-5.
EXAMPLES OF BACTERICIDAL AND BACTERIOSTATIC ANTIMICROBIALS

Bactericidal	Bacteriostatic
Penicillins	Tetracyclines
Cephalosporins	Chloramphenicol
Aminoglycosides	Erythromycin
Vancomycin	Clindamycin
Quinolones	Sulfonamides
Aztreonam	Trimethoprim
Imipenem	Linezolid (staphylococci and enterococci)
Bacitracin	
Polymyxins	
Linezolid (streptococci)	

TABLE 28-6.
EXAMPLES OF NARROW-SPECTRUM AND BROAD-SPECTRUM ANTIMICROBIALS

Narrow-Spectrum Antimicrobials	Broad-Spectrum Antimicrobials
Penicillin G	Ampicillin
Erythromycin	Cephalosporins
Clindamycin	Aminoglycosides
	Tetracyclines
	Chloramphenicol
	Quinolones

TABLE 28-7.
EXAMPLES OF SURGICAL PROCEDURES THAT MAY BENEFIT FROM PROPHYLACTIC ANTIMICROBIALS

Gynecologic surgery
Cesarean section
Hysterectomy (abdominal or vaginal)
Orthopedic surgery
Arthroplasty of joints, including replacement
Open reduction of fractures
General surgery
Cholecystectomy
Colon surgery
Appendectomy
Gastric resection
Penetrating abdominal trauma
Urologic surgery
Oropharyngeal surgery
Cardiothoracic and vascular surgery
Coronary artery bypass graft
Valve annuloplasty or replacement
Pacemaker insertion
Thoracotomy
Peripheral vascular surgery (possible exception: carotid endarterectomy)
Neurosurgery
Shunt procedures
Craniotomy

efficacy of antimicrobial therapy depends on drug delivery to the site of infection. Transport across the blood-brain barrier varies greatly among antimicrobials. Antimicrobial therapy is more likely to be effective if the infected material (foreign body, prosthesis) is removed. Infections behind obstructing lesions such as pneumonia behind a blocked bronchus will not respond to antimicrobials until the obstruction is relieved.

Most bacterial infections can be treated with a single antimicrobial drug. Simultaneous use of multiple antibiotics is avoided because of the risk of drug toxicity and sensitization, microbial superinfections, and antagonism between certain antimicrobials. Initial treatment of life-threatening infections may be initiated with combinations of antimicrobials until the offending organism can be identified.

There has been a dramatic increase in the presence of antimicrobial-resistant organisms. Many factors have contributed to the increase in resistance to antimicrobials but indiscriminate use of broad-spectrum antimicrobials is an important factor. The most problematic mechanism of antimicrobial resistance is the beta-lactamases.

Nosocomial Infections

Nearly 80% of nosocomial infections occur in three sites (urinary tract, respiratory system, and bloodstream). The incidence of nosocomial infections is highly associated with the use of devices such as ventilators, vascular access catheters, and urinary catheters. Intravascular access catheters are the most common causes of bacteremia or fungemia in hospitalized patients (Wenzel and Edmond, 1999). The organism infecting access catheters most commonly comes from the colonized hub or lumen and reflect skin flora (*S. aureus* and *epidermidis)*. Initial therapy of suspected intravascular catheter infection usually includes vancomycin because of the high incidence of methicillin-resistant *S. aureus* and *epidermidis* in the nosocomial environment.

Adverse Reactions

Adverse reactions to antimicrobials can be characterized as hypersensitivity reactions (independent of dose), direct drug toxicity (dose-related), and microbial superinfection. A history of drug allergy is essential before initiation of antimicrobial therapy. More information is available regarding allergies to the penicillins than other antimicrobials, but skin rashes, drug fever, and even anaphylaxis (especially vancomycin) can be caused by many antibiotics. Direct drug toxicity from antimicrobials may manifest as damage to virtually any organ and the potential for toxicity varies greatly from drug to drug (Table 28-8) (Cunha, 2001).

Parturients

Administration of antimicrobials during pregnancy introduces the question of safety for the mother and fetus (Table 28-9). Most antimicrobials cross the placenta and enter maternal milk. The immature fetal liver may lack enzymes necessary to metabolize certain drugs such that pharmacokinetics and toxicities in the fetus are often different from those in older children and adults. Teratogenicity is a concern when any drug is administered during pregnancy. Increases in maternal blood volume, glomerular filtration rate, and hepatic metabolic activity may decrease plasma antimicrobial concentrations (10% to 50%), especially late in pregnancy and in the early postpartum period. In some parturients, delayed gastric emptying may decrease absorption of orally administered antimicrobials.

Elderly Patients

Physiologic changes that occur with increasing age can alter oral absorption (decreased gastric acidity, reduced gastrointestinal motility), distribution (increased total body fat, decreased plasma albumin concentrations), metabolism (decreased hepatic blood flow), and excretion (decreased glomerular filtration rate) of antimicrobials. Penicillins and cephalosporins, because of their high therapeutic index obviate the need for significant changes in dosage schedules in elderly patients who have normal serum creatinine concentrations. Conversely, administration of aminoglycosides and vancomycin to elderly patients may require adjustments in dosing regimens. Measurement of plasma concentrations of antimicrobials and monitoring of renal function may be indicated when administering certain antimicrobials to elderly patients.

PENICILLINS

The basic structure of penicillins is a dicyclic nucleus (aminopenicillanic acid) that consists of a thiazolidine ring connected to a beta-lactam ring (Fig. 28-1). The penicillins may be classified into subgroups because of their structure, beta-lactamase susceptibility, and spectrum of activity (see Fig. 28-1). The bactericidal action of penicillins reflects the ability of these antimicrobials to interfere with the synthesis of peptidoglycan, which is an essential component of cell walls of susceptible bacteria. Penicillins also decrease the availability of an inhibitor of murein hydrolase such that the uninhibited enzyme can then destroy (lyse) the structural integrity of bacterial cell walls. Cell membranes of resistant Gram-negative bacteria prevent penicillins from gaining access to sites where synthesis of peptidoglycan is taking place.

Penicillin G and Penicillin V

Penicillin G (benzylpenicillin) was the first penicillin derivative discovered. This penicillin and its closely related congener, penicillin V (phenoxymethyl penicillin), are highly active against Gram-positive bacteria (streptococci). Both of these penicillins are readily hydrolyzed by bacteria-produced enzymes (penicillinases or beta-lactamases), rendering them ineffective against most strains of *Staphylococcus aureus*. Penicillin V is more expensive than penicillin G.

Clinical Indications

Penicillin is the drug of choice for treatment of pneumococcal, streptococcal, and meningococcal infections. Gonococci have gradually become more resistant to penicillin, requiring higher doses for adequate treatment. Treatment of syphilis with penicillin is highly effective. Penicillin is the drug of choice for treating all forms of actinomycosis and clostridial infections causing gas gangrene.

TABLE 28-8.
DIRECT DRUG TOXICITY ASSOCIATED WITH ADMINISTRATION OF ANTIMICROBIALS

Toxicity	Antimicrobial
Allergic reactions	All antimicrobials but most often with beta-lactam derivatives
Nephrotoxicity	Aminoglycosides Polymyxins Amphotericin B
Neutropenia	Penicillins Cephalosporins Vancomycin
Inhibition of platelet aggregation	Penicillins (high doses)
Prolonged prothrombin time	Cephalosporins
Bone marrow suppression (aplastic anemia, pancytopenia)	Chloramphenicol Flucytosine Linezolid (reversible)
Hemolytic anemia	Chloramphenicol Sulfonamides Nitrofurantoin Primaquine
Agranulocytosis	Macrolides Trimethoprim-sulfamethoxazole
Leukopenia and thrombocytopenia (folate deficiency)	Trimethoprim
Normocytic normochromic anemia	Amphotericin B
Ototoxicity	Aminoglycosides Vancomycin (auditory neurotoxicity) Minocycline (vestibular toxicity)
Seizures	Penicillins and other beta-lactams (high doses, azotemic patients, history of epilepsy) Metronidazole
Neuromuscular blockade	Aminoglycosides
Peripheral neuropathy	Nitrofurantoin (renal failure) Isoniazid (prevent with pyridoxine) Metronidazole
Benign intracranial hypertension	Tetracyclines
Optic neuritis	Ethambutol
Hepatotoxicity	Isoniazid Rifampin Tetracyclines (high doses) Beta-lactam antimicrobials (high doses) Nitrofurantoin Erythromycin Sulfonamides
Increased plasma bilirubin concentrations	Quinupristin-dalfopristin
Gastrointestinal irritation	Erythromycin Tetracyclines
Prolongation of QTc interval	Erythromycin Fluoroquinolones
Exaggerated sympathomimetic effects in patients receiving monoamine oxidase inhibitors	Linezolid
Hyperkalemia	Trimethoprim-sulfamethoxazole
Tendinitis	Fluoroquinolones
Arthralgias and myalgias	Quinupristin-dalfopristin
Photosensitivity	Sulfonamides Tetracyclines Fluoroquinolones
Teratogenicity	Tetracyclines Metronidazole Rifampin Trimethoprim Fluoroquinolones

TABLE 28-9.
ANTIMICROBIALS IN PREGANCY

Drug	Maternal Toxicity	Fetal Toxicity	Excreted in Colostrum
Considered Safe			
Penicillins	Allergic reactions	None known	Trace
Cephalosporins	Allergic reactions	None known	Trace
Erythromycin base	Allergic reactions Gastrointestinal irritation	None known	Yes
Use Cautiously			
Aminoglycosides	Ototoxicity Nephrotroxicity	Ototoxicity	Yes
Clindamycin	Allergic reactions Colitis	None known	Trace
Ethambutol	Optic neuritis	None known	Unknown
Isoniazid	Allergic reactions Hepatotoxicity	Neuropathy Seizures	Yes
Rifampin	Allergic reactions Hepatotoxicity	None known	Yes
Sulfonamides	Allergic reactions	Kernicterus (at term) Hemolysis (G6PD deficiency)	Yes
Avoid			
Metronidazole	Allergic reactions Alcohol intolerance Peripheral neuropathy	None known (teratogenic in animals)	Yes
Contraindicated			
Chloramphenicol	Bone marrow depression	Gray syndrome	Yes
Erythromycin estolate	Hepatotoxicity	None known	Yes
Nalidixic acid	Gastrointestinal irritation	Increased intracranial pressure	Unknown
Fluoroquinolones	Gastrointestianl irritation	Arthropathies (animals)	Unknown
Nitrofurantoin	Allergic reactions Peripheral neuropathy Gastrointestinal irritation	Hemolysis (G6PD deficiency)	Trace
Tetracyclines	Heptatoxicity Nephrotoxicity	Tooth discoloration and dysplasia Impaired bone growth	Yes
Trimethoprim	Allergic reactions	Teratogenicity	Yes

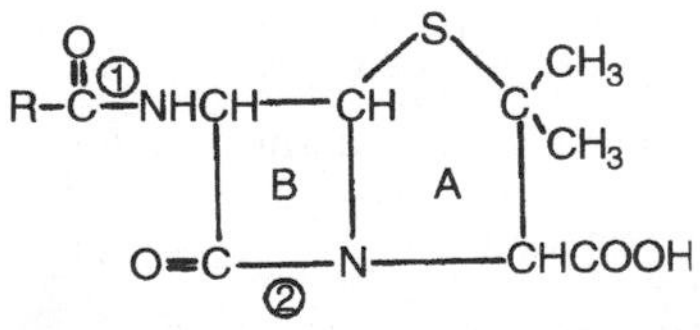

Figure 28-1. The basic structure of penicillins is a thiazolidine ring (**A**) connected to a beta-lactam ring (**B**). The bacterial enzymes amidase and penicillinase cleave the beta-lactam ring (2) or its side chain (1) to form an inactive product. Various synthetic penicillins have been produced by modifying the structure of the side chain (R) that is attached to the penicillin nucleus. This has resulted in penicillins that lack some of the disadvantages of penicillin G, such as poor gastrointestinal absorption, limited spectrum of antimicrobial activity, and inactivation by bacterial enzymes.

Prophylactic administration of penicillin is highly effective against streptococcal infections, accounting for its value in patients with rheumatic fever. Transient bacteremia occurs in the majority of patients undergoing dental extractions, emphasizing the importance of prophylactic penicillin in patients with congenital or acquired heart disease undergoing dental procedures. Transient bacteremia may also accompany surgical procedures, such as tonsillectomy and operations on the genitourinary and gastrointestinal tracts, and vaginal delivery.

Penicillin G and penicillin V have the same spectrum of antimicrobial activity, but penicillin V is more stable in the acid pH of the stomach. Blood levels of penicillin V are more predictable and, on average, are two to five times higher than those achieved by an identical dose of penicillin G. Although all forms of penicillin introduced since the release of penicillin G are prescribed by weight, penicillin

G is still commonly prescribed for parenteral administration as units. For interconversion, 1 mg of penicillin G is equivalent to approximately 1,600 U.

Administration of high doses of penicillin G intravenously (IV) to patients with renal dysfunction may result in neurotoxicity and hyperkalemia (10 million U of penicillin G contains 16 mEq of potassium). If this amount of potassium introduces a risk to the patient, a sodium salt of penicillin G or a sodium salt of a similar penicillin, such as ampicillin or carbenicillin, can be substituted for the aqueous penicillin G.

Other drugs should not be mixed with penicillin, as the combination may inactivate the antimicrobial. Intrathecal administration of penicillins is not recommended, because these drugs are potent convulsants when administered by this route. Furthermore, arachnoiditis and encephalopathy may follow intrathecal penicillin administration.

Excretion

Renal excretion of penicillin is rapid (60% to 90% of an intramuscular [IM] dose is excreted in the first hour), such that the plasma concentration decreases to 50% of its peak value within 1 hour after injection. Approximately 10% is eliminated by glomerular filtration, and 90% is eliminated by renal tubular secretion. Anuria increases the elimination half-time of penicillin G approximately tenfold.

Duration of Action

Methods to prolong the duration of action of penicillin include the simultaneous administration of probenecid, which blocks the renal tubular secretion of penicillin. Alternatively, the IM injection of poorly soluble salts of penicillin, such as procaine or benzathine, delays absorption and thus prolongs the duration of action. Procaine penicillin contains 120 mg of the local anesthetic for every 300,000 U of the antimicrobial. Possible hypersensitivity to procaine must be considered when selecting this form of the antimicrobial for administration.

Penicillinase-Resistant Penicillins

The major mechanism of resistance to the penicillins is bacterial production of beta-lactamase enzymes that hydrolyze the beta-lactam ring, rendering the antimicrobial molecule inactive. Methicillin (dimethoxybenzylpenicillin), oxacillin, nafcillin, cloxacillin, and dicloxacillin are not susceptible to hydrolysis by staphylococcal penicillinases that would otherwise hydrolyze the cyclic amide bond of the beta-lactam ring and render the antimicrobial inactive (see Fig. 28-1). Specific indications for these drugs are infections caused by staphylococci known to produce this enzyme. Penetration of nafcillin into the central nervous system (CNS) is sufficient to treat staphylococcal meningitis. Parenteral methicillin has largely been superseded by oxacillin and nafcillin. Hemorrhagic cystitis and an allergic interstitial nephritis (hematuria, proteinuria) may accompany administration of methicillin. Hepatitis has been associated with high-dose oxacillin therapy. Renal excretion of methicillin, oxacillin, and cloxacillin is extensive. More than 80% of an IV dose of nafcillin is excreted in the bile, which may be an advantage when high-dose therapy is necessary in a patient with impaired renal function.

Oxacillin and nafcillin, unlike methicillin, are relatively stable in an acidic medium, resulting in adequate systemic absorption after oral administration. Nevertheless, variable absorption from the gastrointestinal tract often dictates a parenteral route of administration for treatment of serious infections caused by penicillinase-producing staphylococci. Cloxacillin and dicloxacillin are available only as oral preparations and may be preferable because they produce higher blood levels than do oxacillin and nafcillin.

Penicillinase-Susceptible Broad-Spectrum Penicillins (Second-Generation Penicillins)

Broad-spectrum penicillins, such as ampicillin, amoxicillin, and carbenicillin, have a wider range of activity than other penicillins, being bactericidal against Gram-positive and Gram-negative bacteria. They are, nevertheless, all inactivated by penicillinase produced by certain Gram-negative and Gram-positive bacteria. Therefore, these drugs are not effective against most staphylococcal infections.

Ampicillin

Ampicillin (alpha-aminobenzylpenicillin) has a broader range of activity than penicillin G. Its spectrum encompasses not only pneumococci, meningococci, gonococci, and various streptococci but also a number of Gram-negative bacilli, such as *Haemophilus influenzae* and *Escherichia coli*. Like penicillin G, ampicillin is cleaved by beta-lactamase and is ineffective in the treatment of infections due to *S. aureus* (see Fig. 28-1). Ampicillin is stable in acid and thus is well absorbed after oral administration, although peak plasma concentrations are lower than those achieved after administration of penicillin V. Approximately 50% of an oral dose of ampicillin is excreted unchanged by the kidneys in the first 6 hours, emphasizing that renal function greatly influences the duration of action of this antimicrobial. Ampicillin also appears in the bile and undergoes enterohepatic circulation. Among the penicillins, ampicillin is associated with the highest incidence of skin rash (9%), which typically appears 7 to 10 days after initiation of therapy. Many of these rashes are due to protein impurities in the commercial preparation of the drug and do not represent true allergic reactions.

Amoxicillin

Amoxicillin is chemically identical to ampicillin except for an –OH substituent instead of an –H on the side-chain. Its spectrum of activity is identical to that of ampicillin, but it is more efficiently absorbed from the gastrointestinal tract than ampicillin, and effective concentrations are present in the circulation for twice as long.

Extended-Spectrum Carboxypenicillins (Third-Generation Penicillins)

Carbenicillin

Carbenicillin (alpha-carboxybenzylpenicillin) results from the change from an amino to carboxy substituent on the side-chain of ampicillin (see Fig. 28-1). The principal advantage of carbenicillin is its effectiveness in the treatment of infections caused by *Pseudomonas aeruginosa* and certain *Proteus* strains that are resistant to ampicillin. This antimicrobial is penicillinase susceptible and therefore ineffective against most strains of *S. aureus*. Carbenicillin is not absorbed from the gastrointestinal tract; therefore, it must be administered parenterally. The elimination half-time is approximately 1 hour and is prolonged to approximately 2 hours when there is hepatic or renal dysfunction. Approximately 85% of the unchanged drug is recovered in urine over 9 hours. Probenecid, by delaying renal excretion of the drug, increases the plasma concentration of carbenicillin by approximately 50%.

The sodium load administered with a large dose of carbenicillin (30 to 40 g) is considerable because >10% of carbenicillin is sodium (about 5 mEq/g). Congestive heart failure may develop in susceptible patients in response to this acute drug-produced sodium load. Hypokalemia and metabolic alkalosis may occur because of obligatory excretion of potassium with the large amount of nonreabsorbable carbenicillin. Carbenicillin interferes with normal platelet aggregation such that bleeding time is prolonged but platelet count remains normal.

Extended-Spectrum Acylaminopenicillins (Fourth-Generation Penicillins)

The acylaminopenicillins (mezlocillin, piperacillin, azlocillin) have the broadest spectrum of activity of all the penicillins. Like the carboxypenicillins, the acylaminopenicillins are derivatives of ampicillin. These drugs are ineffective against penicillinase-producing strains of *S. aureus*. The acylaminopenicillins have a lower sodium content than the carboxypenicillins but otherwise the side effects are similar. Clinical studies have not demonstrated that these antimicrobials are superior to the carboxypenicillins.

Penicillin Beta-Lactamase Inhibitor Combinations

Clavulanic acid, sulbactam, and tazobactam are beta-lactam compounds that have little intrinsic antimicrobial activity. However, these compounds bind irreversibly to the beta-lactamase enzymes that are produced by many bacteria, thus inactivating these enzymes and rendering the organisms sensitive to beta-lactamase-susceptible penicillins. Clavulanic acid is available with oral amoxicillin and parenteral ampicillin preparations have been combined with sulbactam.

Allergy to Penicillins

Hypersensitivity is the most common adverse reaction to beta-lactam antimicrobials. Allergic reactions are noted in 1% to 10% of patients treated with penicillins, making these antimicrobials the most allergenic of all drugs (Pallasch, 1988). Most often, the allergic response is a delayed reaction characterized by a maculopapular rash and/or fever. Less often but more serious is immediate hypersensitivity that is mediated by immunoglobulin E antibodies. Manifestations of immediate hypersensitivity may include laryngeal edema, bronchospasm, and cardiovascular collapse. Antibodies to penicillin may also cause hemolytic anemia. Fatal allergic reactions have occurred in patients receiving as little as 1 U of penicillin for skin testing. Allergic reactions may occur in the absence of previous known exposure to any of the penicillins. This may reflect prior unrecognized exposure to penicillin, presumably in ingested foods. Allergic reactions can occur with any dose or route of administration, although severe anaphylactic reactions are more often associated with parenteral than with oral administration. Some patients who experience cutaneous reactions may continue to receive the offending penicillin or receive the same penicillin in the future without experiencing a similar response.

The penicillin molecule itself is probably unable to form a complete antigen, but instead the ring structure of penicillin is opened to form a hapten metabolite, penicilloyl. Approximately 95% of patients allergic to penicillin form this penicilloyl-protein conjugate (the major antigenic determinant); the remaining allergic patients form 6-aminopenicillic acid and benzylpenamaldic acid (minor antigenic determinants). Skin testing with a polyvalent skin test antigen, penicilloyl-polylysine, makes it possible to detect most patients who would develop a life-threatening allergic reaction if treated with a penicillin antimicrobial. Nevertheless, minor antigenic determinants that would not be detected by skin testing may produce severe allergic reactions.

Cross-Reactivity

The presence of a common nucleus (beta-lactam ring) in the structure of all penicillins means that allergy to one penicillin increases the likelihood of an allergic reaction to another penicillin. Furthermore, there would seem to be the potential for cross-reactivity between penicillins and cephalosporins as they both share a common beta-lactam ring. Patients who are allergic to penicillin have an 8% likelihood of having an allergic reaction to cephalosporin antimicrobials (Kelkar and Li, 2001). For this reason, administration of cephalosporins to patients with a history

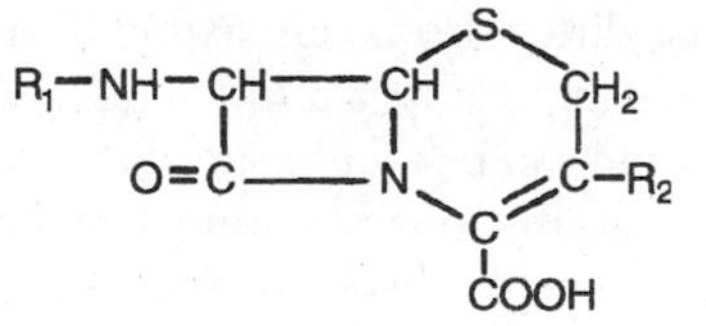

Figure 28-2. Structural formula of cephalosporins.

of allergy to penicillin (hypotension, bronchospasm, laryngeal edema) confirmed by a positive skin test is not recommended.

CEPHALOSPORINS

Cephalosporins, like the penicillins, are bactericidal antimicrobials that inhibit bacterial cell wall synthesis and have a low intrinsic toxicity. These antimicrobials are derived from 7-aminocephalosporanic acid (Fig. 28-2). Resistance to the cephalosporins, as to the penicillins, may be due to an inability of the antimicrobial to penetrate to its site of action. Bacteria can also produce cephalosporinases (beta-lactamases) that disrupt the beta-lactam structure of cephalosporins and thus inhibit their antimicrobial activity. Like the newer penicillins, the new cephalosporins have an extraordinarily broad spectrum of antimicrobial action but are very expensive.

Individual cephalosporins differ significantly with respect to the extent of absorption after oral ingestion, severity of pain produced by IM injection, and protein binding. IV administration of any of the cephalosporins can cause thrombophlebitis. Excretion of cephalosporins is principally by glomerular filtration and renal tubular secretion, emphasizing the need to decrease the dose of these drugs in the presence of renal dysfunction. Diacetyl metabolites of cephalosporins can occur and are associated with decreased antimicrobial activity.

A positive Coombs' reaction frequently occurs in patients who receive large doses of cephalosporins. Hemolysis, however, is rarely associated with this response. Nephrotoxicity owing to cephalosporins, with the exception of cephaloridine, is less frequent than after administration of aminoglycosides or polymyxins.

The incidence of allergic reactions in patients being treated with cephalosporins ranges from 1% to 10%. The majority of the allergic reactions consist of cutaneous manifestations that occur 24 hours after drug exposure. Life-threatening anaphylaxis is estimated to occur in 0.02% of treated patients (Anne and Reisman, 1995). Because the cephalosporins share immunologic cross-reactivity, patients who are allergic to one cephalosporin are likely to be allergic to others. The possibility of cross-reactivity between cephalosporins and penicillins seems to be very infrequent, and cephalosporins are often selected as alternative antimicrobials in patients with a history of penicillin allergy (Anne and Reisman, 1995).

Classification

Cephalosporins are classified as first-, second-, and third-generation because of their antimicrobial spectrum (Table 28-10). In general, activity against Gram-positive cocci decreases, and activity against Gram-negative cocci increases from the first- to third-generation cephalosporins. First-generation cephalosporins are inexpensive, exhibit low toxicity, and are as active as second- and third-generation cephalosporins against staphylococci and nonenterococcal streptococci. For these reasons, first-generation cephalosporins have been commonly selected for antimicrobial prophylaxis in patients undergoing cardiovascular, orthopedic, biliary, pelvic, and intraabdominal surgery (see the section on Antimicrobial Prophylaxis for Surgical Procedures). All cephalosporins can penetrate into joints and can readily cross the placenta.

TABLE 28-10.
CLASSIFICATION OF CEPHALOSPORINS

	First-Generation Cephalosporins	Second-Generation Cephalosporins	Third-Generation Cephalosporins
Oral	Cefadroxil Cephalexin Cephradine	Cefaclor Cefuroxime Cefprozil Cefditoren Loracarbef	Cefixime Cefdinir Cefpodoxime Ceftibuten
Parenteral	Cefazolin Cephapirin Cephradine Cefoperazone	Cefoxitin Cefamandole Cefonicid Cefuroxime	Cefotaxime Ceftizoxime Ceftriaxone

First-Generation Cephalosporins

Cephalothin is the prototype of first-generation cephalosporins. Like most other cephalosporins, cephalothin is excreted largely unaltered by the kidneys, emphasizing the need to decrease the dose in the presence of renal dysfunction. Oral absorption is poor and IM injection is painful, accounting for its common administration by the IV route. Although cephalothin is present in many tissues and fluids, it does not enter the cerebrospinal fluid in significant amounts and is not recommended for treatment of meningitis. Two other first-generation cephalosporins, cephapirin and cephradine, are almost identical to cephalothin in their antimicrobial spectrum, pharmacology, and toxicity. Indeed, cost may be a principal determinant in selecting among these very similar antimicrobials.

Cefazolin has essentially the same antimicrobial spectrum as cephalothin but has the advantage of achieving higher blood levels, presumably due to slower renal elimination. In this regard, cefazolin is viewed as the drug of choice for antimicrobial prophylaxis in the perioperative period. This drug is well tolerated after IM or IV injection.

Second-Generation Cephalosporins

Cefoxitin and cefamandole are examples of second-generation cephalosporins with extended activity against Gram-negative bacteria. Cefoxitin is resistant to cephalosporinases produced by Gram-negative bacteria. Cefamandole is pharmacologically similar to cefoxitin, but its methylthiotetrazole side-chain poses a risk of bleeding and disulfiram-like reactions with concurrent use of alcohol. Both drugs are excreted predominantly unchanged by the kidneys. Cefuroxime is more effective than cefamandole against *H. influenzae* and is the only second-generation cephalosporin effective in the treatment of meningitis.

Third-Generation Cephalosporins

Third-generation cephalosporins have an enhanced ability to resist hydrolysis by the beta-lactamases of many Gram-negative bacilli including *E. coli, Klebsiella, Proteus,* and *H. influenzae*. Unlike older cephalosporins, the third-generation cephalosporins achieve therapeutic levels in the cerebrospinal fluid and can be used to treat meningitis. The third-generation cephalosporins seem to have the same relatively low toxicities as the older cephalosporins.

Cefotaxime was the first third-generation cephalosporin and has been effective in a broad range of infections, including meningitis caused by Gram-negative bacilli other than *Pseudomonas*. The elimination half-time of this antimicrobial is approximately 1 hour, with clearance via the kidneys and hepatic metabolism. An adjustment in dosage or dosing interval is indicated in patients with renal dysfunction who are being treated with this drug. Approximately 30% of cefotaxime is excreted as a desacetyl derivative that has antibacterial activity and is synergistic with the parent compound.

Ceftizoxime differs from cefotaxime in that it depends solely on renal clearance. As a result, it has a longer elimination half-time and can be administered at 8-hour intervals.

Ceftriaxone has the longest elimination half-time of any third-generation cephalosporin and is highly effective against Gram-negative bacilli, especially *Neisseria* and *Haemophilus*.

Cefoperazone is unique among cephalosporins in depending primarily on hepatic elimination for its clearance. Therefore, adjustments in dosage are not necessary for treatment of patients with renal dysfunction. A major asset of cefoperazone is its activity against *P. aeruginosa*. Nevertheless, ceftazidime exceeds all other third-generation cephalosporins in its activity against *P. aeruginosa*.

Cefixime is an orally effective third-generation cephalosporin that is as active as other cephalosporins against pneumococci, group A streptococci, and *H. influenzae* but less active against *S. aureus* and not active against anaerobes such as *Pseudomonas*. The spectrum of activity of cefixime and a single daily dose make it attractive for upper respiratory tract infections, but less expensive alternatives are available.

Moxalactam is a synthetic beta-lactam antimicrobial that, among the third-generation cephalosporins, is the most active against anaerobes. Because of its propensity to produce bleeding from prolongation of the prothrombin time, this antimicrobial has been largely supplanted by other cephalosporins.

OTHER BETA-LACTAM ANTIMICROBIALS

Imipenem

Imipenem is a bactericidal antimicrobial with the broadest antibacterial spectrum of any beta-lactam antimicrobial and is effective against most Gram-positive and Gram-negative bacteria. This antimicrobial is extensively degraded in the renal tubules, resulting in low urinary concentrations. This disadvantage can be prevented by combining imipenem with cilastatin, an inhibitor of the enzyme responsible for the renal tubular metabolism of imipenem. Clearance is by glomerular filtration, and the dose should be decreased in patients with renal dysfunction. There is potential cross-reactivity with other beta-lactam antimicrobials, including the penicillins and cephalosporins. Seizures are a rare complication, and antimicrobial-associated pseudomembranous colitis has occurred. Transient derangements in liver function tests and leukopenia have been described in patients receiving imipenem-cilastatin.

Aztreonam

Aztreonam is a monobactam antimicrobial that lacks the thiazolidine ring present in penicillins and the dihydrothiazine ring found in cephalosporins. The antimicrobial activity of this drug is limited to Gram-negative bacteria. Aztreonam is not absorbed from the gastrointestinal tract, but therapeutic blood levels are achieved after IM or IV administration in most body tissues and fluids, including cerebrospinal fluid. The elimination half-time is about 1.5 hours, and clearance is principally by glomerular filtration. Neither nephrotoxicity nor bleeding disorders have been reported. A unique advantage is the absence of any cross-reactivity between aztreonam and circulating antibodies of penicillin- or cephalosporin-allergic patients (Adkinson, 1990). Because aztreonam combines the activity of the aminoglycosides with the low toxicity of the beta-lactam antimicrobials, it may eventually replace aminoglycosides in the treatment of many Gram-negative infections. A potential disadvantage of aztreonam is the development of enterococcal superinfections. This antimicrobial is significantly more expensive that aminoglycosides.

AMINOGLYCOSIDE ANTIMICROBIALS

Aminoglycosides are poorly lipid-soluble antimicrobials that are rapidly bactericidal for aerobic Gram-negative bacteria. As would be predicted with the poor lipid solubility of these drugs, <1% of an orally administered aminoglycoside is absorbed into the systemic circulation. Negligible binding to proteins is also a predictable characteristic of poorly lipid-soluble drugs. Rapid systemic absorption occurs after IM injection, with peak plasma concentrations occurring in 30 to 90 minutes. Aminoglycosides have a volume of distribution similar to the extracellular fluid volume and undergo extensive renal excretion due almost exclusively to glomerular filtration. There is a linear relationship between the plasma creatinine concentration and the elimination half-time of aminoglycosides. In the presence of normal renal function, the elimination half-time of aminoglycosides is 2 to 3 hours and is prolonged 20- to 40-fold in the presence of renal failure. Determination of the plasma concentration of aminoglycosides is an essential guide to the safe administration of these antimicrobials. The future role of aminoglycosides will be influenced by their toxicity (see the section on Side Effects) and cost-effectiveness relative to new beta-lactams and the fluoroquinolones.

Streptomycin was the first parenterally administered antimicrobial that was active against many Gram-negative bacilli and *Mycobacterium tuberculosis*. Current use of this drug is limited because of the rapid emergence of resistant organisms, the frequent occurrence of vestibular damage during prolonged treatment, and the availability of less toxic antimicrobials. Streptomycin is potentially useful in the treatment of enterococcal infections in which synergism between a penicillin and an aminoglycoside is desired. This antimicrobial remains the drug of choice for the treatment of tularemia and bubonic plague.

Kanamycin has a broader spectrum of activity than streptomycin but has been largely replaced by gentamicin and other aminoglycoside antimicrobials that are less ototoxic and that have a wider range of antibacterial activity.

Gentamicin is active against *P. aeruginosa* as well as the Gram-negative bacilli susceptible to kanamycin. Gentamicin penetrates pleural, ascitic, and synovial fluids in the presence of inflammation. Patients receiving gentamicin or any aminoglycoside should be checked frequently for vestibular or auditory dysfunction. Monitoring plasma concentrations of gentamicin is the best approach for recognizing potentially toxic levels (>9 μg/mL). If plasma concentrations of gentamicin cannot be monitored, the dose can be adjusted based of the plasma creatinine concentration.

Tobramycin is similar to gentamicin with respect to its toxicity and antimicrobial spectrum. This antimicrobial is expensive and appears to offer few advantages over gentamicin.

Amikacin is a semisynthetic derivative of kanamycin that has the advantage of not being associated with the development of resistance. The principal use of amikacin is in the treatment of infections caused by gentamicin- or tobramycin-resistant Gram-negative bacilli. Unlike other aminoglycosides, this drug should not be administered in combination with penicillin, which may result in antagonism of the bactericidal actions of penicillin against some strains of *Enterococcus faecalis*. The incidence of nephrotoxicity and ototoxicity is similar to that produced by gentamicin.

Neomycin is commonly used for topical application to treat infections of the skin (as after burn injury), cornea, and mucous membranes. Allergic reactions occur in 6% to 8% of patients treated with topical neomycin. Continuous irrigation of the bladder with neomycin solution is used to prevent bacteriuria and bacteremia associated with the use of indwelling bladder catheters. Oral neomycin does not undergo systemic absorption and is thus administered to decrease bacterial flora in the intestine before gastrointestinal surgery and as an adjunct to the therapy of hepatic coma (decreases blood ammonia concentrations).

Side Effects

The side effects of aminoglycosides that limit their clinical usefulness include ototoxicity, nephrotoxicity, skeletal muscle weakness, and potentiation of nondepolarizing neuromuscular-blocking drugs. These side effects parallel the plasma concentration of the aminoglycoside, emphasizing the need to decrease the dose of these drugs in patients with renal dysfunction.

Ototoxicity

Ototoxicity manifests as vestibular dysfunction, auditory dysfunction, or both and parallels the accumulation of aminoglycosides in the perilymph of the inner ear. There is drug-induced destruction of vestibular or cochlear sensory hairs that is dose-dependent and most likely occurs with chronic therapy, especially in elderly patients, in whom renal dysfunction is more likely. Furosemide, mannitol, and probably other diuretics seem to accentuate the ototoxic effects of aminoglycosides. Vestibular toxicity manifests as nystagmus, vertigo, nausea, and the acute onset of Ménière's syndrome. Auditory dysfunction manifests as tinnitus or a sensation of pressure or fullness in the ears. Deafness may develop suddenly.

Nephrotoxicity

Aminoglycosides accumulate in the renal cortex and can produce acute tubular necrosis that initially manifests as an inability to concentrate urine and the appearance of proteinuria and red blood cell casts. These changes are usually reversible if the drug is discontinued. Neomycin is the most nephrotoxic of the aminoglycosides, and therefore is not administered by the parenteral route.

Skeletal Muscle Weakness

Skeletal muscle weakness can occur with the intrapleural or intraperitoneal institution of large doses of aminoglycosides. This effect is most likely because of the ability of aminoglycosides to inhibit the prejunctional release of acetylcholine while also decreasing postsynaptic sensitivity to the neurotransmitter. IV administration of calcium overcomes the effect of aminoglycosides at the neuromuscular junction. Patients with myasthenia gravis are uniquely susceptible to skeletal muscle weakness if treated with an aminoglycoside. Administration of a single dose of an aminoglycoside is unlikely to produce skeletal muscle weakness in an otherwise healthy patient.

Potentiation of Nondepolarizing Neuromuscular Blocking Drugs

IV administration of aminoglycosides and the associated high plasma concentrations are likely to potentiate nondepolarizing neuromuscular-blocking drugs (Sokoll and Gergis, 1981). Likewise, irrigation of the peritoneal or pleural cavities with large volumes of aminoglycoside-containing solutions can result in substantial systemic absorption and potentiation of previously administered neuromuscular-blocking drugs. Reappearance of neuromuscular blockade is a possibility if aminoglycosides are administered systemically in the early postoperative period to a patient who has been judged to have adequately recovered from neuromuscular-blocking drugs administered during anesthesia. Furthermore, the neuromuscular-blocking effects of lidocaine are enhanced in the presence of neuromuscular-blocking drugs and aminoglycosides. It is conceivable that administration of lidocaine in the early postoperative period could produce skeletal muscle weakness in a patient who had previously received a neuromuscular-blocking drug and an aminoglycoside (Bruckner et al., 1980).

Neostigmine- or calcium-induced antagonism of aminoglycoside-potentiated neuromuscular blockade may be incomplete or transient (Sokoll and Gergis, 1981). Speculation that reversal of antimicrobial-induced neuromuscular blockade would also antagonize antimicrobial effects, however, has not been documented (Booij et al., 1980). Clinical evaluation, as well as electrophysiologic criteria, is necessary to evaluate aminoglycoside-potentiated neuromuscular blockade. The importance of clinical observation is demonstrated by the fact that neuromuscular blockade in the presence of neomycin can be characterized by a sustained response to continuous electrical stimulation and a train-of-four ratio near 1, despite a greatly decreased single twitch response.

The effects of antimicrobials at the neuromuscular junction probably involve multiple sites of action (Fig. 28-3) (Sokoll and Gergis, 1981). In terms of producing clinically significant skeletal muscle effects with therapeutic doses, the penicillins, cephalosporins, tetracyclines, and erythromycin are devoid of effects at the neuromuscular junction. The mechanism of the neuromuscula-blocking effects of polymyxins is complex but is most likely postsynaptic.

Neomycin and gentamicin decrease the amount of acetylcholine released by the presynaptic motor nerves and decrease the sensitivity of the postsynaptic motor end-plate to the depolarizing action of acetylcholine. Oral neomycin, which is used to decrease the bacterial population of the gastrointestinal tract before abdominal surgery, is unlikely to produce effects at the neuromuscular junction, because this antimicrobial is not absorbed into the systemic circulation. Nevertheless, prolonged oral administration of neomycin has been associated with antimicrobial-induced neuromuscular blockade.

TETRACYCLINES

Tetracyclines are used less extensively because of the availability of more effective antimicrobials (penicillins, cephalosporins, and fluoroquinolones) and the possible occurrence of superinfection in patients treated with high doses of these drugs (Fig. 28-4). These antimicrobials are the drugs of choice in the treatment of rickettsial diseases and are useful in the treatment of mycoplasma pneumonia. Tetracyclines are used as adjuvant therapy in the treatment of severe cystic acne, presumably producing a beneficial effect by decreasing the fatty acid content of sebum. In view of the large number of available tetracyclines, it is reasonable to become familiar with one standard preparation (tetracycline) and one long-acting preparation (doxycycline).

Tetracycline is administered orally, but its absorption is impaired by the presence of mild and particulate antacids, presumably reflecting chelation and an increase in gastric fluid pH. Gastrointestinal distress and the possibility of tetracycline-resistant bacterial enteritis limit the oral dose of these antibiotics. Tetracycline evokes a catabolic response, presumably due to a generalized inhibition of amino acid use for protein synthesis. Topical administration of tetracycline, except for use in the eye, is not recommended

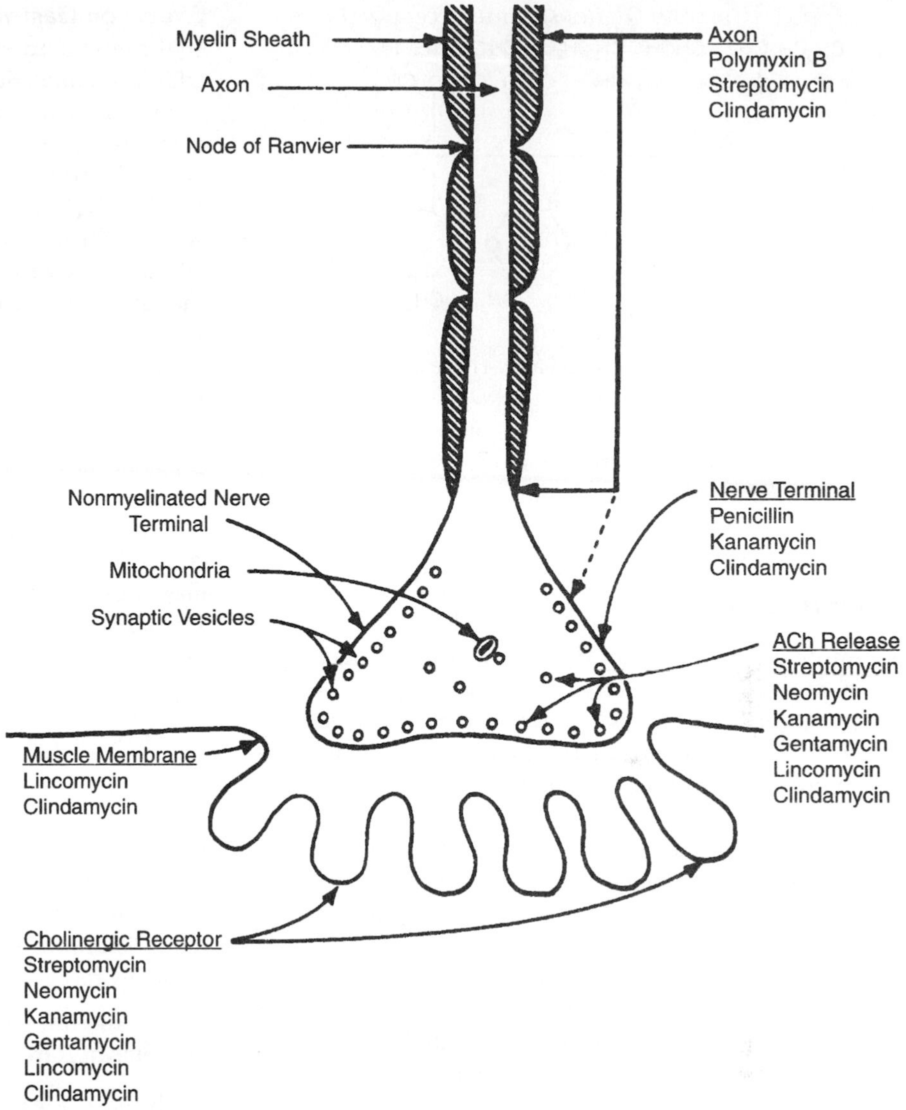

Figure 28-3. Schematic depiction of possible sites of action of antimicrobials at the neuromuscular junction. (ACh, acetylcholine.) (From Sokoll MD, Gergis SD. Antibiotics and neuromuscular function. *Anesthesiology* 1981;55:148–159; with permission.)

because of the high incidence of sensitization. Therapeutic doses cannot be administered satisfactorily by the IM route due to local irritation and poor absorption. Tetracycline is excreted in urine and bile, accumulates in patients with renal dysfunction, and may cause hepatic toxicity. Fatty liver infiltration has been observed; parturients seem particularly susceptible. Tetracyclines should not be administered to parturients or children because they may cause permanent discoloration of the teeth. Deposition of tetracycline in teeth and bones is probably due to its chelating property and the formation of a tetracycline-orthophosphate-calcium complex. Phototoxicity, characterized by increased sensitivity of the skin to sunlight, occurs in patients treated with tetracyclines.

Doxycycline may be administered orally or IV. The elimination half-time after an oral dose is 11 to 22 hours, and administration is needed only every 12 to 24 hours to maintain a therapeutic plasma concentration. An advantage of doxycycline is the presence of an unchanged elimination half-time in the presence of renal dysfunction. The spectrum of antimicrobial activity and toxicity of doxycycline is similar to that of tetracycline.

MACROLIDES

Macrolides are stable in the presence of acidic gastric fluid, and as a result, these antimicrobials are well absorbed from the gastrointestinal tract. Structurally,

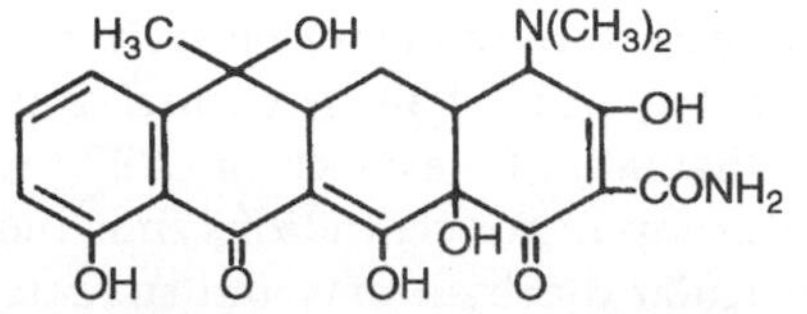

Figure 28-4. Tetracyclines consist of four interconnected carbon rings with side-chains.

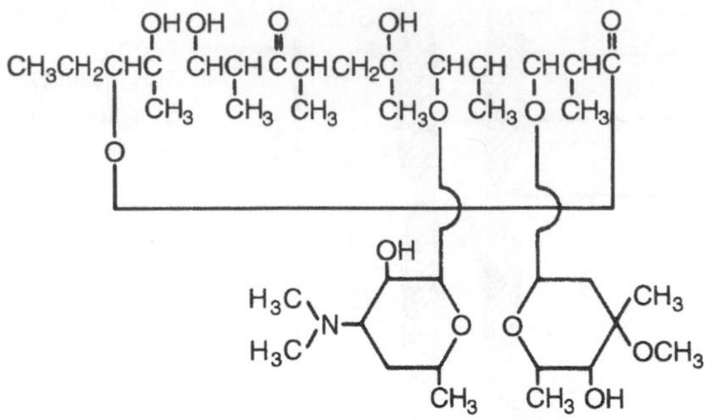

Figure 28-5. Erythromycin.

these antimicrobials are characterized by 14 to 16 carbon atoms joined together in a complex, central molecule that is linked to various side chains (Fig. 28-5).

Erythromycin

Erythromycin has a spectrum of activity that includes most Gram-positive bacteria, *Streptococcus pneumoniae, S. aureus, Moraxella catarrhalis, H. influenzae, Mycoplasma, Chlamydia pneumoniae,* and *Corynebacterium diphtheriae*. It is the preferred drug for treatment of atypical pneumonia. In patients who cannot tolerate penicillins or cephalosporins, erythromycin is an effective alternative for the treatment of streptococcal pharyngitis, bronchitis, and pneumonia. Therapeutic plasma concentrations can only be achieved by oral administration. Because of the occasional occurrence of cholestatic hepatitis after administration of the estolate form, however, erythromycin base or stearate is preferred. Gastrointestinal intolerance is the most common side effect, and enteric-coated preparations are available. IV preparations are available for treatment of severe infections, but prolonged use by this route of administration is limited by the common occurrence of thrombophlebitis at the injection site and development of tinnitus or hearing loss in many patients. Severe nausea and vomiting may accompany infusion of erythromycin. A case of hepatic failure attributed to infusion of erythromycin has been reported (Gholson and Warren, 1990). Erythromycin is excreted largely in bile and only to a minor degree in urine. The dosage need not be altered in the presence of renal failure.

Effects on QTc

Oral erythromycin prolongs cardiac repolarization and is associated with reports of torsades de pointes (Ray et al., 2004). Because erythromycin is extensively metabolized by cytochrome P-450 3A (CYP3A) isozymes, commonly used medications that inhibit the effects of CYP3A may increase plasma erythromycin concentrations thus increasing the risk of ventricular dysrhythmias and sudden death. The concurrent use of erythromycin and strong inhibitors of CYP3A is not recommended.

Effects on Gastric Emptying

Erythromycin in subtherapeutic doses (up to 200 mg) exhibits cholinergic stimulatory properties manifesting as increased lower esophageal sphincter tone, enhanced intraduodenal coordination, and intermittent gastric contractions resulting in accelerated gastric emptying of solids and liquids (Pilot, 1994). When administered orally 1 hour before induction of anesthesia, erythromycin 200 mg significantly decreased gastric fluid pH (Asai et al., 2000). In contrast, when administered 3 hours before induction of anesthesia, erythromycin did not significantly alter gastric acidity. Endoscopic confirmation of total gastric emptying after administration of erythromycin, 100 mg IV, has been described in a patient scheduled for emergency surgery (Kopp et al., 1997). Gastroenterologists have administered erythromycin IV or orally (0.375 to 0.750 mg/kg) to achieve gastric emptying before endoscopy procedures (Lin et al., 1994). These prokinetic properties of erythromycin may be beneficial in the preparation of patients considered at risk for pulmonary aspiration before induction of anesthesia (see Chapter 26).

Clarithromycin

Clarithromycin has a similar antimicrobial spectrum to erythromycin, but its longer elimination half-time permits twice a day oral administration (250 to 500 mg) rather than four times a day as necessary for erythromycin. Gastrointestinal side effects seem to be less than after administration of erythromycin. Clarithromycin is substantially more expensive than erythromycin.

Azithromycin

Azithromycin resembles erythromycin in its antimicrobial spectrum, but an extraordinarily prolonged elimination half-time (68 hours) permits once-a-day dosing for 5 days (500 mg on day 1 and 250 mg on days 2 to 5). Tissue levels of azithromycin can be expected to remain at therapeutic levels for 4 to 7 days after a 5-day treatment course. Unlike clarithromycin, bioavailability of azithromycin is decreased by food such that the drug should be administered 1 hour before or 2 hours after meals. A potential use of azithromycin is treatment of chronic infections in patients with acquired immune deficiency syndrome (AIDS). Azithromycin is substantially more expensive than erythromycin.

CLINDAMYCIN

Clindamycin resembles erythromycin in antimicrobial activity, but it is more active against many anaerobes (Fig. 28-6). Because severe pseudomembranous colitis can be a complication of clindamycin therapy, this drug should be used only to treat infections that cannot be adequately

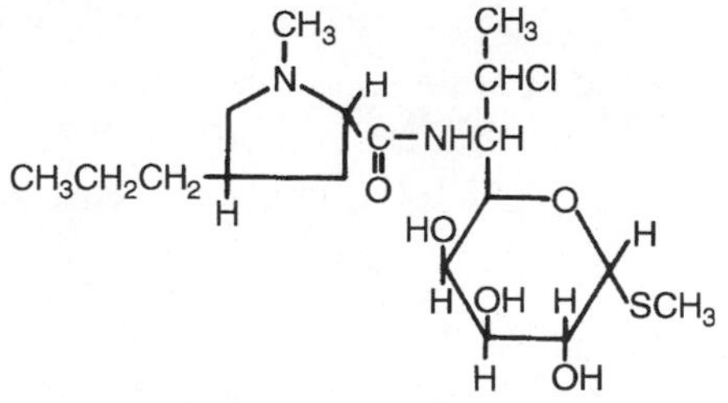

Figure 28-6. Clindamycin.

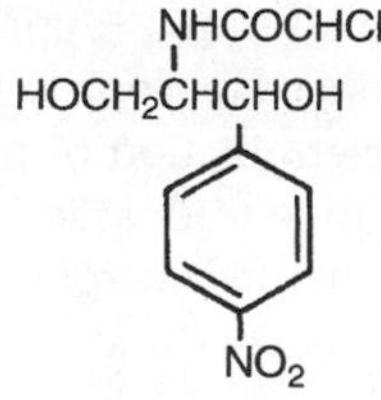

Figure 28-7. Chloramphenicol.

treated by less toxic antimicrobials. Significant diarrhea in patients treated with clindamycin is an indication to discontinue this drug. Clindamycin is indicated in the treatment of serious infections caused by susceptible anaerobes, particularly those originating in the gastrointestinal tract and female genital tract.

Only about 10% of administered clindamycin is excreted in an active form in urine; the remainder is changed into inactive metabolites. In patients with renal dysfunction, the elimination half-time of clindamycin is only slightly prolonged, and little change in dosage is required. In patients with severe liver disease, the dose of clindamycin may need to be decreased.

Side Effects

Clindamycin produces prejunctional and postjunctional effects at the neuromuscular junction, and these effects cannot be readily antagonized with calcium or anticholinesterase drugs. Large doses of clindamycin can induce profound and long-lasting neuromuscular blockade in the absence of nondepolarizing muscle relaxants and after full recovery from the effects of succinylcholine has occurred (Ahdal and Bevan, 1995). Skin rashes occur in about 10% of patients treated with clindamycin.

CHLORAMPHENICOL

Chloramphenicol is unique among antimicrobials in that it contains a nitrobenzene moiety and is a derivative of dichloroacetic acid (Fig. 28-7). Because of the rare occurrence of aplastic anemia (estimated at 1 in 30,000 treated patients), clinical use of chloramphenicol should be limited to serious infections (typhoid fever, salmonellosis) for which alternative antimicrobials may be less effective. An allergic reaction or genetically determined idiosyncratic response to the drug may be responsible for bone marrow depression.

Chloramphenicol is inactivated principally in the liver by glucuronyl transferase. The elimination half-time is 1.5 to 3.5 hours and is prolonged in the presence of liver disease. Over a 24-hour period, 75% to 90% of an orally administered dose of chloramphenicol is excreted in urine. Chloramphenicol can inhibit hepatic microsomal enzymes and prolong the duration of action of drugs such as dicumarol, phenytoin, and tolbutamide. This hepatic microsomal inhibitory effect may protect the liver from toxic effects of known hepatotoxins, such as carbon tetrachloride, by inhibiting metabolism.

VANCOMYCIN

Vancomycin is a bactericidal glycopeptide antimicrobial that impairs cell wall synthesis of Gram-positive bacteria. The oral route of administration is used only for the treatment of staphylococcal enterocolitis and antimicrobial-associated pseudomembranous enterocolitis, taking advantage of the fact that vancomycin is poorly absorbed from the gastrointestinal tract. Vancomycin is administered IV for the treatment of severe staphylococcal infections or streptococcal or enterococcal endocarditis in patients who are allergic to penicillins or cephalosporins. Concomitant administration of an aminoglycoside is often necessary when vancomycin is used in the treatment of enterococcal endocarditis. Vancomycin is the drug of choice in the treatment of infections caused by methicillin-resistant *S. aureus*. Vancomycin can be useful in the therapy of prosthetic heart valve endocarditis caused by *Staphylococcus epidermidis*. In this setting, vancomycin is often administered in combination with gentamicin or rifampin. Vancomycin is also used for prophylaxis against endocarditis in penicillin-allergic patients who have valvular heart disease and are undergoing dental procedures. Likewise, vancomycin is a useful prophylactic antimicrobial in patients undergoing cardiac and orthopedic surgical procedures that involve placement of a prosthetic device (Kaiser, 1986; Dempsey et al., 1988). Vancomycin is used to treat cerebrospinal fluid shunt-related infections due to coagulase-negative staphylococci.

When vancomycin is administered IV, the recommendation is to infuse the calculated dose (10 to 15 mg/kg) over 60 minutes to minimize the occurrence of drug-induced histamine release and hypotension. Infusion over 60 minutes produces sustained plasma concentrations for up to 12 hours. Vancomycin is principally excreted by the kidneys, with 90% of a dose being recovered unchanged in urine. The elimination half-time is approximately 6 hours and may be greatly prolonged (as long as 9 days) in the presence of renal failure. Determination of plasma vancomycin levels is an important guide to dosage (20 to 30 μg/mL is considered ideal) when this antimicrobial must be administered in the presence of renal dysfunction.

Side Effects

Rapid infusion (<30 minutes) of vancomycin has been associated with profound hypotension and even cardiac arrest, though rarely (Lyon and Bruce, 1988; Mayhew and Deutsch, 1985; Southorn et al., 1986; Symons et al., 1985). Hypotension is often accompanied by signs of histamine release characterized by intense facial and truncal erythema ("red man syndrome"). The red man syndrome may occur even with slow infusion of vancomycin and is not always associated with hypotension (Davis et al., 1985). Cardiovascular side effects most likely reflect nonimmunologic histamine release induced by vancomycin (Fig. 28-8) (Levy et al., 1987). Although drug-induced histamine release initially causes increases in myocardial contractility, this effect is promptly followed by venodilation, a sudden decrease in left ventricular filling, and decreased contractility. Histamine produces hypotension in humans by directly dilating peripheral blood vessels. Direct myocardial depression produced by vancomycin does not seem to be important in causing hypotension in humans (Levy et al., 1987). Vancomycin may also produce allergic reactions characterized as anaphylactoid with associated hypotension, erythema, and occasionally bronchospasm (Symons et al., 1985). Plasma tryptase concentrations are not increased following vancomycin-induced anaphylactoid reactions thus permitting a method to distinguish anaphylactic from anaphylactoid reactions (Renz et al, 1998a).

Oral H_1 (diphenhydramine 1 mg/kg) and H_2 (cimetidine 4 mg/kg) receptor antagonists administered 1 hour before induction of anesthesia decreased histamine-related side effects of rapid vancomycin infusion (1 g over 10 minutes) (Renz et al. 1998). In ambulatory anesthesia settings, as for orthopaedic procedures, the time available for vancomycin administration before surgical incision or tourniquet inflation is often limited and may result in inadequate levels of antibiotic in blood and tissues if vancomycin cannot be administered more rapidly than 10 to 15 mg/kg over 60 minutes.

Assertions that anesthesia accentuates vancomycin-induced hypotension are not supported by scientific data. Available data confirm that vancomycin infusion in the presence of anesthesia does not produce adverse hemodynamic responses if the drug is administered over 30 to 60 minutes (von Kaenel et al., 1993). In another report, vancomycin administered over 30 minutes after coronary artery bypass graft surgery was not associated with hemodynamic changes, and there was no correlation between plasma antimicrobial levels and the release of histamine

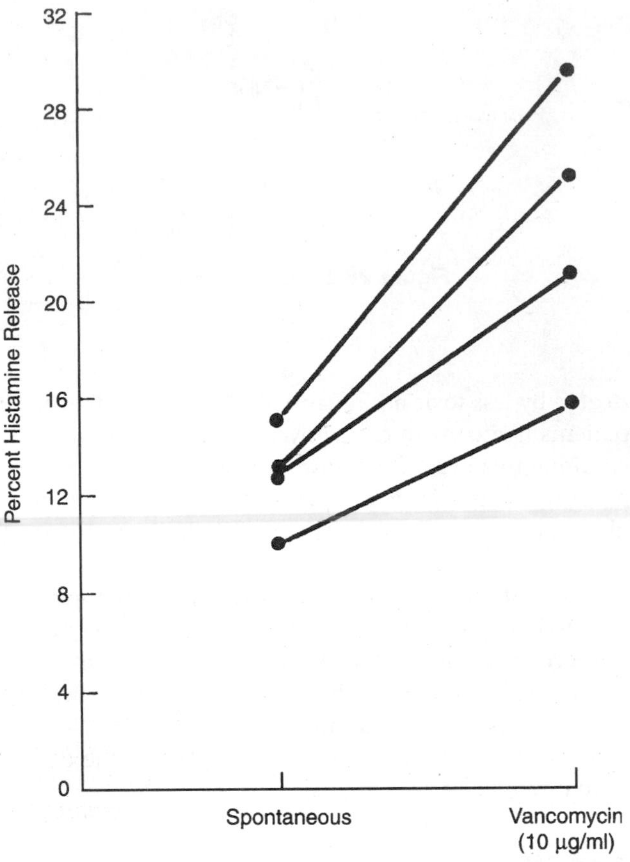

Figure 28-8. Histamine release (%) from dispersed human cutaneous mast cells after the administration of vancomycin. (From Levy JH, Kettlekamp N, Goertz P, et al. Histamine release by vancomycin. A mechanism for hypotension in man. *Anesthesiology* 1987;67:122–125; with permission.)

(Stier et al., 1990). Arterial hypoxemia manifesting as an unexpected decrease in the Spo_2 may occur in association with vancomycin administration, perhaps reflecting drug-induced vasodilation in the lungs leading to an increase in ventilation to perfusion mismatching (Gopalan and Dhandha, 1993). The administration of vancomycin to a patient recovering from succinylcholine-induced neuromuscular blockade has resulted in a return of neuromuscular blockade (Albrecht and Lanier, 1993).

Ototoxicity is likely when persistent high plasma concentrations (>30 μg/mL) are present. The incidence of nephrotoxicity in association with vancomycin treatment is low. Particular attention to ototoxicity and nephrotoxicity is required when vancomycin is administered with an aminoglycoside.

STREPTOGRAMINS

Quinupristin and dalfopristin are two structurally distinct streptogramins that bind to separate sites on the bacterial ribosomal subunit and when combined, act synergistically to inhibit protein synthesis. The principal use for quinupristin-dalfopristin is treatment of vancomycin-resistant infections. This antimicrobial combination is administered IV via a central line to avoid phlebitis. Arthralgias, myalgias, and increased plasma concentrations of bilirubin may accompany treatment. This antimicrobial combination may increase plasma concentrations of drugs (fentanyl) that depend on CYP3A4 for hepatic metabolism.

OXAZOLIDINONES

Linezolid is a synthetic antimicrobial that inhibits protein synthesis by preventing the function of the initiation complex that is required for ribosomal function (Diekema, 2001). Because no other antimicrobial acts in this way, bacteria that have developed resistance to other ribosomally active antimicrobials do not display cross-resistance to linezolid. Linezolid is active against nearly all aerobic Gram-positive cocci including penicillin-resistant pneumococci, methicillin-resistant staphylococci, and vancomycin-resistant enterococci. This antimicrobial is bacteriostatic against staphylococci and enterococci, but it is bacteriocidal against most streptococcal strains.

IV and oral preparations of linezolid are available. The oral preparation is rapidly and completely absorbed. Nonrenal mechanisms account for 65% of the drug's clearance. Patients with mild to moderate renal or hepatic insufficiency do not appear to require decreased doses.

Side Effects

The most common side effects of linezolid are nausea, vomiting, and headache. Reversible bone marrow suppression manifesting as thrombocytopenia, leukopenia, and anemia is a rare side effect. Because linezolid is a reversible inhibitor of monoamine oxidase, patients taking this drug may experience an exaggerated hypertensive response to sympathomimetic drugs. In addition to avoiding decongestants, patients being treated with linezolid should avoid foods (cheeses, soy sauce, and sauerkraut) and beverages (red wine, tap beer) with high tyramine contents. Monoamine oxidase inhibitors and other antidepressants should not be administered to patients receiving linezolid.

POLYMYXIN B AND COLISTIMETHATE

Polymyxin B and colistimethate (polymyxin E) are basic peptides with molecular weights near 1,000 daltons that are effective against Gram-negative bacteria, including *E. coli*, *Klebsiella*, and *P. aeruginosa*. Polymyxin B and colistimethate are used primarily to treat severe urinary tract infections caused by *P. aeruginosa* and other Gram-negative bacteria that are not susceptible to other antimicrobials such as aminoglycosides and carbenicillin. Infections of the skin, mucous membranes, eyes, and ears can be effectively treated with topical application of polymyxin B. *P. aeruginosa* is a common cause of corneal ulcers. These drugs must be administered IM to produce systemic concentrations. Pain after IM injection is common and may follow the distribution of a peripheral nerve. The elimination of these antimicrobials is predominantly by the kidneys, and these drugs accumulate in patients with renal failure.

Side Effects

The polymyxins are the most potent of all the antimicrobials in their actions at the neuromuscular junction. This effect appears to be predominantly prejunctional. Like aminoglycosides, polymyxin B can produce skeletal muscle weakness resembling nondepolarizing neuromuscular blockade, particularly in the presence of high plasma concentrations of drugs as are likely to occur in patients with renal dysfunction. Neostigmine or calcium does not reliably antagonize this drug-induced effect at the neuromuscular junction, which contrasts with the ability of these drugs to reverse aminoglycoside-induced skeletal muscle weakness (Sokoll and Gergis, 1981). This antimicrobial-induced neuromuscular effect may also manifest as marked potentiation of nondepolarizing neuromuscular-blocking drugs.

Nephrotoxicity is a significant risk of treatment with these drugs and alternative antimicrobials are likely to be selected for patients with known renal dysfunction. Polymyxin applied to intact or denuded skin is not absorbed and therefore allergic reactions are unlikely to occur.

BACITRACINS

Bacitracins are a group of polypeptide antibiotics effective against a variety of Gram-positive bacteria. Use of these antimicrobials is limited to topical application in ophthalmologic and dermatologic ointments. Despite a perception that topical application of bacitracin rarely results in allergic reactions there are reports of anaphylactic reactions following bacitracin nasal packing and mediastinal irrigation (Blas et al., 2000; Gail et al., 1999). Established topical uses of bacitracin include treatment of furunculosis, carbuncle, impetigo, suppurative conjunctivitis, and infected corneal ulcer.

SULFONAMIDES

Individual sulfonamides, because of their low cost and efficacy, are used principally to treat uncomplicated urinary tract infections caused by *E. coli* (Fig. 28-9). The emergence of ampicillin-resistant *H. influenzae* is responsible for a return to sulfonamides (in combination with erythromycin or trimethoprim) for treating otitis media in children.

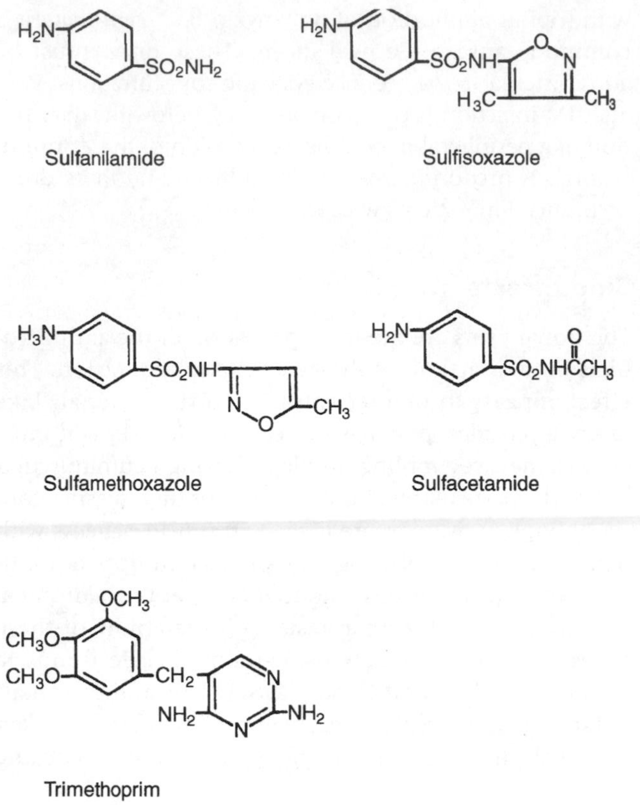

Figure 28-9. Sulfonamides are derivatives of sulfanilamide.

Mechanism of Action

The antimicrobial activity of sulfonamides is due to the ability of these drugs to prevent normal use of paraaminobenzoic acid by bacteria to synthesize folic acid (pteroylglutamic acid). Specifically, sulfonamides act as competitive inhibitors of the bacterial enzyme responsible for the incorporation of paraaminobenzoic acid into the immediate precursor of folic acid. Bacteria that do not require folic acid or normal mammalian cells that can use preformed folic acid absorbed from the gastrointestinal tract are not affected by sulfonamides. The bacteriostatic effects of sulfonamides are countered by paraaminobenzoic acid. For example, ester local anesthetics that are hydrolyzed to paraaminobenzoic acid could theoretically antagonize the antimicrobial effects of sulfonamides.

Pharmacokinetics

Except for sulfonamides that are especially designed for their local effects in the gastrointestinal tract, these antimicrobials are rapidly and extensively absorbed (70% to 100%) primarily from the small intestine. Sulfonamides readily enter pleural, peritoneal, synovial, ocular, and cerebrospinal fluid, reaching concentrations similar to those in the blood. Passage across the placenta is prompt.

Metabolism of sulfonamides is predominantly by acetylation in the liver to pharmacologically inactive compounds. Acetyl metabolites, however, are often less soluble, which increases the likelihood of crystalluria. The magnitude of acetylation varies greatly among the various sulfonamides. Elimination of unchanged and acetylated drug is primarily by glomerular filtration, with renal tubular secretion of variable importance. The elimination half-time depends on renal function.

Side Effects

The side effects that may follow the administration of sulfonamides are numerous and varied. Allergic reactions ranging from skin rash to anaphylaxis are possible with any of the sulfonamides, and cross-sensitivity may or may not occur. Drug fever is a common side effect of sulfonamide treatment. Hepatotoxicity resulting from direct toxicity or sensitization occurs in $<0.1\%$ of patients. Acute hemolytic anemia and agranulocytosis are rare, but possible, adverse effects of treatment with sulfonamides. Formation and deposition of crystalline aggregates in the kidneys and ureter are infrequent with the use of highly soluble sulfonamides. Administration of sulfonamides may increase the effect of oral anticoagulants, methotrexate, sulfonylurea hypoglycemic drugs, and thiazide antidiuretics, probably by displacement of these drugs from binding sites on plasma albumin. Likewise, sulfonamides can compete for the same protein-binding sites as bilirubin, enhancing the risk of jaundice in premature infants. Conversely, indomethacin, probenecid, and salicylates may displace sulfonamides from plasma albumin and increase the concentrations of free drug in the plasma. Hemolytic anemia may occur in patients with glucose-6-phosphate deficiency who receive sulfonamides.

Clinically Useful Sulfonamides

Sulfisoxazole

Sulfisoxazole is a short-acting and highly soluble sulfonamide that has replaced less soluble drugs including sulfadiazine. Oral absorption is rapid and excretion is via the kidneys. Its high water solubility minimizes the hazards of renal toxicity such as crystalluria and hematuria. The usual adult oral dose is 2 to 4 g initially followed by 0.5 to 1.0 g every 4 to 6 hours. Sulfisoxazole is primarily used for treatment of urinary tract infections. In susceptible patients who are allergic to penicillin antimicrobials, sulfisoxazole can be used as prophylaxis against streptococcal infections and recurrences of rheumatic fever.

Sulfamethoxazole

Sulfamethoxazole is an intermediate-acting sulfonamide that is excreted more slowly than sulfisoxazole and requires less frequent administration. Crystalluria is a risk with sulfamethoxazole, and anuria may occur through precipitation of crystals of the acetylated drug in the renal tubules and ureters. Alkalinization of the urine or increased fluid intake is effective in preventing such precipitation.

Sulfasalazine

Sulfasalazine is poorly absorbed from the gastrointestinal tract. For this reason, it is used in the treatment of ulcerative colitis and regional enteritis.

Sulfacetamide

Sulfacetamide is frequently used for topical application as an ointment or solution for treatment of ophthalmic infections. The preparation has a pH of 7.4, is nonirritating, and penetrates into the ocular fluid in high concentrations.

Trimethoprim

Trimethoprim is a pyrimidine analogue that, like sulfonamides, acts to block folic acid synthesis. This drug is well absorbed from the gastrointestinal tract and side effects are uncommon (skin rashes less common than with sulfonamides). Most of the drug is excreted unchanged in the urine. Trimethoprim, 100 mg twice daily, is used for the initial treatment of uncomplicated urinary tract infections.

Trimethoprim-Sulfamethoxazole

Trimethoprim-sulfamethoxazole (cotrimoxazole) combined in a 5:1 ratio results in synergistic antimicrobial action. The antimicrobial activity of this drug combination results from its actions on two sequential steps of the enzymatic pathway for the synthesis of tetrahydrofolic acid. Sulfamethoxazole inhibits the incorporation of paraaminobenzoic acid into folic acid, and trimethoprim prevents the reduction of dihydrofolate to tetrahydrofolate by selectively inhibiting dihydrofolate reductase. The dihydrofolate reductase of the host is far less sensitive to trimethoprim than are the bacterial enzymes, accounting for the selectivity of this drug. Development of resistance to the combination is lower than if either is administered alone. This is predictable, because bacteria that have acquired resistance to one of the components may still be destroyed by the other. Excretion of this drug combination is principally by the kidneys as unchanged drug and metabolites. The antimicrobial spectrum of trimethoprim-sulfamethoxazole includes uncomplicated urinary tract infections caused by organisms other than *E. coli*, prostatitis, acute otitis media, and bronchitis caused by susceptible strains of *H. influenzae* and *S. pneumonia*. It is the treatment of choice for *Pneumocystis carinii* pneumonia and nocardiosis. Treatment with trimethoprim-sulfamethoxazole decreases the incidence of relapses in patients with Wegener granulomatosis (Stegeman et al., 1996).

Side Effects

The most common side effects of this combined preparation are skin rashes, glossitis, and stomatitis. Mild and transient jaundice with histologic features resembling allergic cholestatic hepatitis have been observed. Impairment of renal function may follow administration of this drug combination to patients with renal disease, and a reversible decrease in creatinine clearance has been noted in patients with normal renal function.

There is no evidence that the combination of trimethoprim-sulfamethoxazole induces folate deficiency in normal persons, but the margin between toxicity for bacteria and patients may be narrow when the cells of the patient are already deficient in folate. In this situation, the drug combination may cause or precipitate megaloblastic anemia, leukopenia, or thrombocytopenia. Accordingly, complete blood counts may be recommended for patients who are treated for >2 weeks. Previous or simultaneous administration of diuretics may increase the likelihood of thrombocytopenia, particularly in elderly patients. Patients with AIDS have a high incidence of adverse reactions to this drug combination.

METRONIDAZOLE

Metronidazole is bactericidal against most anaerobic Gram-negative bacilli and *Clostridium* species. If administered orally, the drug is well absorbed and widely distributed in body tissues, including the CNS. As such, this antimicrobial has been useful in treating a variety of CNS, bone and joint infections, abdominal and pelvic sepsis, and endocarditis. Administered orally, metronidazole is useful for treating pseudomembranous colitis. Metronidazole is a useful part of preoperative prophylactic regimens for elective colorectal surgery. For serious anaerobic infections, the drug is administered IV.

Side effects of metronidazole include dry mouth (metallic taste) and nausea. Concurrent ingestion of alcohol may cause a reaction similar to that produced when alcohol is ingested by patients taking disulfiram. Neuropathy and pancreatitis are infrequent.

FLUOROQUINOLONES

The fluoroquinolones are broad-spectrum antimicrobials that are bactericidal against most enteric Gram-negative bacilli (Fig. 28-10) (Hooper and Wolfson, 1991). They are rapidly absorbed from the gastrointestinal tract, and penetration into body fluids and tissues is excellent. Their elimination half-time is prolonged (3 to 8 hours), and the principal route of excretion is via the kidneys, including glomerular filtration and renal tubular secretion. The dose of the fluoroquinolones should be decreased in the presence of renal dysfunction. Side effects are minimal, with mild gastrointestinal disturbances (nausea, vomiting) and CNS disturbances (dizziness, insomnia) occurring in <10% of treated patients. Fluoroquinolones have been

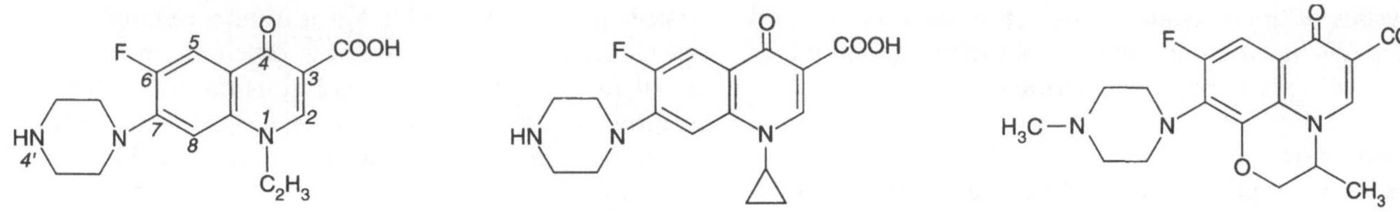

Norfloxacin Ciprofloxacin Ofloxacin

Figure 28-10. Quinolones.

useful clinically in the treatment of genitourinary and gastrointestinal infections, but respiratory tract, soft-tissue, and bone infections have not responded to these drugs. There are several conditions in which these antimicrobials may be preferable to other currently available drugs (Table 28-11) (Hooper and Wolfson, 1991). Fluoroquinolones are bactericidal against most mycobacteria and are useful as part of multidrug regimens (Alangaden and Lerner, 1997).

Norfloxacin

Norfloxacin is highly effective in the treatment of urinary tract infections. A single 800 mg dose is effective for uncomplicated *E. coli* cystitis in women. Although less expensive antimicrobials are available for treatment of uncomplicated urinary tract infections, norfloxacin is especially useful for urinary tract infections caused by resistant organisms such as *P. aeruginosa* and enterococci. Superinfection with resistant Gram-negative organisms is not common, possibly because norfloxacin decreases the aerobic bowel flora but leaves anaerobes intact. The usual dose of norfloxacin is 400 mg every 12 hours. Because food can delay oral absorption, norfloxacin should be administered either 1 hour before or 2 hours after eating, and concurrent use of antacids should be avoided. High fluid intake may help prevent crystalluria.

TABLE 28-11.
CONDITIONS IN WHICH QUINOLONE ANTIMICROBIALS MAY BE THE PREFERRED TREATMENT

Complicated urinary tract infections
Bacterial gastroenteritis
Chronic *Salmonella* carrier state
Respiratory infections related to cystic fibrosis
Osteomyelitis due to Gram-negative bacteria
Invasive external otitis
Mycobacterial infections (as part of multidrug regimens)

Ciprofloxacin

Ciprofloxacin is highly effective in the treatment of urinary and genital tract infections, including prostatitis, and gastrointestinal infections. The major advantage of ciprofloxacin is its greatly enhanced serum concentration and its availability as an IV preparation. Because of high blood levels and good tissue penetration, ciprofloxacin has been useful in the treatment of a variety of systemic infections, including upper and lower respiratory tract infections, skin and soft-tissue infections, and bone and joint infections. Most strains of *M. tuberculosis* are susceptible to ciprofloxacin.

Ofloxacin

Ofloxacin is a tricyclic fluoroquinolone with an antimicrobial spectrum that resembles that of ciprofloxacin but is more active against *Chlamydia*. Absorption from the gastrointestinal tract is excellent, and plasma concentrations are no greater after IV administration. Twice-daily dosing is required for treatment of most susceptible infections.

Lomefloxacin

Lomefloxacin is a difluoroquinolone that resembles other fluoroquinolones, but its longer elimination half-time permits once-daily dosing. A disadvantage of lomefloxacin is its decreased activity against pneumococci and other streptococci.

NITROFURANTOIN

Nitrofurantoin is readily absorbed from the gastrointestinal tract and rapidly excreted such that therapeutic blood levels are not achieved in the blood. The therapeutic utility of this antimicrobial is in the treatment of uncomplicated, mild urinary tract infections. Nausea and vomiting is a common side effect. Chronic active hepatitis is a rare complication. Acute pneumonitis with fever, chills, dyspnea, and chest pain may accompany administration of this drug. Elderly patients are especially susceptible to the pulmonary toxicity of nitrofurantoin. Neuropathies are most likely to occur in patients with impaired renal function.

FOSFOMYCIN

Fosfomycin is a broad-spectrum antibiotic that inhibits cell wall synthesis in *E. coli* and many other common urinary tract pathogens. Diarrhea is the most common side effect. A single dose of fosfomycin is more expensive than a 3-day regimen of comparably effective trimethoprim-sulfamethoxazole or amoxicillin.

DRUGS FOR TREATMENT OF TUBERCULOSIS

Patients with active tuberculosis, in the absence of drug susceptibility data, are treated with daily administration of isoniazid, rifampin, pyrazinamide, and either ethambutol or streptomycin (US Department of Health and Human Services, 1993). After 2 months of such therapy, the regimen for patients with drug-sensitive organisms should be changed to isoniazid and rifampin administered daily or two or three times weekly for an additional 4 months or until sputum cultures are negative for 3 months. Patients with pulmonary tuberculosis who have positive sputum cultures should be treated in an isolation environment until three consecutive sputum samples collected on separate days are negative. As little as 2 weeks of antituberculous chemotherapy greatly decreases the infectiveness of pulmonary tuberculosis, although a few mycobacteria may persist in the sputum cultures. Patients with extrapulmonary tuberculosis are less infectious but prolonged chemotherapy for 6 months with multiple drugs is necessary.

Treatment of HIV-Infected Patients

Human immunodeficiency virus (HIV)-infected patients who do not require antiretroviral therapy can receive standard antituberculous chemotherapy. Although HIV-infected patients respond well to antituberculous therapy, treatment is complicated by drug interactions (US Department of Health and Human Services, 2000). Because rifamycins induce hepatic cytochrome CYP450 enzymes, they decrease plasma concentrations of protease inhibitors and nonnucleoside reverse transcriptase inhibitors. Rifampin is the most potent CYP450 enzyme inducer, followed by rifapentine and rifabutin. Conversely, protease inhibitors are potent CYP450 inhibitors (ritonavir more than saquinavir) and can result in toxic plasma concentrations of rifamycin. Because rifampin is contraindicated in patients receiving protease inhibitors or nonnucleoside reverse transcriptase inhibitors, antituberculous regimens must be modified in the presence of antiretroviral therapy.

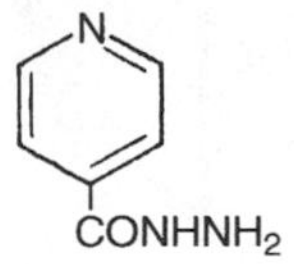

Figure 28-11. Isoniazid.

Antituberculous Drugs

Isoniazid

Isoniazid is the hydrazide of isonicotinic acid and is considered the primary drug for the chemotherapy of tuberculosis (Fig. 28-11). This antimicrobial is the only medication proved efficacious for the prevention of tuberculosis. A congener of isoniazid is the isopropyl derivative, which markedly inhibits the multiplication of the tubercle bacillus and is a potent inhibitor of monoamine oxidase. Isoniazid is both tuberculostatic and tuberculocidal. Resistance during therapy can occur, presumably because of the emergence of strains that do not take up the drug (Gold and Moellering, 1996). Cross-resistance, however, between isoniazid and other tuberculostatic drugs does not occur. The mechanism of action of isoniazid is not known but may reflect drug-induced inhibition of synthesis of mycolic acids, which are important constituents of the mycobacterial cell wall.

Excretion

Isoniazid is readily absorbed when administered orally or parenterally. The drug diffuses into all body fluids and cells. Up to 95% of a dose of isoniazid is excreted in urine over 24 hours, entirely as metabolites. The primary route of metabolism is by hepatic acetylation to acetylisoniazid. There is a genetic determination of the rate of isoniazid acetylation, with patients being categorized as slow or rapid acetylators. Rapid acetylation is inherited as an autosomal dominant trait. Rapid acetylators are homozygous. The average concentration of active isoniazid in the plasma of rapid acetylators is 30 to 50 times less than that present in the plasma of slow acetylators. The elimination half-time of isoniazid averages approximately 1.5 hours in rapid acetylators and 3 hours in patients who are slow acetylators.

The clearance of isoniazid depends only to a small degree on the status of renal function, but patients who are slow acetylators may be susceptible to accumulation of toxic concentrations if renal function is impaired.

Side Effects

The side effects due to isoniazid can be minimized by prophylactic therapy with pyridoxine and careful surveillance of the patient. For example, pyridoxine, 10 mg daily, is administered with isoniazid to minimize the occurrence of

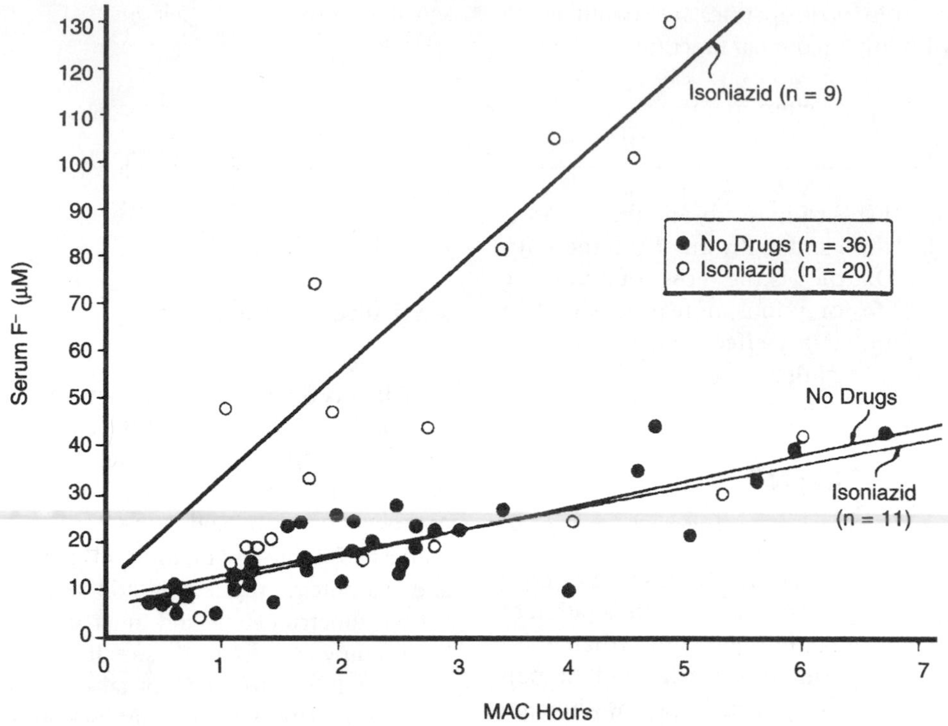

Figure 28-12. Peak serum fluoride after enflurane. Isoniazid enhances defluorination of enflurane in patients who are rapid acetylators. (From Mazze RI, Woodruff RE, Heerdt ME. Isoniazid-induced enflurane defluorination in humans. *Anesthesiology* 1982;57:5–8; with permission.)

peripheral neuropathy and anemia. The protective effect of pyridoxine is because isoniazid increases the excretion of pyridoxine, resulting in a deficiency of this vitamin. Isoniazid may precipitate seizures in patients with epilepsy and, rarely, in patients with no prior history of seizures. Optic neuritis has occurred during therapy with this drug. Mental changes during treatment with isoniazid include euphoria, impairment of memory, and occasionally psychoses. Excessive sedation may occur in slow acetylators and in patients given isoniazid who are also receiving phenytoin, reflecting isoniazid-induced inhibition of anticonvulsant metabolism.

Severe hepatic injury characterized microscopically by bridging and multilobular necrosis (similar to the changes associated with halothane hepatitis) can occur (Garibaldi et al., 1972). The mechanism for hepatotoxicity is not known, although a metabolite of isoniazid, acetylisoniazid, is a known hepatotoxin. Rapid acetylators who produce more acetylisoniazid may be more vulnerable to isoniazid-induced hepatotoxicity than those who are characterized as slow acetylators. Age seems to be an important determinant in the incidence of isoniazid-induced hepatic dysfunction, with an incidence of 0.3% in patients 20 to 34 years old, 1.2% in patients 35 to 49 years old, and 2.3% in patients 50 years old or older. An estimated 10% to 20% of patients treated with isoniazid manifest increased plasma transaminase enzyme levels. A greater than threefold increase in the serum glutamic-oxalacetic transaminase activity is cause for discontinuation of isoniazid.

Isoniazid treatment significantly increases defluorination of volatile anesthetics, presumably by inducing the necessary hepatic microsomal enzymes (Mazze et al., 1982). After enflurane anesthesia, the magnitude of increase in plasma fluoride concentrations in isoniazid-treated patients is variable, presumably reflecting different levels of enzyme induction among rapid and slow acetylators (Fig. 28-12) (Mazze et al., 1982). Plasma fluoride concentrations could reach levels, especially in rapid acetylators, that have been previously associated with nephrotoxicity. Isoniazid interacts with a variety of drugs resulting in increased plasma concentrations of phenytoin, carbamazepine, primidone, and barbiturates and decreased plasma concentrations of ketoconazole (Self et al., 1999). Prednisolone decreases the plasma concentrations of isoniazid.

Rifampin

Rifampin is a complex macrocyclic antimicrobial that inhibits growth of most Gram-positive bacteria as well as many Gram-negative bacteria. Rifampin is bacteriocidal for most mycobacteria and its fat solubility results in penetrations of tissues, including the CNS. This antimicrobial is the drug of choice for prophylaxis against meningococcal disease in household contacts of patients with such infections. Resistance to the antimicrobial effects of rifampin develops rapidly (within 40 hours), emphasizing that this drug must not be used alone in the chemotherapy of tuberculosis. Rifampin is effective because of its ability to inhibit RNA synthesis in bacteria at concentrations far below those that produce this effect in normal cells.

Route of Administration

Oral absorption of rifampin is adequate, but often highly variable. Salicylates may delay absorption and prevent achievement of therapeutic plasma concentrations. Rifampin penetrates tissues and body fluids, including cerebrospinal fluid, imparting a red color to the urine and saliva of patients treated with this drug. An IV preparation of rifampin is also available.

Excretion

Rifampin undergoes hepatic deacetylation, and the resulting metabolite, which has antibacterial activity similar to that of the parent compound, enters bile where enterohepatic circulation occurs. The elimination half-time of rifampin varies from 1.5 to 5.0 hours and is prolonged in patients with hepatic dysfunction. Modification in dosage is not required in patients with renal insufficiency but may be necessary in patients with hepatic insufficiency.

Side Effects

The side effects of rifampin are infrequent but with high doses may include thrombocytopenia, anemia, hepatitis with jaundice, and occasionally hepatorenal syndrome. Hepatitis accompanied by increases in plasma concentrations of liver transaminase enzymes may occur. Hepatic dysfunction rarely occurs in patients with normal hepatic function; it is more likely to occur in elderly patients with preexisting liver disease, especially that related to alcohol abuse.

Rifampin is a potent inducer of hepatic CYP450 oxidative enzymes resulting in accelerated metabolism of many drugs (opioids, warfarin, oral contraceptives, glucocorticoids). Methadone metabolism is accelerated by rifampin, and the likelihood of an opioid withdrawal syndrome may be increased. Accelerated metabolism of oral anticoagulants and contraceptives may jeopardize the reliability of these drugs. CNS and peripheral nervous system effects associated with rifampin administration include fatigue, generalized numbness, skeletal muscle weakness, and pain in the extremities. Biliary excretion of rifampin competes with that of contrast media used for the radiographic study of the gallbladder. Thyroxine clearance is accelerated and rifampin-induced hypothyroidism can occur.

Rifabutin

Rifabutin is structurally and pharmacologically similar to rifampin and possesses a similar antituberculous spectrum. Because it is a much less potent inducer of hepatic cytochrome CYP450, rifabutin is recommended in place of rifampin in the antituberculous treatment of HIV-infected patients receiving antiretroviral therapy.

Rifapentine

Rifapentine is a long-acting analogue of rifampin that has a spectrum of activity and potential toxicities that resemble rifampin. Because of its longer elimination half-time, rifapentine may be administered twice a week during the induction phase of antituberculous chemotherapy and once a week during the continuation phase.

Pyrazinamide

Pyrazinamide is a derivative of nicotinic acid that exhibits bactericidal activity against mycobacteria. It is well absorbed from the gastrointestinal tract and is widely distributed in tissues including the CNS. Excretion of pyrazinamide includes both hepatic and renal mechanisms. Side effects of pyrazinamide include rash, arthralgia, abdominal distress, hyperuricemia, and hepatitis.

Ethambutol

Ethambutol is tuberculostatic to mycobacteria, probably by impairing incorporation of mycolic acids into the cell walls. This drug is useful in combination with isoniazid for the treatment of active tuberculosis as it readily penetrates tissues including the CNS. Absorption after oral administration approaches 85% of the drug.

Excretion

Approximately 50% of an ingested dose of ethambutol is excreted unchanged by the kidneys in 24 hours. The high renal clearance of this drug confirms that excretion is by renal tubular secretion as well as by glomerular filtration. Dosage must be modified when this drug is administered to patients with renal insufficiency. The elimination half-time is 3 to 4 hours. Accumulation of ethambutol is likely in patients with renal dysfunction.

Side Effects

The most important side effect of therapy with ethambutol is optic neuritis, resulting in decreased visual acuity and loss of ability to perceive the color green. The incidence of this complication is dose-related, occurring in approximately 5% of patients treated with 25 mg/kg daily and in $<1\%$ of patients receiving daily doses of <15 mg/kg. There is decreased renal excretion of uric acid, resulting in increased blood concentrations of urate in approximately 50% of patients.

ANTIFUNGAL DRUGS

Nystatin

Nystatin is a polyene antimicrobial that is both fungistatic and fungicidal but lacks effects on bacteria. This drug increases the permeability of the membranes of sensitive fungi such that small molecules escape. Absorption of nystatin via the skin, mucous membranes, or gastrointestinal tract is negligible. Nystatin is used primarily to treat *Candida* infections and is available as oral tablets, vaginal tablets, and ointments. Paronychia, vaginitis, and stomatitis (thrush) caused by *Candida* organisms usually respond to topical therapy. Oral, esophageal, and gastric *Candida* infections are common in patients receiving immunosuppressive therapy and certain antimicrobials such as the tetracyclines. These infections usually respond to oral nystatin. Side effects are rare. For example, allergic reactions have not been reported. Because nystatin has no effect on bacteria, superinfections do not occur.

Amphotericin B

Amphotericin B, like nystatin, is a polyene antimicrobial that exerts maximal antifungal effects between a pH of 6.0 and 7.5. This is the most effective antifungal drug for managing infections due to yeasts and fungi. Cryptococcal infection of the lungs or meninges, histoplasmosis, coccidioidomycosis, blastomycosis, sporotrichosis, and disseminated candidiasis are treated with amphotericin B.

Oral absorption is poor, accounting for the need to administer amphotericin B IV if therapeutic concentrations in infected tissues are to be achieved. The drug does not penetrate into cerebrospinal fluid or vitreous humor. Intrathecal injection may be necessary for treatment of *Coccidioides* meningitis. Renal excretion is slow, with detectable drug being present for up to 8 weeks after discontinuation of therapy.

Side Effects

Side effects are common with the use of amphotericin B. For example, renal function is impaired in >80% of treated patients, and some permanent decrease in glomerular filtration rate is likely. During therapy, plasma creatinine concentrations should be monitored, and the dose of amphotericin B should be decreased when plasma creatinine concentrations are >3.5 mg/dL. Hypokalemia and hypomagnesemia may occur. Fever, chills, dyspnea, and hypotension are common during infusion of amphotericin B. Allergic reactions, seizures, anemia, and thrombocytopenia may occur. Hepatotoxicity is not documented as a side effect of treatment with amphotericin B.

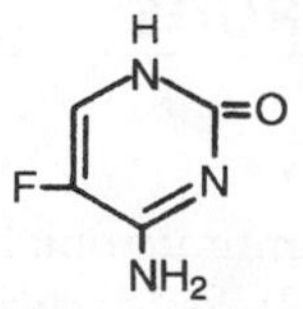

Figure 28-13. Flucytosine.

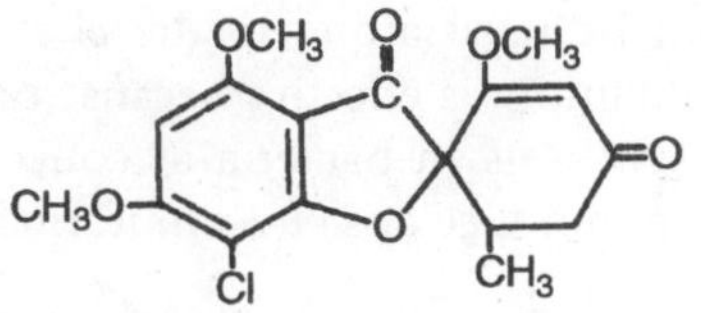

Figure 28-14. Griseofulvin.

Flucytosine

Flucytosine is converted to fluorouracil exclusively in fungal cells by the enzyme cytosine deaminase (Fig. 28-13). This selective effect avoids the cytotoxicity of fluorouracil on normal cells. The drug is well absorbed from the gastrointestinal tract. Penetration into the cerebrospinal fluid and aqueous humor is excellent. Approximately 80% of flucytosine is excreted unchanged in urine by glomerular filtration. The elimination half-time is 3 to 6 hours, but this is greatly prolonged in the presence of renal failure. In approximately 5% of patients, liver transaminase enzymes are increased and hepatomegaly occurs.

Flucytosine is available only for oral administration. It is used predominantly in combination with amphotericin B, because rapid emergence of resistant strains limits the use of flucytosine as a single drug.

Griseofulvin

Griseofulvin inhibits mitosis in certain fungi, accounting for its fungistatic effects, especially in dermatophytes (Fig. 28-14). Mycotic diseases of the skin, hair, and nails respond to griseofulvin. Symptomatic relief of skin infections usually occurs in 48 to 96 hours. There is no effect of this drug on bacteria.

Oral absorption of griseofulvin is adequate but highly variable. Approximately 50% of an oral dose appears in the urine, mostly in the form of metabolites. The drug has greater affinity for cells of diseased skin than of normal skin, accounting for the prompt appearance of new growth of hair or nails.

Headache, which may be severe, occurs in as many as 15% of treated patients. Other nervous system manifestations include peripheral neuritis, fatigue, blurred vision, and syncope. Hepatotoxicity has been observed in patients being treated with griseofulvin. Renal effects of griseofulvin include proteinuria without evidence of renal insufficiency. Griseofulvin appears to decrease the activity of warfarin-like anticoagulants.

ANTIVIRAL DRUGS

The development of antiviral drugs has been hampered by the fact that viruses, in contrast to bacteria, are obligate

TABLE 28-12.
CLASSIFICATION OF VIRUSES AND ASSOCIATED DISEASES

RNA viruses
Picornaviruses: poliomyelitis, encephalitis, common cold
Reoviruses: diarrhea
Togaviruses: encephalitis, rubella
Orthomyxoviruses: influenza
Paramyxoviruses: croup, bronchitis, mumps, measles
Retroviruses: acquired immunodeficiency syndrome, leukemia
DNA viruses
Papovaviruses: warts
Adenoviruses: acute respiratory distress, keratitis
Herpesviruses: cold sores, keratitis, genital lesions, varicella, shingles, cytomegalic inclusion disease, infectious mononucleosis

intracellular parasites that use many of the biochemical mechanisms of the host's cells. Therefore, it is difficult to achieve antiviral activity without also affecting some aspect of normal host cell metabolism and thus causing toxic effects in uninfected host cells. Nevertheless, some host cell surface receptors and enzymes are unique for viruses, providing a mechanism for the development of antiviral drugs with selective activity. Vaccines such as those available for prevention of hepatitis A and B are alternatives to antiviral drugs (Lemon and Thomas, 1996).

Viruses are composed of a nucleic acid core surrounded by a protein-containing outer coat. The viral genome contains either RNA or DNA but never both, and viruses are classified on this basis (Table 28-12) (Melnick, 1980).

Idoxuridine

Idoxuridine is a halogenated pyrimidine that resembles thymidine. After phosphorylation in the cells, the triphosphate derivative is incorporated into both viral and mammalian DNA. As such, the antiviral activity of idoxuridine is mainly limited to DNA viruses, usually of the herpes simplex group. The principal clinical use of this drug is topical treatment of herpes simplex keratitis lesions of the skin, conjunctiva, and mucous membranes. Rapid inactivation of nucleotidases precludes its use by routes other than IV or topical administration. After IV injection, most of the drug disappears from the blood in approximately 30 minutes.

Amantadine

Amantadine is a synthetic tricyclic amine antiviral drug that inhibits replication of strains of influenza A virus. It has no clinical activity against influenza B viruses. Amantadine is almost completely absorbed after oral administration, with 90% of the dose appearing unchanged in urine. Amantadine has prophylactic value when administered to persons who have had contact with an active case of influenza A virus. Approximately 70% of treated patients exposed to influenza A are protected. This drug also has some therapeutic value in the management of patients with Parkinson disease (see Chapter 31).

Amantadine accumulates in patients with impaired renal function. Excessive plasma concentrations are associated with CNS toxicity, including seizures and coma.

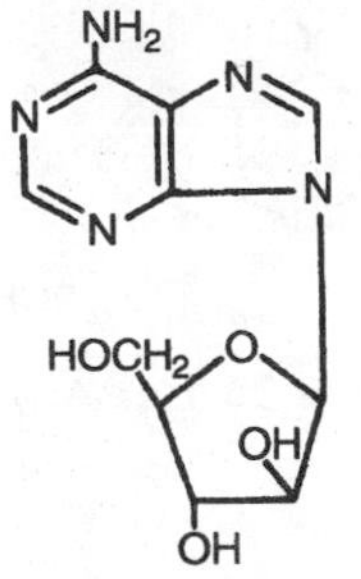

Figure 28-15. Vidarabine.

Vidarabine

Vidarabine is an analogue of adenosine that is effective in the treatment of herpes simplex encephalitis and keratoconjunctivitis (Fig. 28-15) (Whitley et al., 1986). Severe infections with herpes simplex virus in neonates may also respond to vidarabine. This drug is ineffective in the management of patients with varicella, cytomegalic inclusion disease, and recurrent or primary genital herpes. Vidarabine acts by inhibiting viral DNA polymerase, whereas DNA synthesis in noninfected cells is inhibited less. Because vidarabine is poorly soluble in aqueous solutions, large volumes of water (2.5 liters) are needed to dissolve the drug for infusion and treatment of encephalitis. Topical ointment is used for treatment of conjunctivitis. Vidarabine may be both mutagenic and carcinogenic.

Zanamivir

Zanamivir is a sialic acid analogue that acts as a potent inhibitor of influenza virus neuraminidase. This enzyme, essential for replication, cleaves terminal sialic acid residues from glycoconjugates to allow the release of virus from infected cells, prevent the aggregation of virus, and possibly decrease viral inactivation by respiratory mucus. Intranasal or inhaled delivery of zanamivir decreases peak viral titers and the frequency of febrile illness associated with influenza A or B virus infections (Hayden et al., 1997).

Acyclovir

Acyclovir has an antiviral spectrum that is limited to herpes viruses (Fig. 28-16). This drug is administered topically or orally and is effective in the initial and recurrent treatment

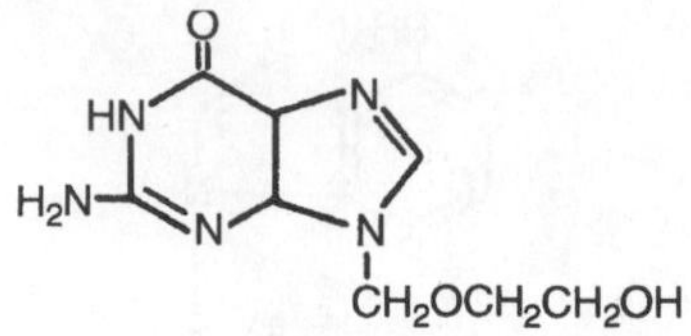

Figure 28-16. Acyclovir.

of genital herpes. IV or oral administration of acyclovir will decrease the duration of viral shedding, decrease pain, and accelerate healing of herpes zoster in immunosuppressed patients. There is no apparent effect, however, on the incidence of postherpetic neuralgia. Patients with chronic fatigue syndrome and persisting antibodies to Epstein-Barr virus fail to experience a beneficial response when treated with acyclovir (Straus et al., 1988).

After IV administration, acyclovir is widely distributed in tissues and body fluids, attaining concentrations in cerebrospinal fluid that are approximately 50% of those in plasma. Excretion of acyclovir is by glomerular filtration and renal tubular secretion, principally of unchanged drug. The elimination half-time of acyclovir is approximately 2.5 hours in the presence of normal renal function.

Increases in blood urea nitrogen and plasma creatinine concentrations have occurred after rapid IV administration of acyclovir. This may reflect crystallization of acyclovir in renal tubules. Thrombophlebitis may occur at the site of IV administration. A frequent nonspecific complaint in patients treated with acyclovir is headache.

Famciclovir

Famciclovir is administered orally for the management of acute herpes zoster. Penciclovir is the active metabolite of famciclovir that results from the actions of the enzyme aldehyde oxidase. No changes in penciclovir pharmacokinetics occur in patients pretreated with cimetidine. The most frequent side effects of treatment with famciclovir are headache, nausea, and fatigue.

Ganciclovir

Ganciclovir is a nucleoside analogue of guanosine, a homologue of acyclovir, and the first antiviral drug effective in the treatment of cytomegalovirus (CMV) disease in humans (Fig. 28-17) (Crumpacker, 1996). In vivo, ganciclovir is converted to ganciclovir triphosphate, which inhibits viral DNA polymerases of CMV by competitively inhibiting the incorporation of deoxyguanosine triphosphate into elongating viral DNA. This drug eliminates CMV excretion in body fluids within 8 days in most patients. Its efficacy in improving vision in patients with CMV retinitis can be preserved by oral maintenance therapy. In patients with AIDS, prolonged oral treatment also decreases excretion of CMV in urine and appears to be effective in preventing CMV disease. Ganciclovir is effective prophylaxis against and therapy for CMV pneumonia in bone marrow transplant recipients.

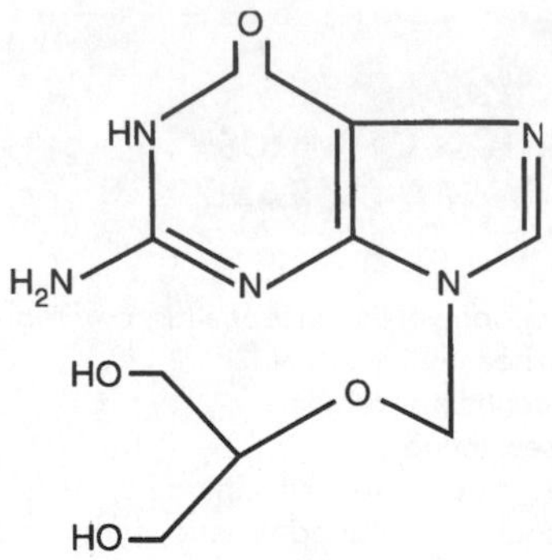

Figure 28-17. Ganciclovir.

Ganciclovir causes granulocytopenia, thrombocytopenia, azoospermia, and an increase in plasma creatinine concentrations. Anemia may also develop with prolonged treatment. Granulocytopenia due to ganciclovir can be prevented by concomitant administration of recombinant granulocyte colony–stimulating factor or granulocyte–macrophage colony–stimulating factor. Azoospermia is due to direct inhibition of sperm-producing cells. The combination of ganciclovir with other drugs that are toxic to bone marrow, such as zidovudine, may result in exaggerated hematologic toxicity, necessitating a decrease in the dose of ganciclovir.

Interferon

Interferon is a general term used to designate glycoproteins produced in response to viral infection. Binding of interferons by specific receptors on cell membranes is the first step in establishing their antiviral effect, which may include degradation of viral RNA. In addition to having antiviral effects, interferons inhibit cell proliferation and enhance tumoricidal activities of macrophages. The immune suppressant effects of volatile anesthetics on natural killer cell function may be attenuated or prevented by prior treatment with interferons (Markovic et al., 1993). Interferon alfa-2b is effective in the treatment of chronic hepatitis B.

Interferons produced by recombinant DNA techniques in bacteria are effective when administered as a nasal spray against rhinovirus infections (Hayden et al., 1986). Treatment with interferons may be associated with influenza-like symptoms (fever, headache, malaise, myalgia, arthralgia), hematologic toxicity (granulocytopenia, leukopenia, thrombocytopenia), neurologic signs (decreased mental concentration, depression, irritability), and immune system disorders (development of autoantibodies, thyroid disease). Nasal irritation may accompany intranasal administration.

Lamivudine

Lamivudine is a nucleoside analogue of interferon that inhibits DNA synthesis and is effective in the treatment of chronic hepatitis B. Surprisingly, the combination of interferon and lamivudine is no more effective than either drug alone. Discontinuation of lamivudine has been associated with return of the hepatitis B virus. Lamivudine therapy may serve as a bridge to liver transplantation for a patient with decompensated cirrhosis while awaiting a donor liver.

Antiretroviral Drugs Effective in the Management of Patients with AIDS

Antiretroviral therapy for AIDS includes nucleoside reverse transcriptase inhibitors (NTRIs), nonnucleoside reverse transcriptase inhibitors (NNRTIs), and protease inhibitors (Table 28-13) (Fauci et al., 2001). The NRTIs structurally resemble the human nucleosides that HIV uses to make viral DNA. The HIV reverse transcriptase enzyme can mistakenly incorporate the synthetic nucleoside analogue into the viral DNA during the reverse transcriptase process and once incorporated into viral DNA, the nucleoside analogues act as chain terminators because they lack the hydroxyl group needed for chain elongation. The NNTRIs do not act as chain terminators but rather directly inhibit the proper functioning of the reverse transcriptase enzyme. The HIV protease inhibitors selectively bind to HIV protease and prevent this enzyme from performing its normal function of cleaving viral polyprotein precursors into individual functional proteins. Successful inhibition of HIV protease causes the formation of deformed HIV particles that are unlikely to replicate.

Antiretroviral regimes that have infrequent dosing schedules, minimal meal restrictions, and the least possible adverse effects are desirable. NRTIs and NNRTIs can be taken without regard to food consumption whereas dosing schedules and food restriction are more complicated with the protease inhibitors. Pharmacologic boosting of protease inhibitor levels is achieved by combining a low dose of ritonavir with another protease inhibitor (saquinavir or lopinavir) also at a decreased dosage.

Initiation of Therapy

Antiretroviral therapy is recommended for patients with acute HIV syndrome, those in whom HIV infection has been diagnosed with 6 months of seroconversion, and those with severe HIV-related symptoms or AIDS. Therapy consists of a potent regimen that includes a combination of three or more drugs that most typically includes (1) two NRTIs plus a protease inhibitor, (2) two NRTIs plus a NNRTI, or (3) two NRTIs plus two protease inhibitors.

Side Effects

Potential adverse side effects can greatly influence the choice of antiretroviral medications (Table 28-13) (Carr

TABLE 28-13. ANTIRETROVIRAL DRUGS USED IN TREATMENT OF HIV

Drug	Side Effects
Nucleoside Reverse Transcriptase Inhibitors	
Abacavir (ABC)	Hypersensitivity reactions (may be fatal) Lactic acidosis (rare)
Didanosine (ddl)	Peripheral neuropathy Pancreatitis Nausea Lactic acidosis (rare)
Lamivudine (3TC)	Lactic acidosis (rare)
Stavudine (d4T)	Peripheral neuropathy Lactic acidosis (rare)
Zalcitabine (ddC)	Peripheral neuropathy Stomatitis Lactic acidosis (rare)
Zidovudine (AZT)	Anemia Neutropenia Gastrointestinal irritation Headache Lactic acidosis (rare)
Nonnucleoside Reverse Transcriptase Inhibitors	
Delavirdine	Rash Increased plasma transaminase concentrations Headache
Efavirenz	Rash Confusion, agitation
Nevirapine	Rash Increased plasma transaminase concentrations (hepatitis can be fatal)
Protease Inhibitors	
Amprenavir	Gastrointestinal irritation Lipid abnormalities Perioral paraesthesias Lipodystrophy
Indinavir	Gastrointestinal irritation Nephrolithiasis Increased indirect serum bilirubin concentrations Headache Lipid abnormalities Lipodystrophy
Lopinavir + ritonavir	Gastrointestinal irritation Lipid abnormalities (including hypertriglyceridemia) Lipodystrophy
Nelfinavir	Diarrhea Lipid abnormalities Lipodystrophy
Ritonavir	Gastrointestinal irritation Perioral paresthesias Taste perversions Hepatitis Lipid abnormalities (including hypertriglyceridemia) Lipodystrophy
Saquinavir	Gastrointestinal irritation Headache Lipid abnormalities Lipodystrophy

and Cooper, 2000). Possible acute life-threatening reactions include didanosine-induced pancreatitis, abacavir-related hypersensitivity syndrome, lactic acidosis secondary to the use of any of the NRTIs, Stevens-Johnson syndrome secondary to the use of any of the NNRTIs, and nevirapine-associated hepatotoxicity. Pancreatitis associated with didanosine can occur without warning and at any time during therapy.

Hypersensitivity

Abacavir hypersensitivity syndrome (fever, rash, nausea, oral lesions, cough) occurs in approximately 2% to 3% of patients typically developing in the first 3 to 4 weeks of therapy. Patients who begin to develop the hypersensitivity syndrome and then stop taking abacavir can have an acute and potentially fatal reaction on resuming abacavir.

Lactic Acidosis

Increased serum lactate concentrations result from NRTIs binding to human mitochondrial DNA polymerase gamma. Serum lactate concentrations are mildly elevated (2 to 5 mmol/liter and serum bicarbonate concentration decreased (<20 mmol/liter) in 10% to 20% of patients receiving antiretroviral therapy. Symptoms associated with increased serum lactate concentrations are vague and may include nausea, abdominal pain, malaise, and anorexia. Life-threatening hyperlactatemia (>5 mmol/liter) occurs in 1% to 2% of treated patients and mortality is approximately 80% in those with serum lactate concentrations >10 mmol/liter.

Increased Insulin Resistance

Protease-inhibitor antiretroviral treatment is associated with insulin resistance but plasma glucose concentrations are generally not increased. Nevertheless, up to 25% of patients will exhibit abnormal glucose tolerance testing.

Hypercholesterolemia

Protease-inhibitor antiretroviral treatment is associated with increases in total serum cholesterol and low-density lipoproteins. In addition, ritonavir has been associated with increases in plasma triglyceride concentrations. It is unclear if these changes predispose treated patients to cardiovascular disease. Among the lipid-lowering statin drugs, pravastatin has the least severe drug interactions with other protease inhibitors and is often used to treat increased plasma cholesterol concentrations. Patients with severe hypertrigly-ceridemia may require treatment with gemfibrozil.

Lipodystrophy

Lipodystrophy (fat redistribution syndrome) is the most problematic long-term complication of antiretroviral treatment. This syndrome typically presents as either central fat distribution (abdomen, breasts, neck) or as peripheral fat wasting (face, buttocks, limbs). Insulin resistance is likely to be important in the etiology of this lipodystrophy. Indeed, the insulin-sensitizing drug metformin may be effective in decreasing central fat distribution (Hadigan, 2000). NRTIs may be associated with lipoatrophy.

Monitoring Treatment

The HIV RNA level is checked before antiretroviral treatment is initiated and then every 4 weeks until the level drops to <50 copies/mL (usually within 16 to 20 weeks). Subsequently, the HIV RNA and $CD4^+$T cell counts are measured about every 3 months. Suppressing HIV levels to <50 copies/mL diminishes the chances that resistant strains will emerge. Measuring $CD4^+$T cells counts reflects the impact of antiretroviral therapy on immune function. The hope that antiretroviral therapy would completely eradicate HIV is not realistic, although treatment does greatly decrease the viral burden. Cellular ($CD4^+$T cells) and anatomic (CNS, male urogenital tract) reservoirs of HIV make it impossible to completely eradicate the infection with antiretroviral treatment. Overall, patient adherence to antiretroviral therapy parallels the likelihood of long-term viral suppression (Paterson et al, 2000).

Drug Interactions

Most of the protease inhibitors are also inhibitors of the cytochrome P-450 (CYP) 3A4 enzymes that are responsible for the metabolism of several drugs thus increasing the risk of pharmocokinetic drug interactions. Among HIV protease inhibitors, ritonavir is the most potent inhibitor of CYP3A4 and CYP2D6. For this reason, ritonavir is expected to produce large increases in the plasma concentration of drugs metabolized by the CYP3A isoform. These drugs include analgesics (fentanyl), lidocaine, antimicrobials, anticonvulsants, anticoagulants, antiemetics (ondansetron), calcium-channel blockers, corticosteroids, and neuroleptics (droperidol, perphenazine) (Olkkola et al., 1999). Although not contraindicated, these drugs should be used with caution in patients being treated with ritonavir. Decreased bioavailability of nonsteroidal antiinflammatory drugs, phenytoin, and oral hypoglycemics may accompany treatment with ritonavir.

Zidovudine

Zidovudine (AZT) has established efficacy in a variety of HIV-1–associated conditions. Beginning zidovudine therapy early in the treatment of AIDS delays the progression of the disease, as manifested by the delayed onset of opportunistic infections, neurologic disease, and tumors. Transmission of HIV from the mother to infant is impaired by zidovudine (Wilfert, 1996). Zidovudine is well absorbed after oral administration. It undergoes glucuronidation during the first pass through the liver, diffuses across cellular membranes, and is converted to the active triphosphate by a series of cellular enzymes. After glucuronidation in the liver, zidovudine is primarily eliminated by the kidneys. An estimated 15% to 20% of the drug is excreted unchanged by the kidneys. Probenecid inhibits both hepatic glucuronidation and renal excretion, thus decreasing total body clearance of zidovudine by an estimated 65%. Other drugs that undergo hepatic glucuronidation and may therefore interfere with the metabolism of zidovudine include nonsteroidal antiinflammatory drugs and opioids (Yarchoan et al., 1989).

Didanosine

Didanosine is a purine dideoxynucleoside that acts as a prodrug for the active intracellular moiety dideoxyadenosine triphosphate. Although the elimination half-time is brief (0.5 hour), the intracellular half-time is prolonged (>12 hours), allowing twice-daily dosing regimens.

Zalcitabine

Zalcitabine is most often administered in combination with zidovudine. Like zidovudine and didanosine, zalcitabine requires intracellular activation to an active triphosphate for activity.

Protease Inhibitors

HIV-1 protease inhibitors are useful in the treatment of individuals with HIV infection (Deeks et al., 1997). HIV-1 protease activity is critical for the terminal maturation of infectious virions. In the presence of HIV-1 protease inhibitors, these infectious virions are unable to mature. As a result, the viral load is greatly decreased and the CD4$^+$T counts increase especially if these drugs are combined with reverse transcriptase inhibitors. Development of protease inhibitors reflects the use of computer modeling to identify compounds that would fit into the substrate-binding pockets of protease enzyme. The development of resistance and the subsequent loss of drug activity is the primary barrier to long-term use of HIV-1 protease inhibitors.

REFERENCES

Adkinson NF. Immunogenicity and cross-allergenicity of aztreonam. *Am J Med* 1990;88:12S–15S.

Ahdal OA, Bevan DR. Clindamycin-induced neuromuscular blockade. *Can J Anaesth* 1995;42:614–617.

Alangaden GJ, Lerner SA. The clinical use of fluoroquinolones for the treatment of mycobacterial diseases. *Clin Infect Dis* 1997;25: 1213–1218.

Albrecht RF, Lanier WL. Potentiation of succinylcholine-induced phase II block by vancomycin. *Anesth Analg* 1993;77:1300–1302.

Asai T, Murao K, Shingu K. Pre-operative oral erythromycin reduces residual gastric volume and acidity. *Br J Anaesth* 2000;85:861–864.

Blas M, Briesacher K, Lobato E. Bacitracin irrigation: A cause of anaphylaxis in the operating room. *Anesth Analg* 2000;91:1027–1028.

Booij LHDJ, Vander Ploeg GCJ, Crul JF, et al. Do neostigmine and 4-aminopyridine inhibit the antibacterial activity of antibiotics? *Br J Anaesth* 1980;52:1097–1099.

Bruckner J, Thomas KC, Bikhazi GH, et al. Neuromuscular drug interactions of clinical importance. *Anesth Analg* 1980;59:678–682.

Carr A, Cooper DA. Adverse effects of antiretroviral therapy. *Lancet* 2000:356:1423–1428.

Classen DC, Evans RS, Pestotnik SL, et al. The timing of prophylactic administration of antibiotics and the risk of surgical-wound infection. *N Engl J Med* 1992;326:281–286.

Crumpacker CS. Ganciclovir. *N Engl J Med* 1996;335:721–729.

Cunha BA. Antibiotic side effects. *Med Clin North Am* 2001;85:149–163.

Davis RL, Smith AL, Koup JR. The "red-man's syndrome" and slow infusion of vancomycin. *N Engl J Med* 1985;313:756–757.

Deeks SG, Smith M, Holodniy M, Kahn JO. HIV-1 protease inhibitors. A review for clinicians. *JAMA* 1997;277:145–153.

Dempsey R, Rapp RP, Young B, et al. Prophylactic parenteral antibiotics in clean neurosurgical procedures: a review. *J Neurosurg* 1988;69:52–57.

Diekema DJ, Jones RN. Oxazolidinone antibiotics. *Lancet* 2001;358: 77–78.

Fauci AS, Bartlett J, Goosby E, et al. Guidelines for the Use of Antiretroviral Agents in HIV-Infected Adults and Adolescents. Department of Health and Human Services and the Henry J. Kaiser Family foundation, San Francisco, 2000 (www.hivatis.org).

Gail R, Blakley B, Warrington R, et al. Intraoperative anaphylactic shock from bacitracin nasal packing after septorhinoplasty. *Anesthesiology* 1999;91:1545–1547.

Garibaldi RA, Drusin RE, Ferebeen SH, et al. Isoniazid-associated hepatitis. Report of an outbreak. *Am Rev Respir Dis* 1972;106: 357–365.

Gholson CF, Warren GH. Fulminant hepatic failure associated with intravenous erythromycin lactobionate. *Arch Intern Med* 1990; 150:215–219.

Gold HS, Moellering RC. Antimicrobial-drug resistance. *N Engl J Med* 1996;335:1445–1453.

Gonzales R, Steiner JF, Sande MA. Antibiotic prescribing for adults with colds, upper respiratory tract infections, and bronchitis by ambulatory care physicians. *JAMA* 1997;278:901–904.

Gopalan K, Dhandha SK. Hypoxia following perioperative administration of vancomycin. *Anesth Analg* 1993;76:200–201.

Hadigan C, Corcoran C, Basgoz N, et al. Metformin in the treatment of HIV lipodystrophy syndrome: A randomized controlled trial. *JAMA* 2000;284:472–476.

Hayden FG, Albrecht JK, Kaiser DL, et al. Prevention of natural colds of contact prophylaxis with intranasal alpha$_2$ interferon. *N Engl J Med* 1986:314:71–75.

Hayden FG, Osterhaus ADME, Treanor JJ, et al. Efficacy and safety of the neuraminidase inhibitor zanamivir in the treatment of influenzavirus infections. *N Engl J Med* 1997;33:874–880.

Hooper DC, Wolfson JS. Fluoroquinolone antimicrobial agents. *N Engl J Med* 1991;324:384–394.

Iseman MD. Treatment of multidrug-resistant tuberculosis. *N Engl J Med* 1993;329:784–791.

Kaiser AB. Antimicrobial prophylaxis in surgery. *N Engl J Med* 1986; 315:1129–1138.

Kelkar PS, Li JT. Cephalosporin allergy. *N Engl J Med* 2001;345: 804–808.

Kopp VJ, Mayer DC, Shaheen NJ. Intravenous erythromycin promotes gastric emptying prior to emergency anesthesia. *Anesthesiology* 1997; 87:703–705.

Lemon SM, Thomas DL. Vaccines to prevent viral hepatitis. *N Engl J Med* 1997;336:196–204.

Levy JH, Kettlekamp N, Goertz P, et al. Histamine release by vancomycin. A mechanism for hypotension in man. *Anesthesiology* 1987;67:122–125.

Lin HC, Sanders SL, Gu YG et al. Erythromycin accelerates solid emptying at the expense of gastric sieving. *Dig Dis Sci* 1994;39: 124–128.

Lyon GD, Bruce DL. Diphenhydramine reversal of vancomycin-induced hypotension. *Anesth Analg* 1988;67:1109–1110.

Markovic SN, Knight PR, Murasko DM. Inhibition of interferon stimulation of natural killer cell activity in mice anesthetized with halothane or isoflurane. *Anesthesiology* 1993;60:700–706.

Mayhew JF, Deutsch S. Cardiac arrest following administration of vancomycin. *Can Anaesth Soc J* 1985;32:65–66.

Mazze RI, Woodruff RE, Heerdt ME. Isoniazid-induced enflurane defluorination in humans. *Anesthesiology* 1982;57:5–8.

Melnick JL. Taxonomy of viruses, 1980. *Prog Med Virol* 1980;26:214–232.

Olkkola KT, Palkama VJ, Neuvonen PJ. Ritonavir's role in reducing fentanyl clearance and prolonging it half-life. *Anesthesiology* 1999; 91:681–685.

Pallasch TJ. Principles of pharmacotherapy: III. drug allergy. *Anesth Prog* 1988;35:178–189.

Paterson DL, Swindells S, Mohr J, et al. Adherence to protease inhibitor therapy and outcomes in patients with HIV infection. *Ann Intern Med* 2000;133:21–26.

Pilot MA. Macrolides in roles beyond antibiotic therapy. *Br J Surg* 1994; 81:1423–1429.

Renz CL, Laroche D, Thurn JD, et al. Tryptase levels are not increased during vancomycin-induced anaphylactoid reactions. *Anesthesiology* 1998;89:620–625.

Renz CL, Thurn JD, Finn HA, et al. Oral antihistamines reduce the side effects from rapid vancomycin infusion. *Anesth Analg* 1998a;87: 681–685.

Self TH, Chrisman CR, Baciewicz AM, et al. Isoniazid drug and food interactions. *Am J Med Sci* 1999;317:304–309.

Sokoll MD, Gergis SD. Antibiotics and neuromuscular function. *Anesthesiology* 1981;55:148–159.

Southorn PA, Plevak DJ, Wilson WR. Adverse effects of vancomycin administered in the perioperative period. *Mayo Clin Proc* 1986;61: 721–724.

Stegeman CA, Cohen Tervaert JWC, de Jong PE, Kallenberg CG. Trimethoprim-sulfamethoxazole (co-trimoxazole) for the prevention of relapses of Wegener's granulomatosis. *N Engl J Med* 1996; 335:16–20.

Stier GR, McGory RW, Spotnitz WD, et al. Hemodynamic effects of rapid vancomycin infusion in critically ill patients. *Anesth Analg* 1990;71:394–399.

Straus SE, Dale JK, Tobi M, et al. Acyclovir treatment of the chronic fatigue syndrome of efficacy in a placebo-controlled trial. *N Engl J Med* 1988;319:1692–1698.

Symons NLP, Hobbes AFT, Leaver HK. Anaphylactoid reactions to vancomycin. *Can Anaesth Soc J* 1985;32:65–66.

Vogt AW, Zollo RA. Long Q-T syndrome associated with oral erythromycin used in preoperative bowel preparation. *Anesth Analg* 1997;85:1011–1013.

US Department of Health and Human Services. Initial therapy for tuberculosis in the era of multidrug resistance: Recommendations of the Advisory Council for the Elimination of Tuberculosis. *MMWR Morb Mortal Wkly Rep* 1993;42:1–7.

US Department of Health and Human Services. Updated guidelines of the use of rifabutin or rifampin for the treatment and prevention of tuberculosis among HIV-infected patients taking protease inhibitors or nonnucleoside reverse transcriptase inhibitors. *MMWR Morb Mortal Wkly Rep* 2000;40:185–190

von Kaenel WE, Bloomfield EL, Amaranath L, Wilde AA. Vancomycin does not enhance hypotension under anesthesia. *Anesth Analg* 1993;76:809–811.

Whitley RJ, Alford C, Hirsch MS, et al. Vidarabine versus acyclovir therapy in herpes simplex encephalitis. *N Engl J Med* 1986;314: 144–149.

Wenzel RP, Edmond MB. The evolving technology of venous access. *N Engl J Med* 1999;340:48–50.

Wilfert CM. Beginning to make progress against HIV. *N Engl J Med* 1996;335:1678–1680.

Yarchoan R, Mitsuya H, Myers CE, Broder S. Clinical pharmacology of 3′-azido-2′,3′-dideoxythymidine (zidovudine) and related dideoxynucleosides. *N Engl J Med* 1989;321:726–738.

Chemotherapeutic Drugs

29

Chemotherapy is the best available therapeutic approach for the eradication of malignant cells that can occur anywhere in the body. The effectiveness of chemotherapy requires that there be complete destruction (total cell-kill) of all cancer cells, because a single surviving clonogenic cell can give rise to sufficient progeny to ultimately kill the host. The recognition for the need of total cell-kill leads to the use of several chemotherapeutic (antineoplastic) drugs concurrently or in a planned sequence. The goal of combination chemotherapy is to administer the largest possible doses of chemotherapeutic drugs, each working by different mechanisms and not sharing similar toxic effects. Using a combination of chemotherapeutic drugs with different mechanisms of action also decreases the chances that drug-resistant tumor cell populations will emerge. Chemotherapeutic drugs used in combination are usually administered over short periods at specific treatment intervals rather than as continuous therapy. This approach is based on the empiric observation that normal cells usually recover more rapidly from a pulse of maximal chemotherapy than do malignant cells. Furthermore, immunosuppression is less with intermittent chemotherapy. With rare exceptions, the optimal dose of chemotherapeutic drugs requires repetitive dosing because even if all cells in a tumor are sensitive to a drug, a single dose of the drug is not sufficient to kill the typically hundreds of millions of cells that are present in patients with cancer.

Malignant cells are often characterized by rapid division and synthesis of deoxyribonucleic acid (DNA). Most chemotherapeutic drugs exert their antineoplastic effects on these cells that are actively undergoing division (mitosis) or DNA synthesis. Slow-growing malignant cells with a slow rate of division, such as in carcinoma of the lung and colon, are often unresponsive to chemotherapeutic drugs. Conversely, rapidly dividing normal cells, as in the bone marrow, gastrointestinal mucosa, skin, and hair follicles, are vulnerable to the toxic effects of chemotherapeutic drugs. It is predictable, therefore, that clinical manifestations of toxicity because of chemotherapeutic drugs may include myelosuppression (leukopenia, thrombocytopenia, or anemia), nausea, vomiting, diarrhea, mucosal ulceration, dermatitis, and alopecia. Often myelosuppression is the dose-limiting factor for chemotherapeutic drugs and is the indication for temporary or permanent withdrawal of therapy. Fortunately, this drug-induced myelosuppression is usually reversible with discontinuation of the chemotherapeutic drug therapy.

DRUG RESISTANCE

Resistance to chemotherapeutic drugs results from induction of drug-metabolizing enzymes in the liver, other tissues or tumor cells. The tenuous blood supply to many tumors prevents therapeutic concentrations from reaching the target, or the chemotherapeutic drugs may find cells that are resistant because of relative hypoxia. Hypoxia causes resistance to both radiation and most chemotherapeutic drugs (exceptions are mitomycins).

Multidrug resistance describes the clinical circumstance in which a tumor is no longer susceptible to several chemotherapeutic drugs. P-glycoprotein spans the plasma membrane and acts to pump chemotherapeutic drugs (anthracyclines, vinca alkaloids, and taxanes but not alkylating drugs, platinating drugs, and antimetabolites) to the extracellular space so an effective intracellular concentration is not reached. In addition to P-glycoprotein, multidrug resistance protein is located on plasma membranes and endoplasmic reticulum and removes drugs from cells (exceptions are taxanes). The breast cancer–resistance protein and mitoxantrone-resistance protein are also involved in resistance to chemotherapeutic drugs.

Topoisomerases are the targets for many chemotherapeutic drugs. Resistance to chemotherapeutic drugs occurs through mutations in the drug-binding domain of the enzyme. Resistance to methotrexate may reflect mutations in the drug target, dihydrofolate reductase. Resistance to alkylating drugs occurs through overexpression of drug-neutralizing substances and metabolizing proteins.

CLASSIFICATION

Chemotherapeutic drugs are classified according to their mechanism of action (Table 29-1) (Rubin and Hait, 2003; Chung, 1982; Selvin, 1981). Knowledge of drug-induced adverse effects and evaluation of appropriate laboratory tests (hemoglobin and platelet count, white blood cell count, coagulation profile, arterial blood gases, blood glucose, plasma electrolytes, liver and renal function tests, electrocardiogram [ECG], and radiograph of the chest) are useful in the preoperative evaluation of patients being treated with chemotherapeutic drugs. Attention to asepsis is essential, because immunosuppression makes these patients susceptible to iatrogenic infections. A history of severe diarrhea may be associated with electrolyte disturbances and decreased intravascular fluid volume. The existence of mucositis makes placement of pharyngeal airways, laryngeal mask airways, and esophageal catheters questionable. The response to inhaled and injected anesthetic drugs may be altered by drug-induced cardiac, hepatic, or renal dysfunction. The response to nondepolarizing neuromuscular-blocking drugs may be altered by impaired renal function. Furthermore, the effects of succinylcholine may be prolonged if plasma cholinesterase activity is decreased by chemotherapeutic drugs.

TOXICITIES

Chemotherapeutic drugs typically target proteins or nucleic acids that are common to malignant and nonmalignant cells and thus possess a narrow therapeutic index. Furthermore, chemotherapeutic drugs are usually administered at maximum tolerated doses. Although toxicities may be unique for specific drugs, many toxicities are shared (nausea and vomiting, myelosuppression, mucositis, alopecia) (Table 29-1) (Rubin and Hait, 2003). Nausea and vomiting result from local gastrointestinal effects as well as activation of the chemoreceptor trigger zone in the central nervous system. Development of serotonin antagonists as effective antiemetics has facilitated the use of emetogenic chemotherapeutic drugs. Mucositis and diarrhea are common gastrointestinal toxicities that reflect the high proliferative rate of gastrointestinal tissues, which makes these tissues more susceptible to the cytotoxic effects of certain chemotherapeutic drugs. Myelosuppression and alopecia reflect similar chemotherapeutic drug effects on highly proliferative tissues. Chemotherapeutic drugs that damage DNA (alkylating drugs, topoisomerases) are associated with secondary malignancies.

DNA ALKYLATING DRUGS

Alkylating drugs include nitrogen mustards, alkyl sulfonates, nitrosoureas, and triazenes. These chemotherapeutic drugs form covalent alkyl bonds with nucleic acid bases, resulting in intrastrand or interstrand DNA cross-links that are toxic to cells undergoing division. By altering the structure of DNA, these drugs inhibit DNA replication and transcription. DNA damage produced by alkylating chemotherapeutic drugs is more likely to kill malignant cells than nonmalignant cells because rates of proliferation are greater for the cancer cells. Acquired resistance to alkylating drugs is a common occurrence, and may reflect decreased cell membrane permeability to the drugs and increased production of nucleophilic substances that can compete with target DNA for alkylation.

Side Effects

Bone marrow suppression is the most important dose-limiting factor in the clinical use of alkylating drugs, especially busulfan. Cessation of mitosis is evident within 6 to 8 hours. Lymphocytopenia is usually present within 24 hours. Variable degrees of depression of platelet and erythrocyte counts may occur. Hemolytic anemia is predictably present.

Treatment with alkylating drugs is often associated with gonadal dysfunction, including oligospermia and amenorrhea. Hemorrhagic cystitis can result from irritation by the acrolein metabolite of cyclophosphamide or ifosfamide. Secondary malignancies may follow treatment with alkylating chemotherapeutic drugs. Gastrointestinal mucosa is sensitive to the effects of alkylating drugs, manifesting as mitotic arrest, cellular hypertrophy, and desquamation of the epithelium. Damage to hair follicles, often leading to alopecia, is a common side effect. Increased skin pigmentation is frequent. All alkylating drugs are powerful central nervous system (CNS) stimulants, manifesting most often as nausea and vomiting. Skeletal muscle weakness and seizures may be present. Pneumonitis and pulmonary fibrosis are potential adverse effects of alkylating drugs. Symptomatic patients may demonstrate a decreased pulmonary diffusing capacity. Inhibition of plasma cholinesterase activity may be responsible for prolonged skeletal muscle paralysis after administration of succinylcholine (Zsigmond and Robins, 1972).

Rapid drug-induced destruction of malignant cells can produce increased purine and pyrimidine breakdown, leading to uric acid nephropathy. To minimize the likelihood of this complication, it is recommended that adequate fluid intake, alkalinization of the urine, and administration of allopurinol be established before drug treatment.

Nitrogen Mustards

The most commonly used nitrogen mustards are mechlorethamine, cyclophosphamide, melphalan, and chlorambucil.

TABLE 29-1.
CLASSIFICATION OF CHEMOTHERAPEUTIC DRUGS AND ASSOCIATED SIDE EFFECTS

Group and *Class*	Therapeutic Uses	Side Effects (Other Than Nausea and Vomiting)
Alkylating Drugs		
Nitrogen Mustards		
Mechlorethamine	Hodgkin disease Non-Hodgkin lymphoma	Myelosuppression Mucositis Alopecia
Cyclophosphamide	Acute lymphocytic leukemia Chronic lymphocytic leukemia Lymphomas Myeloma Neuroblastoma Breast, ovarian, cervical, and testicular cancer Lung cancer Wilms tumor Sarcoma	Myelosuppression Mucositis Alopecia Hemorrhagic cystitis Skin pigmentation Seizures Renal failure Cardiac failure Inappropriate secretion of vasopressin (ADH)
Melphalan	Myeloma Breast cancer	Myelosuppression
Chlorambucil	Hodgkin disease Non-Hodgkin lymphoma Macroglobulinemia	Myelosuppression Secondary leukemias
Ethyleneimine		
Hexamethylmelamine	Ovarian cancer	Myelosuppression
Thiotepa	Bladder, breast and and ovarian cancer	
Alkyl Sulfonates		
Busulfan	Acute myelogenous leukemia Chronic myelogenous leukemia	Myelosuppression Thrombocytopenia
Nitrosoureas		
Carmustine (BCNU)	Hodgkin disease Non-Hodgkin lymphoma Astrocytoma Myeloma Melanoma	Myelosuppression Hepatitis Interstitial pulmonary fibrosis Renal failure Flushing
Lomustine (CCNU)	Hodgkin disease Non-Hodgkin lymphoma Astrocytoma Small cell lung cancer	Myelosuppression
Semustine (methyl-CCNU)	Colon cancer	Myelosuppression
Streptozotocin	Insulinoma Carcinoid tumor	Myelosuppression Hepatitis Renal failure
Triazenes		
Dacarbazine (DTIC)	Hodgkin disease Melanoma Sarcomas	Myelosuppression Flulike syndrome
Temozolomide	Astrocytoma Melanoma	Hepatic toxicity Hyperglycemia Anemia Thrombocytopenia Lymphocytopenia

(Continued)

TABLE 29-1.
(Continued)

Group and *Class*	Therapeutic Uses	Side Effects (Other Than Nausea and Vomiting)
Bioreductive Alkylating Drugs		
Mitomycin-C	Head and neck, breast, lung, gastric, colon, rectal, and cervical cancer	Myelosuppression Mucositis Cardiac failure Interstitial fibrosis Hemolytic-uremic syndrome
Platinating Agents		
Platinum Compounds		
Cisplatin	Head and neck, thyroid, lung, ovarian, endometrial, cervical and testicular cancer Neuroblastoma Osteogenic sarcoma	Myelosuppression Peripheral neuropathy Allergic reactions Renal toxicity Electrolyte abnormalities (hypocalcemia, hypomagnesemia, hypophosphatemia)
Carboplatin	As for Cisplatin	Myelosuppression
Oxaliplatin	Colon cancer	Myelosuppression Peripheral neuropathy
Nucleic Acid Synthetase Inhibitors		
Folate Analogues		
Methotrexate	Head and neck, breast, and lung cancer Acute lymphocytic leukemia Non-Hodgkin lymphoma Osteogenic sarcoma	Myelosuppression Mucositis Pneumonitis Hepatic fibrosis
Pyrimidine Analogues		
Fluorouracil (5-FU)	Head and neck, breast, gastric, pancreatic, bladder, ovarian, cervical, and prostate cancer Hepatoma	Myelosuppression Mucositis Alopecia Pigmentation Chest pain
Cytarabine	Acute lymphocytic leukemia Acute myeloid leukemia Non-Hodgkin lymphoma	Myelosuppression Mucositis Hepatitis
Gemcitabine	Breast, lung, pancreatic, and bladder cancer	Myelosuppression Flulike syndrome
Purine Analogues		
Mercaptopurine	Acute lymphocytic leukemia Acute myeloid leukemia Chronic myeloid leukemia	Myelosuppression Anorexia Jaundice
Thioguanine	As for Mercaptopurine	Myelosuppression Anorexia
Fludarabine	Chronic lymphocytic leukemia Non-Hodgkin lymphoma	Myelosuppression Optic neuritis Peripheral neuropathy Seizures Coma Depletion of CD4 cells
Pentostatin	Chronic lymphocytic leukemia Cutaneous T cell lymphoma Hairy cell leukemia	Myelosuppression Depletion of T cells Hepatitis
Cladribine	Chronic lymphocytic leukemia	Myelosuppression
Cutaneous T cell lymphoma	Tumor lysis syndrome Hairy cell leukemia Waldenstrom macroglobulinemia	Asthenia

TABLE 29-1.
(*Continued*)

Group and *Class*	**Therapeutic Uses**	**Side Effects (Other Than Nausea and Vomiting)**
Hydroxyurea	Chronic myeloid leukemia Polycythemia vera Thrombocytopenia Melanoma	Myelosuppression Dermatologic changes
DNA Topoisomerase Inhibitors		
Anthracyclines		
Doxorubicin	Hodgkin disease Non-Hodgkin lymphoma Acute lymphocytic leukemia Neuroblastoma Thyroid, breast, lung, and gastric cancer	Myelosuppression Cardiomyopathy Mucositis
Daunomycin	Acute myeloid leukemia Acute lymphocytic leukemia	
Idarubicin	As for Daunomycin	
Epirubicin	Hodgkin disease Non-Hodgkin lymphoma Acute lymphocytic leukemia Breast, lung, gastric, and bladder cancer	Myelosuppression Cardiomyopathy Alopecia Phlebitis
Anthracenediones		
Mitoxantrone	Acute myeloid leukemia Breast cancer	Myelosuppression Mucositis
Epipodophyllotoxins		
Etoposide	Hodgkin disease Non-Hodgkin lymphoma Acute myeloid leukemia Kaposi sarcoma Breast, lung, and testicular cancer	Myelosuppression Systemic hypotension Hepatitis Mucositis
Teniposide	Acute lymphocytic leukemia (children) Acute myeloid leukemia (children)	Myelosuppression Systemic hypotension
Dactinomycin	Wilms tumor Rhabdomyosarcoma Choriocarcinoma Kaposi sarcoma Ewing sarcoma Testicular cancer	Myelosuppression Mucositis Cheilitis Glossitis Alopecia Cutaneous erythema
Camptothecins		
Irinotecan	Colon cancer Ovarian cancer	Myelosuppression Alopecia
Topotecan	Lung cancer Ovarian cancer	As for Irinotecan
Other DNA-Damaging Drugs		
Antibiotic		
Bleomycin	Hodgkin disease Non-Hodgkin lymphoma Head and neck cancer Testicular cancer	Interstitial pulmonary fibrosis Allergic reactions Skin pigmentation
Antimicrotubule Drugs		
Vinca Alkaloids		
Vinblastine	Hodgkin disease Non-Hodgkin lymphoma Breast cancer Testicular cancer	Myelosuppression Peripheral neuropathy

(*Continued*)

TABLE 29-1.
(Continued)

Group and *Class*	**Therapeutic Uses**	**Side Effects (Other Than Nausea and Vomiting)**
Vincristine	Hodgkin disease Non-Hodgkin lymphoma Small cell lung cancer Neuroblastoma Wilms tumor Rhabdomyosarcoma Acute lymphocytic leukemia	Myelosuppression Peripheral neuropathy
Vinorelbine	Breast cancer Lung cancer	Myelosuppression Peripheral neuropathy
Taxanes		
Paclitaxel	Breast, lung, bladder, and ovarian cancer	Myelosuppression Peripheral neuropathy Allergic reactions Alopecia totalis
Docetaxel	Breast, lung, bladder, and ovarian cancer	Myelosuppression Peripheral neuropathy Allergic reactions Alopecia totalis Cardiac dysrhythmias Capillary leakage
Signal Transduction Modulators		
Antiestrogens		
Tamoxifen	Breast cancer	Venous thrombosis Weight gain Amenorrhea Hypercalcemia Endometrial cancer Hot flashes
Toremifene	Breast cancer	Venous thrombosis Hot flashes
Raloxifene	Breast cancer	Venous thrombosis Hot flashes
Antiandrogens		
Flutamide	Prostate cancer	Gynecomastia Hot flashes
Bicalutamide	Prostate cancer	Gynecomastia Hot flashes
Nilutamide	Prostate cancer	Gynecomastia Hot flashes Delayed visual adaptation to dark
Monoclonal Antibodies		
Rituximab	Chronic lymphocytic leukemia Non-Hodgkin lymphoma	Infusion-related chills, rash, and fever Noninfusion related myalgias, angioedema, bronchospasm, cardiac dysrhythmias Myelosuppression
Trastuzumab	Breast cancer	Fever and chills
Aromatase Inhibitors		
Aminoglutethimide	Breast cancer	Orthostatic hypotension Glucocorticoid deficiency Cutaneous rash
Anastrazole	Breast cancer	Asthenia Headache Hot flashes
Letrozole	Breast cancer	Headache Heartburn

TABLE 29-1.
(Continued)

Group and *Class*	Therapeutic Uses	Side Effects (Other Than Nausea and Vomiting)
Gonadotropin-Releasing Drugs		
Leuprolide	Breast cancer Prostate cancer	Impotence Hot flashes Pain at sites of bony metastases (tumor flare)
Buserelin	Breast cancer	as for Leuprolide
Progestin		
Megestrol acetate	Breast cancer Prostate cancer Endometrial cancer	Weight gain

Adapted from Rubin EH, Hait WN. Principles of cancer treatment. *Sci Am Med* 2003;12 (IV):1–17.

Mechlorethamine

Mechlorethamine is a rapidly acting nitrogen mustard administered intravenously (IV) to minimize local tissue irritation. This drug must be freshly prepared before each administration. Mechlorethamine and other nitrogen mustards are intensely powerful vesicants, requiring that gloves be worn by personnel handling the drug. A course of therapy with mechlorethamine consists of the injection of a total dose of 0.4 mg/kg. The drug undergoes rapid chemical transformation in tissues such that active drug is no longer present after a few minutes. For this reason, it is possible to prevent tissue toxicity from the drug by isolating the blood supply to that tissue. Alternatively, it is theoretically possible to localize the action of mechlorethamine in a specific tissue by injecting the drug into the arterial blood supply to the tissue.

Clinical Uses

Mechlorethamine produces beneficial effects in the treatment of Hodgkin disease and, less predictably, in other lymphomas. The drug is most often used in combination with vincristine, procarbazine, and prednisone (MOPP regimen) for the treatment of Hodgkin disease.

Side Effects

The major side effects of mechlorethamine include nausea, vomiting, and myelosuppression. Leukopenia and thrombocytopenia constitute the principal limitation on the amount of drug that can be given. Herpes zoster is a type of skin lesion frequently associated with nitrogen mustard therapy. Latent viral infections may be unmasked by treatment with mechlorethamine. Thrombophlebitis is a potential complication, and extravasation of the drug results in severe local tissue reactions, with brawny and tender induration that may persist for prolonged periods.

Cyclophosphamide

Cyclophosphamide is well absorbed after oral administration and is subsequently activated in the liver to aldophosphamide for transport to target tissues. Parenteral administration is also effective. Target cells are able to convert aldophosphamide to highly cytotoxic metabolites, phosphoramide, and acrolein that then alkylate DNA. Maximal plasma concentrations of cyclophosphamide are achieved about 1 hour after oral administration, and the elimination half-time is 6 to 7 hours. Urinary elimination accounts for approximately 14% of this drug in an unchanged form.

Clinical Uses

Cyclophosphamide is one of the most frequently used chemotherapeutic drugs, as it is effective in the treatment of a wide range of cancers and inflammatory diseases. Its versatility is improved because of its effectiveness after oral as well as parenteral administration. Given in combination with other drugs, favorable responses have been shown in patients with Hodgkin disease, lymphosarcoma, Burkitt lymphoma, and acute lymphoblastic leukemia of childhood. Cyclophosphamide is frequently used in combination with methotrexate and fluorouracil as adjuvant therapy after surgery for breast cancer when there is involvement of the axillary nodes. Cyclophosphamide has potent immunosuppressive properties, leading to its use in nonneoplastic disorders associated with altered immune reactivity, including Wegener granulomatosis and rheumatoid arthritis.

Side Effects

Hypersensitivity reactions and fibrosing pneumonitis have been noted in patients treated with cyclophosphamide, although the incidence is $<1\%$, and symptoms may develop months to years after initiation of the drug. Large doses of cyclophosphamide are associated with a high incidence of pericarditis and pericardial effusion, which in some cases has progressed to cardiac tamponade (Gottdiener et al., 1981). Smaller numbers of treated patients develop hemorrhagic myocarditis with symptoms of congestive heart failure, which may not occur for as long as 2 weeks after the last dose of drug.

Cyclophosphamide differs from other nitrogen mustards in that significant degrees of thrombocytopenia are less common but alopecia is more frequent. Nausea and vomiting occur with equal frequency regardless of the route of administration. Mucosal ulcerations, increased skin pigmentation, and hepatotoxicity are possible side effects. Sterile hemorrhagic cystitis occurs in 5% to 10% of patients, presumably reflecting chemical irritation produced by reactive metabolites of cyclophosphamide. Dysuria and hematuria are indications to discontinue the drug. Inappropriate secretion of arginine vasopressin hormone has been observed in patients receiving cyclophosphamide, usually with doses of >50 mg/kg. It is important to consider the possibility of water intoxication because these patients are usually being hydrated to minimize the likelihood that hemorrhagic cystitis will develop. Extravasation of the drug does not produce local reactions, and thrombophlebitis does not complicate IV administration.

Melphalan

Melphalan is a phenylalanine derivative of nitrogen mustard with a range of activity similar to other alkylating drugs. It is not a vesicant. Oral absorption is excellent, resulting in drug concentrations similar to those achieved by the IV route of administration. The elimination half-time is approximately 1.5 hours, and up to 15% of the drug is eliminated unchanged in urine.

Side Effects

The side effects of melphalan are primarily hematologic and are similar to those of other alkylating drugs. It is usually necessary to maintain a significant degree of bone marrow depression (leukocyte count 3,000 to 5,000 cells/mm^3) to achieve optimal therapeutic effects. Pulmonary fibrosis is possible. Nausea and vomiting are not common side effects of melphalan. Alopecia does not occur, and changes in renal or hepatic function have not been reported.

Chlorambucil

Chlorambucil is the aromatic derivative of mechlorethamine. Oral absorption is adequate. The drug has an elimination half-time of approximately 1.5 hours and is almost completely metabolized. Chlorambucil is the slowest-acting nitrogen mustard in clinical use. It is the treatment of choice in chronic lymphocytic leukemia and in primary (Waldenström) macroglobulinemia. A marked increase in the incidence of leukemia and other tumors has been noted with the use of this drug for the treatment of polycythemia vera.

Side Effects

Cytotoxic effects of chlorambucil on the bone marrow, lymphoid organs, and epithelial tissues are similar to those observed with other alkylating drugs. Its myelosuppressive action is usually moderate, gradual, and rapidly reversible. Pulmonary fibrosis is possible. Nausea and vomiting are frequent. CNS stimulation can occur but has been observed only with large doses. Hepatotoxicity may rarely occur.

Alkyl Sulfonates: Busulfan

Busulfan is well absorbed after oral administration. IV administration is also effective. Almost the entire drug is eliminated by the kidneys as methane sulfonic acid. Busulfan produces remissions in up to 90% of patients with chronic myelogenous leukemia. The drug is of no value in the treatment of acute leukemia.

Side Effects

Busulfan can produce progressive pulmonary fibrosis in up to 4% of patients. The prognosis after appearance of clinical symptoms is poor, with a median survival of 5 months (Ginsberg and Comis, 1982). Enhanced toxicity with administration of supplemental oxygen has not been noted. Myelosuppression and thrombocytopenia are important side effects of busulfan. Nausea, vomiting, and diarrhea occur. Hyperuricemia resulting from extensive purine catabolism accompanying the rapid cellular destruction and renal damage from precipitation of urates have been noted. Allopurinol is recommended to minimize renal complications.

Nitrosoureas

Nitrosoureas, represented by carmustine, lomustine, semustine, and streptozocin, possess a wide spectrum of activity for human malignancies including intracranial tumors, melanomas, and gastrointestinal and hematologic malignancies. Indeed, the high lipid solubility results in passage across the blood-brain barrier and efficacy in the treatment of meningeal leukemias and brain tumors. These drugs appear to act by carboxylation and alkylation of nucleic acids. With the exception of streptozocin, the clinical use of nitrosoureas is limited by profound drug-induced myelosuppression.

Carmustine

Carmustine is the nitrosourea in widest clinical use. It is capable of inhibiting synthesis of both RNA and DNA. Although oral absorption is rapid, the drug is injected IV because tissue uptake and metabolism occur quickly. Local burning may accompany infusion. Carmustine disappears from plasma in

5 to 15 minutes. Because of its ability to rapidly cross the blood-brain barrier, carmustine is used to treat meningeal leukemia and primary as well as metastatic brain tumors.

Side Effects

Carmustine has been associated with interstitial pneumonitis and fibrosis much like bleomycin (Weiss et al., 1991). The incidence of pulmonary toxicity is in the range of 20% to 30%, with a mortality in those affected of 24% to 90%. The cumulative dose is the major risk factor, with 50% of patients exhibiting toxicity at doses above the range of 1,200 to 1,500 mg/m^2. A unique side effect of carmustine is a delayed onset (after approximately 6 weeks of treatment) of leukopenia and thrombocytopenia. Active metabolites may be responsible for this toxicity. CNS toxicity, nausea, and vomiting, flushing of the skin and conjunctiva, nephrotoxicity, and hepatotoxicity have been reported.

Lomustine and Semustine

Lomustine and its methylated analogue semustine possess similar clinical toxicity to carmustine, including delayed bone marrow depression manifesting as leukopenia and thrombocytopenia. Lomustine appears to be more effective than carmustine in the treatment of Hodgkin disease.

Streptozocin

Streptozocin has a methylnitrosourea moiety attached to the number 2 carbon atom of glucose. It has a unique affinity for beta cells of the islets of Langerhans and has proved useful in the treatment of human pancreatic islet cell carcinoma and malignant carcinoid. In animals, the drug is used to produce experimental diabetes mellitus.

Side Effects

Approximately 70% of patients receiving this drug develop hepatic or renal toxicity. Renal toxicity may manifest as tubular damage and progress to renal failure and death. Hyperglycemia can occur as a result of selective destruction of pancreatic beta cells and resultant hypoinsulinism (Selvin, 1981). Myelosuppression is not produced by this drug.

Mitomycin

Mitomycin inhibits synthesis of DNA and is of value in the palliative treatment of gastric adenocarcinoma in combination with fluorouracil and doxorubicin. The drug is administered IV and is widely distributed in tissues but does not readily enter the CNS. Metabolism is in the liver, with <10% of mitomycin excreted unchanged in bile or urine.

Side Effects

Myelosuppression is a prominent side effect of mitomycin and is characterized by severe leukopenia and thrombocytopenia, which may be delayed in appearance. Mitomycin is capable of inducing pulmonary fibrosis, with an incidence ranging between 3% and 12% (Gunstream et al., 1983). Like bleomycin, mitomycin appears to act synergistically with thoracic radiation and oxygen therapy, suggesting the need to limit exposure of treated patients to hyperoxia. Nausea, vomiting, gastrointestinal mucositis, and alopecia are recognized toxic effects. Glomerular damage resulting in renal failure is a rare but well-recognized complication.

PLATINATING DRUGS

Cisplatin

Cisplatin contains a platinum atom, two amines, and two chlorides that results in chemotherapeutic effects resembling DNA alkylating drugs by cross-linking adjacent or opposing guanine bases to disrupt DNA. The drug must be administered IV because oral ingestion is ineffective. High concentrations of cisplatin are found in the kidneys, liver, intestines, and testes, but there is poor penetration into the CNS. Cisplatin and its analogue carboplatin are components of the treatment of many nonhematologic malignanceis, including lung, bladder, testicular, and ovarian cancer.

Side Effects

Renal toxicity is prominent and becomes the dose-limiting toxic effect of cisplatin. Decreased glomerular filtration rate and renal tubular dysfunction produced by cisplatin may begin as early as 3 to 5 days after initiating treatment with this drug. Along with increasing blood urea nitrogen and plasma creatinine concentrations, proteinuria, and hyperuricemia, there is a magnesium-wasting defect in as many as 50% of patients manifesting as some degree of cisplatin-induced renal dysfunction. Acute tubular necrosis may progress to acute renal failure, necessitating hemodialysis. Hydration and diuresis induced with mannitol and furosemide may protect against the development of renal toxicity by dilution of the tubular urinary concentration of cisplatin. The hypomagnesemia that is associated with cisplatin's renal tubular injury may predispose to cardiac dysrhythmias and decrease the dose requirements for neuromuscular-blocking drugs.

Ototoxicity caused by cisplatin is manifested by tinnitus and hearing loss in the high-frequency range. Marked nausea and vomiting occur in almost all patients. Mild to moderate myelosuppression may develop, with transient leukopenia and thrombocytopenia. Peripheral sensory neuropathies, paresthesias, and loss of vibratory and position sense are common findings. Most neuropathies are reversible, although symptoms may persist for months. Hyperuricemia, seizures, and cardiac dysrhythmias have been observed. Allergic reactions characterized by facial edema, bronchoconstriction, tachycardia, and hypotension may occur minutes after injection of the drug.

NUCLEIC ACID SYNTHESIS INHIBITORS

Nucleic acid synthesis inhibitors (antimetabolites) include folate analogues, pyrimidine analogues, and purine analogues. These drugs are particularly effective in destroying cells during the S phase of the cell cycle, which is when DNA is synthesized. Selective effects on cancer cells may relate to greater rates of DNA replication in cancer cells than normal cells. Nevertheless, side effects (myelosuppression and mucositis) reflect effects on proliferating but nonmalignant cells.

Folate Analogues

Methotrexate

Methotrexate is a poorly lipid-soluble folate analogue that is effective in the treatment of different hematologic and nonhematologic cancers and is classified as an antimetabolite (folic acid antagonist). This drug inhibits dihydrofolate reductase, which is the enzyme that uses reduced folate as a methyl donor in the synthesis of pyrimidine and purine nucleosides. Inhibition of dihydrofolate reductase by methotrexate prevents the formation of tetrahydrofolic acid and causes disruption of cellular metabolism by producing an acute intracellular deficiency of folate enzymes. As a result, 1-carbon transfer reactions necessary for the eventual synthesis of DNA and RNA cease.

Methotrexate is readily absorbed after oral administration. Significant metabolism of methotrexate does not seem to occur, with more than 50% of the drug appearing unchanged in urine. Renal excretion reflects glomerular filtration and tubular secretion. Toxic concentrations of methotrexate may occur in patients with renal insufficiency. Methotrexate remains in tissues for weeks, suggesting binding of the drug to dihydrofolate reductase.

Clinical Uses

Methotrexate is widely used in the treatment of malignant and some nonmalignant disorders. It is a useful drug in the treatment of acute lymphoblastic leukemia in children but not adults. Choriocarcinoma is effectively treated with this drug. Improvement in the clinical manifestations of psoriasis in patients reflects the effect of methotrexate on rapidly dividing epidermal cells characteristic of this disease. This drug may also be useful in the treatment of rheumatoid arthritis.

Methotrexate is poorly transported across the blood-brain barrier, and neoplastic cells that have entered the CNS probably are not affected by the usual plasma concentrations of the drug. Intrathecal injection is used to treat cerebral involvement with either leukemia or choriocarcinoma.

Acquired resistance to methotrexate develops as a result of (a) impaired transport of methotrexate into cells, (b) production of altered forms of dihydrofolate reductase that have decreased affinity for the drug, and (c) increased concentrations of intracellular dihydrofolate reductase.

Side Effects

The most important side effects of methotrexate occur in the gastrointestinal tract and bone marrow. Leukopenia and thrombocytopenia reflect bone marrow depression. Ulcerative stomatitis and diarrhea are frequent side effects and require interruption of treatment. Hemorrhagic enteritis and death from intestinal perforation may occur. Pulmonary toxicity may take the form of fulminant noncardiogenic edema, or a more progressive inflammation, with interstitial infiltrates and pleural effusions (White et al., 1984). The incidence of pulmonary toxicity attributed to methotrexate is in the range of 8%, but its frequent use in combination with other chemotherapeutic drugs makes this number uncertain (Cooper et al., 1986). Methotrexate is associated with renal toxicity, with an incidence approaching 10% in higher doses (Chabner et al., 1982). Renal insufficiency may be prevented by hydration and urinary alkalinization. Short-term or intermittent therapy with methotrexate results in increases in liver transaminase enzymes. Hepatic dysfunction is usually reversible but may sometimes lead to cirrhosis. It may be useful to measure liver function tests preoperatively in patients who have recently received methotrexate. Encephalopathic syndromes may accompany intrathecal or IV administration of methotrexate and may be transient or permanent (Kaplan and Wienik, 1982). Alopecia and dermatitis may accompany administration of methotrexate. Folic acid antagonists also interfere with embryogenesis, emphasizing the risk in administering these drugs to pregnant patients. Normal cells can be protected from lethal damage by folate antagonists with concomitant administration of leucovorin, thymidine, or both. This approach has been termed the *rescue technique*.

Pyrimidine Analogues

Pyrimidine analogues have in common the ability to prevent the biosynthesis of pyrimidine nucleotides or to mimic these natural metabolites to such an extent that they interfere with vital cellular activities such as the synthesis and functioning of nucleic acids. Examples of antimetabolite chemotherapeutic drugs that function as pyrimidine analogues are fluorouracil and cytarabine.

Fluorouracil

Fluorouracil blocks production of thymine nucleotides by inhibiting thymidylate synthase. This chemotherapeutic drug lacks significant inhibitory activity on cells and must be converted enzymatically to a 5′-monophosphate nucleotide. Administration of fluorouracil is usually by IV injection, because absorption after oral ingestion is unpredictable and incomplete. Metabolic degradation occurs primarily in the liver, with an important metabolite being urea. Only approximately 10% of fluorouracil appears unchanged in urine. Fluorouracil readily enters the cerebrospinal fluid, with therapeutic concentrations being present within 30 minutes after IV administration.

Clinical Uses

Fluorouracil may be of palliative value in certain types of carcinoma, particularly of the breast and gastrointestinal tract. The drug is often used for the topical treatment of premalignant keratoses of the skin and superficial basal cell carcinomas.

Side Effects

Side effects caused by fluorouracil are difficult to anticipate because of their delayed appearance. Fluorouracil-induced myocardial ischemia is a rare cardiac toxicity that may lead to myocardial infarction up to 1 week after treatment (Labianca et al., 1982). The incidence of this side effect is low in patients without underlying heart disease but may increase to 4.5% of treated patients with preexisting coronary artery disease. Stomatitis manifesting as a white patchy membrane that ulcerates and becomes necrotic is an early sign of toxicity and warns of the possibility that similar lesions may be developing in the esophagus and gastrointestinal tract. Myelosuppression, most frequently manifesting as leukopenia between 9 and 14 days of therapy, is a serious side effect. Thrombocytopenia and anemia may complicate treatment with fluorouracil. Loss of hair progressing to total alopecia, nail changes, dermatitis, and increased pigmentation and atrophy of the skin may occur. Neurologic manifestations, including an acute cerebellar syndrome (ataxia), have been reported.

Cepecitabine

Cepecitabine is an orally administerd drug that is metabolized to fluorouracil by thymidine phosphorylase after absorption from the gastrointestinal tract. Because there is more activity of thymidine phosphorylase in cancer cells (especially breast cancer) than in normal cells, cepecitabine has the potential to be more selective than fluorouracil.

Pemetrexed

Pemetrexed is a folate antagonist that is effective in the treatment of mesothelioma and lung cancer. This drug inhibits multiple enzymes involved in the folate pathway, including thymidylate synthase and dihydrofolate reductase.

Cytarabine

Cytarabine (cytosine arabinoside), like other pyrimidine antimetabolites, must be activated by conversion to the 5′-monophosphate nucleotide before inhibition of DNA synthesis can occur. Both natural and acquired resistance to cytarabine develop, reflecting the activity of cytidine deaminase, an enzyme capable of converting cytarabine to the inactive metabolite arabinosyl uracil.

Clinical Uses

In addition to its chemotherapeutic activity, particularly in acute leukemia in children and adults, cytarabine has potent immunosuppressive properties. The drug is particularly useful in chemotherapy of acute granulocytic leukemia in adults. IV administration of cytarabine is recommended, because oral absorption is poor and unpredictable.

Side Effects

Cytarabine is a potent myelosuppressive drug capable of producing severe leukopenia, thrombocytopenia, and anemia. Other side effects include gastrointestinal disturbances, stomatitis, and hepatic dysfunction. Thrombophlebitis at the site of infusion is common. Alternatively, the drug may be given subcutaneously.

Gemcitabine

Gemcitabine resembles cytarabine structurally but yet gemcitabine is active in several nonhematologic cancers, whereas cytarbine is not effective. This most likely reflects unique effects of this chemotherapeutic drug on DNA and RNA metabolism.

Purine Analogues

Antimetabolite chemotherapeutic drugs that function as purine analogues include mercaptopurine, azathioprine, thioguanine, pentostatin (2′-deoxycoformycin), and cladribine (2-chlorodeoxyadenosine). Mercaptopurine and thioguanine are analogues of the natural purines hypoxanthine and guanine, respectively.

Mercaptopurine

Mercaptopurine is incorporated into DNA or RNA strands and either blocks further strand synthesis or causes structural alterations that damage DNA. This drug is useful in the treatment of acute leukemia in children. Oral absorption is prompt, and gastrointestinal epithelium is not damaged. The elimination half-time is brief (about 90 minutes) due to rapid tissue uptake, renal excretion, and hepatic metabolism. One pathway of metabolism is methylation and subsequent oxidation of the methylated derivatives. A second pathway involves the enzyme xanthine oxidase, which oxidizes mercaptopurine to 6-thiouric acid. Allopurinol, as an inhibitor of xanthine oxidase, prevents conversion of mercaptopurine to 6-thiouric acid and thus increases the exposure of cells to mercaptopurine. The dose of mercaptopurine is decreased by about one-third when the drug is combined with allopurinol.

Side Effects

The principal side effect of mercaptopurine is a gradual development of bone marrow depression manifesting as thrombocytopenia, granulocytopenia, or anemia several weeks after initiation of therapy. Anorexia, nausea, and vomiting are common side effects; stomatitis and diarrhea rarely occur. Jaundice occurs in approximately one-third of patients and is associated with bile stasis and occasional hepatic necrosis. Hyperuricemia and hyperuricosuria may occur during treatment with mercaptopurine, presumably reflecting destruction of cells. This effect may require the use of allopurinol.

Thioguanine

Thioguanine is of particular value in the treatment of acute granulocytic leukemia, especially if given with cytarabine. After oral administration, thioguanine appears in the urine as a methylated metabolite and inorganic sulfate. Minimal amounts of 6-thiouric acid are formed, suggesting that deamination is not important in the metabolic inactivation of thioguanine. For this reason, thioguanine may be administered concurrently with allopurinol without a decrease in dosage, unlike mercaptopurine. Toxic manifestations of thioguanine treatment include bone marrow depression and, occasionally, gastrointestinal effects.

Pentostatin and Cladribine

Pentostatin and cladribine are purine analogues that have clinical activity against a variety of indolent lymphoid tumors, with the most dramatic effects occurring in patients with hairy-cell leukemia (Saven and Piro, 1994). These drugs act by irreversibly binding to adenosine deaminase (pentostatin) or by chemical modification of enzyme substrate, rendering it resistant to the action of adenosine deaminase (cladribine). Patients with acute leukemia and cells with high levels of adenosine deaminase activity are most likely to respond to these drugs. Fever, which is likely due to cytokines, is a side effect of treatment with cladribine. Both drugs are capable of producing immunosuppression. The recovery from immunosuppression seems to be more rapid after treatment with cladribine than after treatment with pentostatin, perhaps because of the shorter duration of administration of the former. Indeed, cladribine is emerging as the treatment of choice for hairy-cell leukemia because of its minimal toxicity and its ability to induce a complete and sustained response with a single course of therapy.

Hydroxyurea

Hydroxyurea acts on the enzyme ribonucleoside diphosphate reductase to interfere with the synthesis of DNA. Oral absorption is excellent, and approximately 80% of the drug appears in the urine within 12 hours after oral or IV administration. The primary use of hydroxyurea is in the treatment of chronic granulocytic leukemia. Temporary remissions in patients with metastatic malignant melanoma have been reported.

Side Effects

Myelosuppression manifesting as leukopenia, megaloblastic anemia, and occasionally thrombocytopenia is the major side effect produced by hydroxyurea. Nausea and vomiting may accompany administration of this drug. Hyperpigmentation of the skin, stomatitis, and alopecia occur infrequently.

DNA TOPOISOMERASE INHIBITORS

Topoisomerases are enzymes that correct alterations in DNA that occur during replication and transcription. Certain chemotherapeutic drugs inhibit either topoisomerase I or topoisomerase II. Because cancer cells possess more topoisomerase activity than normal cells, there is more drug-induced DNA damage and resultant cell death. Toxicity reflects effects of inhibition of topoisomerase enzymes on normal proliferating tissues (myelosuppression, mucositis). Topoisomerase II inhibitors which include doxorubicin, daunorubicin, etoposide, and teniposide are part of most combination chemotherapy treatment regimens. Topoisomerase I inhibitors include topotecan and irinotecan. These drugs exhibit a broad spectrum of chemotherapeutic activity being useful in the treatment of leukemia, lung, colon, and ovarian cancer.

Doxorubicin and Daunorubicin

Doxorubicin and daunorubicin are anthracycline antibiotics that are natural products of certain soil fungi. Structurally, they contain a tetracycline ring attached to the sugar daunosamine by a glycosidic linkage. These drugs most likely act by binding to DNA, which results in changes in the DNA helix that inhibit the template activity of the nucleic acid. These drugs are also a likely cause of disruptive effects on cellular membranes. Drug-induced free radicals may overwhelm the heart's antioxidant defenses, leading to the oxidation of critical cardiac proteins and membrane components (unsaturated free fatty acids), leading to cardiotoxicity (Doroshow, 1991). Laboratory studies demonstrate that each subsequent dose of doxorubicin appears to diminish the heart's ability to withstand subsequent oxidant stress. Evidence that free radicals have a role is the protective effect of free radical scavengers.

Daunorubicin and doxorubicin are administered IV, with care taken to prevent extravasation because local vesicant action may result. There is rapid clearance from the plasma into the heart, kidneys, lungs, and liver. These drugs do not cross the blood-brain barrier to any significant extent. The urine may become red for 1 to 2 days after administration of these drugs.

Daunorubicin is metabolized primarily to daunorubiconol, whereas doxorubicin is excreted unchanged and as metabolites, including adriamycinol in the urine. Ultimately, approximately 40% of daunorubicin and doxorubicin are metabolized. Indeed, clinical toxicity may result in patients with hepatic dysfunction.

Clinical Uses

Daunorubicin is used primarily in the treatment of acute lymphocytic and granulocytic leukemia. Doxorubicin, which differs from daunorubicin only by a single hydroxyl group on the number 14 carbon atom, is also effective against a wide range of solid tumors. For example, doxorubicin is one of the most active single drugs for treating metastatic adenocarcinoma of the breast, carcinoma of the bladder, bronchogenic carcinoma, metastatic thyroid carcinoma, oat cell carcinoma, and osteogenic carcinoma.

Resistance is observed to the anthracycline antibiotics, as with other chemotherapeutic drugs. Furthermore, cross-tolerance occurs between daunorubicin and doxorubicin. Cross-resistance also occurs between these antibiotics and the vinca alkaloids, suggesting that an alteration of cellular permeability may be involved.

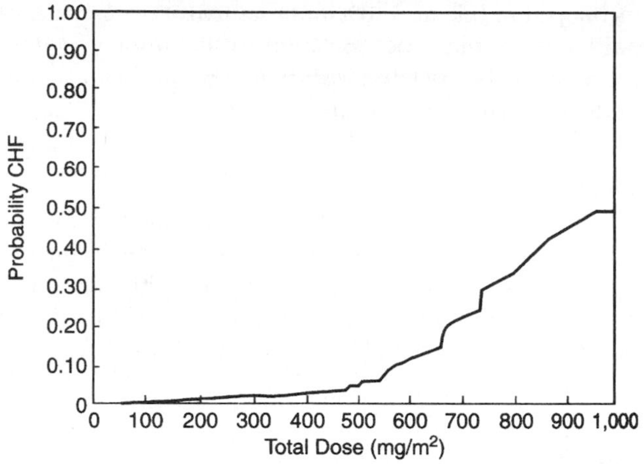

Figure 29-1. The probability of developing doxorubicin-induced congestive heart failure (CHF) versus the total cumulative dose of doxorubicin. (From Von Hoff DD, Layard MW, Basa P, et al. Risk factors for doxorubicin-induced congestive heart failure. *Ann Intern Med* 1979;91:710–707; with permission.)

Side Effects

Cardiomyopathy and myelosuppression are side effects of the chemotherapeutic antibiotics. Leukopenia typically manifests during the second week of therapy. Thrombocytopenia and anemia occur but are usually less pronounced. Stomatitis, gastrointestinal disturbances, and alopecia are common side effects.

Cardiomyopathy

Cardiomyopathy is a unique dose-related and often irreversible side effect of the anthracycline antibiotics. Increased plasma concentrations of troponin T reflect drug-induced injury to myocardial cells. Congestive heart failure develops in <3% of patients with a cumulative dose of doxorubicin of <400 mg/m^2, rising to 18% at 700 mg/m^2 (Fig. 29-1) (Von Hoff et al., 1979). Prior mediastinal radiation or previous treatment with cyclophosphamide increases the subsequent risk of cardiomyopathy in response to administration of an anthracycline antibiotic. Marked impairment of left ventricular function for as long as 3 years after discontinuing doxorubicin has been observed. Previous treatment with anthracycline antibiotics may enhance myocardial depressant effects of anesthetic drugs even in patients withn normal resting cardiac function (Huettemann et al., 2004). Acute left ventricular failure 2 months after cessation of treatment with doxorubicin has been described during general anesthesia (Borgeat et al., 1988).

Two types of cardiomyopathies may occur (Doroshow, 1991; Selvin, 1981). An acute form of cardiomyopathy occurs in approximately 10% of patients and is characterized by relatively benign changes on the ECG that include nonspecific ST-T changes and decreased QRS voltage. Other cardiac changes include premature ventricular contractions, supraventricular tachydysrhythmias, cardiac conduction abnormalities, and left axis deviation. These abnormalities occur during therapy at all dose levels and, except for decreased QRS voltage on the ECG, resolve 1 to 2 months after discontinuation of therapy. There is an associated acute reversible decrease in the ejection fraction within 24 hours after a single dose.

The second form of cardiomyopathy is characterized by the insidious onset of symptoms such as dry nonproductive cough, suggesting bronchitis, followed by rapidly progressive heart failure that is unresponsive to inotropic drugs and mechanical ventricular assistance (Selvin, 1981). This severe form of cardiomyopathy occurs in almost 2% of treated patients and is fatal approximately 3 weeks after the onset of symptoms in nearly 60% of affected patients. Predictive tests to permit early recognition of impending cardiomyopathy are not available, although diminution in QRS voltage on the ECG is consistent with the diffuse character of the myocardial damage. Increased plasma concentrations of cardiac enzymes occur late in the course of cardiac failure and are of limited value in achieving an early diagnosis. Systolic time intervals and echocardiograms have been used to detect cardiotoxicity before the occurrence of clinically significant damage. Dexrazoxane is a free-radical scavenger that protects the heart from doxorubicin-associated damage (Lipshultz et al., 2004).

Dactinomycin

Dactinomycin (actinomycin D) is an antibiotic with chemotherapeutic activity resulting from its ability to bind to DNA, especially in rapidly proliferating cells. As a result of this binding, the function of RNA polymerase, and thus the transcription of the DNA molecule, are blocked. After IV injection, dactinomycin rapidly leaves the circulation. In animals, approximately 50% of an injected dose is excreted unchanged in bile and 10% in urine. There is no evidence that the drug undergoes metabolism. Dactinomycin does not cross the blood-brain barrier in amounts sufficient to produce a pharmacologic effect.

Clinical Uses

The most important clinical use of dactinomycin is the treatment of Wilms tumor in children and of rhabdomyosarcoma. It may be effective in some women with methotrexate-resistant choriocarcinoma. Occasionally, this drug is used to inhibit immunologic responses associated with organ transplantation.

Side Effects

The toxic effects of dactinomycin include the early onset of nausea and vomiting, often followed by myelosuppression manifesting as pancytopenia 1 to 7 days after completion of therapy. Pancytopenia may be preceded by thrombocytopenia as the first manifestation of bone marrow suppression. Glossitis, ulcerations of the oral mucosa, diarrhea, alopecia, and cutaneous erythema are commonly associated with dactinomycin therapy. Extravasation of the drug results in tissue necrosis.

Bleomycin

Bleomycins are water-soluble glycopeptides that differ from one another (there are more than 200 congeners) in their terminal amine moiety. The terminal amine is coupled through an amide linkage to a carboxylic acid. Bleomycin possesses a tripeptide component that binds DNA and a metal-binding region. In the presence of oxygen and either iron or copper, bleomycin produces free radicals that create DNA breaks.

Bleomycin is administered IV, and high concentrations occur in the skin and lungs. The drug accumulates in tumors, suggesting the presence of a lower level of inactivating enzyme. Bleomycin is eliminated primarily by renal excretion, with approximately 50% of the dose is cleared within 4 hours and 70% by 24 hours (Dorr, 1992). Indeed, excessive concentrations of drug occur if usual doses are administered to patients with impaired renal function.

Clinical Uses

Bleomycin is effective in the treatment of testicular carcinoma, particularly if administered in combination with vinblastine. It is also useful in the palliative treatment of squamous cell carcinomas of the head, neck, esophagus, skin, and genitourinary tract.

Side Effects

The most common side effects of bleomycin are mucocutaneous reactions, including stomatitis, alopecia, pruritus, erythema, and hyperpigmentation, which occur in approximately 45% of patients. In contrast to other chemotherapeutic drugs, bleomycin causes minimal myelosuppression. Unexplained exacerbations of rheumatoid arthritis have occurred.

Patients with lymphomas who are receiving bleomycin may develop an acute reaction characterized by hyperthermia, hypotension, and hypoventilation. The likely mechanism is the release of an endogenous pyrogen, presumably from destroyed tumor cells. An initial small test dose of bleomycin is recommended to minimize the occurrence of this syndrome.

Pulmonary Toxicity

The most serious side effect of bleomycin is dose-related pulmonary toxicity (Fig. 29-2) (Ginsberg and Comis, 1982). Indeed, bleomycin is concentrated preferentially in the lungs and is inactivated by hydrolase enzyme, which is relatively deficient in lung tissue. Initially, bleomycin produces pulmonary capillary endothelial damage, progressing to alveolar epithelial injury with necrosis of type 1 and proliferation of type 2 alveolar cells. Interstitial fibrosis develops and may progress to involve the entire lung. It is estimated that some form of pulmonary toxicity (most often pulmonary fibrosis) occurs in 4% of patients treated with bleomycin. Fatal pulmonary toxicity has occurred with bleomycin doses as low as 100 mg but more often in the presence of other risk factors (Table 29-2).

The first signs of pulmonary toxicity are cough, dyspnea, and basilar rales, which progress in one of two directions. A mild form of pulmonary toxicity is characterized by exertional dyspnea and a normal resting PaO_2. A more

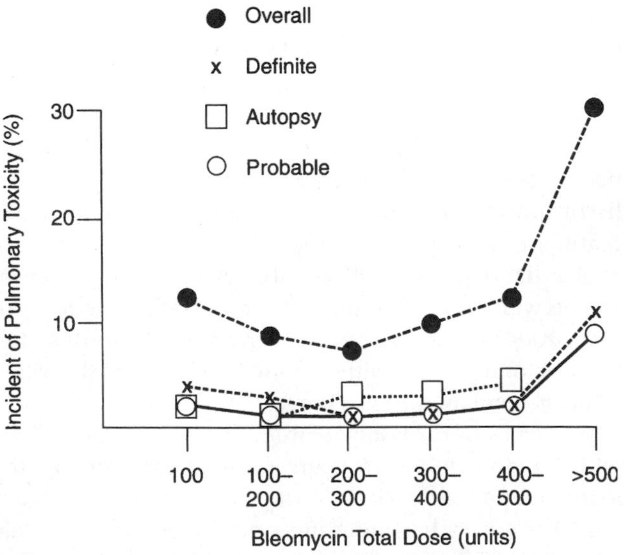

Figure 29-2. The relationship between the total dose of bleomycin and the incidence of pulmonary toxicity. (From Ginsberg SJ, Comis RL. The pulmonary toxicity of antineoplastic agents. *Semin Oncol* 1982;9:34–51; with permission.)

TABLE 29-2.
RISK FACTORS FOR DEVELOPMENT OF CHEMOTHERAPY-INDUCED PULMONARY TOXICITY

Total drug dose
Age
Concurrent or prior chest radiation
Oxygen therapy
Combination chemotherapy
Preexisting pulmonary disease
Genetic predisposition
Cigarette smoking (?)

severe form of arterial hypoxemia at rest is associated with radiographic findings of interstitial pneumonitis and fibrosis. Lesions are found more frequently in lower lobes and subpleural areas, and radiographs of the chest often reveal basilar and perihilar infiltrates. The alveolar-to-arterial difference for oxygen is increased, and pulmonary diffusion capacity may be decreased. Pulmonary function studies have been of no greater value than clinical signs in detecting the onset of pulmonary toxicity.

Early reports of postoperative respiratory failure in bleomycin-treated patients suggested that either arterial hyperoxia or excessive crystalloid administration played a role in the exacerbation of pulmonary fibrosis (Allen et al., 1981; Eigen and Wyszomierski, 1985; Hulbert et al., 1983). One speculation is that acutely increased inhaled concentrations of oxygen facilitate production of superoxide and other free radicals in the presence of bleomycin. For this reason, it has been recommended that inhaled oxygen concentrations be maintained below 30% in bleomycin-treated patients. Animal model literature confirms that the continuous administration of inspired oxygen concentrations of >30% immediately after exposure to bleomycin increases pulmonary damage (Hay et al., 1987). Nevertheless, it is unlikely that patients will present to the operating room immediately after treatment with bleomycin. A more practical question is whether hyperoxia for short periods of time several days after treatment is a risk factor for bleomycin-induced pulmonary damage (Mathes, 1995). In this regard, animal studies have confirmed that delayed exposure to supplemental oxygen after bleomycin treatment is not harmful (Blom-Muilwijk et al., 1988). Nevertheless, there are case reports of respiratory failure with inspired oxygen concentrations >30% in patients last exposed to bleomycin up to 6 to 12 months before hyperoxia. Patients with prior exposure to bleomycin but with no risk factors appear to be at a minimum risk from hyperoxia. In contrast, those patients with one or more major risk factors (preexisting pulmonary damage from bleomycin, which is more likely if the total dose is >450 mg; renal dysfunction, which slows clearance of the drug from the lungs; and/or prior exposure to bleomycin within a 1- to 2-month period) may be at higher risk for the development of bleomycin-induced hyperoxic pulmonary injury in the operating room. It may be prudent to maintain these patients on the minimum inspired oxygen concentration that can be used safely intraoperatively to provide oxygen saturations of >90% by pulse oximetry (Mathes, 1995). The value of corticosteroids as pretreatment in patients with risk factors and in whom >30% oxygen may be needed (cardiopulmonary bypass operations) has not been confirmed by controlled studies. The role of excessive crystalloid administration has not received the same scrutiny as increased delivered oxygen concentrations. A consideration in this regard is replacement of fluids with colloids rather than crystalloids to decrease or prevent pulmonary interstitial edema in bleomycin-treated patients undergoing surgery. Accumulation of interstitial fluid may reflect impaired lymphatic function caused by bleomycin-induced fibrotic changes in the lungs. In the future, bleomycin may be replaced with pleomycin, an analogue of bleomycin that has lower pulmonary toxicity and a broader effectiveness against multiple types of tumors (Comis, 1992).

ANTIMICROTUBULE DRUGS

Microtubules are subcellular structures that are essential for normal function of cells. They form the architecture to maintain cell shape, organize the location of organelles, and mediate intracellular transport and secretion, neurotransmission, axonemal flow, and cell motility (Wilson, 1995). Vinca alkaloids and taxanes are examples of antimitotic chemotherapeutic drugs that disrupt the normal function of microtubules. Vinca alkaloids bind to depolymerized microtubules and inhibit microtubule formation. Taxanes bind to polymerized microtubules and inhibit their breakdown. The result of these interactions is the failure of the cell to undergo normal mitosis leading to cell death.

Vinca Alkaloids

Vinca alkaloids represent the active medicinal ingredients from the pink periwinkle plant and include vincristine, vinblastine, vinorelbine, and vindesine. Vincristine is highly effective against Hodgkin disease, non-Hodgkin lymphoma, and pediatric solid tumors, yet it has little activity against adult solid tumors. Vinorelbine, in constrast, is active against breast and lung cancer. Vinblastine is most often used in the treatment of testicular cancer and non-Hodgkin lymphoma.

Side Effects

Myelosuppression manifesting as leukopenia, thrombocytopenia, and anemia are the most prominent side effects of vinca alkaloids, appearing 7 to 10 days after initiation of treatment. Vincristine is less likely than vinblastine and vinorelbine to cause bone marrow depression.

Symmetric peripheral sensory-motor neuropathy often occurs during administration of therapeutic doses of vincristine and may become the dose-limiting side effect (Postma et al., 1993; Vainionpaa et al., 1995). Clinical manifestations may include several aspects of peripheral nerve function with areflexia (loss of Achilles tendon reflex) being the earliest finding. Paresthesias in the hands and feet, weakness and atrophy of the extremities, and skeletal muscle pain make use of the hands and feet difficult (ataxia). Tremors frequently develop, and neuritic pain and foot drop are common. Autonomic neuropathy with orthostatic hypotension, bowel motility dysfunction, and cranial nerve involvement (laryngeal nerve paralysis with hoarseness, weakness of the extraocular muscles) are present in about 10% of treated patients (Delaney, 1992). CNS effects (confusion, insomnia, seizures, hallucinations) due to vincristine are rare, presumably because of poor penetration of the blood-brain barrier by the drug. The peripheral neuropathy is mainly axonal, but demyelination may also occur as demonstrated by measurement of somatosensory evoked potentials (Vainionpaa et al., 1995). Vincristine peripheral neuropathy is said to be reversible after discontinuing the drug, although this may require months, and in some patients the resolution may be incomplete (Postma et al., 1993).

The syndrome of hyponatremia associated with high urinary sodium and inappropriate secretion of arginine vasopressin hormone has occasionally been observed during vincristine therapy. An effect on the autonomic nervous system may be responsible for paralytic ileus and abdominal pain that commonly develops during vinblastine therapy. Urinary retention, tenderness of the parotid glands, dryness of the mouth, and sinus tachycardia are other occasionally experienced manifestations of altered autonomic nervous system activity. Transient mental depression is most likely to occur on the second or third day of treatment with vinblastine. Alopecia appears to occur more frequently with vincristine than with vinblastine. Vinorelbine may cause chest pain, bronchospasm, dyspnea, and pulmonary infiltrations.

Taxanes

Paclitaxel (active extract from the Pacific yew tree) and docetaxel (more water soluble semisynthetic derivative) share a broad spectrum of similar chemotherapeutic activity against breast, lung, ovarian, and bladder cancer (Rowinsky and Donehower, 1995). Both drugs are also active against lymphoid malignancies. Taxanes block the function of the mitotic apparatus by impeding the normal function of microtubules. Unlike vinca alkaloids, which affect the rates of tubulin polymerization, the taxanes inhibit microtubule depolymerization in a dose-dependent manner. The microtubules formed in the presence of taxanes are extraordinarily stable and dysfunctional, thereby causing the death of the cell by disrupting the normal microtubule dynamics required for cell division.

Taxanes are rapidly cleared from the plasma despite extensive binding to proteins. The volume of distribution is large, suggesting binding to cellular proteins, possibly tubulin. Renal clearance accounts for a small proportion (<10%) of total clearance. Hepatic metabolism, biliary excretion, fecal elimination, or extensive tissue binding appears to be responsible for most of the plasma clearance.

Side Effects

Taxanes are associated with myelosuppression, peripheral neuropathy, and alopecia. Severe neurotoxicity precludes the administration of high doses of taxanes. The peripheral neuropathy is characterized by sensory symptoms such as numbness and paresthesia in a glove-and-stocking distribution. Cardiac effects, including dysrhythmias, myocardial ischemia, and transient asymptomatic bradycardia may be more common with paclitaxes than docetaxel. Docetaxel seems to have unique vascular permeability properties that may result in peripheral edema, pleural effusion, and ascites. Fluid retention produced by docetaxel is dose-dependent and may be decreased by pretreatment with dexamethasone. Docetaxel also produces skin toxicities including an erythematous macrulopapular rash on the forearms and hands. Hypersensitivity reactions (flushing, bronchospasm, dyspnea, systemic hypotension) caused by direct release of histamine or other chemical mediators may occur in 25% to 30% of patients treated with taxanes (Rowinsky and Donehower, 1995).

Estramustine

Estramustine exerts its chemotherapeutic effects by inhibition of microtubule assembly and depolymerization. This drug also binds to an estramustine-binding protein in prostate tissue explaining the possible usefulness of this drug as part of combination therapy of hormone-refractory prostate cancer.

SIGNAL TRANSDUCTION MODULATORS

Signal transduction modulators (hormones) that may be useful in the treatment of neoplastic disease include antiestrogens, antiandrogens, aromatase inhibitors, gonadotropin-releasing drugs, and progestin. Normal cell division results from the interaction of growth factors with specific receptors. This interaction initiates a series of enzyme reactions (signal transduction), culminating in activation of nuclear transcription factors that produce cell proliferation molecules. Mutations in cancer cells result in uncontrolled cell proliferation utilizing activated signaling pathways. Hormonal treatment of cancer represents a disruption of growth factor receptor interactions.

Progestins

Progestational drugs are useful in the management of patients with endometrial carcinoma. Presumably, unopposed overstimulation of the endometrium is responsible for neoplastic changes.

Estrogens and Androgens

Malignant changes in the breast and prostate often depend on hormones for their continued growth. For example, prostatic cancer is stimulated by androgens, whereas orchiectomy or estrogens (diethylstilbestrol) slow the growth of the tumor cells. Eventually, prostatic tumors become insensitive to the lack of androgen or the presence of estrogens, presumably because of the survival of progressively undifferentiated cells that favor the emergence of cell types that no longer depend on androgens for their growth.

Malignant tissues that are responsive to estrogens contain receptors for the hormone, whereas malignant tissues lacking these receptors are unlikely to respond to hormonal manipulation. The onset of action of hormone therapy is slow, requiring 8 to 12 weeks.

Hypercalcemia may be associated with androgen or estrogen therapy, requiring adequate hydration in an attempt to facilitate renal excretion of calcium. Plasma calcium concentrations should be determined in patients receiving treatment with these hormones.

Antiestrogens

Antiestrogens, such as tamoxifen, are useful in the treatment of breast cancer that expresses estrogen or progesterone receptors. The estrogen receptor resides in the cytosol and, upon occupation by estradiol, is transported to the nucleus, where it activates genes (including those genes that encode proliferation molecules) containing estrogen-response elements. Tamoxifen binds to estrogen receptors and disrupts receptor interactions with estrogen in some but not all estrogen-responsive tissues. For example, tamoxifen is antiestrogenic in breast and ovarian tissue but is estrogenic in the uterus, liver, and bone. As a result, tamoxifen is effective in the prevention and treatment of breast cancer but produces undesired estrogen side effects including deep-vein thrombosis ($<1\%$ of patients), endometrial cancer (about 0.3% of patients), and early menopausal symptoms (hot flashes). In addition, tamoxifen lowers plasma cholesterol concentrations and increases bone density.

The response to tamoxifen is proportional to the degree of expression of estrogen receptors in the breast cancer. Tamoxifen is of little benefit in women with breast cancer that does not express hormone receptors. After surgical removal of the primary breast cancer, adjuvant treatment of women with tumors that are hormone-positive decreases the odds of recurrence by more than 30%. Other antiestrogens that may have greater selectivity for breast estrogen receptors include raloxifene, toremifene, and fulvestrant.

Antiandrogens

Antiandrogens such as flutamide, bicalutamide, and nilutamide are competitive antagonists of the interactions between androstenedione and androgen receptors. Flutamide is a nonsteroidal antiandrogenic that possesses pure antiandrogenic activity when metabolized to its hydroxylated derivative. Administered with other drugs that decrease androgen production, flutamide is an effective treatment for hormone-dependent prostate cancer. Androgenic blockade results in feminizing side effects in men, including gynecomastia, hot flashes, and loss of facial hair. Skeletal muscle weakness and development of osteoporosis reflect a male menopause-like state. Flutamide can induce methemoglobinemia (Jackson and Barker, 1995). Pulse oximetry readings in the presence of methemoglobinemia can overestimate the hemoglobin saturation levels. At levels of methemoglobinemia of $>35\%$, the pulse oximetry readings tend to approach a minimal level of 85% (Barker et al., 1989).

Monoclonal Antibodies

Antibody-based therapies for treatment of cancer include the monoclonal antibodies trastuzumab, alemtuzumab, and rituximab that target specific antigen sites on cancer cells (Dillman, 2002). Vaccines are also being developed that may include genetic manipulation of cancer cells to make them more antigenic and thus susceptible to immune responses.

Aromatase Inhibitors

Aromatase is an enzyme complex consisting of two proteins, aromatase cytochrome P-450 (CYP19) and NADPH-cytochrome P-450 reductase. Inhibition of aromatase blocks the conversion of androgens to estrone in peripheral tissues including breast tissue. The high affinity of the aromatase inhibitors anastrozole and letrozole for CYP19, results in intense inhibition of estrogen effects on responsive receptors. Inhibition of aromatase is an effective treatment for postmenopausal women with breast cancer, in which the greatest source of estrone comes from conversion of androstenedione to estrone in liver, skeletal muscles, and fat. Exemestane is a steroidal aromatase inhibitor that binds to the enzyme complex and promotes enzyme degradation.

A medical hypophysectomy is produced by luteinizing hormone-releasing hormone agonists, such as leuprolide, buserelin, and goserelin, which inhibit secretion of follicle-stimulating hormone and luteinizing hormone by down-regulating receptors that respond to these hormones. The result is insignificant plasma concentrations of sex hormones and palliation of breast and prostate cancer.

REFERENCES

Allen SC, Riddell GS, Butchart EG. Bleomycin therapy and anaesthesia: the possible hazards of oxygen administration to patients after treatment with bleomycin. *Anaesthesia* 1981;60:121–124.

Barker SJ, Tremper KK, Hyatt J. Effects of methemoglobinemia on pulse oximetry and mixed venous oximetry. *Anesthesiology* 1989; 70:112–117.

Blom-Muilwijk MC, Vriesendorp R, Veninga TS, et al. Pulmonary toxicity after treatment with bleomycin along or in combination with hyperoxia. Studies in the rat. *Br J Anaesth* 1988;60:91–97.

Borgeat A, Chiolero R, Baylon P, et al. Perioperative cardiovascular collapse in a patient previously treated with doxorubicin. *Anesth Analg* 1988;67:1189–1191.

Chung F. Cancer, chemotherapy, and anaesthesia. *Can Anaesth Soc J* 1982;29:364–371.

Comis RL. Bleomycin pulmonary toxicity: current status and future directions. *Semin Oncol* 1992;19:64–70.

Cooper JA Jr, White DA, Matthay RA. Drug-induced pulmonary disease. Part 1: Cytotoxic drugs. *Am Rev Respir Dis* 1986;133: 321–340.

Delaney P. Vincristine-induced laryngeal nerve paralysis. *Neurology* 1982;32:1285–1288.

Dillman RO. Radiolabled anti-CD20 monoclonal antibodies for the treatment of B-cell lymphoma. *J Clin Oncol* 2002;20:3345–3351.

Doroshow JH. Doxorubicin-induced cardiac toxicity. *N Engl J Med* 1991;324:843–845.

Dorr RT. Bleomycin pharmacology: mechanism of action and resistance, and clinical pharmacokinetics. *Semin Oncol* 1992;19:3–8.

Eigen H, Wyszomierski D. Bleomycin lung injury in children. Pathophysiology and guidelines for management. *Am J Pediatr Hematol Oncol* 1985;7:71–78.

Ginsberg SJ, Comis RL. The pulmonary toxicity of antineoplastic agents. *Semin Oncol* 1982;9:34–51.

Gottdiener JS, Appelbaum FR, Ferrans VJ, et al. Cardiotoxicity associated with high-dose cyclophosphamide therapy. *Arch Intern Med* 1981; 141:758–762.

Gunstream SR, Seidenfeld JJ, Cobonya RE, et al. Mitomycin-associated lung disease. *Cancer Treat Rev* 1983;67:301–304.

Hay JG, Haslam PL, Dewar A, et al. Development of acute lung injury after the combination of intravenous bleomycin and exposure to hyperoxia in rats. *Thorax* 1987;42:374–382.

Huettemann E, Junker T, Chatzinikolaou KP, et al. The influence of anthracycline therapy on cardiac function during anesthesia. *Anesth Analg* 2004:98:941–947.

Hulbert JC, Grossman JE, Cummings KB. Risk factors of anesthesia and surgery in bleomycin-treated patients. *J Urol* 1983;130:163–164.

Jackson SH, Barker SJ. Methemoglobinemia in a patient receiving flutamide. *Anesthesiology* 1995;82:1065–1067.

Kaplan RS, Wienik PH. Neurotoxicity of antineoplastic drugs. *Semin Oncol* 1982;9:103–110.

Labianca R, Beretta G, Clerici M. Cardiac toxicity of 5-fluorouracil: a study of 10,083 patients. *Tumor* 1982;68:505–509.

Lipshultz SE, Rifai N, Dalton VM et al. The effect of dexrazoxane on myocardial injury in doxorubicin-treated children with acute lymphoblastic leukemia. *N Engl J Med* 2004;351:145–153.

Mathes DD. Bleomycin and hyperoxia exposure in the operating room. *Anesth Analg* 1995;81:624–629.

Postma TJ, Benard BA, Huijgens PC, et al. Long term effects of vincristine on the peripheral nervous system. *J Neurooncol* 1993;15: 23–27.

Rowinsky EK, Donehower RC. Paclitaxel (Taxol). *N Engl J Med* 1995; 332:1004–1014.

Rubin EH, Hait WN. Principles of cancer treatment. *Sci Am Med* 2003; 12(IV):1–17.

Saven A, Piro L. Newer purine analogues for the treatment of hairy-cell leukemia. *N Engl J Med* 1994;330:691–697.

Selvin BF. Cancer chemotherapy: implications for the anesthesiologist. *Anesth Analg* 1981;60:425–434.

Vainionpaa L, Kovala T, Tolonen U, et al. Vincristine therapy for children with acute lymphoblastic leukemia impairs conduction in the entire peripheral nerve. *Pediatr Neurol* 1995;13:314–318.

Von Hoff DD, Layard MW, Basa P, et al. Risk factors for doxorubicin-induced congestive heart failure. *Ann Intern Med* 1979;91:710–717.

Weiss HD, Walker MD, Wiernik PH. Neurotoxicity of commonly used antineoplastic agents. *N Engl J Med* 1974;291:75–81.

Weiss RB, Poster DS, Penta JS. The nitrosoureas and pulmonary toxicity. *Cancer Treat Rev* 1981;8:111–125.

White DA, Orenstein M, Godwin TA, Stover DE. Chemotherapy-associated pulmonary toxic reactions during treatment for breast cancer. *Arch Intern Med* 1984;144:953–956.

Wilson L, Jordan MA. Microtubule dynamics: taking aim at a moving target. *Chem Biol* 1995;2:569–575.

Zsigmond EK, Robins G. The effect of a series of anticancer drugs on plasma cholinesterase activity. *Can Anaesth Soc J* 1972;19:75–82.

Antiepileptic Drugs

30

It is estimated that 50 million people (1% to 2% of the population) worldwide have epilepsy (recurrent seizures) (Table 30-1) (Brodie and Dichter, 1996). *Epilepsy* is a collective term used to designate a group of chronic central nervous system (CNS) disorders characterized by the onset of sudden disturbances of sensory, motor, autonomic, or psychic origin. These disturbances are usually transient and are almost always associated with abnormal discharges of the electroencephalogram. About 30% of patients with seizures have an identifiable neurologic or systemic disorder, and the remainder have idiopathic epilepsy.

The goal of pharmacologic treatment of epilepsy is to control seizures without medication-related adverse effects. Approximately 70% of patients with epilepsy will become seizure-free utilizing a single antiepileptic drug (LaRoche and Helmers, 2004). For the remaining 30% of patients, recurrent seizures as well as intolerable adverse drug side effects can have significant impact on the quality of life. The antiepileptic drug selected to treat epilepsy is influenced by the characteristics of the seizure experienced by the patient (Table 30-2) (Brodie and Dichter, 1996; Dichter and Brodie, 1996). Because the efficacies of the antiepileptic drugs overlap, a medication is often chosen because the side-effects profile is most compatible for that particular patient. Indeed, dose-related side effects are common and frequently limit the use of antiepileptic drugs (Table 30-3) (Brodie and Dichter, 1996; Dichter and Brodie, 1996). Although side effects are associated with higher plasma levels of the drug, the specific concentration at which a patient develops toxicity varies (Table 30-4) (Brodie and Dichter, 1996; Dichter and Brodie, 1996). Cognitive impairment (mental slowing, difficulty with concentration, sleepiness) is a dose-related effect common to all antiepileptic drugs. In addition to dose-related side effects, all antiepileptic drugs may be associated with idiosyncratic reactions (see Table 30-3) (Brodie and Dichter, 1996; Ditcher and Brodie, 1996).

PHARMACOKINETICS

All antiepileptic drugs are administered once daily or more frequently. Absorption of these drugs from the gastrointestinal tract occurs slowly over a period of hours and may be incomplete, especially for gabapentin. Protein binding varies greatly (0% for gabapentin to 90% or greater for phenytoin). Except for gabapentin, levetiracetam, and vigabatrin, all antiepileptic drugs are metabolized in the liver before renal excretion.

Antiepileptic drugs clearance and elimination half-time range from hours (carbamazepine, valproate, primidone, gabapentn) to days (phenytoin, lamotrigine, phenobarbital, zonisamide) (Table 30-4). Because of their ability to induce or inhibit drug metabolism, all anetiepileptic drugs (except gabapentin, levetiracetam, vigabatrin) may be associated with pharamacokinetic drug interactions in which plasma drug concentrations and resulting pharmacologic effects of concomitantly administered drugs may be altered. Such drug interactions should be anticipated in all patients receiving antiepileptic drugs and subsequently receiving drugs for other purposes.

Drug Interactions Related to Protein-Binding

Medications that compete for protein-binding sites of highly bound antiepileptic drugs (phenytoin, valproate, carbamazepine) can displace the bound drug and lead to increases in the plasma concentration of pharmacologically active antiepileptic drug. Commonly used medications that are highly protein bound include phenylbutazone, thyroxine, and salicylates. Albumin is the principal binding protein for antiepileptic drugs. Hypoalbuminemia as may accompany renal or hepatic disease, malnutrition, or pregnancy can result in increased plasma concentrations of unbound antiepileptic drug, resulting in toxicity despite therapeutic plasma concentrations.

Drug Interactions Related to Accelerated Metabolism

Enzyme-inducing antiepileptic drugs that accelerate metabolism (carbamazepine, oxcarbazepine, phenobarbital, phenytoin, topiramate) may render oral contraceptives ineffective at usual doses (Mattson et al., 1986). Patients being treated with antiepileptic drugs have increased dose requirements for thiopental, propofol, midazolam, opioids, and

TABLE 30-1.
CLASSIFICATION OF EPILEPTIC SEIZURES

Partial seizures (beginning locally)
Simple partial seizures (consciousness not impaired)
Complex partial seizures (consciousness impaired)
Partial seizures evolving into secondary generalized seizures
Generalized seizures (convulsive or nonconvulsive)
Absence seizures (petit mal)
Myoclonic seizures
Clonic seizures
Tonic seizures
Tonic-clonic seizures
Unclassified seizures

Source: Adapted from Brodie MJ, Dichter MA. Antiepileptic drugs. *N Engl J Med* 1996;334:168–175.

nondepolarizing neuromuscular blocking drug (Tempelhoff et al., 1990). Possible explanations for altered dose requirements for drugs administered during anesthesia include increased hepatic P-450 enzyme activity as a result of stimulating effects of antiepileptic drugs, alterations in the number and/or responsiveness of receptors, and interactions with endogenous neurotransmitters.

PRINCIPLES OF DOSING

The patient's clinical response and, to a lesser extent, plasma concentrations determine the appropriate dose of an antiepileptic drug. An effective dose is one at which seizures cease but side effects do not appear (see Table 30-3) (Brodie and Dichter, 1996; Dichter and Brodie, 1996). A common cause of medication ineffectiveness is failure to achieve a sufficiently high dose. Addition of a second drug is usually not necessary and is complicated by drug interactions and an increased incidence of side effects (Mattson, 1989).

Once the dosage and dosing interval are established, it is important to consider the plasma concentration below which seizures are more likely to occur and above which patients are likely to experience limiting side effects. To maintain plasma drug concentrations in a therapeutic range, equal doses of the antiepileptic drug are often administered at intervals equivalent to less than one elimination half-time of the drug (see Table 30-4) (Brodie and Dichter, 1996; Dichter and Brodie, 1996). Dosing at one-half the drug's elimination half-time ensures that a single missed dose will not result in the plasma concentration decreasing below a therapeutic level.

PLASMA CONCENTRATIONS AND LABORATORY TESTING

Routine monitoring of plasma concentrations of antiepileptic drugs has traditionally been utilized to guide dosage adjustments in patients being treated for epilepsy, despite the fact that "therapeutic ranges" in the literature often do not correlate with a given individual's response (Brodie and Dichter, 1996; Dichter and Brodie, 1996; LaRoche and Helmers, 2004). For this reason, titration to clinical efficacy is recommended for guiding the dosages of all antiepileptic drugs. If a patient does not respond to a particular drug as expected, checking the plasma drug concentration may aid in determining compliance and identifying potential pharmacokinetic interactions.

Since many antiepileptic drugs are associated with rare but potentially life-threatening bone marrow suppression as well as hepatotoxicity, baseline as well as routine monitoring of hematologic and liver function may be recommended. Among the new antiepileptic drugs, the only medication that has been associated with serious organ toxicity is felbamate. Therefore, felmabamte is the only new antiepileptic drug that requires routine monitoring of hematologic and liver function (LaRoche and Helmers, 2004).

MECHANISM OF SEIZURE ACTIVITY

Seizure activity in most patients with epilepsy has a localized or focal origin. The reason for the high frequency and synchronous firing in a seizure focus is unknown. Possible explanations include (a) local biochemical changes, (b) ischemia, (c) loss of cellular inhibitory systems, (d) infections, and (e) head trauma.

Neurons in a chronic seizure focus exhibit a type of denervation hypersensitivity with regard to excitatory stimuli. The spread of seizure activity to neighboring normal cells is presumably restrained by normal inhibitory mechanisms. Factors such as changes in blood glucose concentrations, $Pa{O_2}$, $Pa{CO_2}$, pH, electrolyte balance, endocrine function, stress, and fatigue may result in the spread of a seizure focus into areas of the normal brain. If the spread is sufficiently extensive, the entire brain is activated and a tonic-clonic seizure with unconsciousness ensues. Conversely, if the spread is localized, the seizure produces signs and symptoms characteristic of the anatomic focus. Once initiated, a seizure is most likely maintained by reentry of excitatory impulses in a closed feedback pathway that may not even include the original seizure focus.

MECHANISM OF DRUG ACTION

The mechanism of action of antiepileptic drugs is not completely understood. It is commonly presumed that antiepileptic drugs control seizures by decreasing neuronal excitability or enhancing inhibition of neurotransmission. This is achieved by altering intrinsic membrane ion currents (sodium, potassium, and calcium conductance) or by affecting activity of inhibitory neurotransmitters

TABLE 30-2.
ANTIEPILEPTIC DRUGS USED TO TREAT EPILEPSY

Drug	Principal Mechanism of Action	Targeted Seizure	Dosage Type
Carbamazepine	Sodium ion channel blockade	Partial seizures	10–40 mg/kg/day in 3 to 4 divided doses
Ethosuximide	T-type calcium ion change	Generalized seizures	15–40 mg/kg/day in 2–3 divided doses
Felbamate	Sodium ion channel blockade Glutamate antagonism Calcium ion channel blockade	Partial seizures Generalized seizures	15–45 mg/kg/day in 2–3 divided doses
Gabapentin	Unknown (? increases GABA release)	Partial seizures Generalized seizures	10–60 mg/kg/day
Lamotrigine	Sodium ion channel blockade Calcium ion channel blockade	Partial seizures Generalized seizures	200–500 mg/day in 2 divided doses
Levetiracetam	Unknown (? potassium and calcium ion channel blockade)	Partial seizures Generalized seizures	1,000–3,000 mg/day in 2 divided doses
Oxcarbazepine	Sodium ion channel blockade	Partial seizures Generalized seizures	900–2,400 mg/day in 2 divided doses
Phenobarbital	Chloride ion channels	Partial seizures Generalized seizures	2–5 mg/kg/day every day or in 2 divided doses
Phenytoin	Sodium ion channel blockade Calcium ion channels NMDA receptors	Partial seizures Generalized seizures	3–7 mg/kg/day in 3 divided doses
Primidone	Chloride ion channels GABA uptake	Partial seizures Generalized seizures	500–1500 mg/day in 2–3 divided doses
Tiagabine	Enhanced GABA activity Carbonic anhydrase inhibition	Partial seizures Generalized seizures	32–56 mg/kg/day in 2–4 divided doses
Topiramate	Sodium ion channel blockade Enhanced GABA activity Glutamate antagonism Calcium ion channel blockade	Partial seizures Generalized seizures	500–3,000 mg/day in 2–4 divided doses
Valproate	Sodium ion channel blockade Calcium ion channels	Partial seizures Generalized seizures	500–3,000 mg/day in 2–4 divided doses
Zonisamide	Sodium ion channel blockade Calcium ion channel blockade	Partial seizures Generalized seizures	200–600 mg/day in 2–4 divided doses
Fosphenytoin	Sodium ion channel blockade	Status epilepticus	10–20 mg/kg IV loading dose

(gamma-aminobutyric acid [GABA], glutamate). Ion currents affected by antiepileptic drugs are primarily those involving the voltage-gated sodium and calcium ion channels. Drugs that delay reactivaton of sodium channels (phenytoin, carbamazepine, primidone, valproate, lamotrigine) during high frequency neuronal firing produce an inhibitory effect on creation of action potentials until neuronal discharge is blocked. Some drugs (phenytoin, carbamazepine, valproate, lamotrigine, zonisamide) act at both sodium and calcium ion channels. Other drugs (ethosuximide, phenobarbital) act selectively at calcium ion channels. Ethosuximide selectively blocks the T-type calcium ion current, which is thought to act as a pacemaker for thalamic neurons and may be important in absence seizures.

Drugs (phenobarbital, benzodiazepines) that alter synaptic function act primarily by enhancing GABA-mediated neuronal inhibition. Benzodiazepines increase the frequency of GABA-mediated ion channel openings, whereas barbiturates increase the duration of ion channel openings. Tiagabine delays the reuptake of GABA from synaptic clefts, effectively enhancing GABA-mediated neuronal inhibition after synaptic release of the neurotransmitter.

MAJOR ANTIEPILEPTIC DRUGS

The principal antiepileptic drugs used to treat patients with epilepsy are carbamazepine, ethosuximide, gabapentin, lamotrigine, levetiracetam, oxcarbazepine, phenobarbital, phenytoin, primidone, tiagabine, topiramate, valproate, and zonisamide (see Table 30-2). Prior to 1993, the choice of antiepileptic drugs was limited to phenobarbital, primidone, phenytoin, carbamazepine, and valproate. Since 1993, eight new antiepileptic drugs have been introduced offering potential advantages compared with traditional drugs including fewer drug interactions, broader spectrums of activity, and unique mechanisms of action (Table 30-2) (Fig. 30-1) (LaRoche and Helmers, 2004).

TABLE 30-3.
SIDE EFFECTS OF ANTIEPILEPTIC DRUGS

	Dose-Related	Idiosyncratic
Carbamazepine	Diplopia Vertigo Neutropenia Nausea Drowsiness Hyponatremia	Agranulocytosis Aplastic anemia Allergic dermatitis (rash) Stevens-Johnson syndrome Hepatotoxic effects Pancreatitis Teratogenicity
Ethosuximide	Nausea Anorexia Vomiting Agitation Headache Drowsiness	Agranulocytosis Aplastic anemia Allergic dermatitis (rash) Stevens-Johnson syndrome Lupus-like syndrome
Clonazepam	Sedation Vertigo Hyperactivity (children)	Allergic dermatitis (rash) Thrombocytopenia
Felbamate	Insomnia Anorexia Nausea Headache Irritability	Aplastic anemia Hepatotoxic effects
Gabapentin	Sedation Ataxia Vertigo Gastrointestinal disturbances	
Lamotrigine	Tremor Vertigo Diplopia Ataxia Headache Gastrointestinal disturbances	Stevens-Johnson syndrome
Levetiracetam	Sedation Anxiety Headache	Allergic dermatitis (rash)
Oxcarbazepine		Allergic dermatitis (rash)
Phenobarbital	Sedation Depression Hyperactivity (children)	Agranulocytosis Allergic dermatitis (rash) Stevens-Johnson syndrome Arthritic changes Hepatotoxic effects Teratogenicity
Phenytoin	Nystagmus Ataxia Nausea and vomiting Gingival hyperplasia Depression Megaloblastic anemia Drowsiness	Agranulocytosis Aplastic anemia Allergic dermatitis (rash) Stevens-Johnson syndrome Hepatotoxic effects Pancreatitis Acne Coarse facies Hirsutism Teratogenicity Dupuytren contracture
Primidone	Sedation	Rash Thrombocytopenia Agranulocytosis Lupus-like syndrome Teratogenicity
Tiagabine	Dizziness Aphasia Tremor	Allergic dermatitis (rash)

TABLE 30-3.
(Continued)

Topiramate	Sedation Ataxia Dizziness	Allergic dermatitis (rash)
Valproic acid	Tremor Weight gain Dyspepsia Nausea and vomiting Alopecia Peripheral edema Encephalopathy Teratogenicity	Agranulocytosis Aplastic anemia Allergic dermatitis (rash) Stevens-Johnson syndrome Hepatotoxic effects Pancreatitis
Zonisamide	Sedation Dizziness Ataxia	Allergic dermatitis (rash)
Nephrolithiasis		
	Hyperactivity (children) Mania (adults)	

Source: Adapted in part from Brodie MJ, Dichter MA. Antiepileptic drugs. *N Engl J Med* 1996;334: 168–175; Dichter MA, Brodie MJ. New antiepileptic drugs. *N Engl J Med* 1996;334:1583–1590.

Benzodiazepines (diazepam, lorazepam) are used for short-term treatment of acute seizures or status epilepticus and are usually administered parenterally. Clonazepam can be used to treat epilepsy but most patients develop tolerance to its antiepileptic effects. Felbamate is reserved for use in selected patients with uncontrolled seizures.

Drugs of choice for treatment of partial seizures are carbamazepine and phenytoin, which are highly effective and associated with acceptable adverse side effects (see Table 30-2). Valproate, lamotrigine, and topiramate are the antiepileptic drugs of choice for treatment of patients with generalized seizures. Ethosuximide, lamotrigine, or valproate

TABLE 30-4.
PHARMACOKINETICS OF ANTIEPILEPTIC DRUGS

	Plasma Therapeutic Concentration (μg/mL)	Protein Binding (%)	Elimination Half-Time (hrs)	Route of Elimination
Carbamazepine	6–12	70–80	8–24	Hepatic metabolism (active metabolite)
Clonazepam	0.02–0.08	80–90	30–40	Hepatic metabolism
Diazepam		95	20–35	Hepatic metabolism (active metabolites)
Ethosuximide	40–100	0	20–60	Hepatic metabolism (25% excreted unchanged)
Felbamate		22–25	20–23	Renal excretion
Gabapentin	2–20	0	6	Renal excretion
Lamotrigine		54	25	Hepatic metabolism
Lorazepam		80	14	Hepatic metabolism
Oxcarbazepine		40	8–10	Renal excretion
Phenobarbital	10–40	48–54	72–144	Hepatic metabolism (25% excreted unchanged)
Phenytoin	10–20	90–93	9–40	Saturable hepatic metabolism
Primidone	5–12	20–30	4–12	Hepatic metabolism to active metabolites of which 40% are excreted unchanged
Tiagabine		95	5–8	Hepatic metabolism
Topiramate		10	8–15	Renal excretion and hepatic metabolism
Valproic acid	50–100	88–92	7–17	Hepatic metabolism (active metabolites)
Zonisamide		50	50–70	Hepatic Metabolism

Source: Adapted in part from Brodie MJ, Dichter MA. Antiepileptic drugs. *N Engl J Med* 1996;334:168–175; Dichter MA, Brodie MJ. New antiepileptic drugs. *N Engl J Med* 1996;334:1583–1590.

are effective in treatment of patients with generalized nonconvulsive seizures, especially absence seizures.

Adverse Side Effects

Antiepileptic drugs produce numerous and varied adverse side effect, most of which are tolerated by the patient. Some of the adverse side effects are dose-related (sedation, lethargy, neurotoxicity) whereas other side effects are seem to be idiosyncratic (hepatotoxicity, aplastic anemia) (see Table 30-3).

Maternal Epilepsy

Maternal epilepsy is associated with the risk of fetal malformations and treatment with antiepileptic drugs increases the risk from between 2% to 3% to between 4% to 6% (Yerby, 1994). All of the commonly used antiepileptic drugs cause major malformations including ventricular septal defects and cleft lip and palate. Valproate and carbamazepine treatment are associated with spina bifida. Midface abnormalities, digital hypoplasia, and nail-bed hypoplasia may occur in as many as 30% of infants of mothers treated with antiepileptic drugs. The mechanism of teratogenesis associated with antiepileptic drugs is not known. It is recommended that parturients receive the lowest effective dose of antiepileptic drugs (monotherapy is desirable) and supplemental folate is administered throughout the pregnancy.

Carbamazepine

Carbamazepine is an iminostilbene derivative that is effective for suppression of nonconvulsive and convulsive partial seizures. In addition, this drug is may be useful in the management of patients with trigeminal neuralgia and glossopharyngeal neuralgia. Structurally, carbamazepine is related to the tricyclic antidepressant imipramine. Like phenytoin, carbamazepine alters ionic conductance and thus has a membrane-stabilizing effect.

Pharmacokinetics

This drug is available only as an oral preparation (see Table 30-4). Oral absorption is rapid, with peak plasma concentrations occurring 2 to 6 hours after ingestion. Plasma protein binding is 70% to 80%. The plasma elimination half-time is 8 to 24 hours. The principal metabolite of carbamazepine is an epoxide derivative that has antiseizure effects and may be responsible for many of the dose-limiting side effects of this drug. Because this drug induces its own metabolism, many patients require a dosage increase in 2 to 4 weeks after initiation of therapy. The usual therapeutic plasma concentration of carbamazepine is 6 to 12 μg/mL.

Side Effects

The toxicity of carbamazepine is similar to that produced by phenytoin (see Table 30-3). Sedation, vertigo, diplopia, nausea, and vomiting are the most frequent side effects of this drug. Chronic diarrhea develops in some patients, whereas others experience the syndrome of inappropriate arginine vasopressin hormone (formerly known as antidiuretic hormone) secretion. Aplastic anemia, thrombocytopenia, hepatocellular and cholestatic jaundice, oliguria, hypertension, and cardiac dysrhythmias are rare but potentially life-threatening complications. Chronic suppression of white blood cell counts can occur. For these reasons, it may be prudent to monitor bone marrow, cardiac, hepatic, and renal function in patients being treated with carbamazepine. At high plasma concentrations, carbamazepine has an arginine vasopressin hormone-like action that may result in hyponatremia. Skin rash, often with other manifestations of drug allergy, occurs in approximately 10% of chronically treated patients.

In addition to inducing its own metabolism, carbamazepine can accelerate the hepatic oxidation and conjugation of other lipid-soluble drugs. The most common interaction is with oral contraceptive pills, and most women require an increase in the daily dose of estrogen. Carbamazepine also accelerates the metabolism of valproic acid, ethosuximide, corticosteroids, anticoagulants, and antipsychotic drugs. Drugs that inhibit the metabolism of carbamazepine sufficiently to cause toxic effects include cimetidine, propoxyphene, diltiazem, verapamil, isoniazid, and erythromycin.

Ethosuximide

Ethosuximide is the drug of choice for suppression of absence (petit mal) epilepsy in patients who do not also have tonic-clonic seizures. This drug acts by decreasing voltage-dependent calcium conductance in thalamic neurons. This is consistent with the speculated importance of the thalamocortical system in the etiology of absence seizures.

Pharmacokinetics

This drug is available only as an oral preparation (see Table 30-4). Peak plasma concentrations occur in 1 to 7 hours after oral administration. Ethosuximide is not significantly bound to albumin. Approximately 25% of the drug is excreted unchanged in urine, and the reminder is metabolized to inactive metabolites by hepatic microsomal enzymes. The elimination half-time is 20 to 60 hours. The usual maintenance dose of ethosuximide is 20 to 30 mg/kg. A plasma concentration of 40 to 100 μg/mL is required for satisfactory suppression of absence epilepsy.

Side Effects

Toxicity of ethosuximide is low, manifesting most often as gastrointestinal intolerance (nausea, vomiting) and CNS effects (lethargy, dizziness, ataxia, photophobia). There have been rare reports of bone marrow suppression.

Felbamate

Because of its potential to produce life-threatening side effects, felbamate is not used as a first-line drug for treatment of seizures but rather is reserved for patients with intractable epilepsy. Felbamate is used principally for poorly controlled partial and secondarily generalized seizures. It also decreases the frequency of seizures associated with the Lennox-Gastaut syndrome and myotonic and atonic forms of epilepsy (Dichter and Brodie, 1996). The presumed underlying mechanism of action of felbamate is binding to a glycine regulatory site, causing inhibition of the glycine-enhanced calcium current at the NMDA-induced calcium channels.

Pharmacokinetics

Oral absorption is prompt and the elimination half-time is prolonged (see Table 30-4) (Brodie and Dichter, 1996; Dichter and Brodie, 1996). Felbamate undergoes minimal metabolism with most of the drug being excreted unchanged by the kidneys.

Side Effects

Serious side effects include aplastic anemia and hepatotoxicity (see Table 30-3) (Brodie and Dichter, 1996; Dichter and Brodie, 1996). Monitoring of treated patients with complete blood counts and liver function tests is indicated. Because felbamate is metabolized by hepatic cytochrome P-450 enzymes, its metabolism is affected by concurrent administration of other drugs that are also metabolized by this system. In particular, comcomitant administration of carbamazepine or phenytoin may decrease plasma concentrations of felmabate. Likewise, since felbamate is a potent inhibitor of P-450 enzymes, it can slow the metabolism of phenytoin, phenobarbital, and valproic acid. In this regard, if a patient is receiving phenytoin, carbamazepine, or valproic acid and receives felbamate, the dose of these drugs should be decreased by 20% to 30% to prevent toxic effects.

Gabapentin

Gabapentin as a structural analogue of GABA is a safe and effective antiepileptic drug that is effective as either monotherapy or as an add-on therapy for partial seizures in children or adults. In addition, this drug has been effective in the treatment of a variety of chronic pain syndromes including neuropathic pain associated with diabetic neuropathy, postherpetic neuralgia, and reflex sympathetic dystrophy (Mao and Lucy, 2000; McGraw and Kosek, 1997). Preoperative oral gabapentin decreased pain scores and other analgesic consumption following total abdominal hysterectomy (Turan et al., 2004). The drug's mechanism of action is poorly understood but most likely reflects an increase in the synthesis of GABA independent of any direct drug action on $GABA_A$ receptors or inhibition of reuptake of GABA. Structurally, gabapentin resembles the inhibitory neurotransmitter GABA but the inclusion of a carbon ring greatly enhances its lipid solubility and ability to cross the blood-brain barrier.

The elimination half-time of gabapentin is brief, suggesting that multiple daily doses are necessary (see Table 30-4) (Brodie and Dichter, 1996; Dichter and Brodie, 1996). Gabapentin is well absorbed after oral administration, is not metabolized or bound to plasma proteins, but is excreted unchanged by the kidneys. The dose should be decreased in patients with renal dysfunction. Side effects of gabapentin are limited but may include somnolence, fatigue, ataxia, vertigo, and gastrointestinal disturbances (see Table 30-3) (Brodie and Dichter, 1996; Dichter and Brodie, 1996). Pharmacokinetic drug interactions with other drugs do not seem to occur reflecting the absence of protein binding and any effect on metabolism of other drugs (Dichter and Brodie, 1996). The renal clearance of gabapentin can be slowed by the administration of cimetidine.

Lamotrigine

Lamotrigine is a chemically novel anticonvulsant drug of the phenyltriazine class that most likely acts by stabilizing voltage-sensitive sodium ion channels, thus preventing release of aspartate and glutamate. This drug has a broad spectrum of activity and is effective when used alone or in combination in adults who have partial seizures or generalized seizures and in children with Lennox-Gastaut syndrome (Motte et al., 1997). When administered orally, lamotrigine is well absorbed, and its plasma elimination half-time is about 25 hours (see Table 30-4) (Brodie and Dichter, 1996; Dichter and Brodie, 1996). Drugs that induce hepatic microsomal enzymes (phenobarbital, phenytoin, and carbamazepine) decrease the elimination half-time of lamotrigine by about 50%, necessitating a higher dose (Dichter and Brodie, 1996). Conversely, valproic acid slows the metabolism of lamotrigine and extends its elimination half-time to about 60 hours. The most common side effects of lamotrigine are headache, nausea, vomiting, dizziness, diplopia, and ataxia (see Table 30-3) (Brodie and Dichter, 1996; Dichter and Brodie, 1996). Tremor can be troublesome at higher doses. In approximately 5% of adults, a rash develops, which subsequently disappears in some patients, despite continued therapy. In a few patients, however, the rash is more serious, and fever, arthralgias, and eosinophilia occur. In rare cases, Stevens-Johnson syndrome develops.

Levetiracetam

Levetiracetam is effective in the management of partial-onset seizures in adults. Its mechanism of action is not known. Side effects are considered minor and include sedation, asthenia, anxiety, and headache. The pharmacokinetic profile of levetiracetam is favorable, with the absence of hepatic metabolism and minimal protein binding. No significant drug interactions have been described with coadministration of other antiepileptic drugs.

Oxcarbazepine

Oxcarbazepine is a keto analogue of carbamazepine that provides equivalent seizure control but with fewer adverse side effects. After administration, oxcarbazepine acts as a prodrug being converted to an active metabolite, 10-hydroxycarbazepine. Oxcarbazepine and its active metabolite do not induce hepatic microsomal enzymes nor does it displace other drugs from plasma protein-binding sites.

Phenobarbital

Phenobarbital is a long-acting barbiturate that is effective against all seizure types except nonconvulsive primary generalized seizures. Cognitive and behavioral side effects limit this drug's usefulness in the treatment of epilepsy. Because of these side effects, phenobarbital is considered a second-line drug in the treatment of epilepsy.

Phenobarbital appears to exert its antiepileptic properties partly through modulation of the postsynaptic actions of the inhibitory neurotransmitter GABA and of the excitatory postsynaptic actions of glutamate. These drug-induced effects prolong the duration of chloride channel opening and thus limit the spread of seizure activity and increase the seizure threshold.

Pharmacokinetics

Oral absorption of phenobarbital is slow but nearly complete, with peak concentrations occurring 12 to 18 hours after a single dose (see Table 30-4). Plasma protein binding is 48% to 54%. Approximately 25% of phenobarbital is eliminated by pH-dependent renal excretion, with the remainder inactivated by hepatic microsomal enzymes. The principal metabolite is an inactive parahydroxyphenyl derivative that is excreted in urine as a sulfate conjugate. The elimination half-time of phenobarbital is prolonged.

The usual daily oral dose of phenobarbital is 60 mg in adults or 4 mg/kg in children. Plasma phenobarbital concentrations of 10 to 40 μg/mL are usually necessary for control of seizures. The value of measuring plasma phenobarbital concentrations is limited because the concentration associated with optimal control is highly variable among patients (Brodie and Dichter, 1996). In addition, the development of tolerance to the drug's CNS effects makes the toxic threshold imprecise.

Side Effects

Sedation in adults and children and irritability and hyperactivity in children are the most troublesome side effects when this drug is used to treat epilepsy (see Table 30-3). Tolerance to the sedative effects of phenobarbital may develop with chronic therapy. Depression develops in many adults taking phenobarbital, and confusion may occur in elderly patients. Cognitive effects include slowing of task processing. Scarlatiniform or morbilliform rash occurs in up to 2% of patients. Megaloblastic anemia that responds to folic acid administration and osteomalacia that responds to vitamin D therapy may occur during chronic phenobarbital therapy as well as during treatment with phenytoin. Nystagmus and ataxia are likely if the plasma phenobarbital concentration is >40 μg/mL. Abnormal collagen deposition manifesting as Dupuytren contracture may occur. Congenital malformations may occur when phenobarbital is administered chronically during pregnancy. A coagulation defect and hemorrhage in the neonate must be considered. Interactions between phenobarbital and other drugs usually involve induction of hepatic microsomal enzymes by phenobarbital. In this regard, phenobarbital is the classic example of a hepatic microsomal enzyme inducer that can accelerate the metabolism of many lipid-soluble drugs.

Phenytoin

Phenytoin is the prototype of the hydantoins and is effective for the treatment of partial and generalized seizures. Available in oral and intravenous (IV) preparations, phenytoin may be administered acutely to achieve effective plasma concentrations within 20 minutes. This drug has a high therapeutic index, and its administration is not accompanied by excessive sedation.

Mechanism of Action

Phenytoin regulates neuronal excitability and thus the spread of seizure activity from a seizure focus by regulating sodium and possibly calcium ion transport across neuronal membranes. This stabilizing effect on cell membranes is relatively selective for the cerebral cortex, although the effect also extends to peripheral nerves. In addition to the effect on ion fluxes, phenytoin acts on second messengers such as calmodulin and the cyclic nucleotides.

Pharmacokinetics

Phenytoin is a weak acid (pK 8.3) that is maintained in aqueous solutions as a sodium salt (see Table 30-4) (Brodie and Dichter, 1996; Dichter and Brodie, 1996). The drug precipitates in solutions with a pH of <7.8. Its poor water solubility may result in slow and sometimes variable absorption from the gastrointestinal tract (30% to 97%). The initial daily adult oral dosage is 3 to 4 mg/kg. Doses of >500 mg daily are rarely tolerated. The long duration of action of phenytoin allows a single daily dosage, but gastric intolerance may necessitate divided dosage. After intramuscular (IM) injection, the drug precipitates at the injection site and is slowly absorbed. For this reason, IM administration is not recommended. Infusion of phenytoin should probably not exceed 5 mg per minute.

Plasma Concentrations

Control of seizures is usually obtained when plasma concentrations of phenytoin are 10 to 20 μg/mL. In the control of digitalis-induced cardiac dysrhythmias, phenytoin, 0.5 to

1.0 mg/kg IV, is administered every 15 to 30 minutes until a satisfactory response is achieved or a maximum dose of 15 mg/kg is administered. A plasma phenytoin concentration of 8 to 16 μg/mL is usually sufficient to suppress cardiac dysrhythmias. Adverse side effects of phenytoin such as nystagmus and ataxia are likely when the plasma concentration of drug >20 μg/mL. Nevertheless, the diagnosis of phenytoin toxicity should be made on the basis of clinical symptoms.

Protein Binding

Phenytoin is bound approximately 90% to plasma albumin. A greater fraction of phenytoin remains unbound in neonates, in patients with hypoalbuminemia, and in uremic patients.

Metabolism

Metabolism of phenytoin to inactive metabolites is by hepatic microsomal enzymes that are susceptible to stimulation or inhibition by other drugs. An estimated 98% of phenytoin is metabolized to the inactive derivative parahydroxyphenyl, which appears in urine as a glucuronide. Approximately 2% of phenytoin is recovered unchanged in urine.

When the plasma concentration of phenytoin is <10 μg/mL, metabolism follows first-order kinetics, and the elimination half-time averages 24 hours. At plasma concentrations of >10 μg/mL, the enzymes necessary for metabolism of phenytoin become saturated, and the elimination half-time becomes dose-dependent (zero-order kinetics). At this stage, relatively small increases in dose may result in dramatic increases in the plasma concentration of phenytoin. Zero-order kinetics resembles the metabolism of alcohol.

Side Effects

The side effects of phenytoin include CNS toxicity that manifests clinically as nystagmus, ataxia, diplopia, vertigo (cerebellar-vestibular dysfunction) and is likely when the plasma phenytoin concentration is >20 μg/mL. Peripheral neuropathy has been observed in up to 30% of chronically treated patients. Gingival hyperplasia occurs in approximately 20% of chronically treated patients and is probably the most common manifestation of phenytoin toxicity in children and adolescents. This complication is minimized by improved oral hygiene and does not necessarily require discontinuation of phenytoin therapy. Other reversible cosmetic side effects include acne, hirsutism, and facial coarsening. Administration of phenytoin during pregnancy may result in the fetal hydantoin syndrome, which manifests as wide-set eyes, broad mandible, and finger deformities.

Allergic reactions include morbilliform rash in 2% to 5% of patients. Hyperglycemia and glycosuria may reflect phenytoin-induced inhibition of insulin secretion. Megaloblastic anemia is rare and has been attributed to altered folic acid absorption but probably also involves altered folic acid metabolism. Phenytoin-induced hepatotoxicity, although rare, may occur in genetically susceptible persons who lack the enzyme phenytoin epoxide (Spielberg et al., 1981). This enzyme is necessary to convert an electrophilic intermediate formed after the oxidative metabolism of phenytoin to an inert and nontoxic product. Gastrointestinal irritation is due to alkalinity of the drug; this may be minimized by taking phenytoin after meals.

Phenytoin can induce the oxidative metabolism of many lipid-soluble drugs, including carbamazepine, valproic acid, ethosuximide, anticoagulants, and corticosteroids. Because its metabolism is saturable, inhibitory interactions are particularly likely to have neurotoxic effects. Interactions involving protein-binding displacement are not likely to be clinically significant.

Patients receiving phenytoin chronically have higher dose requirements for nondepolarizing neuromuscular-blocking drugs such as vecuronium compared with untreated patients (Wright et al., 2004). Phenytoin induces hepatic enzymes and it is likely that metabolism and elimination of nondepolarizing neuromuscular-blocking drugs is increased. Phenytoin may also produce mild blocking effects at the neuromusular junction leading to up-regulation of acetylcholine receptors.

Primidone

Primidone is metabolized to phenobarbital and another active metabolite, phenylethylmalonamide. The efficacy of this drug resembles that of phenobarbital, but it is less well tolerated. There is little to recommend this drug over phenobarbital for patients in whom treatment with a barbiturate is contemplated (Brodie and Dichter, 1996).

Tiagabine

Tiagabine is a nipecotic acid moiety that is a potent inhibitor of GABA reuptake. This drug is utilized as adjunctive therapy for complex partial seizures. Possible side effects include dizziness, asthenia, aphasia, and tremor. Mental depression may accompany administration of tigabine perhaps reflecting this drug's ability to increase GABA concentrations. Drug interactions are unlikely despite the high protein binding of tiagabine reflecting the small amount of drug needed to achieve clinical efficacy. Tiagabine has no effect on hepatic enzymes.

Topiramate

Topiramate is a broad-spectrum antiepileptic drug that is indicated as monotherapy or adjunctive therapy in children and adults for the control of partial, generalized tonic-clonic, and absence seizures. Efficacy in treatment of other neurologic and psychiatric disorders has been described including bulimia, migraine headache, and essential tremor. This drug is a monosaccharide that is produced by sulfamate substitution of the R-enantiomer of fructose. Topiramate produces inhibition of voltage-gated sodium ion channels, inhibition of high-voltage activated calcium ion channels, enhancement of $GABA_A$-mediated receptor chloride ion flux, and inhibition of glutamate-mediated neurotransmission at specific receptor subtypes (Brandes et al., 2004). In addition, topiramate is a weak inhibitor of carbonic anhydrase. Minor side effects may include sedation, dizziness, and ataxia. Nephrolithiasis occurs in about 1.5% of treated patients perhaps reflecting this drug's action on carbonic anhydrase. Enzyme-inducing drugs decrease plasma concentrations of topiramate but in contrast, this drug does not affect hepatic P-450 enzymes and undergoes minimal protein binding.

Valproic Acid

Valproic acid is a branched-chain carboxylic acid that is effective in the treatment of all primary generalized epilepsies and all convulsive epilepsies. It is somewhat less effective for the suppression of nonconvulsive partial seizures. This drug acts by limiting sustained repetitive neuronal firing through voltage-dependent sodium channels.

Pharmacokinetics

Valproic acid is available as a syrup and in an enteric-coated formulation, which is preferred because it decreases gastrointestinal side effects. After oral administration, absorption is prompt, with peak plasma concentrations of valproic acid occurring in 1 to 4 hours. Binding to plasma proteins is >80%. More than 70% of the drug can be recovered as inactive glucuronide conjugates. The elimination half-time is 7 to 17 hours. The usual daily dose of valproic acid is 1 to 3 g to achieve a therapeutic plasma concentration of 50 to 100 μg/mL. Nevertheless, the daily variation in plasma concentrations of valproic acid is great, and routine monitoring may not be helpful unless it is correlated with the patient's clinical condition.

Side Effects

Gastrointestinal side effects include anorexia, nausea, and vomiting. Weight gain is common in patients treated chronically with valproic acid. At higher doses, a fine distal tremor may develop. Thrombocytopenia is seen frequently at higher doses. The most serious side effect of valproic acid is hepatotoxicity occurring in about 0.2% of children younger than 2 years of age being treated chronically with this drug. The incidence of this potentially fatal hepatic necrosis decreases dramatically after 2 years of age. Approximately 20% of treated patients have hyperammonemia without hepatic damage. Sedation and ataxia are infrequent side effects of valproic acid.

Because valproic acid is partly eliminated as a ketone-containing metabolite, the urine ketone test may show false-positive results. Valproic acid can displace phenytoin and diazepam from protein-binding sites, resulting in increased pharmacologic effects produced by the displaced drug.

Valproic acid is an enzyme inhibitor. As a result of this enzyme inhibition, the metabolism of phenytoin is slowed by valproic acid. Valproic acid causes the plasma concentration of phenobarbital to increase almost 50%, presumably due to inhibition of hepatic microsomal enzymes. Valproic acid does not interfere with the action of oral contraceptives.

Zonisamide

Zonisamide is a broad spectrum antiepileptic drug utilized as adjunctive therapy for management of partial and secondarily generalized seizures. An effect on voltage-dependent calcium ion channels seems to be an important mechanism for this drugs ability to control seizures. In addition, zonisamide enhances GABA-mediated neuronal inhibition. Adverse side effects include sedation, dizziness, ataxia, anorexia, and behavioral disorders in children and manic responses in adults. Nephrolithiasis may occur in 3% of treated patients. Pharmacokinetic drug interactions are unlikely as zonisamide does not displace other drugs from protein binding sites and effects on metabolism of other drugs is minimal.

Benzodiazepines

Benzodiazepines display anxiolytic, sedative, muscle-relaxant, and anticonvulsant effects (see Chapter 5). Benzodiazepine receptors in the brain are associated with $GABA_A$ receptors. The binding of benzodiazepines to these receptors potentiates GABA-mediated neuronal inhibition, which increases chloride permeability and thereby leads to cellular hyperpolarization and inhibition of neuronal firing. In low doses, benzodiazepines suppress polysynaptic activity in the spinal cord and decrease neuronal activity in the mesencephalic reticular system.

Clonazepam

Clonazepam is generally added to other drug therapy and is the first-line drug only for myoclonic seizures.

Pharmacokinetics

Absorption of clonazepam after oral administration is rapid, with peak plasma concentrations occurring within 2 to 4 hours (see Table 30-4). IV administration of clonazepam results in rapid CNS effects. Approximately 50% of the drug is bound to plasma proteins. Clonazepam is extensively metabolized to inactive products, with <2% of an injected dose appearing unchanged in urine. The elimination half-time of this long-acting drug is 30 to 40 hours. The oral maintenance dose is unlikely to exceed 0.25 mg/kg. Therapeutic plasma concentrations of clonazepam are 0.02 to 0.08 μg/mL.

Side Effects

Sedation is present in approximately 50% of patients but tends to subside with chronic administration (see Table 30-3). Skeletal muscle incoordination and ataxia occur in approximately 30% of patients. Personality changes occur in approximately 25% of patients, manifesting as behavioral disturbances, including hyperactivity, irritability, and difficulty in concentration, especially in children. Elderly patients treated with clonazepam may experience depression. Increased salivary and bronchial secretions may be particularly prominent in children. Generalized seizure activity may be precipitated if the drug is discontinued abruptly. Hypotension and depression of ventilation have been observed after IV administration of clonazepam.

Diazepam

Diazepam is a mainstay for the treatment of status epilepticus and local anesthetic-induced seizures. The typical approach is administration of 0.1 mg/kg IV every 10 to 15 minutes until seizure activity has been suppressed or a maximum dose of 30 mg has been administered (see Chapter 5). Diazepam has a long elimination half-time of 27 to 48 hours. Metabolism of diazepam results in active metabolites.

Lorazepam

Lorazepam has a shorter elimination half-time (8 to 25 hours) than diazepam but a longer duration of antiepileptic action because it is not rapidly redistributed. Lorazepam is metabolized in the liver and has no active metabolites. Lorazepam, which is available in parenteral and oral formulations, is used to treat status epilepticus and as intermittent therapy for seizure clusters.

STATUS EPILEPTICUS

Status epilepticus is defined as continuous seizures or two or more seizures occurring in sequence without recovery of consciousness between seizures. The motor manifestations of convulsive status epilepticus may be symmetrical with tonic and then clonic activity.

Treatment

Treatment begins with life support including ensuring a patent upper airway and maintenance of ventilation that may require tracheal intubation. IV access is obtained in anticipation of administering an antiepileptic drug. If hypoglycemia cannot be excluded, the patient is treated empirically with IV glucose (50 mL of 50% glucose for adults and 2 mL/kg of 25% glucose for children).

Drug therapy of status epilepticus is typically with a benzodiazepine such as diazepam or lorazepam. In the absence of IV access, a rectal gel form of diazepam is available. Ventilatory depression necessitating support of ventilation may accompany administration of benzodiazepines. If diazepam is used to terminate status epilepticus, a long-acting antiepileptic drug such as fosphenytoin (water-soluble prodrug form of phenytoin) is needed (up to 150 mg/min IV or 3 mg/kg IV in children). Hypotension and prolongation of the QT interval on the electrocardiogram may accompany administration of fosphenytoin necessitating a slowing in the rate of IV infusion. Alternatively, phenobarbital 10 to 20 mg/kg IV is useful for treating status epilepticus.

REFERENCES

Brodie MJ, Dichter MA. Antiepileptic drugs. *N Engl J Med* 1996;334:168–175.

Brandes JL, Saper JR, Diamond M, et al. Topiramate for migraine prevention. A randomized controlled trial. *JAMA* 2004;291:965–973.

Dichter MA, Brodie MJ. New antiepileptic drugs. *N Engl J Med* 1996;334:1583–1590.

Mao J, Chen LL. Gabapentin in pain management. *Anesth Analg* 2000;91:680–687.

Mattson RH, Cramer JA, Darney PD, et al. Use of oral contraceptives by women with epilepsy. *JAMA* 1986;256:238–241.

McGraw T, Kosek P. Erythromelalgia pain managed with gabapentin. *Anesthesiology* 1997;86:988–990.

Motte J, Trevathan E, Arvidsson JFV, et al. Lamotrigine for generalized seizures associated with the Lennox-Gastaut syndrome. *N Engl J Med* 1997;337:1807–1812.

Spielberg SP, Gordon GB, Blake DA, et al. Predisposition to phenytoin hepatotoxicity assessed in vitro. *N Engl J Med* 1981;305:722–727.

Tempelhoff R, Modica PA, Jellish WS, et al. Resistance to atracurium-induced neuromuscular blockade in patients with intractable seizure disorders treated with anticonvulsants. *Anesth Analg* 1990;71:665–670.

Turan A, Karamalhoglu B, Memis D, et al. The analgesic effects of gabapentin after total abdominal hysterectomy. *Anesth Analg* 2004;98:1370–1373.

Wright PC, McCarthy G, Szenohradszky J et al. Influence of chronic phenytoin administration on the pharmacokinetics and pharmacodynamics of vecuronium. *Anesthesiology* 2004;100:626–633.

Yerby MS. Pregnancy, teratogenesis, and epilepsy. *Neurol Clin* 1994;12:749–753.

31

Drugs Used for Treatment of Parkinson Disease

Parkinson disease (paralysis agitans) is a neurodegenerative disease that results from a deficiency of dopaminergic innervation of the basal ganglia from the substantia nigra. Degeneration of the nigrostriatal pathway leads to the depletion of the neurotransmitter dopamine. Conceptually, dopamine is thought to act principally as an inhibitory neurotransmitter and acetylcholine as an excitatory neurotransmitter in the extrapyramidal system. Although dopamine is more important, a proper balance with the cholinergic neurotransmitter is also necessary for normal function.

The goal of treating Parkinson disease is to enhance the inhibitory effect of dopamine or to decrease the excitatory effect of acetylcholine by the administration of centrally acting drugs. Often, combinations of drugs with effects on the dopaminergic and cholinergic components of the extrapyramidal nervous system are used. Regardless of the drug or drugs selected, treatment of Parkinson disease is always palliative, emphasizing that therapy does not halt progression of neuronal degeneration. In fact, the gradual loss of responsiveness to drug therapy that occurs over 1 to 5 years may be caused in part by the decreasing capacity of nigrostriatal neurons to synthesize and store dopamine. There is no general agreement on how and when antiparkinsonian drug therapy should be initiated (Calne, 1993).

Approximately 80% of the dopamine in the brain is concentrated in the basal ganglia, mostly in the caudate nucleus and putamen. In patients with Parkinson disease, the basal ganglia content of dopamine is only approximately 10% of normal. As a result, there is an excess of excitatory cholinergic activity, manifesting as progressive tremor, skeletal muscle rigidity, bradykinesia, and disturbances of posture. In addition to these classic peripheral manifestations of Parkinson disease, approximately one-fifth of afflicted patients become mentally depressed and one-third develop cognitive and memory deficits that may progress to delirium. Alzheimer disease is more common in patients with Parkinson disease (Boller et al., 1980).

LEVODOPA

Because dopamine does not readily cross the blood-brain barrier, the major approaches to therapy have involved the administration of its precursor, levodopa, or drugs that mimic the action of dopamine (Fig. 31-1). In this regard, levodopa is the cornerstone of symptomatic therapy of Parkinson disease. Levodopa crosses the blood-brain barrier and is converted to dopamine by aromatic-L-amino-acid decarboxylase (dopa decarboxylase enzyme), acting to replenish dopamine stores in the basal ganglia. Levodopa is usually administered with a peripheral decarboxylase inhibitor (carbidopa or benserazide) to maximize entrance of this precursor into the brain before it is converted to dopamine. Furthermore, side effects associated with increased plasma concentrations of dopamine should be less when it is combined with a decarboxylase inhibitor. Absorption of levodopa from the gastrointestinal tract is efficient, but the brief elimination half-time (1 to 3 hours) requires frequent dosing intervals to maintain a therapeutic concentration. An intravenous (IV) formulation of levodopa is not available.

The beneficial therapeutic response to levodopa typically diminishes after 1 to 5 years of treatment, presumably reflecting progression of the disease process and continuing loss of nigrostriatal neurons with a capacity to store dopamine. Abrupt discontinuation of levodopa therapy may result in a precipitous return of symptoms of Parkinson disease and has been associated with a neuroleptic malignant-like syndrome

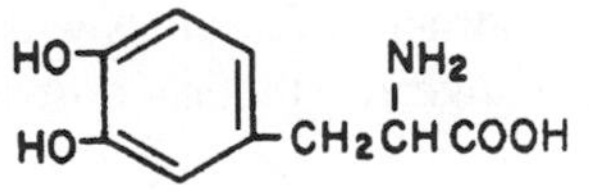

Figure 31-1. Levodopa.

(Smith et al., 1996). For this reason, levodopa should be continued throughout the perioperative period, being included in the preoperative medication.

Metabolism

Approximately 95% of orally administered levodopa is rapidly decarboxylated to dopamine during the initial passage through the liver. The resulting dopamine cannot easily cross the blood-brain barrier to exert beneficial effects, whereas increased plasma concentrations of dopamine often lead to undesirable side effects. In this regard, inhibition of the peripheral activity of the decarboxylase enzyme greatly increases the fraction of administered levodopa that remains intact to cross the blood-brain barrier.

At least 30 metabolites of levodopa have been identified. Most of these metabolites are converted to dopamine, small amounts of which are subsequently metabolized to norepinephrine and epinephrine. Metabolism of dopamine yields 3,4-dihydroxyphenylacetic acid (homovanillic acid). Dietary methionine is necessary as a source of methyl donors to permit continued activity of catechol-O-methyltransferase (COMT), which is necessary for the metabolism of the excess amounts of dopamine that result from high doses of levodopa. Most metabolites of dopamine are excreted by the kidneys.

Side Effects

The most common side effects that occur during the first weeks of therapy with levodopa and dopamine agonists are nausea and hypotension (Calne, 1993). These side effects are associated with peak plasma concentrations of dopamine and may be minimized by taking medications after light meals or snacks. The most common problems that occur during long-term therapy are dyskinesias, fluctuations in mobility, increasing confusion, and psychosis. These problems become progressively more frequent after the first 3 years of therapy.

Gastrointestinal Dysfunction

Nausea and vomiting occur in about 80% of patients during the early period of treatment with levodopa. Presumably, these responses reflect dopamine-induced stimulation of the chemoreceptor trigger zone, which is not protected by the blood-brain barrier. Antiemetic drugs that cross the blood-brain barrier may interfere with the action of dopamine at the basal ganglia and for this reason are not recommended for treatment of nausea associated with levodopa therapy. In contrast, nausea can be effectively prevented by domperidone (10 to 20 mg orally administered 30 to 60 minutes before levodopa), which does not easily cross the blood-brain barrier and is therefore unlikely to exacerbate symptoms of Parkinson disease (Calne, 1993). Domperidone inhibits $dopamine_2$ receptors in the chemoreceptor trigger zone of the medulla oblongata. Antiemetics such as dopamine-receptor antagonists (prochlorperazine, metoclopramide) should be avoided because they significantly worsen symptoms of Parkinson disease. Long-term antiemetic treatment with 5-HT_3 antagonists is not practical due to the expense of these drugs. Gastrointestinal side effects tend to disappear with continuing therapy as tolerance develops.

Cardiovascular Changes

Cardiovascular changes associated with levodopa most likely reflect alpha- and beta-adrenergic responses evoked by increased plasma concentrations of dopamine. Transient flushing of the skin is common during levodopa therapy.

Orthostatic Hypotension

For unknown reasons, approximately 30% of patients develop orthostatic hypotension early in therapy. As a result, some patients experience vertigo and, rarely, syncope. Increased fluid and sodium intake may be useful in decreasing the likelihood of orthostatic hypotension. If symptoms are persistent, administration of fludrocortisone or an alpha-adrenergic agonist may be useful (Calne, 1993). Orthostatic hypotension becomes less prominent with continued therapy. It is of interest that dopamine resulting from levodopa may displace norepinephrine from peripheral sympathetic nerve endings and interfere with adrenergic transmission.

Cardiac Dysrhythmias

Cardiac dysrhythmias, including sinus tachycardia, atrial and ventricular premature contractions, atrial fibrillation, and ventricular tachycardia, although rare, have been associated with levodopa therapy. Presumably, the potential beta-adrenergic effects of dopamine on the heart contribute to cardiac dysrhythmias, although a cause-and-effect relationship has not been documented. Patients with preexisting disturbances of cardiac conduction or coronary artery disease are most likely to develop cardiac dysrhythmias in association with levodopa therapy. Propranolol is an effective treatment when cardiac dysrhythmias occur in these patients.

Abnormal Involuntary Movements

Abnormal involuntary movements in the form of faciolingual tics, grimacing, and rocking movements of the arms, legs, or trunk are the most common side effects of chronic levodopa therapy, developing in about 50% of patients within 1 to 4 months after initiation of therapy. Rarely, exaggerated respiratory movements can produce an irregular gasping pattern, presumably reflecting dyskinesias of the diaphragm and intercostal muscles. Tolerance does not develop to abnormal involuntary movements.

Fluctuations in mobility are characterized by increasing bradykinesia at the end of an interval between doses. High-protein meals are avoided in patients who experience sudden loss of mobility because a large influx of dietary amino acids can interfere with the transport of levodopa into the brain.

Psychiatric Disturbances

Psychiatric disturbances include confusion, visual hallucinations, and paranoia, which may reflect the disease as well as its treatment. Elderly patients are particularly vulnerable to psychotic reactions, especially if treatment includes combinations of levodopa and anticholinergic drugs. Psychiatric disturbances usually begin as nocturnal phenomena, emphasizing the possible value of decreasing or discontinuing the last evening dose of levodopa. Neuroleptic drugs are not recommended for the treatment of psychiatric disturbances because these drugs may cause a protracted exacerbation of symptoms of Parkinson disease. Clonazepam may be useful in some patients, but there is a risk of agranulocytosis with high doses of this drug. Patients who develop drug-induced psychosis with no features of dementia may respond to electroconvulsive therapy.

Endocrine Changes

Dopamine inhibits the secretion of prolactin, presumably by stimulating the release of a prolactin inhibitory factor. The release of growth hormone that occurs in response to the administration of levodopa to normal patients is minimal or absent when levodopa is administered to patients with Parkinson disease. Indeed, signs of acromegaly or diabetes mellitus do not occur in patients treated with levodopa. Large doses of levodopa may cause hypokalemia associated with increased plasma levels of aldosterone.

Laboratory Measurements

Urinary metabolites of levodopa cause false-positive tests for ketoacidosis. These metabolites also color the urine red and then black on exposure to air. Mild, transient increases in the blood urea nitrogen concentration may occur and can usually be controlled by increasing fluid intake. Increased liver transaminase concentrations occasionally occur. Positive Coombs' tests have been attributed to levodopa.

Drug Interactions

Drug interactions may occur in patients being treated with levodopa, resulting in increased or decreased therapeutic effects. Chronic treatment of animals with levodopa does not consistently change anesthetic requirements.

Antipsychotic Drugs

Antipsychotic drugs such as butyrophenones and phenothiazines can antagonize the effects of dopamine. For this reason, these drugs should not be administered to patients with known or suspected Parkinson disease. Indeed, administration of droperidol to patients being treated with levodopa has produced severe skeletal muscle rigidity and even pulmonary edema, presumably reflecting sudden antagonism of dopamine (Ngai, 1972). Droperidol has even produced a Parkinson disease-like syndrome in otherwise healthy patients (Rivera et al., 1975). Metoclopramide may also interfere with dopamine activity.

Monoamine Oxidase Inhibitors

Nonspecific monoamine oxidase inhibitors interfere with the inactivation of catecholamines, including dopamine. As a result, these drugs can exaggerate the peripheral and central nervous system (CNS) effects of levodopa. Hypertension and hyperthermia are side effects associated with the concurrent administration of these drugs.

Anticholinergic Drugs

Anticholinergic drugs act synergistically with levodopa to improve certain symptoms of Parkinson disease, especially tremor. Large doses of anticholinergics, however, can slow gastric emptying such that absorption of levodopa from the gastrointestinal tract is decreased.

Pyridoxine

Pyridoxine, in doses as low as 5 mg as present in multivitamin preparations, can abolish the therapeutic efficacy of levodopa by enhancing the activity of pyridoxine-dependent dopa decarboxylase and thus increasing the metabolism of levodopa in the circulation before it can enter the CNS.

PERIPHERAL DECARBOXYLASE INHIBITORS

Levodopa is usually administered with a peripheral carboxylase inhibitor such as carbidopa or benserazide (Fig. 31-2). As a result, more levodopa escapes metabolism to dopamine in the peripheral circulation and is available to enter the CNS. Furthermore, side effects related to high systemic concentrations of dopamine are decreased when levodopa is

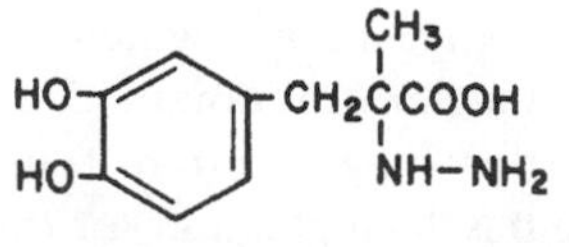

Figure 31-2. Carbidopa.

administered with a peripheral decarboxylase inhibitor. Nausea, vomiting, and cardiac dysrhythmias are diminished or absent. The incidence of abnormal involuntary movements and psychiatric disturbances is not altered by the combination of levodopa with a decarboxylase inhibitor.

Several combinations of levodopa and a peripheral carboxylase inhibitor are available (levodopa augmentation strategies). Sinemet is composed of levodopa and carbidopa in a 10:1 or 4:1 ratio. Madopar is composed of levodopa and benserazide in a 4:1 ratio. Controlled-release preparations of levodopa and carbidopa provide a more constant therapeutic effect, but the onset of action is slower and the bioavailability is decreased compared with the standard combinations. Both carbidopa and benserazide are non-competitive inhibitors of decarboxylase so there is no value in administering progressively higher doses of these enzyme inhibitors. Carbidopa and benserazide do not cross the blood-brain barrier and lack pharmacologic activity when administered alone.

Catechol-O-methyltransferase Inhibitors

COMT is partially responsible for the peripheral breakdown of levodopa. Accordingly, another levodopa augmentation strategy consists of blocking the COMT enzyme activity with tolcapone or entacapone. Administration of either of these drugs slows the elimination of carbidopa-levodopa thus increasing the plasma concentrations by 10% to 15%. In patients treated with tolcapone, the daily dose of carbidopa-levodopa may need to be decreased by 10% to 30% to avoid dyskinesias or other hyperdopaminergic side effects.

Side Effects

Both tolcapone and entacapone worsen levodopa-induced dyskinesias and cause nausea and diarrhea. Tolcapone may cause hepatotoxicity in rare patients empahsizing the need to monitor liver function tests in treated patients. Rhabdomyolysis has been associated with tolcapone therapy. Entacapone can cause the patient's urine to appear orange. Both drugs can cause piloerection.

SYNTHETIC DOPAMINE AGONISTS

Synthetic dopamine agonists require neither transformation or facilitated transport across the blood-brain barrier as they act directly on postsynaptic dopamine receptors (Calne, 1993). Available drugs include bromocriptine and pergolide (tetracyclic ergot alkaloids) and pramipexole and ropinirole (nonergot alkaloids) (Fig. 31-3). After oral administration, the elimination half-time of bromocriptine and pergolide are longer than for levodopa. Absorption of bromocriptine from the gastrointestinal tract is rapid but incomplete. Extensive hepatic first-pass metabolism occurs and >90% of the metabolites are excreted in the bile, whereas <10% of the drug is excreted unchanged or as inactive metabolites in urine. Bromocriptine, 0.5 to 1.0 mg orally, is equivalent to levodopa, 100 mg in combination with either 25 mg of carbidopa or 25 mg of benserazide. The effectiveness of bromocriptine in the treatment of acromegaly reflects the paradoxical inhibitory effect of dopamine agonists on secretion of growth hormone. Bromocriptine also suppresses the excess prolactin secretion that is often associated with growth hormone secretion.

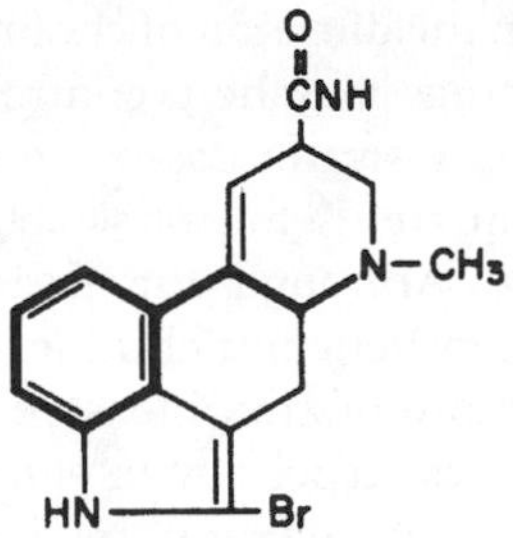

Figure 31-3. Bromocriptine.

Side Effects

Visual and auditory hallucinations, hypotension, and dyskinesia occur more frequently in patients treated with bromocriptine than in those treated with levodopa. Synthetic dopamine agonists occasionally cause pleuropulmonary fibrosis, sometimes with pleural effusions (Bhatt et al., 1991). Depending on the severity of this side effect, the dose of agonist drug should be decreased or the drug discontinued. Another uncommon complication of dopamine agonist therapy is the development of erythromelalgia (red, edematous, tender extremities) (Eisler et al., 1981). If this complication occurs, it is usually necessary to discontinue the dopamine agonist. Asymptomatic increases of serum transaminase and alkaline phosphatase concentrations may occur. Vertigo and nausea are occasionally associated with bromocriptine therapy.

Nonergot alkaloids are supposed to cause less nausea and orthostatic hypotension than the ergot derivatives but this difference appears to be clinically insignificant. Nonergot alkaloids offer no advantage over ergot derivatives with respect to CNS side effects including confusion, hallucinations, and daytime sleep attacks that have been associated with motor vehicle accidents.

ANTICHOLINERGIC DRUGS

Anticholinergic drugs such as trihexyphenidyl and benztropine have modest effects on the clinical manifestations of Parkinson disease (Calne, 1993). These drugs blunt the effects of the excitatory neurotransmitter acetylcholine, thus correcting the balance between dopamine and acetylcholine that is disturbed in the direction of cholinergic dominance. Anticholinergic drugs may help control the tremor and decrease the excess salivation associated with Parkinson disease but seldom are useful for skeletal muscle rigidity and bradykinesia. Although the peripheral and CNS actions of these synthetic anticholinergic drugs are less prominent than those of atropine, side effects, including memory disturbances (especially in elderly patients), hallucinations, confusion, sedation, mydriasis, cycloplegia, adynamic ileus, and urinary retention, may still occur. The mydriatic effect could precipitate glaucoma in a susceptible patient. As more effective drugs have become available, the use of anticholinergic drugs to treat patients with Parkinson disease has diminished (Calne, 1993).

AMANTADINE

Amantadine is an antiviral drug used for prophylaxis against infection with influenza A. This drug was discovered by chance to also produce symptomatic improvement in patients with Parkinson disease. The mode of action of amantadine is not known, although it has been speculated to facilitate the release of dopamine from dopaminergic terminals that remain in the nigrostriatum of patients with this disease. In addition, amantadine may delay uptake of dopamine back into nerve endings, exert anticholinergic effects, is a weak glutamate antagonist, and exhibits noncompetitive antagonist effects at *N*-methyl-D-aspartate receptors. Unlike anticholinergic drugs, amantadine may result in some improvement in skeletal muscle rigidity and bradykinesia. Amantadine is well absorbed after oral administration, and the elimination half-time is approximately 12 hours. More than 90% of the drug is excreted unchanged by the kidneys, necessitating dosage adjustments in patients with renal dysfunction. The side effects are similar to those produced by anticholinergic drugs, but in addition, chronic administration of amantadine tends to induce ankle edema and livedo reticularis of the legs with or without cardiac failure. In older patients, amantadine may aggravate confusion and psychosis.

SELEGILINE

Selegiline is a highly selective and irreversible inhibitor of monoamine oxidase type B enzyme (MAO-B) that has a weak antiparkisnonian effect when used alone and a moderate effect when used as an adjunct to carbidopa-levodopa.

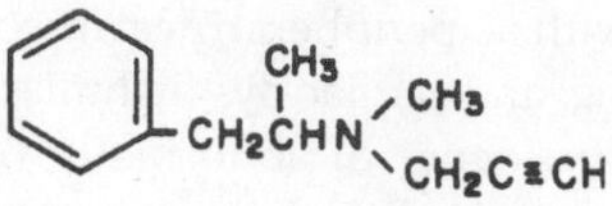

Figure 31-4. Selegiline.

(Fig. 31-4) (Calne, 1993). MAO-B enzyme activity is one of the principal catabolic pathways for dopaine in the central nervous system. Blocking MAO-B enzyme activity increases the intrasynaptic half-time of dopamine leading to improved motor fluctuations and tremor. In contrast to nonspecific monoamine oxidase inhibitors, selegiline does not result in life-threatening potentiation of the effects of catecholamines when administered concurrently with a centrally active amine (Severn, 1988). This reflects the fact that metabolism of norepinephrine in peripheral nerve endings is not altered by selegiline, which minimizes the likelihood of adverse responses during anesthesia in response to sympathomimetics. Insomnia is a significant side effect of sergiline. Other side effects of selegiline include confusion, hallucinations, mental depression, and paranoid ideation.

NONPHARMACOLOGIC TREATMENT

Transplantation of fetal mesencephalic tissue and posteroventral pallidotomy represent surgical approaches to the treatment of patients with Parkinson disease (Calne, 1993). In the future, implantation of cells grown in culture and genetically engineered to produce a desirable profile of biologic activities is likely.

REFERENCES

Bhatt MH, Keenan SP, Feetham JA, et al. Pleuropulmonary disease associated with dopamine agonist therapy. *Ann Neurol* 1991;30:613–616.

Boller F, Mizatani T, Roessmann U, et al. Parkinson disease, dementia and Alzheimer disease: clinicopathological correlations. *Ann Neurol* 1980;7:329–335.

Calne DB. Treatment of Parkinson's disease. *N Engl J Med* 1993;329:1021–1027.

Eisler T, Hall RP, Kalavar KA, et al. Erythromelalgia-like eruption in parkinsonian patients treated with bromocriptine. *Neurology* 1981;31:1368–1370.

Ngai SH. Parkinsonism, levodopa, and anesthesia. *Anesthesiology* 1972;37:344–351.

Rivera VM, Keichian AH, Iliver RE. Persistent parkinsonism following neuroleptanalgesia. *Anesthesiology* 1975;43:635–637.

Severn AM. Parkinsonism and the anaesthetist. *Br J Anaesth* 1988;61:761–770.

Smith MS, Muir H, Hall R. Perioperative management of drug therapy: clinical considerations. *Drugs* 1996;51:238–259.

Drug Treatment of Lipid Disorders

32

Lipoproteins are classified as (a) chylomicrons, (b) very-low-density lipoproteins (VLDLs), (c) intermediate-density lipoproteins (IDLs), (d) low-density lipoproteins (LDLs), and (e) high-density lipoproteins (HDLs) (see Table 58-2). Hypercholesterolemia can occur from increases in the plasma concentrations of any of these forms of lipoproteins). Increased plasma concentrations of total cholesterol and LDL cholesterol, and low plasma concentrations of HDL cholesterol are associated with an increased risk of cardiovascular disease. Lower total and LDL plasma concentrations of cholesterol decreases the risk of coronary events in patients with and without coronary artery disease (CAD) (Downs et al., 1998; Steinberg and Gotto, 1999). Because LDLs are the principal cholesterol-carrying lipoproteins in plasma, there is a predictable relationship between increases in the plasma concentrations of LDL cholesterol and accelerated atherosclerosis. Lowering the plasma cholesterol concentration retards the progression of coronary artery plaques and promotes their regression. Indeed, lowering the plasma cholesterol concentration decreases macrophage activity and the accumulation of cholesterol and improves endothelial integrity and function, making atherosclerotic lesions more stable and less likely to fissure. Plasma concentrations of HDL cholesterol are inversely related to the risk for CAD (Fiedling, 1992). The relationship of plasma concentrations of triglycerides to the risk of CAD are not as well established as for cholesterol (The BIP Group, 2000).

Removal of LDL cholesterol from the plasma, and thus control of the plasma concentration of cholesterol, occurs principally by attachment to LDL receptors on the surfaces of hepatic cells. These receptors invaginate and internalize LDL cholesterol by endocytosis where lysosomal hydrolytic enzymes subsequently exert their effects. Synthesis of these receptors is genetically determined, with one gene from each parent. Inheritance of one nonfunctional and one normal gene (heterozygous) for LDL receptors results in plasma cholesterol levels that are approximately twice the normal level. The incidence of heterozygous familial hypercholesterolemia is approximately 1 in 500 persons, and affected persons are prone to development of premature CAD. Less common is homozygous familial hypercholesterolemia, in which abnormal genes are inherited from both parents, plasma cholesterol concentrations are approximately four times normal, and early atherosclerosis is likely. A high plasma HDL cholesterol concentration is a powerful protective factor against the development of CAD because HDLs are essential for the retrieval of cholesterol from cells and tissues (reverse cholesterol transport) (Fielding, 1992).

It is estimated that 15% to 20% of the population has hypercholesterolemia. Guidelines for the treatment of patients with increased plasma concentrations of total cholesterol focus on interventions to decrease LDL cholesterol (Table 32-1) (Executive Summary, 2001). The choice of drug or drugs to treat lipid disorders is guided by the patient's plasma triglyceride levels (Table 32-2) (Havel and Rapaport, 1995; Fortmann and Maron, 1998). Side effects, cost, and convenience also influence drug selection. Dietary regulation (avoidance of foods high in cholesterol or saturated animal fat), exercise, and weight reduction are important components of any drug therapy designed to lower plasma lipid concentrations.

DRUGS FOR TREATMENT OF INCREASED PLASMA LOW-DENSITY LIPOPROTEIN CHOLESTEROL CONCENTRATIONS

Drugs for treatment of increased plasma LDL cholesterol concentrations act by a variety of mechanisms, including bile acid binding in the intestine, inhibition of the rate-limiting enzyme in cholesterol synthesis (3-hydroxy-3-methylglutaryl coenzyme A reductase [HMG-CoA reductase]), inhibition of lipolysis in adipose tissue, and antioxidant effects (Havel and Rapaport, 1995). Often

TABLE 32-1.
DRUGS AVAILABLE FOR TREATMENT OF LIPID DISORDERS

Bile Acid-Binding Resins
Cholestyramine
Colestipol
Statins (HMG-CoA reductase inhibitors)
Atorvastatin
Fluvastatin
Lovastatin
Pravastatin
Simvastatin
Niacin
Fibrates
Gemfibrozil
Omega-3 fatty acids

there is insufficient efficacy at tolerated doses and sometimes a high incidence of side effects. Dietary regulation and weight reduction must continue, because the effects of diet and drugs are additive.

Bile Acid-Binding Resins

Bile acid-binding resins (sequestrants) are effective for the treatment of lipid disorders in which the primary abnormality is an increased plasma LDL cholesterol concentration with a normal or near normal triglyceride level. The two drugs in this class, cholestyramine and colestipol, are equivalent and may be prescribed because of cost and patient preference. These drugs have a low potential for toxicity, and many patients tolerate these drugs without side effects. Both drugs are available only as powders that must be hydrated

TABLE 32-2.
CHOICE OF DRUGS FOR TREATMENT OF LIPID DISORDERS

Lipid/Lipoprotein Abnormality	Single Drug	Drug Combination
Increased low density lipoproteins	Statin	Statin and Resin
Triglycerides <200 mg/dL	Resin Niacin	Resin and Niacin Statin and Niacin
Increased low density lipoproteins		Statin and Niacin
Triglycerides 200–400 mg/dL	Statin Niacin	Statin and Gemfibrozil Niacin and Resin Niacin and Gemfibrozil
Triglycerides >1,000 mg/dL	Niacin Gemfibrizol Omega-3 fatty Acids	Niacin and Gemfibrozil

Adapted from Fortmann SP and Maron DJ. Diagnosis and treatment of lipid disorders. *Sci Am Med* 1998;9:II:1–20.

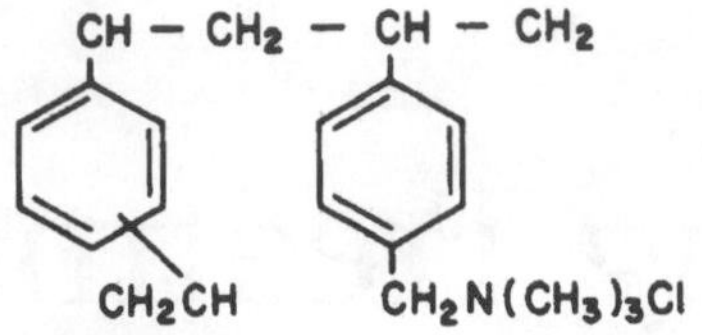

Figure 32-1. Cholestyramine.

before ingestion. There is no systemic absorption of these resins. Administered as monotherapy, bile-acid binding resins decrease plasma concentrations 15% to 30% in a dose-dependent manner. Plasma concentrations of triglycerides may increase 5% to 20% in treated patients owing to increased production of very low-density lipoproteins.

Cholestyramine

Cholestyramine is the chloride salt of an ion exchange resin originally used to control pruritus in patients with increased plasma concentrations of bile acids resulting from cholestasis (Fig. 32-1). This resin binds bile acids in the intestine, interrupting enterohepatic circulation and increasing fecal excretion that increases hepatic bile acid synthesis from cholesterol stores. This increases the production of hepatic LDL receptors that increases the uptake of LDL cholesterol from blood and lowers plasma concentrations of LDL cholesterol. HMG-CoA reductase activity also increases. Bile acid-binding resins may be combined with nicotinic acid, lovastatin, gemfibrozil, or probucol.

Side Effects

Poor palatability and constipation are common complaints in patients being treated with cholestyramine. A high fluid intake is useful in minimizing constipation. The gritty quality of the drug may decrease patient compliance. There may be transient increases in the plasma concentrations of alkaline phosphatase and transaminases. Abdominal pain is an infrequent side effect.

Because cholestyramine is a chloride form of an ion exchange resin, hyperchloremic acidosis can occur, especially in younger and smaller patients in whom the relative dose is larger. Absorption of fat-soluble vitamins may be impaired, and hypoprothrombinemia is a theoretical possibility. Cholestyramine may bind other drugs (thiazides, warfarin, digitalis, beta-blockers) and impair their absorption. For this reason, other drugs should be given at least 1 hour before or 4 hours after administration of cholestyramine.

Colestipol

Colestipol is a bile-sequestering drug with pharmacologic effects similar to those of cholestyramine.

Statins

Statins are drugs that act as inhibitors of HMG-CoA reductase (rate-limiting enzyme) that catalyzes the conversion of substrate, HMG-CoA to mevalonate, which is an early and rate-limiting step in the biosynthesis of cholesterol. The resulting inhibition of the endogenous synthesis of cholesterol is accompanied by decreases (as much as 60%) in the plasma concentrations of LDL cholesterol. The decreased hepatic synthesis of cholesterol also increases the number of LDL receptors on the surfaces of hepatocytes and thereby further enhances the removal of LDL cholesterol from the circulation. A 10% increase in HDL may result from increased synthesis of apolipoprotein A-I. Plasma triglyceride concentrations decrease 10% to 20% in statin-treated patients.

Statins are commonly the first choice when pharmacologic intervention is used to lower plasma concentrations of LDL cholesterol. The drugs in this class (atorvastatin, fluvastatin, lovastatin, pravastatin, simvastatin) are considered equivalent and relatively free of side effects (Fig. 32-2). Randomized clinical trials have shown that statins lower cardiac events (total mortality, death from myocardial infarction, revascularization procedures, stroke, and peripheral vascular disease) in patients with or without atherosclerosis (MRC/BHF Heart Protection Study Collaborative Group, 1999; Sachs et al., 1996; Shepherd et al., 1995). Furthermore, angiographic studies have shown benefit on coronary stenosis in native vessels or grafts in patients treated with statins as well as in patients experiencing acute coronary syndromes (Schwartz et al., 2001). Early initiation of statin therapy following an acute myocardial infarction is recommended (Stenestrand and Wallentin, 2001).

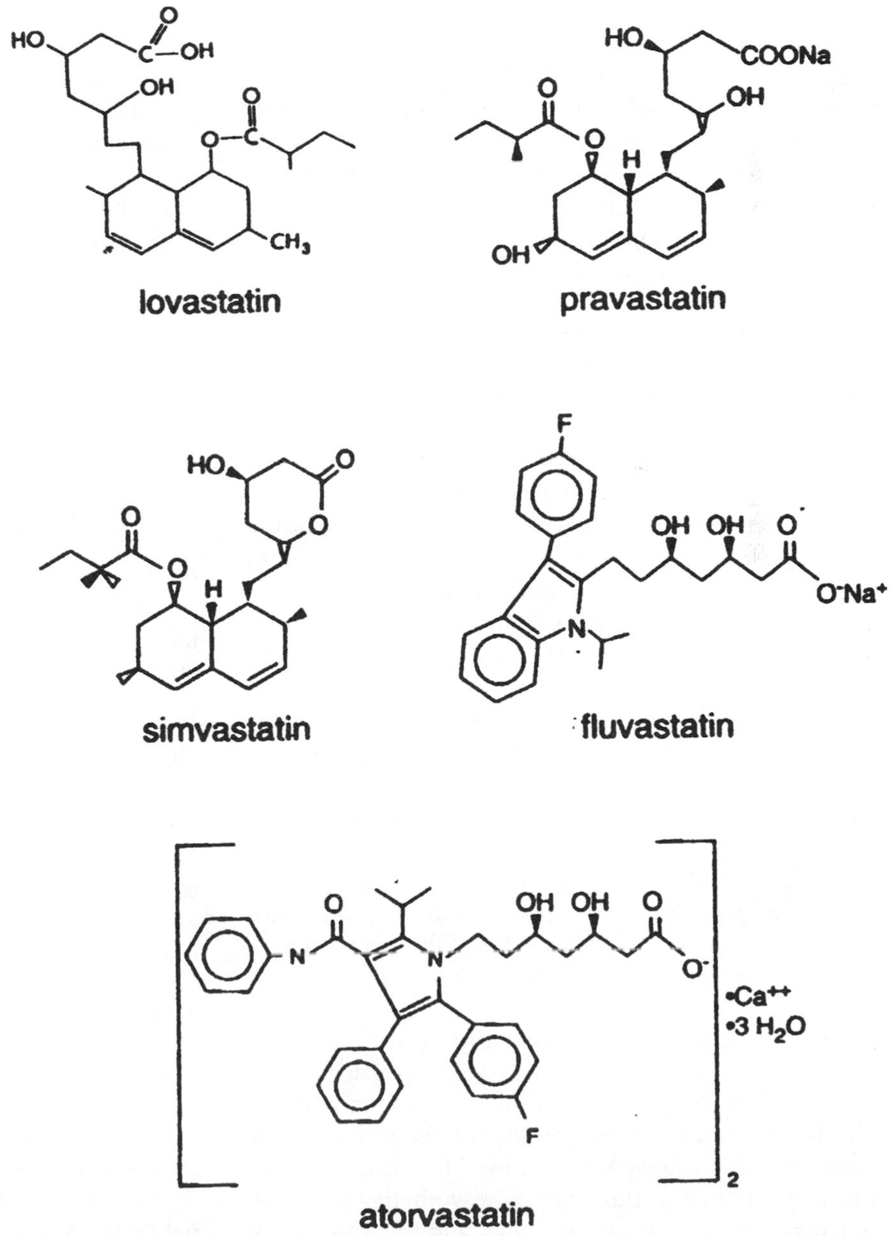

Figure 32-2. Statins.

Side Effects

Statins are usually well tolerated with the most common complaints being gastrointestinal upset, fatigue, and headache. Prothrombin time may be increased in warfarin-treated patients. Peripheral neuropathy and a lupus-like syndrome have been reported (Knopp, 1999). Rare but potential side effects of statin therapy include hepatic dysfunction and myopathy.

Hepatic Dysfunction

Persistent increases in plasma aminotransferase concentrations occur in 0.5% to 2% of treated patients and are dose-dependent. Discontinuation of the drug is recommended if plasma aminotransferase concentrations increase to more than three times normal. Progression to hepatic failure is extremely rare.

Myopathy

Statins and other cholesterol-lowering drugs may cause myopathy (usually reversible) that is characterized by proximal skeletal muscle weakness, myalgia, and increases of the plasma concentrations of creatine phosphokinase and myopathic changes on the electromyogram. Because cholesterol is the principal sterol constituent of skeletal muscle membranes, decreases of the normal cholesterol pool available for membrane synthesis can increase membrane fluidity, leading to unstable sarcolemma, myotonic discharges and, in advanced but rare situations, rhabdomyolysis (Graham et al., 2004). Gradual recovery usually occurs when the offending drug is discontinued. Myopathy is especially likely to occur in patients receiving combination therapy with other drugs including niacin, gemfibrozil, cyclosporine, and erythromycin. Coadministration of cyclosporine and lovastatin to patients with heart or kidney transplants and hyperlipidemia appears to increase the incidence of myopathy with rhabdomyolysis.

Myopathy appears to be most frequent in patients treated with lovastatin (<5% of treated patients) and least common with fluvastatin. Rarely, myopathy can lead to rhabdomyolysis and acute renal failure. Drugs likely to be administered during anesthesia have not been shown to increase the incidence of statin-induced myopathy. Large volumes of grapefruit juice may inhibit intestinal cytochrome P-450 activity but it is unclear if this contributes to the risk of myopathy (Bailey et al., 2001).

Origin and Chemical Structure (Fig. 32-2)

Lovastatin is a naturally occurring product isolated from a strain of *Aspergillus terreus.* Simvastatin is derived synthetically from a fermentation product of the same fungus. Pravastatin is also derived from a fungal fermentation product. Atorvastatin and fluvastatin are synthetic drugs with structures that differ from each other and the three fungal derived statins.

Pharmacokinetics

Statins are variably absorbed from the gastrointestinal tract following oral ingestion. Bile-acid binding resins can decrease the absorption of these drugs. Lovastatin and simvastatin are prodrugs that require metabolism to the open beta-hydroxy acid form to be pharmacologically active. Atorvastatin, fluvastatin, and pravastatin are administered as the active beta-hydroxy acid form. Food intake increases plasma concentrations of lovastatin but has minimal effects on the other statins. All of the statins are highly protein bound with the exception of pravastatin. Except for pravastatin, all of the statins undergo extensive metabolism by hepatic P-450 enzymes. Elimination half-times are 1 to 4 hours for all the statins except atorvastatin that has an elimination half-time of 14 hours (Chong et al., 2001). Despite the short elimination half-times, the duration of pharmacodynamic effects is about 24 hours. This is a consideration in the perioperative period when patients may not be able to ingest oral medications. Atorvastatin and fluvastatin undergo minimal renal excretion and probably do not require dosage adjustments in patients with renal insufficiency. Dosages of pravastatin and to a lesser degree lovastatin and simvastatin may need to be adjusted in patients with renal insufficiency. Statins are teratogenic in animals and thus are not recommended for use during pregnancy.

Niacin

Niacin (nicotinic acid) is a water-soluble B-complex vitamin that inhibits synthesis of VLDLs in the liver by an unknown mechanism. In addition, niacin inhibits release of free fatty acids from adipose tissue and increases the activity of lipoprotein lipase. The result of these effects is a dose-related 15% to 30% decrease in plasma LDL cholesterol concentrations, a 20% to 50% decrease in triglycerides, and a 20% to 30% increase in HDL. Niacin does not produce any detectable changes in synthesis of cholesterol, nor does it alter excretion of bile acids.

Pharmacokinetics

Niacin is readily absorbed from the gastrointestinal tract and undergoes extensive hepatic first-pass metabolism. The primary route of metabolism is methylation to *N*-methylnicotinamide. Niacin also undergoes conjugation with glycine to produce nicotinuric acid. Metabolites undergo renal excretion and at high doses, niacin undergoes renal excretion unchanged.

Side Effects

Niacin, unlike the resins and statins, has many side effects that may limit its usefulness. The most common side effect is intense prostaglandin-induced cutaneous flushing which occurs in about 10% of patients. Aspirin administered 30 minutes before ingestion of niacin decreases flushing, whereas alcohol ingestion potentiates flushing. Abdominal pain, nausea and vomiting, diarrhea, and malaise are common complaints in treated patients.

Hepatic dysfunction manifesting as increased plasma transaminase activity and cholestatic jaundice may be associated with large doses of niacin. Although the mechanism by which niacin or one of its metabolites induces hepatic injury is unknown, evidence suggests a dose-related, direct toxic effect rather than an idiosyncratic drug reaction. Crystalline preparations of niacin are less likely than sustained-release preparations to cause hepatotoxicity. Niacin is not recommended for administration to patients with liver disease.

Hyperglycemia and abnormal glucose tolerance may occur in nondiabetic patients treated with niacin. Plasma concentrations of uric acid are increased, and the incidence of gouty arthritis is increased. Niacin may exaggerate vasodilation and orthostatic hypotension associated with antihypertensive drugs. Peptic ulcer disease may be reactivated by niacin. There seems to be an increased risk of skeletal muscle myopathy when this drug is administered in combination with statins, especially lovastatin. Absorption of niacin is not impaired when combination therapy with bile acid-binding resins is undertaken.

FIBRATES

Fibrates are derivatives of fibric acid and are the most effective drugs for decreasing plasma concentrations of triglycerides. In the postoperative period, treatment with fibrates is restarted when the patient is well hydrated and able to ingest oral medications.

Gemfibrozil

Gemfibrozil is a fibric acid derivative that is the best tolerated drug for the treatment of patients with increased plasma concentrations of triglycerides with or without a concomitant increase in plasma LDL cholesterol concentrations (Fig. 32-3). The drug produces a dose-dependent 40% to 50% decrease in plasma triglycerides, 10% to 35% increase in HDL concentrations, whereas the effect on LDL concentrations is variable. Drug-induced increases in the activity of lipoprotein lipase is the likely mechanism for the triglyceride-lowering effects of gemfibrozil. This action of fibrates may reflect activation of specific transcription factors (peroxisome proliferator-activated receptors) that result in up-regulation of genes for lipoprotein lipase and fatty acid oxidation. Induction of lipoprotein lipase contributes to lipolysis of triglyceride-rich lipoproteins, VLDL, and chylomicrons. When the LDL concentration increases, it is presumed to reflect improved catabolism of VLDLs and hence increased production of LDLs. Niacin or a bile acid-binding resin may be added to the treatment if the increase in plasma LDL cholesterol concentration is higher than viewed to be acceptable.

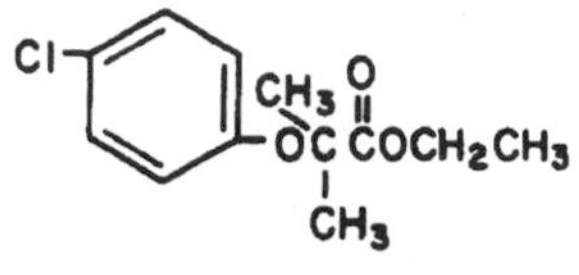

Figure 32-3. Gemfibrozil.

Pharmacokinetics

Gemfibrozil is well absorbed from the gastrointestinal tract following oral administration. Metabolism is by oxidation of a methyl group to form a hydroxymethyl and then a carboxyl metabolite. Protein binding is extensive. The elimination half-time of gemfibrozil is approximately 15 hours, with an estimated 70% of a single dose appearing unchanged in the urine.

Side Effects

The most common side effects of gemfibrozil are gastrointestinal (abdominal pain, nausea) and headache. Gemfibrozil increases the cholesterol content (lithogenicity) of bile and may increase the formation of gallstones. The incidence of skeletal muscle myopathy and risk of rhabdomyolysis is increased when this drug is administered in combination with statins, especially lovastatin. The anticoagulant effect of warfarin is potentiated by gemfibrozil, presumably reflecting its displacement from binding sites on albumin. A mild increase in plasma transaminase enzymes may occur in treated patients. Considering the dependence on renal excretion for elimination and occasional increases in liver function tests, it may be prudent to avoid administration of this drug to patients with preexisting renal or hepatic disease. Noncardiovascular mortality may be increased in treated patients (Gould et al., 1995). For example, low plasma cholesterol concentrations may predispose patients to hemorrhagic stroke, particularly when systemic hypertension is present (Law et al., 1994). Nevertheless, much of the increased mortality at very low plasma concentrations of cholesterol may be attributable to specific diseases that decrease cholesterol concentrations.

Fenofibrate

Fenofibrate is a prodrug that is hydrolyzed by esterases to the active metabolite, fenofibric acid. Fenofibric acid is metabolized by conjugation with glucuronic acid which undergoes extensive renal excretion. The elimination half time of fenofibrate is about 20 hours. Absorption of fenofibrate is increased when the drug is administered with food. Protein binding is approximately 99%. Increased plasma concentrations of liver transaminase enzymes are more likely to occur with fenofibrate than with the other fibrates.

Clofibrate

Clofibrate was the original fibric acid derivative for treatment of increased plasma triglyceride concentrations. This drug is no longer considered the drug of choice, principally because of concern that noncardiovascular adverse events may be increased in treated patients (Gould et al., 1995). Clofibrate is an option in patients with severe hypertriglyceridemia who do not tolerate or respond to niacin and/or gemfibrozil. The side effects of clofibrate resemble those described for gemfibrozil.

OMEGA-3 FATTY ACIDS (FISH OIL)

The type of fat present in marine fish oils is highly unsaturated omega-3 fatty acid. The primary effect of this fatty acid is to decrease plasma concentrations of triglycerides, whereas the effect on the plasma LDL cholesterol concentrations is variable. It is not clear what dose is necessary to cause desirable effects on the plasma concentrations of triglycerides. Fish oil supplements are not regarded as drugs and thus are not regulated by the U.S. Food and Drug Administration. The long-term safety of taking fish oil capsules is not known, and there is no evidence that fish oil supplementation prevents heart disease.

REFERENCES

Bailey DG, Malcolm J, Arnold O, et al. Grapefruit juice-drug interactions. *Br J Clin Pharmacol* 2001;52:216–221.

Chong PH, Seeger JD, Franklin C. Clinically relevant differences between the statins: Implications for therapeutic selection. *Am J Med* 2001;111:390–396.

Downs JR, Clearfield M, Weis S, et al. Primary prevention of acute coronary events with lovastatin in men and women with average cholesterol levels. Results of AFCAPS/TexCAPS. *JAMA* 1998;279: 1615–1621.

Executive Summary of the third report of the National Cholesterol Education Program (NCEP) Expert Panel on detection, evaluation, and treatment of high blood cholesterol in adults (Adult Treatment Panel III). *JAMA* 2001;285:2486–2493.

Fortmann SP, Maron DJ. Diagnosis and treatment of lipid disorders. *Sci Am Med* 1998;9:II:1–20.

Gould AL, Rossouw JE, Santanello NC, et al. Cholesterol reduction yields clinical benefit: a new look at old data. *Circulation* 1995;91: 2274–2278.

Graham DJ, Staffa JA, Shatin D, et al. Incidence of hospitalized rhabdomyolysis in patients treated with lipid-lowering drugs. *JAMA* 2004:292:2585–2590.

Havel RJ, Rapaport E. Management of primary hyperlipidemia. *N Engl J Med* 1995;332:1491–1498.

Knopp RH. Drug treatment of lipid disorders. *N Engl J Med* 1999;341: 498–504.

Law MR, Thompson SG, Wald NJ. Assessing possible hazards of decreasing serum cholesterol. *BMJ* 1994;308:1954–1960.

MRC/BHF Heart Protection Study Collaborative Group: MRC/BHF Heart Protection Study of cholesterol-lowering therapy and of antioxidant vitamin supplementation in a wide range of patients at increased risk of coronary heart disease death: early safety and efficacy experience. *Eur Heart J* 1999;20:725–731.

Sachs FM, Pfeffer MA, Moye LA, et al. The effect of pravastatin on coronary events after myocardial infarction in patients with average cholesterol levels. *N Engl J Med* 1996;339:1001–1006.

Schwartz G, Olsson AD, Ezekowitz MD, et al. Effects of atorvastatin on early recurrent ischemic events in acute coronary syndromes: The MIRACL Study: a randomized controlled trial. *JAMA* 2001;285: 1711–1718.

Shepherd J, Cobbe SM, Ford I, et al. Prevention of coronary heart disease with pravastatin in men with hypercholesterolemia. *N Engl J Med* 1995;333:1301–1307.

Steinberg D, Gotto AM. Preventing coronary artery disease by lowering cholesterol levels. Fifty years from bench to bedside. *JAMA* 1999;282:2043–2050.

Stenestrand U, Wallentin L. Early statin treatment following acute myocardial infarction and 1-year survival. *JAMA* 2001;285:430–436.

The BIP Group. Secondary prevention by raising HDL cholesterol and reducing triglycerides in patients with coronary artery disease. *Circulation* 2000;102:21–28.

Central Nervous System Stimulants and Muscle Relaxants

33

CENTRAL NERVOUS SYSTEM STIMULANTS

Drugs that stimulate the central nervous system (CNS) as their primary action are classified as analeptics or convulsants. Analeptics were previously used in the treatment of generalized CNS depression accompanying deliberate drug overdoses. This practice, however, has been abandoned because these drugs lack specific antagonist properties and their margin of safety is narrow.

The excitability of the CNS reflects a balance between excitatory and inhibitory influences that is normally maintained within relatively narrow limits. Analeptics can increase excitability either by blocking inhibition or by enhancing excitation. Strychnine and picrotoxin selectively block inhibition in the CNS. As such, these drugs lack clinical value but are useful as research tools to study inhibitory neurotransmitters such as gamma-aminobutyric acid (GABA) and corresponding receptors.

Doxapram

Doxapram is a centrally acting analeptic that selectively increases minute ventilation by activating the carotid bodies (Fig. 33-1) (Mitchell and Herbert, 1975). Lack of a direct stimulant effect on the medullary respiratory center is emphasized by the absence of doxapram effect on ventilation when carotid body activity is absent. The stimulus to ventilation produced by administration of doxapram, 1 mg/kg IV, is similar to that produced by a PaO_2 of 38 mm Hg acting on the carotid bodies (Hirsh and Wang, 1974). An increase in tidal volume, more than an increase in breathing frequency, is responsible for the doxapram-induced increase in minute ventilation. Oxygen consumption is increased concomitantly with the increase in minute ventilation.

Doxapram has a large margin of safety as reflected by a 20- to 40-fold difference in the dose that stimulates ventilation and the dose that produces seizures (Sebel et al., 1980). Nevertheless, continuous infusion of doxapram, as required to produce a sustained effect on ventilation, often results in evidence of subconvulsive CNS stimulation (hypertension, tachycardia, cardiac dysrhythmias, vomiting, and increased body temperature). These changes are consistent with increased sympathetic nervous system outflow from the brain.

Doxapram is extensively metabolized, with <5% of an IV dose being excreted unchanged in urine. A single IV dose produces an effect on ventilation that lasts only 5 to 10 minutes.

Clinical Uses

Doxapram administered as a continuous infusion (2 to 3 mg/minute) has been used as a temporary measure to maintain ventilation during administration of supplemental oxygen to patients with chronic obstructive airway disease who otherwise depend on a hypoxic drive to maintain adequate minute ventilation (Fig. 33-2) (Moser et al., 1973). Administered concomitantly with intramuscular meperidine, doxapram prevents the ventilatory depression produced by the opioid without altering analgesia, suggesting a possible benefit in the early postoperative period (Ramamurthy et al., 1975). Because controlled ventilation of the lungs and standard supportive therapy are effective in managing ventilatory failure, doxapram should not be used in patients with drug-induced coma or exacerbation of chronic lung disease. More specific tests (peripheral nerve

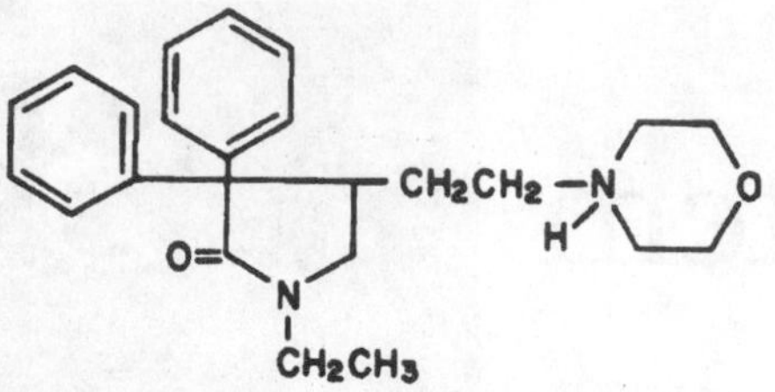

Figure 33-1. Doxapram.

stimulation, airway pressures, head lift) render the diagnostic use of doxapram in postanesthetic apnea or hypoventilation of minimal clinical value. Arousal from residual effects of inhaled anesthetics follows administration of doxapram, but the effect is transient, nonselective, and not recommended.

Amphetamine

Amphetamine and methamphetamine are powerful CNS stimulants. These drugs cause the release and inhibit the reuptake of stimulatory neurotransmitters in the cerebral cortex, motor nuclei, and the reticular activating system. Chronic administration of amphetamines may lower systemic blood pressure owing to metabolism of amphetamine and methamphetamine to false neurotransmitters. Appetite suppression is not a sustained effect of these drugs while tolerance and dependence are likely to develop.

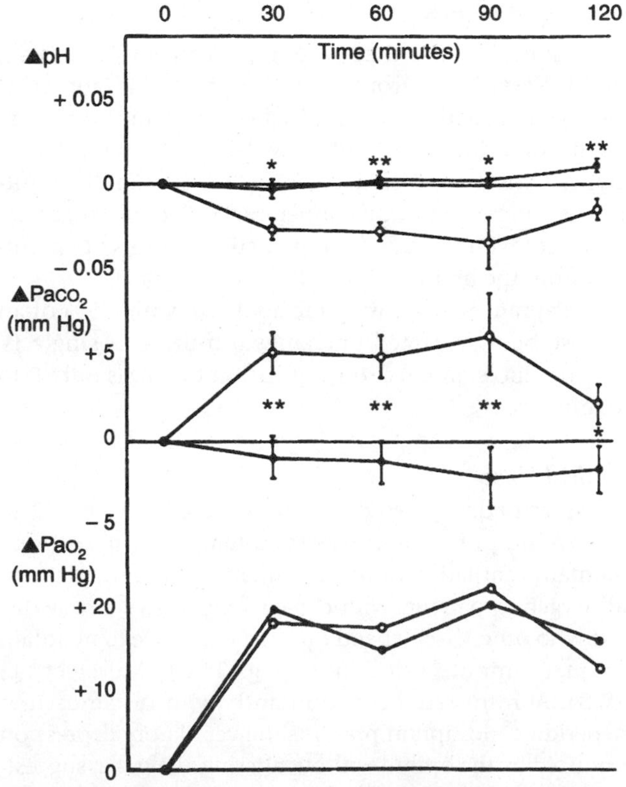

Figure 33-2. Doxapram, as a continuous infusion (*solid circles*), may be used to maintain alveolar ventilation during administration of supplemental oxygen to patients with chronic obstructive airway disease. The open circles represent placebo. (* $P < .05$ compared with placebo infusion; ** $P < .01$ compared with placebo infusion.) (From Moser KM, Luchsinger PC, Adamson JS, et al. Respiratory stimulation with intravenous doxapram in respiratory failure. *N Engl J Med* 1973;288:428–431; with permission.)

Toxicity

Acute intoxication with amphetamines is characterized by restlessness, agitation, irritability, aggressive behavior, and paranoid delusions. Tachycardia and hypertension may be followed by cardiac dysrhythmias and hypotension. Convulsions and circulatory collapse may be fatal terminal events. Hyperpyrexia and disseminated intravascular coagulation have been observed.

Treatment of acute amphetamine intoxication includes acidification of the urine to enhance renal excretion of the drug and administration of medications to treat cardiovascular side effects. Dantrolene is indicated if hyperpyrexia is present.

Methylphenidate

Methylphenidate is structurally related to amphetamine (Fig. 33-3). This drug is a mild CNS stimulant, with more prominent effects on mental than on motor activities. Large doses, however, produce generalized CNS stimulation and seizures. Absorption after oral administration is rapid, and concentrations of methylphenidate in the brain exceed those in the plasma. The abuse potential of methylphenidate is the same as that of amphetamine.

Clinical Uses

Methylphenidate is useful in the treatment of hyperkinetic syndromes in children characterized as having minimal brain dysfunction. Bradycardia, hallucinations, and growth suppression have been described in patients treated with methylphenidate. Methylphenidate may also be effective in the treatment of narcolepsy, either alone or in combination with tricyclic antidepressants.

Methylxanthines

Methylxanthines are represented by caffeine, theophylline, and theobromine (Fig. 33-4). Solubility of methylxanthines is low and is enhanced by formation of complexes as represented by the combination of theophylline with

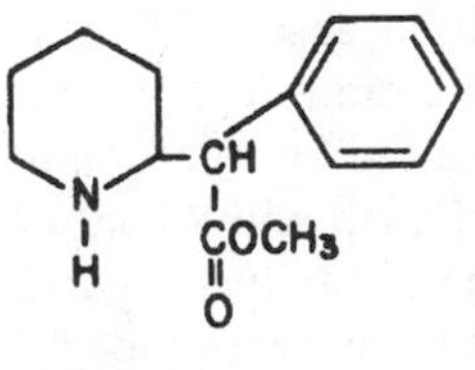

Figure 33-3. Methylphenidate.

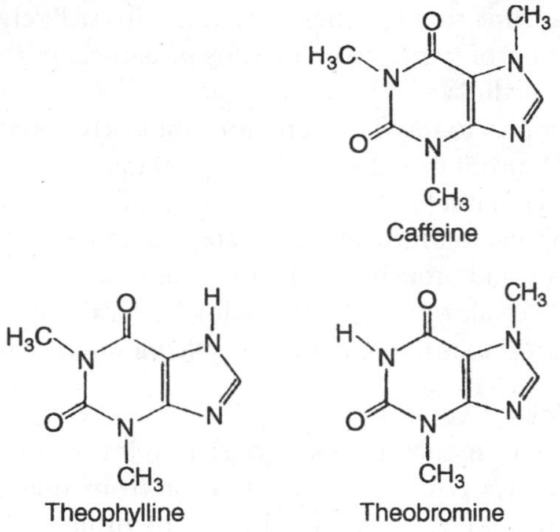

Figure 33-4. Methylxanthines.

ethylenediamine to form aminophylline. Methylxanthines have in common the ability to (a) stimulate the CNS, (b) produce diuresis, (c) increase myocardial contractility, and (d) relax smooth muscle, especially that in the airways (see Chapter 12).

Mechanism of Action

The best-characterized cellular action of methylxanthines is antagonism of receptor-mediated actions of adenosine thus facilitating the release of catecholamines. Theophylline is more active than caffeine or theobromine as an antagonist at these receptors. At high concentrations, theophylline inhibits phosphodiesterase enzymes that are responsible for breakdown of cyclic AMP. Methylxanthines are completely absorbed after oral administration and eliminated primarily by metabolism in the liver. Unlike adults, premature infants metabolize theophylline in part to caffeine. Furthermore, the clearance of methylxanthines is greatly prolonged in the neonate compared with that in the adult.

Clinical Uses

Methylxanthines are used as analeptics to treat primary apnea of prematurity (stimulate medullary respiratory centers by increasing the sensitivity of these centers to carbon dioxide). The slowed metabolism of methylxanthines in neonates compared to adults is a consideration when using theophylline to stimulate ventilation in neonates. Selective beta$_2$-adrenergic agonists delivered by inhalation have largely replaced theophylline preparations in the treatment of bronchospasm associated with asthma. Recognition of theophylline's antiinflammatory effects could be useful for chronic management of asthma, although the narrow therapeutic index and significant side effects are likely to limit its use. Smooth muscle relaxation and bronchodilation produced by theophylline may reflect a combination of effects including catecholamine release, phosphodiesterase inhibition, and inflammation inhibition. The administration of theophylline during maintenance of anesthesia appears to have no added bronchodilator effect over that of the volatile anesthetic alone. Methylxanthines decrease systemic vascular resistance but increase cerebrovascular resistance (associated vasoconstriction may be responsible for relief of postdural puncture headaches).

Toxicity

A single oral dose of theophylline, 5 mg/kg, will produce a peak plasma concentration of 10 μg/mL in adults within 1 to 2 hours following ingestion. Increased levels of unbound drug may result in signs of toxicity despite therapeutic plasma concentrations of drug (10 to 20 μg/mL). Theophylline plasma concentrations only slightly greater than the recommended therapeutic range can produce evidence of CNS stimulation (nervousness, tremors) and at higher concentrations, seizures are a possibility. Vomiting most likely reflecting CNS stimulation is common when plasma concentrations exceed 15 μg/mL. Tachycardia and cardiac dysrhythmias may appear most likely due to drug-induced release of catecholamines from the adrenal medulla.

Drug Interactions

Drugs may enhance (carbamazepine, rifampin) or inhibit (cimetidine, erythromycin) the hepatic metabolism of theophylline. Larger doses of benzodiazepines may be required in the presence of theophylline as benzodiazepines increase the CNS concentrations of adenosine, a potent CNS depressant, whereas theophylline is an adenosine receptor antagonist. Ketamine may decrease the theophylline seizure threshold. Theophylline can antagonize the effects of nondepolarizing neuromuscular-blocking drugs presumably by inhibition of phosphodiesterase.

Caffeine

Caffeine is a methylxanthine-derived phosphodiesterase inhibitor that is present in a variety of beverages and nonprescription medications (Table 33-1) (Bunker and McWilliams, 1979). A prominent effect of caffeine is CNS stimulation. In addition, this substance acts as a cerebral vasoconstrictor and may cause secretion of acidic gastric fluid. Caffeine may increase plasma glucose concentrations.

Pharmacologic uses of caffeine include administration to neonates experiencing apnea of prematurity. Postdural puncture headache may respond to administration of caffeine, 300 mg orally (Camman et al., 1990). Presumably, a cerebral vasoconstriction effect accounts for the occasional efficacy of caffeine in alleviating symptoms of postdural puncture headache as well as migraine headache. Caffeine may be included in common cold remedies in an attempt to offset the sedating effects of certain antihistamines.

Nicotine

Nicotine has no therapeutic action, but its toxicity and presence in tobacco have created medical importance for this

TABLE 33-1.
CAFFEINE CONTENT OF COMMON SUBSTANCES

Substance	Caffeine (mg)
Coffee (150 mL)	
Freeze dried	66
Percolator	107
Drip grind	142
Tea (150 mL)	15–47
Cocoa (150 mL)	13
Coca-Cola (360 mL)	65
Pepsi-Cola (360 mL)	43
Dr. Pepper (360 mL)	61
Mountain Dew (360 mL)	55
Jolt Cola	71
Candy bar (1.2 oz)	5
No-Doze	100

Source: Data from Bunker ML, McWilliams M. Caffeine content of common beverages. *J Am Diet Assoc* 1979;74:28–32.

compound. Smoking is the single most important preventable cause of death, being responsible for more than one in every six fatalities (Rigotti, 1989). The highly addictive nature of nicotine results in a withdrawal syndrome that presents a major barrier to successful cessation of tobacco use. Nicotine is readily absorbed from the respiratory tract and buccal mucous membranes (chewing gum preparation) and through the skin (dermal patch). As an alkaloid, nicotine is absorbed minimally from the acidic environment of the stomach. Nicotine is metabolized in the lungs and liver after inhalation and oral administration, respectively. A principal metabolite is cotinine, which has approximately one-fifth the pharmacologic activity of nicotine. Nicotine and cotinine are rapidly eliminated by the kidneys and, in parturients, in breast milk. The elimination half-time of nicotine is 30 to 60 minutes. Urinary cotinine levels may be used as a marker of cigarette smoke exposure.

Cigarette smoking alters the activity of many drugs, presumably reflecting induction of liver microsomal enzymes by polycyclic hydrocarbons in cigarette smoke. This enzyme activity differs from that produced by phenobarbital. Enzyme activity remains increased for up to 6 months after cessation of cigarette smoking.

Effects on Organ Systems

The complex and often unpredictable pharmacologic effects of nicotine may reflect its stimulant and depressant actions. The primary action of nicotine is an initial stimulation, quickly followed by persistent depression of autonomic ganglia. Nicotine markedly stimulates the CNS, manifesting initially as tremor. Stimulation of ventilation by small doses reflects nicotine-induced excitation of aortic and carotid body chemoreceptors. Nicotine characteristically increases heart rate and systemic blood pressure and evokes peripheral vasoconstriction. These responses most likely reflect stimulation of sympathetic nervous system ganglia and the adrenal medulla.

In contrast to the effects on the cardiovascular system, the effects of nicotine on the gastrointestinal tract are largely due to parasympathetic nervous system stimulation leading to vomiting and diarrhea. Nicotine causes an initial stimulation of salivary and bronchial secretions that is followed by inhibition. Salivation caused by smoking is reflexively produced by irritant smoke rather than by a systemic effect of nicotine.

Overdose

Overdose from nicotine may occur from ingestion of insecticide sprays containing nicotine or from ingestion of tobacco products. The fatal dose of nicotine in adults is approximately 60 mg. Individual cigarettes deliver up to 2.5 mg of nicotine. Gastric absorption of nicotine is minimized by vomiting due to the central emetic effect of the initially absorbed material.

The onset of symptoms of nicotine overdose is rapid and characterized by nausea, salivation, abdominal cramps, vertigo, mental confusion, and skeletal muscle weakness. Hypotension and difficulty in breathing ensue, the heart rate is rapid, and terminal seizures may occur. Paralysis of the intercostal muscles may cause apnea. Treatment is supportive, including attempts to remove any residual nicotine from the stomach.

Almitrine

Almitrine is a peripheral chemoreceptor agonist that increases $Pa{O_2}$ and decreases $Pa{CO_2}$ in patients with chronic respiratory failure associated with obstructive pulmonary disease. Although the mechanism of action is uncertain, two clinical effects have been documented: (a) an improvement of minute ventilation in spontaneously breathing patients resulting in a decrease in $Pa{CO_2}$ owing to stimulation of the chemoreflex and (b) vasoconstriction of pulmonary vessels that predominates in hypoxic zones resulting in better ventilation to perfusion matching, increased $Pa{O_2}$ and decreased venous admixture (Chen et al., 1990). Indeed, continuous IV infusion of almitrene was more successful than placebo in sustaining acceptable oxygen saturation during one lung ventilation (Dalibon et al., 2004). IV administration of almitrine improves $Pa{O_2}$ in patients with acute lung injury but may also induce lactic acidosis and hepatic dysfunction (B'chir et al., 1998). Side effects of prolonged oral almitrine therapy include dyspnea and peripheral neuropathy.

CENTRALLY ACTING MUSCLE RELAXANTS

Centrally acting muscle relaxants act in the CNS or directly on skeletal muscles to relieve spasticity. Spasticity of skeletal muscles occurs when there is an abnormal increase in

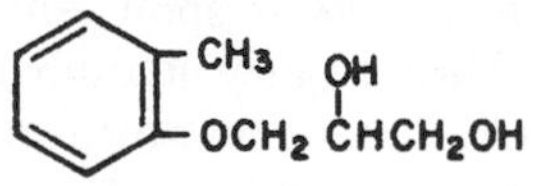

Figure 33-5. Mephenesin.

resistance to passive movement of a skeletal muscle group because of hyperactive proprioceptive or stretch reflexes. Spasticity occurs in a wide variety of neurologic conditions and is highly variable in its etiology and presentation.

Mephenesin

The relative efficacy of centrally acting muscle relaxants that are related to mephenesin has not been determined (Fig. 33-5). As a result, selection of one of these drugs over another remains highly empirical and subjective. These drugs produce skeletal muscle relaxation by an unknown mechanism in the CNS. A prominent effect of centrally acting muscle relaxants is depression of spinal polysynaptic reflexes. Nevertheless, the importance of this effect in the mechanism of skeletal muscle relaxation is not documented. Sedation is not a prominent side effect of these drugs.

Benzodiazepines

Benzodiazepines are widely used as centrally acting skeletal muscle relaxants. These drugs appear to have a more selective action on reticular neuronal mechanisms that control skeletal muscle tone than on spinal interneuronal activity (Tseng and Wang, 1971). Sedation may limit the efficacy of diazepam as a muscle relaxant.

Baclofen

Baclofen is the chlorophenol derivative of GABA that acts as an agonist at $GABA_B$ receptors in the dorsal horn of the spinal cord and is often administered for treatment of spastic hypertonia of cerebral and spinal cord origin (Fig. 33-6). Baclofen relieves spasticity by activating G-protein linked presynaptic $GABA_B$ receptors that hyperpolarize muscle spindle afferent neurons, thereby decreasing the number and amplitude of excitatory postsynaptic potentials along the dendrites of motor neurons. This drug has no effect on the neuromuscular junction. Baclofen is particularly effective in the treatment of flexor spasms and skeletal muscle rigidity associated with spinal cord injury or multiple sclerosis. Intrathecal administration of baclofen may be an effective treatment of spinal spasticity that has not responded to oral administration of the drug (Penn et al., 1989).

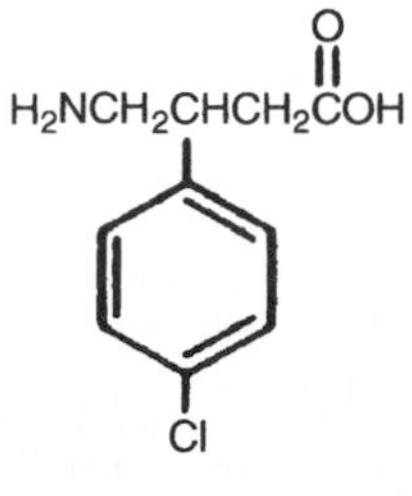

Figure 33-6. Baclofen.

Baclofen is rapidly and almost completely absorbed from the gastrointestinal tract. The elimination half-time is 3 to 6 hours, with approximately 80% of the drug excreted unchanged in urine, emphasizing the need to modify the dose in patients with renal dysfunction. Therapeutic plasma concentrations are 80 to 400 mg/mL (Young and Delwaide, 1981).

Use of baclofen is limited by its side effects, which include sedation, skeletal muscle weakness, and confusion. Sudden discontinuation of chronic baclofen therapy may result in severe withdrawal reactions including evidence of multiple organ system failure, tachycardia, and both auditory and visual hallucinations (Sampathkumar et al., 1998). Vocal cord spasm has been described following abrupt discontinuation of an intrathecal baclofen infusion (Santiago-Palma et al., 2004). Coma, depression of ventilation, and seizures may accompany an overdose of baclofen. The threshold for initiation of seizures may be lowered in patients with epilepsy. Mild hypotension may occur in awake patients being treated with oral baclofen, whereas bradycardia, hypotension, and delayed awakening have been observed when general anesthesia is induced in these patients (Sill et al., 1986). Hemodynamic instability and delayed awakening following general anesthesia have been described in a patient receiving an accidental intrathecal overdose of baclofen (Lyew et al., 2003). A decrease in sympathetic nervous system outflow from the CNS mediated by a GABA-baclofen–sensitive system might contribute to this hemodynamic response. Rarely, increases in liver transaminases and blood glucose levels have occurred.

Cyclobenzaprine

Cyclobenzaprine is related structurally and pharmacologically to tricyclic antidepressants (Fig. 33-7). Its anticholinergic effects are similar to those of tricyclic antidepressants and can include dry mouth, tachycardia, blurred vision, and sedation. The mechanism of skeletal muscle relaxant effects produced by cyclobenzaprine is unknown.

Cyclobenzaprine must not be administered in the presence of monoamine oxidase inhibitors. In view of the potential adverse side effects of some tricyclic antidepressant drugs on the heart, the use of cyclobenzaprine may

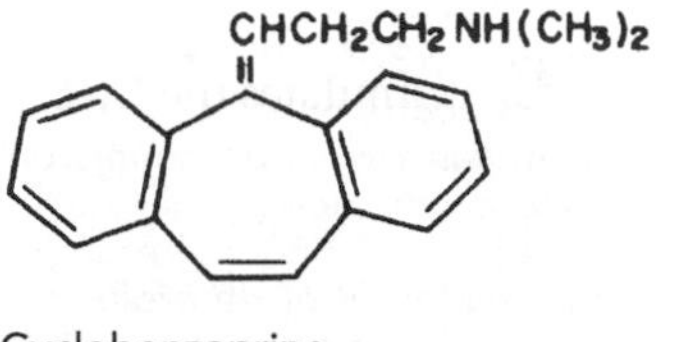

Figure 33-7. Cyclobenzaprine.

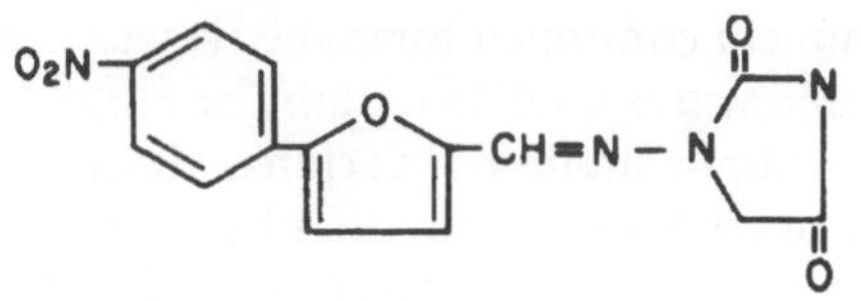

Figure 33-8. Dantrolene.

be questionable in patients with cardiac dysrhythmias or altered conduction of cardiac impulses.

Dantrolene

Dantrolene produces skeletal muscle relaxation by inhibiting calcium release from the endoplasmic reticulum (intracellular storage site of dischargeable calcium in neurons) through ryanodine receptors and inositol 1,4,5-triphosphate receptor channels into cytosol (Fig. 33-8). In addition, dantrolene may stabilize plasma membranes. Neuromuscular transmission and electrical properties of the skeletal muscle membranes are not altered. Unlike nondepolarizing muscle relaxants, dantrolene cannot decrease contractile activity by >80%. Therapeutic doses have little or no effect on cardiac and smooth muscles. In contrast to centrally acting skeletal muscle relaxants, dantrolene does not impair polysynaptic reflexes.

Pharmacokinetics

Absorption of dantrolene from the gastrointestinal tract as well as IV injection provides sustained dose-related concentrations of drug in the plasma (Figs. 33-9 and 33-10) (Allen et al., 1988; Lerman et al., 1989). The IV preparation of dantrolene is alkaline (pH 9.5), and phlebitis may follow its injection. Extravasation of dantrolene may result in tissue necrosis. Diuresis may accompany IV administration, reflecting addition of mannitol to the dantrolene powder to make the solution isotonic. For this reason, it is recommended that patients receiving IV dantrolene also have a urinary catheter in place (Flewellen et al., 1983).

Dantrolene is metabolized in the liver, principally to 5-hydroxydantrolene, which is 30% to 50% as effective in depressing the twitch response. Less than 1% of dantrolene appears unchanged in urine. The elimination half-time of dantrolene is 5 to 8 hours. The minimal effective blood level of dantrolene is not known, although plasma concentrations of 2.8 μg/mL or greater in animals are associated with near-maximal depression of skeletal muscle contractile activity (Allen et al., 1988). For this reason, it seems prudent to maintain blood levels of dantrolene of at least 2.8 μg/mL when the drug is being administered for prophylaxis against or treatment of malignant hyperthermia (Duncan, 1985).

Clinical Uses

Dantrolene is useful in the management of patients with skeletal muscle spasticity due to upper motor neuron lesions. The maximum oral dose is 400 mg administered in four divided doses. Associated dantrolene-induced skeletal muscle weakness, however, often negates any significant improvement, despite decreases in skeletal muscle spasticity.

Dantrolene is effective in the prevention and treatment of malignant hyperthermia (Duncan, 1985). Prophylaxis in malignant hyperthermia–susceptible patients may be with oral administration of dantrolene, 5 mg/kg in three or four divided doses every 6 hours, with the last dose 4 hours preoperatively. This regimen results in plasma levels of

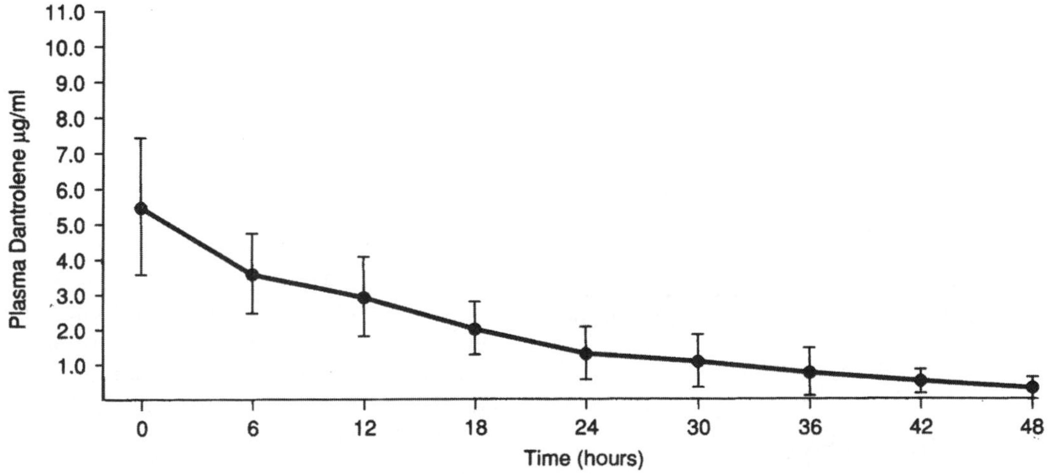

Figure 33-9. Plasma dantrolene concentrations after induction of anesthesia (time 0) and until 48 hours postoperatively in 10 malignant hyperthermia–susceptible patients. The total dose of dantrolene was 5 mg/kg administered orally in three or four divided doses, with the last dose 4 hours before induction of anesthesia. All patients had plasma concentrations of dantrolene of >2.8 μg/mL for at least 6 hours after induction of anesthesia. (From Allen GC, Cattrain CB, Peterson RG, et al. Plasma levels of dantrolene following oral administration in malignant hyperthermia–susceptible patients. *Anesthesiology* 1988;69: 900–904; with permission.)

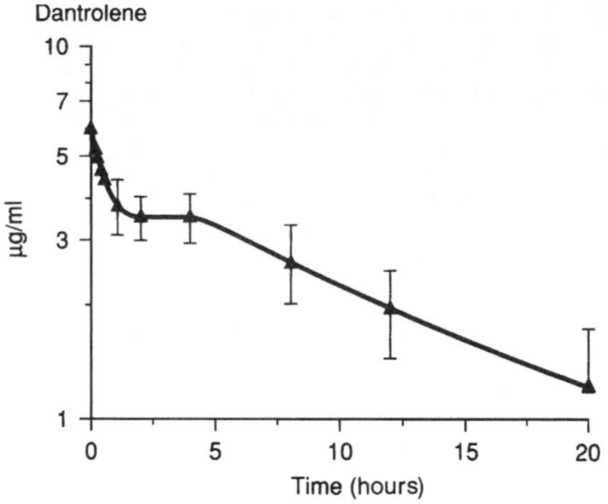

Figure 33-10. Plasma concentrations of dantrolene in venous blood after induction of anesthesia and administration of dantrolene, 2.4 mg/kg intravenously, to ten children. (Mean ± SD.) (From Lerman J, McLeod ME, Strong HA. Pharmacokinetics of intravenous dantrolene in children. *Anesthesiology* 1989;70: 625–629; with permission.)

dantrolene of >2.8 μg/mL at the time of induction of anesthesia and for at least 6 hours (see Fig. 33-9) (Allen et al., 1988). Alternatively, dantrolene, 2.4 mg/kg IV, may be administered over 10 to 30 minutes as prophylaxis just before induction of anesthesia, and for continued protection, one-half the dose is repeated in 6 hours (see Fig. 33-10) (Lerman et al., 1989). For treatment of malignant hyperthermia, the dose of dantrolene is 2 mg/kg IV, with repeated doses until symptoms subside or a cumulative dose of 10 mg/kg IV is reached. Despite the efficacy of dantrolene, it must be recognized that the drug is not 100% effective, and known triggering drugs must be avoided even when dantrolene prophylaxis is used (Fitzgibbon, 1981; Ruhland and Hinkle, 1984).

Side Effects

The most common side effect of dantrolene administration is skeletal muscle weakness. Skeletal muscle weakness may be sufficient to interfere with adequate ventilation or protection of the lungs from aspiration of gastric fluid (Watson et al., 1986). Large doses of dantrolene administered acutely as for prophylaxis against malignant hyperthermia may cause nausea, diarrhea, and blurred vision as well as skeletal muscle weakness. Uterine atony has been observed in a malignant hyperthermia-susceptible patient treated with dantrolene after cesarean section (Weingarten et al., 1987). Dantrolene administered to animals with or without verapamil has been associated with hyperkalemia (San Juan et al., 1988) (see Chapter 18).

Dantrolene produces hepatitis in approximately 0.5% of patients treated for >60 days. Fatal hepatitis occurs in 0.1% to 0.2% of patients treated chronically. For this reason, hepatic function should be monitored when dantrolene therapy is continued for ≥45 days. Pleural effusion may also occur with chronic therapy. Short-term use of dantrolene in preparation or treatment of malignant hyperthermia-susceptible patients is not associated with hepatotoxicity or pleural effusion. Breast feeding can be expected to be safe for the newborn 48 hours after discontinuation of IV dantrolene administration to the mother (Fricke et al., 1998).

REFERENCES

Allen GC, Cattran CB, Peterson RG, et al. Plasma levels of dantrolene following oral administration in malignant hyperthermia-susceptible patients. ***Anesthesiology*** 1988;69:900–904.

B'chir A, Mebazaa A, Lossser M-R et al. Intravenous almitrine bismesylate reversibly induces lactic acidosis and hepatic dysfunction in patients with acute lung injury. ***Anesthesiology*** 1998;89: 823–830.

Bunker ML, McWilliams M. Caffeine content of common beverages. ***J Am Diet Assoc*** 1979;74:28–32.

Camman WR, Murray RS, Mushlin PS, et al. Effects of oral caffeine on postdural puncture headache. A double-blind, placebo-controlled trial. ***Anesth Analg*** 1990;70:181–184.

Chen L, Miller FL, Malmkvist G, et al. Low-dose almitrine bismesylate enhances hypoxic pulmonary vasoconstriction in closed-chest dogs. ***Anesth Analg*** 1990;71:475–483.

Dalibon N, Moutafis M, Liu N et al. Treatment of hypoxemia during one-lung ventilation using intravenous almitrine. ***Anesth Analg*** 2004;98:590–594.

Duncan PG. Availability of dantrolene in Canadian hospitals. ***Can Anaesth Soc J*** 1985;32:205–209.

Fitzgibbon DC. Malignant hyperthermia following preoperative oral administration of dantrolene. ***Anesthesiology*** 1981;54:73–75.

Flewellen EH, Nelson TE, Jones WP, et al. Dantrolene dose response in awake man. Implications for management of malignant hyperthermia. ***Anesthesiology*** 1983;59:275–280.

Fricke RM, Hoerauf KH, Drewe J, et al. Secretion of dantrolene into breast milk after acute therapy of a suspected malignant hyperthermia crisis during cesarean section. ***Anesthesiology*** 1998;89: 1023–1025.

Hirsh K, Wang SC. Selective respiratory stimulating action of doxapram compared to pentylenetetrazol. ***J Pharmacol Exp Ther*** 1974;189:1–11.

Lerman J, McLeod ME, Strong HA. Pharmacokinetics of intravenous dantrolene in children. ***Anesthesiology*** 1989;70:625–629.

Lyew MA, Mondy C, Eagle S, et al. Hemodynamic instability and delayed emergence from general anesthesia associated with inadvertent intrathecal baclofen overdose. ***Anesthesiology*** 2003;98: 265–268.

Mitchell RM, Herbert DA. Potencies of doxapram and hypoxia in stimulating carotid-body chemoreceptors and ventilation in anesthetized cats. ***Anesthesiology*** 1975;42:559–566.

Moser KM, Luchsinger PC, Adamson JS, et al. Respiratory stimulation with intravenous doxapram in respiratory failure. ***N Engl J Med*** 1973;288:428–431.

Penn RD, Savoy SM, Corcos D, et al. Intrathecal baclofen for severe spinal spasticity. ***N Engl J Med*** 1989;320:1517–1521.

Ramamurthy S, Steen SN, Winnie AP. Doxapram antagonism of meperidine-induced respiratory depression. ***Anesth Analg*** 1975; 54:352–356.

Rigotti NA. Cigarette smoking and body weight. ***N Engl J Med*** 1989; 320:931–933.

Ruhland G, Hinkle AJ. Malignant hyperthermia after oral and intravenous pretreatment with dantrolene in a patient susceptible to malignant hyperthermia. ***Anesthesiology*** 1984;60:159–160.

Sampathkumar P, Scanlon PD, Plevak, DJ. Baclofen withdrawal presenting as multiorgan system failure. ***Anesth Analg*** 1998;87: 562–563.

San Juan AC, Wong KC, Port JD. Hyperkalemia after dantrolene and verapamil-dantrolene administration in dogs. ***Anesth Analg*** 1988; 67:759–762.

Santiago-Palma J, Hord D, Vallejo R, et al. Respiratory distress after intrathecal baclofen withdrawal. ***Anesth Analg*** 2004;99: 227–229.

Sebel PS, Kershaw EJ, Rao WS. Effects of doxapram on postoperative pulmonary complications following thoracotomy. ***Br J Anaesth*** 1980;52:81–84.

Sill JC, Schumacher K, Southorn PA, et al. Bradycardia and hypotension associated with baclofen used during general anesthesia. ***Anesthesiology*** 1986;64:255–258.

Tseng TC, Wang SC. Locus of action of centrally acting muscle relaxants, diazepam, and tybamate. ***J Pharmacol Exp Ther*** 1971;178: 350–360.

Watson CB, Reierson N, Norfleet EA. Clinically significant muscle weakness induced by oral dantrolene sodium prophylaxis for malignant hyperthermia. ***Anesthesiology*** 1986;65:312–314.

Weingarten AE, Korsh JI, Neuman GG, et al. Postpartum uterine atony after intravenous dantrolene. ***Anesth Analg*** 1987;66:269– 270.

Young RR, Delwaide PJ. Drug therapy-spasticity. ***N Engl J Med*** 1981; 304:96–99.

Vitamins, Dietary Supplements, and Herbal Remedies

34

VITAMINS

Vitamins are a group of structurally diverse organic substances (water soluble or fat soluble) that must be provided in small amounts in the diet for subsequent synthesis of cofactors that are essential for various metabolic reactions (Table 34-1). Food is the best source of vitamins, and healthy persons consuming an adequate balanced diet will not benefit from supplemental vitamins. Nevertheless, many persons do not consume adequate amounts of vitamin-rich foods, especially the elderly and poor. In addition, antioxidant vitamins can retard atherogenesis, and antioxidants may lower the risk of carcinogenesis. There is a demonstrated relationship between low dietary intake of antioxidants or low plansma concentrations of antioxidants and an increased risk of atherosclerosis and cancer. Studies have linked low plasma concentrations of folic acid, vitamin B_6 and vitamin B_{12} with increased plasma concentrations of homocysteine and increased cardiovascular risks (Wald et al., 2002). A vitamin supplement that combines antioxidants with zinc can slow progression of macular degneration. Individuals who consume multivitamins appear to have a decreased risk of cardiovascular disease and colon cancer, which may represent protection from folic acid (Giovannucci et al., 1998; Rimm et al., 1998). Randomized clinical trials have not confirmed the efficacy of vitamin E in decrasing the risk of myocardial infarction in patients with coronary artery disease (Asplund, 2002). Beta-carotene supplements may increase the risk of lung cancer in individuals who smoke cigarettes and hypervitaminosis is linked to an increased risk of fractures (Michaelsson et al., 2003; Omenn et al., 1996).

It is clear that additional information and studies are necessary to clarify the need for vitamin supplements in the presence of an adequate diet. The present recommendation is for parturients, the elderly, and those individuals receiving a suboptimal nutritional diet to take a single multivitamin tablet daily. Strict vegetarians should take vitamin B_{12} supplements.

Use of megadose vitamin preparations is not encouraged. Brand-name and so-called all-natural preparations are no more effective than generic vitamin preparations. Regardless, vitamin supplements should never be used as a substitute for a balanced healthful diet that provides abundant quantities of vitamin-rich foods.

Water-Soluble Vitamins

Water-soluble vitamins include members of the vitamin B complex (thiamine, riboflavin, nicotinic acid, pyridoxine, pantothenic acid, biotin, cyanocobalamin, folic acid) and ascorbic acid (Fig. 34-1).

Thiamine (Vitamin B_1)

Thiamine is converted to a physiologically active coenzyme known as *thiamine pyrophosphate*. This coenzyme is essential for the decarboxylation of alpha-keto acids such as pyruvate and in the use of pentose in the hexose-monophosphate shunt pathway. Indeed, increased plasma concentrations of pyruvate are a diagnostic sign of thiamine deficiency.

Causes of Deficiency

The requirement for thiamine is related to the metabolic rate and is greatest when carbohydrate is the source of energy. This is important in patients maintained by hyperalimentation in which the majority of calories are

TABLE 34-1.
VITAMINS

	Function	Deficiency	Toxic Effects	Sources
Thiamine (B_1)	Metabolism of carbohydrates, alcohol, amino acids	Beriberi Wernicke-Korsakoff syndrome	None	Grains Legumes Poultry Meat
Riboflavin (B_2)	Cellular oxidation-reduction reactions	Stomatitis Dermatitis Anemia	None	Grains Dairy products Meat Eggs Green vegetables
Nicotinic acid (niacin, B_3)	Oxidative metabolism Decreases LDL cholesterol Increases HDL cholesterol	Pellagra	Flushing Headaches Pruritus Hyperglycemia Hyperuricemia	Meat Poultry Fish Grains Peanuts Tryptophan in Foods
Pyridoxine (B_6)	Amino acid metabolism Heme synthesis Neuronal excitability Decreases blood homocysteine levels	Anemia Cheilosis Dermatitis	Neurotoxicity	Liver Poultry Fish Grains Bananas
Pantothenic acid	Metabolic processes	Rare	None	Many foods
B_{12} (cobalamin, cyanocobalamin)	DNA synthesis Myelin synthesis Decreases blood homocysteine levels	Megaloblastic anemia Peripheral neuropathies	None	Liver Poultry Fish Dairy products
Folic acid	DNA synthesis Decreases blood homocysteine levels	Megaloblastic anemia Birth defects	None	Legumes Grains Fruit Poultry Meat
Ascorbic acid (vitamin C)	Collagen synthesis Possible protection against certain cancers	Scurvy	Nephrolithiasis Diarrhea	Fruits Green vegetables Potatoes Cereals
Vitamin A (retinol, retinoic acid)	Vision Epithelial integrity Possible protection	Night blindness Susceptibility to infection	Teratogenicity Hepatotoxicity Cerebral edema	Liver Dairy products Green vegetables
Vitamin D (calciferol)	Intestinal calcium absorption	Osteomalacia Rickets	Hypercalcemia	Dairy products Fish Eggs Liver
Vitamin E (tocopherol)	Decreases peroxidation of fatty acids Possible protection against atherosclerosis	Rare	Antagonism of vitamin K Headaches	Vegetable oils Wheat germ Nuts
Vitamin K	Synthesis of clotting factors (VII, IX, X)	Hemorrhagic diathesis	None	Green vegetables Intestinal bacteria

provided in the form of glucose. Such patients should receive supplemental amounts of thiamine. Thiamine requirements are also increased during pregnancy and lactation.

Symptoms of Deficiency

Symptoms of mild thiamine deficiency (beriberi) include loss of appetite, skeletal muscle weakness, a tendency to develop peripheral edema, decreased systemic blood pressure, and low body temperature. Severe thiamine deficiency (Korsakoff syndrome), which may occur in alcoholics, is associated with peripheral polyneuritis, including areas of hyperesthesia and anesthesia of the legs, impairment of memory, and encephalopathy. High-output cardiac failure with extensive peripheral edema reflecting hypoproteinemia is often prominent. There is flattening or inversion of the T wave prolongation of the QTc interval on the electrocardiogram (ECG).

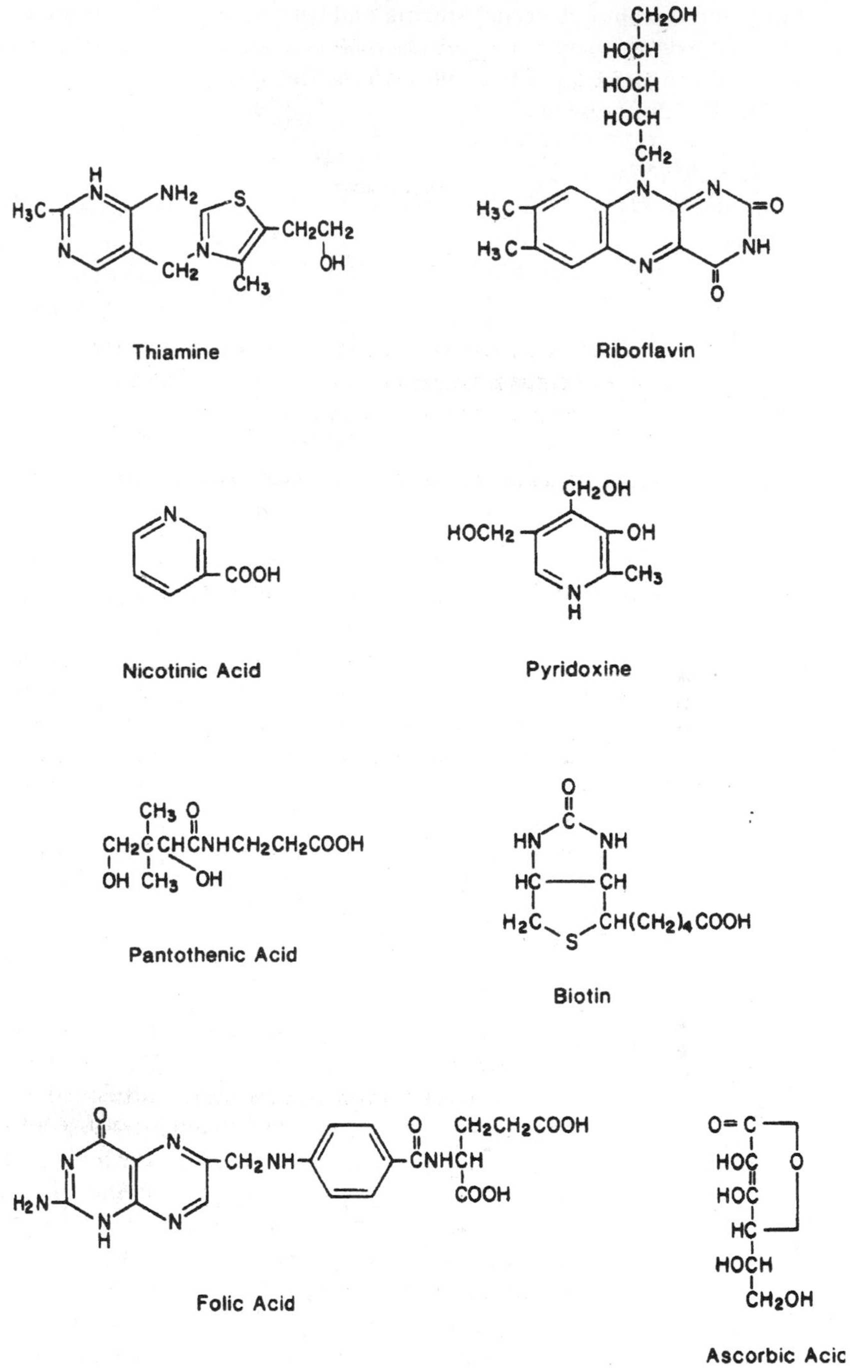

Figure 34-1. Water-soluble vitamins.

Treatment of Deficiency

Severe thiamine deficiency is treated with intravenous (IV) administration of the vitamin. Once severe thiamine deficiency has been corrected, oral supplementation is acceptable.

Riboflavin (Vitamin B_2)

Riboflavin is converted in the body to one of two physiologically active coenzymes: flavin mononucleotide or flavin adenine dinucleotide. These coenzymes primarily influence hydrogen ion transport in oxidative enzyme systems, including cytochrome C reductase, succinic dehydrogenase, and xanthine oxidase. Chlorpromazine and tricyclic antidepressants interfere with the flavokinase reaction necessary to convert riboflavin to its active coenzymes, thus increasing requirements. Tissue storage of this water-soluble vitamin is not extensive.

Symptoms of Deficiency

Pharyngitis and angular stomatitis are typically the first signs of riboflavin deficiency. Later glossitis, red denuded lips, seborrheic dermatitis of the face, and dermatitis over the trunk and extremities occur. Anemia and peripheral neuropathy may be prominent. Corneal vascularization and cataract formation occur in some subjects. Treatment is with oral vitamin supplements that contain riboflavin.

Nicotinic Acid (Niacin, B_3)

Nicotinic acid is converted to the physiologically active coenzyme nicotinamide adenine dinucleotide (NAD) and nicotinamide adenine dinucleotide phosphate (NADP). These coenzymes are necessary to catalyze oxidation-reduction reactions essential for tissue respiration.

Symptoms of Deficiency

Nicotinic acid is an essential dietary constituent, the lack of which leads to dermatitis, diarrhea, and dementia. Pellagra is the all-inclusive term for the symptoms of nicotinic acid deficiency. The skin characteristically becomes erythematous and rough in texture, especially in areas exposed to sun, friction, or pressure. The chief symptoms referable to the digestive tract are stomatitis, enteritis, and diarrhea. The tongue becomes very red and swollen. Salivary secretions are excessive, and nausea and vomiting are common. In addition to dementia, motor and sensory disturbances of the peripheral nerves also occur, mimicking changes that accompany a deficiency of thiamine.

The dietary requirement for niacin can be satisfied not only by nicotinic acid but also by nicotinamide and the amino acid tryptophan. The relationship between nicotinic acid requirements and the intake of tryptophan explains the association of pellagra with tryptophan-deficient corn diets. Carcinoid syndrome is associated with diversion of tryptophan from the synthesis of nicotinic acid to the production of serotonin (5-hydroxytryptamine), leading to symptoms of pellagra. Isoniazid inhibits incorporation of nicotinic acid into NAD and may produce pellagra.

Pellagra is uncommon in the United States, reflecting the supplementation of flour with nicotinic acid. Common causes of pellagra include chronic gastrointestinal disease and alcoholism, which are characteristically associated with multiple nutritional deficiencies. When pellagra is severe, IV administration of nicotinic acid is indicated. In less severe cases, oral administration of nicotinic acid is adequate. The response to nicotinic acid is dramatic, with symptoms waning within 24 hours after initiation of therapy.

Toxic effects of nicotinic acid include flushing, pruritus, hepatotoxicity, hyperuricemia, and activation of peptic ulcer disease. Nicotinic acid has also been prescribed to decrease the plasma concentrations of cholesterol (see Chapter 32).

Pyridoxine (Vitamin B_6)

Pyridoxine is converted to its physiologically active form, pyridoxal phosphate, by the enzyme pyridoxal kinase. Pyridoxal phosphate serves an important role in metabolism as a coenzyme for the conversion of tryptophan to serotonin and methionine to cysteine.

Symptoms of Deficiency

Pyridoxine deficiency is frequent in alcoholics (estimated incidence 30%), manifesting as dermatitis, central nervous system dysfunction, and anemia. Seborrhea-like skin lesions about the eyes, nose, and mouth accompanied by glossitis and stomatitis occur. Seizures accompanying deficiency of pyridoxine and peripheral neuritis such as carpal tunnel syndrome are common. The lowered seizure threshold may reflect decreased concentrations of the inhibitory neurotransmitter gamma-aminobutyric acid, the synthesis of which requires a pyridoxal phosphate-requiring enzyme.

It is presumed that a person with a deficiency of other B vitamins may also have a relative deficiency of pyridoxine. For this reason, pyridoxine is incorporated into many multivitamin preparations for prophylactic use. Pyridoxine is unpredictably effective in the treatment of sideroblastic anemias (deficiency of hemoglobin synthesis and accumulation of iron in the mitochondria).

Drug Interactions

Isoniazid and hydralazine act as potent inhibitors of pyridoxal kinase, thus preventing synthesis of the active coenzyme form of the vitamin. Indeed, administration of pyridoxine decreases the incidence of neurologic side effects associated with the administration of these drugs. Pyridoxine enhances the peripheral decarboxylation of levodopa and decreases its effectiveness for the treatment of Parkinson disease. There is a decrease in the plasma concentration of pyridoxal phosphate in patients taking oral contraceptives.

Pantothenic Acid

Pantothenic acid is converted to its physiologically active form, coenzyme A, which serves as a cofactor for enzyme-catalyzed reactions involving transfer of two carbon (acetyl) groups. Such reactions are important in the oxidative metabolism of carbohydrates, gluconeogenesis, and the synthesis and degradation of fatty acids.

Pantothenic acid deficiency in humans is rare, reflecting the ubiquitous presence of this vitamin in ordinary foods as well as its production by intestinal bacteria. No clearly defined uses of pantothenic acid exist, although it is commonly included in multivitamin preparations and in hyperalimentation solutions.

Biotin

Biotin is an organic acid that functions as a coenzyme for enzyme-catalyzed carboxylation reactions and fatty acid synthesis. In adults, a deficiency of biotin manifests as glossitis, anorexia, dermatitis, and mental depression. Seborrheic dermatitis of infancy is most likely a form of biotin deficiency. For this reason, it is recommended that formulas contain supplemental biotin. Prolonged hyperalimentation may result in a deficiency of biotin.

Cyanocobalamin (Cobalamin, Vitamin B_{12})

Cyanocobalamin and vitamin B_{12} are generic designations that are used interchangeably to describe several cobalt-containing compounds (cobalamins). Dietary vitamin B_{12} in the presence of hydrogen ions in the stomach is released from proteins and subsequently binds to a glycoprotein intrinsic factor. This vitamin-intrinsic factor complex travels to the ileum, where it interacts with a specific receptor and is then transported into the systemic circulation. After systemic absorption, vitamin B_{12} binds to a beta-globulin, transcobalamin II, for transport to tissues, especially the liver, which serves as a storage depot.

Causes of Deficiency

Although humans depend on exogenous sources of vitamin B_{12}, a deficient diet is rarely the cause of a deficiency state. Instead, gastric achlorhydria and decreased gastric secretion of intrinsic factor are more likely causes of vitamin B_{12} deficiency in adults. Antibodies to intrinsic factor may interfere with attachment of the complex to gastrin receptors in the ileum (DeAizpurua et al., 1985). Bacterial overgrowth may prevent an adequate amount of vitamin B_{12} from reaching the ileum. Surgical resection or disease of the ileum predictably interferes with the absorption of vitamin B_{12}. Nitrous oxide irreversibly oxidizes the cobalt atom of vitamin B_{12} such that the activity of two vitamin B_{12}-dependent enzymes, methionine synthetase and thymidylate synthetase, are decreased (see Chapter 2).

Diagnosis of Deficiency

The plasma concentration of vitamin B_{12} (cobalamin) is <200 pg/mL when there is a deficiency state. Measurements of gastric acidity may provide indirect evidence of a defect in gastric parietal cell function, whereas the Schilling test (radioactivity in the urine measured after oral administration of labeled vitamin B_{12}) can be used to quantitate ileal absorption of vitamin B_{12}. Observation of reticulocytosis after a therapeutic trial of vitamin B_{12} confirms the diagnosis.

Symptoms of Deficiency

Deficiency of vitamin B_{12} results in defective synthesis of DNA, especially in tissues with the greatest rate of cell turnover. In this regard, symptoms of vitamin B_{12} deficiency manifest most often in the hematopoietic and nervous systems. Changes in the hematopoietic system are most apparent in erythrocytes, but when vitamin B_{12} deficiency is severe, a pronounced cytopenia may occur. Clinically, the earliest sign of vitamin B_{12} deficiency is megaloblastic (pernicious) anemia. Anemia may be so severe that cardiac failure occurs, especially in elderly patients with limited cardiac reserves.

Encephalopathy is a well-recognized complication of vitamin B_{12} deficiency manifesting as myelopathy, optic neuropathy, and peripheral neuropathy, either alone or in any combination. Neurologic complications do not parallel the presence of megaloblastic anemia. Damage to the myelin sheath is the most obvious symptom of nervous system dysfunction associated with vitamin B_{12} deficiency. Demyelination and cell death occur in the spinal cord and cerebral cortex, manifesting as paresthesias of the hands and feet and diminution of sensation of vibration and proprioception with resultant unsteadiness of gait. Deep tendon reflexes are decreased, and, in advanced states, loss of memory and mental confusion occur. Indeed, vitamin B_{12} deficiency should be considered in elderly patients with psychosis. Folic acid therapy corrects the hematopoietic, but not nervous system, effects produced by vitamin B_{12} deficiency.

Treatment of Deficiency

Vitamin B_{12} is available in a pure form for oral or parenteral use in combination with other vitamins for oral administration. These preparations are of little value in the treatment of patients with deficiency of intrinsic factor or ileal disease. In the presence of clinically apparent vitamin B_{12} deficiency, oral absorption is not reliable; the preparation of choice is cyanocobalamin administered intramuscularly. For example, in the patient with neurologic changes, leukopenia, or thrombocytopenia, treatment must be aggressive. Initial treatment is with intramuscular administration of vitamin B_{12} and oral administration of folic acid. An increase in the hematocrit does not occur for 10 to 20 days. The plasma concentration of iron, however, usually declines within 48 hours, because iron is now used in the formation of hemoglobin. Platelet counts can be expected to reach normal levels within days of initiating treatment; the granulocyte count requires a longer period to normalize. Memory and sense of well-being may improve within 24 hours after initiation of therapy. Neurologic signs and symptoms that have been present for prolonged periods, however, often regress slowly and may never return to completely normal function. Indeed, neurologic damage after pernicious anemia develops that is not reversed after 12 to 18 months of therapy is likely to be permanent. Once initiated, vitamin B_{12} therapy must be continued indefinitely at monthly intervals. It is important to monitor plasma concentrations of vitamin B_{12} and examine the peripheral blood cells every 3 to 6 months to confirm the adequacy of treatment.

Hydroxocobalamin has hematopoietic activity similar to that of vitamin B_{12} but appears to offer no advantage despite its somewhat longer duration of action. Furthermore, some patients develop antibodies to the complex of hydroxocobalamin and transcobalamin II. Large doses of hydroxocobalamin have been proposed for treatment of cyanide poisoning due to nitroprusside (see Chapter 16). Conceptually, cyanide reacts with hydroxocobalamin to form cyanocobalamin.

Folic acid as monotherapy for vitamin B_{12} deficiency masks the anemia and fails to prevent the neurologic complications. Fortification of the food supply with folic acid beginning in 1994 means that anemia may not be evidence of vitamin B_{12} deficiency in the future.

Folic Acid

Folic acid is transported and stored as 5-methylhydrofolate after absorption from the small intestine, principally the jejunum. Conversion to the metabolically active form, tetrahydrofolate, is dependent on the activity of vitamin B_{12}. Tetrahydrofolate acts as an acceptor of 1-carbon units necessary for (a) conversion of homocysteine to methionine, (b) conversion of serine to glycine, (c) synthesis of DNA, and (d) synthesis of purines. Supplies of folic acid are maintained by ingestion of food and by enterohepatic circulation of the vitamin. Virtually all foods contain folic acid, but protracted cooking can destroy up to 90% of the vitamin.

Causes of Deficiency

Folic acid deficiency is a common complication of diseases of the small intestine, such as sprue, that interfere with absorption of the vitamin and its enterohepatic recirculation. Alcoholism reduces intake of folic acid in food, and enterohepatic recirculation may be impaired by the toxic effect of alcohol on hepatocytes. Indeed, alcoholism is the most common cause of folic acid deficiency, with decreases in the plasma concentrations of folic acid manifesting within 24 to 48 hours of continuous alcohol ingestion. Drugs that inhibit dihydrofolate reductase (methotrexate, trimethoprim) or interfere with absorption and storage of folic acid in tissues (phenytoin) may cause folic acid deficiency.

Symptoms of Deficiency

Megaloblastic anemia is the most common manifestation of folic acid deficiency. This anemia cannot be distinguished from that caused by a deficiency of vitamin B_{12}. Folic acid deficiency, however, is confirmed by the presence of a folic acid concentration in the plasma of <4 ng/mL. Furthermore, the rapid onset of megaloblastic anemia produced by folic acid deficiency (1 to 4 weeks) reflects the limited in vivo stores of this vitamin and contrasts with the slower onset (2 to 3 years) of symptoms of vitamin B_{12} deficiency.

Treatment of Deficiency

Folic acid is available as an oral preparation alone or in combination with other vitamins and as a parenteral injection. The therapeutic uses of folic acid are limited to the prevention and treatment of deficiencies. For example, pregnancy increases folic acid requirements, and oral supplementation, usually in a multivitamin preparation, is indicated. In the presence of megaloblastic anemia because of folic acid deficiency, the administration of the vitamin is associated with a decrease in the plasma concentration of iron within 48 hours, reflecting new erythropoiesis. Likewise, the reticulocyte count begins to increase within 48 to 72 hours, and the hematocrit begins to increase during the second week of therapy.

Folate Therapy

Vitamin therapy to lower homocysteine levels has been recommended for the prevention of restenosis after coronary angioplasty. This is based on the belief that homocysteine is thrombogenic and is a risk factor for coronary artery disease. Folate supplementation is an effective treatment of homocystinemia. Nevertheless, folate therapy (combination of folic acid, vitamin B_6, and vitamin B_{12}) may actually increase the risk of in-stent restenosis and the need for revascularization (Lange et al., 2004).

Leucovorin

Leucovorin (citrovorum factor) is a metabolically active, reduced form of folic acid. After treatment with folic acid antagonists, such as methotrexate, patients may receive leucovorin (rescue therapy), which serves as a source of tetrahydrofolate that cannot be formed due to drug-induced inhibition of dihydrofolate reductase (see Chapter 29). It is possible that nitrous oxide, by inhibiting vitamin B_{12}-dependent enzymes, would impair the efficacy of leucovorin as a source for tetrahydrofolate (see Chapter 2) (Ueland et al., 1986).

Ascorbic Acid (Vitamin C)

Ascorbic acid is a six-carbon compound structurally related to glucose. This vitamin acts as a coenzyme and is important in a number of biochemical reactions, mostly involving oxidation. For example, ascorbic acid is necessary for the synthesis of collagen, carnitine, and corticosteroids. Ascorbic acid is readily absorbed from the gastrointestinal tract, and many foods, such as orange juice and lemon juice, have a high content of ascorbic acid. When gastrointestinal absorption is impaired, ascorbic acid can be administered intramuscularly or IV. Apart from its role in nutrition, ascorbic acid is commonly used as an antioxidant to protect the natural flavor and color of many foods.

Despite contrary claims, controlled studies do not support the efficacy of even large doses of ascorbic acid in treating viral respiratory tract infections (Moertel et al., 1985). A risk of large doses of ascorbic acid is the formation of kidney stones resulting from the excessive secretion of oxalate. Excessive ascorbic acid doses can also enhance the absorption of iron and interfere with anticoagulant therapy.

Symptoms of Deficiency

A deficiency of ascorbic acid is known as scurvy. Humans, in contrast to many other mammals, are unable to synthesize ascorbic acid, emphasizing the need for dietary sources of the vitamin to prevent scurvy. Specifically, humans lack the hepatic enzyme necessary to produce ascorbic acid from gluconate (Crandon et al., 1940). Manifestations of scurvy include gingivitis, rupture of the capillaries with formation of numerous petechiae, and failure of wounds to heal. An associated anemia may reflect a specific function of ascorbic acid on hemoglobin synthesis. Scurvy is evident when the plasma concentration of ascorbic acid is <0.15 mg/dL.

Scurvy is encountered among the elderly, alcoholics, and drug addicts. Ascorbic acid requirements are increased during pregnancy, lactation, and stresses such as infection or after surgery. Infants receiving formula diets with inadequate concentrations of ascorbic acid can develop scurvy. Patients receiving hyperalimentation should receive supplemental ascorbic acid. Urinary loss of infused ascorbic acid is large, necessitating daily doses of 200 mg to maintain normal concentrations in plasma of 1 mg/dL. Increased urinary excretion of ascorbic acid is caused by salicylates, tetracyclines, and barbiturates.

Fat-Soluble Vitamins

The fat-soluble vitamins are vitamins A, D, E, and K (Fig. 34-2). They are absorbed from the gastrointestinal tract by a complex process that parallels absorption of fat. Thus, any condition that causes malabsorption of fat, such as obstructive jaundice, may result in deficiency of one or all these vitamins. Fat-soluble vitamins are stored principally in the liver and excreted in the feces. Because these vitamins are metabolized very slowly, overdose may produce toxic effects. Vitamin D, despite its name, functions as a hormone.

Vitamin A (retinol, retinoic acid)

Vitamin A exists in a variety of forms, including retinal and 3-dehydroretinal. This vitamin is important in the function of the retina, integrity of mucosal and epithelial surfaces, bone development and growth, reproduction, and embryonic development. It also has a stabilizing effect on various membranes and regulates membrane permeability. Vitamin A may exert transcriptional control of the production of specific proteins, a process that has important implications with respect to regulation of cellular differentiation and development of malignancies. Limitations in the therapeutic use of vitamin A for antineoplastic uses are the associated hepatotoxicity and its failure to distribute to specific organs.

Major dietary sources of vitamin A are liver, butter, cheese, milk, certain fish, and various yellow or green fruits and vegetables. Fish liver oils contain large amounts of vitamin A. Sufficient vitamin A is stored in the liver of well-nourished persons to satisfy requirements for several months. Plasma concentrations of vitamin A are maintained at the expense of hepatic reserves and thus do not always reflect a person's vitamin A status. Vitamin A may interact with cellular proteins, which function analogously to receptors for estrogens and other steroids.

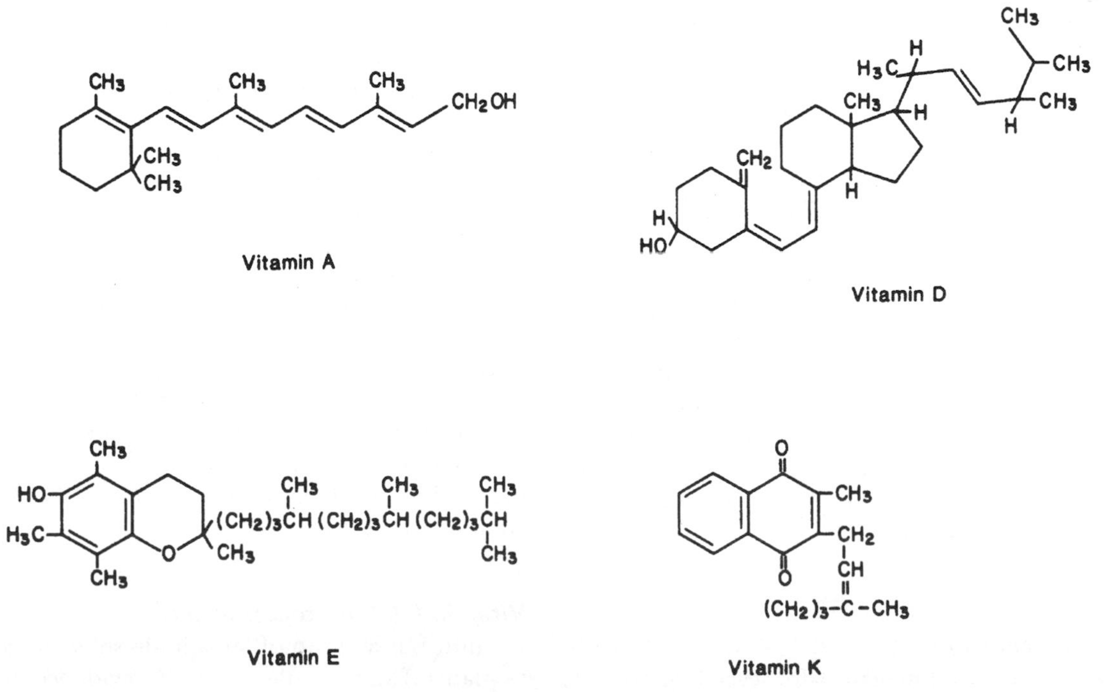

Figure 34-2. Fat-soluble vitamins.

Symptoms of Deficiency

Plasma concentrations of vitamin A of <20 μg/dL indicate the risk of deficiency. Most deficiencies occur in infants or children. Signs and symptoms of mild vitamin A deficiency are easily overlooked. Skin lesions such as follicular hyperkeratosis and infections are often the earliest signs of deficiency. Nevertheless, the most recognizable manifestation of vitamin A deficiency is night blindness (nyctalopia), which occurs only when the depletion is severe. Pulmonary infections are increased as bronchial epithelium for mucous secretion undergoes keratinization. Keratinization and drying of the epidermis occurs. Urinary calculi are frequently associated with vitamin A deficiency, which may reflect epithelial changes that provide a nidus around which a calculus is formed. Abnormalities of reproduction include impairment of spermatogenesis and spontaneous abortion. Impairment of taste and smell is common is patients with vitamin A deficiency, presumably reflecting a keratinizing effect. Decreased erythropoiesis may be masked by abnormal losses of fluids.

Hypervitaminosis A

Hypervitaminosis A is the toxic syndrome that results from excessive ingestion of vitamin A, particularly in children. Typically, high vitamin A intake has resulted from overzealous prophylactic vitamin A therapy. Plasma concentrations of vitamin A of >300 μg/dL are diagnostic of hypervitaminosis A. Treatment consists of withdrawal of the vitamin source, which is usually followed within 7 days by disappearance of the manifestations of excess vitamin A activity.

Early signs and symptoms of vitamin A intoxication include irritability, vomiting, and dermatitis. Fatigue, myalgia, loss of body hair, diplopia, nystagmus, gingivitis, stomatitis, and lymphadenopathy have been observed. Hepatosplenomegaly is accompanied by cirrhosis of the liver, portal vein hypertension, and ascites. Intracranial pressure may be increased, and neurologic symptoms, including papilledema, may mimic those of a brain tumor (pseudotumor cerebri). The diagnosis is confirmed by radiologic demonstration of hyperostoses underlying tender swellings on the extremities and the occipital region of the head. Plasma alkaline phosphatase concentrations are increased, reflecting osteoblastic activity. Hypercalcemia may occur because of bone destruction. Bones continue to grow in length but not in thickness, with increased susceptibility to fractures. Congenital abnormalities may occur in infants whose mothers have consumed excessive amounts of vitamin A during pregnancy. Psychiatric disturbances may mimic mental depression or schizophrenia.

Vitamin D (Calciferol)

Vitamin D is the generic designation for several sterols and their metabolites that act as hormones to maintain plasma calcium concentrations and phosphate ions in an optimal range for neuromuscular function, mineralization of bones, and other calcium-dependent functions. This regulation of the plasma concentrations of calcium and phosphate reflects the ability of vitamin D to facilitate absorption of these ions from the gastrointestinal tract and enhance the mobilization of calcium from bones. In addition, there may be a direct effect of vitamin D on proximal renal tubules that results in increased retention of calcium and phosphate.

The principal provitamin of vitamin D in tissues, 7-dehydrocholesterol, is synthesized in the skin and converted to vitamin D on exposure of the skin to sunlight. Vitamin D is also absorbed from the gastrointestinal tract after oral administration. Bile salts are necessary for this absorption, emphasizing that hepatic or biliary dysfunction may impair passage of vitamin D into the circulation. Absorbed vitamin D is hydroxylated in the liver to calcitriol, the active form of vitamin D. This conversion to calcitriol is regulated in a negative feedback manner by the plasma calcium concentration. The elimination half-time of calcitriol is 3 to 5 days.

Symptoms of Deficiency

A deficiency of vitamin D results in decreased plasma concentrations of calcium and phosphate ions, with the subsequent stimulation of parathyroid hormone secretion. Parathyroid hormone acts to restore plasma calcium concentrations at the expense of bone calcium. In infants and children, this results in failure to mineralize newly formed osteoid tissue and cartilage, causing formation of soft bone, which, with weight bearing, results in deformities known as rickets. In adults, vitamin D deficiency results in osteomalacia. Anticonvulsant therapy with phenytoin increases target organ resistance to vitamin D, resulting in an increased incidence of rickets and osteomalacia. There is evidence that vitamin D supplementation reduces the risk of falling among elderly individuals (Bischoff-Ferrari et al., 2004).

Hypervitaminosis D

Administration of excessive amounts of vitamin D results in hypervitaminosis, manifesting as hypercalcemia, skeletal muscle weakness, fatigue, headache, and vomiting. Early impairment of renal function from hypercalcemia manifests as polyuria, polydipsia, proteinuria, and decreased urine-concentrating ability. In addition to withdrawal of the vitamin, treatment includes increased fluid intake and administration of corticosteroids.

Vitamin E (alpha-tocopherol)

Vitamin E is a group of fat-soluble substances occurring in plants. There is little persuasive evidence that vitamin E is nutritionally significant in humans (Roberts, 1981).

Alpha-tocopherol is the most abundant and important of the eight naturally occurring tocopherols that constitute vitamin E. An important chemical feature of the tocopherols is that they are antioxidants. In acting as an antioxidant, vitamin E presumably prevents oxidation of essential cellular constituents or prevents the formation of toxic oxidation products. There seems to be a relationship between vitamins A and E in which vitamin E facilitates the absorption, hepatic storage, and use of vitamin A. In addition, vitamin E seems to protect against the development of hypervitaminosis A by enhancing the use of the vitamin. Vitamin E is stored in adipose tissue and is thought to stabilize the lipid portions of cell membranes. Other functions attributed to vitamin E are inhibition of prostaglandin production and stimulation of an essential cofactor in corticosteroid metabolism.

Vitamin E requirements may be increased in individuals exposed to high oxygen environments or in those receiving therapeutic doses of iron or large doses of thyroid hormone replacement. Vitamin E may be important in hematopoiesis, with occasional forms of anemia responding favorably to the administration of alpha-tocopherol.

Despite absence of conclusive supportive evidence, vitamin E has been administered to females with a history of recurrent spontaneous abortions and for sterility in both genders. In animals, vitamin E deficiency leads to the development of muscular dystrophy, but there is no evidence that a similar sequence occurs in humans. Changes similar to those observed in skeletal muscles have occurred in cardiac muscle of animals. A necrotizing myopathy with proximal skeletal muscle weakness and increased plasma concentrations of creatine kinase may occur in patients self-medicated with large doses of vitamin E. There are data that support an association between low plasma levels of vitamin E and the risk of developing lung cancer (Menkes et al., 1986).

Epidemiologic studies have provided evidence of an inverse relation between coronary artery disease and antioxidant intake, and vitamin E supplementation in particular (Diaz et al., 1997). This association has been explained because of antioxidants preventing oxidation of lipids in low-density lipoproteins. It is proposed that oxidation of lipids in low-density lipoproteins (lipid peroxidation) initiates the process of atherogenesis. Vitamin C is also an antioxidant but its water-solubility prevents its incorporation into low-density lipoproteins.

Vitamin K

Vitamin K is a lipid-soluble dietary compound that is essential for the biosynthesis of several factors required for normal blood clotting (see Chapter 57). Phytonadione (vitamin K_1) is present in a variety of foods and is the only natural form of vitamin K available for therapeutic use. Vitamin K_2 represents a series of compounds that are synthesized by Gram-positive bacteria in the gastrointestinal tract. Synthesis of vitamin K provides approximately 50% of the estimated daily requirement of vitamin K; the rest is supplied by the diet. Vitamin K is absorbed from the gastrointestinal tract only in the presence of adequate quantities of bile salts. Vitamin K accumulates in the liver, spleen, and lungs, but despite its lipid solubility, significant amounts are not stored in the body for prolonged periods.

Mechanism of Action

Vitamin K functions as an essential cofactor for the hepatic microsomal enzyme that converts glutamic acid residues to gamma-carboxyglutamic acid residues in factors II (prothrombin), VII, IX, and X. The gamma-carboxyglutamic acid residues make it possible for these coagulation factors to bind calcium ions and attach to phospholipid surfaces, leading to clot formation. If vitamin K deficiency occurs, the plasma concentrations of these coagulation factors decrease and a hemorrhagic disorder develops. This disorder is characterized by ecchymoses, epistaxis, hematuria, and gastrointestinal bleeding; postoperative hemorrhage is also a possibility. Prothrombin time is used to monitor vitamin K activity.

Clinical Uses

Vitamin K is administered to treat its deficiency and attendant decrease in plasma concentrations of prothrombin and related clotting factors. Deficiency of vitamin K may be due to (a) inadequate dietary intake, (b) decreased bacterial synthesis due to antibiotic therapy, (c) impaired gastrointestinal absorption resulting from obstructive biliary tract disease and absence of bile salts, or (d) hepatocellular disease. Neonates have hypoprothrombinemia due to vitamin K deficiency until adequate dietary intake of the vitamin occurs and normal intestinal bacterial floras are established. Indeed, at birth, the normal infant has only 20% to 40% of the adult plasma concentrations of clotting factors II, VII, IX, and X. These plasma concentrations decrease even further during the first 2 to 3 days after birth, and then begin to increase toward adult values after approximately 6 days. In premature infants, plasma concentrations of clotting factors are even lower. Human breast milk has low concentrations of vitamin K. Administration of vitamin K, 0.5 to 1.0 mg intramuscularly at birth, to the normal neonate prevents the decrease in concentration of vitamin K dependent clotting factors in the first days after birth but does not increase these concentrations to adult levels.

Vitamin K replacement therapy is not effective when severe hepatocellular disease is responsible for the decreased production of clotting factors. In the absence of severe hepatocellular disease and the presence of adequate bile salts, the administration of oral vitamin K preparations is effective in reversing hypoprothrombinemia. Phytonadione and menadione are the vitamin K preparations most often used to treat hypoprothrombinemia.

Phytonadione

Phytonadione (vitamin K_1) is the preferred drug to treat hypoprothrombinemia, particularly if large doses or prolonged therapy is necessary. Hypoprothrombinemia of the neonate is treated with phytonadione, 0.5 to 1.0 mg intramuscularly, within 24 hours of birth. A frequent indication for phytonadione is to reverse the effects of oral anticoagulants. For example, phytonadione, 10 to 20 mg orally or administered IV at a rate of 1 mg per minute, is usually adequate to reverse the effects of oral anticoagulants (see Chapter 27). The oral and intramuscular routes of administration are less likely than the IV injections of phytonadione to cause side effects and are thus preferred for nonemergency reversal of oral anticoagulants. Even large doses of phytonadione are ineffective against heparin-induced anticoagulation. Vitamin K supplementation is also indicated

TABLE 34-2.
DIETARY SUPPLEMENTS AND HERBAL REMEDIES

	Suggested Uses	Potential Toxicity	Drug Interactions
Black cohosh	Menopausal symptoms	Gastrointestinal discomfort	
Chaste tree berries	Premenstrual symptoms	Pruritus	Dopamine-receptor antagonists
Cranberry	Urinary tract infections	Nephrolithiasis	
Dong quai	Menopausal symptoms	Rash	Warfarin
Echinacea	Upper respiratory infections	Hypersensitivity reactions Hepatic inflammation	
Evening primrose	Eczema Irritable bowel syndrome Premenstrual symptoms Rheumatoid arthritis	Nausea Vomiting Diarrhea Flatulence	Antiepileptic drugs
Feverfew	Prevent migraine Arthritis Allergies	Hypersensitivity reactions Inhibits platelet activity	Warfarin
Garlic	Hypertension Hypertriglyceridemia Hypercholesterolemia	Gastrointestinal discomfort Hemorrhage	Warfarin
Ginger	Motion sickness Vertigo		Warfarin
Ginkgo biloba	Dementia Claudication Tinnitus	Gastrointestinal discomfort Headache Dizziness Bleeding Seizures	Warfarin
Ginseng	Fatigue Diabetes	Tachycardia Hypertension	Warfarin
Goldenseal	Laxative	Hypertension Edema	
Kava kava	Anxiety	Rash Sedation Liver toxicity	Benzodiazepines Alcohol Anesthetic drugs
Kola nut	Fatigue	Irritability Insomnia	Stimulants
Licorice	Gastric ulcers	Hypertension	
Saw palmetto	Prostatic hyperplasia	Gastrointestinal discomfort	
St. John's wort	Depression Anxiety	Headache Insomnia Dizzinesss Gastrointestinal discomfort	Digoxin Oral contraceptives Serotonin antagonists Anesthetic drugs
Valerian	Insomnia	Headaches	Benzodiazepines Anesthetic drugs Antiepileptic drugs

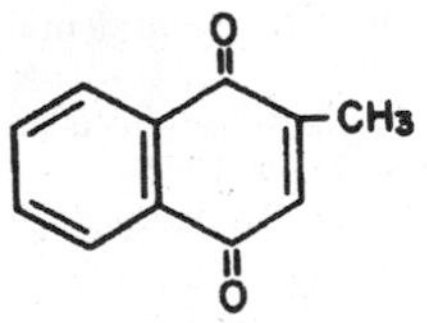

Figure 34-3. Menadione.

for patients receiving prolonged hyperalimentation, especially if antibiotics are concomitantly administered.

IV injection of phytonadione may cause life-threatening allergic reactions characterized by hypotension and bronchospasm. Intramuscular administration may produce local hemorrhage at the injection site in hypoprothrombinemic patients. In neonates, doses of phytonadione of >1 mg may cause hemolytic anemia and increase the plasma concentrations of unbound bilirubin, thus increasing the risk of kernicterus. The occurrence of hemolytic anemia reflects a deficiency of glycolytic enzymes in some neonates.

Menadione

Menadione has the same actions and uses as phytonadione (Fig. 34-3). Water-soluble salts of menadione do not require the presence of bile salts for their systemic absorption after oral administration. This characteristic becomes important when malabsorption of vitamin K is due to biliary obstruction.

Menadione hemolyzes erythrocytes in patients genetically deficient in glucose-6-phosphate dehydrogenase, as well as in neonates, particularly premature infants. This hemolysis and occasionally hepatic toxicity reflect combination of menadione with sulfhydryl groups in tissues. Kernicterus has occurred after menadione administration to neonates. For this reason, menadione is not recommended for treatment of hemorrhagic disease of the neonate. Administration of large doses of menadione or phytonadione may depress liver function, particularly in the presence of preexisting liver disease.

DIETARY SUPPLEMENTS

Dietary supplements (vitamins, minerals, herbs, amino acids, enzymes) are products ingested orally and intended to supplement the diet. Herbs include flowering plants, shrubs, seaweed, and algae. It is estimated that 25% of patients use alternative therapies characterized as dietary supplements or herbal remedies (more than 3 billion doses). These products are not subject to FDA approval (do not undergo scientific testing to prove efficacy and plants and parts of plants are not patent-eligible) although they cannot be promoted specifically for treatment, prevention, or cure of disease. Nevertheless, these products can be labeled with statements describing their alleged effects. The FDA has no control over the herbal industry in terms of safety guidelines that would regulate purity and consistency of therapeutic medications.

Adverse Effects and Drug Interactions (Tables 34-2 and 34-3)

Individuals who take dietary supplements and/or herbal remedies in combination with prescription drugs may be at risk for adverse interactions (Tables 34-2 and 34-3) (Cupp, 1999). The most serious side effects associated with these substances include cardiovascular instability, bleeding tendency particularly in conjunction with other anticoagulants such as warfarin, and delayed awakening from anesthesia.

Ephedra (ma huang) is a common ingredient in herbal weight-loss products, stimulants, decongestants, and bronchodilators. The active moiety in ephedra is ephedrine, a sympathomimetic amine structurally related to amphetamines. Serious adverse reactions, including hypertension, cardiac dysrhythmias, prolonged QTc interval on the ECG, myocardial infarction, stroke, and death have been described in patients taking ephedra (McBride et al., 2004). The chances of experiencing an adverse reaction when taking ephedra are estimated to be 100-fold greater than with any other dietary supplement or herbal remedy. Although

TABLE 34-3.
NONHERBAL DIETARY SUPPLEMENTS

	Suggested Uses	Potential Toxicity	Drug Interactions
Coenzyme Q10	Congestive heart failure Hypertension	Dyspepsia Nausea Diarrhea	Warfarin
Glucosamine	Osteoarthritis	Gastrointestinal discomfort	Warfarin
Melatonin	Insomnia Jet lag	Fatigue Sedation	
S-adenosylmethionine	Osteoarthritis Depression	Nausea Gastrointestinal discomfort	Tricyclic antidepressants

tachycardia and vasoconstriction can occur in healthy patients, those with heart disease or systemic hypertension, or those who engage in strenuous physical exercise seem to be at greatest risk for ephedra-related side effects. Based on the risk of adverse reactions it was concluded by the FDA that dietary supplements containing ephedra present an unreasonable risk of illness or injury. Sales of dietary supplements containing ephedra were banned by the FDA in April 2004.

Ginseng may cause tachycardia or systemic hypertension particularly in combinations with other cardiac stimulant drugs. In addition, ginseng may decrease the anticoagulant effects of warfarin. Feverfew may enhance bleeding by inhibition of platelet activity. Warfarin may also be potentiated by concomitant use garlic, ginkgo biloba, and ginger. Ginkgo biloba has been suggested to possess antiplatelet effects, and spontaneous hemorrhage has been reported (Matthews, 1998). St. John's wort that is alleged to be a natural antidepressant has been shown to inhibit serotonin, dopamine, and norepinephrine reuptake and thus present the possibility of interactions with monoamine oxidase inhibitors and other serotoninergic drugs (Haller and Benowitz, 2000). Valerian, kava-kava, and possibly St. John's wort may delay awakening from anesthesia by prolonging sedative effects of anesthetic drugs.

REFERENCES

Asplund K. Antioxidant vitamins in the prevention of cardiovascular disease: A systematic review. *J Intern Med* 2002;251:372–376.

Bischoff-Ferrari HA, Dawson-Hughes B, Willett WC, et al. Effect of vitamin D on falls. A meta-analysis. *JAMA* 2004;291:1999–2006.

Crandon JH, Lund CC, Dill DB. Experimental human scurvy. *N Engl J Med* 1940;223:353–369.

Cupp MJ. Herbal remedies: adverse effects and drug interactions. *Am Fam Physician* 1999;59:1239–1245.

DeAizpurua HJ, Ungar B, Toh BH. Autoantibody to the gastrin receptor in pernicious anemia. *N Engl J Med* 1985;313:479–483.

Diaz MN, Frei B, Vita JA, et al. Antioxidants and atherosclerotic heart disease. *N Engl J Med* 1997;337:408–416.

Giovannucci E, Stampfer MJ, Colditz GA, et al. Multivitamin use, folate, and colon cancer in women in the Nurses' Health Study. *Ann Intern Med* 1998;129:517–521.

Haller CA, Benowitz NL. Adverse cardiovascular and central nervous system events associated with dietary supplements containing ephedra alkaloids. *N Engl J Med* 2000;343:1833–1837.

Lange H, Surapranata H, De Luca G, et al. Folate therapy and in-stent restenosis after coronary stenting. *N Engl J Med* 2004;350: 2673–2681.

Matthews MK. Association of Ginkgo biloba with intracerebral hemorrhage (letter). *Neurology* 1998;50:1933–1937.

McBride BF, Karapanos AK, Krudysz A, et al. Electrocardiographic and hemodynamic effects of a multicomponent dietary supplement containing ephedra and caffeine. A randomized controlled trial. *JAMA* 2004:291:216–221.

Menkes MS, Comstock GW, Vuilleumier JP, et al. Serum beta-carotene, vitamins A and E, selenium, and the risk of lung cancer. *N Engl J Med* 1986;315:1250–1254.

Michaelsson K, Lithell H, Vessby B, et al. Serum retinol levels and the risk of fracture. *N Engl J Med* 2003;348:287–291.

Moertel CG, Fleming TR, Creagan ET, et al. High-dose vitamin C versus placebo in the treatment of patients with advanced cancer that have had no prior chemotherapy. *N Engl J Med* 1985;312:137–141.

Rimm EB, Willett WC, Hu FB, et al. Folate and vitamin B6 from diet and supplements in relation to risk of coronary heart disease among women. *JAMA* 1998;279:359–362.

Roberts HJ. Perspective on vitamin E as therapy. *JAMA* 1981;246: 129–131.

Ueland PM, Refsum H, Wesenberg F, et al. Methotrexate therapy and nitrous oxide anesthesia. *N Engl J Med* 1986;314:1514.

Wald DS, Law M, Morris JK. Homocysteine and cardiovascular disease: evidence on causality from a meta-analysis *BMJ* 2002:323: 1202–1205.

Minerals and Electrolytes

35

Many minerals function as essential constituents of enzymes and regulate a variety of physiologic functions, including (a) maintenance of osmotic pressure, (b) transport of oxygen, (c) skeletal muscle contraction, (d) integrity of the central nervous system, (e) growth and maintenance of tissues and bones, and (f) hematopoiesis. Elements present in the body in large amounts include calcium, phosphorus, sodium, potassium, magnesium, sulfur, and chloride. Iron, cobalt in vitamin B_{12}, copper, zinc, chromium, selenium, manganese, and molybdenum are present in trace amounts. Nickel, tin, silicon, and arsenic also are considered essential elements. In the absence of absorption abnormalities, severe mineral deficiency is unlikely because most minerals, with the exception of zinc, are present in foods. Nevertheless, iron deficiency is common especially in infants and menstruating females consuming inadequate diets. Modest zinc and copper deficiencies also occur frequently.

A balanced and varied diet supplies adequate amounts of trace elements, and dietary supplements containing minerals, should be used only if evidence of deficiency exists or if demands are known to be increased (during pregnancy lactation). Mineral deficiencies may develop during prolonged hyperalimentation, emphasizing the importance of monitoring plasma concentrations of trace metals in these patients.

CALCIUM

Calcium is present in the body in greater amounts than any other mineral. The plasma concentration of calcium is maintained between 4.5 and 5.5 mEq/L (8.5 to 10.5 mg/dL) by an endocrine control system that includes vitamin D, parathyroid hormone, and calcitonin (see Chapter 52). Total plasma calcium consists of (a) calcium bound to albumin, (b) calcium complexed with citrate and phosphorus ions, and (c) freely diffusible ionized calcium. It is the ionized fraction of calcium that produces physiologic effects.

The ionized fraction of calcium represents approximately 45% of the total plasma concentration. Therefore, a normal plasma ionized calcium concentration is 2 to 2.5 mEq/L. Symptoms due to altered concentrations of calcium reflect changes in the plasma level of ionized calcium. It must be remembered that the ionized concentration of calcium depends on arterial pH, with acidosis increasing and alkalosis decreasing the concentration. Likewise, the plasma albumin concentration must be considered when interpreting plasma calcium concentrations. For example, albumin in plasma binds nonionized calcium. If the serum albumin concentration is decreased, there will be less calcium bound to protein. As a result, nonionized calcium is free to return to storage sites such as bone. Therefore, the total plasma calcium concentration can be decreased in the presence of hypoalbuminemia, but symptoms of hypocalcemia do not occur unless the ionized calcium concentration is also decreased. For example, hypocalcemia due to hypophosphatemia is not accompanied by signs of hypocalcemia unless the ionized fraction of calcium in the plasma is also decreased. For this reason, accurate interpretation of the plasma concentration of calcium is not possible without knowledge of the plasma albumin concentration.

Role of Calcium

Calcium is important for (a) neuromuscular transmission, (b) skeletal muscle contraction, (c) cardiac muscle contractility, (d) blood coagulation, and (e) exocytosis necessary for release of neurotransmitters and autocoids. In addition, calcium is the principal component of bone. The cytoplasmic concentration of ionized calcium is maintained at low levels by extrusion from the cells and sequestration of this ion within cellular organelles, particularly mitochondria, and in the sarcoplasmic reticulum of skeletal muscles. The large gradient for calcium across cell membranes contributes to the use of this ion for transmembrane signaling in response to various electrical or chemical stimuli.

Cardiovascular Effects

Calcium is recognized as a positive inotropic drug. Increasing the plasma concentrations of ionized calcium with exogenous administration of calcium chloride or calcium gluconate is commonly used to treat cardiac depression as may accompany delivery of volatile anesthetics, transfusion of citrated blood, and following termination of cardiopulmonary bypass. Calcium is necessary for excitation-contraction coupling in vascular smooth muscle and may result in a vasoconstricting effect on coronary arteries that impairs coupling of coronary blood flow to augment myocardial oxygen demand (Crystal et al., 1998).

Hypocalcemia

The most common cause of hypocalcemia (plasma concentration of calcium <4.5 mEq/L) is a decreased plasma concentration of albumin. Other causes of hypocalcemia include hypoparathyroidism, acute pancreatitis, vitamin D deficiency, and chronic renal failure associated with hyperphosphatemia. Malabsorption states resulting in deprivation of calcium and vitamin D readily lead to hypocalcemia.

Citrate binding of calcium can result in hypocalcemia, but this is unlikely in adults because the rate of whole blood infusion must exceed 50 ml/70 kg/minute before a decrease in the plasma concentration of ionized calcium occurs (Fig. 35-1) (Denlinger et al., 1976). This reflects mobilization of calcium from bone and the ability of the liver to rapidly metabolize citrate to bicarbonate ions. Therefore, the arbitrary IV administration of supplemental calcium to adults receiving stored blood is not indicated in the absence of objective evidence for hypocalcemia. Supplemental IV administration of calcium, however, is indicated to prevent citrate-induced hypocalcemia in neonates receiving stored blood. Furthermore, in the presence of hypothermia or severe liver dysfunction, the ability of the liver to convert citrate to bicarbonate may be decreased and the administration of supplemental calcium may be indicated.

Symptoms

Symptoms of hypocalcemia include (a) tetany, (b) circumoral paresthesias, (c) increased neuromuscular excitability, (d) laryngospasm, and (e) seizures. Abrupt decreases in the ionized portion of the total plasma concentration of calcium are associated with hypotension and increased left ventricular end-diastolic pressure. The QTc interval on the electrocardiogram (ECG) may be prolonged, but this is not a consistent observation. For this reason, monitoring the QTc interval on the ECG may not be a clinically reliable guide to the presence or absence of hypocalcemia.

Treatment

Treatment of hypocalcemia is with commercially available preparations of calcium (calcium chloride, calcium gluconate, calcium gluceptate) administered IV. In this regard, equal elemental doses of calcium chloride and calcium gluconate are approximately 1:3 (Cote et al., 1987). For example, calcium chloride contains 27 mg/mL of calcium and calcium gluconate contains 8 mg/mL of calcium. Administered IV over 5 to 15 minutes, equivalent doses of calcium chloride (3 to 6 mg/kg) and calcium gluconate (7 to

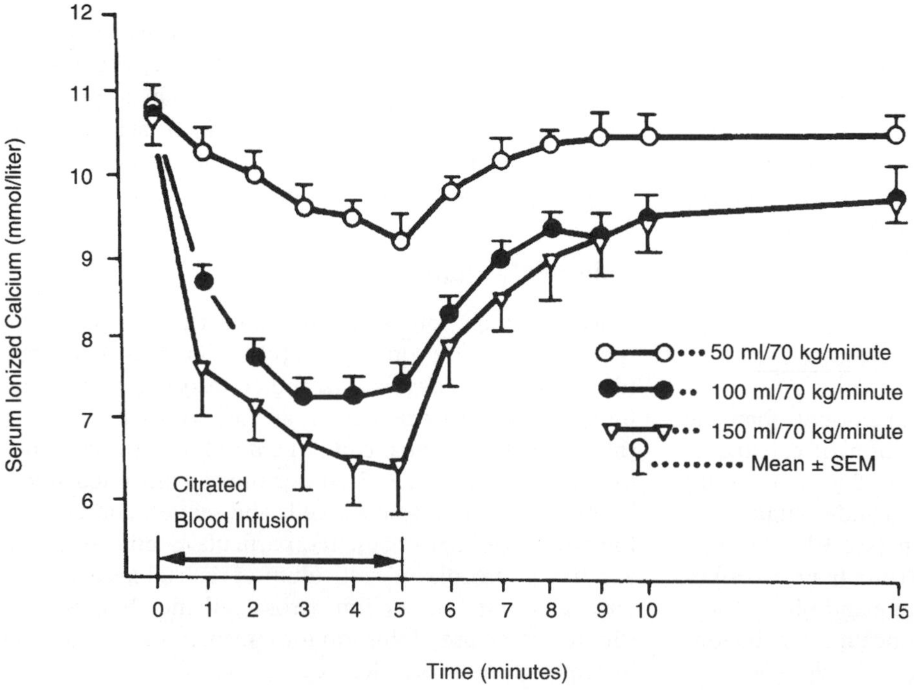

Figure 35-1. Citrate-induced decreases in serum ionized calcium concentrations do not occur unless the rate of whole blood infusion is >50 mL/70 kg per minute. (From Denlinger JK, Kaplan JA, Lecky JH, et al. Cardiovascular responses to calcium administered intravenously to a man during halothane anesthesia. *Anesthesiology* 1975;42:390–397; with permission.)

14 mg/kg) produce similar effects on the plasma concentration of calcium. Calcium chloride is irritating to veins and may cause discomfort in an awake patient. Calcium gluceptate contains 23 mg/mL of calcium and may be injected intramuscularly (IM) as well as IV.

Hypercalcemia

Cancer is the most common cause of life-threatening hypercalcemia (plasma calcium concentration >5.5 mEq/L), presumably reflecting activation of osteoclasts by various cytokines (interleukin-1, interleukin-6, tumor necrosis factor) secreted by tumor cells in the microenvironment of the bone marrow. Indeed, malignancy accounts for about one-half of the cases of hypercalcemia seen in hospitalized patients and about 5% of hospitalized patients with cancer have hypercalcemia (Heath, 1989). Hypoalbuminemia that frequently accompanies malignancy will mean the total plasma concentration of calcium underestimates the severity of the hypercalcemia. The most common cause of mild hypercalcemia is hyperparathyroidism. Hyperparathyroidism due to chronic renal failure may persist as hypercalcemia after successful renal transplantation. Sarcoidosis is associated with hypercalcemia in approximately 20% of patients.

Symptoms

Early symptoms of hypercalcemia include sedation and vomiting. When the plasma concentration of calcium is >10 mEq/L, cardiac conduction disturbances, characterized on the ECG as a prolonged P-R interval, a wide QRS complex, and a shortened QTc interval, occur. The most serious adverse effect of persistent hypercalcemia is renal damage.

Treatment

The goal of treatment of hypercalcemia is to correct dehydration and to prescribe a drug that will return the calcium concentration to near normal within 24 to 48 hours. More rapid correction of hypercalcemia may be dangerous. Treatment of hypercalcemia of malignancy is with IV administration of saline (2 to 3 liters daily) combined with administration of a bisphosphonate (disodium etidronate, 7.5 mg/kg IV for 3 days) (Heath, 1989). Furosemide-induced diuresis may contribute to the speed of renal excretion of calcium. Other bisphosphonates administered IV to treat hypercalcemia caused by cancer include clodronate, pamidronate, and ibandronate (Delmas, 1997).

Although corticosteroids and calcitonin have been recommended, there are few data supporting their use. Except in some hematologic malignancies, corticosteroids are ineffective, and calcitonin has only a modest early effect in some patients (Hosking and Gilson, 1984). Corticosteroids, such as prednisone, decrease the absorption of calcium from the gastrointestinal tract by antagonizing the actions of vitamin D. The onset of calcium-lowering effects by this mechanism, however, is often slow (7 to 14 days) and unpredictable.

Bone Composition

Bone is composed of an organic matrix that is strengthened by deposits of calcium salts. The organic matrix is >90% collagen fibers, and the remainder is a homogenous material called *ground substance*. Ground substance is composed of proteoglycans that include chondroitin sulfate and hyaluronic acid. Salts deposited in the organic matrix of bone are composed principally of calcium and phosphate ions in a combination known as *hydroxyapatites*. Many different ions can conjugate to these bone crystals, explaining deposition of radioactive substances in bone that may lead to an osteogenic sarcoma from a prolonged radiation effect.

The initial stage of bone production is the secretion of collagen and ground substance of osteoblasts. Calcium salts precipitate on the surfaces of collagen fibers, forming nidi that develop into hydroxyapatite crystals. Bone is continually being deposited by osteoblasts and is constantly being absorbed where osteoclasts are active. Parathyroid controls the bone-absorptive activity of osteoclasts. Except in growing bones, the rate of bone deposition and absorption are equal, so the total mass of bone remains constant.

Bone is deposited in proportion to the compressional load that the bone must carry. For example, continual physical stress stimulates new bone formation. The deposition of bone at points of compression may be caused by a piezoelectric effect. Indeed, small amounts of electrical current flowing in bone cause osteoblastic activity at the negative end of current flow. Fracture of a bone maximally activates osteoblasts involved in the break. The resulting bulge of osteoblastic tissue and new bone matrix is known as the *callus*.

Osteoblasts secrete large amounts of alkaline phosphatase when they are actively depositing bone matrix. As a result, the rate of new bone formation is mirrored by measurement of the plasma concentration of alkaline phosphatase. Alkaline phosphatase concentrations are also increased by any disease process that causes destruction of bone (metastatic cancer, osteomalacia, and rickets).

Calcium salts almost never precipitate in normal tissues other than bone. A notable exception, however, is atherosclerosis, in which calcium precipitates in the walls of large arteries. Calcium salts are also frequently deposited in degenerating tissues or in old blood clots.

Exchangeable Calcium

Exchangeable calcium is the calcium in the body that is in equilibrium with calcium in the extracellular fluid. Most of this exchangeable calcium is in bone, providing a rapid buffering mechanism to keep the calcium concentration in the extracellular fluid from changing excessively in either direction. The movement of exchangeable calcium in either direction is so rapid that a single passage of blood containing excess calcium through bone will remove almost all the excess calcium. It is estimated that approximately 5% of the cardiac output flows through bone.

Teeth

The major functional parts of teeth are enamel, dentine, cementum, and pulp (Fig. 35-2) (Guyton and Hall, 2000). The tooth can also be divided into the (a) crown, which is the portion that protrudes above the gum; (b) root, which protrudes into the bony sockets of the mandible and maxilla; and (c) neck, which separates the crown from the root.

Structure

Dentine is the main body of the tooth and is composed principally of hydroxyapatite crystals similar to those in bone. In contrast to those in bone, dentine lacks osteoblasts, osteoclasts, or spaces for nerves and blood vessels. The outer surface of the tooth is covered by a layer of enamel that is formed before eruption of the tooth by special epithelial cells. Once the tooth has erupted, no more enamel is formed. Enamel is a protein that is extremely hard and resistant to corrosive agents such as acids or enzymes. Cementum is a body substance secreted by cells that line the socket of the tooth. This substance is important in holding the tooth in place in the body socket. Cementum has characteristics similar to normal bone including the presence of osteoblasts and osteoclasts. The interior of each tooth is filled with pulp containing nerves, blood vessels, and lymphatics.

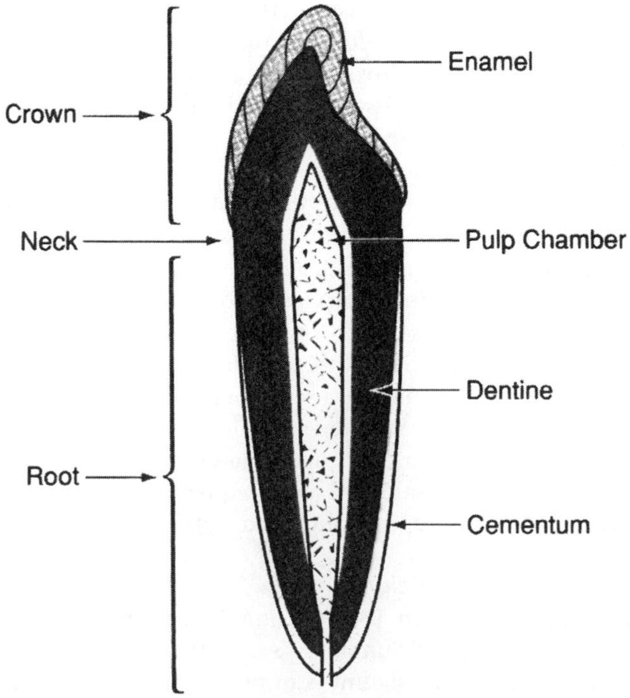

Figure 35-2. Schematic depiction of the functional parts of a tooth. (From Guyton AC, Hall JE. *Textbook of medical physiology*, 10th ed. Philadelphia: Saunders, 2000; with permission.)

Dental Caries

Dental caries result from the action of bacteria, the most common of which are streptococci. The first event in the development of caries is deposition of plaque, which is a film of precipitated products of saliva and food. Bacteria inhabit this plaque, setting the stage for the development of caries. Formation of acids by bacteria is the most important event leading to the development of caries. Enamel is very resistant to demineralization by acids and thus serves as a primary barrier to the development of caries. Once the carous process has penetrated through the enamel of dentine, it proceeds rapidly, reflecting the high solubility of dentine salts.

Bacteria depend on carbohydrates for survival, explaining the association between caries and the frequent ingestion of food containing glucose. If carbohydrates are ingested in small amounts though the day, such as in the form of candy, bacteria are supplied with their preferential metabolic substrate for many hours of the day. Conversely, ingestion of carbohydrates only at meals followed by brushing of the teeth limits the availability of metabolic substrate to the bacteria and thus decreases the likelihood of caries formation.

Teeth formed in children who drink fluorinated water develop enamel that is approximately three times more resistant than normal to the formation of caries. Fluorine does not make the enamel harder than usual, but instead displaces hydroxyl ions in the hydroxyapatite crystals; this in turn makes the enamel less soluble.

Dental Injury

Dental injuries in the perioperative period are commonly attributed to trauma caused by the laryngoscope blade during tracheal intubation. However, only 20% of the described cases of dental injury are associated with difficult intubation (Warner et al., 1999). This questions the assumption that the application of large forces with the laryngoscope blade is the usual cause of injury. In fact, involuntary biting (bruxism) on the endotracheal tube or oral airway in the postoperative period may be an underappreciated cause of dental injury (Quinn et al., 2005).

Bisphosphonates in the Treatment of Bone Diseases

Bisphosphonates are drugs with a phosphorus-carbon-phosphorus (P-C-P) chemical structure in which the hydrogen atoms bound to the carbon atom are replaced by various groups (Fig. 35-3) (Delmas, 1996; Delmas and Meunier, 1997; Rosen and Kessenich, 1996). The main action of bisphosphonates is to induce marked and

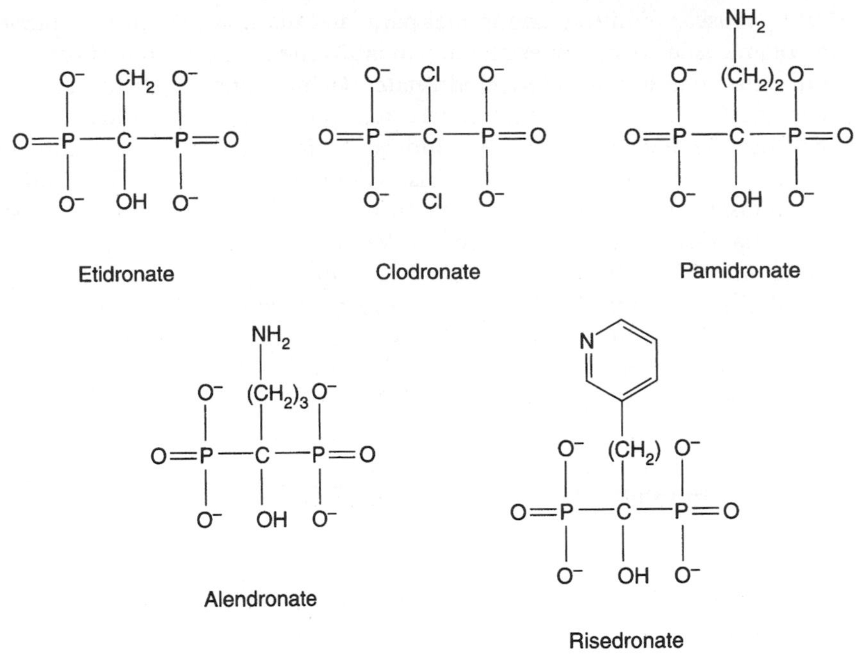

Figure 35-3. Bisphosphonates.

prolonged inhibition of bone resorption by decreasing osteoclastic activity (Delmas and Meunier, 1997). In addition, these compounds decrease the number of osteoclasts by decreasing their recruitment and by stimulating the production of osteoblasts. Bisphosphonates bind to bone minerals through the P-C-P structure and inhibit both the formation and dissolution of calcium phosphate crystals. These compounds remain in bone until it is resorbed. Decreased bone resorption also allows bone formation to match bone dissolution.

Clinical Uses

Bisphosphonates, because of their favorable benefit-to-risk ratio, are the preferred alternative to estrogen-replacement therapy in women with postmenopausal osteoporosis and are the treatment of choice for patients with Paget disease, corticosteroid-induced bone loss, and hypercalcemia due to malignancy (Table 35-1) (Delmas 1996; Delmas and Meunier, 1997; Rosen and Kessenich, 1996). During a 10-year treatment period, alendronate produced sustained increases in bone mineral density (decreased risk of fracture) that disappeared when treatment was discontinued (Bone et al., 2004). Bisphosphonates are useful as adjuvant therapy in patients with multiple myeloma and bone metastases to decrease bone pain and the risk of fractures and hypercalcemia. Monthly infusions of pamidronate may protect against skeletal muscle complications in women with metastatic breast cancer. Likewise, IV administration of pamidronate may be more cost-effective than continuous oral therapy in the treatment of Paget disease. Serum alkaline phosphatase concentrations and urinary excretion of hydroxyproline are likely to decrease in treated patients by an average of 50% (Delmas and Meunier, 1997).

Side Effects

The toxicity of bisphosphonates is low, with relatively few side effects outside the skeleton (Rosen and Kessenich,

TABLE 35-1.
PHARMACOKINETICS AND CLINICAL USES OF BISPHOSPHONATES

	Etidronate	Clodronate	Pamidronate	Alendronate
Route of administration	Oral IV	Oral IV	IV	Oral IV
Oral bioavailability (%)	1–10	1–10	1–10	1–10
Clinical uses				
Paget's disease	++	+	+++ (IV)	+++
Osteoporosis	+++	+	++	++++

IV, intravenous; +, possible benefit.

1996). Nausea, vomiting, abdominal pain, and diarrhea are possible side effects, especially in patients treated with etidronate, alendronate, and clodronate (Delmas and Meunier, 1997). Osteomalacia has occurred with chronic high-dose therapy with etidronate. Indeed, etidronate is not recommended in patients with a history of osteomalacia. A transient acute influenza-like syndrome may accompany initial treatment with pamidronate. Venous irritation may accompany the IV administration of pamidronate.

Oral bisphosphonates increase tubular reabsorption of phosphate, which, in turn, can lead to secondary hyperparathyroidism. Nevertheless, hypocalcemia induced by these drugs is unusual, except in cases of treatment of malignant hypercalcemia. The inhibition of bone resorption by IV pamidronate decreases the outflow of calcium from bone, and the early effects of treatment include a decrease in plasma calcium concentrations and an increase in the secretion of parathyroid hormone. Calcium should be given to blunt the increase in the serum level of parathyroid hormone.

Pharmacokinetics

All bisphosphonates share some pharmacokinetic features, including poor systemic absorption after oral administration, especially in the presence of food (bioavailability 1% to 10%) (see Table 35-1) (Delmas and Meunier, 1997; Rosen and Kessenich, 1996). After a brief period in the circulation, most bisphosphonates are cleared rapidly, entering bone (20% to 50% of an orally absorbed dose) where it is tightly bound to hydroxyapatite, whereas the remaining drug is excreted unchanged by the kidneys. The rate of entry of etidronate into bone approximates that of calcium and phosphate, and the drug has a volume of distribution of between 0.3 to 1.3 liters/kg. A history of renal failure may influence the decision to administer bisphosphonates.

POTASSIUM

Potassium is the second most common cation in the body and the principal intracellular cation (Tetzlaff et al., 1993). Approximately 3,500 mEq of potassium are present in the body of a 70-kg patient (40 to 50 mEq/kg). The concentration in the extracellular fluid is about 4 mEq/L, and the intracellular concentration is 150 mEq/L, with only 2% of total body potassium being extracellular. Estimation of total body potassium concentration from serum potassium values is not accurate because of the predominance of intracellular potassium, although the majority (>90%) is readily exchangeable between compartments.

Role of Potassium

Potassium has an important influence on the control of osmotic pressure and is a catalyst of numerous enzymatic reactions. This cation is involved in the function of excitable cell membranes (nerves, skeletal muscles, cardiac muscle) and is directly involved in the function of the kidneys. Disturbances of potassium homeostasis are reflected as cardiac dysrhythmias, skeletal muscle weakness, and acid-base disturbances.

The kidneys are the principal organ involved in potassium homeostasis. Most renal regulation of potassium is governed by active secretion, which is different from that of other electrolytes, which are regulated by distal reabsorption. A number of hormones influence renal potassium secretion including aldosterone, glucocorticoids, catecholamines, and arginine vasopressin. Aldosterone acts at the collecting duct to increase reabsorption of sodium ions, which favors potassium secretion. Arginine vasopressin also increases secretion of potassium at the distal collecting tubule. Glucocorticoids influence renal potassium secretion by a direct action in the renal parenchyma. Catecholamines decrease renal secretion of potassium by an effect on the distal collecting system. Acidosis opposes and alkalosis favors potassium secretion. When uremia develops, gastrointestinal secretion of potassium increases, and when creatinine clearance is <20% of normal, gastrointestinal potassium loss can approach 20% of uptake.

Hypokalemic Drug Effects

Numerous drugs alter the intracellular and extracellular distribution of potassium. For example, catecholamines shift potassium intracellularly, predominantly into the liver and skeletal muscles. Hypokalemia may also occur after administration of beta-adrenergic agonists as for the treatment of bronchial asthma or premature labor. Indeed, hypokalemic effects of beta agonists may be useful in the treatment of hyperkalemia. Theophylline causes potassium movement intracellularly, and hypokalemia should be anticipated in the presence of theophylline toxicity. Insulin favors movement of potassium into cells. Gastrointestinal potassium losses can be related to chronic laxative abuse as well as aggressive bowel preparation for abdominal surgery.

The largest group of drugs that induce renal potassium loss are diuretics (see Chapter 25). Large doses of penicillin and its synthetic derivatives are kaliuretic. Aminoglycoside antibiotics are kaliuretic reflecting drug-induced magnesium loss and by direct nephrotoxicity.

Hyperkalemic Drug Effects

Drugs that increase serum potassium concentrations do so by redistribution, suppression of aldosterone secretion, inhibition of potassium secretion in the distal collecting duct, or by direct cell destruction. Extracellular movement of potassium can result in plasma hyperkalemia without an increase in total body potassium. For example, succinylcholine causes a release of potassium from skeletal muscle cells, resulting in an increase of the serum potassium concentration by as much as 0.5 mEq/L. Digitalis toxicity can cause hyperkalemia by preventing potassium entry into cells. Beta-adrenergic antagonists can cause a modest increase in the serum potassium concentration by virtue of an extracellular shift. Although this shift is modest, it can be additive with other hyperkalemic effects such as cardiopulmonary bypass and renal failure. Nonsteroidal anti-inflammatory drugs may cause hyperkalemia by preventing aldosterone release. Potassium-sparing diuretics inhibit the secretion of potassium in the distal collecting duct to cause clinical hyperkalemia. Chemotherapy for treatment of acute blood cell proliferative malignancies can result in abrupt cell lysis and hyperkalemia.

Hypokalemia

The clinical significance of the physiologic effects of hypokalemia on cardiac and skeletal muscles is controversial. Failure to confirm an increased incidence of serious cardiac dysrhythmias in chronically hypokalemic patients has resulted in less acute potassium replacement therapy and a decrease in the frequency of cancellation of elective operations on the basis of arbitrary serum potassium concentrations (Tetzlaff et al., 1993). Active intervention with supplemental potassium is still recommended for select patients, including those receiving digitalis preparations or who have evidence of acute myocardial ischemia.

Symptoms

Skeletal muscle weakness and a predisposition to cardiac dysrhythmias are recognized symptoms of clinically significant hypokalemia. At the cellular level, hypokalemia results in enhanced cardiac automaticity and a decreased rate of myocardial repolarization that predisposes to tachydysrhythmias. The cellular changes resemble those produced by digitalis or beta-adrenergic agonists. However, there is no serum potassium value below which there is an undisputed risk of serious cardiac dysrhythmias (Atlee, 1997).

Treatment

It is important to determine the cause of hypokalemia before aggressive potassium replacement is initiated. For example, if serum potassium concentrations are acutely decreased due to redistribution into the intracellular space and potassium therapy is initiated, potentially serious hyperkalemia could occur, especially if the cause of the redistribution were to abruptly reverse. If total body depletion is the cause of hypokalemia, the amount of increase in the plasma concentration of potassium produced by supplementation may be small due to rapid redistribution into intracellular sites.

Life-threatening hypokalemia, presenting as malignant cardiac dysrhythmias, acute digitalis intoxication, or extreme neuromuscular collapse, requires supplemental IV potassium administration. The rate of potassium infusion depends on the urgency of the indication, with a common recommendation being administration of 40 mEq/hour. If the starting serum potassium concentration is >2.5 mEq/L, administration of 0.5 mEq/kg of potassium chloride would be expected to increase the serum potassium concentration 0.6 mEq/L (Tetzlaff et al., 1993). If the patient was receiving beta-adrenergic antagonists, the serum potassium concentration increase would be 0.9 mEq/L, but during endogenous catecholamine therapy, the increase would be only 0.1 mEq/L. Correction of hypomagnesemia may be needed to avoid increased renal losses of potassium.

Morbidity associated with supplemental potassium therapy is not trivial. Patients with diminished internal potassium regulation, especially diabetics and renal failure patients, are at risk for accidental treatment-induced hyperkalemia. The lack of demonstrated perioperative risk from chronic hypokalemia in patients without clinical symptoms should influence the decision to treat chronic hypokalemia acutely.

Hyperkalemia

The earliest sign of hyperkalemia is usually an ECG change such as a peaked T wave, which typically occurs when the serum potassium concentration reaches 6 mEq/L. As the extracellular concentration increases further, the transmembrane gradient is decreased, with prolongation of the P-R interval and QRS widening on the ECG. At this point, the risk of ventricular fibrillation or asystole due to cardiac conduction blockade increases dramatically. Asystole may also occur due to decreased automaticity in the sinoatrial node. Occasionally, the clinical presentation of hyperkalemia can be neuromuscular, with paresthesias and skeletal muscle weakness.

Treatment

The decision to treat hyperkalemia, in contrast to hypokalemia, is easier and based on the degree of increase in the serum potassium concentration and the symptoms that are present. If ECG changes other than peaked T waves occur, or if the serum potassium concentration is >6.5 mEq/L, the incidence of serious cardiac compromise is high and rapid intervention is indicated.

Calcium is indicated to rapidly offset the adverse effects of potassium on cardiac conduction and contractility. Calcium activates calcium ion channels so that ion flux through these channels generates an action potential and restores myocardial contractility. The IV administration of 10 to 20 mL of a 10% calcium chloride solution restores myocardial contractility in 1 to 2 minutes. This effect lasts 15 to 20 minutes. Calcium gluconate may be recommended over the chloride form on the basis that this preparation induces more potassium secretion acutely by the renal tubules. The IV administration of calcium must be slowed in patients on digitalis preparations, because acute hypercalcemia can precipitate digitalis toxicity. Serum potassium concentrations are not significantly changed by IV administration of calcium.

Other measures to treat hyperkalemia include IV administration of sodium bicarbonate and glucose-insulin mixtures. Sodium bicarbonate, 0.5 to 1.0 mEq/kg IV, causes a shift of potassium into cells in approximately 5 minutes. The serum potassium concentration remains decreased for as long as the arterial pH is increased. Glucose-insulin infusion (50 mL of 50% glucose plus 10 U of regular insulin) produces a sustained transfer of potassium into cells, resulting in a 1.5 to 2.5 mEq/L decrease in the serum potassium concentration after approximately 30 minutes. Epinephrine and beta agonists—especially beta$_2$-selective agonists—decrease serum potassium concentrations by redistribution intracellularly.

PHOSPHATE

Inorganic phosphate exists in two forms in the plasma. Because it is difficult to measure the exact amounts of each ion, it is common to express the total quantity of phosphate as mg/dL of phosphorus. The total quantity of inorganic phosphorus represented by both phosphate ions is 3.0 to 4.5 mg/dL.

Phosphate is important in energy metabolism and maintenance of acid-base balance. For example, phosphate ions are the most abundant buffer in the distal renal tubules, allowing excretion of large quantities of hydrogen ions. These ions are also important intracellular buffers. Vitamin D stimulates the systemic absorption of phosphate from the gastrointestinal tract. This absorbed phosphate is almost entirely excreted by the kidneys because parathyroid hormone blocks reabsorption from the renal tubules. Conversely, vitamin D facilitates reabsorption of phosphate from the proximal renal tubules.

A decrease in the plasma concentration of phosphate permits the presence of a higher plasma concentration of calcium and inhibits deposition of new bone salts. Hypophosphatemia (phosphorus concentration <1.5 mg/dL) causes a decrease in the concentration of adenosine triphosphate and 2,3-diphosphoglycerate in erythrocytes. Profound skeletal muscle weakness sufficient to contribute to hypoventilation may be a manifestation of hypophosphatemia (Aubier et al., 1985). Central nervous system dysfunction and peripheral neuropathy may accompany hypophosphatemia. Alcohol abuse and prolonged parenteral nutrition are causes of phosphorus deficiency.

MAGNESIUM

Magnesium is the fourth most prevalent cation in the body and the second most prevalent intracellular cation after potassium (James, 1992). Only 1% of magnesium is present in the extracellular fluid compartment and 30% of this is bound to protein. Approximately one-half of total body magnesium is present in bone and 20% in skeletal muscles.

Normal plasma concentrations of magnesium are achieved and maintained by absorption from the small intestine and renal excretion. Abnormalities of plasma and cellular magnesium concentrations frequently accompany other electrolyte abnormalities. For example, there is a strong correlation between hypomagnesemia and hypokalemia. Including measurement of plasma magnesium concentrations with that of other electrolytes has been recommended on the basis that >8% of patients who have hypomagnesemia or hypermagnesemia are currently clinically unrecognized (Whang and Ryder, 1990). Plasma magnesium concentrations may remain normal despite significant intracellular deficits because only 5% of the available magnesium pool is extracellular.

Role of Magnesium

Magnesium strongly influences cardiac cell membrane ion transport function and is essential for activating approximately 300 enzyme systems, including most of the enzymes involved in energy metabolism. Adenosine triphosphate (ATP) is fully functional when chelated to magnesium. This ion is an essential regulator of calcium access into cells and the actions of calcium within cells. Magnesium regulates intracellular calcium levels by activating membrane pumps in cells that extrude calcium and by competing with calcium for transmembrane channels by which extracellular calcium gains access to the interior of cells. Magnesium is the natural physiologic antagonist of calcium. Presynaptic release of acetylcholine depends on the actions of magnesium. Magnesium may exert analgesic effects by acting as an antagonist of *N*-methyl-D-aspartate (NMDA) receptors. Nevertheless, perioperative IV administration of magnesium (50 mg/kg IV followed by 15 mg/kg/hour) had no effect on postoperative pain (Ko et al., 2001). Magnesium produces systemic and coronary vasodilation, inhibits platelet function, and decreases reperfusion injury.

Hypomagnesemia

Hypomagnesemia (serum magnesium concentration <1.6 mEq/L) may be the most common unrecognized electrolyte deficiency (Gambling et al., 1988). Emergency treatment of life-threatening hypomagnesemia is infusion of magnesium, 10 to 20 mg/kg, administered over 10 to 20 minutes.

Causes

Patients at increased risk for hypomagnesemia include chronic alcoholics (magnesium-poor diets, increased renal magnesium losses due to alcohol) and those in critical care units maintained on hyperalimentation solutions containing minimal amounts of magnesium. Malabsorption syndromes and protracted vomiting or diarrhea may also lead to hypomagnesemia. Patients undergoing cardiac surgery requiring cardiopulmonary bypass may be vulnerable to hypomagnesemia due to dilutional effects from pump-priming solutions or preexisting effects of diuretic therapy. In addition, secondary aldosteronism associated with chronic congestive heart failure increases renal excretion of magnesium. Increased fluxes of magnesium may occur in organ donors due to large-volume infusion of nonelectrolyte solutions to prevent hypernatremia that can occur secondary to diabetes insipidus. In this regard, organ transplant recipients may experience cyclosporine-induced loss of magnesium via the kidneys, resulting in hypomagnesemia. There is a strong correlation between hypomagnesemia and hypokalemia. Repletion of intracellular potassium concentrations is impaired in the presence of unrecognized and untreated hypomagnesemia, perhaps reflecting impaired ion pump activity. A low serum magnesium concentration is almost always due to a total body depletion of this cation.

Symptoms

Chronic hypomagnesemia is less likely to be symptomatic than an acute hypomagnesemia, suggesting a normalization of the intracellular to extracellular magnesium ratio with time similar to that with chronic hypokalemia. Neuromuscular manifestations (Chvostek and Trousseau signs, carpopedal spasm, stridor, skeletal muscle weakness) resemble hypocalcemia. Severe magnesium deficiency may lead to seizures, coma, or both. Manifestations of hypomagnesemia on the ECG are nonspecific and mimic those associated with hypokalemia and digitalis toxicity (Atlee, 1997). Ventricular dysrhythmias are a frequent symptom of hypomagnesemia that may manifest for the first time during anesthesia. Magnesium (1 to 2 g IV over 5 to 60 minutes, or a continuous infusion, 0.5 to 1.0 g/hour) is recommended for treatment of torsades de pointes with QTc interval prolongation or as adjunct management for cardiac dysrhythmias in the presence of hypomagnesemia, hypokalemia, or digitalis toxicity (Atlee, 1997).

Hypermagnesemia

Hypermagnesemia is present when the plasma concentration of magnesium is >2.6 mEq/L. Treatment of life-threatening hypermagnesemia is with calcium gluconate, 10 to 15 mg/kg IV, followed by fluid loading and drug-induced diuresis.

Causes

Increased serum magnesium levels are rare in clinical situations, as this ion is poorly absorbed from the gastrointestinal tract and the renal elimination of any excess magnesium is extremely rapid. The most common cause of hypermagnesemia is parenteral administration of magnesium to treat pregnancy-induced hypertension. Patients with chronic renal dysfunction are at an increased risk for developing hypermagnesemia because excretion of magnesium depends on glomerular filtration.

Symptoms

Symptoms of hypermagnesemia include sedation, myocardial depression, and suppression of peripheral neuromuscular function due to decreases in acetylcholine release from motor nerve endings, as well as decreased responsiveness of the postjunctional membrane to acetylcholine (James, 1992). Furthermore, magnesium exerts a direct relaxant effect on skeletal muscles. Deep tendon reflexes diminish when the plasma concentration of magnesium is 10 mEq/L. Paralysis of muscles of ventilation and heart block may appear at plasma magnesium concentrations of >12 mEq/L. Magnesium enhances the effects of nondepolarizing neuromuscular-blocking drugs, emphasizing the need to decrease the usual dose of these drugs by one-half to one-third in patients being treated with magnesium sulfate (see Chapter 8). Potentiation of succinylcholine by magnesium sulfate therapy is not a consistent observation (Gambling et al., 1988). Patients treated with magnesium sulfate do not demonstrate fasciculations after administration of succinylcholine. Calcium administered IV is not predictably effective in the antagonism of magnesium-enhanced neuromuscular blockade. Magnesium may precipitate skeletal muscle weakness in patients with the Lambert-Eaton syndrome or myasthenia gravis.

Clinical Uses

The clinical uses of magnesium reflect its antiadrenergic properties that are accompanied by minimal myocardial depression (James, 1992). Magnesium is a physiologic antagonist of calcium. The potential value of magnesium as a bronchodilator in the management of asthma awaits confirmation. The only major toxic effect of magnesium is neuromuscular weakness and the potential for accumulation in the presence of renal dysfunction.

Pregnancy-Induced Hypertension

Magnesium is primarily used in obstetrics for prophylaxis and treatment of convulsions in the management of the parturient with gestational proteinuric hypertension (Gomez, 1998). Magnesium has a large volume of distribution, and this characteristic coupled with rapid renal elimination means that a large initial dose (40 to 60 mg/kg IV) and a continuous infusion (15 to 30 mg/kg/hour) of magnesium sulfate is likely to be necessary to maintain serum magnesium concentrations in a therapeutic range of 4 to 6 mEq/L. Magnesium is widely regarded as a central nervous system depressant, largely because of its anticonvulsant properties in gestational proteinuric hypertension. Nevertheless, magnesium poorly penetrates the blood-brain barrier, and its level in the cerebrospinal fluid is well controlled, probably by an active transport mechanism. The most likely explanation for its anticonvulsant effects in vulnerable parturients is cerebral vasodilation, which reverses cerebral vasospasm thought to cause seizures. Despite acting as a calcium antagonist, the evidence for cardiac depression produced by clinically useful levels of hypermagnesemia is not clear (James, 1992). Magnesium has no effect on ventilatory drive, and its only depressant effects on breathing are related to neuromuscular blockade. Bronchodilation has been alleged to occur after administration of magnesium, suggesting this drug might be useful in the management of asthma-induced bronchospasm (James, 1992).

Cardiac Dysrhythmias and Hypertension

Magnesium is a useful cardiac antidysrhythmic, particularly for dysrhythmias associated with digitalis, hypokalemia, alcoholism, myocardial infarction, cardiac surgery, and catecholamine release (England et al., 1992). It has been recommended for intractable ventricular tachycardia and fibrillation, torsades de pointes, and multifocal atrial tachycardia (James, 1992). An initial dose of magnesium sulfate, 2 g IV administered over 5 minutes, is often recommended, followed by a continuous infusion, 1 to 2 g/hour, to maintain a therapeutic concentration. The vasodilator and antidysrhythmic effects of magnesium have been presumed to protect against hypertensive responses to direct laryngoscopy and tracheal intubation, management of patients undergoing resection of pheochromocytoma, and cross-clamping of the abdominal aorta.

Cardioprotective Effects

Magnesium may act as a cardioprotective drug by attenuating the increase in intracellular calcium ion flux that accompanies myocardial ischemia followed by reperfusion (Gomez 1998). Significant decreases in the size of an acute myocardial infarction are present in animal models that receive magnesium during the interval following coronary occlusion and extending through the period of initial reperfusion. Magnesium is useful for patients who develop torsades de pointes-type ventricular tachycardia following acute myocardial infarction.

IRON

Iron present in food is absorbed from the proximal small intestine, especially the duodenum, into the circulation, where it is bound to transferrin. Transferrin is a glycoprotein that delivers iron to specific receptors on cell membranes. Approximately 80% of the iron in plasma enters the bone marrow to be incorporated into new erythrocytes. In addition to bone marrow, iron is incorporated into reticuloendothelial cells of the liver and spleen. Iron is also an essential component of many enzymes necessary for energy transfer. A normal range for the plasma iron concentration is 50 to 150 μg/dL.

Iron that is stored in tissues is bound to protein as ferritin or in an aggregated form known as *hemosiderin*. Hemoglobin synthesis is the principal determinant of the plasma iron turnover rate. When blood loss occurs, hemoglobin concentration is maintained by mobilization of tissue iron stores. Indeed, hemoglobin concentrations become chronically decreased only after these iron reserves are depleted. For this reason, the presence of a normal hemoglobin concentration is not a sensitive indicator of tissue iron stores. The infant, parturient, and menstruating female may have iron requirements that exceed amounts available in the diet. Absorption of iron from the gastrointestinal tract is increased by ascorbic acid or the presence of iron deficiency. Antacids bind iron and impair its systemic absorption.

Iron Deficiency

Iron deficiency is estimated to be present in 20% to 40% of menstruating females and fewer than 5% of adult males and postmenopausal females. Attempts to achieve better iron balance in large parts of the population are evidenced by addition of iron to flour, use of iron-fortified formulas for infants, and the prescription of iron-containing vitamin supplements during pregnancy.

Causes

Causes of iron-deficiency anemia include inadequate dietary intake of iron (nutritional) or increased iron requirements due to pregnancy, blood loss, or interference with absorption from the gastrointestinal tract. Most nutritional iron deficiency in the United States is mild. Severe iron deficiency is usually the result of blood loss, either from the gastrointestinal tract or, in females, from the uterus. Partial gastrectomy and sprue are causes of inadequate iron absorption.

Diagnosis

Iron deficiency initially results in a decrease in iron stores and a parallel decrease in the erythrocyte content of iron. Depleted iron stores are indicated by decreased plasma concentrations of ferritin and the absence of reticuloendothelial hemosiderin in the bone marrow aspirate. Plasma ferritin concentrations of <12 μg/dL are diagnostic of iron deficiency. Iron-deficiency anemia is present when depletion of total body iron is associated with a recognizable decrease in the blood concentration of hemoglobin. The large physiologic variation in hemoglobin concentration, however, makes it difficult to reliably identify all individuals with iron-deficiency anemia.

The frequency of iron-deficiency anemia in infants and in menstruating females or parturient makes an exhaustive search for the cause of mild anemia less important. Conversely, in males and postmenopausal females, in whom iron balance should be favorable, it becomes more important to pursue the search for the site of bleeding whenever anemia is present.

Treatment

Prophylactic use of iron preparations should be reserved for individuals at high risk for developing iron deficiency, such as pregnant and lactating females, low-birth-weight infants, and females with heavy menses. The inappropriate prophylactic use of iron should be avoided in adults because of excessive accumulation of iron, which may damage tissues.

Administration of medicinal iron is followed by an increased rate of erythrocyte production that manifests as an improved hemoglobin concentration within 72 hours. If the concentration of hemoglobin before treatment is decreased by >3 g/dL, an average daily incremental increase of 0.2 g/dL of hemoglobin is achieved with the usual therapeutic doses of oral or parenteral iron. An increase of 2 g/dL or more in the plasma concentration of hemoglobin within 3 weeks is evidence of a positive response to iron. If a positive response does not occur within this time, the presence of (a) continuous bleeding, (b) an infectious process, or (c) impaired gastrointestinal absorption of iron should be considered.

There is no justification for continuing iron therapy beyond 3 weeks if a favorable response in the hemoglobin concentration has not occurred. Once a response to iron therapy is demonstrated, the medication should be continued until the hemoglobin concentration is normal. Iron therapy may be continued beyond this point for 4 to 6 weeks if it is desired to reestablish iron stores. The replenishment of tissue iron stores requires several months of therapy.

Oral Iron

Ferrous sulfate administered orally is the most frequently used approach for the treatment of iron-deficiency anemia. Ferric salts are less efficiently absorbed than ferrous salts from the gastrointestinal tract. Ferrous sulfate is available as syrup, pills, or tablets. Although other salts of the ferrous form of iron are available, they offer little or no advantage over sulfate preparations. The usual therapeutic dose of iron for adults to treat iron-deficiency anemia is 2 to 3 mg/kg (200 mg daily) in three divided doses. Prophylaxis and treatment of mild nutritional iron deficiency can be achieved with modest dosages of iron, such as 15 to 30 mg daily, if the object is the prevention of iron deficiency in parturients.

Nausea and upper abdominal pain are the most frequent side effects of oral iron therapy, particularly if the dosage is >200 mg daily. Hemochromatosis is unlikely to result from oral iron therapy that is administered to treat nutritional anemia. Fatal poisoning from overdose of iron is rare, but children 1 to 2 years of age are most vulnerable. Symptoms of severe iron poisoning may manifest within 30 minutes as vomiting, abdominal pain, and diarrhea. In addition, there may be sedation, hyperventilation due to acidosis, and cardiovascular collapse. Hemorrhagic gastroenteritis and hepatic damage are often prominent at autopsy. If iron overdose is suspected, a plasma concentration of >0.5 mg/dL confirms the presence of a life-threatening situation that should be treated with deferoxamine.

Parenteral Iron

Parenteral iron acts similarly to oral iron but should be used only if patients cannot tolerate or do not respond to oral therapy (continuing loss is greater than can be replaced because of limitations of oral absorption). For example, parenteral iron therapy is necessary if disease processes such as sprue impair gastrointestinal absorption of iron. In addition, tissue iron stores may be rapidly restored by administration of parenteral iron in contrast to the slow response with oral therapy. There is no evidence, however, that the therapeutic response to parenteral iron is more prompt than that achieved with oral iron.

Iron dextran injection contains 50 mg/mL of iron and is available for IM or IV use. After absorption, the iron must be split from the glucose molecule of dextran before it becomes available to tissues. IM injection is painful, and there is concern about malignant changes at the injection site. For these reasons, IV administration of iron is preferred over IM injection. A dose of 500 mg of iron can be infused over 5 to 10 minutes.

The principal side effect of parenteral iron therapy is the rare occurrence of a severe allergic reaction, presumably due to the presence of dextran. Less severe reactions include headache, fever, generalized lymphadenopathy, and arthralgias. Hemosiderosis is more likely to occur with parenteral iron therapy that bypasses gastrointestinal absorptive regulatory mechanisms.

COPPER

Copper is present in ceruloplasmin and is a constituent of other enzymes, including dopamine beta-hydroxylase and cytochrome C oxidase. It is bound to albumin and is an essential component of several proteins. Copper is thought to act as a catalyst in the storage and release of iron from hemoglobin. It is believed to be essential for the formation of connective tissues, hematopoiesis, and function of the central nervous system. Copper deficiency is rare in the presence of an adequate diet. Supplements of copper should be given during prolonged hyperalimentation.

ZINC

Zinc is a cofactor of enzymes and is essential for cell growth and synthesis of nucleic acid, carbohydrates, and proteins.

Adequate zinc is provided by a diet containing sufficient animal protein. Diets in which protein is obtained primarily from vegetable sources may not supply adequate zinc.

Zinc deficiency may occur in elderly or debilitated patients or during periods of increased requirements as in growing children, pregnancy, lactation, or infection. Severe zinc deficiency occurs most often in the presence of malabsorption syndromes. Based on animal evidence, it has been suggested that maternal zinc deficiency during pregnancy may have teratogenic effects. Cutaneous manifestations of zinc deficiency may occur during prolonged hyperalimentation, emphasizing the need for zinc supplements in these patients. During hemodialysis, zinc chloride may be added to the dialysis bath. Symptoms of zinc deficiency include disturbances in taste and smell, suboptimal growth in children, hepatosplenomegaly, alopecia, cutaneous rashes, glossitis, and stomatitis.

CHROMIUM

Chromium is important in a cofactor complex with insulin and thus is involved in normal glucose utilization. Deficiency has been accompanied by a diabetes-like syndrome, peripheral neuropathy, and encephalopathy.

SELENIUM

Selenium is a constituent of several metabolically important enzymes. A selenium-dependent glutathione peroxidase is present in human erythrocytes. There seems to be a close relationship between vitamin E and selenium. Deficiency of selenium has been associated with cardiomyopathy, suggesting the need to add this trace element to supplements administered during prolonged hyperalimentation.

MANGANESE

Manganese is concentrated in mitochondria, especially in the liver, pancreas, kidneys, and pituitary. It influences the synthesis of mucopolysaccharides, stimulates hepatic synthesis of cholesterol and fatty acids, and is a cofactor in many enzymes. Deficiency is unknown clinically, but supplementation is recommended during prolonged hyperalimentation.

MOLYBDENUM

Molybdenum is an essential constituent of many enzymes. It is well absorbed from the gastrointestinal tract and is present in bones, liver, and kidneys. Deficiency is rare, whereas excessive ingestion has been associated with a gout-like syndrome.

REFERENCES

Atlee JL. Perioperative cardiac dysrhythmias: diagnosis and management. *Anesthesiology* 1997;86:1397–1424.

Aubier M, Murciano D, Lecocguic Y, et al. Effect of hypophosphatemia on diaphragmatic contractility in patients with acute respiratory failure. *N Engl J Med* 1985;313:420–424.

Bone HG, Hosking D, Devogelaer J-P et al. Ten years' experience with alendronate for osteoporosis in postmenopausal women. *N Engl J Med* 2004;350:1189–1199.

Cote CJ, Drop LJ, Daniels AL, et al. Calcium chloride versus calcium gluconate: comparison of ionization and cardiovascular effects in children and dogs. *Anesthesiology* 1987;66:465–470.

Crystal GJ, Zhouq X, Salem MR. Is calcium a coronary vasoconstrictor in vivo? *Anesthesiology* 1998;88:735–743.

Delmas PD. Bisphosphonates in the treatment of bone diseases. *N Engl J Med* 1996;335:1836–1837.

Delmas PD, Meunier PJ. The management of Paget's disease of bone. *N Engl J Med* 1997;336:558–566.

Denlinger JK, Nahrwold ML. Cardiac failure associated with hypocalcemia. *Anesth Analg* 1976;55:34–36.

Denlinger JK, Nahrwold ML, Gibbs PS, et al. Hypocalcemia during rapid transfusion in anesthetized man. *Br J Anaesth* 1976;48:995–1000.

England MR, Gordon G, Salem M, et al. Magnesium administration and dysrhythmias after cardiac surgery: a placebo-controlled, double-blind, randomized trial. *JAMA* 1992;268:2395–2402.

Gambling DR, Birmingham CL, Jenkins LC. Magnesium and the anaesthetist. *Can J Anaesth* 1988;35:644–654.

Gomez MN. Magnesium and cardiovascular disease. *Anesthesiology* 1998;89:222–40.

Guyton AC, Hall JE. *Textbook of medical physiology,* 10th ed. Philadelphia: WB Saunders, 2000.

Heath DA. Hypercalcaemia in malignanacy: fluids and bisphosphonates are best when life is threatened. *BMJ* 1989;298:1468–1469.

Hosking DJ, Gilson D. Comparison of the renal and skeletal actions of calcitonin in the treatment of severe hypercalcaemia of malignancy. *Q J Med* 1987;211:359–369.

James MFM. Clinical use of magnesium infusions in anesthesia. *Anesth Analg* 1992;74:129–136.

Ko S-H, Lim H-R, Kim D-C, et al. Magnesium sulfate does not reduce postoperative analgesic requirements. *Anesthesiology* 2001;95: 640–646.

Quinn JB , Schultheis LW, Schumacher GE. A tooth broken after laryngoscopy: unlikely to be caused by the force applied by the anesthesiologist. *Anesth Analg* 2005;100:594–596.

Rosen CJ, Kessenich CR. Comparative clinical pharmacology and therapeutic use of bisphosphonates in metabolic bone diseases. *Drugs* 1996;51:537–551.

Warner ME, Benefield SM, Marner MA, et al. Perianesthetic dental injuries: frequency, outcomes and risk factors. *Anesthesiology* 1999;90:1302–1305.

Whang R, Ryder KW. Frequency of hypomagnesemia and hypermagnesemia. *JAMA* 1990;263:3063–3304.

Blood Components, Substitutes and Hemostatic Drugs

36

Blood components and certain drugs are most often administered systemically to improve oxygenation and decrease bleeding due to specific coagulation defects (Practice Guidelines for Blood Component Therapy, 1996; Nuttall et al., 2003; Roberts et al., 2004). It is estimated that more than 22 million blood components are transfused annually in the United States and ≥60% of these transfusions are administered to surgical and obstetric patients (Wallace et al., 1993). The transmission of infectious diseases (hepatitis C, hepatitis B, human immunodeficiency virus [HIV], cytomegalovirus), hemolytic and nonhemolytic transfusion reactions, and immunosuppression are potential adverse sequelae of blood component therapy. For example, despite rigorous screening for infectious disease, there is a modest (1:3,000) risk of hepatitis C transmission and a smaller (1:100,000 to 1:1,000,000) risk of HIV transmission (Dietz et al., 1996). The risk of dying from an allogeneic blood transfusion is estimated to be 0.0001% annually (risk of dying in an automobile accident is approximately 0.002% annually) (Donahue et al., 1992; Graham, 1993). The cost associated with blood component therapy is great but can be decreased by following transfusion guidelines (Practice Guidelines for Blood Component Therapy, 1996; Nuttall et al., 2003).

Topical application of hemostatics is used to control surface bleeding and capillary oozing. Blood substitutes lack coagulation activity but are administered systemically to replace and maintain intravascular fluid volume.

BLOOD COMPONENTS

The advantages of blood components include (a) replacement of only the deficient blood procoagulant, cell, or protein, (b) minimization of the likelihood for circulatory overload, and (c) avoidance of transfusion of unnecessary donor plasma, which may contain undesirable antigens or antibodies. Administration of specific components is recommended in all circumstances other than acute hemorrhage. In the presence of acute hemorrhage, whole blood is indicated to replace both oxygen-carrying capacity and intravascular fluid volume. A unit of whole blood can be divided into several components (Table 36-1).

Packed Erythrocytes

Packed erythrocytes are prepared by removing most of the plasma from whole blood at any time during the acceptable storage period. The resulting volume is about 300 mL, and the hematocrit is 70% to 80%. Preparation of packed erythrocytes from whole blood just before transfusion results in the infusion of fewer sodium and potassium ions and less ammonia, citrate, and lactic acid. As a result, packed erythrocytes so prepared are useful for administration to patients with renal or hepatic dysfunction. The decreased amounts of plasma infused with packed erythrocytes decreases the likelihood of allergic transfusion reactions compared with whole blood.

Packed erythrocytes are stored at 1° to 6°C. The expiration date for these cells is not different from that of whole blood from which they are derived. The addition of adenine to the citrate-phosphate dextrose preservative (CPDA-1) increases storage time from 28 days to 35 days. As reflected by the fact that at least 70% of the erythrocytes remain viable at the time of transfusion. Adenine increases erythrocyte survival by allowing cells to resynthesize adenosine triphosphate (ATP) needed to fuel metabolic reactions. Glucose is added to maintain glycolysis during prolonged storage with

TABLE 36-1.
COMPONENTS AVAILABLE FOR WHOLE BLOOD

Component	Content	Approximate Volume (mL)	Shelf-Life
Packed erythrocytes	Erythrocytes Leukocytes Plasma clotting factors	300	35 days in CPDA-1 42 days in Adsol
Platelet concentrates	Leukocytes (limited) Plasma Erythrocytes (limited)	50	1–5 days
Fresh frozen plasma	Clotting factors	225	Frozen: 1 yr Thawed: 6 hrs
Cryoprecipitate	Factor VIII	Lyophilized powder	Determined by manufacturer
Factor IX concentrate	Factor IX Factors II, VII and X (limited)	Lyophilized powder	Determined by manufacturer
Granulocyte concentrates	Leukocytes Platelets Erythrocytes (limited)	50–300	24 hrs
Albumin	5% albumin 25% albumin	250 or 500 50 or 100	3 yrs
Plasma protein fraction	Albumin Alpha globulins Beta globulins	500	3 yrs
Immune globulins	Gamma globulin	1–2	3 yrs

Adsol, adenine-glucose-mannitol-sodium chloride; CPDA-1, citrate-phosphate dextrose preservative.

adenine. Nephrotoxicity from precipitation of a metabolite of adenine in the renal tubules is unlikely considering the estimated amount of CPDA-1 blood (60 units) that would be required before toxic levels occurred. Addition of extra nutrients to citrate-phosphate-dextrose (adenine, glucose, mannitol, sodium chloride) results in Adsol and an increased storage time to 42 days. Adsol contains about 100 mL of additional saline, making the hematocrit of packed erythrocytes stored in Adsol 55% rather than 70%.

The expiration date for frozen erythrocytes stored at 65°C is 3 years. Once the unit has been thawed and deglycerolized or saline washed, however, it is outdated in 24 hours. The normal function of frozen packed erythrocytes after prolonged storage reflects the maintenance of concentrations of 2,3-diphosphoglycerate and ATP in the erythrocyte at levels near those present at the time the cells were frozen. The major indication for frozen erythrocytes is as a source of rare blood types (Chaplin, 1984). Otherwise, the cost of frozen erythrocytes is too great to justify their more frequent use. Furthermore, transmission of viral hepatitis still can occur after administration of frozen erythrocytes (Alter et al., 1978).

Clinical Uses

Packed erythrocytes are selected when the goal is to increase oxygen-carrying capacity in the absence of preexisting hypovolemia. Many clinicians believe that packed erythrocytes may be used to replace blood loss that is <1,500 mL in an adult. One unit of packed erythrocytes typically increases the hematocrit 3% or hemoglobin concentration 1 g/dL in a 70-kg nonbleeding adult. Controlled studies have not been performed to determine the hemoglobin concentration at which erythrocyte administration improves outcome. Erythrocyte transfusion is rarely indicated when the hemoglobin concentration is >10 g/dL and is almost always indicated when it is <6 g/dL, especially when anemia is acute (Practice Guidelines for Blood Component Therapy, 1996). The determination of whether intermediate hemoglobin concentrations (6 to 10 g/dL) justify or require erythrocyte transfusion should be based on the patient's risk for complications from inadequate oxygenation.

Administration of packed erythrocytes is facilitated by reconstituting them with crystalloid solutions (5% glucose in 0.9% saline, 0.9% saline, Normosol) to decrease viscosity. Lactated Ringer's solution should probably not be used for this purpose because the calcium ions present could induce clotting. A diluent that is hypotonic with respect to plasma (glucose solutions) may cause osmotic lysis of infused erythrocytes.

Platelet Concentrates

Platelets can be provided as platelet concentrates either from multiple donors or from a single donor (continuous apheresis process that removes platelets and returns all other blood components). Platelet concentrates are prepared by centrifugation of citrated whole blood within 8 hours after collection. An average single unit of platelets contains 5.5 to 10 million platelets, which is too small for an adequate therapeutic effect in an adult with thrombocytopenia; therefore, platelet concentrates from four to ten donors are customarily combined (pooled concentrates). A single donor plateletpheresis unit contains approximately 40 million platelets and is considered to be equivalent to about 6 units derived from whole blood. The volume of plasma from either 6 random units or 1 plateletpheresis unit is 250 to 300 mL. One unit of platelet concentrate will increase the platelet count 5,000 to 10,000 cells/mL^3. The usual therapeutic dose is one platelet concentrate per 10 kg of body weight. Platelets lose their ability to aggregate when stored in a refrigerator. For this reason, platelets are stored at room temperature and are constantly agitated to facilitate gas exchange. Room temperature facilitates bacterial growth, and sepsis is a potentially fatal complication of platelet transfusion (Kruskall, 1997). To minimize the risk of sepsis, platelet storage is limited to 5 days.

Although platelet concentrates contain only a few erythrocytes, they do contain large amounts of plasma (leukocytes) and administration based on ABO compatibility is desirable. Likewise, the small quantity of erythrocytes present can cause Rh immunization if platelets from an Rh-positive donor are administered to an Rh-negative recipient. For this reason, Rh-compatible platelets should be used in females of child-bearing age. Platelets possess human leukocyte antigen (HLA) antigens on their cell membranes, and patients sensitized to these antigens will destroy infused platelets, thus manifesting as the absence of a therapeutic response. In these patients, the administration of type-specific HLA platelets is the only effective treatment. Ultraviolet irradiation of platelet concentrates lowers the incidence of immune-mediated refractoriness to platelet transfusions.

Clinical Uses

Surgical and obstetric patients usually require platelet transfusion if the platelet count is <50,000 cells/mL^3 and rarely require therapy if it is >100,000 cells/mL^3 (Practice Guidelines for Blood Component Therapy, 1996). With intermediate platelet counts (50,000 to 100,000 cells/mL^3), the determinant is based on the patient's risk for more significant bleeding. Nevertheless, the platelet count at which surgical and obstetric patients are likely to experience increased bleeding is unknown. In nonsurgical patients, spontaneous bleeding is uncommon with platelet counts of >10,000 cells/mL^3 (Rebulla et al., 1997). Platelet transfusion may be indicated despite an apparently adequate platelet count if there is known platelet dysfunction and microvascular bleeding. The bleeding time is a test of overall platelet function but it has not been found to be a predictor of surgical bleeding (Rogers and Levin, 1990). In contrast, the thromboelastogram reliably reflects qualitative and quantitative abnormalities of platelets (Fig. 36-1) (Mallett and Cox, 1992).

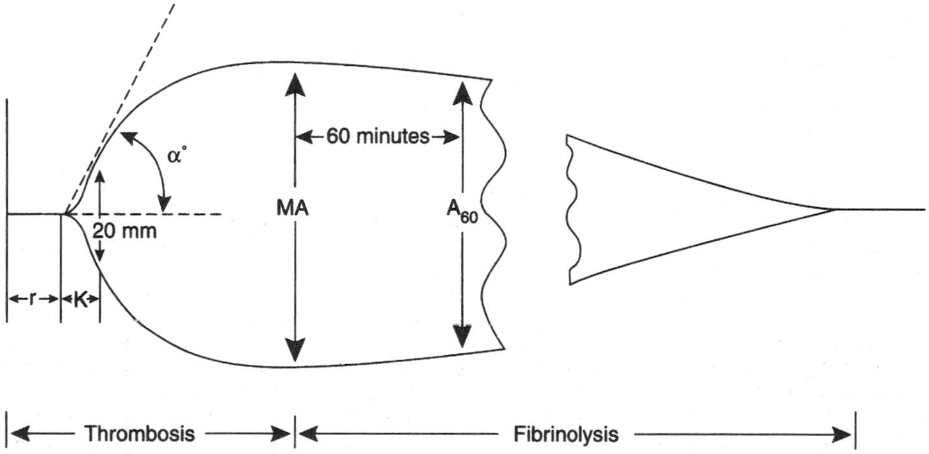

Figure 36-1. Quantification of thromboelastograph (TEG) variables. r = reaction time (time from sample placement in the curette until TEG amplitude reaches 2 mm). The normal r time is 6 to 8 minutes and represents the rate of initial fibrin formation. Prolongation of the r time may be the result of coagulation factor deficiencies, anticoagulation (heparin), or severe hypofibrinogenemia. A short r time may be present in hypercoagulability syndromes. K = clot formation time (normal range 3 to 6 minutes) as measured from the r time to the point where the amplitude of the tracing reaches 20 mm. This is influenced by the activity of the intrinsic clotting factors, fibrinogen, and platelets. The alpha angle (normal range 50 to 60 degrees) is the angle formed by the slope of the TEG tracing from the r to the K value. It denotes the speed at which solid clot forms. Decreased values may occur with hypofibrinogenemia and thrombocytopenia. The maximum amplitude (MA) (normal range 50 to 60 mm) is the greatest amplitude on the TEG trace and is a reflection of the absolute strength of the fibrin clot. Platelet abnormalities alter the MA. A_{60} (normal range = MA – 5 mm) is the amplitude of the tracing 60 minutes after MA is achieved. This is a measure of clot lysis or retraction. (From Mallett SV, Cox DJ. Thrombelastography. *Br J Anaesth* 1992;69:307–313; with permission.)

Thrombocytopenia has virtually no effect on the incidence of postpartum bleeding because hemostasis after placental separation is largely mechanical. Mild thrombocytopenia is detected in approximately 15% of women with pregnancy-induced hypertension. With the HELLP syndrome (*h*emolysis, *e*levated *l*iver enzymes, *l*ow *p*latelet count), the thrombocytopenia is more severe, but spontaneous resolution usually occurs by the fourth postpartum day.

Fresh Frozen Plasma

Fresh frozen plasma is plasma separated from erythrocytes and platelets of whole blood donations and placed at −18°C or below within 8 hours after collection. It may be stored at −18°C for up to 12 months. After thawing in a water bath at 37°C, the unit must be administered within a few hours. Fresh frozen plasma contains all procoagulants except platelets in a concentration of 1 unit/mL, as well as naturally occurring inhibitors. Four to five units of platelet concentrates, one unit of single-donor apheresis platelets, or one unit of whole blood provide a quantity of coagulation factors similar to that contained in one unit of fresh frozen plasma.

One unit of fresh frozen plasma contains approximately 200 to 250 mL. Larger volumes of fresh frozen plasma (approximately 400 to 600 mL) prepared by plasmapheresis from a single donor are preferable for use instead of two units of fresh frozen plasma from different donors. A substantial sodium load is associated with administration of fresh frozen plasma. Compatibility for ABO antigens is desirable, but cross-matching is not necessary. Life-threatening allergic reactions may occur, and transmission of diseases, including hepatitis and HIV, is possible (Bove, 1985).

Clinical Uses

The usual starting dose of fresh frozen plasma is two units (400 to 500 mL) or one plasmapheresis unit to treat active bleeding due to a congenital or acquired deficiency of coagulation factors as confirmed by a (a) prothrombin time >1.5 times normal (usually >18 s), (b) partial thromboplastin time >1.5 times normal (usually >55 to 60 s), or (c) coagulation factor assay of <25% activity (Practice Guidelines Development Task Force of the College of American Pathologists, 1994). Thromboelastography offers a unique method of monitoring coagulation that provides information about fibrinolytic activity and platelet function that may not be generally available from routine coagulation screens (see Fig. 36-1) (Mallett and Cox, 1992). In determining the need for repeated fresh frozen plasma transfusions, the half-times of the coagulation factors must be considered. Because factor VII has a shorter half-time (5 to 6 hours) than other factors, the prothrombin time may become prolonged sooner than the activated plasma thromboplastin time. The patient's clinical bleeding must also be assessed. There are data that suggest the relationship between a clinical coagulopathy, laboratory tests of coagulation, and the need for fresh frozen plasma remains unclear (Murray et al., 1988; Miller, 1995).

Fresh frozen plasma (5 to 8 mL/kg) is recommended for urgent reversal of warfarin therapy as may be needed before emergency surgery. An infrequent use of fresh frozen plasma is for management of patients with antithrombin deficiency who require heparin for surgery or treatment of thrombosis. Consistent with the ability of fresh frozen plasma to provide supplemental antithrombin is the observation that infusion of this material potentiates the effects of systemic heparinization (Fig. 36-2) (Barnette et al., 1988). Fresh frozen plasma may be considered for treatment of continued bleeding in patients

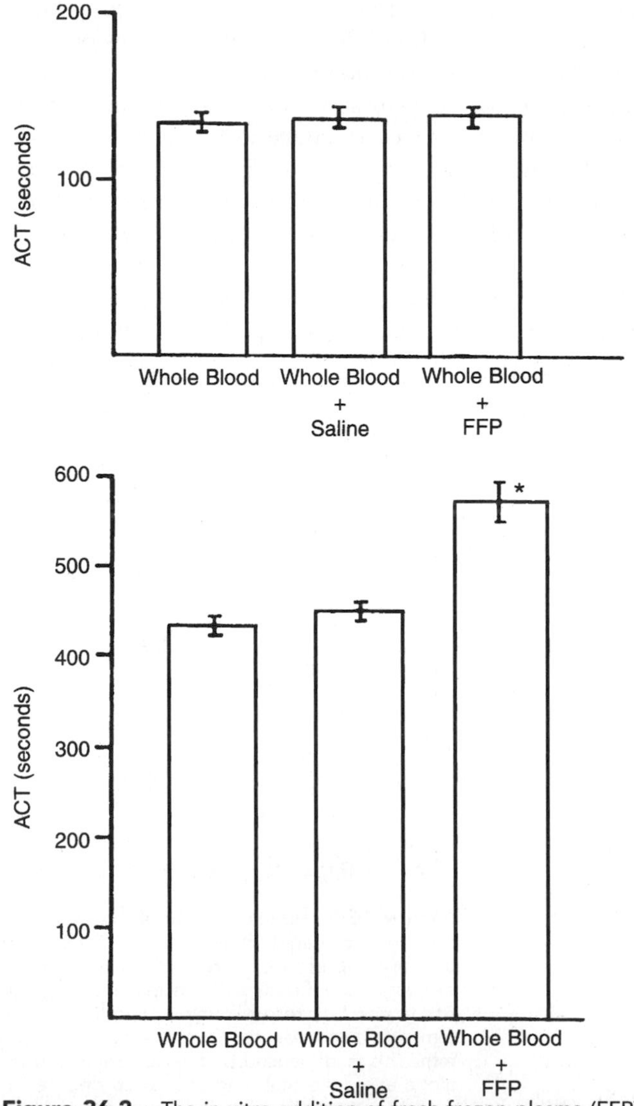

Figure 36-2. The in vitro addition of fresh frozen plasma (FFP) to blood containing heparin significantly (*P <.05) prolongs the activated coagulation time (ACT). (From Barnette RB, Shupak RC, Pontius J, et al. In vitro effect of fresh frozen plasma on the activated coagulation time in patients undergoing cardiopulmonary bypass. *Anesth Analg* 1988;67: 57–60; with permission.)

receiving massive blood transfusions (>5,000 mL in an adult), especially when measurement of the prothrombin time or activated partial thromboplastin time cannot be promptly obtained (Practice Guidelines for Blood Component Therapy, 1996). It has not been possible to document a beneficial effect of fresh frozen plasma when used as part of the transfusion management strategy in patients with massive hemorrhage in the absence of a documented clotting deficiency (Bove, 1985). Even when packed erythrocytes are used to replace blood loss equivalent to one blood volume, clotting factors in the form of fresh frozen plasma may not be necessary to maintain the prothrombin time or activated plasma thromboplastin time at normal levels (Murray et al., 1988). Fresh frozen plasma is not recommended for treatment of hypovolemia or hypoalbuminemia.

Cryoprecipitated Antihemophiliac Factor

Cryoprecipitated antihemophiliac factor (factor VIII) is that fraction of plasma that precipitates when fresh frozen plasma is thawed (Hoyer, 1981). This precipitate is generally resuspended in a minimal volume of residual supernatant plasma (9 to 16 mL), refrozen, and stored at −18°C for up to 1 year. Cryoprecipitate should be kept at room temperature after thawing and used within 3 hours. The major portion of transfused cryoprecipitate remains in the intravascular space with an elimination half-time of about 12 hours. Multiple transfusions of cryoprecipitate may result in hyperfibrinogenemia, emphasizing the substantial fibrinogen content of these preparations.

Commercial factor VIII concentrates, in contrast to single-donor cryoprecipitate, contain a standardized amount of antihemophiliac factor (Hoyer, 1981). These preparations, however, are more expensive than cryoprecipitated antihemophiliac factor and have a potentially greater risk for transmitting viral diseases because they are prepared from pooled plasma derived from a large number of donors. Indeed, hepatitis is the most common adverse side effect of pooled plasma products, reflecting the multiple donor sources of the fibrinogen that are present. Hemolytic anemia may occur when cryoprecipitated antihemophiliac factor is administered to individuals with group A, B, or AB erythrocyte antigens. These patients should be treated with cryoprecipitate from type-specific or type O donors who have low liters of antibodies.

Clinical Uses

Cryoprecipitate is useful for treatment of hemophilia A because it contains high concentrations of factor VIII (80 to 120 units) in a volume of only about 10 mL (Practice Guidelines Development Task Force of the American College of Pathologists, 1994). About 10% to 15% of patients with hemophilia A develop an immunoglobulin inhibitor that inactivates infused antihemophiliac factor. Assay for this inhibitor may be recommended before cryoprecipitate infusion to hemophiliacs, especially preoperatively. Hemophilia A patients with factor VIII levels of >5% of normal usually do not experience spontaneous bleeding. Effective hemostasis during and after major surgery, however, requires maintenance of factor VIII levels of ≥40% of normal for 7 to 10 days (Ellison, 1977).

Cryoprecipitate is recommended for prophylaxis in nonbleeding perioperative or peripartum patients with congenital fibrinogen deficiencies or von Willebrand's disease that is unresponsive to desmopressin (Practice Guidelines for Blood Component Therapy, 1996). Cryoprecipitate is recommended for treatment of bleeding patients with von Willebrand's disease and for correction of bleeding in massively transfused patients with fibrinogen concentrations of <80 to 100 mg/dL. Most cases of hypofibrinogenemia are associated with conditions that cause consumption coagulopathy requiring treatment with other blood components as well. Cryoprecipitate is the only approved blood component that contains fibrinogen in a concentrated form.

Desmopressin

Desmopressin, a synthetic analogue of arginine vasopressin hormone (formerly known as antidiuretic hormone), greatly increases factor VIII activity in patients with mild to moderate hemophilia and von Willebrand's disease (see Chapter 23). Doses of 0.3 to 0.5 μg/kg administered intravenously (IV) before and soon after dental surgery have prevented abnormal bleeding. Even cholecystectomy and tonsillectomy have been performed successfully in hemophiliac patients treated with desmopressin. This drug has been administered to improve hemostasis after complex cardiopulmonary bypass procedures, perhaps reflecting desmopressin-induced release of von Willebrand factor necessary for adequate activity of factor VIII and optimal adhesion of platelets (Czer et al., 1987; Salzman et al., 1986). Nevertheless, routine administration of desmopressin to patients undergoing elective cardiac surgery does not alter blood loss after cardiopulmonary bypass (Hackman et al., 1989). Decreases in systemic blood pressure associated with evidence of peripheral vasodilation may occur in association with infusion of desmopressin (D'Alauro and Johns, 1988). In contrast to blood components, desmopressin administration does not introduce the risk of transmission of viral diseases.

Factor IX Concentrate

Factor IX concentrate (prothrombin complex, plasma thromboplastin component) is prepared from pooled plasma. Cryoprecipitated antihemophiliac factor preparations do not contain factor IX. Factor IX concentrates can be infused without typing or cross-matching. Hypervolemic reactions do not occur because of the concentrated nature of these products and the small amount of fluid needed for administration. Factor IX concentrates are stable for at least 12 hours at room temperature after reconstitution.

Factor IX concentrates have significant potential to cause hepatitis because of the pooled origin of these products. In addition, there is a high risk of thrombotic complications associated with infusion, presumably reflecting the high concentrations of prothrombin and factor X that result from factor IX administration (Fuerth and Mahrer, 1981). This complication seems particularly likely and severe in patients with preexisting liver disease.

Fibrin Glue

Fibrin glue, or cryoprecipitated fibrinogen, is prepared from bovine thrombin and human fibrinogen, which form a clot when combined. This glue has been used for sealing suture holes as associated with vascular anastomoses. An allergic reaction to fibrin glue has been reported (Milde, 1989).

Antifibrinolytics

Synthetic (aminocaproic acid, tranexamic acid) and natural (aprotinin) antifibrinolytics decrease postoperative bleeding and the need for transfusions after cardiopulmonary bypass, scoliosis surgery, orthotopic liver transplantation, and lower urinary tract surgery (Fig. 36-3) (see Chapter 22) (Casati et al., 2001; Dowd et al., 2002; Kluger et al., 2003; Neilipovitz et al., 2001; Pleym et al., 2003). The antifibrinolytic effect of these drugs is due to formation of a reversible complex with plasminogen thus preventing fibrinolysis that would normally occur with activation of plasminogen to plasmin. As a result of this inhibition, fibrin is not lysed, which allows for formation of a more stable clot and decreased risk of recurrent bleeding. Fibrinolysis is a putative mechanism of bleeding following cardiopulmonary bypass. Treatment with fibrinolytic inhibitors is associated with a theoretical risk of an increased thrombotic tendency. Fatal aortic thrombosis has been described in patients treated with aminocaproic acid during aortic valve replacement (Fanashawe et al., 2001). Administration of aminocaproic acid in the presence of renal or ureteral bleeding is not recommended because ureteral clot formation and possible obstruction may result. Indeed, unchanged aminocaproic acid is rapidly excreted by the kidneys. Aminocaproic acid does not control hemorrhage caused by thrombocytopenia or most other coagulation defects.

Granulocyte Concentrates

Leukapheresis is continuous or intermittent flow centrifugation to obtain granulocytes for subsequent infusion to treat infection (Higby and Burnett, 1980). Granulocytes have been beneficial in patients recovering from bone marrow transplants. Phagocytic and microbicidal functions of collected granulocytes persist for about 48 hours.

Fever often accompanies granulocyte transfusion and can be ameliorated by administration of an antihistamine and an antipyretic. Granulocytes should be administered slowly to avoid pulmonary insufficiency that may be caused by sequestration of these cells in the pulmonary capillaries. Acute dyspnea, arterial hypoxemia, and interstitial infiltrates may be more likely when patients treated with amphotericin B receive granulocyte transfusions (Wright et al., 1981). Cytomegalovirus infections frequently are observed after granulocyte transfusions because the virus is concentrated in granulocytes.

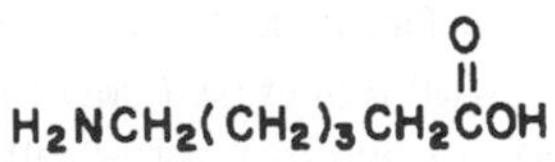

Figure 36-3. Aminocaproic acid.

Albumin

Albumin is obtained by fractionating human plasma that is nonreactive for hepatitis. Coagulation factors and blood group antibodies are not present. In fact, an albumin-induced increase in the intravascular fluid volume may actually dilute the plasma concentrations of coagulant factors. Albumin is heated for 10 hours at 60°C, which appears to remove the hazard of transmission of viral diseases. Albumin preparations contain sodium caprylate, acetyltryptophanate, or both as stabilizers, allowing storage for about 3 years.

Albumin, 25 g, is equivalent osmotically to about 500 mL of plasma but contains only about one-seventh the amount of sodium present in the same volume of plasma. Hypoalbuminemia is the most frequent indication for the administration of albumin. Albumin also binds bilirubin and has been administered during exchange transfusions to treat hyperbilirubinemia. Administration of hypertonic 25% albumin will draw 3 to 4 mL of fluid from the interstitial space into the intravascular fluid space for every 1 mL of albumin administered. This is the reason 25% albumin is not recommended for administration to patients in cardiac failure or in the presence of anemia. The 5% solution of albumin is isotonic with plasma and is most often administered undiluted at a rate of 2 to 4 mL/minute. In patients in an intensive care unit, administration of either albumin or normal saline for fluid resuscitation results in similar outcomes at 28 days (The SAFE Study Investigators, 2004; Boldt, 2000).

Antioxidant Activity

Albumin possesses potential free radical scavenging characteristics and is the principal intravascular source of reduced sulfhydryl groups. These sulfhydryl groups are avid scavengers of reactive oxygen and nitrogen molecules (Stratford, 1997). Antioxidants may have therapeutic value in reducing cellular damage, particularly during local and systemic inflammatory responses. Nonprotein-containing IV solutions (mannitol, hydroxyethyl starch) lack antioxidant activity.

Plasma Protein Fraction

Plasma protein fraction is a 5% pooled solution of stabilized human plasma proteins in saline containing at least 83% albumin and no more than 17% globulins, of which <1% are gamma globulins. Each 100 mL of solution provides 5 g of proteins. The preparation is equivalent osmotically to an equal volume of plasma. Although plasma protein fraction is prepared from large pools of normal human plasma, transmission of viral diseases is not a hazard because of heating to 60°C for 10 hours. It must be recognized that plasma protein fraction does not contain any coagulation factors and may even dilute the plasma concentration of existing coagulants.

Clinical Uses

Plasma protein fraction is administered to treat hypovolemic shock and to provide protein to patients with hypoproteinemia. It is also effective for the initial treatment of shock in infants and small children with dehydration, hemoconcentration, and electrolyte deficiency caused by diarrhea. Although dosage is guided by individual response, the usual treatment of hypovolemia or hypoproteinemia is with 20 to 30 mL/kg IV of plasma protein fraction (75 to 100 g of protein). An important deterrent to the use of plasma protein fraction to treat hypovolemia is its high cost and limited availability compared with blood substitutes.

Hypotension that may accompany rapid infusion of plasma protein fraction has been attributed to the presence of prekallikrein activator that leads to production of bradykinin with resulting peripheral vasodilation (Bland et al., 1973; Isbister and Fisher, 1980). The level of prekallikrein activator in plasma protein fraction has been decreased since these reports, and hypotension no longer seems to occur.

Signs of hypervolemia may occur when plasma protein fraction is administered to patients with increased intravascular fluid volumes. Administration of large quantities of plasma protein fraction to patients with impaired renal function has been reported to cause electrolyte imbalances and metabolic alkalosis (Rahilly and Berl, 1979).

Immune Globulin

Immune globulin is a concentrated solution of globulins, primarily immunoglobulins, prepared from large pools of human plasma. This preparation protects against clinical manifestations of hepatitis A when administered before or within 2 weeks after exposure. Replacement therapy for patients with hypogammaglobulinemia is another use of immune globulin. Immune globulin prevents or modifies rubeola, rubella, and varicella. Low concentrations of immunoglobulin A are present in immune globulin, emphasizing the need to avoid administration of this preparation to patients with antiimmunoglobulin A. Hepatitis B immune globulin is a special preparation with a high antibody titer that delays the onset of hepatitis B and ameliorates the severity of the disease (Prince, 1978).

TOPICAL HEMOSTATICS

Topical hemostatics include absorbable gelatin sponge or film, oxidized cellulose, microfibrillar collagen and hemostat, and thrombin. These substances may help to control surface bleeding and capillary oozing as associated with biliary tract surgery; partial hepatectomy; resection or injuries of the pancreas, spleen, or kidneys; and oral, neurologic, and otolaryngologic surgery. Although usually innocuous, the presence of bacterial contamination at the site of application of topical hemostatics may exacerbate infections.

Absorbable Gelatin Sponge (Gelfoam®)

Gelfoam is a sterile gelatin-base surgical sponge that controls bleeding in highly vascular areas that are difficult to suture. The preparation may be left in place after closure of the surgical wound. Absorption is complete in 4 to 6 weeks, and scar formation or cellular reaction is minimal. When this material is placed into closed tissue spaces, it must be remembered that the material absorbs fluid and expands, which could cause pressure on neighboring structures.

Absorbable Gelatin Film (Gelfilm®)

Gelfilm is sterile, thin film used primarily in neurologic and thoracic surgery for nonhemostatic purposes to repair defects in the dura and pleural membranes. It is also used in ocular surgery. Absorption is complete within 6 months of implantation.

Oxidized Cellulose (Oxycel®) and Oxidized Regenerated Cellulose (Surgicel®)

Oxycel and oxidized regenerated cellulose do not enter into the normal clotting cascade, but when exposed to blood, they expand and are converted to a reddish brown or black gelatinous mass that forms an artificial clot. Oxidized cellulose has a low pH, which contributes to a local cauterizing action. The hemostatic action of these celluloses is not enhanced by other hemostatic agents, and thrombin is destroyed by the low pH. Absorption of these products may require 6 weeks or longer. Some stenosis of arterial anastomoses may occur, apparently from cicatricial contraction. These products should not be used for permanent packing or implantation in fractures because they may interfere with bone regeneration and cause cyst formation.

Microfibrillar Collagen Hemostat (Avitene®)

When applied directly onto a bleeding surface, this water-insoluble, fibrous material attracts and entraps platelets to initiate formation of a platelet plug and development of a natural clot. Absorption without cellular reaction occurs in about 7 weeks. This topical hemostatic appears to retain its effectiveness in heparinized patients, in those receiving oral anticoagulants, and in the presence of moderate thrombocytopenia. Microfibrillar collagen hemostat is a useful adjunct to therapy in the oral cavity of patients with hemophilia. This material can be used on skin graft donor sites, around a vascular anastomosis where only minimal suturing is possible, and to control oozing from cancellous bone. It should not, however, be used on bone surfaces to which prosthetic materials are to be attached with methylmethacrylate adhesives.

As a foreign protein, microfibrillar collagen hemostat may exacerbate infection, abscess formation, and dehiscence of cutaneous incisions. Use of this hemostatic is not recommended for skin incisions because healing of the wound edges is impaired. Despite its protein structure, allergic reactions have not been described.

Thrombin

Thrombin is a sterile protein derived from bovine prothrombin. It is applied topically as a powder or in a solution to control capillary oozing in operative procedures and to shorten effectively the duration of bleeding from puncture sites in heparinized patients. Thrombin may be combined with gelatin sponge but should not be used to moisten microfibrillar collagen hemostat. Thrombin alone does not control arterial bleeding.

When applied to denuded tissue, thrombin is inactivated by antithrombins and by absorption onto fibrin. A pH of <5 also inactivates thrombin. Systemic absorption is unlikely, and direct IV injection is not recommended because resulting thrombosis could be fatal. Allergic reactions are a theoretical possibility when thrombin is used.

BLOOD SUBSTITUTES

Blood substitutes may be viewed as oxygen-carrying volume expanders that, in contrast to blood products, have a prolonged shelf life and do not introduce the risk for disease transmission or need for compatibility testing (Dietz et al., 1996; Jones, 1995). A projected short-fall in available blood with the increasing number of elderly patients (at present, patients ≥65 years of age consume half of the erythrocytes transfused) would be obviated by blood substitutes. In contrast to blood, blood substitutes do not contain any coagulant factors. Furthermore, available blood substitutes tend to have short intravascular half-times, undesirable routes of elimination (nephrotoxicity), physiologic side effects (hypertension, coagulopathy), and interactions with coexisting diseases.

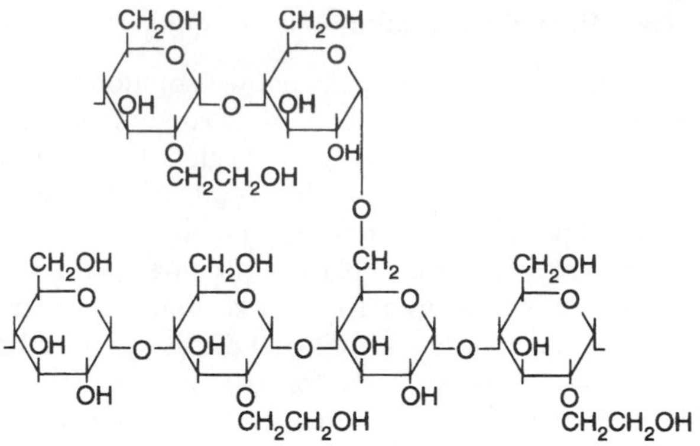

Figure 36-4. Hydroxyethyl starch.

Hydroxyethyl Starch

Hydroxyethyl starch (hetastarch) is a complex polysaccharide (average molecular weight 450,000 daltons) that is available in 6% and 10% aqueous solutions for intravascular volume expansion (plasma substitute in place of 5% albumin) during the perioperative period (Fig. 36-4) (Beyer et al., 1997; Warren and Durieux, 1997). In fact, hydroxyethyl starch and albumin expand intravascular fluid volume equally effectively. In addition to volume replacement, hydroxyethyl starch is useful for acute normovolemic hemodilution and to improve blood rheology by decreasing blood viscosity. The advantages of hydroxyethyl starch as an artificial colloid include its oncotic properties, its long duration of hemodynamic effects due to its long elimination half-time, its low antigenicity and infrequent anaphylactoid reactions, the absence of disease transmission, and the low cost compared with albumin (Dieterich et al., 1998). The potential for hydroxyethyl starch to produce a coagulopathy (dose-dependent decrease in factor VIII and von Willebrand factor and interference with platelet function) is cited as a reason to use caution in transfusing this solution to neurosurgical patients (Baldassarre and Vincent, 1997). This synthetic colloid is not recommended for use as a cardiac bypass pump prime, while the patient is on cardiopulmonary bypass, or in the immediate period following separation from bypass because of the risk of increasing coagulation abnormalities and bleeding in patients whose coagulation status is already impaired (see the section, Side Effects). Disruption of the blood-brain barrier due to hemorrhage or trauma does not result in passage of hydroxyethyl starch molecules into the brain (Dieterich et al., 2003; Neff et al., 2003).

Pharmacokinetics

Hydroxyethyl starch is removed from the circulation by renal excretion and redistribution (Wilkes et al., 2002).

Reversible swelling of renal tubular cells may reflect reabsorption of hydroxyethyl starch macromolecules. The duration of volume expansion approximates 24 hours, which is similar to that produced by albumin. In contrast to albumin, hydroxyethyl starch does not act as a carrier protein for drugs. The solution administered clinically consists of 6 g or 10 g of hydroxyethyl starch in 100 mL of saline with an osmolarity of 310 mOsm/L and a pH of 3.5 to 7.

Side Effects

Hydroxyethyl starch may interfere with coagulation and accumulate in tissues. Serum macroamylasemia may follow transfusion of hydroxyethyl starch. For this reason, serum amylase concentrations as a diagnostic marker of pancreatic disease should not be relied on for 3 to 5 days after hydroxyethyl starch infusion. Pruritus associated with deposition of hydroxyethyl starch in the skin may be treated with topical capsaicin (Szelmies et al., 1994). An adverse influence on immune function may accompany administration of hydroxyethyl starches (Boldt et al. 1996).

Coagulopathy

Hydroxyethyl starch has been associated with a prolongation of the activated partial thromboplastin time and a decrease in the plasma concentrations of factor VIII, von Willebrand factor, and fibrinogen plus decreased platelet function that appears to be independent of the dose administered (Egli et al., 1997; Warren and Durieux, 1997). Low-molecular-weight hydroxyethyl starch compromises blood coagulation slightly less than high-molecular-weight hydroxyethyl starch but the difference is not likely to be significant (Jamnicki et al., 2000). The maximum amplitude of the thromboelastogram is depressed in patients receiving hydroxyethyl starch, indicating formation of a clot with decreased strength (Kuitunen et al., 1993). Hydroxyethyl starch solutions, when administered in doses of 20 mL/kg with the cardiopulmonary bypass prime compromise hemostasis after cardiac surgery (Kuitunen et al., 2004). This effect appears related to formation of a less stable thrombus. It is hypothesized that this complex polysaccharide precipitates certain coagulation factors, making them unavailable to the coagulation cascade. Hydroxyethyl starch has been suggested to decrease platelet function by coating the platelet surface or inducing platelet damage.

Dextran

Dextran-70 is a water-soluble glucose polymer (polysaccharide) synthesized by certain bacteria from sucrose. The mean molecular weight of dextran-70 is about 70,000 daltons and a colloid osmotic pressure of about 350 mOsm/L. This high-molecular-weight dextran is treated to yield low-molecular-weight dextran (dextran-40) with a molecular weight of about 40,000 daltons and a higher colloid osmotic pressure. Dextrans are eliminated largely through the kidneys although small amounts are metabolized. The renal threshold for dextran is a molecular weight of about 55,000 daltons. Therefore, more dextran-40 than dextran-70 is filtered by the glomeruli. Dextran-70 may persist in the circulation for 72 hours and interfere with platelet activation. Ultimately, dextran-70 is degraded enzymatically to glucose.

Clinical Uses

High-molecular-weight dextrans remain in the intravascular space for about 12 hours. For this reason, they may be suitable alternatives to blood or plasma for expansion of intravascular fluid volume. For replacement of intravascular fluid volume, the recommended maximum dose during the first 24 hours is 20 mL/kg IV and then 10 mg/kg IV on subsequent days. Therapy should not be continued for longer than 5 days. A special solution of dextran (32% dextran-70) is used in hysteroscopy to help distend and irrigate the uterine cavity and to decrease the likelihood of tubal adhesions after reconstructive tubal surgery for infertility. Because this dextran may be absorbed, adverse reactions are the same as those encountered after IV administration. For example, vascular absorption of this solution may be sufficient to produce pulmonary edema (Mangar et al., 1991). Dextran-40 remains intravascular for only 2 to 4 hours and is used most often to prevent thromboembolism by decreasing blood viscosity. Dextrans may also influence leukocyte adherence that suggests a possible role in ischemia/reperfusion injury (Steinbauer et al., 1998).

Side Effects

The potential side effects of dextran must be considered before the blood substitute is selected in lieu of safer, though more expensive, products such as albumin or plasma protein fraction.

Allergic Reactions

Dextran allergic reactions are caused by circulating dextran-reactive immunoglobulin G antibodies that are present in most adults (Dieterich et al., 1998). The incidence of allergic reactions after infusion of high- or low-molecular-weight dextrans appears to be approximately 1:3,000 administrations (Isbister and Fisher, 1980). Nevertheless, low-molecular-weight dextran probably has considerably less antigenic potential than high-molecular-weight dextran. Histamine release may manifest as urticaria, angioedema, hypotension, and bronchospasm. Discontinuation of the dextran infusion is usually sufficient treatment but, in rare cases, life-threatening allergic reactions require aggressive therapy. Indeed, fatal allergic reactions have occurred after IV administration of as little as 10 mL of dextran-70 (Isbister and Fisher, 1980).

Increased Bleeding Time

Increased bleeding time caused by decreased platelet adhesiveness occurs, especially when high-molecular-weight dextran is infused and the dose is >1,500 mL. This impairment of coagulation may not appear for 6 to 9 hours after the infusion. Plasma levels of fibrinogen and factors V, VIII, and IX may be decreased.

Rouleaux Formation

Dextran solutions, regardless of their molecular weight, may induce rouleaux formation and therefore interfere with subsequent cross-matching of blood. For this reason, blood for cross-matching should be obtained before dextran infusion. Dextrans may also interfere with certain tests of renal and hepatic function and cause factitious increases in the blood glucose concentrations.

Noncardiogenic Pulmonary Edema

Systemic absorption of 32% dextran-70 used as irrigation fluid during hysteroscopy may be sufficient to produce pulmonary edema (Mangar et al., 1989; Mangar et al., 1991). For this reason, it is recommended that the dose of this irrigation solution as used for diagnostic procedures be limited to 500 mL. In addition, a direct toxic effect of 32% dextran-70 on pulmonary capillaries after systemic absorption may be responsible for pulmonary edema (Mangar et al., 1989).

Gelatin

Gelatin solutions (Hemaccel®, Gelofusin®) have average molecular weights of about 35,000 daltons and are approximatley isotonic. These inexpensive solutions have a relatively short intravascular half-time although it exceeeds that of colloid solutions. Metabolism is in the liver and the gelatin is completely eliminated via the kidneys resulting in an osmotic diuresis. Coagulation problems are unlikely and when they occur are probably related to hemodilution. There is a small risk (<1%) for immune-mediated hypersensitivity. Gelatin-induced histamine release has been associated with hypotension, bronchospasm, and cutaneous rashes.

Hemoglobin Solutions

Pure solutions of hemoglobin (stroma-free) provide oxygen-carrying capacity but have a limited duration of action due to their rapid clearance from the circulation. For example, free hemoglobin has an elimination half-time of 10 to 30 minutes, reflecting its passage into the phagocyte system and rapid renal excretion (Jones, 1995). The high colloid osmotic pressure of hemoglobin solutions prohibits their administration at concentrations of >7 g/dL. Hemoglobin in solution is gradually oxidized to methemoglobin and so must be stored in an oxygen-free environment. Large-scale manufacture of a hemoglobin product from human erythrocytes is probably not feasible because blood donors are in short supply.

Hemoglobin-based oxygen carriers combine oxygen transport with volume expanding properties and thus may be useful for treatment of anemia and hemorrhagic shock. In the presence of increasing levels of these solutions in the plasma, measurement of serum lactate concentrations may be underestimated leading to undertreatment of the patient (Jahr et al., 2005).

Recombinant Human Hemoglobin

Recombinant human hemoglobin is a genetically engineered protein produced in *Escherichia coli* that yields a pure solution of hemoglobin (P_{50} in a normal range) without remnants of red blood cell stroma (Dietz et al., 1996). Synthetic genes encoding the human alpha- and beta-globin polypeptides result in a fully assembled tetrameric molecule. The intravascular half-time of these products is short and they are cleared from the circulation by the reticuloendothelial system. Infusion of recombinant hemoglobin does not produce evidence of nephrotoxicity. Nevertheless, manufacture of recombinant hemoglobin has been discontinued (Winslow, 2000).

Perfluorocarbons

Perfluorocarbons are inert synthetic compounds that dissolve large amounts of carbon dioxide and oxygen molecules (oxygen carrying colloid) (Dietz et al., 1996; Tremper, 1999). The oxygen content of perfluorocarbons is directly proportional to the oxygen partial pressure. Since perfluorocarbons exchange gases by simple diffusion, they load and unload oxygen two times faster than hemoglobin. Because perfluorocarbons are highly hydrophobic they require emulsification with a surfactant to create a formulation suitable for IV administration. Intravascularly administered fluorocarbons are excreted intact by exhalation and are also cleared from the circulation by phagocytosis and subsequent uptake into the reticuloendothelial system, from which they are progressively excreted through the lungs. The reticuloendothelial system mechanism of excretion results in a temporary increase in the weight of the liver and spleen and a slight increase in liver enzymes. Although second-generation fluorocarbons have increased oxygen-carrying capacity, their dissolved oxygen contents at ambient partial pressures are still limited. Short intravascular persistence, poor shelf-life, temperature instability, and side effects, which include uptake by the reticuloendothelial system and disruption of normal pulmonary surfactant mechanisms, restrict widespread use of these solutions. Perfluorocarbons do not affect coagulation but do appear as platelets in automated cell counters, which may result in an overestimate of platelet counts especially in thrombocytopenic blood samples (Cuignet et al., 2000; Leese et al., 2000). Fluosol-DA 20% is licensed only for oxygen delivery (not as a erythrocyte substitute) during coronary angioplasty when the ballon is inflated.

REFERENCES

Alter HJ, Tabor E, Meryman HT, et al. Transmission of hepatitis B virus infection by transfusion of frozen-deglycerolized red blood cells. *N Engl J Med* 1978;298:637–642.

Baldassarre S, Vincent JL. Coagulopathy induced by hydroxyethyl starch. *Anesth Analg* 1997;84:451–453.

Barnette RE, Shupak RC, Pontius J, Rao AK. In vitro effect of fresh frozen plasma on the activated coagulation time in patients undergoing cardiopulmonary bypass. *Anesth Analg* 1988;67:57–60.

Beyer R, Harmening U, Rittmeyer O, et al. Use of modified fluid elastin and hydroxyethyl starch for colloidal volume replacement in major orthopaedic surgery. *Br J Anaesth* 1997;78:44–50.

Bland JHL, Laver MB, Lowenstein E. Vasodilator effect of commercial 5% plasma protein fraction solutions. *JAMA* 1973;224:1721–1724.

Boldt J, Heesen M, Padbewrg W, et al. The influence of volume therapy and pentoxifylline infusion on circulating adhesion molecules in trauma patients. *Anaesthesia* 1996;51:529–535.

Boldt J. The good, the bad, the ugly: Should we completely banish human albumin from our intensive care units? *Anesth Analg* 2000;91:887–895.

Bove JR. Fresh frozen plasma: too few indications—too much use [editorial]. *Anesth Analg* 1985;64:849–850.

Casati V, Bellotti F, Gerli C, et al. Tranexamic acid administration after cardiac surgery; a prospective, randomized, double-blind, placebo-controlled study *Anesthesiology* 2001;94:8–14.

Cuignet OY, Wood BL, ChandLer WL, et al. A second-generation blood substitute (perfluorodichlorooctane emulsion) generates spurious elevations in platelet counts from automated hematology analyzers. *Anesth Analg* 2000;90:517–522.

Czer LS, Bateman TM, Gray RJ, et al. Treatment of severe platelet dysfunction and hemorrhage after cardiopulmonary bypass: reduction in blood product usage with desmopressin. *J Am Coll Cardiol* 1987;9:1139–1147.

D'Alauro F, Johns RA. Hypotension related to desmopressin administration following cardiopulmonary bypass. *Anesthesiology* 1988; 69:962–963.

Dieterich H-J, Kraft D, Cirtl, C, et al. Hydroxyethyl starch antibodies in humans: incidence and clinical relevance. *Anesth Analg* 1998;86: 1123–1126.

Dieterich H-J, Reutershan J, Felbinger TW, et al. Penetration of intravenous hydroxethyl starch into the cerebrospinal fluid in patients with impaired blood-brain barrier function. *Anesth Analg* 2003; 96:1150–1154.

Dietz NM, Joyner MJ, Warner MA. Blood substitutes: fluids, drugs, or miracle solutions? *Anesth Analg* 1996;82:390–405.

Donahue JG, Munoz A, Ness PM, et al. The declining risk of post-transfusion hepatitis C virus infection. *N Engl J Med* 1992;327:369–373.

Dowd NP, Karski JM, Cheng DC, et al. Pharmacokinetics of tranexamic acid during cardiopulmonary bypass. *Anesthesiology* 2002; 97:390–399.

Egli GA, Zollinger A, Seifert B, et al. Effect of progressive haemodilution with hydroxyethyl starch, gelatin and albumin on blood coagulation. *Br J Anaesth* 1997;78:684–689.

Ellison N. Diagnosis and management of bleeding disorders. *Anesthesiology* 1977;47:171–180.

Fanashawe MP, Shore-Lesserson L, Reich DL. Two cases of fatal thrombosis after aminocaproic acid therapy and deep hypothermic circulatory arrest. *Anesthesiology* 2001;95:1525–1527.

Fuerth JH, Mahrer P. Myocardial infarction after factor IX therapy. *JAMA* 1981;245:1455–1456.

Graham JD. Injuries from traffic crashes: meeting the challenge. *Annu Rev Public Health* 1993;14:515–543.

Hackmann T, Gascoyne RD, Naiman SC, et al. A trial of desmopressin (1-desamino-8-D-arginine vasopressin) to reduce blood loss in uncomplicated cardiac surgery. *N Engl J Med* 1989;321: 1437–1443.

Higby DJ, Burnett D. Granulocyte transfusions: current status. *Blood* 1980; 55:2–8.

Hoyer LW. Factor VIII complex: structure and function. *Blood* 1981; 58:1–13.

Isbister JP, Fisher MM. Adverse effects of plasma volume expanders. *Anaesth Intensive Care* 1980;8:145–151.

Jahr JS, Osgood S, Rothenberg SJ, et al. Lactate measurement interference by hemoglobin-based oxygen carriers (Oxyglobin®, Hemopure®, and Hemolink®). *Anesth Analg* 2005;100:431–436.

Jamnicki M, Bombeli T, Seifert B, et al. Low- and medium-molecular-weight hydroxyethyl starches. *Anesthesiology* 2000;93:1231–1237.

Jones JA. Red blood cell substitutes: current status. *Br J Anaesth* 1995; 74:697–703.

Kluger R, Olive DJ, Stewart AB, et al. Epsilon-aminocaproic acid in coronary artery bypass graft surgery: preincision or postheparin? *Anesthesiology* 2003;99:1263–1269.

Kruskall MS. The perils of platelet transfusions. *N Engl J Med* 1997; 337:1914–1915.

Kuitunen A, Hynynen M, Salmenpera M, et al. Hydroxyethyl starch as a prime for cardiopulmonary bypass: effects of two different solutions on hemostasis. *Acta Anaesthesiol Scand* 1993;37:652–658.

Kuitunen AH, Hynynen MK, Vahtera E, et al. Hydroxyethyl starch as a priming solution for cardiopulmonary bypass impairs hemostasis after cardiac surgery. *Anesth Analg* 2004;98:291–297.

Leese PT, Noveck RJ, Shorr JS, et al. Randomized safety studies of intravenous perflubron emulsion. 1. Effects on coagulation function in healthy volunteers. *Anesth Analg* 2000;91:804–811.

Mallett SV, Cox DJ. Thrombelastography. *Br J Anaesth* 1992;69:307–313.

Mangar D, Gerson JI, Baggish MS, et al. Serum levels of hyskon during hysteroscopic procedures. *Anesth Analg* 1991;73:186–189.

Mangar D, Gerson JI, Constantine RM, et al. Pulmonary edema and coagulopathy due to hyskon (32% dextran-70) administration. *Anesth Analg* 1989;68:686–687.

Milde LN. An anaphylactic reaction to fibrin glue. *Anesth Analg* 1989; 69:684–686.

Miller RD. Coagulation and packed red blood cell transfusions. *Anesth Analg* 1995;80:215–216.

Murray DJ, Olson J, Strauss R, et al. Coagulation changes during packed red cell replacement of major blood loss. *Anesthesiology* 1988;69:839–845.

Neff TA, Doelberg M, Jungheinrich C, et al. Repetitive large-dose infusion of the novel hydroxethyl starch 130/0.4 in patients with severe head injury. *Anesth Analg* 2003;96:1453–1459.

Neilipovitz DT, Murto K, Hall L, et al. A randomized trial of tranexamic acid to reduce blood transfusion for scoliosis surgery. *Anesth Analg* 2001;93:82–87.

Nuttall GA, Stehling LC, Beighley CM et al. Current transfusion practices of members of the American Society of Anesthesiologists. *Anesthesiology* 2003;99:1433–1443.

Pleym H, Senseth R, Wahba A, et al. Single-dose tranexamic acid reduces postoperative bleeding after coronary surgery in patients treated with aspirin until surgery. *Anesth Analg* 2003;96: 923–928.

Practice Guidelines Development Task Force of the College of American Pathologists. Practice parameter for use of fresh-frozen plasma, cryoprecipitate, and platelets. *JAMA* 1994;271:777–781.

Practice Guidelines for Blood Component Therapy. *Anesthesiology* 1996;84:732–746.

Prince AM. Use of hepatitis B immune globulin: reassessment needed. *N Engl J Med* 1978;299:198–199.

Rahilly GT, Berl T. Severe metabolic alkalosis caused by administration of plasma protein fraction in end-stage renal failure. *N Engl J Med* 1979; 301:824–826.

Rebulla P, Finazzi G, Marangoni F, et al. The threshold for prophylactic platelet transfusions in adults with acute myeloid leukemia. *N Engl J Med* 1997;337:1870–1875.

Roberts HR, Monroe DM, Esacobar MA. Current concepts of hemostasis. Implications for therapy. *Anesthesiology* 2004;100:722–730.

Rogers RP, Levin J. A critical reappraisal of the bleeding time. *Semin Thromb Hemost* 1990;16:1–20.

Salzman EW, Weinstein MJ, Weintraub RM, et al. Treatment with desmopressin acetate to reduce blood loss after cardiac surgery: a double-blind randomized trial. *N Engl J Med* 1986;314: 1402–1406.

Stratford N. Antioxidant potential of i.v. fluids. *Br J Anaesth* 1997;78: 757–759.

Steinbauer M, Harris AG, Leiderer R, et al. Impact of dextran on microvascular disturbances and tissue injury following ischemia/ reperfusion in striated muscle. *Shock* 1998;9: 345–351.

Szeimies RM, Stolz W, Wlotzke U, et al. Successful treatment of hydroxyethyl starch-induced pruritus with topical capsaicin. *Br J Dermatol* 1994;131:380–382.

The SAFE Study Investigators. A comparison of albumin and saline for fluid resuscitation in the intensive care unit. *N Engl J Med* 2004; 350:2247–2256.

Tremper KK. Perfluorochemical "blood substitutes" Indications for an oxygen-carrying colloid. *Anesthesiology* 1999;91:1185–1187.

Wallace EL, Surgenor DM, Hao HS, et al. Collection and transfusion of blood and blood components in the United States, 1989. *Transfusion* 1993;33:139–144.

Warren BB, Durieux ME. Hydroxyethyl starch: safe or not? *Anesth Analg* 1997;84:206–212.

Wilkes NJ, Woolf RL, Popwanda MC, et al. Hydroxyethyl starch in balanced electrolyte solution (Hextend®)-pharmacokinetic and pharmacodynamic profiles in healthy volunteers. *Anesth Analg* 2002;94:538–544.

Winslow RM. Blood substitutes. *Adv Drug Deliv Rev* 2000;40:131–142.

Wright DG, Robichaud KJ, Rizzo PA, et al. Lethal pulmonary reactions associated with combined use of amphotericin B and leukocyte transfusion. *N Engl J Med* 1981;304:1185–1189.

Enteral and Parenteral Nutrition

37

Enteral nutrition is defined as providing nourishment to a patient utilizing a liquid diet of specific composition that is delivered directly into the gastrointestinal tract (nasogastric tube, nasointestinal tube, gastrostomy tube, jejunostomy tube). Parenteral nutrition is defined as delivery of nutrients directly into the venous circulation (peripheral vein, central vein). Total parenteral nutrition (TPN) is being utilized when the only source of nutrient supply is via the parenteral route. Nutritional support is characterized as the use of enteral or parenteral nutrition rather than an oral diet. TPN should be continued during the perioperative period, whereas enteral nutrition should be discontinued about 6 hours before surgery (reflecting recommendations for food ingestion prior to elective surgery) and a glucose infusion initiated to minimize the risk of hypoglycemia.

HYPERALIMENTATION

Hyperalimentation is intended to supply all the essential inorganic and organic nutritional elements necessary to maintain optimal body composition as well as positive nitrogen balance. Alimentation by the gastrointestinal tract (enteral nutrition) is preferred to intravenous (IV) alimentation (parenteral nutrition) because it avoids catheter-induced sepsis, maintains gut integrity by providing luminal nutrients (especially glutamine) and thus lessening the translocation of bacteria from the gastrointestinal tract, and maintains the absorptive activity of the small intestine (Braunschweig et al., 2001). Indeed, the route of feeding is more important than the amount of nutrition provided, and the outcome correlates with the enteral protein intake in injured patients. Thus, even if the patient's caloric and nitrogen requirements cannot be met with luminal nutrition, the enteral route of feeding should be used unless it is contraindicated (bowel obstruction, inadequate bowel surface area, intractable diarrhea). The enteral and parenteral routes may be used simultaneously to meet nutritional requirements.

Most patients do not need nutritional support, and clear-cut benefits of this expensive intervention have been established for only a select group of patients (Table 37-1) (Souba, 1997). For example, data suggest that preoperative nutritional support should be reserved for malnourished patients undergoing major elective surgery. Patients not expected to resume adequate oral feedings within 7 to 10 days of surgery should begin nutritional support within 2 to 4 days postoperatively. Elderly patients, especially those with weight loss, may benefit from nutritional supplementation during their hospitalization. Although the benefits of parenteral nutrition in the perioperative period are controversial, randomized trials of postoperative enteral feeding have shown decreased complication rates in malnourished patients although mortality rates are unchanged (Heyland et al., 1998; Lewis et. al., 2001).

Nutritional support can improve outcome in bone marrow transplant patients (Weisdorf et al., 1987). Likewise, severely injured patients, burn patients, and those with sepsis often are hypermetabolic, so aggressive early nutritional support is beneficial. For example, energy requirements may double and protein requirements may triple in severely burned patients. Conversely, the increase in basal metabolic rate that occurs during and soon after major uncomplicated elective surgery is $<10\%$, so that providing glucose solutions (approximately 500 kcal/day) in the postoperative period is sufficient, and further nutritional support does not improve outcome.

Critically ill patients metabolize glucose at decreased rates, so the exogenous glucose load should not exceed approximately 500 g/day. Minimally stressed patients require about 25 to 30 cal/kg and 1 g/kg of protein daily to remain in nitrogen and energy equilibrium. Mildly catabolic patients usually gain weight with a daily provision of 35 to 45 cal/kg, whereas patients in severe catabolic states

TABLE 37-1.
ESTABLISHED INDICATIONS FOR USE OF NUTRITIONAL SUPPORT

Major elective surgery in severely malnourished patients
Major trauma (blunt or penetrating injury, head injury)
Burns
Hepatic dysfunction
Renal dysfunction
Bone marrow transplant recipients undergoing intensive chemotherapy
Patients unable to eat or absorb nutrients for an indefinite period (neurologic impairment, or pharyngeal dysfunction, short bowel syndrome)
Well-nourished, minimally stressed patients unable to eat for 7 to 10 days

Source: Adapted from Souba WW. Nutritional support. *N Engl J Med* 1997;336:41–48.

may require up to 80 cal/kg daily. Adequate caloric intake is essential for efficient use of amino acids. Lipid calories from infusions of propofol may be significant and should be included when calculating caloric intake (Lowrey et al., 1996).

ENTERAL NUTRITION

A variety of enteral solutions containing various amounts of protein (amino acids), carbohydrates (glucose), fat micronutrients, and electrolytes are available. No single formulation has been found to be ideal for all patients (Souba, 1997). Carbohydrates are the source of up to 90% of the calories, emphasizing the increased osmolarity of these solutions. Fat has a higher caloric density than carbohydrates, does not increase the osmolarity of the formula as much as carbohydrates, and improves palatability. The amount of fat in enteral solutions varies. Unless the patient has maldigestion or malabsorption of fat, formulas with a normal range of fat content are preferred. In patients with hepatic cirrhosis or portocaval shunts, excessive plasma concentrations of fatty acids may act synergistically with high levels of ammonia and other toxins to exacerbate or cause hepatic encephalopathy. Selection of a formula that provides sufficient total nitrogen as protein or amino acids is essential for all patients. Low-protein formulations, however, are indicated for patients with severe renal dysfunction. Specialized crystalline amino acid supplements are available for nutritional deficiencies associated with liver or renal disease. Increased amounts of protein or amino acids are indicated when the nitrogen requirement is increased, as in patients with trauma, burns, or sepsis. The efficient use of amino acids for tissue synthesis depends on adequate caloric intake. Addition of glutamine to parenteral nutrition solutions results in an improvement in nitrogen balance and gastrointestinal barrier function, a decrease in infections, and a reduction in the number of days of mechanical ventilation (Byrne et al., 1995).

Enteral Tube Feeding

Enteral tube feeding may be necessary when patients are unable to consume nutritionally complete, liquefied food orally. Commercial formulations of natural foods can be so finely suspended that they pass through small-bore tubes. Defined-formula diets are necessary when luminal hydrolysis or absorption is impaired, as in malabsorption syndromes. An important consideration when utilizing enteral nutrition is placement and positioning of the small bore (8 to 12 French) silastic delivery tube. Most often patients receive continuous infusions of enteral nutrition through a nasoenteric tube positioned in the stomach, duodenum, or jejunum. Dislodgement of the tip especially in the presence of gastroparesis can result in pulmonary aspiration. In patients likely to have gastroparesis (critically ill patients), it is common to place the tip of the feeding tube distal to the ligament of Treitz in an effort to prevent pooling of fluids in the stomach with the attendant risk of pulmonary aspiration. Nevertheless, it is not confirmed that jejunal feeding decreases the risk of pulmonary aspiration (Esparza et al., 2001). In addition, long-term use of nasoenteric tubes may result in sinusitis and otitis media.

Surgical placement of an esophagostomy or gastrostomy tube may be indicated for long-term feeding. For slow-drip feeding, an automated infusion pump to control the rate of administration is useful. Indeed, absorption and tolerance are improved and the incidence of side effects is decreased by slow, constant feeding over several hours. The rate of infusion is typically 100 to 120 mL/hour. This slow rate of infusion prevents the dumping syndrome, which may occur when hyperosmolar solutions are introduced rapidly into the small intestine.

Side Effects

Gastric retention, diarrhea, and abdominal distension can limit patient acceptance of enteral feeding. Hypovolemia due to osmotic diuresis induced by glycosuria may occur. These side effects are most likely related to osmolar load and can be decreased by slowing the rate of administration. Hyperosmolar dehydration progressing to nonketotic coma results from administration of a high glucose load. Caution is necessary if enteral nutrition is administered to patients prone to developing hyperglycemia (diabetics, treatment with glucocorticoids or adrenergic drugs). Cutaneous rashes that occur after prolonged enteral nutrition are thought to be caused by fatty acid deficiency.

Pulmonary aspiration is always a danger when enteral tube feeding is used. Patients should be maintained in a semi-sitting position (head of bed elevated 30 degrees) during feeding and for 1 hour after feeding. Preparations

TABLE 37-2.
CONTENTS OF VARIOUS CRYSTALLOID SOLUTIONS

	Glucose (mg/dl)	Sodium (mEq/L)	Chloride (mEq/L)	Potassium (mEq/L)	Magnesium (mEq/L)	Calcium (mEq/L)	Lactate (mEq/L)	pH	Osmolarity (mOsm/L)
5% glucose in water	5,000	0	0	0	0	0	0	5.0	253
5% glucose in 0.45% sodium chloride	5,000	77	77	0	0	0	0	4.2	407
5% glucose in 0.9% sodium chloride	0	154	154	0	0	0	0	4.2	561
0.9% sodium chloride	0	154	154	0	0	0	0	5.7	308
Lactated Ringer's solution	0	130	109	4	0	3	28	6.7	273
5% glucose in lactated Ringer's solution	5,000	130	109	4	0	3	28	5.3	527
Normosol-R	0	140	98	5	3	0	*	7.4	295

*Contains 27 mEq/liter of acetate and 23 mEq/liter of gluconate.

containing large amounts of electrolytes should be administered cautiously to patients with cardiovascular, renal, or hepatic disease. Many commercial formulas contain large amounts of sodium. Dry preparations mixed with water become excellent culture media unless they are kept sterile and refrigerated.

PARENTERAL NUTRITION

Parenteral nutrition is indicated for patients who are unable to ingest or digest nutrients or to absorb them from the gastrointestinal tract. Parenteral nutrition using isotonic solutions delivered through a peripheral vein is acceptable when the patient requires <2,000 calories daily and the anticipated need for nutritional support is brief. Peripheral veins do not tolerate infusion of solutions with an osmolarity that exceeds 750 mOsm/L (equivalent to 12.5% glucose) thus limiting the number of calories that can be administered. When nutritional requirements are >2,000 calories daily or prolonged nutritional support is required, a catheter is placed in the central venous system to permit infusion of a hypertonic (1,900 mOsm/L) nutrition solution.

Short-Term Parenteral Therapy

Short-term parenteral therapy (3 to 5 days in patients without nutritional deficits) after uncomplicated surgical procedures is most often provided by hypocaloric, nonnitrogen glucose-electrolyte solutions. For example, glucose solutions, 5% to 10%, with supplemental sodium, chloride, and other electrolytes are commonly administered for short-term therapy (Table 37-2). These solutions provide total fluid and electrolyte needs and sufficient calories to decrease protein catabolism and prevent ketosis. For example, daily infusion of approximately 150 g of glucose maintains brain and erythrocyte metabolism and decreases protein catabolism from skeletal muscles and viscera.

Amino acids may have a greater protein-sparing effect than glucose, but amino acids without glucose do not prevent negative nitrogen balance completely after major surgery. The higher cost of amino acid solutions relative to potential benefit has prevented their popularity for use in place of glucose for short-term therapy.

Peripheral infusion of fat emulsions may be administered as a nonprotein source of calories to augment those supplied by glucose. Thrombosis of the peripheral vein used for infusion of the fat emulsion is a potential complication.

Long-Term (Total) Parenteral Nutrition

Total parenteral nutrition (IV hyperalimentation) is the technique of providing total nutrition needs by infusion of amino acids combined with glucose and varying amounts of fat emulsion. Lean body mass is preserved, wound healing may be enhanced, and there may even be improvement of an impaired immune response mechanism.

Total parenteral nutrition solutions contain a large proportion of calories from glucose and thus are hypertonic.

For this reason, these solutions must be infused into a central vein with a high blood flow to provide rapid dilution. A catheter is often placed percutaneously into the subclavian vein and guided into the right atrium. The parenteral nutrition solution may be infused continuously or intermittently over a 12- to 16-hour period. When intermittent administration is used, the infusion must be decreased gradually during the 60 to 90 minutes preceding discontinuation to avoid hypoglycemia. The daily volume of infusion is about 40 mL/kg.

The efficacy of nutritional support is reflected by body weight measurements that confirm a maintenance or increase of lean body mass. Daily weight gains of >0.5 kg, however, may signify fluid retention. Serum electrolytes, blood glucose concentrations, and blood urea nitrogen should be measured periodically during total parenteral nutrition. Tests of hepatic and renal function are also recommended but can be performed at less frequent intervals.

Side Effects

The side effects of total parenteral nutrition are numerous and include an increased incidence of pneumonia, catheter-related sepsis, and metabolic abnormalities resulting from the administered nutrients (Table 37-3) (Michel et al., 1981; Souba, 1997). Pneumothorax may occur as a complication of placement of a central venous catheter while thrombophlebitis is a risk of peripheral venous catheter placement.

Sepsis

Total parenteral nutrition solutions infused through an IV catheter can support the growth of bacteria and fungi. Indeed, infection at the infusion site, as well as systemic infection, is a serious side effect of parenteral nutrition therapy.

A spiking temperature most likely reflects contamination via the delivery system or catheter. The catheter should be removed and the tip cultured to determine the appropriate antibiotic therapy. In view of the hazard of contamination, the use of a central venous hyperalimentation catheter for administration of medications, as during the perioperative period, or for sampling of blood, is not recommended.

Fatty Acid Deficiency

Fatty acid deficiency may develop during prolonged total parenteral nutrition. Exogenous lipids (lipid emulsions) are necessary to prevent free fatty acid deficiency during TPN. Possible immunosuppressive effects of lipid emulsions and an increased incidence of infections has led to recommendations to limit fat calories to about 30% of total TPN calories (Chan et al., 1999).

Hyperglycemia

Blood glucose concentrations should be monitored until glucose tolerance is demonstrated, which usually occurs after 2 to 3 days of therapy as endogenous insulin production increases. In addition, blood glucose concentrations should be periodically monitored during the perioperative period. The degree of hyperglycemia accompanying TPN is directly related to the rate of glucose infusion, and elderly patients seem more vulnerable to this complication (Watters et al., 1996). Persistent hyperglycemia (may require insulin therapy) can lead to osmotic diuresis with resulting hypovolemia. Nonketotic hyperosmolar hyperglycemic coma is a potential complication of total parenteral nutrition solutions.

Hypoglycemia

Accidental, sudden discontinuation of the infusion of total parenteral nutrition solutions containing large amounts of glucose (catheter kink or disconnection) may cause hypoglycemia. Indeed, TPN infusion should be discontinued gradually over 60 to 90 minutes. Hypoglycemia occurs because the pancreatic insulin response does not always cease in parallel with discontinuation of the parenteral nutrition solution. As a result, a high plasma concentration of insulin may persist in the absence of continued infusion of glucose. If administration of the total parenteral nutrition solution must be stopped abruptly, exogenous glucose should be infused for up to 90 minutes to prevent hypoglycemia. The incidence of hypoglycemia has decreased with the use of total parenteral nutrition solutions containing lower glucose to lipid ratios (50:50) (Nirula et al., 2002).

Hepatobiliary Complications

Large glucose loads may be associated with hepatic steatosis and steatohepatitis. Intrahepatic cholestasis with increased alkaline phosphatase and serum bilirubin concentrations may occur when total parenteral nutrition duration exceeds 3 to 6 weeks. Large lipid loads may result in cholestasis.

TABLE 37-3.
SIDE EFFECTS ASSOCIATED WITH TOTAL PARENTERAL NUTRITION

Sepsis
Pneumonia
Fatty acid deficiency
Hyperglycemia
Nonketotic hyperosmolar hyperglycemic coma
Hypoglycemia
Hepatobiliary complications
Metabolic acidosis
Hypercarbia
Fluid overload
Renal dysfunction
Hepatic dysfunction
Thrombosis of central veins

Metabolic Acidosis

Hyperchloremic metabolic acidosis may occur because of the liberation of hydrochloric acid during the metabolism of amino acids in the parenteral nutrition solution. A decrease in the plasma bicarbonate concentration suggests the presence of metabolic acidosis.

Hypercarbia

Increased production of carbon dioxide resulting from the metabolism of large quantities of glucose may result in the need to initiate artificial ventilation of the patient's lungs or in failure to successfully wean the patient from long-term mechanical ventilation support (Askanazi et al., 1981).

Monitoring During Total Parenteral Nutrition

Acutely ill patients receiving TPN must be followed closely for the development of treatment-related complications. It is important to quantify the actual caloric intake, as it is unlikely that all caloric needs can be met with only the enteral route. Access sites are observed for signs of infection. Substitution of sodium or potassium acetate (metabolized to bicarbonate) for sodium or potassium chloride may be helpful should signs of metabolic acidosis appear. Plasma triglyceride concentrations may increase in patients with diabetes mellitus, sepsis, and impaired hepatic or renal function. Additional vitamin K may be indicated based on measurement of prothrombin and plasma thromboplastin times. Increases in aminotransferases and alkaline phosphatase suggest the development of hepatic steatosis. Careful maintenance of fluid intake and output is needed as critically ill patients often experience significant fluid shifts.

Preparation of Total Parenteral Nutrition Solutions

TPN solutions are prepared from commercially available solutions by mixing hypertonic glucose with an amino acid solution. Sodium, potassium, phosphorus, calcium, magnesium, and chloride are added to TPN solutions. Trace elements including zinc, copper, manganese, and chromium must also be added if the need for parenteral therapy is prolonged. Requirements for vitamins may be increased, emphasizing the need to add a multivitamin preparation to TPN solutions. Vitamin B_{12} and folic acid may be administered as components of a multivitamin preparation or separately. Vitamin D should be used sparingly because metabolic bone diseases may be associated with use of this vitamin in some patients on long-term parenteral nutrition. Vitamin K is administered separately once every week. The serum albumin concentration will usually increase in patients receiving TPN if adequate amino acids and calories are provided. Therefore, the routine administration of supplemental albumin is not necessary in the absence of signs or symptoms of hypoalbuminemia.

Fat emulsions are not mixed with the TPN solutions. Instead, these isotonic emulsions are administered IV through a separate peripheral vein or by a Y-connector into the same vein. Drugs should not be added to TPN solutions unless compatibility has been determined. To decrease the possibility of bacterial contamination, TPN solutions are prepared aseptically under a laminar air-flow hood, refrigerated, and administered within 24 to 48 hours.

Immunonutrition

Cellular immunity decreases during acute stress as may accompany multiple organ system failure, sepsis, and shock. Immunonutrition is an attempt to enhance immunity and cellular integrity by incorporating specific additives (omega-3 fatty acids, arginine to enhance lymphocyte cytotoxicity, purine as a precursor of RNA and DNA) into enteral diets. A risk of immunonutrition may be an enhanced inflammatory response especially in critically ill patients whereas less severely stressed postoperative patients may benefit from immunonutrition (Beale et al., 2000).

REFERENCES

Askanazi J, Nordenstrom J, Rosenbaum SH, et al. Nutrition for the patient with respiratory failure: glucose vs. fat. *Anesthesiology* 1981; 54:373–377.

Beale RJ, Bryd DJ, Bihari DJ. Immunonutrition in the critically ill: a systematic review of clinical outcome. *Crit Care Med* 1999;27: 2799–2805.

Braunschweig CL, Levy P, Sheean PM, et al. Enteral compared with parenteral nutrition: a meta-analysis. *Am J. Clin Nutr* 2001;74:534–539.

Byrne TA, Persinger RL, Young LS, et al. A new treatment for patients with short-bowel syndrome: growth hormone, glutamine, and modified diet. *Ann Surg* 1995;222:243–255.

Chan S, McCowen KC, Blackburn GL. Nutritional management in the ICU. *Chest* 1999;115:145S–148S.

Esparza J, Boivin MA, Hartshorne MF, et al. Equal aspiration rates in gastrically and transpylorically fed critically ill patients. *Intensive Care Med* 2001;27:660–604.

Heyland DK, Macdonald S, Keele L et al. Total parenteral nutrition in the critically ill patient. *JAMA* 1998;5:175–176.

Lewis SJ, Egger M, Sylvester PA, et al. Early enteral feeding versus "nil by mouth" after gastrointestinal surgery: systematic review and meta-analysis of controlled trials. *BMJ* 2001;323:771–777.

Lowrey TS, Dunlap AW, Brown RO, et al. Pharmacologic influence on nutrition support therapy: use of propofol in a patient receiving combined enteral and parenteral nutrition support. *Nutr Clin Pact* 1996;11:147–149.

Michel L, Serrano A, Malt RA. Nutritional support of hospitalized patients. *N Engle J Med* 1981;304:1147–1152.

Nirula R, Yamada K, Waxman K. The effect of abrupt cessation of total parenteral nutrition on serum glucose: a randomized trial. *Am Surg* 2002;66:866–869.

Souba WW. Nutritional support. *N Engle J Med* 1997;336:41–48.

Watters JM, Kirkpatrick SM, Hipbath D, et al. Aging exaggerates the blood glucose response to total parenteral nutrition. *Can J Surg* 1996;39:481–485.

Weisdorf SA, Lysine J, Wind D, et al. Positive effect of prophylactic total parenteral nutrition on long-term outcome of bone marrow transplantation. *Transplantation* 1987;43:833–838.

Antiseptics and Disinfectants

38

Antiseptics and disinfectants are of obvious importance in the preoperative preparation of the patient and surgeon. Substances that are applied topically to living tissues to kill or prevent the growth of microorganisms are antiseptics. A disinfectant is an agent that is applied topically to an inanimate object to destroy pathogenic microorganisms and thus prevent transmission of infection. Antiseptics most often used include (a) ethyl and isopropyl alcohols, (b) cationic surface-active quaternary ammonium compounds, (c) the biguanide chlorhexidine, (d) iodine compounds, and (e) hexachlorophene. Disinfectants most often used are (a) the aldehydes—formaldehyde and glutaraldehyde, (b) the phenolic compound cresol, and (c) elemental chlorine.

Sterilization is the complete and total destruction of all microbial life, including vegetative bacteria, spores, fungi, and viruses. Ethylene oxide is the only chemical available that is approved for sterilization of objects that cannot be heated or sterilized by other physical methods such as radiation.

ALCOHOLS

Alcohols are applied topically to decrease local cutaneous bacterial flora (immediate antisepsis and quick drying) before penetration of the skin with needles. Their antiseptic action can be enhanced by prior mechanical cleansing of the skin with water and a detergent and gentle rubbing with sterile gauze during application.

Ethyl alcohol is an antiseptic of low potency but moderate efficacy, being bactericidal to many bacteria. On the skin, 70% ethyl alcohol kills nearly 90% of the cutaneous bacteria within 2 minutes, provided the area is kept moist. Greater than a 75% decrease in cutaneous bacterial count is unlikely with a single wipe of an ethyl alcohol–wetted sponge followed by evaporation of the residual solution. Isopropyl alcohol has a slightly greater bactericidal activity than ethyl alcohol due to its greater depression of surface tension. Neither of the alcohols, however, is fungicidal or virucidal.

Fire Risks

It is important to recognize that alcohol-based preps are flammable until all the liquid has evaporated (Barker and Polson, 2001; ECRI Hazard Report, 2003). Alcohol-based surgical prep solutions can create a fire hazard (flash fire) especially if the prep solution is allowed to pool (umbilicus) or the patient is draped before the prep is completely dry resulting in trapped alcohol vapors being channeled to the surgical site where a heat source may be used. Sterile towels may be used to absorb excess prep solution.

QUATERNARY AMMONIUM COMPOUNDS

Quaternary ammonium compounds are bactericidal in vitro to a wide variety of Gram-positive and Gram-negative bacteria. Many fungi and viruses are also susceptible. *Mycobacterium tuberculosis*, however, is relatively resistant. Alcohol enhances the germicidal activity of quaternary ammonium compounds so that tinctures are more effective than aqueous solutions.

The major site of action of quaternary ammonium compounds appears to be the cell membrane, where these solutions cause a change in permeability.

Benzalkonium and cetylpyridinium (mouthwash) are examples of quaternary ammonium compounds. These compounds may be used preoperatively to decrease the number of microorganisms on intact skin. There is a rapid onset of action, but the availability of more efficacious solutions has decreased their frequency of use. Quaternary ammonium compounds have been widely used for the sterilization of instruments. Endoscopes and other instruments

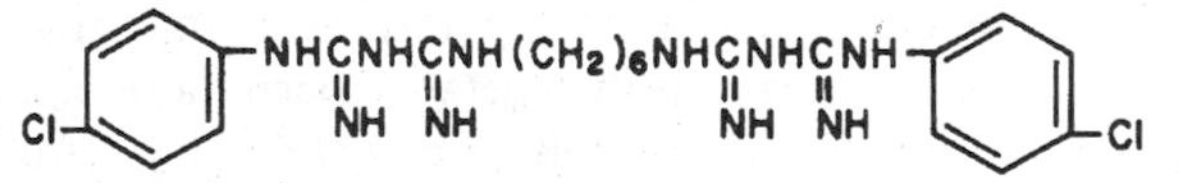

Figure 38-1. Chlorhexidine.

made of polyethylene or polypropylene, however, absorb quaternary ammonium compounds, which may decrease the concentration of the active ingredient to below a bactericidal concentration.

CHLORHEXIDINE

Chlorhexidine (Hibiclens®) is a colorless chlorophenol biguanide solution that disrupts cell membranes of the bacterial cells and is effective against both Gram-positive and Gram-negative bacteria (Fig. 38-1). It persists on the skin to provide continued antibacterial protection. As a hand wash or surgical scrub, 2% chlorhexidine causes a greater initial decrease in the number of normal cutaneous bacteria than does povidone-iodine or hexachlorophene, and it has a persistent effect equal to or greater than that of hexachlorophene. 2% chlorhexidine is superior to povidone iodine for skin preparation and and prevention of catheter-related blood stream infections due to placement of invasive intravascular catheters (Chaiyakunapruk et al, 2002). A chlorhexidine-impregnated split dressing may reduce colonization of epidural catheters (Kinirons et al. 2001). Chlorhexidine is mainly used for the preoperative cutaneous preparation of the surgeon and patient. It is also used to treat superficial infections caused by Gram-positive bacteria and to disinfect wounds. As an antiseptic, chlorhexidine is rapid acting, has considerable residual adherence to the skin, has a low potential for producing contact sensitivity and photosensitivity, and is poorly absorbed even after many daily hand washings. Chlorhexidine solutions in an alcohol base are not appropriate for instillation into the eye (corneal injury) or middle ear (deafness).

IODINE

Iodine is a rapid-acting antiseptic that, in the absence of organic material, kills bacteria, viruses, and spores. For example, on the skin, 1% tincture of iodine will kill 90% of the bacteria in 90 seconds, whereas a 5% solution achieves this response in 60 seconds. In the presence of organic matter, some iodine is bound covalently, diminishing the immediate but not eventual effect. Nevertheless, commercial preparations contain iodine in such excess that organic matter usually does not adversely influence immediate efficacy. The local toxicity of iodine is low, with cutaneous burns occurring only with concentrations of >7%. In rare instances, an individual may be allergic to iodine and react to topical application. An allergic reaction usually manifests as fever and generalized skin eruption.

The most important use of iodine is disinfection of the skin, for which it is probably superior to any other antiseptic. For this use, it is best used in the form of a tincture of iodine because the alcohol vehicle facilitates spreading and penetration. Iodine may also be used in the treatment of wounds and abrasions. Applied to abraded tissue, 0.5% to 1.0% iodine aqueous solutions are less irritating than the tinctures.

Iodophors

An iodophor is a loose complex of elemental iodine with an organic carrier that not only increases the solubility of iodine but also provides a reservoir for sustained release. The most widely used iodophor is povidone-iodine, in which the carrier molecule is polyvinylpyrrolidone. A 10% solution contains 1% available iodine, but the free iodine concentration is <1 ppm. This is sufficiently low that little, if any, staining of the skin occurs. Because of the low concentrations, the immediate bactericidal action is only moderate compared with that of iodine solutions.

Clinical Uses

The iodophors have a broad antimicrobial spectrum and are widely used as hand washes, including surgical scrubs; preparation of the skin before surgery or needle puncture; and treatment of minor cuts, abrasions, and burns. A standard surgical scrub with 10% povidone-iodine solutions (Betadine®) will decrease the usual cutaneous bacterial population by >90%, with a return to normal in about 6 to 8 hours. Compared with with povodine-iodine, a disinfectant which contains an iodophor in isopropyl alcohol (DuraPrep®) is more effective than povidone-iodine in decreasing the number of positive skin cultures immediately after disinfection as well as in bacterial regrowth and colonization of epidural catheters (Birnbach et al, 2003).

As vaginal disinfectants, iodophors may be absorbed, introducing the risk of fetal hypothyroidism if used in a parturient (Vorherr et al., 1980). For the disinfection of endoscopes and other instruments, povidone-iodine is superior to 3% hexachlorophene.

Corneal Toxicity

Chemical burns to the cornea may follow exposure (accidental splashes) to a variety of disinfectant solutions (chlorhexidine, hexachlorophene, iodine, alcohol, detergents containing iodine-based solutions). Povidone iodine solution without detergent appears to be least toxic to the cornea (Rae et al, 1984).

HEXACHLOROPHENE

Hexachlorophene (pHisoHex®) is a polychlorinated bisphenol that exhibits bacteriostatic activity against Gram-positive but not Gram-negative organisms (Fig. 38-2). Immediately

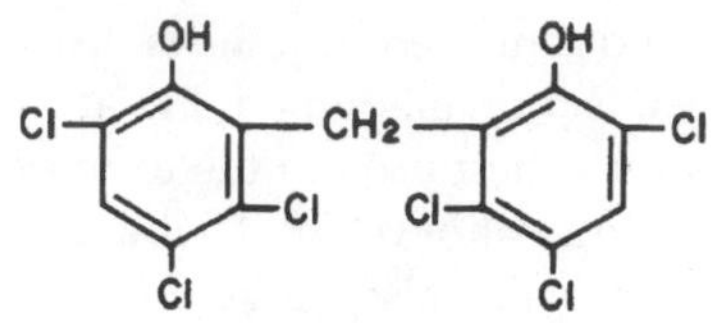

Figure 38-2. Hexachlorophene.

after a hand scrub with hexachlorophene, the cutaneous bacterial population may be decreased by only 30% to 50% compared with >90% following use of an iodophor. Nevertheless, 60 minutes later, the bacterial population surviving a hexachlorophene scrub will have decreased further to about 4%, whereas with the iodophor scrub, the bacterial population will have recovered to about 16% of normal.

Because most of the potentially pathogenic bacteria on the skin are Gram-positive, 3% hexachlorophene is commonly used by physicians and nurses to decrease the spread of contaminants from caregiver's hands. This antiseptic is also used to cleanse the skin of patients scheduled for certain surgical procedures. Hexachlorophene may be absorbed through intact skin in sufficient amounts to produce neurotoxic effects, including cerebral irritability. Thus, the routine use of hexachlorophene by health care providers who are pregnant may be questionable.

FORMALDEHYDE

Formaldehyde is a volatile, wide-spectrum disinfectant that kills bacteria, fungi, and viruses by precipitating proteins. A 0.5% concentration requires 6 to 12 hours to kill bacteria and 2 to 4 days to kill spores. A 2% to 8% concentration is used to disinfect inanimate objects such as surgical instruments.

GLUTARALDEHYDE

Glutaraldehyde is superior to formaldehyde as a disinfectant because it is rapidly effective against all microorganisms, including viruses and spores. This disinfectant also possesses tuberculocidal activity. Glutaraldehyde is less volatile than formaldehyde and hence causes minimal odor and irritant fumes. A period of 10 hours is necessary to sterilize dried spores, whereas an acid-stabilized solution kills dried spores in 20 minutes. Neither alkaline nor acidic solutions are damaging to most surgical instruments and endoscopes. As a sterilizing solution for endoscopes, glutaraldehyde is superior to iodophors and hexachlorophene.

PASTEURIZATION

Pasteurization (hot water disinfection) is a process that destroys microorganisms in a liquid medium by application of heat. Pasteurizing water temperatures in the range of 55° to 75°C will destroy all vegetative bacteria of significance in human disease, as well as many fungi and viruses. Pasteurization kills bacteria by coagulating cell proteins, and water acts as a very effective medium for transferring the heat required to destroy organisms. This is the rationale for maximizing direct water contact with surfaces to be disinfected. Water temperatures of >75°C may cause some plastic parts to deform. Equipment (respiratory therapy breathing circuits, anesthesia breathing circuits) should be submerged in water at 68°C for a minimum of 30 minutes. With respect to breathing circuits, pasteurization is effective against Gram-negative rods, *M. tuberculosis*, and most fungi and viruses. Pasteurization may be a cost-effective alternative to other disinfecting solutions such as glutaraldehyde.

CRESOL

Cresol is bactericidal against common pathogenic organisms including *M. tuberculosis*. It is widely used for disinfecting inanimate objects. Cresol should not be used to disinfect materials that can absorb this solution because burns could result from subsequent tissue contact.

SILVER NITRATE

Silver nitrate is used as a caustic, antiseptic, and astringent. A solid form is used for cauterizing wounds and removing granulation tissue. It is conveniently dispensed in pencils that should be moistened before use. Solutions of silver nitrate are strongly bactericidal, especially for gonococci, accounting for its frequent use as prophylaxis for ophthalmia neonatorum.

Silver sulfadiazine or nitrate is used in the treatment of burns. With this use, hypochloremia may occur, reflecting the combination of silver ions with chloride. Hyponatremia also may result because the sodium ions are attracted by chloride ions into the exudate. Furthermore, absorbed nitrate can cause methemoglobinemia.

MERCURY

Organic mercurial compounds are nonirritating but lack bactericidal activity. In fact, these compounds possess only weak bacteriostatic activity and are less effective than ethyl alcohol. Serum and tissue proteins decrease antimicrobial activity, and skin sensitization is common.

ETHYLENE OXIDE

Ethylene oxide is a readily diffusible gas that is noncorrosive and antimicrobial to all organisms at room temperature. This gaseous alkylating material is widely used as an alternative to heat sterilization. It reacts with chloride and water to produce two additional active germicides, ethylene chlorohydrin and ethylene glycol. Special sterilizing chambers are required because the gas must remain in contact with the objects for several hours. Adequate airing of sterilized materials, such as tracheal tubes, is essential to ensure removal of residual ethylene oxide and thus minimize tissue irritation. Ethylene oxide sensitization has been described in children with spina bifida experiencing preoperative anaphylactic reactions, always in association with latex sensitization (Porri et al., 1997).

REFERENCES

Barker SJ, Polson JS. Fire in the operating room: a case report and laboratory study. *Anesth Analg* 2001;93:960–965.

Birnbach DJ, Meadows W, Stein DJ, et al. Comparison of povidone iodine and DuraPrep, an iodophor-in-isopropyl alcohol solution, for skin disinfection prior to epidural catheter insertion in parturients. *Anesthesiology* 2003;98:164–169.

Chaiyakunapruk N, Veenstra DL, Lipsky, BA et al. Chlorhexidine compared with povidone-iodine solutions for vascular catheter-site care: a meta-analysis. *Ann Intern Med* 2002;136:792–801.

ECRI Hazard Report, Improper use of alcohol-based skin preps can cause surgical fires. *Health Devices* 2003;32:441–443.

Kinirons B, Mimoz O, Lafendi L, et al. Chlorhexidine versus povidone iodine in preventing colonization of continuous epidural catheters in children. *Anesthesiology* 2001;94:239–244.

Porri F, Pradal M, Lemiere C, et al. Association between latex sensitization and repeated latex exposure in children. *Anesthesiology* 1997; 86:599–602.

Rae SCC, Brown B, Edelhauser HF. The corneal toxicity of presurgical skin antiseptics. *Am J Ophthalmol* 1984;97:221–232.

Stetson JB, Whitbourne BS, Eastman C. Ethylene oxide degassing of rubber and plastic materials. *Anesthesiology* 1976;44:174–180.

Vorherr H, Vorherr UF, Mehta P, Ulrich JA, Messer RH. Vaginal absorption of povidone-iodine. *JAMA* 1980;244:2628–2629.

Physiology

II

Cell Structure and Function

39

The basic living unit of the body is the cell. It is estimated that the entire body consists of 100 trillion or more cells, of which 25 trillion are red blood cells (Guyton and Hall, 2000). Each organ is a mass of cells held together by intracellular supporting structures. A common characteristic of all cells is dependence on oxygen to combine with nutrients (carbohydrates, lipids, proteins) to release energy necessary for cellular function. Almost every cell is within 25 to 50 μm of a capillary, assuring prompt diffusion of oxygen to cells. All cells exist in nearly the same composition of extracellular fluid (*milieu interieur*), and the organs of the body (lungs, kidneys, gastrointestinal tract) function to maintain a constant composition (homeostasis) of extracellular fluid.

CELL ANATOMY

The principal components of cells include the nucleus and the cytoplasm, which contains structures known as *organelles* (Fig. 39-1) (Junqueira et al., 1992). The nucleus is separated from the cytoplasm by a nuclear membrane, and the cytoplasm is separated from surrounding fluids by a cell (plasma) membrane.

Cytoplasm

Cytoplasm consists of water, electrolytes, and proteins including enzymes, lipids, and carbohydrates. About 70% to 80% of the cell substance is water. Cellular chemicals are dissolved in the water, and these substances can diffuse to all parts of the cell in this fluid medium. Proteins are, next to water, the most abundant substance in most cells, accounting for 10% to 20% of the cell mass.

Cell Membrane

Each cell is surrounded by a cell membrane that acts as a permeability barrier, allowing the cell to maintain a cytoplasmic composition different from extracellular fluid. Proteins and phospholipids are the most abundant constituents of cell membranes (Table 39-1). A model of cell membrane structure envisions the membrane as a lipid bilayer (two molecules thick) that is interspersed with large globular proteins (Fig. 39-2) (Lodish and Rothman, 1979). The lipid bilayer of cell membranes is nearly impermeable to water and water-soluble substances, such as ions and glucose. Conversely, fat-soluble substances, such as oxygen and carbon dioxide, readily cross cell membranes.

There are several types of proteins in the cell membrane (see Table 39-1). In addition to structural proteins (microtubules), there are transport proteins (sodium-potassium adenosine triphosphatase [ATPase]) that function as pumps, actively transporting ions across cell membranes. Other proteins function as passive channels for ions that can be opened or closed by changes in the conformation of the protein. There are proteins that function as receptors to bind ligands (hormones or neurotransmitters), thus initiating physiologic changes inside cells. Another group of proteins function as enzymes (adenylate cyclase), catalyzing reactions at the surface of cell membranes. The protein structure of cell membranes, especially the enzyme content, varies from cell to cell.

Cell membranes are usually dynamic fluid structures, reflecting the ability of the lipid bilayer to flow to other areas of the membrane and carry proteins or other dissolved substances with it. An example of a membrane component that is not free to diffuse in the plane of the membrane is the acetylcholine receptor, which is sequestered at the motor end plate of skeletal muscle.

Nucleus

The nucleus is made up, in large part, of chromosomes that carry the blueprint for heritable characteristics of the cell. Each chromosome consists of a molecule of DNA that is covered with proteins. The ultimate units of heredity are genes on the chromosomes, and each gene is a portion of the DNA

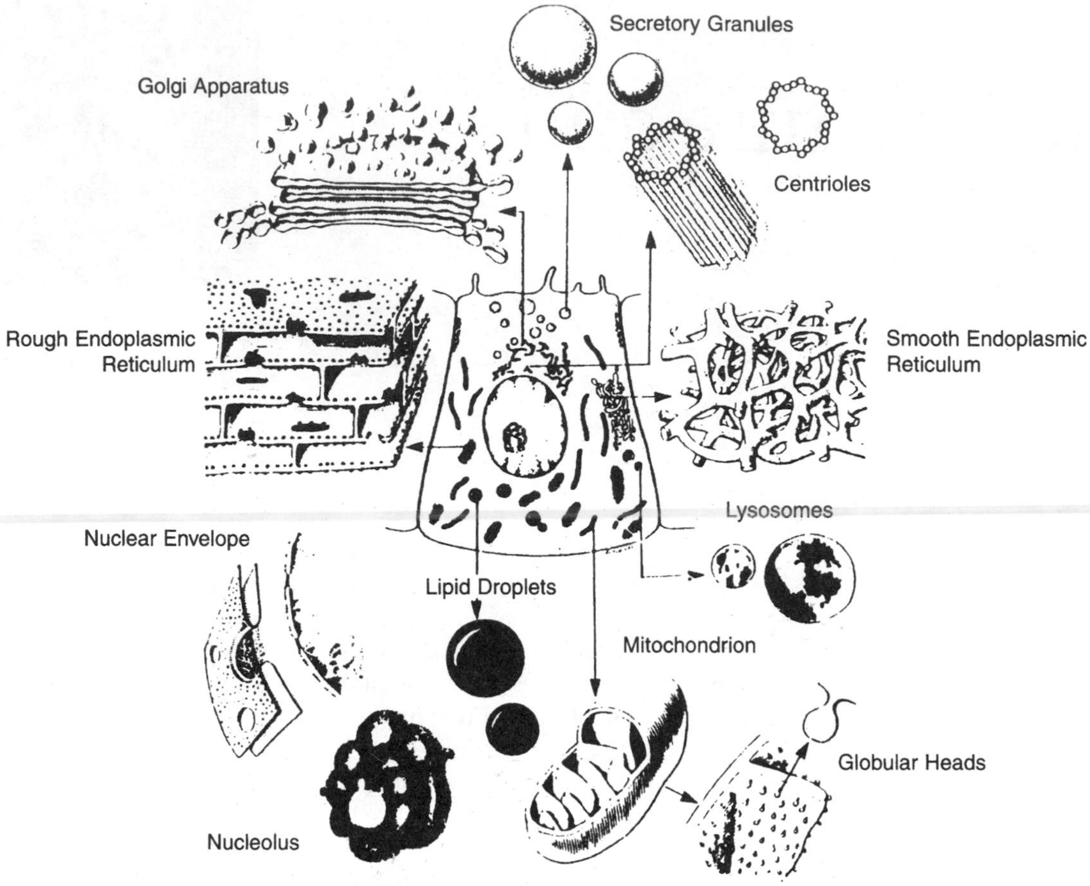

Figure 39-1. Schematic diagram of a hypothetical cell (*center*) and its organelles. (From Junqueira LC, Carneiro J, Kelley RO. *Basic histology*, 7th ed. Norwalk, CT: Appleton & Lange, 1992; with permission.)

molecule. The nucleus is surrounded by a membrane that separates its contents from the cytoplasm. This membrane consists of a bilayer of lipid molecules and protein channels through which dissolved suspended substances, including RNA, can pass from the nucleus to the cytoplasm.

During normal cell division by mitosis, the chromosomes duplicate themselves and then divide in such a way that each daughter cell receives a full complement (diploid number) of 46 chromosomes. Mature sperm and ova contain half the number (haploid number) of chromosomes. When a sperm and ovum unite, the resultant cell (zygote) has a full (diploid) complement of 46 chromosomes.

TABLE 39-1.
CELL MEMBRANE COMPOSITION

Phospholipids
Lecithins (phosphatidylcholines)
Sphingomyelins
Amino phospholipids (phosphatidylethanolamine)
Proteins
Structural proteins (microtubules)
Transport proteins (sodium-potassium ATPase)
Ion channels
Receptors
Enzymes (adenylate cyclase)

ATPase, adenosine triphosphatase.

Structure and Function of Deoxyribonucleic Acid and Ribonucleic Acid

DNA consists of two nucleotide chains containing adenine, guanine, thymine, and cytosine (Fig. 39-3) (Murray et al., 1988). The genetic message is determined by the sequence of these amino acids in the nucleotide chains. DNA determines the type of RNA that is formed; RNA is responsible for transferring the genetic message to the site of protein synthesis (ribosomes) in cytoplasm. Cell reproduction (mitosis) is determined by the DNA-genetic system. If there is an insufficient number of some types of cells in the body, these cells will grow and reproduce rapidly until appropriate numbers are again present. For example, nearly all of the liver can be removed surgically and the remaining cells will reproduce until liver mass is returned to almost normal. Similar reproduction occurs for glandular cells, cells of the bone marrow, and gastrointestinal epithelium. Highly differentiated cells such as nerve and muscle cells, however, are not

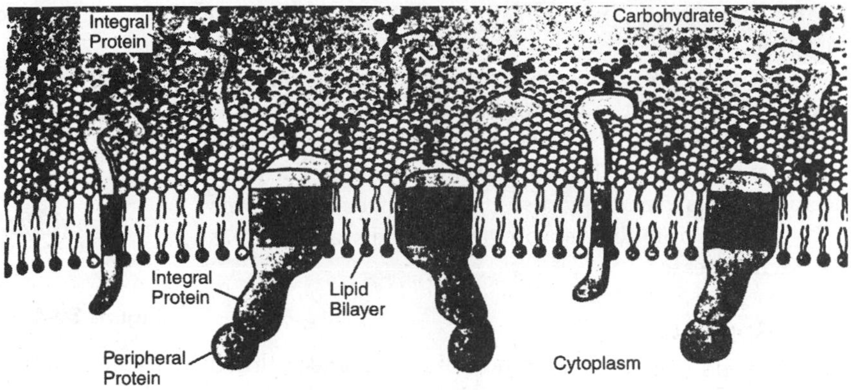

Figure 39-2. The cell membrane is a two molecule–thick lipid bilayer containing protein molecules that extend through the bilayer. (From Lodish HF, Rothman JE. The assembly of cell membranes. *Sci Am* 1979;240:48–63; with permission.)

capable of reproduction to replace lost cells. Mutations occur when the amino acid sequence in the DNA structure is altered by mutagenic chemicals or radiation.

Regulation of Gene Expression

Genes may be activated by steroids and by proteins manufactured by other genes in the cell. Oncogenes are genes that, when activated, produce uncontrolled cell reproduction (tumors). These genes may alter receptors such that they are continuously stimulated by ligands or alter second messenger systems in the cell so that the response to normal stimulation is excessive. Still other genes may stimulate cells to produce growth factors that act on cells themselves.

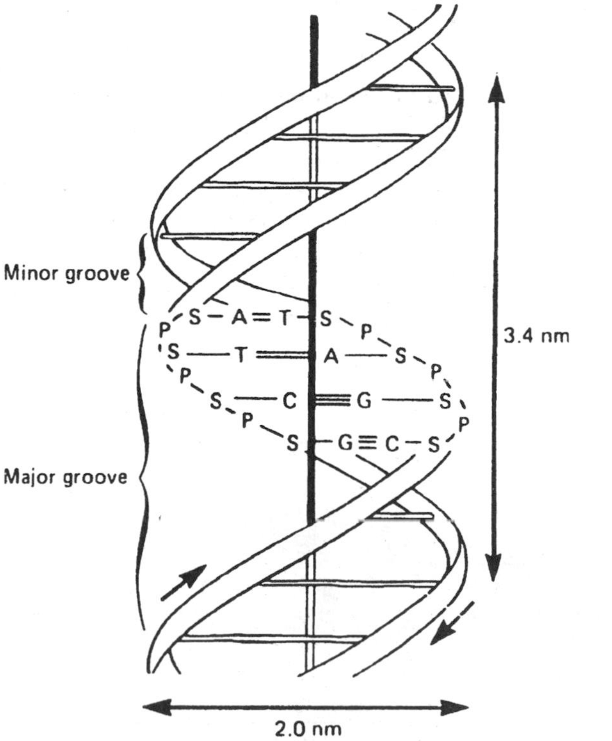

Figure 39-3. Double helical structure of DNA with adenine (A) bonding to thymine (T) and cytosine (C) to guanine (G). (From Murray RK, Granner DK, Mayes PA, et al. *Harper's biochemistry*, 21st ed. Norwalk, CT: Appleton & Lange, 1988; with permission.)

Organelles

Organelles are structures in the cytoplasm that have specific roles in cellular function.

Mitochondria

Mitochondria are the power-generating units of cells containing the enzymes and substrates of the tricarboxylic acid cycle (Krebs cycle). As a result, oxidative phosphorylation and synthesis of adenosine triphosphate (ATP) are localized to mitochondria. ATP leaves the mitochondria and diffuses throughout the cell, providing energy for cellular functions. Increased need for ATP in the cell leads to an increase in the number of mitochondria. In the absence of mitochondria, the cell is unable to extract sufficient energy from nutrients and oxygen, leading to cessation of cellular function.

Endoplasmic Reticulum

The endoplasmic reticulum is a complex series of tubules in the cytoplasm. Ribosomes, composed mainly of RNA, attach to the outer portions of many parts of the endoplasmic reticulum membranes, serving as the sites for protein synthesis (hormones, hemoglobin). The portion of the membrane containing these ribosomes is known as the *rough endoplasmic reticulum*. The part of the membrane that lacks ribosomes is the *smooth endoplasmic reticulum*. This smooth portion of the endoplasmic reticulum membrane functions in the synthesis of lipid substances and enzymatic processes.

Lysosomes

Lysosomes are scattered throughout the cytoplasm, provid ing an intracellular digestive system. Structurally, lysosomes are surrounded by bilayer lipid membranes and are filled with digestive (hydrolytic) enzymes. When cells are damaged or die, these digestive enzymes cause autolysis of the remnants. Bactericidal substances in the lysosome kill phagocytized bacteria before they can cause cellular damage. These bactericidal substances include (a) lysozyme, which dissolves the cell membranes of bacteria; (b) lysoferrin, which binds iron and other metals that are essential for bacterial growth; (c) acid that has a pH of <4, and (d) hydrogen peroxide, which can disrupt some bacterial metabolic systems.

In the presence of gout, release of lysosomal enzymes may contribute to the inflammatory response in joints. Congenital absence of a lysosomal enzyme results in engorgement of the lysosome with material normally degraded. This eventually disrupts the defective lysosome and is responsible for lysosomal storage diseases such as Tay-Sachs disease.

Golgi Apparatus

The Golgi apparatus is a collection of membrane-enclosed sacs that are responsible for storing proteins to serve specific functions. Proteins synthesized in the endoplasmic reticulum are transported to the Golgi apparatus, where they are stored in highly concentrated packets (secretory vesicles) for subsequent release into the cell's cytoplasm. These vesicles may also diffuse to the surface of cell membranes and discharge their contents (often neurotransmitters) to the exterior by the process of exocytosis.

Specialized portions of the Golgi apparatus form lysosomes, and other portions form peroxisomes. Peroxisomes can both form and destroy hydrogen peroxide. Destruction of hydrogen peroxide, which is formed by many metabolic reactions, is essential, as accumulation of high concentrations has a toxic effect on important enzyme systems.

Nucleus

The nucleus contains granules rich in RNA and is the site of synthesis of ribosomes. RNA enters the cytoplasm and controls the formation of specific proteins, usually enzymes that control different cellular actions. The specific type of RNA formed and, thus, the protein synthesized is determined by DNA, which functions as a gene.

Centrioles

Centrioles are present in the cytoplasm near the nucleus and are concerned with the movement of chromosomes during cell division.

TRANSFER OF MOLECULES ACROSS CELL MEMBRANES

Endocytosis and exocytosis are examples of processes that transfer molecules such as nutrients across but not through cell membranes. The uptake of particulate matter (bacteria, damaged cells) by cells is *phagocytosis*, whereas uptake of materials in solution in the extracellular fluid is *pinocytosis* (Fig. 39-4) (Berne et al., 2004). The process of phagocytosis is initiated when antibodies attach to damaged tissue and foreign substances (opsonization), which results in acquisition of a positive charge. Typically, objects that have a negative charge are repelled by cell membranes and thus are not vulnerable to phagocytosis. Fusion of phagocytic or pinocytic vesicles with lysosomes allows intracellular digestion of materials to proceed. Molecules such as neurotransmitters are ejected from cells by exocytosis, a process that requires calcium ions and resembles endocytosis in reverse.

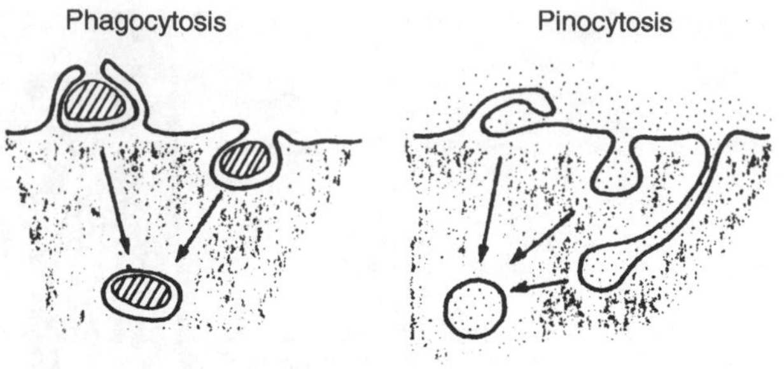

Figure 39-4. Schematic depiction of phagocytosis (ingestion of solid particles) and pinocytosis (ingestion of dissolved particles). (From Berne RM, Levy MN, Koeppen BM, et al. *Physiology*, 5th ed. St. Louis: Mosby, 2004; with permission.)

TRANSFER OF MOLECULES THROUGH CELL MEMBRANES

Some molecules (oxygen, carbon dioxide, nitrogen) move through cell membranes by diffusion among the molecules that make up the membrane, whereas the passage of other molecules (glucose, amino acids) requires the presence of specific transport proteins in cell membranes.

Diffusion

Diffusion is the process whereby molecules intermingle because of their random thermal motion. The diffusion rate across cell membranes is proportional to the area available for diffusion and the difference in concentration of the diffusing substances on the two sides of the membrane. Because of the slowness of diffusion over macroscopic distances, organisms have developed circulatory systems to deliver nutrients within reasonable diffusion ranges of cells (Table 39-2). Substances can diffuse through cell membranes by becoming dissolved in the lipid bilayer or by passing through protein channels.

Lipid Bilayer

The lipid bilayer of cell membranes is the principal barrier to substances that permeate membranes by simple diffusion.

TABLE 39-2.
PREDICTED RELATIONSHIP BETWEEN DIFFUSION DISTANCE AND TIME

Diffusion Distance (mm)	Time Required for Diffusion
0.001	0.5 ms
0.01	50 ms
0.1	5 s
1	498 s
10	14 hrs

The positive correlation between lipid solubility and cell membrane permeability suggests that lipid-soluble molecules can dissolve in and diffuse across cell membranes. Highly lipid-soluble oxygen and carbon dioxide diffuse readily. Conversely, cell membranes are impermeable to charged water-soluble molecules, especially those with molecular weights of >200 daltons.

Protein Channels

Ion channels constitute a class of proteins that is ultimately responsible for generating and orchestrating the electrical signals passing through the brain, heart, and skeletal muscles (Fig. 39-5) (Ackerman and Clapham, 1997). These ion channels are macromolecular protein tunnels that span the lipid bilayer of the cell membrane. Approximately 30% of the energy expended by cells is used to maintain the gradient of sodium and potassium ions across cell membranes. Ion channels use this stored energy much as a switch releases the electrical energy of a battery. They are more efficient than enzymes as small conformational alterations change (gate) a single channel from closed to open, allowing up to 10 million ions to flow into or out of the cell each second.

Genes encoding the protein ion channels may be defective, leading to diseases such as cystic fibrosis (chloride channel defects), long Q-T interval syndrome (mutant sodium channels), hereditary nephrolithiasis, hereditary myopathies including myotonia congenita, and malignant hyperthermia (calcium channel defects) (Ackerman and Clapham, 1997). Drugs that target ion channels include calcium channel blockers, antiseizure medications, and cardiac antidysrhythmic drugs.

Because of their charge, most ions are relatively insoluble in cell membranes such that their passage across these membranes is thought to occur through protein channels. These channels are likely to be intermolecular spaces in proteins that extend through the entire cell membrane. Some channels are highly specific with respect to ions allowed to pass (sodium, potassium), whereas other channels allow all ions below a certain size to pass (Table 39-3). Tetrodotoxin is a specific blocker of sodium ion channels as a result of binding to the extracellular side of the channel, whereas tetraethylammonium blocks potassium ion channels by attaching to the inside surface of the membrane.

Some channels are continuously open, whereas others are gated (gates open or closed). Some channels are gated

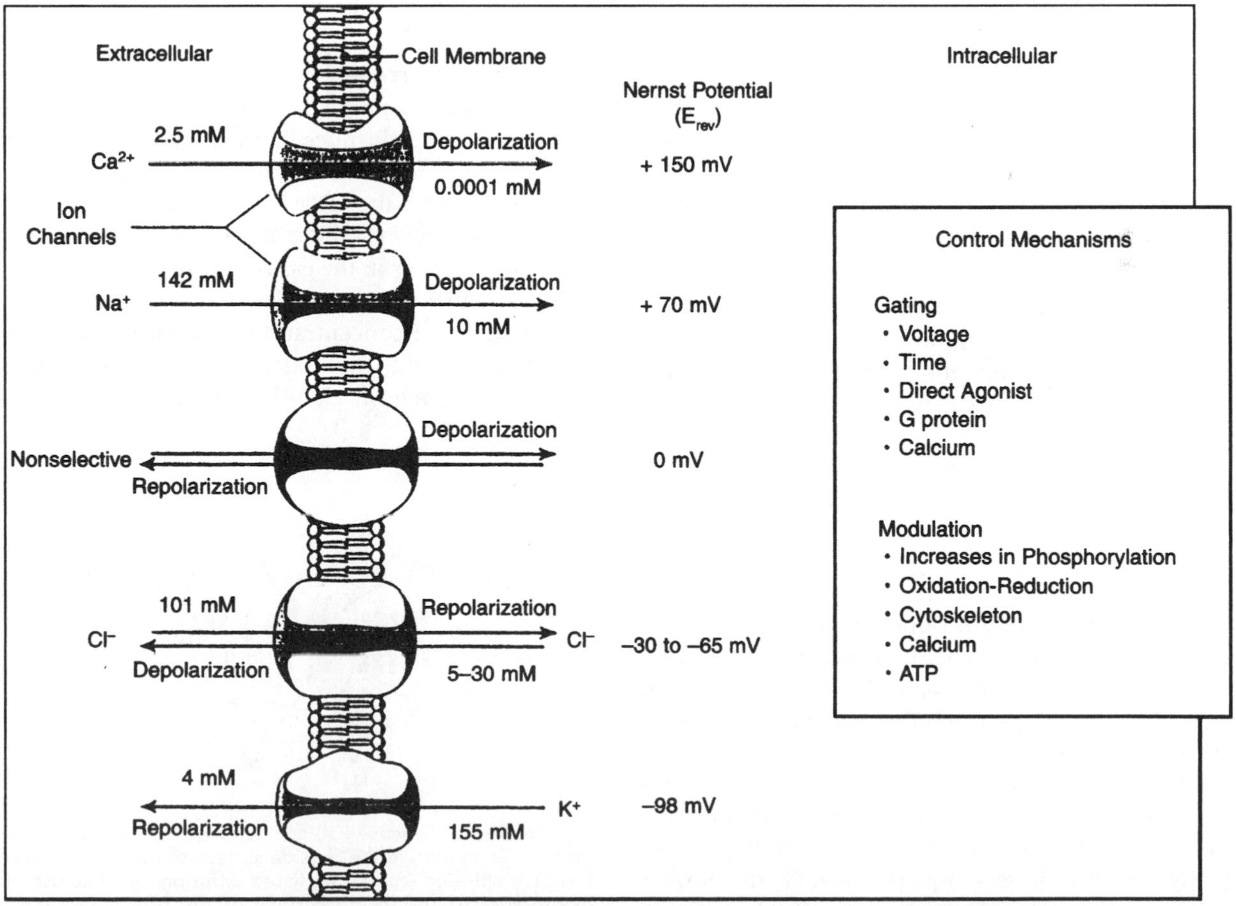

Figure 39-5. The five major types of protein ion channels are calcium, sodium, nonselective, chloride, and potassium. Flow of ions through these channels (calcium and sodium into cells and potassium outward) determines the transmembrane potential of cells. (From Ackerman MJ, Clapham DE. Ion channels—basic science and clinical disease. *N Engl J Med* 1997;336:1575–1586; with permission.)

TABLE 39-3.
DIAMETERS OF IONS, MOLECULES, AND CHANNELS

	Diameter (nm)*
Channel (average)	0.80
Water	0.30
Sodium (hydrated)	0.51
Potassium (hydrated)	0.40
Chloride (hydrated)	0.39
Glucose	0.86

*1 nm = 10 Å.

by alterations in membrane potential (voltage-gated sodium ion channels), whereas others are opened or closed when they bind a ligand such as a neurotransmitter or a hormone (chemically or ligand-gated acetylcholine receptors). For example, one end of the sodium ion channel may become blocked by the presence of a positive charge at its external opening. This charge is designated the *gate* because it repels sodium ions and interferes with passage of these ions through the protein channel.

Permeability of cell membranes to sodium and potassium ions may change as much as 50- to 5,000-fold during the course of nerve impulse transmission. These changes most likely reflect rapid alterations in the electrical charges lining the channels or guarding their entrances. Extracellular fluid concentrations of calcium ions influence the permeability of protein ion channels. For example, decreased calcium ion concentrations greatly increase channel permeability, manifesting as exaggerated activity of nerves throughout the body. Conversely, increased calcium ion concentrations in extracellular fluid decreases channel permeability and activity of nerves is greatly reduced. In the kidneys, the presence of arginine vasopressin hormone enlarges pores in cells lining the collecting ducts, allowing water and other substances to diffuse from the renal tubules back into peritubular capillaries.

Aquaporins

Small, nonpolar molecules such as oxygen and nitrogen and small uncharged polar molecules such as carbon dioxide diffuse across lipid cell membranes. Lipid cell membranes have limited permeability to other substances (glucose, urea, amino acids) which depend on endocytosis and exocytosis as well as passage through highly specific protein channels. This limited permeability applies even to water with simple diffusion being facilitated by highly specific protein channels known as aquaporins that are responsive only to water (Agre et al., 2002). In the absence of aquaporins, diffusion of water may not be sufficiently rapid for many physiologic processes. Aquaporins may be contributory to numerous disorders involving fluid transport including cerebral edema, cirrhosis of the liver, congestive heart failure, and glaucoma (Kozono et al., 2002).

Protein-Mediated Transport

Protein-mediated transport is responsible for movement of certain substances into or out of cells by way of specific carriers or channels that are intrinsic proteins of cell membranes. Transport across cell membranes may be facilitated (carrier-mediated diffusion) or active, with the principal distinction being that active transport is capable of moving a substance across cell membranes against a concentration gradient, whereas facilitated transport tends to equilibrate substances across the membrane.

Facilitated Diffusion

Poorly lipid-soluble substances, such as glucose and amino acids, may pass through lipid bilayers by facilitated diffusion. For example, glucose combines with a carrier to form a complex that is lipid soluble. This lipid-soluble complex can diffuse to the interior of the cell membrane where glucose is released into the cytoplasm, and the carrier moves back to the exterior of the cell membrane, where it becomes available to transport more glucose from the extracellular fluid (Fig. 39-6) (Guyton and Hall, 2000). As such, the carrier renders glucose soluble in cell membranes that otherwise would prevent its passage. Insulin greatly speeds facilitated diffusion of glucose and some amino acids across cell membranes.

Active Transport

Active transport requires energy that is most often provided by hydrolysis of ATP. Indeed, carrier molecules are enzymes known as *ATPases* that catalyze the hydrolysis of ATP. The most important of the ATPases is sodium-potassium ATPase, which is also known as the *sodium pump*. There are hydrogen-potassium ATPases in the gastric mucosa and renal tubules. Substances that are actively transported through cell membranes against a concentration gradient include sodium, potassium, calcium, hydrogen, chloride, and magnesium ions; iodide (thyroid gland); carbohydrates; and amino acids.

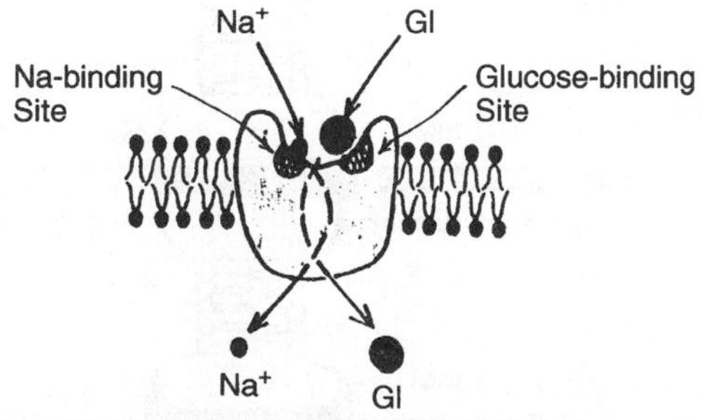

Figure 39-6. Glucose (Gl) can combine with a sodium cotransport carrier system at the outside surface of the cell membrane to facilitate diffusion (carrier-mediated diffusion) of Gl across the cell membrane. At the inside surface of the cell membrane, Gl is released to the interior of the cell and the carrier again becomes available for reuse. (From Guyton AC, Hall JE. *Textbook of medical physiology*, 10th ed. Philadelphia: Saunders, 2000; with permission.)

Sodium-Potassium ATPase

Sodium-potassium ATPase is present in all cells and is responsible for providing the energy (catalyzes conversion of ATP to adenosine diphosphate [ADP]) necessary for extruding three sodium ions from the cell while two potassium ions enter the cell for each mole of ATP hydrolyzed to ADP (Fig. 39-7) (Guyton and Hall, 2000). As a result, there is net movement of positive charges out of the cell, which creates a potential (voltage) difference across cell membranes, with the interior of the cell being negative with respect to the exterior. Maintenance of this electrical potential difference is essential to nerve conduction and skeletal muscle contraction.

Sodium-potassium ATPase opposes the tendency of cells to swell by continually transporting sodium ions to the exterior, which initiates an opposite osmotic tendency to move water out of the cell. This enzyme provides sufficient energy to transport sodium ions against concentration gradients as great as 20 to 1 and potassium ions against concentration gradients as great as 30 to 1. When the metabolism of the cell ceases so that energy from ATP is not available to maintain enzyme activity, the cell begins to swell. Activity of sodium-potassium ATPase is also inhibited by cardiac glycosides, resulting in decreased intracellular extrusion of calcium ions. The subsequent increase in intracellular calcium ion concentration is consistent with the positive inotropic effect of cardiac glycosides.

Sodium Ion Cotransport of Glucose

Despite the widespread presence of sodium-potassium ATPase, the active transport of sodium ions in some tissues is coupled to the transport of other substances. For example, a carrier system present in the gastrointestinal tract and renal tubules will transport sodium ions only in combination with a glucose molecule. As such, glucose is returned to the circulation, thus preventing its excretion.

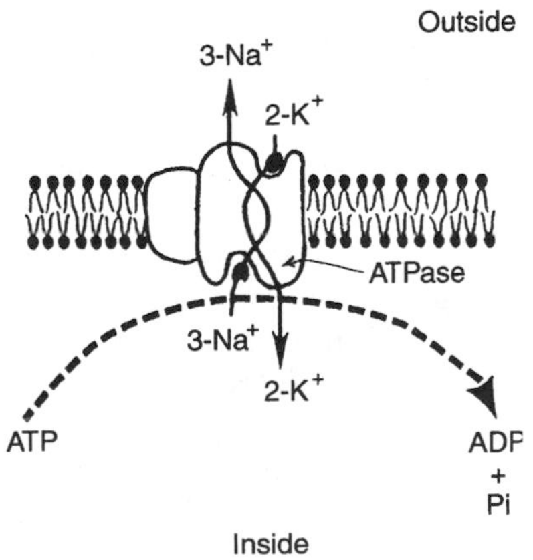

Figure 39-7. Sodium-potassium adenosine triphosphatase is an enzyme present in all cells that catalyzes the conversion of adenosine triphosphate (ATP) to adenosine diphosphate (ADP). The resulting energy is used by the active transport carrier system (sodium pump) that is responsible for the outward movement of three sodium ions across the cell membrane for every two potassium ions that pass inward. (From Guyton AC, Hall JE. *Textbook of medical physiology*, 10th ed. Philadelphia: Saunders, 2000; with permission.)

Sodium Ion Cotransport of Amino Acids

Sodium ion cotransport of amino acids is an active transport mechanism that supplements facilitated diffusion of amino acids into cells. Epithelial cells lining the gastrointestinal tract and renal tubules are able to reabsorb amino acids into the circulation by this mechanism, thus preventing their excretion. Other substances, including insulin, steroids, and growth hormone, influence amino acid transport by the sodium ion cotransport mechanism. For example, estradiol facilitates transport of amino acids into the musculature of the uterus, which promotes development of this organ. The effect of steroids on skeletal muscle development is a widely publicized controversy as it relates to body building.

Calcium ATPase

Calcium ATPase is present in cell membranes to maintain the large gradient between calcium ion concentrations in the cytoplasm and extracellular fluid. This cell membrane ATPase is different from the calcium ATPase that is responsible for sequestering calcium ions in the sarcoplasmic reticulum of skeletal muscles. In keeping with the vital role of calcium as a controller of cellular responses, the activity of calcium ATPase is highly regulated by calmodulin, an intracellular regulatory protein that increases the affinity of this enzyme for calcium ions at the inner surface of cell membranes.

ELECTRICAL POTENTIALS ACROSS CELL MEMBRANES

Electrical potentials exist in nearly all cell membranes, reflecting principally the difference in transmembrane concentrations of sodium and potassium ions. This unequal distribution of ions is created and maintained by the membrane-bound enzyme sodium-potassium ATPase, which causes a net transfer of positive charges out of the cell (three sodium ions out for two potassium ions in), resulting in the establishment of a voltage difference across cell membranes known as the *resting membrane potential*. The cytoplasm is usually electrically negative (about −70 mv) relative to the extracellular fluid (Fig. 39-8) (Berne et al., 2004). The number of ions responsible for the membrane potential is a small fraction of the total number present.

Action Potential

An action potential is the rapid change in transmembrane potential followed by a return to the resting membrane

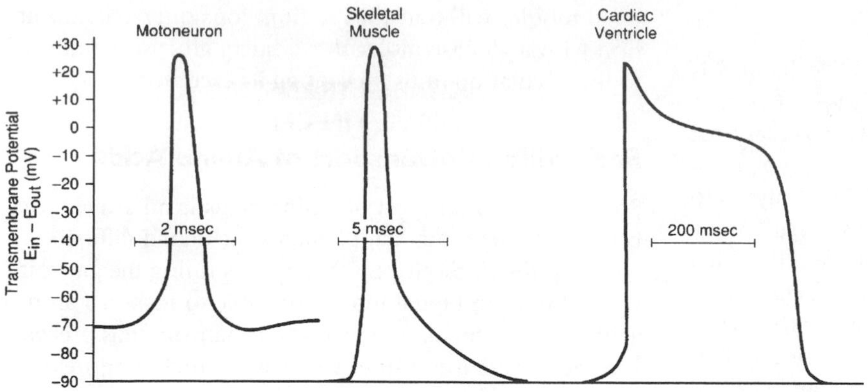

Figure 39-8. The transmembrane potential and duration of the action potential varies with the tissue site. (From Berne RM, Levy MN, Koeppen B, et al. *Physiology*, 5th ed. St. Louis: Mosby, 2004; with permission.)

potential. Propagation of the action potential along the entire length of a nerve axon or muscle cell is the basis of signal-carrying ability of nerve cells and allows muscle cells to contract simultaneously. The size and shape of the action potential varies among excitable tissues (see Fig. 39-8) (Berne et al., 2004).

An action potential is triggered when successive conductance increases to sodium and potassium ions cause a threshold potential (about −50 mv) to be reached. Acetylcholine, as an endogenous neurotransmitter, is the most important chemical substance that is capable of enlarging sodium ion channels and increasing permeability of cell membranes to sodium up to 5,000-fold. The initial, sudden, inward rush of sodium ions leads to a positive charge inside the cell, corresponding to the phase of the action potential known as *depolarization*. Subsequent increased permeability of the cell membrane to potassium allows loss of this positive ion, tending to return the electrical charge inside the cell toward the resting membrane potential. This phase of the action potential is known as *repolarization*.

Properties of Ion Channels

Ion channels may be voltage-gated (regulated by membrane potentials) or chemically-gated (regulated by binding of a neurotransmitter). During an action potential, voltage-gated sodium ion channels open briefly, allowing a small quantity of extracellular sodium to flow into the cell, thus depolarizing the cell membrane. A more slowly developing outward current—often potassium ions flowing through voltage-gated potassium ion channels—helps to repolarize the cell membrane. Sodium ion channels undergo transitions between ion-conducting states (open) and one of two nonconducting states known as the *resting* and *inactivated* forms. Resting ion channels may activate to open ion channels, whereas inactivated channels must first undergo transition to the resting state.

Measurement of Current

Current flowing through individual ion channels can be measured by patch-clamping electrophysiology (Ackerman and Clapham, 1997). Currents carried through different ion-selective channels can be separated by the use of specific inhibitors. For example, tetraethylammonium blocks many, but not all, types of potassium ion channels, whereas tetradotoxin blocks nearly all types of sodium ion channels.

Properties of Action Potentials

During much of the action potential, the cell membrane is completely refractory to further stimulation. This is termed the *absolute refractory period* and is due to the presence of a large fraction of inactivated sodium ion channels. During the last portion of the action potential, a stronger than normal stimulus can evoke a second action potential. This relative refractory period reflects the need to activate a critical number of sodium ion channels to trigger an action potential.

A deficiency of calcium ions in the extracellular fluid prevents the sodium ion channels from closing between action potentials. The resulting continuous leak of sodium contributes to sustained depolarization or repetitive firing of cell membranes (tetany). Conversely, high calcium ion concentrations decrease cell membrane permeability to sodium and thus decrease excitability of nerve membranes. Low potassium ion concentrations in extracellular fluid increase the negativity of the resting membrane potential, resulting in hyperpolarization and decreased cell membrane excitability. Skeletal muscle weakness that accompanies hypokalemia presumably reflects hyperpolarization of skeletal muscle membranes. Local anesthetics decrease permeability of nerve cell membranes to sodium ions, preventing achievement of a threshold potential that is necessary for generation of an action potential. Blockage of cardiac sodium ion channels by local anesthetics may result in altered conduction of cardiac impulses and decreases in myocardial contractility.

Conduction of Action Potentials

Action potentials are conducted along nerve or muscle fibers by local current flow that produces depolarization of adjacent areas of the cell membrane (Fig. 39-9). These propagated action potentials travel in both directions along the entire extent of the fiber. The transmission of the depolarization process along nerve or muscle fibers is

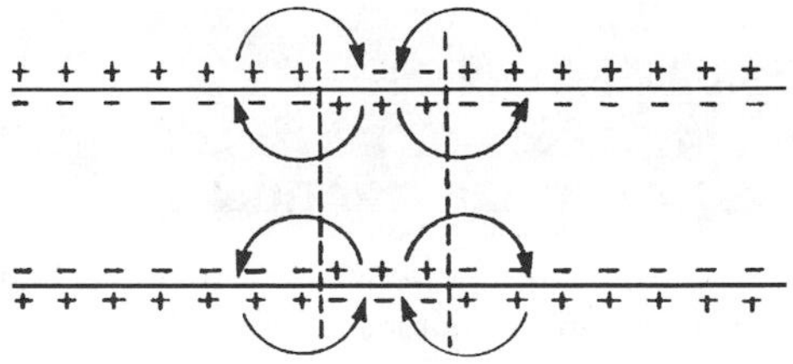

Figure 39-9. Depolarization spreads in both directions along cell membranes, resulting in propagation of an action potential.

called a *nerve* or *muscle impulse*. The entire action potential usually occurs in <1 ms.

Conduction velocity is greatly increased by myelination, which decreases capacitance of the axon and permits an action potential to be generated only at the nodes of Ranvier. Myelination reflects wrapping of Schwann cell membranes around the axon, and nodes of Ranvier represent the lateral spaces (1 to 2 mm apart) between cells. Myelinated nerves are more efficient metabolically than nonmyelinated axons because ion exchange is restricted to the nodes of Ranvier and less ion pumping is thus required to maintain sodium and potassium ion gradients. Another property of conduction in myelinated fibers that enhances conduction velocity is called *saltatory conduction* because the impulse jumps from one node of Ranvier to the next.

INTRACELLULAR COMMUNICATION

Cells communicate (transfer biologic information) with their environments in different ways that include stimulation or inhibition of cytoplasmic receptors, transmembrane receptors, and enzyme systems (Fig. 39-10) (Schwinn,

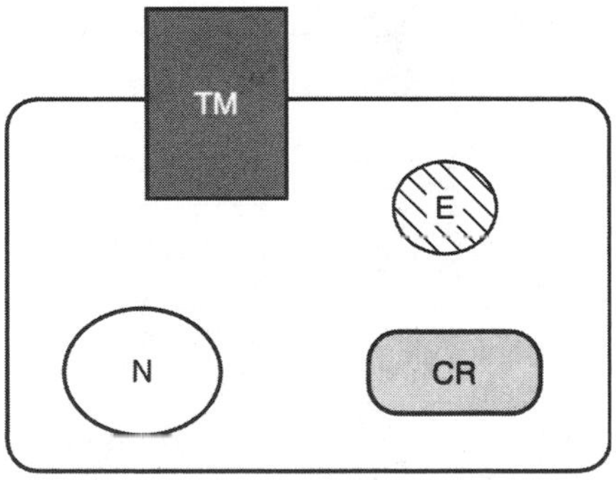

Figure 39-10. Cell communication that manifests as cellular (physiologic), and ultimately as clinical responses, occurs via cytoplasmic receptors (CR), stimulation or inhibition of enzyme systems (E), and excitable transmembrane (TM) proteins. The location of each system is illustrated schematically in relation to the cell nucleus (N) and cell membrane. Examples of CRs may be steroid receptors, whereas E may be represented by phosphodiesterase inhibitors. Most clinically useful drugs and endogenously secreted hormones mediate their effects via excitable TM proteins. (From Schwinn DA. Adrenoceptors as models for G protein–coupled receptors: structure, function, and regulation. *Br J Anaesth* 1993;71: 77–85; with permission.)

TABLE 39-4.
TYPES OF EXCITABLE TRANSMEMBRANE PROTEINS INVOLVED IN CELL COMMUNICATION

	Examples
Voltage-sensitive ion channels	Sodium Potassium Calcium Chloride
Ligand-gated ion channels	Nicotinic cholinergic receptors Amino acid receptors Gamma-aminobutyric acid *N*-methyl-D-aspartate
Transmembrane receptors (signal transduction)	Adrenoceptors (alpha, beta) Muscarinic cholinergic Opioid Serotonin Dopamine

Source: Adapted from Schwinn DA. Adrenoceptors as models for G protein–coupled receptors: structure, function, and regulation. *Br J Anaesth* 1993;71:77–85.

1993). Most clinically useful drugs and endogenously secreted hormones mediate their effects via one of three types of excitable transmembrane proteins (Table 39-4) (Schwinn, 1993). Transmembrane receptors located in lipid cell membranes interact with endogenous chemical messengers (hormones, neurotransmitters) or exogenous compounds (drugs), resulting in the initiation of a cascade of biochemical changes that lead to cellular responses (physiologic effects) (see Fig. 39-10) (Schwinn, 1993). Translation of information encoded in hormones, neurotransmitters, and drugs into a cellular response (most often a change in transmembrane voltage and excitability) is known as *signal transduction*. Chemical messengers (first messengers, ligands) generally exert their effects by increasing the concentrations of second messengers (cyclic adenosine monophosphate [cAMP], calcium ions) in target cells (Tables 39-5 and 39-6). Steroids and thyroid hormones are examples of chemical messengers that produce their effects by altering RNA in the cell's cytoplasm. Many of the chemical messengers are polypeptides to which antibodies can be produced, thus allowing measurement of messengers in body fluids or tissues by radioimmunoassay.

Receptors

Receptors can be classified by their cellular localization. Most signaling molecules are hydrophobic and interact with cell surface receptors that are directly or indirectly coupled to effector molecules. There are three known classes of cell surface receptors as defined by thier signal transduction mechanisms: G protein coupled receptors, ligand-gated ion channels, and receptor-linked enzymes.

TABLE 39-5.
LIGANDS THAT ACT BY ALTERING INTRACELLULAR CYCLIC ADENOSINE MONOPHOSPHATE (cAMP) CONCENTRATIONS

Increase cAMP
Adrenocorticotrophic hormone
Catecholamines (beta$_1$ and beta$_2$ receptors)
Glucagon
Parathyroid hormone
Thyroid-stimulating hormone
Follicle-stimulating hormone
Vasopressin
Decrease cAMP
Catecholamines (alpha$_2$ receptors)
Dopamine (dopamine$_2$ receptors)
Somatostatin

TABLE 39-6.
LIGANDS THAT INCREASE INTRACELLULAR CALCIUM ION CONCENTRATION

Catecholamines (alpha$_1$ receptors)
Acetylcholine (muscarinic receptors)
Serotonin
Substance P
Vasopressin (V$_1$ receptors)
Oxytocin

These cell surface receptor proteins act as signal transducers by binding the extracellular signal molecule and converting this information into an intracellular signal that alters target cell function. G protein coupled receptors interact with specific G proteins in the plasma membrane, which in turn activates or inhibits enzymes or ion channels. G protein coupled receptors constitute the largest family of cell surface receptors. A number of different isoforms of G protein subunits (alpha, beta, gamma) are present and mediate stimulation or inhibition of functionally diverse effector enzymes and ion channels. Most hormones and neurotransmitters are water soluble signaling molecules that interact with G protein coupled cell-surface receptors to translate informaton encoded in neurotransmitters and hormones into cellular responses (Fig. 39-11) (Gelman, 1987; Maze, 1990; Schwinn, 1993). The resulting response is most often a change in transmembrane voltage and thus excitability. There is great diversity in the number of G protein coupled receptors for the same ligand as reflected by multiple receptors for catecholamines and opioids. Intracellular receptors represented by steroid receptors act by directly regulating the transcription of specific genes.

Ligand-gated ion channels (ionotropic receptors) are involved principally with fast synaptic transmission between excitable cells in which binding of signaling molecules to receptors causes an immediate conformational change in receptor-ion channels. Specific neurotransmitters bind to these receptors and transiently open or close the associated ion channels to alter ion permeability of plasma membranes and thereby membrane potentials. An example of an ion channel whose conductance is

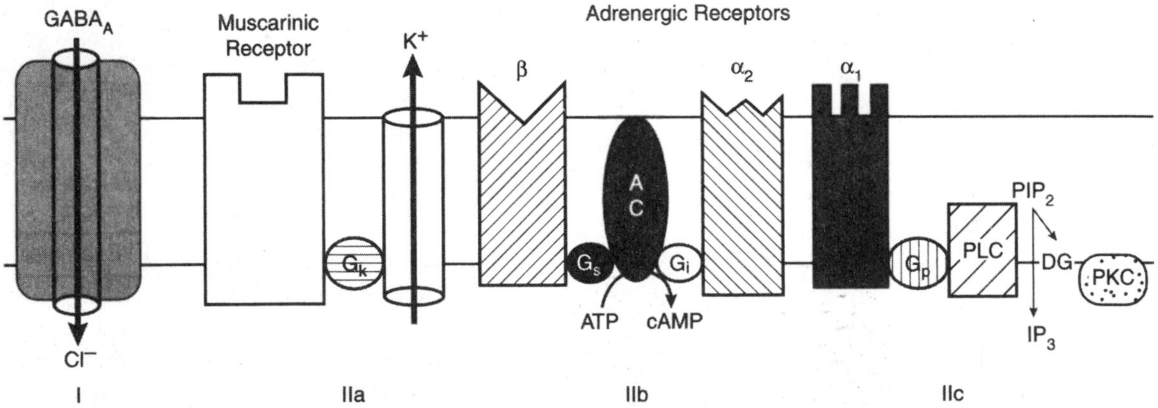

Figure 39-11. Schematic depiction of receptors on cell surfaces. Stimulation of the gamma-aminobutyric acid (GABA) receptor by an agonist results in flow of chloride ions into the cell along the protein ion channel (I). Stimulation of the muscarinic receptor by an agonist (acetylcholine) causes the coupling guanine (G) protein (G_k) to facilitate conductance of potassium ions to the exterior of the cell (IIa). Adenylate cyclase (AC) activity can be enhanced via a stimulatory G protein (G_s) on activation of a beta-adrenergic receptor by an agonist ligand, whereas the enzyme's activity can be attenuated via an inhibitory G protein (G_i) that is coupled with an alpha$_2$-adrenergic receptor, thus controlling the conversion of adenosine triphosphate (ATP) to cyclic adenosine monophosphate (cAMP) (IIb). On stimulation of the alpha$_1$-adrenergic receptor by an agonist ligand, the coupling G protein (G_p) activates phospholipase C (PLP) to hydrolyze phosphatidylinositol biphosphate (PIP_2) into inositol triphosphate (IP_3) and diacylglycerol (DG), which then activates protein kinase C (PKC) (IIc). (From Maze M. Transmembrane signalling and the Holy Grail of anesthesia. *Anesthesiology* 1990;72:959–961; with permission.)

regulated by receptor activation is the gamma-aminobutyric acid receptor, in which chloride ion conductance through the associated ion channel is the effector mechanism (see Fig. 39-11) (Maze, 1990). A second type of receptor involves the coupling of at least three separate components—a receptor protein, a guanine nucleotide binding protein (G protein), and an effector mechanism. Nicotinic acetylcholine receptors at the neuromuscular junction is an example of ligand-gated ion channels. Conceptually, the receptor protein functions as a recognition site that is stimulated or inhibited by a ligand. Stimulatory or inhibitory G proteins link the recognition site to the effector mechanism (catalytic site). These G proteins are the most prevalent proteins in the brain. The recognition site faces the exterior of the lipid cell membrane to facilitate access of water-soluble endogenous ligands and exogenous drugs, whereas the catalytic site faces the interior of the cell. In this type of receptor, a second messenger may or may not be generated. For example, when the muscarinic receptor is stimulated, the activated coupling G protein increases conductance of potassium ions through a discrete ion channel (see Fig. 39-11) (Maze, 1990). Alternatively, the activity of an enzyme may be changed to generate a second messenger. Such a receptor may regulate the activity of adenylate cyclase in a positive manner (beta-adrenergic receptor) through a stimulatory G protein or in a negative manner (alpha$_2$-adrenergic receptor) through an inhibitory G protein, thereby controlling the intracellular concentration of cAMP (see Fig. 39-11) (Maze, 1990). In contrast to the immediate cellular responses associated with ion channels, signals that use G protein coupled receptors are involved in functions that operate with time courses of seconds to minutes as occur with slow synaptic transmission or neuromodulation.

Another membrane-associated enzyme, similar to adenylate cyclase, is phospholipase C, which catalyzes reactions that result in production of second messengers (diacylglycerol and inositol triphosphate). Phospholipase C–coupled receptors (alpha$_1$-adrenergic receptors) are physiologically important because the resulting second messengers activate protein kinase and calcium ion release from intracellular sites (see Fig. 39-11) (Maze, 1990).

Receptor Concentration

Receptors in cell membranes are not static components of cells. Excess circulating concentrations of ligand (norepinephrine due to a pheochromocytoma) results in a decrease in the density of beta-adrenergic receptors in cell membranes (down-regulation). Drug-induced antagonism of beta-adrenergic receptors results in an increased density of receptors in cell membranes (up-regulation) and the possibility of exaggerated sympathetic nervous system activity if the beta-adrenergic antagonist drug is abruptly discontinued, as in the preoperative period. Desensitization of receptor responsiveness is the waning of a physiologic response over time despite the presence of a constant stimulus (Fig. 39-12) (Schwinn, 1993).

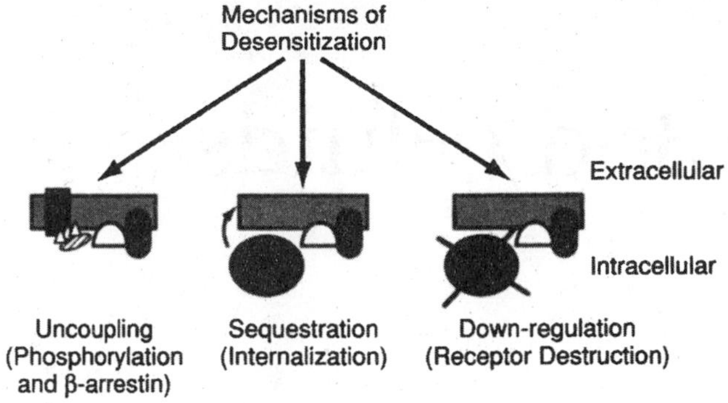

Figure 39-12. Three basic mechanisms for desensitization of receptors are uncoupling (preventing receptor interaction with G proteins), sequestration (mobilization of the receptor to intracellular vesicles over minutes to hours and recycling it back to the cell membrane surface once agonist stimulation terminates), and down-regulation (destruction of sequestered receptors over a period of hours to days). (From Schwinn DA. Adrenoceptors as models for G protein–coupled receptors: structure, function, and regulation. *Br J Anaesth* 1993;71:77–85; with permission.)

Receptor Diseases

Failure of parathyroid hormone and arginine vasopressin to produce increases in cAMP in target organs manifests as pseudohypoparathyroidism and nephrogenic diabetes insipidus, respectively. Grave disease and myasthenia gravis reflect development of antibodies against thyroid-stimulating hormone and nicotinic acetylcholine receptors, respectively.

REFERENCES

Ackerman MJ, Clapham DE. Ion channels—basic science and clinical disease. *N Engl J Med* 1997;336:1575–1586.

Agre P, King LS, Yasui M, et al. Aquaporin water channels—from atomic structure to clinical medicine. *J Physiol* 2002;542:3–16.

Berne RM, Levy MN, Koeppen BM, Stanton BA.. *Physiology*, 5th ed. St. Louis: Mosby, 2004.

Gelman AC. G proteins: transducers of receptor-generated signals. *Ann Rev Biochem* 1987;56:615–649.

Guyton AC, Hall JE. *Textbook of medical physiology*, 10th ed. Philadelphia: Saunders, 2000.

Junqueira LC, Carneiro J, Kelley RO. *Basic histology*, 7th ed. Norwalk, CT: Appleton & Lange, 1992.

Kozono D, Yasui M, King LS, et al. Aquaporin water channels: Atomic structure and molecular dynamics meet clinical medicine. *J Clin Invest* 2002;109: 1395–1399.

Lodish HF, Rothman JE. The assembly of cell membranes. *Sci Am* 1979;240:48–63.

Maze M. Transmembrane signaling and the Holy Grail of anesthesia. *Anesthesiology* 1990;72:959–961.

Murray RK, Granner DK, Mayes PA, et al. *Harper's biochemistry*, 21st ed. Norwalk, CT: Appleton & Lange, 1988.

Schwinn DA. Adrenoceptors as models for G protein–coupled receptors: structure, function, and regulation. *Br J Anaesth* 1993;71:77–85.

Body Fluids

40

Body fluids can be divided into intracellular and extracellular fluid depending on their location relative to the cell membrane (Fig. 40-1) (Gamble, 1954). Approximately 28 liters of the total body fluid (about 42 liters) present in an adult are contained inside the estimated 100 trillion cells of the body. The fluid in these cells, despite individual differences in constituents, is collectively designated *intracellular fluid*. The 14 liters of fluid outside the cells is referred to as extracellular fluid. Extracellular fluid is divided into interstitial fluid and plasma (intravascular fluid) by the capillary membrane (see Fig. 40-1) (Gamble, 1954).

Interstitial fluid is present in the spaces between cells. An estimated 99% of this fluid is held in the gel structure of the interstitial space. Plasma is the noncellular portion of blood. The average plasma volume is 3 liters. Plasma communicates continuously with the interstitial fluid through pores in the capillaries. Interstitial fluid is also in dynamic equilibrium with the plasma, serving as an available reservoir from which water and electrolytes can be mobilized into the circulation. Loss of plasma from the intravascular space is minimized by colloid osmotic pressure exerted by the plasma proteins.

Other extracellular fluid that may be considered as part of the interstitial fluid includes cerebrospinal fluid, gastrointestinal fluid, and fluid in potential spaces (pleural space, pericardial space, peritoneal cavity, synovial cavities). Excess amounts of fluid in the interstitial space manifest as peripheral edema.

Water is the most abundant single constituent of the body and is the medium in which all metabolic reactions occur. The total amount of water in a man weighing 70 kg is about 42 liters, accounting for nearly 60% of total body weight (see Fig. 40-1) (Gamble, 1954). In a neonate, total body water may represent 70% of body weight. Total body water is less in women and in obese individuals, reflecting the decreased water content of adipose tissue. For example, total body water represents about 50% of the body weight in women. Advanced age is also associated with increased fat content and decreased total body water (Table 40-1).

The normal daily intake of water (drink and internal product of food metabolism) by an adult averages 2.5 liters, of which about 1.5 liters is excreted as urine, 100 mL is lost in sweat, and 100 mL is present in feces. The remaining water intake is lost by evaporation from the respiratory tract and diffusion through the skin (insensible water loss not perceived by the individual). The cornified layer of the skin acts as a protector against greater insensible water loss through the skin. When the cornified layer becomes denuded, as after burn injury, the outward diffusion of water is greatly increased.

All gases that are inhaled become saturated with water vapor (47 mm Hg at 37°C). This water vapor is subsequently exhaled, accounting for an average daily water loss through the lungs of 300 to 400 mL. The water content of inhaled gases decreases with decreases in ambient air temperature such that more endogenous water is required to achieve a saturated water vapor pressure at body temperature. As a result, insensible water loss from the lungs is greatest in cold environments and least in warm temperatures. This is consistent with the dry feeling perceived in the respiratory passages when the ambient air temperature is cold.

BLOOD VOLUME

Blood contains extracellular fluid, as represented by plasma, and intracellular fluid, as represented by fluid in erythrocytes. The main priority of the body is to maintain intravascular fluid volume. Acute decreases in blood volume, as occur with (a) fluid deprivation in the perioperative period, (b) blood loss, or (c) surgical trauma that results in tissue edema, elicit the release of renin and arginine vasopessin (previously known as antidiuretic hormone). These hormones evoke changes in the renal tubules that lead to restoration of intravascular fluid volume (see Chapter 53).

The average blood volume of an adult is 5 liters, of which about 3 liters is plasma and 2 liters is erythrocytes. These volumes, however, vary greatly with age, weight, and gender. For example, in nonobese individuals, the blood volume varies in direct proportion to the body weight, averaging 70 mL/kg for lean men and women. The greater the ratio of fat to body weight, however, the less is the blood

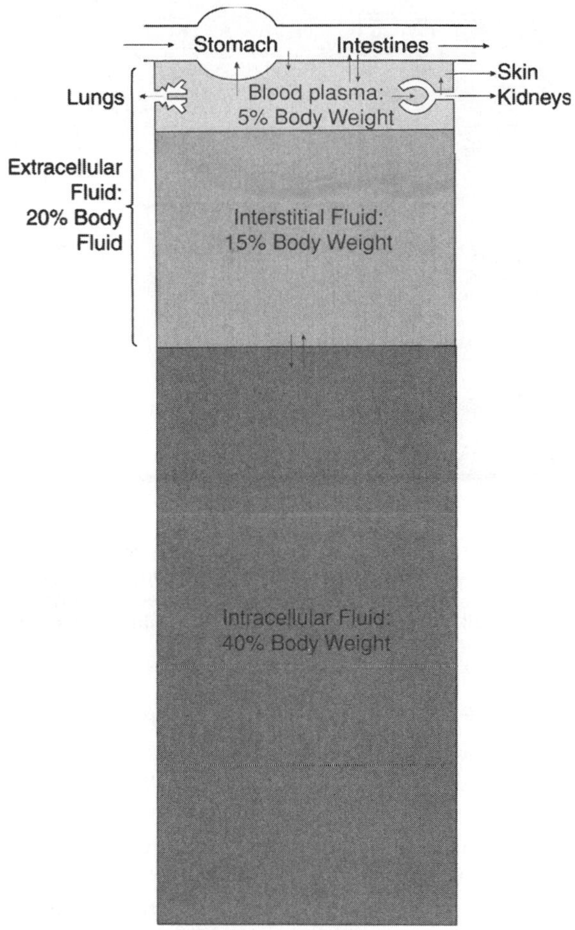

Figure 40-1. Body fluid compartments and the percentage of body weight represented by each compartment. The location relative to the capillary membrane divides extracellular fluid into plasma or interstitial fluid. Arrows represent fluid movement between compartments. (From Gamble JL. *Chemical anatomy, physiology, and pathology of extracellular fluid*, 6th ed. Boston: Harvard University Press, 1954; with permission.)

volume in ml/kg because adipose tissue has a decreased vascular supply.

Hematocrit

The true hematocrit is about 96% of the measured value because 3% to 8% of plasma remains entrapped among the erythrocytes even after centrifugation. The measured hematocrit is about 40% for men and 36% for women. The hematocrit of blood in arterioles and capillaries is lower than that in large arteries and veins. This reflects axial streaming of erythrocytes in small vessels. Specifically, erythrocytes tend to migrate to the center of vessels, whereas a large portion of the plasma remains near the vessel walls. In large blood vessels, the ratio of wall surface to total volume is near 1, so that the accumulation of plasma near the walls does not significantly affect the hematocrit. In small blood vessels, however, this ratio of wall surface to volume is larger, causing the ratio of plasma to cells to be greater than in large vessels.

TABLE 40-1.
TOTAL BODY WATER BY AGE AND GENDER

	Total Body Water	
Age (yrs)	**Men (%)**	**Women (%)**
18–40	61	51
40–60	55	47
>60	52	46

MEASUREMENT OF COMPARTMENTAL FLUID VOLUMES

The volume of a fluid compartment can be measured by the indicator dilution principle, in which a known amount of substance is placed in the compartment and the resulting concentration of this material is then determined after complete mixing has occurred. Using this principle, blood volume, extracellular fluid volume, and total body water can be measured, whereas interstitial fluid volume is calculated as extracellular fluid volume minus plasma volume.

Blood Volume

Substances used for measuring blood volume must be capable of dispersing throughout the blood with ease and then must remain in the circulation for a sufficient time for measurements to be completed. Most often, a small amount of the patient's blood is removed and mixed with radioactive chromium. After determining the total content of chromium with a scintillation counter, the tagged blood sample is injected into the patient. After mixing in the systemic circulation for about 10 minutes, the chromium concentration in blood is determined. Using the dilution principle, the total blood volume is calculated.

CONSTITUENTS OF BODY FLUID COMPARTMENTS

The constituents of plasma, interstitial fluid, and intracellular fluid are identical, but the quantity of each substance varies among the compartments (Fig. 40-2) (Leaf and Newburgh, 1955). The most striking differences are the low protein content in interstitial fluid compared with intracellular fluid and plasma and the fact that sodium and chloride ions are largely extracellular, whereas most of the potassium ions (approximately 90%) are intracellular. This unequal distribution of ions results in establishment of a potential (voltage) difference across cell membranes.

The constituents of extracellular fluid are carefully regulated by the kidneys so that cells remain bathed continually

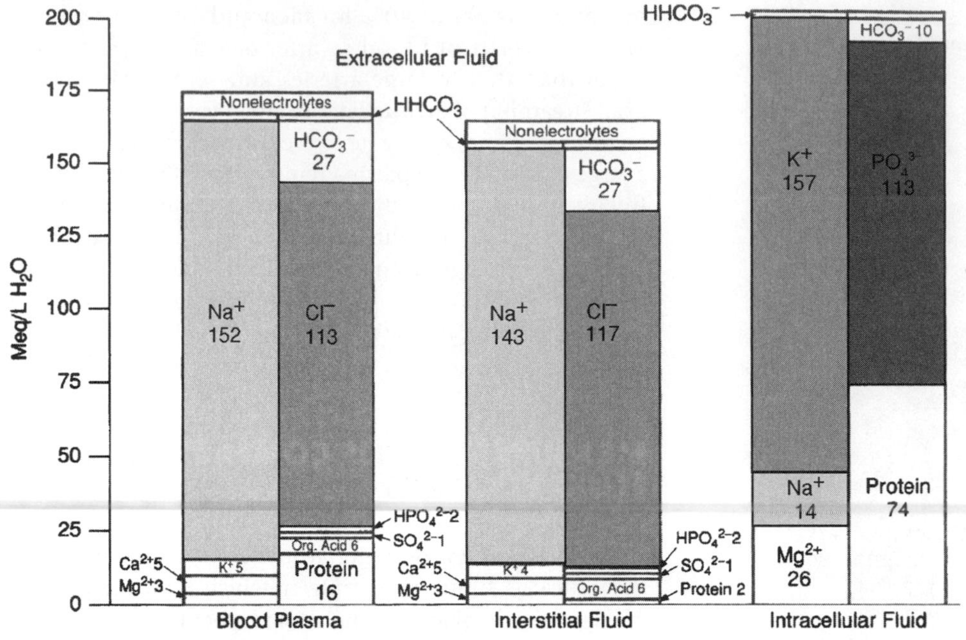

Figure 40-2. Electrolyte composition of body fluid compartments. (From Leaf A, Newburgh LH. *Significance of the body fluids in clinical medicine*, 2nd ed. Springfield, IL: Thomas, 1955; with permission.)

in a fluid containing the proper concentrations of electrolytes and nutrients for continued optimal function of the cells. The normal amount of sodium and potassium in the body is about 58 mEq/kg and 45mEq/kg, respectively. Trauma is associated with progressive loss of potassium through the kidneys. For example, a patient undergoing surgery excretes about 100 mEq of potassium in the first 48 hours postoperatively and, after this period, about 25 mEq daily. Plasma potassium concentrations are not good indicators of total body potassium content because most potassium is intracellular. There is a correlation, however, between the potassium and hydrogen ion content of plasma, the two increasing and decreasing together.

OSMOSIS

Osmosis is the movement of water (solvent molecules) across a semipermeable membrane from a compartment in which the nondiffusible solute (ion) concentration is lower to a compartment in which the solute concentration is higher (Fig. 40-3) (Ganong, 2003). A membrane is semipermeable when water can diffuse freely but sodium and potassium ions cannot diffuse freely.

Osmotic Pressure

Osmotic pressure is the pressure on one side of the semipermeable membrane that is just sufficient to keep water from moving to a region of higher solute concentration (see Fig. 40-3) (Ganong, 2003). The osmotic pressure exerted by nondiffusible particles in a solution is determined by the number of particles in the solution (degree of ionization) and not the type of particles (molecular weight). Thus a 1-mol solution of glucose or albumin and 0.5-mol solution of sodium chloride (dissociates into two ions) should exert the same osmotic pressure. Osmole is the unit used to express osmotic pressure in solutes. Milliosmole (1/1000 Osm) is commonly used to express the osmotic activity of solutes in the body.

The osmole concentration of a solution is called its *osmolality* when the concentration is expressed in osmole per kilogram of water. *Osmolarity* is the correct terminology when osmole concentrations are expressed in liters. In the dilute solutions of the body, these terms are frequently used interchangeably. Furthermore, because it is much easier to express body fluids in liters rather than kilograms of

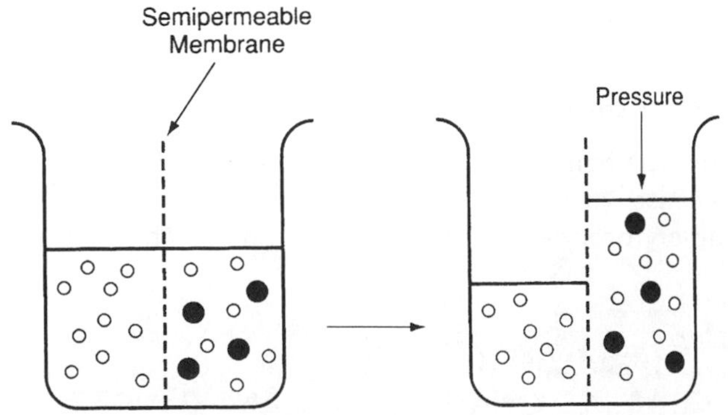

Figure 40-3. Diagrammatic representation of osmosis depicting water molecules (*open circles*) and solute molecules (*solid circles*) separated by a semipermeable membrane. Water molecules move across the semipermeable membrane to the area of higher concentration of solute molecules. Osmotic pressure is the pressure that would have to be applied to prevent continued movement of water molecules. (From Ganong WF. *Review of medical physiology*, 21st ed. New York: Lange Medical Books/McGraw-Hill, 2003.)

water, almost all physiology calculations are based on osmolarity rather than osmolality.

Moles and Equivalents

A mole is the molecular weight of a substance in grams, and each mole contains about 6.10^{23} molecules. A 1-mol solution of sodium chloride is 58.5 g and 1 mmol is 58.5 mg. An equivalent is 1 mol of an ionized substance divided by its valence. The mole is the standard unit for expressing concentrations in the International System of Units (SI) system.

Osmolarity of Body Fluids

The freezing point of plasma averages 0.54 °C, which corresponds to a plasma osmolarity of about 290 mOsm/L. All but about 20 mOsm of the 290 mOsm in each liter of plasma are contributed by sodium ions and their accompanying anions, principally chloride and bicarbonate ions. Proteins normally contribute <1 mOsm/L. The major nonelectrolytes of plasma are glucose and urea, and these substances can contribute significantly to plasma osmolarity when hyperglycemia or uremia is present (Table 40-2). Plasma osmolarity is important in evaluating dehydration, overhydration, and electrolyte abnormalities. The transfer of water through cell membranes by osmosis occurs so rapidly that any lack of osmotic equilibrium between two fluid compartments in a given tissue is corrected, usually within seconds.

Tonicity of Fluids

Tonicity is the term used to describe the osmolarity of a solution relative to plasma. Solutions that have the same osmolarity as plasma are said to be *isotonic* (no transfer of fluid into or out of cells occurs), those with higher osmolarity are *hypertonic* (cells shrink), and those with a lower osmolarity are *hypotonic* (cells swell) (Fig. 40-4) (Guyton and Hall, 2000). This reflects the fact that most cell membranes are relatively impermeable to many solutes but are highly permeable to water. For example, packed erythrocytes must be suspended in isotonic solutions to avoid damage to the cells before infusion. A 0.9% solution of sodium chloride is isotonic and remains so because there is no net movement of the osmotically active particles in the solution into cells, and the particles are not metabolized. A solution of 5% glucose in water is initially isotonic when infused, but glucose is metabolized, so the net effect is that of infusing a

TABLE 40-2.
CALCULATION OF PLASMA OSMOLARITY

Plasma osmolarity = 2 (Na+) + 0.055 (glucose) + 0.36 (blood urea nitrogen)

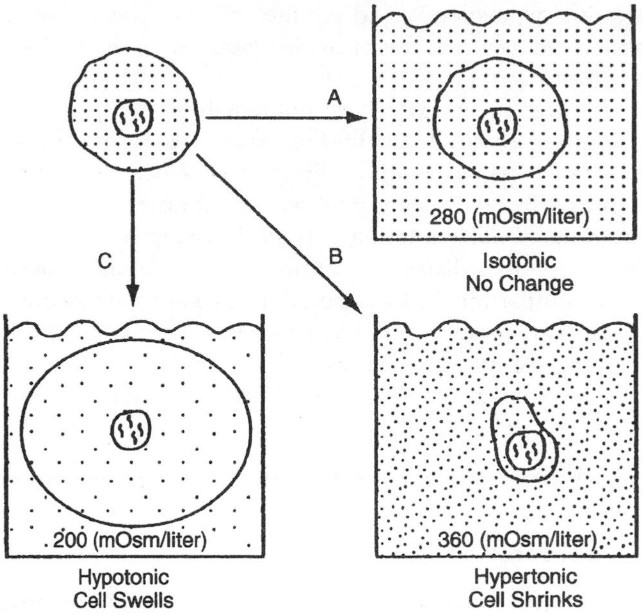

Figure 40-4. Effects of isotonic (A), hypertonic (B), and hypotonic (C) solutions on cell volume. (From Guyton AC, Hall JE. *Textbook of medical physiology*, 10th ed. Philadelphia: W.B. Saunders, 2000.)

hypotonic solution. Lactated Ringer's solution plus 5% glucose is initially hypertonic (about 560 mOsm/L), but as glucose is metabolized, the solution becomes less hypertonic. The maintenance of a normal cell volume and pressure depends on sodium-potassium adenosine triphosphatase (sodium pump), which, if absent, would permit sodium and chloride ions to enter cells along their concentration gradients and water would follow among the osmotic gradient, causing the cells to swell.

CHANGES IN VOLUMES OF BODY FLUID COMPARTMENTS

Factors that may alter extracellular fluid or intracellular fluid volumes significantly include infusion of fluids and dehydration from gastrointestinal fluid loss, diaphoresis, and fluid loss by the kidneys. As a rule, chronic diseases are characterized by a decline in intracellular fluid volume and concomitant expansion of extracellular fluid volume.

Intravenous Fluids

The goal of fluid management is to maintain normovolemia characterized by hemodynamic stability. Crystalloids consist of water, electrolytes, and occasionally glucose that freely distribute along a concentration gradient between the two extracellular spaces. After 20 to 30 minutes, an estimated 75% to 80% of an isotonic saline or a lactate-containing solution will have distributed outside the confines of the circulation, thus limiting the efficacy of these solutions in treating hypovolemia. Indeed, the ability of crystalloids to restore perfusion in the microcirculation is doubtful (Funk and Baldinger, 1995).

Intravenous fluids that do not remain in the circulation can dilute extracellular fluid, causing it to become hypotonic with respect to intracellular fluid. When this occurs, osmosis begins instantly at cell membranes, with large amounts of water entering cells. Within a few minutes, this water becomes distributed almost evenly among all body fluid compartments. Increased intracellular fluid volume is particularly undesirable in patients with intracranial masses or increased intracranial pressure. Protection from excessive fluid accumulation in the interstitium (extravascular lung water) is mediated by lympahtic flow, which can increase as much as tenfold.

Hypertonic Saline

Hypertonic saline solutions (7.5% sodium chloride) have been useful for rapid intravascular fluid repletion during resuscitation as during hemorrhagic and septic shock. Hyertonic saline solutions compare favorably with mannitol for lowering inctracranial pressure (Qureshi and Suaarez, 2000). The primary effect of hypertonic saline solutions (increase systemic blood pressure and decrease intracranial pressure) most likely reflects increased intravascular fluid volume because of fluid shifts and movement of water away from uninjured region of the brain. The use of hypertonic saline solutions is viewed as short-term treatment as hypertonicity and hypernatremia are likely with sustained administration. Furthermore, patients with hypotension due to traumatic brain injury who received prehospital resuscitation with hypertonic saline solutions have similar neurologic outcomes to those treated with conventional fluids after 6 months (Cooper et al., 2004).

Dehydration

Loss of water by gastrointestinal or renal routes or by diaphoresis is associated with an initial deficit in extracellular fluid volume. At the same instant, intracellular water passes to the extracellular fluid compartment by osmosis, thus keeping the osmolarities in both compartments equal despite decreased absolute volume (dehydration) of both compartments. The ratio of extracellular fluid to intracellular fluid is greater in infants than adults, but the absolute volume of extracellular fluid is obviously less, explaining why dehydration develops more rapidly and is often more severe in the very young. Clinical signs of dehydration are likely when about 5% to 10% (severe dehydration) of total body fluids have been lost in a brief period of time. Physiologic mechanisms can usually compensate for acute loss of 15% to 25% of the intravascular fluid volume, whereas a greater loss places the patient at risk for hemodynamic decompensation.

REFERENCES

Cooper DJ, Myles PS, McDermott FT, et al. Prehospital hypertonic saline resuscitation of patients with hypotension and severe traumatic brain injury. A randomized controlled trial. *JAMA* 2004; 291:1350–1357.

Funk W, Baldinger V. Microcirculatory perfusion during volume therapy. A comparative studyusing crystalloid or colloid in awake animals. *Anesthesiology* 1995;82: 975–982.

Gamble JL. *Chemical anatomy, physiology, and pathology of extracellular fluid*, 6th ed. Boston: Harvard University Press, 1954.

Ganong WF. *Review of medical physiology*, 21st ed. New York: Lange Medical Books/McGraw-Hill, 2003.

Guyton AC, Hall JE. *Textbook of medical physiology*, 10th ed. Philadelphia: W.B. Saunders, 2000.

Leaf A, Newburgh LH. *Significance of the body fluids in chemical medicine*, 2nd ed. Springfield, IL: Charles C Thomas, 1955.

Qureshi AI, Suarez JI. Use of hypertonic saline solutions in treatment of cerebral edema and intracranial hypertension. *Crit Care Med* 2000;28:3301–3313.

Central Nervous System

41

The brain is a complex collection of neural systems that regulate their own and each other's activity. For example, activity of the central nervous system (CNS) reflects a balance between excitatory and inhibitory influences that are normally maintained within relatively narrow limits. Anatomic divisions of the brain reflect the distribution of brain functions. The three components of the CNS are the cerebral hemispheres, brainstem, and spinal cord. The two cerebral hemispheres constitute the cerebral cortex, where sensory, motor, and associational information is processed. The limbic system lies beneath the cerebral cortex and integrates the emotional state with motor and visceral activities. The thalamus lies in the center of the brain beneath the cerebral cortex and basal ganglia and above the hypothalamus. The neurons of the thalamus are arranged in nuclei that act as relays between the incoming sensory pathways and the cerebral cortex, hypothalamus, and basal ganglia. The hypothalamus is the principal integrating region for the autonomic nervous system (ANS) and regulates other functions, including systemic blood pressure, body temperature, water balance, secretions of the pituitary gland, emotions, and sleep.

The brainstem connects the cerebral cortex to the spinal cord and contains most of the nuclei of the cranial nerves and the reticular activating system. The reticular activating system is essential for regulation of sleep and wakefulness. The cerebellum arises from the posterior pons and is responsible for maintenance of body posture.

The spinal cord extends from the medulla oblongata to the lower lumbar vertebrae. Ascending and descending tracts are located within the white matter of the spinal cord, whereas intersegmental connections and synaptic contacts are concentrated in the gray matter. Sensory information flows into the dorsal portion of the gray matter, and motor outflow exits from the ventral portion. Preganglionic neurons of the ANS are found in the intermediolateral portions of the gray matter.

CEREBRAL HEMISPHERES

The two cerebral hemispheres, known as the *cerebral cortex*, constitute the largest division of the human brain. Regions of the cerebral cortex are classified as *sensory*, *motor*, *visual*, *auditory*, and *olfactory*, depending on the type of information that is processed. *Frontal*, *temporal*, *parietal*, and *occipital* designate anatomic positions of the cerebral cortex. For each area of the cerebral cortex, there is a corresponding and connecting area to the thalamus such that stimulation of a small portion of the thalamus activates the corresponding and much larger portion of the cerebral cortex. Indeed, the cerebral cortex is actually an outgrowth of the lower regions of the nervous system, especially the thalamus. The functional part of the cerebral cortex is comprised mainly of a 2- to 5-mm layer of neurons covering the surface of all the convolutions. It is estimated that the cerebral cortex contains 50 to 100 billion neurons.

Anatomy of the Cerebral Cortex

The sensorimotor cortex is the area of the cerebral cortex responsible for receiving sensation from sensory areas of the body and for controlling body movement (Fig. 41-1) (Guyton and Hall, 2000). The premotor cortex is important for controlling the functions of the motor cortex. The motor cortex lies anterior to the central sulcus. Its posterior portion is characterized by the presence of large, pyramid-shaped (pyramidal or Betz) cells.

Topographic Areas

The area of the cerebral cortex to which the peripheral sensory signals are projected from the thalamus is designated the *somesthetic cortex* (see Fig. 41-1) (Guyton and Hall, 2000). Each side of the cerebral cortex receives sensory information exclusively from the opposite side of the body. The size of these areas is directly proportional to the number of specialized sensory receptors in each respective area of the body. For example, a large number of specialized nerve endings are present in the lips and the thumbs, whereas only a few are present in the skin of the trunk.

In the motor cortex, there are various topographic areas from which skeletal muscles in different parts of the body can be activated. In general, the size of the area in the motor cortex is proportional to the preciseness of the skeletal muscle movement required. As such, the digits,

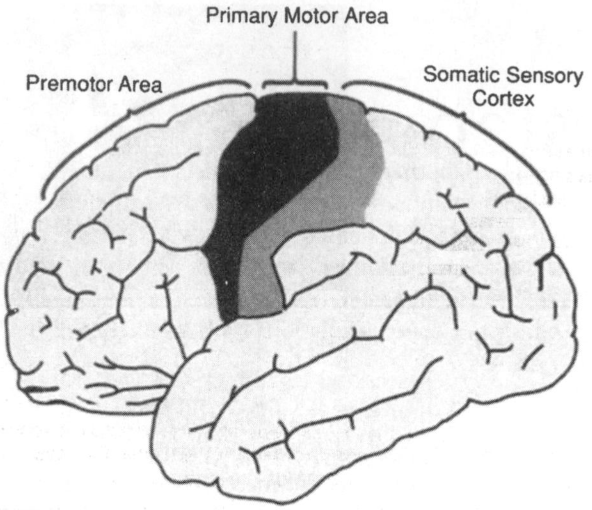

Figure 41-1. The sensorimotor cortex consists of the motor cortex, pyramidal (Betz) cells, and somatic sensory cortex. (From Guyton AC, Hall JE. *Textbook of medical physiology*, 10th ed. Philadelphia. Saunders, 2000; with permission.)

lips, tongue, and vocal cords have large representations in humans. The various topographic areas in the motor cortex were originally determined by electrical stimulation of the brain during local anesthesia and observation of the evoked skeletal muscle response. Such stimulation can be used intraoperatively to identify the location of the motor cortex and thus avoid damage to this area. The motor cortex is commonly damaged by loss of blood supply as occurs during a stroke. The spatial organization of the somatic sensory cortex is similar to the motor areas of the cerebral cortex.

Corpus Callosum

The two hemispheres of the cerebral cortex, with the exception of the anterior portions of the temporal lobes, are connected by fibers in the corpus callosum. The anterior portions of the temporal lobes, including the amygdala, are connected by fibers that pass through the anterior commissure. One of the functions of the corpus callosum and anterior commissure is to make information stored in one hemisphere available to the other hemisphere.

Dominant versus Nondominant Hemisphere

Language function and interpretation depend more on one cerebral hemisphere (dominant hemisphere) than the other, whereas spatiotemporal relationships (ability to recognize faces) depend on the other nondominant hemisphere. Based on genetic determinations, 90% of individuals are right-handed and the left hemisphere is dominant. Likewise, the left hemisphere is dominant in about 70% of persons who are left-handed. For reasons that are not clear, dyslexia is more common in left-handed persons. Destruction of the dominant cerebral hemisphere results in loss of nearly all intellectual function, whereas destruction of the prefrontal areas of the frontal lobes is less harmful.

Failure to document an important role of prefrontal lobes in intellectual function is surprising because the principal difference between the brains of humans and monkeys is the prominence of human prefrontal areas. It seems that the function of the prefrontal areas in humans is to provide additional cortical area in which cerebration can occur. Furthermore, selection of behavior patterns for different situations may be an important role of the prefrontal areas that transmit signals to the limbic areas of the brain. Persons without prefrontal lobes may react precipitously in response to incoming signals, manifesting undue anger at slight provocations. Ability to maintain a sustained level of concentration is lost in the absence of the prefrontal lobes.

Memory

The cerebral cortex, especially the temporal lobes, serves as a storage site for information that is often characterized as memory (Budson and Price, 2005). The mechanisms for short-term and long-term memory are not documented.

Short-Term Memory

Short-term memory may involve the presence of reverberating circuits. As the reverberating circuit fatigues or as new signals interfere with the reverberations, the short-term memory fades. Evidence in favor of a reverberating theory of short-term memory is the ability of a general disturbance of brain function (fright, loud noise) to erase short-term memory immediately.

An alternative explanation for short-term memory is the phenomenon of posttetanic potentiation. For example, tetanic stimulation of a synapse for a few seconds causes increased excitability of the synapse that lasts for seconds to hours. This change in excitability of the synapse could function as short-term memory. Another change that often occurs in neurons after a prolonged period of excitation is a sustained decrease in the resting transmembrane potential of the neuron. This change in excitability of the neuron could also result in short-term memory.

Long-Term Memory

Long-term memory does not depend on continued activity of the nervous system, as evidenced by total inactivation of the brain by hypothermia or anesthesia without detectable significant loss of long-term memory. Nevertheless, postoperative cognitive dysfunction (impaired memory) persisting after 3 months has been described in 10% of elderly patients receiving general anesthesia without arterial hypoxemia or systemic hypotension (Moller et al., 1998). It is assumed that long-term memory results from physical or chemical alterations in the size and conductivities of the dendrites. These anatomic changes could cause permanent or semipermanent increases in the degree of facilitation of specific neuronal circuits. The entire facilitated circuit is called a *memory engram* or *memory trace*. If memory is to persist, these synapses must be permanently facilitated (consolidated). Maximum consolidation requires at least 1 hour. For example, if a strong sensory impression is made on the brain but is followed within a few seconds by a disruptive signal, such as an electrically induced convulsion or institution of deep general anesthesia, the sensory experience is erased. An obvious analogy is the lightly anesthetized patient who reacts purposefully to a painful stimulus but later has no recall if the depth of anesthesia is increased after the purposeful movement. Conversely, the same sensory stimulus allowed to persist for 5 to 10 minutes may result in at least partial establishment of a memory trace. If the sensory stimulus is unopposed for 60 minutes, it is likely the memory will have become fully consolidated. Indeed, intraoperative awareness with or without associated pain is a recognized phenomenon, especially when minimal amounts of anesthetic drugs are combined with neuromuscular-blocking drugs (see the section on Awareness during Anesthesia).

Rehearsal of the same information accelerates and potentiates the process of consolidation, thus converting short-term memory to long-term memory. This explains why a person can remember small amounts of information studied in depth better than large amounts of information studied only superficially. Each time a memory is recalled, a more indelible memory trace develops that may last a lifetime. An important feature of consolidation is that long-term memory is encoded into different categories. Thus, during consolidation, new memories are not stored randomly in the brain but rather are stored in association with previously encoded and similar information. This form of storage is necessary to permit scanning of the memory store to retrieve desired information at a later date.

Awareness during Anesthesia

Awareness, defined as conscious memory of events during anesthesia, has been a recurrent problem since the introduction of neuromuscular-blocking drugs (Ghoneim, 2000). Memory may be considered to be conscious (explicit) or unconscious (implicit). Conscious memory includes spontaneous recall and recognition memory, both of which occur with the aid of a specific cue. Unconscious memory is manifest by altered performance or behavior due to unremembered experiences. By definition, general anesthesia abolishes conscious memory, but whether it also abolishes unconscious memory of verbal information is controversial.

The incidence of awareness with recall (conscious memory) following general anesthesia is estimated to be 0.13% (Sebel et al., 2004). Although the incidence of conscious recall of intraoperative events is rare and the development of posttraumatic stress disorder is even more uncommon, the fact that approximately 20 million general anesthetics are administered annually in the United States corresponds to 26,000 cases of awareness (0.13% of approximately 20 million) each year. The incidence of awareness in patients undergoing cesarean section was 0.4% and for cardiac surgery was 1.14% to 1.50% (Lyons and MacDonald, 1991; Ranta et al., 1996). A higher incidence of awareness has been described for major trauma cases (11% to 43%) (Bogetz and Katz, 1984). Many cases of conscious awareness during surgery can be attributed to physician error and/or equipment malfunction.

Subanesthetic doses of inhaled anesthetics have powerful inhibitory effects on short-term memory, and the decrease in the transfer of information from the periphery to the cerebral cortex associated with general anesthesia prevents the recall of intraoperative events (Hudspith, 1997). Excitatory amino acid neurotransmitters are important in the pharmacology of learning and memory, especially in the hippocampus. With respect to absence of memory for intraoperative events, it is important to recognize that inhibition of excitatory amino acid neurotransmitters is a common property of inhaled anesthetics.

Isoflurane (and presumably other volatile anesthetics) and nitrous oxide suppress memory in a dose-dependent manner, and isoflurane is more potent than equivalent concentrations of nitrous oxide (Fig. 41-2) (Dwyer et al., 1992a). For example, conscious memory was prevented by 0.45 MAC isoflurane or 0.6 MAC nitrous oxide. Isoflurane concentrations of ≥0.6 MAC prevent conscious recall and unconscious learning of factual information and behavioral suggestions (Dwyer et al., 1992b).

Recognizing Awareness

Monitoring patients during general anesthesia for the presence of awareness is challenging. Despite a variety of monitoring methods, awareness is difficult to recognize in real time. Indicators of awareness (heart rate, blood pressure

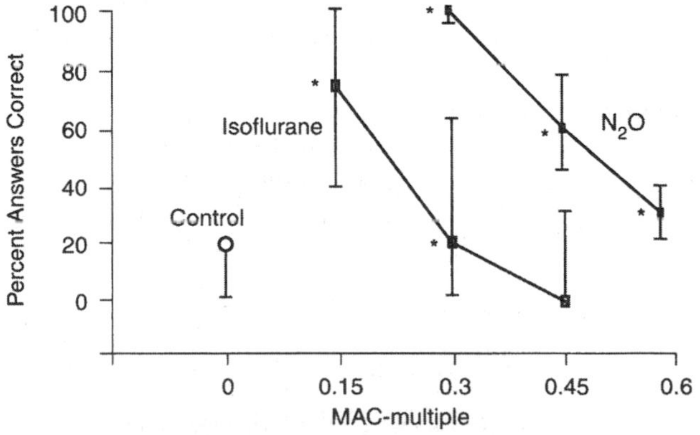

Figure 41-2. Percentage of correct answers for each anesthetic at increasing anesthetic concentrations. (From Dwyer R, Bennett HL, Eger EI, et al. Effects of isoflurane and nitrous oxide in subanesthetic concentrations on memory and responsiveness in volunteers. *Anesthesiology* 1992;77:888–898; with permission.)

and skeletal muscle movement) are often masked by anesthetic and adjuvant drugs (beta-adrenergic blockers) and/or neuromuscular-blocking drugs. Methods to recognize awareness that are less affected by drugs include brain wave monitors such as the Bispectral Index (BIS). Based on published studies, the Food and Drug Administration has determined that use of BIS monitoring to guide anesthetic administration may be associated with a reduction of the incidence of awareness with recall in adults during general anesthesia and sedation (Ekman et al., 2004; Lennmarken and Sandin, 2004; Myles et al., 2004).

Pyramidal and Extrapyramidal Tracts

A major pathway for transmission of motor signals from the cerebral cortex to the anterior motor neurons of the spinal cord is through the pyramidal (corticospinal) tracts (Fig. 41-3) (Guyton and Hall, 2000). All pyramidal tract fibers pass downward through the brainstem and then cross to the opposite side to form the pyramids of the medulla. After crossing the midline at the level of the medulla, these fibers descend in the lateral corticospinal tracts of the spinal cord and terminate on motor neurons in the dorsal horn of the spinal cord. A few fibers do not cross to the opposite side of the medulla but rather descend in the ventral corticospinal tracts. In addition to these pyramidal fibers, a large number of collateral fibers pass from the motor cortex into the basal ganglia, forming the extrapyramidal tracts. Extrapyramidal tracts are all those tracts beside the pyramidal tracts that transmit motor impulses from the cerebral cortex to the spinal cord.

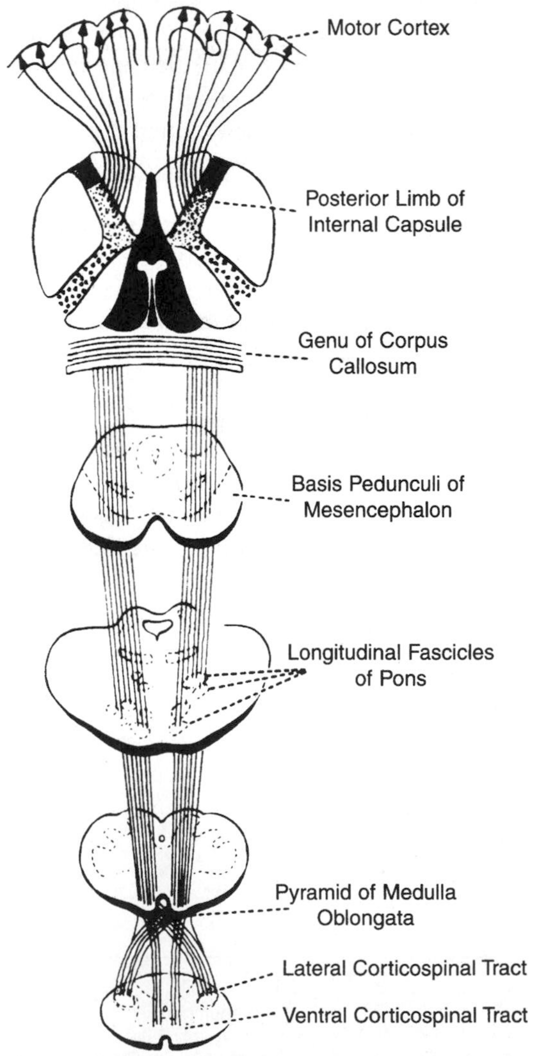

Figure 41-3. The pyramidal tracts are major pathways for transmission of motor signals from the cerebral cortex to the spinal cord. (From Guyton AC, Hall JE. *Textbook of medical physiology*, 10th ed. Philadelphia. Saunders, 2000; with permission.)

The pyramidal and extrapyramidal tracts have opposing effects on the tone of skeletal muscles. For example, the pyramidal tracts cause continuous facilitation and therefore a tendency to produce increases in skeletal muscle tone. Conversely, the extrapyramidal tracts transmit inhibitory signals through the basal ganglia with resultant inhibition of skeletal muscle tone. Selective or predominant damage to one of these tracts manifests as spasticity or flaccidity.

Babinski Sign

A positive Babinski sign is characterized by upward extension of the first toe and outward fanning of the other toes in response to a firm tactile stimulus applied to the dorsum of the foot. A normal response to the same tactile stimulus is downward motion of all the toes. A positive Babinski sign reflects damage to the pyramidal tracts. Damage to the extrapyramidal tracts does not cause a positive Babinski sign.

Thalamocortical System

The thalamocortical system serves as the pathway for passage of nearly all afferent impulses from the cerebellum; basal ganglia; and visual, auditory, taste, and pain receptors as they pass through the thalamus on the way to the cerebral cortex. Signals from olfactory receptors are the only peripheral sensory signals that do not pass through the thalamus. Overall, the thalamocortical system controls the activity level of the cerebral cortex.

BRAINSTEM

Subconscious activities of the body (intrinsic life processes) are controlled in the brainstem. The brainstem includes the medulla, pons, thalamus, limbic system, basal ganglia, reticular activating system, and cerebellum. Examples of subconscious activities of the body regulated by the brainstem include control of systemic blood pressure and breathing in the medulla. The thalamus serves as a relay station for most afferent impulses before they are transmitted to the cerebral cortex. The hypothalamus receives fibers from the thalamus and is also closely associated with the cerebral cortex.

Limbic System and Hypothalamus

Behavior associated with emotions is primarily a function of structures known as the *limbic system* (hippocampus, basal ganglia) located in the basal regions of the brain. The hypothalamus functions in many of the same roles as the limbic system and is considered by some to be part of the limbic system rather than a separate structure. In addition, the hypothalamus controls many internal conditions of the body, such as core temperature, thirst, and appetite. These internal functions represent responses whose control is closely related to behavior. In addition, the hypothalamus indirectly affects cerebral function, and thus behavior, by activation or inhibition of the reticular activating system.

Basal Ganglia

The basal ganglia include the caudate nucleus, putamen, globus pallidus, substantia nigra, and subthalamus. Many of the impulses from basal ganglia are inhibitory, and the inhibitory neurotransmitters are dopamine and gamma-aminobutyric acid (GABA). The balance between agonist and antagonist skeletal muscle contractions is an important role of the basal ganglia. A general effect of diffuse excitation of the basal ganglia is inhibition of skeletal muscles, reflecting transmission of inhibitory signals from the basal ganglia to both the motor cortex and the lower brainstem. Therefore, whenever destruction of the basal ganglia occurs, there is associated skeletal muscle rigidity. For example, damage to the caudate and putamen nuclei that normally secrete GABA results in random and continuous uncontrolled movements designated as *chorea*. Destruction of the substantia nigra and loss of dopamine result in a predominance of the excitatory neurotransmitter acetylcholine, manifesting as skeletal muscle rigidity that is characterized as Parkinson disease. Indeed, dopamine precursors or anticholinergic drugs are used in the treatment of Parkinson disease in an attempt to restore the balance between excitatory and inhibitory impulses traveling from the basal ganglia (see Chapter 31).

Reticular Activating System

The reticular activating system is a polysynaptic pathway that is intimately concerned with electrical activity of the cerebral cortex. Neurons of the reticular activating system are both excitatory and inhibitory, and the presumed neurotransmitter is acetylcholine. The reticular activating system determines the overall level of CNS activity, including wakefulness and sleep. Selective activation of certain areas of the cerebral cortex by the reticular activating system is crucial for the direction of the attention of certain aspects of mental activity. It is likely that many of the clinically used, injected and inhaled anesthetics, exert depressant effects on the reticular activating system.

Sleep and Wakefulness

Sleep is a state of unconsciousness from which an individual can be aroused by sensory stimulation. Therefore, depression of the reticular activating system by anesthetics or as present in comatose individuals cannot be defined as sleep. Sleep can occur from decreased activity of the reticular activating system (slow-wave sleep) or it can result from abnormal channeling of signals in the brain, even though activity of the reticular activating system may not be depressed (desynchronized sleep). Depletion of CNS catecholamine stores by antihypertensive drugs is associated with sedation and decreases in anesthetic requirements (MAC) for inhaled drugs (Miller et al., 1968).

Slow-Wave Sleep

Most of the sleep that occurs each night is slow-wave sleep. The electroencephalogram (EEG) is characterized by the presence of high-voltage delta waves occurring at a frequency of <4 cycles per second. Presumably, decreased activity of the reticular activating system that accompanies sleep permits an unmasking of this inherent rhythm in the cerebral cortex. Slow-wave sleep is restful and devoid of dreams. During slow-wave sleep, sympathetic nervous system activity decreases, parasympathetic nervous system activity increases, and skeletal muscle tone is greatly decreased. As a result, there is a 10% to 30% decrease in systemic blood pressure, heart rate, breathing frequency, and basal metabolic rate.

Desynchronized Sleep

Periods of desynchronized sleep typically occur for 5 to 20 minutes during each 90 minutes of sleep. These periods tend to be shortest when the person is extremely tired. This form of sleep is characterized by active dreaming, irregular heart rate and breathing, and a desynchronized pattern of low-voltage beta waves on the EEG similar to those that occur during wakefulness. This brain wave pattern emphasizes that desynchronized sleep is associated with an active cerebral cortex, but this activity is not channeled in a direction that permits persons to be aware of their surroundings and thus be awake. Despite the inhibition of skeletal muscle activity, the eyes are an exception, exhibiting rapid movements. For this reason, desynchronized sleep is also referred to as *paradoxical sleep* or *rapid eye movement sleep*.

Cerebellum

The cerebellum operates subconsciously to monitor and elicit corrective responses in motor activity caused by stimulation of other parts of the brain and spinal cord. Rapid skeletal muscle activities, such as typing, playing musical instruments, and running, require intact function of the cerebellum. Loss of function of the cerebellum causes incoordination of fine skeletal muscle activities even though paralysis of the skeletal muscles does not occur. The cerebellum is also important in the maintenance of equilibrium and postural adjustments of the body. For example, sensory signals are transmitted to the cerebellum from receptors in muscle spindles, Golgi tendon organs, and receptors in skin joints. These spinocerebellar pathways can transmit impulses at velocities of >100 m per second, which is the most rapid conduction of any pathway in the CNS. This extremely rapid conduction is important for instantaneous appraisal by the cerebellum of changes that take place in the positional status of the body.

Dysfunction of the Cerebellum

In the absence of cerebellar function, a person cannot predict prospectively how far movements will go; this results in overshoot of the intended mark (past pointing). This overshoot is known as *dysmetria*, and the resulting incoordinate movements are called *ataxia*. Dysarthria is present when rapid and orderly succession of skeletal muscle movements of the larynx, mouth, and chest do not occur. Failure of the cerebellum to dampen skeletal muscle movements results in intention tremor when a person performs a voluntary act. Cerebellar nystagmus is associated with loss of equilibrium, presumably because of dysfunction of the pathways that pass through the cerebellum from the semicircular canals. In the presence of cerebellar disease, a person is unable to activate antagonist skeletal muscles that prevent a certain portion of the body from moving unexpectedly in an unwanted direction. For example, a person's arm that was previously contracted but restrained by another person will move back rapidly when it is released rather than automatically remain in place.

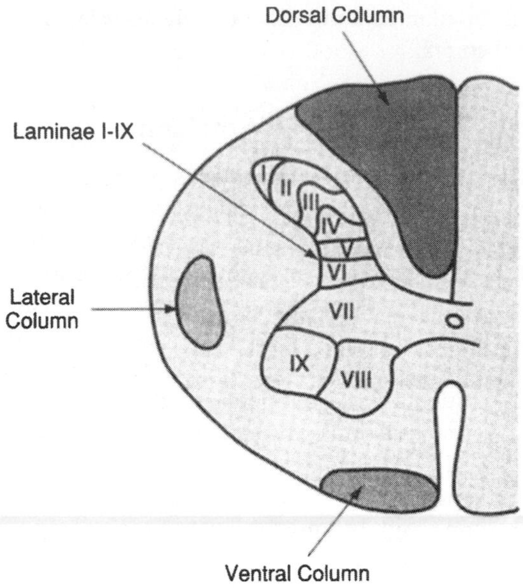

Figure 41-4. Schematic diagram of a cross-section of the spinal cord depicting anatomic laminae I to IX of the spinal cord gray matter and the ascending dorsal, lateral, and ventral sensory columns of the spinal cord white matter.

SPINAL CORD

The spinal cord extends from the medulla oblongata to the lower border of the first and, occasionally, the second lumbar vertebra. Below the spinal cord, the vertebral canal is filled by the roots of the lumbar and sacral nerves, which are collectively known as the *cauda equina*. The spinal cord is composed of gray and white matter, spinal nerves, and covering membranes.

Gray Matter

The gray matter of the spinal cord functions as the initial processor of incoming sensory signals from peripheral somatic receptors and as a relay station to send these signals to the brain. In addition, this area of the spinal cord is the site for final processing of motor signals that are being transmitted downward from the brain to skeletal muscles. Anatomically, the gray matter of the spinal cord is divided into anterior, lateral, and dorsal horns consisting of nine separate laminae that are H shaped when viewed in cross-section (Fig. 41-4). The anterior horn is the location of alpha and gamma motor neurons that give rise to nerve fibers that leave the spinal cord via the anterior (ventral) nerve roots and innervate skeletal muscles. Cells of Renshaw in the anterior horn are intermediary neurons, providing nerve fibers that synapse in the gray matter with anterior motor neurons. These cells inhibit the action of anterior motor neurons to limit excessive activity. Cells of the preganglionic neurons of the sympathetic nervous system are located in the lateral horns of the thoracolumbar portions of the spinal cord. Cells of the intermediate neurons located in the portion of the dorsal horns of the spinal cord known as the *substantia gelatinosa* (laminae II to III) transmit afferent tactile, temperature, and pain impulses to the spinothalamic tract. The dorsal horn serves as a gate where impulses in sensory nerve fibers are translated into impulses in ascending tracts (see Chapter 43).

White Matter

The white matter of the spinal cord is formed by the axons of intermediate neurons and their respective ascending and descending tracts. This area of the spinal cord is divided into dorsal, lateral, and ventral columns (see Fig. 41-4). The dorsal column of the spinal cord is composed of spinothalamic tracts that transmit touch and pain impulses to the brain.

Imaging of the Nervous System

Until the introduction of computed tomography (CT), imaging studies of the brain included skull radiography, cerebral angiography, and pneumoencephalography (Gilman,

1992). These techniques allowed only examination of the skull, the cerebral blood vessels, and the fluid-containing spaces of the brain. CT and subsequently magnetic resonance imaging (MRI) provide images of brain tissue directly and discrimination between gray and white matter. Positron emission tomography (PET) and single photon emission computed tomography (SPECT) permit imaging of both structure and functional characteristics (blood flow, metabolism, concentrations of neurochemicals) of the brain.

Comparative studies indicate that MRI is superior to CT in evaluating most cerebral parenchymal lesions (Gilman, 1992). Nevertheless, CT is preferable for patients with acute trauma who are accompanied by cumbersome life-support equipment or patients who cannot voluntarily remain immobile (uncooperative, movement disorders, children) as required for MRI. CT is used in patients who cannot undergo MRI because of the presence of artificial cardiac pacemakers, mechanical heart valves, or magnetizable intracranial metal clips and in individuals who experience claustrophobia. CT is the imaging procedure of choice after injuries to the head or spine because of its rapidity. CT is also useful in visualizing intracranial blood that may be present in patients with subdural hematomas or cerebral hemorrhage.

Spinal Nerve

A pair of spinal nerves arises from each of 31 segments of the spinal cord. Spinal nerves are made up of fibers of the anterior and dorsal (posterior) roots. Efferent motor fibers travel in the anterior roots that originate from axons in the anterior and lateral horns of the spinal cord gray matter. Sensory fibers travel in the dorsal nerve roots that originate from axons that arise from cell bodies in the spinal cord ganglia. These cell bodies send branches to the spinal cord and to the periphery. The anterior and dorsal nerve roots each leave the spinal cord through an individual intervertebral foramen enclosed in a common dural sheath that extends just past the spinal cord ganglia where the spinal nerve originates.

Each spinal nerve innervates a segmental area of skin designated a *dermatome* and an area of skeletal muscle known as a *myotome*. A dermatome map is useful in determining the level of spinal cord injury or level of sensory anesthesia produced by a regional anesthetic (Fig. 41-5) (Guyton and Hall, 2000). Despite common depictions of dermatomes as having distinct borders, there is extensive overlap between segments. For example, three consecutive dorsal nerve roots need to be interrupted to produce complete denervation of a dermatome. The scrotum has considerable sensory overlap, with innervation coming from T1 (variable) and L1 to L2 and S2 to S4 despite common depictions on dermatome charts as being limited to sacral innervation (Sprung et al., 1993). Segmental innervation of myotomes is even less well defined than that of der-

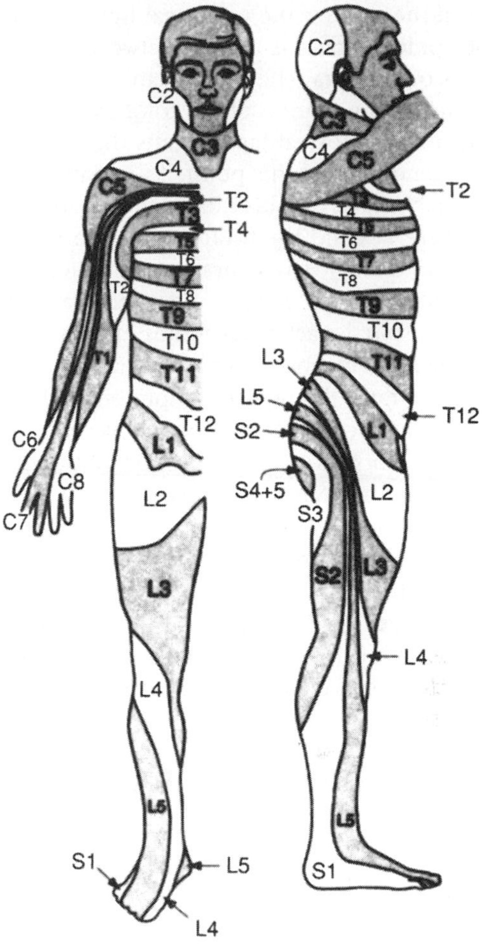

Figure 41-5. Dermatome map that may be used to evaluate the level of sensory anesthesia produced by regional anesthesia. (From Guyton AC, Hall JE. *Textbook of medical physiology*, 10th ed. Philadelphia. Saunders, 2000; with permission.)

matomes, emphasizing that skeletal muscle groups receive innervation from several anterior nerve roots.

Sensory signals from the periphery are transmitted through spinal nerves into each segment of the spinal cord, resulting in automatic motor responses that occur instantly (muscle stretch reflex, withdrawal reflex) in response to sensory signals. Spinal cord reflexes are important, causing emptying of the bladder and rectum. Segmental temperature reflexes allow localized cutaneous vasodilation or vasoconstriction in response to changes in skin temperature. The function of the spinal cord component of the CNS and spinal cord reflexes is particularly apparent in patients with transection of the spinal cord.

Covering Membranes

The spinal cord is enveloped by membranes (dura, arachnoid, pia) that are direct continuations of the corresponding membranes surrounding the brain. The dura consists of an inner and an outer layer. The outer periosteal layer in the cranial cavity is the periosteum of the skull, whereas this layer in the spine is the periosteal lining of the spinal cord. The epidural space is located between the inner and outer layers of the dura. The fact that the inner layer of the dura adheres to the margin of the foramen magnum and blends with the periosteal layer means the epidural space does not extend beyond this point. As a result, drugs such as local anesthetics or opioids cannot travel cephalad in the epidural space beyond the foramen magnum. The inner layer of the dura extends as a dural cuff that blends with the perineurium of spinal nerves. The cerebral arachnoid extends as the spinal arachnoid, ending at the second sacral vertebra. The pia is in close contact with the spinal cord.

CT demonstrates the occasional presence of a connective tissue band (dorsomedian connective tissue band or plica mediana dorsalis) that divides the epidural space at the dorsal midline (Savolaine et al., 1988). This band binds the dura mater and the ligamentum flavum at the midline, making it difficult to feel loss of resistance during attempted midline identification of the epidural space. The band may also explain the occasional occurrence of unilateral analgesia after injection of local anesthetic solutions into the epidural space (Gallart et al., 1990).

PATHWAYS FOR PERIPHERAL SENSORY IMPULSES

Sensory information from somatic segments of the body enter the gray matter of the spinal cord via the dorsal nerve roots. After entering the spinal cord, these neurons give rise to long, ascending fiber tracts that transmit sensory information to the brain. These sensory signals are transmitted to the brain by the dorsal-lemniscal system, which includes dorsal column pathways and spinocervical tracts, and by anterolateral spinothalamic tracts (Figs. 41-6 and 41-7) (Guyton and Hall, 2000). Impulses in the dorsal column pathways cross in the spinal cord to the opposite side before passing upward to the thalamus. Synapses in the thalamus are followed by neurons that extend into the somatic sensory area of the cerebral cortex. Nerve fibers of the anterolateral spinothalamic system cross in the anterior commissure to the opposite side of the spinal cord, where they turn upward toward the brain as the ventral and lateral spinothalamic tracts. Sensory signals from the anterolateral spinothalamic system are relayed from the thalamus to the somatic sensory area of the cerebral cortex. All sensory information that enters the cerebral cortex, with the exception of the olfactory system, passes through the thalamus.

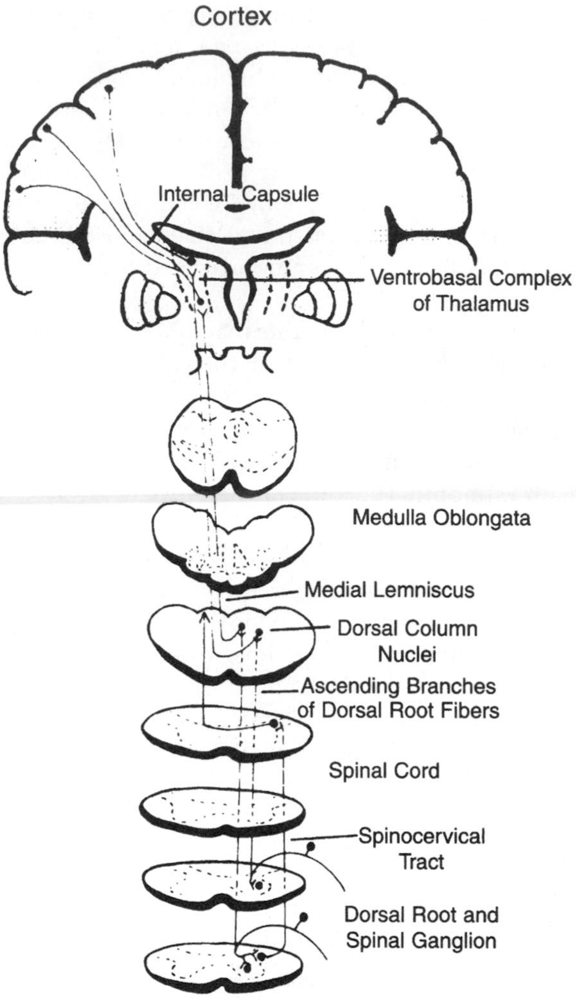

Figure 41-6. Sensory signals are transmitted to the brain by the dorsal column pathways and spinocervical tracts of the dorsal-lemniscal system. (From Guyton AC, Hall JE. *Textbook of medical physiology*, 10th ed. Philadelphia. Saunders, 2000; with permission.)

PATHWAYS FOR PERIPHERAL MOTOR RESPONSES

Sensory information is integrated at all levels of the nervous system and causes appropriate motor responses, beginning in the spinal cord with relatively simple reflex responses. Motor responses originating in the brainstem are more complex, whereas the most complicated and precise motor responses originate from the cerebral cortex.

Anterior motor neurons in the anterior horns of the spinal cord gray matter give rise to A-alpha fibers, that leave the spinal cord by way of anterior nerve roots and innervate skeletal muscles. Skeletal muscles and tendons contain muscle spindles and Golgi tendon organs that operate at a subconscious level to relay information to the spinal cord and brain relative to changes in length and tension of skeletal muscle fibers. The stretch reflex is reflex contraction of the skeletal muscle whenever stretch results in stimulation of the muscle spindle. Tapping the patellar tendon elicits a knee jerk, which is a stretch reflex of the quadriceps femoris muscle. The ankle jerk is due to reflex contraction of the gastrocnemius muscle. Transmission of large numbers of facilitatory impulses from upper regions of the CNS to the spinal cord results in exaggerated stretch reflex responses. For example, lesions in the contralateral

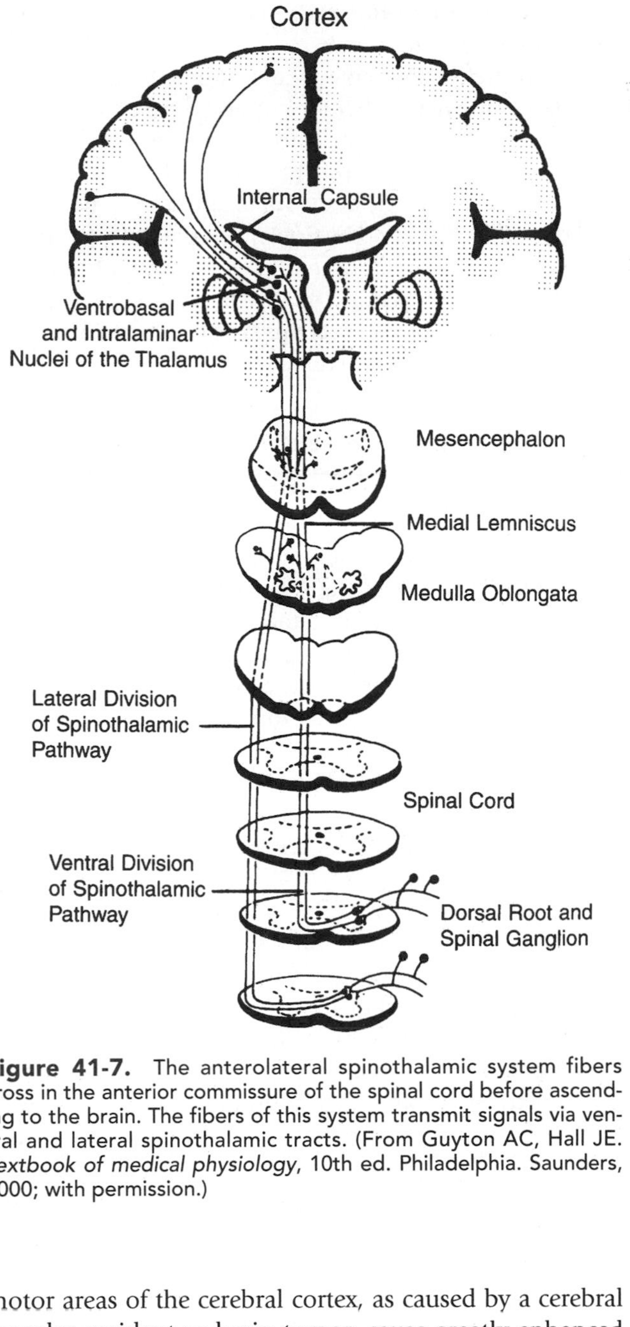

Figure 41-7. The anterolateral spinothalamic system fibers cross in the anterior commissure of the spinal cord before ascending to the brain. The fibers of this system transmit signals via ventral and lateral spinothalamic tracts. (From Guyton AC, Hall JE. *Textbook of medical physiology*, 10th ed. Philadelphia. Saunders, 2000; with permission.)

motor areas of the cerebral cortex, as caused by a cerebral vascular accident or brain tumor, cause greatly enhanced stretch reflexes. Clonus occurs when evoked muscle jerks oscillate. This phenomenon typically occurs when the stretch reflex is sensitized by facilitatory impulses from the brain, resulting in exaggerated facilitation of the spinal cord. When associated with recovery from general anesthesia, clonus as initiated by abrupt dorsiflexion of the foot can be eliminated by flexing the knees and keeping them in a flexed position (Azzam, 1987).

Transection of the brainstem at the level of the pons (isolates the spinal cord from the rest of the brain) results in spasticity known as *decerebrate rigidity*. Decerebrate rigidity reflects diffuse facilitation of stretch reflexes.

The motor system is often divided into upper and lower motor neurons. Lower motor neurons are those from the spinal cord that directly innervate skeletal muscles. A lower motor neuron lesion is associated with flaccid paralysis, atrophy of skeletal muscles, and absence of stretch reflex responses. Spastic paralysis with accentuated stretch reflexes in the absence of skeletal muscle paralysis is due to destruction of upper motor neurons in the brain.

Withdrawal flexor reflexes are most often elicited by a painful stimulus. Associated with withdrawal of the stimulated limb is extension of the opposite limb (cross-extensor reflex) that occurs 0.2 to 0.5 s later and serves to push the body away from the object causing the painful stimulus. The delayed onset of the cross-extensor reflex is due to the time necessary for the signal to pass through the additional neurons to reach the opposite side of the spinal cord.

Spasm of skeletal muscles surrounding a broken bone seems to result from nociceptive impulses initiated from the broken edges of bone. Relief of pain and skeletal muscle spasm is provided by infiltration of a local anesthetic at the injured site. In some instances, general anesthesia may be necessary to relieve skeletal muscle spasm and permit proper alignment of the two ends of the bone. Abdominal muscle spasm caused by irritation of the parietal peritoneum by peritonitis is an example of local skeletal muscle spasm caused by a spinal cord reflex. Similar spasm of the abdominal skeletal muscles occurs during surgical operations in which stimulation of the parietal peritoneum causes the abdominal muscles to contract with subsequent extrusion of intestines through the surgical wound. During surgical operations in the abdomen, this skeletal muscle spasm is attenuated by volatile anesthetics and abolished by regional anesthesia or neuromuscular-blocking drugs.

Autonomic Reflexes

Segmental autonomic reflexes occur in the spinal cord and include changes in vascular tone, diaphoresis, and evacuation reflexes from the bladder and colon. Simultaneous excitation of all the segmental reflexes is the mass reflex (denervation hypersensitivity or autonomic hyperreflexia) (see Chapter 43). The mass reflex typically occurs in the presence of spinal cord transection when a painful stimulus to the skin below the level of the spinal cord transection or distension of a hollow viscus, such as the bladder or gastrointestinal tract, occurs. This mass reflex is analogous to seizures that involve the CNS. The principal manifestation of the mass reflex is systemic hypertension due to intense peripheral vasoconstriction, reflecting an inability of vasodilating inhibitory impulses from the CNS to pass beyond the site of spinal cord transection. Carotid sinus baroreceptor-mediated reflex bradycardia accompanies the systemic hypertension associated with the mass reflex.

Spinal Shock

Spinal shock is a manifestation of the abrupt loss of spinal cord reflexes that immediately follows transection of the spinal cord. It emphasizes the dependence of spinal cord reflexes on continual tonic discharges from higher centers. The immediate manifestations of spinal shock are hypotension due to loss of vasoconstrictor tone and absence of all skeletal muscle reflexes. Within a few days to weeks, spinal cord neurons gradually regain their intrinsic excitability. Sacral reflexes for control of bladder and colon evacuation are completely suppressed for the first few weeks after spinal cord transection, but these spinal cord reflexes also eventually return.

ANATOMY OF NERVE FIBERS

Nerve fibers are afferent if they transmit impulses from peripheral receptors to the spinal cord and efferent if they relay signals from the spinal cord and CNS to the periphery.

Neurons

The principal function of neurons is to relay information between the periphery and the CNS. A neuron consists of a cell body or soma, dendrites, and a nerve fiber or axon (Fig. 41-8). Dendrites are extensions of the cell body. The axon of one neuron terminates (synapses) near the cell body or dendrites of another neuron. The end areas of an axon are called *presynaptic terminals*. The space between the presynaptic terminals and the cell body or dendrites of the next neuron is known as the *presynaptic cleft*. Transmission of impulses between responsive neurons at a synapse is mediated by presynaptic release of a chemical mediator (neurotransmitter), such as norepinephrine or acetylcholine. This chemically mediated response differs from electrical transmission of impulses along axons. Nerve membranes of postsynaptic neurons are speculated to contain receptors that bind neurotransmitters released from presynaptic nerve terminals.

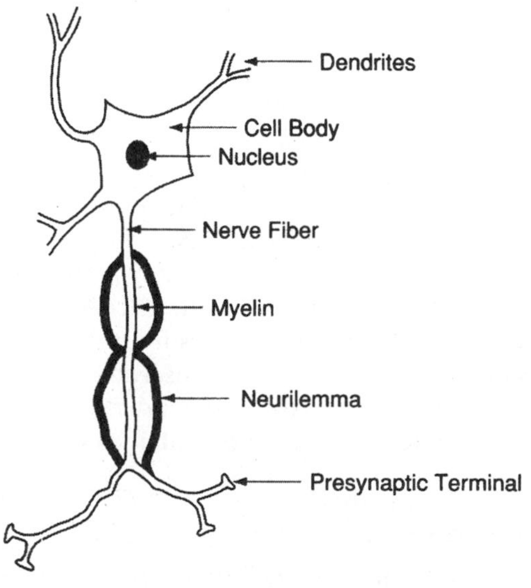

Figure 41-8. Anatomy of a neuron.

Functionally, the nerve membrane is the most important part of the nerve fiber for impulse conduction. Indeed, removal of the axoplasm from the nerve fiber does not alter conduction of impulses. Nerve fibers derive their nutrition from the cell body. Interruption of a nerve fiber causes the peripheral portion to degenerate (wallerian degeneration). The central part of the neuron, however, is able to regenerate, as does the myelin sheath. Nevertheless, lack of neurilemma prevents this type of regeneration from occurring in the brain or spinal cord.

Classification of Afferent Nerve Fibers

Afferent nerve fibers are classified as A, B, and C on the basis of fiber diameter and velocity of conduction of nerve impulses (Table 41-1). The largest-diameter A fibers are subdivided into alpha, beta, gamma, and delta. Type A-alpha fibers innervate skeletal muscles. Tactile sensory receptors (Meissner's corpuscles, hair receptors, pacinian corpuscles) transmit signals in type A-beta fibers. Type A-gamma fibers are distributed to skeletal muscle spindles. Touch and fast pain are transmitted by type A-delta fibers (see Chapter 44). Type C fibers transmit slow pain, pruritus, and temperature impulses. Type A and B fibers are myelinated, whereas type C fibers are unmyelinated.

Myelin that surrounds type A and B nerve fibers acts as an insulator that prevents flow of ions across nerve membranes. The myelin sheath, however, is interrupted approximately every millimeter by the nodes of Ranvier (Fig. 41-9) (Guyton and Hall, 2000). Ions can flow freely between nerve fibers and extracellular fluid at the nodes of Ranvier. Action potentials are conducted from node to node by the myelinated nerve rather than continuously along the entire fiber as occurs in unmyelinated nerve fibers. This successive excitation of nodes of Ranvier by an impulse that jumps between successive nodes is termed *saltatory excitation* (see Fig. 41-9) (Guyton and Hall, 2000). Saltatory conduction greatly increases velocity of nerve transmission in myelinated fibers and also conserves energy because only the nodes of Ranvier depolarize, resulting in less loss of ions than would otherwise occur. Furthermore, because depolarization is limited to only the nodes of Ranvier, little additional energy for reestablishing sodium and potassium ion concentration differences across nerve membranes is necessary.

Evaluation of Peripheral Nerve Function

Peripheral nerves may be injured by ischemia of the intraneural vasa nervorum that accompanies stretch of the nerve or external compression of the nerve. Nerve conduction studies are useful in the localization and assessment of peripheral nerve dysfunction. Focal demyelination of nerve fibers causes slowing of conduction and decreased

TABLE 41-1.
CLASSIFICATION OF PERIPHERAL NERVE FIBERS

	Myelinated	Fiber Diameter (mm)	Conduction Velocity (m/s)	Function	Sensitivity to Local Anesthetic (Subarachnoid, Procaine, %)
A-alpha	Yes	12–20	70–120	Innervation of skeletal muscles Proprioception	1
A-beta	Yes	5–12	30–70	Touch Pressure	1
A-gamma	Yes	3–6	15–30	Skeletal muscle tone	1
A-delta	Yes	2–5	12–30	Fast pain Touch Temperature	0.5
B	Yes	3	3–15	Preganglionic autonomic fibers	0.25
C	No	0.4–1.2	0.5–2.0	Slow pain Touch Temperature Postganglionic sympathetic fibers	0.5

amplitudes of compound muscle and sensory action potentials. Electromyography studies are an adjunct to nerve conduction studies. The presence of denervation potentials in a skeletal muscle indicates axon or anterior horn cell loss, and changes in motor unit potentials arise from reinnervation of skeletal muscle fibers by surviving axons. Signs of denervation on the electromyogram after acute nerve injury requires 18 to 21 days to develop (Perreault et al., 1992).

NEUROTRANSMITTERS

Neurotransmitters are chemical mediators that are released into the synaptic cleft in response to the arrival of an action potential at the nerve ending. Release of all neurotransmitters is voltage dependent and requires the influx of calcium ions into the presynaptic terminals. Synaptic vesicles of the cell body and dendrites of neurons are the sites of continuous synthesis and storage of neurotransmitters. These vesicles may contain and release more than one neurotransmitter simultaneously, so a single agonist or antagonist drug might not produce total reversal of the anticipated response. Neurotransmitters may be excitatory or inhibitory, depending on the configurational change produced in the protein receptor by its interaction with the neurotransmitter. Specifically, permeability to most ions is increased by interaction of an excitatory neurotransmitter and receptor, whereas inhibitory responses typically reflect selective increased permeability to chloride and potassium ions. A postsynaptic receptor may be excited or inhibited, reflecting the existence of both types of receptors in the same postsynaptic neuron. Furthermore, the same neurotransmitter may be inhibitory at one site and cause excitation at another. Some neurotransmitters function as neuromodulators in that they influence the sensitivity of receptors to other neurotransmitters. General anesthetics produce a broad spectrum of actions, as reflected by their ability to modify both inhibitory and excitatory neurotransmission at presynaptic and postsynaptic loci within the CNS. Nevertheless, the precise mechanism of these effects remains uncertain, and it is likely that general anesthetics interact with multiple neurotransmitter systems by a variety of mechanisms (Hudspith, 1997). For example, general anesthetics may depress excitable tissues at all levels of the nervous system by stabilizing neuronal membranes, resulting in a decreased release of neurotransmitters

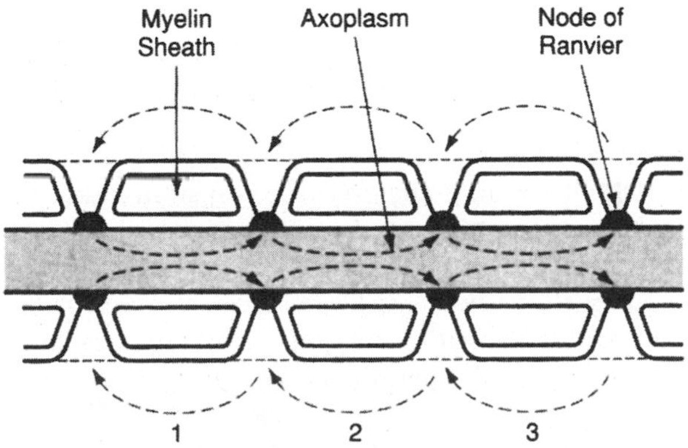

Figure 41-9. Saltatory conduction is transmission of nerve impulses that jump between successive nodes of Ranvier of myelinated nerves. (From Guyton AC, Hall JE. *Textbook of medical physiology*, 10th ed. Philadelphia. Saunders, 2000; with permission.)

and transmission of impulses at synapses as well as a general depression of postsynaptic responsiveness and ion movement.

Types of Neurotransmitters

The list of chemical mediators functioning as excitatory or inhibitory neurotransmitters continues to increase (Table 41-2). Glutamate is the major excitatory amino acid neurotransmitter in the CNS, whereas GABA is the major inhibitory neurotransmitter (Hudspith, 1997). Acetylcholine, dopamine, and norepinephrine are widely and unevenly distributed, suggesting these substances are important neurotransmitters in the CNS. Neuromodulators coexist in presynaptic terminals with neurotransmitters but do not themselves cause substantive voltage or conductance changes in postsynaptic cell membranes. They can, however, amplify, prolong, decrease, or shorten the postsynaptic response to selected neurotransmitters. There is evidence that the state of anesthesia is associated with inhibition of excitatory amino acid neurotransmission throughout the CNS.

Glutamate

Glutamate is the major excitatory amino acid neurotransmitter in the CNS. Glutamate-responsive receptors are distributed widely in the CNS but are particularly concentrated in the hippocampus, the outer layer of the cerebral cortex, and the substantia gelatinosa of the spinal cord. Within these areas, glutamate and other excitatory neurotransmitters play key roles in learning and memory (including awareness during anesthesia), central pain transduction, and pathologic processes such as excitotoxic neuronal injury as may follow CNS trauma or ischemia.

TABLE 41-2.
CHEMICALS THAT ACT AT SYNAPSES AS NEUROTRANSMITTERS

Glutamate
Acetylcholine
Norepinephrine
Glycine
Endorphins
Serotonin
Histamine
Oxytocin
Cholecystokinin
Gastrin
Gamma-aminobutyric acid
Dopamine
Epinephrine
Substance P
Vasopressin
Prolactin
Vasoactive intestinal peptide
Glucagon

Glutamate is synthesized by the deamination of glutamine via the tricarboxylic acid cycle and then released into the synaptic cleft in response to depolarization of the presynaptic nerve terminal. The release of glutamate from presynaptic terminals as well as that of other neurotransmitters is a calcium ion-dependent process regulated by multiple types of calcium channels. In common with many other central neurotransmitter systems, the actions of glutamate within the synaptic cleft are terminated by high affinity sodium-dependent uptake.

The two main subgroups of excitatory amino acid receptors have been categorized as *inotropic* and *metabotropic* receptors (Hudspith, 1997). Ionotropic glutamate receptors (includes *N*-methyl-D-aspartate receptors) are ligand-gated ion channels, and a change in membrane permeability to specific cations occurs in response to binding of the agonist. When activated, ionotropic receptors undergo a conformational change that results in the opening of their ligand-operated channels and a transmembrane flux of cations (mainly sodium), resulting in depolarization of postsynaptic membranes. Metabotropic glutamate receptors are transmembrane receptors that are linked to guanine (G) proteins that modulate intracellular second messengers such as inositol phosphates and cyclic nucleotides.

Gamma-Aminobutyric Acid

GABA is the major inhibitory neurotransmitter in the CNS, being present in diverse areas including the cerebral cortex, basal ganglia, cerebellum, and spinal cord. It is estimated that as many as one-third of the synapses in the brain are GABAergic. When two molecules of GABA bind to the receptor, the chloride ion channel opens and allows chloride ions to flow into the neuron, causing it to become hyperpolarized. A hyperpolarized cell membrane is more resistant to neuronal excitation, accounting for the inhibitory effects of GABA. The alpha and beta subunits of the GABA receptor constitute the chloride ion channel.

There is an increase in the amount of GABA released in the brain when the EEG manifests a slow-wave sleep pattern. Nonselective CNS stimulants may act as selective antagonists of GABA (see Chapter 33). Life cannot be sustained without GABAergic neurotransmission to counterbalance the influence of excitatory amino acid neurotransmitters.

Acetylcholine

Acetylcholine is an excitatory neurotransmitter that interacts with muscarinic and nicotinic receptors in the CNS. This excitatory effect on the CNS contrasts with the inhibitory effects (increased potassium permeability leading to hyperpolarization of postsynaptic membranes) of acetylcholine on the peripheral parasympathetic nervous system.

Dopamine

Dopamine represents >50% of the CNS content of catecholamines, with high concentrations especially in the basal ganglia. It is most likely that dopamine is an inhibitory neurotransmitter, perhaps by acting on dopamine-sensitive adenylate cyclase.

Norepinephrine

Norepinephrine is present in large amounts in the reticular activating system and the hypothalamus. Neurons responding to norepinephrine send predominantly inhibitory impulses to widespread areas of the brain, such as the cerebral cortex.

Epinephrine

Epinephrine-containing neurons are present in the reticular activating system, where its presumed effect is that of an inhibitory neurotransmitter.

Glycine

Glycine is the principal inhibitory neurotransmitter in the spinal cord, acting to increase chloride ion conductance. Strychnine and tetanus toxin result in seizures because they antagonize the effects of glycine on postsynaptic inhibition. Visual disturbances after transurethral resection of the prostate in which glycine is the irrigating solution may reflect the role of this substance as an inhibitory neurotransmitter in the retina (Ovassapian et al., 1982). Amplitude and latency of visual evoked potentials are triggered by infusions of glycine (Wang et al., 1989).

Substance P

Substance P is an excitatory neurotransmitter presumed to be released by terminals of pain fibers that synapse in the substantia gelatinosa of the spinal cord (see Chapter 44).

Endorphins

Endorphins are secreted by nerve terminals in the thalamus, hypothalamus, brainstem, and spinal cord, where they most likely act as excitatory neurotransmitters for descending pathways that inhibit the transmission of pain.

Serotonin

Serotonin is present in high concentrations in the brain, where it is believed to act as an inhibitory neurotransmitter, exerting profound effects on mood and behavior. Lysergic acid diethylamide (LSD) is a serotonin antagonist. The similarities of the effects of ketamine and LSD on behavior suggest a common effect on serotonin.

Histamine

Histamine is present in high concentrations in the hypothalamus and the reticular activating system, where it is presumed to act as an inhibitory neurotransmitter. Cyclic adenosine monophosphate may serve as a second messenger to mediate the actions of histamine in the CNS.

ELECTRICAL EVENTS DURING NEURONAL EXCITATION

Resting transmembrane potentials of neurons in the CNS are about −70 mv, which is less than the −90 mv in large peripheral nerve fibers and skeletal muscles. This decreased magnitude of the resting transmembrane potential is important for controlling the responsiveness of neurons. At inhibitory synapses, a neurotransmitter increases the permeability of postsynaptic receptors to potassium and chloride ions. Receptors responding to inhibitory neurotransmitters are associated with protein channels that are too small to allow passage of larger hydrated sodium ions. The predominant outward diffusion of potassium ions increases the negativity of the resting transmembrane potential, and the neuron is hyperpolarized (functions as an inhibitory neuron). GABA is most likely the presynaptic inhibitory neurotransmitter in the brain, whereas glycine may be the presynaptic inhibitory neurotransmitter in the spinal cord. In addition to postsynaptic inhibition caused by inhibitory synapses at neuron cell membranes, there is also presynaptic inhibition.

Permeability changes evoked by excitatory neurotransmitters decrease the negativity of the resting transmembrane potential, bringing it nearer threshold potential. As a result, these neurons function in the excitatory mode. Glutamate is the likely excitatory amino acid neurotransmitter in the CNS.

Synaptic Delay

Synaptic delay is the 0.3 to 0.5 s necessary for the transmission of an impulse from the synaptic varicosity to the postsynaptic neuron. This synaptic delay reflects the time for release of the neurotransmitter from the synaptic varicosity, diffusion of the neurotransmitter to the postsynaptic receptor, and the subsequent change in permeability of the postsynaptic membrane to various ions.

Synaptic Fatigue

Synaptic fatigue is a decrease in the number of discharges by the postsynaptic membrane when excitatory synapses are repetitively and rapidly stimulated. For example, synaptic fatigue decreases excessive excitability of the brain as may accompany a seizure, thus acting as a protective mechanism against excessive neuronal activity. The mechanism of synaptic fatigue is presumed to be exhaustion of the stores of neurotransmitter in the synaptic vesicles.

Posttetanic Facilitation

Posttetanic facilitation is increased responsiveness of the postsynaptic neuron to stimulation after a rest period that was preceded by repetitive stimulation of an excitatory synapse. This phenomenon may reflect increased release of neurotransmitters due to enhanced permeability of synaptic varicosities to calcium. Posttetanic facilitation may be a mechanism for short-term memory.

Factors That Influence Neuron Responsiveness

Neurons are highly sensitive to changes in the pH of the surrounding interstitial fluids. For example, alkalosis enhances neuron excitability. Indeed, voluntary hyperventilation can evoke a seizure in a susceptible individual. Conversely, acidosis depresses neuron excitability, with a decrease in arterial pH to 7.0 potentially causing coma. Lack of oxygen can cause total inexcitability of neurons within 3 to 5 s as reflected by the onset of unconsciousness due to cessation of cerebral blood flow.

Inhaled anesthetics may increase cell membrane threshold for excitation and thus decrease neuron activity throughout the body. This concept is based on the speculation that most lipid-soluble volatile anesthetics may change the permeability characteristics of cell membranes, making the neuron less responsive to excitatory neurotransmitters.

CEREBRAL BLOOD FLOW

Cerebral blood flow averages 50 mL/100g/minute of brain tissue. For an adult, this is equivalent to 750 mL/minute, or about 15% of the resting cardiac output, delivered to an organ that represents only about 2% of the body's mass. The gray matter of the brain has a higher cerebral blood flow (80 mL/100g/minute) than the white matter (20 mL/100g/minute). As in most other tissues of the body, cerebral blood flow parallels cerebral metabolic requirements for oxygen (3 to 5 mL/100g/minute). $Paco_2$ and Pao_2 influence cerebral blood flow, whereas sympathetic and parasympathetic nerves play little or no role in the regulation of cerebral blood flow (Fig. 41-10). Changes in the $Paco_2$ between about 20 and 80 mm Hg produce corresponding changes in cerebral blood flow. For example, in this range, a 1-mm Hg increase in the $Paco_2$ evokes a 1 to 2 mL/100g/minute increase in cerebral blood flow (Table 41-3) (Brian, 1998).

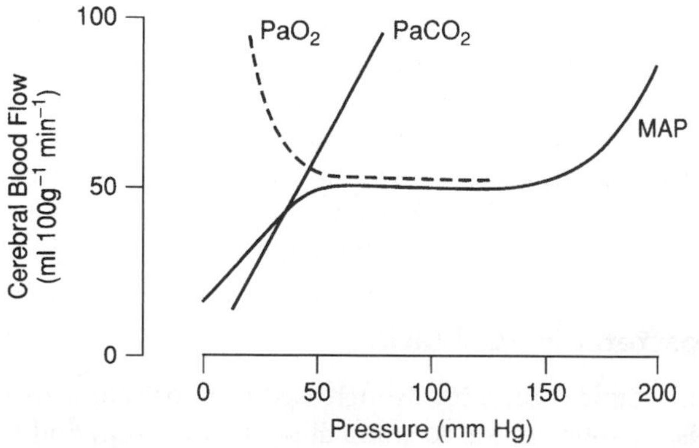

Figure 41-10. Cerebral blood flow is influenced by Pao_2, $Paco_2$, and mean arterial pressure (MAP).

TABLE 41-3.
CARBON DIOXIDE AND CEREBRAL PHYSIOLOGY

Cerebral blood flow (CBF)
Changes 1-2 mL/100g/minute for each 1 mm Hg change in $Paco_2$ between 20 and 80 mm Hg
Slope of the response depends on normocapnic CBF
CBF returns to baseline over several hours during sustained alterations in $Paco_2$ (reflects correction of brain extracellular fluid pH)
Response to hypocapnia not altered by aging if CBF is maintained
Response to changes in $Paco_2$ not altered by untreated hypertension
Hypothermia decreases normocapnic CBF and the response of CBF to changes in $Paco_2$
Cerebral blood volume (CBV)
Changes 0.05 mL/100g for each 1 mm Hg change in $Paco_2$
Returns to baseline during sustained alterations in $Paco_2$
Cerebral autoregulation
Modest hypercapnia impairs and marked hypercapnia abolishes
Hypotension below the lower limit of autoregulation abolishes hypocapnic cerebral vasoconstriction
Carbon dioxide response and anesthetics
Maintained during inhaled and intravenous anesthetics
Relative response to hypocapnia depends on normocapnic CBF (anesthetics that increase CBF enhance the reduction of CBF by hypocapnia)
Carbon dioxide response in presence of disease or injury
Hypercapnic response intact with hypertension
Hypocapnia response present with brain injury (subarachnoid hemorrhage) but may be attenuated if vasospasm is present

Carbon dioxide increases cerebral blood flow by combining with water in body fluids to form carbonic acid, with subsequent dissociation to form hydrogen ions. Hydrogen ions produce vasodilation of cerebral vessels that is proportional to the increase in hydrogen ion concentration.

Any other acid that increases hydrogen ion concentration, such as lactic acid, also increases cerebral blood flow. Increased cerebral blood flow in response to increases in $Paco_2$ serves to carry away excess hydrogen ions that would otherwise greatly depress neuronal activity.

Unlike the continuous response of cerebral blood flow to changes in $Paco_2$, the response to Pao_2 is a threshold phenomenon (see Fig. 41-10). If the $Paco_2$ is maintained, cerebral blood flow begins to increase when the Pao_2 decreases below 50 mm Hg or the cerebral venous PO_2 decreases from its normal value of 35 mm Hg to about 30 mm Hg.

Autoregulation

Cerebral blood flow is closely autoregulated between a mean arterial pressure of about 60 and 140 mm Hg (see

Fig. 41-10). As a result, changes in systemic blood pressure within this range will not significantly alter cerebral blood flow. Chronic systemic hypertension shifts the autoregulation curve to the right such that decreases in cerebral blood may occur at a mean arterial pressure of >60 mm Hg. Autoregulation of cerebral blood flow is attenuated or abolished by hypercapnia, arterial hypoxemia, and volatile anesthetics. Furthermore, autoregulation is often abolished in the area surrounding an acute cerebral infarction. For example, reactivity of blood vessels in areas surrounding cerebral infarcts and tumors is abolished. These blood vessels are maximally vasodilated, presumably reflecting accumulation of acidic metabolic products. As a result, cerebral blood flow to this area is already maximal (luxury perfusion), and changes in $Paco_2$ have no effect on its local blood flow. If $Paco_2$ should increase, however, it is theoretically possible that resulting vasodilation in normal blood vessels would shunt blood flow away from the diseased area (intracerebral steal syndrome). Conversely, a decrease in $Paco_2$ that constricts normal cerebral vessels could divert blood flow to diseased areas ("Robin Hood" phenomenon). Increases in mean arterial pressure above the limits of autoregulation can cause leakage of intravascular fluid through capillary membranes, resulting in cerebral edema. Because the brain is enclosed in a solid vault, the accumulation of edema fluid increases intracranial pressure and compresses blood vessels, decreasing cerebral blood flow and leading to destruction of brain tissue.

Measurement of Cerebral Blood Flow

Cerebral blood flow can be measured by injecting a radioactive substance, usually xenon, into the carotid artery and measuring the rate of decay of the radioactivity in each tissue segment using scintillation detectors. Using this technique, it can be demonstrated that cerebral blood flow changes within seconds in response to changes in local neuronal activity. For example, clasping the hand can be shown to cause an immediate increase in blood flow in the motor cortex of the opposite cerebral hemisphere. Reading increases blood flow in the occipital cortex and the language areas of the temporal cortex. This measuring procedure can be used to localize the origin of epilepsy because blood flow increases acutely at the site of origin of the seizure.

ELECTROENCEPHALOGRAM

The EEG is a recording of the brain waves that result from the continuous electrical activity in the brain. The intensity of the electrical activity recorded from the surface of the scalp ranges from 0 to 300 μv, and the frequency may exceed 50 cycles/s. The character of the waves greatly depends on the level of activity of the cerebral cortex and the degree of wakefulness. There is a direct relationship between the degree of cerebral activity and the frequency of brain waves. Furthermore, during periods of increased mental activity, brain waves become asynchronous rather than synchronous, so the voltage decreases despite greater cortical activity.

Classification of Brain Waves

Brain waves are classified as alpha, beta, theta, and delta waves depending on their frequency and amplitude (Fig. 41-11). The classic EEG is a plot of voltage against time, usually recorded by 16 channels on paper moving at 30 mm per second. One page of recording is 10 s of data.

Alpha Waves

Alpha waves occur at a frequency of 8 to 12 cycles/s and a voltage of about 50 μv. These waves are typical of an awake, resting state of cerebration with the eyes closed. During sleep, alpha waves disappear. Because alpha waves do not occur when the cerebral cortex is not connected to the thalamus, it is assumed these waves result from spontaneous activity in the thalamocortical system.

Beta Waves

Beta waves occur at a frequency of 13 to 30 cycles/s and a voltage usually of <50 μv. These high-frequency and low-voltage asynchronous waves replace alpha waves in the presence of increased mental activity or visual stimulation.

Theta Waves

Theta waves occur at a frequency of 4 to 7 cycles/s. These waves occur in healthy children during sleep and also during general anesthesia.

Delta Waves

Delta waves include all the brain waves with a frequency of <4 cycles/s. These waves occur (a) in deep sleep, (b) during general anesthesia, and (c) in the presence of organic brain

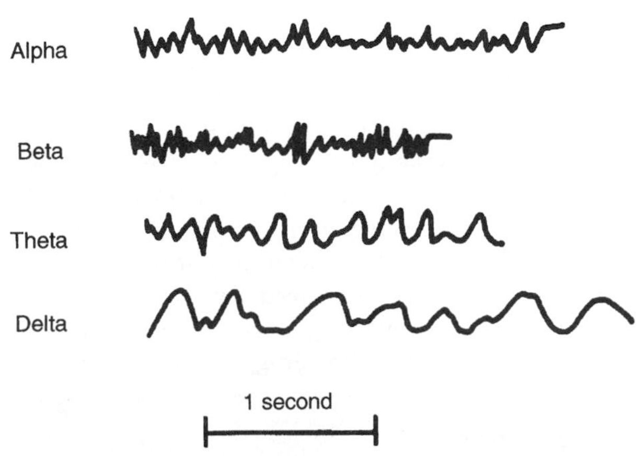

Figure 41-11. The electroencephalogram consists of alpha, beta, theta, and delta waves.

disease. Delta waves occur even when the connections of the cerebral cortex to the reticular activating system are severed, indicating these waves originate in the cerebral cortex independently of lower brain structures. Occurrence of delta waves during sleep suggests that the cerebral cortex is released from the activating influences of the reticular activating system.

Clinical Uses

The EEG is useful in diagnosing different types of epilepsy and for determining the focus in the brain causing seizures. Brain tumors, which compress surrounding neurons and cause abnormal electrical activity, may be localized using the EEG. Monitoring of the EEG during carotid endarterectomy, cardiopulmonary bypass, or controlled hypotension may provide an early warning of inadequate cerebral blood flow. In this regard, the EEG may be influenced by anesthetic drugs, depth of anesthesia, and hyperventilation of the patient's lungs (see Chapter 2).

Brain Wave Monitors

Bispectral Index

The Bispectral Index (BIS) is a variable derived from the EEG that is a quantifiable measure of the sedative and hypnotic effects of anesthetic drugs on the CNS (Sigl and Chamoun, 1994) BIS is a processed EEG descriptor that predicts depth of consciousness. Bispectral analysis is based on the correlation of the phase between different frequency components of the EEG in which the EEG signal is converted into its component sine waves using Fourier transformation. A set of bispectral features is calculated by analyzing the phase relations between the component waves. These bispectral features are combined with other EEG features into a single measurement, the BIS expressed as a dimensionless numerical index from 0 to 100. Decreasing numerical values correlate with sedation and predict the response of patients to surgical stimulation (values of <60 are associated with a low probability of recall and a high probability of unresponsiveness during surgery) (Fig. 41-12) (Flaishon et al., 1997; Kearse et al., 1994). Titrating desflurane and sevoflurane using the BIS monitor to maintain a numerical value of 60 results in decreased use of drug and faster awakening (Song et al., 1997). Likewise, titration of propofol to maintain a numerical value of 45 to 60 and then permitting an increase to 60 to 75 during the last 15 minutes of the operation results in decreased propofol use and more rapid recovery (Gan et al., 1997). In this regard, BIS monitoring may serve as a useful intraoperative monitor for guiding drug administration.

Spectral Entropy

Spectral entropy represents an alternative concept to bispectral analysis for quantifying the EEG. Spectral entropy

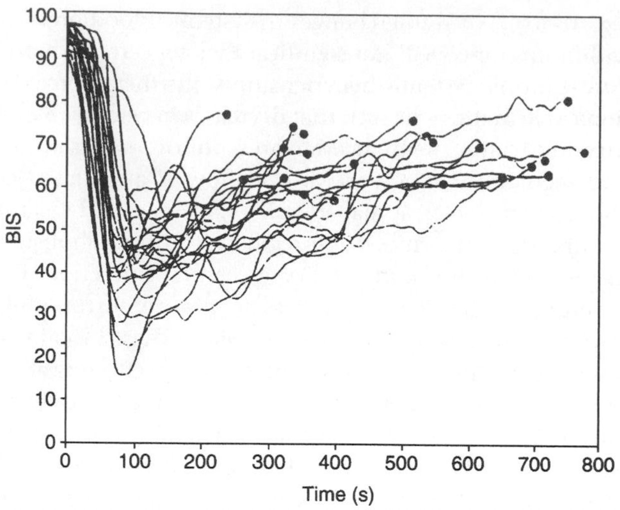

Figure 41-12. Plot of bispectral index (BIS) against time from induction of anesthesia to recovery of consciousness after administration of propofol. (Flaishon R, Windsor A, Sigl J, Sebel PS. Recovery of consciousness after thiopental or propofol. Bispectral index and the isolated forearm technique. *Anesthesiology* 1997; 86:613–619; with permission.)

(SE) and response entropy (RE) are computed over specific frequency ranges of the EEG. RE includes electromyographic activity. SE, RE, and BIS reveal similar information about the level of sedation (Schmidt et al., 2004).

Epilepsy

Epilepsy is characterized by excessive activity of either a part or all of the CNS. Grand mal epilepsy is characterized by intense neuronal discharges in multiple areas of the cerebral and reticular activating system. These impulses are transmitted to the spinal cord, resulting in alternating skeletal muscle contractions known as *tonic-clonic seizures*. Signals to the viscera often result in defecation and urination. The grand mal seizure lasts from a few seconds to several minutes and is followed by generalized depression of the entire CNS. The EEG during a grand mal seizure reveals high-voltage, synchronous brain wave discharges over the entire cerebral cortex. Synaptic fatigue is a likely mechanism that contributes to spontaneous cessation of a grand mal seizure and postictal depression.

Status epilepticus is present when grand mal seizure activity is sustained. Diazepam, administered intravenously, is an often recommended treatment to stop seizures and permit resumption of effective breathing. Drugs such as thiopental are also effective, but their depressant effect on the CNS is generalized and nonspecific and may be associated with lingering sedative effects. In the rare instance in which conventional drug therapy is ineffective, volatile anesthetics such as isoflurane may be administered in an attempt to stop status epilepticus (Kofke et al., 1989). When volatile anesthetics are administered for this purpose, it is likely that systemic blood pressure will need to be supported with intravenous administration of fluids and/or sympathomimetics. Evidence that volatile anesthetics do not reverse the underlying cause of seizures is the predictable reappearance of seizure activity when administration of the anesthetic is discontinued.

EVOKED POTENTIALS

Evoked potentials are the electrophysiologic responses of the nervous system to sensory, motor, auditory, or visual stimulation. The waveforms resulting from sensory stimulation reflect transmission of impulses through specific sensory pathways. Poststimulus latency is the time in milliseconds from application of the stimulus to a peak in the recorded waveform. The amplitude and latency of evoked potentials may be influenced by a number of events, especially volatile anesthetics. Evoked potentials are used to monitor (a) spinal cord function during operations near or on the spinal cord, and (b) auditory nerve and brainstem function, as during operations on pituitary tumors or other lesions that impinge on the optic nerves or optic chiasm. The modes of sensory stimulation used to produce evoked potentials in the operating room are somatosensory, auditory, and visual.

Somatosensory Evoked Potentials

Somatosensory evoked potentials are produced by application of a low-voltage electrical current that stimulates a peripheral nerve such as the median nerve at the wrist or the posterior tibial nerve at the ankle. The resulting evoked potentials reflect the integrity of sensory neural pathways from the peripheral nerve to the somatosensory cortex. Somatosensory stimulation follows the dorsal column pathways of proprioception and vibration. These pathways are supplied by the posterior spinal artery, leaving the motor pathway, which is supplied by the anterior spinal artery, unmonitored. Indeed, postoperative paraplegia has been described in patients despite the preservation of somatosensory evoked potentials intraoperatively (Ginsburg et al., 1985). Inhaled anesthetics, especially volatile anesthetics, produce dose-dependent depression of somatosensory evoked potentials (see Chapter 2). Although less so than volatile anesthetics, morphine and fentanyl also produce depressant effects on somatosensory evoked potentials, with a low-dose continuous infusion of the opioid producing less depression than intermittent injections (Fig. 41-13) (Pathak et al., 1987). Ketamine or etomidate may increase the amplitude of somatosensory evoked potentials (see Chapter 4). Acute hyperventilation of the patient's lungs to produce a Pa_{CO_2} near 20 mm Hg does not significantly alter the amplitude or latencies of somatosensory evoked potentials (Schubert and Drummond, 1986).

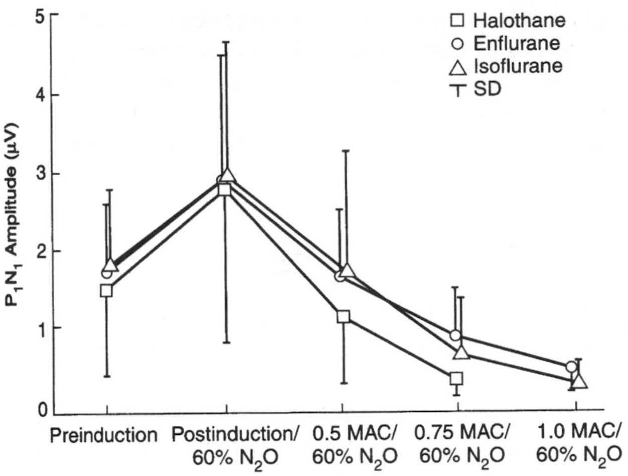

Figure 41-13. Peak-to-peak amplitudes (and latencies—*not shown*) decrease significantly with increasing MAC levels. (From Pathak KS, Ammadio M, Kalamchi A, et al. Effects of halothane, enflurane, and isoflurane on somatosensory evoked potentials during nitrous oxide anesthesia. *Anesthesiology* 1987;66:753–757; with permission.)

Motor Evoked Potentials

The use of motor evoked potentials remains limited, as their recording requires direct (epidural) or indirect (transosseous) stimulation of the brain or spinal cord (Adams et al., 1993). These evoked potentials reflect the integrity of motor neural pathways from the peripheral nerve to the motor cerebral cortex. Motor evoked potentials are extremely sensitive to depression by anesthetics. Furthermore, it is not possible to monitor motor evoked potentials in the presence of significant drug-induced neuromuscular blockade. During scoliosis surgery or other operations that place spinal cord motor function at risk, the use of motor evoked potentials obviates the need for an intraoperative wake-up test. In many instances, it is useful to monitor both motor and sensory evoked potentials to fully evaluate the functional integrity of both motor and sensory pathways. As an alternative to motor evoked potentials, transcranial motor stimulation may be used to monitor spinal cord function during spinal surgery.

Auditory Evoked Potentials

Auditory evoked potentials arise from brainstem auditory pathways. Volatile anesthetics produce dose-dependent depression of auditory evoked potentials. Auditory evoked potentials may provide an objective electrophysiological alternative to the clinical assessment of sedation (Haenggi et al., 2004).

Visual Evoked Potentials

Visual evoked potentials are produced by flashes from light-emitting diodes that are mounted on goggles placed over the patient's closed eyes. During neurosurgical procedures involving visual pathways (transphenoidal or anterior fossa surgery), the monitoring of visual evoked potentials has been used. Volatile anesthetics produce dose-dependent depression of visual evoked potentials, especially above concentrations equivalent to about 0.8 MAC (Chi and Field, 1986).

CEREBROSPINAL FLUID

Cerebrospinal fluid (CSF) is present in the (a) ventricles of the brain, (b) cisterns around the brain, and (c) subarachnoid space around the brain and spinal cord (Fig. 41-14). The total volume of CSF is about 150 mL, and the specific gravity is 1.002 to 1.009. A major function of CSF is to cushion the brain in the cranial cavity. A blow to the head moves the entire brain simultaneously, causing no one portion of the brain to be selectively contorted by the blow. When a blow to the head is particularly severe, it usually does not damage the brain on the ipsilateral side, but instead damage manifests on the opposite side. This phenomenon is known as *contrecoup* and reflects the creation of a vacuum between the brain and skull opposite the blow caused by sudden movement of the brain at this site away from the skull. When the skull is no longer being accelerated by the blow, the vacuum suddenly collapses and the brain strikes the interior of the skull.

Formation

The choroid plexuses (cauliflower-like growths of blood vessels covered by a thin layer of epithelial cells) in the four cerebral ventricles are the major site of formation of CSF, which continually exudes from the surface of the choroid plexus at a rate of about 30 mL/hour. The rate of CSF production is increased by enflurane but not isoflurane, halothane, or fentanyl (see Chapters 2 and 3).

In comparison with other extracellular fluids, the concentration of sodium and chloride in CSF is 7% greater and the concentration of glucose and potassium is 30% and 40% less, respectively. This difference in composition from other extracellular fluids emphasizes that CSF is a choroid secretion and not a simple filtrate from the capillaries. The pH of CSF is closely regulated and maintained at 7.32. Changes in $Paco_2$, but not arterial pH, promptly alter CSF pH, reflecting the ability of carbon dioxide, but not hydrogen ions, to cross the blood-brain barrier easily. As a result, acute respiratory acidosis or alkalosis produces corresponding changes in CSF pH. Active transport of bicarbonate ions eventually returns CSF pH to 7.32, despite the persistence of alterations in arterial pH.

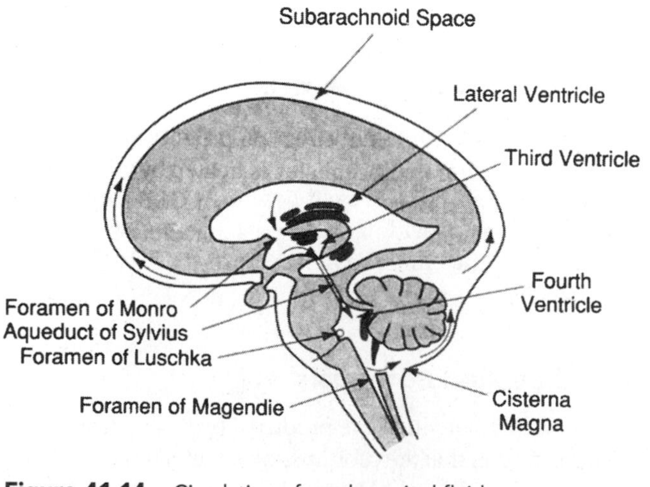

Figure 41-14. Circulation of cerebrospinal fluid.

Reabsorption

Almost all the CSF formed each day is reabsorbed into the venous circulation through special structures known as *arachnoid villi* or *granulations*. These villi project the subarachnoid spaces into the venous sinuses of the brain and occasionally into veins of the spinal cord. Arachnoid villi are actually trabeculae that protrude through venous walls, resulting in highly permeable areas that permit relatively free flow of CSF into the circulation. The magnitude of reabsorption depends on the pressure gradient between the CSF and the venous circulation. Enflurane, but not isoflurane, increases resistance to the reabsorption of CSF (see Chapter 2).

Circulation

CSF formed in the lateral cerebral ventricles passes into the third ventricle through the foramen of Monro (see Fig. 41-14). In the third ventricle, the CSF mixes with that secreted in the lateral ventricle and then passes along the aqueduct of Sylvius into the fourth cerebral ventricle, where still more CSF is formed. The CSF then passes into the cisterna magna through the lateral foramen of Luschka and via a middle foramen of Magendie. From this point, CSF flows through the subarachnoid spaces upward toward the cerebrum, where most of the arachnoid villi are located.

Hydrocephalus

Obstruction to free circulation of CSF in the neonate results in hydrocephalus. For example, blockage of the aqueduct of Sylvius results in expansion of the lateral and third cerebral ventricles and compression of the brain (see Fig. 41-14). This type of obstruction producing a noncommunicating type of hydrocephalus is treated by surgical creation of an artificial pathway for flow of CSF between the cerebral ventricular system and the subarachnoid space.

Intracranial Pressure

Normal intracranial pressure (ICP) is <15 mm Hg. This pressure is regulated by the rate of CSF formation and resistance to CSF reabsorption through arachnoid villi as determined by venous pressure. In addition, increases in cerebral blood flow, as during inhalation of volatile anesthetics, can cause the ICP to increase because of the concomitant increase in cerebral blood flow and cerebral blood volume. Systemic blood pressure does not alter ICP within the range of normal autoregulation. Phasic variations in systemic blood pressure, however, are transmitted as variations in ICP.

Papilledema

Anatomically, the dura of the brain extends as a sheath around the optic nerve and then connects with the sclera of the eye. When ICP increases, it is also reflected in the optic nerve sheath. Increased pressure in the optic sheath impedes blood flow in the retinal veins, leading to increases in the retinal capillary pressure and retinal edema. The tissues of the optic disc are more distendible than the rest of the retina, so the disc becomes more edematous than the remainder of the retina and swells into the cavity of the eye. This swelling of the optic disc is termed *papilledema*.

Blood-Brain Barrier

The blood-brain barrier reflects the impermeability of capillaries in the CNS, including the choroid plexuses, to circulating substances such as electrolytes and exogenous drugs or toxins. As a result, the internal consistency of the environment to which brain neurons are exposed is maintained over a narrow limit. An anatomic explanation for the blood-brain barrier is the tight junction between endothelial cells of brain capillaries and envelopment of brain capillaries by glial cells, which further decreases their permeability. The blood-brain barrier is less developed in the neonate and tends to break down in areas of the brain that are irradiated or infected or are the site of tumors. The exception of the existence of a blood-brain barrier is the area around the posterior pituitary and the chemoreceptor trigger zone.

VISION

The eye is optically equivalent to a photographic camera in that it contains a lens system, a variable aperture system (pupil), and the retina that corresponds to the film (Fig. 41-15) (Ganong, 2003). The lens system of the eye focuses an image on the retina. Relaxation and contraction of the ciliary muscles are responsible for altering the tension of ligaments attached to the lens, causing its refractive power to change. One diopter is equivalent to the ability of a lens to converge parallel light rays to a focal point 1 meter beyond the lens (59 diopters equals the total refractive power of the eye). Stimulation of parasympathetic nervous system fibers to the ciliary muscle causes this muscle to

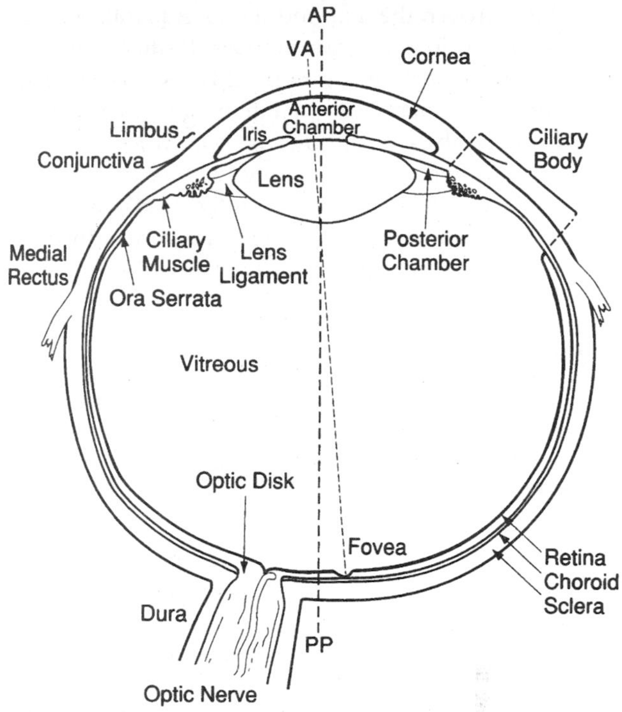

Figure 41-15. Schematic diagram of the eye. (AP, anterior pole; PP, posterior pole; VA, visual axis.) (From Ganong WF. *Review of medical physiology*, 21st ed. New York. Lange Medical Books/McGraw-Hill, 2003; with permission.)

relax, which in turn relaxes the ligaments of the lens and increases its refractive power. This increased refractive power allows the eye to focus on objects that are nearby. Interference with this process of accommodation may be noted by patients in the postoperative period who have received an anticholinergic drug in the preoperative medication or as part of the pharmacologic reversal of nondepolarizing neuromuscular blockade. The principal function of the pupil is to increase or decrease the amount of light that enters the eye. For example, the pupil may vary from 1.5 to 8.0 mm in diameter, permitting a 30-fold variation in the amount of light that enters the eye.

The lens loses its elastic nature with aging because of progressive denaturation of the len's proteins. As a result, the ability to accommodate is almost totally absent by 45 to 50 years of age. This lack of ability to accommodate is known as *presbyopia*.

Progressive denaturation of the proteins in the lens leads to the formation of a cataract. In later stages, calcium is often deposited in the coagulated proteins, thus further increasing the opacity. When the cataract impairs vision, the lens is surgically removed and replaced by an artificial convex lens that compensates for the loss of refractive power created by removal of the lens.

Intraocular Fluid

Intraocular fluid consists of aqueous humor, which lies in front and at the sides of the lens, and vitreous humor, which lies between the lens and retina. Aqueous humor is freely flowing fluid that is continuously formed (2 to 3 mL/minute) and reabsorbed. This fluid is secreted by ciliary processes of the ciliary body in a manner similar to formation of CSF by the choroid plexus. After flowing into the anterior chamber, aqueous humor enters the Schlemm canal, a thin vein that extends circumferentially around the eye. Vitreous humor is a gelatinous mass into which substances can diffuse slowly, but there is little flow of fluid.

Intraocular Pressure

Intraocular pressure is normally 15 to 25 mm Hg. This pressure is measured clinically by tonometry, in which the amount of displacement of the tonometer is calibrated in terms of intraocular pressure. It is believed that intraocular pressure is regulated primarily by resistance to outflow of aqueous humor from the anterior chamber into the Schlemm canal. Glaucoma is associated with increased intraocular pressure sufficient to compress retinal artery inflow to the eye, leading to ischemic pain and eventually blindness. When medical control of glaucoma fails, it may be necessary to surgically create an artificial outflow tract for aqueous humor.

Retina

The retina is the light-sensitive portion of the eye containing the cones, which are responsible for color vision, and the rods, which are mainly responsible for vision in the dark. When the cones and rods are stimulated, impulses are transmitted through successive neurons in the retina and optic nerve before reaching the cerebral cortex. The presence of melanin in the pigment layer of the retina prevents reflection of light throughout the globe. Without this pigment, light rays would be reflected in all directions within the globe, causing visual acuity to be impaired. Indeed, albinos, who lack melanin, have greatly decreased visual acuity.

The nutrient blood supply for the retina is largely derived from the central retinal artery, which accompanies the optic nerve. This independent retinal blood supply prevents rapid degeneration of the retina should it become detached from the pigment epithelium and allows time for surgical correction of a detached retina. The main arterial supply to the globe and orbital contents is from the ophthalmic artery, which is a branch of the internal carotid artery (Johnson, 1995).

Ischemic Optic Neuropathy

Ischemic optic neuropathy (ION) results from infarction of the optic nerve and is the most frequently reported cause of vision loss following general anesthesia (Williams et al., 1995). ION is classified as *anterior ION* (nonarteritic or arteritic) and *posterior ION*. Nonarteritic anterior ION occurs more often in patients with congenitally small optic discs. It is presumed that the small cross-sectional area of the optic disc results in little room for expansion of optic nerve fibers in response to ischemia-induced edema.

Posterior ION has been reported after diverse surgical procedures (prolonged spinal fusion surgery, cardiac operations requiring cardiopulmonary bypass, radical neck surgery) and its etiology appears to be multifactorial—including intraoperative anemia and hypotension combined with at least one other factor (congenital absence of the central retinal artery, increased venous pressure owing to venous obstruction; large amounts of fluid administration; prolonged head-down position; administration of vasopressors) (Janicki et al., 2001; Myers et al., 1997; Roth and Barach, 2001; Williams et al., 1995). Prone positioning increases IOP during anesthesia and could contribute to decreases in ocular perfusion pressure (Fig. 41-16) (Cheng et al., 2001). Despite the multifactorial etiology of ION, some cases do not have any of the speculated associated factors (anemia, hypotension), except perhaps for a large amount of intravenous fluids (Lee and Lam, 2001).

Other Causes of Postoperative Blindness

Cortical blindness, retinal occlusion, and ophthalmic venous obstruction need to be excluded when postoperative blindness occurs and ION is a consideration. Cortical blindness is characterized by loss of visual sensation with retention of pupillary reaction to light and normal funduscopic examination results. CT or MRI abnormalities in the parietal or occipital lobe confirm the diagnosis. A rare cause of cortical blindness is cyclosporine-induced neurotoxicity that is usually reversible (Janicki et al., 2001). Central retinal artery occlusion presents as painless, monocular blindness. Ophthalmoscopic examination of

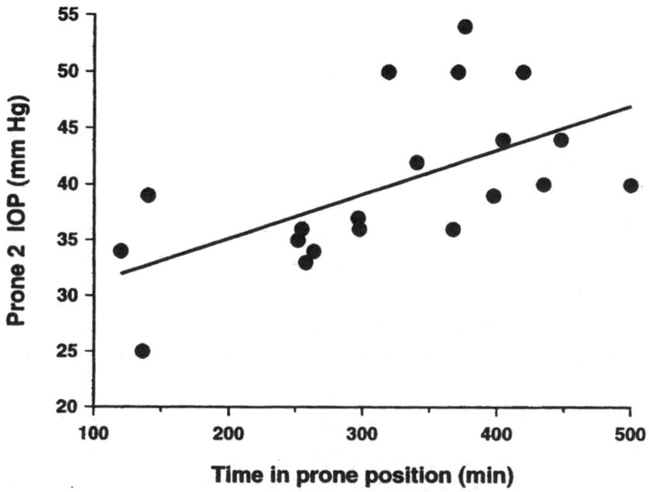

Figure 41-16. Intraocular pressure (IOP) at the conclusion of prone positioning (prone 2) is correlated with the total time spent in the prone position (minutes). (From Cheng MA, Todorov A, Tempelhoff R, et al. The effect of prone positioning on intraocular pressure in anesthetized patients. *Anesthesiology* 2001;95: 1351–1355; with permission.)

the eyes with retinal artery occlusion shows a pale edematous retina, a cherry-red spot at the fovea, and platelet-fibrin or cholesterol emboli in the narrowed retinal arteries. Obstruction of venous drainage from the eye may occur intraoperatively when patient positioning results in external pressure on the eyes.

Photochemicals

The light-sensitive photochemical continuously synthesized in rods is rhodopsin. Cones contain photochemicals that resemble rhodopsin. Vitamin A is an important precursor of photochemicals, which explains the occurrence of night blindness when this vitamin becomes deficient. Photochemicals in rods and cones decompose on exposure to light and in the process stimulate fibers in the optic nerve. Decomposition of rhodopsin decreases conductance of the membranes of rods for sodium ions. The resulting hyperpolarization in rods is opposite to the effect that occurs in almost all other sensory receptors. The intensity of the hyperpolarization signal is proportional to the logarithm of light energy, in contrast to the more linear response of most other receptors. This logarithmic response is important to vision because it allows the eyes to detect contrasts on the image even when light intensities vary several thousandfold.

If a person is in bright light for a prolonged period, large proportions of photochemicals in the rods and cones are depleted, resulting in decreased sensitivity of the eye to light (light adaptation). Conversely, during total darkness, the sensitivity of the retina is increased, reflecting conversion of photochemicals to rhodopsin (dark adaptation). The eye can also adapt to changes in light intensity by changing the size of the pupillary opening up to 30-fold.

Color Blindness

Red-green color blindness is present when red or green types of cones are absent. Color blindness is a sex-linked recessive trait that will not appear as long as one X chromosome carries the genes necessary for the development of color-receptor cones. Because males have only one X chromosome, all three color genes must be present in this single chromosome to prevent color blindness. In about 1 in 50 times, the X chromosome lacks the gene from the red cone and, in about 1 in 16 times, the gene for the green cone is absent. As a result, about 2% of males are color blind. Color blindness is rare in females because they possess two X chromosomes.

Visual Pathway

Impulses from the retina pass backward through the optic nerve (Fig. 41-17) (Ganong, 2003). The macula is a small area in the center of the retina that is composed mainly of cones to permit detailed vision. The fovea is the central portion of the macula and is the site of the clearest vision. At the optic chiasm, all the fibers from the nasal halves of the retina cross to the opposite side to join fibers from the opposite temporal retina to form the optic tracts. Fibers of the optic tract synapse in the lateral geniculate body before passing into the visual (occipital) area of the cerebral cortex. Specific points of the retina connect with specific points of the visual cortex, which results in the detection of lines, borders, and colors.

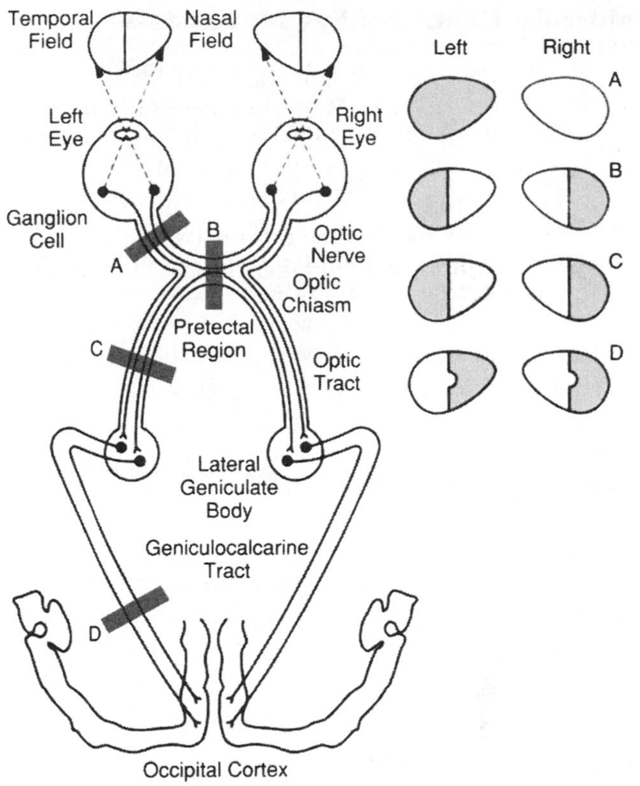

Figure 41-17. Visual impulses from the retina pass to the optic chiasm, where fibers from the nasal halves of the retina cross to the opposite side to join temporal fibers and form the optic tract. These fibers synapse in the lateral geniculate body before passing to the visual (occipital) area of the cerebral cortex. Visual field defects reflect lesions at various sites (A–D) in the nerve pathways. (From Ganong WF. *Review of medical physiology*, 21st ed. New York. Lange Medical Books/McGraw-Hill, 2003; with permission.)

Field of Vision

The field of vision is the area seen by the eye at a given instant. The area seen to the nasal side is called the *nasal field of vision*, and the area seen to the lateral side is called the *temporal field of vision* (see Fig. 41-17) (Ganong, 2003). Blind spots called *scotomata* are due to the lack of rods and cones in the retina. An important use of visual fields is localization of lesions in the visual neural pathway. For example, anterior pituitary tumors may compress the optic chiasm, causing blindness in both temporal fields of vision (called *bitemporal hemianopia*). Thrombosis of the posterior cerebral artery is a cause of infarction of the visual cortex.

Muscular Control of Eye Movements

The cerebral control system for directing the eyes toward the object to be viewed is as important as the cerebral system for interpretation of the visual signals. Movements of the eyes are controlled by three pairs of skeletal muscles designated as the (a) medial and lateral recti, (b) superior and inferior recti, and (c) superior and inferior obliques. The medial and lateral recti contract reciprocally to move the eyes from side to side; the superior and inferior recti move the eyes upward or downward; and rotation of the globe is accomplished by the superior and inferior obliques. Each of the three sets of eye muscles is reciprocally innervated by cranial nerves III, IV, and VI so that one muscle of the pair contracts while the other relaxes.

Simultaneous movement of both eyes in the same directions is called *conjugate movement of the eyes*. Occasionally, abnormalities occur in the control system for eye movements that cause continuous nystagmus. Nystagmus is likely to occur when one of the vestibular apparatuses is damaged or when deep nuclei in the cerebellum are damaged.

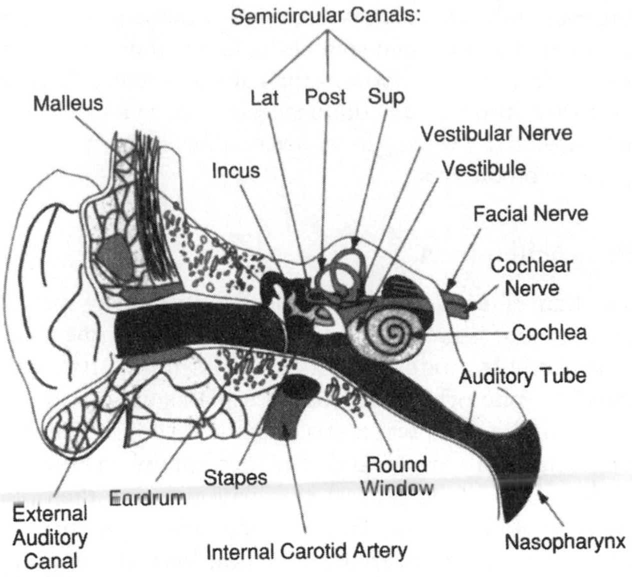

Figure 41-18. Schematic diagram of the outer and inner ear. (Lat, lateral; Post, posterior; Sup, superior.) (From Ganong WF. *Review of medical physiology*, 21st ed. New York. Lange Medical Books/McGraw-Hill, 2003; with permission.)

Innervation of the Eye

The eyes are innervated by the sympathetic and parasympathetic nervous system. The preganglionic fibers of the parasympathetic nervous system arise in the Edinger-Westphal nucleus of cranial nerve III and then pass to the ciliary ganglion, which gives rise to nerve fibers that innervate the ciliary muscle and sphincter of the iris. Sympathetic nervous system fibers innervate the radial fibers of the iris as well as several extraocular structures. Stimulation of the parasympathetic nervous system fibers to the eye excites the ciliary sphincter, causing miosis. Conversely, stimulation of sympathetic nervous system fibers to the eye excites the radial fibers of the iris and causes mydriasis.

Horner Syndrome

Interruption of the superior cervical chain of the sympathetic nervous system innervation to the eye results in miosis, ptosis, and vasodilation with absence of sweating on the ipsilateral side of the body. These findings are known as *Horner syndrome* and characteristically occur after performance of a stellate ganglion block. Miosis occurs because of interruption of sympathetic nervous system innervation to the radial fibers of the iris. Ptosis reflects the normal innervation of the superior palpebral muscle by the sympathetic nervous system.

HEARING

Receptors for hearing and equilibrium are housed in the ear (Fig. 41-18) (Ganong, 2003). The external ear, middle ear, and cochlea of the inner ear are concerned with hearing based on mechanical vibrations of sound waves in air. Transmission of sound from the tympanic membrane to the cochlea uses an ossicle system.

Ossicle System

The middle ear is an air-filled cavity containing the ossicle system that includes the malleus, incus, and stapes. The handle of the malleus is attached to the tympanic membrane, whereas the other end is bound by ligaments to the incus. The opposite end of the incus articulates with the stapes, which lies against the membranous labyrinth in the opening of the oval window, where sound waves are transmitted to the cochlea. The handle of the malleus is constantly pulled inward by ligaments and by the tensor tympanic membrane muscle, which keeps the tympanic membrane tensed. This allows vibrations on any portion of the tympanic membrane to be transmitted to the malleus. The eustachian tube allows pressures on both sides of the tympanic membrane to be equalized during chewing or swallowing. Nitrous oxide may increase middle ear pressure and has been associated with rupture of the tympanic membrane when inflammation or scarring of the eustachian tube opening into the nasopharynx prevents spontaneous decompression of middle ear pressures (Owens et al., 1978).

Cochlea

The cochlea is a system of coiled tubes embedded in a bony cavity in the temporal bone. The organ of Corti contains hair cells that function as end organs to generate nerve impulses in response to sound vibrations. These hair cells synapse with cochlear nerve endings, which enter the CNS for transmission to the auditory cerebral cortex.

Deafness

Nerve deafness is due to an abnormality of the cochlear or auditory nerve. Conversely, conduction deafness is present when an abnormality exists in the middle ear mechanisms for transmitting sounds into the cochlea. Certain drugs such as streptomycin, kanamycin, and chloramphenicol may damage the organ of Corti, causing nerve deafness. Conduction deafness is often caused by fibrosis of the structures in the middle ear after repeated infections in the middle ear by the hereditary disease known as *osteosclerosis*.

Perioperative Hearing Impairment

Perioperative hearing impairment is often subclinical and may go unnoticed unless audiometry is performed (Sprung et al., 2003). Hearing loss (incidence may be as high as 50%) after dural puncture in the low-frequency range is most likely due to CSF leak and should resolve completely within days. Hearing loss following general anesthesia for surgery not requiring cardiopulmonary bypass does not appear to have a uniform prognosis being more a function of the specific etiology-CSF leak after ENT and neurosurgery, middle ear barotrauma (nitrous oxide), embolism, or vascular. Any recovery in hearing appears to be independent of treatment. Unilateral hearing loss following cardiopulmonary bypass is often permanent and probably due to embolism and subsequent ischemic injury to areas of the organ of Corti.

EQUILIBRIUM

Semicircular canals—the utricle and saccule of the inner ear—are important for maintaining equilibrium (see Fig. 41-18) (Ganong, 2003). The utricle and saccule contain cilia that transmit nerve impulses to the brain necessary for maintaining orientation of the head in space. Endolymph present in the semicircular canals flows with changes in head position, causing signals to be transmitted via the vestibular nerve nuclei and the cerebellum. The semicircular canals predict ahead of time that loss of equilibrium is going to occur, leading to initiation of preventive responses.

A simple test of the integrity of the equilibrium mechanisms is to have the individual stand motionless with the eyes closed. In the absence of a functioning static equilibrium system of the utricles, the person will tend to fall to one side. Nevertheless, proprioceptive mechanisms (joint receptors) may be sufficiently developed to maintain balance even with the eyes closed. Separate testing of the semicircular canals is accomplished by placing ice water in the external auditory canal. The external semicircular canal is adjacent to the tympanic membrane such that selective cooling of the endolymph occurs. This cooling causes nystagmus in the presence of normally functioning semicircular canals.

CHEMICAL SENSES

Chemical senses are manifest as taste and smell.

Taste

Taste is mainly a function of taste buds located principally in the papillae of the tongue. Sweet, sour, salty, and bitter are the four primary sensations of taste. Sour taste is caused by acids, and the taste sensation is approximately proportional to the logarithm of the hydrogen ion concentration. The bitter taste of alkaloids causes the individual to reject these substances. This is probably protective because many toxins in poisonous plants are alkaloids. Adaptation to taste sensations is almost complete in 1 to 5 minutes of continuous stimulation. Individuals with upper respiratory tract infections complain of loss of taste sensation when, in fact, taste bud function is normal, emphasizing that most of what is considered taste is actually smell. Taste preference is presumed to be a CNS phenomenon.

Smell

Olfactory hairs, or cilia, are believed to sense odors in the air, causing stimulation of olfactory cells. It is presumed that olfactory cells initiate impulses in olfactory nerve fibers. A substance must be volatile and lipid soluble to stimulate olfactory cells. The importance of upward air movement in smell acuity is the reason sniffing improves the sense of smell, whereas holding one's breath prevents the sensation of unpleasant odors. Olfactory receptors adapt rapidly such that smell sensation may become extinct in about 60 seconds. Compared with lower animals, the sense of smell in humans is almost rudimentary. Nevertheless, the threshold for smell is low as reflected by the detection of trace concentrations of methyl mercaptan that is mixed with odorless natural gas to alert one to a gas leak.

NAUSEA AND VOMITING

Nausea is the conscious recognition of excitation of an area in the medulla that is associated with the vomiting (emetic) center (Fig. 41-19) (Watcha and White, 1992). Impulses are transmitted by afferent fibers of the parasympathetic and sympathetic nervous system to the vomiting center. Motor impulses transmitted via cranial nerves V, VII, IX, X, and XII to the gastrointestinal tract and through the spinal nerves to

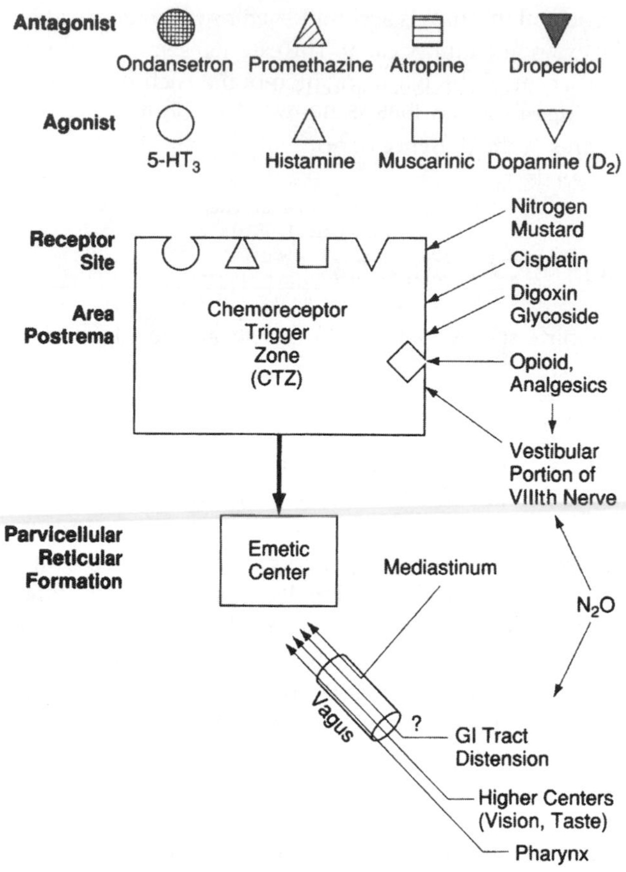

Figure 41-19. The chemoreceptor trigger zone and emetic center respond to a variety of stimuli resulting in nausea and vomiting. (5-HT_3, 5-hydroxytryptamine; GI, gastrointestinal.) (From Watcha MR, White PF. Postoperative nausea and vomiting. Its etiology, treatment, and prevention. *Anesthesiology* 1992;77:162–184; with permission.)

the diaphragm and abdominal muscles are required to cause the mechanical act of vomiting. Psychic stimuli, including unpleasant visual input or odors, most likely cause vomiting by stimulating the vomiting center.

The medullary vomiting center is located close to the fourth cerebral ventricle and receives afferents from the (a) chemoreceptor trigger zone, (b) cerebral cortex, (c) labyrinthovestibular center, and (d) neurovegetative system. Impulses from these afferents lead to nausea and vomiting. The chemoreceptor trigger zone includes receptors for serotonin, dopamine, histamine, and opioids. Stimulation of the chemoreceptor trigger zone located on the floor of the fourth cerebral ventricle initiates vomiting independent of the vomiting center. The chemoreceptor trigger zone is not protected by the blood-brain barrier and thus this zone can be activated by chemical stimuli received through the systemic circulation as well as the CSF. The cerebral cortex is stimulated by smell and physiologic stresses. Motion can stimulate equilibrium receptors in the inner ear, which may also stimulate the chemoreceptor trigger zone. The neurovegetative system is sensitive principally to gastrointestinal stimulation. Blocking of impulses from the chemoreceptor trigger zone does not prevent vomiting due to irritative stimuli (ipecac) arising in the gastrointestinal tract.

REFERENCES

Adams DC, Emerson RG, Heyer EJ, et al. Monitoring of intraoperative motor-evoked potentials under condition of controlled neuromuscular blockade. *Anesth Analg* 1993;77:913–918.

Azzam FJ. A simple and effective method for stopping post-anesthesia clonus. *Anesthesiology* 1987;66:98.

Bogetz MS, Katz JA. Recall of surgery for major trauma. *Anesthesiology* 1984;61:6–9.

Brian JE. Carbon dioxide and the cerebral circulation. *Anesthesiology* 1998;88:1365–1386.

Budson AE, Price BH. Memory dysfunction. *N Engl J Med* 2005;352: 692–699.

Cheng MA, Todorov A, Tempelhoff R, et al. The effect of prone positioning on intraocular pressure in anesthetized patients. *Anesthesiology* 2001;95:1351–1355.

Chi OZ, Field C. Effects of isoflurane on visual evoked potentials in humans. *Anesthesiology* 1986;65:328–330.

Dwyer R, Bennett HL, Eger EI, et al. Effects of isoflurane and nitrous oxide in subanesthetic concentrations on memory and responsiveness in volunteers. *Anesthesiology* 1992a;77:888–898.

Dwyer R, Bennett HL, Eger EI, et al. Isoflurane anesthesia prevents unconscious learning. *Anesth Analg* 1992b;75:107–112.

Ekman A, Lindholm M-L, Lennmarken C, et al. Reduction in the incidence of awareness using BIS monitoring. *Acta Anesthesiol Scand* 2004;48:20–26.

Flaishon R, Windsor A, Sigl J, Sebel PS. Recovery of consciousness after thiopental or propofol. Bispectral index and the isolated forearm technique. *Anesthesiology* 1997;86:613–619.

Gallart L, Blanco D, Samso E, et al. Clinical and radiologic evidence of the epidural plica medina dorsalis. *Anesth Analg* 1990;71:698–701.

Gan TJ, Glass PS, Windsor A, et al. Bispectral index monitoring allows faster recovery from propofol, alfentanil, and nitrous oxide anesthesia. *Anesthesiology* 1997;87:808–815.

Ganong WF. *Review of medical physiology*, 21st ed. New York. Lange Medical Books/McGraw-Hill, 2003.

Ghoneim MM. Awareness during anesthesia. *Anesthesiology* 2000;92: 597–602.

Gilman S. Advances in neurology. *N Engl J Med* 1992;326:1608–1616.

Ginsburg HH, Shetter AG, Raudzens PA. Postoperative paraplegia with preserved intraoperative somatosensory evoked potentials. *J Neurosurg* 1985;63:296–299.

Guyton AC, Hall JE. *Textbook of medical physiology*, 10th ed. Philadelphia. Saunders, 2000.

Haenggi M, Ypparila H, Takala J, et al. Measuring depth of sedation with auditory evoked potentials during controlled infusion of propofol and remifentanil in health volunteers. *Anesth Analg* 2004; 99:1728–1736.

Hudspith MJ. Glutamate: a role in normal brain function, anaesthesia, analgesia and CNS injury. *Br J Anaesth* 1997;78:731–747.

Janicki PK, Pai R, Wrights JK, et al. Ischemic optic neuropathy after liver transplantation. *Anesthesiology* 2001:94:361–363.

Johnson RW. Anatomy for ophthalmic anaesthesia. *Br J Anaesth* 1995; 75:80–87.

Kearse LA, Manberg P, Chamoun N, et al. Bispectral analysis of the electroencephalogram correlates with patient movement to skin incision during propofol/nitrous oxide anesthesia. *Anesthesiology* 1994;81:1365–1370.

Kofke WA, Young RSK, Davis P, et al. Isoflurane for refractory status epilepticus: a clinical series. *Anesthesiology* 1989;71:653–659.

Lee LA, Lam AM. Unilateral blindness after prone lumbar spine surgery. *Anesthesiology* 2001;95:793–795.

Lennmarken C, Sandin R. Neuromonitoring for awareness during surgery. *Lancet* 2004;363:1747–1748.

Lyons G, MacDonald R. Awareness during cesarean section. *Anaesthesia* 1991;46:62–64.

Miller RD, Way WL, Eger EI. The effects of alpha-methyldopa, reserpine, guanethidine, and iproniazid on minimal alveolar anesthetic requirement (MAC). *Anesthesiology* 1968;29:1153–1158.

Moller JT, Cluitmans P, Rasmussen LS, et al. Long-term postoperative cognitive dysfunction in the elderly. *Lancet* 1998;351:857–861.
Myers MA, Hamilton SR, Bogosian AJ, et al. Visual loss as a complication of spine surgery. *Spine* 1997;22:1325–1329.
Myles PS, Leslie K, McNeil J, et al. Bispectral index monitoring to prevent awareness during anaesthesia: the B-Aware randomized controlled trial. *Lancet* 2004;363:1757–1763.
Ovassapian A, Joshi CW, Brunner EA. Visual disturbances: an unusual symptom of transurethral prostatic resection reaction. *Anesthesiology* 1982;57:332–334.
Owens WD, Gustave F, Schlaroff A. Tympanic membrane rupture with nitrous oxide anesthesia. *Anesth Analg* 1978;57:283–286.
Pathak KS, Ammadio M, Kalamchi A, et al. Effects of halothane, enflurane, and isoflurane on somatosensory evoked potentials during nitrous oxide anesthesia. *Anesthesiology* 1987;66:753–757.
Perreault L, Drolet P, Farny J. Ulnar nerve palsy at the elbow after general anaesthesia. *Can J Anaesth* 1992;39:499–503.
Ranta S, Jussila J, Hynyen M. Recall of awareness during cardiac anaesthesia: influence of feedback information to the anaesthesiologist. *Acta Anaesthesiol Scand* 1996;40:554–560.
Roth S, Barach P. Postoperative visual loss. Still no answers—Yet. *Anesthesiology* 2001;95:575–577.
Rubenstein E, Federman D, eds. *Scientific American Medicine*. New York: Scientific American, 1992.
Schmidt GN, Bischoff P, Standl T, et al. Comparative evaluation of the Datex-Ohmeda S/5 entropy module and the Bispectral Index® monitor during propofol-remifentanil anesthesia. *Anesthesiology* 2004;101:1283–1290.
Savolaine ER, Pandya JB, Greenblatt SH, Conover SR. Anatomy of the human lumbar epidural space. New insights using CT-epidurography. *Anesthesiology* 1988;68:217–220.
Schubert A, Drummond JC. The effect of acute hypocapnia on human median nerve somatosensory evoked responses. *Anesth Analg* 1986;65:240–244.
Sebel PS, Bowdle TA, Ghoneim MM, et al. The incidence of awareness during anesthesia: A multicenter United States study. *Anesth Analg* 2004;99:833–839.
Sigl J, Chamoun N. An introduction to bispectral analysis for the electroencephalogram. *J Clin Monit* 1994;10:392–404.
Song D, Joshi G, White PF. Titration of volatile anesthetics using bispectral index facilitates recovery after ambulatory anesthesia. *Anesthesiology* 1997;87:842–848.
Sprung J, Wilt S, Bourke D, et al. Is it time to correct the dermatome chart of the anterior scrotal region? *Anesthesiology* 1993;79: 381–383.
Sprung J, Bourke DL, Contreras MG, et al. Perioperative hearing impairment. *Anesthesiology* 2003;98:241–257.
Wang JML, Creel DJ, Wong KC. Transurethral resection of the prostate: serum glycine levels and ocular evoked potentials. *Anesthesiology* 1989;70:36–41.
Watcha MR, White PF. Postoperative nausea and vomiting. Its etiology, treatment, and prevention. *Anesthesiology* 1992;77:162–184.
Williams EL, Hart WM, Tempelhoff R. Postoperative ischemic optic neuropathy. *Anesth Analg* 1995;80:1018–1029.

Thermoregulation

42

Body temperature is determined by the relationship between heat production and heat dissipation. Heat is continually being produced in the body as a product of metabolism. As heat is produced, it is also continuously being lost to the environment. Both heat generation and heat loss are adjusted in order to regulate body temperature within narrow limits. Normal core body temperatures range from about 36°C to 37.5°C and undergo circadian fluctuations, being lowest in the morning and highest in the evening. This is consistent with a 10% to 15% decrease in basal metabolic rate during physiologic sleep; presumably reflecting decreased activity of skeletal muscles and the sympathetic nervous system. An estimated 55% of the energy in nutrients is converted to heat during the formation of adenosine triphosphate. The average daily caloric requirement for basal function is approximately 2,000 calories.

HEAT LOSS

The important mechanisms of heat loss from the body include: *radiation, conduction, convection, and evaporation*. Their relative contributions vary, and depend upon the environmental circumstances (Buggy and Crossley, 2000). The skin is the most important route for heat dissipation, while the lungs account for only about 10% of heat loss. Under typical circumstances, most heat (about 60%) is lost by radiation. A warm object emits energy in the form of radiation, predominantly in the infrared range. Infrared radiation allows heat transfer from a warm object to a cooler object, independent of the temperature of the intervening air. The unclothed human is an excellent source of radiant heat. Significant radiant losses can occur from the patient to the walls of an operating room. In infant incubators, radiant heat losses occur between the infant and the relatively cold walls of the incubator despite active warming of the air between them. Double walled incubators are intended to reduce radiant heat loss because of the presence of warm air on both sides of the inner wall of the incubator. In this way, the influence of the ambient temperature of the nursery on the temperature of the infant is significantly reduced. Space blankets reduce radiant heat loss by reflecting infrared radiation back towards the patient. Radiant heat transfer *to* the patient can also occur when radiant warmers are used for active warming. *Conduction* of heat from the body occurs by direct contact with a cooler object, for example between the patient and an adjacent mattress. The area of the conducting surfaces, their temperature difference, and the presence or absence of insulation affects conductive heat transfer. Reductions in core temperature during the administration of cold intravenous fluids and blood products are attributable to conductive losses. Conductive loss to still air is limited because a stationary layer of air next to the skin acts as a good insulator. Air has a very low heat capacity and warms quickly, thus promptly eliminating the temperature gradient. In humans, piloerection reduces heat loss by trapping a layer of air next to the skin. Although pure conduction accounts for <5% of heat loss, conductive heat loss to air is greatly facilitated by air movement and is termed *convection* or *facilitated conduction*. The rate of convective loss depends on both the air temperature and its velocity (the "wind-chill" phenomenon). Convection accounts for approximately 15% to 30% of heat loss in the operating room but increases significantly in high "wind-chill" environments such as a laminar flow unit. However, significant convective heat losses occur even in a draft-free environment because warmed air has a low density and will rise to be replaced by denser cold air, thus maintaining cutaneous airflow. *Evaporative* heat losses are important because significant energy is required to vaporize water. Evaporation accounts for about 20% of total heat losses, most of these occurring via the skin. The magnitude of evaporative loss depends upon environmental humidity, exposed skin surface area, presence of diaphoresis, wound and bowel exposure, and application of fluid to the skin (prep solutions). Evaporation is the only mechanism by which the body can eliminate excess heat when the temperature of the surroundings is higher than that of the skin. Paradoxically, the use of radiant warmers may increase both evaporative and convective heat losses. Diaphoresis occurs in response to stimulation of the preoptic area of the hypothalamus. A normal unacclimatized individual has a maximal sweat production of about 700 mL/hour. With continued exposure to a warm environment, sweat production may increase to 1,500 mL/hour. Evaporation of this amount of sweat can remove heat from the body at a rate of >10 times the normal basal rate of heat production. Evaporation accounts for two-thirds of the heat loss from the respiratory tract.

REGULATION OF BODY TEMPERATURE

Central regulation of body temperature is by feedback mechanisms that operate predominantly through the preoptic nucleus of the anterior hypothalamus (Simon, 2003). This area integrates afferent input from thermoreceptors in the skin, deep tissues, and spinal cord. However, it is now known that considerable modulation of afferent thermoregulatory input occurs in the brain stem and spinal cord before arrival in the hypothalamus. The preoptic area also contains heat-sensitive neurons and receives additional thermal input from extra-hypothalamic areas of the brain. The reflex responses to cold (vasoconstriction, piloerection, shivering, and nonshivering thermogenesis) originate in the posterior hypothalamus. The reflex responses to heat (vasodilatation, sweating) originate in the anterior hypothalamus. The hypothalamic thermostat detects body temperature changes and initiates autonomic, somatic, and endocrine thermoresponses when the various set points are reached. However, in the awake individual, behavioral responses usually occur before the core temperature reaches the set points. In the case of hypothermia, if the behavioral responses fail or are abolished by anesthesia, the hypothalamic thermostat stimulates vasoconstriction. As a result, the rate of heat transfer to the skin is decreased and body temperature increases. Conversely, hypothalamic-induced vasodilation of the cutaneous blood vessels will decrease body temperature. Thermoregulatory responses are graded and each particular response is characterized by a threshold temperature at which it is initiated. For example, vasoconstriction in response to cold occurs at 36.5°C whereas shivering does not occur until core temperature decreases 36.2°C. In the awake individual, there is a narrow range of normal core temperature, the interthreshold range (36.7°C–37.1°C), within which thermoregulatory responses are not triggered. During general anesthesia, the threshold temperatures for activation of responses to cold are decreased and the threshold temperatures for activation of warm responses are increased. Thus, the interthreshold range is significantly larger during general anesthesia. Maintenance of body temperature at a value close to the optimum for enzyme activity assures a constant rate of metabolism, optimal nervous system conduction, and skeletal muscle contraction. Protein denaturation begins at about 42°C, whereas ice crystals form in cells at about −1°C.

Nonshivering Thermogenesis

Nonshivering thermogenesis (alternatively called chemical thermogenesis) is an increase in the rate of cellular metabolism in brown adipose tissue evoked by sympathetic nervous system stimulation or by circulating catecholamines. In adults, who have almost no brown fat, it is rare that chemical thermogenesis increases the rate of heat production by >15%. In infants, however, chemical thermogenesis in brown fat located in the interscapular space and around the great vessels in the thorax and abdomen can increase the rate of heat production by as much as 200%. In contrast to other fat depots, brown fat contains large numbers of mitochondria, and has extensive sympathetic innervation. Within these mitochondria, the generation of adenosine triphosphate is uncoupled as oxidative phosphorylation is short-circuited to generate heat. This process is dependent upon an uncoupling protein (UCP 1). Lipolysis and heat generation in brown fat is mediated via beta-adrenergic receptors.

Shivering

Skeletal muscle activity is a major source of heat. Shivering increases body heat production in response to decreased core temperature. The posterior hypothalamic area responsible for the response to hypothermia controls reflex shivering. Shivering occurs due to both increased motor traffic via anterior motor neurons and to upregulation of the muscle stretch reflex.

Causes of Increased Body Temperature

A variety of disorders can increase body temperature. Those disorders resulting from thermoregulatory failure (excessive metabolic production of heat, excessive environmental heat, and impaired heat dissipation) are properly characterized as *hyperthermia*, whereas those resulting from intact homeostatic responses are categorized as *fever* (Table 42-1) (Simon, 2003).

In hyperthermic states, the hypothalamic set-point is normal but peripheral mechanisms are unable to maintain body temperature that matches the set-point. In contrast, fever occurs when the hypothalamic set-point is increased by the action of circulating pyrogenic cytokines, causing intact peripheral mechanisms to conserve and generate heat until the body temperature increases to the elevated set-point. Despite their physiologic differences, hyperthermia and fever cannot be differentiated clinically based on the height of the temperature or its pattern. However, the clinical management of hyperthermia and fever require differing approaches. The treatment of hyperthermia should be directed at promoting heat dissipation, whereas the treatment of fever should be directed at identification and eradication of pyrogens and lowering the thermoregulatory set-point with antipyretic drugs such as aspirin, acetaminophen, and other cyclooxygenase inhibitors.

TABLE 42-1.
CAUSES OF HYPERTHERMIA

Disorders associated with excessive heat production	
	Malignant hyperthermia
	Neuroleptic malignant syndrome
	Thyrotoxicosis
	Delirium tremens
	Pheochromocytoma
	Salicylate intoxication
	Drug abuse (cocaine, amphetamine)
	Status epilepticus
	Exertional hyperthermia
Disorders associated with decreased heat loss	
	Autonomic nervous system dysfunction
	Anticholinergics
	Drug abuse (cocaine)
	Dehydration
	Occlusive dressings
	Heat stroke
Disorders associated with dysfunction of the hypothalamus	
	Trauma
	Tumors
	Idiopathic hypothalamic dysfunction
	Cerebrovascular accidents
	Encephalitis
	Neuroleptic malignant syndrome

Fever

Pyrogens are bacterial toxins that indirectly cause the set-point of the hypothalamic thermostat to increase. Bacterial pyrogens stimulate host inflammatory cells (mononuclear phagocytes) to generate endogenous pyrogens, including interleukins and tumor necrosis factor. Similarly, viruses do not release pyrogens directly, but stimulate infected cells to release interferons alpha and beta that act as endogenous pyrogens. All known endogenous pyrogens are polypeptides and are therefore unlikely to cross the blood brain barrier. However, endogenous pyrogens have actions in the organum vasculosum of the lamina terminalis (OVLT), which is a structure adjacent to the lateral ventricles that lies outside the blood brain barrier. It is likely that endogenous pyrogens acting in the OVLT evoke the release of prostaglandins, leading to stimulation of the preoptic nucleus and generation of the febrile response (Ganong, 2003).

Chills

Sudden resetting of the hypothalamic thermostat to a higher level because of tissue destruction, pyrogens, or dehydration, results in a lag between blood temperature and the new hypothalamic set point. During this period, the person experiences chills and feels cold even though body temperature may be increased. The skin is cold because of cutaneous vasoconstriction. Chills continue until the body temperature increases to the new set point of the hypothalamic thermostat. As long as the process causing the hypothalamic thermostat to be set at a higher level is present, the body's core temperature will remain increased above normal. Sudden removal of the factor that is causing the body temperature to remain increased is accompanied by intense diaphoresis and feeling of warmth because of generalized cutaneous vasodilation.

Cutaneous Blood Flow

Cutaneous blood flow is a major determinant of heat loss. The cutaneous circulation is among the most variable in the body, reflecting its primary role in regulation of body temperature in response to alterations in the rate of metabolism and the temperature of the external surroundings. Nutritional requirements are so low for skin that this need does not significantly influence cutaneous blood flow. For example, at ordinary skin temperature, cutaneous blood flow is about ten times that needed to supply nutritive needs of the skin.

Cutaneous blood flow is largely regulated by the sympathetic nervous system and not local regulatory mechanisms that reflect tissue oxygen needs. Vascular structures concerned with heat loss from skin consist of subcutaneous venous plexuses than can hold large quantities of blood. Furthermore, the cutaneous circulation of the fingers, palms, toes, and earlobes has richly innervated arteriovenous anastomoses that facilitate heat loss via significant increases in blood flow. In an adult, typical total cutaneous blood flow is about 400 mL/minute. This flow can decrease to as little as 50 mL/minute in severe cold and may increase to as much as 2,800 mL/minute in extreme heat. Indeed, patients with borderline cardiac function may become symptomatic in hot environments, emphasizing the increase in cardiac output necessitated by marked increases in cutaneous blood flow. During acute hemorrhage, the sympathetic nervous system can produce sufficient cutaneous vasoconstriction to transfer large amounts of blood into the central circulation. As such, the cutaneous veins act as an important blood reservoir that can supply 5% to 10% of the blood volume in times of need. Indeed, acute hemorrhage may be less well tolerated in a warm environment because the hypothalamic vasodilator response may override the vasoconstrictor response to hypovolemia. Inhaled anesthetics increase cutaneous blood flow, perhaps by inhibiting the temperature-regulating center of the hypothalamus (Heistad and Abboud, 1974).

Skin Color

Skin color in light-skinned individuals is principally due to the color of blood in the cutaneous capillaries and veins. The skin has a pinkish hue when arterial blood is flowing rapidly through these tissues. Conversely, when the skin is cold and blood is flowing slowly, the removal of oxygen for nutritive purposes gives the skin the bluish hue (cyanosis) of deoxygenated blood. Severe vasoconstriction of the skin forces most of this blood into the central circulation, and skin takes on the whitish hue (pallor) of underlying connective tissue, which is composed primarily of collagen fibers.

PERIOPERATIVE TEMPERATURE CHANGES

The thermoregulatory system contains three key elements: afferent input, central processing, and the efferent response. General anesthesia affects all three elements and regional anesthesia affects both the afferent and efferent components. Thus, anesthesia and surgery in a cool environment makes perioperative hypothermia a likely occurrence (Table 42-2) (Giesbrecht, 1994; Sessler, 2000). General anesthesia (inhaled and injected drugs) and regional anesthesia (epidural and spinal) widen the interthreshold range to 4.0°C, a value approximately 20 times the normal range. Typically, the threshold for sweating and vasodilation is increased about 1°C, and the threshold for vasoconstriction and shivering is decreased about 3°C. As a result, anesthetized patients are relatively poikilothermic, with body temperatures determined by the environment. Anesthetics inhibit thermoregulation in a dose-dependent manner and inhibit vasoconstriction and shivering about three times as much as they restrict sweating (Fig. 42-1) (Sessler, 1997).

TABLE 42-2.
EVENTS THAT CONTRIBUTE TO DECREASES IN BODY TEMPERATURE DURING SURGERY

Resetting of the hypothalamic thermostat
Ambient temperature <21°C
Administration of unwarmed intravenous fluids
Drug-induced vasodilation
Basal metabolic rate decreased
Attenuated shivering response
Core compartment exposed to ambient temperature
Heat required to humidify inhaled dry gases

Alfentanil and propofol similarly lower the threshold for vasoconstriction and sweating. Volatile anesthetics such as isoflurane and desflurane decrease the threshold temperatures for cold responses in a nonlinear fashion. Nonshivering thermogenesis does not occur during general anesthesia in adults or infants.

Sequence of Temperature Changes during Anesthesia

In the awake individual, body heat is unevenly distributed. Tonic thermoregulatory vasoconstriction maintains a temperature gradient between the core and periphery of 2°C to 4°C. The core compartment which is insulated from

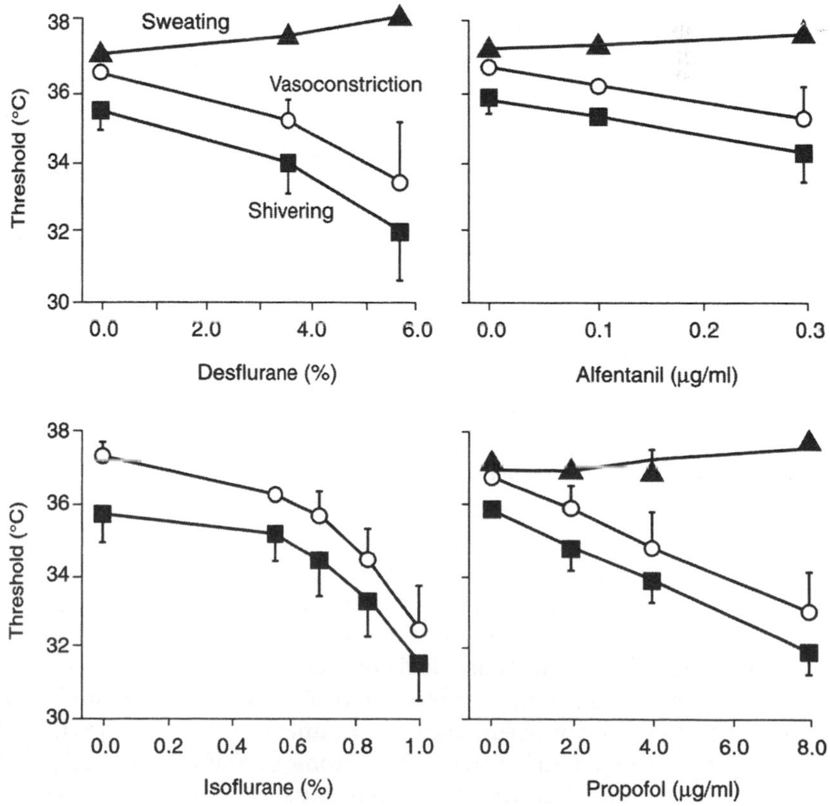

Figure 42-1. Changes in the thermoregulatory threshold for sweating, vasoconstriction, and shivering in the presence of increasing concentrations of inhaled or injected anesthetics. (From Sessler DI. Mild perioperative hypothermia. *N Engl J Med* 1997;336:1630–1637; with permission.)

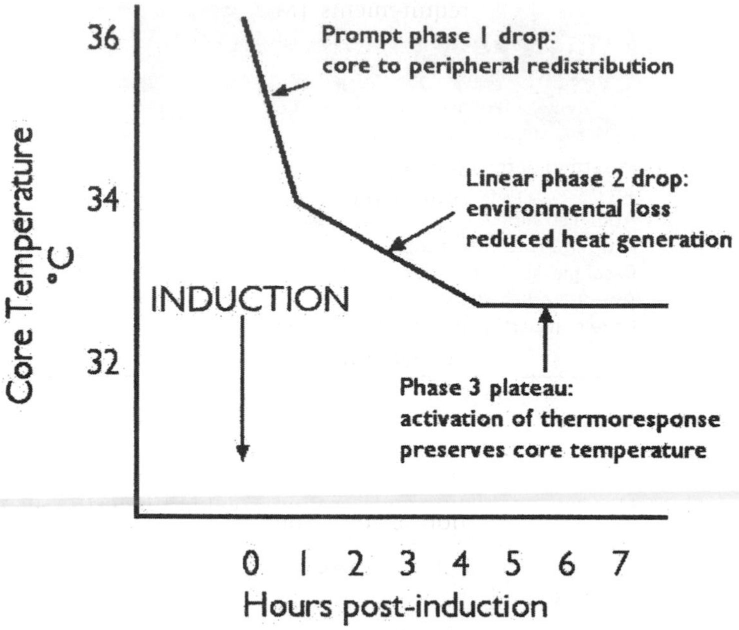

Figure 42-2. Graphic representation of the typical triphasic core temperature pattern that occurs after induction of anesthesia. Note that the phase 3 plateau may not occur, particularly during regional anesthesia or during combined regional and general anesthesia. Although core temperature is preserved during the phase 3 plateau, heat will continue to be lost to the environment from the peripheral compartment.

the environment by the peripheral compartment, consists of the major viscera, and includes the head, chest, abdomen, and pelvis. Under general anesthesia, tonic vasoconstriction is attenuated and heat contained in the core compartment will move to the periphery, thus allowing the core temperature to decrease towards the anesthetic-induced lowered threshold for vasoconstriction. This core to peripheral heat redistribution is responsible for the 1 °C to 5 °C decrease in core temperature that occurs during the first hour of general anesthesia (Fig. 42-2). The loss of heat from the body to the environment contributes little to this initial decrease (Fig. 42-3) (Sessler, 1997).

After the first hour of general anesthesia, the core temperature usually decreases at a slower rate. This decrease is nearly linear and occurs because continuing heat loss to the environment exceeds the metabolic production of heat. After 3 to 5 hours of anesthesia, the core temperature often stops decreasing (see Fig. 42-2). This thermal plateau may reflect a steady state in which heat loss equals heat production. This type of thermal steady state is especially likely in patients who are well insulated or effectively warmed. However, if a patient becomes sufficiently hypothermic, activation of thermoregulatory vasoconstriction will occur, decreasing cutaneous heat loss and retaining heat in the core compartment. Intraoperative vasoconstriction thus reestablishes the normal core-to-periphery temperature gradient by preventing the loss of centrally generated metabolic heat to peripheral tissues. Although vasoconstriction may effectively maintain the core temperature plateau, mean body temperature and the total heat content of the body continue to decrease as continued loss of heat occurs from the peripheral compartment to the environment. Because reflex vasoconstriction is usually effective in maintaining core temperature, the intraoperative

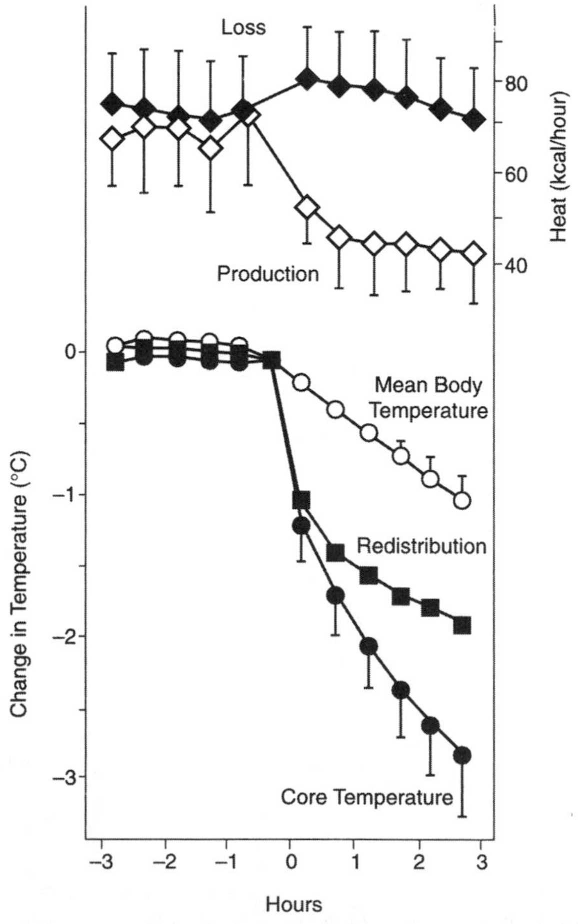

Figure 42-3. Changes in heat loss and heat production and changes in temperature (mean, redistribution, core) from 3 hours before to 3 hours after the induction of anesthesia. (From Sessler DI. Mild perioperative hypothermia. *N Engl J Med* 1997;336:1630–1637; with permission.)

core temperature rarely decreases the additional 1°C necessary to trigger shivering during general anesthesia (Sessler, 2000).

Although regional anesthesia is thought to have minimal effect upon the central processing and integration of the thermoregulatory response, afferent cold input from the lower body may be overridden by a sense of warmth from cutaneous vasodilatation. Decreases in core temperature of a similar or greater magnitude to those experienced during general anesthesia may occur during spinal or epidural techniques. The initial redistributive temperature drop may be less precipitous during regional anesthesia because vasodilatation is restricted to the blocked area. However, because reflex vasoconstriction is abolished below the level of the block, the plateau phase seen during general anesthesia may not occur during regional anesthesia (see Fig. 42-2). Indeed, core temperature may decrease sufficiently during regional anesthesia to trigger the shivering response. However, the ability of reflex shivering to generate heat is markedly attenuated because it is restricted to the unblocked upper body. The risk of significant core hypothermia during regional anesthesia strongly supports the routine use of core temperature monitoring. Combined general and regional anesthetic techniques predispose the patient to a greater degree of heat loss than either technique used alone.

Adverse Consequences of Perioperative Hypothermia

Perioperative hypothermia may predispose to several significant complications (Table 42-3). These include postoperative shivering (significantly increasing metabolic rate and cardiac work) and impaired coagulation (impaired platelet function, decreased activation of the coagulation cascade). Indeed, hypothermia-induced coagulopathy is associated with increased transfusion requirements. A 1°C decrease in temperature is associated with a 5% reduction in anesthetic requirements (MAC) and an increase in volatile anesthetic blood/gas solubility. Drug metabolism is also decreased by hypothermia, particularly of nondepolarizing neuromuscular-blocking drugs. These factors all conspire to delay emergence from anesthesia and delay recovery room discharge. Hypothermia also impairs wound healing and is associated with decreased resistance to surgical wound infection (Sessler, 1997). The underlying mechanism is thought to be hypothermia-induced vasoconstriction, which decreases wound perfusion and local tissue oxygen partial pressure. Perioperative hypothermia is also associated with delayed hospital discharge and an increased catabolic state. Shivering occurs in approximately 40% of unwarmed patients who are recovering from general anesthesia and is associated with substantial sympathetic nervous system activation and discomfort from the sensation of cold. Core hypothermia equal to a 1.5°C decrease triples the incidence of ventricular tachycardia and morbid cardiac events (Frank et al., 1997).

TABLE 42-3.
IMMEDIATE ADVERSE CONSEQUENCES OF PERIOPERATIVE HYPOTHERMIA

Adverse Outcome	Mechanism
Increased operative blood loss	Coagulopathy and platelet dysfunction
Increased morbid cardiac events	Increased myocardial work load
Dysrhythmias and myocardial ischemia	Increased sympathetic activity
Wound infection	Sympathetic mediated cutaneous vasoconstriction
Delayed wound healing	
Delayed anesthetic emergence	Decreased drug metabolism and increased volatile agent solubility, decreased MAC
Delayed recovery room discharge	Post-anesthetic shivering, delayed recovery

BENEFICIAL EFFECTS OF HYPOTHERMIA

Oxygen consumption is decreased by approximately 5% to 7% per °C of cooling. Thus even moderate decreases in

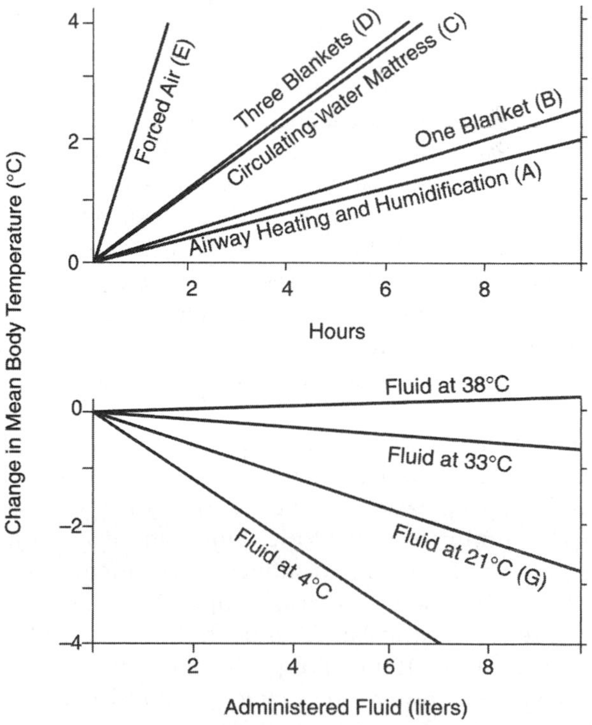

Figure 42-4. The effects of different warming techniques on mean body temperature plotted according to the elapsed hours of treatment (*top*) and changes in mean body temperature according to the volume of fluid administered (*bottom*). (From Sessler DI. Mild perioperative hypothermia. *N Engl J Med* 1997;336:1630–1637; with permission.)

core temperature of 1°C to 3°C below normal provide substantial protection against cerebral ischemia and arterial hypoxemia. Indeed, induced hypothermia to 28°C, as used during cardiopulmonary bypass, will reduce cerebral metabolic rate by 50%. Mild hypothermia (33°C–36°C) may be recommended during operations likely to be associated with cerebral ischemia such as carotid endarterectomy, aneurysm clipping, and cardiac surgery. Operations involving aortic cross-clamping can jeopardize spinal cord perfusion and may also benefit from the increased margin of safety afforded by mild hypothermia. Mild hypothermia also slows the triggering of malignant hyperthermia (Iaizzo et al., 1996). Outside the operating room, there has been renewed interest in mild hypothermia during the resuscitation of survivors of cardiac arrest, stroke, traumatic brain injury, and acute myocardial infarction (Zviman et al., 2004). The main benefit of mild hypothermia accrues from a reduction in metabolic demand. Typical approaches to achieve mild hypothermia often include surface cooling. However, surface cooling will induce shivering, which will delay core cooling.

MEASUREMENT OF BODY TEMPERATURE

The significant adverse physiologic effects of changes in body temperature are a compelling reason to monitor body temperature during anesthesia. Unless hypothermia is specifically indicated, as for protection against tissue ischemia, it is recommended that intraoperative core temperature be maintained at ≥36°C (Sessler, 1997). Measuring the temperature of the lower 25% of the esophagus (about 24 cm beyond the corniculate cartilages or site of the loudest heart sounds heard through an esophageal stethoscope) gives a reliable approximation of blood and cerebral temperature. Readings elsewhere in the esophagus are more likely to be influenced by the temperature of inhaled gases. A nasopharyngeal temperature probe positioned behind the soft palate gives a less reliable measure of cerebral temperature than a correctly positioned esophageal probe. Leakage of gases around the tracheal tube may also influence nasopharyngeal temperature measurements. Heat-producing bacteria in the gastrointestinal tract, cold blood returning from the lower limbs, and insulation of the probe by feces, can all influence rectal temperature. Bladder temperature is also subject to a prolonged response time, particularly if urine flow is <270 mL/hour (Imrie and Hall, 1990). Tympanic membrane and aural canal temperatures provide a rapidly responsive and accurate estimate of hypothalamic temperature and correlate well with esophageal temperature. Potential damage to the tympanic membrane has limited the acceptance of tympanic membrane probes. However, infrared thermometers allow nontraumatic measurement of tympanic temperature. Thermistors in pulmonary artery catheters provide the best continuous estimate of body temperature but are invasive. Skin temperature gives no information other than the temperature of that area of the skin.

PREVENTION OF PERIOPERATIVE HYPOTHERMIA

Passive or active airway heating and humidification contribute little to perioperative thermal management because <10% of metabolic heat is lost via ventilation (Sessler, 1997). Each liter of intravenous fluid at ambient temperature that is infused into adult patients, or each unit of blood at 4°C decreases the mean core body temperature about 0.25°C. In this regard, the administration of unwarmed fluids can markedly decrease body temperature. Warming fluids to near 37°C is useful for preventing hypothermia, especially if large volumes of fluid are being infused.

The skin is the predominant source of heat loss during anesthesia and surgery, although evaporation from large surgical incisions may also be important. A high ambient temperature maintains normothermia in anesthetized patients, but temperatures of >25°C are uncomfortable for operating room personnel.

Covering the skin with surgical drapes or blankets can decrease cutaneous heat loss. A single layer of insulator decreases heat loss by approximately 30%, but additional layers do not proportionately increase the benefit (Sessler and Schroeder, 1993). For this reason, active warming is needed to prevent intraoperative hypothermia. Forced-air warming is probably the most effective method available, although any method or combination of methods that maintains core body temperature near 36°C is acceptable (Fig. 42-4) (Sessler, 1997). Circulating warm water mattresses are generally ineffective because cutaneous blood flow to the back is limited in the supine position. Patients undergoing minor operations in a warm environment may not require active warming, whereas forced-air warming, alone or combined with fluid warming, is helpful for maintaining normal intraoperative core temperature in most other instances.

REFERENCES

Buggy DJ, Crossley AWA. Thermoregulation, mild perioperative hypothermia, and post-anaesthetic shivering. *Br J Anaesth* 2000; 84:615–628.

Frank SM, Fleisher LA, Breslow MJ, et al. Perioperative maintenance of normothermia reduces the incidence of morbid cardiac events: a randomized clinical trial. *JAMA* 1997;277:1127–1134.

Ganong WF. *Review of medical physiology,* 21st ed. Norwalk, CT: Appleton & Lange, 2003.

Giesbrecht GG. Human thermoregulatory inhibition by regional anesthesia. *Anesthesiology* 1994;81:277–281.

Heistad DD, Abboud FM. Factors that influence blood flow in skeletal muscle and skin. *Anesthesiology* 1974;41:139–156.

Iaizzo PA, Kehler CH, Carr RJ, et al. Prior hypothermia attenuates malignant hyperthermia in susceptible swine. *Anesth Analg* 1996; 82:803–809.
Imrie MM, Hall GM. Body temperature and anaesthesia. *Br J Anaesth* 1990;64:346–354.
Sessler DI. Mild perioperative hypothermia. *N Engl J Med* 1997;336: 1630–1637.
Sessler DI. Perioperative heat balance. *Anesthesiology* 2000;92:578–599.
Sessler DI, Schroeder M. Heat loss in humans covered with cotton hospital blankets. *Anesth Analg* 1993;77:73–77.
Simon HB. Hyperthermia, fever and fever of undetermined origin. In: Rubenstein E, Federman D, eds. *ACP medicine*. WebMD, Inc. 2003.
Zviman MM, Roguin A, Jacobs A, et al. A new method for inducing hypothermia during cardiac arrest. *Crit Care Med* 2004;32: S369–S373.

Autonomic Nervous System

43

The autonomic nervous system (ANS) controls the visceral functions of the body. In addition, the ANS exerts partial control over systemic blood pressure, gastrointestinal motility and secretion, urinary bladder emptying, sweating, and body temperature. Activation of the ANS occurs principally via centers located in the hypothalamus, brainstem, and spinal cord (see Chapter 41). The ANS is divided into the sympathetic, parasympathetic, and enteric nervous systems.

The sympathetic and the parasympathetic nervous systems usually function as physiologic antagonists such that the activity of organs innervated by other divisions of the ANS represents a balance of the influence of each component (Table 43-1). The sympathetic nervous system functions as an amplification response whereas the parasympathetic nervous system evokes discrete and narrowly targeted responses. The enteric nervous system is arranged nontopographically and it's neurons and cells are located in the walls of the gastrointestinal tract. Although the gastrointestinal tract is influenced by sympathetic and parasympathetic nervous system activity, it is the enteric nervous system through the myenteric and submucous plexi that regulates digestive activity even in the presence of spinal cord transection.

An understanding of the anatomy and physiology of the ANS is useful for predicting the pharmacologic effects of drugs that act on either the sympathetic nervous system or the parasympathetic nervous system (Table 43-2).

ANATOMY OF THE SYMPATHETIC NERVOUS SYSTEM

Nerves of the sympathetic nervous system arise from the thoracolumbar (T1 to L2) segments of the spinal cord (Fig. 43-1) (Guyton and Hall, 2000). These nerve fibers pass to the paravertebral sympathetic chains located lateral to the spinal cord. From the paravertebral chain, nerve fibers pass to tissues and organs innervated by the sympathetic nervous system.

Each nerve of the sympathetic nervous system consists of a preganglionic neuron and a postganglionic neuron (Fig. 43-2). Cells bodies of preganglionic neurons are located in the intermediolateral horn of the spinal cord. Fibers from these preganglionic cell bodies leave the spinal cord with anterior (ventral) nerve roots and pass via white rami into one of 22 pairs of ganglia composing the paravertebral sympathetic chain. Axons of preganglionic neurons are mostly myelinated, slow-conducting type B fibers (see Table 41-1). In the ganglia of the paravertebral sympathetic chain, the preganglionic fibers can synapse with cell bodies of postganglionic neurons or pass cephalad or caudad to synapse with postganglionic neurons (mostly unmyelinated type C fibers) in other paravertebral ganglia. Postganglionic neurons then exit from paravertebral ganglia to travel to various peripheral organs. Other postganglionic neurons return to spinal nerves by way of gray rami and subsequently travel with these nerves to influence vascular smooth muscle tone and the activity of piloerector muscles and sweat glands.

Fibers of the sympathetic nervous system are not necessarily distributed to the same part of the body as the spinal nerve fibers from the same segments. For example, fibers from T1 usually ascend in the paravertebral sympathetic chain into the head, T2 into the neck, T3 to T6 into the chest, T7 to T11 into the abdomen, and T12 and L1 to L2 into the legs. The distribution of these sympathetic nervous system fibers to each organ is determined in part by the position in the embryo from which the organ originates. In this regard, the heart receives many sympathetic nervous system fibers from the neck portion of the paravertebral sympathetic chain because the heart originates in the neck of the embryo. Abdominal organs receive their sympathetic nervous system innervation from the lower thoracic segments, reflecting the origin of the gastrointestinal tract from this area.

TABLE 43-1.
RESPONSES EVOKED BY AUTONOMIC NERVOUS SYSTEM STIMULATION

	Sympathetic Nervous System Stimulation	Parasympathetic Nervous System Stimulation
Heart		
Sinoatrial node	Increase heart rate	Decrease heart rate
Atrioventricular node	Increase conduction velocity	Decrease conduction velocity
His-Purkinje system	Increase automaticity, conduction velocity	Minimal effect
Ventricles	Increase contractility, conduction velocity Automaticity	Minimal effects, slight decrease in contractility (?)
Bronchial smooth muscle	Relaxation	Contraction
Gastrointestinal tract		
Motility	Decrease	Increase
Secretion	Decrease	Increase
Sphincters	Contraction	Relaxation
Gallbladder	Relaxation	Contraction
Urinary bladder		
Smooth muscle	Relaxation	Contraction
Sphincter	Contraction	Relaxation
Uterus	Contraction	Variable
Ureter	Contraction	Relaxation
Eye		
Radial muscle	Mydriasis	
Sphincter muscle		Miosis
Ciliary muscle	Relaxation for far vision	Contraction for near vision
Liver	Glycogenolysis Gluconeogenesis	Glycogen synthesis
Pancreatic beta cell secretion	Decrease	
Salivary gland secretion	Increase	Marked increase
Sweat glands	Increase*	Increase
Apocrine glands	Increase	
Arterioles		
Coronary	Constriction (alpha) Relaxation (beta)	Relaxation (?)
Skin and mucosa	Constriction	Relaxation
Skeletal muscle	Constriction (alpha) Relaxation (beta)	Relaxation
Pulmonary	Constriction	Relaxation

*Postganglionic sympathetic fibers to sweat glands are cholinergic.

ANATOMY OF THE PARASYMPATHETIC NERVOUS SYSTEM

Nerves of the parasympathetic nervous system leave the central nervous system (CNS) through cranial nerves III, V, VII, IX, and X (vagus) and from the sacral portions of the spinal cord (Fig. 43-3) (Guyton and Hall, 2000). About 75% of all parasympathetic nervous system fibers are in the vagus nerves passing to the thoracic and abdominal regions of the body. As such, the vagus nerves supply parasympathetic nervous system innervation to the heart, lungs, esophagus, stomach, small intestine, liver, gallbladder, pancreas, and upper portions of the uterus. Fibers of the parasympathetic nervous system in cranial nerve III pass to the eye. The lacrimal, nasal, and submaxillary glands receive parasympathetic nervous system fibers via cranial nerve VII, whereas the parotid gland receives parasympathetic nervous system innervation via cranial nerve IX.

The sacral part of the parasympathetic nervous system consists of the second and third sacral nerves, and, occasionally, the first and fourth sacral nerves. Sacral nerves form the sacral plexus on each side of the spinal cord. These nerves distribute fibers to the distal colon, rectum, bladder, and lower portions of the uterus. In addition, parasympathetic nervous system fibers to the external genitalia transmit impulses that elicit various sexual responses.

In contrast to the sympathetic nervous system, preganglionic fibers of the parasympathetic nervous system pass

TABLE 43-2.
MECHANISM OF ACTION OF DRUGS THAT ACT ON THE AUTONOMIC NERVOUS SYSTEM

Mechanism	Site	Drug
Inhibition of neurotransmitter synthesis	SNS	Alpha-methyldopa
False neurotransmitter	SNS	Alpha-methyldopa
Inhibition of uptake of neurotransmitter	SNS	Tricyclic antidepressants, cocaine, ketamine (?)
Displacement of neurotransmitter from storage sites	SNS	Amphetamine
	PNS	Carbachol
Prevention of neurotransmitter release	SNS	Bretylium
	PNS	Botulinum toxin
Mimic action of neurotransmitter at receptor	SNS	
	$Alpha_1$	Phenylephrine, methoxamine
	$Alpha_2$	Clonidine dexmedetomidine
	$Beta_1$	Dobutamine
	$Beta_2$	Terbutaline, albuterol
Inhibition of action of neurotransmitter on postsynaptic receptor	SNS	
	$Alpha_1$	Prazosin
	$Alpha_2$	Yohimbine
	$Alpha_1$ and $alpha_2$	Phentolamine
	$Beta_1$	Metoprolol, esmolol
	$Beta_1$ and $beta_2$	Propranolol
	PNS	
	M_1	Pirenzepine
	M_1, M_2	Atropine
	N_1	Hexamethonium
	N_2	*d*-Tubocurarine
Inhibition of metabolism of neurotransmitter	SNS	Monoamine oxidase inhibitors
	PNS	Neostigmine, pyridostigmine, edrophonium

PNS, parasympathetic nervous system; SNS, sympathetic nervous system.

uninterrupted to ganglia near or in the innervated organ (see Fig. 43-3) (Guyton and Hall, 2000). Postganglionic neurons of the parasympathetic nervous system are short because of the location of the corresponding ganglia. This contrasts with the sympathetic nervous system, in which postganglionic neurons are relatively long, reflecting their origin in the ganglia of the paravertebral sympathetic chain, which is often distant from the innervated organ. Furthermore, unlike the amplified and diffuse discharges characteristic of sympathetic nervous system responses, activation of the parasympathetic nervous system is tonic and discrete. The vasodilatory effects of acetylcholine depend on the integrity of the vascular endothelium because muscarinic receptors on the endothelium release nitric oxide (Johns, 1991).

PHYSIOLOGY OF THE AUTONOMIC NERVOUS SYSTEM

Postganglionic fibers of the sympathetic nervous system secrete norepinephrine as the neurotransmitter (Fig. 43-4). These norepinephrine-secreting neurons are classified as *adrenergic fibers*. Postganglionic fibers of the parasympathetic nervous system secrete acetylcholine as the neurotransmitter (see Fig. 43-4). These acetylcholine-secreting neurons are classified as *cholinergic fibers*. In addition, innervation of sweat glands and some blood vessels is by postganglionic sympathetic nervous system fibers that release acetylcholine as the neurotransmitter. All preganglionic neurons of the sympathetic and parasympathetic nervous system release acetylcholine as the neurotransmitter and are thus classified as *cholinergic fibers*. For this reason, acetylcholine release at preganglionic fibers activates both sympathetic and parasympathetic postganglionic neurons.

Norepinephrine as a Neurotransmitter

Synthesis

Synthesis of norepinephrine involves a series of enzyme-controlled steps that begin in the cytoplasm of postganglionic sympathetic nerve endings (varicosities) and are completed in the synaptic vesicles (Fig. 43-5). For example, the initial enzyme-mediated steps leading to the formation of dopamine take place in the cytoplasm. Dopamine then

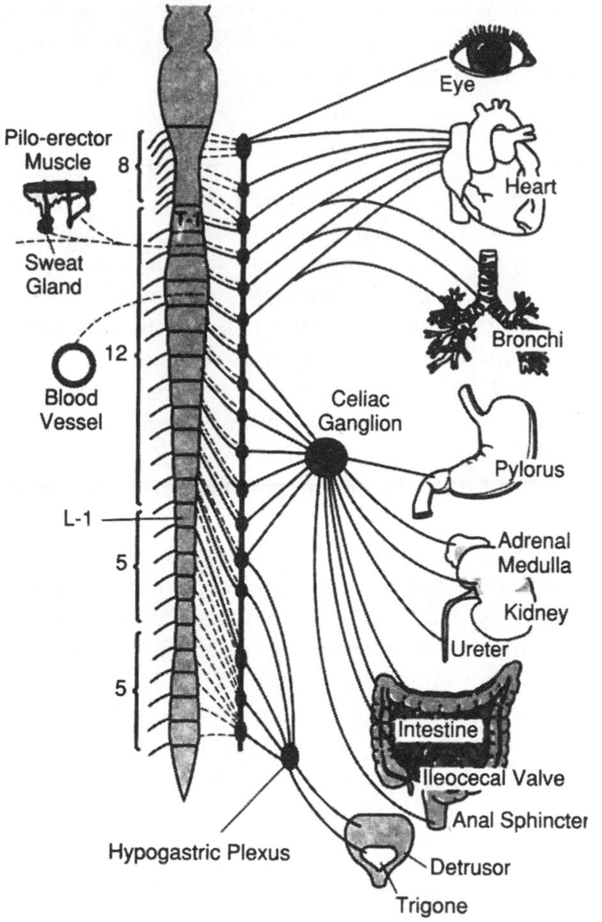

Figure 43-1. Anatomy of the sympathetic nervous system. Dashed lines represent postganglionic fibers in gray rami leading to spinal nerves for subsequent distribution to blood vessels and sweat glands. (From Guyton AC, Hall JE. *Textbook of medical physiology*, 10th ed. Philadelphia. Saunders, 2000; with permission.)

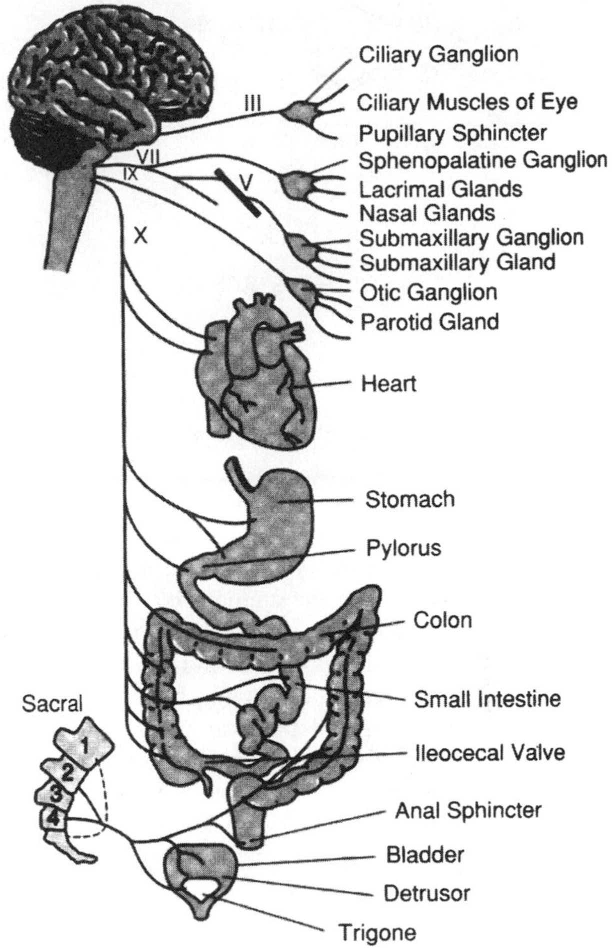

Figure 43-3. Anatomy of the parasympathetic nervous system. (From Guyton AC, Hall JE. *Textbook of medical physiology*, 10th ed. Philadelphia. Saunders, 2000; with permission.)

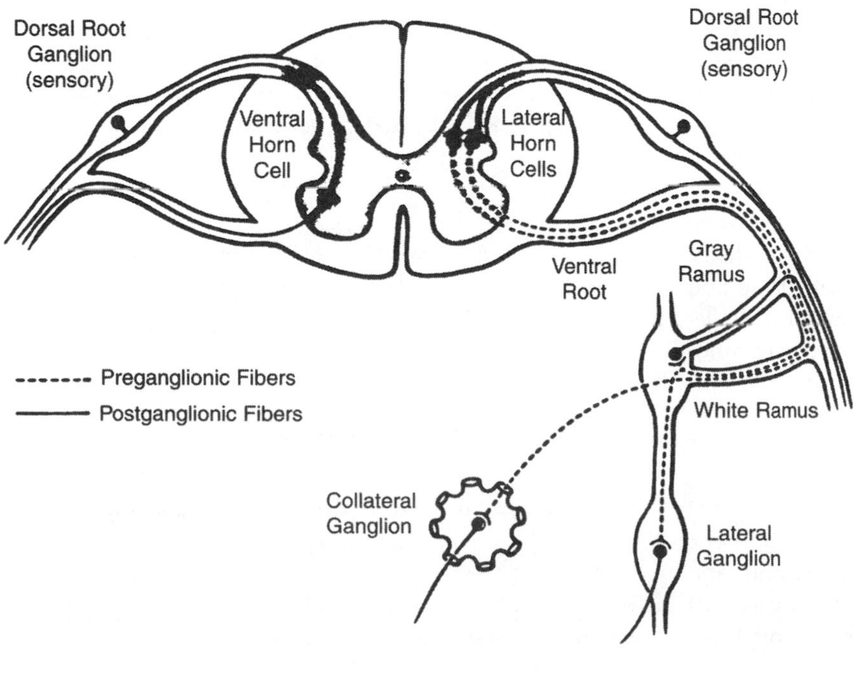

Figure 43-2. Anatomy of a sympathetic nervous system nerve. Preganglionic fibers pass through the white ramus to a paravertebral ganglia, where they may synapse, course up the sympathetic chain to synapse at another level, or exit the chain without synapsing to pass to an outlying collateral ganglion.

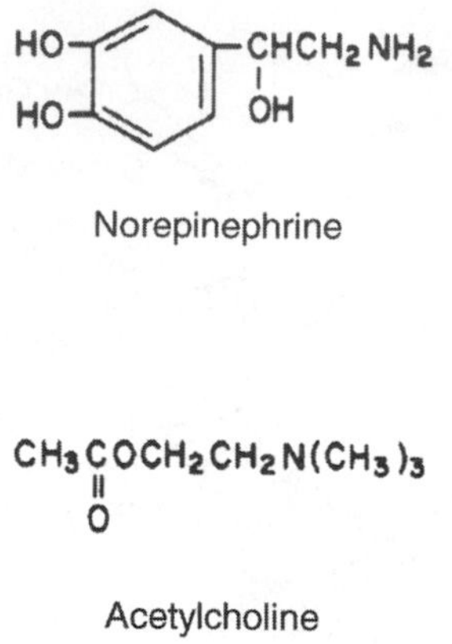

Figure 43-4. Neurotransmitters of the autonomic nervous system.

enters the synaptic vesicle, where it is converted to norepinephrine by dopamine beta-hydroxylase. It is likely that the enzymes that participate in the synthesis of norepinephrine are produced in postganglionic sympathetic nerve endings. These enzymes are not highly specific, and other endogenous substances, as well as certain drugs, may be acted on by the same enzyme. For example, dopa-decarboxylase can convert the antihypertensive drug alpha-methyldopa to alpha-methyldopamine, which is subsequently converted by dopamine beta-hydroxylase to the weakly active (false) neurotransmitter alpha-methylnorepinephrine (see Chapter 15).

Storage and Release

Norepinephrine is stored in synaptic vesicles for subsequent release in response to an action potential (Sudhof, 2000). Calcium ions are important in coupling the nerve impulse to the subsequent release of norepinephrine from postganglionic sympathetic nerve endings into the extracellular fluid. Evidence that exocytosis is the primary event in the release of norepinephrine from synaptic vesicles in the nerve terminals is the observation that increased activity of the sympathetic nervous system is accompanied by increased circulating concentrations of dopamine beta-hydroxylase and norepinephrine. This should occur only if the entire contents of the synaptic vesicles are released.

Adrenergic fibers can sustain output of norepinephrine during prolonged periods of stimulation. Tachyphylaxis, which may accompany administration of ephedrine and other indirect-acting sympathomimetics, may reflect depletion of the limited pool of neurotransmitter at these binding sites in contrast to the large total amount of norepinephrine stored in sympathetic nerve endings.

Termination of Action

Termination of the action of norepinephrine is by (a) uptake (reuptake) back into postganglionic sympathetic nerve endings, (b) dilution by diffusion from receptors, and (c) metabolism by the enzymes monoamine oxidase (MAO) and catechol-O-methyltransferase (COMT). Norepinephrine released in response to an action potential exerts its effects at receptors for only a brief period, reflecting the efficiency of these termination mechanisms.

Uptake

Uptake of previously released norepinephrine back into postganglionic sympathetic nerve endings is probably the most important mechanism for terminating the action of this neurotransmitter on receptors. Indeed, it is estimated that as much as 80% of released norepinephrine undergoes uptake. Furthermore, this uptake provides a source for reuse of norepinephrine in addition to synthesis.

It is likely that two active transport systems are involved in uptake of norepinephrine, with one system responsible for uptake into the cytoplasm of the varicosity and a second system for passage of norepinephrine into the synaptic vesicle for storage and reuse. The active transport system for norepinephrine uptake can concentrate the neurotransmitter 10,000-fold in postganglionic sympathetic nerve endings. Magnesium and adenosine triphosphate are essential for function of the transport system necessary for the transfer of norepinephrine from the cytoplasm into the synaptic vesicle. The transport system for uptake of norepinephrine into cytoplasm is blocked by numerous drugs, including cocaine and tricyclic antidepressants.

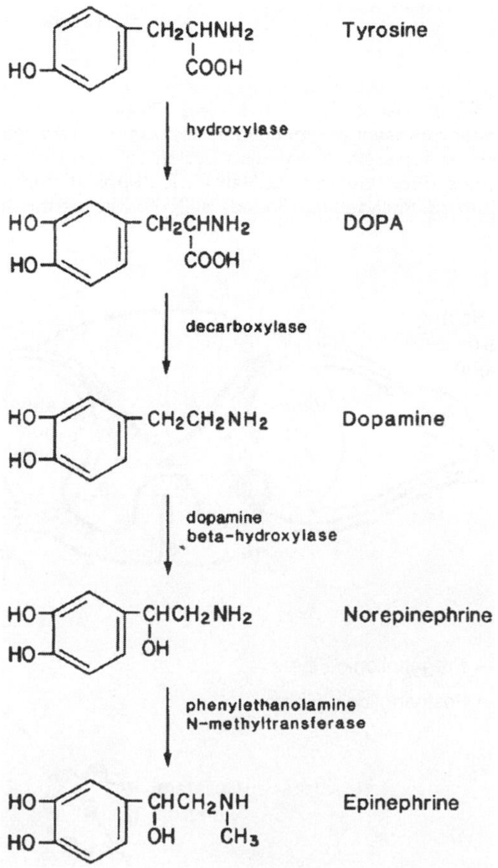

Figure 43-5. Steps in the enzymatic synthesis of endogenous catecholamines and neurotransmitters.

Metabolism

Metabolism of norepinephrine is of relatively minor significance in terminating the actions of endogenously released norepinephrine. The exception may be at some blood vessels, where enzymatic breakdown and diffusion account for the termination of action of norepinephrine. Norepinephrine that undergoes uptake is vulnerable to metabolism in the cytoplasm of the varicosity by MAO. Any neurotransmitter that escapes uptake is vulnerable to metabolism by COMT, principally in the liver. Inhibitors of MAO cause an increase in tissue levels of norepinephrine and may be accompanied by a variety of pharmacologic effects (see Chapter 19). Conversely, no striking pharmacologic change accompanies inhibition of COMT.

The primary urinary metabolite resulting from metabolism of norepinephrine by MAO or COMT is 3-methoxy-4-hydroxymandelic acid (Fig. 43-6). This metabolite is also referred to as *vanillylmandelic acid*. Normally the 24-hour urinary excretion of 3-methoxy-4-hydroxymandelic acid is 2 to 4 mg, representing primarily norepinephrine that is deaminated by MAO in the cytoplasm of the varicosity of the postganglionic sympathetic nerve endings.

Acetylcholine as a Neurotransmitter

Synthesis

Synthesis of acetylcholine occurs in the cytoplasm of varicosities of the preganglionic and postganglionic parasympathetic nerve endings. The enzyme choline acetyltransferase is responsible for catalyzing the combination of choline with acetyl coenzyme A to form acetylcholine. Choline enters parasympathetic nerve endings from the extracellular fluid through an active transport system. Acetyl coenzyme A is synthesized in mitochondria present in high concentrations in parasympathetic nerve endings.

Storage and Release

Acetylcholine is stored in synaptic vesicles for release in response to an action potential. Arrival of an action potential at a parasympathetic nerve ending results in the release of 100 or more vesicles of acetylcholine. It is estimated that a single nerve ending contains >300,000 synaptic vesicles.

Preceding arrival of the action potential is the initial depolarization that permits the influx of calcium ions. Conceptually, calcium ions bind to sites on axonal and vesicular membranes, resulting in the extrusion of the contents of the synaptic vesicles. Thus, the presence of calcium in the extracellular fluid is essential to the subsequent release of acetylcholine in response to an action potential. The effect of calcium is antagonized by magnesium.

Metabolism

Acetylcholine has a brief effect at receptors (<1 ms) because of its rapid hydrolysis by acetylcholinesterase (true cholinesterase) to choline and acetate. Choline is transported back into parasympathetic nerve endings, where it is used for synthesis of new acetylcholine. Plasma cholinesterase (pseudocholinesterase) is an enzyme found in low concentrations around acetylcholine receptors, being present in the highest amounts in plasma. The physiologic significance of plasma cholinesterase is unknown. Indeed, the enzyme hydrolyzes acetylcholine too slowly to be physiologically important. Furthermore, absence of plasma cholinesterase produces no detectable clinical signs or symptoms until a drug such as succinylcholine or mivacurium is administered.

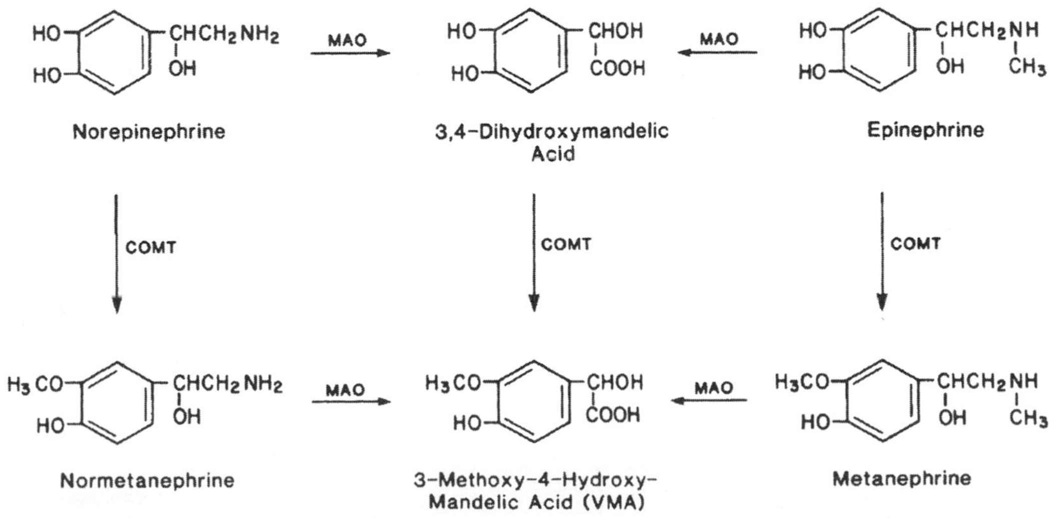

Figure 43-6. Norepinephrine and epinephrine are initially deaminated by monoamine oxidase (MAO) or, alternatively, they are first methylated by catechol-*O*-methyltransferase (COMT). The resulting metabolites are then further metabolized by the other enzyme (MAO or COMT) to form the principal end-metabolite, 3-methoxy-4-hydroxymandelic acid (vanillylmandelic acid, or VMA).

INTERACTIONS OF NEUROTRANSMITTERS WITH RECEPTORS

Norepinephrine and acetylcholine, acting as neurotransmitters, interact with receptors (protein macromolecules) in lipid cell membranes (Table 43-3) (see Chapter 39). This receptor-neurotransmitter interaction most often activates or inhibits effector enzymes, such as adenylate cyclase, or alters flux of sodium and potassium ions across cell membranes via protein ion channels. The net effect of these changes is transduction of external stimuli into intracellular signals.

Norepinephrine Receptors

The pharmacologic effects of catecholamines led to the original concept of alpha- and beta-adrenergic receptors (Ahlquist, 1948). Subdivision of these receptors into $alpha_1$ (postsynaptic), $alpha_2$ (presynaptic), $beta_1$ (cardiac), and $beta_2$ (noncardiac) allows an understanding of drugs that act as either agonists or antagonists at these sites (see Table 43-2) (see Chapter 12). Dopamine receptors are also subdivided as $dopamine_1$ (postsynaptic) and $dopamine_2$ (presynaptic). Activation of $dopamine_1$ receptors is responsible for vasodilation of the splanchnic and renal circulations. Presynaptic alpha and $dopamine_2$ receptors function as a negative feedback loop such that their activation inhibits subsequent release of neurotransmitter (Table 43-4). Postsynaptic $alpha_2$ receptors are also present on platelets, where they mediate platelet aggregation by influencing platelet adenylate cyclase concentrations. In the CNS, stimulation of postsynaptic $alpha_2$ receptors by drugs such as clonidine or dexmedetomidine results in enhanced potassium ion conductance and membrane hyperpolarization manifesting as decreased anesthetic requirements (see Chapter 1).

Signal Transduction

Signal transduction is the process by which the extracellular signal created by adrenergic receptor stimulation is transformed into an intracellular signal. In this process, $alpha_1$ and beta-receptors are coupled to G proteins. Activated G proteins modulate either the synthesis or availability of intracellular cytoplasmic messengers and ultimately the activation of protein kinases and phosphorylation of target proteins. G proteins consist of alpha, beta, and gamma subunits and are capable of greatly amplifying signals that are characteristic of the sympathetic nervous system stimulation. The alpha subunit determines the activity of G proteins (G_s [stimulatory], G_o [inhibitory] or G_{q11}) (see Table 43-3).

Adrenergic receptors link to different subfamilies of G proteins that are subsequently linked to different effectors.

TABLE 43-3.
CLASSIFICATION AND CHARACTERIZATION OF ADRENERGIC AND CHOLINERGIC RECEPTORS

Classification	Molecular Pharmacology	Signal Transduction	Effectors
Adrenergic Receptors			
$alpha_1$	$alpha_{1A1D}$	G_{q11}	Activates phospholipase C
	$alpha_{1B}$	G_{q11}	Activates phospholipase C
	$alpha_{1C}$	G_{q11}	Activates phospholipase C
$alpha_2$	$alpha_{2A}$	G_i and G_o	Inhibits adenylate cyclase, calcium and potassium ion channels
	$alpha_{2B}$	G_i and G_o	Inhibits adenylate cyclase, calcium and potassium ion channels
	$alpha_{2C}$	G_i and G_o	Inhibits adenylate cyclase, calcium and potassium ion channels
$beta_1$	$beta_1$	G_s	Stimulates adenylate cyclase and calcium ion channels
$beta_2$	$beta_2$	G_s	Stimulates adenylate cyclase and calcium ion channels
$beta_3$	$beta_3$	G_s	Stimulates adenylate cyclase and calcium ion channels
Cholinergic Receptors			
Nicotinic	Autonomic ganglia Neuromuscular junction Central nervous system	Ion channels	
Muscarinic	M_1	G_q	Phospholipase activation
	M_3	G_q	Phospholipase activation
	M_5	G_q	Phospholipase activation
	M_2	G_1 and G_o	Inhibits adenylate cyclase
	M_4	G_1 and G_o	Inhibits adenylate cyclase

TABLE 43-4.
RESPONSES EVOKED BY SELECTIVE STIMULATION OF ADRENERGIC RECEPTORS

$Alpha_1$ (postsynaptic) receptors
Vasoconstriction
Mydriasis
Relaxation of gastrointestinal tract
Contraction of gastrointestinal sphincters
Contraction of bladder sphincter
$Alpha_2$ (presynaptic) receptors
Inhibition of norepinephrine release
$Alpha_2$ (postsynaptic) receptors
Platelet aggregation
Hyperpolarization of cells in the central nervous system
$Beta_1$ (postsynaptic) receptors
Increased conduction velocity
Increased automaticity
Increased contractility
$Beta_2$ (postsynaptic) receptors
Vasodilation
Bronchodilation
Gastrointestinal relaxation
Uterine relaxation
Bladder relaxation
Glycogenolysis
Lipolysis
$Dopamine_1$ (postsynaptic) receptors
Vasodilation
$Dopamine_2$ (presynaptic) receptors
Inhibition of norepinephrine release

Activation of alpha subunits and binding to effector sites initiates a cascade of intracellular events reflecting activation of second messengers. For example, catecholamines encountering beta-adrenergic receptors results in dramatic increases in intracellular cyclic adenosine monophosphate (cAMP). The resulting increased intracellular concentration of cAMP then initiates a series of intracellular events (cascading protein phosphorylation reactions and stimulation of the sodium-potassium pump), resulting in the metabolic and pharmacologic effects considered typical of beta-adrenergic or dopaminergic receptor stimulation by norepinephrine, epinephrine, dopamine, or agonist drugs. The number of G protein molecules greatly exceeds the number of beta-adrenergic receptors resulting in amplification of agonist signals. In contrast to beta receptors, $alpha_1$ receptors facilitate calcium ion movement into cells and stimulate hydrolysis of polyphosphoinositides. $Alpha_2$ and $dopamine_2$ receptors inhibit adenylate cyclase.

Adrenergic Receptor Concentrations

Concentrations of beta-adrenergic receptors are not fixed but parallel concentrations of norepinephrine present in the synaptic cleft and plasma. Desensitization reflects the rapid waning of responses to hormones and neurotransmitters despite continuous exposure to adrenergic agonists (Insel, 1996). Down-regulation is different from the rapid appearance of desensitization occurring only hours after exposure to agonists. During down-regulation, receptors are destroyed and new receptors must be synthesized before a return to baseline is possible. Changes in adrenergic receptor activity is consistent with rebound tachycardia and myocardial ischemia that may accompany sudden discontinuation of chronic beta-adrenergic receptor blockers.

Chronic congestive heart failure (CHF) results in depletion of catecholamines in the myocardium and compensatory increases in plasma concentrations of norepinephrine to maintain systemic vascular resistance and perfusion pressure. Accompanying decreases in the concentrations of $beta_1$ receptors in the heart are likely responsible for the failure of beta agonists to effectively treat CHF (Lefkowitz et al., 2000).

Acetylcholine Receptors

Cholinergic receptors are classified as *nicotinic* and *muscarinic*. The links between stimulus and response are different in nicotinic and muscarinic receptors (see Table 43-3).

Nicotinic Receptors

Acetylcholine can affect nicotinic receptors at either the neuromuscular junction or autonomic ganglia. Nicotinic receptors are designated N_1 and N_2. N_1 receptors are present at autonomic ganglia, and N_2 receptors are present at the neuromuscular junction. Hexamethonium produces blockade at N_1 receptors, whereas the nondepolarizing neuromuscular-blocking drug *d*-tubocurarine, in high doses, produces some degree of autonomic ganglia blockade, although the effects at N_2 receptors still predominate.

Nicotinic receptors belong to the superfamily of ligand-gated ion channels that includes glutamate and glycine receptors. Nicotinic receptors are membrane proteins (two alpha subunits, beta, epsilon and delta) that form nonselective ion channels (Martyn et al., 1992). In humans, the gamma subunit is replaced by the epsilon subunit within the first two weeks of life. This change in structure converts the receptor from one with low conductance and long duration to a receptor with high conductance and brief duration of opening. When acetylcholine occupies both alpha subunits, the channel opens and ions flow. If only one site is occupied, the channel remains closed and there is no flow of ions or change in electrical potential. Unlike adrenergic receptors that react promptly to changes in catecholamine concentrations, changes in nicotinic receptor numbers take days.

Muscarinic Receptors

In contrast to ligand-gated nicotinic receptors, muscarinic receptors belong to the superfamily of G protein coupled receptors and are more homologous to adrenergic receptors than to nicotinic receptors. Five muscarinic receptors have been identified. These receptors are coupled to second messenger systems such as cyclic nucleotides or phosphoinositides, which are in turn coupled to ion channels. The specific response is determined by the cation involved. M_2 receptors are present in the heart and salivary glands and M_3 receptors are present in airway smooth muscles. M_3 receptors mediate contractile and secretory processes. Pirenzepine is an example of a drug that is a selective antagonist at M_1 receptors, whereas atropine is a nonselective antagonist at M_1 and M_2 receptors.

Signal Transduction

Muscarinic receptors exhibit different signal transduction mechanisms. Odd numbered muscarinic receptors (M_1, M_3, and M_5) work predominantly through hydrolysis of phosphoinositide and release of intracellular calcium, whereas even number receptors (M_2 and M_4) work primarily through G_i proteins to regulate adenylate cyclase (Hosey, 1992). M_2 receptors in cardiac pacemaker cells oppose increased myocardial contractility evoked by beta-adrenergic stimulation and activate potassium channels through G_i proteins, causing hyperpolarization and decreasing heart rate. Like other G-protein coupled receptors, the response of muscarinic receptors to changes in concentrations is slow.

RESIDUAL AUTONOMIC NERVOUS SYSTEM TONE

The sympathetic and parasympathetic nervous systems are continually active, and this basal rate of activity is referred to as *sympathetic* or *parasympathetic tone*. The value of this tone is that it permits alterations in sympathetic or parasympathetic nervous system activity to either increase or decrease responses at innervated organs. For example, sympathetic nervous system tone normally keeps blood vessels about 50% constricted. As a result, increased or decreased sympathetic nervous system activity produces corresponding changes in systemic vascular resistance. If sympathetic tone did not exist, the sympathetic nervous system could only cause vasoconstriction.

In addition to continual direct sympathetic nervous system stimulation, a portion of overall sympathetic tone reflects basal secretion of norepinephrine and epinephrine by the adrenal medulla. The normal resting rate of secretion of norepinephrine is about 0.05 μg/kg/minute, and epinephrine is about 0.2 μg/kg/minute. These secretion rates are nearly sufficient to maintain systemic blood pressure in a normal range even if all direct sympathetic nervous system innervation to the cardiovascular system is removed.

Determination of Autonomic Nervous System Function

Autonomic dysfunction associated with aging and diabetes mellitus may increase operative risk and can be associated with increased morbidity and mortality (Charlson et al., 1994). Diagnosis of autonomic neuropathy in patients with diabetes mellitus is facilitated by tests of cardiovascular function (Table 43-5). Tests involving changes in heart rate, measure injury to the parasympathetic nervous system and precede changes in the measures of blood pressure that reflect the sympathetic nervous system. In addition to clinical tests of autonomic function, sensitive techniques for measuring plasma catecholamines are available. Interpretation of these data is confounded by other influences. Plasma epinephrine concentrations (normally 100 to 400 pg/mL) reflect adrenal release but vary greatly with psychologic and physical stress. Plasma norepinephrine concentrations (normally 100 to 400 pg/mL) reflect both sympathetic nervous system and adrenal activity. Unlike plasma epinephrine levels, plasma norepinephrine concentrations reflect spillover from neuroeffector junctions, which may represent 10% to 20% of total release and vary among various organ systems.

Aging and Autonomic Nervous System Dysfunction

Common clinical manifestations of ANS dysfunction in elderly patients are orthostatic hypotension, postprandial hypotension, hypothermia and heat stroke. These responses reflect limited ability of elderly patients to adapt to stresses with vasoconstriction and vasodilation as mediated by the ANS (see Chapter 60). Decreased ANS function in elderly patients is due to fewer prejunctional terminals as plasma epinephrine concentrations and the numbers of beta-adrenergic receptors are unchanged with aging. Plasma norepinephrine concentrations increase with age, suggesting a primary physiologic deficit in uptake (reuptake) mechanisms (Veith et al., 1986).

Clinically, there is attenuation of physiologic responses to beta-adrenergic stimulation in the elderly. Exogenous beta-adrenergic agonists have less profound effects on heart rate (Lakatta, 1993). This decreased response to adrenergic stimulation seems to reflect decreased affinity (number of receptors unchanged) of beta receptors for the neurotransmitter and decreases in coupling of stimulatory G proteins and adenylate cyclase units.

Diabetic Autonomic Neuropathy

Diabetic autonomic neuropathy is present in 20% to 40% of insulin-dependent diabetic patients. Common manifestations of diabetic autonomic neuropathy include impotence, diarrhea, postural hypotension, sweating abnormalities, and gastroparesis. When impotence or diarrhea are the sole manifestations of autonomic neuropathy, there is little impact on survival. Conversely, 5-year mortality rates may exceed 50% when postural hypotension or gastroparesis are present. Anesthetic risk is increased in diabetic patients with autonomic neuropathy based on gastroparesis (aspiration hazard) and postural hypotension (hemodynamic instability) (Burgos et al., 1989).

Chronic Sympathetic Nervous System Stimulation

Chronic sympathetic nervous system stimulation may increase morbidity and mortality. Pheochromocytoma is

TABLE 43-5.
CLINICAL ASSESSMENT OF AUTONOMIC NERVOUS SYSTEM FUNCTION

Clinical Observation	Method of Measurement	Normal Value
Parasympathetic Nervous System		
Heart rate response to Valsalva	Patient blows into a mouthpiece maintaining a pressure of of 40 mm Hg for 15 seconds.	
	The Valsalva ratio is the ratio of the longest R-R interval on the electrocardiogram immediately after release to the shortest R-R interval during the maneuver.	Ratio >1.21
Heart rate response to standing	Heart rate is measured as the patient changes from the supine to standing position (increase maximal around 15th beat after standing and slowing maximal around 30th beat).	
	The response to standing is expressed as the "30:15" ratio and is the ratio of the longest R-R interval (around 30th beat) to the shortest R-R interval (around 15th beat).	Ratio >1.04
Heart response to deep breathing	Patient takes six deep breaths in 1 minute.	
	The maximum and minimum heart rates during each cycle are measured and the mean of the differences (maximum heart rate–minimum heart rate) during three successive breathing cycles is taken as the maximum–minimum heart rate.	Mean difference >15 bpm
Sympathetic Nervous System		
Blood pressure response to standing	The patient changes from the supine to standing position and the standing systolic blood pressure is subtracted from the supine systolic blood pressure.	Difference <10 mm Hg
Blood pressure response to sustained handgrip	The patient maintains a handgrip of 30% of maximum squeeze for up to 5 minutes.	Difference >16 mm Hg
	The blood pressure is measured every minute and the initial diastolic blood pressure is subtracted from the diastolic blood pressure just prior to release.	

characterized by explosive and uncontrolled release of catecholamines. Even physiologic responses and surgical stress that lead to sustained ANS hyperactivity can result in metabolic and endocrine responses. Interventions that attenuate stress responses during the entire perioperative period (continuous epidural infusions of local anesthetics, perioperative administration of beta-adrenergic blocking drugs, $alpha_2$ agonists) may influence morbidity and mortality rates (Kehlet, 2000; Mangano et al., 1996; Wallace et al., 2004). Inhaled anesthetics and adjuvants that interfere with stress responses in the perioperative period may also be beneficial in long-term outcomes following surgery (Ebert et al., 1998).

Acute Denervation

Acute removal of sympathetic nervous system tone, as produced by a regional anesthetic or spinal cord transection, results in immediate maximal vasodilation of blood vessels (spinal shock). Over several days, however, intrinsic tone of vascular smooth muscle increases, usually restoring almost normal vasoconstriction. Similar intrinsic parasympathetic nervous system compensation occurs, but return of an organ to basal function may require several months.

Denervation Hypersensitivity

Denervation hypersensitivity is the increased responsiveness (decreased threshold) of the innervated organ to norepinephrine or epinephrine that develops during the first week or so after acute interruption of ANS innervation (see Chapter 41). The presumed mechanism for denervation hypersensitivity is the proliferation of receptors (upregulation) on postsynaptic membranes that occurs when norepinephrine or acetylcholine is no longer released at synapses. As a result, more receptor sites become available to produce an exaggerated response when circulating neurotransmitter does become available.

ADRENAL MEDULLA

The adrenal medulla is innervated by preganglionic fibers that bypass the paravertebral ganglia. As a result, these fibers pass directly from the spinal cord to the adrenal medulla. Cells of the adrenal medulla are derived embryologically from neural tissue and are analogous to postganglionic neurons. Stimulation of the sympathetic nervous system causes release of epinephrine (80%) and norepinephrine from the adrenal medulla. Epinephrine and norepinephrine released by the adrenal medulla function as hormones and not as neurotransmitters.

Synthesis

In the adrenal medulla, most of the formed norepinephrine is converted to the hormone epinephrine by the action of phenylethanolamine-*N*-methyltransferase (see Fig. 43-5). Activity of this enzyme is enhanced by cortisol, which is carried by the intraadrenal portal vascular system directly to the adrenal medulla. For this reason, any stress that releases glucocorticoids also results in increased synthesis and release of epinephrine.

Release

The triggering event in the release of epinephrine and norepinephrine from the adrenal medulla is the liberation of acetylcholine by preganglionic cholinergic fibers. Acetylcholine acts on specific receptors, resulting in a change in permeability (localized depolarization) that permits entry of calcium ions. Calcium ions result in extrusion, by exocytosis, of synaptic vesicles containing epinephrine.

Norepinephrine and epinephrine released from the adrenal medulla evoke responses similar to direct stimulation of the sympathetic nervous system. The difference, however, is that effects are greatly prolonged (10 to 30 seconds) compared with the brief duration of action on receptors that is produced by norepinephrine released as a neurotransmitter from postganglionic sympathetic nerve endings. The prolonged effect of circulating epinephrine and norepinephrine released by the adrenal medulla reflects the time necessary for metabolism of these substances by COMT.

Circulating norepinephrine from the adrenal medulla causes vasoconstriction of blood vessels, inhibition of the gastrointestinal tract, increased cardiac activity, and dilatation of the pupils (see Table 43-1). The effects of circulating epinephrine differ from those of norepinephrine in that the cardiac and metabolic effects of epinephrine are greater, whereas relaxation of blood vessels in skeletal muscles reflects a predominance of beta- over alpha-effects at low concentrations of epinephrine. Circulating norepinephrine and epinephrine released by the adrenal medulla and acting as hormones can substitute for sympathetic nervous system innervation of an organ. Another important role of the adrenal medulla is the ability of circulating norepinephrine and epinephrine to stimulate areas of the body that are not directly innervated by the sympathetic nervous system. For example, the metabolic rate of all cells can be influenced by hormones released from the adrenal medulla, even though these cells are not directly innervated by the sympathetic nervous system.

REFERENCES

Ahlquist RP. A study of adrenotropic receptors. *Am J Physiol* 1948;53:586–606.

Burgos LG, Ebert TJ, Asiddao C, et al. Increased intraoperative cardiovascular morbidity in diabetics with autonomic neuropathy. *Anesthesiology* 1989;70:591–599.

Charlson ME, MacKenzie CR, Gold JP. Preoperative autonomic function abnormalities in patients with diabetes mellitus and patients with hypertension. *J Am Coll Surg* 1994;179:1–6.

Ebert TJ, Perez F, Uhrich TD, et al. Desflurane-mediated sympathetic activation occurs in humans despite preventing hypotension and baroreceptor unloading. *Anesthesiology* 1998;88:1227–1235.

Guyton AC, Hall JE. *Textbook of medical physiology*, 10th ed. Philadelphia. Saunders, 2000.

Hosey MM. Diversity of structure, signaling and regulation within the family of muscarinic cholinergic receptors. *FASEB J* 1992;6:845–851.

Insel PA. Adrenergic receptors-evolving concepts and clinical implications. *N Engl J Med* 1996;334:580–589.

Johns RA. EDRF/nitric oxide. the endogenous nitrovasodilator and a new cellular messenger. *Anesthesiology* 1991;75:927–933.

Kehlet H. Manipulation of the metabolic response in clinical practice. *World J Surg* 2000.24:690–698.

Lakatta ED. Deficient neuroendocrine regulation of the cardiovascular system with advancing age in healthy humans. *Circulation* 1993;87:631–637.

Lefkowitz RJ, Rockman HA, Koch WJ. Catecholamines, cardiac beta-adrenergic receptors, and heart failure. *Circulation* 2000;101:1634–1640.

Linder ME, Gilman AG. G proteins. *Sci Am* 1992;267:56–65.

Mangano DT, Layug EL, Wallace A, et al. Effect of atenolol on mortality and cardiovascular morbidity after noncardiac surgery. *N Engl J Med* 1996;335:1713–1719.

Martyn JA, White DA, Gronert GA, et al. Up-and-down regulation of skeletal muscle acetylcholine receptors. Effects on neuromuscular blockers. *Anesthesiology* 1992;76:822–830.

Sudhof TC. The synaptic vesicle cycle revisited. *Neuron* 2000;28:317–323.

Veith RC, Featherstone JA, Linares OA, et al. Age differences in plasma norepinephrine kinetics in humans. *J Gerontol* 1986;41:319–325.

Wallace AW, Galindez D, Salahieh A, et al. Effect of clonidine on cardiovascular morbidity and mortality after noncardiac surgery. *Anesthesiology* 2004;101:284–293.

Pain

44

Pain is a complex phenomenon and includes both sensory-discriminative and motivational-affective components (Galer et al., 2002). The sensory-discriminative component of pain depends upon ascending projections of tracts (includes the spinothalamic and trigeminothalamic tracts) into the cerebral cortex. Sensory processing at these higher levels results in the perception of the quality of pain (pricking, burning, aching), the location of the painful stimulus, the intensity of the pain, and the duration of the pain. The motivational-affective responses to painful stimuli include attention and arousal, somatic and autonomic reflexes, endocrine responses, and emotional changes. These account collectively for the unpleasant nature of painful stimuli.

The definition of pain as accepted by the International Association for the Study of Pain emphasizes the complex nature of pain as a physical, emotional, and psychological condition. It is recognized that pain does not necessarily correlate with the degree of tissue damage that is present. Failure to appreciate the complex factors that affect the experience of pain and reliance entirely upon physical examination findings and laboratory tests may lead to misunderstanding and inadequate treatment of pain. Oversimplified anatomic concepts predispose to simplistic therapeutic interventions, such as neurectomy or rhizotomy, that may intensify pain or create new and often more distressing pain.

In reality, the nociceptive system is highly complex and highly adaptable. Sensitivity of most of its components can be reset by a variety of physiologic and pathologic conditions. Innovative medications are being developed that target the causes of pain by actions on pain transduction, transmission, interpretation, and modulation in both the peripheral nervous system (PNS) and the central nervous system (CNS) (Table 44-1).

SOCIAL IMPACT

Pain (low back pain, headache, arthritis) is one of the most common reasons for visiting a physician. It is estimated that chronic pain may affect as many as 40% of the adult population (Glajchen, 2001). The prevalence of low back pain ranges from 8% to 37% and is particularly prominent in patients between 45 and 60 years of age. It is estimated that 40 million persons experience musculoskeletal pain conditions (Helmick et al., 1995). Patients with malignant disease often experience increasing pain as their disease progresses. The costs to society related to chronic pain are immense with an estimate that the annual cost attributed to back pain, migraine headache, and arthritis is 40 billion dollars (does not include surgical procedures to treat pain, lost workdays) (Anand and Craig, 1996).

NEUROBIOLOGY OF PAIN

The experience of pain involves a series of complex neurophysiologic processes that reflect four distinct components: transduction, transmission, modulation, and perception. Transduction is the process by which a noxious stimulus is converted to an electrical impulse in sensory nerve endings. Transmission is the conduction of these electrical impulses to the CNS with the major connections for these nerves being in the dorsal horn of the spinal cord and thalamus with projections to the cingulate, insular and somatosensory cortexes. Modulation of pain is the process of altering pain transmission. It is likely that both inhibitory and excitatory mechanisms modulate pain (nociceptive) impulse transmission in the PNS and CNS. Pain perception is thought to occur at the thalamus with the cortex being important for discrimination of specific sensory experiences (Anand and Craig, 1996).

Pain may occur in the absence of the occurrence of these four steps. For example pain from trigeminal neuralgia occurs in the absence of transduction of a chemical stimulus at a nociceptor reflecting axonal discharges initiated at the site of a compressed or demyelinated nerve. Modulation of pain impulses may not occur if specific nervous system tracts are injured. For example, phantom-limb pain occurs in the absence of nociception or nociceptors (pain receptors).

MODULATION OF NOCICEPTION

Modulation of nociceptive stimuli can occur in the periphery or at any point where synaptic transmission occurs.

TABLE 44-1.
TREATMENT OF NEUROPATHIC PAIN WITH ADJUVANT DRUGS

Drug	Mechanism of Action
Carbamazepine	Sodium ion channel blockade
Gabapentin	Effects on calcium ion channels (?)
Lidocaine patch	Sodium ion channel blockade Mechanical protection of allodynic skin
Mexiletine	Sodium ion channel blockade
Phenytoin	Sodium ion channel blockade
Nortriptyline	Neurotransmitter reuptake inhibitor
Desipramine	Neurotransmitter reuptake inhibitor
Corticosteroids	Antiinflammatory effects Sodium ion channel blockade Decreased capillary permeability
Clonidine	Alpha-adrenergic blockade

Peripheral Modulation

Peripheral modulation of nociceptive stimuli occurs by either liberation or elimination of chemicals near the nociceptor. Tissue injury activates nociceptors in the periphery by causing the release of neurotransmitters such as substance P and glutamate that directly activate nociceptors. Other mediators (bradykinin, histamine, prostaglandins, serotonin, potassium and hydrogen ions, lactic acid) further sensitize and excite nociceptors and act as mediators of inflammation. The sources of these substances include ischemic damaged cells and mast cells in the area of injury, as well as plasma and platelets in the environment surrounding the nociceptors. Aspirin, nonsteroidal antiinflammatory drugs, and specific cyclooxygenase inhibitors exert analgesic effects by inhibiting prostaglandin synthesis.

Spinal Modulation

Modulation in the spinal cord results from the action of neurotransmitter substances in the dorsal horn or from spinal reflexes, which convey efferent impulses back to the peripheral nociceptive field. The excitatory amino acid transmitters glutamate and aspartate and several neuropeptides (vasoactive intestinal peptide, calcitonin, neuropeptide Y) modulate transmission of nociceptive afferent signals. Substance P is also an important neuromodulator than can enhance or aggravate pain. Inhibitory substances involved in the regulation of afferent impulses in the dorsal horn include gamma-aminobutyric acid, glycine, enkephalins, endorphins, norepinephrine, dopamine and adenosine.

Supraspinal Modulation

Descending inhibitory tracts at the brainstem level originate from cell bodies located in the region of the periaqueductal gray matter. These inhibitory tracts descend into the dorsolateral fasciculus and synapse in the dorsal horn. Neurotransmitters act presynaptically on first-order neurons and postsynaptically on second-order neurons in the spinothalamic tract. Nerve fibers identified as participants in inhibitory modulation include the opioid system and associated neurotransmitters (endorphins, enkephalins, other neuropeptides). Analgesia is produced during electrical stimulation of the periaqueductal gray matter. Neurotransmitters released from these projections hyperpolarize A-delta and C fibers that serve to negate depolarizing currents that approach terminal endplates thus diminishing the release of neurotransmitters such as substance P. In addition to opioid descending inhibitory pathways, a monoamine pathway originates from locations in the periaqueductal gray matter. Stimulation of this pathway inhibits synaptic transmission in the dorsal horn, similar to inhibition produced by the opioid system. Hyperpolarization of nerves results in decreased transmission of action potentials and decreased release of stored neurotransmitters. Hyperpolarization of nerves most likely occurs because of the opening of potassium ion channels and inhibition of calcium ion movement.

Cognitive Modulation

Cognitive modulation of pain involves the patient's ability to relate a painful experience to another event. For example, pain experienced in a pleasant environment elicits a less intense response than pain experienced in a setting of depression. Another area of perception is attention that presumes that only a fixed number of afferent impulses can reach cortical centers. If a patient in pain concentrates on separate and unrelated images, it is possible to decrease the effects of painful sensations (biofeedback or hypnosis).

Neuroplasticity

Neuroplasticity describes the dynamic modulation of neural impulses. As peripheral nerve firing increases, other changes also occur in the excitability of spinal cord neurons, altering their response to afferent impulses. Central sensitization to afferent impulses results from a functional change in spinal cord processing termed neuroplasticity. The temporal summation of the number and duration of action potentials elicited per stimulus that occurs in dorsal horn neurons has been referred to as the "wind-up phenomenon." The wind-up phenomena results in a persistence of action potentials for up to 60 seconds after the discontinuance of the stimulus, and results in a change in spinal cord processing that can last for 1 to 3 hours.

Spinal cord synaptic plasticity involves the binding of glutamate to the N-methyl-D-aspartate (NMDA) receptors as well as binding of substance P and neurokinins. Binding of glutamate to NMDA receptors alters a magnesium-dependent block of ion channels, subsequently increasing cellular permeability to all cations, especially calcium and sodium ions. Glutamate also activates alpha-amino-3-hydroxy-5-methyl-4-isoxazoleproprionate (AMPA) receptors that control depolarization primarily through modulation of sodium influx into cells. In addition to modulating augmented excitability, these transmitter and cellular mechanisms mediate changes in postsynaptic cells, leading to more permanent changes in nerve conduction.

PERIPHERAL NERVE PHYSIOLOGY

Nociceptors (Pain Receptors)

Nociceptors are free nerve ending receptors present in skin, muscles, joints, viscera, and vasculature. These nociceptors are responsible for detecting the presence of noxious stimuli resulting from chemical, thermal (heat, cold), or mechanical changes. In normal tissues, nociceptors are inactive until they are stimulated by sufficient energy to overcome their stimulus (resting) threshold (Galer et al., 2002). Thus, nociceptors prevent random signal propagation (screening function) to the CNS for the interpretation of pain.

Nociceptive neurons synapse in the dorsal horn of the spinal cord with both local interneurons and projection neurons that carry nociceptive information to higher centers in the brainstem and thalamus. In contrast to other sensory receptors, pain receptors do not adapt. Failure of pain receptors to adapt is protective because it allows the individual to remain aware of continued tissue damage. After damage has occurred, pain is usually minimal. The onset of pain in a tissue rendered acutely ischemic is related to its rate of metabolism. For example, pain occurs in exercising ischemic skeletal muscles in 15 to 20 seconds but not for 20 to 30 minutes in ischemic skin.

Specific types of nociceptors react to different types of stimuli. Certain C-nociceptors and A-delta nociceptors react only to heat or cold stimuli, whereas others react to multiple stimuli (chemical, heat, cold) (Galer et al., 2002). Some A-beta receptors have nociceptor-like activity. A-beta mechanoreceptor sensory fibers can be recruited to transmit signals that will be interpreted as painful when their environment is changed by inflammation and its byproducts. Mechanical allodynia (painful or burning sensation caused by light touching) results from A-beta mechanoreceptor recruitment (Bennett, 2000).

Visceral nociceptors, unlike cutaneous nociceptors, are not designed solely as pain receptors because internal organs are infrequently exposed to potentially damaging events. Many damaging stimuli (cutting, burning, clamping) produce no pain when applied to visceral structures. Rather, inflammation, ischemia, mesenteric stretching, dilation, or spasm of hollow viscera may produce severe spasm. These stimuli are usually associated with pathologic processes, and the pain they induce may serve a survival function by promoting immobility.

Transduction

Mechanical, thermal, or chemical energy is converted into an electrical action potential (transduction) capable of propagating (transmission) along the nerve fiber toward the spinal cord when the resting threshold of a nociceptor is exceeded. Action potential propagation occurs via the opening and closing of sodium and potassium ion channels. Nociceptors may detect a stimulus (touching a hot object) and generate an action potential that results in perception of pain before tissue damage occurs (protective).

In addition to the generation of an action potential, there are a number of other events that occur after detection of a noxious stimulus (Galer et al., 2002). Acute inflammation that develops in response to tissue injury serves to protect injured tissues and promote healing. Several inflammatory mediators (bradykinin, prostaglandins, serotonin, histamine, cytokines) are released in response to tissue injury. Bradykinin is viewed as the first mediator to cause activation of second messengers resulting in increased sodium ion channel conductance and sensitization. Prostaglandins enhance activity of bradykinin and contribute to inflammatory responses.

Exposure to these inflammatory mediators causes A-delta fibers and C-fibers to undergo peripheral sensitization such that their stimulus thresholds are decreased and their firing and intensity is increased and prolonged. This results in an increase in the frequency of pain signals arriving in the CNS. In the majority of cases of acute inflammation, the process naturally resolves as tissues heal and peripheral sensitization diminishes and nociceptors return to their original resting threshold. Chronic pain, however, occurs when for unknown reasons the conditions associated with inflammation do not resolve, resulting in persistent pain sensations because of normally painful stimuli (hyperalgesia) and the occurrence of pain sensations in response to normally nonpainful stimuli (allodynia).

Hyperalgesia

Hyperalgesia is a decrease in the pain threshold in an area of inflammation such that even trivial stimuli cause pain. It is most likely due to local release of chemical mediators from injured cells in the inflamed area, resulting in the sensitization of pain receptors. The metabolites of arachidonic acid and bradykinin appear to play an important role in sensitization of pain receptors (Fig. 44-1) (Dahl and Kehlet, 1991).

Transmission

Pain signals are transmitted from nociceptors along myelinated A-delta fibers (rapid conduction for early response) and unmyelinated C fibers (slow conduction for more delayed response). These afferent fibers enter the spinal cord through the dorsal nerve roots and terminate on cells in the dorsal horn.

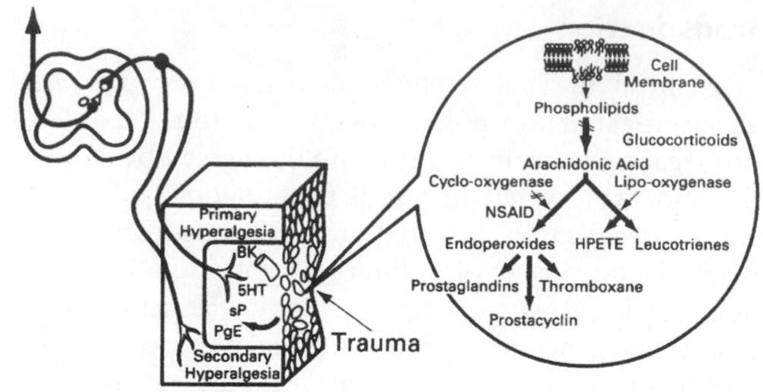

Figure 44-1. Trauma to tissue leads to the local release of multiple chemical substances [substance P (sP), bradykinin (BK), serotonin (5-HT), prostaglandins (PgE) from a cascade of arachidonic acid metabolites] from afferent nerve endings resulting in vasodilation, increased vascular permeability (inflammation), and sensitization of nociceptors (primary hyperalgesia). (From Dahl JB, Kehlet H. Nonsteroidal antiinflammatory drugs: rationale for use in severe postoperative pain. *Br J Anaesth* 1991;66:703–712; with permission.)

Fast and Slow Pain

Two qualitatively different types of pain can be readily appreciated (Figs. 44-2 and 44-3) (Guyton and Hall, 2000). *Fast* pain is a short, well-localized, stabbing sensation that is matched to the stimulus, such as a pinprick or surgical skin incision. This pain starts abruptly when the stimulus is applied and ends promptly when the stimulus is removed. Fast pain results from stimulation of small, myelinated type A-delta nerve fibers with conduction velocities of 12 to 30 m/s. Myelination of the axon provides junctions that permit the electrical pain signal to jump, resulting in rapid pain signal transmission. The second type of pain sensation, *slow* pain, is characterized as a throbbing, burning, or aching sensation that is poorly localized and less specifically related to the stimulus. This pain may continue long after the removal of the stimulus. Slow pain results from stimulation of more primitive, unmyelinated type C nerve fibers with conduction velocities of 0.5 to 2 m/s. The farther from the brain the stimulus originates, the greater is the temporal distinction of the two components. It is the immediate, stabbing pain that instantly tells the person that tissue damage is occurring, whereas burning pain becomes the source of sustained discomfort. Nerve fibers for temperature follow the same pathways as fibers for pain. Indeed, artificially applied pain in the form of a heat stimulus causes pain in almost all individuals when skin temperature exceeds 43 °C (pain threshold).

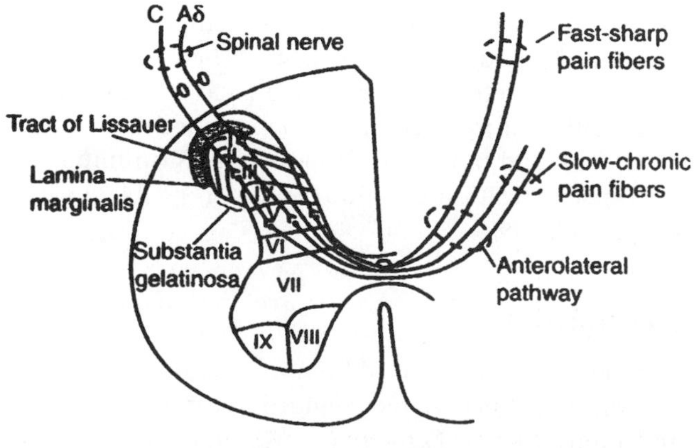

Figure 44-2. Transmission of both fast-sharp and slow-chronic pain signals into and through the spinal cord on their way to the brain. (Guyton AC, Hall JE. *Textbook of medical physiology.* 10th edition. Saunders. Philadelphia, 2000; with permission.)

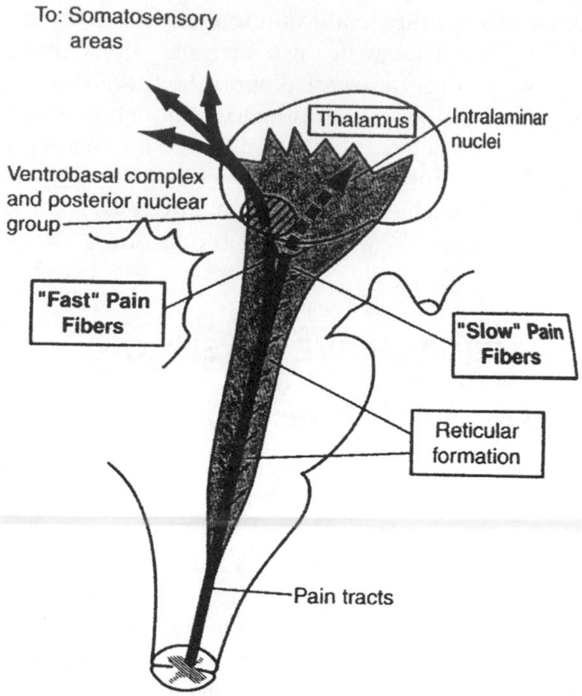

Figure 44-3. Transmission of pain signals into the brainstem, thalamus, and cerebral cortex by way of the fast conducting pain (sharp) fibers and the slow conducting pain (burning) fibers. (Guyton AC, Hall JE. *Textbook of medical physiology.* 10th edition. Saunders. Philadelphia, 2000; with permission.)

Neuropathic Pain

Neuropathic pain of a peripheral origin is a distinct type of chronic pain that occurs in the complete absence of an inflammatory reaction. Direct damage to a peripheral nerve results in a continual ectopic spontaneous discharge of pain signals (neuropathic pain). In addition, the involved anatomic region becomes sensitive to stimulation (mechanical, thermal) resulting in severe chronic pain, hyperalgesia, and allodynia (Bennett, 2000). This peripheral sensitization can contribute to secondary hyperalgesia and central sensitization.

CENTRAL NERVOUS SYSTEM PHYSIOLOGY

Pain transmission from peripheral nociceptors to the spinal cord and higher structures of the CNS is a dynamic

TABLE 44-2.
FACTORS THAT INFLUENCE THE ACTIVATION OF ASCENDING PAIN SYSTEMS

Degree of activation of activation of segmental and descending inhibitory neurons in the dorsal horn
Preexisting concentrations of excitatory neurotransmitters
Level of activation of inhibitory neurotransmitters
Intensity of noxious stimulus
Degree of sensitization of nociceptors in the periphery

process involving several pathways, numerous receptors, neurotransmitters and secondary messengers (Galer et al., 2002). The dorsal horn functions as a relay center for nociceptive and other sensory activity. The degree of activation of ascending pain projection systems depends on multiple factors (Table 44-2).

Dorsal Horn and Ascending Nociceptive Pathway

Primary afferent fibers with their cell bodies in the dorsal root ganglion, connect with a second neuronal cell, located in the dorsal horn of the spinal cord. Afferent fibers from peripheral nociceptors enter the spinal cord in the dorsal root and ascend or descend several segments in the Lissauer tract before synapsing in the dorsal horn.

The dorsal horn consists of six laminae (see Fig. 44-2) (Guyton and Hall, 2000). Laminae I and II are the sites of termination of afferent C-fibers and these two laminae are known as the substantia gelatinosa. The substantia gelatinosa is important for integration and modulation of incoming nociceptive information. Lamina V is the site of second-order wide dynamic range (WDR) and nociceptive-specific (NS) neurons that receive input from nociceptive and nonnociceptive neurons. The NS neurons respond only to noxious stimuli in their peripheral environment, whereas WDR neurons respond to innocuous and noxious stimuli of many types. Both types of neurons are believed to be important in the perception of nociceptive information. Often chronic pain states may be explained in terms of the inputs to these cells and their supraspinal connections.

Transmission and Modulation

The dorsal horn and its laminae serve as the receiving site for activity initiated on the arrival of action potentials from the periphery via primary afferent neurons. These primary afferent neurons terminate in the dorsal horn and synapse with secondary afferent neurons. These secondary neurons act as gate cells providing initial modulation of action potentials in the dorsal horn. The two main classes of neurotransmitters associated with primary afferent nociceptive transmission in the dorsal horn—excitatory amino acids are glutamate and neurokinin peptides such as substance P.

Thalamus and Cerebral Cortex

After leaving the dorsal horn and ascending via spinothalamic and other pain pathways, nociceptive action potentials reach higher brain centers (reticular formation, midbrain, hypothalamus, cerebral cortex). Each area of the brain contributes to the development of the pain experience and subsequent reaction to it. These areas act to alert the individual to the pain and its accompanying dangers, alleviate pain through pain modulation and prevent further tissue damage. In addition, autonomic function, motor function and descending modulating pain pathways respond as a result of activity in this central area. It is likely that multiple complex brain systems are involved when a pain signal reaches the brain. The cingulate cortex is important in processing nociceptive information.

Cells in laminae I and V are spinothalamic cells, and about 75% of fibers originating from these cells cross to the contralateral spinothalamic tract. The phylogenetically newer portion of the spinothalamic tract (neospinothalamic tract) projects to the posterior portions of the thalamus and is considered connected to the spatial and temporal aspects of pain perception. The phylogenetically older portion of the spinothalamic (paleospinothalamic) tract projects to the medial thalamus and is responsible for initiation of unpleasant aspects of pain as well as autonomic nervous system responses to pain. Other pathways involved in cephalad transmission of pain impulses include the spinocervical tracts, spinoreticular tracts, and spinomesencephalic tracts. Pain impulses travel from the thalamus to the somatosensory areas of the cerebral cortex. Complete removal of these cortical areas does not destroy the individual's ability to perceive pain, suggesting that the thalamus participates in the conscious perception of pain. It is speculated that the cerebral cortex is important for interpreting the intensity of pain even though perception of pain seems predominantly to be a function of lower brain centers.

Afferent fibers conducting burning and aching types of pain terminate in the reticular area of the brainstem. This area transmits activating signals into most areas of the brain, especially through the thalamus to the cerebral cortex and hypothalamus. Stimulation of the reticular activating system by burning and aching pain awakens the individual from sleep and produces generalized activation of the nervous system. These signals are poorly localized and only alert the individual to continuing tissue damage. Even weak pain signals via this pathway may summate with time, converting initially tolerable discomfort into intolerable pain.

Both tactile and thermal afferent stimulation has inhibitory influences on pain perception. The basis of the gate control theory is that A-delta fiber stimulation activates interneurons in the dorsal horn that inhibit the activity of nociceptive transmission neurons. This inhibition is the basis of transcutaneous electrical nerve stimulation, as well as spinal cord stimulation and thalamic stimulation for pain control.

Gate Cells

Gate cells screen action potentials by determining which ones are transmitted to the CNS for perception. These cells also are involved in determining which action potentials result in reflex responses that serve to move the tissue away from the noxious stimulus and avoid further injury. Involvement of inhibitory interneurons that release neurotransmitters such as gamma-aminobutyric acid (GABA), which also have receptors on these secondary afferent neurons and produce inhibitory postsynaptic action potentials, counteract the transmission of excitatory action potentials received from the primary afferent neurons. This gate cell function determines the nature of excitation and inhibition action potentials and the resulting effect on further signal transmission.

Under normal conditions, secondary afferent neurons are not spontaneously active but rather are activated by action potentials generated in the periphery. Similar to peripheral nociceptors, these gate cells have a specific physiologic role (regulate incoming action potentials) and a stimulus threshold that must be reached for depolarization to occur.

Glutamate

Several types of excitatory amino acid receptors are involved in the initiation of excitation that leads to transmission of pain information. Glutamate is an excitatory amino acid that is released from presynaptic endings of the primary afferent neurons terminating in the dorsal horn (Hudspith, 1997). This excitatory amino acid activates receptors including kainate, AMPA, and NMDA receptors. The action of glutamate on AMPA receptors causes a rapid depolarization of secondary afferent neurons and generation of an action potential. In addition, binding of glutamate can result in the activation of cascades of enzymatic processes and second-messenger systems that may be involved in nociception and responsible for the initial pain modulation than can occur in the spinal cord. Much like peripheral modulators (bradykinin), glutamate acts as a central pain mediator at nearly all secondary afferent neurons involved in nociceptive processing (Woolf and Mannion, 1999).

NMDA Receptors

NMDA receptors are postsynaptic to the primary afferent neuron being located on the secondary afferent neuron. The NMDA ion channel is blocked by magnesium ions and under normal circumstances the secondary afferent neurons are not depolarized long enough to permit magnesium ions to be dislodged and calcium ions to cross. Glutamate is rapidly removed from the synaptic cleft and thus there is no activity at NMDA receptors in normal nociceptive transmission processes. However, in the presence of persistent pain arising from abnormal conditions (peripheral sensitization, neuropathic pain, chronic pain), the frequency of pain signal transmission increases resulting in increased amounts of glutamate available in synaptic clefts. As a result, secondary afferent neurons are depolarized long enough for magnesium ions blocking NMDA receptors to be dislodged. Subsequent activation of NMDA receptors serves to activate secondary messengers and enzymatic processes and generation of various substances (nitric oxide) that are believed to contribute to enhanced neuronal sensitivity known as central sensitization.

Protein kinase C activated by activity of excitatory amino acids on NMDA receptors is capable of uncoupling the opioid receptor mechanism resulting in decreased responsiveness to opioids. As a result, prolonged opioid administration can lead to spinal sensitization and sustained excitatory amino acid release, (occurs with neuropathic states) and reduced responsiveness to opioids (Pockett, 1995).

Central Sensitization

Central sensitization is believed to be the origin of many chronic pain conditions, especially those classified as neuropathic (Woolf and Mannion, 1999). Central sensitization describes increased excitability of secondary afferent neurons evoked by neurochemical changes resulting from activation of NMDA receptors (Petrenko et al., 2003). The increased excitability of secondary afferent neurons changes the subsequent responses of these neurons to future input. An increase in the number of action potentials generated by peripheral C-fiber input is referred to as central wind-up or central sensitization. Prolonged input from sensitized nociceptors resulting from inflammation or spontaneous discharge associated with nerve injury can cause a chronic state of central sensitization (Bennett, 2000). It is likely that many chronic pain conditions reflect central sensitization resulting from sustained sensory input from the sustained sensory PNS into the spinal cord and activation of NMDA receptors. Furthermore, the gatekeeping function of secondary afferent neurons is compromised, leaving the excitatory effects of pain transmission unopposed. This results in spontaneous generation of pain signals and exaggerated nervous system responses to sensory stimuli (Woolf and Mannion, 1999). Persistent pain can also lead to anatomic changes in both the PNS and CNS. Following nerve injury, a variety of neuronal plasticity changes occur, such as sprouting of dendrites on neurons projecting to the dorsal horn or ingrowth of sympathetic fibers into the dorsal root ganglia. These anatomic changes likely produce functional changes characteristic of chronic pain states (Baron et al., 2002).

Because the higher levels of the brain cannot discern the origin of the pain signals, the patient is in a continual state of pain. It is not known when normal events associated with acute pain become transformed to produce pathologic pain and the point at which activity occurring at the dorsal horn causes secondary afferent neurons to become chronically sensitized. What is known is that NMDA receptors are important in facilitating central sensitization and development of opioid tolerance.

Emotional or physical stress exacerbates central neuropathic pain in up 50% of cases but seldom accompanies peripheral neuropathic pain. Cold evoked allodynia is more common with central neuropathic pain. The most common description of spontaneous pain of central neuropathic pain is burning or scalding. Oral gabapentin, administered to healthy volunteers in a regimen similar to that used in treating chronic neuropathic pain, reduces measures of central sensitization evoked by intradermal capsaicin (Gottrup et al. 2004). This suggests that the pain-relieving effect in chronic neuropathic pain is linked to the effect of gabapentin on central sensitization.

Glial Cells

Glial cells (microglia, astrocytes, oligodendrocytes) represent nearly three quarters of all of the cells in the CNS and have historically been viewed as providing physical support for neurons. It is now known that glial cells have important neuromodulatory and neurotrophic effects and that they are critically important in providing immune function following injury, inflammation or infection. Following nerve injury, there is rapid activation of glial cells within the CNS with release of substances that activate astrocytes. Microglia initiate the immune response while astrocytes maintain it. Both types of cells produce proinflammatory cytokines including the interleukins IL-1 and IL-6 and tumor necrosis factor that can diffuse through the surrounding cellular environment and produce functional changes in neuronal cells. Inflammatory substances play a part in the modulation of pain by interfering with nociceptive transduction, conduction, and transmission of nociceptive signals resulting in prolonged or permanent signaling to the brain's cognitive centers in the absence of a painful noxious or nonnoxious stimulus (Dugong et al., 2003). This modulation may result from alteration of the transcription rate and/or posttranslational changes in proteins involved in pain pathways.

Cytokines are important in acute and chronic pain as they induce the release of a variety of substances that participate in the sensitization of sensory neurons. These include cyclooxygenase-2, inducible nitric oxide synthase, and substance P. Activated glial cells also release glutamate, nitric oxide, reactive oxygen species, eicosanoids, and other substances that act via NMDA receptors to produce spinal sensitization. IL-6 is a cytokine that is synthesized after nerve injury in peripheral nerves, dorsal root ganglions, and in the spinal cord.

Preemptive Analgesia

Preemptive analgesia is based on the concept that blocking nociceptive afferent inputs or their effects on dorsal horn neurons before the start of tissue injury would delay or halt the process of central sensitization (Woolf and Chong, 1993). Clinically, it is speculated that postoperative pain would be decreased by preemptive analgesia. However, the efficacy of preemptive analgesia is dependent on the extent by which afferent impulses are controlled during the whole perioperative period. Therefore, comprehensive preemptive strategies must start before the painful stimulus (surgical incision) and be maintained during the entire period of intense nociceptive stimulation. This approach is more correctly viewed as perioperative analgesia rather than preemptive analgesia (Katz, 2000).

ENDOGENOUS PAIN SUPPRESSION PATHWAYS

There is great interindividual variation in the response to pain which in part reflects the capability of the brain to suppress input of pain signals to the nervous system by activating endogenous pain suppression pathways (Fig. 44-4) (Guyton and Hall, 2000). This endogenous pain suppression system consists of three major components

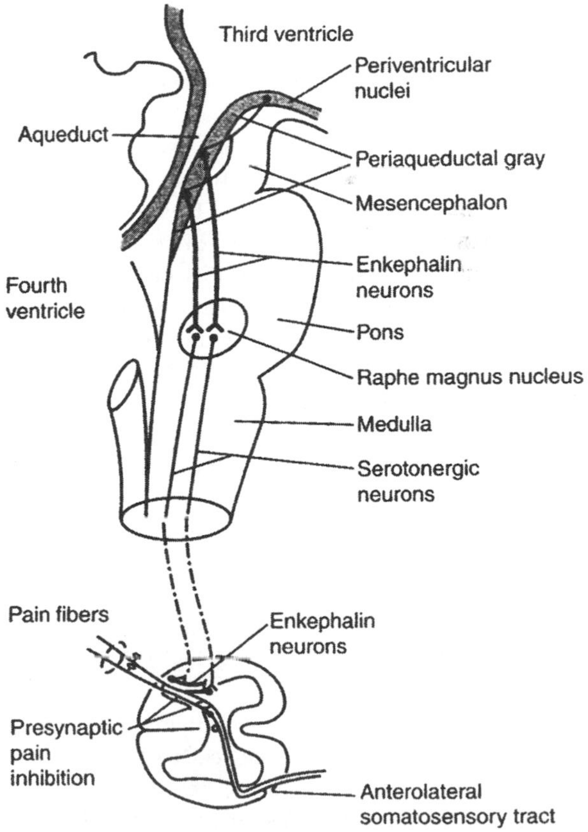

Figure 44-4. Analgesia system of the brain and spinal cord demonstrating inhibition of incoming pain signals at the cord level and the presence of enkephalin-secreting neurons that suppress pain signals in both the spinal cord and brainstem. (Guyton AC, Hall JE. *Textbook of medical physiology*. 10th edition. Saunders. Philadelphia, 2000; with permission).

TABLE 44-3.
COMPONENTS OF THE ENDOGENOUS PAIN SUPPRESSION SYSTEM

Periaqueductal gray and periventricular areas surrounding the aqueduct of Sylvius and portions of the third and fourth ventricles (transmit signals to next component of endogenous pain suppression system)
Raphe magnus nucleus (lower pons and upper medulla) and nucleus reticularis paragigantocellularis (medulla) (transmit signals to next component of the endogenous pain suppression system)
Dorsal horns of the spinal cord (analgesia signals can be blocked at this area before being relayed to brain)

(Table 44-3). Electrical stimulation either in the periaqueductal gray area or in the raphe magnus nucleus can almost completely suppress pain signals entering by way of the dorsal spinal roots. Neurotransmitters, especially enkephalins and serotonin are involved in the endogenous pain suppression system. Enkephalins are believed to cause presynaptic inhibition and postsynaptic inhibition of incoming type C and type A-delta pain fibers where they synapse in the dorsal horns. Presynaptic inhibition is probably achieved by blocking calcium ion channels and calcium ions cause the release of neurotransmitters at the synapses. Descending pain pathways are activated as a result of pain detection, discrimination, and perception at the higher levels of the CNS. Inhibitory and excitatory neuroanatomic pathways originate in the brainstem and descend in the dorsal longitudinal fasciculus to modulate nociception and pain perception (Basbaum and Fields, 1978). When activated these pathways inhibit nociceptive stimuli. Neurotransmitters identified in descending pathways include norepinephrine, serotonin, and endogenous opioids. Inhibitory pathways are activated by opioids and excitatory pathways are inhibited by opioids thus providing the mechanism of analgesia induced by drugs such as morphine (also tricyclic antidepressants and alpha$_2$-adrenergic agonists). Tricyclic antidepressants block the presynaptic reuptake of serotonin and norepinephrine and thus augment their postsynaptic actions in descending pain suppression pathways.

CLASSIFICATION OF PAIN

Pain experience is unique to each individual patient even when the physical injury is identical to that present in another patient. The presence of fear, anger, anxiety, depression, and fatigue can affect the way in which pain is perceived. The subjectivity of pain makes it difficult to categorize pain and to understand pain mechanisms. One approach is to classify pain with regard to duration (acute versus chronic) and pathophysiology (nociceptive versus neuropathic pain) (Table 44-4) (Galer et al., 2002).

TABLE 44-4.
PHYSIOLOGIC PAIN CATEGORIES

	Example	Mechanism
Nociceptive	Arthritis Bone fracture Bone metastasis Cellulitis	Activation of nociceptors
Visceral	Pancreatic Peptic ulcer Myocardial infarction	Activation of nociceptors
Neuropathic	Posthepatic neuralgia	Ectopic discharges in the nervous system
	Diabetic neuropathy	Spontaneous activity in nerves
	Poststroke pain Trigeminal neuralgia	Neuroma formation
Complex regional pain syndrome	Persistent focal pain after trauma with or without evidence of sympathetic nervous system involvement	Sensitization of spinal neurons

Adapted from Galer B, Gammaitoni A, Alvarez NA. Pain. *Sci Am Med* 2002:11:XIV:1–27.

Acute and Chronic Pain

Acute pain is generally associated with well-defined tissue damage and is of limited duration after which nociceptors return to a normal resting stimulus threshold. Treatment approaches include common analgesic medications (opioids and nonopioids). Chronic pain can be categorized as malignant or nonmalignant. Malignant chronic pain usually has pathology present and is indicative of a life-limiting disease such as cancer, end-stage organ dysfunction, or HIV infection. Chronic pain may have both nociceptive and neuropathic elements. Chronic nonmalignant pain (back pain, migraine headaches, arthritis, diabetic neuropathy) often has no detectable pathology and neuroplastic changes that have occurred in remote locations (dorsal horn of the spinal cord) make treatment difficult.

Patients with acute pain or chronic pain may exhibit autonomic nervous system signs and symptoms (tachycardia, increased blood pressure, diaphoresis, rapid breathing) when pain is present. Guarding is more common in patients with chronic pain who manifest allodynia. Nevertheless, the presence or absence of autonomic signs and symptoms does not confirm that pain is present or not present.

Nociceptive and Neuropathic Pain

Organic pain may be subdivided into nociceptive or neuropathic pain. Nociceptive pain includes visceral and somatic pain and refers to pain owing to peripheral stimulation of nociceptors in visceral or somatic structures (Portenoy and Hagen, 1990). Nociceptive pain is usually responsive to opioid or nonopioid analgesics. Neuropathic pain involves peripheral or central afferent neural pathways and commonly is described as burning or lancinating pain. Patients experiencing neuropathic pain often respond poorly to opioid analgesics.

Visceral Pain

Pain receptors in viscera are similar to those in the skin but are more sparsely distributed than in somatic structures. Indeed, highly localized damage to a viscus, as produced by a surgical incision, is not associated with intense pain. Nevertheless, the liver capsule is highly sensitive to direct trauma and stretch, and the bile ducts are sensitive to pain. Any event that causes stimulation of nerve endings throughout a viscus causes intense pain that is diffuse, poorly localized, and often associated with nausea and signs of autonomic nervous system activation. Visceral pain typically radiates and may be referred to surface areas of the body far removed from the painful viscus but with the same dermatome origin as the diseased viscus. Often, visceral pain occurs as rhythmic contractions of smooth muscles. A cramping type of visceral pain frequently accompanies gastroenteritis, gallbladder disease, ureteral obstruction, menstruation, and distension of the uterus during the first stage of labor. Visceral pain, like deep somatic pain, initiates reflex contraction of nearby skeletal muscles, which makes the abdominal wall rigid when inflammatory processes involve the peritoneum. Visceral pain due to malignant invasion of a hollow or solid viscus is often described as diffuse, gnawing, or cramping if a hollow viscus is involved and as sharp or aching if a solid viscus is involved (Ashburn and Lipman, 1993).

Causes of visceral pain include ischemia, stretching of ligament attachments, spasm of smooth muscles, or distension

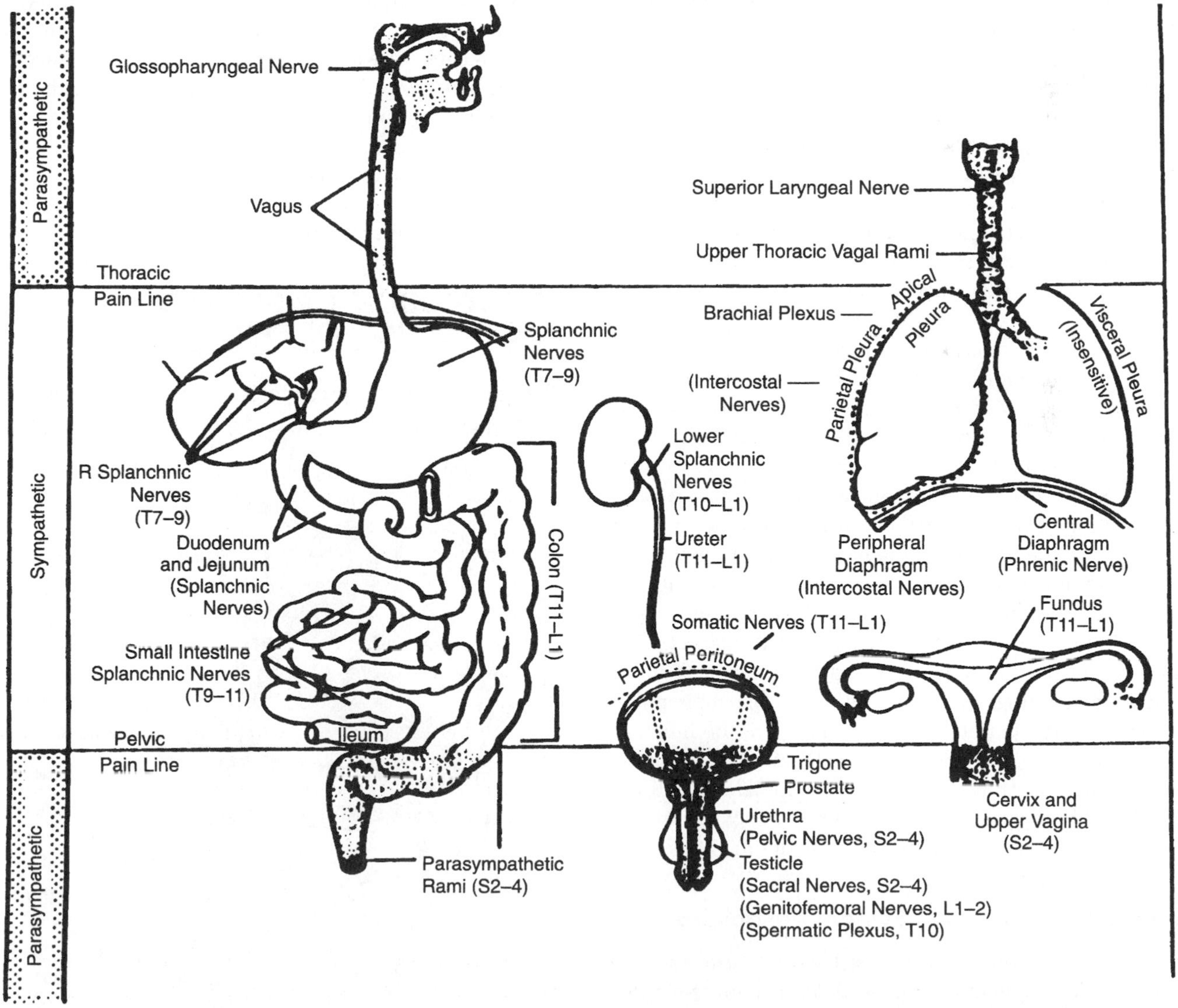

Figure 44-5. Pain innervation of the viscera. Pain afferents from structures above the thoracic pain line and below the pelvic pain line traverse parasympathetic pathways. (Ganong WF. *Review of medical physiology*, 21st ed. Lange Medical Books/McGraw-Hill. New York, 2003).

of a hollow structure such as the gallbladder, common bile duct, or ureter. Distension of a hollow viscus results in pain due to stretch of the tissues and possibly ischemia due to compression of blood vessels by overdistension of the tissue.

Pain impulses from most of the abdominal and thoracic viscera are conducted through afferent fibers that travel with the sympathetic nervous system, whereas impulses from the esophagus, trachea, and pharynx are mediated via vagal and glossopharyngeal afferents, and impulses from structures deep in the pelvis are transmitted via the sacral parasympathetic nerves (Fig. 44-5) (Ganong, 2003). Pain impulses from the heart are conducted through sympathetic nervous system nerves to the middle cervical ganglia, stellate ganglion, and the first four or five thoracic ganglia of the sympathetic chain. These impulses enter the spinal cord through the second, third, fourth, and fifth thoracic nerves. The cause of pain impulses from the heart is almost always myocardial ischemia. Parenchyma of the brain, liver, and alveoli of the lungs are devoid of pain receptors. Nevertheless, the bronchi and parietal pleura are very sensitive to pain.

Somatic Pain

Somatic pain is described as sharp, stabbing, well-localized pain that typically arises from the skin, skeletal muscles, and peritoneum (Ashburn and Lipman, 1993). Pain from a surgical incision, the second stage of labor, or peritoneal irritation is somatic pain. Disease of a viscus that spreads to the parietal wall, elicits stabbing pain transmitted by spinal nerves. In this respect, the parietal wall resembles the skin in being extensively innervated by spinal nerves. Indeed, a surgical incision through parietal peritoneum is exquisitely painful, whereas incision of visceral peritoneum is not painful. In contrast to diffuse and poorly localized visceral pain, parietal pain is usually localized directly over the damaged area.

The presence of both visceral and parietal pain pathways can result in localization of pain from viscera to dual surface areas of the body at the same time. For example, pain impulses from an inflamed appendix pass through the sympathetic nervous system visceral pain fibers into the sympathetic chain and then into the spinal cord at T10 to T11. This pain is referred to an area around the umbilicus and is aching or cramping in character. In addition, pain impulses originate in the parietal peritoneum where the inflamed appendix touches the abdominal wall, and these impulses pass through the spinal nerves into the spinal cord at L1 to L2. This stabbing pain is localized directly over the irritated peritoneal surface in the right lower quadrant.

Sympathetic Nervous System Responses

Painful stimulation may evoke reflex increases in sympathetic nervous system efferent activity. It is possible that associated vasoconstriction leads to acidosis, tissue ischemia, and release of chemicals that further activate pain receptors. Resulting sustained, painful stimulation produces further increases in sympathetic nervous system activity, and the vicious cycle termed reflex sympathetic dystrophy (complex regional pain syndrome) may develop.

After certain types of nerve injury, pain may occur without activation of pain receptors. Spontaneous firing that occurs from injured peripheral nerves, especially in response to sympathetic nervous system stimulation, may reflect a proliferation of alpha-adrenergic receptors on the increased number of neuroma sprouts (Devor, 1983). Spontaneous firing may also occur from dorsal root ganglia whose peripheral projections have been interrupted, as after nerve transection or limb amputation.

Sites Amenable to Surgical Section of Pain Pathways

Multiple sites in the peripheral and central nervous systems are amenable to surgical ablative procedures to relieve pain. Surgical section through the anterolateral quadrant of the spinal cord (cordotomy) at the thoracic level interrupts the anterolateral spinothalamic tract and relieves pain from the limb on the side opposite the cord transection. Cordotomy may be unsuccessful because some pain fibers do not cross to the opposite side of the spinal cord until they have reached the brain. Furthermore, pain that is more intense than the original pain may develop several months after the cordotomy.

EMBRYOLOGIC ORIGIN AND LOCALIZATION OF PAIN

The position in the spinal cord to which visceral afferent fibers pass for each organ depends on the segment

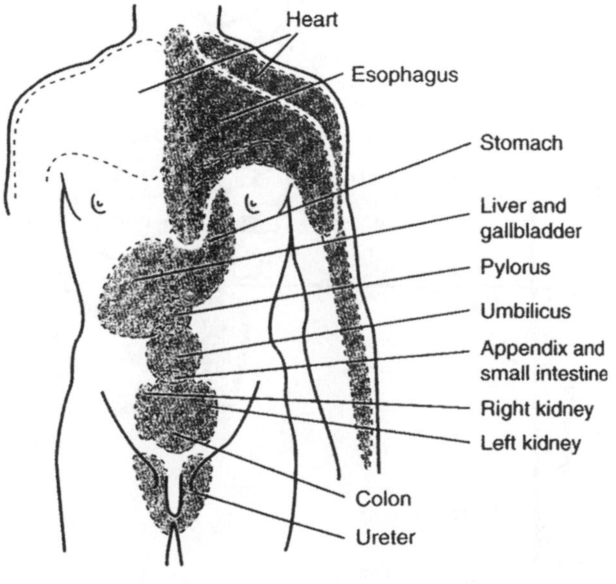

Figure 44-6. Surface area of referred pain from different visceral organs. (Guyton AC, Hall JE. *Textbook of medical physiology*. 10th edition. Saunders. Philadelphia, 2000; with permission.)

(dermatome) of the body from which the organ developed embryologically. This explains the phenomenon of referred pain to a site distal from the tissue causing the pain (Fig. 44-6) (Guyton and Hall, 2000). For example, the heart originates in the neck and upper thorax such that visceral afferents enter the spinal cord at C3 to C5. As a result, the referred pain of myocardial ischemia is to the neck and arm. The gallbladder originates from the ninth thoracic segment, so visceral afferents from the gallbladder enter the spinal cord at T9. Skeletal muscle spasm caused by damage in adjacent tissues may also be a cause of referred pain. For example, pain from the ureter can cause reflex spasm of the lumbar muscles.

REFERENCES

Anand JKS, Craig KD. New perspectives on the definition of pain. *Pain* 1996;67:3–7.

Ashburn MA, Lipman AG. Management of pain in the cancer patient. *Anesth Analg* 1993;76:402–416.

Basbaum AI, Fields HL. Endogenous pain control mechanisms: Review and hypothesis. *Ann Neurol* 1978;4:451–460.

Baron R, Fields HL, Janig W, et al. National Institutes of Health Workshop: reflex sympathetic dystrophy/complex regional pain syndromes-state of the-science. *Anesth Analg* 2002;95:1812–1816.

Bennett GJ. Update on the neurophysiology of pain transmission and modulation: focus on the NMDA-receptor. *J Pain Symptom Manage* 2000;19:S2–S10.

Dahl JB, Kehlet H. Nonsteroidal antiinflammatory drugs: rationale for use in severe postoperative pain. *Br J Anaesth* 1991;66:703–712.

DeJongh RF, Vissers KC, Meert TF, et al. The role of interleukin-6 in nociception and pain. *Anesth Analg* 2003;96:1096–1103.

Devor M. Nerve pathophysiology and mechanisms of pain in causalgia. *J Auton Nerv Syst* 1983;7:371–385.

Galer B, Gammaitoni A, Alvarez NA. Pain. *Sci Am Med* 2002:11:XIV:1–27.

Ganong WF. *Review of medical physiology*, 21st ed. Lange Medical Books/McGraw-Hill. New York, 2003.

Glajchen M. Chronic pain: treatment barriers and strategies for clinical practice. *J Am Board Fam Pract* 2001;14:211–215.

Gottrup H, Juhl G, Kristensen AD, et al. Chronic oral gabapentin reduces elements of central sensitization in human experimental hyperalgesia. *Anesthesiology* 2004;101:1400–1408.

Guyton AC, Hall JE. *Textbook of medical physiology*. 10th edition. Saunders. Philadelphia, 2000.

Helmick CG, Lawrence RC, Pollard RA, et al. Arthritis and other rheumatic conditions: who is affected now and will be affected later. *Arthritis Care Res* 1995;8:203–208.

Hudspith MJ. Glutamate: a role in normal brain function, anaesthesia, analgesia and CNS injury. *Br J Anaesth* 1997;78:731–747.

Katz J. Preemptive analgesia: where do we go from here? *J Pain* 2000;1:89–92.

Petrenko AB, Yamakura T, Baba H, et al. The role of *N*-methyl-D-aspartate (NMDA) receptors in pain: a review. *Anesth Analg* 2003;97:1108–1116.

Pockett S. Spinal cord plasticity and chronic pain. *Anesth Analg* 1995; 80:173–178.

Portenoy RK, Hagen NA. Breakthrough pain: definition, prevalence and characteristics. *Pain* 1990;41:273–281.

Woolf CJ, Chong MS. Preemptive analgesia—treating postoperative pain by preventing the establishment of central sensitization. *Anesth Analg* 1993;77:362–379.

Woolf CJ, Mannion RJ. Neuropathic pain: aetiology, symptoms, mechanisms and management. *Lancet* 1999;353:1959–1965.

Systemic Circulation

45

The systemic circulation supplies blood to all the tissues of the body except the lungs. Important considerations in understanding the physiology of the systemic circulation include (a) components of the systemic circulation, (b) physical characteristics of the systemic circulation, (c) physical characteristics of blood, (d) determinants and control of tissue blood flow, (e) regulation of systemic blood pressure, and (f) regulation of cardiac output and venous return. In addition, the fetal circulation possesses many unique features that distinguish it from the systemic circulation after birth.

ENDOTHELIAL FUNCTION

The entire vascular system is lined by endothelial cells. Thus, the endothelium is a large and widely distributed structure. Indeed, it is estimated that the adult endothelium is composed of ten trillion cells and weighs approximately 1 kg (Galley, 2004). It is now widely appreciated that the endothelium is not simply an inert lining layer of the circulation, but is an important "organ" that is involved in many physiologic and processes in health and disease (Table 45-1 and Table 45-2). The healthy endothelium promotes vasodilatation and confers antithrombotic and antiadhesive properties to the vessel wall. The endothelium also regulates vascular permeability, smooth muscle proliferation, and has an important role in the regulation of glucose and lipid metabolism. Endothelial dysfunction is an important element of cardiovascular disease and aging. Cardiovascular risk factors including smoking, diabetes mellitus, hyperlipidemia, obesity, and systemic hypertension are related to their adverse effects upon endothelial function.

Endothelial Function and Regulation of Vascular Tone

Endothelial synthesis and release of vasoactive mediators are important elements in the regulation of vascular tone. Substances are released by the endothelium in response to both mechanical and humoral stimuli and generally have an immediate effect upon the adjacent vascular smooth muscle tone. However, there may also be endothelium-induced long-term effects from vascular remodeling and smooth muscle hypertrophy. Under physiologic conditions, local vascular pressure and flow are the primary stimuli for endothelial vasoactive substance release. Nitric oxide and prostacyclin are powerful vasodilators released by endothelial cells and both also inhibit platelet aggregation and thrombosis. Continuous nitric oxide production maintains vascular tone in a normally low state. This minute-to-minute regulation of local vascular tone is controlled by type 3 constitutive nitric oxide synthase (cNOS). Constitutive NOS is a rapidly responding endothelial enzyme that catalyses the local conversion of L-arginine into small quantities of nitric oxide in response to endothelial shear stress during normal pulsatile flow. On the other hand, type 2 inducible NOS (iNOS) is a relatively slow responding enzyme that catalyses the production of large amounts of nitric oxide in response to inflammatory cytokines. The widespread generation of large amounts of nitric oxide via iNOS is responsible for the low systemic vascular resistance and hypotension encountered in septic shock (Young, 2004). Endothelin-1 (ET-1) is a potent vasoactive compound released by the endothelium. Its predominant effect is vasoconstriction via smooth muscle ET_A receptors. However, ET-1 can also cause vasodilation through its effect on endothelial ET_B receptors. ET-1 stimulates smooth muscle proliferation and is an important factor in the development of vascular structural changes in systemic and pulmonary hypertension.

COMPONENTS OF THE SYSTEMIC CIRCULATION

The components of the systemic circulation are the arteries, arterioles, capillaries, venules, and veins.

Arteries

The function of the arteries is to transport blood under high pressure to tissues. Therefore, arteries have strong vascular walls and blood flows rapidly through their lumens.

TABLE 45-1.
PHYSIOLOGIC ROLES OF ENDOTHELIAL FUNCTION

Endothelial Function	Example
Regulation of vascular tone	Vasodilator release (nitric oxide, prostacyclin) Vasoconstrictor release (thromboxane A_2, leukotriene, endothelia, angiotensin) converting enzyme
Regulation of coagulation	Procoagulant release Anticoagulant release
Vascular growth regulation (angiogenesis)	Growth factor synthesis and release
Lipid clearance	LDL-receptor expression Lipoprotein lipase synthesis
Inflammatory regulation and defense	Inflammatory mediator synthesis and release
Vascular support matrix elaboration	Synthesis of collagen, laminin, fibronectin proteoglycans, proteases
Regulation of molecular transport	Transport of glucose, amino acid, and albumin

Arterioles

Arterioles are the last small branches of the arterial system, having diameters of <200 μm. Arterioles have strong muscular walls that are capable of dilating or contracting and thus controlling blood flow into the capillaries. Indeed, blood flow to each tissue is controlled almost entirely by resistance to flow in the arterioles. Metarterioles arise at right angles from arterioles and branch several times, forming 10 to 100 capillaries.

Capillaries

Capillaries are the sites for transfer of oxygen and nutrients to tissues and receipt of metabolic byproducts (see Chapter 46).

Venules and Veins

Venules collect blood from capillaries for delivery to veins, which act as conduits for transmitting blood to the right

TABLE 45-2.
PATHOLOGIC PROCESSES ASSOCIATED WITH ENDOTHELIAL DYSFUNCTION

Systemic hypertension
Pulmonary hypertension
Atherosclerosis
Sepsis and inflammation
Multisystem organ failure
Metastatic tumor spread
Thrombotic disorders

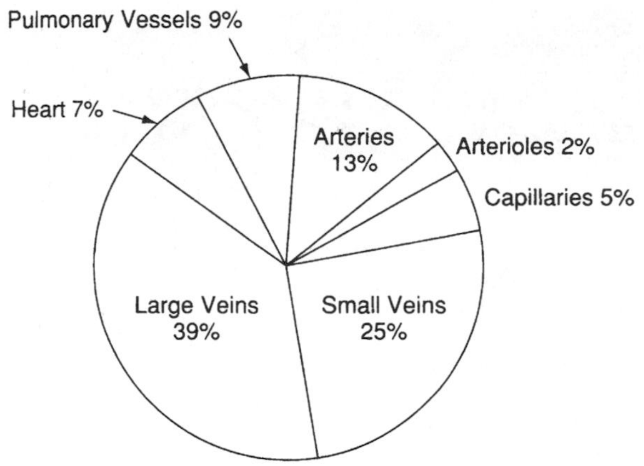

Figure 45-1. Distribution of blood volume in the systemic and pulmonary circulation. (From Guyton AC, Hall JE. *Textbook of medical physiology*, 10th ed. Philadelphia: Saunders, 2000; with permission.)

atrium. Because the pressure in the venous system is low, venous walls are thin. Nevertheless, walls of veins are muscular, which allows these vessels to contract or expand and thus store varying amounts of blood, depending on physiologic needs. As a result, veins serve an important storage function as well as being conduits to return blood to the right atrium. A venous pump mechanism is important for propelling blood forward to the heart.

PHYSICAL CHARACTERISTICS OF THE SYSTEMIC CIRCULATION

The systemic circulation contains about 80% of the blood volume, with the remainder present in the pulmonary circulation and heart (Fig. 45-1) (Guyton and Hall, 2000). Of the blood volume in the systemic circulation, about 64% is in veins and 7% is in the cardiac chambers. The heart ejects blood intermittently into the aorta such that blood pressure in the aorta fluctuates between a systolic level of about 120 mm Hg and a diastolic level of about 80 mm Hg (Table 45-3) (Fig. 45-2) (Guyton and Hall, 2000).

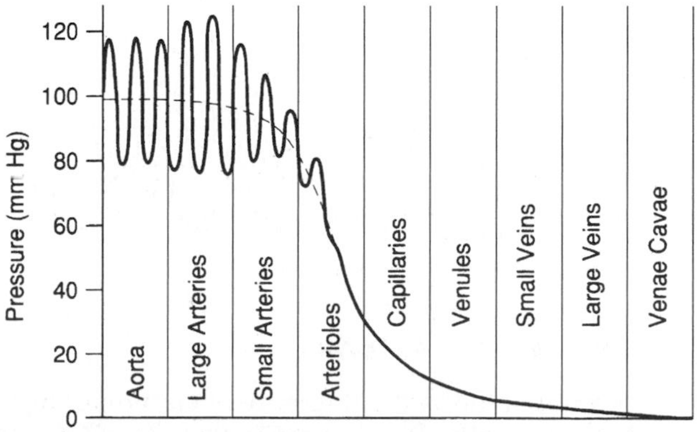

Figure 45-2. Systemic blood pressure decreases as blood travels from the aorta to large veins. (From Guyton AC, Hall JE. *Textbook of medical physiology*, 10th ed. Philadelphia: Saunders, 2000; with permission.)

TABLE 45-3.
NORMAL PRESSURES IN THE SYSTEMIC CIRCULATION

	Mean value (mm Hg)	Range (mm Hg)
Systolic blood pressure*	120	90–140
Diastolic blood pressure*	80	70–90
Mean arterial pressure	92	77–97
Left ventricular end-diastolic pressure	6	0–12
Left atrium		
a wave	10	2–12
v wave	13	6–20
Right atrium		
a wave	6	2–10
c wave	5	2–10
v wave	3	0–8

*Measured in the radial artery.

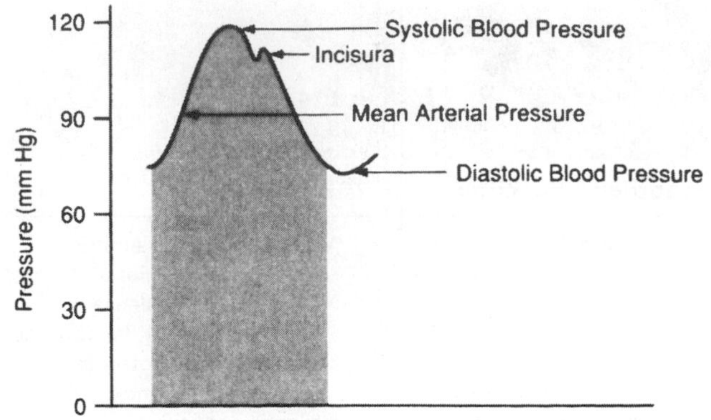

Figure 45-3. Schematic depiction of systemic blood pressure recorded from a large systemic artery. Mean arterial pressure is equal to the area under the blood pressure curve divided by the duration of systole.

Progressive Declines in Systemic Blood Pressure

As blood flows through the systemic circulation, perfusion pressure decreases progressively to nearly 0 mm Hg by the time blood reaches the right atrium (see Fig. 45-2) (Guyton and Hall, 2000). The decrease in systemic blood pressure in each portion of the systemic circulation is directly proportional to the resistance to flow in the vessels. Resistance to blood flow in the aorta is minimal, and mean arterial pressure decreases only 3 to 5 mm Hg as blood travels into arteries as small as 3 mm in diameter. Resistance to blood flow begins to increase rapidly in small arteries, causing the mean arterial pressure to decrease to about 85 mm Hg at the beginning of the arterioles. It is in the arterioles that resistance to blood flow is the highest, accounting for about 50% of the resistance in the entire systemic circulation. As a result, systemic blood pressure decreases to about 30 mm Hg at the point where blood enters the capillaries. At the venous end of the capillaries, the intravascular pressure has decreased to about 10 mm Hg. The decrease in systemic blood pressure from 10 mm Hg to nearly 0 mm Hg as blood traverses veins indicates that these vessels impart far more resistance to blood flow than would be expected for vessels of their large sizes. This resistance to blood flow is caused by compression of the veins by external forces that keep many of them, especially the venae cavae, partially collapsed.

Pulse Pressure in Arteries

Pulse pressure reflects the intermittent ejection of blood into the aorta by the heart (see Table 45-3). The difference between systolic and diastolic blood pressure is the pulse pressure. A typical systemic blood pressure curve recorded from a large artery is characterized by a rapid decline in pressure during ventricular systole followed by a maintained high level of blood pressure for 0.2 to 0.3 s (Fig. 45-3). This plateau is followed by the dicrotic notch (incisura) at the end of systole and a subsequent, more gradual decrease of pressure back to the diastolic level. The dicrotic notch reflects a decrease in the intraventricular pressure and a backflow of blood in the aorta that causes the aortic valve to close.

Factors That Alter Pulse Pressure

The principal factors that alter pulse pressure in the arteries are the left ventricular stroke volume, velocity of blood flow, and compliance of the arterial tree. The larger the stroke volume, the greater the volume of blood that must be accommodated in the arterial vessels with each contraction, resulting in an increased pulse pressure. Pulse pressure also increases when systemic vascular resistance decreases and flow of blood from arteries to veins is accelerated. Indeed, pulse pressure is increased in the presence of patent ductus arteriosus and aortic regurgitation, reflecting rapid runoff of blood into the pulmonary circulation or left ventricle, respectively. In this regard, attempts have been made to predict systemic vascular resistance by the position of the dicrotic notch relative to the diastolic pressure. A controlled study, however, failed to confirm a correlation between the position of the dicrotic notch and the calculated systemic vascular resistance (Fig. 45-4) (Gerber et al., 1987). An increase in heart rate while the cardiac output remains constant causes the stroke volume and pulse pressure to decrease. Pulse pressure is inversely proportional to the compliance (distensibility) of the arterial system. For example, with aging, the distensibility of the arterial walls often decreases (elastic and muscular tissues are replaced by fibrous tissue) and pulse pressure increases.

Transmission of the Pulse Pressure

There is often enhancement of the pulse pressure as the pressure wave is transmitted peripherally (Fig. 45-5) (Guyton and Hall, 2000). Part of this augmentation results

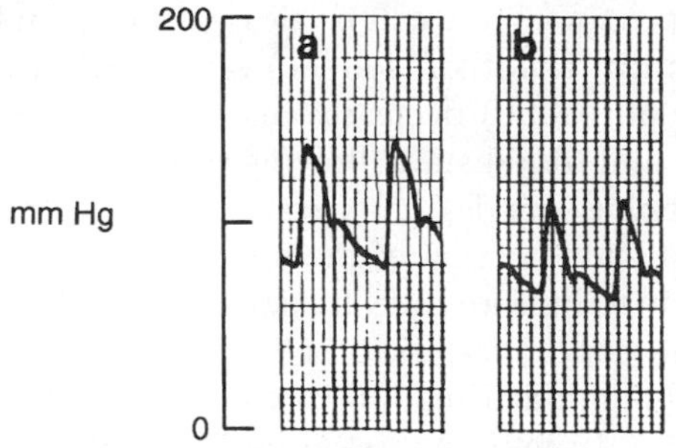

Figure 45-4. Despite a different height of the dicrotic notch (measured from baseline to the peak of the notch), the calculated systemic vascular resistance is similar for tracings a and b. (From Gerber MJ, Hines RL, Barash PG. Arterial waveforms and systemic vascular resistance: is there a correlation? *Anesthesiology* 1987;66:823–825; with permission.)

from the progressive decrease in compliance of the more distal portions of the large arteries. Second, pressure waves are reflected to some extent by the peripheral arteries. Specifically, when a pulsatile pressure wave enters the peripheral arteries and distends them, the pressure on these peripheral arteries causes the pulse wave to begin traveling backward. If the returning pulse wave strikes an oncoming wave, the two summate, causing a much higher pressure than would otherwise occur. These changes in the contour of the pulse wave are most pronounced in young patients, whereas in elderly patients with less compliant arteries, the pulse wave may be transmitted virtually unchanged from the aorta to peripheral arteries.

Augmentation of the peripheral pulse pressure must be identified whenever systemic blood pressure measurements are made in peripheral arteries. For example, systolic pressure in the radial artery is sometimes as much as 20% to 30% higher than that pressure present in the central aorta, and diastolic pressure is often decreased as much as 10% to 15%. Mean arterial pressures are similar regardless of the site of blood pressure measurement in a peripheral artery.

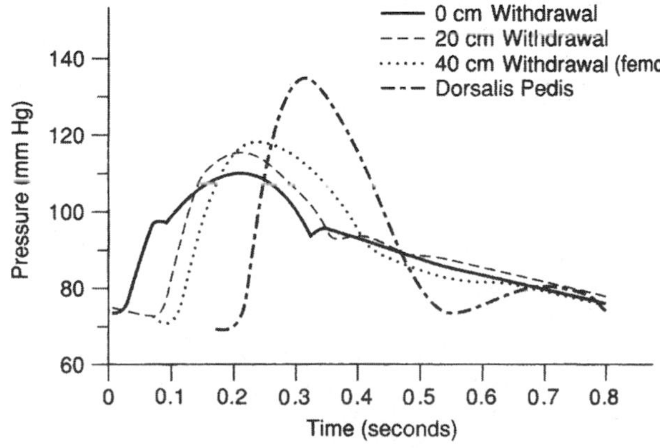

Figure 45-5. There is enhancement of the pulse pressure as the systemic blood pressure is transmitted peripherally. (From Guyton AC, Hall JE. *Textbook of medical physiology*, 10th ed. Philadelphia: Saunders, 2000; with permission.)

Pulse pressure becomes progressively less as blood passes through small arteries and arterioles until it becomes almost absent in capillaries (see Fig. 45-2) (Guyton and Hall, 2000). This reflects the extreme distensibility of small vessels such that the small amount of blood that is caused to flow during a pulsatile pressure wave produces progressively less pressure increase in the more distal vessels. Furthermore, resistance to blood flow in these small vessels is such that flow of blood and, consequently, the transmission of pressure are greatly impeded.

Systemic Blood Pressure Measurement during and after Cardiopulmonary Bypass

Reversal of the usual relationship between aortic and radial artery blood pressures can occur during the late period of hypothermic cardiopulmonary bypass and in the early period after termination of cardiopulmonary bypass (Fig. 45-6) (Pauca et al., 1989; Stern et al., 1985). One mechanism proposed for this unpredictable and transient disparity (usually persists for 10 to 60 minutes after discontinuation of cardiopulmonary bypass) is a high blood flow in the forearm and hand after rewarming on cardiopulmonary bypass, causing an increased pressure drop along the normal resistance pathway provided by the arteries leading to the radial site. Conversely, others describe the appearance of this gradient with initiation of cardiopulmonary bypass, suggesting that the etiology is associated with events such as cross-clamping of the aorta occurring during initiation of cardiopulmonary bypass rather than rewarming or discontinuing cardiopulmonary bypass (Fig. 45-7) (Baba et al., 1997; Rich et al., 1992). Failure to

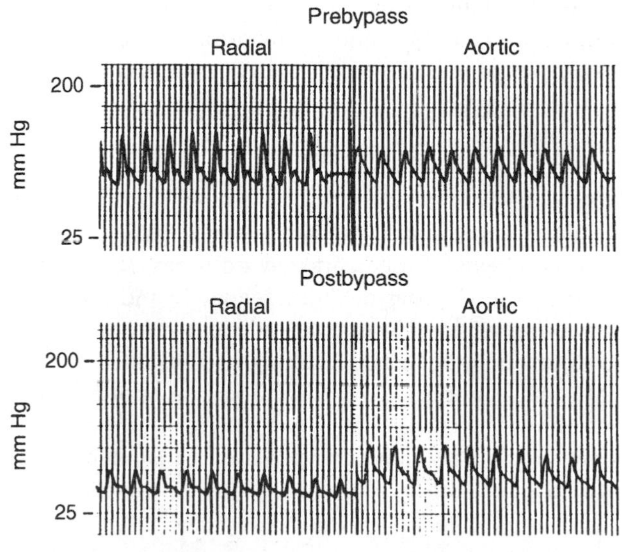

Figure 45-6. There may be a reversal of the usual relationship of simultaneous recordings of radial and aortic blood pressures (Prebypass) in the early period after separation from cardiopulmonary bypass (Postbypass). (From Stern DH, Gerson JI, Allen FB, et al. Can we trust the direct radial artery pressure immediately following cardiopulmonary bypass? *Anesthesiology* 1985;62:557–561; with permission.)

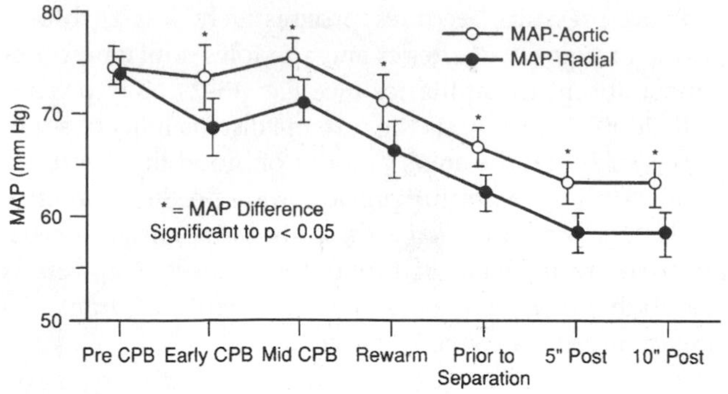

Figure 45-7. Comparison of mean arterial pressure (MAP) as measured from the aorta or radial artery before, during, and after cardiopulmonary bypass (CPB). (From Rich GF, Lubanski RE, McLoughlin TM. Differences between aortic and radial artery pressure associated with cardiopulmonary bypass. *Anesthesiology* 1992;77:63–66; with permission.)

recognize this disparity may lead to an erroneous diagnosis and unnecessary treatment. Systemic blood pressure measured in the brachial artery is more accurate and reliable during the periods surrounding cardiopulmonary bypass, which are most likely to be associated with disparities between the aortic and radial artery blood pressures (Bazaral et al., 1990).

Pulsus Paradoxus

Pulsus paradoxus is an exaggerated decrease in systolic blood pressure (>10 mm Hg) during inspiration in the presence of increased intrapericardial pressures (cardiac tamponade).

Pulsus Alternans

Pulsus alternans is alternating weak and strong cardiac contractions causing a similar alteration in the strength of the peripheral pulse. Digitalis toxicity and varying degrees of atrioventricular heart block are commonly associated with pulsus alternans.

Pulse Deficit

In the presence of atrial fibrillation or ectopic ventricular beats, two beats of the heart may occur so close together that the ventricle does not fill adequately and the second cardiac contraction ejects an insufficient volume of blood to create a peripheral pulse. In this circumstance, a second heart beat is audible with a stethoscope applied on the chest directly over the heart, but a corresponding pulsation in the radial artery cannot be palpated. This phenomenon is called a *pulse deficit.*

Measurement of Blood Pressure by Auscultation

Measurement of blood pressure by auscultation uses the principle that blood flow in large arteries is laminar and not audible. If blood flow is arrested by an inflated cuff and the pressure in the cuff is released slowly, audible tapping sounds (Korotkoff sounds) can be heard when the pressure of the cuff decreases just below systolic blood pressure and blood starts flowing in the brachial artery. These tapping sounds occur because flow velocity through the constricted portion of the blood vessel is increased, resulting in turbulence and vibrations that are heard through the stethoscope. Diastolic blood pressure correlates with the onset of muffled auscultatory sounds. The auscultatory method for determining systolic and diastolic blood pressure usually gives values within 10% of those determined by direct measurement from the arteries.

Right Atrial Pressure

Right atrial pressure is regulated by a balance between venous return and the ability of the right ventricle to eject blood. Normal right atrial pressure is about 5 mm Hg, with a lower limit of about −5 mm Hg, which corresponds to the pressure in the pericardial and intrapleural spaces that surround the heart. Right atrial pressure approaches these low values when right ventricular contractility is increased or venous return to the heart is decreased by hemorrhage. Poor right ventricular contractility or any event that increases venous return (hypervolemia, venoconstriction) tends to increase right atrial pressure. Pressure in the right atrium is commonly designated the *central venous pressure.*

Jugular Venous Pressure

Jugular venous pressure, which mirrors the central venous pressure, may be monitored in the perioperative period to provide information about intravascular volume and ventricular function. The normal jugular venous pressure reflects phasic changes in the right atrium and consists of three positive waves and three negative troughs (Fig. 45-8) (Cook et al., 1996). Abnormalities of these venous waveforms may be useful in the diagnosis of various cardiac conditions (Table 45-4) (Cook et al., 1996).

Peripheral Venous Pressure

Large veins offer little resistance to blood flow when they are distended. Most large veins, however, are compressed at multiple extrathoracic sites. For example, pressure in the

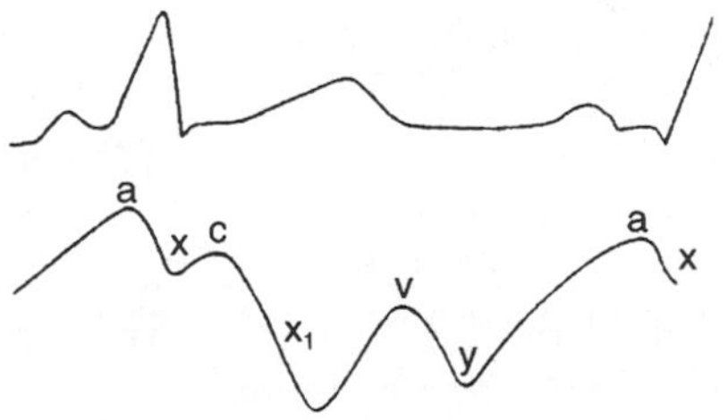

Figure 45-8. Simultaneous recording of the electrocardiogram (*top tracing*) and jugular venous pressure waves (*bottom tracing*). (From Cook DJ, Simel DL. Does this patient have abnormal venous pressure? *JAMA* 1996;275:630–634; with permission.)

TABLE 45-4.
ABNORMALITIES OF JUGULAR VENOUS PRESSURE WAVEFORMS

Waveform	Cardiac abnormality
Absent a wave	Atrial fibrillation
	Sinus tachycardia
Flutter waves	Atrial flutter
Prominent a waves	First-degree atrioventricular heart block
Large a wave	Tricuspid stenosis
	Pulmonary hypertension
	Pulmonic stenosis
	Right atrial myxoma
Cannon a waves	Atrioventricular dissociation
	Ventricular tachycardia
Absent x wave descent	Tricuspid regurgitation
Large cv waves	Tricuspid regurgitation
	Constrictive pericarditis
Slow y wave descent	Tricuspid stenosis
	Right atrial myxoma
Rapid y wave descent	Tricuspid regurgitation
	Atrial septal defect
	Constrictive pericarditis
Absent y wave descent	Cardiac tamponade

Source: Adapted from Cook DJ, Simel DL. Does this patient have abnormal central venous pressure? *JAMA* 1996;275:630–634.

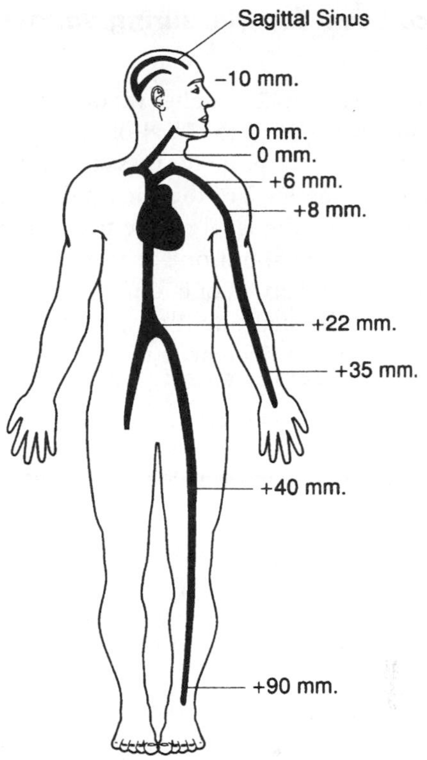

Figure 45-9. Effect of hydrostatic pressure on venous pressures throughout the body. (From Guyton AC, Hall JE. *Textbook of medical physiology*, 10th ed. Philadelphia: Saunders, 2000; with permission.)

external jugular vein is often so low that atmospheric pressure on the outside of the neck causes it to collapse. Veins coursing through the abdomen are compressed by intraabdominal pressure, which may increase 15 to 20 mm Hg as a result of pregnancy or ascites. When this occurs, pressure in leg veins must increase above abdominal pressure. It is important to recognize that veins inside the thorax are not collapsed because of the distending effect of negative intrathoracic pressure.

Effect of Hydrostatic Pressure

Pressure in veins below the heart is increased and that in veins above the heart is decreased by the effect of gravity (Fig. 45-9) (Guyton and Hall, 2000). As a guideline, pressure changes 0.77 mm Hg for every centimeter the vessel is above or below the heart. For example, in a standing human, pressure in the veins of the feet is 90 mm Hg because of the distance from the heart to the feet. Conversely, veins above the heart tend to collapse, with the exception being veins inside the skull, where they are held open by surrounding bone. As a result, negative pressure can exist in the dural sinuses and air can be entrained immediately if these sinuses are entered during surgery.

Hydrostatic pressure affects peripheral pressure in arteries and capillaries as well as veins. For example, a standing human who has a systemic blood pressure of 100 mm Hg at the level of the heart has a blood pressure of about 190 mm Hg in the feet.

Venous Valves and the Pump Mechanism

Valves in veins are arranged so that the direction of blood flow can be only toward the heart. In a standing human, movement of the legs compresses skeletal muscles and veins so blood is directed toward the heart. This venous pump or skeletal muscle pump is usually sufficient to maintain venous pressure below 25 mm Hg in a walking human. If an individual stands immobile, the venous pump does not function. As a result, pressures in the veins and capillaries of the legs can increase rapidly, resulting in leakage of fluid from the intravascular space. Indeed, as much as 15% of the blood volume can be lost from the intravascular space in the first 15 minutes of quiet standing.

Varicose Veins

Valves of the venous system can be destroyed when the veins are chronically distended by increased venous pressure as occurs during pregnancy or in an individual who stands most of the day. The end result is varicose veins characterized by bulbous protrusions of the veins beneath the skin of the legs. Venous and capillary pressures remain increased because of the incompetent venous pump, and this causes constant edema in the legs of these individuals. Edema interferes with diffusion of nutrients from the capillaries to tissues, so there is often skeletal muscle discomfort and the skin may ulcerate.

Reference Level for Measuring Venous Pressure

Hydrostatic pressure does not alter venous or arterial pressures that are measured at the level of the tricuspid valve. As a result, the reference point for pressure measurement is considered to be the level of the tricuspid valve. External reference points for the level of the tricuspid valve in a supine individual are about one-third the distance from the anterior chest and about one-fourth the distance above the lower end of the sternum. A precise hydrostatic point to which pressures are referenced is essential for accurate interpretation of venous pressure measurements. For example, each centimeter below the hydrostatic point adds 0.77 mm Hg to the measured pressure, whereas 0.77 mm Hg is subtracted for each centimeter above this point. The potential error introduced by measuring pressures above or below the tricuspid valve is greatest with venous pressures that are normally low. For example, an error introduced by 5 cm of hydrostatic pressure has a much greater influence on the clinical interpretation of central venous pressure than arterial pressure.

The reason for lack of hydrostatic effects at the tricuspid valve is the ability of the right ventricle to act as a regulator of pressure at this site. For example, if the pressure at the tricuspid valve increases, the right ventricle fills to a greater extent, thereby decreasing the pressure at the tricuspid valve toward normal. Conversely, if the pressure decreases at the tricuspid valve, the right ventricle does not fill optimally and blood pools in the veins until pressure at the tricuspid valve again increases to a normal value.

Measurement of right atrial pressure is accomplished by using a transducer or a fluid-filled manometer referenced to the level of the tricuspid valve. A venous pressure measurement in mm Hg can be converted to cm H_2O by multiplying the pressure by 1.36, which adjusts for the density of mercury relative to water (10 mm Hg equals 13.6 cm H_2O). Conversely, dividing the central venous pressure measurement in cm H_2O by 1.36 converts this value to an equivalent pressure in mm Hg.

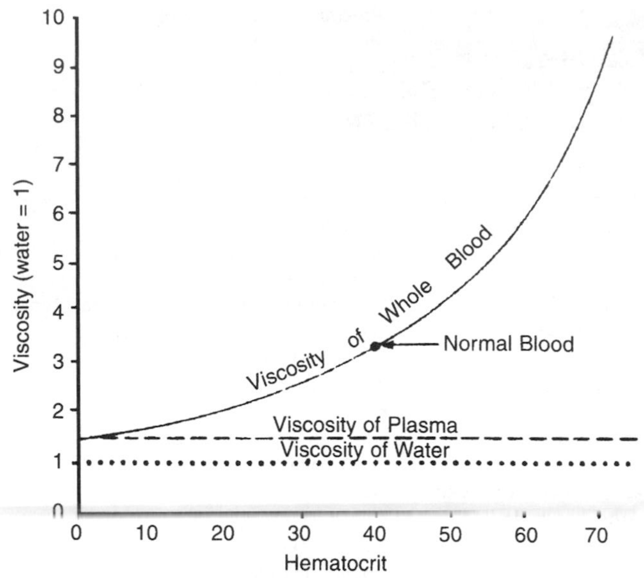

Figure 45-10. Hematocrit greatly influences the viscosity of blood. (From Guyton AC, Hall JE. *Textbook of medical physiology*, 10th ed. Philadelphia: Saunders, 2000; with permission.)

Viscosity exerts fewer effects on blood flow in capillaries than in larger vessels. This most likely reflects alignment of erythrocytes as they pass through small blood vessels rather than the random arrangement characteristic of flow through larger vessels. This alignment of erythrocytes, which greatly decreases the viscous resistance that occurs normally between cells, is largely offset by a decreased velocity of flow that greatly increases viscosity. The net effect may be that viscous effects in small blood vessels are similar to those that occur in large blood vessels.

Plasma is considered extracellular fluid that is identical to interstitial fluid except for the greater concentrations of proteins (albumin, globulin, fibrinogen) in plasma. These greater concentrations reflect the inability of plasma proteins to pass easily through capillaries into the interstitial spaces. Indeed, the primary function of albumin is to create colloid osmotic pressure, which prevents fluid from leaving the capillaries.

PHYSICAL CHARACTERISTICS OF BLOOD

Blood is a viscous fluid composed of cells and plasma. More than 99% of the cells in plasma are erythrocytes. As a result, leukocytes exert a minimal influence on the physical characteristics of blood. The percentage of blood comprising erythrocytes is the hematocrit, which to a large extent determines the viscosity of blood (Fig. 45-10) (Guyton and Hall, 2000). When the hematocrit increases to 60% to 70%, viscosity of blood is increased about tenfold compared with water, and flow through blood vessels is greatly decreased. Plasma protein concentrations influence blood viscosity only minimally.

DETERMINANTS OF TISSUE BLOOD FLOW

Tissue blood flow is directly proportional to the pressure difference between two points (not absolute pressure) and inversely proportional to resistance to flow through the vessel. This relationship between flow, pressure, and resistance can be expressed mathematically as a variant of Ohm's law, in which blood flow (amperes) is directly proportional to the pressure drop across two points (voltage) and inversely proportional to resistance (Fig. 45-11). Rearrangement of this formula emphasizes that pressure is directly proportional to flow times resistance. Likewise,

$$\text{Blood Flow (Q)} = \frac{\text{Pressure Difference Between Two Points (P)}}{\text{Resistance to Flow (R)}}$$

$$\Delta P = Q \times R$$

$$R = \Delta P / Q$$

Figure 45-11. The relationship between blood flow, pressure, and resistance to flow can be expressed as a variant of Ohm's law.

resistance is directly proportional to pressure and inversely proportional to flow. Furthermore, resistance is directly proportional to viscosity of blood and the length of the vessel and inversely proportional to the fourth power of the radius of the vessel (doubling the radius of the vessel or intravenous catheter size decreases resistance to flow 16-fold [Poiseuille's law]).

It is important to understand that resistance to blood flow cannot be measured but rather is a calculated value based on measurement of driving pressures and the cardiac output. For example, systemic vascular resistance is calculated as the difference between mean arterial pressure and right atrial pressure divided by cardiac output. Pulmonary vascular resistance is calculated as the difference between mean pulmonary artery pressure and left atrial pressure divided by the cardiac output. Resistance is expressed in dynes/s/cm^{-5} if the calculated value is multiplied by 80. Conductance is the reciprocal of resistance and is a measure of the amount of blood flow that can pass through a blood vessel in a given time for a given pressure gradient.

Vascular Distensibility

Blood vessels are distendible such that increases in systemic blood pressure cause the vascular diameter to increase, which in turn decreases resistance to blood flow. Conversely, decreases in intravascular pressure increase the resistance to blood flow. The ability of blood vessels to distend as intravascular pressure increases varies greatly in different parts of the circulation. Anatomically, the walls of arteries are stronger than those of veins. As a result, veins are 6 to 10 times as distendible as arteries. Systemic blood pressure can eventually decrease to a level where intravascular pressure is no longer capable of keeping the vessel open. This pressure averages 20 mm Hg and is defined as the *critical closing pressure*. When the heart is abruptly stopped, the pressure in the entire circulatory system (mean circulatory pressure) equilibrates at about 7 mm Hg.

Vascular Compliance

Vascular compliance is defined as the increase in volume (capacitance) of a vessel produced by an increase in intravascular pressure. The compliance of the entire circulatory system is estimated to be 100 mL for each 1 mm Hg increase in intravascular pressure (Guyton and Hall, 2000). The compliance of veins is much greater than that of arteries. For example, the volume of blood normally present in all veins is about 2,500 mL, whereas the arterial system contains only about 750 mL of blood when the mean arterial pressure is 100 mm Hg. Sympathetic nervous system activity can greatly alter the distribution of blood volume. Enhancement of sympathetic nervous system activity to the blood vessels, especially the veins, decreases the dimensions to the circulatory system, and the circulation continues to function almost normally even when as much as 25% of the total blood volume has been lost. *Vasoconstriction* or *vasodilation* refers to resistance changes in arterioles, whereas changes in the caliber of veins is described as *venoconstriction* or *venodilation*.

CONTROL OF TISSUE BLOOD FLOW

Control of blood flow to different tissues includes (a) local mechanisms, (b) autonomic nervous system responses, and (c) release of hormones. Total tissue blood flow or cardiac output is about 5 L/minute, with large amounts being delivered to the heart, brain, liver, and kidneys (Table 45-5) (Guyton and Hall, 2000). A high cerebral blood flow limits excessive accumulation of hydrogen ions and carbon dioxide in the brain. Hepatic blood flow parallels the high level of metabolic activity in this organ. In contrast, skeletal muscles represent 35% to 40% of body mass but receive only about 15% of the total cardiac output, reflecting the low metabolic rate of inactive skeletal muscles.

Local Control of Blood Flow

Local control of blood flow is most often based on the need for delivery of oxygen or other nutrients such as glucose or

TABLE 45-5.
TISSUE BLOOD FLOW

	Approximate Blood Flow		Cardiac Output
	(mL/minute)	(mL/100 g/minute)	(% of Total)
Brain	750	50	15
Liver	1,450	100	29
Portal vein	1,100		
Hepatic artery	350		
Kidneys	1,000	320	20
Heart	225	75	5
Skeletal muscles (at rest)	750	4	15
Skin	400	3	8
Other tissues	425	2	8
Total	5,000		100

Source: Adapted from Guyton AC, Hall JE. *Textbook of medical physiology*, 10th ed. Philadelphia: Saunders, 2000.

fatty acids to the tissues. The response to decreased oxygen delivery may reflect the local release of vasodilatory substances (adenosine, lactic acid, carbon dioxide, potassium ions), which results in increased tissue blood flow and oxygen delivery.

Autoregulation of Blood Flow

Autoregulation is a local mechanism of control of blood flow in which a specific tissue is able to maintain a relatively constant blood flow over a wide range of mean arterial pressures. Conceptually, when the mean arterial pressure increases, the associated increase in tissue blood flow delivers too many nutrients or flushes out vasodilatory substances, either of which causes the blood vessels to constrict. As a result, increased perfusion pressure does not increase blood flow because of the modifying effect of vasoconstriction. Conversely, decreases in mean arterial pressure result in decreased delivery of nutrients to tissues such that vasodilation occurs to maintain an unchanged tissue blood flow despite a decreased perfusion pressure. Autoregulatory responses to sudden changes in mean arterial pressure occur within 60 to 120 seconds. The ability of autoregulation to return local tissue blood flow to normal is incomplete.

Long-Term Control of Blood Flow

Long-term regulatory mechanisms that return local tissue blood flow to normal involve a change in vascularity of tissues. For example, sustained increases in mean arterial pressure to specific tissues, as occurs with coarctation of the aorta, is accompanied by a decrease in the size and number of blood vessels. Likewise, if metabolism in a tissue becomes chronically increased, vascularity increases, or, if metabolism is decreased, vascularity decreases. Indeed, inadequate delivery of oxygen to a tissue is the stimulus for the development of collateral vessels. Neonates exposed to increased concentrations of oxygen may manifest cessation of new vascular growth in the retina. Subsequent removal of the neonate from a high-oxygen environment causes an overgrowth of new vessels to offset the abrupt decrease in availability of oxygen. There may be so much overgrowth that the new vessels cause blindness (retrolental fibroplasia).

Autonomic Nervous System Control of Blood Flow

Autonomic nervous system control of blood flow is characterized by a rapid response time (within 1 second) and an ability to regulate blood flow to certain tissues at the expense of other tissues. The sympathetic nervous system is the most important component of the autonomic nervous system in the regulation of blood flow. Release of norepinephrine stimulates alpha-adrenergic receptors to produce vasoconstriction characteristic of sympathetic nervous system stimulation. Constriction of small arteries influences resistance to blood flow through tissues, whereas venoconstriction alters vascular capacitance and distribution of blood in the peripheral circulation. Sympathetic nervous system innervation is prominent in the kidneys and skin and minimal in the cerebral circulation.

Vasomotor Center

The vasomotor center, which is located in the pons and medulla, transmits sympathetic nervous system impulses through the spinal cord to all blood vessels. Evidence for a continuous, sustained state of partial vasoconstriction (vasomotor tone) is the abrupt decrease in systemic blood pressure that occurs when sympathetic nervous system innervation to the vasculature is abruptly interrupted, as by traumatic spinal cord transection or regional anesthesia. Activity of the vasomotor center can be influenced by impulses from a number of sites, including diffuse areas of the reticular activating system, hypothalamus, and cerebral cortex. Sympathetic nervous system impulses are transmitted to the adrenal medulla at the same time they are transmitted to the peripheral vasculature. These impulses stimulate the adrenal medulla to secrete epinephrine and norepinephrine into the circulation, where they act directly on adrenergic receptors in the walls of vascular smooth muscle.

The medial and lower portions of the vasomotor center do not participate in transmission of vasoconstrictor impulses but rather function as an inhibitor of sympathetic nervous system activity, which allows blood vessels to dilate. Conceptually, this portion of the vasomotor center is functioning as the parasympathetic nervous system.

Mass Reflex

The mass reflex is characterized by stimulation of all portions of the vasomotor center, resulting in generalized vasoconstriction and an increase in cardiac output in an attempt to maintain tissue blood flow. The alarm reaction resembles the mass reflex, but associated skeletal muscle vasodilation and psychic excitement are intended to prepare the individual to confront a life-threatening situation.

Syncope

Emotional fainting (vasovagal syncope) may reflect profound skeletal muscle vasodilation such that systemic blood pressure decreases abruptly and syncope occurs. Associated vagal stimulation results in bradycardia. This phenomenon may occur in patients who have an intense fear of needles, resulting in syncope during placement of an intravenous catheter.

Hormone Control of Blood Flow

Vasoconstrictor hormones that may influence local tissue blood flow include epinephrine, norepinephrine, angiotensin, and arginine vasopressin (formerly known as antidiuretic hormone). Bradykinin, serotonin, histamine, prostaglandins, and low circulating concentrations of epinephrine are vasodilating substances. Local chemical factors, such as accumulation of hydrogen ions, potassium ions, and carbon dioxide, relax vascular smooth muscle and cause vasodilation. Carbon dioxide also has an indirect vasoconstrictor effect because it stimulates the outflow of sympathetic nervous system impulses from the vasomotor center.

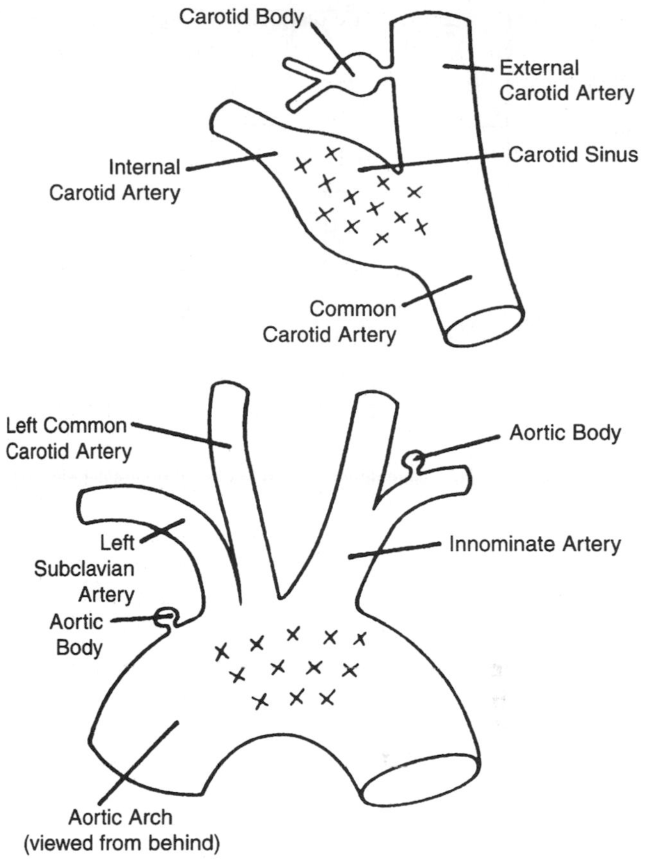

Figure 45-12. Baroreceptors are represented by the carotid sinus and receptors in the arch of the aorta. Chemoreceptors are located in the carotid and aortic bodies. (From Ganong WF. *Review of medical physiology*, 21st ed. New York, Lange Medical Books/McGraw Hill, 2003; with permission.)

REGULATION OF SYSTEMIC BLOOD PRESSURE

Systemic blood pressure is maintained over a narrow range by reciprocal changes in cardiac output and systemic vascular resistance. The autonomic nervous system and baroreceptors play a key role in moment-to-moment regulation of systemic blood pressure. Long-term regulation of blood pressure depends on control of fluid balance by the kidneys, adrenal cortex, and central nervous system to maintain a constant blood volume.

Systolic, diastolic, and mean arterial pressure tend to increase progressively with age. Because a greater portion of the cardiac cycle is nearer the diastolic blood pressure, it follows that mean arterial pressure is not the arithmetic average of the systolic and diastolic blood pressures. Mean arterial blood pressure is the most important determinant of tissue blood flow because it is the average, tending to drive blood through the systemic circulation.

Rapid-Acting Mechanisms for the Regulation of Systemic Blood Pressure

Rapid-acting mechanisms for regulation of systemic blood pressure involve nervous system responses as reflected by the (a) baroreceptor reflexes, (b) chemoreceptor reflexes, (c) atrial reflexes, and (d) central nervous system ischemic reflex. These reflex mechanisms respond almost immediately to changes in systemic blood pressure. Furthermore, within about 30 minutes, these nervous system reflex responses are further supplemented by activation of hormonal mechanisms and shift of fluid into the circulation to readjust the blood volume. These short term mechanisms can return systemic blood pressure toward but never entirely back to normal. Indeed, the impact of many of the rapid-acting regulatory mechanisms, such as the baroreceptor reflexes, diminish with time as these mechanisms adapt to the new level of systemic blood pressure.

Baroreceptor Reflexes

Baroreceptors are nerve endings in the walls of large arteries in the neck and thorax, especially in the internal carotid arteries just above the carotid bifurcation and in the arch of the aorta (Fig. 45-12) (Ganong, 2003). These nerve endings respond rapidly to changes in systemic blood pressure and are crucial for maintaining normal blood pressure when an individual changes from the supine to standing position. An increase in mean arterial pressure produces stretch of baroreceptor nerve endings, and increased numbers of nerve impulses are transmitted to the depressor portion of the vasomotor center, leading to a relative decrease in the central nervous system outflow of sympathetic nervous system (vasoconstrictive) impulses (Fig. 45-13) (Ganong, 2003). The net effects are vasodilation throughout the peripheral circulation, decreased heart rate, and decreased myocardial contractility, which all act to decrease systemic blood pressure back toward normal. Conversely, decreases in systemic blood pressure reflexively produce changes likely to increase blood pressure. Baroreceptors adapt in 1 to 3 days to whatever systemic blood pressure level they are exposed to, emphasizing that these reflexes are probably of no importance in long-term regulation of blood pressure. Volatile anesthetics, particularly halothane, inhibit the heart rate response portion of the baroreceptor reflex that occurs in response to changes in systemic blood pressure (see Chapter 2).

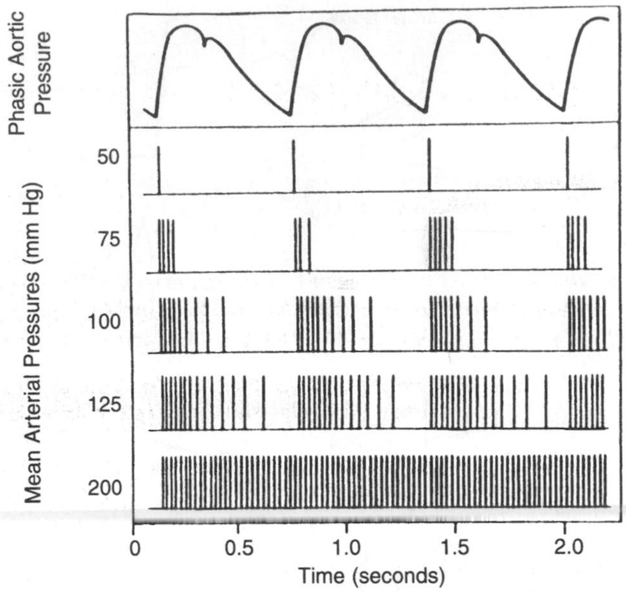

Figure 45-13. Discharges (*vertical lines*) in a single afferent nerve fiber from the carotid sinus at various arterial pressures, plotted against changes in aortic pressure with time. (From Ganong WF. *Review of medical physiology*, 21st ed. New York, Lange Medical Books/McGraw Hill, 2003; with permission.)

Chemoreceptor Reflexes

Chemoreceptors are chemosensitive cells located in the carotid bodies and aortic body (see Fig. 45-12) (Ganong, 2003). Each carotid or aortic body is supplied with an abundant blood flow through a nutrient artery so that the chemoreceptors are always exposed to oxygenated blood. Whenever the systemic blood pressure, and thus the blood flow, decrease below a critical level, chemoreceptors are stimulated by decreased availability of oxygen and also because of excess carbon dioxide and hydrogen ions that are not removed by the sluggish blood flow. Impulses from the chemoreceptors are transmitted to the vasomotor center, which results in reflex changes that tend to increase systemic blood pressure back toward the normal level. Nevertheless, chemoreceptors do not respond strongly until systemic blood pressure decreases below 80 mm Hg. Instead, chemoreceptors are more important in stimulating breathing when the PaO_2 decreases below 60 mm Hg (ventilatory response to arterial hypoxemia). The ventilatory response to arterial hypoxemia is inhibited by subanesthetic concentrations of most of the volatile anesthetics (0.1 MAC) as well as injected drugs such as barbiturates and opioids (see Chapters 2 to 4).

Atrial Reflexes

The atria contain low-pressure atrial stretch receptors similar to baroreceptors in large arteries. Stretching of the atria evokes reflex vasodilation and decreases the systemic blood pressure back toward the normal level. An increase in atrial pressure also causes an increase in heart rate due to a direct effect of the increased atrial volume on stretch of the sinoatrial node, as well as the Bainbridge reflex. The increase in heart rate evoked by stretching of the atria prevents accumulation of blood in the atria, veins, or pulmonary circulation.

Central Nervous System Ischemic Reflex

The central nervous system ischemic reflex response occurs when blood flow to the medullary vasomotor center is decreased to the extent that ischemia of this vital center occurs. As a result of this ischemia, there is an intense outpouring of sympathetic nervous system activity, resulting in profound increases in systemic blood pressure. It is believed that this reflex response is caused by failure of slowly flowing blood to remove carbon dioxide from the vasomotor center. The central nervous system reflex response does not become highly active until mean arterial pressure decreases to <50 mm Hg and reaches its greatest degree of stimulation at systemic blood pressures of 15 to 20 mm Hg. This reflex response is not useful for regulation of normal blood pressure but rather acts as an emergency control system to prevent further decreases in systemic blood pressure when cerebral blood flow is dangerously decreased.

Cushing Reflex

The Cushing reflex is a special type of central nervous system ischemic reflex response that results from increased intracranial pressure. When intracranial pressure increases to equal arterial pressure, the Cushing reflex acts to increase systemic blood pressure above intracranial pressure.

Respiratory Variations in Systemic Blood Pressure

Systemic blood pressure usually increases and decreases 4 to 6 mm Hg in a wavelike manner during quiet spontaneous breathing. Typically, systemic blood pressure is increased during end-inspiration and the beginning of exhalation and decreased during the remainder of the breathing cycle. Positive pressure ventilation of the lungs produces a different sequence because the initial positive airway pressure pushes more blood toward the left ventricle followed by impaired venous return. As a result, systemic blood pressure becomes maximal during the early phases of the mechanically produced inspiration.

Systemic Blood Pressure Vasomotor Waves

Cyclic increases and decreases in systemic blood pressure lasting 7 to 10 s are referred to as *vasomotor* or *Traube-Hering waves*. The presumed cause of vasomotor waves is oscillation in the reflex activity of baroreceptors. For example, increased systemic blood pressure stimulates baroreceptors, which then inhibit the sympathetic nervous system, causing a decrease in systemic blood pressure. Decreased systemic blood pressure decreases baroreceptor activity and allows the vasomotor center to become active once again, increasing the systemic blood pressure to a higher value.

Moderately Rapid-Acting Mechanisms for the Regulation of Systemic Blood Pressure

There are at least three hormonal mechanisms that provide either rapid or moderately rapid control of systemic blood pressure. These hormonal mechanisms are (a) catecholamine-induced vasoconstriction, (b) renin-angiotensin–induced vasoconstriction, and (c) vasoconstriction induced by arginine vasopressin, all of which increase systemic blood pressure by increasing systemic vascular resistance. Circulating catecholamines may even reach parts of the circulation that are devoid of sympathetic nervous system innervation, such as metarterioles. Renin-angiotensin-induced vasoconstriction manifests to a greater degree on arterioles than veins and requires about 20 minutes to become fully active.

In addition to hormonal mechanisms, there are two intrinsic mechanisms (capillary fluid shift and stress-relaxation of blood vessels), which begin to react within minutes of changes in systemic blood pressure. For example, changes in systemic blood pressure produce corresponding changes in capillary pressure, thus allowing fluid to enter or leave the capillaries to maintain a constant blood volume. Stress-relaxation is the gradual change in blood vessel size to adapt to changes in systemic blood pressure and the amount of blood that is available. The stress-relaxation mechanism has definite limitations such that increases in blood volume greater than about 30% or decreases of more than about 15% cannot be corrected by this mechanism alone.

Long-Term Mechanisms for the Regulation of Systemic Blood Pressure

Long-term mechanisms for the regulation of systemic blood pressure, unlike the short-term regulatory mechanisms, have a delayed onset but do not adapt, providing a sustained regulatory effect on systemic blood pressure. The renal-body fluid system plays a predominant role in long-term control of systemic blood pressure because it controls both the cardiac output and systemic vascular resistance. This crucial role is supplemented by accessory mechanisms, including the renin-angiotensin system, aldosterone, and arginine vasopressin.

Renal-Body Fluid System

Increased systemic blood pressure, as provoked by modest increases in blood volume, results in sodium ion and water excretion by the kidneys. The resultant decrease in blood volume leads to decreases in cardiac output and systemic blood pressure. After several weeks, the cardiac output returns toward normal, and systemic vascular resistance decreases to maintain the lower but more acceptable blood pressure. Conversely, a decrease in systemic blood pressure stimulates the kidneys to retain fluid. A special feature of this regulatory mechanism is its ability to return systemic blood pressure completely back to normal values. This contrasts with rapid-acting to moderately rapid-acting mechanisms, which cannot return systemic blood pressure entirely back to normal.

Renin-Angiotensin System

Aldosterone secretion that results from the action of angiotensin II on the adrenal cortex exerts a long-term effect on systemic blood pressure by stimulating the kidneys to retain sodium and water. The resulting increase in extracellular fluid volume causes cardiac output, and subsequently systemic blood pressure, to increase.

REGULATION OF CARDIAC OUTPUT AND VENOUS RETURN

Cardiac output is the amount of blood pumped by the left ventricle into the aorta each minute (product of stroke volume and heart rate), and venous return is the amount of blood flowing from the veins into the right atrium each minute. Because the circulation is a closed circuit, the cardiac output must equal venous return. Cardiac output for the average person weighing 70 kg and with a body surface area of 1.7 m^2 is about 5 L/minute. This value is about 10% less in women.

Determinants of Cardiac Output

Venous return is more important than myocardial contractility in determining cardiac output. In essence, the metabolic requirements in tissues control cardiac output through alterations in resistance to tissue blood flow. For example, increased local metabolic needs lead to regional vasodilation, with a resulting increase in tissue blood flow and thus venous return. Cardiac output is increased by an amount equivalent to the venous return.

Any factor that interferes with venous return can lead to decreased cardiac output. Hemorrhage decreases blood volume such that venous return decreases and cardiac output decreases. Acute venodilation, such as that produced by spinal anesthesia and accompanying sympathetic nervous system blockade, can so increase the capacitance of peripheral vessels that venous return is reduced and cardiac output declines. Indeed, the definitive therapy for hypotension resulting from spinal anesthesia is appropriate positioning of the patient and intravenous infusion of fluids to improve venous return. Positive-pressure ventilation of the lungs, particularly in the presence of a decreased blood volume, causes a decrease in venous return and cardiac output.

Factors that increase cardiac output are associated with decreases in systemic vascular resistance. For example, anemia decreases the viscosity of blood, leading to a decrease in systemic vascular resistance and increase in venous return. An increased blood volume increases cardiac output by increasing the gradient for flow to the right atrium and by distending blood vessels, which decreases resistance to blood flow. Increased cardiac output caused by an increased blood volume lasts only 20 to 40 minutes because increased capillary pressures causes fluid to enter tissues, thereby returning blood volume to normal. Furthermore, increased pressure in veins caused by the increased blood volume causes the veins to distend (stress-relaxation). Cardiac output increases during exercise, in hyperthyroidism, and in the presence of arteriovenous shunts associated with hemodialysis, reflecting decreases in systemic vascular resistance.

Sympathetic nervous system stimulation increases myocardial contractility and heart rate to increase cardiac output beyond that possible from venous return alone. Maximal stimulation by the sympathetic nervous system can double cardiac output. Nevertheless, this sympathetic nervous system-induced increase of cardiac output is only transient, despite sustained increases in nervous system activity. A reason for this transient effect is autoregulation of tissue blood flow, which manifests as vasoconstriction to decrease venous return and thus decrease cardiac output back toward normal. In addition, increased systemic blood pressure associated with increases in the cardiac output causes fluid to leave the capillaries, thereby decreasing blood volume, venous return, and cardiac output.

Heart muscle is sensitive to calcium and a number of hormones and drugs that increase myocardial contractility at a constant preload and heart rate. Positive inotropic drugs increase myocardial contractility for a given preload whereas negative inotropic interventions (volatile anesthetics) decrease myocardial contractility at a constant preload. Typically, inotropic interventions evoke responses through increases in myoplasmic calcium concentrations and less often by increasing the sensitivity of the contractile components to calcium. It is difficult to separate changes in myocardial contractility from changes in preload. Regardless of the mechanism for increased myocardial contractility, the effects of positive inotropic interventions are additive to the effects of increasing the preload.

Ventricular Function Curves

Ventricular function curves (Frank-Starling curves) depict the cardiac output at different atrial (ventricular end-diastolic) filling pressures (Fig. 45-14). Clinically, ventricular function curves are used to estimate myocardial contractility. Improved cardiac function (sympathetic nervous system stimulation) is characterized by a shift of the cardiac output curve to the left of the normal curve (greater cardiac output for a given filling pressure), whereas a shift of the curve to the right of normal (myocardial infarction, valvular heart disease) reflects decreased cardiac function. In this regard, in patients with coronary artery disease, the appearance of a new wall motion abnormality as observed by transesophageal echocardiography is most likely due to acute myocardial ischemia or infarction. Even with a normal ventricular function curve, a point is reached where further stretching of the cardiac muscle results in a decrease in cardiac output.

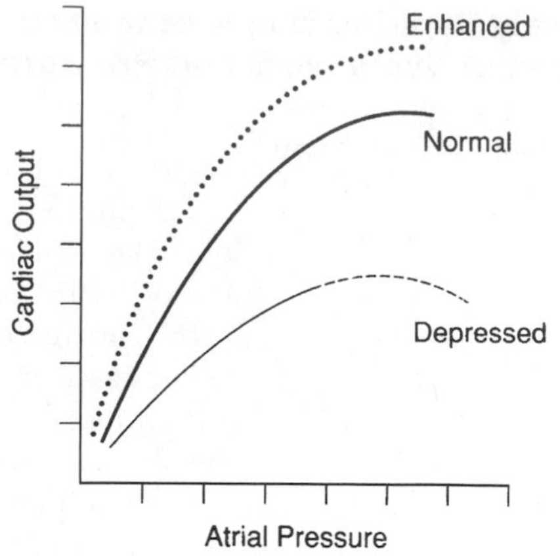

Figure 45-14. Ventricular function curves (Frank-Starling curves) depict the volume of forward ventricular ejection (cardiac output) at different atrial filling pressures and varying degrees of myocardial contractility.

Pressure-Volume Loops

Pressure-volume loops describe the dynamic characteristics of cardiac function (Fig. 45-15). If ventricular pressure is plotted against ventricular volume, each cardiac cycle can be depicted by a pressure-volume loop.

Shock Syndromes

Circulatory shock is characterized by inadequate tissue blood flow and oxygen delivery to cells, resulting in generalized

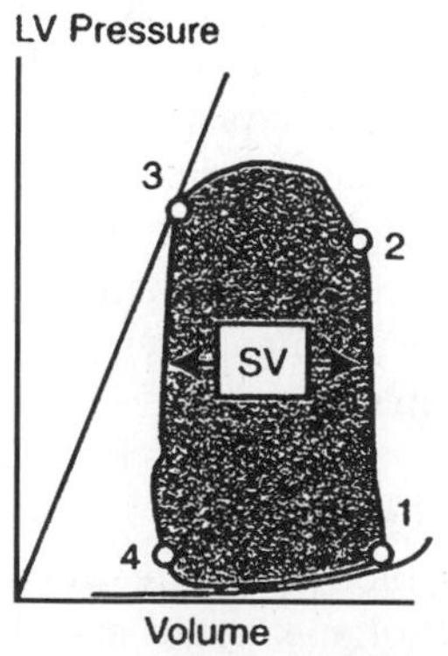

Figure 45-15. Pressure-volume loop representing the cardiac cycle. The end-diastolic and the end-systolic pressure-volume relationships represent the boundaries for the loops. The width of the pressure-volume loop represents the stroke volume (SV). Increases or decreases in myocardial contractility make the end-systolic pressure volume relationship steeper or shallower. The four segments of the loop (isovolumic contraction, ejection, isovolumic relaxation, ventricular filling) for the left ventricle are depicted in succession by mitral valve closure (1), aortic valve opening (2), aortic valve closure (3), mitral valve opening (4).

deterioration of organ function. The usual cause of inadequate tissue perfusion is inadequate cardiac output due to decreased venous return or myocardial depression. Decreased cardiac output associated with shock decreases tissue oxygen delivery, which in turn decreases the level of metabolism that can be maintained by different cells of the body. Skeletal muscle weakness is prominent, reflecting inadequate delivery of oxygen to these tissues. Metabolism is depressed, and the amount of heat liberated is decreased. As a result, body temperature tends to decrease, especially in the presence of a cold ambient environment. In the early stages of shock, consciousness is usually maintained, although mental clarity may be impaired. Consciousness is likely to be lost as shock progresses. Low cardiac output greatly decreases urine output or even causes anuria because glomerular pressure decreases below the critical value required for filtration of fluid into Bowman's capsule. Furthermore, the kidneys have such a high rate of metabolism and require such a large amount of nutrients that decreased renal blood flow may cause acute tubular necrosis (see Chapter 54). An important feature of persistent shock is eventual progressive deterioration of the heart. In addition to myocardial depression caused by decreased coronary artery blood flow, the myocardium can also be depressed by lactic acid, bacterial endotoxins, and myocardial depressant factor released from an ischemic pancreas.

Hemorrhagic Shock

Hemorrhage is the most common cause of shock due to decreased venous return. Any decrease in systemic blood pressure initiates powerful baroreceptor-mediated increases in sympathetic nervous system activity, manifesting as arterial constriction, venoconstriction, and direct myocardial stimulation. Venoconstriction is particularly important for sustaining venous return to the heart and, thus, maintaining cardiac output. Arterial constriction is responsible for initially maintaining systemic blood pressure despite decreases in cardiac output. This maintenance of systemic blood pressure sustains cerebral and coronary artery blood flow because significant vasoconstriction does not occur in these organs. In other organs, such as the kidneys, intense sympathetic nervous system-mediated vasoconstriction may decrease blood flow dramatically.

Nonhemorrhagic Shock

Loss of plasma from the circulation in the absence of blood loss can result in shock similar to that produced by hemorrhage. Intestinal obstruction results in extreme loss of plasma volume into the gastrointestinal tract. Severe burns may also be associated with sufficient plasma loss to result in shock. Hypovolemic shock that results from plasma loss has the same clinical characteristics as hemorrhagic shock except that selective loss of plasma greatly increases viscosity of blood and exacerbates sluggishness of blood flow.

Neurogenic Shock

Neurogenic shock occurs in the absence of blood loss when vascular capacity increases so greatly that even a normal blood volume is not capable of maintaining venous return and cardiac output. A classic cause of loss of vasomotor tone and subsequent neurogenic shock is traumatic transection of the spinal cord or acute blockade of the peripheral sympathetic nervous system by spinal or epidural anesthesia.

Septic Shock

Septic shock is characterized by profound peripheral vasodilation, increased cardiac output secondary to decreased systemic vascular resistance, and development of disseminated intravascular coagulation. Causes of septic shock are most often the release of endotoxins from ischemic portions of the gastrointestinal tract or bacteremia owing to extension of urinary tract infections. The septic response is likely to reflect a systemic inflammatory response produced by exposure to bacterial cell products that ultimately lead to a progressively dysfunctional host response and multisystem organ failure. Immunosuppressed and elderly patients are vulnerable to the development of sepsis and associated septic shock. The end-stages of septic shock are not greatly different from the end-stages of hemorrhagic shock, even though the initiating factors are markedly different. Mortality approaches 50% in septic shock despite significant improvements in supportive care (Baxter, 1997).

Measurement of Cardiac Output

The management of patients in the operating room and intensive care unit involves therapeutic interventions intended to optimize tissue oxygen delivery. Common interventions include fluid administration, blood transfusion, inotrope and vasoactive pharmacotherapy, heart rate and rhythm manipulation, mechanical assist devices, nitric oxide administration, and mechanical ventilation. Ideally, these interventions should be guided by the measurement of cardiac output. However, cardiac output determination has traditionally required invasive techniques such as the insertion of pulmonary artery catheters. Recent advances in microprocessor technology, a greater awareness of the limitations and hazards of pulmonary artery catheter insertion, and a need to measure cardiac output in nonoperating room settings such as the emergency department, have led to the development of newer monitoring techniques. The general trend has been to develop techniques that are less invasive and allow more frequent, or even continuous, measurement of cardiac output (Tibby and Murdoch, 2002). Nevertheless, the pulmonary artery thermodilution technique represents the clinical standard against which new techniques are compared (Moise et al., 2002). Currently utilized methods of cardiac output measurement include (a) Fick methods, (b) indicator dilution methods, (c) thermodilution,

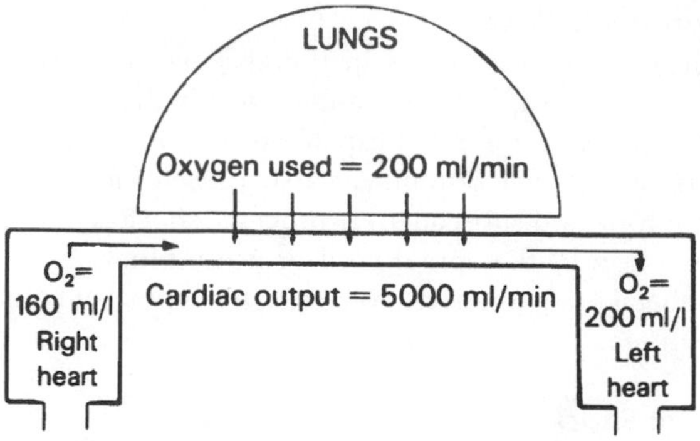

Figure 45-16. The Fick method calculates cardiac output as oxygen consumption divided by the arteriovenous difference for oxygen. (From Ganong WF. *Review of medical physiology*, 21st ed. Lange Medical Books, New York: McGraw Hill, 2003; with permission.)

(d) echocardiographic techniques, (e) impedance cardiography, and (f) pulse contour analysis.

Fick Method

Fick first described this method the "Fick principle" to estimate cardiac output in 1870. Cardiac output is estimated by dividing the oxygen consumption by the arteriovenous difference for oxygen (Fig. 45-16) (Guyton and Hall, 2000). Oxygen consumption is usually measured by a respirometer containing a known oxygen mixture. The patient's exhaled gases are collected in a Douglas bag. The volume and oxygen concentrations of the exhaled gases allow calculation of oxygen consumption. Venous blood for calculation of oxygen content must be obtained from the right ventricle, or, ideally, the pulmonary artery to ensure adequate mixing. Blood from the right atrium may not yet be adequately mixed to provide a true mixed venous sample. Blood used for determining the oxygen saturation in arterial blood can be obtained from any artery because all arterial blood is thoroughly mixed before it leaves the heart and therefore, has the same concentration of oxygen. The Fick principle can also be applied to carbon dioxide elimination from the lung (Berton and Cholley, 2002).

The NICO (Novametrix Medical Systems, Inc., Wallingford, CT) is a continuous noninvasive monitor of cardiac output. By intermittently adding an additional dead space to the breathing circuit, CO_2 elimination is reduced thus increasing end-tidal CO_2. The change in end-tidal CO_2 is used to estimate the change in arterial CO_2 content. This proprietary system uses these data in a modified Fick equation to calculate cardiac output.

Indicator Dilution Method

In measuring the cardiac output by the indicator dilution method, a nondiffusible dye (indocyanine green) is injected into the right atrium (or central venous circulation), and the concentration of dye is subsequently measured continuously in the arterial circulation by a spectrophotometer. The area under the resulting time-concentration curve before recirculation of the dye occurs, combined with knowing the amount of dye injected, allows calculation of the pulmonary blood flow, which is the same as the cardiac output. It is necessary to extrapolate the dye curve to zero because recirculation of the dye occurs before the down slope of the curve reaches baseline. Early recirculation of the dye may indicate the presence of a right-to-left intracardiac shunt (foramen ovale), permitting direct passage of a portion of the dye to the left side of the heart without first passing through the lungs.

Thermodilution Method

A bolus of cold fluid may also be considered an indicator and used in the indicator dilution technique. A pulmonary artery catheter with ports in the right atrium and pulmonary artery and a temperature sensor on the distal port is used to measure thermodilution cardiac outputs. Thermodilution cardiac outputs are determined by measuring the change in blood temperature between two points (right atrium and pulmonary artery) after injection of a known volume of cold saline solution at the proximal right atrial port. The change in blood temperature as measured at the distal pulmonary artery port is inversely proportional to pulmonary blood flow (the extent to which the cold saline solution is diluted by blood), which is equivalent to cardiac output. A computer converts the area under the temperature-time curve to its equivalent in cardiac output. Advantages of this technique compared with the indicator dilution method include dissipation of cold in tissues so recirculation is not a problem, and safety of repeated and frequent measurements because saline is innocuous. Recent advances in thermodilution techniques include semicontinuous cardiac output determination using a heat generating thermal filament incorporated into the pulmonary artery catheter. It is necessary to utilize sophisticated signal processing strategies to measure the downstream temperature because the thermal filament must generate only a modest level of heat for safety.

Echocardiographic techniques

Echocardiography can be used to estimate cardiac output by combining the Doppler principle to determine the velocity of blood in the aorta with two-dimensional views to determine aortic diameter (Tibby and Murdoch, 2002). Conventional transesophageal or transthoracic echocardiographic techniques have the advantage that systolic and diastolic function, volume status, regional wall abnormalities, valve function, and the presence of pericardial effusion may also be evaluated. However, this technique requires significant operator expertise. More recently, Doppler techniques have been developed utilizing transesophageal probes designed solely for the purpose of estimating cardiac output. Aortic dimensions are not measured but are estimated from a nomogram. Transesophageal Doppler estimates of cardiac output require minimal operator training and allow rapid cardiac output estimation.

Impedance Cardiography

The thorax is a conductor whose impedance is altered by changes in blood volume and velocity with each cardiac cycle. Impedance cardiography is based on the principle of thoracic electrical bioimpedance and involves the placement of electrodes to allow the transmission of current and measurement of voltage across the chest (Summers et al., 2003). Thus, thoracic electrical bioimpedance techniques can be used to noninvasively estimate cardiac output. However, the validity of this technique is limited under several circumstances including; patient movement, poor ECG signal quality, cardiac tachydysrhythmias, excessive thoracic fluid, and open chest wounds with metal retractors.

Pulse contour analysis

The first attempt to determine cardiac output from analysis of the pulse contour was made in 1904. The aortic pressure waveform is a function of the stroke volume and its interaction with the vascular tree. The arterial pulse contour can be modeled in manner analogous to an electrical circuit that has specific values for resistance, compliance, and impedance (Berton and Cholley, 2002). Thus, the flow within that system can be estimated from the pressure waveform that is generated. The validity of this system is improved by calibration using a separate cardiac output estimation technique. However, in clinical practice, reliable use of this technique requires frequent recalibration because the peripheral circulation undergoes significant changes in arteriolar tone in response to physiologic and pharmacologic stimuli.

FETAL CIRCULATION

Fetal circulation is considerably different from circulation after birth. For example, in utero, the placenta acts as the fetal lung, and oxygenated blood (saturation about 80%) from the placenta passes through a single umbilical vein to the fetus. This blood flows predominantly through the ductus venosus and into the inferior vena cava, thus bypassing the liver (Fig. 45-17) (Ganong, 2003). Most of the oxygenated blood entering the right atrium from the inferior vena cava preferentially passes through the foramen ovale into the left atrium, thus bypassing the lungs. Passage of this oxygenated blood directly to the left atrium allows perfusion of the fetal brain with maximal available concentrations of oxygen. Fetal hemoglobin differs from adult hemoglobin in binding oxygen less avidly, thus maximizing oxygen transfer to tissues despite low hemoglobin saturations with oxygen.

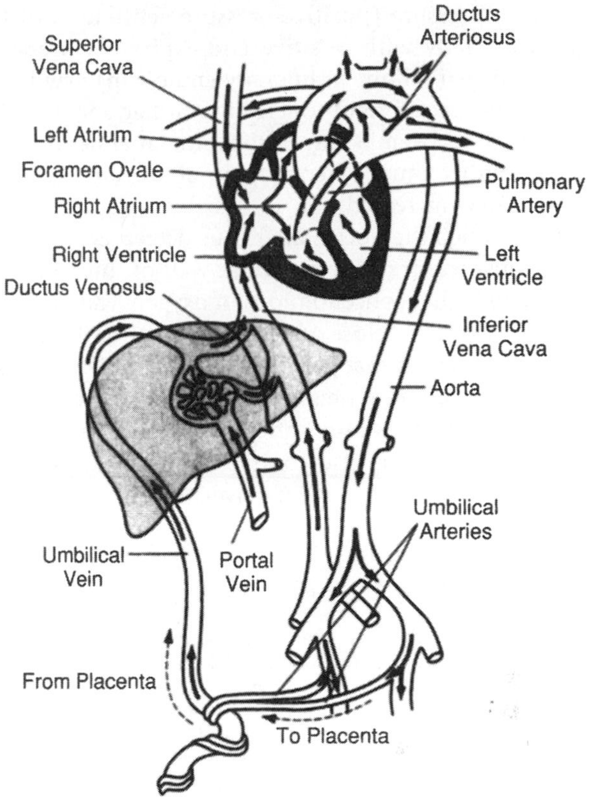

Figure 45-17. The placenta acts as the lungs for the fetus. Most of the oxygenated blood reaching the fetal heart via the umbilical vein and inferior vena cava is diverted through the foramen ovale and pumped out the aorta to the head. Deoxygenated blood returned via the superior vena cava is mostly pumped through the pulmonary artery and ductus arteriosus to the feet and the umbilical arteries. (From Ganong WF. *Review of medical physiology*, 21st ed. Lange Medical Books, New York: McGraw Hill, 2003; with permission.)

Blood entering the right atrium from the superior vena cava is mainly oxygenated blood from the fetal head regions. This blood enters the right ventricle for delivery into the pulmonary artery and then to the descending thoracic aorta via the ductus arteriosus. As a result, this deoxygenated blood is delivered distal to the blood vessels that supply the fetal brain. Blood is returned to the placenta by two umbilical arteries for oxygenation.

The principal changes in the fetal circulation at birth are increased systemic vascular resistance and systemic blood pressure due to cessation of blood flow through the placenta. In addition, pulmonary vascular resistance decreases dramatically with expansion of the lungs, leading to a marked increase in pulmonary blood flow. These alterations in pulmonary and systemic vascular resistances change the pressure gradient across the foramen ovale, causing the flaplike valve that is present on the left atrial septum to occlude the opening and prevent continued right-to-left shunting of blood at this site. In about two-thirds of individuals, this valve becomes adherent over the foramen ovale in a few months. In the absence of permanent closure of the foramen ovale, sudden increases in right atrial pressure (positive-pressure ventilation of the lungs, especially with positive end-expiratory pressure, right ventricular failure, pulmonary embolism) may introduce an unexpected right-to-left intracardiac shunt at this site. Arterial hypoxemia may be the initial manifestation of this intracardiac shunt when right atrial pressure is acutely and selectively increased.

Flow through the ductus arteriosus decreases after birth due to constriction of the muscular wall of this vessel on exposure to higher concentrations of oxygen. Failure of the ductus arteriosus to close after birth results in reversal of flow compared with that present before birth. This reversal of flow occurs because pressure in the aorta exceeds pressure in the pulmonary artery after birth. The muscular wall of the ductus venosus also contracts after birth, diverting portal venous blood through the liver.

REFERENCES

Baba T, Goto T, Yoshitake A, et al. Radial artery diameter decreases with increased femoral to radial arterial pressure gradient during cardiopulmonary bypass. *Anesth Analg* 1997;85:252–258.

Baxter F. Septic shock. *Can J Anaesth* 1997;44:59–72.

Bazaral MG, Welch M, Golding LAR, et al. Comparison of brachial and radial arterial pressure monitoring in patients undergoing coronary artery bypass surgery. *Anesthesiology* 1990;73:38–45.

Berton C, Cholley B. Equipment review: New techniques for cardiac output measurement–oesophageal Doppler, Fick principle using carbon dioxide, and pulse contour analysis. *Critical Care* 2002;6:216–221.

Cook DJ, Simel DL. Does this patient have abnormal central venous pressure? *JAMA* 1996;275:630–634.

Galley HF, Webster NR. Physiology of the endothelium. *Br J Anaesth* 2004;93:105–113.

Ganong WF. *Review of medical physiology*, 21st ed. Lange Medical Books, New York: McGraw Hill, 2003.

Gerber MJ, Hines RL, Barash PG. Arterial waveforms and systemic vascular resistance: is there a correlation? *Anesthesiology* 1987;66:823–825.

Guyton AC, Hall JE. *Textbook of medical physiology*, 10th ed. Philadelphia: Saunders, 2000.

Moise SF, Sinclair CJ, Scott DHT. Pulmonary artery blood temperature and the measurement of cardiac output by thermodilution. *Anaesthesia* 2002;57:562–566.

Pauca AL, Hudspeth AS, Wallenhaupt SL, et al. Radial artery-to-aorta pressure difference after discontinuation of cardiopulmonary bypass. *Anesthesiology* 1989;70:935–941.

Rich GF, Lubanski RE, McLoughlin TM. Differences between aortic and radial artery pressure associated with cardiopulmonary bypass. *Anesthesiology* 1992;77:63–66.

Stern DH, Gerson JI, Allen FB, Parker FB. Can we trust the direct radial artery pressure immediately following cardiopulmonary bypass? *Anesthesiology* 1985;62:557–561.

Summers RL, Shoemaker WC, Peacock WF et al. Bench to bedside: electrophysiologic and clinical principles of noninvasive hemodynamic monitoring using impedance cardiography. *Acad Emerg Med* 2003;10:669–680.

Tibby SM, Murdoch IA. Measurement of cardiac output and tissue perfusion. *Curr Opin Pediatr.* 2002;14:303–309.

Young JD. The heart and circulation in severe sepsis. *Br J Anaesth* 2004;93:114–120.

Microcirculation and Lymphatics

46

The circulation exists to supply tissues with blood in amounts commensurate with their needs for oxygen and nutrients (Guyton and Hall, 2000). Capillaries whose walls consist of a single layer of endothelial cells, serve as the site for the rapid transfer of oxygen and nutrients to tissues and receipt of metabolic byproducts. There are an estimated 10 billion capillaries providing a total surface area that exceeds 6,300 m^2 for nutrient exchange. Capillary density varies from tissue to tissue. Capillaries are numerous in metabolically active tissues, such as cardiac and skeletal muscles, whereas in less active tissues, capillary density is low. Nevertheless, it is unlikely that any functional cell is >50 μm away from a capillary. The muscular arterioles serve as the major resistance vessels and regulate regional blood flow to the capillary beds. Venules act primarily as collecting channels and storage vessels.

The lymphatic system is composed of lymph vessels, nodes and lymphoid tissue. Fluid and proteins that have escaped from the circulation are retuned to the venous circulation by the lymphatic system.

MICROCIRCULATION

The microcirculation is defined as the circulation of blood through the smallest vessels of the body-arterioles, capillaries, and venules.

Anatomy of the Microcirculation

Arterioles give rise to metarterioles, which give rise to capillaries (Table 46-1) (Fig. 46-1) (Ganong, 2003). Other metarterioles serve as thoroughfare channels to the venules, bypassing the capillary bed. Capillaries drain via short collecting venules to the venules. Blood flow through capillaries is regulated by muscular precapillary sphincters present at the capillary opening. The arterioles, metarterioles, and venules contain smooth muscle. As a result, the arterioles serve as the major resistance vessels and regulate regional blood flow to the capillary beds, whereas the venules and veins serve primarily as collecting channels and storage or capacitance vessels.

Capillary walls are about 1 μm thick, consisting of a single layer of endothelial cells surrounded by a thin basement membrane on the outside (Fig. 46-2) (Ganong, 2003). The structure of the capillary wall varies from tissue to tissue, but in many organs, including those in skeletal, cardiac, and smooth muscle, the interdigitated junction between endothelial cells allows passage of molecules up to 10 nm in diameter. In addition, the cytoplasm of endothelial cells is attenuated to form gaps or pores that are 20 to 100 nm in diameter. These pores permit the passage of relatively large molecules. It also appears that plasma and its dissolved proteins are taken up by endocytosis, transported across endothelial cells, and discharged by exocytosis into the interstitial fluid. In the brain, the capillaries resemble those in skeletal muscles, except the interdigitated junctions between endothelial cells are tighter (blood-brain barrier), permitting passage of only small molecules.

The diameter of capillary pores is about 25 times the diameter of water molecules (0.3 nm), which are the smallest molecules that normally pass through capillary channels. Plasma proteins have diameters that exceed the width of capillary pores. Other substances, such as sodium, potassium, and chloride ions and glucose, have intermediate diameters (0.39 to 0.86 nm) such that permeability of capillary pores for different substances varies according to their molecular weights (Table 46-2). Oxygen and carbon dioxide are both lipid soluble and readily pass through endothelial cells.

True capillaries are devoid of smooth muscle and are therefore incapable of active constriction. Nevertheless, the endothelial cells that form them contain actin and myosin and can alter their shape in response to certain chemical stimuli. The diameter of capillaries (7 to 9 μm)

TABLE 46-1.
ANATOMY OF THE VARIOUS TYPES OF BLOOD VESSELS

Vessel	Lumen Diameter	Approximate Cross-Sectional Area (cm^2)	Percentage of Blood Volume Contained
Aorta	2.5 cm	2.5	
Artery	0.4 cm	20	13
Arteriole	30 μm	40	1
Capillary	5 μm	2,500	6
Venule	20 μm	250	
Vein	0.5 cm	80	64*
Vena cava	3 cm	8	
Heart			7
Pulmonary circulation		18	9

*Blood volume contained in venules, veins, and vena cava.

is just sufficient to permit erythrocytes to squeeze through in single file. The thin walls of capillaries are able to withstand high intraluminal pressures because their small diameter prevents excessive wall tension (Laplace law).

Blood Flow in Capillaries

Blood flow in capillaries is approximately 1 mm/s and is intermittent rather than continuous. This intermittent blood flow reflects contraction and relaxation of metarterioles and precapillary sphincters in alternating cycles 6 to 12 times per minute (Welsch and Segal, 1998). The phenomenon of alternating contraction and relaxation is known as *vasomotion*. Oxygen is the most important determinant of the degree of opening and closing of metarterioles and precapillary sphincters. A low PO_2 allows more blood to flow through capillaries to supply tissues. In this regard, the impact of oxygen on capillary blood flow provides a form of autoregulation of tissue blood flow.

In addition to nutritive blood flow through tissues that is regulated by oxygen, there is also nonnutritive (shunt) blood flow regulated by the autonomic nervous system. The nonnutritive blood flow is characterized by direct vascular connections between arterioles and venules. Some of these arteriovenous connections have muscular coverings so blood flow can be altered over a wide range. In some parts of the skin, these arteriovenous anastomoses provide a mechanism to permit rapid inflow of arterial blood to warm the skin and dissipate the heat.

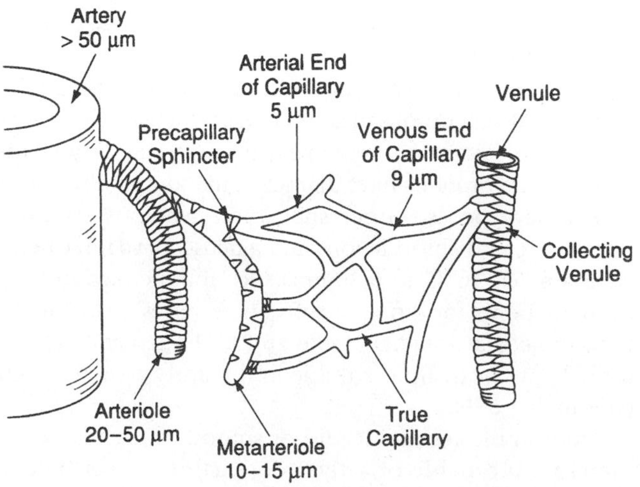

Figure 46-1. Anatomy of the microcirculation. (From Ganong WF. *Review of medical physiology*, 21st ed. Lange Medical Books, New York: McGraw-Hill, 2003; with permission.)

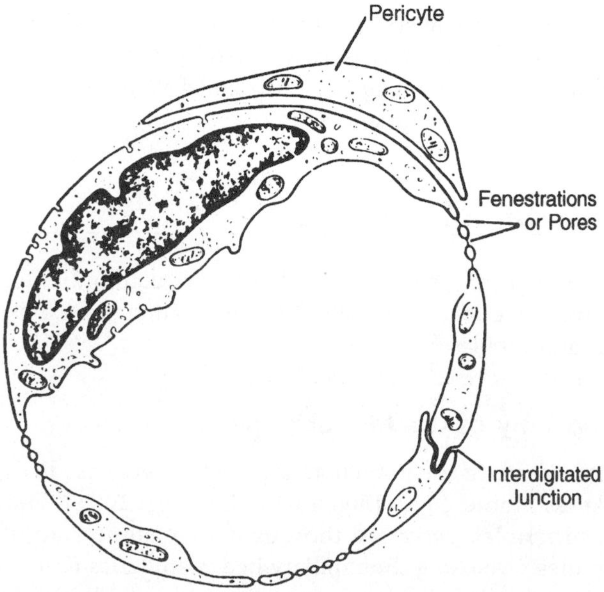

Figure 46-2. Capillaries include interdigitated junctions and pores to facilitate passage of lipid-insoluble ions and molecules. (From Ganong WF. *Review of medical physiology*, 21st ed. Lange Medical Books, New York: McGraw-Hill, 2003; with permission.)

TABLE 46-2.
PERMEABILITY OF CAPILLARY MEMBRANES

	Molecular Weight (Daltons)	Relative Permeability
Water	18	1.0
Sodium chloride	58.5	0.96
Glucose	180	0.6
Hemoglobin	66,700	0.01
Albumin	69,000	0.0001

TABLE 46-3.
FILTRATION OF FLUID AT THE ARTERIAL ENDS OF CAPILLARIES

Pressure favoring outward movement	
Capillary pressure	25 mm Hg
Interstitial fluid pressure	−6.3 mm Hg
Interstitial fluid colloid osmotic pressure	5 mm Hg
Total	36.3 mm Hg
Pressure favoring inward movement	
Plasma colloid osmotic pressure	28 mm Hg
Net filtration pressure	**8.3 mm Hg**

Vasoactive Role of the Capillary Endothelium

The notion that the endothelium of capillaries is an inert single layer of cells serving only as a passive filter to permit passage of water and small molecules across the blood vessel wall is no longer considered valid (Berne et al., 2004). Rather, the endothelium is now recognized as an important source of substances that cause contraction or relaxation of vascular smooth muscle.

One of these substances is prostacyclin that can relax vascular smooth muscle via an increase in cyclic adenosine monophosphate (cAMP) concentration. Prostacyclin is formed in the endothelium from arachidonic acid and the reaction is catalyzed by prostacyclin synthase. The principal function of prostacyclin is to inhibit platelet adherence to the endothelium and platelet aggregation and thus prevent intravascular clot formation.

The formation and release of nitric oxide (NO) is also important in the endothelium-mediated vascular dilation (Feng and Hedner, 1990). NO is released when endothelial cells are stimulated by acetylcholine or other vasodilator substances (adenosine triphosphate, bradykinin, serotonin, substance P, and histamine). NO release can be stimulated by the shear stress of blood flow on the endothelium. A vasoconstrictor peptide synthesized by the capillary endothelium is endothelin. Endothelin may affect vascular tone and blood pressure.

Fluid Movement across Capillary Membranes

Solvent and solute movement across capillary endothelial cells occurs by filtration, diffusion, and pinocytosis via endothelial vesicles (Michel and Neal, 1999). Diffusion is the most important process for transcapillary exchange and pinocytosis is the least important. It is important to distinguish between filtration and diffusion through capillary membranes. Filtration is the net outward movement of fluid at the arterial end of capillaries. Diffusion of fluid occurs in both directions across capillary membranes.

Filtration

The four pressures that determine whether fluid will move outward across capillary membranes (filtration) or inward across capillary membranes (reabsorption) are (a) capillary pressure, (b) interstitial fluid pressure, (c) plasma colloid osmotic pressure, and (d) interstitial fluid colloid osmotic pressure. The net effect of these four pressures is a positive filtration pressure at the arterial end of capillaries, causing fluid to move outward across cell membranes into interstitial fluid spaces (Table 46-3). At the venous end of capillaries, the net effect of these four pressures is a positive reabsorption pressure causing fluid to move inward across capillary membranes into capillaries (Table 46-4). Overall, the mean values of the four pressures acting across capillary membranes are nearly identical such that the amount of fluid filtered nearly equals the amount reabsorbed (Table 46-5). Any fluid that is not reabsorbed enters the lymph vessels.

Traditionally, filtration has been considered to occur at the arterial end of the capillary and absorption to occur at the venous end because of the gradient of hydrostatic pressure along the capillary. Nevertheless, many capillaries only filter, whereas others only absorb. In some vascular beds such as the renal glomerulus, hydrostatic pressure in the capillary is high enough to cause filtration along the entire length of the capillary.

Capillary Pressure

Capillary pressure tends to move fluid outward across the arterial ends of capillary membranes. It is estimated that

TABLE 46-4.
REABSORPTION OF FLUID AT THE VENOUS ENDS OF CAPILLARIES

Pressure favoring outward movement	
Capillary pressure	10 mm Hg
Interstitial fluid pressure	−6.3 mm Hg
Interstitial fluid colloid osmotic pressure	5 mm Hg
Total	21.3 mm Hg
Pressure favoring inward movement	
Plasma colloid osmotic pressure	28 mm Hg
Net reabsorption pressure	**6.7 mm Hg**

TABLE 46-5.
MEAN VALUES OF PRESSURES ACTING ACROSS CAPILLARY MEMBRANES

Pressure favoring outward movement	
Capillary pressure	17 mm Hg
Interstitial fluid pressure	−6.3 mm Hg
Interstitial fluid colloid osmotic pressure	5 mm Hg
Total	28.3 mm Hg
Pressure favoring inward movement	
Plasma colloid osmotic pressure	28 mm Hg
Net overall filtration pressure	**0.3 mm Hg**

capillary pressure at the arterial end of capillaries is 25 mm Hg, whereas pressure at the venous end of capillaries is 10 mm Hg, corresponding to the pressure in venules. The mean capillary pressure is about 17 mm Hg. Changes in arterial pressure have little effect on capillary pressure and flow becase of adjustments of precapillary resistance vessels. Autoregulation describes the maintenance of unchanged tissue blood flow despite changes in perfusion pressure.

Interstitial Fluid Pressure

Interstitial fluid pressure tends to move fluid outward across capillary membranes. It is estimated that average interstitial fluid pressure is −6.3 mm Hg. This negative pressure acts as a vacuum to hold tissues together and maintain a minimal distance for diffusion of nutrients. Under normal conditions, almost all of the interstitial fluid is held in a gel that fills the spaces between cells. This gel contains large quantities of mucopolysaccharides, the most abundant of which is hyaluronic acid. Loss of negative interstitial fluid pressure allows fluid to accumulate in tissue spaces as edema.

Plasma Colloid Osmotic Pressure

Plasma proteins are principally responsible for the plasma colloid osmotic (oncotic) pressure that tends to cause movement of fluid inward through capillary membranes. Each gram of albumin exerts twice the colloid osmotic pressure of a gram of globulin. Because there is about twice as much albumin as globulin in the plasma, about 70% of the total colloid osmotic pressure results from albumin and only about 30% from globulin and fibrinogen.

A special phenomenon known as *Donnan equilibrium* causes the colloid osmotic pressure to be about 50% greater than that caused by proteins alone. This reflects the negative charge characteristic of proteins that necessitates the presence of an equal number of positively charged ions, mainly sodium ions, on the same side of the capillary membrane as the proteins. These extra positive ions increase the number of osmotically active substances and thus increase the colloid osmotic pressure. Indeed, about one-third of the normal plasma colloid osmotic pressure of 28 mm Hg is caused by positively charged ions held in the plasma by proteins. This is the reason that plasma proteins cannot be replaced by inert substances, such as dextran, without some decrease in plasma colloid osmotic pressure.

Interstitial Fluid Colloid Osmotic Pressure

Proteins present in the interstitial fluid are principally responsible for the interstitial fluid colloid osmotic pressure of about 5 mm Hg, which tends to cause movement of fluid outward across capillary membranes. Albumin, because of its small size, normally leaks 1.6 times as readily as globulins through capillaries, causing the proteins in interstitial fluids to have a disproportionately high albumin to globulin ratio. The total protein content of interstitial fluid is similar to the total protein content of plasma, but because the volume of the interstitial fluid is four times the volume of plasma, the average interstitial fluid protein content is only one-fourth that in plasma, or about 1.8 g/dL. Interstitial fluid protein content also remains low because proteins cannot readily diffuse across capillary membranes, and any that crosses is likely to be removed by lymph vessels.

Diffusion

Diffusion is the most important mechanism for transfer of nutrients between the plasma and the interstitial fluid. Oxygen, carbon dioxide, and anesthetic gases are examples of lipid-soluble molecules that can diffuse directly through capillary membranes independently of pores. Sodium, potassium, and chloride ions and glucose are insoluble in lipid capillary membranes and therefore must pass through pores to gain access to interstitial fluids. The diffusion rate of lipid-soluble molecules across capillary membranes in either direction is proportional to the concentration difference between the two sides of the membrane. For this reason, large amounts of oxygen move from capillaries toward tissues, whereas carbon dioxide moves in the opposite direction. Typically, only slight partial pressure differences suffice to maintain adequate transport of oxygen between the plasma and interstitial fluid.

Pinocytosis

Pinocytosis is the process by which capillary endothelial cells ingest small amounts of plasma or interstitial fluid followed by migration to the opposite surface where the fluid is released. Transport of high-molecular-weight substances such as plasma proteins, glycoproteins, and polysaccharides (dextran) most likely occurs principally by pinocytosis.

LYMPHATICS

Lymph vessels represent an alternate route by which excess fluids can flow from interstitial fluid spaces into the blood (Aukland and Reed, 1993). The most important function of the lymphatic system is return of protein into the circulation and maintenance of a low-protein concentration in the interstitial fluid. The small amount of protein that escapes from the arterial end of the capillary cannot undergo reabsorption at the venous end of the capillary. If lymph vessels were not available, this protein would be progressively concentrated in the interstitial fluid, resulting in increases in interstitial fluid colloid osmotic pressure that, within a few hours, would produce life-threatening edema. Only cartilage, bone, epithelium, and tissues of the central nervous system are devoid of lymphatic vessels.

Anatomy

The terminal lymph vessels are the thoracic duct and the right lymphatic duct (Fig. 46-3). The thoracic duct is the larger of the two (2 mm in diameter), entering the venous system in the angle of the junction of the left internal jugular and subclavian veins. The right lymphatic duct is not always present, and if it is, it rarely exists as such because the three vessels that occasionally unite to form it usually open separately into the right internal jugular, subclavian, and innominate veins. Avoidance of possible damage to the thoracic duct is often the reason to select the right side of the neck as the site for percutaneous placement of venous catheters into the right internal jugular vein.

Lymph vessels contain flaplike valves between endothelial cells that open toward the interior, allowing the unimpeded entrance of interstitial fluid and proteins. Backflow out of the lymph vessel is not possible because any flow in this direction causes the flaplike valves to close.

Formation

Lymph is interstitial fluid that flows into lymphatic vessels. As such, the protein concentration of lymph is about

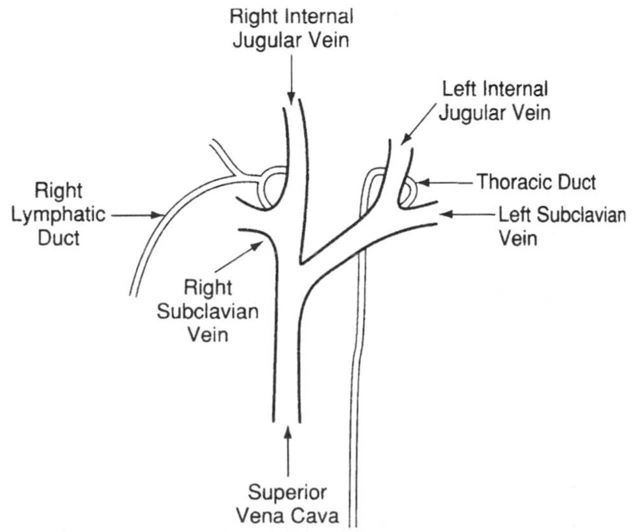

Figure 46-3. Depiction of the thoracic duct and right lymphatic duct as they enter the venous system.

1.8 g/dL, with the exception of lymph from the gastrointestinal tract and liver, which contains two to three times this concentration of protein. The lymphatic system is also one of the major channels for absorption of nutrients, especially fat, from the gastrointestinal tract. Bacteria that enter lymph vessels are removed and destroyed by lymph nodes.

Flow

Flow of lymph through the thoracic duct is about 100 mL/hour. A decrease in the negative value of interstitial fluid pressure increases the flow of interstitial fluid into terminal lymph vessels and consequently increases the rate of lymph flow. For example, at 0 mm Hg interstitial fluid pressure, the rate of lymph flow is increased 10 to 50 times compared with flow at an average interstitial fluid pressure of −6.3 mm Hg. Skeletal muscle contraction and passive movements of the extremities facilitate flow of lymph. For example, during exercise, lymph flow is increased up to 14 times that present at rest.

Edema

Edema is the presence of excess interstitial fluid in peripheral tissues that results in positive pressure in interstitial fluid spaces and exceeds the ability of lymph vessels to transport the excess fluid. When this occurs, external pressure in one area will displace fluid to another area, resulting in pitting edema. In addition, fluid flows downward in tissues because of gravity, resulting in dependent edema. Coagulation of edema fluid may occur with infection or trauma and manifest as nonpitting or brawny edema.

Edema may also be accompanied by the presence of fluid in potential spaces such as the pleural cavity, pericardial space, peritoneal cavity, and synovial spaces. Fluid that collects in these spaces is called *transudate* if it is sterile and *exudate* if it contains bacteria. Excessive fluid in the peritoneal space—one of the spaces most prone to develop edema fluid—is called *ascites*. The peritoneal cavity is susceptible to the development of edema fluid because any increased pressure in the liver, as owing to cirrhosis or cardiac failure, causes transudation of protein-containing fluids from the surface of the liver into the peritoneal cavity.

Causes of increased interstitial fluid volume that manifests as edema include (a) increased capillary pressure, (b) decreased plasma protein concentrations, (c) obstruction to lymph vessels, and (d) increased permeability of capillaries. Renal dysfunction leading to excessive retention of fluid is also a cause of edema.

Increased Capillary Pressure

Increased capillary pressure, as accompanies impaired venous return because of cardiac failure, results in filtration of fluid from capillaries that exceeds reabsorption. Local edema, as associated with allergic reactions, reflects histamine-induced smooth muscle relaxation of arterioles and constriction of veins. Angioneurotic edema reflects activation of the complement cascade and release of vasoactive substances that increase capillary permeability.

Decreased Plasma Protein Concentrations

Decreased plasma protein concentrations reduce the colloid osmotic pressure such that capillary pressure predominates and excess fluid leaves the circulation. It is estimated that edema begins to appear when the plasma colloid osmotic pressure decreases below 11 mm Hg. Albumin may be lost from the plasma in large quantities when the skin is burned. Renal disease may be associated with urinary loss of albumin sufficient to lower the plasma colloid osmotic pressure. Nutritional edema occurs when dietary intake is not adequate to support formation of sufficient amounts of protein.

Obstruction of Lymph Vessels

Obstruction of lymph vessels results in accumulation of protein in interstitial fluid. The subsequent increase in interstitial fluid colloid osmotic pressure causes excess fluid to collect in the interstitial fluid space. Obstruction of lymph vessels with associated edema may follow operations such as radical mastectomy in which it is necessary to remove lymph nodes as part of the procedure. Edema as a result of this cause typically regresses over 2 to 3 months as new lymph vessels develop.

REFERENCES

Aukland K, Reed RK. Interstitial-lymphatic mechanisms in the control of extracellular fluid volume. *Physiol Rev* 1993;73:1–5.

Berne RM, Levy MN, Koeppen BM. *Physiology*. 5th edition. St Louis. Mosby, 2004.

Feng Q, Hedner T. Endothelium-derived relaxing factor (EDRF) and nitric oxide. II. Physiology, pharmacology, and pathophysiological implications. *Clin Physiol* 1990;10:503–510.

Ganong WF. *Review of medical physiology*, 21st ed. New York. Lange Medical Books/McGraw Hill, 2003.

Guyton AC, Hall JE. *Textbook of medical physiology*, 10th ed. Philadelphia. Saunders, 2000.

Michel CC, Neal CR. Openings through endothelial cells associated with increased permeability. *Microcirculation* 1999;6:45–51.

Welsch DG, Segal SS. Endothelial and smooth muscle cell conduction in arterioles controlling blood flow. *Am J Physiol* 1998;274: H323–H328.

Pulmonary Circulation

47

The pulmonary circulation is a low-pressure, low-resistance system in series with the systemic circulation. The volume of blood flowing through the lungs and systemic circulation is essentially identical. Blood passes through pulmonary capillaries in about 1 s, during which time it is oxygenated and excess carbon dioxide is removed. Increasing the cardiac output tends to shorten capillary transit time towards the estimated 0.3 s required for complete oxygenation of red cells.

ANATOMY

Anatomically, the right ventricle is wrapped halfway around the left ventricle. The semilunar shape of the right ventricle allows it to pump with minimal shortening of its muscle fibers. The thickness of the right ventricle is one-third that of the left ventricle, reflecting the difference in pressures between the two ventricles. The wall of the right ventricle is typically only about three times as thick as the atrial walls.

The pulmonary artery extends only about 4 cm beyond the apex of the right ventricle before division into the right and left main pulmonary arteries. The pulmonary artery is a thin structure with a wall thickness about twice that of the venae cavae and one-third that of the aorta. The large diameter and distensibility of the pulmonary arteries allows the pulmonary circulation to easily accommodate the stroke volume of the right ventricle. Pulmonary veins, like pulmonary arteries, are large in diameter and highly distendible. Pulmonary capillaries supply the estimated 300 million alveoli, providing a gas-exchange surface of 70 m^2.

Pulmonary blood vessels are innervated by the sympathetic nervous system, but the density of these fibers is less than in systemic vessels. Alpha-adrenergic stimulation from norepinephrine produces vasoconstriction of the pulmonary vessels, whereas beta-adrenergic stimulation, as produced by isoproterenol, results in vasodilation. Parasympathetic nervous system fibers from the vagus nerves release acetylcholine, which produces vasodilation of pulmonary vessels. Despite the presence of autonomic nervous system innervation, the resting vasomotor tone is minimal, and the larger pulmonary vessels are almost maximally dilated in the normal resting state. Indeed, overall regulation of pulmonary blood flow is passive, with local adjustments of perfusion relative to ventilation being determined by local oxygen tension.

The diameter of thin-walled alveolar vessels changes in response to alterations in the transmural pressure (intravascular pressure minus alveolar pressure). If alveolar pressure exceeds intravascular pressure as during positive-pressure ventilation of the lungs, pulmonary capillaries collapse and blood flow ceases. The size of larger vessels embedded in the lung parenchyma (extra-alveolar vessels) largely depends on lung volume. For example, resistance to flow through these vessels decreases as lung volumes increase because these vessels are tethered to the surrounding tissue (Fig. 47-1A and Fig. 47-1B). However, the largest pulmonary vessels, those at the hilum of the lung, vary in size in response to changes in intrapleural pressure.

Bronchial Circulation

Bronchial arteries from the thoracic aorta supply oxygenated blood to supporting tissues of the lungs, including connective tissue and airways. After bronchial arterial blood has passed through supporting tissues, the majority of it empties into pulmonary veins and enters the left atrium rather than passing back to the right atrium. The entrance of deoxygenated blood into the left atrium dilutes oxygenated blood and accounts for an anatomic shunt that is equivalent to an estimated 1% to 2% of the cardiac output. This anatomic shunt is the reason that the cardiac output of the left ventricle exceeds that of the right ventricle by an amount approximately equal to the bronchial blood flow.

Pulmonary Lymph Vessels

Pulmonary lymph vessels extend from all the supportive tissues of the lung to the hilum of the lung and then to the thoracic duct. Pulmonary lymphatic flow facilitates the removal of edema fluid from alveolar spaces. Particulate matter entering the alveoli is also eventually removed by lymph vessels.

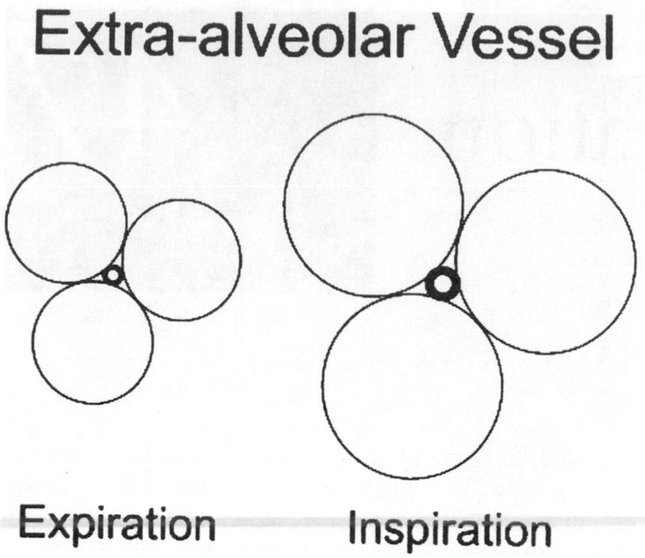

Figure 47-1A. Schematic illustration of the effect of lung inflation on an extra-alveolar vessel surrounded by three alveoli. Extra-alveolar vessels are tethered by surrounding lung parenchyma and increase in caliber with lung inflation.

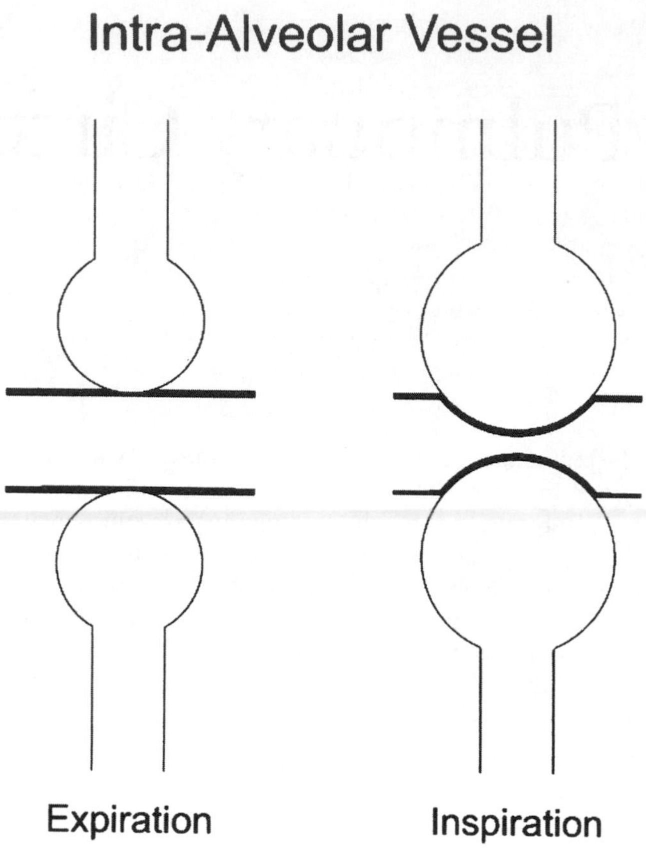

Figure 47-1B. Schematic illustration of an intra-alveolar vessel adjacent to two alveoli. Intra-alveolar vessels are compressed during lung inflation.

INTRAVASCULAR PRESSURES

Pressures in the pulmonary circulation are about one-fifth those present in the systemic circulation (Fig. 47-2) (Guyton and Hall, 2000). The normal pressure in the pulmonary artery is about 22/8 mm Hg, with a mean pulmonary artery pressure of 13 mm Hg. The mean pulmonary capillary pressure is about 10 mm Hg, and the mean pressure in the pulmonary veins is about 4 mm Hg, such that the pressure gradient across the pulmonary circulation is only 9 mm Hg.

The atria contract approximately 0.16 s before the ventricles, completing ventricular filling. Immediately after priming by atrial contraction, the right ventricle contracts, increasing the right ventricular pressure until it exceeds the pressure in the pulmonary artery. At this time, pulmonary valve opening allows blood to flow into the pulmonary artery. When the right ventricular pressure begins to decline, the pulmonary valve closes and the right ventricular pressure continues to fall to a diastolic pressure near 0 mm Hg.

At low pulmonary artery pressures, the resistance to blood flow is increased due to compression of vessels by extravascular structures. Once pressure in the vessels is sufficient to overcome this compression, pulmonary vessels distend, and resistance to blood flow decreases to low values. Overall, the resistance to blood flow in the pulmonary circulation is about one-tenth the resistance in the systemic circulation.

Pulmonary artery pressure is not typically influenced by left atrial pressures of <7 mm Hg. However, when left atrial pressure exceeds ~7 mm Hg, previously collapsed pulmonary veins are expanded, and pulmonary artery pressure increases in parallel with increases in left atrial pressure. In

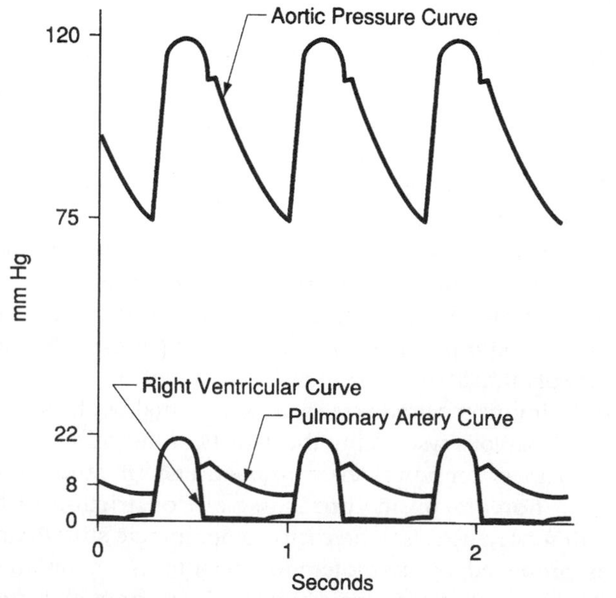

Figure 47-2. Comparison of intravascular pressures in the systemic and pulmonary circulations. (From Guyton AC, Hall JE. *Textbook of medical physiology*, 10th ed. Philadelphia: Saunders, 2000; with permission.)

the absence of left ventricular failure, even marked increases in systemic vascular resistance do not cause the left atrial pressure to increase significantly. Consequently, the right ventricle continues to eject its stroke volume against a normal pulmonary artery pressure despite increased workloads imposed on the left ventricle. Accordingly, the right ventricular stroke volume is not measurably altered by changes in systemic vascular resistance unless the left ventricle fails.

Should the left ventricle fail, left atrial pressures can increase to >15 mm Hg. Mean pulmonary artery pressures also increase, placing an increased workload on the right ventricle. Provided that the mean pulmonary artery pressure is <30 to 40 mm Hg, the right ventricle continues to eject its normal stroke volume, accompanied by only a slight increase in right atrial pressure. However, when the mean pulmonary artery pressure exceeds 30 to 40 mmHg, the right ventricle may begin to fail, so that further increases in pulmonary artery pressure cause exaggerated increases in right atrial pressure and associated decreases in stroke volume.

Measurement of Left Atrial Pressure

The left atrial pressure can be estimated by inserting a balloon tipped catheter into a small pulmonary artery. When the balloon is temporarily inflated and the vessel is completely occluded, a stationary column of blood is created distal to the catheter tip. As a result, the pressure measured immediately distal to the balloon is equivalent to that downstream in the pulmonary veins. This measurement is termed the pulmonary artery occlusion pressure (wedge pressure), and is usually 2 to 3 mm Hg higher than left atrial pressure. If the balloon is deflated, flow will resume and the pulmonary artery end-diastolic pressure can be measured. This measurement correlates with the pulmonary artery occlusion pressure in the absence of pulmonary hypertension.

INTERSTITIAL FLUID SPACE

The interstitial fluid space in the lung is minimal, and a continual negative pulmonary interstitial pressure of about minus 8 mm Hg dehydrates interstitial fluid spaces of the lungs and keeps the alveolar epithelial membrane in close approximation to the capillary membranes. As a result, the diffusion distance between gas in the alveoli and the capillary blood is minimal, averaging about 0.4 μm. Another consequence of negative pressure in pulmonary interstitial spaces is that it pulls fluid from alveoli through alveolar membranes and into interstitial fluid spaces, keeping the alveoli dry. Mean pulmonary capillary pressure is about 10 mm Hg, whereas plasma colloid osmotic pressure is about 28 mm Hg. This net pressure gradient of about 18 mm Hg discourages the movement of fluid out of capillaries, decreasing the likelihood of pulmonary edema.

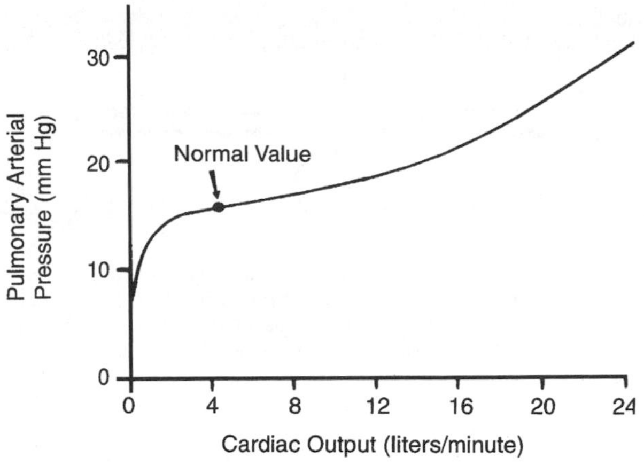

Figure 47-3. Cardiac output can increase nearly fourfold without greatly increasing the pulmonary arterial pressure. (From Guyton AC, Hall JE. *Textbook of medical physiology*, 10th ed. Philadelphia: Saunders, 2000; with permission.)

PULMONARY BLOOD VOLUME

Blood volume in the lungs is about 450 mL. Of this amount, about 70 mL is in capillaries and the remainder is divided equally between pulmonary arteries and veins. Cardiac failure or increased resistance to flow through the mitral valve causes pulmonary blood volume to increase.

Cardiac output can increase nearly four times before pulmonary artery pressure becomes increased (Fig. 47-3) (Guyton and Hall, 2000). This reflects the distensibility of the pulmonary arteries and opening of previously collapsed pulmonary capillaries. The ability of the lungs to accept greatly increased amounts of pulmonary blood flow, as during exercise, without excessive increases in pulmonary artery pressures is important in preventing development of pulmonary edema or right ventricular failure.

Pulmonary blood volume can increase up to 40% when an individual changes from the standing to the supine position. This sudden shift of blood from the systemic circulation to pulmonary circulation is responsible for the decrease in vital capacity in the supine position and the occurrence of orthopnea in the presence of left ventricular failure.

PULMONARY BLOOD FLOW AND DISTRIBUTION

Optimal oxygenation depends on matching ventilation to pulmonary blood flow (West, 1974). Shunt occurs in lung areas that are perfused but inadequately ventilated, whereas dead space ventilation occurs in lung areas that are ventilated but inadequately perfused (Fig. 47-4). Although the lungs are innervated by the autonomic nervous system, it is doubtful that neural influences exert a major effect in the normal control of pulmonary blood flow. There is no

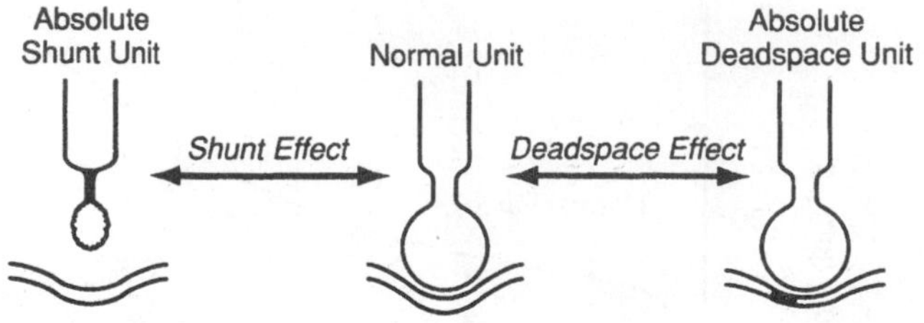

Figure 47-4. Gas exchange is maximally effective in normal lung units with optimal ventilation to perfusion ($\dot{V}/\dot{Q}$) relationships. The continuum of $\dot{V}/\dot{Q}$ relationships is depicted by the ratios between normal and absolute shunt or dead space units.

doubt, however, that decreases in Pa_{O_2} cause increases in pulmonary artery and right ventricular pressures.

Clinically, segmental pulmonary blood flow can be studied by intravenous injection of radioactive xenon while monitoring is performed externally over the chest with radiation detectors. Xenon rapidly diffuses from capillaries into alveoli and radioactivity is detected early in well-perfused regions of the lung.

Endothelial Regulation of Pulmonary Blood Flow

Active vasodilation is crucial to the maintenance of the low resting tone of the normal pulmonary circulation. The pulmonary vascular endothelium is responsible for the synthesis and secretion of various compounds that regulate smooth muscle activity in the pulmonary circulation. The primary vasodilatory compounds are nitric oxide (NO) and prostacyclin. The predominant influence of a healthy pulmonary endothelium is to reduce pulmonary vascular tone. Indeed pulmonary endothelial injury, as following cardiopulmonary bypass, is associated with increased pulmonary vascular resistance. Endothelin is also released by the pulmonary endothelium and may have both a constrictive or dilatory effect depending upon the circumstances. There are several negative feedback mechanisms in effect that regulate vascular tone. The synthesis and release of NO, prostacyclin, endothelin-1, and other vasoactive compounds are integrated into a system that optimizes pulmonary vascular tone and facilitates local control of ventilation to perfusion (V/Q) matching.

Nitric Oxide

NO is synthesized in endothelial cells by NO synthase (NOS). There are several isoforms of NOS, but it is likely that constitutive NOS (cNOS, also termed endothelial NOS or eNOS) is responsible for the normal regulation of pulmonary vascular tone. The activity of cNOS is rapidly up- or down-regulated and produces picomolar amounts of NO in response to stimuli such as shear stress and local oxygen tension. In pathologic states another NOS isoform, inducible NOS (iNOS), produces considerably larger quantities of NO, but takes longer to up-regulate and down-regulate. Inducible NOS is located in vascular smooth muscle cells and inflammatory macrophages. Inflammatory mediators are potent up-regulators of iNOS activity. NO diffuses from its site of production, usually endothelial cells, into adjacent pulmonary vascular smooth muscle cells. NO induces vasorelaxation by stimulating the production of cyclic guanosine monophosphate (cGMP) by the enzyme guanylate cyclase. Cyclic GMP is promptly metabolized by phosphodiesterases. Increased cGMP production appears to stimulate phosphodiesterase upregulation, thus causing accelerating cGMP clearance. Indeed, phosphodiesterase up-regulation may be partly responsible for suboptimal responses to inhaled NO and for rebound pulmonary hypertension after NO withdrawal. Type V phosphodiesterase is the predominant enzyme type in the pulmonary circulation. Selective inhibitors of type V phosphodiesterase such as sildenafil and zaprinast can both selectively decrease pulmonary vascular resistance when given alone and significantly potentiate the effects of iNO and prostacyclin.

Endothelin

Endothelin-1 is a potent endogenous peptide vasoconstrictor that also promotes smooth muscle proliferation. Endothelin has been implicated in the pathogenesis of pulmonary hypertension because some patients have both increased expression and reduced clearance of endothelin-1 in lung tissue and plasma. There are two endothelin receptors: vascular smooth muscle endothelin A and endothelial endothelin B. Smooth muscle endothelin A receptor stimulation causes vasoconstriction, whereas endothelial endothelin B receptor stimulation causes both vasoconstriction and relaxation. Endothelin-1 release is increased as part of the inflammatory response to cardiopulmonary bypass, thereby increasing the potential for pulmonary hypertension after cardiovascular surgery. Exposure to inhaled NO significantly increases endothelin-1 levels, suggesting that endothelin-1 may be partly responsible for rebound pulmonary hypertension after withdrawal of inhaled NO. Endothelin antagonists may prove to be useful in the treatment of pulmonary hypertension. Bosentan is an oral, nonselective endothelin antagonist that is being investigated for use in pulmonary hypertension. Sitaxsentan is an endothelin antagonist that has a 6,000-fold selectivity for the endothelin A receptors versus endothelin B receptors. However, both sitaxsentan and bosentan have adverse effects on liver function, including fatal acute hepatitis.

Prostacyclin

Prostacyclin is a potent vasodilatory prostaglandin released by the pulmonary endothelium. Other prostaglandins, such as thromboxane A_2, have potent vasoconstrictive effects. Pulsatile flow and local shear stress are important stimuli for prostacyclin release. Prostacyclin receptor binding causes the activation of adenylate cyclase, thereby increasing local adenosine-3,5 cyclic monophosphate release. The adenyl cyclase pathway, regulated by prostacyclin, and the guanylate cyclase pathway, regulated by NO, are parallel pathways that converge to reduce vascular smooth muscle tone. Prostacyclin is also an extremely potent inhibitor of platelet aggregation and vascular smooth muscle proliferation. The chronic intravenous administration of prostacyclin is an established treatment for pulmonary hypertension and was first described more than 20 years ago. However, intravenous prostacyclin is not a selective pulmonary vasodilator and can cause significant systemic side effects, including hypotension, and will worsen V/Q matching in the pulmonary circulation. Both the positive and negative hemodynamic effects of prostacyclin are potentiated by the coadministration of phosphodiesterase inhibitors. Of particular interest to anesthesiologists are the encouraging findings with the inhaled aerosolized prostacyclin analogue iloprost. This drug has physical characteristics that make it better suited to nebulization and has a longer duration of action than intravenous prostacyclin.

Hypoxic Pulmonary Vasoconstriction

Alveolar hypoxia (Pa_{O_2} <70 mm Hg) evokes vasoconstriction in the pulmonary arterioles supplying these alveoli. The net effect is to divert blood flow away from poorly ventilated alveoli. As a result, the shunt effect is minimized, and the resulting Pa_{O_2} is maximized. The mechanism for hypoxic pulmonary vasoconstriction is presumed to be locally mediated, as this response occurs in isolated and denervated lungs as well as intact lungs. Indeed, this vasoconstrictor response is apparent in isolated pulmonary artery strips and isolated smooth muscle cells. There are probably multiple mechanisms responsible for hypoxic pulmonary vasoconstriction and these mechanisms probably differ during acute and chronic responses. The suppression of endothelial release of the potent vasodilator NO is probably an important element of both the acute and chronic response. A crucial component of the acute response is the inhibition of potassium channels that leads to membrane depolarization. Membrane depolarization increases calcium influx, which in turn activates the intracellular contractile response. Chronic vascular responses to hypoxia may be, in part, mediated by endothelin release and eventually involve vascular remodeling, eventually leading to irreversible increases in pulmonary vascular resistance (pulmonary hypertension).

Drug-induced inhibition of hypoxic pulmonary vasoconstriction could result in unexpected decreases in Pa_{O_2} in the presence of lung disease. Indeed, potent vasodilating drugs, such as nitroprusside and nitroglycerin, may be accompanied by decreases in Pa_{O_2} that have been attributed to inhibition of hypoxic pulmonary vasoconstriction (Colley et al., 1979). Although animal studies suggest that potent inhaled anesthetic agents inhibit hypoxic vasoconstriction in a dose-dependent manner, in clinically relevant concentrations, these findings have not been supported by clinical studies in patients (Fig. 47-5) (Rogers and Benumof, 1985; Carlsson et al., 1987). The present consensus is that potent volatile anesthetics are acceptable choices for thoracic surgery requiring one-lung ventilation, particularly in view

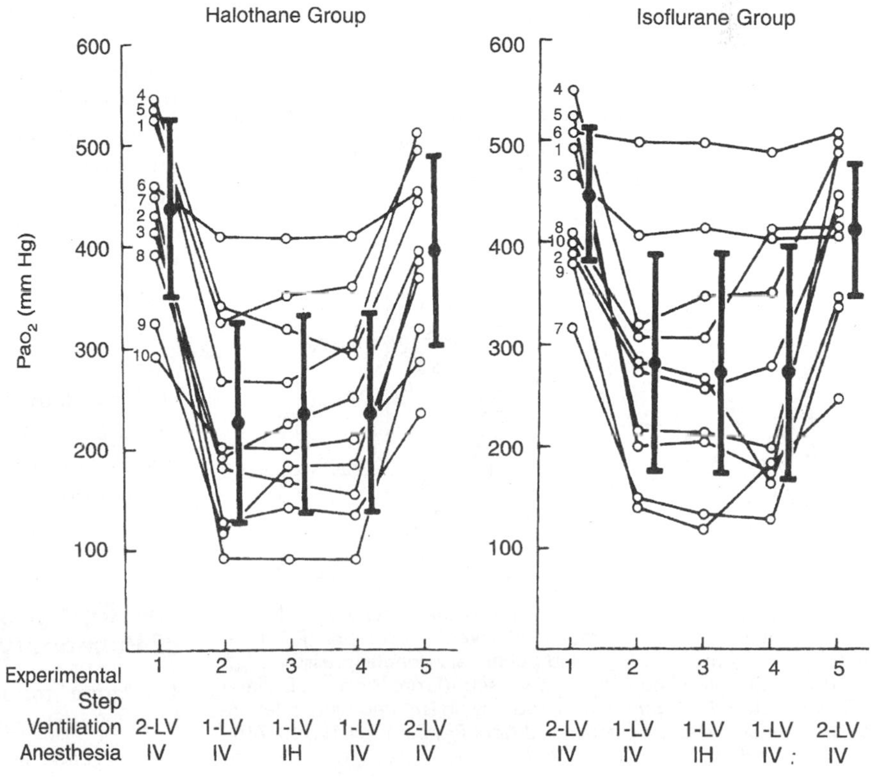

Figure 47-5. Pa_{O_2} was measured during two-lung ventilation (2-LV) and then during one-lung ventilation (1 LV) in patients anesthetized with fentanyl and diazepam without halothane or isoflurane (experimental steps 2 and 4) and with halothane or isoflurane (experimental step 3). Addition of halothane or isoflurane (about 1.2 MAC) does not alter the Pa_{O_2}, suggesting these drugs do not inhibit hypoxic pulmonary vasoconstriction. Clear circles are individual patient data and closed circles are mean ± SD for each group. (From Rogers SN, Benumof JL. Halothane and isoflurane do not decrease Pa_{O_2} during one-lung ventilation in intravenously anesthetized patients. *Anesth Analg* 1985;64: 946–954; with permission.)

of the beneficial effects of these drugs on bronchomotor tone and their high potency that permits delivery of maximal concentrations of oxygen (Eisenkraft, 1990).

Effect of Breathing

During spontaneous respiration, venous return to the heart is increased due to contraction of the diaphragm and abdominal muscles, which decreases intrathoracic pressure. The resulting augmented blood flow to the right atrium increases right ventricular stroke volume. In contrast to spontaneous breathing, positive pressure ventilation increases intrathoracic pressure and thus impedes venous return to the heart and decreases right ventricular stroke volume.

Hydrostatic Pressure Gradients

Blood flow to the lungs in the upright position is to a certain extent gravity dependent. Pressure in the pulmonary artery decreases by about 1.25 mm Hg for every centimeter of vertical distance traveled up the lung. The amount of blood flow to the various areas of the lung along this vertical axis depends on the relationship between pulmonary artery pressure, alveolar pressure, and pulmonary venous pressure (Permutt and Riley, 1963). Traditionally, the lung is divided into three blood flow zones, reflecting the impact of alveolar pressure, pulmonary artery pressure, and pulmonary venous pressure on the caliber of pulmonary blood vessels (Fig. 47-6) (West et al., 1964). The limits of these zones are not fixed and vary with physiologic or pathologic changes.

Zone 1

Zone 1 is the upper part of the lung, where alveolar pressure exceeds pulmonary artery pressure, leading to collapse of the pulmonary capillaries. The absence of pulmonary blood flow to this area means that ventilation to corresponding alveoli represents dead space or wasted ventilation. Normally, zone 1 is of limited extent, but when pulmonary artery pressure decreases (hypovolemia, decreased cardiac output) or alveolar pressure increases (positive-pressure ventilation of the lungs, positive end-expiratory pressure), zone 1 may extend, causing a wide discrepancy between $PaCO_2$ and $PETCO_2$. Indeed, it is not uncommon for the gradient between arterial and exhaled PCO_2 to increase during general anesthesia, presumably reflecting changes in perfusion pressures, effects of positive-pressure ventilation, or both.

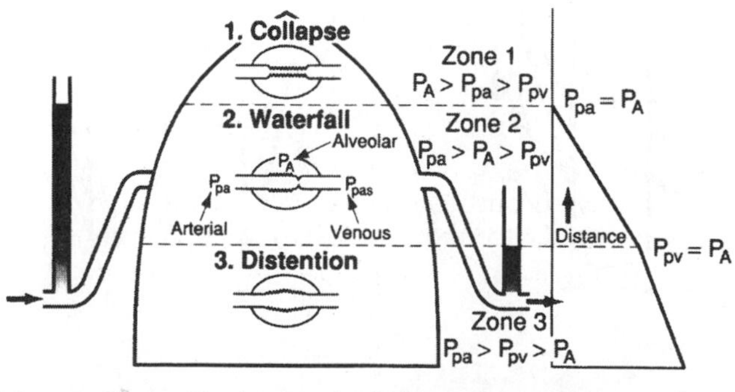

Figure 47-6. The lung is divided into three pulmonary blood flow zones reflecting the impact of alveolar pressure (P_A), pulmonary artery pressure (P_{pa}), and pulmonary venous pressure (P_{pv}) on the caliber of pulmonary blood vessels. (From West JB, Dollery CT, Naimark A. Distribution of blood flow in isolated lung: relation to vascular and alveolar pressures. *J Appl Physiol* 1964;19:713–718; with permission.)

Zone 2

Flow in zone 2 is increased compared to zone 1 but may be intermittent because pulmonary artery pressure exceeds alveolar pressure during systole but not diastole. In a standing patient, zone 2 begins 7 to 10 cm above the level of the heart and extends to the uppermost portions of the lungs. Blood flow increases toward the more dependent portions of zone 2 because it is the difference between the arterial and alveolar pressures that determine flow. The downstream pressure (venous pressure) has no influence upon the flow unless it exceeds the alveolar pressure. Thus, zone 2 is referred to as a *Starling resistor* or *waterfall zone* by analogy to a waterfall over a dam, where the height of the dam has little influence on the water flow.

Zone 3

Zone 3 is termed the *distension zone* because pulmonary artery pressure always exceeds alveolar pressure, and pulmonary blood flow is continuous. This zone extends from about 7 to 10 cm above the heart to the lowermost portions of the lungs. In the supine position, all portions of the lungs become zone 3, with pulmonary blood flow being more evenly distributed. Increases in pulmonary artery pressure, as with exercise, recruit previously underperfused capillaries, converting most of the lungs to a zone 3 pattern of pulmonary blood flow where flow is determined by the difference between the arterial and venous pressures.

Zone 4

Under certain circumstances there may also be a region of reduced blood flow near the bottom of the lung (zone 4, not shown in Fig. 47-6). Flow in zone 4 is diminished by gravitational compression of the lung parenchyma or by interstitial edema formation.

The Topographic Distribution of Pulmonary Blood Flow

The "zone" model of the lung predicts there will be greater blood flow in areas of the lung that are below the level of the heart and less flow in areas above the level of the heart.

This model also suggests that pulmonary blood flow will be uniform in gravitationally level planes (isogravitational levels). Measurements confirm that the first prediction is correct; on average, pulmonary blood flow is greater in areas of the lung below the heart as compared to those above the heart. (Glenny et al., 1999). However, the second part of the prediction, that pulmonary blood flow is uniform in isogravitational planes, turns out to be incorrect. Measurements demonstrate greater variation from spot to spot in any isogravitational plane than there is on average from the top of the lung to the bottom. Indeed, only 25% of the variability in pulmonary blood flow is accounted for by gravitational effects. Furthermore, the local differences in flow at any isogravitational level are fairly constant over time, suggesting that approximately 75% of the distribution of pulmonary blood flow is determined by the branching structure of the pulmonary vascular tree. Therefore, while the West "zonal" model adds to the understanding of pulmonary blood flow, other factors predominate over gravitational effects on pulmonary blood flow distribution.

PULMONARY EDEMA

Pulmonary edema is present when there are excessive quantities of fluid either in pulmonary interstitial spaces or in alveoli. Mild degrees of pulmonary edema may be limited to only an increase in the interstitial fluid volume. The alveolar epithelium, however, is not able to withstand more than a modest increase in interstitial fluid pressure before fluid spills into alveoli. Dehydrating forces of the colloid osmotic pressure of the blood in the lungs provide a large safety factor against development of pulmonary edema. In humans, plasma colloid osmotic pressure is about 28 mm Hg, so pulmonary edema rarely develops below a pulmonary capillary pressure of 30 mm Hg. The most common cause of acute pulmonary edema is greatly increased pulmonary capillary pressure resulting from left ventricular failure and pooling of blood in the lungs.

During chronic increases of left atrial pressure, pulmonary edema may not occur despite pulmonary capillary pressures as high as 45 mm Hg. Enlargement of the pulmonary lymph vessels allowing lymph flow to increase up to 20 times is the most likely reason pulmonary edema does not occur in the presence of chronically increased left atrial pressures.

Pulmonary edema can also result from local capillary damage that occurs with inhalation of acidic gastric fluid or irritant gases, such as smoke. The result is rapid transudation of fluid and proteins into alveoli and interstitial spaces. This is called "permeability" pulmonary edema to distinguish it from "hydrostatic" pulmonary edema, which is due to increased pulmonary capillary pressure. Both "permeability" and "hydrostatic" pulmonary edema cause impaired gas exchange because of V/Q mismatch. In pulmonary edema, fluid-filled alveoli decrease lung compliance, which markedly increases the work of breathing.

EVENTS THAT INFLUENCE PULMONARY BLOOD FLOW

Causes of obstruction to pulmonary blood flow include gaseous or particulate emboli. Less dramatic increases in resistance to pulmonary blood flow may occur with conditions such as atelectasis, pulmonary emphysema, and anthracosis, and in which there is loss of functioning lung tissues or surface area.

Pulmonary Embolism

Total blockage of one of the major branches of the pulmonary artery by an embolus is usually not immediately fatal because the opposite lung is able to accommodate all the pulmonary blood flow. As the blood clot extends, however, death ensues because of right ventricular failure due to excessive increases in pulmonary artery pressure. Tachypnea and dyspnea are characteristic responses in awake patients experiencing pulmonary embolism. Tachypnea may reflect stimulation of pulmonary deflation receptors that are innervated by the vagus nerves. Anticoagulation is recommended to prevent extension of the clot, and in some patients, surgical removal of the embolus may be life saving.

Diffuse pulmonary emboli, as occurs with fat, air, or clot produces increased pulmonary artery pressures similar to those that occur with an isolated embolus. In addition, reflex-mediated pulmonary vasospasm initiated by pulmonary emboli further increases resistance to blood flow. This vasospasm may reflect reflex sympathetic nervous system stimulation or local release of chemical mediators, such as histamine or serotonin.

Atelectasis

Atelectasis most commonly occurs when pulmonary blood flow absorbs air from unventilated alveoli, as occurs when secretions plug bronchi. Continued perfusion in the absence of ventilation removes oxygen from the alveolar air space. Subsequent collapse of these alveoli increases local resistance to pulmonary blood flow and the addition of hypoxic pulmonary vasoconstriction diverts pulmonary blood flow to better ventilated alveoli. This response will tend to restore V/Q matching and hence oxygenation towards normal.

Pulmonary Emphysema

Destruction of alveoli that characterizes pulmonary emphysema is accompanied by a concomitant loss of pulmonary vasculature, thus decreasing the cross-sectional area of the pulmonary circulation and increasing pulmonary artery pressures. Pulmonary hypertension is further exaggerated by arterial hypoxemia, which stimulates hypoxic pulmonary vasoconstriction. Hypoxia-induced increases in cardiac output further increase pulmonary artery pressure. Patients with long-standing emphysema will develop hypertrophy of the right ventricle. Modest increases in the inhaled concentrations of oxygen may be sufficient to lower pulmonary artery pressures in these patients and attenuate the adverse effects on right ventricular function.

Anthracosis

Anthracosis is an example of a condition in which there is fibrosis of the supportive tissues in the lungs. Pulmonary artery pressures may remain normal at rest. However, even modest activity may evoke dramatic increases in pulmonary artery pressures because vessels surrounded by fibrous tissue cannot expand with increases in pulmonary blood flow. In chronic situations, pulmonary artery pressures remain increased, and right ventricular failure eventually occurs.

REFERENCES

Carlsson AJ, Bindsley L, Hedenstierna G. Hypoxia-induced pulmonary vasoconstriction in the human lung: the effect of isoflurane anesthesia. *Anesthesiology* 1987;66:312–316.

Colley PS, Cheney FW, Hlastala MP. Ventilation-perfusion and gas exchange effects of sodium nitroprusside in dogs with normal and edematous lungs. *Anesthesiology* 1979;50:489–495.

Eisenkraft JB. Effects of anaesthetics on the pulmonary circulation. *Br J Anaesth* 1990;65:63–78.

Glenny RW, Bernard S, Robertson HT, et al. Gravity is an important but secondary determinant of regional pulmonary blood flow in upright primates. *J. Appl. Physiol.* 1999;86:623–632.

Guyton AC, Hall JE. *Textbook of medical physiology*, 10th ed. Philadelphia: Saunders, 2000.

Permutt S. Riley RL. Hemodynamics of collapsible vessels with tone: the vascular waterfall. *J. Appl. Physiol.* 1963;18:924–32.

Rogers SN, Benumof JL. Halothane and isoflurane do not decrease Pa_{O_2} during one-lung ventilation in intravenously anesthetized patients. *Anesth Analg* 1985;64:946–954.

West JB. Blood flow to the lung and gas exchange. *Anesthesiology* 1974; 41:124–138.

West JB, Dollery CT, Naimark A. Distribution of blood flow in isolated lung: relation to vascular and alveolar pressures. *J Appl Physiol* 1964;19:713–718.

Heart

48

CARDIAC PHYSIOLOGY

The heart can be characterized as a pulsatile four-chamber pump composed of two atria and two ventricles. The atria function primarily as conduits (primer pumps) to the ventricles, but they also contract weakly to facilitate movement of blood into the ventricles. The ventricles serve as power pumps to supply the main force that propels blood through the systemic and pulmonary circulations. *Systole* means contraction and is the time interval between closure of the tricuspid and mitral valves and closure of the pulmonary and aortic valves. *Diastole* is a period of relaxation corresponding to the interval between closure of the pulmonary and aortic valves and closure of the tricuspid and mitral valves. Special mechanisms in the heart maintain cardiac rhythm and transmit action potentials through cardiac muscle to initiate contraction. Because the heart is coupled to two circulations, its function is influenced by the characteristics of these two circulations. During normal physiologic conditions, the systemic circulation plays a dominant role in the function of the heart by modifying its venous return and its resistance to ejection through changes in vasomotor tone reflecting changes in metabolic requirements.

Cardiac Muscle

Cardiac muscle is a syncytium in which the cells are so tightly bound together that when one of these cells becomes excited, the action potential spreads to all of them. As a result, stimulation of a single atrial or ventricular cell causes the action potential to travel over the entire muscle mass such that the atria or ventricles contract as a single unit. The atrial syncytium is separated from the ventricular syncytium by the fibrous tissues surrounding the valvular rings. The cardiac action potential is conducted from the atrial syncytium to the ventricular syncytium by a specialized conduction pathway known as the *atrioventricular bundle*. Cardiac muscle, like skeletal muscles, is striated and contains actin and myosin filaments. These filaments interdigitate and slide along each other during contraction in the same manner as occurs in skeletal muscles.

Cardiac Action Potential

The normal cardiac action potential results from time-dependent changes in the permeability of cardiac muscle cell membranes to sodium, potassium, calcium, and chloride ions during phases 0 to 4 of the action potential (Table 48-1) (Fig. 48-1). The resting transmembrane potential of normal cardiac muscle cell membranes is about −90 mv and is designated phase 4. Depolarization and reversal of the transmembrane potential is designated phase 0, whereas the three phases of repolarization are labeled 1, 2, and 3. In nonpacemaker contractile atrial and ventricular cardiac cells, phase 4 is constant during diastole, and these cells remain at rest until activated by a propagated cardiac impulse or an external stimulus. In contrast, pacemaker cardiac cells exhibit spontaneous phase 4 depolarization until threshold potential is reached (about −70 mv), resulting in self-excitation and propagation of a cardiac action potential. Indeed, the principal distinguishing feature of pacemaker cells is the presence of spontaneous phase 4 depolarization in the absence of external stimulation. Compared with the transmembrane potential recorded from ventricular myocardial cells, the resting potential of sinoatrial node pacemaker cells is usually less (about −60 mv), the upstroke of phase 0 has a slower velocity, a plateau is absent, and repolarization (phase 3) is more gradual (see Fig. 48-1).

Phase 0 of the cardiac action potential is generated by the brief but intense inward movement of sodium ions through specific protein ion channels that are activated when spontaneous phase 4 depolarization reaches threshold potential. The rate of depolarization during phase 0 is referred to as V_{max}. V_{max} is a reflection of myocardial contractility. During phase 0, the resting transmembrane potential across cardiac cells relative to extracellular fluid changes from about −90 mv to a peak spike potential of about 20 mv (see Fig. 48-1). Repolarization that follows phase 0 includes a brief phase 1 followed by a plateau lasting up to 150 ms. Phase 2 reflects closure of sodium ion channels and inward flux of calcium ions through specific slow calcium ion channels. The plateau characterizing phase 2 of the cardiac action potential of ventricular contractile

TABLE 48-1.
ION MOVEMENT DURING PHASES OF THE CARDIAC ACTION POTENTIAL

Phase	Ion	Movement across Cell Membranes
0	Sodium	In
1	Potassium	Out
	Chloride	In
2	Calcium	In
	Potassium	Out
3	Potassium	Out
4	Sodium	In

cells provides the sustained contraction of ventricular muscle fibers necessary to eject blood and distinguishes these cardiac action potentials from those developed by skeletal muscle cells. Phase 3 is due principally to a return to normal of cardiac cell membrane permeability to sodium ions and a sudden increase in permeability to potassium ions, allowing rapid loss of these ions so as to restore the transmembrane potential to −90 mv.

The frequency of discharge of cardiac pacemaker cells is determined by the rate of phase 4 depolarization, the threshold potential, and the resting transmembrane potential (Fig. 48-2). When the rate of spontaneous phase 4 depolarization increases, the threshold potential is reached sooner and the heart rate increases. A similar response occurs when the rate of spontaneous phase 4 depolarization remains constant but the threshold potential becomes more negative or the resting transmembrane potential becomes less negative. Norepinephrine increases heart rate by increasing the rate of spontaneous phase 4 depolarization. Conversely, vagal stimulation through the release of acetylcholine diminishes the heart rate by hyperpolarizing cardiac pacemaker cells and decreasing the slope of spontaneous phase 4 depolarization.

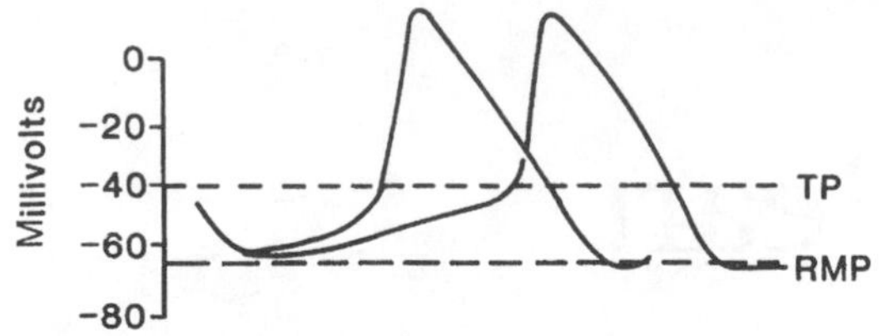

Figure 48-2. The rate of pacemaker discharge is dependent on the slope of spontaneous phase 4 depolarization, negativity of the threshold potential (TP), and negativity of the resting transmembrane potential (RMP).

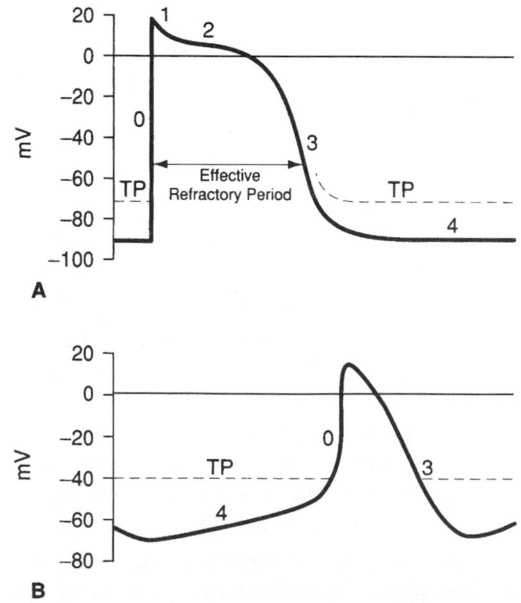

Figure 48-1. Cardiac action potential recorded from a ventricular contractile cell (**A**) or an atrial pacemaker cell (**B**). (TP, threshold potential.)

Cardiac muscle, like other excitable tissues, is refractory to stimulation during the action potential. The absolute refractory period of ventricular cells extends through phases 1, 2, and part of phase 3 of the cardiac action potential. During the remainder of phase 3, ventricular cells respond to stimuli of greater than normal intensity (relative refractory period). The absolute refractory period of atrial muscle is shorter than that of ventricular muscle such that the rhythmic rate of contraction of the atria can be much faster than that of the ventricles.

Cardiac Cycle

The cardiac cycle consists of a period of relaxation (diastole) followed by a period of contraction (systole) (Fig. 48-3) (Guyton and Hall, 2000). Each cardiac cycle is initiated by the spontaneous generation of an action potential in the sinoatrial node. Delay of transmission of this action potential for 0.1 s in the atrioventricular node allows the atria to contract before the ventricles, thereby pumping blood into the ventricles before forceful ventricular contraction. As such, the atria act as primer pumps for the ventricles, and the ventricles then provide the major source of power for forcing blood through the systemic and pulmonary circulations. Excessive increases in heart rate may so shorten diastole that insufficient time is available for complete filling of the cardiac chambers before systole.

Atrial Pressure Curves

Atrial pressure curves exhibit characteristic waveforms that may reflect specific cardiac abnormalities (see Fig. 48-3) (see Table 45-2 and Fig. 45-8) (Guyton and Hall, 2000). Ordinarily, right atrial pressure is 4 to 6 mm Hg, and left atrial pressure is 6 to 8 mm Hg during atrial contraction. The c wave occurs when the ventricles begin to contract and is caused by bulging of the tricuspid and mitral valves backward toward the atria because of increasing pressure in

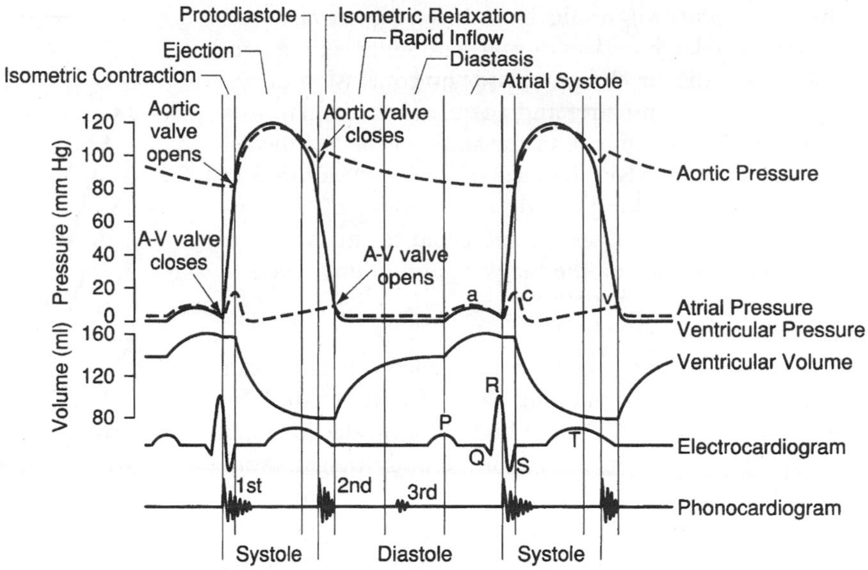

Figure 48-3. Events of the cardiac cycle, including changes in intravascular pressures, ventricular volume, electrocardiogram, and phonocardiogram. (A-V, atrioventricular.) (From Guyton AC, Hall JE. *Textbook of medical physiology*, 10th ed. Philadelphia: Saunders, 2000; with permission.)

the ventricles. In addition, pulling on atrial muscle by the contracting ventricles contributes to the c wave. Atrial contraction is responsible for the a wave, explaining the absence of this wave in the presence of atrial fibrillation. The v wave occurs toward the end of ventricular contraction and is due to accumulation of blood in the atria. Retrograde flow into the atria through an incompetent tricuspid or mitral valve will manifest as a large v wave. Likewise, acute mitral regurgitation secondary to papillary muscle ischemia due to coronary artery disease (CAD) may be first recognized by the appearance of a large v wave on the recording of left atrial pressure from a pulmonary artery catheter.

Atria as Pumps

During ventricular systole, large amounts of blood accumulate in the atria because of the closed tricuspid and mitral valves. At the conclusion of ventricular systole and when ventricular pressures decrease rapidly, the higher pressures in the atria force the valves open and allow blood to flow rapidly into the ventricles. This period of rapid ventricular filling lasts for the first one-third of diastole and accounts for about 70% of the blood that enters the ventricles. During the latter portion of diastole, the atria contracts to deliver about 30% of the blood that normally enters the ventricle during each cardiac cycle. This component of ventricular filling is lost during atrial fibrillation and contributes to the decrease in stroke volume that accompanies this cardiac dysrhythmia.

Ventricles as Pumps

The start of ventricular systole causes an abrupt increase in intraventricular pressure, resulting in closure of the tricuspid and mitral valves (see Fig. 48-3) (Guyton and Hall, 2000). An additional 0.02 to 0.03 s is required for each ventricle to develop sufficient pressure to open the pulmonary and aortic valves, which are kept closed by the back pressure of blood in the pulmonary artery and aorta. During this brief period of isovolemic contraction, there is no blood ejection from the ventricles. When intraventricular pressures are sufficient, the pulmonary and aortic valves open and about 60% of the total ventricular ejection of blood occurs during the first one-fourth of systole. At the end of systole, intraventricular pressures decrease rapidly, allowing higher pressures in the arteries to close the pulmonary and aortic valves.

During diastole, filling of the ventricles with blood from the atria normally increases the volume of blood in each ventricle to about 130 mL. This volume is known as the *end-diastolic volume*. Subsequent ventricular ejection creates a stroke volume of about 70 mL. The remaining volume in the ventricle is called the *end-systolic volume*. The ejection fraction (ratio of stroke volume to end-diastolic volume) is a clinically useful measurement of left ventricular function (Robotham et al., 1991). For example, ejection fraction is decreased (<0.4) in patients with left ventricular dysfunction as due to myocardial ischemia or myocardial infarction (MI). Conversely, an ejection fraction of >0.8 may accompany intense sympathetic nervous system stimulation or the presence of hypertrophic cardiomyopathy. Angiographic techniques and echocardiography are used to make the measurements necessary to calculate the ejection fraction.

Function of the Heart Valves

Heart valves open passively along a pressure gradient and close when a backward pressure gradient develops due to high pressure in the pulmonary artery and aorta. Papillary muscles are attached to the tricuspid and mitral valves by chordae tendineae. These papillary muscles prevent the valves from bulging too far backward into the atria during ventricular systole. Rupture of a chorda tendineae or dysfunction of a papillary muscle, as may accompany myocardial ischemia or acute MI, results in an incompetent valve and appearance of large v waves during ventricular contraction.

High pressures in the arteries at the conclusion of systole cause the pulmonary and aortic valves to snap to a closed position in contrast to the softer closure of the tricuspid and mitral valves. Because of the rapid closure and rapid velocity of blood ejection, the edges of the pulmonary and aortic valves are subjected to much greater mechanical trauma than the tricuspid and mitral valves.

Work of the Heart

The work of the heart is the amount of energy that the heart converts to work while pumping blood into the arteries. The heart accounts for 12% of total body heat production even though it represents only 0.5% of the body weight. Work required to increase the pressure for ejection of blood is calculated as stroke volume times ejection pressure. Right ventricular work output is usually about one-seventh the work output of the left ventricle because of the difference in systolic pressure against which the two ventricles must pump. The energy required for the work of the heart is derived mainly from metabolism of fatty acids and, to a lesser extent, of other nutrients, especially lactate and glucose.

Intrinsic Autoregulation of Cardiac Function

The intrinsic ability of the heart to adapt to changing venous return (preload) reflects the increased stretch of cardiac muscle produced by increased filling of the ventricles from the atria and is called the *Frank-Starling* law of the heart. Indeed, the most important factor determining cardiac output is the atrial pressure created by venous return. When cardiac muscle becomes stretched, it contracts with greater force (analogous to increased stretch of a rubber band), thereby pumping additional blood into the arteries. The ability of stretched cardiac muscle to contract with increased force is characteristic of all striated muscle, not just cardiac muscle. The increased force of contraction is probably caused by the fact that actin and myosin filaments are brought to a more nearly optimal degree of interdigitation for achieving contraction. A plot of cardiac output with changes in atrial filling pressures (ventricular function curves) reflects the degree of stretch applied to cardiac muscle (see Fig. 45-12). In the presence of ventricular dysfunction, the heart may not be able to pump all the blood it receives and filling pressures increase.

Neural Control of the Heart

The atria are abundantly innervated by the sympathetic and parasympathetic nervous systems, but the ventricles are supplied principally by the sympathetic nervous system (Fig. 48-4) (Guyton and Hall, 2000). These nerves affect cardiac output by changing the heart rate and strength of myocardial contraction. Sympathetic nervous system fibers to the heart continually discharge at a slow rate that maintains a strength of ventricular contraction about 20% to

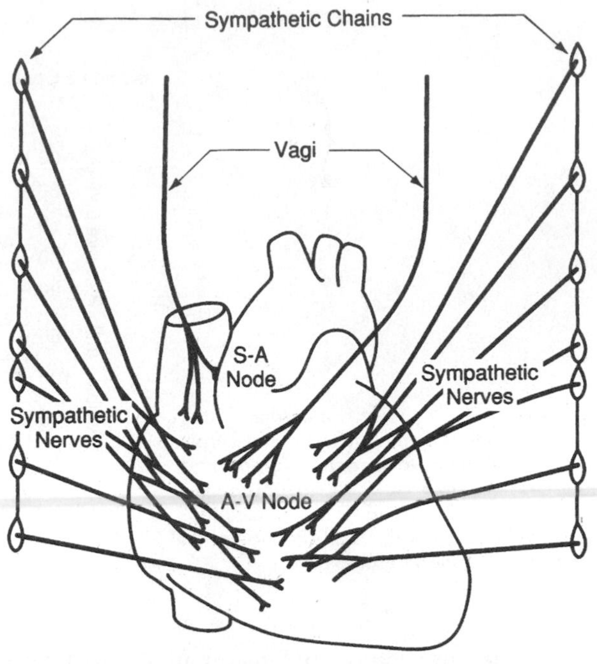

Figure 48-4. Innervation of the atria is from the sympathetic and parasympathetic (vagi) nervous systems, whereas the ventricles are innervated principally by the sympathetic nervous system. A-V, atrioventricular; S-A, sinoatrial. (From Guyton AC, Hall JE. *Textbook of medical physiology*, 10th ed. Philadelphia: Saunders, 2000; with permission.)

25% above its strength in the absence of sympathetic nervous system stimulation. Maximal sympathetic nervous system stimulation can increase cardiac output by about 100% above normal. Conversely, maximal parasympathetic nervous system stimulation decreases ventricular contractile strength and subsequent cardiac output only by about 30%, emphasizing that parasympathetic nervous system stimulation of the heart is small compared with the effect of sympathetic nervous system stimulation. Increased myocardial contractility associated with sympathetic nervous system stimulation of the heart is most likely due to norepinephrine-induced increases in the permeability of cardiac muscle cell membranes to calcium ions.

CORONARY BLOOD FLOW

Unique features of coronary blood flow include interruption of blood flow during systole due to mechanical compression of vessels by myocardial contraction and the absence of anastomoses between the left and right coronary arteries. Another characteristic of the coronary circulation is the maximal oxygen extraction (approximately 70%) that occurs, resulting in a coronary venous oxygen saturation of about 30%.

Anatomy of the Coronary Circulation

The two coronary arteries that supply the myocardium arise from the sinuses of Valsalva located behind the cusps

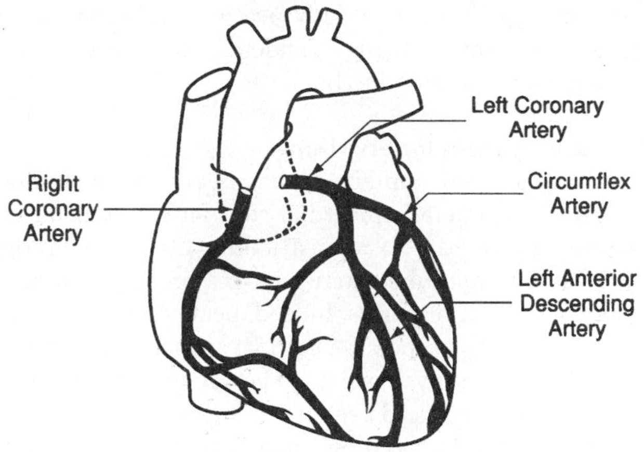

Figure 48-5. Anatomy of the coronary circulation.

of the aortic valve at the root of the aorta (Fig. 48-5). Resting coronary blood flow is 225 to 250 mL/minute, or 4% to 5% of the cardiac output. Assuming the normal adult heart weighs about 280 g, this is equivalent to a blood flow of 75 mL/100 g/minute.

Resting myocardial oxygen consumption is 8 to 10 mL/100 g/minute, or about 10% of the total body consumption of oxygen. Oxygen consumption of the arrested, nondistended, and normothermic heart is 1 mL/100 g/minute compared with 5 mL/100 g/minute in both the arrested distended and beating but empty heart. Lowering myocardial temperature from 37 °C to 11 °C produces only a modest (5%) further decrease in myocardial oxygen consumption compared with the arrested and nondistended heart (Noble et al., 1991). This may be an important consideration if hypothermic-induced damage to cellular membranes during cardiopulmonary bypass is a consideration.

The left coronary artery divides shortly after its origin into the left anterior descending and circumflex arteries, which supply the anterior part of the left ventricle. The right coronary artery supplies the right ventricle and the posterior portion of the left ventricle. In about 50% of individuals, more blood flows through the right coronary artery than the left, in about 30% the flow in both arteries is similar, and in about 20% the left coronary artery is dominant. These large coronary arteries lie predominantly on the epicardial surface of the heart and serve principally as conductance vessels that offer little resistance to coronary blood flow. The second type of vessels are small coronary arterioles that ramify throughout the cardiac muscle. These arterioles impose a highly variable resistance and regulate distribution of blood flow in the myocardium. Atherosclerosis characterized as coronary artery disease (CAD) involves the epicardial coronary arteries and not the coronary arterioles.

Coronary blood flow, especially to the left ventricle, occurs predominantly during diastole when cardiac muscle relaxes and no longer obstructs blood flow through ventricular capillaries (Fig. 48-6) (Berne et al., 2004). It is

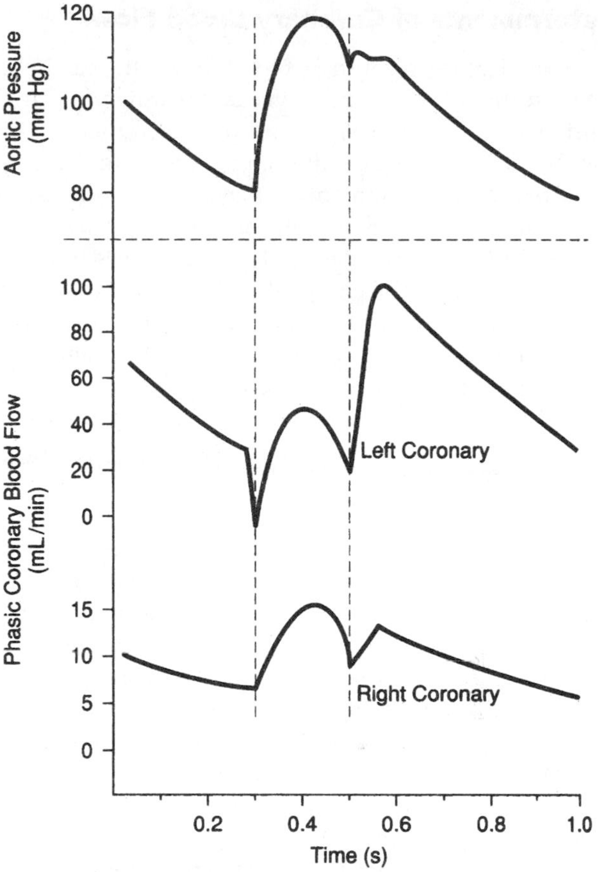

Figure 48-6. Phasic left and right coronary artery blood flow in relation to aortic pressures. (From Berne RM, Levy MD, Koeppen BM. *Physiology*, 5th ed. St Louis, Mosby, 2004; with permission.)

estimated that at least 75% of total coronary blood flow occurs during diastole. During systole, blood flow through subendocardial arteries of the left ventricle decreases to almost zero, which is consistent with the observation that the subendocardial region of the left ventricle is the most common site for myocardial infarction (MI). Tachycardia, with an associated decrease in the time for coronary blood flow to occur during diastole, further jeopardizes the adequacy of myocardial oxygen delivery, particularly if coronary arteries are narrowed by atherosclerosis. The impact of systole on coronary blood flow through the right ventricle is minimal. This reflects the fact that systemic pressure in the coronary arteries is greater than the cavitary pressure developed in the right ventricle.

Most of the venous blood that has perfused the left ventricle enters the right atrium via the coronary sinus. This accounts for about 75% of the total coronary blood flow. Most of the coronary blood flow to the right ventricle enters anterior cardiac veins that empty into the right atrium independent of the coronary sinus. A small amount of coronary blood flows back into the heart through thebesian veins that can empty into any cardiac chamber. Thebesian veins that empty into the left side of the heart contribute to the inherent anatomic shunt.

Determinants of Coronary Blood Flow

A striking feature of coronary blood flow is the parallelism between the local metabolic needs of cardiac muscle for nutrients, especially oxygen, and the magnitude of coronary blood flow. This parallelism is present in the denervated heart and presumably reflects the local release of vasodilator substances that dilate coronary arteries. The most potent local vasodilator substance released by cardiac cells is adenosine. The endothelium of the coronary circulation is capable of releasing endothelium-dependent vasodilator substances such as prostacyclin and nitric oxide. Increased extraction of oxygen is not likely to offset local increases in oxygen needs because even in the normal resting state, oxygen extraction by cardiac cells is nearly maximal (approaches 70%). This means that increases in myocardial oxygen consumptions must be met by commensurate increases in coronary blood flow, because there is little additional oxygen extraction that can occur.

Arterial blood pressure acts as the perfusion pressure to drive blood through coronary arteries. For example, an increase in perfusion pressure increases coronary blood flow. This increased flow, however, is transient, as autoregulation of coronary artery tone acts to return blood flow toward normal. Perfusion pressure is particularly important in maintaining coronary blood flow through atherosclerotic arteries that cannot dilate in response to autoregulatory mechanisms (pressure-dependent perfusion).

Myocardial Oxygen Consumption

Sympathetic nervous system stimulation with associated increases in heart rate, systemic blood pressure, and myocardial contractility results in increased myocardial oxygen consumption. Increases in heart rate that shorten diastolic time for coronary blood flow are likely to increase myocardial oxygen consumption more than increases in systemic blood pressure, which are likely to offset increased oxygen demands by enhanced pressure-dependent coronary blood flow. This is the reason that the absolute value of the rate-pressure product (product of heart rate and systolic blood pressure) is less important as an estimation of myocardial oxygen consumption than the absolute value of the individual components used to calculate the product. Furthermore, the validity of maintaining the rate-pressure product below a certain value (usually $<12,000$) has not been proved to be efficacious in anesthetized patients.

Increasing venous return (volume work) is the least costly means of increasing cardiac output in terms of myocardial oxygen consumption. This emphasizes that the most important aspect of hemodynamic management is to first optimize venous return by appropriate adjustments in the intravascular fluid volume. Usually, increases in myocardial oxygen consumption are paralleled by increases in coronary blood flow, resulting in a remarkably constant coronary sinus oxygen saturation of about 30% (Po_2 18 to 20 mm Hg). When myocardial oxygenation is inadequate, the heart produces lactate, with increases in coronary sinus lactate concentration being considered a conclusive indicator of global myocardial ischemia.

Nervous System Innervation

Coronary arteries contain alpha, beta, and histamine receptors. In general, epicardial coronary arteries have a preponderance of vasoconstricting alpha receptors, whereas intramuscular arteries have a preponderance of vasodilating beta receptors. Indeed, beta-adrenergic antagonists are likely to increase coronary vascular resistance, but decreases in myocardial oxygen requirements occur because of drug-induced decreases in heart rate and myocardial contractility. H_1 receptors mediate coronary artery vasoconstriction, whereas H_2 receptors are responsible for coronary artery vasodilation. It is conceivable that H_2 antagonists administered preoperatively could allow H_1 vasoconstrictor effects to become predominant in the coronary arteries in the same manner as described for changes in bronchomotor tone. In some individuals, alpha-vasoconstrictor effects seem to be excessive, resulting in vasospastic myocardial ischemia (Prinzmetal angina). Venous smooth muscle contains alpha receptors, emphasizing the potential for venoconstriction after coronary artery bypass operations using venous grafts. This venoconstriction is readily offset by nitroglycerin. The distribution of parasympathetic nervous system fibers to the coronary arteries in the ventricles is sparse, and any direct effect on coronary blood flow as a result of vagal-induced vasodilation is likely to be modest.

Coronary Artery Steal

Coronary artery steal is an absolute decrease in collateral-dependent myocardial perfusion at the expense of an increase in blood flow to a normally perfused area of

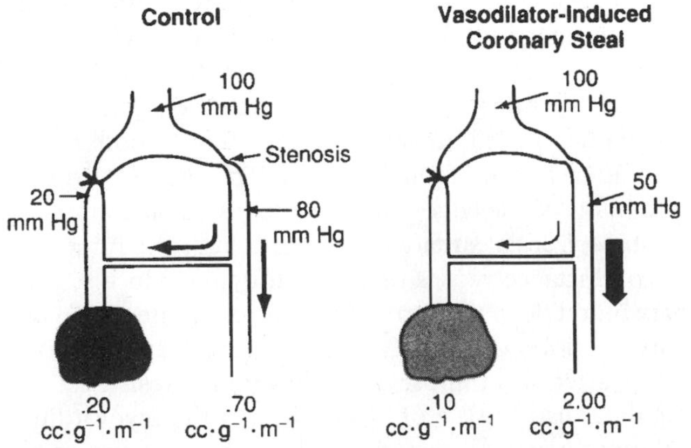

Figure 48-7. Schematic depiction of vasodilatory-induced coronary steal. After distal coronary artery vasodilation, flow increases to the normally perfused area and there is a significant pressure decrease across the stenosis that reduces the pressure gradient across the collateral bed. (From Cason BA, Verrier ED, London MJ, et al. Effects of isoflurane and halothane on coronary vascular resistance and collateral myocardial blood flow: their capacity to induce coronary steal. *Anesthesiology* 1987;67:665–675; with permission.)

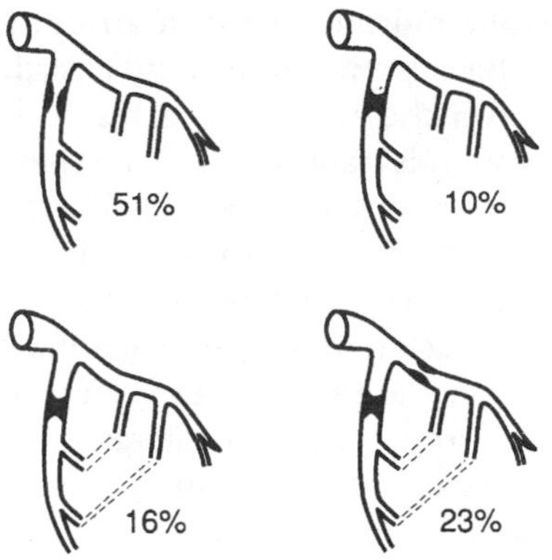

Figure 48-8. Anatomic variants of CAD and the incidence on coronary angiograms. Steal-prone anatomy is present on 23% (*lower right*) of the angiograms because arteriolar dilation decreases pressure distal to the stenosis and decreases flow through the high-resistance collaterals. (From Buffington CW, Davis KB, Gillespie S, et al. The prevalence of steal-prone coronary anatomy in patients with CAD: an analysis of the coronary artery surgery registry. *Anesthesiology* 1988;69:721–727; with permission.)

myocardium, as may follow drug-induced vasodilation of coronary arterioles (Fig. 48-7) (Becker, 1978; Cason et al., 1987). Conceptually, diseased coronary arterioles might be fully dilated to compensate for the increased resistance imposed by narrowed atherosclerotic vessels. Drug-induced vasodilation of normal coronary arterioles might then divert (steal) blood flow from potentially ischemic areas of myocardium being perfused by atherosclerotic vessels. There is evidence that drugs that produce arteriolar vasodilation (nitroprusside and isoflurane but not desflurane and sevoflurane) can redistribute coronary blood flow under certain conditions leading to myocardial ischemia in patients with CAD (see Chapter 2) (Priebe, 1989). Coronary artery steal is most likely to occur in those patients with steal-prone anatomy. Steal-prone anatomy is characterized by one or more total occlusions of a coronary artery and a concomitant, hemodynamically significant stenosis (>90%) of the collateral supply vessel. An estimated 23% of patients with CAD have a zone of collateral-dependent myocardium that is supplied by a vessel with proximal stenosis (steal-prone anatomy) (Fig. 48-8) (Buffington et al., 1988).

DYNAMICS OF HEART SOUNDS

Closure of the heart valves creates sudden pressure differentials such that blood vibrates, creating a sound that travels in all directions through the chest. In contrast, opening of heart valves is a relatively slow-developing process that makes no audible sound.

First and Second Heart Sounds

Closure of the mitral and tricuspid valves produces the first heart sound, whereas the second heart sound is due to closure of the aortic and pulmonary valves (see Fig. 48-3) (Guyton and Hall, 2000). An audible sound is produced by vibration of the taut valves immediately after closure as well as vibration of the adjacent blood, walls of the heart, and major vessels around the heart. These vibrations then travel to the chest wall, where they can be heard as sound by a stethoscope (Fig. 48-9) (Guyton and Hall, 2000). The optimal areas for auscultation of heart sounds on the chest are not directly over the specific valve; emphasizing that sounds caused by closure of the mitral and tricuspid valves are transmitted to the chest wall through each respective ventricle. Sounds from the aortic and pulmonary valves are transmitted along the courses of the respective vessels leading from the heart.

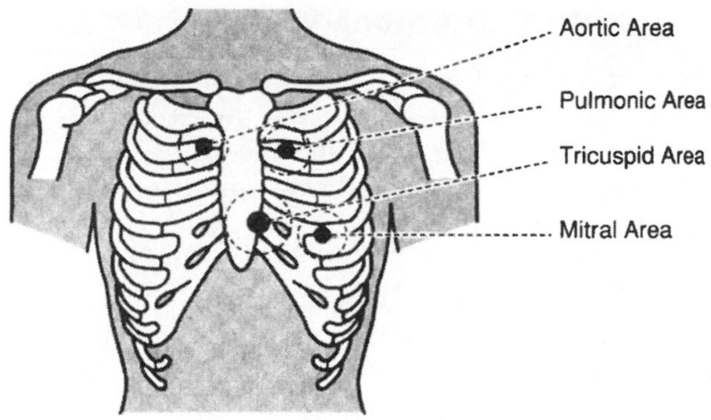

Figure 48-9. Optimal sites for auscultation of heart sounds due to opening or closure of specific cardiac valves. (From Guyton AC, Hall JE. *Textbook of medical physiology*, 10th ed. Philadelphia: Saunders, 2000; with permission.)

The loudness of the first heart sound is almost directly proportional to the rate of development of pressure differences across the mitral and tricuspid valves. For example, when the force of ventricular contraction is enhanced, the first heart sound is accentuated. Conversely, in a weakened heart in which the onset of contraction is sluggish, the intensity of the first heart sound is diminished. The loudness of the second heart sound is determined by the rate of ventricular pressure decrease at the end of systole. For this reason, the intensity of the second heart sound is accentuated in the presence of systemic or pulmonary hypertension. Conversely, when systemic blood pressure is decreased, as in shock or cardiac failure, the second heart sound as heard through a stethoscope is diminished in intensity.

Third Heart Sound

Occasionally, a third heart sound is heard at the beginning of the middle third of diastole. This sound is of such low frequency that it usually cannot be detected with a stethoscope but can be recorded on the phonocardiogram (see Fig. 48-3) (Guyton and Hall, 2000). This third heart sound is presumed to reflect the flaccid and inelastic condition of the heart during diastole.

TABLE 48-2.
HEART MURMURS

	Timing of Murmur*
Aortic stenosis	Systole
Aortic regurgitation	Diastole
Mitral stenosis	Diastole
Mitral regurgitation	Systole
Patent ductus arteriosus	Continuous
Atrial septal defect	Systole
Ventricular septal defect	Systole

*Pulmonary and tricuspid stenosis or regurgitation produces murmurs during the cardiac cycle corresponding to the similar aortic or mitral valve abnormality.

Fourth Heart Sound

The fourth heart sound is caused by rapid inflow of blood into the ventricles due to atrial contraction. The auditory frequency of this heart sound is so low that it rarely can be heard using a stethoscope.

Abnormal Heart Sounds

Abnormal heart sounds known as *murmurs* occur in the presence of abnormalities of the cardiac valves or congenital anomalies (Table 48-2).

Murmur of Aortic Stenosis

Resistance to ejection of blood through a stenotic aortic valve causes pressures in the left ventricle to increase to values as high as 350 mm Hg, whereas pressures in the aorta remain normal. Thus, a nozzle effect is created during systole, with blood jetting at a high velocity through the small opening of the aortic valve. This turbulent flow causes vibrations, and a systolic murmur is transmitted throughout the upper aorta and even into the carotid arteries.

Murmur of Aortic Regurgitation

Turbulence created by blood jetting backward into blood already in the left ventricle produces the diastolic murmur characteristic of aortic regurgitation. This murmur is not as loud as that of aortic stenosis because the pressure differential between the aorta and left ventricle is not nearly as great as it is in aortic stenosis.

Murmur of Mitral Stenosis

In the presence of mitral stenosis, a low-intensity murmur occurs in diastole. The abnormal sounds produced by mitral stenosis are of low intensity because, except for brief periods, the pressure differential forcing blood from the left atrium into the left ventricle rarely exceeds 35 mm Hg.

Murmur of Mitral Regurgitation

Backward flow of blood through an incompetent mitral valve during left ventricular contraction produces a loud, swishing systolic murmur. The left atrium is located so deeply in the chest that it is difficult to auscultate the murmur directly over the atrium. As a result, the sound of mitral regurgitation is transmitted to the chest wall mainly through the left ventricle and typically is heard maximally at the apex of the heart. Presumably, the murmur of mitral regurgitation is caused by vibrations from the turbulence of blood ejected backward through the mitral valve against the atrial wall or into blood already in the atrium. The quality of the murmur of mitral regurgitation is similar to that of aortic regurgitation, but it occurs during systole rather than diastole.

Murmur of Patent Ductus Arteriosus

In the presence of a patent ductus arteriosus, blood flows backward from the aorta into the pulmonary artery, producing a continuous (machinery) murmur. This murmur is most audible in the pulmonic area, being more intense during systole when pressure in the aorta is increased and less intense during the low-pressure phase of diastole. This accounts for a murmur that waxes and wanes with each heartbeat. At birth, the amount of reversed blood flow may be inadequate to cause a murmur.

Murmur of Atrial Septal Defect

Increased flow through the pulmonary valve in the presence of an atrial septal defect produces a characteristic pulmonary systolic ejection murmur. The pulmonary valve closes late, causing a wide splitting of the second heart sound.

Murmur of Ventricular Septal Defect

A ventricular septal defect is characterized by blood flow from the left ventricle to right ventricle resulting in a systolic murmur. This systolic murmur contrasts with the continuous murmur of patent ductus arteriosus.

CONDUCTION OF CARDIAC IMPULSES

Cardiac impulses are transmitted over a specialized conduction system in the heart, with normal impulses being spontaneously generated at the sinoatrial node so as to maintain resting heart rate at about 70 beats/minute (Fig. 48-10). The self-excitatory impulse travels from the sinoatrial node to the atrioventricular node, where it is delayed before passing into the ventricles. In the ventricles, the cardiac impulse travels via the atrioventricular bundle (bundle of His), which divides initially into the left and right bundle branches. Bundle branches then divide into a complex network of conducting fibers known as *Purkinje fibers*, which ramify over the subendocardial surfaces of both ventricles.

The role of the conduction system in the generation of cardiac dysrhythmias, is exemplified by the antidysrhythmic effects of adenosine that transiently blocks conduction

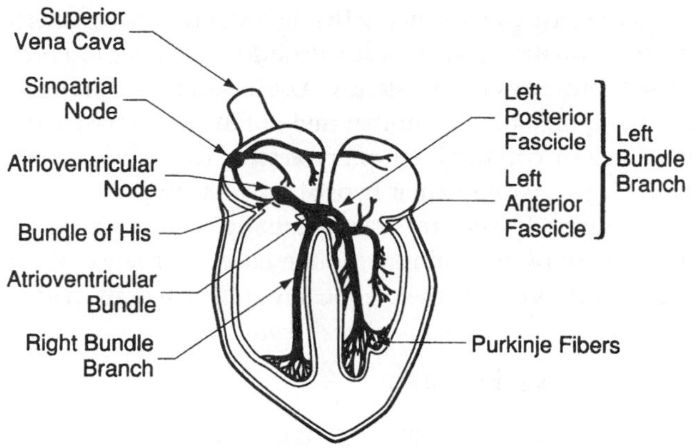

Figure 48-10. Anatomy of the conduction system for transmission of cardiac impulses.

within the atrioventricular node. This characteristic feature makes adenosine an effective treatment for terminating supraventricular tachycardia that originates in the atrioventricular node. Conversely, atrial flutter or atrial fibrillation that originate in tissues above the atrioventricular node respond to adenosine with transient slowing of the ventricular response rate reflecting slowing of passage of cardiac impulses through the atrioventricular node.

Sinoatrial Node

The sinoatrial node is a specialized cardiac muscle (15 mm long, 5 mm wide, 2 mm thick) located on the posterior surface of the heart at the site where the superior vena cava joins the right atrium. The fibers of the sinoatrial node are continuous with atrial fibers such that a cardiac action potential that begins in the sinoatrial node spreads immediately into the atria. Sinoatrial fibers exhibit a resting transmembrane potential of only about −60 mv in comparison with −90 mv in most other cardiac fibers (see Fig. 48-1). This lower resting transmembrane potential is caused by increased leakiness of the membranes of sinoatrial fibers to sodium ions and is responsible for the self-excitation and rhythmic repetitiveness of the action potential from the sinoatrial node. Immediately after the cardiac action potential ends, the sinoatrial transmembrane potential reaches its greatest degree of negativity (hyperpolarization), reflecting diffusion of potassium ions (positive charges) from the interior of the cells. As the sinoatrial membrane becomes less permeable to potassium ions and the natural leakiness of the membrane to sodium ions returns, the transmembrane potential slowly drifts back toward a less negative value (spontaneous phase 4 depolarization) until it reaches the threshold potential for self-excitation of the fiber.

Internodal Pathways

Action potentials originating in the sinoatrial node spread through the entire atrial muscle mass on their way to the atrioventricular node. There are, however, internodal pathways that conduct cardiac impulses from the sinoatrial to atrioventricular node more rapidly than in the general mass of atrial muscle.

Atrioventricular Node

The atrioventricular node is a specialized cardiac muscle (20 mm long, 10 mm wide, 3 mm thick) located on the right side of the interatrial septum near the opening of the coronary sinus. There is a delay of transmission of cardiac impulses in the atrioventricular node that allows the atria to empty blood into the ventricles before ventricular systole is initiated. Cardiac impulses originating in the sinoatrial node typically reach the atrioventricular node in about 0.04 s. Between this time and the time each impulse emerges from the atrioventricular node, another 0.11 s. elapses. Slow conduction of cardiac impulses through the atrioventricular node is related to the small size of the conducting fibers and the presence of fewer points of tight fusion between cardiac muscle cells in this node.

Purkinje Fibers

Purkinje fibers originating in the atrioventricular node form the atrioventricular bundle (bundle of His), which passes subendocardially between the valves of the heart into the ventricular muscle. This bundle divides almost immediately into left and right bundle branches, with the left bundle dividing into the left anterior and left posterior fascicle. These branches descend toward the apex of each ventricle, dividing into smaller branches that spread around each ventricle. Purkinje fibers that pass from the atrioventricular node through the atrioventricular bundle and into the ventricles are large fibers that transmit cardiac impulses so rapidly that both ventricles contract at almost exactly the same time. Any delay in transmission of cardiac impulses through the ventricle can make it possible for impulses from the last excited ventricular muscle fiber to reenter the first muscle fiber and produce ventricular fibrillation. Ordinarily, rapid transmission of cardiac impulses means the first stimulated fibers are still refractory at the time the last fibers are stimulated.

Cardiac Pacemakers

A cardiac pacemaker cell is one that undergoes spontaneous phase 4 depolarization to reach threshold potential and thus undergoes self-excitation. The role of the sinoatrial node as the normal cardiac pacemaker reflects the higher intrinsic discharge rate of this node relative to other potential cardiac pacemakers. For example, atrioventricular node fibers discharge at an intrinsic rate of 40 to 60 beats/minute, and Purkinje fibers discharge at a rate of 15 to 40 beats/minute compared with an intrinsic sinoatrial node rate of 70 to 80 beats/minute. A cardiac pacemaker other than the sinoatrial node is called an *ectopic pacemaker*.

Stimulation of the parasympathetic nervous system results in the release of acetylcholine, which depresses the intrinsic discharge rate of the sinoatrial node and slows the transmission rate of cardiac impulses through atrial internodal pathways to the atrioventricular node. Acetylcholine also depresses the activity of the atrioventricular node. The mechanism of these effects is the ability of acetylcholine to hyperpolarize cell membranes, rendering excitable tissues less excitable. Intense stimulation of the parasympathetic nervous system can totally suppress cardiac pacemaker activity, making the individual dependent on a ventricular escape pacemaker to survive.

Stimulation of the sympathetic nervous system results in the release of norepinephrine, which speeds the rate of spontaneous phase 4 depolarization and thus increases the intrinsic rate of discharge of the sinoatrial node. It is likely that norepinephrine results in increased permeability of cardiac muscle cell membranes to sodium and calcium ions. A similar increase in permeability to sodium ions in the atrioventricular node decreases conduction time for cardiac impulses to travel to the ventricles.

CIRCULATORY EFFECTS OF HEART DISEASE

Valvular heart disease produces circulatory effects related to volume overload (regurgitant lesions) or pressure overload (stenotic lesions) of the atria or ventricles. Exercise tolerance is a valuable clinical indicator of both the presence and severity of valvular heart disease. During exercise, large quantities of venous blood are returned to the heart from the peripheral circulation, resulting in exacerbation of all the circulatory abnormalities associated with valvular heart disease.

Congenital heart disease produces circulatory effects predominantly due to the presence of a left-to-right or right-to-left intracardiac shunt. Pulmonary blood flow is greatly increased in the presence of a left-to-right intracardiac shunt, necessitating an increased cardiac output that often leads to cardiac failure. Right-to-left intracardiac shunts are characterized by decreased pulmonary blood flow, direct return of venous blood to the systemic circulation, and chronic arterial hypoxemia. Congenital heart defects are often associated with other congenital defects elsewhere in the body.

Aortic Valve Disease

Aortic stenosis or aortic regurgitation results in a decrease in forward left ventricular stroke volume. Compensatory responses to offset this decreased cardiac output include left ventricular hypertrophy (four to five times normal size) and an increased circulating blood volume that facilitates venous return. Myocardial ischemia is often present, reflecting inadequate coronary blood flow due to higher intraventricular pressures (aortic stenosis) or low diastolic pressures (aortic regurgitation). Another cause of myocardial ischemia is failure of collateral coronary vessels to develop to the same degree as ventricular hypertrophy. Many patients with aortic valve disease are asymptomatic, emphasizing the importance of determining the presence or absence of cardiac murmurs during the preoperative physical examination.

Mitral Valve Disease

Mitral stenosis or mitral regurgitation results in accumulation of blood in the left atrium and accompanying increases in left atrial pressure. Pulmonary edema is likely when left atrial pressure exceeds 30 mm Hg, although pulmonary lymphatics may efficiently remove excess fluid at even greater pressures. Increased left atrial pressure predisposes to atrial fibrillation because the associated enlargement of the left atrium increases the distance cardiac impulses must travel, thus increasing the likelihood of reentry. There is intense constriction of pulmonary arterioles with resulting pulmonary hypertension and right ventricular hypertrophy.

Patent Ductus Arteriosus

The ductus arteriosus remains patent in about 1 of every 5,500 neonates, resulting in backward flow of blood from the aorta into the pulmonary artery. As the child grows, the pulmonary blood flow may become two to three times greater than systemic blood flow. Because cardiac output is increased at rest, these patients exhibit decreased exercise tolerance. Increased pulmonary blood flow results in increased pulmonary artery pressures and right ventricular hypertrophy. Cyanosis does not occur unless cardiac failure develops.

Atrial Septal Defect

Increased pulmonary blood flow due to an atrial septal defect via a patent foramen ovale or a defect in the atrial septum eventually results in pulmonary hypertension, right ventricular hypertrophy, and right ventricular failure. In about one-third of patients, the flaplike opening covering the foramen ovale does not adhere to the atrial septum such that events that selectively increase right atrial pressure over left atrial pressure (positive-pressure ventilation of the lungs with or without positive end-expiratory pressure) can produce an unexpected right-to-left intracardiac shunt and arterial hypoxemia (Moorthy and LoSasso, 1974).

Ventricular Septal Defect

A ventricular septal defect produces a left-to-right intracardiac shunt, reflecting the fact that pressure in the left ventricle is about six times that in the right ventricle. Blood flow through the intracardiac shunt increases right ventricular pressure and pulmonary blood flow leading to right ventricular hypertrophy and, ultimately, pulmonary hypertension. The presence of oxygenated blood in the right ventricle is consistent with the presence of this congenital defect.

Tetralogy of Fallot

Tetralogy of Fallot is the classic cause of right-to-left intracardiac shunt. Abnormalities associated with tetralogy of Fallot include an aorta that overrides the interventricular septum, pulmonary artery narrowing, a ventricular septal defect, and right ventricular hypertrophy. The major physiologic derangement caused by tetralogy of Fallot is shunting of as much as 75% of returning venous blood through the ventricular septal defect directly to the aorta, resulting in decreased pulmonary blood flow and profound arterial hypoxemia, even at birth.

MYOCARDIAL INFARCTION

Humans with CAD have few collateral communications between the large epicardial coronary arteries. Consequently, acute occlusion of an epicardial coronary artery leads rapidly to transmural infarction. Within 1 hour after an acute MI, the muscle fibers in the center of the ischemic area die. During the next few days, collateral channels growing into the outer rim of the infarcted area cause the nonfunctional area of cardiac muscle to become smaller. Maximal collateral development after an infarct may be present within 1 month. Fibrous tissue develops among the infarcted fibers, and the resulting scarring contracts the size of the infarcted area and usually prevents any aneurysmal effect. Technetium pyrophosphate is taken up selectively by areas of recent myocardial necrosis, providing a so-called hot-spot. The ability of the heart to increase its cardiac output after recovery from a MI is often less than in a normal, undamaged heart.

The magnitude of cardiac cell death after a MI is determined by the product of the degree of ischemia and metabolism of the heart muscle. This emphasizes the need to avoid sympathetic nervous system stimulation after an acute MI. The four major causes of mortality after a MI are (a) decreased cardiac output, (b) pulmonary edema, (c) ventricular fibrillation, and, rarely, (d) rupture of the heart.

Decreased Cardiac Output

Decreased cardiac output occurs immediately after a MI, reflecting the impaired contractility associated with ischemic or infarcted fibers. Cardiogenic shock is likely when >40% of the left ventricular muscle is infarcted. In some instances, when normal portions of the ventricle contract, the damaged muscle is forced outward (aneurysmal) by the intracavitary pressure (Fig. 48-11) (Guyton and Hall, 2000). As a result, much of the pumping force dissipates into the area of the ventricular aneurysm.

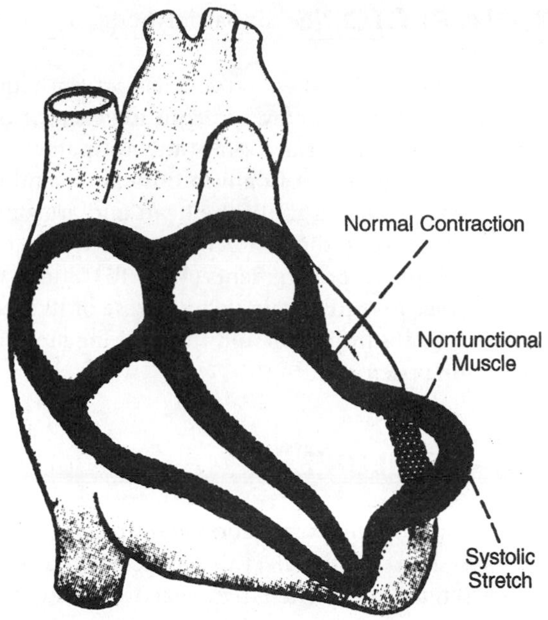

Figure 48-11. Aneurysmal dilatation of ischemic left ventricular muscles may follow a myocardial infarction, leading to decreases in cardiac output. (From Guyton AC, Hall JE. *Textbook of medical physiology*, 10th ed. Philadelphia: Saunders, 2000; with permission.)

Pulmonary Edema

Decreased cardiac output leads to pooling of blood in pulmonary capillaries with associated increases in capillary pressure. Furthermore, decreased cardiac output causes decreased renal blood flow with subsequent retention of fluid. Pulmonary edema may develop suddenly several days after MI in patients who previously had been recovering without complications.

Ventricular Fibrillation

Ventricular fibrillation is a common cause of sudden death related to acute MI, especially in the first few minutes after the infarction. This potentially fatal cardiac dysrhythmia may reflect increased irritability due to depletion of potassium ions from damaged cardiac muscles or altered pathways for conduction of cardiac impulses necessitated by infarcted tissues.

Rupture of the Infarcted Area

Rupture of an area of acute MI is unlikely in the first few days after the event. Several days later, however, the infarcted cardiac muscle may degenerate and increase the likelihood of cardiac rupture with subsequent acute cardiac tamponade.

ANGINA PECTORIS

Angina pectoris occurs when myocardial oxygen requirements exceed delivery, as may occur during exercise or an event associated with stimulation of the sympathetic nervous system. Distribution of pain into the arms and neck reflects the embryonic origin of the heart and arms in the neck such that both of these structures receive pain fibers from the same spinal cord segments (T2 to T5). Stimulation of nerve endings in cardiac muscle by release of lactic acid, histamine, or kinins from ischemic muscle is the most likely cause of angina pectoris.

CARDIAC FAILURE

Cardiac failure manifests as decreased cardiac output or pulmonary edema, with selective left ventricular failure occurring 30 times more often than selective right ventricular failure. The weakened ventricle is unable to pump the blood delivered to it such that venous pressure is increased and ventricular end-diastolic pressure increases. Dyspnea reflects increased left atrial pressure and accumulation of fluid in the lungs, whereas selective increases in right atrial pressure manifest as hepatomegaly, ascites, and peripheral edema. Chronic decreases in cardiac output result in renal-induced retention of fluid in an effort to improve venous return to the heart. Any increased stress, such as exercise, sepsis, or trauma, may unmask decreased cardiac reserve in patients vulnerable to cardiac failure. Inhaled anesthetics produce exaggerated decreases in myocardial contractility when administered in the presence of cardiac failure (Kemmotsu et al., 1973).

Diastolic Heart Failure

Diastolic ventricular function is an important determinant of overall cardiovascular performance. The initial isovolemic myocardial relaxation phase of diastole is accompanied by a rapid fall in ventricular pressure. When the ventricular pressures fall below the atrial pressures, the mitral and tricuspid valves open, and ventricular filling commences. The rapid early phase of filling is related to ventricular relaxation, which is an active, energy consuming, process. The late diastolic filling phase is largely dependent upon active atrial contraction. Diastolic dysfunction is an important cause of heart failure, particularly in the elderly population. The typical preoperative evaluation of cardiac function is focused upon the evaluation of systolic function. However, more than 40% of patients with symptomatic congestive cardiac failure have normal systolic function that is accompanied by diminished diastolic function (Redfield et al., 2003). Congestive heart failure is associated with increased adverse perioperative outcomes. Diastolic ventricular dysfunction is accompanied by abnormal increases in atrial and ventricular filling pressures and is not simply a result of ventricular hypertrophy and poor ventricular compliance, but is related to failure of active ventricular relaxation (Philip et al., 2003). In contrast to animal data that demonstrates significant anesthetic-induced diastolic dysfunction, human studies suggests that sevoflurane does not impair left ventricular relaxation or reduce early diastolic ventricular filling when administered in 1 MAC doses during spontaneous ventilation (Filipovic et al., 2005). However, propofol is associated with mild impairment of diastolic function. It is thought that anesthetics interfere with diastolic calcium reuptake from the cytosol into the sarcoplasmic reticulum (Lee and Woodruff, 1996). Propofol impairs calcium uptake by the sarcoplasmic reticulum via a separate effect on sarcolemmal calcium channels and alters myocardial muscle phosphorylation (Kanaya et al., 2003). Anesthetic drugs may also impair filling in late diastole by decreasing atrial contractility. Perioperative diastolic dysfunction may reduce the patients` ability to tolerate perioperative changes in blood volume, heart rate and rhythm, and positive pressure ventilation. Diastolic dysfunction is more common in patients with hypertension, CAD, cardiomyopathies, aortic stenosis, diabetes mellitus, and chronic renal disease (Philip et al., 2003).

REFERENCES

Becker L. Conditions for vasodilatory-induced coronary steal in experimental myocardial ischemia. *Circulation* 1978;57:1103–1110.

Berne RM, Levy MD, Koeppen BM. *Physiology*, 5th ed. St Louis, Mosby, 2004.

Buffington CW, Davis KB, Gillespie S, et al. The prevalence of steal-prone coronary anatomy in patients with CAD: an analysis of the coronary artery surgery registry. *Anesthesiology* 1988;69:721–727.

Cason BA, Verrier ED, London MJ, et al. Effects of isoflurane and halothane on coronary vascular resistance and collateral myocardial blood flow: their capacity to induce coronary steal. *Anesthesiology* 1987;67:665–675.

Filipovic M, Wang J, Michaux I, et al. Effects of halothane, sevoflurane, and propofol on left ventricular function in humans during spontaneous and controlled ventilation. *Br J Anaesth*. 2005;94:186–192.

Guyton AC, Hall JE. *Textbook of medical physiology*, 10th ed. Philadelphia: Saunders, 2000.

Kanaya N, Gable B, Murray PA, et al. Propofol increases phosphorylation of troponin 1 and myosin light chain 2 via protein kinase C activation in cardiomyocytes. *Anesthesiology* 2003;98:1363–1371.

Kemmotsu O, Hashimoto Y, Shimosati S. Inotropic effects of isoflurane on mechanics of contraction in isolated cat papillary muscles from normal and failing hearts. *Anesthesiology* 1973;39:470–477.

Lee DL, Woodruff AC. Mechanisms of myocardial depression by volatile anaesthetics. *Anaesth Pharmacol Physiol Rev* 1996;4:74–87.

Moorthy SS, LoSasso AM. Patency of the foramen ovale in the critically ill patient. *Anesthesiology* 1974;41:405–407.

Noble WH, Lichtenstein SV, Mazer CD. Cardioplegia controversies. *Can J Anaesth* 1991;38:1–6.

Philip BK, Pastor D, Bellows W et al. The prevalence of preoperative diastolic filling abnormalities in geriatric surgical patients. *Anesth Analg* 2003;97:1214–1221.

Priebe HJ. Isoflurane and coronary hemodynamics. *Anesthesiology* 1989;71:960–976.

Redfield M, Jacobsen S, Burnett JC Jr, et al. Burden of systolic and diastolic ventricular dysfunction in the community: Appreciating the scope of the heart failure epidemic. *JAMA* 2003;289:194–202.

Robotham JL, Takata M, Berman M, Harasawa Y. Ejection fraction revisited. *Anesthesiology* 1991;74:172–183.

The Electrocardiogram and Analysis of Cardiac Dysrhythmias

49

ELECTROCARDIOGRAM

Body fluids are good conductors, making it possible to record the sum of the action potentials of all myocardial cells on the surface of the body as the electrocardiogram (ECG) that is biased toward the activity of the left ventricle because of its greater mass. The normal ECG consists of a P-wave (atrial systole), a QRS complex (ventricular systole), and a T-wave (ventricular repolarization) (Fig. 49-1). Ventricular repolarization is prolonged, explaining the low voltage of the T-wave compared with the QRS complex. The atrial T-wave, which reflects repolarization of the atria, is obscured on the ECG by the larger QRS complex. A U-wave, if present, may reflect slow repolarization of the papillary muscles.

Recording the Electrocardiogram

Paper used for recording the ECG is designed such that each horizontal line corresponds to 0.1 mv and each vertical line corresponds to 0.04 second, assuming proper calibration and paper speed of the recording device (see Fig. 49-1). Electric currents generated by cardiac muscle during each cardiac cycle can change potentials, and polarity is <0.01 second. An oscilloscope display of the ECG, with or without the ability to provide a paper recording, is commonly used for clinical monitoring. Indeed, continuous monitoring of the ECG during anesthesia is considered to be a standard of monitoring for all patients under the anesthesiologist's care.

The duration of events during conduction of the cardiac impulse can be calculated from a recording of the ECG (Table 49-1). The interval between the beginning of atrial contraction and the beginning of ventricular contraction is the P-R interval (actually the P-Q interval, but the Q-wave is frequently absent). The P-R interval depends on heart rate, averaging 0.18 second at a rate of 70 beats/minute and 0.14 second at a rate of 130 beats/minute. The QRS complex reflects ventricular depolarization, whereas the Q-T interval represents the time necessary for complete depolarization and repolarization of the ventricle. Like the P-R interval, the Q-T interval depends on heart rate. The Q-T interval corrected for heart rate (QTc) may be calculated as the Q-T interval in seconds divided by the square root of the R-R interval in seconds (prolongation of the Q-T interval is present when the QTc is ≥440 msec) (Booker et al., 2003). Using a small portable tape recorder (Holter monitor), it is possible to record the ECG for prolonged periods in ambulatory individuals.

Electrocardiogram Leads

The ECG is recorded using a unipolar lead (an exploring electrode connected to an indifferent electrode at zero potential) or bipolar leads (two active electrodes). Depolarization moving toward an active electrode produces a positive deflection, whereas depolarization moving in the opposite direction produces a negative deflection. Electric current flow is normally from the base of the heart toward the apex during most of the depolarization phase with the exception being at the extreme end of the wave. Therefore, an electrode nearer the base of the heart will record a negative potential with respect to an electrode placed nearer the apex of the heart. The usual 12-lead ECG consists of three bipolar standard limb leads, six unipolar chest leads, and three unipolar augmented limb leads.

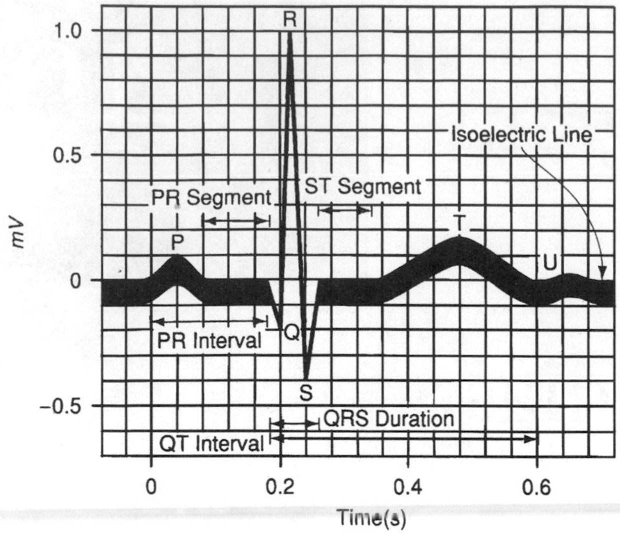

Figure 49-1. The normal waves and intervals on the electrocardiogram.

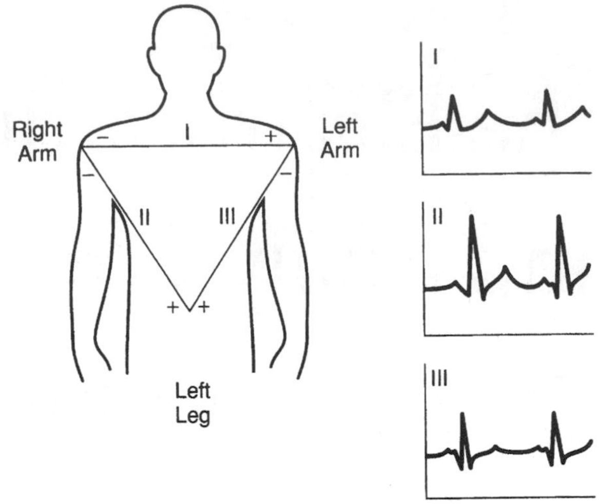

Figure 49-2. Standard limb leads of the electrocardiogram and typical recordings.

Standard Limb Leads

Standard limb leads are placed on the left and right arms and the left leg (Fig. 49-2). These leads record the potential difference between two points on the body. Polarity is positive for the ECG recorded from these standard limb leads. The legs of the three standard limb leads form the arms of an equilateral (Einthoven) triangle. The direction of depolarization of the atria parallels lead II. For this reason, P-waves are prominent in this lead.

Chest Leads

Precordial unipolar leads (V_1 through V_6) are recorded by placing an electrode on the anterior surface of the chest over one of six separate points (Table 49-2). Each chest lead records mainly the electrical potential of the cardiac muscle immediately beneath the electrode. The nearness of the heart surface to the electrode means that relatively small abnormalities in the ventricles, particularly in the anterior ventricular wall, can produce marked changes in the corresponding ECG. In leads V_1 and V_2, the normal QRS recordings are mainly negative because the chest electrode in these leads is nearer the base of the heart than the apex. Conversely, the QRS complexes in V_4 through V_6 are mainly positive because the chest electrode in these leads is nearer the apex of the heart, which is the direction of the electropositivity during depolarization.

Augmented Limb Leads

Augmented limb leads are similar to the standard limb leads except that the recording from the right-arm lead (aVR) is inverted. When the positive terminal is on the right arm, the lead is aVR; when on the left arm, the lead is aVL; and when on the left leg, the lead is aVF.

Interpretation of the Electrocardiogram

Abnormalities of the heart can be detected by analyzing the contours of the different waves in the various ECG leads. The electrical axis of the heart can be determined from the standard limb leads of the Einthoven triangle. In a normal heart, the average direction of the vector during spread of

TABLE 49-1.
INTERVALS AND CORRESPONDING EVENTS ON THE ELECTROCARDIOGRAM

	Average	Range	Events in Heart
P-R interval* (s)	0.18	0.12–0.20	Atrial depolarization and conduction through the atrioventricular node
QRS duration (s)	0.08	0.05–0.10	Ventricular depolarization
Q-T interval* (s)	0.40	0.26–0.45	Ventricular depolarization and repolarization
S-T segment (s)	0.32		

*Dependent on heart rate.

TABLE 49-2.
PLACEMENT OF PRECORDIAL LEADS

V_1	Fourth intercostal space at the right sternal border
V_2	Fourth intercostal space at the left sternal border
V_3	Equidistant between V_2 and V_4
V_4	Fifth intercostal space in the left midclavicular line
V_5	Fifth intercostal space in the left anterior axillary line
V_6	Fifth intercostal space in the left midaxillary line

the depolarization wave is approximately 59 degrees (Fig. 49-3). When one ventricle of the heart hypertrophies, the axis of the heart shifts toward the enlarged ventricle. The predominant direction of the vector through the heart during depolarization and repolarization of the ventricles is from the base to the apex. As a result, the T-waves and most of the QRS complexes in the normal ECG are positive. The vector of current flow during depolarization in the atria is similar to that in the ventricles. As a result, the P-waves recorded from the three standard limb leads are positive.

Abnormalities of the QRS Complex

The QRS complex is considered to be prolonged when it lasts >0.1 second. Hypertrophy of the ventricles prolongs the duration of the QRS complex, reflecting the longer pathway the ventricular depolarization wave must travel. Blockade of the Purkinje fibers necessary for conduction of the cardiac impulse greatly slows conduction and prolongs the duration of the QRS complex. Multiple peaks in an abnormally prolonged QRS complex most often reflect multiple local blocks in conduction of the cardiac impulse along Purkinje fibers as may occur from scar tissue formed at sites of myocardial infarction (MI).

Voltage of the QRS interval in the standard limb leads of the ECG varies between 0.5 and 2.0 mv, with lead III usually recording the lowest voltage and lead II the greatest. High-voltage QRS complexes are considered to be present when

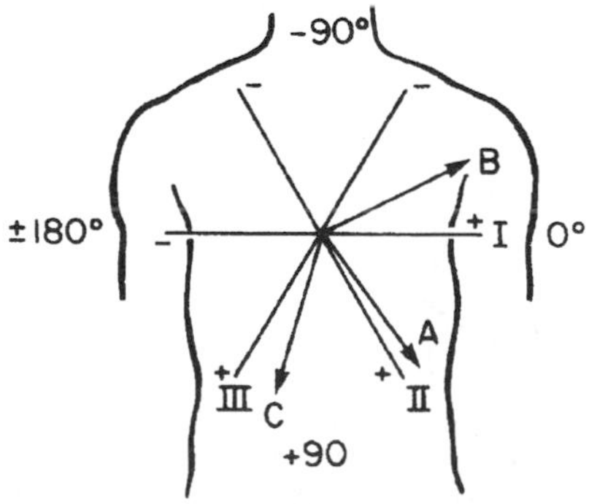

Figure 49-3. Electrical axis of the heart as determined from the standard limb leads of the electrocardiogram. In the normal heart, the electrical axis is approximately 59 degrees (A). Left axis deviation shifts the electrical axis to <0 degrees (B); right axis deviation is associated with an electrical axis of >100 degrees.

the sum of the voltages of all the QRS complexes of the three standard limb leads is >4 mv. The most frequent cause of high-voltage QRS complexes is ventricular hypertrophy.

Decreased Voltage in the Standard Limb Leads

Causes of decreased voltage on the ECG recorded from standard limb leads are (a) multiple small MIs that prevent generation of large quantities of electrical currents, (b) rotation of the apex of the heart toward the anterior chest wall, and (c) abnormal conditions around the heart so electric currents cannot be easily conducted from the heart to the surface of the body. For example, pericardial fluid diminishes voltage recorded from standard limb leads due to the ability of this fluid to rapidly conduct electrical currents to multiple sites. Pulmonary emphysema is associated with decreased conduction of electrical current through the lungs caused by the effects of excessive amounts of air in the lungs.

Current of Injury

A current of injury is due to the inability of damaged areas of the heart to undergo repolarization during diastole. The current of injury results when electrical current flows between the pathologically depolarized (negative) and normally polarized (positive) areas. The most common cause of a current of injury is myocardial ischemia or infarction. Mechanical trauma to the heart and infectious processes that damage cardiac muscle membranes (pericarditis or myocarditis) may also be responsible for a current of injury. In these conditions, a current of injury occurs when the depolarization period of some cardiac muscle is so long that the muscle fails to repolarize completely before the next cardiac cycle begins.

Specific leads of the ECG are more likely than others to reflect myocardial ischemia that develops in areas of the myocardium supplied by an individual coronary artery (Table 49-3). An estimated 80% to 90% of S-T segment information contained in the conventional 12-lead ECG is present on lead V_5. Lead II has special value in the diagnosis of inferior wall myocardial ischemia and the origin of cardiac dysrhythmias. Complete interruption of a coronary artery with infarction of the cardiac muscle results in a deep Q-wave in the ECG leads recording from the infarcted area. The Q-wave occurs because there is no electrical activity in the infarcted area. A Q-wave whose amplitude is more than one-third of the corresponding R-wave and whose duration is >0.04 second is diagnostic of MI. In the presence of an old anterior wall MI, a Q-wave develops in lead I because of loss of muscle mass in the anterior wall of the left ventricle. Conversely, in posterior wall MI, a Q-wave develops in lead III because of the loss of cardiac muscle in the posterior apical part of the ventricles.

Abnormalities of the T-Wave

The T-wave is normally positive in the standard limb leads, reflecting repolarization of the apex of the heart before the

TABLE 49-3.
RELATIONSHIP OF THE ELECTROCARDIOGRAM LEAD REFLECTING MYOCARDIAL ISCHEMIA TO THE AREAS OF MYOCARDIUM INVOLVED

Electrocardiogram Lead	Coronary Artery Responsible for Ischemia	Area of Myocardium Supplied by Coronary Artery
II, III, aVF	Right coronary artery	Right atrium Interatrial septum Right ventricle Sinoatrial node Atrioventricular node Inferior wall of left ventricle
V_3–V_6	Left anterior descending coronary artery	Anterior and lateral wall of left ventricle
I, aVL	Circumflex coronary artery	Lateral wall of left ventricle Sinoatrial node Atrioventricular node

endocardial surfaces of the ventricles. The direction in which repolarization spreads over the heart is backward to the direction in which depolarization occurs. The T-wave becomes abnormal when the normal sequence of repolarization does not occur. For example, delay of conduction of cardiac impulses through the ventricles (prolonged depolarization), as occurs with left or right bundle branch block or ventricular premature contractions, results in a T-wave with a polarity opposite the QRS complex.

Myocardial ischemia is the most common cause of prolonged depolarization of cardiac muscle. When myocardial ischemia occurs in only one area of the heart, the duration of depolarization in this area increases disproportionately to that in other areas, resulting in abnormalities (inversion or biphasic) of the T-wave. Myocardial ischemia also leads to elevation of the S-T segment on the ECG. To be clinically significant, the S-T elevation should be at least 1 mm above the baseline. Artifactual S-T elevation or depression may be introduced by filters incorporated in some ECG monitors to eliminate baseline drift due to movement such as that produced by breathing. For this reason, it is important to verify that the monitor is in the diagnostic mode before concluding that S-T changes represent myocardial ischemia. During exercise, the development of any change in T-wave or S-T segments is evidence that some portion of ventricular muscle has become ischemic and is manifesting an increased period of depolarization out of proportion to the rest of the heart.

His Bundle Electrogram

The His bundle electrogram is recorded from an electrode inserted through a vein and positioned near the tricuspid valve (Fig. 49-4) (Ganong, 2003). The A deflection reflects activation of the atrioventricular node, the H spike is transmission through the His bundle, and the V deflection occurs during ventricular depolarization. Using the standard ECG and His bundle electrogram, it is possible to accurately measure conduction time from the sinus node to the atrioventricular node (AH interval), conduction time through the atrioventricular node, and conduction time through the bundle of His and bundle branches (HV interval) (see Fig. 49-4) (Ganong, 2003). As such, the His bundle electrogram permits detailed analysis of the block site when there is a defect in the system for conduction of cardiac impulses through the heart.

CARDIAC DYSRHYTHMIAS

The incidence of intraoperative cardiac dysrhythmias depends on the definition (any dysrhythmia versus only potentially dangerous dysrhythmias), continuous surveillance versus intermittent observation, patient characteristics, and the nature of the surgery (Atlee, 1997). For example, the incidence of cardiac dysrhythmias may exceed 90% with continuous monitoring of patients undergoing cardiothoracic surgery.

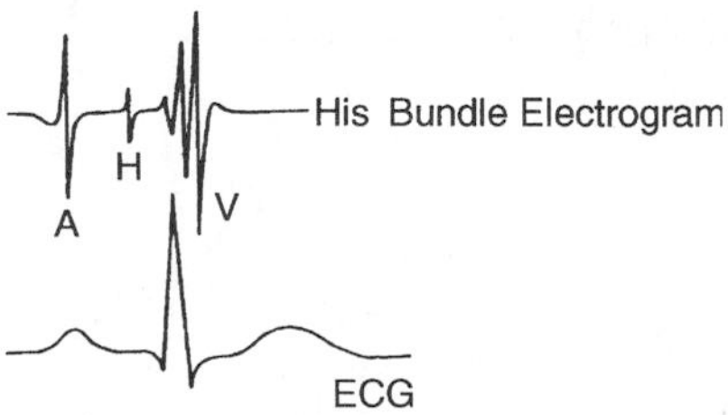

Figure 49-4. A normal His bundle electrogram and the corresponding electrocardiogram (ECG). (From Ganong WF. *Review of medical physiology*, 21st ed. Lange Medical Books, New York: McGraw Hill, 2003.)

TABLE 49-4.
DIAGNOSIS OF CARDIAC DYSRHYTHMIAS FROM THE ELECTROCARDIOGRAM

Are P-waves present and what is their relationship to the QRS complexes?
Are the amplitudes, durations, and contours of the P-waves, P-R intervals, QRS complexes, and Q-T intervals normal?
During tachycardia, is the R-P long and P-R interval short (or vice versa)?
What are the atrial and ventricular discharge rates (same or different)?
Are the P-P and R-R intervals regular or irregular?

Source: Adapted from Atlee JL. Perioperative cardiac dysrhythmias: diagnosis and management. *Anesthesiology* 1997;86:1397–1424.

A systematic approach to the ECG improves the accuracy of diagnosis and effectiveness of treatment (Table 49-4) (Atlee, 1997). Especially important are the rate and regularity of cardiac rhythm, appearance of P-waves, relation of P-waves to the QRS complexes, and determining the cause of widened or bizarre QRS complexes (ventricular aberration reflecting abnormal ventricular conduction of supraventricular beats).

Mechanisms

Perioperative cardiac dysrhythmias are most likely to occur in patients with preexisting heart disease (coronary artery disease, valvular heart disease, cardiomyopathies) in the presence of a transient physiologic imbalance (ischemia, catecholamines, electrolyte abnormalities, laryngoscopy, and tracheal intubation) (Atlee, 1997). Cardiac dysrhythmias may be caused by altered automaticity of pacemaker cardiac cells, altered excitability of myocardial cells, and altered conduction of cardiac impulses through the specialized conduction systems of the heart. Manifestations of these alterations may be the appearance of an ectopic cardiac pacemaker, development of heart block, or appearance of a reentry circuit.

Automaticity

Automaticity depicts the ability of pacemaker cardiac cells to undergo spontaneous phase 4 depolarization. Under normal circumstances, automaticity is exhibited by cells in the sinoatrial node, atrioventricular node, and specialized conducting fibers of the atria and ventricles.

Activation of the sympathetic nervous system by events such as arterial hypoxemia, acidosis, or release of catecholamines is the most common cause of enhanced automaticity. In addition, enhanced automaticity occurs when the threshold potential becomes more negative such that the difference between the threshold potential and resting transmembrane potential is less.

Decreased automaticity is produced by increased parasympathetic nervous system activity, which decreases responsiveness of sinoatrial and atrioventricular node cells by increasing outward flux of potassium ions. This increased outward movement of potassium ions evoked by acetylcholine hyperpolarizes cardiac cell membranes and prevents them from depolarizing. Vagal stimulation may decrease the vulnerability of the heart to develop ventricular fibrillation, especially in the presence of sympathetic nervous system stimulation. Carotid sinus stimulation decreases the frequency of premature ventricular contractions and can abolish ventricular tachycardia.

Ectopic Pacemaker

An ectopic cardiac pacemaker (focus) manifests as a premature contraction of the heart that occurs between normal beats. A depolarization wave spreads outward from the ectopic pacemaker and initiates the premature contraction. The usual cause of an ectopic pacemaker is an irritable area of cardiac muscle resulting from a local (focal) area of myocardial ischemia or use of stimulants such as caffeine or nicotine. Sometimes an ectopic pacemaker becomes persistent and assumes the role of a pacemaker in place of the sinoatrial node. The most common point for development of an ectopic pacemaker is the atrioventricular node or atrioventricular bundle.

Excitability

Excitability is the ability of a cardiac cell to respond to a stimulus by depolarizing. A measure of excitability is the difference between the resting transmembrane potential and threshold potential of cardiac cell membranes. The smaller the difference between these potentials, the more excitable, or irritable, are the cells. Although epinephrine enhances excitability, this is somewhat offset by a concomitant small increase in the negativity of the resting transmembrane potential. Once a cell depolarizes, it is no longer excitable, being refractory to all stimuli. After this absolute refractory period, cardiac cells enter a relative refractory period during which greater than normal stimuli can cause cardiac cell membranes to depolarize.

Conduction

Conduction of cardiac impulses proceeds through specialized conduction systems of the heart such that coordinated contractions occur (see Fig. 48-10). Abnormalities of conduction of cardiac impulses manifest as development of heart block, reentry circuits, or preexcitation syndromes.

Heart Block

The most frequent sites of heart block are at the atrioventricular bundle or one of the bundle branches. Causes of heart block at these sites include (a) excessive parasympathetic nervous system stimulation, (b) drug-induced (digitalis, beta-adrenergic antagonists such as propranolol) depression of cardiac impulse conduction, (c) MI, (d) pressure on the conduction system by atherosclerotic plaques, and (e) age-related degeneration of the conduction system.

Reentry

Reentry (circus movements) implies reexcitation of cardiac tissue by return of the same cardiac impulse using a circuitous pathway (Fig. 49-5) (Akhtar, 1982). This contrasts with automaticity, in which a new cardiac impulse is generated each time to excite the heart. Reentry circuits can develop at any place in the heart where there is an imbalance between conduction and refractoriness. Causes of this imbalance include (a) elongation of the conduction pathway such as occurs in dilated hearts (especially a dilated left atrium associated with mitral stenosis), (b) decreased velocity of conduction of cardiac impulses as occurs with myocardial ischemia or hyperkalemia, and (c) a shortened refractory period of cardiac muscle as produced by epinephrine or electric shock from an alternating current. Each of these conditions creates a situation in which cardiac impulses conducted by normal Purkinje fibers can return retrograde through abnormal Purkinje fibers, which are not in a refractory state (a reentry circuit). A reentry circuit is the most likely mechanism for supraventricular tachycardia, atrial flutter, atrial fibrillation, premature ventricular contractions, ventricular tachycardia, and ventricular fibrillation. Reentry circuits can be eliminated by speeding conduction through normal tissues so cardiac impulses reach their initial site of origin when the fibers are still refractory, or by prolonging the refractory period of normal cells so the returning impulses cannot reenter.

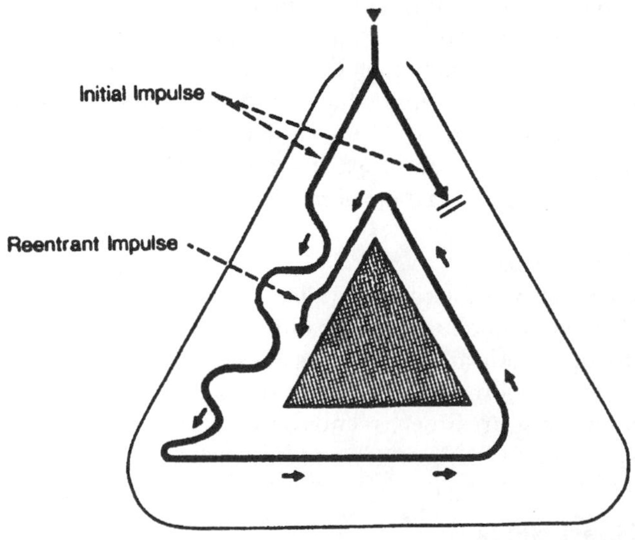

Figure 49-5. The essential requirement for initiation of a reentry circuit is a unilateral block that prevents uniform anterograde propagation of the initial cardiac impulse. This same cardiac impulse, under appropriate conditions, can traverse the area of block in a retrograde direction and become a reentrant cardiac impulse. (From Akhtar M. Management of ventricular tachyarrhythmias. *JAMA* 1982;247:671–674; with permission.)

TABLE 49-5.
ACCESSORY PATHWAYS AND PREEXCITATION SYNDROMES

	Connections
Kent's bundle	Atrium to ventricle
Mahaim bundle	Atrioventricular node to ventricle
Atriohisian fiber	Atrium to His bundle
James fiber	Atrium to atrioventricular node

Preexcitation Syndromes

A preexcitation syndrome is present when atrial impulses bypass the atrioventricular node to produce early excitation of the ventricle. The most common accessory conduction pathway providing a direct connection (anatomic loop) of the atrium to the ventricle is known as *Kent's bundle* (usually left atrium to left ventricle) (Table 49-5) (Wellens et al., 1987). Conduction via this accessory pathway produces the Wolff-Parkinson-White syndrome (P-R interval <0.12 s, delta wave), most often manifesting as intermittent bouts of supraventricular tachydysrhythmias. Normally, the ventricles are protected from rapid atrial rhythms by the refractory period of the atrioventricular node. Propranolol has no specific effect on the accessory pathways, whereas digitalis preparations and verapamil may enhance conduction through these pathways.

Anesthesia

The ability of halogenated anesthetics to evoke atrioventricular junctional (nodal rhythms) and/or increase ventricular automaticity may be related to altered potassium and calcium ion translocation dynamics across cardiac cell membranes (Atlee and Bosnjak, 1990). Halothane, enflurane, and isoflurane slow the rate of sinoatrial node discharge and prolong His-Purkinje and ventricular conduction times. Perioperative increases in the QTc interval can predispose certain individuals to ventricular tachydysrhythmias, most importantly torsades des pointes. Propofol has little effect on the duration of the QTc (Whyte et al., 2005). However, potent inhaled drugs, most notably sevoflurane, increase the duration of myocardial repolarization and thus significantly prolongs QTc duration (Whyte et al., 2005). Changes in Pa_{CO_2} dramatically alter autonomic nervous system effects on the sinoatrial and atrioventricular node depolarization as well as reentry. Autonomic nervous system imbalance due to drugs (anticholinergics, anticholinesterases, exogenous catecholamines, beta-adrenergic antagonists) or minimal concentrations of anesthetic drugs in the presence of intense surgical stimulation, may be responsible for the initiation of cardiac dysrhythmias during anesthesia and surgery.

Type of Cardiac Dysrhythmias

Initial management of perioperative cardiac dysrhythmias does not differ from other acute circumstances (Atlee, 1997). When life-threatening circulatory compromise occurs, prompt interventions with artificial cardiac pacing or electrical cardioversion is recommended. Recognized physiologic imbalances should be corrected and management provided for underlying heart disease. Specific antidysrhythmic drugs are used to suppress cardiac dysrhythmias and prevent recurrences (see Chapter 17).

Complex tachydysrhythmias may require more than two simultaneous leads for diagnosis (Atlee, 1997). At least one of these leads should maximize P-waves (II, III, aVF, V_1) so as to determine the relationship between atrial and ventricular depolarizations. P-waves are best seen when recording from esophageal, transvenous, or epicardial pacing leads.

Sinus Tachycardia

Sinus tachycardia is usually defined as a heart rate of >100 beats/minute. A common cause of sinus tachycardia is sympathetic nervous system stimulation such as may occur during a noxious stimulus in the presence of low concentrations of anesthetic drugs. Increased body temperature increases heart rate approximately 18 beats/minute for every degree Celsius increase. Fever causes tachycardia because increased temperature accelerates the rate of metabolism in the sinoatrial node. Carotid sinus-mediated reflex stimulation of the heart rate accompanies decreases in systemic blood pressure as produced by vasodilator drugs or acute hemorrhage.

Sinus Bradycardia

Sinus bradycardia is usually defined as a heart rate of <60 beats/minute. Heart rate slowing accompanies parasympathetic nervous system stimulation of the heart. Bradycardia that occurs in physically conditioned athletes reflects the ability of their hearts to eject a greater stroke volume with each contraction compared with the less conditioned heart.

Sinus Dysrhythmias

Sinus dysrhythmias are present during normal breathing with heart rate (R-R intervals) varying approximately 5% during various phases of the resting breathing cycle (Fig. 49-6). This variation may increase to 30% during deep breathing. These variations in heart rate with breathing most likely reflect baroreceptor reflex activity and changes in the negative intrapleural pressures that elicit a waxing and waning Bainbridge reflex. Variation in heart rate that is not related to breathing (nonphasic sinus dysrhythmias) is abnormal and is a result of sinoatrial node dysfunction, aging, or digitalis intoxication. The absence of phasic changes suggests autonomic nervous system dysfunction as may accompany diabetes mellitus. In perioperative settings, sinus dysrhythmias are usually transient and often caused by autonomic nervous system imbalance as the result of an intervention (spinal or epidural anesthesia, laryngoscopy, surgical stimulation) or by the effects of drugs on the sinoatrial node.

Atrioventricular Heart Block

First-degree atrioventricular heart block is considered to be present when the P-R interval is >0.2 second at a normal heart rate. Second-degree atrioventricular heart block is classified as Wenckebach phenomenon (type I) or Mobitz (type II) heart block. Wenckebach phenomenon is characterized by a progressive prolongation of the P-R interval until conduction of the cardiac impulse is completely interrupted and a P-wave is recorded without a subsequent QRS complex. After this dropped beat, the cycle is repeated. Mobitz heart block is the occurrence of a nonconducted atrial impulse without a prior change in the P-R interval.

Third-degree atrioventricular heart block occurs during complete block of the transmission of cardiac impulses from the atria to the ventricles. The P-waves are dissociated from the QRS complexes and the heart rate depends on the intrinsic discharge rate of the ectopic pacemaker beyond the site of conduction block. If the ectopic pacemaker is near the atrioventricular node, the QRS complexes appear normal and the heart rate is typically 40 to 60 beats/minute (Fig. 49-7). When the site of the block is infranodal, the escape ventricular pacemaker often has a discharge rate of <40 beats/minute and the QRS complexes are wide, resembling a bundle branch block (Fig. 49-8). Patients may experience syncope (Stokes-Adams syndrome) at the onset of third-degree heart block, reflecting the 5- to 10-second period of asystole that may precede ventricular escape and appearance of an ectopic ventricular pacemaker. Occasionally, the interval of ventricular standstill at the onset of third-degree heart block is so long that death occurs. Treatment of patients with third-degree heart block is by insertion of a permanent artificial cardiac pacemaker. Temporary cardiac pacing may be provided with

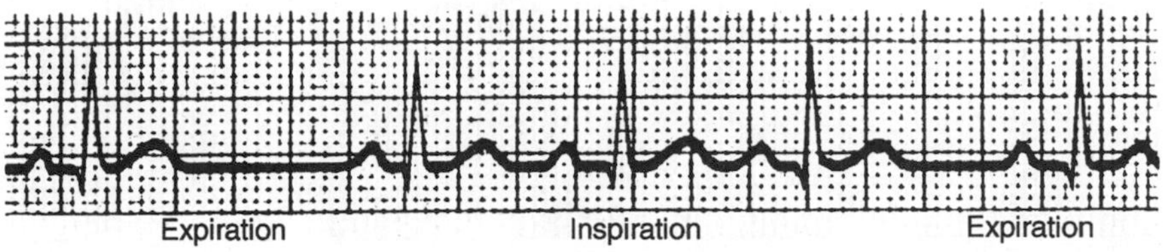

Figure 49-6. Sinus dysrhythmia reflecting changes in sinoatrial pacemaker activity with the breathing cycle.

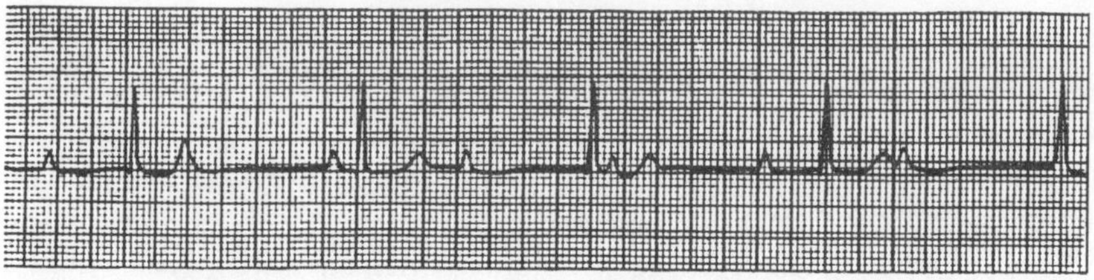

Figure 49-7. Third-degree atrioventricular heart block occurring at the level of the atrioventricular node (QRS complexes are narrow). There is no relation between the P-waves and QRS complexes.

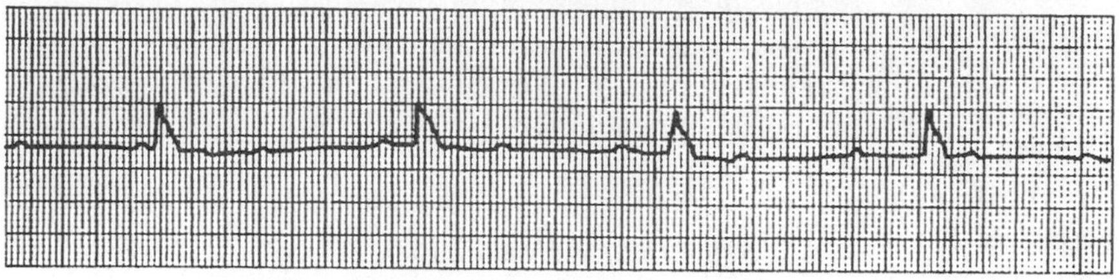

Figure 49-8. Third-degree atrioventricular heart block occurring at an infranodal level (QRS complexes are wide).

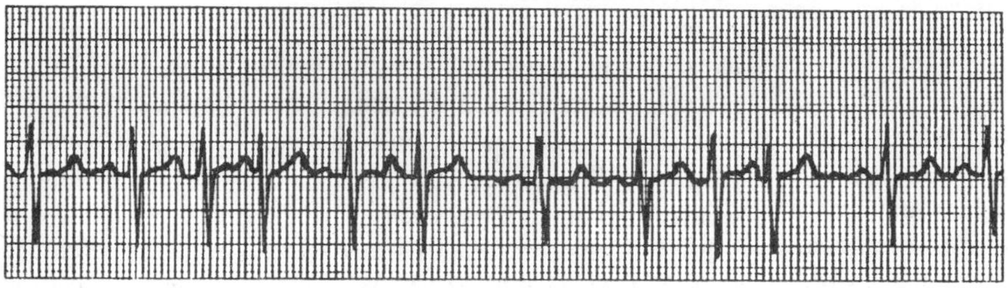

Figure 49-9. Premature atrial contractions resulting in an irregular rhythm.

intravenous infusion of isoproterenol (chemical cardiac pacemaker) or a transvenous artificial cardiac pacemaker. The safe perioperative management of patients with implanted rhythm control devices requires a basic understanding of the classification, function, and emergency management of these devices (Atlee and Bernstein, 2001a; Atlee and Bernstein, 2001b).

Premature Atrial Contractions

Premature atrial contractions are recognized by an abnormal P-wave and a shortened P-R interval (Fig. 49-9). The QRS complex of the premature atrial contraction has a normal configuration. Also, the interval between the premature atrial contraction and the next succeeding contraction is usually not prolonged. Premature atrial contractions are usually benign and often occur in individuals without heart disease.

Premature Nodal Contractions

Premature nodal contractions are characterized by the absence of P-waves preceding the QRS complexes. The P-wave is obscured by the QRS complex of the premature contraction because the cardiac impulse travels retrograde into the atria at the same time it travels forward into the ventricles.

Premature Ventricular Contractions

Premature ventricular contractions result from an ectopic pacemaker in the ventricles. The QRS complex of the ECG is typically prolonged because the cardiac impulse is

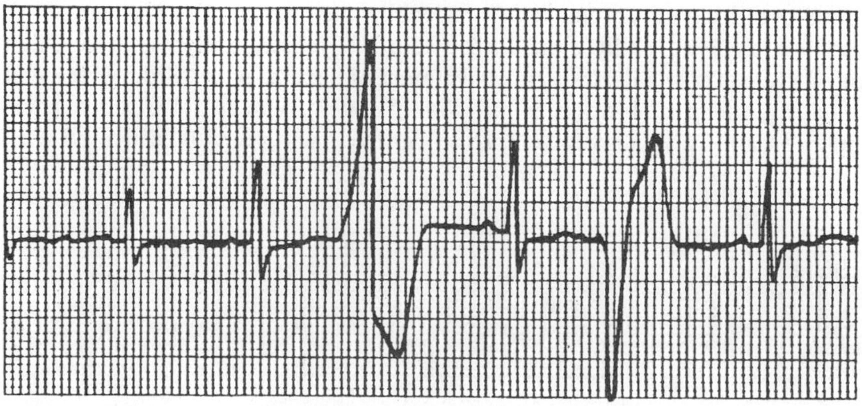

Figure 49-10. Multifocal premature ventricular contractions.

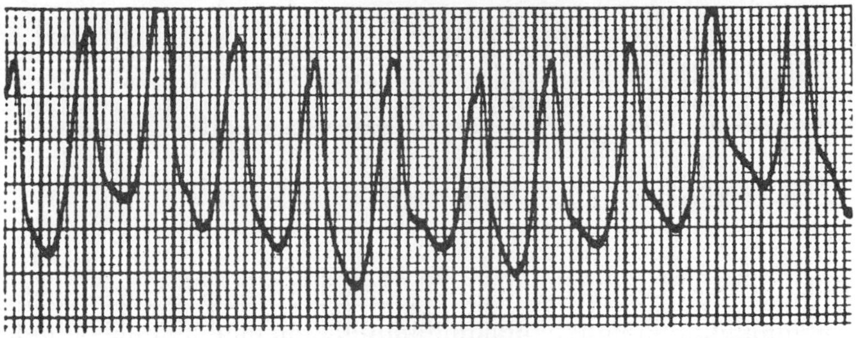

Figure 49-11. Ventricular tachycardia.

conducted mainly through the slowly conducting muscle of the ventricle rather than the Purkinje fibers (Fig. 49-10). The voltage of the QRS complex of the premature ventricular contraction is increased, reflecting the absence of the usual neutralization that occurs when a normal cardiac impulse passes through both ventricles simultaneously. After almost all premature ventricular contractions, the T-wave has an electrical potential opposite that of the QRS complex. A compensatory pause after a premature ventricular contraction occurs because the first impulse from the sinoatrial node reaches the ventricle during its refractory period. When a premature ventricular contraction occurs, the ventricle may not have filled adequately with blood and the stroke volume resulting from this contraction fails to produce a detectable pulse. The subsequent stroke volume, however, may be increased due to added ventricular filling that occurs during the compensatory pause that typically follows a premature ventricular contraction.

Premature ventricular contractions often reflect significant cardiac disease. For example, myocardial ischemia may be responsible for initiation of premature ventricular contractions from an irritable site in poorly oxygenated ventricular muscle. Treatment of premature ventricular contractions includes supplemental oxygen and intravenous administration of lidocaine.

Atrial Paroxysmal Tachycardia

Atrial paroxysmal tachycardia, which often occurs in otherwise healthy young individuals, is caused by rapid rhythmic discharges of impulses from an ectopic atrial pacemaker. The rhythm on the ECG is perfectly regular and the P-waves are abnormal, often inverted, indicating a site of origin other than the sinoatrial node. The rapid discharge rate of this ectopic focus causes it to become the pacemaker. Typically, the onset of atrial paroxysmal tachycardia is abrupt (a single beat) and may end just as suddenly with the pacemaker shifting back to the sinoatrial node. Atrial paroxysmal tachycardia can be terminated by producing parasympathetic nervous system stimulation at the heart with drugs or by unilateral external pressure applied to the carotid sinus. Drugs that increase refractoriness of the atrioventricular node (adenosine, calcium channel blockers, esmolol) are preferred initial therapy for any narrow QRS paroxysmal supraventricular tachycardia.

Nodal Paroxysmal Tachycardia

Nodal paroxysmal tachycardia resembles atrial paroxysmal tachycardia except P-waves are not identifiable on the ECG. P-waves are obscured by QRS complexes because the atrial impulse travels backward from the atrioventricular node at the same time the ventricular impulse travels through the ventricles.

Ventricular Tachycardia

Ventricular tachycardia on the ECG resembles a series of ventricular premature contractions that occur at a rapid and regular rate without any normal supraventricular beats interspersed (Fig. 49-11). Stroke volume is often severely depressed during ventricular tachycardia because the ventricles have insufficient time for cardiac filling. Sustained ventricular tachycardia may necessitate termination with electrical cardioversion. This cardiac dysrhythmia predisposes to ventricular fibrillation.

Atrial Flutter

Atrial flutter on the ECG is characterized by 2:1, 3:1, or 4:1 conduction of atrial impulses to the ventricle (Fig. 49-12). This occurs because the functional refractory period of Purkinje fibers and ventricular muscle is such that no more than 200 impulses per minute can be transmitted to the ventricles. P-waves have a characteristic saw-toothed appearance, especially in leads II, III, aVF, and V_1. Atrial flutter is

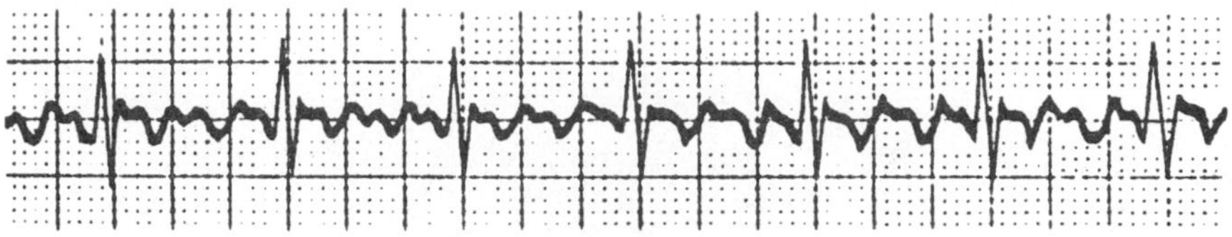

Figure 49-12. Atrial flutter.

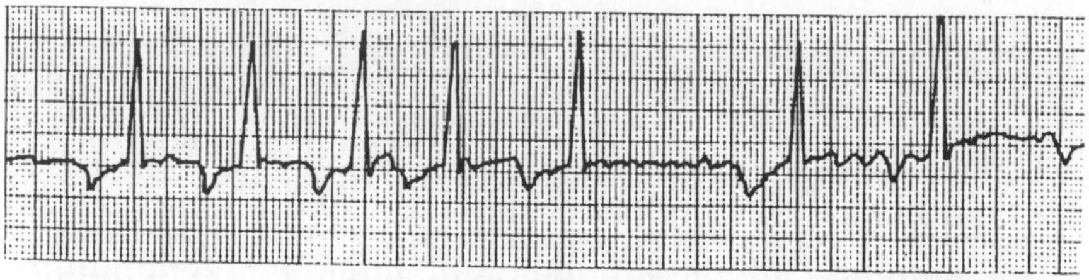

Figure 49-13. Atrial fibrillation.

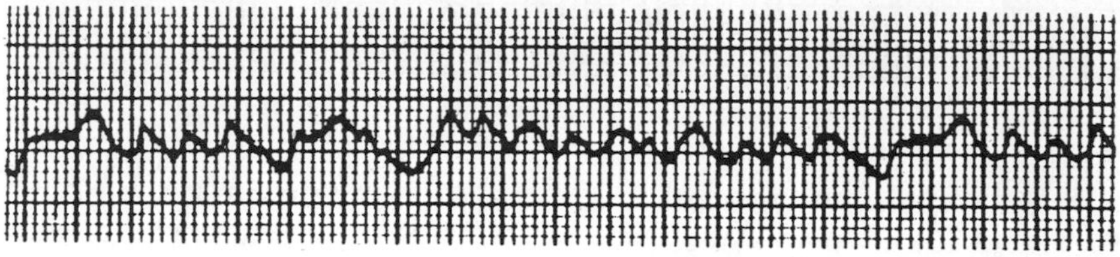

Figure 49-14. Ventricular fibrillation.

seen commonly in patients with chronic pulmonary disease, dilated cardiomyopathy, myocarditis, ethanol intoxication, and thyrotoxicosis. This dysrhythmia lasts only minutes to hours before changing to sinus rhythm or atrial fibrillation.

Atrial Fibrillation

Atrial fibrillation is characterized by normal QRS complexes occurring at a rapid and irregular rate in the absence of identifiable P-waves (Fig. 49-13). The irregular ventricular response reflects arrival of atrial impulses at the atrioventricular node at times that may or may not correspond to the refractory period of the node from a previous discharge. Stroke volume is decreased during atrial fibrillation because the ventricles do not have sufficient time to fill optimally between cardiac cycles. A pulse deficit (heart rate by palpation is less than that calculated from the ECG) reflects the inability of each ventricular contraction to eject a sufficient stroke volume to produce a detectable peripheral pulse. Treatment of atrial fibrillation is classically with digitalis, which prolongs the refractory period of the atrioventricular node. This prolongation decreases the ventricular response rate, which improves stroke volume by permitting additional time for filling the ventricles between cycles. There is an estimated 5% annual risk of thromboembolism in patients with atrial fibrillation who are not treated with anticoagulants.

Ventricular Fibrillation

Ventricular fibrillation on the ECG is characterized by an irregular wavy line with voltages that range from 0.25 to 0.5 mv (Fig. 49-14). There is total incoordination of contractions with cessation of any effective pumping activity and disappearance of detectable systemic blood pressure. Flutter or fibrillation is usually confined to either the atria or ventricles because the two masses of muscle are electrically insulated from each other by the rings of fibrous tissue around the heart valves. Most instances of atrial or ventricular fibrillation are due to a reentry mechanism. The only effective treatment of ventricular fibrillation is the delivery of direct electric current through the ventricles (defibrillation), which simultaneously depolarizes all ventricular muscle. This depolarization allows the reestablishment of a cardiac pacemaker at a site other than the irritable focus that was responsible for ventricular fibrillation.

REFERENCES

Akhtar M. Management of ventricular tachyarrhythmias. *JAMA* 1982; 247:671–674.

Atlee JL. Perioperative cardiac dysrhythmias: diagnosis and management. *Anesthesiology* 1997;86:1397–1424.

Atlee JL, Bernstein AD. Cardiac rhythm management devices (Part I): indications, device selection, and function. *Anesthesiology* 2001a; 95:1265–1280.

Atlee JL, Bernstein AD. Cardiac rhythm management devices (Part I): indications, device selection, and function. *Anesthesiology* 2001b; 95:1492–1506.

Atlee JL, Bosnjak ZJ. Mechanisms for cardiac dysrhythmias during anesthesia. *Anesthesiology* 1990;72:347–374.

Booker PD, Whyte SD, Laudusans EJ. Long QT syndrome and anaesthesia. *Br J Anaesth* 2003;90:349–366.

Ganong WF. *Review of medical physiology*, 21st ed. Lange Medical Books, New York: McGraw Hill, 2003.

Kies SJ, Pabelick CM, Hurley HA, et al. Anesthesia for patients with congenital long QT syndrome. *Anesthesiology* 2005;102:204–210.

Wellens HJJ, Brugada P, Penn OC. The management of preexcitation syndromes. *JAMA* 1987;257:2325–2333 .

Whyte SD, Booker PD, Buckley DG. The effects of propofol and sevoflurane on the QT interval and transmural dispersion of repolarization in children. *Anesth Analg* 2005;100:71–77.

The Lungs

50

ANATOMY

The thoracic cage is composed of 12 thoracic vertebral bodies, the ribs, and the sternum. This structure is sufficiently rigid to protect the organ systems contained within but pliable enough to allow the lungs to inflate and deflate. The articulation of the ribs with their respective vertebral bodies allows them to move in a bucket handle fashion. The sternum, consisting of the manubrium, body, and xiphoid process, is the most important anterior supporting skeletal chest wall structure. The suprasternal notch (upper border of the manubrium between the sternoclavicular joints) is in the same horizontal plane as the midportion of the second thoracic vertebra. The second thoracic vertebra is a useful radiologic landmark because it corresponds to the midportion of the trachea, which is a desirable location for the distal tip of a tracheal tube. External palpation of tracheal tube cuff inflation in the suprasternal notch is an indirect method for confirming that the distal end of a tracheal tube is properly positioned above the carina.

The adult trachea is a fibromuscular tube approximately 10 to 12 cm in length with a diameter of approximately 20 mm and a capacity of approximately 30 mL. The trachea begins at the level of the sixth cervical vertebra, just below the cricoid cartilage. The trachea extends downward until it bifurcates at the carina opposite the fifth thoracic vertebra. The mucosal lining of the trachea consists of ciliated columnar epithelium and mucus-secreting cells. Each ciliated cell has approximately 200 cilia beating 12 to 20 times per minute and moving mucus toward the pharynx at a rate of 0.5 to 1.5 cm/minute.

The bifurcation of the trachea at the carina gives rise to the right and left main stem bronchus. The right main stem bronchus extends approximately 2.5 cm before its initial division into the bronchus to the right upper and middle lobes with a continuation as the right lower lobe bronchus. The left main stem bronchus extends approximately 5 cm before its initial division into branches to the left upper lobe and lingula and continuation as the bronchus to the left lower lobe. The short length of the right main stem bronchus increases the technical difficulty in placing a right endobronchial tube (double-lumen tube) without obstructing the orifice to the right upper lobe. For this reason, it is common to select a left endobronchial tube when a double-lumen tube is placed (Benumof et al., 1987). The observation that an anomalous right upper lobe bronchus from the trachea (above the carina) is present in approximately 1 in 250 individuals is a further complication to the placement of an endobronchial tube. This anomaly may occur as frequently as 1 in 50 in patients with congenital heart disease (Atwell, 1967; Benumof et al., 1987). A right upper lobe originating at the level of the carina (trifurcation) has also been described (Stene et al., 1994).

The takeoff of the right bronchus from the long vertical axis of the trachea is approximately 25 degrees in adults, whereas the angle for the left bronchus is approximately 45 degrees. Thus, in the adult, accidental endobronchial intubation or aspiration of foreign material is likely to enter the right main stem bronchus. In children <3 years of age, the bifurcations of both the right and left bronchi are approximately equal, with takeoff angles of approximately 55 degrees.

Continued division of the right and left main stem bronchus gives rise to bronchioles, characterized by the absence of cartilage, and ultimately to respiratory bronchioles, which mark the transitional zone between the bronchioles and alveolar ducts. Continued division of bronchi into successive, more distal, airway generations is associated with a decrease in the caliber of the individual airways. However, there is a dramatic increase in the combined cross-sectional area of the airway because the total number of airways increases at each division.

Alveoli arise from alveolar ducts as well as alveolar sacs. Collateral ventilation may occur via pores of Kohn located in the interspaces between capillary networks as well as pathways directly communicating between terminal respiratory bronchioles and neighboring alveoli.

In health the lungs are expanded to completely fill the pleural cavity. Therefore, the visceral pleura of the lungs are in contact with the parietal pleura lining the chest wall. The two pleural surfaces are separated by a fluid film that helps to keep the lung and chest wall closely approximated. The isolated lung will recoil and collapse if not supported. Conversely, the isolated chest wall tends to recoil outwards

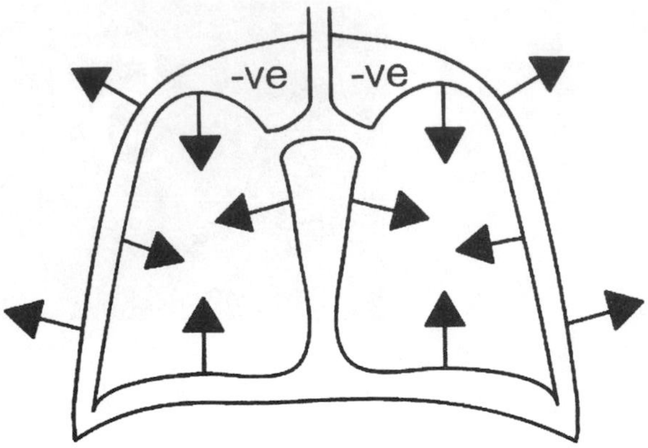

Figure 50-1. The respiratory system is at an elastic equilibrium at functional residual capacity. The outward recoil of the chest wall is counterbalanced by the inward recoil of the lungs. These opposing forces generate the negative (subatmospheric) intrapleural pressure.

if not constrained. In the intact thorax, the opposing recoil forces of the lung and chest wall are balanced and produce a stable system that generates optimal lung inflation (Fig. 50-1). These opposing recoil forces generate a subatmospheric pressure of approximately −4 mm Hg in the potential space between the visceral and parietal pleura (intrapleural pressure) during quiet breathing. This pressure can be estimated by measurement of pressure in the lumen of the flaccid esophagus using an esophageal balloon catheter. The intrapleural pressure is not uniform, becoming progressively higher (closer to atmospheric pressure) in dependent areas and lower (lower than atmospheric) in non-dependent areas (Fig. 50-2). Local variations in intrapleural pressure are an important determinant of regional ventilation.

Regulation of Airway Caliber

In health, airway caliber is determined actively by the state of contraction of airway smooth muscle and passively by

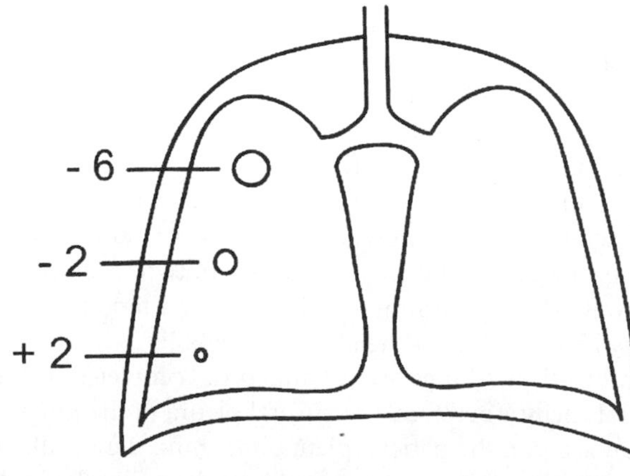

Figure 50-2. The intrapleural pressure is more negative (more subatmospheric) in the nondependent areas of the chest. Thus, alveoli in the nondependent zones are exposed to a greater distending force and are larger. Conversely, alveoli located in dependent areas are smaller and more prone to collapse.

the state of inflation of the lung. However, in the presence of obstructive airways disease, mucosal edema, secretions, smooth muscle hypertrophy, and airway remodeling affect airway caliber.

Increases in lung volume are accompanied by increases in airway diameter because the airways are tethered by the surrounding lung parenchyma. This phenomenon is most apparent in airways <1 mm in diameter because these structures lack intrinsic supporting cartilage. Passive stretching causes relatively minor changes in airway resistance at lung volumes greater than functional residual capacity (FRC). Conversely, as lung volumes decrease below FRC there are significant increases in airway resistance. Indeed, small airway closure may occur in the dependent areas of the lung at low lung volumes. Airway smooth muscle is under both neural and humeral influence. There is rich parasympathetic innervation of the bronchi and bronchioles via the vagus nerves. These nerves release acetylcholine onto M_3 muscarinic receptors on airway smooth muscle, which leads to contraction of the muscle and bronchoconstriction, especially in conducting airways >1 mm in diameter (Pereira et al., 1996). Pharmacologic blockade of parasympathetic nervous system pathways or surgical transection of the vagus nerves causes bronchodilation, demonstrating that airway smooth muscle is tonically contracted by the parasympathetic nerves. In addition to M_3 receptors on the airway smooth muscle, there are also inhibitory presynaptic M_2 receptors on the parasympathetic nerves in the lungs. Stimulation of these M_2 receptors inhibits acetylcholine release by as much as 80% thus attenuating bronchoconstriction. Beta$_2$-adrenergic receptors are present in higher concentrations in peripheral lung tissue in contrast to M_3 receptors that predominate in larger airways. Sympathetic nervous system innervation is sparse in human airways, thus sympathetic influence on bronchial tone is mediated via circulating catecholamines. Activation of beta$_2$-adrenergic receptors causes bronchodilation. Circulating catecholamines may also influence parasympathetic tone via alpha-adrenergic receptors located in parasympathetic ganglia. Alpha-receptor activation in this location reduces parasympathetic transmission and therefore decreases bronchoconstriction. Airway muscle tone is also influenced by nonadrenergic, noncholinergic (NANC) innervation of the bronchioles (Hlastala and Berger, 2001). There are two NANC systems, inhibitory NANC (iNANC) causing bronchodilation via release of vasoactive intestinal peptide (VIP), and excitatory NANC (eNANC) causing bronchoconstriction via the release of tachykinins such as substance P. Histamine stimulates H_1 receptors (bronchoconstriction) and H_2 receptors (bronchodilation), but the predominant effect is bronchoconstriction. Histamine is released in response to inflammation, irritant challenge, and during allergic and anaphylactic responses. Histamine may also indirectly stimulate eNANC activity.

Inhaled gases are warmed, filtered, and humidified by the vascular surfaces of the nasal turbinates and septum, which comprise approximately 160 cm^2 of mucosal surface area in adults. Room air is warmed to within 1 °C of body temperature and almost completely saturated with water vapor before entering the trachea. Bypassing the nasal passageways with an endotracheal tube, laryngeal mask airway, or tracheostomy impairs delivery of humidified gases to the lungs. The filtering function of the nose is a result of its internal structure that causes turbulent flow. Inhaled particles are forced to strike and adhere to the mucosal lining of the nose (turbulent precipitation). This system is sufficient to remove almost all particles >6 μm in diameter before they reach the lungs. Cilia move mucus containing foreign particles and dust toward the pharynx, where it is swallowed. Anesthetic drugs depress the velocity of mucus flow by diminishing ciliary activity. Inhaled particles that reach the airways often accumulate in smaller bronchioles because of gravitational precipitation. For example, bronchiolar disease is common in coal miners, reflecting the presence of settled dust particles. Particles that are even smaller (<0.5 μm), such as those present in cigarette smoke, travel deeper into the lung and may be precipitated in the alveoli. Particles that are trapped in alveoli may eventually cause fibrous tissue growth in alveolar septa, leading to irreversible damage.

Innervation of the Larynx

A working knowledge of the innervation of the larynx is important when performing topical laryngeal anesthesia, such as in preparation for awake tracheal intubation. The sensory innervation of the larynx is derived from the branches of the glossopharyngeal nerve (posterior tongue, pharynx, and tonsils) and the superior laryngeal nerve branch of the vagus nerve (epiglottis and mucous membranes of the larynx to the level of the false vocal cords). The vocal cords and upper trachea receive sensory innervation from the recurrent laryngeal nerve branch of the vagus nerves. Motor innervation of the laryngeal muscles is from the recurrent laryngeal nerves with the exception of the cricothyroid muscles (vocal cord tensors), which are innervated by the superior laryngeal nerves.

Cough Reflex

Cough is the mechanism by which the airways are cleared of foreign material and secretions. Administration of general anesthesia, local anesthesia to the airway, opioids, and benzodiazepines, all cause cough reflex suppression. Thus, clearance of secretions and foreign material from the airway is likely to be impaired during the perioperative period. The rapidly adapting "irritant" receptors of the upper and lower airway are particularly sensitive to stimulation by light touch, dust, cold air, and chemical stimuli. The mucosa of the larynx is the most sensitive to irritant stimuli, followed by the carina, trachea, and central bronchi. Lower airway irritant receptor activation may trigger bronchospasm.

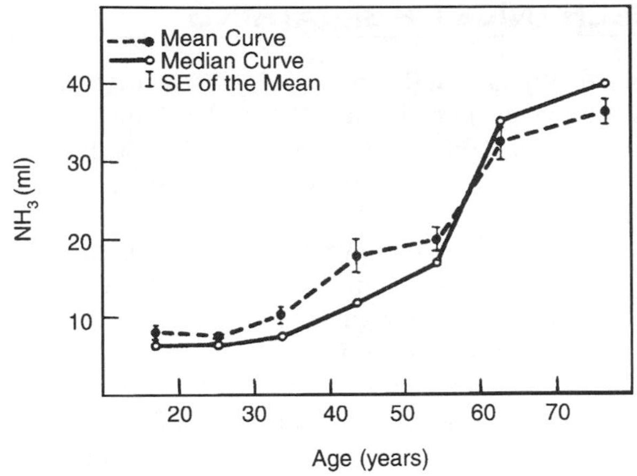

Figure 50-3. Volume of inhaled ammonia necessary to cause breath holding increases noticeably after 60 years of age, suggesting a decline in the sensitivity of protective airway reflexes with increasing age. (From Pontoppidan H, Beecher HK. Progressive loss of protective reflexes in the airway with the advance of age. *JAMA* 1960;174:2209–2213; with permission.)

However, cough and bronchospasm may occur independently and it is unclear why some stimuli cause bronchospasm or cough, and others may cause both. Irritant receptor stimulation results in the transmission of afferent stimuli via the vagus nerves to the medulla. The medulla initiates a series of responses characterized by a deep inhalation followed by closure of the glottis. The efferent response continues with forceful contraction of the expiratory muscles (diaphragm, abdominal, intercostal, and accessory muscles of respiration). The result is an increase in intrapulmonary pressures such that air is forced outward when the glottis opens abruptly. This rapidly moving air usually carries with it any foreign matter that is present in the larger airways below the glottis. There may be a series of several coughs during each expiration. Airflow during a cough may only transiently exceed that observed during a forced expiratory maneuver, due to the elevated intrapleural pressure and resulting dynamic airway compression. However, although expiratory flow is limited during a cough by airway narrowing, the velocity of airflow is markedly increased at the site of narrowing, generating the shear forces necessary to dislodge foreign material. Increasing age is associated with depression of the cough reflex (Fig. 50-3) (Pontoppidan and Beecher, 1960). Surgical incisional pain, and processes that limit muscle strength, such as neuromuscular disease and malnutrition, will also diminish the effectiveness of cough.

Sneeze Reflex

The sneeze reflex is similar to the cough reflex except that it facilitates clearance of secretions from the nasal passageways rather than passageways below the nose. The initiating stimulus for the sneeze reflex is stimulation of the nasal passageways.

MECHANICS OF BREATHING

The diaphragm is the principal muscle of breathing, accounting for approximately 75% of the air that enters the lungs during spontaneous inspiration. Contraction of the diaphragm forces abdominal contents downward and forward. During quiet breathing diaphragmatic excursion is approximately 1 cm. However, during forced breathing diaphragmatic excursion increases to approximately 10 cm. The action of the diaphragm is similar to that of a piston in a cylinder. Diaphragmatic activity causes gas flow into the chest by decreasing intrathoracic pressure to less than atmospheric pressure. Motor innervation of the diaphragm is via the phrenic nerves, which originate from the 3rd, 4th, and 5th cervical segments. Diaphragmatic muscle is predominantly of the slow twitch variety. Slow twitch fibers are high endurance-fatigue resistant, densely populated by mitochondria, myoglobin rich, utilize predominantly aerobic energy pathways, and have very dense capillary networks. During quiet breathing, the contribution of intercostal muscle contraction to inspiration is small. The intercostals muscles are responsible for the "bucket handle" like movement of the ribs, which increases the diameter of the thoracic cavity. Intercostal motor innervation is via their corresponding thoracic segments. Overall, the oxygen cost of breathing is usually <5% of minute oxygen consumption. More than two-thirds of the work of quiet breathing is spent in overcoming the elastic recoil of the lungs and thorax. When the rate of breathing increases or airways are narrowed, a large proportion of work is spent in overcoming the resistance to gas flow.

In contrast to inspiration, normal exhalation is a passive event, utilizing the elastic recoil of the lungs, chest wall, and abdominal structures. Elastic recoil returns the thoracic wall and lungs to their resting equilibrium, which corresponds to the FRC, the lung volume at the end of a normal expiration. The inherent tendency for the lungs to collapse (recoil away from the chest wall) is due to elastic fibers that are stretched by lung inflation and therefore attempt to return to their resting length. An important additional deflating force is the surface tension of the fluid lining the alveoli (see the section on Surface Tension and Pulmonary Surfactant). Elastic fibers in the lungs normally account for approximately one-third of the recoil tendency, and surface tension accounts for the remainder. These elastic recoil properties of stretched tissues lead to an increase in the alveolar pressure to above atmospheric and gas is forced outward. Abdominal muscles are the important muscles of exhalation during exertion. These muscles of exhalation are active only during forced exhalation maneuvers (cough to clear secretions) or obstruction to the flow of gas. Indeed, paralysis of abdominal muscles produced by regional anesthesia does not influence resting alveolar ventilation, but the patient's ability to cough and clear secretions may be compromised.

Elastic coil of the lungs and of the chest wall is responsible for the average negative intrapleural pressure of approximately −4 mm Hg. Intrapleural pressure varies depending upon the location within the thoracic cavity (see Fig. 50-2). Expansion of the lungs during maximum inspiration creates an intrapleural pressure of −12 mm Hg or greater.

Alveolar Volume and Distribution of Ventilation

Alveolar volume is not uniform throughout the lungs because of differences in distending pressures to which alveoli are subjected. Pleural pressure is most negative at the apices of the lungs and becomes progressively less negative toward the lung bases. These regional differences in transalveolar pressure (alveolar pressure minus pleural pressure) means that alveoli in lung apices are more expanded than those at the lung bases (see Fig. 50-2). Although alveoli at the apices are more expanded than those at the base, regional ventilation at the apex is not increased compared to the base. Indeed, basal ventilation is generally increased compared to ventilation at the apex. This occurs because basal alveoli lie on the optimal portion of the alveolar pressure-volume curve. There is a relatively large change in volume in basal alveoli for a given change in pressure compared to apical alveoli. Regional ventilation is determined by the *change* in alveolar size, not by the absolute alveolar size. However, in some circumstances, the lowermost regions of the lungs may have markedly reduced ventilation. If the local intrapleural pressure exceeds atmospheric pressure the transalveolar pressure will favor small airway and alveolar collapse in that region.

Distribution of ventilation in the lungs and the volume at which airways in lung bases begin to close can be assessed by the single-breath nitrogen washout test. After exhaling to residual volume, the subject takes a single breath of oxygen to total lung capacity. During the subsequent slow exhalation from total lung capacity to residual volume, the concentration of nitrogen in the exhaled air is plotted against the exhaled volume (Fig. 50-4). The first

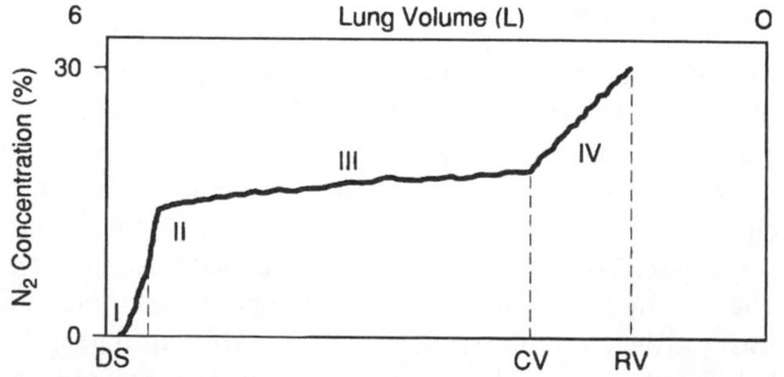

Figure 50-4. Single-breath nitrogen washout curve reflecting dead space volume (phase I), exhalation of alveolar gas (phases II and III), and airway closure in the lung bases (phase IV). (CV, closing volume; DS, dead space; RV, residual volume.)

gases exhaled from large airways are considered to represent dead space gases (phase I) and contain little nitrogen (see the section on Dead Space). The beginning of alveolar gas exhalation is reflected by an increase in the exhaled nitrogen concentration (phase II), followed by a plateau (phase III) if ventilation is distributed fairly evenly. If the nitrogen concentration continues to increase during phase III, it can be assumed that alveoli are filling and emptying at different rates. Phase IV reflects higher nitrogen concentrations in alveoli of the lung spaces that continue to empty at low lung volumes that are associated with airway closure.

Pneumothorax

When air enters the pleural space via a rupture in the lung or a hole in the chest wall, the lung on the affected side collapses because of its elastic recoil. The intrapleural pressure on the affected side is now atmospheric, thus shifting the mediastinum towards the normal side, which has a subatmospheric pressure. Mediastinal shift may cause kinking of the great vessels and hemodynamic compromise. If the communication between the pleural space and the atmosphere remains open (open pneumothorax), air will preferentially flow into the pleural cavity from the atmosphere during inspiration rather than into the lung via the airway (Fig. 50-5). Under these circumstances respiration becomes labored and inefficient. There is marked stimulation of breathing due to arterial hypoxemia, hypercarbia, and activation of pulmonary deflation receptors.

Occasionally, the defect in the lung or chest wall will act as a flutter valve. Under this circumstance, air is allowed to enter during inspiration but cannot exit during exhalation. The pressure in the pleural space will increase above atmospheric (tension pneumothorax). As with an open pneumothorax, there is a shift of the mediastinum toward the intact lung with kinking of the great vessels and development of arterial hypoxemia. Life-saving treatment is decompression of the pneumothorax by insertion of a chest tube and removing the air. Spontaneous pneumothorax is due to rupture of a bleb or blebs on the surface of the visceral pleura. Air from a closed pneumothorax diffuses along a partial pressure gradient into venous blood, being completely absorbed in 1 to 2 weeks.

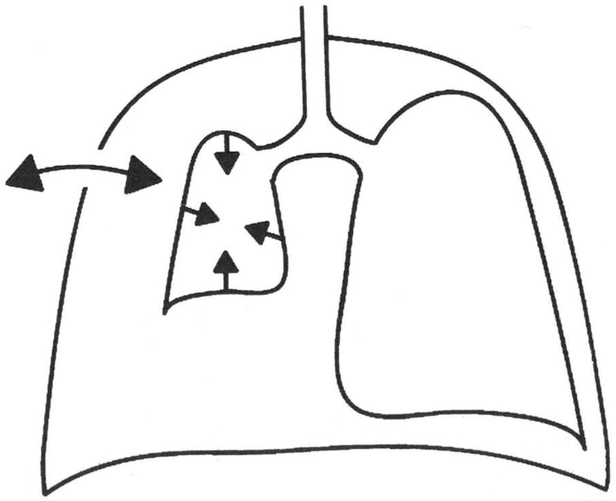

Figure 50-5. Schematic depiction of an open pneumothorax. Air enters the pleural space via a rupture in the lung or a hole in the chest wall, the lung on the affected side collapses because of its elastic recoil. Air will preferentially flow into the pleural cavity from the atmosphere during inspiration rather than into the lung via the airway.

SURFACE TENSION AND PULMONARY SURFACTANT

Surface tension greatly influences the mechanical properties of the lung. Surface tension results from the attraction between the molecules of the fluid film that lines the alveoli. The fluid molecules have a greater attraction for each other than they have for the adjacent air. Therefore, the fluid film will tend to occupy the smallest area possible. The forces of attraction between the fluid molecules are greater when the molecules are closer together. Surface tension forces tend to reduce alveolar diameter. Furthermore, because the surface tension forces increase as the alveolus becomes smaller, an inherently unstable situation is created whereby alveoli are subjected to ever increasing surface tension forces as they get smaller, causing eventual collapse of small alveoli. Surface tension also encourages the movement of fluid into the alveolus, facilitating the development of pulmonary edema. The alveolar fluid–air interface is critical for the development of surface tension. This is illustrated by the finding that when lungs are inflated with saline, eliminating the air–fluid interface, the pressure required for inflation is markedly reduced. Surface tension properties are mathematically described by Laplace law, that states that the pressure inside a bubble (or alveolus) necessary to keep it expanded is directly proportional to the tension on the wall of the bubble, which tends to collapse it, divided by the radius of the bubble. As the radius of the alveolus is diminished, the collapsing pressure in the alveolus will increase, eventually emptying its contents into an adjacent larger alveolus.

From the above, it can be predicted that if alveolar surface tension properties were not modified by the presence of surfactant (see the Section on Surfactant) the lungs would eventually become collapsed, stiff, and fluid filled.

Surfactant

In health, alveolar surface tension is very low because of the presence of surfactant. Pulmonary surfactant is a lipoprotein secreted by type II alveolar cells (pneumocytes) lining the alveoli. These cells begin to appear at approximately 21 weeks of gestation, and surfactant is first produced between 28 and 32 weeks. When premature delivery of an infant is anticipated, formation of pulmonary surfactant may be hastened by administration of corticosteroids to the parturient. The phospholipid component of pulmonary surfactant, dipalmitoyl phosphatidylcholine (DPPC), decreases surface tension of fluids lining the alveoli. DPPC is dispersed over the surface of the alveolar fluid lining. The DPPC molecule contains a hydrophilic portion, which is located within the alveolar lining fluid, and a hydrophobic portion that projects into the alveolar lumen. DPPC molecules tend to repel each other, thus counteracting the surface tension forces of the alveolar lining fluid. The intermolecular repulsive forces of DPPC are greatest when the DPPC molecules are close to each other. Therefore, alveoli with small diameters have a lower surface tension because DPPC molecules densely populate the lining fluid. Furthermore, as an alveolus increases in size, the pulmonary surfactant becomes diluted at the surface of the alveolar lining fluid, thus diminishing its surface tension reducing effect. Thus, pulmonary surfactant helps to stabilize the sizes of alveoli, reducing surface tension in larger alveoli to a lesser extent than in smaller alveoli. The net effect is the maintenance of consistent alveolar diameter and stability.

Absence or inadequate amounts of pulmonary surfactant is characteristic of respiratory distress syndrome of the neonate in which a large number of alveoli are filled with fluid. In the absence of surfactant, lung expansion is difficult, requiring intrapleural pressures often approaching −30 mm Hg to overcome the collapsing tendency of the alveoli. The average alveolar diameter of the premature infant may be as little as a quarter of that of the adult alveolus. Laplace law predicts that diminished alveolar diameters potentiate the adverse effects of surfactant deficiency on alveolar stability in the premature infant. Delivery of commercially available surfactant into the lungs of neonates is effective in decreasing morbidity and mortality from respiratory distress syndrome (Jobe, 1993).

Pulmonary surfactant may be diminished after cardiopulmonary bypass, after prolonged inhalation of 100% oxygen, and in persons who inhale tobacco smoke. When the surface area of the surfactant film is kept small, a rearrangement of molecules occurs, causing surface tension to increase with time. Therefore, peripheral alveoli tend to collapse during prolonged periods of shallow breathing. A single large breath, vital capacity maneuver, or sigh, reexpands these alveoli, increasing their surface area, thus restoring normal surface tension.

COMPLIANCE

Compliance is expressed as the increase in the gas volume of the lungs for each unit increase of alveolar pressure. The combined compliance of normal lungs and thorax is 0.13 liters/cm H_2O. This means that the lungs expand 130 mL for every 1 cm H_2O pressure increase in the alveoli. Any condition that destroys lung tissue or blocks bronchioles causes decreased pulmonary compliance. Deformities of the thoracic cage such as kyphosis or scoliosis decrease thoracic compliance.

TABLE 50-1.
LUNG VOLUMES AND CAPACITIES

	Abbreviation	Normal Adult Value
Tidal volume	VT	500 (6–8 mL/kg)
Inspiratory reserve volume	IRV	3,000 mL
Expiratory reserve volume	ERV	1,200 mL
Residual volume	RV	1,200 mL
Inspiratory capacity	IC	3,500 mL
Functional residual capacity	FRC	2,400 mL
Vital capacity	VC	4,500 mL (60–70 mL/kg)
Forced exhaled volume in 1 second	FEV_1	80%
Total lung capacity	TLC	5,900 mL

LUNG VOLUMES AND CAPACITIES

The amount of gas in the lungs has been subdivided into four different volumes and capacities (Table 50-1) (Fig. 50-6). A lung capacity is the sum of two or more lung volumes (see Fig. 50-6). In normal persons, the volume of gas in the lungs depends primarily on body size and build. For example, large and athletic persons have larger lung volumes than small and asthenic individuals. Lung volumes

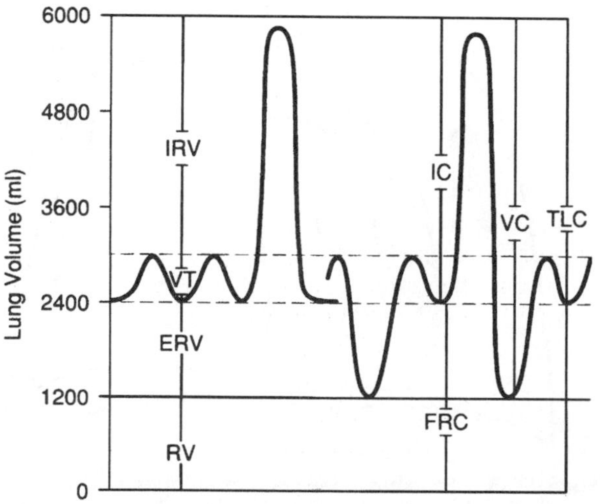

Figure 50-6. Schematic diagram of breathing excursions at rest and during maximal inhalation and/or exhalation (see Table 50-1 for definition of abbreviations). Lung capacities are the sum of two or more lung volumes.

and capacities are approximately 25% less in females than in males. Lung volumes and capacities also change with body position, most of them decreasing when the patient is supine and increasing when the patient is standing. Decreases in lung volumes in the recumbent position reflect the tendency for abdominal contents to press upward against the diaphragm and an increase in thoracic blood volume, both of which decrease the space available in the thoracic cavity for gas.

In diseases associated with airway obstruction, such as asthma and emphysema, it is usually more difficult to exhale than to inhale. Expiratory obstruction occurs because expiration is associated with a higher intrapleural pressure, which tends to compress intrathoracic airways. Conversely, the negative intrapleural pressure of inspiration tends to increase intrathoracic airway diameter. As a result, asthma, bronchitis, and emphysema are associated with gas trapping, leading to an increased residual volume and total lung capacity.

Functional Residual Capacity

FRC is the volume remaining in the lungs at the end of a normal quiet expiration and is determined by the elastic properties of the lung and chest wall. If expiration is active and is continued past FRC, the residual volume (RV) will eventually be reached (the volume in the lung after maximal expiration). The normal FRC is 35 mL/kg, or approximately 2.5 liters in an adult male. The FRC is effectively the volume of distribution for each tidal breath and buffers alveolar gas tensions against abrupt alterations in Pa_{O_2} and Pa_{CO_2} during the respiratory cycle. In the presence of a decreased FRC, transient interruptions in breathing, as during direct laryngoscopy, may result in rapid changes in Pa_{O_2}. Breathing 100% oxygen offsets the effect of apnea on Pa_{O_2}, especially when the FRC is decreased, as in the parturient.

Effects of Anesthesia

After induction of anesthesia and placement of a tracheal tube, there is a decrease in the FRC of approximately 450 mL that occurs whether or not neuromuscular blockade is present (Nunn, 1990). The decrease in FRC is thought to be caused by several factors, including, cephalad movement of the diaphragm, a decrease in the cross-sectional area of the rib cage, and movement of blood into or out of the thorax. The decrease in FRC has important functional consequences that include changes in airway caliber, distribution of ventilation, gas exchange, airway closure, and atelectasis (Magnusson and Spahn, 2003). For example, changes in lung volume decrease airway caliber, especially in dependent parts of the lungs. This effect is to a certain extent, offset by the bronchodilator effect of inhaled anesthetics such that airway resistance does not usually change after induction of anesthesia. Airway closure, especially in patients at the extremes of age, is likely if FRC decreases below closing capacity. Reductions in FRC alter the distribution of ventilation such that regional ventilation will be diverted toward the nondependent portions of the lung. Because perfusion remains distributed in a gravity-dependent manner toward the dependent regions, there will be ventilation/perfusion mismatching. These factors, combined with alveolar collapse in dependent regions, are responsible for the right-to-left shunt equivalent to approximately 10% of the cardiac output that typically accompanies general anesthesia. Indeed, it is estimated that airway closure and atelectasis contribute equally to the increased ventilation to perfusion mismatching that occurs during general anesthesia (Wahba, 1996). Positive end-expiratory pressure decreases this shunt by reinflating previously collapsed areas of the lung. However, the beneficial effect on Pa_{O_2} may be offset by decreases in cardiac output induced by the decreased venous return associated with increased intrathoracic pressures.

Vital Capacity

Other than the anatomic build of an individual, the major factors that determine vital capacity (VC) are respiratory muscle conditioning and the compliance of the lungs and chest wall. A tall, thin person usually has a larger VC than an obese person. A well-conditioned athlete may have a VC 30% to 40% above normal. Fibrotic changes in the lungs produced by chronic bronchial asthma or chronic bronchitis decrease pulmonary compliance and thus decrease VC. Any excess fluid in the lungs, such as pulmonary edema or pleural effusions associated with heart failure, decreases pulmonary compliance and thus the VC. Indeed, an improvement in VC may reflect a decrease in pulmonary edema as associated with an improvement in left ventricular dysfunction.

Forced Exhaled Vital Capacity

The forced exhaled VC is the volume of gas that can be rapidly and maximally exhaled starting from total lung capacity. It is customary to measure the volume of exhaled gases after 1 second (FEV_1) and 3 seconds (FEV_3). The FEV_1 and FEV_3 are also expressed as a percentage of the VC. In normal individuals, the FEV_1 is >80% of the VC (Fig. 50-7). In the presence of obstructive airway disease, this value is <50%.

Measurement of the mean airflow rate over the middle half of the forced VC is the forced midexpiratory flow rate ($MEFR_{25\%-75\%}$). Reduction in this flow rate is a sensitive index of airway obstruction. Measurement of $MEFR_{25\%-75\%}$ is attractive because this value is remarkably effort-independent. Forced expiratory flow is limited because forced expiration is associated with significant increases in intrapleural pressure. Increased intrapleural pressure results in airflow limitation by causing airway compression (greater expiratory effort is associated with greater airway compression).

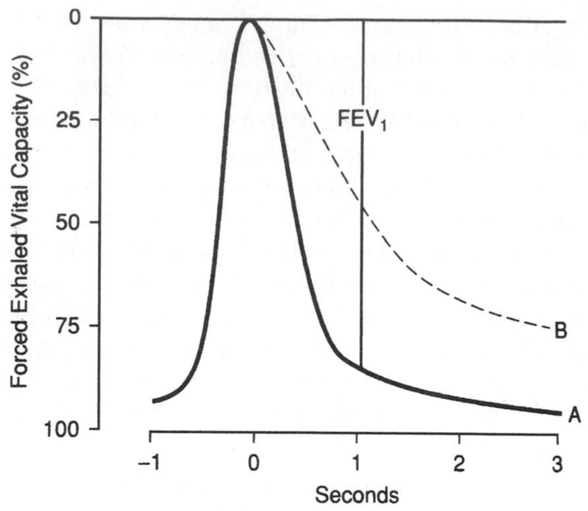

Figure 50-7. Schematic diagram of forced exhaled volume in normal individuals (A) and in individuals with obstructive airway disease (B). A normal individual can exhale approximately 80% of the vital capacity in 1 s (FEV$_1$) compared with approximately 50% in 1 s in individuals with obstructive airway disease.

MINUTE VENTILATION

The minute ventilation represents the total amount of gas moved into the lungs each minute (tidal volume times breathing frequency). The average minute ventilation is approximately 6 liters.

Alveolar Ventilation

Alveolar ventilation is the volume of gas each minute that enters areas of the lungs capable of participating in gas exchange with pulmonary capillary blood. Alveolar ventilation is less than minute ventilation because a portion of inhaled gases resides in portions of the airway that do not participate in gas exchange with pulmonary capillary blood (see the Section on Dead Space). As such, alveolar ventilation is equal to tidal volume, from which dead space volume is subtracted (estimate 150 mL), multiplied by the frequency of breathing. The average alveolar ventilation is approximately 4.2 liters/minute. The $PaCO_2$, and to a lesser extent the PaO_2, are determined by alveolar ventilation. The frequency of breathing and tidal volume are the primary determinants of alveolar ventilation.

Dead Space

Anatomic dead space includes those areas of the respiratory tract (nasal passageways, pharynx, trachea, and bronchi) that do not normally participate in gas exchange with pulmonary capillary blood. Physiologic dead space is the gas volume of alveoli that are not functional or only partially functional because of absent or poor blood flow through corresponding pulmonary capillaries (wasted ventilation). The volume of dead space is determined by measuring the exhaled concentration of nitrogen after a single breath of oxygen. Gas being exhaled from dead space (2 mL/kg or approximately 150 mL in an adult) contains no nitrogen (see Fig. 50-4). Normally, the contributions of anatomic and physiologic dead space are nearly equal. Chronic lung disease is associated with the maldistribution of ventilation relative to pulmonary capillary blood flow, which will increase physiologic dead space.

During exhalation, gas in dead space is exhaled before gas coming from the alveoli. This is why anesthetic breathing systems are designed to preferentially conserve dead space gas (oxygen and anesthetic not removed and devoid of carbon dioxide) and to eliminate alveolar gas (oxygen and anesthetic depleted and carbon dioxide added). Conceptually, rebreathing dead space gas is similar to delivering fresh gases from the anesthesia machine.

CONTROL OF VENTILATION

Many of the drugs used in the perioperative period to provide anesthesia, amnesia, and analgesia have profound effects upon the control of ventilation (Dahan and Teppema, 2003). Respiratory depression is an important life-threatening side-effect of anesthetic and opioid administration.

Control of ventilation is designed to make adjustments in alveolar ventilation so as to maintain optimal PaO_2, $PaCO_2$, and hydrogen ion concentrations. Fine control of ventilation is provided by the respiratory center under the influence of chemical stimuli from chemoreceptors. The major factor in regulation of alveolar ventilation is the $PaCO_2$ rather than the PaO_2. For example, a 50% increase in $PaCO_2$ evokes a tenfold increase in alveolar ventilation, and a PaO_2 of 40 mm Hg evokes a 1.5-fold increase in alveolar ventilation. At the onset of exercise, an increase in alveolar ventilation occurs immediately due to direct stimulation of the respiratory center by the cerebral cortex (anticipatory stimulation) and indirect stimulation of the respiratory center by proprioceptors that are activated by joint movement. The respiratory center is depressed by inhaled anesthetics and other centrally acting depressant drugs such as barbiturates and opioids. Cerebrovascular accidents may damage the respiratory center, leading to abnormalities of the breathing pattern (see the section on Periodic Breathing). Stimulation of the medullary vasomotor center is associated with spillover of impulses to the nearby respiratory center. As a result, decreases in systemic blood pressure that evoke increases in sympathetic nervous system activity from the vasomotor center also evoke increases in alveolar ventilation due to increased activity of the respiratory center. Increased body temperature directly stimulates the respiratory center in addition to the indirect stimulation provided by increases in carbon dioxide production. Voluntary control of alveolar ventilation is mediated through the cerebral cortex rather than the respiratory center.

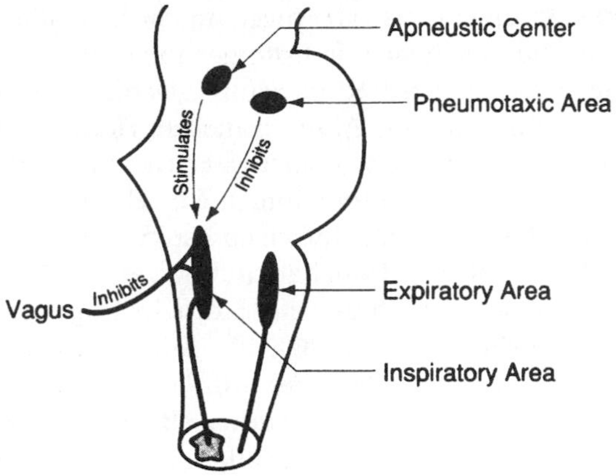

Figure 50-8. The respiratory center is located bilaterally in the reticular substance of the medulla oblongata and pons. (From Guyton AC, Hall JE. *Textbook of medical physiology*, 10th ed. Philadelphia: Saunders, 2000; with permission.)

Respiratory Center

The respiratory center is a widely dispersed group of neurons located bilaterally in the reticular substance of the medulla oblongata and pons (Fig. 50-8) (Guyton and Hall, 2000). This center is divided into four areas: (a) inspiratory area, (b) pneumotaxic area, (c) expiratory area, and (d) apneustic center.

Inspiratory Area

Rhythmic inspiratory cycles are generated in the inspiratory area located bilaterally in the dorsal portion of the medulla. After contraction of the diaphragm, the neurons of the inspiratory area become dormant until intrinsic rhythmic activity again occurs. Afferent input from peripheral chemoreceptors travels to the inspiratory area via the vagus and glossopharyngeal nerves. In addition, the vagus nerves transmit sensory signals from the lungs that provide data about lung inflation and regulate the frequency of breathing.

Pneumotaxic Area

The pneumotaxic area is located in the upper dorsal pons. Signals from the pneumotaxic area are transmitted to the inspiratory area and trigger the termination of inspiration, limiting lung inflation. However, by determining the duration of inspiration, the pneumotaxic center influences the rate of breathing. For example, a strong pneumotaxic signal generates a rapid shallow breathing pattern. A weak pneumotaxic signal results in a slow rate of breathing accompanied by large tidal volumes.

Inflation Reflex

Stretch receptors in the walls of bronchi transmit signals via the vagus nerves to the inspiratory area during maximal lung inflation. These signals limit the duration of inspiration in the same way as signals from the pneumotaxic area and tend to increase the respiratory rate in a similar manner. However, stretch receptor stimulation also increases the duration of expiration and the final effect upon respiratory rate may be unpredictable. The mechanism to limit inspiration is designated the *inflation reflex* or *Hering-Breuer reflex*. It seems unlikely that the inflation reflex is important in controlling normal lung inflation because it becomes activated only when the tidal volume is >1.5 liters. The rapid, shallow breathing that is observed during inhalation of volatile anesthetics is not likely to be related to the inflation reflex. Conversely, in situations of decreased pulmonary compliance, such as pulmonary fibrosis, the pattern of breathing becomes shallow and rapid, thus minimizing elastic work. This response has been ascribed to stretch receptor activation.

Deflation Reflex

Stretch receptors also respond to lung deflation by initiating inspiratory activity and shortening the expiratory period. This response is termed the *Hering-Breuer deflation reflex*.

Apneustic Center

The apneustic center is located in the lower pons. The apneustic center transmits signals to the inspiratory center that prolong inspiratory activity. However, in the presence of normal pneumotaxic area activity, the apneustic center has little influence upon the inspiratory center. When apneustic center activity is unmasked because of damage to the pneumotaxic area, the pattern of breathing is maximal lung inflation with occasional brief expiratory gasps (apneuses).

Expiratory Area

The expiratory area in the ventral portion of the medulla is normally inactive during quiet respiration. At rest, exhalation results from passive recoil of the elastic structure of the lungs and surrounding chest wall and requires no motor activity. However, when alveolar ventilation is increased the expiratory area becomes active, providing signals that evoke forceful and frequent contraction of the diaphragm and abdominal muscles.

Chemical Control

Chemical control of breathing adjusts respiration to maintain P_{CO_2} constant, to defend against excessive changes in hydrogen ion concentration, and to prevent dangerous decreases in P_{O_2}. Chemoreceptors respond to changes in carbon dioxide, oxygen, and hydrogen ion concentrations, and are located in the chemosensitive area of the medulla or in peripheral chemoreceptors. Minute ventilation is proportional to metabolic rate and determined primarily by carbon dioxide production. Signals from the chemoreceptors are integrated in the respiratory center.

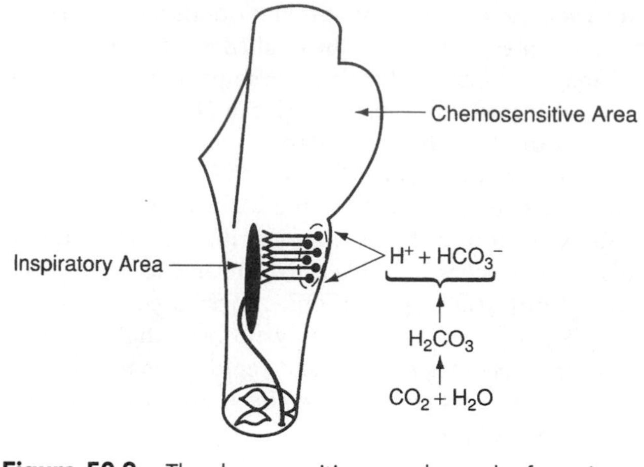

Figure 50-9. The chemosensitive area, located a few microns below the ventral surface of the medulla, transmits stimulatory impulses to the inspiratory area. This chemosensitive area is highly responsive to hydrogen ions (H^+) in the cerebrospinal fluid that result from hydration of carbon dioxide. (From Guyton AC, Hall JE. *Textbook of medical physiology*, 10th ed. Philadelphia: Saunders, 2000; with permission.)

Chemosensitive Area

The chemosensitive area (also known as medullary chemoreceptors) is located a few microns below the surface of the medulla (Fig. 50-9) (Guyton and Hall, 2000). Hydrogen ions are the most important stimulus of the chemosensitive area, but these ions do not easily cross the blood-brain barrier to enter the cerebrospinal fluid. For this reason, changes in blood pH have less effect on stimulating the chemosensitive area than does carbon dioxide, which readily crosses the blood-brain barrier. Carbon dioxide stimulates the chemosensitive area through its reaction with water in the cerebrospinal fluid to form carbonic acid and subsequent dissociation to hydrogen ions (see Fig. 50-9) (Guyton and Hall, 2000). In normal individuals, the average ventilatory response to inhaled carbon dioxide is approximately 2.5 liters/minute for every millimeter of mercury increase in $Paco_2$. It is estimated that 70% to 80% of the ventilatory response to carbon dioxide reflects activation of the chemosensitive area and a subsequent increase in transmission of signals to the inspiratory area of the respiratory center. The remainder of the ventilatory response to carbon dioxide is mediated via the peripheral chemoreceptors.

An advantage of a cerebrospinal fluid system in the control of ventilation is the rapidity with which changes in $Paco_2$ are reflected in the cerebrospinal fluid. This change occurs within seconds compared with at least 1 minute required for changes in the $Paco_2$ to be reflected in interstitial fluid. Hydrogen ions formed in the cerebrospinal fluid are able to rapidly diffuse to the chemosensitive area neurons located only a few microns below the surface of the medulla. The limited buffering capacity of cerebrospinal fluid facilitates relatively large changes in hydrogen ion concentration in response to changes in carbon dioxide production. In contrast, the protein-rich interstitial fluid promptly buffers changes in hydrogen ion concentration.

The effect of increased $Paco_2$ on alveolar ventilation peaks within 1 minute. After several hours, however, the stimulant effect wanes, reflecting active transport (ion pump) of bicarbonate ions into the cerebrospinal fluid from the blood to return the cerebrospinal fluid pH to a normal value of 7.32 (Mitchell and Berger, 1975). These bicarbonate ions combine with excess hydrogen ions in the cerebrospinal fluid, and thus stimulation of the chemosensitive area decreases with time. Therefore, a change in $Paco_2$ has an intense initial effect on the control of ventilation but only a weak effect after several hours during which time adaptation occurs (cerebrospinal fluid pH returns to 7.32) by active transport of bicarbonate ions.

Peripheral Chemoreceptors

The carotid and aortic bodies are chemoreceptors located outside the central nervous system that are responsive to changes in Po_2, Pco_2, and concentration of hydrogen ions. The hypoxic ventilatory response is potent and is predominantly mediated via the carotid body chemoreceptors. Peripheral chemoreceptors transmit signals via the glossopharyngeal nerves (carotid bodies) and vagus nerves (aortic bodies) to the respiratory center in the medulla. Blood flow through the peripheral chemoreceptors is the highest of any tissue in the body, which means that the metabolic needs of chemoreceptor tissues can be met almost entirely by dissolved oxygen. Therefore, it is the Pao_2 and not the arterial hemoglobin saturation with oxygen (Sao_2) that determines the stimulation level of the peripheral chemoreceptors. This is the reason that anemia or carbon monoxide poisoning, in which the amount of dissolved oxygen and thus Po_2 remains normal, do not stimulate alveolar ventilation via the chemoreceptors. Nevertheless, when mean arterial pressure decreases below 60 mm Hg, blood flow through chemoreceptors may decrease sufficiently to lower tissue Po_2 and stimulate alveolar ventilation as well as evoke peripheral vasoconstriction in an attempt to restore perfusion pressure.

The carotid bodies are more involved with ventilatory responses than are the aortic bodies. Conversely, aortic bodies are more prominent than carotid bodies in influencing cardiovascular responses. Removal or denervation of the carotid bodies as that may occur during carotid endarterectomy results in loss of the ventilatory response to arterial hypoxemia and approximately a 30% decrease in the ventilatory response to carbon dioxide. Normally, peripheral chemoreceptors become strongly stimulated when Pao_2 decreases below approximately 60 mm Hg. Conversely, the stimulating effect of increased $Paco_2$ or hydrogen ion concentration on the peripheral chemoreceptors is much less than the effect of these changes on the respiratory center via changes in the pH of the cerebrospinal fluid.

The normal response to hypoxia is a prompt increase in minute ventilation caused by carotid body chemoreceptor activation. However, the ventilatory response of peripheral chemoreceptors to arterial hypoxemia, metabolic acidosis, or both is greatly attenuated by injected and inhaled anesthetics. The concentration of volatile agents associated with depression of hypoxic ventilatory response is much lower than that required for loss of consciousness. For this reason, arterial hypoxemia in the postanesthetic period is unlikely to trigger an increase in alveolar ventilation. Conversely, subanesthetic doses of desflurane do not have a detectable effect on the normocapnic hypoxic ventilatory response, although carbon dioxide-induced augmentation of the hypoxic response is decreased, confirming that this volatile anesthetic also depresses the carotid bodies at subanesthetic doses (Dahan et al., 1996). In addition to their effects upon respiratory control, volatile anesthetics also depress ventilation by suppression of intercostal, diaphragmatic, and upper airway muscle function.

EFFECTS OF SLEEP ON BREATHING

Approximately 30% of the human lifespan is spent sleeping. Sleep has important effects upon respiratory function. Decreases in the level of environmental stimulation during sleep are associated with modest increases in Pa_{CO_2}, and the ventilatory response to carbon dioxide is decreased. The ventilatory response to hypoxia is better maintained during sleep than are responses to carbon dioxide. Persons with depressed ventilatory responses to hypercapnia and hypoxia while awake breathe even less during sleep compared to those who show normal awake responses. The different phases of sleep have varying effects upon respiratory function. Rapid eye movement sleep (REM sleep) is associated with loss of activity in upper airway muscles while diaphragmatic function is relatively preserved. Because of the relative loss of tone in the upper airway, the negative airway pressure created by the diaphragm during inspiration may be sufficient to occlude the upper airway. Indeed, brief periods of upper airway obstruction occur even in normal individuals during REM sleep. Respiratory rhythm is irregular during REM sleep. Nonrapid eye movement sleep (NREM sleep) is characterized by a regular breathing pattern. Minute ventilation is decreased to a greater extent during NREM sleep than REM sleep.

APNEIC PERIODS DURING SLEEP

Apneic periods occur during sleep in approximately one-third of normal individuals and are particularly common among elderly males. Apnea may last for >10 s and may be associated with decreases in Sa_{O_2} to 75% or less. Apneic spells are also common in premature infants.

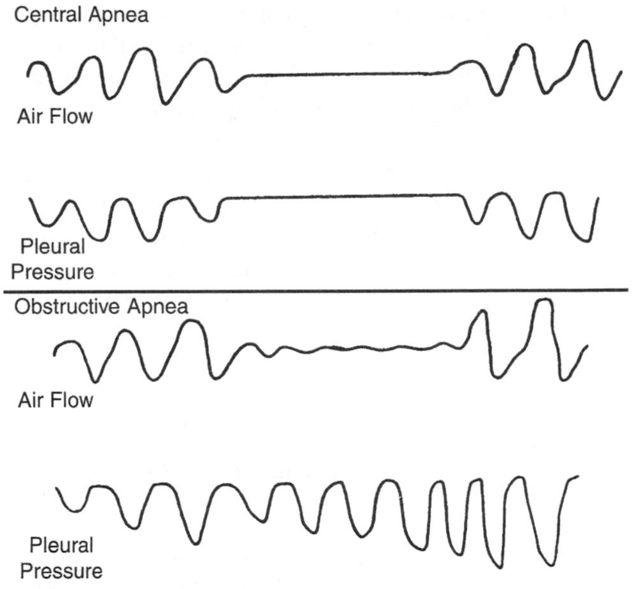

Figure 50-10. Central sleep apnea is characterized by cessation of air flow as a result of suspension of all expiratory efforts. Obstructive sleep apnea is characterized by cessation of air flow despite persistent respiratory efforts as reflected by pleural pressure changes. (From Berne RM, Levy MN, Koeppen BM. *Physiology*, 5th ed. St. Louis: Mosby, 2004; with permission.)

Sleep apneas are classified as *central* (cessation of respiratory efforts) or *obstructive* (despite respiratory efforts, air flow ceases because of total upper airway obstruction) (Fig. 50-10) (Berne and Levy, 2004). Mixed apnea occurs when both obstructive and central apnea are present. Sleep apnea is defined as cessation of airflow at the mouth and nostril for >10 seconds occurring more than 15 times per hour. Snoring is a manifestation of partial obstruction of the upper airway at sites including the pharynx and oropharynx. This may reflect failure of the genioglossus muscles to contract during inspiration, thus permitting the tongue to fall back and obstruct the upper airway. Indeed, genioglossal muscle tone is markedly depressed during REM sleep. Arousal is evoked by chemoreceptor activation due to arterial hypoxemia. Hypercarbia may also be an important factor in terminating sleep apnea. Recurrent episodes of arterial hypoxemia and hypercarbia may lead to polycythemia and pulmonary hypertension.

PERIODIC BREATHING

Cheyne-Stokes breathing, which is characterized by a waxing and waning pattern of ventilation, is the most common form of periodic breathing. There may be apneic periods that last for up to 20 seconds followed by periods of hyperventilation. This pattern of respiration is unusual in healthy individuals except at high altitude during sleep. Cheyne-Stokes breathing is seen most often in patients with brain injury, congestive cardiac failure, and uremia. Cyclic increases and decreases in Pa_{CO_2} are associated with periodic breathing. The normal absence of Cheyne-Stokes breathing reflects the rapid lung-to-brain circulation time, minimizing the time that is required for changes in $Paco_2$ to be detected by central chemoreceptors. When there is a delay in blood flow from the lungs to the brain as in congestive heart failure, however, the respiratory center may lag behind the $Paco_2$, causing cyclic variations in the alveolar ventilation. Brainstem damage may increase the feedback gain control of the respiratory center such that a small change in $Paco_2$ causes a large change in alveolar ventilation.

NONVENTILATORY FUNCTIONS OF THE LUNGS

Nonventilatory functions of the lungs include a number of metabolic functions as reflected by synthesis, release and removal of biologically active substances (Table 50-2) (Bakhle, 1990). For example, prostaglandins are removed from the circulation during passage through the lungs, and they are also synthesized in the lungs and released into the blood when the lung tissue is stretched. Inhaled anesthetics may interfere with the removal of norepinephrine from the blood by the lungs (Bakhle, 1990). Endothelial cells of the pulmonary capillaries contain the converting enzyme responsible for conversion of angiotensin I to angiotensin II. Halothane, but not enflurane, undergoes metabolism in the lungs (Blitt et al., 1981). The lungs contain a fibrinolytic system that lyses clots in the pulmonary vessels. Indeed, the pulmonary capillaries, by receiving the entire cardiac output, act as filters for emboli and air. This filter effect is lost in the presence of a right-to-left intracardiac shunt or during cardiopulmonary bypass. The majority of exogenous substances removed by passage through the pulmonary circulation are not metabolized but instead are bound to components of lung tissue. Drugs most effectively bound to lung tissue are lipid soluble, with pK values of >8.0. Drug extraction by metabolism or binding to tissues may prevent delivery of toxic concentrations of local anesthetics to the systemic circulation. Conversely, first-pass pulmonary uptake of some injected drugs, especially opioids, is sufficient to influence the peak arterial concentration of these drugs (see Chapters 1 and 3).

TABLE 50-2.
METABOLIC FUNCTIONS OF THE LUNGS

Synthesized and used in the lungs
Surfactant
Synthesized and released into the blood
Prostaglandins
Histamine
Kallikrein
von Willebrand factor
Tissue plasminogen activator
Partially removed from the blood
Prostaglandins
Bradykinin
Serotonin
Norepinephrine
Acetylcholine
Fentanyl
Propranolol
Lidocaine
Atrial natriuretic factor
Adenosine
Imipramine
Not removed from the blood
Epinephrine
Dopamine
Prostacyclin
Morphine
Histamine
Angiotensin II
Vasopressin
Activated in the lungs
Angiotensin I
Arachidonic acid

REFERENCES

Atwell SW. Major anomalies of the tracheobronchial tree. *Chest* 1967; 52:611–615.

Bakhle YS. Pharmacokinetic and metabolic properties of the lung. *Br J Anaesth* 1990;65:79–93.

Benumof JL, Partridge BL, Salvatierra C, et al. Margin of safety in positioning modern double-lumen endotracheal tubes. *Anesthesiology* 1987;67:729–738.

Berne RM, Levy M, Koeppen BM, et al. *Physiology*, 5th ed. St. Louis: Mosby, 2004.

Blitt CD, Gandolfi AJ, Soltis JJ, et al. Extrahepatic biotransformation of halothane and enflurane. *Anesth Analg* 1981;60:129–132.

Dahan A, Sarton E, van den Elsen M, et al. Ventilatory response to hypoxia in humans: influences of subanesthetic desflurane. *Anesthesiology* 1996;85:60–68.

Dahan A, Teppema LJ. Influence of anaesthesia on the control of breathing. *Br J Anaesth* 2003; 91:40–49.

Guyton AC, Hall JE. *Textbook of medical physiology*, 10th ed. Philadelphia: Saunders, 2000.

Hlastala MP, Berger AJ. *Physiology of respiration*, 2nd ed. Oxford University Press, 2001.

Jobe AH. Pulmonary surfactant therapy. *N Engl J Med* 1993;328: 861–868.

Magnusson L, Spahn DR. New concepts of atelectasis during general anaesthesia. *Br J Anaesth*, 2003;91:61–72.

Mitchell RA, Berger AJ. Neural regulation of respiration. *Am Rev Respir Dis* 1975;111:206–224.

Nunn JF. Effects of anaesthesia on respiration. *Br J Anaesth* 1990;65: 54–62.

Pereira LMP, Orrett FA, Balbirsingh M. Physiological perspectives of therapy in bronchial hyperreactivity. *Can J Anaesth* 1996;43:700–713.

Pontoppidan H, Beecher HK. Progressive loss of protective reflexes in the airway with the advance of age. *JAMA* 1960;174:2209–2213.

Stene R, Rose M, Weinger MB, et al. Bronchial trifurcation at the carina complicating use of a double-lumen tracheal tube. *Anesthesiology* 1994;80:1162–1164.

Wahba RM. Airway closure and intraoperative hypoxemia: twenty-five years later. *Can J Anaesth* 1996;43:1144–1149.

51

Pulmonary Gas Exchange and Blood Transport of Gases

PULMONARY GAS EXCHANGE

The primary function of the lungs is to provide for the optimal exchange of oxygen and carbon dioxide between the ambient environment and pulmonary capillaries. This gas exchange process is termed *external respiration*. Gas transport between the atmosphere and the alveolus consists of (a) convection (bulk flow of gases within the airways) and (b) diffusion (random molecular motion leading to complete mixing of all gases beginning at the terminal bronchioles). The transition from convective flow to diffusion at the terminal bronchioles occurs because the cross-sectional area of the airway increases rapidly in this region, thus there is an abrupt decrease in the velocity of convective flow. The third component of gas transport is alveolar-capillary gas exchange, which is greatly dependent on the matching of regional alveolar ventilation with pulmonary capillary perfusion (V/Q). Oxygen leaves alveoli to enter pulmonary capillary blood and carbon dioxide enters alveoli from pulmonary capillary blood by the process of diffusion. Diffusion of molecules occurs from areas of high partial pressure to areas of low partial pressure.

Partial Pressure

The partial pressure (P) that a gas exerts is due to the constant impact of molecules in motion against a surface. The higher the concentration of gas molecules or the higher the temperature, the greater the sum of the forces of all the molecules striking the surface at any instant. As a result, the partial pressure of a gas is directly proportional to its concentration and temperature.

In a mixture of gases, the partial pressure that each gas contributes to the total pressure is directly proportional to its relative concentration (Table 51-1). For example, at sea level, 79% of the total atmospheric pressure (P_B) of 760 mm Hg is due to nitrogen (PN_2 597 mm Hg) and 21% is due to oxygen (Po_2 159 mm Hg). The P_B is the sum of all the individual partial pressures of the component gases. Partial pressure may also be expressed in kilopascals (1 kPa equals 7.6 mm Hg or 10 cm H_2O).

When a gas is exposed to an adjoining liquid or tissue interface, gas molecules dissolve in the liquid or tissue until equilibrium is achieved. Equilibrium is present when the number of molecules leaving the gas phase equals the number returning to the gas phase. At equilibrium, the partial pressure of the gas dissolved in the liquid phase is equal to the partial pressure of the gas in the gas phase and there is no net movement of gas across the interface.

The concentration of a gas in liquid is determined not only by the partial pressure the gas exerts but also by the solubility coefficient of the gas. For example, some molecules are physically or chemically attracted to water (hydrophilic), whereas others are repelled (hydrophobic). Hydrophilic molecules dissolve readily in water without exerting a large partial pressure in the solution. Conversely, hydrophobic molecules exert high partial pressure and are poorly soluble in an aqueous solution. Henry law states that the concentration of a dissolved gas is equal to the partial pressure of that gas multiplied by its solubility coefficient.

Vapor Pressure of Water

Water in tissues has a tendency to escape into an adjoining gas phase just as molecules in the gas phase pass into the water. The pressure that water molecules exert to escape to the surface is the vapor pressure of water (47 mm Hg at 37°C). The higher the temperature, the greater the kinetic

TABLE 51-1.
PARTIAL PRESSURES OF RESPIRATORY GASES AT SEA LEVEL (760 mm Hg)

Respiratory Gas	Inhaled Air (mm Hg)	Alveolar Gases (mm Hg)	Exhaled Gases (mm Hg)
Oxygen	159	104	120
Carbon dioxide	0.3	40	27
Nitrogen	597	569	566
Water	3.7	47	47

activity of the molecules and thus the greater the likelihood that water molecules will escape from the surface into the gas phase (vapor pressure of water is >47 mm Hg).

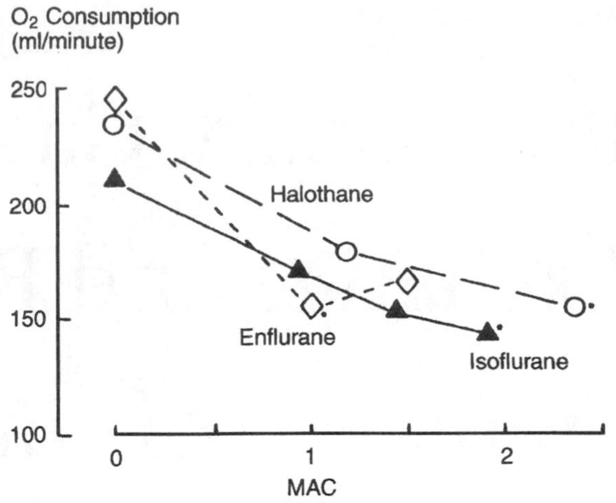

Figure 51-1. Potent inhaled anesthetics decrease oxygen consumption with the greatest change occurring in the transition from wakefulness to sleep. (From Eger EI. *Isoflurane [Forane]: a compendium and reference.* Madison, WI: Ohio Medical Products, 1984; with permission.)

Composition of Alveolar Gases

The composition of alveolar gases is different from the composition of inhaled (atmospheric) gases because (a) oxygen is constantly being absorbed from the alveoli, (b) carbon dioxide is constantly being added to the alveoli, and (c) dry inhaled gases are humidified by the addition of water vapor (see Table 51-1). Because the total partial pressure of gases in the alveoli remains unchanged, the addition of water vapor and carbon dioxide and removal of oxygen from the inhaled gases alters the delivered Po_2 from 159 mm Hg to 104 mm Hg and the PN_2 from 597 mm Hg to 569 mm Hg.

Alveolar Partial Pressure of Oxygen

The alveolar partial pressure of oxygen (PAO_2) is determined by the rate of delivery of new oxygen by alveolar ventilation and the rate of absorption of oxygen into pulmonary capillary blood. The normal rate of oxygen absorption in the resting state is 250 mL/minute. Exercise increases and anesthesia decreases oxygen consumption (Fig. 51-1) (Eger, 1984).

The inspired partial pressure of oxygen (PIO_2) is diluted by the vapor pressure of water (47 mm Hg) and the diffusion of carbon dioxide into the alveolus ($PACO_2$ 40 mm Hg). Both of these processes are essentially independent of the P_B. Thus, the impact of this dilution on the PAO_2 is magnified when the PIO_2 is decreased by a low P_B (high altitude). Breathing supplemental oxygen offsets the dilutional effect of carbon dioxide and water vapor as well as the effect of altitude on PIO_2.

Alveolar Partial Pressure of Carbon Dioxide

The $PACO_2$ is determined by the rate of carbon dioxide delivery to the alveoli from pulmonary capillary blood and the rate of removal of this carbon dioxide from the alveoli by alveolar ventilation. The normal rate of delivery of carbon dioxide to alveoli by blood is 200 mL/minute. In the presence of a constant delivery of carbon dioxide to alveoli, the $PACO_2$ is directly proportional to alveolar ventilation.

The Alveolar Gas Equation

A simplified version of the alveolar gas equation can be used to predict the PAO_2 if the $PACO_2$, FiO_3, and respiratory quotient (R) are known.

$Paco_2$ is typically substituted for the $PACO_2$. Although the alveolar gas equation is not accurate under all circumstances, it remains a useful tool that can be used to illustrate the factors that determine PAO_2. The alveolar gas equation may be used clinically to calculate the gradient (or difference) between alveolar and arterial Po_2 (Δ A-a Po_2), which may provide an approximate indication of the efficiency of oxygenation in the presence of lung disease. The healthy individual has an A-a Po_2 difference of approximately 5 mm Hg. The alveolar to arterial oxygen gradient will increase as V/Q matching deteriorates. The alveolar gas equation may also predict the effects of changes in $PACO_2$ on the PAO_2.

Composition of Exhaled Gases

The composition of exhaled gases is determined by the proportion that is alveolar gas and the proportion that is dead space gas. The first portion of exhaled gas is from the large conducting airways (no gas exchange occurs) and is designated *dead space gas*. Because gas exchange does not occur in conducting airways, the composition of dead space gas resembles the composition of inhaled gas. Later in expiration, more and more alveolar gas becomes mixed with dead space gas until all the dead space gas has been exhaled and only alveolar gas remains. For this reason, analysis of the last portion of exhaled alveolar gas (end-tidal sample) is commonly used in the operating room to determine the composition of alveolar gas, including anesthetic concentrations. Indeed, minimum alveolar concentration (MAC) uses the alveolar concentration of the inhaled anesthetic as an index of anesthetic depth and to compare equally potent concentrations of inhaled anesthetics. Contamination of the end-tidal sample with inhaled gases invalidates the interpretation of the obtained values. Pure end-tidal samples are most reliably obtained from the tracheas of intubated patients.

Gas Diffusion from Alveoli to Blood

At birth, there are an estimated 12 million alveoli in each lung, and this number increases to approximately 150 million in each lung by 8 to 9 years of age. Each alveolus has a diameter of approximately 0.25 mm. Alveolar walls are extremely thin (0.5 μm) and contain a network of interconnecting capillaries. The average diameter of the pulmonary capillaries is only 8 μm, which means that erythrocytes must squeeze through vessels in single file such that the distance for diffusion of oxygen and carbon dioxide is minimized. The total surface area available for gas exchange is an estimated 70 m^2. The pulmonary capillary blood volume is about 60 mL at rest but can increase to approximately 140 mL during exercise and is spread as a thin sheet over the alveolar surface.

In addition to the thickness of the membrane and its surface area, the rate of gas diffusion across the alveolar-capillary membrane is determined by the solubility of the gas in the constituents of the membrane and the partial pressure difference across the membrane. Carbon dioxide diffuses across the membrane approximately 20 times as rapidly as oxygen, and oxygen diffuses about twice as rapidly as nitrogen. The partial pressure gradient between capillary blood and alveoli determines the direction of diffusion (oxygen into blood from alveoli and carbon dioxide from blood into alveoli). Any factor that increases the thickness of the membrane (pulmonary edema) interferes with the diffusion of oxygen more than with that of carbon dioxide. When the total surface area of the membrane is decreased to approximately one-fourth of normal as by emphysema (alveoli coalesce into large sacs), exchange of gases through the respiratory membrane is inadequate, even under resting conditions.

Ventilation to Perfusion Ratio

The matching of ventilation to perfusion within the lung is crucial to the efficiency of gas exchange. The V/Q ratio determines the composition of the alveolar gas and the effectiveness of gas exchange across the alveolar–capillary membrane. In the presence of optimal V/Q matching, the Pa_{O_2} is approximately 104 mm Hg and the Pa_{CO_2} is 40 mm Hg. A V/Q ratio of 0 is present when there is no ventilation to an alveolus that continues to be perfused by pulmonary capillary blood (shunt). A V/Q ratio equal to infinity means that there is ventilation but no pulmonary capillary blood flow to the alveolus (wasted ventilation). The topographic distribution of ventilation is an important element of the V/Q concept. V/Q ratios can be applied to the whole lung or to regions of all sizes including individual alveoli. For example, the V/Q ratio of a whole lung may be 1, implying optimal matching of ventilation and perfusion to that lung. However, if ventilation is directed primarily to the upper zones and perfusion to the lower zones then gas exchange will be severely limited even though the total ventilation and perfusion to that lung is the same. This concept is illustrated by the clinical use of inhaled nitric oxide (iNO). Nitric oxide is an ultra short-acting vasodilator that may be administered by inhalation. Low dose iNO (<2 parts per million [ppm]) is occasionally used to improve oxygenation in patients with acute respiratory distress syndrome (ARDS), a disease characterized by severe V/Q mismatch causing refractory hypoxemia. The administration of iNO causes dilation of vessels that supply well ventilated alveoli, thus diverting blood flow from poorly ventilated regions and improving regional V/Q matching and oxygenation. Thus local V/Qs will improve even though the total lung V/Q may not change significantly. If the dose of iNO is increased (>5 ppm) in an attempt to produce greater vasodilatation, gas exchange and oxygenation may worsen as NO begins to diffuse into poorly ventilated alveoli and increases blood flow to these regions, stealing blood from better ventilated areas and worsening local V/Q matching. In contrast, the administration of intravenous vasodilators, such as nitroprusside, will frequently worsen oxygenation in patients with intrapulmonary disease. Intravenous vasodilators cause vasodilation in all perfused regions regardless of their ventilatory status. This effect tends to divert blood flow away from well-ventilated regions and increases flow to poorly ventilated areas.

Physiologic Shunt

Physiologic shunt designates the 2% to 5% of the cardiac output that normally bypasses the lungs by flowing through bronchial veins into pulmonary veins or through thebesian and anterior cardiac veins into the left side of the heart. Physiologic shunt is calculated from measurements of the oxygen concentration of mixed venous and arterial blood (Table 51-2).

Physiologic Dead Space

Conducting airways that do not participate in gas exchange (anatomic dead space) and unperfused alveoli that are

TABLE 51-2.
CALCULATION OF PHYSIOLOGIC SHUNT FRACTION

$$Q_S/Q_T = \frac{CcO_2 - CaO_2}{CcO_2 - CvO_2}$$

Q_S = amount of pulmonary blood flow not exposed to ventilated alveoli
Q_T = total pulmonary blood flow
CcO_2 = O_2 content of pulmonary capillary blood, mL/dL
CaO_2 = O_2 content of arterial blood, mL/dL
CvO_2 = O_2 content of mixed venous blood, mL/dL

ventilated but do not participate in gas exchange, are designated as *physiologic dead space*. In health, the physiologic dead space is accounted for almost entirely by the anatomic dead space. The ratio of physiologic dead space to tidal volume is calculated by measuring the tidal volume, the $PaCO_2$, and $PETCO_2$ (Table 51-3). Approximately one-third of a typical breath is dead space ventilation. In contrast to shunting, increased dead space tends to impair carbon dioxide elimination rather than oxygenation. During anesthesia, breathing systems may add additional dead space (apparatus dead space). Although it is important to avoid excessive apparatus dead space in all patients, infants are particularly vulnerable to respiratory compromise because their tidal volumes are relatively small compared to breathing circuit volumes. For example, an additional 10 mL of apparatus dead space will have little impact on a healthy adult receiving a tidal volume of 500 mL. However, a newborn with a tidal volume of 30 mL may be severely compromised by the addition of 10 mL of apparatus dead space.

BLOOD TRANSPORT OF OXYGEN AND CARBON DIOXIDE

After diffusion from alveoli into pulmonary capillary blood, oxygen is transported principally in combination with hemoglobin to tissue capillaries, where it diffuses down a partial pressure gradient into cellular mitochondria. Carbon dioxide, formed in the cells from oxygen-dependent metabolic pathways, diffuses into tissue capillaries along its partial pressure gradient and is transported to the alveoli.

TABLE 51-3.
CALCULATION OF THE PHYSIOLOGIC DEAD SPACE TO TIDAL VOLUME RATIO

$$V_D/V_T = \frac{PaCO_2 - PETCO_2}{PaCO_2}$$

V_D/V_T = ratio of physiologic dead space to V_T
$PaCO_2$ = arterial partial pressure of CO_2, mm Hg
$PETCO_2$ = mixed exhaled partial pressure of CO_2, mm Hg

Oxygen Uptake into the Blood

The mixed venous oxygen tension ($P\bar{v}O_2$) is approximately 40 mm Hg. This value corresponds to a hemoglobin-oxygen saturation of 75%, reflecting the approximate 25% of delivered oxygen that has been removed from the blood as it passes through various tissues (Fig. 51-2) (Guyton and Hall, 2000). This mixed venous blood is exposed to a PAO_2 of approximately 104 mm Hg, causing rapid diffusion of oxygen down a about a 60 mm Hg partial pressure gradient into pulmonary capillary blood. Indeed, the PO_2 of pulmonary capillary blood is nearly equal to the PAO_2 after passing through only the first one-third of the capillary (see Fig. 51-2) (Guyton and Hall, 2000). This rapid equilibration of pulmonary capillary blood with the PAO_2 provides an important safety factor for transfer of oxygen when blood flow through the lungs is accelerated as during exercise. Severe exercise is accompanied by a large increase in cardiac output, which tends to decrease alveolar capillary transit time towards the critical time (0.3s) that it takes for an erythrocyte to become fully oxygenated. Fortunately, pulmonary capillary blood volume is increased during exercise by the combination of capillary distension and recruitment of previously unperfused vessels, thus increasing gas exchange surface area to facilitate oxygen uptake. The increase in pulmonary capillary cross-sectional area attenuates the increase in erythrocyte velocity that would otherwise occur with such a significant increase in cardiac output and prevents erythrocytes from crossing the alveolar capillaries in less time (0.3s) than required for complete oxygenation. Indeed, pulmonary venous blood remains fully oxygenated, even during severe exertion, in healthy individuals at sea level.

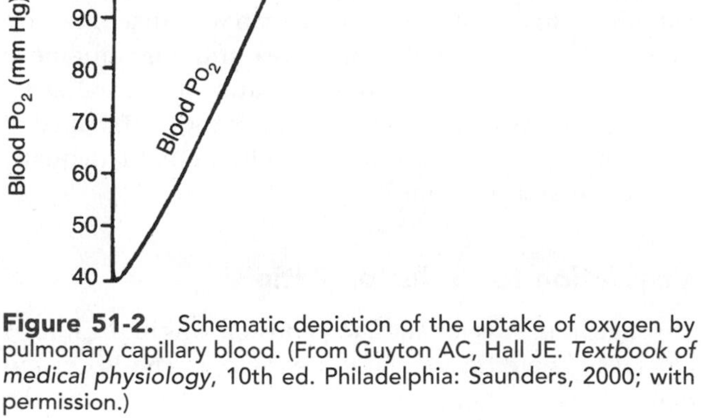

Figure 51-2. Schematic depiction of the uptake of oxygen by pulmonary capillary blood. (From Guyton AC, Hall JE. *Textbook of medical physiology*, 10th ed. Philadelphia: Saunders, 2000; with permission.)

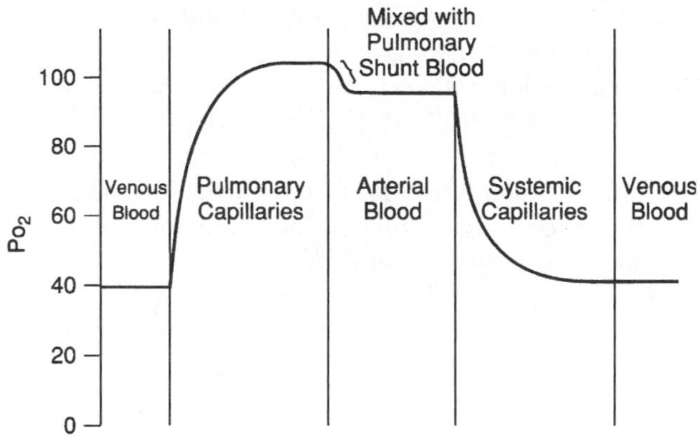

Figure 51-3. Changes in the Po_2 as blood traverses the systemic and pulmonary circulation. (From Guyton AC, Hall JE. *Textbook of medical physiology*, 10th ed. Philadelphia: Saunders, 2000; with permission.)

Blood leaving the pulmonary capillaries has a Po_2 of approximately 104 mm Hg, whereas the arterial blood, which is diluted by contributions from bronchial blood flow, has a Pao_2 of approximately 95 mm Hg (Fig. 51-3) (Guyton and Hall, 2000).

Diffusion of Oxygen from the Capillaries

Interstitial fluid Po_2 averages approximately 40 mm Hg, providing a large initial partial pressure gradient for diffusion of oxygen from tissue capillaries with a Pao_2 near 95 mm Hg (Fig. 51-4) (Guyton and Hall, 2000). At the end of the capillary, the Po_2 in blood and the interstitial fluid have nearly equilibrated such that the $P\bar{v}o_2$ is also approximately 40 mm Hg. Because nearly 97% of the oxygen transported in blood is carried by hemoglobin, a decrease in the concentration of hemoglobin has the same effect on interstitial fluid Po_2 as does a decrease in tissue blood flow.

Diffusion of Carbon Dioxide from the Cells

Continuous formation of carbon dioxide in cells maintains a partial pressure gradient for its diffusion into capillary blood (Fig. 51-5) (Guyton and Hall, 2000). Diffusion of carbon dioxide from cells into capillaries is rapid

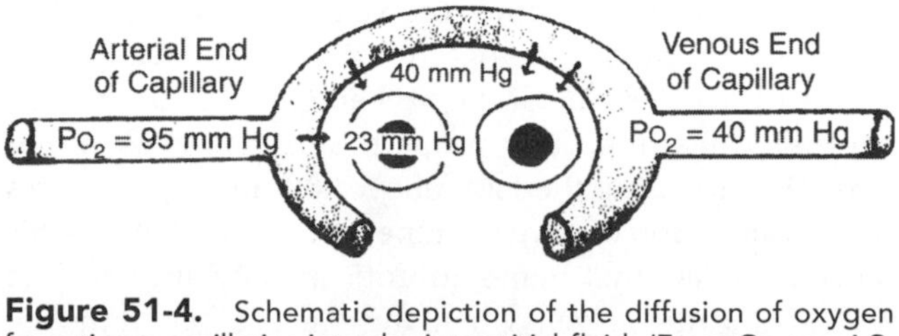

Figure 51-4. Schematic depiction of the diffusion of oxygen from tissue capillaries into the interstitial fluid. (From Guyton AC, Hall JE. *Textbook of medical physiology*, 10th ed. Philadelphia: Saunders, 2000; with permission.)

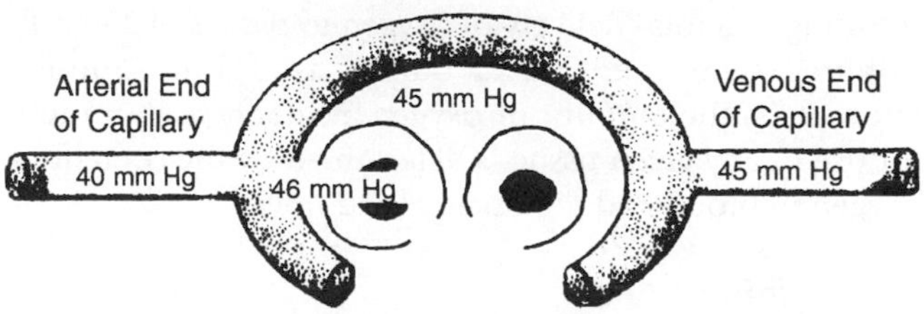

Figure 51-5. Schematic depiction of uptake of carbon dioxide by capillary blood. (From Guyton AC, Hall JE. *Textbook of medical physiology*, 10th ed. Philadelphia: Saunders, 2000; with permission.)

despite a partial pressure gradient of only 1 to 6 mm Hg compared with approximately 64 mm Hg for oxygen. On arrival at alveoli, the $P\bar{v}o_2$ is only 5 to 6 mm Hg greater than the $PACO_2$. Nevertheless, passage from the capillaries to blood like that from tissues into capillaries is rapid, reflecting the fact that the diffusion coefficient for carbon dioxide is 20 times that for oxygen.

Blood Transport for Oxygen

Approximately 97% of oxygen transported from alveoli to tissues is carried to tissues in chemical combination with hemoglobin, whereas approximately 3% of oxygen is transported in the dissolved state in plasma. A single molecule of hemoglobin can combine with four molecules of oxygen. When the Po_2 in pulmonary capillaries is increased, oxygen binds with hemoglobin. Conversely, when the Po_2 is low in tissue capillaries, oxygen is released from hemoglobin. This reaction occurs independently of enzyme action and is not associated with a change in the ferrous state of iron in the hemoglobin molecule. Therefore, this uptake of oxygen by hemoglobin is termed *oxygenation* rather than *oxidation*.

Each gram of hemoglobin can combine with approximately 1.34 mL of oxygen. This combination is rapid, requiring approximately 10 ms. In the presence of a normal hemoglobin concentration of 15 g/dL; blood will carry approximately 20 mL of oxygen when the hemoglobin is 100% saturated. Approximately 5 mL of this 20 mL passes to tissues, decreasing the hemoglobin saturation with oxygen to approximately 75%, corresponding to a $P\bar{v}o_2$ of about 40 mm Hg.

The amount of oxygen dissolved in plasma is a linear function of the Po_2 (0.003 mL/mm Hg corresponding to 0.3 mL/100 mL when the Po_2 is 100 mm Hg). Approximately 0.29 mL of oxygen is dissolved in 100 mL of blood when the Po_2 is 95 mm Hg. When the Po_2 of blood decreases to 40 mm Hg in tissue capillaries, approximately 0.12 mL of oxygen remains dissolved. This means that approximately 0.17 mL of oxygen is delivered to tissues in the dissolved state in 100 mL of blood compared with approximately 5 mL of oxygen attached to hemoglobin in the same amount of blood. Under resting conditions, approximately 5 mL of oxygen is released to the tissues for every 100 mL of blood, resulting in a total delivery of oxygen to tissues of 250 mL/minute when the cardiac output is 5 liters/minute. Ultimately, the amount of oxygen available each minute for use in any given tissue is determined by the content of oxygen in blood and the tissue blood flow.

Hemoglobin

Hemoglobin is a conjugated protein with a molecular weight of 66,700. The four heme molecules, each with a central iron atom, combine with globin, a globular protein synthesized in the ribosomes of the endoplasmic reticulum to form hemoglobin. The globin portion of the hemoglobin molecule comprises four polypeptide chains of more than 700 amino acids. The genetically determined sequences of these amino acids influence the binding affinity of hemoglobin for oxygen.

Types of Hemoglobin

Hemoglobin types are designated as A through S, depending on the sequence of amino acids in the polypeptide chains. Normal adult hemoglobin A consists of two identical alpha and beta polypeptide chains. Fetal erythrocytes contain hemoglobin F, which has a low concentration of 2,3-diphosphoglycerate (2,3-DPG) and a resulting high affinity for oxygen, which facilitates transfer of oxygen from the placenta to the fetus. Indeed, at a normal umbilical vein PO_2 of 28 mm Hg, hemoglobin F is 80% saturated with oxygen (oxyhemoglobin dissociation curve shifted to the left), whereas hemoglobin A would only be approximately 50% saturated with oxygen at this same PO_2 (Fig. 51-6). After birth, the presence of hemoglobin F impairs release of oxygen to tissues. However, hemoglobin F is replaced by adult hemoglobin A by 4 to 6 months of age.

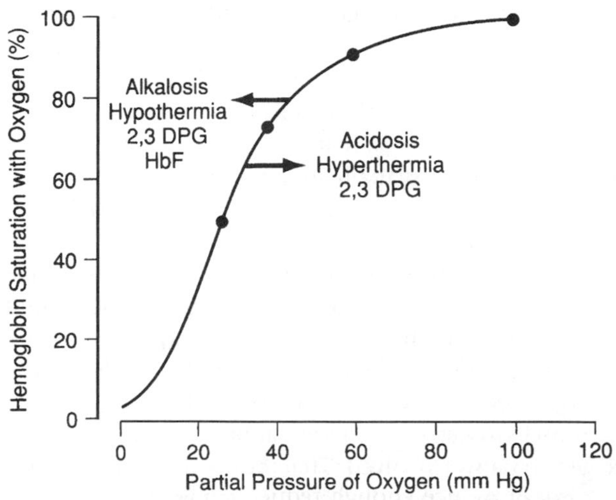

Figure 51-6. Oxyhemoglobin dissociation curve for hemoglobin A at pH 7.4 and 37°C. Changes in pH, body temperature, concentration of 2,3-diphosphoglycerate (2,3-DPG), and the presence of different types of hemoglobin (HbF) shift the oxyhemoglobin dissociation curve to the left or right of its normal position.

With the exception of hemoglobin A and hemoglobin F, all other forms of hemoglobin are considered abnormal. The oxyhemoglobin dissociation curve for abnormal hemoglobin types is typically shifted to the right, which interferes with transfer of oxygen from alveoli to hemoglobin. Abnormal hemoglobin results from changes in the amino acid sequences of the polypeptide chains of globin. For example, substitution of valine for glutamic acid in two of the four polypeptide chains of hemoglobin A results in hemoglobin S. Erythrocytes containing hemoglobin S become elongated and inflexible when exposed to low concentrations of oxygen and are known as *sickle cells*.

Other Heme-containing Compounds

Myoglobin is an iron-containing pigment resembling hemoglobin that is present in skeletal muscles. Unlike hemoglobin, myoglobin binds only one molecule of oxygen. However, the affinity of myoglobin for oxygen is greater than that of hemoglobin A, thus facilitating the transfer of oxygen from blood to muscle. Thus oxygen continues to be available in exercising muscle, particularly during sustained contraction when blood flow and local PO_2 have decreased to very low values.

Neuroglobin, another oxygen binding globin helps supply oxygen to neurons and is found within the brain. Cytochrome c is a heme-containing respiratory chain enzyme that is involved in mitochondrial oxidative phosphorylation.

Preoxygenation

Preoxygenation of the patient's lungs prior to induction of anesthesia and tracheal intubation is intended to increase oxygen reserves in the lungs and thus delay the onset of arterial hypoxemia during apnea as may occur during the period of time needed for direct laryngoscopy to place a tracheal tube. It is particularly advantageous when difficult intubation or ventilation is anticipated. Maximum alveolar preoxygenation in an adult during tidal volume breathing (100% oxygen via a face mask using a circle absorption system) requires at least 2.5 minutes (Nimmagadda et al., 2000).

Oxyhemoglobin Dissociation Curve

The percentage of hemoglobin saturation with oxygen at different partial pressures of oxygen in the blood is described by the oxyhemoglobin dissociation curve (see Fig. 51-6). The S shape of the oxyhemoglobin dissociation curve explains important properties of hemoglobin. For example, increasing the PaO_2 above 100 mm Hg increases the concentration of oxygen in the blood only slightly. This reflects the fact that hemoglobin is already at least 97% saturated with oxygen when the PaO_2 is 100 mm Hg. Likewise, decreasing the PaO_2 to 60 mm Hg maintains at least 90% saturation of hemoglobin with oxygen, reflecting the flat aspect of the oxyhemoglobin dissociation curve over this range. At tissue capillaries where the Po_2 is 20 to 40 mm Hg, the oxyhemoglobin dissociation curve is steep such that small changes in the Pao_2 result in transfer of large amounts of oxygen from hemoglobin to tissues.

Shift of the Oxyhemoglobin Dissociation Curve

Factors that influence the position of the oxyhemoglobin dissociation curve include (a) hydrogen ion concentration of the blood, (b) body temperature, (c) concentration of 2,3-DPG, and (d) type of hemoglobin (see Fig. 51-6). For unknown reasons, inhaled anesthetics may produce a modest rightward shift of the oxyhemoglobin dissociation curve (Kambam, 1982).

Partial Pressure of Oxygen at 50% Saturation

A convenient indicator of the position of the oxyhemoglobin dissociation curve is the Po_2 that produces 50% saturation of hemoglobin with oxygen, which is designated the P_{50}. In the normal adult at a pH of 7.4 and body temperature of 37°C, the P_{50} is approximately 26 mm Hg (see Fig. 51-6). A shift of the oxyhemoglobin dissociation curve to the right is reflected by an increase in the P_{50} to >26 mm Hg, whereas the P_{50} is <26 mm Hg when the oxyhemoglobin dissociation curve is shifted to the left. A shift of the oxyhemoglobin dissociation curve to the left means the Po_2 must decrease further before oxygen is released from hemoglobin to tissues.

Bohr Effect

The shift in the position of the oxyhemoglobin dissociation curve caused by carbon dioxide entering or leaving the blood is the *Bohr effect.* For example, at tissues, carbon dioxide enters blood, causing the pH to decrease (acidosis), and the oxyhemoglobin dissociation curve shifts to the right, facilitating the release of oxygen from hemoglobin. The reverse change at the lungs results in alkalosis with a leftward shift of the oxyhemoglobin dissociation curve, thus enhancing the affinity of hemoglobin for oxygen. The related effect of oxygenation on the buffering capacity of hemoglobin is called the *Haldane effect.*

2,3-Diphosphoglycerate

The effect of 2,3-DPG is to decrease the affinity of hemoglobin for oxygen (shifts the oxyhemoglobin dissociation curve to the right), causing oxygen to be released to tissues at a higher Pao_2 than in the absence of this substance. Increases in the erythrocyte content of 2,3-DPG are evoked by anemia and arterial hypoxemia as produced by ascent to altitude. Storage of whole blood is associated with a progressive decrease in erythrocyte content of 2,3-DPG. This decrease is less in blood preserved in citrate-phosphate-dextrose than in acid-citrate-dextrose.

Exercise

During exercise, the oxyhemoglobin dissociation curve for skeletal muscles is shifted to the right, reflecting release of carbon dioxide by exercising muscles. In addition, the temperature of exercising muscles may increase 3°C to 4°C. These changes, and the presence of muscle myoglobin, facilitate the release of oxygen from hemoglobin to exercising muscles even when the Po_2 in the blood has decreased to as low as 40 mm Hg.

Carbon Monoxide

Carbon monoxide competes with oxygen for binding at the same location on the hemoglobin molecule. Furthermore, the strength of the carboxyhemoglobin bond is approximately 230 times greater than that exhibited by oxygen. Therefore, a carbon monoxide partial pressure of 0.4 mm Hg is equivalent to a Po_2 of 92 mm Hg. At this partial pressure of carbon monoxide, approximately half the hemoglobin is bound with this gas rather than oxygen. A carbon monoxide partial pressure of 0.7 mm Hg can bind nearly all the hemoglobin sites normally occupied by oxygen. The Pao_2 remains normal despite the absence of oxyhemoglobin, reflecting the fact that dissolved oxygen determines the Po_2. Chemoreceptors that would otherwise increase alveolar ventilation in response to hypoxemia are not stimulated because the Pao_2 remains normal. The primary treatment of carbon monoxide poisoning is administration of oxygen in order to elevate the Pao_2 thus displacing carbon monoxide from hemoglobin. This is the rationale for the use of a hyperbaric oxygen chamber in the treatment of severe carbon monoxide poisoning.

Carbon monoxide results from incomplete combustion of organic matter and is an abundant pollutant in the lower atmosphere. The automobile is the greatest source of carbon monoxide. Another source of carboxyhemoglobin is cigarette smoking. Most victims of fires die from acute carbon monoxide poisoning. Carbon monoxide formation also results from degradation of volatile anesthetics (desflurane>enflurane>isoflurane) by strong bases in certain carbon dioxide absorbents. (see Chapter 2). There is no excretion of carbon monoxide without alveolar ventilation. Therefore, valid measurements of carboxyhemoglobin concentrations can be obtained long after death. Carboxyhemoglobin does not influence the readings obtained by pulse oximetry.

Cyanosis

Blueness of the skin caused by excessive amounts of reduced hemoglobin in cutaneous capillaries is designated *cyanosis.* More than 5 g of reduced hemoglobin causes cyanosis regardless of the overall concentration of oxyhemoglobin. Therefore, patients with polycythemia may appear cyanotic despite adequate arterial concentrations of oxygen, whereas the anemic patient may lack sufficient hemoglobin to produce enough reduced hemoglobin to cause cyanosis even in the presence of profound tissue hypoxia. The degree of cyanosis is influenced by the rate of blood flow through the skin. If cutaneous blood flow is sluggish, even low skin metabolism may result in production of sufficient

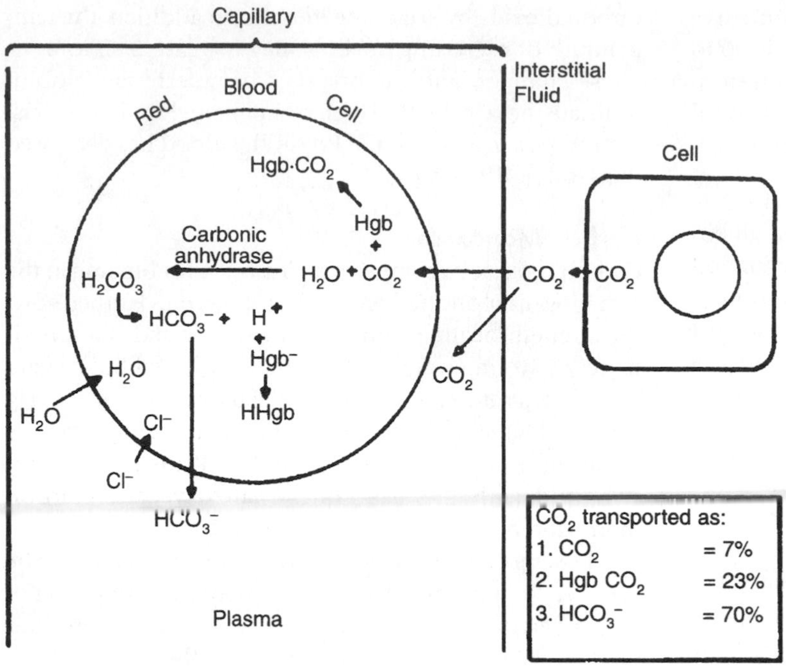

Figure 51-7. Schematic depiction of transport of carbon dioxide in blood. (From Guyton AC, Hall JE. *Textbook of medical physiology*, 10th ed. Philadelphia: Saunders, 2000; with permission.)

reduced hemoglobin to cause cyanosis. This explains the occurrence of peripheral cyanosis in cold weather, particularly when the skin permits transmission of the color of reduced hemoglobin from the deeper vascular structures.

Blood Transport of Carbon Dioxide

Carbon dioxide formed as a result of metabolic processes in cells readily diffuses across cell membranes into capillary blood. Despite a small partial pressure difference between tissues and blood (1 to 6 mm Hg), the high solubility of carbon dioxide (20 times more soluble than oxygen) permits rapid transfer. An average of 4 mL of carbon dioxide in each 100 mL of blood is transported to the lungs as (a) dissolved carbon dioxide, (b) bicarbonate ions, and (c) carbaminohemoglobin (Fig. 51-7) (Guyton and Hall, 2000).

Approximately 0.3 mL of the 4 mL of carbon dioxide in every 100 mL of blood is transported to the lungs in the dissolved state. The $P\bar{v}O_2$ is approximately 5 mm Hg greater than the $PaCO_2$, reflecting the addition of carbon dioxide from the tissues. This increase in the $P\bar{v}O_2$ lowers the venous blood pH to 7.36 compared with a pH of 7.4 in arterial blood and a $PaCO_2$ of 40 mm Hg. The ratio of dissolved carbon dioxide to bicarbonate ions is normally 20:1.

Approximately 2.8 mL of the 4 mL of carbon dioxide in every 100 mL of blood enters erythrocytes, where it reacts with water to form carbonic acid (see Fig. 51-7) (Guyton and Hall, 2000). This reaction in erythrocytes is almost instantaneous in the presence of the enzyme carbonic anhydrase. Carbonic anhydrase is essentially absent in the plasma. Immediately after its formation, there is dissociation of carbonic acid into hydrogen and bicarbonate ions. Most of the hydrogen ions combine with reduced hemoglobin, which acts as a powerful buffer. Bicarbonate ions diffuse from erythrocytes into plasma, accompanied by the opposite movement of chloride ions into the cells to maintain electrochemical neutrality (chloride shift). The increase in osmotically active ions such as chloride and bicarbonate in venous erythrocytes encourages the entry of water, thus increasing their volume. This explains why the venous hematocrit is approximately 3% higher than the arterial hematocrit.

Haldane Effect

Approximately one-tenth of the carbon dioxide transported from the tissues to the lungs is carried in the form of carbaminohemoglobin. Within the lungs, the combination of oxygen with hemoglobin causes hemoglobin to become a stronger acid, which inhibits carbon dioxide-hemoglobin binding to form carbaminohemoglobin. The dissociation of carbaminohemoglobin liberates carbon dioxide, which diffuses from pulmonary capillary blood into alveoli. This displacement of carbon dioxide from hemoglobin by oxygen that occurs at the lungs is known as the Haldane effect. The Haldane effect at the tissues facilitates the passage of carbon dioxide into the blood. The Haldane effect explains in part the greater carbon dioxide carrying capacity of venous blood.

Body Stores of Carbon Dioxide

In contrast to total body oxygen stores of approximately 1.5 liters (approximately 1 liter in arterial blood), there are an estimated 120 liters of carbon dioxide dissolved in the body. In the presence of apnea but provision of oxygen (apneic oxygenation), the $PaCO_2$ increases 5 to 10 mm Hg during the first minute of apnea (Eger and Severinghaus, 1961). This initial rapid increase in the $Paco_2$ represents equilibration of the alveolar gas with the $P\bar{v}o_2$. After the first minute of apnea, the $Paco_2$ increases approximately 3 mm Hg/minute, reflecting metabolic production of carbon dioxide.

Respiratory Quotient

The ratio of carbon dioxide output to oxygen uptake is the *respiratory quotient*. During resting conditions, the amount of oxygen added to blood (5 mL/dL) exceeds the amount of carbon dioxide that is removed from the blood (4 mL/dL), resulting in a respiratory quotient of 0.8. The respiratory quotient varies with different metabolic conditions, being 1 when carbohydrates are used exclusively for metabolism and decreasing to 0.7 when fat is the primary source of metabolic energy. The reason for this difference is the formation of one molecule of carbon dioxide for every molecule of oxygen consumed when carbohydrates are metabolized. When oxygen reacts with fats, a substantial amount of oxygen combines with hydrogen ions to form water instead of carbon dioxide, thus decreasing the respiratory quotient to near 0.7. Consumption of a normal diet consisting of carbohydrates, fats, and proteins results in a respiratory quotient of approximately 0.83.

CHANGES ASSOCIATED WITH HIGH ALTITUDE

The total partial pressure of all gases in the atmosphere (P_B) decreases progressively as distance above sea level increases (Table 51-4) (Fig. 51-8) (Ganong, 2003). For example, the P_B is 760 mm Hg at sea level and 523 mm Hg at 3,300 m (10,000 feet) above sea level. Because the concentration of oxygen remains constant at approximately 21%, the decrease in the P_B above sea level is associated with a progressive decrease in the ambient Po_2. For example, the Po_2 at sea level is 159 mm Hg (21% × 760 mm Hg) and 110 mm Hg at 3,300 m (21% × 523 mm Hg). The decrease in the P_B with increasing altitude is not linear because air is compressible (see Fig. 51-8) (Ganong, 2003).

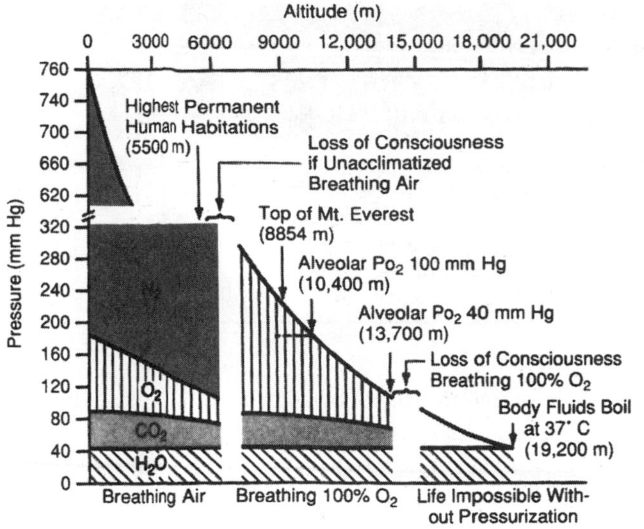

Figure 51-8. Composition of alveolar gases breathing air (0 to 6,100 m) and 100% oxygen (6,100 to 13,700 m). (From Ganong WF. *Review of medical physiology*, 21st ed. New York, Lang Medical Books/McGraw Hill, 2003; with permission.)

The pharmacologic effect of inhaled anesthetics is decreased as P_B is reduced. For example, 60% inhaled nitrous oxide produces a partial pressure of 456 mm Hg at sea level compared with 314 mm Hg at 3,300 m. The inhaled concentration of nitrous oxide at 3,300 m elevation would have to be 87% to produce the same partial pressure produced by breathing 60% nitrous oxide at sea level. Likewise, 1% isoflurane producing 7.6 mm Hg at sea level would have to be increased to nearly 1.5% to produce the same partial pressure at 3,300 m.

Mental function remains intact up to 2,700 to 3,300 m above sea level. The frequency of breathing ordinarily does not increase until one ascends above 2,400 m; at which point the peripheral chemoreceptors are stimulated.

Acclimatization to Altitude

Acclimatization to altitude occurs because of several compensatory responses (Table 51-5). The initial increase in alveolar ventilation lowers the $Paco_2$, which blunts the magnitude of this compensatory response. Within a few days,

TABLE 51-4.
EFFECTS OF ALTITUDE ON RESPIRATORY GASES WHILE BREATHING AIR

Altitude (m/ft)	P_B (mm Hg)	Pio_2 (mm Hg)	PAo_2 (mm Hg)	$PAco_2$ (mm Hg)	Sao_2 (%)
Sea level	760	159	104	40	97
3,300/10,000	523	110 (436)*	67	36	90
6,600/20,000	349	73	40	24	70
9,900/30,000	226	47	21	24	20

*Breathing 100% oxygen.

TABLE 51-5.
COMPENSATORY RESPONSES EVOKED BY ASCENT TO ALTITUDE

Increased alveolar ventilation
Increased hemoglobin production
Increased 2,3-diphosphoglycerate concentrations
Increased diffusing capacity of the lungs
Increased vascularity of the tissues
Increased cellular use of oxygen

however, active transport of bicarbonate ions returns the cerebrospinal fluid pH to normal and alveolar ventilation again increases despite a low Pa_{CO_2}. Increased production of hemoglobin requires several months to reach its maximal effect, during which time the hemoglobin concentration may increase to >20 g/dL. In addition, the plasma volume may increase as much as 30%. Cardiac output often increases as much as 30% immediately after ascent to altitude, but this increase is transient, returning to normal in a few days. Chronic exposure to altitude is associated with an increased number of mitochondria and certain cellular oxidative systems, presumably reflecting an improved ability to use available oxygen.

Acute Mountain Sickness

Acute mountain sickness is a syndrome of headache, insomnia, dyspnea, anorexia, and fatigue that has been described on rapid ascent to even intermediate altitude (2,000 m) (Montgomery et al., 1989). Symptoms usually develop 8 to 24 hours after arrival at altitude and last 4 to 8 days. It is speculated that the low P_{O_2} at high altitude causes arteriolar dilation, and if cerebral autoregulation does not compensate, there is an increase in capillary pressure that favors transudation of fluid into brain tissue. Alkalosis produced by treatment with acetazolamide is effective in decreasing symptoms.

High-altitude pulmonary edema and cerebral edema are serious forms of acute mountain sickness. Pulmonary edema is apt to occur in individuals who ascend to altitudes above 2,500 m and engage in strenuous physical activity during the first 3 days after arrival. Pulmonary hypertension is prominent and the protein content of pulmonary edema fluid is high, implying that there is increased pulmonary capillary permeability.

Chronic Mountain Sickness

An occasional sea level native who remains for prolonged periods at high altitude may develop chronic mountain sickness characterized by polycythemia, pulmonary hypertension, and right ventricular failure. Presumably, the increased hemoglobin concentration so increases the viscosity of blood that tissue blood flow becomes inadequate; at the same time, chronic arterial hypoxemia causes constriction of pulmonary vessels. Recovery is usually prompt when these individuals return to sea level, provided that pulmonary vascular remodelling has not caused an irreversible increase in pulmonary vascular resistance.

CHANGES ASSOCIATED WITH EXCESSIVE BAROMETRIC PRESSURE

The P_B increases the equivalent of 1 atm for every 10 m below the surface of sea water (10.4 m for fresh water). For example, a person 10 m beneath the water surface is exposed to 2 atm, reflecting the 1 atm of pressure caused by the weight of air above the water and the second atmosphere by the weight of water. At 20 m below the water surface, the P_B is equivalent to 3 atm.

Another important effect of increased P_B below the surface of the water is compression of gases in the lungs to smaller volumes. High P_B produces nitrogen narcosis when the inhaled gases are air. Presumably, the PN_2 at an increased P_B causes sufficient absorption and deposition of nitrogen molecules in lipid membranes to produce an anesthetic effect. Helium can be substituted for nitrogen to avoid narcosis associated with absorption of nitrogen. In addition to a lesser sedative effect, helium is less soluble, thus decreasing the quantity of bubbles that result with return to normal P_B.

Nitrogen that is absorbed at high P_B remains dissolved in the tissues until the PN_2 decreases. Decompression sickness (caisson disease) occurs when sudden decreases in the P_B allow nitrogen bubbles to develop in body tissues and fluids. Nitrogen bubbles develop because pressure on the outside of the body is insufficient to keep the excess gas that was absorbed during exposure to the high P_B in solution. As a result, nitrogen can escape from the dissolved state and form bubbles in the tissues. The most frequent sign of nitrogen bubble formation is pain in the extremities; the most serious sequelae are seizures and cerebral ischemia that occur as a result of bubble formation in the central nervous system. Nitrogen bubbles that form in the blood block pulmonary blood flow, manifesting as dyspnea ("chokes"). Symptoms of decompression sickness usually appear within minutes but may also be delayed for as long as 6 hours or more after decompression. The time

TABLE 51-6.
INDICATIONS FOR HYPERBARIC OXYGEN THERAPY

Decompression sickness
Air embolism
Carbon monoxide poisoning
Clostridial gangrene
Refractory osteomyelitis
Radiation necrosis
Profound anemia

TABLE 51-7.
COMPLICATIONS OF HYPERBARIC OXYGEN THERAPY

Tympanic membrane rupture
Nasal sinus trauma
Pneumothorax
Air embolism
Central nervous system toxicity
Oxygen toxicity

period for which a diver must be decompressed depends on the depth of submersion and duration of exposure. For example, submersion at 60 m for 1 hour requires approximately 3 hours for decompression.

Hyperbaric Oxygen Therapy

Hyperbaric oxygen therapy involves intermittent inhalation of 100% oxygen. Indications for hyperbaric oxygen therapy are evolving, with primary treatment for decompression sickness and massive air embolism being accepted uses of this modality (Table 51-6) (Grim et al., 1990). Patients with carbon monoxide poisoning improve rapidLy after treatment with hyperbaric oxygen. For example, the elimination half-time of carboxyhemoglobin is decreased from 320 minutes breathing room air to 80 minutes with 100% oxygen and 23 minutes with 100% oxygen at 3 atm. Most hyperbaric oxygen treatments are performed at 2 to 3 atm. In treatment of decompression sickness and air embolism, where a mechanical reduction in bubble size by an increase in ambient pressure is crucial to the therapeutic effect, treatments often are initiated at 6 atm. For example, at 6 atm, a bubble is reduced to 20% of its original volume and 60% of its original diameter.

Complications of hyperbaric oxygen therapy reflect barometric pressure changes or oxygen toxicity (Table 51-7) (Grim et al., 1990). The most common complications involve cavity trauma due to changes in pressure. Any air-filled cavity that cannot equilibrate with ambient pressure, such as the middle ear when the eustachian tube is blocked, nasal sinuses, or lungs, is subject to barotrauma during hyperbaric oxygen therapy (Melamed et al., 1992). Almost all patients develop symptoms of oxygen toxicity after 6 continuous hours of 100% oxygen at 2 atm. No hyperbaric oxygen therapy protocol requires this length of continuous exposure. Even 80% to 100% oxygen inhaled at 1 atm for 8 hours or more causes the respiratory passages to become irritated, manifesting as substernal distress, nasal congestion, pharyngitis, and coughing. Exposure to 100% oxygen for 24 to 48 hours at 1 atm may cause damage to capillary endothelium with exudation of fluid into the interstitial spaces of the lungs and development of pulmonary edema.

REFERENCES

Eger EI. *Isoflurane (Forane). A compendium and reference.* Madison, WI: Ohio Medical Products, 1984.

Eger EI, Severinghaus JW. The rate of rise of $PaCO_2$ in the apneic anesthetized patient. *Anesthesiology* 1961;44:419–425.

Ganong WF. *Review of medical physiology*, 21st ed. New York, Lange Medical Books/McGraw Hill, 2003.

Grim PS, Gottlieb LJ, Boddie A, et al. Hyperbaric oxygen therapy. *JAMA* 1990;263:2216–2220.

Guyton AC, Hall JE. *Textbook of medical physiology*, 10th ed. Philadelphia: Saunders, 2000.

Kambam JR. Isoflurane and oxy-hemoglobin dissociation. *Anesthesiology* 1982;57:A496.

Melamed Y, Shupak A, Bitterman H. Medical problems associated with underwater diving. *N Engl J Med* 1992;326:30–35.

Montgomery AB, Mills J, Lee JM. Incidence of acute mountain sickness at intermediate altitude. *JAMA* 1989;261:732–734.

Nimmagadda U, Ramez SM, Ninos J, et al. Efficacy of preoxygenation with tidal volume breathing: comparison of breathing systems. *Anesthesiology* 2000;93:693–698.

Acid-Base Balance

52

Hydrogen ion concentrations in the various compartments are precisely regulated in the face of enormous variations in local production and clearance. Deviations in hydrogen ion concentrations from the normal range can cause marked alterations in protein structure and function, enzyme activity, and cellular function. Although hydrogen ions are continuously produced in the hydrolysis of adenosine triphosphate, the largest contribution of metabolic acids arises from the oxidation of carbohydrates, principally glucose, to produce carbon dioxide (volatile acid, approximately 24,000 mEq/day). By comparison, the average net production of nonvolatile metabolic acid, such as lactate, is relatively small (approximately 60 mEq/day).

The hydrogen ion concentration is regulated to maintain the arterial pH between 7.35 and 7.45. The pH is equivalent to the negative logarithm of the hydrogen ion concentration expressed in nmol/liter. The pH notation is useful for expressing physiologic hydrogen ion concentrations because hydrogen ion concentrations are low relative to other cations. For example, a normal pH of 7.4 is equivalent to a hydrogen ion concentration of 40 nmol/liter, whereas the normal plasma concentration of sodium ions is 1 million times greater (140,000,000 nmol/liter, or 140 mEq/liter). Compared with the osmotic effect of sodium, the osmotic effect of hydrogen ions is negligible. However, expression of the hydrogen ion concentration as pH masks large variations in hydrogen ion concentration despite small changes in pH. For example, a pH range of 7.0 to 7.7 is associated with a fivefold change (100 nmol/liter to 20 nmol/liter) in hydrogen ion concentration (Table 52-1). A decrease in pH of 0.3 represents a doubling of the hydrogen ion concentration and an increase in pH of 1.0 represents a tenfold decrease in hydrogen ion concentration. The pH of venous blood and interstitial fluid is lower than that of arterial blood, approximately 7.35.

MECHANISMS FOR REGULATION OF HYDROGEN ION CONCENTRATION

Regulation of pH over a narrow range is a complex physiologic process that depends on (a) buffer systems, (b) ventilatory responses, and (c) renal responses. The buffer system mechanism is local and immediate, but incomplete. Ventilatory and renal responses are systemic, develop less rapidly, but can produce nearly complete pH correction.

Buffer Systems

Body fluids contain acid-base buffer systems that immediately combine with acid or alkali to prevent excessive changes in the hydrogen ion concentration. This ability to neutralize excess protons maintains the local pH near 7.4 in the face of continuous acid generation. The most important buffer systems are (a) bicarbonate and carbonic acid in plasma, interstitial and intracellular fluid and bone, (b) hemoglobin and other proteins in intracellular fluid, (c) plasma proteins, and (d) phosphates in intracellular and extracellular fluid and the kidney (Fig. 52-1). By convention, an acid is any substance that increases the hydrogen ion concentration (proton donor), and an alkali is any substance that decreases the hydrogen ion concentration (proton acceptor). A strong acid, such as hydrochloric acid, is fully dissociated to hydrogen and chloride ions, whereas carbonic acid, which is a weaker acid, dissociates only partially to hydrogen and bicarbonate ions.

Bicarbonate Buffering System

The bicarbonate buffering system consists of carbonic acid and sodium bicarbonate. Bicarbonate buffer is primarily a product of the approximately 200 mL of carbon dioxide produced per minute, of which considerably less than 1% dissolves to become carbonic acid. Carbonic acid is a weak acid because of its limited degree of dissociation (<5% at physiologic pH) into hydrogen and bicarbonate ions (Fig. 52-2). Most carbonic acid in solution almost immediately dissociates into carbon dioxide and water, the net result being a very high concentration of dissolved carbon dioxide compared to the concentration of bicarbonate ions. This relationship is described mathematically by the Henderson-Hasselbach equation, which can be used to calculate the pH of a solution if the concentration of bicarbonate ions and dissolved carbon dioxide is known (Fig. 52-3).

The addition of a strong acid such as hydrochloric acid to the bicarbonate buffering system results in conversion of

TABLE 52-1.
RELATION OF HYDROGEN ION CONCENTRATION TO pH

Hydrogen Ions (nmol/L)	pH
100	7.0
80	7.10
63	7.20
50	7.30
42	7.38
40	7.40
38	7.42
32	7.50
25	7.60
20	7.70

the strong acid to weak carbonic acid (Fig. 52-4). Therefore, a strong acid lowers the pH of body fluids only slightly. The addition of a strong base, such as potassium hydroxide, to the bicarbonate buffering system results in the formation of a weak base and water. Buffers are most effective when they operate at a pH that is close to their pKa (under these circumstances the buffer system is approximately 50% dissociated). The bicarbonate buffering system is not a powerful buffer because its pKa of 6.1 differs greatly from the normal pH of 7.4. However, the bicarbonate system is important because (a) bicarbonate is present in significant quantities in nearly all fluid compartments, (b) the concentration of its components is ultimately regulated by the lungs and kidneys, and (c) in severe acidosis the pH approaches the pKa of the buffer system thus increasing its efficiency.

The bicarbonate buffer system accounts for >50% of the total buffering capacity of blood. Approximately one-third of the bicarbonate buffering capacity of blood occurs within erythrocytes. The electrical charge of bicarbonate ions limits their diffusion into cells other than erythrocytes.

Hemoglobin Buffering System

Hemoglobin is a particularly effective buffer because it is localized in quantity in erythrocytes, it has a pKa of 6.8, which is close to physiologic pH, and has a buffering capacity that varies with oxygenation. The imidazole ring of the amino acid histidine has a pKa that is close to the physiologic pH. Thus, hemoglobin and other histidine-containing

$$HHb \rightleftharpoons H^+ + Hb^-$$

$$HProt \rightleftharpoons H^+ + Prot^-$$

$$H_2PO_4^- \rightleftharpoons H^+ + HPO_4^{2-}$$

$$H_2CO_3 \rightleftharpoons H^+ + HCO_3^-$$

Figure 52-1. Buffering systems present in the body.

$$pH = 6.10 + \log \frac{HCO_3^-}{Paco_2\ (0.03)}$$

Figure 52-2. The Henderson-Hasselbalch equation can be used to calculate the pH of a solution.

proteins are excellent physiologic buffers. Furthermore, deoxygenated hemoglobin is a weaker acid (better proton acceptor) than oxyhemoglobin. Thus, in the systemic capillaries, dissociation of oxyhemoglobin to deoxyhemoglobin facilitates the binding of hydrogen ions produced by the dissociation of carbonic acid. This situation is reversed in the pulmonary circulation where the conversion of deoxyhemoglobin to oxyhemoglobin facilitates the release of hydrogen ions.

Protein Buffering System

Like hemoglobin, other histidine-containing proteins are important intracellular buffers. Proteins are localized in high concentrations within the cell where it is estimated that approximately 75% of all the buffering of body fluids occurs, mostly by proteins. Of particular importance is the local buffering of hydrogen ions by proteins in the mitochondria. Although the relatively low concentration of plasma proteins limits their role as extracellular buffers, hypoproteinemia will further reduce buffering capacity, especially in the critically ill patient.

Phosphate Buffering System

The phosphate buffering system is important in most fluid compartments but is especially important in renal tubules, where phosphate is concentrated. Renal tubular fluid is more acidic than extracellular fluid, bringing the pH of renal tubular fluid closer to the pKa (6.8) of the phosphate buffering system. Phosphate is a very important intracellular buffer because it is the most abundant intracellular anion. Furthermore, the relatively acidic pH of intracellular fluid is closer to the pKa of the phosphate buffering system than is the pH of extracellular fluid.

Intracellular pH regulation

Although blood pH is commonly measured clinically, it is the intracellular pH (pHi) that is of functional importance. The routine measurement and manipulation of intracellular pH is not possible in current practice. Indeed, during hypothermic cardiopulmonary bypass and hibernation, the intracellular pH in heart and brain tissue appears to be highly regulated despite significant deviations in systemic

$$CO_2 + H_2O \rightleftharpoons H_2CO_3 \rightleftharpoons HCO_3^- + H^+$$

Figure 52-3. Hydration of carbon dioxide results in carbonic acid, which can subsequently dissociate into bicarbonate and hydrogen ions.

$HCL + NaHCO_3 \rightarrow H_2CO_3 + NaCl$

Figure 52-4. The addition of a strong acid (hydrochloric acid) to the bicarbonate buffering system results in the formation of weak carbonic acid.

pH. Cellular metabolism, transmembrane transport, membrane potential generation, cell growth and division, cytoskeletal structure, and contractile function are processes that are crucially dependent upon pHi (Table 52-2). Furthermore, the optimal function of several organelles, including lysosomes and mitochondria, require that their local pH is significantly different from the general intracellular pHi. Thus there are highly regulated mechanisms to maintain local pHi including intracellular buffer systems and membrane bound proton transporters. Indeed, the pHi (7.0) is higher than is predicted by the −90mV transmembrane potential (pH 6.8). As in the extracellular compartment, intracellular protons are rapidly bound to weak acids and bases resulting in a low free proton concentration.

Ventilatory Responses

Ventilation is quantitatively the most important mechanism of acid removal, given the enormous daily production of volatile acid compared to nonvolatile acid. Ventilatory responses for regulation of pH manifest as alterations in activity of the respiratory center within 1 to 5 minutes of the change in hydrogen ion concentration. As a result, alveolar ventilation increases or decreases to produce appropriate changes in the concentration of carbon dioxide. In the presence of a constant carbon dioxide production, the dissolved concentration of carbon dioxide is inversely proportional to alveolar ventilation.

Doubling alveolar ventilation eliminates sufficient carbon dioxide to increase pH to approximately 7.6. Conversely, decreasing alveolar ventilation to one-fourth of normal results in retention of carbon dioxide sufficient to decrease the pH to approximately 7.0.

TABLE 52-2.
INTRACELLULAR FUNCTIONS AFFECTED BY LOCAL pH

Cellular metabolism
Cytoskeletal structure
Muscle contractility
Cell-cell coupling
Membrane conductance
Intracellular messengers
Cell activation, growth, and proliferation
Cell volume regulation
Intracellular membrane flow

Degree of Ventilatory Response

Ventilatory responses cannot return pH to 7.4 when a metabolic abnormality is responsible for the acid-base disturbance. This reflects the fact that the intensity of the stimulus responsible for increases or decreases in alveolar ventilation will begin to diminish as pH returns toward 7.4. As a buffer, ventilatory responses are able to buffer up to twice the amount of acids or bases as all the chemical buffers combined. However, compensation for extreme metabolic acidosis imposes a significant respiratory burden. If the bicarbonate is reduced to 10 mmol/liter, the carbon dioxide tension must be reduced to 15 mm Hg in order to normalize the pH. Most patients will not hyperventilate to below 20 mm Hg. Further, it is likely that the insult causing severe metabolic acidosis will also adversely affect respiratory muscle function thus compromising the respiratory response.

Renal Responses

The day-to-day renal contribution to acid-base regulation is directed toward the conservation of bicarbonate and the excretion of hydrogen ions.

Bicarbonate Conservation

Plasma bicarbonate is freely filtered at the glomerulus. Almost all filtered bicarbonate must be reabsorbed from the glomerular filtrate to maintain the normal plasma bicarbonate concentration (25 mEq/liter) and plasma pH. Most bicarbonate reabsorption occurs in the proximal convoluted tubule and is facilitated by the presence of carbonic anhydrase in the luminal fluid and is driven by the sodium-potassium-ATPase pump in the peritubular cell membrane. Active sodium ion extrusion from the renal tubular cell into the peritubular circulation favors sodium diffusion from the tubular lumen into the tubular cell in exchange for hydrogen ions. Hydrogen in the renal tubular fluid then combines with filtered bicarbonate to form carbonic acid. Carbonic anhydrase facilitates the dissociation of carbonic acid into water and carbon dioxide that both enter the renal tubular cell. Carbon dioxide and water generate bicarbonate, which enters the peritubular circulation accompanied by sodium. The remaining hydrogen ions are secreted into the lumen in exchange for sodium (Fig. 52-5). Inhibition of carbonic anhydrase by acetazolamide interferes with the reabsorption of bicarbonate ions from renal tubular fluid. As a result, excess bicarbonate ions are lost in the urine and the plasma bicarbonate concentration is decreased.

Renal Tubular Secretion of Hydrogen Ions

Hydrogen ions are secreted into renal tubules by epithelial cells lining proximal renal tubules, distal renal tubules, and collecting ducts. At the same time, sodium ions are reabsorbed in exchange for the secreted hydrogen ions and combine with bicarbonate ions in the peritubular capillaries.

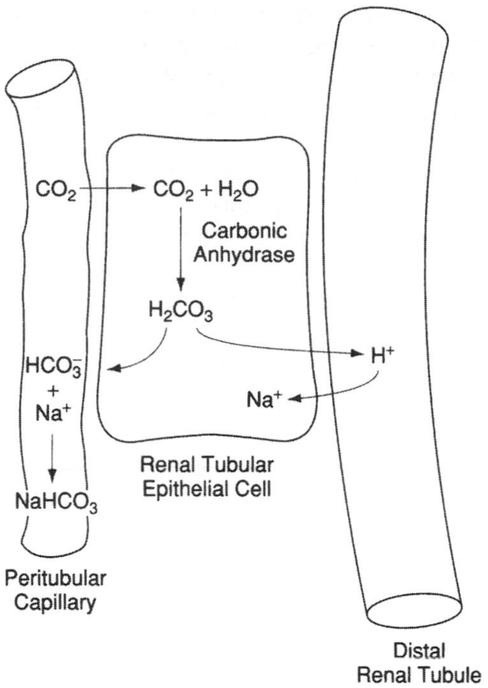

Figure 52-5. Schematic depiction of the renal tubular secretion of hydrogen ions, which are formed from the dissociation of carbonic acid in renal tubular epithelial cells.

This process is facilitated by aldosterone (see Fig. 52-5). As a result, the amount of sodium bicarbonate in the plasma is increased during the secretion of hydrogen ions into renal tubules. Active hydrogen ion transport is inhibited when the urinary pH drops below 4.0. Thus, hydrogen ions must combine with ammonia and phosphate buffers in the renal tubular lumen to prevent the pH from decreasing below this critical level. Ammonia is generated in the mitochondria of the proximal tubule. Ammonia combines with hydrogen ions to form ammonium, which is excreted in the urine in combination with chloride ions as the weak acid ammonium chloride (Fig. 52-6). In renal insufficiency the capacity to generate urinary ammonia is impaired thus reducing hydrogen ion excretion.

Renal responses that regulate hydrogen ion concentrations do so by acidification or alkalinization of the urine. In the presence of acidosis, the rate of hydrogen ion secretion exceeds the net loss of bicarbonate ion into the renal tubules. As a result, an excess of hydrogen ions is excreted into the urine. In the presence of alkalosis, the effect of the titration process in the renal tubules is to increase the number of bicarbonate ions filtered into the renal tubules relative to the secretion of hydrogen ions. Excess bicarbonate ions are excreted into the urine accompanied by cations, most often sodium.

Regulation of Chloride

Extracellular fluid is electroneutral such that the sum of the positive charges of all cations must equal the sum of negative charges of all anions. In the process of altering the plasma concentration of bicarbonate ions, it is mandatory to remove some other anion each time the concentration of bicarbonate ions is increased or to increase some other anion when the bicarbonate concentration is decreased. Typically, the anion that follows changes in the concentration of bicarbonate ions is chloride. As the most abundant extracellular anion, physiologic manipulation of chloride appears to be an important element of pH control. Conceptually, when bicarbonate ions are replaced by chloride ions, the pH will generally tend to decrease as a weak acid (carbonic acid) is replaced by a *strong acid (hydrochloric acid)*.

Degree of Renal Compensation

Renal responses for regulation of acid-base balance are slow to act (hours) but continue until the pH returns to almost 7.4. Thus, unlike ventilatory responses that are rapid but incomplete, the value of renal regulation of hydrogen ion concentration is not its rapidity but instead its ability to nearly completely neutralize any excess acid or alkali that enters the body fluids. Ordinarily, the kidneys can remove up to 500 mmol of acid or alkali each day. If greater quantities than this are generated the kidneys are unable to maintain normal acid-base balance, and acidosis or alkalosis occurs. Even when the plasma pH is 7.4, a small amount of acid is still lost each minute. This reflects the daily production of 50 to 80 mmol of more acid than alkali. Indeed, the normal urine pH of approximately 6.4 rather than 7.4 is due to the presence of this excess acid in the urine.

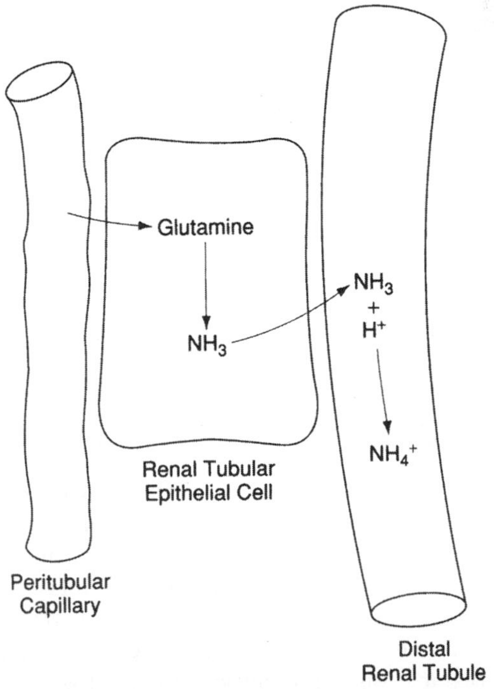

Figure 52-6. Ammonia formed in renal tubular epithelial cells combines with hydrogen ions in the renal tubules to form ammonium.

TABLE 52-3.
CLASSIFICATION OF ACID-BASE DISTURBANCES

	pH	$Paco_2$	Bicarbonate
Respiratory acidosis			
Acute	−−	+++	+
Chronic	NC	+++	++
Respiratory alkalosis			
Acute	++	−−−	−
Chronic	NC	−−−	−−
Metabolic acidosis			
Acute	−−−	−	−−−
Chronic	−	−−−	−−−
Metabolic alkalosis			
Acute	+++	+	+++
Chronic	++	++	+++

+, increase; −, decrease; NC, no change from normal.

ACID-BASE DISTURBANCES

Acid-base disturbances are categorized as respiratory or metabolic acidosis (pH <7.35) or alkalosis (pH >7.45) (Table 52-3) (Black, 2001). An acid-base disturbance that results primarily from changes in alveolar ventilation is described as respiratory acidosis or alkalosis. An acid-base disturbance unrelated to changes in alveolar ventilation is designated as metabolic acidosis or alkalosis. Compensation describes the secondary renal or ventilatory responses that occur as a result of the primary acid-base disturbance. These compensatory changes tend to return the pH toward a normal value.

The principal manifestation of respiratory or metabolic acidosis is depression of the central nervous system. For example, coma is a characteristic of severe diabetic acidosis or renal dysfunction leading to uremia. The principal manifestation of respiratory or metabolic alkalosis is increased excitability of the peripheral nervous system and central nervous system. As a result, there may be repetitive stimulation, causing skeletal muscles to undergo sustained contraction known as *tetany*. Tetany of respiratory muscles may interfere with adequate ventilation of the lungs. Central nervous system excitability may manifest as seizures.

Respiratory Acidosis

Any event (drug or disease) that decreases alveolar ventilation results in an increased concentration of dissolved carbon dioxide in the plasma (increased $PACO_2$), which in turn leads to formation of carbonic acid and hydrogen ions (see Fig. 52-3). By convention, carbonic acid resulting from dissolved carbon dioxide is considered a respiratory acid, and respiratory acidosis is present when the pH is <7.35. It is important to note that although an increase in dissolved carbon dioxide generates an equivalent increase in both the hydrogen ion and bicarbonate ion concentrations, the pH will fall. This is because the *relative* increase in hydrogen ions is significantly greater than the *relative* increase in bicarbonate ions. For example, an increase in carbon dioxide sufficient to reduce the pH from 7.4 to 7.1 will increase the hydrogen ion concentration from 40 to 79 nmol/liter, compared to an increase in the bicarbonate ion concentration from 24.000000 to 24.000039 mEq/liter.

Respiratory Alkalosis

Respiratory alkalosis is present when increased alveolar ventilation removes sufficient carbon dioxide from the body to decrease the hydrogen ion concentration to the extent that pH becomes >7.45. A physiologic cause of respiratory alkalosis is hyperventilation due to stimulation of chemoreceptors by a low Po_2 associated with ascent to altitude. Kidneys compensate with time for this loss of carbon dioxide by excreting bicarbonate ions in association with sodium and potassium ions. This renal compensation is evident in individuals residing at altitude who have a nearly normal pH despite a low $Paco_2$. A frequent cause of acute respiratory alkalosis is iatrogenic hyperventilation of the lungs as during anesthesia. Tetany that accompanies alkalosis reflects hypocalcemia due to the greater affinity of plasma proteins for calcium ions in an alkaline, compared with an acidic, solution.

Metabolic Acidosis

Any acid formed in the body other than carbon dioxide is considered a metabolic acid, and its accumulation results in metabolic acidosis.

Lactic Acidosis

Under normal circumstances lactate is produced at a rate of approximately 1 mmol/kg/hour. Normal clearance of lactate maintains its serum concentration between 0.5 and 1.0 mmol/liter. Most lactate is cleared by the liver, where it undergoes oxidation, gluconeogenesis, and eventual conversion to bicarbonate. Lactate undergoes both passive diffusion and active transport into the liver via a monocarboxylate transporter. However, active transportation becomes saturated at serum lactate concentrations that exceed 2.5 mmol/liter. Severe reductions in hepatic blood flow, which occur during shock, will decrease hepatic lactate clearance. Lactic acid is a strong acid and therefore dissociates almost completely under physiologic conditions into the lactate anion and a proton. Although lactate accumulation has classically been taught to occur mainly during anaerobic glycolysis, it is now clear that significant lactate generation occurs under normoxic conditions. Indeed, lactate is an important gluconeogenic precursor and is involved in cell-to-cell signaling. However, in the critically ill patient, both lactate production may increase while lactate clearance is impaired and lactic acidosis may occur. Point-of-care testing allows almost instantaneous lactate determinations to be performed in the operating room and intensive care unit. A serum lactate >1.5 mmol/liter upon admission is an independent predictor of mortality in critically ill patients. Furthermore, failure to decrease lactate concentration to ≤1.0 mmol/liter 24 hours after admission is also associated with significant mortality.

The investigational drug dichloroacetate (DCA) decreases lactate concentration in cardiogenic shock, burns, diabetic ketoacidosis, and malaria. DCA activates the mitochondrial pyruvate dehydrogenase complex, thus accelerating the irreversible oxidation of lactate via pyruvate to acetyl CoA, which then enters the Krebs cycle.

Metabolic Acidosis

Metabolic acidosis impairs myocardial contractility and the responses to endogenous or exogenous catecholamines (Hindman, 1990). Hemodynamic deterioration is usually minimal when the pH remains >7.2 due to compensatory increases in sympathetic nervous system activity. Of great clinical importance are the accentuated detrimental effects of metabolic acidosis in individuals with underlying left ventricular dysfunction or myocardial ischemia or in those in whom sympathetic nervous system activity may be impaired, as by drug-induced beta-adrenergic blockade or general anesthesia. Respiratory acidosis may produce more rapid and profound myocardial dysfunction than does metabolic acidosis, reflecting the ability of carbon dioxide to freely diffuse across cell membranes and exacerbate intracellular acidosis.

Acute metabolic acidosis has been treated with intravenous administration of an exogenous buffer, usually sodium bicarbonate, in the hope that normalizing pH will attenuate the detrimental effects of acidosis. Nevertheless, use of sodium bicarbonate to treat metabolic acidosis is questionable (Graf et al., 1985; Hindman, 1990). For example, sodium bicarbonate administration increases the carbon dioxide load to the lungs, leading to further increases in arterial and intracellular P_{CO_2} if alveolar ventilation is not concomitantly increased. It is estimated that 1 mEq/kg sodium bicarbonate, given intravenously, produces approximately 180 mL of carbon dioxide and necessitates a transient doubling of alveolar ventilation to prevent hypercarbia. In the presence of increased dead space ventilation, even greater increases in alveolar ventilation are required for carbon dioxide elimination to equal production. Even if Pa_{CO_2} is maintained normal, it is likely that tissue pHi and the risk of ventricular defibrillation will not be altered by administration of sodium bicarbonate during cardiopulmonary resuscitation.

Renal failure prevents excretion of acids formed by normal metabolic processes, and metabolic acidosis occurs. Severe diarrhea and associated loss of sodium bicarbonate rapidly leads to metabolic acidosis, especially in the pediatric age group. Lack of insulin secretion or starvation impairs glucose utilization, forcing tissues to metabolize fat to meet energy needs. As a result, the plasma concentration of acetoacetic acid often increases sufficiently to cause metabolic acidosis.

Dilutional Acidosis

Dilutional acidosis occurs when the plasma pH is decreased by extracellular volume expansion with solutions such as normal saline. Clinically, a hyperchloremic metabolic acidosis may accompany large-volume infusion of isotonic saline (Mathes et al., 1997). Although the term *dilutional acidosis* is often used, the precise mechanism of this phenomenon is disputed. Dilution of extracellular bicarbonate is unlikely because acid should be diluted to a similar degree. Furthermore, bicarbonate should be regenerated from carbonic acid. Although normal saline is commonly thought of as being "physiologic," it has a pH (5.7) that is more acidic than plasma and contains significantly more chloride (154 versus 100 mmol/liter) and slightly more sodium (154 versus 140 mmol/liter). Thus, infusion of a large volume of normal saline will increase plasma chloride concentration to a relatively greater degree than sodium concentration. Chloride can be thought of as a strong acid, (hydrochloric acid-proton donor), just as sodium can be thought of as a strong base (sodium hydroxide-hydroxyl donor) (Levetown, 2002). Measurement of the plasma lactic acid concentration and calculation of the anion gap from sodium, chloride, and bicarbonate permits differentiation of dilutional acidosis from acidosis due to tissue hypoperfusion.

Metabolic Alkalosis

Causes of metabolic alkalosis include vomiting with excess loss of hydrochloric acid, nasogastric suction, chronic administration of thiazide diuretics, and excess secretion of aldosterone. Excess administration of sodium bicarbonate may be an iatrogenic cause of metabolic alkalosis.

Compensation of Acid-Base Disturbances

Respiratory acidosis is compensated for within 6 to 12 hours by increased renal secretion of hydrogen ions, with a resulting increase in the plasma bicarbonate concentration. After a few days, the pH will be normal despite persistence of an increased Pa_{CO_2}. Sudden correction of chronic respiratory acidosis, by iatrogenic hyperventilation, may result in acute metabolic alkalosis because increased plasma bicarbonate is not promptly eliminated by the kidneys.

Respiratory alkalosis is compensated for by decreased reabsorption of bicarbonate ions from renal tubules. As a result, more bicarbonate ions are excreted in the urine, which decreases the plasma concentration of bicarbonate and returns the pH toward normal despite persistence of a decreased Pa_{CO_2}.

Metabolic acidosis stimulates alveolar ventilation, which causes rapid removal of carbon dioxide from the body and decreases the hydrogen ion concentration toward normal. This respiratory compensation for metabolic acidosis, however, is only partial because pH remains somewhat below normal.

Metabolic alkalosis diminishes alveolar ventilation, which in turn causes accumulation of carbon dioxide and a subsequent increase in hydrogen ion concentration. As with metabolic acidosis, the respiratory compensation for metabolic alkalosis is only partial. Renal compensation for metabolic alkalosis is increased by reabsorption of hydrogen ions. This metabolic compensation is limited by the availability of sodium, potassium, and chloride ions. During prolonged vomiting, there may be excessive loss of chloride ions along with sodium and potassium. When this occurs, the kidneys preferentially conserve sodium and potassium ions and the urine becomes paradoxically acidic. Indeed, the presence of paradoxical aciduria indicates electrolyte depletion.

TABLE 52-4.
MEASURED AND UNMEASURED IONS COMMONLY USED IN ANION GAP CALCULATION

Cations		Anions	
Electrolyte	Value (mEq/L)	Electrolyte	Value (mEq/L)
Sodium	140	Chloride	104
		Bicarbonate	24
Calcium	5	Phosphate	2
Magnesium	1.5	Sulphate	1
Potassium	4.5	Organic Acids	5
		Proteins	15
Total Measured Cations	140	Total Measured Anions	128
Total Cations	**151**	**Total Anions**	**151**

The Anion Gap

Calculation of the anion gap may assist in the evaluation of acid-base disorders. However, the availability of rapid bedside lactic acid measurements may decrease the utility of the anion gap. The anion gap is a derived value based upon the principle of electrochemical neutrality such that the sum of the positive (cationic) charges in a solution must equal the sum of the negative (anionic) charges (Table 52-4). The major extracellular anions are chloride and bicarbonate. Other significant anions include proteins, phosphate, sulfate, and organic acids (including lactate). The latter are less commonly measured in routine practice and are referred to as "unmeasured anions". The predominant extracellular cation is sodium. Although potassium is now routinely measured, its inclusion in the anion gap calculation is inconsistent and varies from institution to institution. Potassium is often grouped with the other "unmeasured cations", calcium, and magnesium. Under normal circumstances the concentration of the predominant cation (sodium) exceeds that of the combined predominant anions (chloride and bicarbonate) by 9 to 13 mEq/liter. For electroneutrality to occur, the concentration of the combined unmeasured anions must therefore exceed that of the unmeasured cations by the same amount (Fig. 52-7).

The term anion gap refers solely to the difference in concentration between the traditionally *measured* anions and cations (Fig. 52-8). The anion gap does not imply a true discrepancy between the total positive and negative charges in physiologic solution.

Metabolic acidosis is most often associated with an increase in the anion gap. A decrease in the concentration of unmeasured cations or an increase in the concentration of unmeasured anions will increase the anion gap. Lactic acidosis, ketoacidosis, and renal failure increase the concentration of unmeasured endogenous anions. Exogenous anions will also increase the concentration of unmeasured anions (salicylate toxicity, ethylene glycol, and methanol ingestion).

Effects of Temperature on Acid-Base Status

Temperature changes have several effects on blood and tissue pH and P_{CO_2}. As blood is cooled, carbon dioxide becomes more soluble. Therefore, for a given carbon dioxide content, the partial pressure will decrease as the temperature falls. The magnitude of this change is approximately 4.5% per °C and will tend to increase the pH. The blood pH is further increased as the dissociation of water into protons and hydroxyl ions decreases with cooling, thus decreasing hydrogen ion concentration. In addition, proton buffering by hemoglobin alpha-imadazole groups is enhanced by hypothermia. The sum of these effects is an increase of 0.015 pH units per °C decrease in temperature. These changes are probably insignificant within the physiologic temperature range but are important when interpreting blood-gas and acid-base data during induced cooling during cardiopulmonary bypass. If the blood temperature is decreased by 10°C to 27°C the pH will increase to 7.6. Two alternate blood-gas management strategies, alpha-stat and pH-stat,

TOTAL CATION CHARGE = TOTAL ANION CHARGE

$$Na^+ + \text{unmeasured cations} = (HCO_3^- + C1^-) + \text{unmeasured anions}$$

Figure 52-7. Calculation of electrochemical neutrality.

$$\text{Anion Gap} = Na^+ - (HCO_3^- + Cl^-)$$

Figure 52-8. Calculation of the anion gap.

are utilized during hypothermia in the operating room (Table 52-5). Although there is debate concerning the two strategies, each are thought to have important beneficial effects under particular clinical circumstances (Table 52-5).

pH Stat Management

During hypothermic conditions blood pH is increased and P_{CO_2} is decreased. The pH stat strategy seeks to return the pH and P_{CO_2} of hypothermic blood to normal. During hypothermic cardiopulmonary bypass, this strategy usually involves the addition of carbon dioxide via the oxygenator. A purported advantage of this strategy is that cerebral blood flow will be increased because carbon dioxide is a potent cerebral vasodilator. However, delivery of microemboli to the brain may also be increased. Temperature correction of blood gas samples is required to interpret the values obtained from a hypothermic patient but measured at 37°C. The pH stat strategy is used more often in surgery for congenital heart disease, especially during cooling prior to profound hypothermic circulatory arrest. Under these circumstances enhanced cerebral perfusion that facilitates brain cooling is thought to be desirable. Cerebral injury secondary to global hypoperfusion is thought to be a greater threat than delivery of microemboli in this patient population. Hypothermia, hypocarbia (via the Bohr effect), and alkalosis, all shift the oxyhemoglobin dissociation curve to the left and impair tissue oxygen delivery. The addition of carbon dioxide during pH stat management will counter these effects and facilitate oxygen unloading from hemoglobin.

Alpha-stat management

The alpha-stat strategy seeks to replicate the alkalinization of blood that occurs during cooling in ectothermic mammals. This strategy seeks to optimize enzyme function during hypothermia. The alpha of alpha-stat refers to the charged portion of the histidine imidazole residue. The objective is to maintain biologic neutrality by preserving the alpha imadazole and protein charge state, the OH^-/H^+ ratio, and therefore enzyme function, even though the pH will increase. This strategy is most often used during adult cardiopulmonary bypass and does not generally encourage the delivery of microemboli to the brain because supplemental carbon dioxide is not generally administered. This strategy does not require temperature correction of blood gas results.

There are examples of both strategies in nature. Homeotherms have homeostatic mechanisms for maintaining the temperature of the internal environment within very narrow limits. Homeotherms and hibernating animals both hypoventilate in order to maintain blood pH at 7.4 as their body temperature decreases (pH stat). However, pHi is low in most tissues under these circumstances and suppresses metabolism and conserves energy stores in nonfunctioning tissues. However, the brain and heart of these animals employ alpha-stat strategies to maintain pHi at alpha-stat values and to maintain near normal function. Poikilotherms have not developed mechanisms for regulating the temperature of their internal environment that changes with that of the external environment. Poikilotherms use the alpha-stat strategy and allow their blood pH to increase and P_{CO_2} to decrease with cooling in order to preserve cellular and enzyme function over wide temperature ranges.

TABLE 52-5.
COMPARISON OF ALPHA STAT AND pH STAT BLOOD GAS MANAGEMENT STRATEGIES

	Alpha Stat	pH Stat
Carbon dioxide added to oxygenator	No	Yes
Enzyme function	Near normal	Decreased
Cerebral blood flow	Normal	Increased
Blood gas temperature correction required	No	Yes
$Hb\text{-}O_2$ dissociation curve	Marked left shift	Less marked left shift

GASTRIC INTRAMUCOSAL pH

Tissue acid-base balance is determined primarily by the balance between the protons released and buffered during the production of energy by adenosine triphosphate (ATP) hydrolysis and the protons consumed by resynthesis of ATP by oxidative phosphorylation (Fiddian-Green, 1995). When tissue oxygen delivery decreases, the resynthesis of ATP necessary to meet the energy demands of the tissue is jeopardized. If the rate of ATP hydrolysis exceeds the rate of synthesis, the tissue pH will decrease. During hemorrhage and shock, vasoconstriction is most pronounced in the cutaneous, skeletal muscle, and splanchnic beds. Hypovolemia may be accompanied by significant splanchnic ischemia despite relative preservation of systemic blood pressure. Thus, acid-base changes in the gut may precede systemic changes in early shock. It has been proposed that measurement of gastric intramucosal pH (indirect tonometric method by measuring P_{CO_2} in the lumen of the stomach and the bicarbonate concentration in arterial blood) provides a more specific measure of the degree of unreversed ATP hydrolysis than does systemic measurement of acid-base balance and blood lactate, which may provide only delayed and dampened signals of tissue oxygenation (Fiddian-Green, 1995).

REFERENCES

Black RM. Disorders of acid-base and potassium balance. In ACP Medicine, Section 10 Nephrology, WebMD Professional Publishing, Danbury CT. December 2001.

Aduen J, Bernstein WK, Khastgir T, et al. The use and clinical importance for a substrate-specific electrode for rapid determination of blood lactate concentrations. *JAMA* 1994;272:1678–1685.

Fiddian-Green RG. Gastric intramucosal pH, tissue oxygenation and acid-base balance. *Br J Anaesth* 1995;74:591–606.

Graf H, Leach W, Arieff AI. Metabolic effects of sodium bicarbonate in hypoxic lactic acidosis in dogs. *Am J Physiol* 1985;249:F630–F635.

Hindman BJ. Sodium bicarbonate in the treatment of subtypes of acute lactic acidosis: physiologic considerations. *Anesthesiology* 1990;72:1064–1066.

Levetown, M. Saline-induced hyperchloremic metabolic acidosis. *Crit Care Med* 2002;30:259–261.

Mathes DD, Morell RC, Rohr MS. Dilutional acidosis: is it a real clinical entity? *Anesthesiology* 1997;86:501–503.

Endocrine System

53

The principal organs of communication for the responses to exogenous and endogenous stimuli (surgery, diseases) are the nervous system and endocrine system. Neural responses to stress involve intercelluair communication over minuscule distances and utilize neurotransmitters. Response times are the period before another response can occur and are measured in milliseconds. In contrast, endocrine responses involve hormones that cirulate in the blood and response times (latency) are measured in minutes to hours. The hypothalamic-pituitary axis provides for convergence of neural and hormonal adaptive responses. The hypothalamus is outside the blood-brain barrier (can sense and respond to circulating concentrations of glucose, cortisol, sodium) and is also the site for major homeostatic controls (thirst, hunger, osmolarity, blood pressure, breathing, temperature). The hypothalamus is also the source of stimulatory and inhibitory humoral communication with the anterior pituitary.

Glands of the endocrine system are primarily concerned with regulating different metabolic functions of the body. Endocrine glands secrete hormones into the blood for delivery to distant sites where a response is evoked. Hormone output is typically regulated by a negative feedback system in which increased circulating plasma concentrations of the hormone decrease its subsequent release from the parent gland. Tumors that secrete hormones, however, usually escape from this negative-feedback control, and excess plasma concentrations of the hormone occur. Unrecognized endocrine dysfunction is unlikely if it can be established that (a) body weight is unchanged, (b) heart rate and systemic blood pressure are normal, (c) glycosuria is absent, (d) sexual function is normal, and (e) there is no history of recent endocrine system–related medication.

MECHANISM OF HORMONE ACTION

Hormones typically exert their physiologic effects by attaching to specific receptors on cell membranes. The combination of the hormone and receptor activates adenylate cyclase, leading to the conversion of adenosine triphosphate (ATP) to cyclic adenosine monophosphate (cAMP). The resulting increased intracellular concentration of cAMP is responsible for initiating cellular responses attributed to the effects of hormones. Examples of hormones that lead to production of cAMP are anterior pituitary and posterior pituitary hormones and hypothalamic-releasing hormones. An alternative mechanism of action of hormones is illustrated by corticosteroids that stimulate genes in cells to form specific intracellular proteins. These proteins then function as enzymes or carrier proteins, which, in turn, activate other functions of cells.

PITUITARY GLAND

The pituitary gland lies in the sella turcica at the base of the brain and is connected to the hypothalamus by the pituitary stalk. Physiologically, the gland is outside the blood-brain barrier and is divided into the anterior pituitary (adenohypophysis) and posterior pituitary (neurohypophysis). The anterior pituitary synthesizes, stores, and secretes six tropic hormones. Adrenocorticotrophic hormone (ACTH), prolactin, and human growth hormone (HGH) are polypeptides, whereas thyroid-stimulating hormone (TSH), luteinizing hormone (LH), and follicle-stimulating hormone (FSH) are glycoproteins. In addition, the anterior pituitary secretes beta-lipotropin, which contains the amino acid sequences of several endorphins that bind to opioid receptors. The posterior pituitary stores and secretes two hormones—arginine vasopressin (AVP), formerly designated antidiuretic hormone (ADH) and oxytocin—that are initially synthesized in the hypothalamus and subsequently transported to the posterior pituitary (Table 53-1).

Hormones designated as hypothalamic-releasing hormones and hypothalamic-inhibitory hormones originating in the hypothalamus control secretions from the anterior pituitary (Table 53-2). These hormones travel via hypothalamic-hypophyseal portal vessels to react with cell membrane receptors in the anterior pituitary, leading to increases in the intracellular concentrations of calcium ions and cAMP.

TABLE 53-1.
PITUITARY HORMONES

Hormone	Cell Type	Principal Action
Anterior pituitary		
Human growth hormone (HGH, somatotrophin)	Somatotropes	Accelerates body growth
Prolactin	Mammotropes	Stimulates secretion of milk and maternal behavior, inhibits ovulation
Luteinizing hormone (LH)	Gonadotropes	Stimulates ovulation in females and testosterone secretion in males
Follicle-stimulating hormone (FSH)	Gonadotropes	Stimulates ovarian follicle growth in females and spermatogenesis in males
Adrenocorticotrophic hormone (ACTH)	Corticotropes	Stimulates adrenal cortex secretion and growth
Thyroid-stimulating hormone (TSH)	Thyrotropes	Stimulates thyroid secretion and growth
Beta-lipotropin	Corticotropes	Precursor of endorphins
Posterior pituitary		
Arginine vasopressin	Supraoptic nuclei	Promotes water retention and regulates plasma osmolarity
Oxytocin	Paraventricular nuclei	Causes ejection of milk and uterine contraction

Synthesis and release of releasing and inhibitory hormones is controlled by many factors, including adrenergic and dopaminergic receptors, pain signals, emotions, and olfactory sensations. As such, the hypothalamus is a collecting center for information and provides a link between the central nervous system and endocrine system and the response to the environment. Hypothalamic and pituitary secretion is pulsatile rather than tonic and these pulses are superimposed on broader biologic rhythms such as the circadian release of ACTH, the sleep-entrained release of HGH, and the monthly cycle of gonadotropins in females.

Anterior Pituitary

Anterior pituitary cells have been traditionally classified on the basis of their staining characteristics as agranular chromophobes and granular chromophils. Chromophils are subdivided into acidophils and basophils depending on their staining response to acidic or basic dyes. With more modern techniques, including electron microscopy and immunochemistry, it is possible to identify at least five types of cells, some of which secrete more than one tropic hormone (see Table 53-1).

TABLE 53-2.
HYPOTHALAMIC HORMONES

Hormone	Target Anterior Pituitary Hormone
Human growth hormone–releasing hormone	HGH
Human growth hormone–inhibiting hormone (somatostatin)	HGH, prolactin, TSH
Prolactin-releasing factor	Prolactin
Prolactin-inhibiting factor	Prolactin
Luteinizing hormone–releasing hormone	LH, FSH
Corticotropin-releasing hormone	ACTH, beta-lipotropins, endorphins
Thyrotropin-releasing hormone	TSH

ACTH, adrenocorticotrophic hormone; FSH, follicle-stimulating hormone; HGH, human growth hormone; LH, luteinizing hormone; TSH, thyroid-stimulating hormone.

Human Growth Hormone

HGH stimulates growth of all tissues in the body and evokes intense metabolic effects (Fig. 53-1) (Ganong, 2003). The most striking and specific effect is stimulation of linear bone growth that results from HGH action on the epiphyseal cartilage plates of long bones. Excess secretion of HGH before epiphyseal closure occurs results in giantism. Acromegaly occurs when excess HGH secretion occurs after epiphyseal closure and long bones can no longer increase in length but can increase in thickness. The metabolic effects of HGH include increased rates of protein synthesis (anabolic effect), increased mobilization of free fatty acids (ketogenic effect), and decreased rate of glucose use (diabetogenic effect). Many of the activities of HGH require the prior generation of a family of peptides known as *somatomedins.*

Secretion of HGH is regulated by releasing and inhibitory (somatostatin) hormones secreted by the hypothalamus as well as physiologic and pharmacologic events (Table 53-3). For example, anxiety and stress associated with anesthesia evoke the release of HGH. Plasma concentrations of HGH characteristically increase during physiologic sleep. Drugs may influence the secretion of HGH, presumably via effects on the hypothalamus. In this regard, large doses of corticosteroids suppress secretion of HGH, which may be responsible for the inhibitory effects on growth observed in children receiving high doses of corticosteroids for prolonged periods as required for

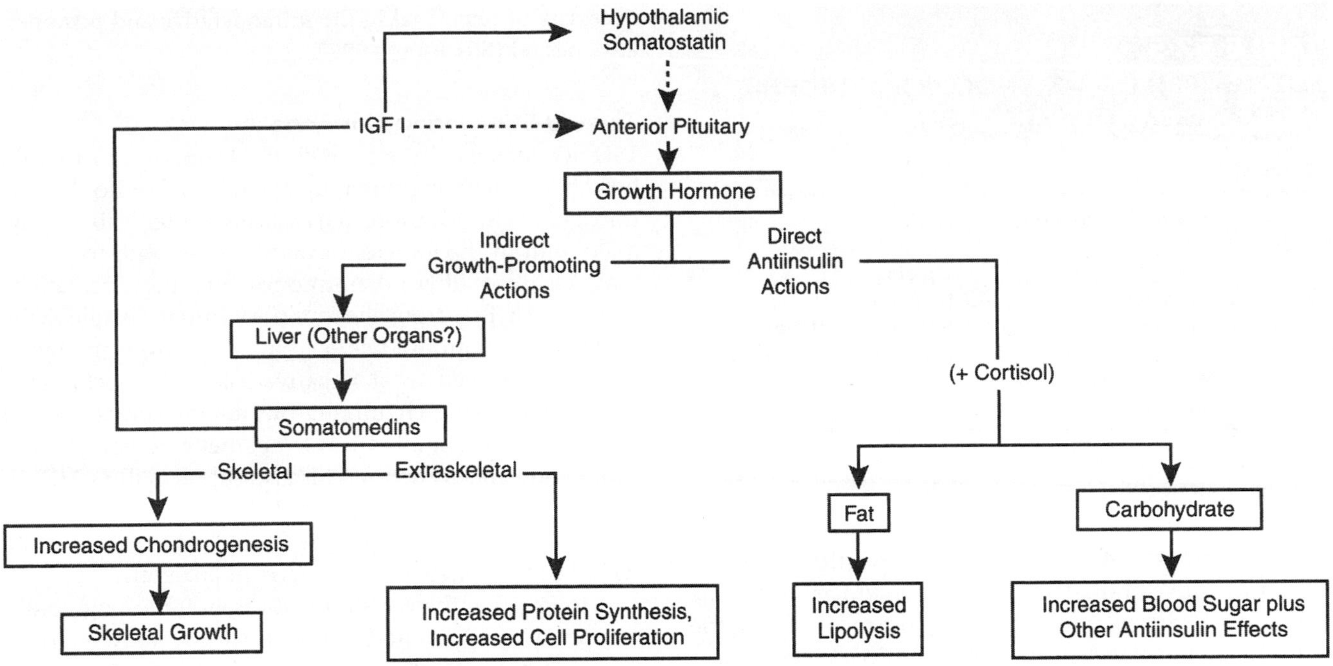

Figure 53-1. Effects of human growth hormone manifesting as direct effects or via production of somatomedins in the liver. (From Ganong WF. *Review of medical physiology*, 21st ed. Lange Medical Books. New York: McGraw Hill, 2003; with permission.)

immunosuppression after organ transplantation. Conversely, dopaminergic agonists acutely increase the secretion of HGH.

Prolactin

Prolactin is responsible for growth and development of the breast in preparation for breast-feeding. Pregnancy is the principal event responsible for stimulating the release of prolactin; dopamine inhibits release of this hormone (Table 53-4). Preoperative anxiety is often accompanied by increased plasma concentrations of prolactin. Prolactin secretion in response to suckling is a potent inhibitor of ovarian function, explaining the usual lack of ovulation and resulting infertility during breast-feeding.

Gonadotropins

LH and FSH are gonadotropins responsible for pubertal maturation and secretion of steroid sex hormones by the gonads of either sex. These hormones presumably bind to cell membrane receptors in the ovaries or testes to stimulate the synthesis of cAMP.

Adrenocorticotrophic Hormone

ACTH is principally responsible for regulating secretions of the adrenal cortex, especially cortisol. In addition, ACTH stimulates the formation of cholesterol in the

TABLE 53-3.
REGULATION OF HUMAN GROWTH HORMONE (HGH) SECRETION

Stimulation	Inhibition
HGH-releasing hormone	HGH-inhibiting hormone
Stress	HGH
Physiologic sleep	Pregnancy
Hypoglycemia	Hyperglycemia
Free fatty acid decrease	Free fatty acid increase
Amino acid increase	Cortisol
Fasting	Obesity
Estrogens	
Dopamine	
Alpha-adrenergic agonists	

TABLE 53-4.
REGULATION OF PROLACTIN SECRETION

Stimulation	Inhibition
Prolactin-releasing factor	Prolactin-inhibiting factor
Pregnancy	Prolactin
Suckling	Dopamine
Stress	L-dopa
Physiologic sleep	
Metoclopramide	
Cimetidine	
Opioids	
Alpha-methyldopa	

TABLE 53-5.
REGULATION OF ADRENOCORTICOTROPHIC HORMONE (ACTH) SECRETION

Stimulation	Inhibition
Corticotropin-releasing hormone	ACTH
Cortisol decrease	Cortisol increase
Stress	Opioids
Sleep-wake transition	Etomidate
Hypoglycemia	Suppression of the hypothalamic-pituitary axis
Trauma	
Alpha-adrenergic agonists	
Beta-adrenergic antagonists	

adrenal cortex. Cholesterol is the initial building block for the synthesis of corticosteroids. Secretion of ACTH responds most dramatically to stress and is under the control of corticotropin-releasing hormone from the hypothalamus, as well as a negative-feedback mechanism that depends on the circulating plasma concentration of cortisol (Table 53-5) (Taylor and Fishman, 1988). Secretory rates of corticotropin-releasing hormone and ACTH are high in the morning and low in the evening. This diurnal variation results in high plasma cortisol concentrations in the morning (approximately 20 μg/dL) and low levels (approximately 5 μg/dL) around midnight. For this reason, plasma concentrations of cortisol must be interpreted in terms of the time of day the measurement was made.

In the absence of ACTH, the adrenal cortex undergoes atrophy, but the zona glomerulosa, which secretes aldosterone, is least affected. Indeed, hypophysectomy has minimal effects on electrolyte balance, reflecting the continued release of aldosterone from the adrenal cortex. Pigmentary changes that may accompany certain endocrine diseases most likely reflect changes in plasma concentrations of ACTH, emphasizing the melanocyte-stimulating effects of this hormone. For example, pallor is a hallmark of hypopituitarism. Conversely, hyperpigmentation occurs in patients with adrenal insufficiency due to primary adrenal gland disease, reflecting increased circulating plasma concentrations of ACTH as the anterior pituitary attempts to stimulate corticosteroid secretion.

Chronic administration of corticosteroids leads to functional atrophy of the hypothalamic-pituitary axis. Several months may be required for recovery of this axis after removal of the suppressive influence. In such patients, it is conceivable that stressful events during the perioperative period might evoke life-threatening hypotension. For this reason, it is a common practice to administer supplemental exogenous corticosteroids to patients considered at risk based on suppression of the hypothalamic-pituitary axis. There is no evidence, however, that supplemental corticosteroids in excess of normal daily physiologic secretion are necessary or beneficial in the intraoperative and postoperative period (Stoelting, 1997).

Thyroid-Stimulating Hormone

TSH accelerates all the steps in the formation of thyroid hormones, including initial uptake of iodide into the thyroid gland. In addition, TSH causes proteolysis of thyroglobulin in the follicles of thyroid cells, with the resultant release of thyroid hormones into the circulation. Secretion of TSH from the anterior pituitary is under the control of thyrotropin-releasing hormone from the hypothalamus as well as a negative-feedback mechanism, depending on the circulating plasma concentrations of thyroid hormones. Likewise, sympathetic nervous system stimulation and corticosteroids also suppress the secretion of TSH and thus diminish activity of the thyroid gland. Thyrotropin-releasing hormone is widely distributed in the central nervous system and is a potent analeptic.

A long-acting thyroid stimulator is an immunoglobulin A antibody that can bind to receptor sites on thyroid cells. Presumably, the binding of these antibodies can mimic the effects of TSH and account for hyperthyroidism. Indeed, patients with hyperthyroidism often have detectable circulating concentrations of these proteins. Hypothyroidism with increased plasma concentrations of TSH indicates a primary defect at the thyroid gland and an attempt by the anterior pituitary to stimulate hormonal output by releasing TSH. A defect at the hypothalamus or anterior pituitary is indicated by low circulating plasma concentrations of both TSH and thyroid hormones.

Posterior Pituitary

The posterior pituitary is composed of cells that act as supporting structures for terminal nerve endings of fibers from the supraoptic and paraventricular nuclei of the hypothalamus. AVP is synthesized in the supraoptic nuclei and oxytocin in the paraventricular nuclei. These hormones are transported in secretory granules along axons from corresponding nuclei in the hypothalamus to the posterior pituitary for subsequent release in response to appropriate stimuli.

Arginine Vasopressin

AVP is responsible for conserving body water and regulating the osmolarity of body fluids. Release of AVP is influenced by a number of factors, especially decreases in blood volume (Table 53-6). Painful stimulation and hemorrhage as associated with surgery are potent events for evoking the release of AVP. Hydration and establishment of an adequate blood volume before induction of anesthesia serve to maintain urine output, presumably by blunting the release of AVP associated with painful stimulation or fluid deprivation before surgery. Concentrations of AVP in the plasma in response to acute decreases in extracellular fluid

TABLE 53-6.
REGULATION OF ARGININE VASOPRESSIN SECRETION

Stimulation	Inhibition
Increased plasma osmolarity	Decreased plasma osmolarity
Hypovolemia	Ethanol
Pain	Alpha-adrenergic agonists
Hypotension	Cortisol
Hyperthermia	Hypothermia
Stress	
Nausea and vomiting	
Opioids (?)	

volume may be sufficient to exert direct pressor effects on arterioles and thus contribute to maintenance of systemic blood pressure. Administration of morphine, and presumably other opioids, in the absence of painful stimulation does not evoke the release of AVP. Ethanol inhibits the secretion of AVP. Decreased urine output and fluid retention previously attributed to release of AVP during positive pressure ventilation of the lungs are more likely due to changes in cardiac filling pressures that impair the release of atrial natriuretic hormone (see Chapter 54).

AVP is transported in the blood to the kidneys, where it attaches to receptors on the capillary side of epithelial cells lining the distal convoluted renal tubules and collecting ducts of the renal medulla. This receptor-hormone interaction results in the formation of large amounts of cAMP, which causes pores on the cell membranes to open and allow free permeability to water. Fluoride resulting from the metabolism of enflurane and sevoflurane interferes with normal receptor responses to AVP and may result in high-volume output of dilute urine. Hypokalemia, hypercalcemia, cortisol, and lithium also interfere with renal responsiveness to AVP.

Diabetes insipidus results when there is destruction of neurons in or near the supraoptic and paraventricular nuclei of the hypothalamus. It will not occur when the posterior pituitary alone is damaged because the transected fibers of the pituitary stalk can still continue to secrete AVP. Diabetes insipidus, which develops in association with pituitary surgery, typically is due to trauma to the posterior pituitary and is usually transient.

Oxytocin

The primary role of oxytocin is to eject milk from the lactating mammary gland. In this regard, oxytocin causes contraction of the myoepithelial cells that surround the alveoli of the mammary glands, making milk available in response to suckling. In addition, oxytocin exerts a contracting effect on the pregnant uterus by lowering the threshold for depolarization of uterine smooth muscle. Large amounts of oxytocin cause sustained uterine contraction as necessary for postpartum hemostasis. Oxytocin has only 0.5% to 1.0% the antidiuretic activity of AVP and can be released abruptly and independently of AVP.

THYROID GLAND

The thyroid gland is responsible for maintaining the level of metabolism in tissues that is optimal for their normal function (Bennett-Guerrero et al., 1997). The principal hormonal secretions of the thyroid gland are thyroxine (T_4) and triiodothyronine (T_3) (Fig. 53-2). T_4 is a prohormone synthesized from tyrosine and represents 80% of the body's thyroid hormone production. T_3 is the most biologically active form of thyroid hormone (five times more active than T_4) and is produced directly from tyrosine metabolism or from conversion of T_4 in peripheral tissues. Two distinct deiodases located in the liver, kidneys, and central nervous system metabolize T_4 and T_3 to inactive compounds. The half-lives of endogenously or exogenously administered T_3 and T_4 are 1.5 and 7 days, respectively. T_3 and T_4 are both highly protein bound to albumin, thyroid-binding prealbumin, and thyroid-binding globulin with only 0.2% of T_3 and 0.3% of T_4 freely circulating unbound and pharmacologically active (Bennett-Guerrero et al., 1997). It is of interest that iodine present in thyroid hormones is not necessary for biologic activity (see Fig. 53-2). In addition to thyroid hormones, the thyroid gland secretes calcitonin, which is important for calcium ion use. The plasma concentration of T_4 is the standard screening test for thyroid gland function.

The most obvious effect of thyroid hormones is to increase minute oxygen consumption in nearly all tissues, with the brain being an important exception. Failure of thyroid hormones to greatly alter the minute oxygen consumption of the brain is consistent with the minimal changes in anesthetic requirements (MAC) that accompany hyperthyroidism or hypothyroidism (Babad and Eger, 1968). Cardiovascular changes are often the earliest clinical manifestations of abnormal thyroid hormone

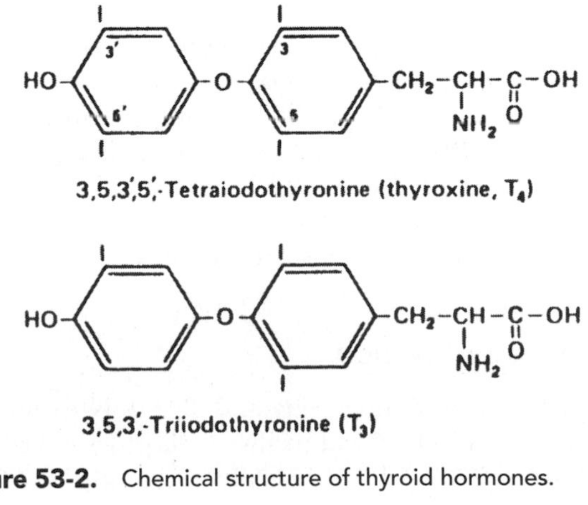

3,5,3',5'-Tetraiodothyronine (thyroxine, T_4)

3,5,3'-Triiodothyronine (T_3)

Figure 53-2. Chemical structure of thyroid hormones.

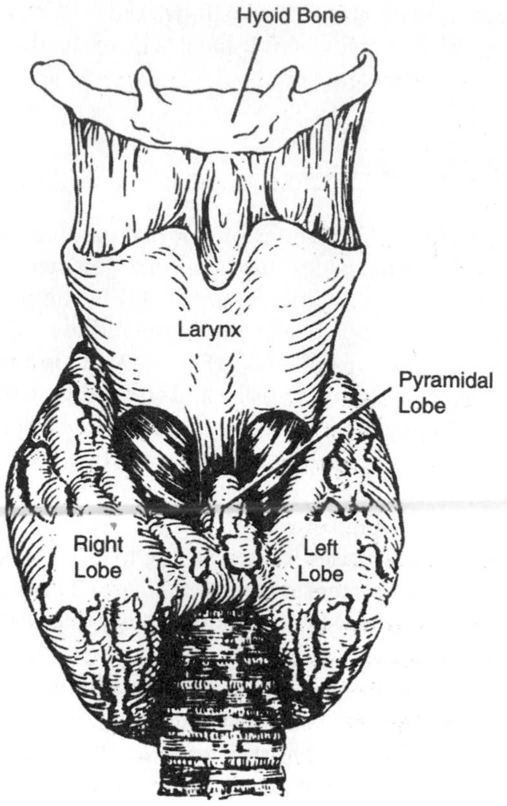

Figure 53-3. The two lobes of the thyroid and their relationship to the larynx and trachea.

levels. Absence of thyroid gland hormones causes minute oxygen consumption to decrease to approximately 40% less than normal, whereas excesses of these hormones can increase minute oxygen consumption as much as 100% more than normal. Thyroid hormones stimulate all aspects of carbohydrate metabolism and facilitate the mobilization of free fatty acids. Despite the latter effect, plasma concentrations of cholesterol usually decrease, reflecting stimulation of low-density lipoprotein receptor synthesis by thyroid hormones.

Anatomically, the thyroid gland consists of two lobes connected by a bridge of tissues known as the *thyroid isthmus* (Fig. 53-3). The gland is highly vascularized and receives innervation from the autonomic nervous system. Structurally, the gland consists of multiple follicles (acini) that are filled with colloid, which consists principally of thyroglobulin. Thyroid hormones are stored in combination with thyroglobulin. Stimulation of proteases by TSH results in cleavage of hormones from thyroglobulin and their release into the systemic circulation.

Mechanism of Action

Thyroid hormones enter cells and T_3 binds to nuclear receptors. T_4 can also bind to these receptors but not as avidly. Indeed, T_4 serves principally as a prohormone for T_3, emphasizing that the biologic effects of T_4 are largely a result of its intracellular conversion to T_3.

It is generally believed that thyroid hormones exert most, if not all, of their effects through control of protein synthesis. This most likely reflects the ability of thyroid hormones to activate the DNA transcription process in the cell nucleus, with resulting formation of new cell proteins, including enzymes. Sympathomimetic effects that accompany thyroid hormone stimulation most likely reflect an increased number and sensitivity of beta-adrenergic receptors in response to release of T_4 and T_3. It has been proposed that thyroid hormones modulate conversion of alpha-adrenergic to beta-adrenergic receptors. Cardiac cholinergic receptor numbers are decreased by thyroid hormones, which is consistent with an increase in heart rate that is out of proportion to the increase in cardiac output.

Increased metabolism produced by thyroid hormones causes vasodilation in tissues to provide the required blood flow to deliver necessary oxygen and carry away metabolites and heat. As a result, cardiac output often increases but systemic blood pressure is unchanged as peripheral vasodilation offsets the impact of increased blood flow. Excess protein catabolism associated with increased secretion of thyroid hormones is the presumed mechanism of skeletal muscle weakness characteristic of hyperthyroidism. The fine muscle tremor that accompanies hyperthyroidism is probably due to increased sensitivity of neuronal synapses in the area of the spinal cord that controls skeletal muscle tone. Diarrhea reflects increased gastrointestinal tract motility that accompanies excess thyroid gland activity.

Calcitonin

Calcitonin, a polypeptide hormone secreted by the thyroid gland, causes a decrease in the plasma concentration of calcium ions. This effect is due to a decrease in the activity of osteoclasts and an increase in osteoblastic activity. Calcitonin is most important in the early moments after ingestion of high-calcium meals. Nevertheless, a total thyroidectomy and subsequent absence of calcitonin does not measurably influence regulation of the plasma concentration of calcium, emphasizing the predominant role of parathyroid hormone.

PARATHYROID GLANDS

The four parathyroid glands secrete an amino and acid polypeptide that constitutes parathyroid hormone. This hormone is responsible for regulating the plasma concentration of calcium ions. Secretion of parathyroid hormone is inversely related to the plasma ionized calcium concentration. Small decreases in the plasma concentration of calcium ions are potent stimulants for the release of parathyroid hormone. Overall, the effect of parathyroid hormone is to increase the plasma concentration of calcium and to decrease the plasma concentration of phosphate by acting on bones, kidneys, and the gastrointestinal tract. The most prominent effect of parathyroid hormone is to promote mobilization of calcium from bones, reflecting stimulation of osteoclastic activity. At the kidneys, parathyroid hormone increases renal tubular reabsorption of calcium ions and inhibits renal reabsorption of phosphate.

Parathyroid hormone is likely to exert its effect on target cells in bones, renal tubules, and the gastrointestinal tract by stimulating the formation of cAMP. Indeed, a portion of cAMP synthesized in the kidneys escapes into the urine, and its assay serves as a measure of parathyroid gland activity. It is likely that parathyroid hormone functions in bones in the same way that it works in the kidneys and gastrointestinal tract by causing the conversion of vitamin D to its active form, 1,25-dihydroxycholecalciferol.

ADRENAL CORTEX

The two major classes of corticosteroids are mineralocorticoids and glucocorticoids. In addition, the adrenal cortex secretes sex steroids. The precursor of all corticosteroids is cholesterol. Mineralocorticoids influence the plasma concentrations of sodium and potassium ions, whereas glucocorticoids influence carbohydrate, fat, and protein metabolism as well as exhibiting antiinflammatory effects. More than 30 different corticosteroids have been isolated from the adrenal cortex, but only two are of major importance: aldosterone, a mineralocorticoid, and cortisol, the principal glucocorticoid (Table 53-7). These corticosteroids are not stored in the adrenal cortex, emphasizing that the rate of synthesis determines the subsequent plasma concentration. Anatomically, the adrenal cortex is divided into three zones designated the (a) *zona glomerulosa* that secretes mineralocorticoids, (b) *zona fasciculata* that secretes glucocorticoids, and (c) *zona reticularis* that secretes androgens and estrogens.

Mineralocorticoids: Aldosterone

Aldosterone accounts for approximately 95% of the mineralocorticoid activity produced by corticosteroids. Desoxycorticosterone is the other naturally occurring mineralocorticoid, but it has only 3% of the sodium ion-retaining potency of aldosterone. Cortisol induces sodium ion retention and potassium ion secretion, but much less effectively than aldosterone.

Physiologic Effects

The principal functions of aldosterone are to sustain extracellular fluid volume by conserving sodium and to maintain a normal plasma concentration of potassium. In this regard, aldosterone causes absorption of sodium ions and simultaneous secretion of potassium ions by the lining of renal tubular epithelial cells of the distal renal tubules and collecting ducts. As a result, aldosterone causes sodium to be conserved in the extracellular fluid, whereas potassium is excreted in the urine. Water follows sodium such that extracellular fluid volume tends to change in proportion to the rate of aldosterone secretion. Indeed, in the presence of excess aldosterone secretion, the extracellular fluid volume, cardiac output, and systemic blood pressure are increased. When the plasma concentration of potassium is decreased approximately 50% due to excess secretion of aldosterone, skeletal muscle weakness or even paralysis occurs, reflecting hyperpolarization of nerve and muscle membranes, which prevents transmission of action potentials.

Aldosterone has effects on sweat glands and salivary glands that are similar to its effects on the renal tubules. For example, aldosterone increases the reabsorption of sodium and secretion of potassium by sweat glands. This effect is important for conserving sodium in hot environments, or when excess salivation occurs. Aldosterone also enhances sodium ion reabsorption by the gastrointestinal tract.

Mechanism of Action

Aldosterone diffuses to the interior of renal tubular epithelial cells, where it induces DNA to form messenger RNA (mRNA) necessary for the transport of sodium and potassium ions. It is speculated that this mRNA is a specific adenosine triphosphatase (ATPase) that catalyzes energy from cytoplasmic ATP to the sodium ion transport mechanism of cell membranes. It takes as long as

TABLE 53-7.
PHYSIOLOGIC EFFECTS OF ENDOGENOUS CORTICOSTEROIDS (mg)

	Daily Secretion	Sodium Retention*	Glucocorticoid Effect*	Antiinflammatory Effect*
Aldosterone	0.125	3,000	0.3	Insignificant
Desoxycorticosterone	—	100	0	0
Cortisol	20	1	1	1
Corticosterone	Minimal	15	0.35	0.3
Cortisone	Minimal	0.8	0.8	0.8

*Relative to cortisol

30 minutes before the new mRNA appears and approximately 45 minutes before the rate of sodium ion transport begins to increase.

Regulation of Secretion

The most important stimulus for aldosterone secretion is an increase in the plasma potassium concentration. For example, an increase in plasma potassium concentration of <1 mEq/liter will triple the rate of aldosterone secretion. This increase establishes a powerful negative-feedback system that maintains the plasma concentration of potassium ions in a normal range. The renin-angiotensin system is also an important determinant of aldosterone secretion (see Chapter 22). The elimination half-time of aldosterone is approximately 20 minutes, with nearly 90% of the hormone being cleared by the liver in a single passage. Mineralocorticoid secretion is not under the primary control of ACTH. For this reason, hypoaldosteronism does not accompany loss of ACTH secretion from the anterior pituitary.

Glucocorticoids: Cortisol

At least 95% of the glucocorticoid activity results from the secretion of cortisol. In addition, a small amount of glucocorticoid activity is provided by corticosterone and an even smaller amount by cortisone. Cortisol is one of the few hormones essential for life.

Physiologic Effects

The most important physiologic effects of cortisol are (a) increased gluconeogenesis, (b) protein catabolism, (c) fatty acid mobilization, and (d) antiinflammatory effects. Cortisol may improve cardiac function by increasing the number or responsiveness of beta-adrenergic receptors. In addition to sustaining cardiac function and maintaining systemic blood pressure, cortisol permits normal responsiveness of arterioles to the constrictive action of catecholamines. Cortisol inhibits bone formation.

Developmental Changes

Plasma concentrations of cortisol increase progressively during the last trimester of pregnancy to reach a peak plasma concentration at term, permitting maturation of a number of systems that are critical for survival with the onset of extrauterine life. These systems include production of pulmonary surfactant, maturation of various enzyme systems in the liver, and the expression of phenylethanolamine *N*-methyltransferase, the enzyme necessary for the synthesis of epinephrine from norepinephrine.

Gluconeogenesis

Cortisol stimulates gluconeogenesis by the liver as much as tenfold, reflecting principally mobilization of amino acids from extrahepatic sites and transfer to the liver for conversion to glucose. This increased rate of gluconeogenesis, in addition to a moderate decrease in the rate of glucose use caused by cortisol, results in increased blood glucose concentrations. The resulting adrenal diabetes is responsive to the administration of insulin.

Protein Catabolism

Cortisol decreases protein stores in nearly all cells except hepatocytes, reflecting mobilization of amino acids for gluconeogenesis. In the presence of sustained excesses of cortisol, skeletal muscle weakness may become profound.

Fatty Acid Mobilization

Cortisol promotes mobilization of fatty acids from adipose tissue and enhances oxidation of fatty acids in cells. Despite these effects, excess amounts of cortisol cause deposition of fat in the neck and chest regions, giving rise to a "buffalo-like" torso. This peculiar distribution of fat reflects deposition of fat at these sites at a rate that exceeds its mobilization.

Antiinflammatory Effects

Cortisol in large amounts has antiinflammatory effects, reflecting its ability to stabilize lysosomal membranes and to decrease migration of leukocytes into the inflamed area. Stabilization of lysosomal membranes decreases the release of inflammation-causing lysosomes. Other antiinflammatory effects of cortisol reflect decreased capillary permeability, which prevents loss of plasma into tissues. Even after inflammation has been well established, the administration of cortisol can decrease its manifestations. This effect of cortisol is important in attenuating inflammation associated with disease states such as rheumatoid arthritis and acute glomerulonephritis.

Cortisol decreases the number of eosinophils and leukocytes in the blood within a few minutes after its administration. In addition, there is atrophy of lymphoid tissue throughout the body, which results in decreased production of antibodies. As a result, the level of immunity against bacterial or viral infection is decreased, and fulminating infection can occur. Conversely, this ability of cortisol to suppress immunity is useful in decreasing the likelihood of immunologic rejection of transplanted tissues.

The beneficial effect of cortisol in the treatment of allergic reactions reflects prevention of inflammatory responses that are responsible for many of the life-threatening effects of an allergic reaction such as laryngeal edema. Cortisol may also interfere with complement pathway activation and formation of chemical mediators derived from arachidonic acid, such as leukotrienes. Cortisol does not, however, alter the antigen–antibody interaction or histamine release associated with allergic reactions.

Mechanism of Action

Cortisol stimulates DNA-dependent synthesis of mRNA in the nuclei of responsive cells, leading to the synthesis of appropriate enzymes.

Regulation of Secretion

The most important stimulus for the secretion of cortisol (13 to 20 mg daily) is the release of ACTH from the anterior pituitary (see Table 53-5). The secretion of ACTH in the anterior pituitary is determined by two hypothalamic neurohormones (diurnal release of corticotropin-releasing hormone and AVP) that act synergistically. Circulating cortisol also exerts a direct negative-feedback effect on the hypothalamus and anterior pituitary to decrease the release of corticotropin-releasing hormone and ACTH from these respective sites. Immediately following release from the adrenal gland, cortisol is bound to the alpha-globulin, transcortin (cortisol-binding globulin). Plasma concentrations of cortisol are higher in females than males with additional increases accompanying the menstrual cycle just before ovulation. Stress as associated with the intraoperative period can override the normal negative-feedback control mechanisms, and plasma concentrations of cortisol are increased. The beneficial effect of an increased plasma concentration of cortisol and other hormones in response to stressful stimuli may be the acute mobilization of cellular proteins and fat stores for energy and synthesis of other compounds, including glucose

Cortisol is secreted and released by the adrenal cortex at a basal rate of approximately 20 mg daily. In response to maximal stressful stimuli (sepsis, burns), the output of cortisol is increased to approximately 150 mg daily (Hume et al., 1962). Therefore, this amount should be sufficient replacement when provided to patients who lack adrenal function and who are acutely ill or undergoing major surgery. The peak plasma cortisol concentration of 8 to 25 μg/dL occurs in the morning shortly after awakening. Stress-induced changes in the plasma concentration of cortisol are superimposed on the circadian tone and vary in onset, magnitude, and duration depending on the intensity of the stress. In the systemic circulation, 80% to 90% of cortisol is bound to a specific globulin known as *transcortin*. It is the relatively small amount of unbound cortisol that exerts a biologic effect. The elimination half-time of cortisol is approximately 70 minutes. Degradation of cortisol occurs mainly in the liver with the formation of inactive 17-hydroxycorticosteroids that appear in the urine. Cortisol is also filtered at the glomerulus and may be excreted unchanged in urine.

Effect of Anesthesia and Surgery

Plasma cortisol concentrations typically increase (two- to tenfold) following the induction of anesthesia, during surgery, and in the postoperative period (Udelsman and Chrousos, 1988). As with other types of stress, the episodic release of cortisol remains intact but the amplitude of these episodic releases is increased. The increase in plasma cortisol concentrations occurring in the postoperative period may in part be due to baroreceptor and spinal reflexes that signal the hypothalamus of tissue injury associated with surgery (Udelsman and Holbrook, 1994). Other factors that activate the hypothalamic-pituitary-adrenal axis to release cortisol include proinflammatory mediators released by damaged tissues and the presence of postoperative pain.

Plasma cortisol concentrations typically return to normal levels within 24 hours postoperatively but may remain elevated for as long as 72 hours depending on the severity of the surgical trauma. In addition, disturbances in the circadian rhythm may be associated with postoperative fatigue and debility. Return of plasma cortisol concentrations to normal following surgery is initially characterized by increased plasma concentrations of ACTH and cortisol (consistent with sustained, stress-induced stimulation of the hypothalamus) followed by a second phase in which plasma ACTH concentrations are low and increased plasma cortisol concentrations presumably are independent of the hypothalamic-pituitary system. It is possible that cytokines released from traumatized tissue stimulate synthesis of cortisol directly despite low plasma concentrations of ACTH. Alternatively, prior increases in plasma ACTH concentrations may stimulate production of ACTH receptors in the adrenal glands resulting in increased cortisol production.

Plasma cortisol concentrations in the perioperative period reflect a response designed to provide protection during and after surgery. Supportive animal evidence is the observation that adrenalectomized animals receiving sub-physiologic doses of cortisol experienced hemodynamic instability and increased mortality following surgery, whereas those animals treated with physiologic or supra-physiologic doses of cortisol were indistinguishable from control animals (Udelsman et al., 1987).

In addition to surgical trauma, the choice of anesthetic drugs and techniques may influence the hypothalamic-pituitary-adrenal response. For example, large doses of opioids may attenuate the cortisol response to surgical stimulation (Bovill et al., 1983; Sebel et al., 1981). Volatile anesthetics provide less suppression to this stress-induced endocrine response. Etomidate is unique among drugs administered to induce anesthesia with respect to its ability to inhibit cortisol synthesis even in the absence of surgical stimulation (see Chapter 6). The effect of regional anesthesia on cortisol response to surgical trauma is consistent with the concept that neural mechanisms that link the operative site with the spinal cord are essential for the stress-induced release of cortisol. This mechanism is also consistent with the view that proinflammatory mediators (cytokines) released from damaged tissue activate the hypothalamic-pituitary-adrenal axis. The marked increase in plasma cortisol concentrations in the postoperative period often parallels the waning effects of regional anesthesia.

Suppression of the hypothalamic-pituitary axis as produced by chronic administration of corticosteroids also prevents the release of cortisol in response to stressful stimuli.

REPRODUCTIVE GLANDS

In both sexes, the reproductive glands (testes and ovaries) are responsible for production of germ cells and steroid sex hormones.

Testes

The testes secrete male sex hormones, which are collectively designated *androgens*. All androgens are steroid compounds that can be synthesized from cholesterol. Testosterone is the most potent and abundant of the androgens, being responsible for the development and maintenance of male sex characteristics. Skeletal muscle growth is an anabolic effect of testosterone in the male. Testosterone is produced in the testes only when stimulation occurs from LH, and FSH is necessary for spermatogenesis. Puberty occurs when the production of testosterone increases rapidly in response to hypothalamic-releasing hormones that evoke the release of LH and FSH. Hypertrophy of the laryngeal mucosa accompanies secretion of testosterone, leading to the characteristic changes in voice at puberty. Testosterone increases secretion of sebaceous glands, leading to acne. Beard growth is the last manifestation of puberty. Testosterone production continues throughout life, although the amount produced decreases beyond the age of 40 years to become approximately one-fifth the peak value at 80 years of age.

At most sites of action, testosterone is not the active form of the hormone being converted in target tissues to the more active dihydrotestosterone by a reductase enzyme. Dihydrotestosterone binds to a cytoplasmic protein receptor that results in increased synthesis of specific mRNA protein. In the absence of sufficient reductase enzyme, external genitalia fail to develop (pseudohermaphroditism) despite secretion of adequate amounts of testosterone. Not all target tissues, however, require the conversion of testosterone to dihydrotestosterone for activity. For example, effects of testosterone on skeletal muscles and bone marrow are mediated by the hormone or a metabolite other than dihydrotestosterone.

The adrenal cortex also secretes androgens, but the effects of these hormones are usually inconsequential unless a hormone-secreting tumor develops. For example, in males, approximately 10% of androgens are produced in the adrenal cortex. This is an insufficient amount to maintain spermatogenesis or secondary sexual features in an adult male. In abnormal conditions, such as the adrenogenital syndrome, the adrenal cortex can secrete large quantities of steroids and androgenic precursors.

Ovaries

The two ovarian hormones, estrogen and progesterone, are secreted in response to LH and FSH, which are released from the anterior pituitary in response to hypothalamic-releasing hormones. In postpubertal females, an orderly secretion of LH and FSH is necessary for the occurrence of menstruation, pregnancy, and lactation. The Stein-Leventhal syndrome is characterized by virilization resulting from excessive ovarian secretion of androgens.

Estrogens

Estrogens are responsible for the development of female sexual characteristics. In the nonpregnant female, most of the estrogen comes from the ovaries, although small amounts are also secreted by the adrenal cortex. The three most important estrogens are beta-estradiol, estrone, and estriol. These estrogens are conjugated in the liver to inactive metabolites that appear in urine.

Progesterone

Progesterone is necessary for preparation of the uterus for pregnancy and the breasts for lactation. Almost all of the progesterone in the nonpregnant female is secreted by the corpus luteum during the lateral phase of the menstrual cycle. The adrenal cortex forms small amounts of progesterone. Progesterone is metabolized to pregnanediol, which appears in the urine, providing a valuable index of the secretion and metabolism of this hormone.

Menstruation

The overall duration of a normal menstrual cycle is 21 to 35 days and consists of three phases designated as follicular, ovulatory, and luteal. The follicular phase begins with the onset of menstrual bleeding, reflecting a decrease in the plasma concentration of progesterone. After a variable length of time, the follicular phase is followed by the ovulatory phase lasting 1 to 3 days and culminating in ovulation. The increase in body temperature (approximately 0.5°C) that accompanies ovulation most likely reflects a thermogenic effect of progesterone. The luteal phase follows ovulation and is characterized by the development of a corpus luteum that secretes progesterone and estrogen. The corpus luteum degenerates after a fairly constant period of 13 to 14 days and the menstrual cycle repeats.

Pregnancy

During pregnancy, the placenta forms large amounts of estrogens, progesterone, chorionic gonadotropin, and chorionic somatomammotropin. Chorionic gonadotropin prevents the usual involution of the corpus luteum, which would lead to the onset of menstrual bleeding. This placental hormone is the first key hormone of pregnancy and can be detected in the maternal plasma within 9 days after conception, thus providing the basis for pregnancy tests.

After approximately 12 weeks, the placenta secretes sufficient amounts of progesterone and estrogens to maintain pregnancy and the corpus luteum involutes. Chorionic somatomammotropin has important metabolic effects, including decreased insulin activity, making more glucose available to the fetus.

Increased circulating concentrations of estrogen cause enlargement of the breasts and uterus, whereas progesterone is necessary for development of decidual cells in the uterine endometrium and for suppression of uterine contractions that could result in spontaneous abortion. Increased plasma concentrations of progesterone and associated sedative effects during pregnancy may be the explanation for decreases in anesthetic requirements (MAC) for volatile anesthetics in gravid animals. Nevertheless, anesthetic requirements in animals return to nonpregnant values within 5 days postpartum, whereas the plasma concentration of progesterone remains increased, suggesting that the decrease in MAC cannot be attributed entirely to progesterone (Strout and Nahrwold, 1981). Increased plasma concentrations of progesterone are presumed to be the stimulus for increased alveolar ventilation that accompanies pregnancy. Near term, the ovaries secrete a hormone designated as relaxin, which relaxes pelvic ligaments so the sacroiliac joints become limber and the symphysis pubis becomes elastic.

The parturient with asthma may experience unpredictable changes in airway reactivity. Exacerbation of asthma may reflect bronchoconstriction evoked by prostaglandins of the F series, which are present in all trimesters of pregnancy but especially during labor (see Chapter 20). Conversely, prostaglandins of the E series are bronchodilators and predominate during the third trimester. A role of corticosteroids in altered airway responsiveness is questionable, because increased plasma concentrations of cortisol associated with pregnancy are offset by concomitant increases in the carrier protein transcortin, with the net effect being an unchanged level of available cortisol.

Menopause

The ovaries gradually become unresponsive to the stimulatory effects of LH and FSH, resulting in the disappearance of sexual cycles between the ages of 45 and 55 years. Because the negative-feedback control of estrogen and progesterone on the anterior pituitary is decreased, there is increased output of LH and FSH, manifesting as increased circulating plasma concentrations of these gonadotropins. Sensations of warmth spreading from the trunk to the face (hot flashes) coincide with surges of LH secretion and are prevented by exogenous administration of estrogens.

PANCREAS

The pancreas secretes digestive substances into the duodenum as well as four hormones (insulin, glucagon, somatostatin, pancreatin peptide) that are secreted by the islets of Langerhans and released into the systemic circulation. Somatostatin regulates islet cell secretion, acting as a profound inhibitor of both insulin and glucagon release. This peptide hormone is the same as growth hormone-releasing inhibitory hormone that is secreted by the hypothalamus. The role of pancreatic peptide hormone is not known.

The pancreas contains 1 to 2 million islets, which, based on staining characteristics and morphology, are classified as alpha, beta, and delta cells. Beta cells account for about 60% of the islet cells and are the site of insulin production as a part of a larger preprohormone. Alpha cells account for 25% of the islet cells and are the site of glucagon production. Each islet receives a generous blood supply, which, like the gastrointestinal tract but unlike any other endocrine organ, drains into the portal vein.

Insulin

Insulin is an anabolic hormone promoting the storage of glucose, fatty acids, and amino acids (Fig. 53-4) (Berne et al., 2004). The amount of insulin secreted daily is equivalent to approximately 40 units. In the systemic circulation, insulin has an elimination half-time of approximately 5 minutes, with >80% degraded in the liver and kidneys. Insulin binds to receptor proteins in cell membranes, leading to activation of the glucose transport system (Fig. 53-5) (Ganong, 2003). Activation of sodium-potassium ATPase in cell membranes by insulin results in movement of potassium ions into cells and a decrease in the plasma concentration of potassium.

Regulation of Secretion

The principal control of insulin secretion is via a negative-feedback effect of the blood glucose concentration of the pancreas (Table 53-8). Virtually no insulin is secreted by the pancreas when the blood glucose concentrations are <50 mg/dL, and maximum stimulation for release of insulin occurs when blood glucose concentrations are >300 mg/dL. This feedback system provides prompt responses that maintain blood glucose concentrations within a narrow range. The pancreas is richly innervated by the autonomic nervous system, with insulin release occurring in response to beta-adrenergic stimulation or release of acetylcholine. Conversely, alpha-adrenergic stimulation or beta-adrenergic blockade results in inhibition of insulin release. Oral glucose is more effective than glucose administered intravenously in evoking the release of insulin, suggesting the presence of an anticipatory signal from the gastrointestinal tract to the pancreas. Consistent with this is the more likely occurrence of glycosuria after intravenous rather than oral glucose administration. This observation has obvious implications for the intravenous infusion of fluids containing glucose during the perioperative period. Glucagon, HGH, and corticosteroids can potentiate glucose-induced stimulation of insulin secretion. Prolonged

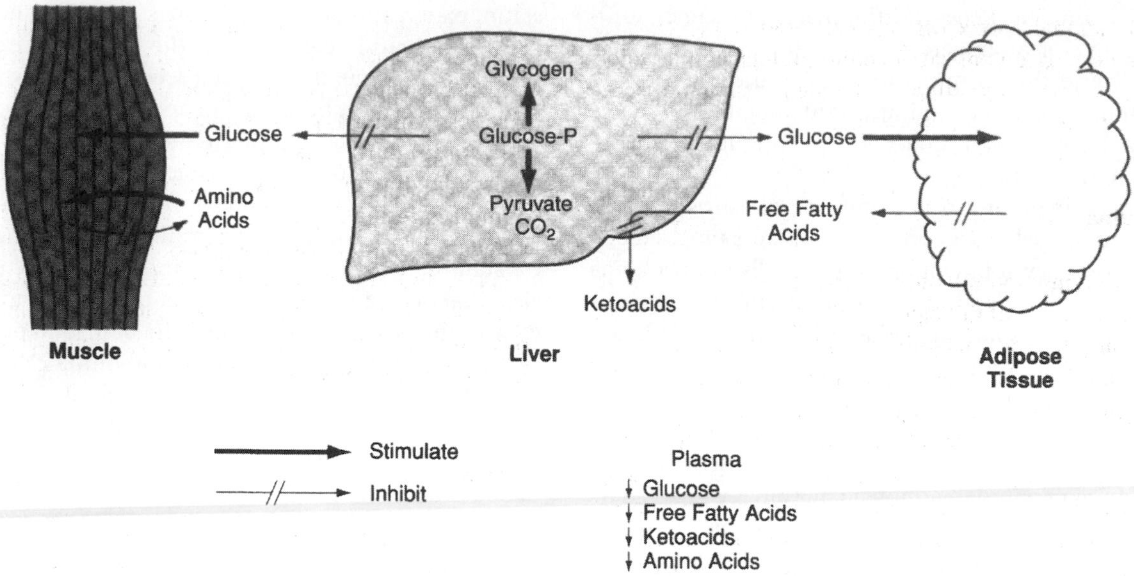

Figure 53-4. Insulin stimulates tissue uptake of glucose and amino acids, whereas release of fatty acids is inhibited. As a result, the plasma concentrations of glucose, free fatty acids, amino acids, and ketoacids decrease. (From Berne RM, Levy MN, Koeppen BM, et al. *Physiology*, 5th ed. St. Louis: Mosby, 2004; with permission.)

secretion of these hormones or their exogenous administration can lead to the exhaustion of pancreatic beta cells and the development of diabetes mellitus. Indeed, diabetes mellitus often occurs in patients who develop acromegaly or in those persons with a diabetic tendency who are treated with corticosteroids.

Physiologic Effects

Insulin promotes the use of carbohydrates for energy while depressing the use of fats and amino acids. For example, insulin facilitates storage of fat in adipose cells by inhibiting lipase enzyme, which normally causes hydrolysis of triglycerides in fat cells. In the liver, insulin inhibits enzymes necessary for gluconeogenesis, thus conserving amino acid stores.

Insulin facilitates glucose uptake and storage in the liver by its effects on specific enzymes. Enhanced uptake of glucose into liver cells reflects insulin-induced increases in the activity of glucokinase. Glucokinase is the enzyme that causes initial phosphorylation of glucose after it diffuses into hepatocytes. Once phosphorylated, glucose is trapped and unable to diffuse back through cell membranes. Storage is further enhanced by insulin-induced inhibition of phosphorylase enzyme, which normally causes liver glycogen to split into glucose. The net effects of these actions of insulin on enzymes is to increase hepatic stores of glycogen up to a maximum of approximately 100 g. Ordinarily, approximately 60% of the glucose in a meal is stored in the liver as glycogen.

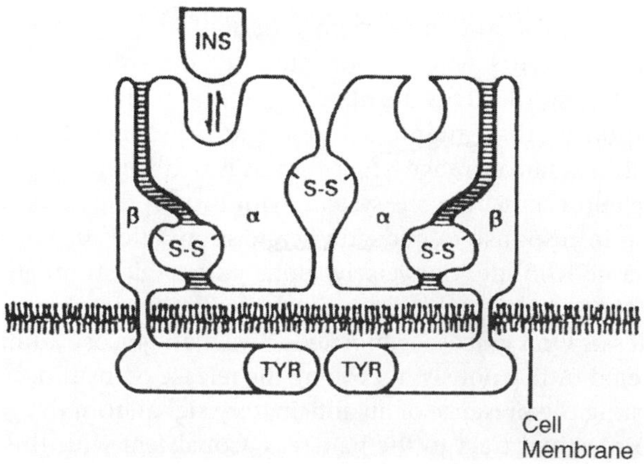

Figure 53-5. Schematic depiction of the insulin receptor consisting of two alpha and two beta subunits joined by disulfide bonds (-S-S-). Insulin (INS) attaches to the alpha subunits, which triggers autophosphorylation of the tyrosine kinase (TYR) portions of the beta subunits inside the cell and the resultant effects of insulin. (From Ganong WF. *Review of medical physiology*, 21st ed. New York, Lange Medical Books/McGraw Hill, 2003; with permission.)

TABLE 53-8.
REGULATION OF INSULIN SECRETION

Stimulation	Inhibition
Hyperglycemia	Hypoglycemia
Beta-adrenergic agonists	Beta-adrenergic antagonists
Acetylcholine	Alpha-adrenergic agonists
Glucagon	Somatostatin
	Diazoxide
	Thiazide diuretics
	Volatile anesthetics
	Insulin

Resting skeletal muscles are almost impermeable to glucose except in the presence of insulin. Glucose that enters resting skeletal muscles under the influence of insulin is stored as glycogen for subsequent use as energy. The amount of glycogen that can be stored in skeletal muscles, however, is much less than the amount that can be stored in the liver. Furthermore, glycogen in skeletal muscles, in contrast to that stored in the liver, cannot be reconverted to glucose and released into the systemic circulation. This occurs because skeletal muscles lack glucose phosphatase enzyme, which is necessary for splitting glycogen. Exercise increases the permeability of skeletal muscle membranes to glucose, perhaps reflecting the release of insulin from within the skeletal muscle itself or its vasculature.

Brain cells are unique in that the permeability of their membranes to glucose does not depend on the presence of insulin. This characteristic is crucial because brain cells use only glucose for energy, and it emphasizes the importance of maintaining blood glucose concentrations above a critical level of approximately 50 mg/dL. Indeed, lack of insulin causes the use mainly of fat to the exclusion of glucose except by brain cells.

Diabetes Mellitus

Diabetes mellitus is a metabolic disease characterized by hyperglycemia that results from defects in insulin secretion and/or action of insulin. Abnormalties of fat and protein metabolism are also present but the diagnosis of diabetes mellitus is based on the presence of hyperglycemia. The presence of chronic hyperglycemia is associated wth long-term damage and dysfunction of the kidneys, eyes, autonomic nervous system, heart, vessles, and microcirculation. The vast majority of cases of diabetes are either type 1 (insulin-dependent) or type 2 (noninsulin dependent) in an approximate ratio of 1 to 9 (Table 53-9). Even in the absence of overt diabetes, patients with latent disease release less insulin in response to glucose stimulation.

TABLE 53-9.
ETIOLOGIC CLASSIFICATION OF DIABETES MELLITUS

Type 1 diabetes mellitus (absolute insulin deficiency owing to pancreatic beta cell destruction)
Type 2 diabetes mellitus (insulin resistance vs. insulin deficiency)
Endocrinopathies (acromegaly, Cushing syndrome)
Drug-induced (glucocorticoids, thiazides)
Gestational diabetes mellitus
Genetic defects in pancreatic beta cell function
Genetic defects in insulin action (resistance)

In the absence of sufficient insulin, there is a marked decrease in the rate of transport of glucose across certain cells membranes, resulting in hyperglycemia. The formation of glucose from protein accounts for the observation that glucose lost in urine may exceed oral intake. Much of the protein used for glucose formation comes from skeletal muscles; glucose loss may manifest in extreme cases as skeletal muscle wasting. Increased free fatty acid concentrations in the plasma of diabetic patients reflects loss of insulin-induced inhibition of the lipase enzyme system such that mobilization of fatty acids proceeds unopposed. The insulin-deficient liver is likely to use fatty acids to produce ketones, which can serve as an energy source for skeletal muscles and cardiac muscle. Production of ketones can lead to ketoacidosis, whereas urinary excretion of these anions contributes to the depletion of electrolytes, especially potassium. Hypokalemia, however, may not be apparent, because intracellular potassium ions are exchanged for extracellular ions to compensate for the acidosis.

Low plasma concentrations of insulin, although inadequate to prevent hyperglycemia, may be quite effective in blocking lipolysis. This differential effect of insulin explains the frequent observation in patients with diabetes

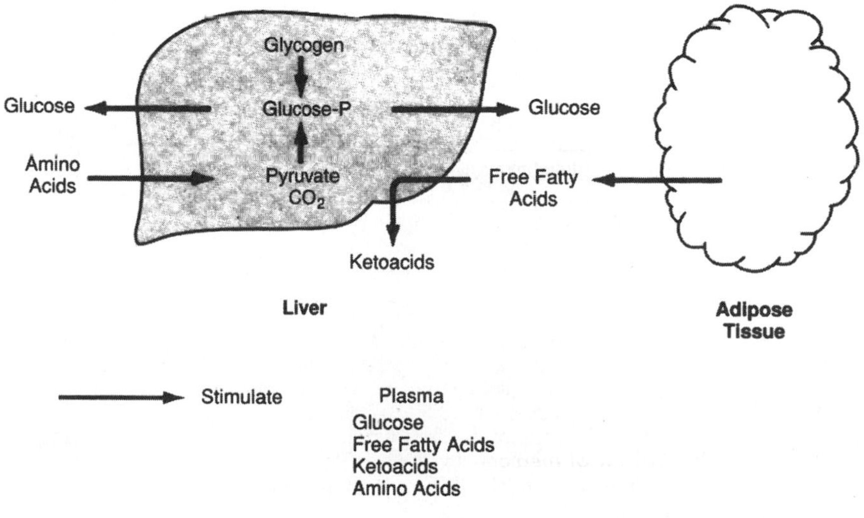

Figure 53-6. Glucagon stimulates tissue release of glucose, free fatty acids, and ketoacids and hepatic uptake of amino acids. (From Berne RM, Levy MN, Koeppen BM, et al. *Physiology*, 5th ed. St. Louis: Mosby, 2004; with permission.)

TABLE 53-10.
REGULATION OF GLUCAGON SECRETION

Stimulation	Inhibition
Hypoglycemia	Hyperglycemia
Stress	Somatostatin
Sepsis	Insulin
Trauma	Free fatty acids
Beta-adrenergic agonists	Alpha-adrenergic agonists
Acetylcholine	
Cortisol	

mellitus that hyperglycemia can exist without the presence of ketone bodies. Ketosis can be reliably prevented by continuously providing all diabetic patients with glucose and insulin (Hirsch et al., 1991). This is uniquely important in the perioperative period when nutritional intake is altered.

Glucagon

Glucagon is a catabolic hormone acting to mobilize glucose, fatty acids, and amino acids into the systemic circulation (Fig. 53-6) (Berne et al., 2004). These responses are the reciprocal of the insulin effects, emphasizing that these two hormones are also reciprocally secreted (Table 53-10). Indeed, the principal stimulus for secretion of glucagon is hypoglycemia. Glucagon is able to abruptly increase the blood glucose concentration by stimulating glycogenolysis in the liver. This reflects activation of adenylate cyclase by glucagon and the subsequent formation of cAMP. In this regard, the metabolic effects of glucagon at the liver mimic those produced by epinephrine. Indeed, the study of the mechanism by which glucagon and epinephrine acted as hyperglycemics led to the discovery of cAMP (Rall and Sutherland, 1958). Glucagon also causes hyperglycemia by stimulating gluconeogenesis in hepatocytes. Other effects of glucagon such as enhanced myocardial contractility and increased secretion of bile probably occur only when exogenous administration increases plasma concentrations of this hormone far above those levels that occur normally (see Chapter 13). Amino acids enhance the release of glucagon and thus prevent hypoglycemia that would occur from ingestion of a pure protein meal and associated stimulation of insulin secretion. Glucagon undergoes enzymatic degradation to inactive metabolites in the liver and kidneys and at receptor sites in cell membranes. The elimination half-time of glucagon is brief—only 3 to 6 minutes.

REFERENCES

Babad AA, Eger EI II. The effects of hyperthyroidism and hypothyroidism on halothane and oxygen requirements in dogs. *Anesthesiology* 1968;29:1087–1093.

Bennett-Guerrero E, Kramer DC, Schwinn DA. Effect of chronic and acute thyroid hormone reduction on perioperative outcome. *Anesth Analg* 1997;85:30–36.

Berne RM, Levy MN, Koeppen BM, et al. *Physiology*, 5th ed. St. Louis: Mosby, 2004.

Bovill JG, Sebel PS, Fiolet JW, et al. The influence of sufentanil on endocrine and metabolic responses to cardiac surgery. *Anesth Analg* 1983;62:391–397.

Ganong WF. *Review of medical physiology*, 21st ed. New York, Lange Medical Books/McGraw Hill, 2003.

Hirsch IB, McGill JB, Cryer PE, et al. Perioperative management of surgical patients with diabetes mellitus. *Anesthesiology* 1991;74:346–359.

Hume DM, Bell CC, Bartter FC. Direct measurement of adrenal secretion during operative trauma and convalescence. *Surgery* 1962;52: 174–187.

Rall TW, Sutherland EW. Formation of a cyclic adenine ribonucleotide by tissue particles. *J Biol Chem* 1958;232:1065–1076.

Sebel PS, Bovill JG, Schellekens APM, et al. Hormonal responses to high-dose fentanyl anesthesia. *Br J Anaesth* 1981;53:941–948.

Stoelting RK. Perioperative management of the patient receiving glucocorticoids. *Curr Opin Anesth* 1997;10:227–228.

Strout CD, Nahrwold ML. Halothane requirement during pregnancy and lactation in rats. *Anesthesiology* 1981;55:322–323.

Taylor AL, Fishman LM. Corticotropin-releasing hormone. *N Engl J Med* 1988;319:213–221.

Udelsman R, Chrousos GP. Hormonal responses to stress. *Adv Exp Med Biol* 1988;245:265–271.

Udelsman R, Goldstein DS, Loariaus DL, et al. Catecholamine-glucocorticoid interactions during surgical stress. *J Surg Res* 1987;43: 539–545.

Udelsmann R, Holbrook NJ. Endocrine and molecular responses to surgical stress. *Curr Prob Surg* 1994;31:653–658.

Kidneys

54

The principal function of the kidneys is to stabilize the composition of the extracellular fluid as reflected by electrolyte and hydrogen ion concentrations. End-products of protein metabolism such as urea are excreted, whereas essential body nutrients including amino acids and glucose are retained. The kidneys also secrete hormones for the regulation of systemic blood pressure (angiotensin II, prostaglandins, kinins) and the production of erythrocytes (erythropoietin). Anatomically, the kidneys are paired organs weighing 115 to 160 g each and located retroperitoneally just beneath the diaphragm. Each kidney consists of a cortical (outer) and medullary (inner) portion, with the mid-portion of each kidney corresponding to approximately the level of L2. The kidneys receive an estimated 20% of the cardiac output.

NEPHRON

The functional unit of the kidney is the nephron, which is composed of capillaries known as the *glomerulus* and a long tubule in which the fluid filtered through the glomerular capillaries is converted to urine on its way to the renal pelvis (Fig. 54-1) (Pitts, 1974). Each kidney contains approximately 1.2 million nephrons; this number does not change after birth.

Glomerulus

The glomerulus is formed only in the renal cortex by a tuft of capillaries that invaginate into the dilated blind end of the renal tubule known as *Bowman's capsule*. Capillaries that form the glomerulus are unique anatomically in being interposed between two sets of arterioles. Blood enters the glomerular capillaries through afferent arterioles and leaves through efferent arterioles. Pressure in glomerular capillaries can be altered by changing the vascular activity of either the afferent or the efferent arterioles. The pressure in glomerular capillaries causes water and low-molecular-weight substances to filter into Bowman's capsule, which is in direct continuity with the proximal renal tubule.

Renal Tubule

Components of the renal tubule are the proximal convoluted tubule, the loop of Henle, and the distal convoluted tubule. From the proximal renal tubule, glomerular filtrate passes into the loop of Henle. Those loops of Henle that extend into the renal medulla are termed *juxtamedullary nephrons*; those that lie close to the surface of the kidneys are designated as *cortical nephrons* (see Fig. 54-1) (Pitts, 1974). From the loop of Henle, fluid flows back into the renal cortex by way of the distal renal tubule. Finally, the glomerular filtrate enters the collecting duct, which delivers fluid from several nephrons into the renal pelvis.

As the glomerular filtrate travels along the renal tubule, most of its water and varying amounts of solutes are reabsorbed from the renal tubular lumen into peritubular capillaries (Table 54-1) (Ganong, 2003). In addition, small amounts of other solutes are secreted by renal tubular epithelial cells into the lumens of the renal tubules. Unwanted metabolic waste products are filtered through glomerular capillaries but, unlike water and electrolytes, are not reabsorbed as the glomerular filtrate progresses through the renal tubules (see Table 54-1) (Ganong, 2003).

Ultimately, the urine that is formed is composed mainly of substances filtered through the glomerular capillaries in addition to small amounts of substances secreted by the renal tubular epithelial cells into the lumens of the renal tubules.

RENAL BLOOD FLOW

The kidneys have an enormous blood supply, receiving 20% to 25% of the cardiac output despite representing only about 0.5% of the total body weight (Lote et al., 1996). The renal blood flow is about 400 mL/100 g/minute compared with 70 mL/100 g/minute for the heart and liver. The kidneys also have very high oxygen consumption, but because of the high renal blood flow, the arteriovenous difference across the kidneys is small. For example, the Po_2 decreases from about 95 mm Hg in the renal artery to about 70 mm Hg in the renal venous blood. Despite this high oxygen delivery via renal blood flow, renal ischemia and acute

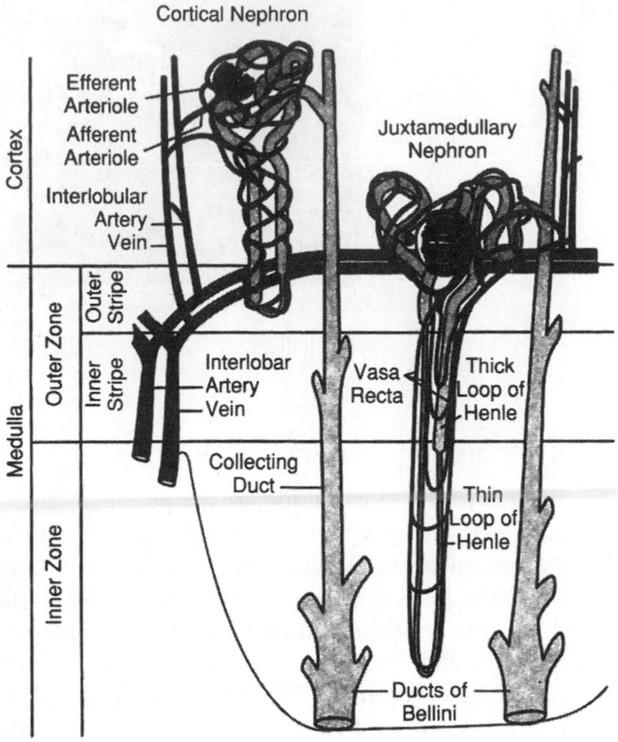

Figure 54-1. Schematic depiction of the nephron and accompanying blood supply. (From Pitts RF. *Physiology of the kidney and body fluids*, 3rd ed. Chicago: Year Book, 1974; with permission.)

renal failure are prominent clinical problems, especially in severely injured patients and elderly patients undergoing major vascular surgery (Lote et al., 1996).

Although the kidneys receive a disproportionate share of the cardiac output, there is a marked discrepancy between blood flow to the renal cortex compared with the renal medulla. Normally, renal blood flow is approximately 90% to 95% delivered to the renal cortex, with the remainder to the renal medulla. The Po_2 in the renal cortex is about 50 mm Hg compared with about 10 mm Hg in the renal medulla. The apparent overabundance of renal blood flow to the renal cortex is designed to maximize flow-dependent functions such as glomerular filtration and tubular reabsorption. In the renal medulla, the blood flow and oxygen consumption are restricted by a renal tubular vascular anatomy that is specifically designed for concentration of urine (*countercurrent circulation*) (Brezis et al., 1987).

Influence of Anesthesia and Surgery

All anesthetic drugs, whether inhaled or injected, have the potential to alter renal function by changing systemic blood pressure and cardiac output such that renal blood flow is redistributed away from the outer renal cortex. There is evidence, however, that epidural anesthesia (T6 sensory level) administered to healthy volunteers with normal renal function does not significantly decrease renal blood flow (Suleiman et al., 1997). Nevertheless, redistribution of blood flow from the renal cortex to the inner renal medulla as may occur during anesthesia and surgery is accompanied by sodium and water conservation manifesting as decreased urine output. Anesthetic-induced decreases in cardiac output are accompanied by release of arginine vasopressin (AVP) (previously known as antidiuretic hormone) and by increased activity of the sympathetic nervous system and renin-angiotensin-aldosterone system. Renal blood flow is decreased by hypovolemia and sympathetic nervous system stimulation associated with surgical stimulation that increases renal vascular resistance (kidneys are richly innervated by the sympathetic nervous system) and shunts blood to nonrenal sites. In this regard, renal ischemia may be prominent despite the absence of systemic hypotension, emphasizing that systemic blood pressure may not be a good guide to the adequacy of renal perfusion. Furthermore, intraoperative urine output does not correlate with postoperative changes in renal function as reflected by plasma creatinine concentrations (Fig. 54-2) (Alpert et al., 1984).

TABLE 54-1.
MAGNITUDE AND SITE OF SOLUTE REABSORPTION OR SECRETION IN THE RENAL TUBULES

	Filtered (24 hrs)	Reabsorbed (24 hrs)	Secreted (24 hrs)	Excreted (24 hrs)	Percent Reabsorbed	Location
Water (liters)	180	179		1	99.4	P,L,D,C
Sodium (mEq)	26,000	25,850		150	99.4	P,L,D,C
Potassium (mEq)	600	560	50	90	93.3	P,L,D,C
Chloride (mEq)	18,000	17,850		150	99.2	P,L,D,C
Bicarbonate (mEq)	4,900	4,900		0	10	P,D
Urea (mM)	870	460		410	53	P,L,D,C
Uric acid (mM)	50	49	4	5	98	P
Glucose (mM)	800	800		0	100	P

C, convoluted tubule; D, distal tubule; L, loop of Henle; P, proximal tubule.

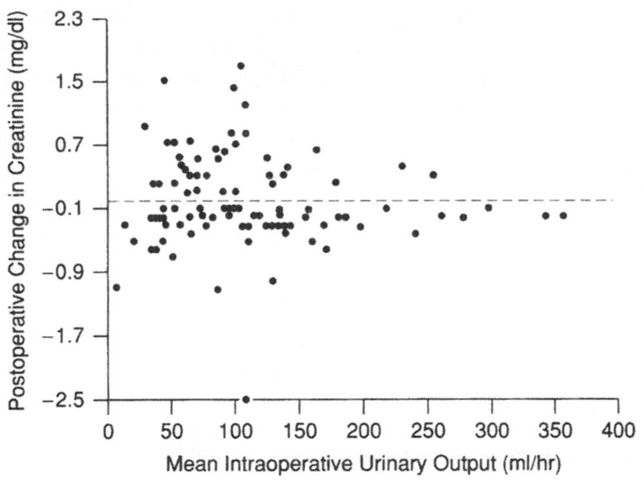

Figure 54-2. Mean intraoperative urine output does not correlate with postoperative changes in the plasma concentrations of creatinine. (From Alpert RA, Roizen MF, Hamilton WK, et al. Intraoperative urinary output does not predict postoperative renal function in patients undergoing abdominal aortic revascularization. *Surgery* 1984;95:707–711; with permission.)

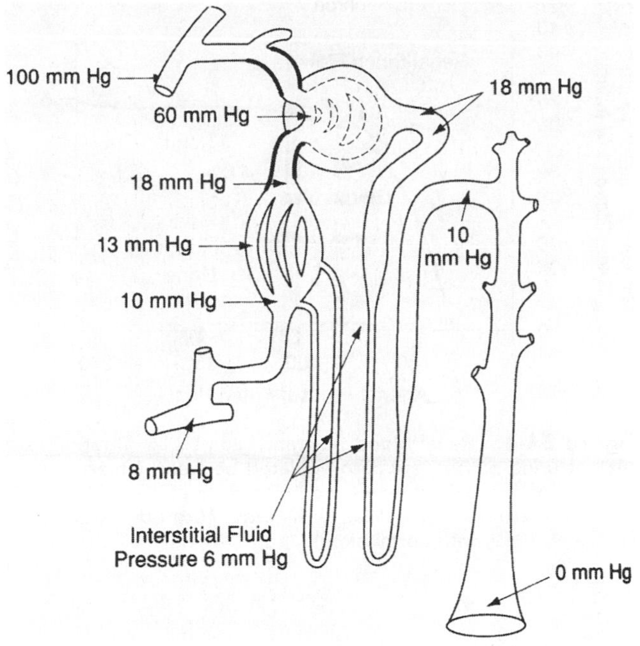

Figure 54-3. Intravascular pressures in the renal circulation. (From Guyton AC, Hall JE. *Textbook of medical physiology*, 10th ed. Philadelphia: Saunders, 2000; with permission.)

Prostaglandins

Prostaglandins have renal tubular and renal vascular actions that are important in the renal response to ischemia. In this regard, nonsteroidal antiinflammatory drugs that inhibit cyclooxygenase have little or no effect on renal blood flow or glomerular filtration rate in healthy subjects but cause marked decreases in these parameters when the renal circulation is compromised as by hemorrhage (see Chapter 20). This emphasizes that vasodilator prostaglandins are important in maintaining renal blood flow and glomerular filtration rate in these circumstances. In addition to these vasodilator actions, prostaglandin E_2 decreases sodium ion reabsorption in the renal tubules, which decreases oxygen consumption.

Glomerular Capillaries

Blood enters the renal artery, which divides and ramifies, eventually providing the afferent arteriole of the glomerulus. This afferent arteriole is separated from the efferent arteriole by the glomerular capillaries (see Fig. 54-1) (Pitts, 1974). The efferent arteriole offers significant resistance to blood flow, causing the glomerular capillaries to be a high-pressure system (Fig. 54-3) (Guyton and Hall, 2000). High pressure in the glomerular capillaries causes them to function in the same manner as arterial ends of tissue capillaries, with fluid moving continuously out of the glomerular capillaries into Bowman's capsule.

Peritubular Capillaries (Renal Cortex Blood Flow)

In the renal cortex, blood flows from the efferent arteriole into a second capillary network known as *peritubular capillaries*. These efferent arterioles, by virtue of linking two sets of capillaries (glomerular capillaries to the peritubular capillaries), are viewed as portal arterioles. In contrast to the high-pressure glomerular capillaries, the peritubular capillaries are a low-pressure system, which allows these capillaries to function in much the same way as the venous ends of tissue capillaries (see Fig. 54-2) (Guyton and Hall, 2000). As a result, fluid from the renal tubules is absorbed continually into the low-pressure peritubular capillaries. Indeed, of the 180 liters of fluid filtered daily through the glomerular capillaries, all but approximately 1.5 liter is reabsorbed from the renal tubules back into the peritubular capillaries, which eventually empty into the inferior vena cava.

Vasa Recta (Renal Medulla Blood Flow)

The function of the renal medulla is to maintain a high osmolarity (produced by solute transport out of the ascending limb of the loop of Henle) to allow the tubular fluid to be concentrated by the osmotic absorption of water from the collecting ducts. This function depends on a unique blood supply reflected by the countercurrent arrangement of a specialized portion of the peritubular capillaries known as the *vasa recta*. This specialized vascular arrangement minimizes washout of solutes from the medullary interstitium, which is critical to the formation of concentrated urine.

The vasa recta capillaries descend with the thin loops of Henle into the renal medulla before returning to the renal cortex to empty into the veins. Only 1% to 2% of renal

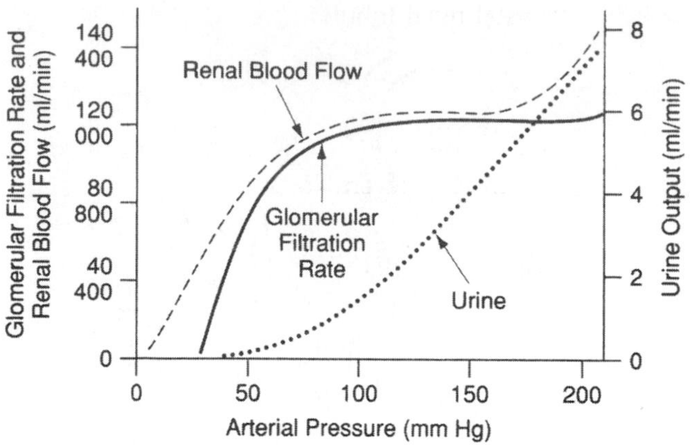

Figure 54-4. Renal blood flow and glomerular filtration rate, but not urine output, are autoregulated between a mean arterial pressure of approximately 60 and 160 mm Hg. (From Guyton AC, Hall JE. *Textbook of medical physiology*, 10th ed. Philadelphia: Saunders, 2000; with permission.)

blood flow passes through the vasa recta, emphasizing that blood flow through the medulla of the kidneys is sluggish compared with the rapid blood flow that occurs in the renal cortex. For the vasa recta countercurrent exchange to function properly, it is important that the hematocrit of the entering blood be low (about 10%). If this were not the case, the osmotic removal of water from the descending vasa recta would dramatically increase blood viscosity.

Autoregulation of Renal Blood Flow

Changes in mean arterial pressure between approximately 60 and 160 mm Hg simultaneously autoregulate both renal blood flow and glomerular filtration rate (Fig. 54-4) (Guyton and Hall, 2000). The mechanism for autoregulation is controversial (Steinhausen et al., 1990). One explanation is a myogenic response, whereby the increased wall tension in the afferent arterioles, due to an increase in perfusion pressure, causes automatic contraction of the smooth muscle fibers in the vessel wall, thereby increasing resistance to flow, and keeping flow constant despite the increase in perfusion pressure (Lote et al., 1996). An alternative hypothesis is that a tubuloglomerular feedback mechanism is responsible for autoregulation, whereby increased perfusion pressure will increase filtration, increasing the tubular fluid delivery to the macula densa, which then releases a factor or factors that cause vasoconstriction.

The concept of autoregulation can be very misleading (Lote et al., 1996). For example, when effective circulating volume decreases, there is a decrease in renal blood flow regardless of the perfusion pressure and the presence of autoregulation. This reflects sympathetic nervous system vasoconstriction and shunting of cardiac output and renal blood flow to extrarenal sites. As such, there may be underperfusion of the kidneys, even though mean arterial pressure is in the range for autoregulation of renal blood flow. Thus, systemic blood pressure may not be a good guide to the adequacy of renal perfusion, especially when vasoconstriction is responsible for maintaining blood pressure in the presence of hypovolemia.

Autoregulation of renal blood is not abolished during administration of most anesthetic drugs. Conversely, autoregulation is impaired in severe sepsis, in the presence of acute renal failure and during cardiopulmonary bypass. Autoregulation of renal blood flow is not sustained in the presence of persistent changes in mean arterial pressure (approximately 10 minutes), which contrasts with sustained effects of autoregulation on glomerular filtration rate. This allows the glomerular filtration rate to remain near normal despite marked decreases in renal blood flow, which can be redistributed to other vital organs during prolonged periods of hypotension.

Juxtaglomerular Apparatus

Anatomically, the juxtaglomerular apparatus is the site where the distal renal tubule passes in the angle between renal afferent and efferent arterioles. Epithelial cells of the distal renal tubules that actually contact these arterioles are designated *macula densa cells*, whereas corresponding cells in the arterioles are known as *juxtaglomerular cells*. These juxtaglomerular cells release renin into the circulation in response to decreased renal blood flow as may accompany hypovolemia, systemic hypotension, renal ischemia, or sympathetic nervous system stimulation (Fig. 54-5) (Lote et al., 1996). This is an effort by the kidneys to maintain normal renal blood flow and glomerular filtration rate. For example, formation of angiotensin II causes vasoconstriction of the efferent renal arterioles, which increases the glomerular capillary pressure to increase the glomerular filtration rate toward normal.

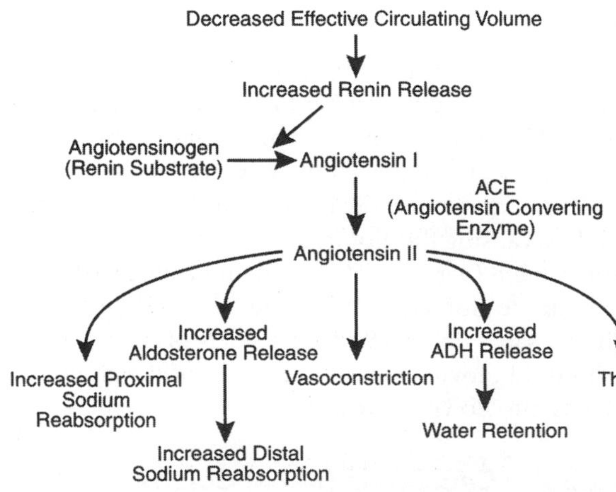

Figure 54-5. The role of the renin-angiotensin system in the maintenance of effective circulating volume. (From Lote CJ, Harper L, and Savage COS. Mechanisms of acute renal failure. *Br J Anaesth* 1996;77:82–89; with permission.)

GLOMERULAR FILTRATE

Fluid that filters across glomerular capillaries into the renal tubules is designated *glomerular filtrate*. The permeability of glomerular capillaries is 100 to 1,000 times as great as that of the usual tissue capillary. This increased capillary permeability reflects the presence of pores in the endothelial cells of the glomerular capillary membrane. These pores are of sufficient size to allow rapid filtration of fluid and small molecular weight substances with diameters of <8 nm, while excluding plasma proteins that have high molecular weights (albumin is the smallest protein, with a molecular weight of 69,000 daltons). For all practical purposes, glomerular filtrate is plasma without proteins.

Glomerular Filtration Rate

Glomerular filtration rate is the amount of glomerular filtrate formed each minute by all the nephrons. In normal persons, glomerular filtration rate averages 125 mL/minute, or approximately 180 liters/day. Reabsorption of approximately 99% of this 180 liters of glomerular filtrate occurs during its passage through the renal tubule, resulting in a daily urine output of 1 to 2 liters. Urinary sodium ion excretion parallels glomerular filtration rate, with approximately 1% of the filtered sodium being excreted in the urine (see Table 54-1) (Ganong, 2003).

Mechanisms of Glomerular Filtration

Glomerular filtration occurs by the same mechanism by which fluid filters out of any tissue capillary. Specifically, pressure inside glomerular capillaries causes filtration of fluid through capillary membranes into renal tubules. Normal filtration pressure is approximately 10 mm Hg, which is calculated as glomerular capillary pressure (60 mm Hg) minus colloid osmotic pressure (32 mm Hg) and pressure in Bowman's capsule (18 mm Hg). Normal glomerular filtrate rate is 12.5 mL/minute/mm Hg of filtration pressure, resulting in a glomerular filtration rate of 125 mL/minute when the net filtration pressure is 10 mm Hg.

Filtration pressure responsible for glomerular filtration rate is influenced by mean arterial pressure, cardiac output, and sympathetic nervous system activity. Anesthetic-induced changes in these factors can exert profound effects on glomerular filtration rate and urine output. Indeed, virtually all anesthetic drugs and techniques are associated with decreases in glomerular filtration rate and urine output.

Mean Arterial Pressure

The impact of mean arterial pressure on glomerular filtration rate is blunted by autoregulation. Tubuloglomerular feedback, which probably occurs at the juxtaglomerular apparatus, is responsible for autoregulation of glomerular filtration rate. Specifically, signals from the macula densa cells in the distal renal tubules cause efferent or afferent renal arterioles to vasodilate or vasoconstrict and thus adjust the capillary pressure in the glomerulus to maintain an almost constant glomerular filtration rate, regardless of changes in mean arterial pressure, between approximately 60 and 160 mm Hg. Nevertheless, even a 5% change in glomerular filtration rate can result in substantial increases or decreases in urine output.

Cardiac Output

Because glomerular filtration rate parallels renal blood flow, it is clear that changes in cardiac output, including those produced by anesthetics, will have an important impact on glomerular filtrate rate.

Sympathetic Nervous System

Innervation of the kidneys is principally from T4 to T12. Sympathetic nervous system stimulation as may occur in the perioperative period or with exogenous administration of catecholamines results in preferential constriction of afferent renal arterioles, decreased pressure in glomerular capillaries, and a decrease in glomerular filtration rate. Excessive sympathetic nervous system stimulation can decrease glomerular blood flow such that urine output decreases to almost zero.

RENAL TUBULAR FUNCTION

Glomerular filtrate flows through renal tubules and collecting ducts, during which time substances are selectively reabsorbed from tubules into peritubular capillaries or secreted into tubules by tubular epithelial cells. The resulting glomerular filtrate entering the renal pelvis is urine. The reabsorptive capabilities of various portions of renal tubules are different (see Table 54-1) (Ganong, 2003). Reabsorption is more important than secretion in the overall formation of urine. Secretion, however, is particularly important in determining the amounts of potassium and hydrogen ions that appear in urine. Secretion of hydrogen ions by renal tubular cells is analogous to that which occurs in the stomach. Approximately two-thirds of all reabsorption and secretory processes in renal tubules take place in proximal renal tubules. As a result, only approximately one-third of the original glomerular filtrate normally passes the entire distance through proximal renal tubules to reach the loops of Henle. The major physiologic determinants of the reabsorption of sodium and water are aldosterone, AVP, renal prostaglandins, and atrial natriuretic factor.

Active transport is responsible for the movement of sodium ions against a concentration gradient from the lumens of proximal renal tubules and then into peritubular capillaries. Energy necessary for reabsorption of sodium ions is supplied by the sodium-potassium adenosine triphosphatase (ATPase) system. Other transport processes along the nephron (glucose reabsorption, amino acid reabsorption, organic acid secretion) share a common carrier (cotransport) with sodium to pass from renal tubules. Thus, there would be almost no transport across renal tubular cells without sodium-potassium ATPase activity. The proximal convoluted renal tubules have the highest sodium-potassium ATPase activity, and approximately 80% of renal oxygen consumption is used to drive this ATPase enzyme system for sodium reabsorption (Lote et al., 1996). Aldosterone promotes reabsorption of sodium and secretion of hydrogen and potassium in the distal convoluted tubule.

More than 99% of the water in the glomerular filtrate is reabsorbed into peritubular capillaries as it passes through renal tubules. Nevertheless, lining epithelial cells in some portions of the renal tubule are more permeable to water, regardless of the concentration gradient for osmosis. For example, osmosis of water through proximal renal tubules is so rapid that the osmolar concentration of solutes on the peritubular capillary side of cell membranes is almost never more than a few milliosmoles greater than in the lumens of the tubules. Conversely, distal renal tubules are almost completely impermeable to water, which is important for controlling the specific gravity of urine. The permeability of the epithelial cells lining the collecting ducts is determined by AVP. AVP works by activating adenylate cyclase in the lining epithelial cells, leading to formation of cyclic adenosine monophosphate and increased permeability of the cell membranes to water. As a result, when AVP levels are increased, most of the water is reabsorbed from the collecting ducts and returned to peritubular capillaries, resulting in excretion of minimal amounts of highly concentrated urine. In the absence of large amounts of AVP, little water is reabsorbed and large volumes of dilute urine are excreted. Painful stimulation as produced by surgery may evoke the release of AVP. Conversely, anesthetic drugs and opioids in the absence of surgical stimulation do not predictably cause the release of AVP. Likewise, positive end-expiratory pressure-induced antidiuresis is not associated with changes in the circulating plasma concentrations of AVP (Payen et al., 1987).

Aquaporins

Aquaporins are protein water channels (tetramers) that facilitate rapid passage of water across lipid cell membranes at a velocity that exceeds that possible by simple diffusion (Agre et al., 2002; Kozono et al., 2002). Five aquaporins (aquaporin-1, 2, and 3 in the kidneys, aquaporin-4 in the brain, and aquaporin-5 in the salivary and lacrimal glands and in the respiratory tract) have been characterized in humans Aquaporin-1 is localized in the proximal renal tubules and the vasopressin-responsive water channel in renal collecting ducts (aquaporin-2) is present in the renal

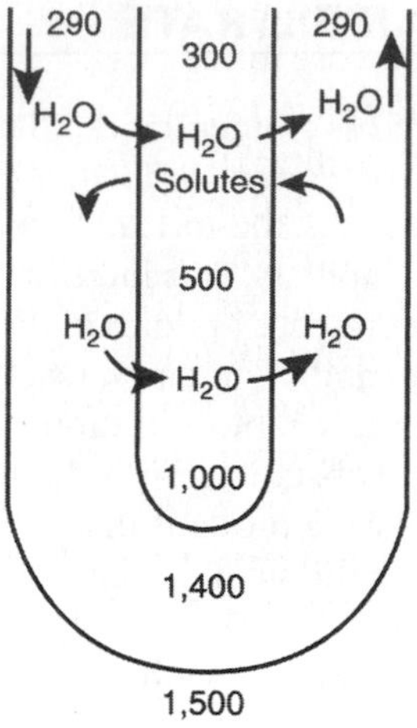

Figure 54-6. Countercurrent exchange of water and solutes in the vasa recta. (From Lote CJ, Harper L, and Savage COS. Mechanisms of acute renal failure. *Br J Anaesth* 1996;77:82–89; with permission.)

collecting ducts. Aquaporin-2 is stored in vesicles in the cytoplasm and vasopressin causes rapid transcription of these vesicles into the luminal membranes of renal tubular collecting duct cells.

Countercurrent System

A *countercurrent system* is one in which blood inflow runs parallel and in the opposite direction to outflow. In the kidneys, the U-shaped anatomic arrangement of peritubular capillaries known as the vasa recta to those loops of Henle that extend into the renal medulla make the countercurrent system possible. As a result, the kidneys are able to eliminate solutes with minimal excretion of water. The first step in the excretion of excess solutes in urine is the formation of a high osmolarity renal medullary interstitial fluid. Indeed, osmolarity increases from approximately 300 mOsm/liter in the renal cortex to approximately 1,400 mOsm/liter in the pelvic tip of the renal medulla (Fig. 54-6) (Lote et al., 1996). In addition, a sluggish medullary blood flow minimizes removal of solutes from the interstitial fluid of the renal medulla.

TUBULAR TRANSPORT MAXIMUM

Tubular transport maximum (Tm) is the maximal amount of a substance that can be actively reabsorbed from the lumens of renal tubules each minute. The Tm depends on the amounts of carrier substance and enzyme available to the specific active transport system in the lining epithelial cells of renal tubules.

The Tm for glucose is approximately 220 mg/minute. When the amount of glucose that filters through the glomerular capillary exceeds this amount, the excess glucose cannot be reabsorbed, but instead passes into urine. The usual amount of glucose in the glomerular filtrate entering proximal renal tubules is 125 mg/minute, and there is no detectable loss into urine. When the tubular load, however, exceeds approximately 220 mg/minute (threshold concentration), glucose first begins to appear in urine. A blood glucose concentration of 180 mg/dL in the presence of a normal glomerular filtration rate results in delivery of 220 mg/minute of glucose into the renal tubular fluid. Loss of glucose in urine occurs at concentrations above the Tm for glucose. The presence of large amounts of unreabsorbed solutes in the urine such as glucose (or mannitol) produces osmotic diuresis.

REGULATION OF BODY FLUID CHARACTERISTICS

The kidneys are the most important organs for regulating the characteristics of body fluids. This regulation is apparent in the control of (a) blood volume, (b) extracellular fluid volume, (c) osmolarity of body fluids, and (d) plasma concentration of various ions, including hydrogen ions, and the resulting pH of body fluids. Thirst also plays a vital role in controlling some characteristics of body fluids.

Blood Volume

Blood volume is maintained over a narrow range despite marked daily variations in fluid and solute intake or loss. The basic mechanism for the control of blood volume is the same feedback loop that also influences systemic blood pressure, cardiac output, and urine output. Specifically, an increase in blood volume increases cardiac output, which increases blood pressure. Increased systemic blood pressure subsequently leads to renal changes (increased renal blood flow and glomerular filtrate rate) that cause an increased urine output and a return of blood volume to normal. The reverse sequence occurs when the blood volume is decreased. The effect of changes in systemic blood pressure on urine output seems to be sustained indefinitely.

The effects of blood volume on systemic blood pressure, cardiac output, and urine output are slow to develop, requiring several hours to produce a full effect. This process, however, can be accelerated by (a) volume receptor reflexes, (b) AVP, (c) aldosterone, and (d) the inherent vascular capacity of the circulation. For example, increased blood volume causes increased pressure in the atria, and the resultant stretch of the volume receptors initiates reflex responses that facilitate renal excretion of fluid and speed the return of blood volume toward normal. Increased circulating concentrations of AVP (water reabsorption is facilitated), aldosterone (sodium reabsorption leads to osmotic reabsorption of water), or both produce a decrease in urine volume and a tendency to restore blood volume. Persistent stimulation of the sympathetic nervous system and associated vasoconstriction as may occur in the presence of a pheochromocytoma leads to a decrease in blood volume, reflecting the inherent vascular capacity of the circulation. A similar decrease in blood volume may accompany chronic systemic blood pressure increases associated with essential hypertension. Conversely, blood volume may be increased by chronic drug-induced vasodilation or the effects of severe varicose veins.

Extracellular Fluid Volume

Control of extracellular fluid volume by the kidneys occurs by the same mechanisms and at the same time as control of blood volume. It is not possible to alter blood volume without simultaneously changing extracellular fluid volume. Indeed, extracellular fluid becomes a reservoir for excess fluid that may be administered intravenously during the perioperative period.

Osmolarity of Body Fluids

Osmolarity of body fluids is determined almost entirely by the concentration of sodium in the extracellular fluid. Control of sodium ion concentration and, thus, osmolarity of body fluids is under the influence of the osmoreceptor-AVP mechanism and the thirst reflex. In contrast, the effects of aldosterone on plasma sodium concentration and the resulting plasma osmolarity are insignificant (Fig. 54-7) (Guyton and Hall, 2000). This is because aldosterone-induced reabsorption of sodium is accompanied by a simultaneous reabsorption of water. Indeed, patients with primary aldosteronism often manifest an increased extracellular fluid volume, but the plasma sodium concentration rarely increases more than 2 to 3 mEq/liter.

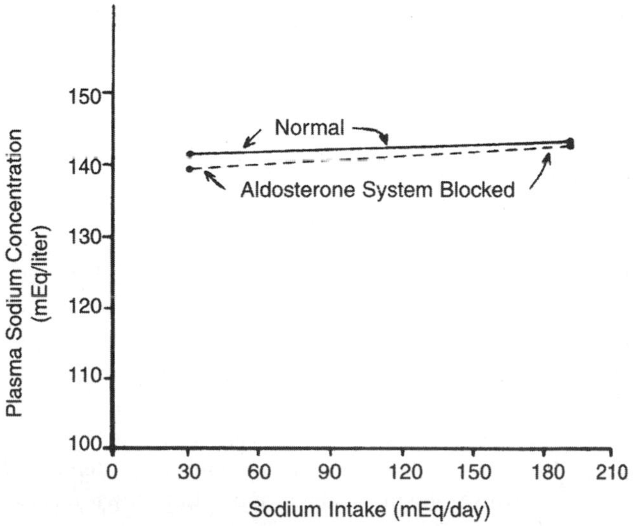

Figure 54-7. In the absence of aldosterone, the plasma concentration of sodium varies <2% over a sixfold range in sodium intake. (From Guyton AC, Hall JE. *Textbook of medical physiology*, 10th ed. Philadelphia: Saunders, 2000; with permission.)

Osmoreceptor-Arginine Vasopressin Hormone

An increase in osmolarity of extracellular fluid due to excess sodium ions causes osmoreceptors in the supraoptic nuclei of the hypothalamus to shrink and thereby increase the discharge rate of impulses through the pituitary stalk to the posterior pituitary where AVP is released. The resulting AVP-induced retention of water dilutes the plasma sodium concentration and returns osmolarity downward toward a normal value. Conversely, when extracellular fluid becomes too dilute, the osmoreceptors inhibit the release of AVP, and more water than solute is excreted by the kidneys, thus concentrating sodium and returning osmolarity upward toward normal. Changes in osmolarity of 1% to 5% evoke substantial alterations in the circulating concentration of AVP. In contrast, changes in blood volume must usually exceed 10% to evoke changes in AVP release by the osmoreceptors. For all practical purposes, osmoreceptors may be considered as sodium concentration receptors.

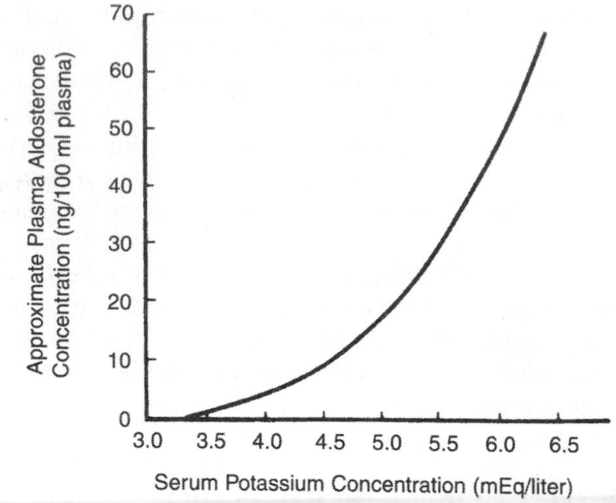

Figure 54-8. Small changes in the plasma concentrations of potassium evoke large changes in the plasma concentration of aldosterone. (From Guyton AC, Hall JE. *Textbook of medical physiology*, 10th ed. Philadelphia: Saunders, 2000; with permission.)

Thirst Reflex

The most common cause for thirst is an increased sodium concentration in the extracellular fluid. Any change in circulation that leads to increased production of angiotensin II, such as acute hemorrhage or congestive heart failure, also leads to thirst. Although the sensation of a dry mouth is often associated with the thirst reflex, the blockade of salivary secretions, as by anticholinergic drugs, does not cause humans to drink excessively. The thirst reflex is activated when the plasma concentration of sodium increases approximately 2 mEq/liter above normal or when the plasma osmolarity increases approximately 4 mOsm/liter. Humans typically drink the correct amount of water, allowing precise maintenance of the osmolarity of extracellular fluid. Indeed, relief from thirst occurs almost immediately after drinking water, even before this water has been absorbed from the gastrointestinal tract.

Plasma Concentration of Ions

Potassium

The role of the kidneys in controlling the plasma concentration of potassium is mediated principally by the effects of aldosterone on the renal tubules. Indeed, small changes in the plasma concentration of potassium evoke large changes in the plasma concentration of aldosterone (Fig. 54-8) (Guyton and Hall, 2000). In the presence of aldosterone, there is increased secretion of potassium ions into renal tubules, leading to increased loss of this ion into urine. Excessive amounts of aldosterone in patients with primary aldosteronism produce hypokalemia with associated skeletal muscle weakness due to nerve transmission failure because of hyperpolarization of nerve membranes. When aldosterone activity is blocked, as by certain diuretics, the plasma potassium concentration parallels intake of potassium, making hypokalemia or hyperkalemia possible (Fig. 54-9) (Guyton and Hall, 2000). Absence of aldosterone, such as is associated with Addison disease, may result in hyperkalemia.

In addition to aldosterone, the plasma concentration of hydrogen and sodium ions may exert modest effects on potassium elimination in urine. For example, hydrogen ions compete with potassium ions for secretion into the renal tubules. In the presence of acidosis, hydrogen ions

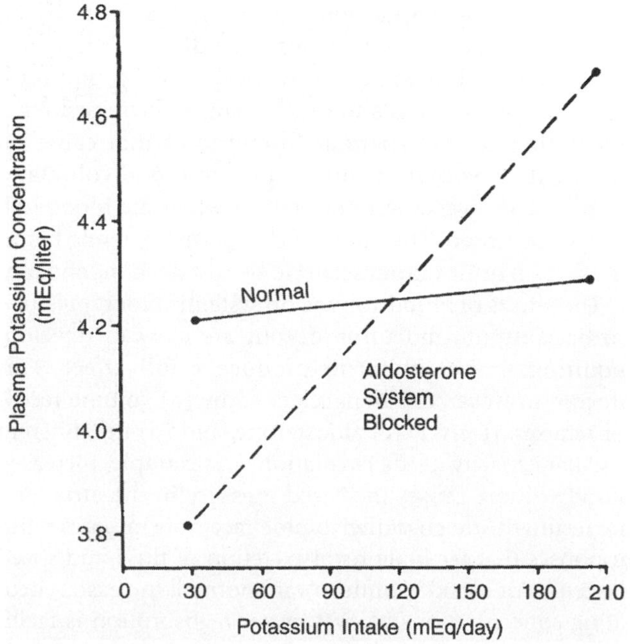

Figure 54-9. Plasma concentrations of potassium parallel intake when aldosterone activity is impaired. (From Guyton AC, Hall JE. *Textbook of medical physiology*, 10th ed. Philadelphia: Saunders, 2000; with permission.)

are preferentially secreted into the renal tubules and plasma potassium concentrations may increase. Conversely, alkalosis is associated with hypokalemia. The level of sodium intake may influence plasma concentrations of potassium because sodium is transported through renal tubular epithelial cells in exchange for potassium.

Sodium

The role of the kidneys in controlling the plasma concentration of sodium reflects active transport of sodium ions across renal tubular epithelial cells into peritubular capillaries. Approximately two-thirds of sodium is reabsorbed from the proximal renal tubules and no more than 10% of sodium that initially enters the glomerular filtrate is likely to reach the distal renal tubule. Aldosterone influences reabsorption of sodium from the distal renal tubules and collecting ducts. In the presence of large amounts of aldosterone, almost all the remaining sodium is reabsorbed, and urinary excretion of sodium approaches zero. Aldosterone acts by entering the lining epithelial cells of the renal tubules, where it combines with a receptor protein. This receptor protein activates DNA molecules to form messenger RNA, which subsequently causes the formation of the carrier proteins or protein enzymes necessary for the sodium and potassium transport process. The formation of these substances requires approximately 45 minutes after the release of aldosterone.

Hydrogen

The kidneys secrete excess hydrogen ions by exchanging a hydrogen ion for a sodium ion, thus acidifying the urine, and by the synthesis of ammonia, which combines with hydrogen to form ammonium.

Calcium

Calcium ion concentration is controlled principally by the effect of parathyroid hormone on bone reabsorption. For example, a decrease in the plasma concentration of calcium evokes the release of parathyroid hormone, which causes the release of calcium from bone. When plasma calcium concentrations are increased, the secretion of parathyroid hormone is decreased to the point at which almost no release of calcium from bone occurs. In addition to effects on bone, parathyroid hormone increases reabsorption of calcium from the distal renal tubules, collecting ducts, and gastrointestinal tract.

Magnesium

Magnesium is reabsorbed by all portions of the renal tubules. Urinary excretion of magnesium parallels the plasma concentration of this ion.

Urea

Urea is the most abundant of the metabolic waste products that must be excreted in urine to prevent excess accumulation in body fluids. The major factors in determining the rate of urea excretion are the plasma concentration of urea (blood urea nitrogen [BUN]) and the glomerular filtration rate. Typically, approximately 50% of the urea that initially enters the renal tubules appears in the urine.

When the glomerular filtration rate is low, the glomerular filtrate remains in the renal tubules for prolonged periods before it becomes urine. The longer the period that the filtrate remains in the renal tubules, the greater is the reabsorption of urea. As a result, the amount of urea that reaches the urine is decreased and the BUN is increased. Conversely, when the glomerular filtration rate is increased, glomerular filtrate passes through renal tubules so rapidly that very little urea is reabsorbed into peritubular capillaries.

ATRIAL AND RENAL NATRIURETIC FACTORS

Cardiac atria synthesize, store, and secrete via the coronary sinus an amino acid hormone known as *atrial natriuretic peptide* (ANP). The renal analogue of ANP is renal natriuretic peptide (urodilatin), which is synthesized in renal cortical nephrons. High-affinity binding sites for these peptides are present in the renal collecting ducts, and binding results in increased intracellular cyclic guanine monophosphate concentrations and inhibition of sodium transport. It is likely that ANP is primarily a cardiovascular regulator and relatively unimportant for sodium excretion, whereas renal natriuretic peptide is more likely to participate in the intrarenal regulation of sodium excretion (Lote et al., 1996; Shirakami et al., 1997). As a potent vasodilator, ANP decreases systemic blood pressure and elicits renal artery vasodilation.

Circulating plasma concentrations of ANP are linearly related to right and left atrial pressure and are proportional to atrial diameter. Inhibition of ANP release diminishes urine output and urinary sodium excretion while increasing plasma renin activity. Positive end-expiratory pressure-induced decreases in atrial distension result in decreased ANP release, which may mediate in part the antidiuretic and antinatriuretic effects of positive end-expiratory pressure.

ACUTE RENAL FAILURE

Acute renal failure is characterized by an abrupt deterioration of renal function with a decrease in glomerular filtration rate occurring over a period of hours to days, resulting in the failure of the kidneys to excrete nitrogenous waste products (urea and creatinine) and to maintain fluid and electrolyte homeostasis (Lote et al., 1996; Thadhani et al., 1996). Loss of urinary concentrating ability is an early and precise manifestation of acute tubular necrosis (aminoglycoside antibiotics a potential cause), most likely reflecting failure of the energy-requiring

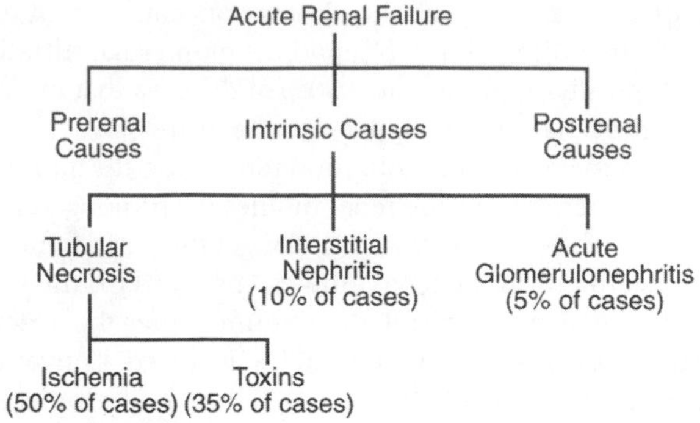

Figure 54-10. Classification of acute renal failure. (From Thadhani R, Pascual M, Bonventre JV. Acute renal failure. *N Engl J Med* 1996;334:1448–1460; with permission.)

sodium-potassium ATPase pump in the renal tubules. Acute interstitial nephritis is not as common as prerenal azotemia or acute tubular necrosis as a cause of acute renal failure and is most often due to drug-induced damage (beta-lactam antibiotics especially methicillin, and nonsteroidal antiinflammatory drugs). Medication-related acute interstitial nephritis is often preventable or reversible by discontinuing the offending medication.

Classification

A traditional classification of acute renal failure is prerenal, intrarenal, and postrenal (Fig. 54-10) (Thadhani et al., 1996).

Prerenal Azotemia

Prerenal azotemia denotes a disorder in the systemic circulation that causes renal hypoperfusion. Implicit in this explanation is that correction of the underlying circulatory disorder (improved cardiac output or repletion of intravascular fluid volume) will restore glomerular filtration. Elderly patients are particularly susceptible to prerenal azotemia because of their predisposition to hypovolemia and high prevalence of renal artery atherosclerosis. Nonsteroidal antiinflammatory drugs can precipitate prerenal azotemia principally in patients who are dependent on prostaglandins for renal vasodilatory effects. Among hospitalized patients, prerenal azotemia is the single most common cause of acute renal failure and is often due to congestive heart failure, hypovolemia, septic shock, or administration of radiocontrast media (especially patients with preexisting renal disease, diabetes, hypovolemia, and concomitant exposure to other nephrotoxins).

Intrinsic Renal Failure

Intrinsic renal failure generally includes renal tubular necrosis, which may be due to ischemia or nephrotoxins. Acute tubular necrosis reflects destruction of epithelial cells lining the renal tubules and is most often due to nephrotoxins or renal ischemia as produced by prolonged decreases in systemic blood pressure and renal blood flow (shock). This renal tubular injury is likely due to an imbalance of the oxygen supply and demand of renal medullary ascending limb tubular cells (Byrick and Rose, 1990). High oxygen demand of these renal tubular cells is secondary to active reabsorption of solute, especially sodium, which is increased in the presence of hypovolemia. In the presence of decreased renal blood flow, injury to ascending limb renal tubular cells is exacerbated by arterial hypoxemia and endothelial cell swelling, which decreases further the perfusion of these metabolically active cells.

Acute tubular necrosis due to ischemia of the renal medullary ascending tubular cells is the most likely cause of acute renal failure in the perioperative period. In this regard, hypoperfusion of the kidneys is the most frequently recognized single insult leading to acute renal failure in the setting of trauma, surgery, hemorrhage, or dehydration. There is no correlation between urine volume and histologic evidence of acute tubular necrosis, glomerular filtration rate, or renal function tests in patients who are severely traumatized, undergo cardiovascular surgery, or experience shock (Kellen et al., 1994).

Postrenal Obstructive Nephropathy

Obstructive postrenal failure (renal stones, prostatic hypertrophy, mechanical kinking of catheters) may be a cause of acute renal failure in some patients. Sudden acute oliguria in the perioperative period warrants evaluation of possible mechanical obstruction to urinary drainage devices.

Oliguric versus Nonoliguric Renal Failure

Acute renal failure may be oliguric (urine output $<$400 mL/day) or nonoliguric ($>$400 mL/day). Patients with nonoliguric acute renal failure have a better prognosis than those with oliguric renal failure, probably due to the decreased severity of the causative insult and the fact that many of these patients have drug-associated nephrotoxicity or interstitial nephritis. The percentage of patients with acute renal failure who require dialysis ranges from 20% to 60%. On average, mortality for patients on chronic renal dialysis is 20% per year.

Mortality

Mortality rates in acute renal failure range from approximately 7% among patients with prerenal azotemia to $>$80% among patients with postoperative renal failure (Thadhani et al., 1996). Despite dramatic improvements in dialysis and intensive care, the mortality rate among patients with severe acute renal failure (ischemic in origin) requiring dialysis has not decreased appreciably over the past 50 years. This may be explained by an increased predominance of elderly patients and associated coexisting diseases in this age group. When acute renal failure occurs in the setting of multiorgan failure, especially in patients with severe hypotension or the acute respiratory distress syndrome, mortality rates range from 50% to 80% (Thadhani et al., 1996).

Diagnosis

Urine indexes, which measure urine osmolarity, urine sodium concentration, and fractional excretion of sodium, help differentiate between prerenal azotemia, in which the reabsorptive capacity of renal tubular cells and the concentrating ability of the kidneys are preserved, and tubular necrosis, in which both of these functions are impaired. One of the earliest functional defects seen with renal tubular damage is loss of the ability to concentrate urine. Patients with oliguria and acute renal failure due to prerenal causes tend to have a urine osmolarity of >500 mOsm/liter, a urinary sodium concentration of <20 mEq/liter, and a fractional excretion of sodium of <1%. In contrast, in patients with acute tubular necrosis, urine osmolarity is <350 mOsm/liter, the urinary sodium concentration is >40 mEq/liter, and the fractional excretion of sodium is >1%. Renal ultrasound examination is a useful means of diagnosing postrenal obstruction, but its sensitivity may be <85%.

Treatment

The initial treatment of patients with acute renal failure is focused on reversing the underlying cause and correcting fluid and electrolyte imbalances (Fig. 54-11). Although restoration of renal blood flow with intravenous volume resuscitation is ineffective in restoring renal function once tubular necrosis is established, volume replacement remains the most effective prophylactic strategy (Conger, 1995). Aggressive and early treatment of perioperative oliguria is most important for those patients at increased risk for developing acute renal failure (Table 54-2) (Noris et al., 1994). The occurrence of transient oliguria during elective operations in young patients without preexisting renal disease does not require the same aggressive treatment as does oliguria in elderly patients with preexisting renal disease.

The presumption that early therapy modifies the prognosis of perioperative renal dysfunction remains an untested hypothesis. Conceptually, dopamine could protect the renal tubules from ischemia by suppressing sodium pump energy requirements, decreasing oxygen consumption, and increasing renal tubular flow. Nevertheless, a renoprotective effect of dopamine is unproven (see Chapter 12). Furthermore, dopamine can cause cardiac tachydysrhythmias, pulmonary shunting, and gastrointestinal necrosis. Mannitol and furosemide have not been shown to be effective in patients for the prevention or treatment of ischemic or toxic acute renal failure. Both mannitol and loop diuretics, if administered early in the course of ischemic acute renal failure, can convert an oliguric state to a nonoliguric state. Although nonoliguric acute renal failure is generally associated with lower morbidity there is little evidence that a chemically-induced conversion from an oliguric to a nonoliguric state decreases the mortality rate. At present, the use of loop diuretics can only be justified to increase urine output for fluid management with no expectation that these drugs will improve outcome.

Dialysis has remained the standard therapy for severe acute renal failure (see the section on Dialytic Therapy). Common indications for acute dialysis include volume overload, hyperkalemia, metabolic acidosis, and signs of severe uremia.

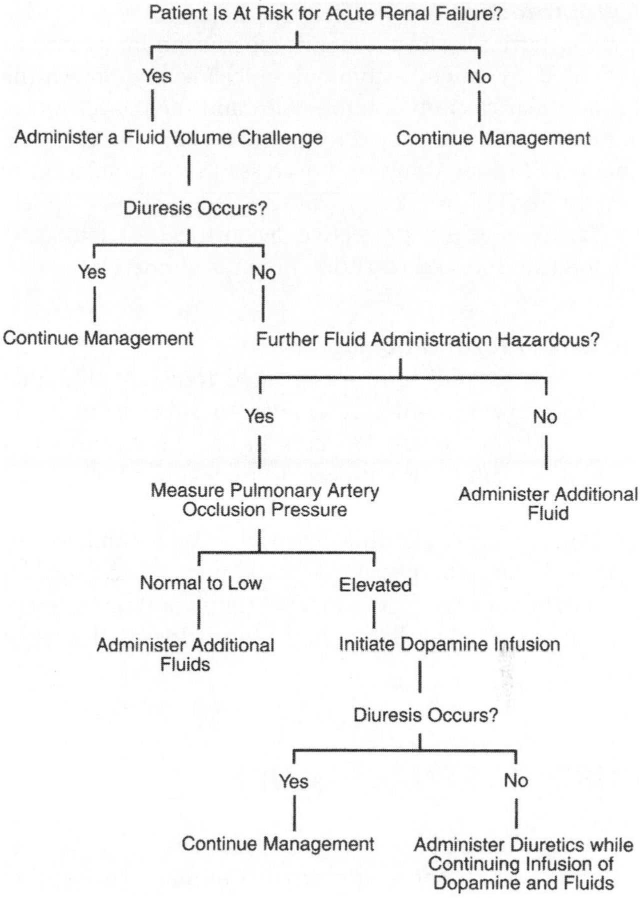

Figure 54-11. Treatment diagram for a patient who develops acute oliguria in the perioperative period.

TABLE 54-2.
CHARACTERISTICS OF PATIENTS AT INCREASED RISK FOR DEVELOPING ACUTE RENAL FAILURE IN THE POSTOPERATIVE PERIOD

Preexisting renal disease
Congestive heart failure
Advanced age
Prolonged renal hypoperfusion
High-risk surgery (abdominal aneurysm resection, cardiopulmonary bypass)
Sepsis
Jaundice

Cytoprotection

Cytoprotection against ischemic reperfusion injury may be provided by calcium-channel blockade. By preventing intracellular calcium accumulation and the conversion of xanthine dehydrogenase to xanthine oxidase, calcium-channel blocking drugs may decrease the accumulation of oxygen free radicals. Furthermore, calcium-channel blocking drugs may be protective by virtue of attenuating angiotensin-induced constriction in the glomeruli.

Ischemic Preconditioning

Ischemic preconditioning (repeated transient sublethal ischemic events confer resistance to subsequent more severe ischemic insults) occurs in an animal model of acute renal failure and appears to be mediated by adenosine (Lee and Emala, 2000). Adenosine is important in regulating intrarenal distribution of blood flow and adenosine receptor subtypes A_{1a} and A_{2a} may protect against renal ischemic reperfusion injury. Stimulation of A_{2a} receptors increases medullary renal blood flow and oxygen delivery.

CHRONIC RENAL FAILURE

Despite different causes (chronic glomerulonephritis or pyelonephritis), the common denominator present in patients who develop chronic renal failure is progressive loss of nephron function and decline in glomerular filtration rate (Table 54-3). Renal reserve is decreased, but patients remain asymptomatic when at least 40% of the nephrons continue to function. Renal insufficiency is present when only 10% to 40% of nephrons are functioning. These patients are compensated, but there is no renal reserve such that excess catabolic loads or toxic substances (aminoglycosides) can exacerbate renal insufficiency. Polyuria and nocturia in these patients most likely reflect decreased urine concentrating ability. Loss of >90% of functioning nephrons results in uremia (urine in the blood) and the need for dialytic therapy.

TABLE 54-4.
MANIFESTATIONS OF CHRONIC RENAL FAILURE

- Accumulation of metabolic waste products in blood
- Excretion of fixed specific gravity urine
- Metabolic acidosis
- Hyperkalemia
- Anemia (less common with introduction of recombinant erythropoietin)
- Platelet dysfunction
- Fluid overload and systemic hypertension
- Nervous system dysfunction
- Osteomalacia

Manifestations of Chronic Renal Failure

Chronic renal failure is associated with multiple derangements affecting several organ systems (Table 54-4). It has been estimated that 5% of the adult population has preexisting renal disease that may contribute to perioperative morbidity. A comprehensive preoperative evaluation must include assessment of these multiple physiologic derangements and review of renal function tests, keeping in mind that most of these tests are imprecise and insensitive indicators of the degree of renal dysfunction (Table 54-5) (Kellen et al., 1994). Furthermore, normal values for renal function tests as established in healthy individuals may not be applicable during anesthesia (Mazze, 1998).

Specific gravity of the urine approaches the glomerular filtrate (approximately 1.008) as progressively more nephrons are lost and the countercurrent system fails. Anemia is severe but usually well tolerated, reflecting its slow onset and compensatory increases in tissue blood flow and rightward shift of the oxyhemoglobin dissociation curve in response to acidosis and increased concentrations of 2,3-diphosphoglycerate. It is presumed that anemia associated with chronic renal failure reflects decreased renal secretion of the enzyme that splits erythropoietin from a plasma protein. Erythropoietin normally stimulates

TABLE 54-3.
STAGES OF CHRONIC RENAL FAILURE

	Number of Functioning Nephrons (% of Total)	Glomerular Filtration Rate (mL/min)	Signs	Laboratory Changes
Normal	100	125	None	None
Decreased renal reserve	40	50–80	None	None
Renal insufficiency	10–40	12–50	Polyuria, nocturia	Increased BUN and creatinine
Uremia	10	<12	See Table 53-4	

BUN, blood urea nitrogen.

TABLE 54-5.
RENAL FUNCTION TESTS

	Normal Value	Factors That Influence Interpretation
Blood urea nitrogen	8–20 mg/dL	Dehydration Variable protein intake Gastrointestinal bleeding Catabolism
Creatinine	0.5–1.2 mg/dL	Age Skeletal muscle mass Catabolism
Creatinine clearance	120 mL/min	Accurate urine volume measurement

bone marrow to produce erythrocytes. Inability of the kidneys to eliminate hydrogen ions produced by metabolic processes of the body predictably results in metabolic acidosis. Hyperkalemia reflects inability of diseased kidneys to eliminate potassium and has important anesthetic implications, especially with respect to cardiac rhythm and responses at the neuromuscular junction. Accumulation of metabolic waste products in the blood interferes with platelet aggregation whereas prothrombin time and plasma thromboplastin time usually remain normal. Retention of sodium and water results in fluid overload that may manifest as congestive heart failure and hypertension. Neurologic complications occur in the central nervous system (confusion or coma), peripheral nervous system (neuropathy), and autonomic nervous system. Uremic coma is most likely due to decreases in systemic pH, whereas rapid and deep breathing during uremic coma is presumed to reflect an attempt to compensate for metabolic acidosis. Dialytic therapy is useful in correcting electrolyte, fluid, and platelet function. Alternatively, an analogue of vasopressin, DDAVP, is effective in shortening bleeding time within 1 hour after its infusion.

Dialytic Therapy

Indications for initiating dialytic therapy are (a) hyperkalemia and/or acidosis that are not controlled by medical management, and (b) fluid overload that is not responsive to fluid restriction and/or diuretic therapy. In the absence of these indications, many nephrologists recommend dialysis when the blood urea nitrogen (BUN) reaches 80 to 100 mg/dL, because the goal is to avoid the occurrence of uremic symptoms. The patient undergoes dialysis as frequently as necessary to keep the BUN <80 mg/dL. Monitoring of the plasma concentrations of drugs being administered to the patient is an important adjunct to effective dialytic therapy. Infection remains the main cause of death despite aggressive dialytic therapy. In this regard, meticulous aseptic care of intravenous catheters and wounds and avoidance of the use of indwelling urinary catheters are important.

TABLE 54-6.
COMPLICATIONS OF DIALYTIC THERAPY

Infection
Activation of complement system
Hypotension
Arterial hypoxemia
Skeletal muscle cramping
Protein depletion
Anticoagulation
Access failure

Chronic dialytic therapy is a complex technical challenge associated with multiple side effects (Table 54-6). The choice of dialysis technique (intermittent, continuous, and peritoneal) is often based on preferences of the nephrologist, availability of local resources, and the hemodynamic stability of the patient.

Intermittent Hemodialysis

Hemodialysis is based on diffusive transport of solute down an osmotic gradient across a semipermeable membrane. Cuprophane (cellulose-based) membranes have been used since the 1960s, and it is recognized that these membranes may interact with blood to activate the alternate complement pathway (Thadhani et al., 1996). This activation is associated with up-regulation of certain leukocyte adhesion molecules, which are responsible for pulmonary sequestration of leukocytes, arterial hypoxemia, and transient neutropenia. These neutrophils may preferentially localize in the ischemic portions of the kidneys and aggravate tissue damage. Synthetic membranes (polymethylmethacrylate, polyacrylonitrile, polysulfone) activate complement to a lesser extent than cellulose-based membranes, but they may activate other humoral pathways and cellular elements. Intermittent hemodialysis with biocompatible membranes (polyacrylonitrile or polymethylmethacrylate) may be preferable, especially in patients with acute renal failure who require dialysis.

The dialysate should contain little or none of the substance to be removed from the patient's blood such that there will be a net transfer of solutes from the plasma into the dialyzing fluid. During hemodialysis, blood flows continually from an artery through the artificial kidney and back into a vein. Heparin is added to the blood as it enters the artificial kidney and protamine is added before the blood is returned to the patient. The need to maintain chronic vascular access via a surgically created arteriovenous fistula is a major cause of morbidity in patients with chronic renal failure.

Continuous Hemodialysis

Continuously administered (venovenous or arteriovenous) hemodialysis is an alternative form of dialysis for critically ill patients with renal failure (Bellomo et al., 1993). The advantages of continuous dialysis over intermittent dialysis include more precise fluid and metabolic control, decreased hemodynamic instability, and, in patients with sepsis or multiorgan failure, an enhanced possibility of removing injurious cytokines. Another possible advantage of continuous dialysis is the associated ability to administer unlimited nutritional support. The disadvantages of continuous dialysis techniques are the needs for both prolonged anticoagulation and constant surveillance.

Peritoneal Dialysis

Peritoneal dialysis is effective in patients with acute renal failure associated with hemodynamic instability or when technical support is limited (Howdieshell et al., 1992). The capillary network present in the peritoneal cavity provides a large surface area for contact of the patient's blood with the dialysate and is the basis for peritoneal dialysis. Surgical placement of an indwelling peritoneal catheter (Tenckhoff catheter) is necessary. Peritonitis is the major complication associated with peritoneal dialysis.

TRANSPORT OF URINE TO THE BLADDER

Urine is transported to the bladder through the ureters, which originate in the pelvis of each kidney. Each ureter is innervated by the sympathetic and parasympathetic nervous system. As urine collects in the renal pelvis, the pressure in the pelvis increases and initiates a peristaltic contraction that travels downward along the ureter to force urine toward the bladder. Parasympathetic nervous system stimulation increases the frequency of peristalsis, whereas sympathetic nervous system stimulation decreases peristalsis. At its distal end, the ureter penetrates the bladder obliquely such that pressure in the bladder compresses the ureter, thereby preventing reflux of urine into the ureter when bladder pressure increases during micturition.

Ureters are well supplied with nerve fibers such that obstruction of a ureter by a stone causes intense reflex constriction and pain. In addition, pain is likely to elicit a sympathetic nervous system reflex (ureterorenal reflex) that causes vasoconstriction of the renal arterioles and a concomitant decrease in urine formation in the kidney served by the obstructed ureter.

As the bladder fills with urine, stretch receptors in the bladder wall initiate micturition contractions. Sensory signals are conducted to the sacral segments of the spinal cord through the pelvic nerves and then back again to the bladder through parasympathetic nervous system fibers. The micturition reflex is a completely automatic spinal cord reflex that can be inhibited (tonic contraction of the external urinary sphincter) or facilitated by centers in the brain. Spinal cord damage above the sacral region leaves the micturition reflex intact but is no longer controlled by the brain.

REFERENCES

Agre P, King LS, Yasui M, et al. Aquaporin water channels-from atomic structure to clinical medicine. *J Physiol* 2002;542:3–16.

Alpert RA, Roizen MF, Hamilton WK, et al. Intraoperative urinary output does not predict postoperative renal function in patients undergoing abdominal aortic revascularization. *Surgery* 1984;95:707–711.

Bellomo R, Parkin G, Love J, et al. A prospective comparative study of continuous arteriovenous hemodiafiltration and continuous venovenous hemodiafiltration in critically ill patients. *Am J Kidney Dis* 1993;21:400–404.

Byrick RJ, Rose DK. Pathophysiology and prevention of acute renal failure: the role of the anaesthetist. *Can J Anaesth* 1990;37:457–467.

Conger JD. Interventions in clinical acute renal failure: what are the data? *Am J Kidney Dis* 1995;26:565–576.

Ganong WF. *Review of medical physiology*, 21st ed. Lange Medical Books, New York: McGraw Hill, 2003.

Guyton AC, Hall JE. *Textbook of medical physiology*, 10th ed. Philadelphia: W.B. Saunders, 2000.

Howdieshell TR, Blalock WE, Bowen PA, et al. Management of posttraumatic acute renal failure with peritoneal dialysis. *Am Surg* 1992;58:378–382.

Kellen M, Aronson S, Roizen MF, et al. Predictive and diagnostic tests of renal failure: a review. *Anesth Analg* 1994;78:134–142.

Kozono D, Yasui M, King LS, et al. Aquaporin water channels: atomic structure and molecular dynamics meet clinical medicine. *J Clin Invest* 2002;109:1395–1399.

Lee HT, Emala CW. Protective effects of renal ischemic preconditioning and adenosine pretreatment: Role of A(1) and A(3) receptors. *Am J Physiol Renal Physiol* 2000;278:F380–387.

Lote CJ, Harper L, Savage COS. Mechanisms of acute renal failure. *Br J Anaesth* 1996;77:82–89.

Mazze RI. No evidence of sevoflurane-induced renal injury in volunteers. *Anesth Analg* 1998;86:228.

Norris BF, Roizen MF, Aronson S, et al. Association of preoperative risk factors with postoperative acute renal failure. *Anesth Analg* 1994;78:143–149.

Pitts RF. *Physiology of the kidney and body fluids*, 3rd ed. Chicago: Year Book, 1974.

Shirakami G, Segawa H, Shingu K, et al. The effects of atrial natriuretic peptide infusion on hemodynamic, renal, and hormonal responses during gastrectomy. *Anesth Analg* 1997;85:907–912.

Steinhausen M, Endlich K, Wiegman DL. Glomerular blood flow. *Kidney Int* 1990;38:769–784.

Suleiman MY, Passannante AN, Onder RL, et al. Alteration of renal blood flow during epidural anesthesia in normal subjects. *Anesth Analg* 1997;84:1076–1080.

Thadhani R, Pascual M, Bonventre JV. Acute renal failure. *N Engl J Med* 1996;334:1448–1460.

Liver and Gastrointestinal Tract

55

LIVER

The liver lies in the right upper quadrant of the abdominal cavity and is attached to the diaphragm. It is the largest organ in the body, weighing approximately 1,500 g and representing 2% of body weight. In the neonate, the liver accounts for approximately 5% of body weight. Hepatocytes represent approximately 80% of the cytoplasmic mass within the liver. These cells perform diverse and complex functions (Table 55-1). The ability of hemopoietic stem cells to differentiate into hepatocytes introduces the possibility of treating inherited disorders of metabolism (reflecting absent to altered enzymes due to a single or multiple genetic defect) a possibility in the future (Alison et al., 2000).

Anatomy

The liver is divided into four lobes consisting of 50,000 to 100,000 individual hepatic lobules (Fig. 55-1) (Bloom and Fawcell, 1975). Blood flows past hepatocytes via sinusoids from branches of the portal vein and hepatic artery to a central vein. There is usually only one layer of hepatocytes between sinusoids so the total area of contact with plasma is great. Central veins join to form hepatic veins, which drain into the inferior vena cava. Each hepatocyte is also located adjacent to bile canaliculi, which coalesce to form the common hepatic duct. This duct and the cystic duct from the gallbladder join to form the common bile duct, which enters the duodenum at a site surrounded by the sphincter of Oddi (Fig. 55-2) (Bell et al., 1976). The main pancreatic duct also unites with the common bile duct just before it enters the duodenum.

Hepatic lobules are lined by macrophages (derived from circulating monocytes) known as Kupffer cells, which phagocytize 99% or more of bacteria in the portal venous blood. This is crucial because the portal venous blood drains the gastrointestinal tract and usually contains colon bacteria.

Endothelial cells that line the hepatic lobules contain large pores, permitting easy diffusion of certain substances, including plasma proteins, into extravascular spaces of the liver that connect with terminal lymphatics. The extreme permeability of the lining of endothelial cells allows large quantities of lymph to form, which contain protein concentrations that are only slightly less than the protein concentration of plasma. Indeed, approximately one-third to one-half of all the lymph is formed in the liver (see Chapter 46).

Hepatic Blood Flow

The liver receives a dual afferent blood supply from the hepatic artery and portal veins (Fig. 55-3). Total hepatic blood flow is approximately 1,450 mL/minute or approximately 29% of the cardiac output. Of this amount, the portal vein provides 75% of the total flow but only 50% to 55% of the hepatic oxygen supply because this blood is partially deoxygenated in the preportal organs and tissues (gastrointestinal tract, spleen, pancreas). The hepatic artery provides only 25% of total hepatic blood flow but provides 45% to 50% of the hepatic oxygen requirements. Hepatic artery blood flow maintains nutrition of connective tissues and walls of bile ducts. For this reason, loss of hepatic artery blood flow can be fatal because of ensuing necrosis of vital liver structures. An increase in hepatic oxygen requirements is met by an increase in oxygen extraction rather than a further increase in the already high hepatic blood flow.

Control of Hepatic Blood Flow

Portal vein blood flow is controlled primarily by the arterioles in the preportal splanchnic organs. This flow, combined with the resistance to portal vein blood flow within the liver, determines portal venous pressure (normally 7 to 10 mm Hg) (see the section on Portal Venous Pressure).

TABLE 55-1.
FUNCTIONS OF HEPATOCYTES

Absorb nutrients from portal venous blood
Store and release carbohydrates, proteins, and lipids
Excrete bile salts
Synthesize plasma proteins, glucose, cholesterol, and fatty acids
Metabolize exogenous and endogenous compounds

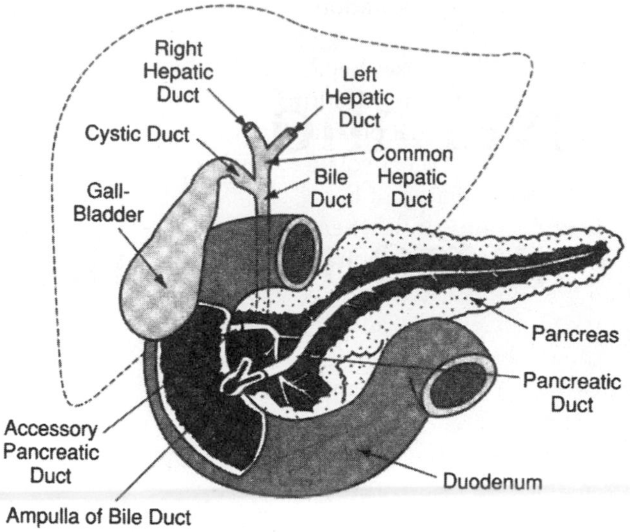

Figure 55–2. Connections of the ducts of the gallbladder, liver, and pancreas. (From Bell GH, Emslie-Smith D, Paterson CR. *Textbook of physiology and biochemistry*, 9th ed. New York: Churchill Livingstone, 1976; with permission.)

Sympathetic nervous system innervation is from T3 to T11 and is mediated via alpha-adrenergic receptors. This innervation is principally responsible for resistance and compliance of hepatic venules. Changes in hepatic venous compliance play an essential role in overall regulation of cardiac output and the reservoir function of the liver (see the section on Reservoir Function).

Fibrotic constriction characteristic of hepatic cirrhosis (most often due to chronic alcohol abuse and hepatitis C) can increase resistance to portal vein blood flow as evidenced by portal venous pressures of 20 to 30 mm Hg (portal hypertension). The resulting increased resistance to portal vein blood flow may result in development of shunts (varices) to allow blood flow to bypass the hepatocytes. Conversely, congestive heart failure and positive pressure ventilation of the lungs impair outflow of blood from the liver because of increased central venous pressure, which is transmitted to hepatic veins. Ascites results when increased portal venous pressures cause transudation of protein-rich fluid through the outer surface of the liver capsule and gastrointestinal tract into the abdominal cavity. Hepatic artery blood flow is influenced by arteriolar tone that reflects local and intrinsic mechanisms (autoregulation). For example, a decrease in portal vein blood flow is accompanied by an increase in hepatic artery blood flow by as much as 100%. Presumably, a vasodilating substance such as adenosine accumulates in the liver when portal vein blood flow decreases, leading to subsequent

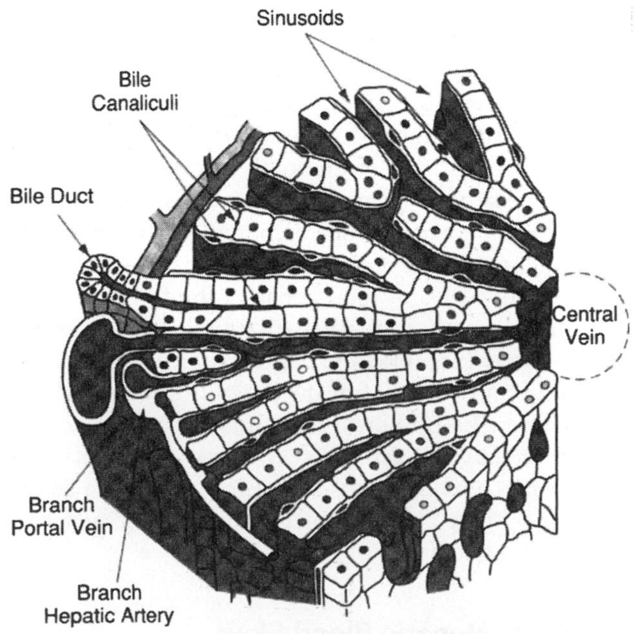

Figure 55–1. Schematic depiction of a hepatic lobule with a central vein and plates of hepatic cells extending radially. Blood from peripherally located branches of the hepatic artery and vein perfuses the sinusoids. Bile ducts drain the bile canaliculi that pass between the hepatocytes. (From Bloom W, Fawcell DW. *A textbook of histology*, 10th ed. Philadelphia: Saunders, 1975; with permission.)

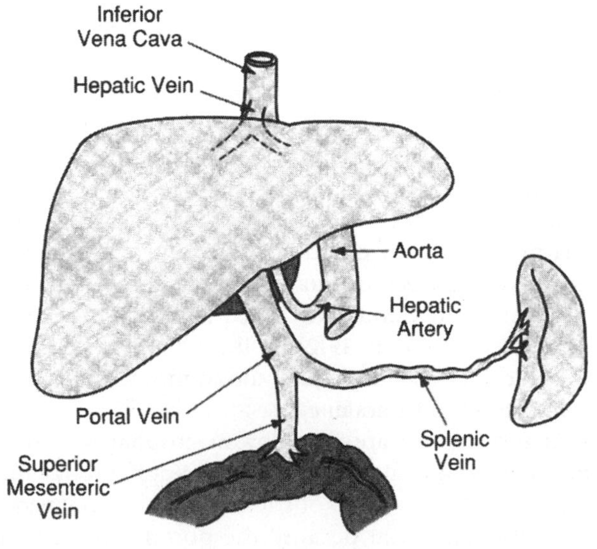

Figure 55–3. Schematic depiction of the dual afferent blood supply to the liver provided by the portal vein and hepatic artery.

hepatic arterial vasodilation and washout of the vasodilating material.

Halothane decreases hepatic oxygen supply more than isoflurane, enflurane, desflurane, or sevoflurane when administered in equal potent doses (Gelman et al., 1984). In contrast to the other volatile anesthetics, halothane preserves autoregulation of hepatic blood flow only to a limited extent and only when used in doses that do not decrease systemic blood pressure >20%. Surgical stimulation may further decrease hepatic blood flow, independent of the anesthetic drug administered. The greatest decreases in hepatic blood flow occur during intraabdominal operations, presumably due to mechanical interference of blood flow produced by retraction in the operative area, as well as the release of vasoconstricting substances such as catecholamines.

Reservoir Function

The liver normally contains approximately 500 mL of blood or approximately 10% of the total blood volume. An increase in central venous pressure causes back pressure, and the liver, being a distendible organ, may accommodate as much as 1 liter of extra blood. As such, the liver acts as a storage site when blood volume is excessive, as in congestive heart failure, and is capable of supplying extra blood when hypovolemia occurs. Indeed, the large hepatic veins and sinuses are constricted by stimulation from the sympathetic nervous system, discharging up to 350 mL of blood into the circulation. Therefore, the liver is the single most important source of additional blood during strenuous exercise or acute hemorrhage.

Bile Secretion

Hepatocytes continually form bile (500 mL daily) and then secrete it into bile canaliculi, which empty into progressively larger ducts ultimately reaching the common bile duct (see Fig. 55-2) (Bell et al., 1976). Between meals, the tone of the sphincter of Oddi, which guards the entrance of the common bile duct into the duodenum, is high. As a result, bile flow is diverted into the gallbladder, which has a capacity of 35 to 50 mL. The most potent stimulus for emptying the gallbladder is the presence of fat in the duodenum, which evokes the release of the hormone cholecystokinin by the duodenal mucosa. This hormone enters the circulation and passes to the gallbladder, where it causes selective contraction of the gallbladder smooth muscle. As a result, bile is forced from the gallbladder into the duodenum. When adequate amounts of fat are present, the gallbladder empties in approximately 1 hour.

The principal components of bile are bile salts, bilirubin, and cholesterol.

Bile Salts

Bile salts combine with lipids in the duodenum to form water-soluble complexes (micelles) that facilitate gastrointestinal absorption of fats (triglycerides) and fat-soluble vitamins. Once absorbed, bile salts return to the liver via the portal vein where they enter hepatocytes (enterohepatic circulation). In the absence of bile secretion, steatorrhea and a deficiency of vitamin K develop in a few days. Vitamin K is necessary for activation of several of the clotting factors that contain glutamic acid residues.

Bilirubin

After approximately 120 days, the cell membranes of erythrocytes rupture and the released hemoglobin is converted to bilirubin in reticuloendothelial cells (Fig. 55-4) (Guyton and Hall, 2000). The resulting bilirubin is released into the circulation and transported in combination with albumin to the liver. In hepatocytes, bilirubin dissociates from albumin and conjugates principally with glucuronic acid. Unlike conjugated bilirubin, unconjugated bilirubin may be neurotoxic and may even cause a rapidly fatal encephalopathy. In the gastrointestinal tract, bilirubin is converted by bacterial action mainly into urobilinogen.

Jaundice

Jaundice is the yellowish tint of body tissues that accompanies accumulation of bilirubin in extracellular fluid. Skin

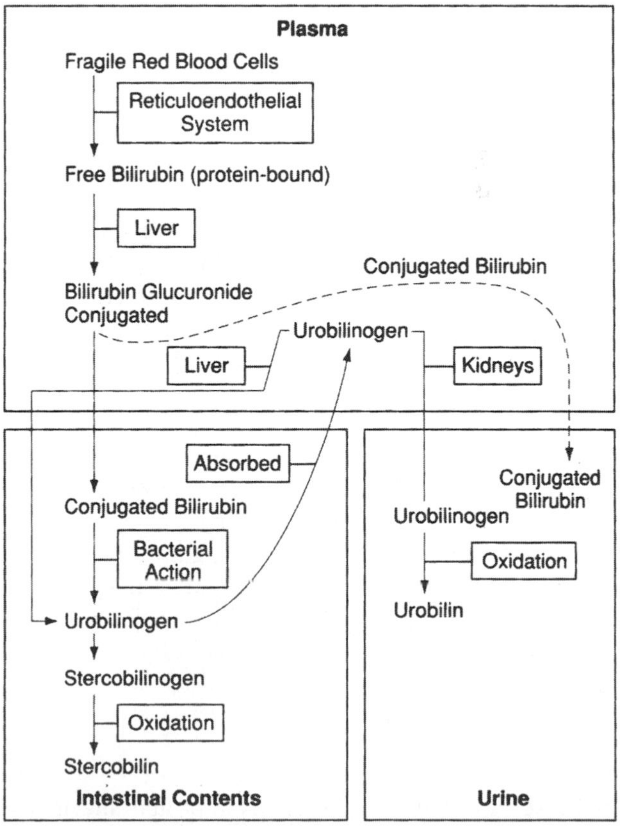

Figure 55–4. Schematic depiction of bilirubin formation and excretion. (From Guyton AC, Hall JE. *Textbook of medical physiology*, 10th ed. Philadelphia: Saunders, 2000; with permission.)

color usually begins to change when the plasma concentration of bilirubin increases to approximately three times normal. The most common types of jaundice are hemolytic jaundice, due to increased destruction of erythrocytes, and obstructive jaundice, due to obstruction of bile ducts.

Cholesterol

Cholesterol is an important component of cell walls (synthesized in tissues from acetate in a reaction catalyzed by beta-hydroxy beta-methylglutaryl coenzyme A) and is transported from the periphery to the liver as high density lipoproteins (HDL). Once cholesterol has reached the liver, it can be excreted in the bile in association with bile acids. Cholesterol in the bile may precipitate as gallstones if there is excess absorption of water in the gallbladder or the diet contains too much cholesterol. Gallstones occur in 10% to 20% of individuals; 85% are cholesterol stones.

Metabolic Functions

Metabolism of carbohydrates, lipids, and proteins depends on normal hepatic function (see Chapter 59). Furthermore, the liver is an important storage site for vitamins and iron (see Chapter 34). Degradation of certain hormones (catecholamines and corticosteroids), as well as drugs, is an important function of the liver. Hepatocytes are the principal site for synthesis of all the coagulation factors with the exception of von Willebrand factor and factor VIIIC. Because the half-life of clotting factors produced in the liver is short, coagulation is particularly sensitive to acute hepatocellular damage.

Carbohydrates

Regulation of blood glucose concentration is an important metabolic function of the liver. When hyperglycemia is present, glycogen is deposited in the liver, and when hypoglycemia occurs, glycogenolysis provides glucose. Amino acids can be converted to glucose by gluconeogenesis when the blood glucose concentration is decreased.

Lipids

The liver is responsible for beta-oxidation of fatty acids and formation of acetoacetic acid. Triglycerides are formed from the esterification of glycerol with three molecules of fatty acid. Pancreatic lipases and esterases are important in facilitating the absorption of dietary fats. After absorption, fat may be stored as triglycerides (reserve energy) or metabolized to energy. Lipoproteins, cholesterol, and phospholipids, such as lecithin, are formed in the liver. Synthesis of fats from carbohydrates and proteins also occurs in the liver.

Proteins

The most important liver functions in protein metabolism are oxidative deamination of amino acids, formation of urea for removal of ammonia, formation of plasma proteins and coagulation factors, and interconversions (transfer of one amino group to another amino acid) among different amino acids. Albumin formed in the liver is critically important for maintaining plasma oncotic pressure as well as providing an essential transport role. The half-time for albumin is about 21 days; therefore, plasma albumin concentrations are unlikely to be significantly altered in acute hepatic failure. Deamination of amino acids is required before these substances can be used for energy or converted into carbohydrates or fats. Decreases in portal vein blood flow, as may occur with the surgical creation of a portocaval shunt to treat esophageal varices, can result in fatal hepatic coma because of accumulation of ammonia.

GASTROINTESTINAL TRACT

The primary function of the gastrointestinal tract is to provide the body with a continual supply of water, electrolytes, and nutrients. To achieve this goal, the contents of the gastrointestinal tract must move through the entire system at an appropriate rate for digestive and absorptive functions to occur. Each part of the gastrointestinal tract is adapted for specific functions such as (a) passage of food in the esophagus, (b) storage of food in the stomach or fecal matter in the colon, (c) digestion of food in the stomach and small intestine, and (d) absorption of the digestive end-products and fluids in the small intestine and proximal parts of the colon. Overall, approximately 9 liters of fluid and secretions enters the gastrointestinal tract daily, and all but approximately 100 mL is absorbed by the small intestine and colon (Fig. 55-5) (Berne et al., 2004). The pH of gastrointestinal secretions varies widely (Table 55-2).

Anatomy

The smooth muscle of the gastrointestinal tract is a syncytium such that electrical signals originating in one smooth muscle fiber are easily propagated from fiber to fiber. Mechanical activity of the gastrointestinal tract is enhanced by stretch and parasympathetic nervous system stimulation, whereas sympathetic nervous system stimulation decreases mechanical activity to almost zero.

TABLE 55-2.
pH AND GASTROINTESTINAL SECRETIONS

Secretions	pH
Saliva	6–7
Gastric fluid	1.0–3.5
Bile	7–8
Pancreatic fluid	8.0–8.3
Small intestine	6.5–7.5
Colon	7.5–8.0

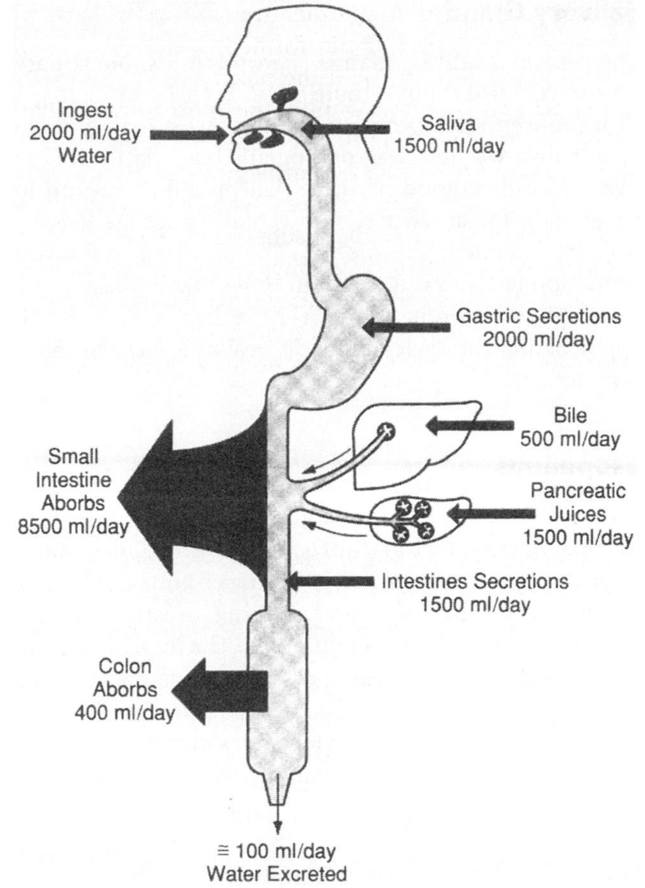

Figure 55–5. Overall fluid balance in the human gastrointestinal tract. Approximately 2 liters of water are ingested each day and approximately 7 liters of various secretions enter the gastrointestinal tract. Of this 9 liters, about 8.5 liters are absorbed from the small intestine. Approximately 0.5 liter passes to the colon, which normally absorbs 80% to 90% of the water presented to it. (Berne RM, Levy M, Koeppen BM, et al. *Physiology*, 5th ed. St Louis: Mosby, 2004; with permission.)

Tonic contraction of gastrointestinal smooth muscle at the pylorus, ileocecal valve, and anal sphincter helps regulate the rate at which materials move through the gastrointestinal tract. In these parts of the gastrointestinal tract, rhythmic movements (peristalsis) occur 3 to 12 times per minute to facilitate mixing and movement of food.

Blood Flow

Most of the blood flow to the gastrointestinal tract is to the mucosa to supply energy needed for producing intestinal secretions and absorbing digested materials. Blood flow parallels digestive activity of the gastrointestinal tract. Approximately 80% of portal vein blood flow originates from the stomach and gastrointestinal tract, with the remainder coming from the spleen and pancreas.

Stimulation of the parasympathetic nervous system increases local blood flow at the same time it increases glandular secretions. Conversely, stimulation of the sympathetic nervous system causes vasoconstriction of the arterial supply to the gastrointestinal tract. The decrease in blood flow, however, is transient, because local metabolic vasodilator mechanisms elicited by ischemia return blood flow toward normal. The importance of this transient sympathetic nervous system-induced vasoconstriction is that it permits shunting of blood from the gastrointestinal tract for brief periods during exercise, or when increased blood flow is needed by skeletal muscles or the heart.

Portal Venous Pressure

The liver offers modest resistance to blood flow from the portal venous system. As a result, the pressure in the portal vein averages 7 to 10 mm Hg, which is considerably higher than the almost zero pressure in the inferior vena cava. Cirrhosis of the liver, most frequently caused by alcoholism, is characterized by increased resistance to portal vein blood flow due to replacement of hepatic cells with fibrous tissue that contracts around the blood vessels. The gradual increase in resistance to portal vein blood flow produced by cirrhosis of the liver causes large collateral vessels to develop between the portal veins and the systemic veins. The most important of these collaterals are from the splenic veins to the esophageal veins. These collaterals may become so large that they protrude into the lumen of the esophagus, producing esophageal varicosities. The esophageal mucosa overlying these varicosities may become eroded, leading to life-threatening hemorrhage.

In the absence of the development of adequate collaterals, sustained increases in portal vein pressure may cause protein-containing fluid to escape from the surface of the mesentery, gastrointestinal tract, and liver into the peritoneal cavity. This fluid, known as *ascites,* is similar to plasma, and its high protein content causes an increased colloid osmotic pressure in the abdominal fluid. This high colloid osmotic pressure draws additional fluid from the surfaces of the gastrointestinal tract and mesentery into the peritoneal cavity.

Splenic Circulation

The splenic capsule in humans, in contrast to that in many lower animals, is nonmuscular, which limits the ability of the spleen to release stored blood in response to sympathetic nervous system stimulation. A small amount (150 to 200 mL) of blood is stored in the splenic venous sinuses and can be released by sympathetic nervous system-induced vasoconstriction of the splenic vessels. Release of this amount of blood into the systemic circulation is sufficient to increase the hematocrit 1% to 2%.

The spleen functions to remove erythrocytes from the circulation. This occurs when erythrocytes reenter the venous sinuses from the splenic pulp by passing through pores that may be smaller than the erythrocyte. Fragile cells do not withstand this trauma, and the released hemoglobin that results from their rupture is ingested by the reticuloendothelial cells of the spleen. These same reticuloendothelial cells also function, much like lymph nodes, to remove bacteria and parasites from the circulation. Indeed, asplenic patients are more prone to bacterial infections.

During fetal life, the splenic pulp produces erythrocytes in the same manner as does the bone marrow in the adult. As the fetus reaches maturity, however, this function of the spleen is lost.

Innervation

The gastrointestinal tract receives innervation from both divisions of the autonomic nervous system as well as from an intrinsic nervous system consisting of the myenteric plexus, or Auerbach plexus, and the submucous plexus, or Meissner plexus. In the absence of sympathetic nervous system or parasympathetic nervous system innervation, the motor and secretory activities of the gastrointestinal tract continue, reflecting the function of the intrinsic nervous system. Signals from the autonomic nervous system influence the activity of the intrinsic nervous system. For example, impulses from the parasympathetic nervous system increase intrinsic activity, whereas signals from the sympathetic nervous system decrease intrinsic activity. A large number of neuromodulatory substances act in the gastrointestinal tract.

The cranial component of parasympathetic nervous system innervation to the gastrointestinal tract (esophagus, stomach, pancreas, small intestine, colon to the level of the transverse colon) is by way of the vagus nerves. The distal portion of the colon is richly supplied by the sacral parasympathetics via the pelvic nerves from the hypogastric plexus. Fibers of the sympathetic nervous system destined for the gastrointestinal tract pass through ganglia such as the celiac ganglia.

Motility

The two types of gastrointestinal motility are mixing contractions and propulsive movements characterized as *peristalsis*. The usual stimulus for peristalsis is distension. Peristalsis occurs only weakly in portions of the gastrointestinal tract that have congenital absence of the myenteric plexus. Peristalsis is also decreased by increased parasympathetic nervous system activity and anticholinergic drugs.

Ileus

Trauma to the intestine or irritation of the peritoneum as follows abdominal operations causes adynamic (paralytic) ileus. Peristalsis returns to the small intestine in 6 to 8 hours, but colonic activity may take 2 to 3 days. Adynamic ileus can be relieved by a tube placed into the small intestine and aspiration of fluid and gas until the time when peristalsis returns.

Salivary Glands

The principal salivary glands (parotid and submaxillary) produce 0.5 to 1.0 mL/minute of saliva (pH 6 to 7), largely in response to parasympathetic nervous system stimulation. Saliva washes away pathogenic bacteria in the oral cavity as well as food particles that provide nutrition for bacteria. In the absence of saliva, oral tissues are likely to become ulcerated and infected. The bicarbonate ion concentration in saliva is two to four times that in plasma, and the high potassium content of saliva can result in hypokalemia and skeletal muscle weakness if excess salivation persists.

Esophagus

The esophagus serves as a conduit for passage of food from the pharynx to the stomach. The swallowing or deglutition center located in the medulla and lower pons inhibits the medullary ventilatory center, halting breathing at any point to allow swallowing to proceed. The upper and lower ends of the esophagus function as sphincters to prevent entry of air and acidic gastric contents, respectively, into the esophagus. The sphincters are known as the *upper esophageal (pharyngoesophageal) sphincter* and *lower esophageal (gastroesophageal) sphincter*.

Lower Esophageal Sphincter

The lower esophageal sphincter regulates the flow of food between the esophagus and the stomach. The sphincter mechanism at the lower end of the esophagus consists of the intrinsic smooth muscle of the distal esophagus and the skeletal muscle of the crural diaphragm (Mittal and Balaban, 1997). Under normal circumstances, the lower esophageal sphincter is approximately 4 cm long. The crural diaphragm, which forms the esophageal hiatus, encircles the proximal 2 cm of the sphincter. The intraluminal pressure of the esophagogastric junction is a measure of the strength of the antireflux barrier and is typically quantified with reference to the intragastric pressure (normal <7 mm Hg). Both the lower esophageal sphincter and the crural diaphragm contribute to the intragastric pressure. Muscle tone in the lower esophageal sphincter is the result of neurogenic and myogenic mechanisms. A substantial part of the neurogenic tone in humans is due to cholinergic innervation via the vagus nerves. The presynaptic neurotransmitter is acetylcholine, and the postsynaptic neurotransmitter is nitric oxide.

The normal lower esophageal sphincter pressure is 10 to 30 mm Hg at end-exhalation (Mittal and Balaban, 1997). Transient relaxation of the lower esophageal sphincter is a neural reflex mediated through the brainstem. Gastric barrier pressure is calculated as lower esophageal sphincter pressure minus intragastric pressure. This barrier pressure is considered the major mechanism in preventing reflux of gastric contents into the esophagus. Gastric distension, meals

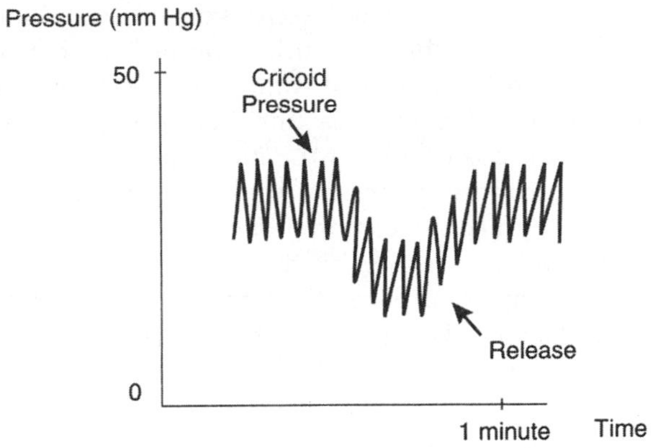

Figure 55–6. Application of cricoid pressure causes the lower esophageal sphincter pressure to decrease. (From Chassard D, Tournadre JP, Berrada KR, et al. Cricoid pressure decreases lower esophageal sphincter tone in anaesthetized pigs. *Can J Anaesth* 1996;43:414–417; with permission.)

high in fat, and pharyngeal stimulation are two possible mechanisms by which the afferent stimulus that initiates transient relaxation of the lower esophageal sphincter may originate (Mittal et al., 1995). Cricoid pressure decreases lower esophageal sphincter pressure, presumably reflecting stimulation of mechanoreceptors in the pharynx created by the external pressure on the cricoid cartilage (Fig. 55-6) (Brimacombe and Berry, 1997; Chassard et al., 1996; Tournadre et al., 1997). General anesthesia decreases lower esophageal sphincter pressure 7 to 14 mm Hg depending on the degree of skeletal muscle relaxation (Vanner et al., 1992). Normally, upper esophageal sphincter pressure prevents regurgitation into the pharynx in the awake state. The administration of anesthetic drugs may decrease upper esophageal sphincter pressure even before the loss of consciousness (Vanner et al., 1992).

The influence, if any, of changes in lower esophageal sphincter tone and barrier pressure (lower esophageal sphincter tone minus gastric pressure) and subsequent inhalation of gastric fluid during anesthesia remains undocumented (Hardy, 1988). Despite decreases in lower esophageal sphincter pressure associated with anesthesia, the incidence of gastroesophageal reflux as reflected by decreases in esophageal fluid pH is rare in patients undergoing elective operations (Illing et al., 1992; Joshi et al., 1996).

Gastroesophageal Reflux Disease

Transient relaxation of the lower esophageal sphincter, rather than decreased lower esophageal sphincter pressure, is the major mechanism of gastroesophageal reflux disease (GERD). Transient relaxation of the lower esophageal sphincter is associated with simultaneous inhibition of the sphincter and crural diaphragm. Some patients with gastroesophageal reflux have a weak lower esophageal sphincter, some have a weak crural diaphragm, and some have both. In GERD, the reflux of gastric fluid into the esophagus or oropharynx causes symptoms (esophagitis characterized as "heartburn") and/or tissue injury (esophageal strictures). It is estimated that approximately 20% of adults in the United States experience symptoms of GERD at least weekly and many patients with severe GERD have a hiatal hernia.

Atropine and morphine decrease the frequency of transient relaxation of the lower esophageal sphincter in normal patients through an unknown mechanism (Mittal and Balaban, 1997). Antisecretory drugs such as histamine (H_2) receptor antagonists or proton-pump inhibitors may be useful in treating gastroesophageal reflux. Therapy with a prokinetic drug such as metoclopramide may be effective. Patients with severe gastroesophageal reflux may benefit from surgical fundoplication of the esophagus via a laparoscopic technique.

Hiatal Hernia

The majority of patients with moderate-to-severe gastroesophageal reflux have a hiatal hernia in which a portion of the stomach herniates into the chest (Mittal and Balaban, 1997). Hiatal hernia may promote gastroesophageal reflux by trapping gastric acid in the hernia sac, which may then flow backward into the esophagus when the lower esophageal sphincter relaxes during swallowing. Hiatal hernia can also cause gastroesophageal reflux when contraction of the crural diaphragm during inspiration and other physical maneuvers lead to a compartmentalization of the stomach between the lower esophageal sphincter and the diaphragm. The presence of acid in the esophagus causes esophagitis, which decreases the lower esophageal sphincter pressure and impairs esophageal contractility.

Achalasia

Achalasia is the best characterized of all esophageal motility disorders reflecting degeneration of neurons in the wall of the esophagus, especially the nitric oxide-producing inhibitory neurons that affect the relaxation of esophageal smooth muscle necessary for opening the lower esophageal sphincter. The loss of inhibitory innervation in the lower esophageal sphincter causes basal sphincter pressure to increase and interferes with sphincter relaxation. In the body of the esophagus, the loss of intramural neurons manifests as aperistalsis. Dysphagia for both solid foods and liquids is the primary symptom of achalasia. A substantial number of patients complaining of heartburn and achalasia may be confused with GERD.

Achalasia can be confirmed with radiographic (barium swallow shows dilatation of the esophagus with a beaklike narrowing of esophagogastric junction), manometric, and endoscopic evaluation (often performed utilizing drugs to produce sedation). The diagnosis may be suggested by a routine radiograph of the chest that shows widening of the mediastinum from the dilated esophagus and the absence of the normal gastric air bubble, because lower esophageal sphincter contraction prevents swallowed air from entering the stomach.

Nitrates and calcium channel blockers relax the smooth muscle of the lower esophageal sphincter and may produce limited success in treating patients with achalasia. Pneumatic dilation therapy for achalasia (a large deflated balloon is passed through the mouth to the lower esophageal sphincter and then rapidly inflated) may be helpful. Esophageal perforation is a risk of this treatment. Surgical myotomy of the lower esophageal sphincter performed laparoscopically often results in excellent relief but may be followed by GERD. For this reason, the myotomy may be combined with an antireflux procedure (fundoplication). Endoscopic injection of botulinum toxin into the area of the lower esophageal sphincter blocks the excitatory (acetylcholine-releasing) neurons that contribute to lower esophageal sphincter tone. Unfortunately, the effect is usually short-lived (less than 6 to 12 months).

A patient with achalasia presenting for surgery unrelated to the underlying esophageal motility disorder represents a potential risk for pulmonary aspiration during the perioperative period.

Stomach

The stomach is a specialized organ of the digestive tract that stores and processes food for absorption (Fig. 55-7). The ability to secrete hydrogen ions in the form of hydrochloric acid is a hallmark of gastric function. The secretory unit of gastric mucosa is the oxyntic glandular mucosa. The stomach is richly innervated by the vagus nerves and celiac plexus.

Gastric Secretions

Total daily gastric secretion is approximately 2 liters with a pH of 1.0 to 3.5. The stomach secretes only a few milliliters of gastric fluid each hour during the periods between digestion. Strong emotional stimulation, such as occurs preoperatively, can increase interdigestive secretion of highly acidic gastric fluid to >50 mL/hour. The major secretions are hydrochloric acid, pepsinogen, intrinsic factor, and mucus. Mucous secretion protects the gastric mucosa from mechanical and chemical destruction. Substances that disrupt the mucosal barrier and cause gastric irritation include ethanol and drugs that inhibit prostaglandin synthesis (aspirin, nonsteroidal antiinflammatory drugs).

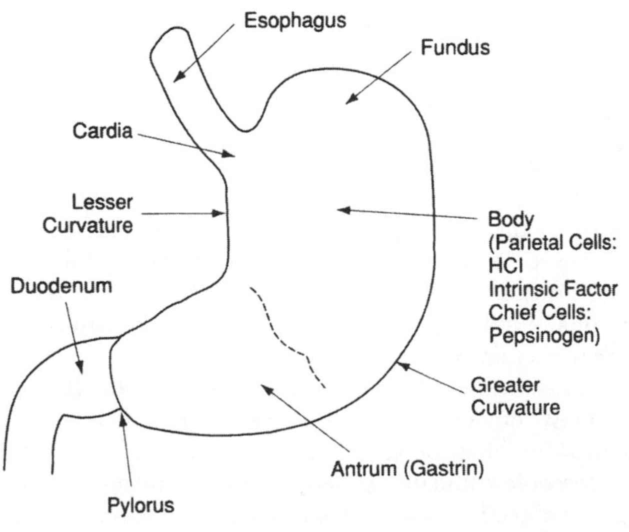

Figure 55–7. Anatomy of the stomach indicating the site of production of secretions. Mucus is secreted in all parts of the stomach.

Parietal Cells

Parietal cells secrete an hydrogen ion-containing solution with a pH of approximately 0.8. At this pH, the hydrogen ion concentration is approximately 3 million times that present in the arterial blood. Hydrochloric acid kills bacteria, aids protein digestion, provides the necessary pH for pepsin to start protein digestion, and stimulates the flow of bile and pancreatic juice.

Secretion of hydrochloric acid depends on stimulation of receptors in the membrane of parietal cells by histamine, acetylcholine (vagal stimulation), and gastrin (Wolfe and Soll, 1988). All of these receptors increase the transport of hydrogen ions into the gastric lumen by the hydrogen-potassium adenosine triphosphatase (ATPase) enzyme system (Fig. 55-8) (Ganong, 2003). Activation of one receptor type potentiates the response of the other receptors to stimulation. Blockade of receptors with specific antagonist drugs produces effective decreases in acid transport responses

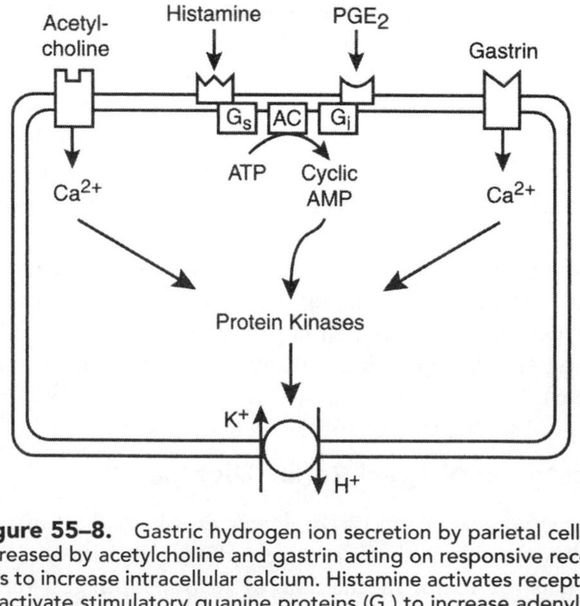

Figure 55–8. Gastric hydrogen ion secretion by parietal cells is increased by acetylcholine and gastrin acting on responsive receptors to increase intracellular calcium. Histamine activates receptors to activate stimulatory guanine proteins (G_s) to increase adenylate cyclase (AC) activity, whereas prostaglandins (PGE_2) activate inhibitory guanine proteins (G_i) to decrease AC activity. Cyclic adenosine monophosphate (cyclic AMP) and calcium act via protein kinases to increase transport of hydrogen ions into the gastric lumen. (Ganong WF. *Review of medical physiology*, 21st ed. New York, Lange Medical Books/McGraw Hill, 2003; with permission.)

by removing the potentiating effect of stimulation of these receptors on the responses to other stimuli (see Chapter 21). Blockade of muscarinic receptors is produced by atropine or the more specific anticholinergic pirenzepine. Gastrin receptors can be inhibited by proglumide. Alternatively, the hydrogen-potassium ATPase enzyme system can be inhibited by omeprazole. Pharmacologic manipulation of gastric fluid pH has special implications in the management of patients considered to be at risk for pulmonary aspiration during the perioperative period.

Intrinsic factor, which is essential for absorption of vitamin B_{12} from the ileum, is secreted by parietal cells. For this reason, destruction of parietal cells as associated with chronic gastritis produces achlorhydria and often pernicious anemia.

Chief Cells

Pepsinogens secreted by chief cells undergo cleavage to pepsins in the presence of hydrochloric acid. Pepsins are proteolytic enzymes important for the digestion of proteins.

G Cells

Gastrin is secreted by gastric antral cells (G cells) into the circulation, which carries this hormone to responsive receptors in parietal cells to stimulate gastric hydrogen ion secretion. Gastrin also increases the tone of the lower esophageal sphincter and relaxes the pylorus.

Gastric Fluid Volume and Rate of Gastric Emptying

Neural and humoral mechanisms greatly influence gastric fluid volume and gastric-emptying time (Houghton et al., 1988; Minami and McCallum, 1984; Read and Houghton, 1989). In general, parasympathetic nervous system stimulation enhances gastric fluid secretion and motility, whereas sympathetic nervous system stimulation has an opposite effect. The elimination of nonnutrient liquids is an exponential process (volume of liquid emptied per unit of time is directly proportional to the volume present in the stomach), whereas the emptying of solids is a linear process (Fig. 55-9) (Minami and McCallum, 1984). In this regard, emptying of liquids from the stomach begins within 1 minute of ingestion, whereas emptying of solids typically begins after a lag time of 15 to 137 minutes (median 49 minutes) (Houghton et al., 1988). Gastric emptying in healthy, term, nonobese parturients is not delayed after ingestion of 300 mL of water (Wong et al., 2002). Contraction of the gastric fundus is responsible for facilitating the emptying of liquids, whereas antral contractions control the emptying of solids (Read and Houghton, 1989). It is generally thought that the delay in gastric emptying of solids is caused by the time necessary for antral contractions to break solids down into small enough particles to exit

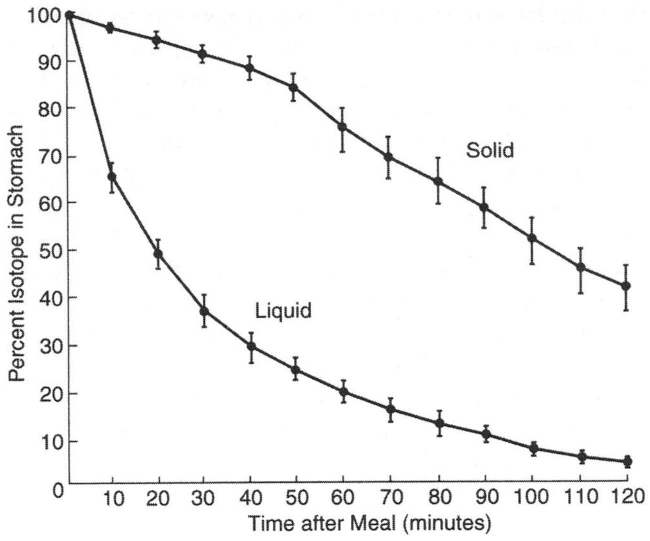

Figure 55–9. Gastric emptying of liquids is exponential, whereas emptying of solids is a linear process. (From Minami H, McCallum RW. The physiology of gastric emptying in humans. *Gastroenterology* 1984;86:1592–1610; with permission.)

through the pylorus. Clinical manifestations of delayed gastric emptying include anorexia, persistent fullness after meals, abdominal pain, and nausea and vomiting.

Several factors affect the rate of gastric emptying (Minami and McCallum, 1984). The primary determinant of the emptying of liquids from the stomach is volume. In addition to volume, another factor that influences the rate of gastric emptying is the composition of the liquids. Emptying of neutral, isoosmolar, and calorically inert solutions is rapid (250 mL of 500 mL of normal saline is emptied in 12 minutes). A small amount of water (up to 150 mL) to facilitate administration of oral medications shortly before the induction of anesthesia does not produce sustained increases in gastric fluid volume and could even contribute to gastric emptying (Soreide et al., 1993). Solutions that are hypertonic or contain acid, fat, or certain amino acids all retard gastric emptying. High lipid and/or caloric content (glucose) slows the emptying of solids from the stomach (Collins et al., 1983; Houghton et al., 1988).

The basic defect of diabetic gastroparesis appears to be one of impaired neural control. Delayed gastric emptying of solids is the most consistent abnormality in diabetics with gastroparesis and is the most predictably responsive to pharmacologic manipulation. Nevertheless, as diabetes progresses, it is possible that gastric retention of liquids will also occur (Minami and McCallum, 1984). Patients with GERD and documented slowing of gastric emptying of solids have been shown to have normal gastric-emptying rates for liquids. Most patients with slowed gastric emptying of solids in association with GERD do not demonstrate symptoms such as nausea and vomiting, which are usually associated with gastric stasis. The existence of delayed gastric emptying in gastric ulcer disease is controversial. Some data suggest a slowing of gastric emptying of solids but not liquids in the presence of gastric ulcers. Although obesity and pregnancy are often assumed to slow gastric emptying, there are also data that fail to confirm this slowing, whereas other data suggest accelerated gastric emptying in obese individuals (Macfie et al., 1991; O'Sullivan et al., 1987; Sandhar et al., 1992; Wisen and Johansson, 1992). Gastrointestinal transit time has been shown to vary during the menstrual cycle, with prolongation occurring during the luteal phase when progesterone levels are increased. Acute viral gastroenteritis has been associated with delayed gastric emptying.

Certain drugs, including opioids, beta-adrenergic agonists, and tricyclic antidepressants, may slow gastric emptying. Aluminum hydroxide antacid may slow gastric emptying. Alcohol, at least in concentrations present in wine, does not significantly affect gastric emptying of liquids or solids. Higher concentrations of alcohol, such as present in whiskey, do cause slowing of gastric emptying. The mechanism of this slowing is not clear but may be due to hyperosmolarity, changes in gastric acid secretion, or damage to gastric mucosa. Total parenteral nutrition may cause gastric stasis. Elemental diets, probably due to their high concentration of amino acids and hyperosmolarity, take longer to empty from the stomach than does blenderized food of comparable caloric composition. Cigarette smoking has been shown to delay emptying of solids although it may accelerate emptying of liquids. Gastric prokinetic drugs such as metoclopramide may speed the emptying of solids and liquids.

Gastric Emptying Prior to Elective Surgery

Clear liquids can be administered to adult patients scheduled for elective operations until 2 hours before induction of anesthesia without increasing gastric fluid volume. It takes 3 to 4 hours for the stomach to empty following a light breakfast (one slice of white bread with butter and jam, 150 mL of coffee without milk or sugar, 150 mL of pulp-free orange juice) (Soreide et al., 1996). These data are consistent with the recommendation that a 6-hour fast should be enforced after a light breakfast (Warner et al., 1999).

Opioid-Induced Slowing of Gastric Emptying

Opioid peptides and their receptors are found throughout the gastrointestinal system with particularly high concentrations in the gastric antrum and proximal duodenum. Central and peripheral mu opioid receptors can regulate gastric emptying, and opioid-induced delay in gastric emptying can be reversed with naloxone, which acts simultaneously at both central and peripheral sites. The demonstration that methylnaltrexone, a selective peripheral-acting opioid antagonist, attenuates morphine-induced changes in the rate of gastric emptying indicates that peripheral opioid receptors modulate this response in humans (see Chapter 3) (Murphy et al., 1997).

Measurement of the Rate of Gastric Emptying

The rate of gastric emptying can be evaluated by a noninvasive electrical bioimpedance method (epigastric impedance method) and indirectly by the acetaminophen absorption technique (McClelland and Sutton, 1985). Dye dilution techniques and scintigraphy also have been used to assess the rate of gastric emptying in humans (Sutton et al., 1985).

Electrical Bioimpedance Technique

The basis of the bioimpedance technique is that after ingestion of fluids with a different conductivity from body tissues, the impedance to an electrical current through the upper abdomen changes. Electrodes are placed on the abdomen and back, and a constant current is applied. Impedance increases as the stomach fills and decreases as it empties. The slope of the plot of impedance versus time, allows calculation of the emptying half-time of a meal.

The principal benefit of the bioimpedance method is that it is noninvasive and avoids gastric intubation or exposure to radioactivity. A limitation is that the subject must not move because alterations in body posture may alter baseline impedance readings and thus invalidate the recording. Another possible source of error is that gastric secretions might decrease the conductivity of gastric contents, thus reducing total surface impedance and producing inaccurate emptying rates. For this reason, deionized water may be used as the "test meal" because it does not appear to provoke sufficient gastric secretions to alter impedance (Murphy et al., 1997).

Acetaminophen Absorption Test

The appearance of acetaminophen in the systemic circulation is an indirect method of determining the rate of gastric emptying. The area under the plasma concentration curve of acetaminophen after oral administration is determined by the rate of gastric emptying, because acetaminophen is not absorbed from the stomach but is rapidly absorbed from the small intestine.

Absorption from the Stomach

The stomach is a poor absorptive area of the gastrointestinal tract because it lacks the villus structure characteristic of absorptive membranes. As a result, only highly lipid-soluble liquids such as ethanol and some drugs such as aspirin can be significantly absorbed from the stomach.

Vomiting

Vomiting is coordinated by the vomiting center in the medulla. This center receives input from multiple sites including the chemoreceptor trigger zone in the floor of the fourth ventricle, from the vestibular apparatus, from cortical centers and the gastrointestinal tract. The blood-brain barrier is poorly developed around the chemoreceptor trigger zone and emetic substances present in the circulation are readily accessible to this site. Serotonin acting at 5-hydroxytryptamine receptors (5-HT_3) is an important emetic signal via neural pathways from the gastrointestinal tract ending at the chemoreceptor trigger zone. Likewise, dopamine and acetylcholine may provide emetic signals to the chemoreceptor trigger zone. Pharmacologic antagonism of these emetic signals results in antiemetic effects. The role of specific opioid receptors in emetic responses is unresolved. Following stimulation of the vomiting center (directly or indirectly via neural pathways), vomiting is mediated by efferent pathways including the vagus and phrenic nerves, and innervation of the abdominal musculature. The initial manifestation of vomiting often involves nausea in which gastric peristalsis is reduced or absent and the tone of the upper small intestine is increased and gastric reflux occurs. Ultimately, the upper portion of the stomach relaxes while the pylorus constricts and the coordinated contraction of the diaphragm and abdominal muscles leads to expulsion of gastric contents. Risk factors for postoperative nausea and vomiting include female gender, young age (children), and obesity (perhaps reflecting emetic anesthetic drugs stored in adipose tissue) (Borgeat et al., 2003).

Small Intestine

The small intestine consists of the duodenum (from the pylorus to the ligament of Treitz), the jejunum, and the ileum (ending at the ileocecal valve). There is no distinct anatomic boundary between the jejunum and ileum, but the first 40% of small intestine after the ligament of Treitz is often considered the jejunum. The small intestine is presented with approximately 9 liters of fluid daily (2 liters from the diet and the rest representing gastrointestinal secretions), but only 1 to 2 liters of chyme enters the colon. The small intestine is the site of most of the digestion and absorption of proteins, fats, and carbohydrates (Table 55-3).

Chyme moves through the 5 m of small intestine at an average rate of 1 cm/minute. As a result, it takes 3 to 5 hours for chyme to pass from the pylorus to the ileocecal valve. On reaching the ileocecal valve, chyme may remain in place for several hours until the person eats another meal. An inflamed appendix can increase the tone of the ileocecal valve to the extent that emptying of the ileum ceases. Conversely, gastrin causes relaxation of the ileocecal valve. When more than 50% of the small intestine is resected, the absorption of nutrients and vitamins is so compromised that development of malnutrition is likely.

Secretions of the Small Intestine

Mucus glands (Brunner glands) present in the first few centimeters of the duodenum secrete mucus to protect the duodenal wall from damage by acidic gastric fluid. Stimulation of the sympathetic nervous system inhibits the protective mucus-producing function of these glands, which may be one of the factors that causes this area of the gastrointestinal tract to be the most frequent site of peptic ulcer disease.

The crypts of Lieberkühn contain epithelial cells that produce up to 2 liters daily of secretions that lack digestive enzymes and mimic extracellular fluid, having a pH of 6.5 to 7.5. This fluid provides a watery vehicle for absorption of substances from chyme as it passes through the small intestine. The most important mechanism for regulation of small intestine secretions is local neural reflexes, especially those initiated by distension produced by the presence of chyme.

The epithelial cells in the crypts of Lieberkühn continually undergo mitosis, with an average life cycle of approximately 5 days. This rapid growth of new cells allows prompt repair of any excoriation that occurs in the mucosa. This rapid turnover of cells also explains the vulnerability of the gastrointestinal epithelium to chemotherapeutic drugs (see Chapter 29).

The epithelial cells in the mucosa of the small intestine contain digestive enzymes that most likely are responsi-

TABLE 55-3.
SITE OF ABSORPTION

	Duodenum	Jejunum	Ileum	Colon
Glucose	++	+++	++	0
Amino acids	++	+++	++	0
Fatty acids	+++	++	+	0
Bile salts	0	+	+++	0
Water–soluble vitamins	+++	++	0	0
Vitamin B_{12}	0	+	+++	0
Sodium	+++	++	+++	+++
Potassium	0	0	+	++
Hydrogen	0	+	++	++
Chloride	+++	++	+	0
Calcium	+++	++	+	?

ble for digestion of food substances because they are absorbed across the gastrointestinal epithelium. These enzymes include peptidases for splitting peptides into amino acids, enzymes for splitting disaccharides into monosaccharides, and intestinal lipases.

Absorption from the Small Intestine

Mucosal folds (valvulae conniventes), microvilli (brush border), and epithelial cells provide an absorptive area of approximately 250 m^2 in the small intestine for nearly all the nutrients and electrolytes as well as approximately 95% of all the water. Daily absorption of sodium is 25 to 35 g, emphasizing the rapidity with which total body sodium depletion can occur if excessive intestinal secretions are lost as occurs with extreme diarrhea. Active transport of sodium ions in the small intestine is important for the absorption of glucose, which is the physiologic basis for treating diarrhea by oral administration of saline solutions containing glucose. Bacterial toxins as from cholera and staphylococci can stimulate the chloride-bicarbonate ion exchange mechanism, resulting in life-threatening diarrhea consisting of loss of sodium, bicarbonate, and an isosmotic equivalent of water.

Colon

The functions of the colon are absorption of water and electrolytes from the chyme and storage of feces. A test meal reaches the cecum in approximately 4 hours and then passes slowly through the colon during the next 6 to 12 hours, during which time 1 to 2 liters of chyme are converted to 200 to 250 g of feces (Fig. 55-10). The circular muscle of the colon constricts and, at the same time, strips of longitudinal muscle (tinea coli) contract, causing the unstimulated portion of the colon to bulge outward into baglike sacs, or haustrations. Vagal stimulation causes segmental contractions of the proximal part of the colon and stimulation of the pelvic nerves causes explosive movements. Activation of the sympathetic nervous system inhibits colonic activity. Bacteria are predictably present in the colon.

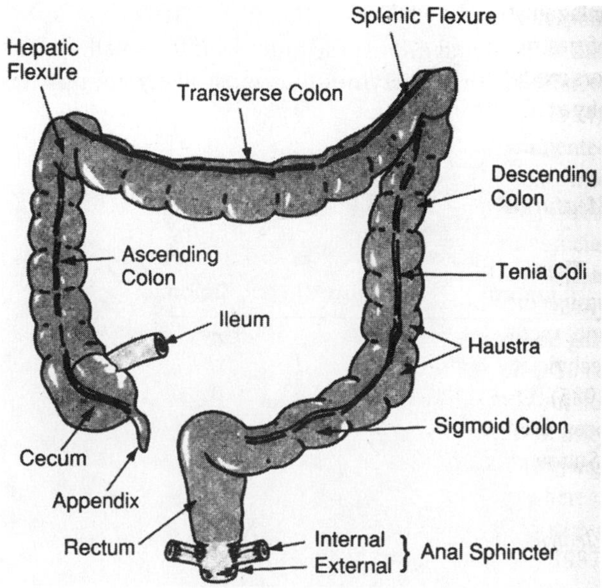

Figure 55–10. Anatomy of the colon.

Secretions of the Colon

Epithelial cells lining the colon secrete almost exclusively mucus, which protects the intestinal mucosa against trauma. The alkalinity of the mucus due to the presence of large amounts of bicarbonate ions provides a barrier to keep acids that are formed in the feces from attacking the intestinal wall. Irritation of a segment of colon as occurs with bacterial infection causes the mucosa to secrete large quantities of water and electrolytes in addition to mucus, diluting the irritating factors, and causing rapid movement of feces toward the anus. The resulting diarrhea may result in dehydration and cardiovascular collapse.

Pancreas

The pancreas lies parallel to and beneath the stomach, serving as both an endocrine (insulin or glucagon) and exocrine gland. Exocrine secretions (approximately 1.5 liters daily) are rich in bicarbonate ions to neutralize duodenal contents and digestive enzymes to initiate breakdown of carbohydrates, proteins, and fats.

Regulation of Pancreatic Secretions

Pancreatic secretions are regulated more by hormonal than neural mechanisms. For example, secretin is released by duodenal mucosa in response to hydrochloric acid. This hormone enters the circulation and causes the pancreas to produce large amounts of alkaline fluid necessary to neutralize the acidic pH of gastric fluid. In addition to the release of secretions, the presence of food in the duodenum causes the release of a second polypeptide hormone, cholecystokinin. Cholecystokinin also enters the circulation and causes the pancreas to secrete digestive enzymes (trypsins, amylase, lipases). Trypsins are activated in the gastrointestinal tract by the enzyme enterokinase, which is secreted by the gastrointestinal mucosa when chyme is exposed to the mucosa. Damage to the pancreas or blockade of a pancreatic duct may cause pooling of proteolytic enzymes, resulting in acute pancreatitis due to autodigestion by these enzymes. In general, pancreatic secretions are stimulated by the parasympathetic nervous system and inhibited by the sympathetic nervous system.

REFERENCES

Alison MR, Poulsom R, Jeffery R, et al. Hepatocytes from non-hepatic adult stem cells. *Nature* 2000;406:257–60.

Bell GH, Emslie-Smith D, Paterson CR. *Textbook of physiology and bio-*

chemistry, 9th ed. New York: Churchill Livingstone, 1976.

Berne RM, Levy M, Koeppen BM, et al. *Physiology*, 5th ed. St Louis: Mosby, 2004.

Bloom W, Fawcell DW. *A textbook of histology*, 10th ed. Philadelphia: Saunders, 1975.

Borgeat A, Ekatodramis G, Schenker CA. Postoperative nausea and vomiting in regional anesthesia. *Anesthesiology* 2003;98:530–547.

Brimacombe JR, Berry AM. Cricoid pressure. *Can J Anaesth* 1997;44: 414–425.

Chassard D, Tournadre JP, Berrada KR, et al. Cricoid pressure decreases lower oesophageal sphincter tone in anaesthetized pigs. *Can J Anaesth* 1996;43:414–417.

Collins PJ, Horowitz M, Cook DJ, et al. Gastric emptying in normal subjects—a reproducible technique using a single scintillation camera and computer system. *Gut* 1983;24:1117–1125.

Ganong WF. *Review of medical physiology*, 21st ed. Lange Medical Books, New York: McGraw Hill, 2003.

Gelman SI, Fowler KC, Smith LR. Liver circulation and function during isoflurane and halothane anesthesia. *Anesthesiology* 1984;61: 726–730.

Guyton AC, Hall JE. *Textbook of medical physiology*, 10th ed. Philadelphia: W.B. Saunders, 2000.

Hardy JF. Large volume gastroesophageal reflux: a rationale for risk reduction in the perioperative period. *Can J Anaesth* 1988;35: 162–173.

Houghton LA, Read NW, Horowitz HM, et al. Relationship of the motor activity of the antrum, pylorus, and duodenum to gastric emptying of a solid-liquid mixed meal. *Gastroenterology* 1988;94: 1285–1291.

Illing L, Ducan PG, Yip R. Gastroesophageal reflux during anaesthesia. *Can J Anaesth* 1992;39:466–470.

Joshi GP, Morrison SG, Okonkwo NA, et al. Continuous hypopharyngeal pH measurements in spontaneously breathing anesthetized outpatients: laryngeal mask airway versus tracheal intubation. *Anesth Analg* 1996;82:254–257.

Macfie AG, Magide AD, Richmond MN, et al. Gastric emptying in pregnancy. *Br J Anaesth* 1991;67:54–57.

MacGregor IL, Gueller R, Watts HD, et al. The effect of acute hyperglycemia on gastric emptying in man. *Gastroenterology* 1976;70: 190–196.

McClelland GR, Sutton JA. Epigastric impedance: a noninvasive method for the assessment of gastric emptying and motility. *Gut* 1985;26:607–614.

Minami H, McCallum RW. The physiology and pathophysiology of gastric emptying in humans. *Gastroenterology* 1984;86:1592–1610.

Mittal RK, Balaban DH. The esophagogastric junction. *N Engl J Med* 1997;336:924–932.

Mittal RK, Holloway RH, Penagini R, et al. Transient lower esophageal sphincter relaxation. *Gastroenterology* 1995;109:601–610.

Murphy DB, Sutton JA, Prescott LF, et al. Opioid-induced delay in gastric emptying: a peripheral mechanism in humans. *Anesthesiology* 1997; 87:765–770.

O'Sullivan GM, Sutton AJ, Thompson SA, et al. Noninvasive measurement of gastric emptying in obstetric patients. *Anesth Analg* 1987; 66:505–511.

Read NW, Houghton LA. Physiology of gastric emptying and pathophysiology of gastroparesis. *Gastroenterol Clin North Am* 1989;18: 359–373.

Sandhar BK, Elliott RH, Windram I, et al. Peripartum changes in gastric emptying. *Anaesthesia* 1992;47:196–198.

Soreide E, Holst-Larsen K, Reite K, et al. Effects of giving water 20–450 mL with oral diazepam premedication 1–2 h before operation. *Br J Anaesth* 1993;71:503–506.

Soreide E, Hausken T, Soreide A, Steen PA. Gastric emptying of a light hospital breakfast. A study using real time ultrasonography. *Acta Anaesthesiologica Scandinavica* 1996;40:549–553.

Sutton JA, Thompson S, Sobnack R. Measurement of gastric emptying rates by radioactive isotope scanning and epigastric impedance. *Lancet* 1985;1:898–900.

Tournadre JP, Chassard D, Berrada KR, et al. Cricoid cartilage pressure decreases lower esophageal sphincter tone. *Anesthesiology* 1997; 86:7–9.

Vanner RG, O'Dwyer JP, Pryle BJ, et al. Upper oesophageal sphincter pressure and the effect of cricoid pressure. *Anaesthesia* 1992;47: 95–100.

Warner MA, Caplan RA, Epstein BS, et al. Practice guidelines for preoperative fasting and the use of pharmacologic agents to reduce the risk of pulmonary aspiration: application to healthy patients undergoing elective procedures. *Anesthesiology* 1999;90: 896–905.

Wisen O, Johansson C. Gastrointestinal function in obesity: motility, secretion, and absorption following a liquid test meal. *Metabolism* 1992;41:390–395.

Wolfe MM, Soll AH. The physiology of gastric acid secretion. *N Engl J Med* 1988;319:1707–1715.

Wong CA, Loffredi M, Ganchiff JN, et al. Gastric emptying of water in term pregnancy. *Anesthesiology* 2002;96:1395–1400.

Skeletal and Smooth Muscle

56

Muscle is generally classified as skeletal, smooth, or cardiac. Skeletal muscle is responsible for voluntary actions, whereas smooth muscle and cardiac muscle subserve functions related to the cardiovascular, respiratory, gastrointestinal, and genitourinary systems. Muscle composes 45% to 50% of total body mass, with skeletal muscles accounting for approximately 40% of body mass. An estimated 250 million cells are present in the more than 400 skeletal muscles of humans. Muscle cells are highly specialized cells for the conversion of chemical energy into mechanical energy. Inappropriate activity of smooth muscle is involved in many illnesses including hypertension, atherosclerosis, asthma, and disorders of the gastrointestinal tract.

SKELETAL MUSCLE

Skeletal muscle is made up of individual muscle fibers; each fiber being a single cell. There are no syncytial bridges between cells. Cross striations characteristic of skeletal muscles are due to differences in the refractive indexes of the various parts of the muscle fiber. Each skeletal muscle fiber comprises thousands of fibrils that consist of the contractile proteins known as *myosin, actin, tropomyosin,* and *troponin*. Myofibrils are suspended inside skeletal muscle fibers in a matrix known as *sarcoplasm*. The sarcoplasm contains mitochondria, enzymes, potassium ions, and extensive endoplasmic reticulum known as the *sarcoplasmic reticulum*. The cell membrane of the muscle fiber is known as the *sarcolemma*. At the ends of skeletal muscle fibers, surfaces of the sarcolemma fuse with tendon fibers, which form tendons that insert into bones. *Hypertrophy* is synthesis of new myofibrils; *hyperplasia* is formation of more cells. Skeletal muscle has only limited capacity to form new cells.

Excitation-Contraction Coupling

The process by which depolarization of the sarcolemma and propagation of an action potential initiates skeletal muscle contraction is described as *excitation-contraction coupling*. An action potential occurs only in response to motor nerve activity and reflects opening of fast channels in the membrane, allowing rapid inward movement of sodium ions followed by outward movement of potassium ions and depolarization. The resting membrane potential of skeletal muscle is approximately −90 mv. The action potential lasts 2 to 4 ms and is conducted along the muscle fiber at approximately 5 m/s, which is slower than the velocity of conduction in large myelinated nerve fibers.

Motor neurons initiate contracton of skeletal muscle fibers by producing action potentials in the fibers. The action potential is transmitted deep into skeletal muscle to all myofibrils by way of transverse (T) tubules. As action potentials pass down T-tubules, dihydropyridine receptors in the T-tubules undergo conformational changes that result in the opening of sarcoplasmic calcium channels (ryanodine receptors) which in turn causes release of calcium ions from the sarcoplasmic reticulum into the immediate vicinity of all myofibrils. The calcium ions bind to troponin, thus abolishing the inhibitory effect of troponin on the interaction between myosin and actin. As a result, the head of a myosin molecule links to an actin molecule (cross-bridging), producing movement of myosin on actin, which is repeated in serial fashion to produce contraction of the muscle fiber (Fig. 56-1) (Ganong, 2003). The immediate source of chemical energy for contraction is provided by adenosine triphosphate (ATP). Hydrolysis of ATP to adenosine diphosphate (ADP) is provided by adenosine triphosphatase (ATPase) activity present in the heads of the myosin molecules where they are in contact with actin. Each interaction of myosin with actin results in hydrolysis of ATP. The amount of ATP present in a skeletal muscle fiber is sufficient to maintain full contraction for <1 s. This emphasizes the importance of rephosphorylation of ADP to form ATP.

Shortly after releasing calcium, the sarcoplasmic reticulum begins to reaccumulate this ion by an active transport

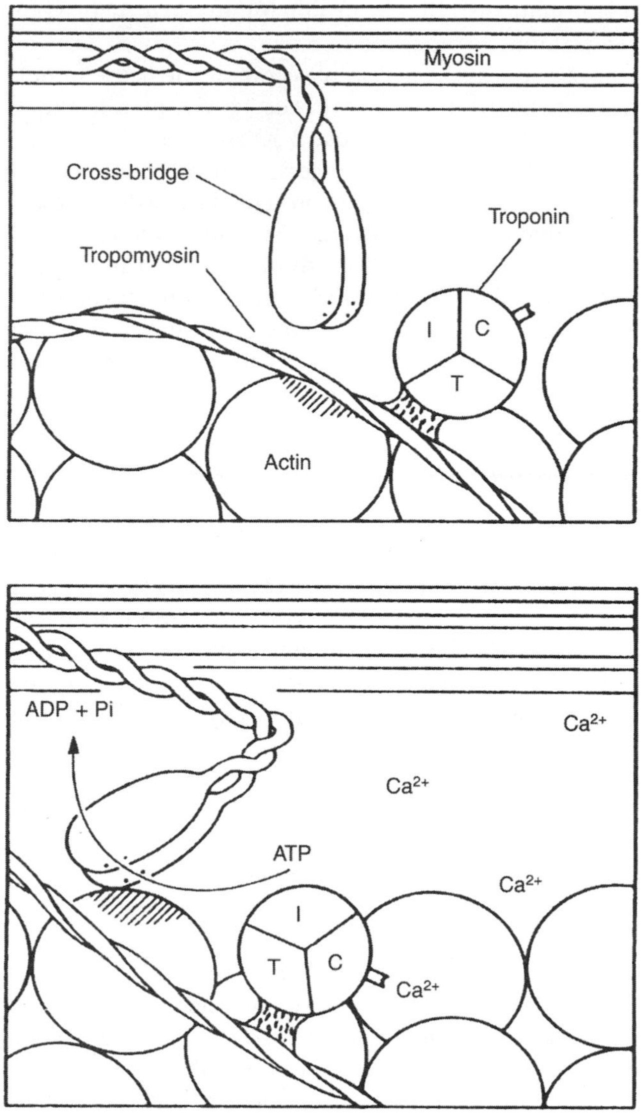

Figure 56-1. Contraction of skeletal muscle is initiated by attachment of calcium ions (Ca^{2+}) to troponin, leading to hydrolysis of adenosine triphosphate (ATP) and cross-bridging between actin and myosin. (From Ganong WF. *Review of medical physiology*, 21st ed. Lange Medical Books, New York: McGraw-Hill, 2003; with permission.)

process (calcium pump). This transport mechanism can concentrate calcium up to 2,000-fold inside the sarcoplasmic reticulum. ATP provides the energy for calcium ion transport. Once the calcium concentration in the sarcoplasm has been lowered sufficiently, cross-bridging between myosin and actin ceases and the skeletal muscle relaxes. Failure of the calcium ion pump results in sustained skeletal muscle contraction and marked increases in heat production, leading to malignant hyperthermia. The gene for this calcium ion channel (ryanodine receptor) is on chromosome 19 (McCarthy et al., 1990). A mutation in this gene is speculated to be responsible for malignant hyperthermia susceptibility in some patients.

Rigor mortis reflects ATP depletion and failure of the calcium ion transport mechanism, leading to permanent cross-bridging between myosin and actin. Skeletal muscles remain rigid until muscle proteins are destroyed. This occurs 15 to 25 hours after death and is due to autolysis caused by enzymes released from lysosomes.

Neuromuscular Junction

The *neuromuscular junction* is the site at which presynaptic motor nerve endings meet the postsynaptic membranes of skeletal muscles (motor end plates) (see Fig. 8-5). The motor nerve ending branches to form a complex of nerve terminals that invaginate into the skeletal muscle fiber but lie outside the sarcolemma. The space between the nerve terminal and the sarcolemma is known as the *synaptic cleft* and is filled with extracellular fluid. Acetylcholine is synthesized in the cytoplasm of the nerve terminal and stored in synaptic vesicles. A nerve impulse arriving at the nerve ending causes the release of approximately 60 vesicles, each containing an estimated 10,000 molecules of acetylcholine (Ganong, 2003). In the absence of calcium ions or in the presence of excess magnesium ions, the release of acetylcholine is greatly decreased. Acetylcholine diffuses across the synaptic cleft to excite skeletal muscles, but within 1 ms, the neurotransmitter is hydrolyzed by acetylcholinesterase enzyme (true cholinesterase) in the folds of the sarcolemma. This rapid inactivation of acetylcholine prevents reexcitation after skeletal muscle fibers have recovered from the first action potential.

Mechanism of Acetylcholine Effects

Nicotinic acetylcholine receptors comprise five subunits arranged in a nearly symmetric fashion that extend through the cell membrane (see Fig. 8-6). An average end-plate contains an estimated 50 million nicotinic acetylcholine receptors. Binding of two acetylcholine molecules (one molecule at each alpha subunit) causes a conformation change in the receptor such that sodium ions enter into the interior of the cell. As a result, the resting transmembrane potential increases in this local area of the motor end-plate, creating a local action potential known as the end-plate potential. This end-plate potential initiates an action potential that spreads in both directions along the skeletal muscle fiber. The threshold potential at which skeletal muscle fibers are stimulated to contract is approximately 50 mv. The duration of the action potential in skeletal muscles is <5 ms, which contrasts with the duration of the action potential in cardiac muscle, which is approximately 200 ms. The short duration of skeletal muscle action potentials allows for rapid contraction of muscle fibers.

Altered Responses to Acetylcholine

Nondepolarizing neuromuscular-blocking drugs compete with acetylcholine at alpha subunits of the receptor and thus prevent changes in the permeability of skeletal muscle membranes (see Chapter 8). As a result, an end-plate potential does not occur and neuromuscular transmission is effectively prevented. Anticholinesterase drugs inhibit acetylcholinesterase enzyme, allowing accumulation of acetylcholine at receptors and subsequent displacement of nondepolarizing neuromuscular-blocking drugs from the alpha subunits (see Chapter 9). Myasthenia gravis is characterized by a decrease in the number of nicotinic acetylcholine receptors; the resulting end-plate potentials are too weak to initiate a propagated action potential.

Blood Flow

Skeletal muscle blood flow can increase more than 20 times (a greater increase than in any other tissue of the body) during strenuous exercise. At rest, only 20% to 25% of the capillaries are open, and skeletal muscle blood flow is 3 to 4 mL/100 g/minute. During strenuous exercise, almost all skeletal muscle capillaries become patent. Opening of previously collapsed capillaries diminishes the distance that oxygen and other nutrients must diffuse from capillaries to skeletal muscle fibers and contributes an increased surface area through which nutrients can diffuse from blood. Presumably, exercise lowers the local concentration of oxygen, which in turn causes vasodilation because the vessel walls cannot maintain contraction in the absence of adequate amounts of oxygen. Alternatively, oxygen deficiency may cause release of vasodilator substances such as potassium ions and adenosine. The increase in cardiac output that occurs during exercise results principally from local vasodilation in active skeletal muscles and subsequent increased venous return to the heart. Among inhaled anesthetics, isoflurane is a potent vasodilator, producing marked increases in skeletal muscle blood flow.

Exercise is associated with a centrally mediated stimulation of the sympathetic nervous system manifesting as vasoconstriction in nonmuscular tissues and increases in systemic blood pressure. Excessive increases in systemic blood pressure, however, are prevented by vascular vasodilation that occurs in the large tissue mass represented by skeletal muscles. Exceptions to nonmuscular tissue vasoconstriction induced by exercise are the coronary and cerebral circulations. This is teleologically understandable because the heart and brain are essential to the response to exercise, as are the skeletal muscles.

Innervation

Skeletal muscles are innervated by large myelinated alpha motor neurons that originate from cell bodies in ventral (anterior) horns of the spinal cord (Fig. 56-2) (Berne et al., 2004). The nerve axon exits via the ventral root and reaches the muscle through a mixed peripheral nerve. Motor nerves branch in the skeletal muscle with each nerve terminal innervating a single muscle cell. A motor unit consists of the motor nerve and all of the muscle fibers innervated by that nerve. The motor unit is the functional contractile unit. Skeletal muscle tone is a residual degree of skeletal muscle contraction that persists even at rest. Presumably, skeletal muscle tone reflects nerve impulses that are emitted continuously from the spinal cord.

Denervation Hypersensitivity

Denervation of skeletal muscle causes atrophy of the involved muscle and development of abnormal excitability of the skeletal muscle to its neurotransmitter acetylcholine.

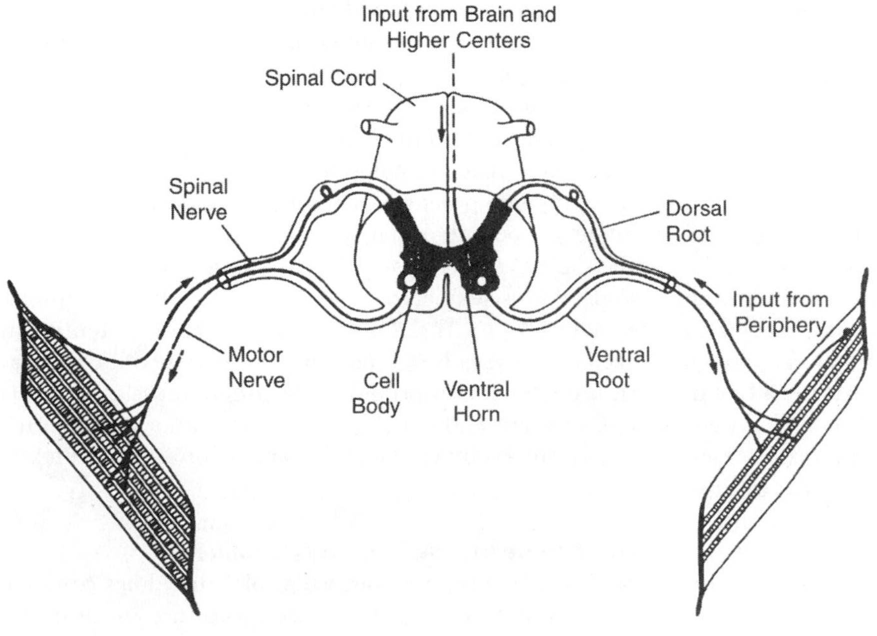

Figure 56-2. Schematic depiction of skeletal muscle innervation. (From Berne et al. *Physiology*, 5th ed. St. Louis: Mosby, 2004; with permission.)

Initially, after the motor nerve is interrupted, fasciculations occur due to the release of acetylcholine from the terminals of the degenerating distal portion of the axon. Approximately 3 to 5 days after denervation, skeletal muscle fibrillation appears, reflecting spread of cholinergic receptors over the entire skeletal muscle membrane and development of increased sensitivity (denervation hypersensitivity) to acetylcholine. After several weeks, atrophy of skeletal muscle fibers is so severe that fibrillation impulses cease. An *electromyogram* is the recording from skin electrodes of the electrical current that spreads from skeletal muscles to skin during simultaneous contraction of numerous skeletal muscle fibers.

SMOOTH MUSCLE

Smooth muscle is distinguished anatomically from skeletal and cardiac muscle because it lacks visible cross-striations (actin and myosin are not arranged in regular arrays). Smooth muscle is categorized as *multiunit* or *visceral* smooth muscle. Multiunit smooth muscle contraction is controlled almost exclusively by nerve signals, and spontaneous contractions rarely occur. Examples of multiunit smooth muscles are the ciliary muscles of the eye, iris of the eye, and smooth muscles of many large blood vessels. Smooth muscle must develop force or shorten to provide motility or to alter the dimensions of an organ.

Smooth muscle cells lack T-tubules that provide electrical links to sarcoplasmic reticulum. However, the sarcolemma of smooth muscle contains saclike inpocketings (caveoli) that may be sites where calcium ions enter the cells through voltage-gated calcium ion channels. Calcium ions are released from the sarcoplasmic reticulum into the myoplasm when stimulatory neurotransmitters, hormones, or drugs bind to receptors on the sarcolemma. Calcium ion channels on the sarcoplasmic reticulum of smooth muscles includes ryanodine receptors (similar to that present in skeletal muscles) and inositol 1,4,5-triphosphate (IP_3)-gated calcium ion channels. Neurotransmitters or hormones that act via receptors in the sarcolemma can activate phospholipase C followed by the generation of the second messenger IP_3. IP_3 channels are activated when hormones bind to calcium-mobilizing receptors in the sarcoplasmic reticulum in smooth muscle cells.

Visceral smooth muscle is characterized by cell membranes that contact adjacent cell membranes, forming a functional syncytium that often undergoes spontaneous contractions as a single unit in the absence of nerve stimulation. These spontaneous action potentials are particularly prominent in tubular structures, accounting for peristaltic motion in sites such as the bile ducts, ureters, and gastrointestinal tract, especially when they are distended. Plateaus in the action potentials of visceral smooth muscle lasting up to 30 seconds may occur in the ureters and uterus. The normal resting transmembrane potential is approximately −60 mv, which is approximately 30 mv less negative than in skeletal muscles.

In addition to stimulation in the absence of extrinsic innervation, smooth muscles are unique in their sensitivity to hormones or local tissue factors. For example, smooth muscle spasm may persist for hours in response to norepinephrine or antidiuretic hormone, whereas local factors such as lack of oxygen or accumulation of hydrogen ions cause vasodilation. It is believed that local factors and hormones cause smooth muscle contraction by activating the calcium ion transport mechanism. Drugs relax smooth muscle by increasing the intracellular concentration of cyclic adenosine monophosphate or cyclic guanosine monophosphate.

Mechanism of Contraction

Smooth muscles contain both actin and myosin but, unlike skeletal muscles, lack troponin. In contrast to skeletal muscles, in which calcium binds to troponin to initiate cross-bridging, in smooth muscle the calcium-calmodulin complex activates the enzyme necessary for phosphorylation of myosin. This myosin has ATPase activity, and actin then slides on myosin to produce contraction.

The source of calcium in smooth muscle differs from that in skeletal muscle because the sarcoplasmic reticulum of smooth muscle is poorly developed. Most of the calcium that causes contraction of smooth muscles enters from extracellular fluid at the time of the action potential. The time required for this diffusion is 200 to 300 ms, which is approximately 50 times longer than for skeletal muscles. Subsequent relaxation of smooth muscles is achieved by a calcium ion transport system that pumps these ions back into extracellular fluid or into the sarcoplasmic reticulum. This calcium ion pump is slow compared with the sarcoplasmic reticulum pump in skeletal muscles. As a result, the duration of smooth muscle contraction is often seconds rather than milliseconds as is characteristic of skeletal muscles.

Smooth muscles, unlike skeletal muscles, do not atrophy when denervated, but they do become hyperresponsive to the normal neurotransmitter. This denervation hypersensitivity is a general phenomenon that is largely due to synthesis or activation of more receptors.

Neuromuscular Junction

A neuromuscular junction similar to that present on skeletal muscles does not occur in smooth muscles. Instead, nerve fibers branch diffusely on top of a sheet of smooth muscle fibers without making actual contact. These nerve fibers secrete their neurotransmitter into an interstitial fluid space a few microns from the smooth muscle cells. Two different neurotransmitters, acetylcholine and norepinephrine, are secreted by the autonomic nervous system nerves that innervate smooth muscles. Acetylcholine is an excitatory neurotransmitter for smooth muscles at some sites and functions as an inhibitory neurotransmitter at other sites. Norepinephrine exerts the reverse effect of acetylcholine. It is believed that the presence of specific excitatory or inhibitory receptors in the membranes of smooth muscle fibers determines the response to acetylcholine or norepinephrine. When the neurotransmitter interacts with an inhibitory receptor instead of an excitatory receptor, the membrane potential of the smooth muscle fiber becomes more negative (hyperpolarized).

Uterine Smooth Muscle

Uterine smooth muscle is characterized by a high degree of spontaneous electrical and contractile activity. Unlike the heart, there is no pacemaker, and the contraction process spreads from one cell to another at a rate of 1 to 3 cm/s. Contractions of labor result in peak intrauterine pressures of 60 to 80 mm Hg in the second stage. Resting uterine pressure during labor is approximately 10 mm Hg. Movement of sodium ions appears to be the primary determinant in depolarization, whereas calcium ions are necessary for excitation-contraction coupling. Availability of calcium ions greatly influences the response of uterine smooth muscle to physiologic and pharmacologic stimulation or inhibition. Alpha excitatory and beta inhibitory receptors are also present in the myometrium.

REFERENCES

Berne RM, Levy MN, Koeppen BM, et al. *Physiology*, 5th ed. St Louis: Mosby, Year Book, 2004.

Ganong WF. *Review of medical physiology*, 21st ed. Lange Medical Books, New York: McGraw-Hill, 2003.

McCarthy TV, Healy JMS, Heffron JJA, et al. Localization of the malignant hyperthermia susceptibility locus to human chromosome. *Nature* 1990;343:562–564.

Erythrocytes and Leukocytes

57

ERYTHROCYTES

Erythrocytes (red blood cells, RBCs) are the most abundant of all cells in the body (25 trillion of the estimated total 100 trillion cells), and they have an irreplaceable role in delivery of oxygen to tissues. Indeed, the major function of RBCs is to transport hemoglobin, which, in turn, carries oxygen from the lungs to tissues. In addition to transporting hemoglobin, RBCs contain large amounts of carbonic anhydrase. This enzyme speeds the reaction between carbon dioxide and water, making it possible to transport carbon dioxide from tissues to the lungs for elimination. In addition, hemoglobin in RBCs is an excellent acid–base buffer, providing approximately 70% of the buffering power of whole blood.

Anatomy

RBCs are biconcave disks with a mean diameter of 8 μ. The shape of these cells can change, conforming to the capillaries through which they must pass. The average number of RBCs in each milliliter of plasma, and thus the hemoglobin concentration and hematocrit, varies with the individual, gender, and barometric pressure (Table 57-1). Each RBC contains approximately 29 pg of hemoglobin, and each gram of hemoglobin is capable of combining with 1.34 mL of oxygen.

Bone Marrow

In the adult, RBCs, platelets, and many of the leukocytes are formed in bone marrow. Normally, approximately 75% of the cells in the bone marrow belong to the leukocyte-producing myeloid series and only 25% are maturing RBCs, even though there are more than 500 times as many RBCs in the circulation as there are leukocytes. This difference reflects the short half-time of leukocytes compared with RBCs. In the fetus, RBCs are also produced in the liver and spleen. The marrow of long bones, except for the proximal portions of the humerus and tibia, becomes fatty and produces few or no RBCs after approximately 20 years of age. After 20 years, most RBCs are produced in the marrow of membranous bones, including the vertebrae, sternum, ribs, and pelvis. When the bone marrow produces RBCs at a rapid rate, many of the cells are released into the blood before they are mature. For example, during rapid RBC production, the number of circulating reticulocytes may increase from <1% to as great as 30% to 50%. Overall, the bone marrow is one of the largest organs of the body, approaching the size and weight of the liver.

Control of Production

The total mass of RBCs in the circulation is regulated within narrow limits so that the number of cells is optimal to provide tissue oxygenation without an excessive number that would adversely increase viscosity of blood and decrease tissue blood flow (Fig. 57-1) (Ganong, 2003). It is not the concentration of RBCs in the blood that controls the rate of their production but rather the ability of cells to transport oxygen to tissues in relation to tissue demand for oxygen. Any event that causes the amount of oxygen transported to tissues to decrease, as in anemia, chronic pulmonary disease, or cardiac failure, will stimulate production of RBCs by the bone marrow. Destruction of bone marrow by radiation, drugs, or inadequate amounts of iron predictably results in anemia (see Fig. 57-1) (Ganong, 2003).

Erythropoietin

Erythropoietin is a glycoprotein synthesized in response to arterial hypoxemia as produced by ascent to altitude or chronic pulmonary disease. It is speculated that arterial hypoxemia evokes release of renal erythropoietic factor into the circulation from the kidneys. This enzyme acts on a globulin to split away the erythropoietin molecule.

TABLE 57-1.
ERYTHROCYTES IN THE PLASMA

	Contents
Erythrocytes (mL)	
Male	$4.3–5.9 \times 10^6$
Female	$3.5–5.5 \times 10^6$
Hematocrit (%)	
Male	39–55
Female	36–48
Hemoglobin (g/dL)	
Male	13.9–16.3
Female	12.0–15.0

Erythropoietin stimulates RBC production in the bone marrow, with the peak effect occurring in approximately 5 days. After this peak is reached, RBCs continue to be produced at an increased rate as long as arterial hypoxemia persists. When arterial hypoxemia is corrected, erythropoietin production decreases to zero almost immediately, followed in a few days by a similar decrease in RBC production. RBC production in the bone marrow remains at a low level until enough cells have lived out their life spans, thus decreasing the number of circulating RBCs to a level consistent with normal tissue oxygenation (negative-feedback mechanism). The absence of kidneys removes the source of renal erythropoietic factor, which in the absence of an exogenous source of erythropoietin, such as recombinant erythropoietin, results in anemia. Indeed, before the availability of recombinant erythropoietin, severe anemia was considered an unavoidable result of chronic renal failure.

Despite advances in the safety of the blood supply, the search for therapeutic alternatives to blood continues. Therapy with recombinant human erythropoietin is an alternative to blood transfusion if the clinical condition of the patient permits sufficient time for stimulation of erythropoiesis to correct anemia. Four weekly subcutaneous doses of erythropoietin are usually sufficient to produce a reticulocyte response (Goodnough et al., 1997).

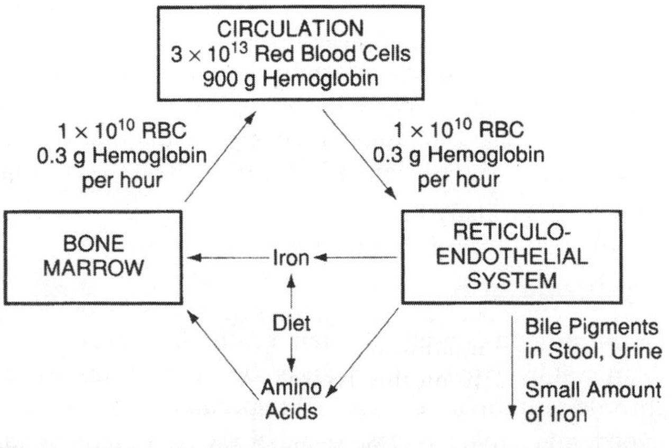

Figure 57-1. Erythrocyte formation and destruction. (From Ganong WF. *Review of medical physiology*, 21st ed. Lange Medical Books/McGraw-Hill, 2003; with permission.)

Vitamins Necessary for Formation

Vitamin B_{12} (cyanocobalamin) is necessary for the synthesis of DNA. Lack of this vitamin results in failure of nuclear maturation and division, which is particularly evident in rapidly proliferating cells such as RBCs. In addition, maturation failure is reflected by formation of megaloblasts and macrocytes. The amount of vitamin B_{12} required each day to maintain normal RBC maturation is 1 μg, and the normal store in the liver is approximately 1,000 times this amount. As a result, many months of impaired vitamin B_{12} absorption are necessary before maturation failure macrocytic anemia manifests. Macrocytes have a weak cell membrane, causing them to exhibit a shorter life span than normal erythrocytes.

Folic acid, like vitamin B_{12}, is necessary for formation of DNA and maturation of RBCs. Deficiency of this vitamin predictably leads to a macrocytic anemia.

Destruction

RBCs normally circulate an average of 120 days after leaving the bone marrow. With increasing RBC age, the metabolic system of RBCs declines (cytoplasmic enzymes capable of metabolizing glucose to form adenosine triphosphate) and cell membranes become fragile. Many fragile RBCs rupture in the spleen. Hemoglobin released from ruptured RBCs is rapidly phagocytized by reticuloendothelial cells (see Fig. 57-1) (Ganong, 2003). Iron is released from hemoglobin back into the blood to be carried by transferrin either to bone marrow for production of new RBCs or to the liver and other tissues for storage as ferritin. The heme portion of the hemoglobin molecule is converted by the reticuloendothelial cells into bilirubin.

BLOOD GROUPS

Genetically determined antigens (agglutinogens) are present on the cell membranes of RBCs. The most antigenic are the A, B, and Rh agglutinogens; other agglutinogens (Kell, Duffy, Lewis, M, N, and P) are less antigenic. A and B antigens are glycoproteins that differ in composition by only a single substitution. Blood is divided into different groups and types on the basis of the antigen present on RBC membranes.

ABO Antigen System

Blood is grouped for transfusion as A, B, AB, or O on the basis of the ABO antigen system (Table 57-2). A and B antigens can occur alone or in combination on RBC membranes, and in some individuals, both antigens are absent. There are six genotypes (see Table 57-2). In addition to RBCs, A and B antigens are present in many other tissues

TABLE 57-2.
ABO ANTIGEN SYSTEM

Blood Type	Incidence (%)	Genotype	Antigens (Agglutinogens)	Antibodies (Agglutinins)
O	47	OO		anti-A, anti-B
A	41	OA,AA	A	anti-B
B	9	OB,BB	B	anti-A
AB	3	AB	A,B	

(kidneys, liver, testes, salivary glands) and fluids (saliva, semen, amniotic fluid).

In the absence of the A or B antigens, the opposite antibody (agglutinin) is present in the circulation (see Table 57-2). These antibodies are gamma globulins, most often being immunoglobulin M (IgM) or IgG molecules. It seems paradoxical that antibodies are produced in the absence of the respective antigen on RBC membranes. It is likely that small amounts of A and B antigens enter the body by way of food or bacteria, thus initiating the development of corresponding antibodies. Indeed, immediately after birth, the circulating level of antibodies to A or B antigens is almost zero. It is only at 2 to 8 months of age that an individual begins to produce antibodies to the antigen not present on RBC membranes. A maximum titer of antibodies is usually reached by 8 to 10 years of age and then gradually decreases with increasing age.

Blood Typing

Blood typing is the in vitro mixing of a drop of the patient's blood with plasma containing antibodies against the A or B antigen. This mixture is observed under a microscope for the presence or absence of agglutination (Fig. 57-2) (Ganong, 2003). Using this procedure, blood can be typed as O, A, B, or AB. Cross-matching is the procedure that determines the compatibility of the patient's blood with the donor's RBCs and plasma. Failure of agglutination when the RBCs from the donor and plasma from the recipient are mixed and when the RBCs of the recipient are mixed with plasma from the donor confirms compatibility. In the past, blood typing was used to determine parentage, although it could only prove that a specific individual was not the father.

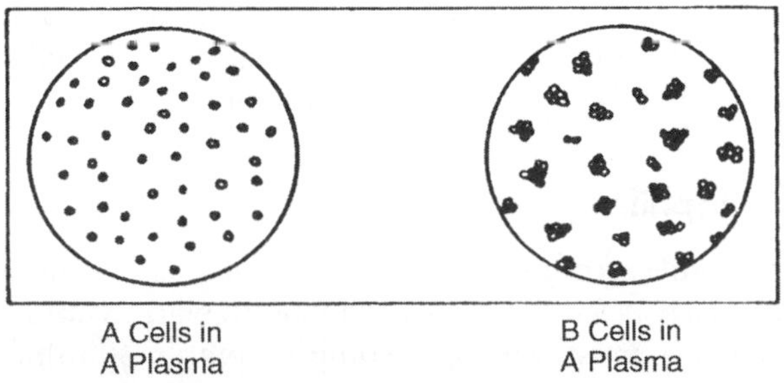

Figure 57-2. Erythrocyte agglutination in incompatible plasma. (From Ganong WF. *Review of medical physiology*, 21st ed. Lange Medical Books/McGraw-Hill, 2003; with permission.)

Rh Blood Types

There are six common types of Rh antigens—designated C, D, E, c, d, and e—that are collectively known as the *Rh factor*. Only the C, D, and E antigens are sufficiently antigenic to cause development of anti-Rh antibodies capable of causing transfusion reactions. An individual with C, D, or E antigens on RBC membranes is Rh-positive, and an individual with c, d, or e antigens is Rh-negative. Approximately 85% of Caucasian Americans are Rh-positive. Typing for Rh factors is performed in a manner similar to that for typing A and B antigens.

An individual who is Rh-negative develops anti-Rh antibodies only when exposed to RBCs containing the C, D, or E antigens. This exposure may occur with transfusion of Rh-positive blood to an Rh-negative patient, or during pregnancy, when an Rh-negative mother is sensitized to the Rh-positive factor in her child. The development of anti-Rh antibodies is usually slow, and these antibodies are less potent agglutinogens than are antibodies to the A and B antigens. Nevertheless, multiple exposures of an Rh-negative person to Rh-positive blood results in exaggerated responses.

If an Rh-negative individual is transfused with Rh-positive blood, there is often no immediate reaction. In some individuals, however, anti-Rh antibodies develop in sufficient amounts after 2 to 4 weeks to cause agglutination of any transfused cells that are still circulating. These cells are then hemolyzed in the reticuloendothelial system, producing a delayed and usually mild transfusion reaction. On subsequent transfusion of Rh-positive blood to this same individual, however, the severity of the transfusion reaction is greatly increased and can be similar to reactions resulting from ABO incompatibility.

An Rh-negative mother typically becomes sensitized to the Rh-positive factor in her child during the first few days after delivery, when degenerating products of the placenta release Rh-positive antigens into the maternal circulation. If these Rh antigens are destroyed at this time before an anti-Rh antibody response occurs, the mother will not become sensitized for subsequent pregnancies. This goal is achieved by injecting antibodies (Rh [D] immune globulin) against the antigen before it can evoke the formation of antibodies. If anti-Rh antibodies form, any subsequent pregnancy in which the fetus is Rh-positive may result in erythroblastosis fetalis.

Hemolytic Transfusion Reactions

Transfusion of ABO type blood that is different from that of the recipient, results in agglutination of the transfused RBCs by antibodies present in the plasma of the recipient. Agglutination of the recipient's RBCs is less likely because antibodies in the incompatible blood are rapidly diluted in the recipient's plasma. In addition to agglutination, this antigen-antibody interaction may result in immediate hemolysis of the transfused RBCs. Hemolysis reflects activation of the complement system, which releases proteolytic enzymes that result in lysis of RBCs. Indeed, blockade of blood vessels by agglutinated RBCs and concomitant intravascular hemolysis are well-recognized hazards of transfusion of incompatible blood. Nevertheless, immediate intravascular hemolysis is less common than agglutination, presumably reflecting the need for very high titers of antibody to evoke hemolysis. Ultimately, however, even agglutination leads to hemolysis of agglutinated RBCs. When the rate of hemolysis is rapid, the plasma concentration of hemoglobin may exceed the binding capacity of haptoglobin, and free hemoglobin continues to circulate. This free hemoglobin is converted to bilirubin, and jaundice may occur. Nevertheless, if liver function is normal, jaundice does not appear unless >300 to 500 mL of blood is hemolyzed in <24 hours. Acute renal failure often accompanies a severe transfusion reaction.

LEUKOCYTES

Leukocytes are classified as granulocytes (polymorphonuclear leukocytes), monocytes, and lymphocytes (Table 57-3).

TABLE 57-3.
CLASSIFICATION OF LEUKOCYTES

	Cells per mL of Plasma (Range)	% of Total (Range)
Granulocytes		
Neutrophils	3,000–6,000	55–65
Eosinophils	0–300	1–3
Basophils	0–100	0–1
Monocytes/macrophages	300–500	3–6
Lymphocytes	1,500–3,500	25–35
Total leukocytes	4,000–11,000	

Granulocytes are further subdivided as neutrophils, eosinophils, and basophils based on the staining characteristics of granules contained in these cells. Acting together, leukocytes provide an important defense against invading organisms (bacterial, viral, or parasitic) and are necessary for immune responses. Normally, each milliliter of blood contains 4,000 to 11,000 leukocytes, the most numerous being neutrophils. Granulocytes and monocytes are formed from stem cells in the bone marrow. After birth, some lymphocytes are formed in bone marrow, but most are produced in the thymus, lymph nodes, and spleen from precursor cells that came originally from the bone marrow. Lymphocytes enter the circulation via the lymphatic system.

Neutrophils

Neutrophils are the most numerous leukocytes in the blood, representing approximately 60% of the circulating leukocytes. These cells seek out, ingest, and kill bacteria (phagocytosis) and thus represent the body's first line of defense against bacterial infection. Neutrophils contain lysosomes filled with proteolytic enzymes capable of digesting bacteria. Eventually, neutrophils are killed by toxins produced and released by lysosomes. Hydrogen peroxide produced by neutrophils also exerts an antibacterial effect. Neutrophils also release thromboxanes (vasoconstriction and platelet aggregation) and leukotrienes (increased vascular permeability).

Once neutrophils are released from bone marrow into the circulation, they have a life span of 6 to 8 hours. To maintain a normal circulating blood level of neutrophils, it is necessary for the bone marrow to produce >100 billion neutrophils daily. In the presence of infection, the need for neutrophils is even greater because these cells are destroyed in the process of phagocytosis. Indeed, a marked increase (up to fivefold) in the number of circulating neutrophils (leukocytosis) occurs within a few hours after bacterial infection or onset of inflammation. Leukocytosis is stimulated by release of a chemical substance from inflamed tissues known as *leukocytosis-inducing factor*. This factor is believed to dilate venous sinusoids of bone marrow, thus facilitating release of stored neutrophils. A similar increase in circulating neutrophils may accompany nonbacterial tissue injury such as myocardial infarction. Even intense exercise lasting only 1 minute can cause the number of circulating neutrophils to increase threefold (physiologic neutrophilia).

Eosinophils

Eosinophils account for approximately 20% of circulating leukocytes. After release from the bone marrow into the circulation, most eosinophils migrate within 30 minutes into extravascular tissues where they survive 8 to 12 days. These cells are weak phagocytes but enter the circulation in increased numbers after ingestion of foreign proteins. The most common chronic cause of increases in the circulating concentration of eosinophils is the presence of parasites in the blood, perhaps reflecting the role of eosinophils in detoxifying foreign proteins. Eosinophils show a special propensity to collect at sites of antigen-antibody reactions in tissues, most likely in response to a chemotactic stimulus. The effect of this accumulation is to dampen the host's response by limiting antigen-induced release of chemical mediators from mast cells and basophils. The total number of circulating eosinophils increases during allergic reactions, presumably because tissue reactions release products that selectively increase the production of eosinophils in the bone marrow.

Basophils

Basophils in the blood are similar to mast cells in tissues in that both types of cells contain histamine and heparin. Release of heparin into the blood inhibits coagulation and speeds removal of fat particles after a meal. Degranulation of these cells occurs when IgE selectively attaches to the membranes of previously sensitized basophils or mast cells. The subsequent release of histamine and perhaps other chemical mediators is responsible for the manifestations of allergic reactions.

Tryptase

Tryptase is a neutral protease that is stored in granules of mast cells present in tissues. Mast cell degranulation results in increased plasma concentrations of tryptase as evidence of anaphylaxis (Laroches et al., 1991). Because tryptase is present in low concentrations in leukocytes, hemolysis and blood clotting have little influence on the measured plasma concentration. Furthermore, the plasma half-life of tryptase is approximately 2 hours, and immunoreactive tryptase is stable in plasma, allowing for delayed sampling and measurement. When measurement of plasma tryptase concentrations is intended to be a biochemical marker of the occurrence of an allergic reaction after the intravenous administration of a drug, it is recommended that sampling be 15 to 20 minutes after the onset of symptoms (Laroches et al., 1991). In contrast, increased plasma concentrations of histamine as evidence of basophil and/or mast cell degranulation are difficult to measure accurately as the half-life of histamine in plasma is brief.

Monocytes

Monocytes enter the circulation from the bone marrow but, after approximately, 24 hours migrate into tissues to become macrophages. These macrophages, like neutrophils, contain peroxidase and lysosomal enzymes and are actively phagocytic. Macrophages constitute the reticuloendothelial system. In addition to bacteria, these cells phagocytize large particles including RBCs, necrotic tissue, and dead neutrophils. Macrophages in different tissues are designated by different names; for example, macrophages in the liver are known as *Kupffer cells;* in lymph nodes, spleen, and bone marrow, as *reticulum cells;* in alveoli of the lungs as *alveolar macrophages;* in subcutaneous tissue as *histiocytes;* and in the brain as *microglia.*

Kupffer Cells

Kupffer cells line the hepatic sinuses and serve as a filtration system to remove bacteria that have entered the portal blood from the gastrointestinal tract. Indeed, these tissue macrophages are capable of removing almost all bacteria from the portal blood.

Reticulum Cells

Reticulum cells line the sinuses of lymph nodes. These macrophages effectively phagocytize foreign particles as they pass through lymph nodes. Invading organisms that manage to find their way into the general circulation are vulnerable to phagocytosis by reticulum cells in the bone marrow and spleen. The spleen is similar to lymph nodes except that blood rather than lymph flows through the substance of the spleen. The spleen is also important for the removal of abnormal platelets and RBCs.

Alveolar Macrophages

Alveolar macrophages are present in alveolar walls and can phagocytize invading organisms that are inhaled. If the phagocytized particles are digestible, the resulting products are released into the lymph. If the particles are not digestible (carbon), the macrophages often form a giant cell capsule around the particles.

Histiocytes

Histiocytes are tissue macrophages present in subcutaneous tissues. These cells phagocytize invading organisms that gain access when the skin is broken. When local inflammation occurs in the subcutaneous tissues, histiocytes are stimulated to divide and form additional macrophages.

Cytokines

Cytokines are a heterogeneous group of proteins (also termed *interleukins, lymphokines, interferons*) that are synthesized by activated macrophages and lymphocytes (Table 57-4) (Levy and Kelly, 1993; Sheeran and Hall, 1997). These proteins act as secondary messengers and induce the synthesis and expression of specific adhesion molecules on endothelial cells and leukocytes that promote attachment and transmigration of leukocytes (chemoattractants and leukocyte activators). The term *interleukin* was intended to emphasize that these proteins facilitate communication between/among (inter) leukocytes (leukin).

Cytokines are involved in immunity and inflammatory responses and regulate the magnitude and duration of the response. For example, liberation of interleukin-1 and tumor necrosis factor produces multiple inflammatory

TABLE 57-4.
EXAMPLES OF CYTOKINES AND THEIR CLINICAL RELEVANCE

Cytokine	Cellular Sources	Clinical Effects	Clinical Impact
Interleukin-1	Macrophages	Activation of T cells and macrophages Promotion of inflammation	Implicated in the pathogenesis of septic shock, rheumatoid arthritis, and atherosclerosis
Interleukin-2	Type 1 helper T cells	Activation of lymphocytes, and macrophages	Used to induce lymphokine-activated killer cells Used in the treatment of renal-cell carcinoma
Interleukin-4	Type 2 helper T cells,	Activation of lymphocytes Activation of monocytes	Stimulates IgE production (allergy)
Interleukin-5	Type 2 helper T cells	Differentiation of eosinophils	Monoclonal antibody against Interleukin-5
Interleukin-6	Type 2 helper T cells	Activation of lymphocytes Differentiation of B cells Production of acute-phase proteins	Acts as an autocrine growth factor
Interleukin-8	T cells and macrophages	Chemotaxis of neutrophils, basophils, and T cells	Increased in diseases accompanied by neutrophilia
Interleukin-11	Bone marrow stromal cells	Production of acute-phase proteins	Decrease chemotherapy-induced thrombocytopenia
Interleukin-12	Macrophages and B cells	Production of interferon	Adjuvant for vaccines

effects including fever, neuropeptide release, endothelial cell activation, increased adhesion molecular expression, hypotension, myocardial depression, and a catabolic state. Overall, the interleukins are considered to be a group of regulatory proteins that act to control many aspects of the immune and inflammatory response. Secretion of interleukin by monocytes promotes the proliferation and maturation of T lymphocytes.

Release of cytokines is one of the earliest cellular responses to tissue injury and is also associated with the release of other inflammatory mediators including arachidonic acid metabolites, complement-split products, lysosomal enzymes, and oxygen-free radicals. Interleukin-6 is the principal cytokine released after surgery (Hall and Desborough, 1992). The other principal stimulus to the metabolic response to injury is afferent neuronal input from the injured or operative site.

Cytokines, in common with other polypeptide hormones, initiate their action by binding to specific receptors on the surface of target cells. Cytokines tend to be paracrine (act on nearby cells) or autocrine (act on the same cell), rather than endocrine (secreted into the circulation to act on distant cells). Most cytokines are synthesized as they are needed and not stored. Alternatively, some cytokines (tumor necrosis factor, transforming growth factor, endothelial growth factor, platelet factor 4) are presynthesized and stored in cytoplasmic granules.

Lymphocytes

Lymphocytes account for approximately 30% of circulating leukocytes. These cells play a prominent role in immunity (see the section on Immunity).

Agranulocytosis

Agranulocytosis is the acute cessation of leukocyte production by the bone marrow. Within 2 to 3 days, ulcers appear in the mouth and colon, reflecting the uninhibited growth of bacteria that normally populate these areas. Irradiation of the body by gamma rays associated with a nuclear explosion or exposure to drugs or chemicals containing benzene or anthracene rings (sulfonamides, chloramphenicol, thiouracil) can cause acute bone marrow aplasia in which neither RBCs nor leukocytes are produced. Usually sufficient stem cells (hemocytoblasts) remain after injury to allow recovery of bone marrow function if fatal infection is prevented by appropriate antibiotic therapy. This regeneration, however, may require several months.

Bacterial Destruction

Leukocytes participate in destruction of bacteria by the processes of diapedesis, chemotaxis, and phagocytosis. Opsonization also makes bacteria susceptible to phagocytosis.

Diapedesis

Neutrophils and monocytes can squeeze through pores in blood vessels by diapedesis. Specifically, even though the pore is smaller than the leukocyte, a small portion of the cell slides through the pore at a time, the portion sliding through being momentarily constricted to the size of the pore.

Chemotaxis

Chemotaxis is the phenomenon by which different chemical substances in tissues cause neutrophils and monocytes to move either toward or away from the chemical. For example, inflamed tissue may contain substances (leukotrienes, C5a, bacterial toxins, products of coagulation) that cause neutrophils and monocytes to move toward (chemotaxis) the inflamed area. Chemotaxis is effective up to 100 μm away from an inflamed tissue. Because almost no tissue is more than 30 to 50 μm away from a capillary, the chemotactic signal can rapidly attract large numbers of leukocytes to the inflamed area. Chemotaxis may be inhibited by inhaled anesthetics (see Chapter 2).

Opsonization

Opsonization is the coating of bacteria by IgG and complement proteins (opsonins), thus making the microorganisms susceptible to phagocytosis.

Phagocytosis

Neutrophils and monocytes are known as *phagocytes*. On approaching a particle to be phagocytized, the neutrophil projects pseudopodia around the particle. These pseudopodia fuse, creating a chamber containing the ingested particle. Phagocytosis is likely to occur when (a) the surface of the particle is rough, (b) the particle is electropositive, and (c) the particle is recognized as foreign. Most natural substances of the body, including neutrophils and monocytes, have electronegative surfaces. Conversely, necrotic tissues and foreign particles are often electropositive and thus are attracted to phagocytes.

INFLAMMATION

Inflammation is a series of sequential changes that occur in tissues in response to injury. Tissue injury, whether it is due to bacterial infection or trauma, causes the release of local substances (histamine, bradykinin, serotonin) into the surrounding fluid. These substances, particularly histamine, increase local blood flow as well as the local permeability of capillaries, allowing fibrinogen to leak into tissues. Local extracellular edema results, and the extracellular fluid and lymphatic fluid coagulate because of the coagulating effects of fibrinogen present in extravasated fluid. As a result, brawny edema develops in the spaces surrounding damaged tissues.

Tissue spaces and lymphatics in the inflamed area are blocked by clots of fibrinogen; thus, blood flow through the area is minimal. This effectively isolates the injured area from normal tissues and minimizes the dissemination of bacteria or toxic products. Staphylococci liberate potent cellular toxins, causing the rapid onset of inflammation and isolation of the infected area. In contrast, streptococci cause less intense local destruction, such that the walling-off process develops slowly, allowing streptococci to spread extensively. As a result, streptococci have a greater tendency to produce disseminated and life-threatening infection than do staphylococci, even though staphylococci produce more intense local tissue damage.

Soon after inflammation begins, the inflamed area is invaded by neutrophils and macrophages. These cells immediately begin their function of phagocytosis. Products of inflamed tissues also stimulate movement of neutrophils into the inflamed area from the circulation. When neutrophils and macrophages engulf large numbers of bacteria and necrotic tissue, almost all the neutrophils and many of the macrophages die. The collection of dead leukocytes and necrotic tissue is known as pus. The pus cavity may digest its way to the exterior or into an internal cavity and thus discharge its contents. Alternatively, the pus cavity may remain closed, and eventually its contents will undergo autolysis and absorption into surrounding tissues.

IMMUNITY

Immunity is the ability to resist all types of organisms or toxins that could damage tissues or organs. Cell-mediated immunity and humoral immunity are the two types of immune defense systems designed to protect the body against organisms or toxins that cause tissue damage (Fig. 57-3) (Guyton and Hall, 2000; Stevenson et al., 1990). The principal defense against bacterial infection is provided by humoral immunity due to circulating antibodies in the gamma globulin fraction of plasma proteins. Cellular immunity is responsible for delayed allergic reactions, rejection of foreign tissue, and destruction of early cancer cells. Cellular immunity also serves as a major defense against infections due to viruses, fungi, and bacteria such as *Mycobacterium tuberculosis*. Signals mediating interactions

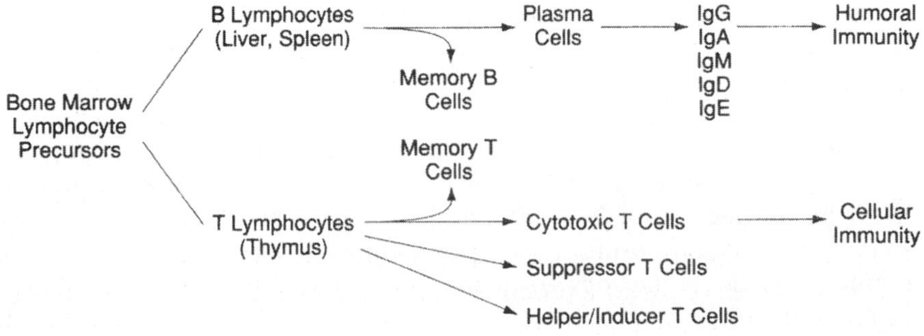

Figure 57-3. Schematic depiction of the immune system.

between immune system effector cells are termed *biologic response modifiers*. Substances responsible for these signals are polypeptides as represented by cytokines (see the section on Cytokines). Short-term anesthesia has not been shown to adversely impact the immune system although high doses of anesthetics (as used for long-term sedation) may reach tissue concentrations sufficient to cause suppression of cellular immune mechanisms. For example, an increased incidence of bacterial pneumonia may occur in patients with severe head trauma who receive high doses of thiopental (Nadal et al., 1995).

B Lymphocytes and T Lymphocytes

Lymphocytes responsible for humoral immunity are designated *B lymphocytes* and those responsible for cellular immunity are *T lymphocytes* (see Fig. 57-3). The designation as B lymphocytes reflects the original discovery in birds, in which the formation of these cells occurs in the bursa of Fabricius, whereas the T designation emphasizes the role of the thymus gland in the origin of these cells. Morphologically, B lymphocytes and T lymphocytes are indistinguishable.

B lymphocytes differentiate into memory B cells and plasma cells. Plasma cells are the source of gamma globulin antibodies responsible for humoral immunity. T lymphocytes are categorized as helper/inducer T cells, suppressor T cells, cytotoxic T cells, and memory T cells. Helper/inducer T cells and suppressor T cells are involved in the regulation of antibody production by B lymphocyte derivatives, and cytotoxic T cells destroy foreign cells as represented by organ transplants. Helper/inducer T cells may be designated T4 cells because they often have on their surface a glycoprotein marker called *T4*; cytotoxic and suppressor T cells may be designated T8 cells for a similar reason.

Most of the preprocessing of B lymphocytes that prepares them to manufacture antibodies occurs before and shortly after birth. In humans, it is likely that this preprocessing occurs predominantly in the lymphoid tissue in the fetal liver, and to a lesser extent in bone marrow and gastrointestinal mucosa. Most of the preprocessing of T lymphocytes occurs in the thymus shortly before birth and for a few months after birth. Removal of the thymus gland after this time usually will not interfere with cellular immunity. After formation of processed B and T lymphocytes, these cells are delivered by the circulation to lymphoid tissues, where they are trapped. The location of lymphoid tissues (gastrointestinal tract, spleen, tonsils, adenoids) is optimal for intercepting ingested or inhaled antigens as well as those that reach the circulation.

It is believed that during the processing of B and T lymphocytes, all those clones of lymphocytes capable of destroying the body's own tissues are self-destroyed because of their continued exposure to the body's antigens. This immune tolerance to the body's own tissues may diminish, resulting in autoimmune diseases such as thyroiditis, rheumatic fever, glomerulonephritis, myasthenia gravis, and systemic lupus erythematosus. Likewise, selective suppression of T lymphocytes as with cyclosporine may interfere with early destruction of cancer cells, manifesting as an increased incidence of cancer as in patients who are chronically immunosuppressed, so as to improve acceptance of organ transplants. The human immunodeficiency virus specifically attacks helper/inducer T lymphocytes (T4 cells), with eventual loss of immune function and death from cancer or infections due to normally nonpathogenic bacteria.

Antigens

Antigens are foreign proteins or chemicals that evoke the production of antibodies. Bacteria or toxins contain unique chemical structures that differ from normal body constituents, resulting in their role as antigens. For a substance to be antigenic, it typically must have a molecular weight of >8,000 daltons. Nevertheless, immunity against low-molecular-weight substances can occur if the material acts as a hapten and binds to a protein, the combination resulting in an antigenic response. Haptens that elicit such an immune response are usually drugs, chemical constituents in dust, or shed breakdown products of animal skin.

The critical event in the initiation of the complex immune process that leads to the destruction of foreign pathogens or self-antigens is antigen-induced activation, proliferation, and differentiation of T lymphocytes. The interaction between antigens and T-cell receptors results in activation of T cells, which involves signal transduction mechanisms leading to up-regulation of T-cell derived cytokines. Cytokines in turn initiate events leading to proliferation of T cells to helper and effector cells which with B-cell mediated humoral responses leads to destruction of the antigen.

Antibodies

Before exposure to a specific antigen, clones of B lymphocytes remain dormant in lymphoid tissue. Entry of antigens into lymphoid tissues causes clones of B lymphocytes to form plasma cells capable of producing gamma globulin antibodies specific for activity against that antigen (primary response) (Fig. 57-4) (Guyton and Hall, 2000). Each antibody that is specific for a particular antigen has a different organization of amino acids that lends steric shape. This steric shape fits the antigen and results in a rapid and tight chemical or physical bond between the antibody and antigen. Some B lymphocytes, however, remain dormant in the lymphoid tissue, functioning as B memory cells. Subsequent exposure to the antigen causes these memory cells to participate in an exaggerated antibody response (secondary response) compared with the primary response (see Fig. 57-4) (Guyton and Hall, 2000). The increased intensity and duration of the secondary response is the

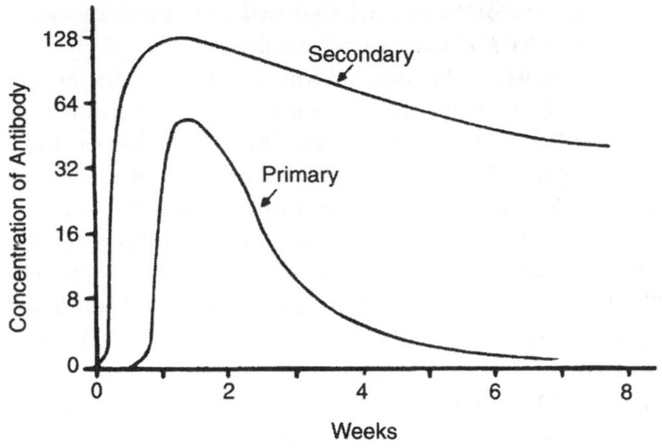

Figure 57-4. Time course of antibody response after primary and secondary injection of antigen. (From Guyton AC, Hall JE. *Textbook of medical physiology*, 10th ed. Philadelphia: Saunders, 2000; with permission.)

reason why vaccination is often achieved by injection of the antigen in multiple small doses several weeks apart.

Structure

Plasma cells form gamma globulin antibodies, which are grouped into five classes of immunoglobulins: IgG, IgA, IgM, IgD, and IgE (Table 57-5). IgG can cross the placenta to enter the fetal circulation and is the principal antibody that reacts with bacteria and probably viruses. IgA is elaborated by plasma cells localized to secretory tissues (tears, saliva, respiratory mucosa, gastrointestinal mucosa, cervical mucosa), thus providing a topical and localized defense against infection. IgM is the most prominent immunoglobulin on the surface of lymphocytes and is the first type of antibody synthesized after initial exposure to an antigen. Natural antibodies against antigens on RBC membranes are IgM. IgD is important in antigen recognition by B cells. IgE antibodies are uniquely important in evoking degranulation of mast cells and basophils, resulting in release of chemical mediators, especially histamine, that are responsible for the symptoms of an allergic reaction.

Mechanism of Action

Antibodies act by (a) direct effects on the antigen, (b) activation of the complement system, or (c) initiation of an anaphylactic reaction. Examples of direct effects of antibodies that destroy antigens are (a) agglutination such as occurs with transfusion of incompatible blood, (b) precipitation, (c) neutralization, and (d) lysis. More important, however, than these direct effects are the amplifying effects of the complement system on anaphylactic reactions.

Complement System

Complement is a system of enzyme precursors that are normally present in the plasma in an inactive form. These enzymes are designated C1 through C9 for the classical pathway and B, D, H, I, and P (properdin) for the alternative pathway (Fig. 57-5) (Frank, 1987). Complement activation proceeds in a sequential fashion comparable to the blood coagulation cascade. Classical pathway activation occurs when IgG or IgM binds to an antigen on the cell membrane of mast cells and basophils. This antigen-antibody complex initiates a sequential cascading process by initially activating the normally quiescent C1. Hereditary angioedema is periodic swelling due to decreased functional activity of the C1 esterase inhibitor. Activation of the alternative pathway occurs via nonimmunologic mechanisms (endotoxins, bubble oxygenator membranes, radiographic contrast media, protamine) independent of antibodies. Activation of C3 and C5 occurs via either pathway, leading to the formation of active fragments known as anaphylatoxins (C3a, C5a). These active fragments evoke changes characterized by (a) lysis of bacterial cell membranes, (b) facilitation of phagocytosis by the phenomenon

TABLE 57-5.
PROPERTIES OF IMMUNOGLOBULINS

	IgG	IgA	IgM	IgD	IgE
Location	Plasma Amniotic fluid	Plasma Saliva Tears	Plasma	Plasma	Plasma
Plasma concentration (mg/dL)	600–1,500	85–380	50–400	<15	0.01–0.03
Plasma half-time (days)	21–23	6	5	2–8	1–5
Function					
Complement activation	+	−	+	−	−
Degranulation of mast cells	−	−	−	−	+
Bacterial lysis	+	−	+	−	−
Opsonization	+	?	−	−	−
Agglutination	+	+	+	−	−
Virus inactivation	+	+	+	−	−

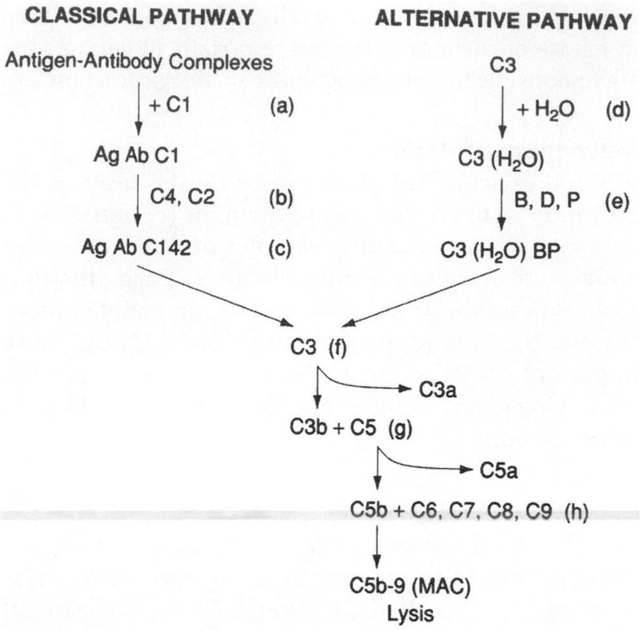

Figure 57-5. Diagram depicting the classical and alternative pathways of the complement system. (From Frank MM. Complement in the pathophysiology of human disease. *N Engl J Med* 1987;316: 1525–1530; with permission.)

of opsonization, (c) attraction of leukocytes to the site of injury (chemotaxis), and (d) degranulation of mast cells and basophils manifesting as an allergic reaction. Activation of the complement system by endotoxin may be important in the development of renal failure and vasodilation in Gram-negative sepsis. Protamine and heparin-protamine complexes can activate the complement cascade.

Anaphylactic Reaction

An anaphylactic reaction occurs when an antigen attaches to IgE antibodies on the cell membranes of circulating basophils or tissue mast cells. This antigen-antibody interaction changes the permeability of the cell membrane, leading to degranulation and release of chemical mediators (histamine, leukotrienes, prostaglandins) into the circulation. These chemical mediators are responsible for the symptoms (hypotension, bronchoconstriction, edema) of an anaphylactic reaction. Chemotactic factors are also released during degranulation, serving to attract neutrophils, eosinophils, and platelets to the site of the antigen-antibody interaction. It is important to recognize that an anaphylactic reaction requires prior exposure to the antigen causing production of IgE antibodies that attach to cell membranes, rendering that cell sensitized should a repeat exposure to that antigen occur.

In some highly sensitized individuals, the degranulation resulting from the antigen-antibody interaction may be so explosive that life-threatening hypotension or bronchoconstriction occurs. Less explosive reactions are characterized by urticaria in which an antigen enters the skin and evokes the local release of histamine. Hay fever results when the antigen-antibody reaction occurs in the nose in contrast to asthma, in which the reaction occurs in the bronchioles of the lungs. Histamine seems to be primarily responsible for the symptoms of hay fever, whereas bronchospasm characteristic of asthma may be mainly due to leukotrienes. Indeed, antihistamines have beneficial effects in the treatment of hay fever; however, less effect is seen in their use for the prevention and treatment of asthma.

TISSUE TYPING

Tissue typing is possible in much the same way that blood is typed. For example, the most important antigens that cause rejection of transplanted tissue are the human leukocyte antigens (HLAs). HLAs are also present on the cell membranes of leukocytes. As a result, tissue typing can be accomplished by determining the types of antigens on the recipient's lymphocyte membranes. Some HLA antigens are poorly antigenic, negating the need for precise tissue matching of all antigens.

REFERENCES

Frank MM. Complement in the pathophysiology of human disease. *N Engl J Med* 1987;316:1525–1530.

Ganong WF. *Review of medical physiology*, 21st ed. Lange Medical Books/McGraw-Hill, 2003.

Goodnough LT, Monk TG, Andriole GL. Erythropoietin therapy. *N Engl J Med* 1997;336:333–338.

Guyton AC, Hall JE. *Textbook of medical physiology*, 10th ed. Philadelphia: Saunders, 2000.

Hall GM, Desborough JP. Interleukin-6 and the metabolic response to surgery. *Br J Anaesth* 1992;69:337–338.

Laroches D, Vergnaud MC, Sillard B, et al. Biochemical markers of anaphylactoid reactions to drugs: comparison of plasma histamine and tryptase. *Anesthesiology* 1991;75:945–949.

Levy JH, Kelly AB. Inflammation and cardiopulmonary bypass. *Can J Anaesth* 1993;40:1009–1015.

Nadal P, Nicolas JM, Font C, et al. Pneumonia in ventilated head trauma patients: The role of thiopental therapy. *Eur J Emerg Med* 1995;2:14–16.

Sheeran P, Hall GM. Cytokines in anaesthesia. *Br J Anaesth* 1997;78: 201–219.

Stevenson GW, Hall SC, Rudnick S, et al. The effect of anesthetic agents on the human immune response. *Anesthesiology* 1990;72:542–552.

Hemostasis and Blood Coagulation

58

Blood consists of components derived from many different sources, including the bone marrow, vascular endothelium, and reticuloendothelial system. Under normal circumstances, the blood remains a liquid system permitting flow and delivery of vital nutrients to tissues. When vascular injury occurs, however, components of this liquid coagulate in a complex cascade of reactions involving multiple enzymes and inhibitor systems designed to transform blood into a solid clot, localized to the site of vascular injury. Once tissue repair has occurred, the blood clot liquefies, restoring normal blood flow through the vessel. This transformation of liquid blood into a solid clot and back again into a liquid is controlled by the hemostatic mechanism, which must regulate the procoagulant as well as the fibrinolytic and antifibrinolytic forces within the blood.

HEMOSTATIC MECHANISM

Normally, the intact endothelial layer of the blood vessel prevents activation of the hemostatic mechanism. When the endothelial lining of the blood vessel is disrupted, however, the hemostatic mechanism sets in motion a series of reactions that culminate in the formation of a fibrin blood clot. The hemostatic response involves three processes characterized as (a) primary hemostasis, (b) coagulation, and (c) fibrinolysis.

Primary Hemostasis (Platelet Plug)

Primary hemostasis takes place within seconds of vascular endothelial injury and is characterized by formation of a platelet plug. Within seconds after the endothelial lining of the blood vessel is disrupted, receptors on the surfaces of platelets interact with exposed collagen and adhere to the site of injury. Factor VIII:vWF and thrombin are also important in platelet activation and adhesion. Contents of cytoplasmic granules (alpha granules) of these platelets are extruded into the circulation, providing the stimulus to attract other platelets (aggregation) to the site of vascular disruption and to further enhance the platelet plug. Substances extruded from platelets include adenosine diphosphate (ADP) and thromboxane A_2. It is likely that platelets can aggregate onto surface receptors that only become available after the platelets are activated by ADP, thrombin, or collagen. Aspirin inhibits the platelet release reaction and subsequent aggregation by irreversibly acetylating cyclooxygenase. Prostacyclin, presumed to come primarily from the vessel wall, allows a clot to form in the wall of the vessel without extending into the vessel lumen. Primary hemostasis is controlled by the balance between thromboxane A_2 and prostacyclin.

The platelet plug mechanism is very important for closing minute breaks in small blood vessels that occur hundreds of times daily. Together, aggregated platelets, fibrinogen, trapped thrombin, and plasminogen form the platelet plug, which temporarily arrests bleeding. Formation of this initial friable platelet plug by the actions of platelets and blood vessels occurs within approximately 5 minutes of vascular damage. When the number of platelets is decreased, small hemorrhagic areas appear under the skin (purpura) and internally.

Vascular Spasm

In addition to the steps that initiate formation of a platelet plug, the wall of the cut blood vessel immediately contracts, which serves to decrease blood loss from the damaged vessel. This contraction results from neural reflexes initiated by pain impulses from the traumatized vessel and release of vasoconstricting substances such as serotonin from platelets. Vascular spasm is most intense in severely traumatized or crushed blood vessels. The sharply cut or transected blood vessel, as occurs during surgery, undergoes less vascular spasm, and blood loss is greater than following surgical trauma. Vascular spasm lasts 20 to 30 minutes, providing time for additional mechanisms of hemostasis to become active.

Megakaryocytes

Megakaryocytes are giant cells in the bone marrow from which cytoplasmic fragments are pinched off and extruded into the circulation as nuclear platelets. It is estimated that each megakaryocyte gives rise to 1,000 to 1,500 platelets. Thrombopoietin is a circulating substance that stimulates the formation of megakaryocytes and thus regulates the production of platelets. There are normally approximately 150,000 to 350,000 platelets in each milliliter of blood, with an average life span of 8 to 12 days. Aged platelets are removed by the reticuloendothelial system and spleen.

Clot Formation

The fundamental reaction in blood clotting is conversion of fibrinogen to fibrin by the action of activated thrombin. Activator substances from the traumatized vascular wall and platelets initiate this process within 15 to 20 s, and after 3 to 6 minutes the cut end of a blood vessel is filled with clot. If whole blood is allowed to clot and the clot is removed, the remaining fluid is serum. Serum is thus plasma with factors I, II, V, and VII removed.

Growth of Fibrous Tissue

Invasion of blood clot by fibroblasts causes formation of connective tissue throughout the clot. Conversion of the clot to fibrous tissue is complete in 7 to 10 days.

Coagulation

Coagulation takes place in three essential steps. In response to rupture of the vessel or damage to the blood itself, a complex cascade of chemical reactions occurs in the blood involving more than a dozen blood coagulation factors. The net result is formation of a complex of activated substances collectively called prothrombin activator (Fig. 58-1) (Guyton and Hall, 2000). The prothrombin activator catalyzes the conversion of prothrombin into thrombin. The thrombin acts as an enzyme to convert fibrinogen into fibrin fibers that enmesh platelets, blood cells, and plasma to form the clot.

The coagulation process is closely intertwined with primary hemostasis and fibrinolysis. At the same time that platelets are adhering to the denuded endothelial surfaces and becoming activated, the coagulation cascade provides thrombin, which is incorporated into the platelet plug along with fibrinogen and plasminogen. The completion of the coagulation process converts fibrinogen into fibrin and the platelet plug is transformed into a fibrin clot. Plasminogen is incorporated into the forming fibrin clot and will ultimately initiate the fibrinolytic process that dissolves the blood clot.

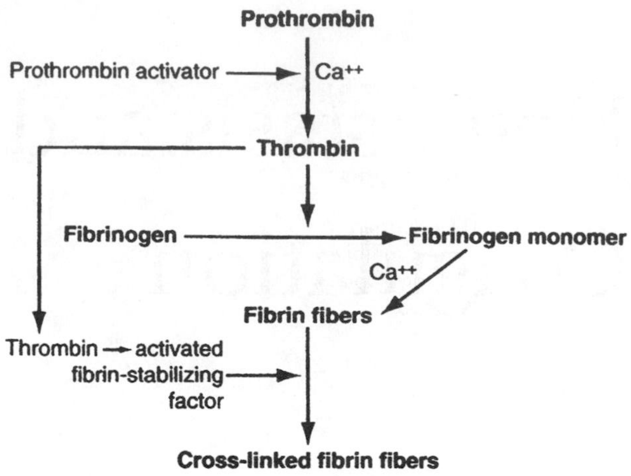

Figure 58-1. Pathway for conversion of prothrombin to thrombin and polymerization of fibrinogen from fibrin fibers (From Guyton AC, Hall JE. *Textbook of medical physiology*, 10th ed. Philadelphia: Saunders, 2000; with permission.)

Clotting Factors

More than 50 different substances that promote (procoagulants) or inhibit (anticoagulants) coagulation have been identified in blood and tissues (Table 58-1) (Guyton and Hall, 2000). Normally anticoagulants (antithrombin, protein C, protein S) predominate and blood does not coagulate. When a blood vessel is transected or damaged, activity of the procoagulants in the area of the damage becomes predominant and clot formation occurs. During the process of coagulation, a portion of the protein procoagulant molecule is cleaved and the "activated clotting factor" is designated by a lowercase *a* after the Roman numeral of the factor. Most of the coagulation proteins are synthesized in the liver with the exception of von Willebrand (vWF) factor VIII, which is synthesized by endothelial cells and megakaryocytes and serves as a carrier protein for the procoagulant factor VIII. Factor VIII:vWF is important for enhancing adhesion of platelets to vascular endothelial surfaces. The smaller subcomponent (factor VIII:C) is most likely synthesized in the liver, and its deficiency or absence is responsible for hemophilia A. The plasma concentration of factor VIII is precisely controlled, with increases in the circulating level of this factor being evoked by epinephrine, vasopressin, and estrogens.

Continued clot formation occurs only where blood is not flowing. This is true because the flow of blood dilutes thrombin and other procoagulants released during the clotting process, thus preventing their concentration from increasing sufficiently to sustain continued formation of clot. Furthermore, activated clotting factors are preferentially removed from the circulation by the liver and reticuloendothelial system.

Within a few minutes after the clot is formed, it begins to contract and typically expresses most of the fluid from itself after 30 to 60 minutes. Platelets are necessary for this clot retraction to occur. Indeed, failure of clot retraction is

TABLE 58-1.
NOMENCLATURE OF BLOOD CLOTTING FACTORS

Factor	Synonyms	Plasma Concentration (μg/ml)	Half-Time (hrs)	Stability in Stored Whole Blood
I	Fibrinogen	2,000–4,000	95–120	No change
II	Prothrombin	150	65–90	No change
III	Thromboplastin			
IV	Calcium			
V	Proaccelerin	10	15–24	Labile
VII	Proconvertin	0.5	4–6	No change
VIII	Antihemophilic factor	50–100	10–12	Labile
VIII:vWF		50–100		
VIII:C		0.05–0.10		
IX	Christmas factor	3	18–30	No change
X	Stuart-Prower factor	15	40–60	No change
XI	Plasma thromboplastin factor	5	45–60	Labile
XII	Hageman factor			
XIII	Fibrin-stabilizing factor			

an indication that the number of circulating platelets is inadequate. Normally, as the blood clot retracts, the edges of the broken blood vessels are pulled together, restoring the integrity of the vascular lumen.

Pathway for Coagulation

The classic depiction of coagulation as an intrinsic and extrinsic pathway that converged with the formation of activated factor X has been replaced by the concept that integrates all of the factors into a single coagulation pathway. In this model, coagulation is triggered by the exposure of blood to "tissue factor" that is extrinsic to blood. The pathway is designated the *tissue factor pathway of coagulation.*

Tissue Factor Pathway of Coagulation

Coagulation is initiated when damage to blood vessels exposes tissue factor (thromboplastin) to circulating factor VII. Tissue factor is a protein embedded in association with phospholipid in the surface membranes of fibroblasts and pericytes in blood vessel walls and in a variety of other tissue cells. Tissue factor is considered the in vivo trigger for coagulation.

Exposure of factor VII to tissue factor results in formation of factor VIIa/tissue factor complex. This newly formed complex reacts with factors X and XI to result in activation of these procoagulants. Once formed, factor Xa binds together with its cofactor, factor Va, on the platelet phospholipid surface (PF3), and together they activate prothrombin (factor II) to thrombin (IIa). Prothrombin as well as factors VII, IX, and X depends on the presence of vitamin K for synthesis in the liver. Lack of vitamin K resulting from absence of bile salts or the presence of severe liver disease may prevent normal prothrombin formation. Failure of the liver to synthesize prothrombin leads to a decrease in its plasma concentration below normal levels in 24 hours.

Recombinant activated factor VII is approved for treatment of patients with congenital hemophilia and inhibitors of factor VIII or IX, as well as for patients with acquired hemophilia. Administration of recombinant activated factor VII may be the only remaining therapeutic option to stop life-threatening coagulopathic bleeding (Haas et al., 2005).

Thrombin is a proteolytic enzyme that acts on fibrinogen to remove two low-molecular-weight peptides from each molecule of fibrinogen, resulting in a fibrin monomer that can polymerize with other fibrin monomers. A large number of fibrin monomers polymerize within seconds into long fibrin threads that form the reticulum of the clot. Ultimately, the blood clot comprises a meshwork of cross-linked fibrin threads that adhere to the damaged surfaces of blood vessels, entrapping platelets, erythrocytes, and plasma. Because of its large molecular weight, little fibrinogen normally leaks into interstitial fluids, accounting for the lack of coagulation in this fluid. When capillary permeability increases, however, as in the presence of inflammation, fibrinogen can enter interstitial fluids and initiate coagulation.

Endogenous Anticoagulants

Antithrombin is a circulating substance that binds to thrombin, thus preventing its conversion to fibrin. The binding of antithrombin to thrombin is greatly facilitated by heparin. Heparin is present in circulating basophils and mast cells located in tissues around capillaries. Mast cells are particularly abundant in tissues surrounding capillaries of the lungs and, to a lesser extent, those of the liver. This is important because capillaries of the lungs and liver receive many embolic clots formed in the slowly moving venous blood. Heparin may prevent further growth of these clots. Protein C is a circulating substance that inhibits the activity of factors VIII:C and V. Protein S enhances the effect of protein C. There is an increased incidence of thrombosis in patients with deficient amounts of antithrombin, protein C, or protein S. Furthermore, heparin is not an effective anticoagulant when administered to patients with deficient antithrombin levels.

Drotrecogin Alfa (Activated)

Drotrecogin alfa (activated) is a recombinant form of human-activated protein C. Infusions of drotrecogin alfa are indicated for reduction of mortality in adult patients with severe sepsis associated with acute organ dysfunction. The risk of bleeding in increased and this drug should not be administered to patients with active internal hemorrhage. Drotrecogin alfa is inactivated by endogenous plasma protease inhibitors.

Impact of Progressive Blood Loss

It is likely that stress, tissue trauma with release of tissue thromboplastin, and increases in the plasma concentrations of catecholamines offset any hypocoagulable tendency resulting from hemodilution and loss of coagulation factors during progressive blood loss. These offsetting factors are probably responsible for the increase in coagulability seen in many surgical patients experiencing moderate to massive blood loss (Tuman et al., 1987).

Fibrinolysis

The process of fibrinolysis leads to the dissolution of fibrin clots and restores normal blood flow through blood vessels. The fibrinolytic system involves the conversion of plasminogen to plasmin, the active fibrinolytic enzyme. Plasmin is formed in response to thrombin and tissue plasminogen activator, leading to the lysis of fibrin clots and production of fibrin split products. Urokinase, which is secreted by the kidneys, is capable of converting plasminogen to plasmin. Likewise, certain bacteria such as streptococci secrete substances (streptokinase) capable of converting plasminogen to plasmin. The therapeutic use of plasminogen activators is dissolution of intravascular clots by plasmin without a major effect on circulating fibrinogen. The principal importance of the endogenous fibrinolysin system is the removal of minute clots from small peripheral vessels that otherwise would become occluded. Conversely, opening of large blood vessels by this process rarely occurs. Excess activity of plasmin causes destruction of clotting factors I, II, V, VIII, and XII. As a result, lysis of clots may also be associated with hypocoagulability of the blood.

THROMBOEMBOLISM

Formation of clot inside a blood vessel is called *thrombus* to distinguish it from normal extravascular clotting of blood. An embolus is a fragment of the thrombus that breaks off and travels in the blood until it lodges at a site of vascular narrowing. For this reason, an embolus originating in an artery usually occludes a more distal and smaller artery. Conversely, an embolus originating in a vein commonly lodges in the lungs causing pulmonary vascular obstruction.

Thromboembolism is likely to occur in the presence of (a) any condition that causes a roughened endothelial vessel wall, such as arteriosclerosis, infection, or trauma, and (b) a slowing of blood flow. Slow or sluggish blood flow means activated clotting factors are less diluted and carried away slowly, thus increasing the likelihood of localized clotting. Indeed, vascular stasis in leg veins associated with pregnancy or postoperative immobility is a common precipitating event for the formation of a venous thrombus and subsequent pulmonary embolism.

DISSEMINATED INTRAVASCULAR COAGULATION

Disseminated intravascular coagulation (DIC) reflects entrance of substances into the circulation that cause elaboration of thrombin, leading to widespread thrombosis in small blood vessels. Hypofibrinogenemia occurs when fibrinogen is consumed in formation of these thrombi. Other clotting factors along with platelets may also be consumed. Spontaneous hemorrhage is likely while the presence of fibrin-split products reflects activity of plasmin in dissolving (lysing) intravascular clots. Examples of events that may provoke DIC include complications of pregnancy and childbirth, sepsis, prolonged hypotension, incompatible blood transfusions, and cancer.

REFERENCES

Guyton AC, Hall JE. *Textbook of medical physiology*, 10th ed. Philadelphia: Saunders, 2000.

Haas T, Innerhofer P, Kuhbacher G, et al. Successful reversal of deleterious coagulopathy by recombinant factor VIIa. *Anesth Analg* 2005;100:54–58.

Tuman KJ, Spiess BD, McCarthy RJ, et al. Effects of progressive blood loss on coagulation as measured by thrombelastography. *Anesth Analg* 1987;66:856–863.

Metabolism of Nutrients

59

Metabolism refers to all the chemical and energy transformations that occur in the body. Oxidation of nutrients (carbohydrates, fats, and proteins) results in production of carbon dioxide, water, and high-energy phosphate bonds necessary for life processes. The most important high-energy phosphate bond is adenosine triphosphate (ATP) (Fig. 59-1). This ubiquitous molecule is the energy storehouse for the body, providing the energy necessary for essentially all physiologic processes and chemical reactions. Probably the most important intracellular process that requires energy from hydrolysis of ATP is formation of peptide linkages between amino acids during protein synthesis. Skeletal muscle contraction cannot occur without energy from ATP hydrolysis. ATP from metabolism of nutrients is necessary to provide energy for transport of ions across cell membranes and thus to maintain the distribution of these ions, which is necessary for propagation of nerve impulses. In renal tubules, as much as 80% of ATP is used for membrane transport of ions. In addition to its function in energy transfer, ATP is also the precursor of cyclic adenosine monophosphate (cAMP).

For adults, total energy expenditure averages 39 kcal/kg in males and 34 kcal/kg in females. Approximately 20 kcal/kg is expended as basal metabolism necessary to maintain energy-requiring tasks essential for life. In the resting state, the necessary basal expenditure of calories is equivalent to approximately 1.1 kcal/minute, which requires use of 200 to 250 mL/minute of oxygen. Activities increase caloric requirements in proportion to the energy expenditure required (Table 59-1). The caloric values of carbohydrates, fats, and proteins are approximately 4.1 kcal/g, 9.3 kcal/g, and 4.1 kcal/g, respectively. Fat forms the major energy storage depot because of its greater mass and high caloric value (Fig. 59-2) (Berne et al., 2004). Indeed, the primary form in which potential chemical energy is stored in the body is fat (triglyceride). The high caloric density and hydrophobic nature of triglycerides permit efficient energy storage without adverse osmotic consequences.

CARBOHYDRATE METABOLISM

The liver is the site of carbohydrate metabolism where regulation of production and storage of glucose takes place based on metabolic needs. At least 99% of all the energy derived from carbohydrates is used to form ATP in the cells. The final products of carbohydrate digestion in the gastrointestinal tract are glucose, fructose, and galactose. After absorption into the circulation, fructose and galactose are rapidly converted to glucose. As a result, glucose is the predominant molecule in carbohydrate metabolism. This glucose must be transported through cell membranes into cellular cytoplasm before it can be used by cells. This transport uses a protein carrier known as *carrier-mediated diffusion*, which is enhanced by insulin. Immediately upon entering cells, glucose is converted to glucose-6-phosphate under the influence of the enzyme glucokinase. This phosphorylation of glucose prevents escape of glucose from cells back into the circulation.

The fetus derives almost all its energy from glucose obtained by means of the maternal circulation. Immediately after birth, the infant stores of glycogen are sufficient to supply glucose for only a few hours. Furthermore, gluconeogenesis is limited in the neonate. As a result, the neonate is vulnerable to hypoglycemia.

Glycogen

After entering cells, glucose can be used immediately for release of energy to cells or it can be stored as a polymer of glucose known as *glycogen*. Although all cells can store at least some glucose as glycogen, the liver and skeletal muscles are particularly capable of storing large amounts of glycogen. The ability to form glycogen makes it possible to

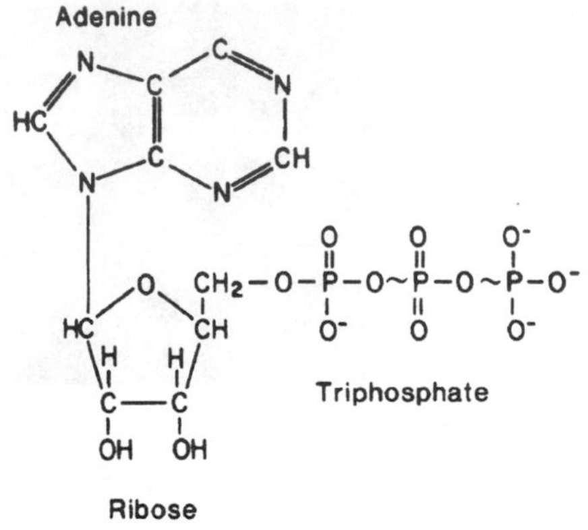

Figure 59-1. Metabolism of nutrients in cells is directed toward the ultimate synthesis of adenosine triphosphate (ATP). Energy necessary for physiologic processes and chemical reactions is derived from the high-energy phosphate bonds of ATP.

TABLE 59-1. ESTIMATES OF ENERGY EXPENDITURE IN ADULTS

Activity	Calorie Expenditure (kcal/Minute)
Basal	1.1
Sitting	1.8
Walking (2.5 miles/hr)	4.3
Walking (4 miles/hr)	8.2
Climbing stairs	9.0
Swimming	10.9
Bicycling (13 miles/hr)	11.1

store substantial quantities of carbohydrates without significantly altering the osmotic pressure of intracellular fluids. Glycogen breakdown is catalyzed by activation of phosphorylase in the liver and skeletal muscles by the action of epinephrine on beta receptors.

Gluconeogenesis

Gluconeogenesis is the formation of glucose from amino acids and the glycerol portion of fat. This process occurs when body stores of carbohydrates decrease below normal levels. An estimated 60% of the amino acids in the body's proteins can be converted easily to carbohydrates, whereas the remaining 40% have chemical configurations that make this conversion difficult.

Gluconeogenesis is stimulated by hypoglycemia. In addition, simultaneous release of cortisol mobilizes proteins, making these available in the form of amino acids for gluconeogenesis, especially in the liver. Thyroxine is also capable of increasing the rate of gluconeogenesis.

Energy Release from Glucose

Glucose is progressively broken down, and the resulting energy is used to form ATP. For each mole of glucose that is completely degraded to carbon dioxide and water, a total of 38 moles of ATP is ultimately formed. The most important means by which energy is released from the glucose molecule is by glycolysis and the subsequent oxidation of the end-products of glycolysis. Glycolysis is the splitting of the glucose molecule into two molecules of pyruvate, which enter the mitochondria. In the mitochondria, pyruvate is converted to acetyl-coenzyme A (CoA), which enters the citric acid cycle (tricarboxylic acid cycle or Krebs cycle) and is converted to carbon dioxide and hydrogen ions with the formation of large quantities of ATP (oxidative phosphorylation) (Fig. 59-3). Oxidative phosphorylation occurs only in the mitochondria and in the presence of adequate amounts of oxygen.

Anaerobic Glycolysis

In the absence of adequate amounts of oxygen, a small amount of energy can be released to cells by anaerobic

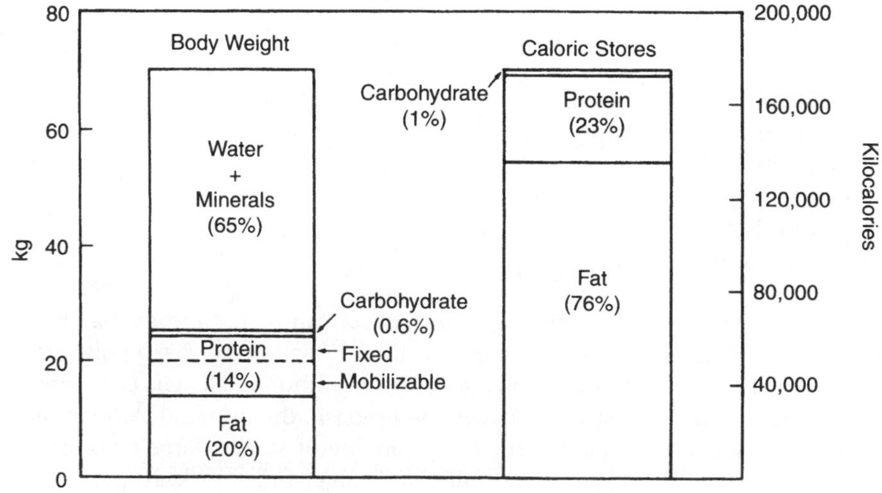

Figure 59-2. Comparison of the composition of body weight to caloric stores. (From Berne RM, Levy MN, Koeppen BM, et al. *Physiology*, 5th ed. St. Louis: Mosby, 2004; with permission.)

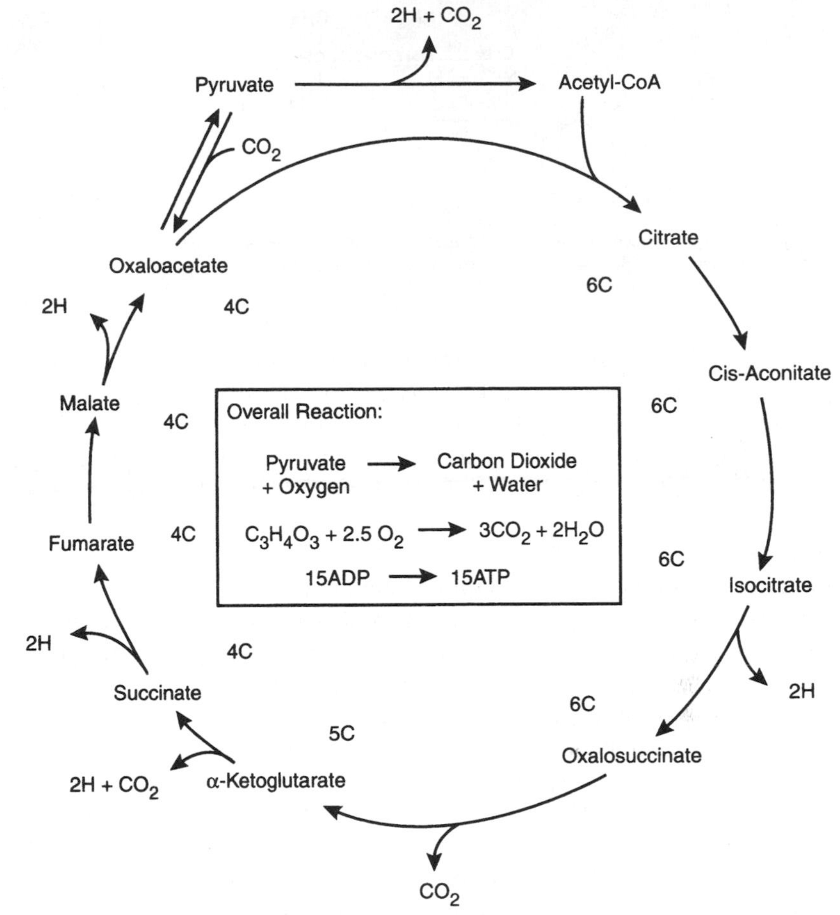

Figure 59-3. Citric acid cycle resulting in production of 15 moles of adenosine triphosphate (ATP) by oxidative phosphorylation.

glycolysis because conversion of glucose to pyruvate does not require oxygen. Indeed, carbohydrates are the only nutrient that can form ATP without oxygen. This release of glycolytic energy to cells can be lifesaving for a few minutes should oxygen become unavailable.

During anaerobic glycolysis, most pyruvic acid is converted to lactic acid, which diffuses rapidly out of cells into extracellular fluid. When oxygen is again available, this lactic acid can be reconverted to glucose. This reconversion occurs predominantly in the liver. Indeed, severe liver disease may interfere with the ability of the liver to convert lactic acid to glucose, leading to metabolic acidosis.

LIPID METABOLISM

Lipids include phospholipids, triglycerides, and cholesterol. The basic lipid moiety of phospholipids and triglycerides is fatty acids. Fatty acids are long-chain hydrocarbon organic acids that, when bound to albumin, are known as *free fatty acids* (Fig. 59-4). An important role of free fatty acids is as precursors for prostaglandins. Phospholipids include lecithins, cephalins, and sphingomyelins, which are formed principally in the liver and are important in the formation of myelin and cell membranes. The basic structure of the triglyceride molecule is three long-chain fatty acids bound with one molecule of glycerol (Fig. 59-5). Triglycerides, after absorption from the gastrointestinal tract, are transported in the lymph and then, by way of the thoracic duct, into the circulation in droplets known as *chylomicrons.* Chylomicrons are rapidly removed from the circulation and stored as they pass through capillaries of adipose tissue and skeletal muscles. Triglycerides are used in the body mainly to provide energy for metabolic processes similar to those fueled by carbohydrates. Cholesterol does not contain fatty acids, but its sterol nucleus is synthesized

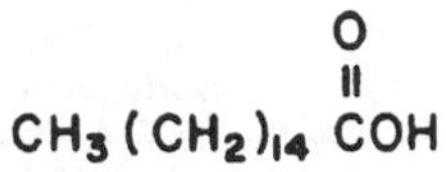

Figure 59-4. Palmitic acid.

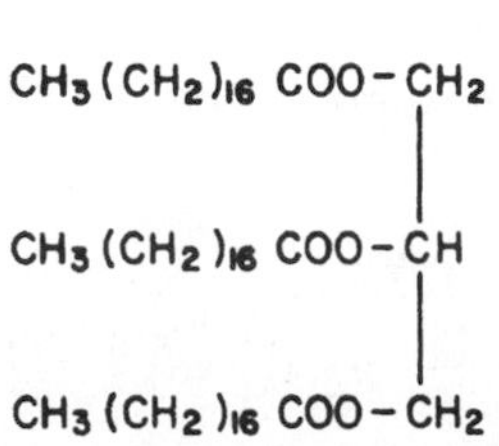

Figure 59-5. The basic structure of the triglyceride molecule is three long-chain fatty acids bound with one molecule of glycerol.

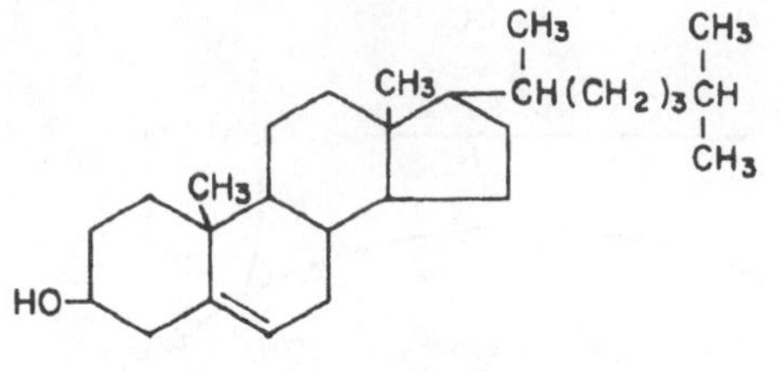

Figure 59-6. Cholesterol contains a sterol nucleus that is synthesized from degradation products of fatty acid molecules.

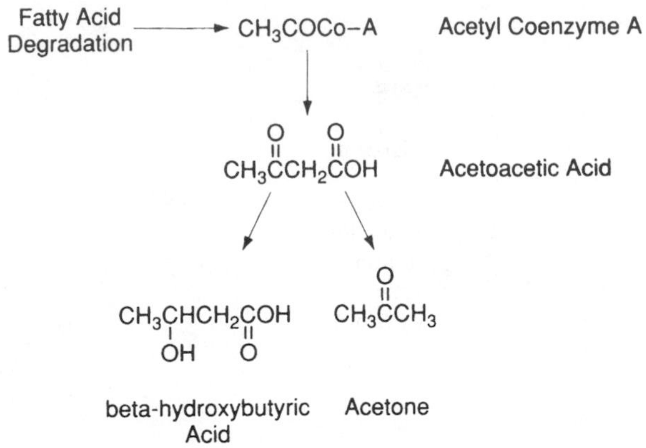

Figure 59-7. Fatty acid degradation in the liver leads to the formation of acetyl-CoA. Two molecules of acetyl-CoA combine to form acetoacetic acid, which, in large part, is converted to beta-hydroxybutyric acid, and in lesser amounts, to acetone.

from degradation products of fatty acid molecules, thus giving it many of the physical and chemical properties characteristic of lipids (Fig. 59-6).

Lipoproteins are synthesized principally in the liver and are mixtures of phospholipids, triglycerides, cholesterol, and proteins (Table 59-2). The presumed function of lipoproteins is to provide a mechanism of transport for lipids throughout the body. Lipoproteins are classified according to their density, which is inversely proportional to their lipid content (see Table 58-2) (see Chapter 32). All the cholesterol in plasma is in lipoprotein complexes, with low-density lipoproteins (LDL) representing the major cholesterol component in plasma. These LDLs provide cholesterol to tissues, where it is an essential component of cell membranes and is used in the synthesis of corticosteroids and sex hormones. In the liver, LDLs are taken up by receptor-mediated endocytosis. An intrinsic feedback control system increases the endogenous production of cholesterol when exogenous intake is decreased, explaining the relatively modest lowering effect on plasma cholesterol concentrations produced by low-cholesterol diets. If this endogenous increase in cholesterol synthesis is blocked by drugs that inhibit hydroxymethylglutaryl coenzyme A (HMG-CoA) reductase, then there is an appreciable decrease in the plasma cholesterol concentration.

Drugs that selectively inhibit HMG-CoA are known as statins. Statins effectively lower plasma LDL cholesterol concentrations and seem to provide protection against acute cardiac events, perhaps reflecting antiinflammatory effects. In addition, statins lower plasma triglyceride concentrations and modestly increase HDL cholesterol concentrations. Drugs that bind bile salts (cholestyramine, colestipol) prevent cholesterol from reentering the circulation as part of the enterohepatic circulation. A disadvantage of using drugs that bind bile salts to lower plasma cholesterol concentrations is an associated increase in plasma triglyceride concentrations.

The first step in the use of triglycerides for energy is hydrolysis into fatty acids and glycerol and subsequent transport of these products to tissues, where they are oxidized. Almost all cells, except for brain cells, can use fatty acids interchangeably with glucose for energy. Degradation and oxidation of fatty acids occur only in mitochondria, resulting in progressive release of two carbon fragments (beta-oxidation) in the form of acetyl-CoA (Fig. 59-7). These acetyl-CoA molecules enter the citric acid cycle in the same manner as acetyl-CoA formed from pyruvate during the metabolism of glucose, ultimately leading to formation of ATP. In the liver, two molecules of acetyl-CoA formed from the degradation of fatty acids can combine to form acetoacetic acid (see Fig. 59-7). A substantial amount of acetoacetic acid is converted to beta-hydroxybutyric acid

TABLE 59-2.
COMPOSITION OF LIPIDS IN THE PLASMA

	Phospholipid (%)	Triglyceride (%)	Free Cholesterol (%)	Cholesterol Esters	Protein (%)	Density
Chylomicrons	3	90	2	3	2	0.94
LDL	21	6	7	46	20	1.019–1.063
HDL	25	5	4	16	50	1.063–1.21
IDL	20	40	5	25	10	1.006–1.019
VLDL	17	55	4	18	8	0.94–1.006

HDL, high-density lipoprotein; IDL, intermediate-density lipoprotein; LDL, low-density lipoprotein; VLDL, very-low-density lipoprotein.

TABLE 59-3.
TYPES OF PROTEINS

Globular	Fibrous	Conjugated
Albumin	Collagen	Mucoprotein
Globulin	Elastic fibers	Structural components of cells
Fibrinogen	Keratin	
Hemoglobin	Actin	
Enzymes	Myosin	
Nucleoproteins		

and small amounts of acetone. In the absence of adequate carbohydrate metabolism (starvation or uncontrolled diabetes mellitus), large quantities of acetoacetic acid, beta-hydroxybutyric acid, and acetone accumulate in the blood to produce ketosis because almost all the energy of the body must come from metabolism of lipids.

In contrast to glycogen, large amounts of lipids can be stored in adipose tissue and in the liver. A major function of adipose tissue is to store triglycerides until they are needed for energy. Epinephrine and norepinephrine activate triglyceride lipase in cells, leading to mobilization of fatty acids.

PROTEIN METABOLISM

Approximately 75% of the solid constituents of the body are proteins (Table 59-3). All proteins are composed of the same 20 amino acids, and several of these must be supplied in the diet because they cannot be formed endogenously (essential amino acids) (Table 59-4). Endogenous synthesis of amino acids depends first on the formation of appropriate alpha-keto acids. For example, pyruvate formed during the glycolytic breakdown of glucose is the keto acid precursor of alanine. Each amino acid has an acidic group (COOH) and a nitrogen radical, usually represented by an

TABLE 59-4.
AMINO ACIDS

Essential	Nonessential
Arginine	Alanine
Histidine	Asparagine
Isoleucine	Aspartic acid
Leucine	Cysteine
Lysine	Glutamic acid
Methionine	Glutamine
Phenylalanine	Glycine
Threonine	Proline
Tryptophan	Serine
Valine	Tyrosine

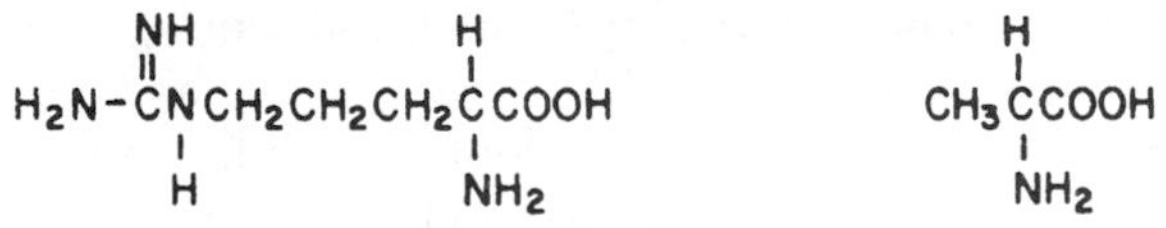

Arginine Alanine

Figure 59-8. Examples of amino acids containing an acidic group (COOH) or an amino group (NH_2).

amino group (Fig. 59-8). In proteins, amino acids are connected into long chains by peptide linkages. Even the smallest proteins characteristically contain more than 20 amino acids connected by peptide linkages, whereas complex proteins have as many as 100,000 amino acids. In addition, more than one amino acid chain in a protein may be bound together by hydrogen bonds, hydrophobic bonds, and electrostatic forces. The type of protein formed by the cell is genetically determined.

Amino acids are relatively strong acids and exist in the blood principally in the ionized form. Even after a meal, the blood amino acid concentration increases only a few milligrams, reflecting rapid tissue uptake, especially by the liver. Passage of amino acids into cells requires active transport mechanisms, because these substances are too large to pass through channels in cell membranes. In proximal renal tubules, amino acids that have entered the glomerular filtrate are actively transported back into the blood. These transport mechanisms have maximums above which amino acids appear in the urine. In the normal person, however, loss of amino acids in the urine each day is negligible.

Storage of Amino Acids

Immediately after entry into cells, amino acids are conjugated under the influence of intracellular enzymes into cellular proteins. As a result, concentrations of amino acids inside cells remain low. Indeed, storage of large amounts of amino acids does not occur, but rather these substances are stored as actual proteins in the liver, kidneys, and gastrointestinal mucosa. Nevertheless, these proteins can be rapidly decomposed again into amino acids under the influence of intracellular liposomal digestive enzymes. The resulting amino acids can then be transported out of cells into blood to maintain optimal plasma amino acid concentrations. Tissues can synthesize new proteins from amino acids in blood. This response is especially apparent in relation to protein synthesis in cancer cells. Cancer cells are prolific users of amino acids, and, simultaneously, the proteins of other tissues become markedly depleted.

Plasma Proteins

Plasma proteins are represented by (a) albumin, which provides colloid osmotic pressure; (b) globulins necessary for natural and acquired immunity; and (c) fibrinogen, which polymerizes into long fibrin threads during coagulation of blood. Essentially, all plasma albumin and fibrinogen and 60% to 80% of the globulins are formed in the liver. The remainder of the globulins are formed in lymphoid tissues and other cells of the reticuloendothelial system. The rate of plasma protein formation by the liver can be greatly increased in situations, such as severe burns, where there is loss of large amounts of fluid and protein through denuded tissues. The synthesis rate of plasma proteins by the liver depends on the blood concentration of amino acids. Even during starvation or severe debilitating diseases, the ratio of total tissue proteins to total plasma proteins in the body remains relatively constant at approximately 33:1. Because of the reversible equilibrium between plasma proteins and other proteins of the body, one of the most effective of all therapies for acute protein deficiency is the intravenous administration of plasma proteins. Within hours, amino acids of the administered protein become distributed throughout cells of the body to form proteins where they are needed.

Albumin

Albumin is the most abundant plasma protein and is principally responsible for maintaining plasma osmotic pressure. In addition, albumin is important as a transporter of plasma bound substances often including exogenously administered drugs. Normal daily synthesis of albumin is about 10 g and the half-time for this protein may be as long as 22 days. Therefore, serum albumin concentrations may not be noticeably decreased in early states of acute hepatic failure. Cytokines associated with sepsis may interfere with the hepatic production of albumin.

Coagulation Factors

Hepatocytes are the site of synthesis of all protein coagulation factors with the exception of von Willebrand factor and factor VIIIC. Coagulation may be rapidly impaired by acute liver failure reflecting the short plasma half-time (factor VII 100 to 300 minutes). Vitamin K (uptake dependent on bile salts) is necessary for modification of several of the clotting factors (prothrombin, antithrombin, protein S, and protein C).

Use of Proteins for Energy

After cells contain a maximal amount of protein, any additional amino acids are either deaminated (oxidative deamination) to keto acids that can enter the citric acid cycle to become energy or are stored as fat. Deamination of surplus amino acids may also be coupled with the transfer of an amino acid group from one amino acid to another amino acid (transamination). Ammonia resulting from transamination is converted to urea in the liver for excretion by the kidneys. Indeed, acute hepatic failure manifests by accumulation of toxic concentrations of ammonia. Certain deaminated amino acids are similar to the breakdown products that result from glucose and fatty acid metabolism. For example, deaminated alanine is pyruvic acid, which can be converted to glucose or glycogen, or it can become acetyl-CoA, which is polymerized to fatty acids. The conversion of amino acids to glucose or glycogen is *gluconeogenesis*, and the conversion of amino acids into fatty acids is *ketogenesis*. In the absence of protein intake, approximately 20 to 30 g of endogenous protein are degraded into amino acids daily. In severe starvation, cellular functions deteriorate because of protein depletion. Carbohydrates and lipids spare protein stores because they are used in preference to proteins for energy.

Growth hormone and insulin promote the synthesis rate of cellular proteins, possibly by facilitating the transfer of amino acids into cells. Glucocorticoids increase the breakdown rate of extrahepatic proteins, thereby making increased amino acids available to the liver. This allows the liver to synthesize increased amounts of cellular proteins and plasma proteins. Testosterone increases protein deposition in tissues, particularly the contractile proteins of skeletal muscles.

EFFECT OF STRESS ON METABOLISM

Carbohydrate, lipid, and protein metabolism are significantly altered by stress. Stress increases secretion of cortisol, catecholamines, and glucagon resulting in increased endogenous glucose production (hepatic gluconeogenesis) and hyperglycemia (provides glucose to cells involved in wound healing and inflammatory responses). Increased lipolysis reflects stress-induced beta-adrenergic stimulation. A predictable response to stress is catabolism of proteins in skeletal muscles.

Exogenous glucose administered to injured or septic patients has a minimal effect on gluconeogenesis and lipolysis. Conversely, administration of glucose in the presence of starvation decreases gluconeogenesis and lipolysis. Total parenteral nutrition including lipid emulsions are utilized to provide nutrition to severely stressed patients.

OBESITY

Given the importance of energy stores to individual survival and reproductive capacity, the ability to conserve energy in the form of adipose tissue would at one time have conferred a survival advantage (Rosenbaum et al., 1997). For this reason, human genes that favor energy intake and storage are presumed to be present although not yet identified. Nevertheless, the combination of easy access to calorically dense foods and a sedentary lifestyle has made the metabolic consequences of these presumed genes maladaptive. In addition, certain medications are commonly associated with weight gain (Table 59-5) (Purnell and Weyer, 2003).

TABLE 59-5.
DRUGS COMMONLY ASSOCIATED WITH WEIGHT GAIN

Classification	Drug	Alternative Drug
Antidepressants	Tricyclic antidepressants Monoamine oxidase inhibitors	Selective serotonin reuptake inhibitors
Antidiabetics	Insulin Sulfonylureas Thiazolidinediones	Metformin, acarbose
Antiepileptics	Gabapentin Valproic acid	Lamotrigine Topiramate
Antipsychotics	Clozapine	Haloperidol
Steroids	Glucocorticoids	

Obesity is the most common and costly nutritional problem in the United States. Based on body mass index (BMI) (weight in kilograms divided by the square of the height in meters), 67% of adult males and 62% of adult females are overweight (BMI ≥25) and 27.5% of adult males and 34% of adult females (BMI ≥30) are obese (Flegal et al., 2002). The prevalence of obesity peaks between 60 and 69 years of age. BMI of >28 is associated with a three to four times increase in the risk of ischemic heart disease, stroke, and diabetes mellitus compared with the general population. Increased waist circumference (>102 cm in adult males and >88 cm in adult females) is associated with an increased risk for ischemic heart disease, diabetes mellitus, and systemic hypertension. In this regard, an overweight person with a predominant abdominal fat distribution (most likely in males, elderly, and impaired glucose tolerance) may be at high risk for these diseases even if not considered obese by body mass index criteria. The increased risk for morbidity and mortality extend beyond measurements of BMI and fat distribution as reflected by the diagnosis of *Metabolic Syndrome* (syndrome X, insulin-resistance syndrome) (Table 59-6) (Executive Summary of the NCEP Expert Panel, 2001). Risk of anesthesia may be increased in morbidly obese patients reflecting mechanical (airway, positioning, ventilation) and comorbid conditions (diabetes mellitus, systemic hypertension).

TABLE 59-6.
CRITERIA FOR DIAGNOSIS OF METABOLIC SYNDROME (ANY THREE OF THE FOLLOWING CHARACTERISTICS)

Characteristic	Specific Finding
Waist circumference	Males >102 cm (40 inches) Females >88 cm (35 inches)
Blood glucose concentration (fasting)`	>110 mg/dL
Increased systemic blood pressure	Systolic >130 mm Hg Diastolic >85 mm Hg
Serum triglyceride concentration	>150 mg/dL
High density lipoprotein cholesterol concentration	Males <40 mg/dL Females <50 mg/dL

Treatment (see the section, Pharmacologic Treatment) of obesity directed toward the long-term decrease in body weight is largely ineffective, and 90% to 95% of persons who lose weight subsequently regain it (Wadden, 1993). Both proteins and carbohydrates can be metabolically converted to fat, and there is no evidence that changing the relative proportions of protein, carbohydrate, and fat in the diet without decreasing caloric intake will promote weight loss (Leibel et al., 1992). However, fat has a higher caloric density than protein and carbohydrate, and its contribution to the palatability of foods promotes the ingestion of calories.

Pharmacologic Treatment

Phentermine is an appetite suppressant that is utilized for short-term therapy intended to induce weight loss. In the past, this drug was frequently used in combination with fenfluramine. Central nervous system activation may manifest as anxiety, tachycardia, and insomnia. Long-term pharmacologic therapy intended to induce weight loss utilizes sibutramine or orlistat. Sibutramine-induced weight loss may be associated with decreased plasma triglyceride concentrations, increased HDL cholesterol concentrations, and improved glycemic control in patients with diabetes mellitus (Dujovne et al., 2001). Side effects of sibutramine include cardiovascular stimulation (monitor blood pressure and heart rate) and this drug is not recommended in patients with untreated systemic hypertension or coronary artery disease. Orlistat inhibits lipases in the gastrointestinal lumen thus antagonizing triglyceride hydrolysis and decreasing fat absorption by about 30%. Since orlistat is not absorbed, its ability to cause weight loss likely reflects the resulting low-fat diet and lower caloric intake. Gastrointestinal side effects (abdominal discomfort, flatus, fecal urgency) occur in the majority of patients treated with orlistat. It is recommended that orlistat not be prescribed for patients with known malabsorptive conditions, and daily multivitamins are useful. Sibutramine and orlistat treatment may be continued as long as patients continue to experience weight loss in the absence of significant side effects.

REFERENCES

Berne RM, Levy MN, Koeppen BM, et al. *Physiology*, 5th ed. St Louis: Mosby, 2004.

Dujovne CA, Zavoral JH, Rowe E, et al. Effects of sibutramine on body weight and serum lipids: A double-blind, randomized, placebo-controlled study in 322 overweight and obese patients with dyslipidemia. *Am Heart J* 2001;142:489–495.

Executive Summary of the Third Report of the National Cholesterol Education Program (NCEP) Expert panel on the detection, evaluation, and treatment of high blood cholesterol in adults (Adult Treatment Panel III). *JAMA* 2001;285:2486–2490.

Flegal KM, Carroll MD, Ogden CL, et al. Prevalence and trends in obesity among US adults, 1999–2000. *JAMA* 2002;288:1723–1726.

Kuczmarski RJ, Glegal KM, Campbell SM. Increasing prevalence of overweight among US adults. *JAMA* 1994;272:205–211.

Leibel RL, Hirsch J, Appel BE, et al. Energy intake required to maintain body weight is not affected by wide variation in diet composition. *Am J Clin Nutr* 1992;55:350–355.

Purnell JY, Weyer C. Body weight effects of current and experimental drugs for diabetes mellitus. *Treat Endocrinonl* 2003;2:23–29.

Rosenbaum M, Leibel RL, Hirsch J. Obesity. *N Engl J Med* 1997;337:396–407.

Wadden TA. Treatment of obesity by moderate and severe caloric restriction: results of clinical research trials. *Ann Intern Med* 1993;229:688–693.

Physiology of the Newborn and Elderly

60

The physiology of both the neonatal and the elderly patient can be characterized by decreased functional reserve. In both groups of patients, physiologic function is usually adequate to meet the needs of normal daily activity. However, the additional demands commonly encountered in the perioperative period may place a significant burden on organ systems that already have little functional reserve. In both populations, the presence of coexisting disease severely limits their ability to tolerate significant perioperative stresses.

NEONATAL PHYSIOLOGY

The relatively high metabolic rate of the neonate is the crucial determinant of cardiopulmonary function. Neonatal oxygen consumption is approximately 6 mL/kg/minute versus 3 mL/kg/minute in the adult. Even under normal physiologic circumstances, the immature cardiac, and respiratory systems must function near the edge of their functional reserve to support this metabolic demand. Multisystem immaturity creates important developmental differences in drug handling and response when compared to the older child or adult (Hillier et al., 2004).

Neonatal Cardiovascular Physiology

The newborn infant is in a state of transition from the fetal to the extrauterine circulatory pattern. The fetal circulation is characterized by high pulmonary vascular resistance, low systemic vascular resistance (placenta), and right-to-left shunting via the foramen ovale and ductus arteriosus. Aeration of the lungs at birth causes a rapid decline in pulmonary vascular resistance and an increase in pulmonary blood flow. The decrease in pulmonary vascular resistance at birth is mediated by the endogenous production of nitric oxide. Increasing blood return to the heart via the pulmonary veins raises the pressure of the left atrium above that of the right, causing a functional closure of the foramen ovale. Anatomic closure of the foramen ovale usually occurs between 3 months and 1 year of age. The functional closure of the ductus arteriosus is, in part, mediated by an increase in arterial oxygen partial pressure and is complete within the first 10 to 15 hours. However, anatomic closure does not occur until 2 months of age.

Because the foramen ovale and ductus arteriosus are only functionally closed in the neonatal period, the neonatal circulation is able to readily revert to the fetal pattern, particularly in response to physiologic stresses occasionally encountered in the perioperative period. The neonatal pulmonary circulation is very reactive. Hypoxemia, hypercarbia, or acidosis cause both pulmonary vasoconstriction and dilation of the ductus arteriosus. Increases in pulmonary vascular resistance result in right-to-left shunting across the foramen ovale and ductus arteriosus. Right-to-left shunting, by causing arterial hypoxemia, causes a further increase in pulmonary vascular resistance, thus creating a vicious circle. Persistent pulmonary hypertension may be seen in neonates with diaphragmatic hernia, meconium aspiration, infection, congenital heart disease, and polycythemia.

The neonatal myocardium contains immature contractile elements and is less compliant than the adult myocardium. The Frank-Starling relationship is functional only within a very narrow range of left ventricular end diastolic pressure. Thus, there is a limited increase in cardiac output to be gained from aggressive volume loading in the normovolemic newborn. However, if preload is reduced by hypovolemia or dehydration, normalization of volume status will generally restore cardiac output. However, because stroke volume cannot be significantly augmented by volume loading, and because contractile reserve is limited, neonatal cardiac output is exquisitely heart rate dependent.

Although adrenergic receptors are thought to be mature at birth, sympathetic innervation is incomplete. After birth, neurotransmitter concentrations increase progressively, reflecting the maturation of sympathetic innervation.

When compared to the adult, neonatal myocardium is more sensitive to norepinephrine. This phenomenon is a reflection of the relatively denervated status of neonatal myocardium. Dopamine is an indirectly acting inotrope that depends, in part, upon endogenous norepinephrine release for its action. Neonatal myocardium, being deficient in sympathetic innervation, is therefore less responsive to dopamine.

To meet the elevated metabolic demand, neonatal cardiac output, relative to body weight, is twice that of the adult. This is achieved by a relatively rapid heart rate (140 beats/minute) because stroke volume cannot be significantly increased. The neonatal circulation is characterized by centralization (increased peripheral vascular resistance and distribution of cardiac output primarily to vital organs), a situation comparable to an adult in compensated shock. Because neonatal baroreflex activity is impaired, the response to hemorrhage produces little increase in heart rate or change in total peripheral resistance. Thus, even a modest (10%) reduction in blood volume will cause a 15% to 30% decrease in mean blood pressure in the newborn infant. The structural and functional immaturity of the neonatal cardiovascular system severely limits the reserve that is available in the face of common perioperative insults such as hypovolemia, anesthetic-induced depression of contractility, relative bradycardia, and positive pressure ventilation-induced decreases in venous return. The marginal cardiovascular reserve of the neonate and leftward shift of the fetal hemoglobin dissociation curve are the rationale underlying the recommendation that the hematocrit be maintained at 30% or higher.

Respiratory Physiology of the Newborn

The respiratory system of a term neonate at birth is immature and postnatal development continues through early childhood. Although the conducting airways are fully developed by 16 weeks of gestation, the number of alveoli is reduced at birth. A premature infant born at 24 to 28 weeks of gestation is just beginning to alveolarize the distal saccules of the lung. Indeed, complete alveolar maturation does not occur until 8 to 10 years of age. Thus, the ratio of alveolar surface area to body surface area is one-third that of the adult. At birth, the infant possesses approximately one-tenth of the adult population of alveoli. To satisfy increased oxygen demand, neonatal alveolar minute ventilation is twice that of the adult. Increasing respiratory rate rather than tidal volume is the most efficient means to increase alveolar ventilation in the newborn. The diaphragm is the primary muscle of respiration in the neonate but has fewer high-oxidative muscle fibers and is thus less fatigue-resistant than in the adult. Ventilation-perfusion imbalance occurs as a result of distal airway closure during normal tidal breathing in the neonate. This phenomenon is responsible for an increase in the alveolar-arterial oxygen tension gradient compared to adults.

Adequate gas exchange depends upon adequate alveolar recruitment and thus surfactant function. Production of surfactant begins by 23 to 24 week of gestation and reaches maturity at approximately 35 weeks of gestation. Surfactant deficient preterm infants have decreased lung compliance and are at risk for the development of respiratory distress syndrome (RDS). Administration of corticosteroids to mothers in preterm labor may accelerate lung maturation. Furthermore, the instillation of intratracheal exogenous surfactant in preterm babies has considerably improved the outcome of premature infants.

The neonatal chest wall is more compliant and has less outward recoil than that of the adult. Thus, the neonatal lung has a greater tendency to collapse and the infant is obliged to utilize active mechanisms to maintain normal lung volumes (Table 60-1). First, by breathing at a relatively rapid rate, the duration of expiration is limited. In this way, inspiration is initiated before the lung has completed recoiling to its end-expiratory volume. Second, the neonate utilizes intercostal muscle activity during expiration to stabilize the chest wall, thus retarding the decline in lung volume during expiration. Last, the neonate exhales through a partially closed glottis, also retarding expiratory flow and maintaining end-expiratory lung volume. Thus, the awake neonate has a functional residual capacity (FRC) that is similar, when normalized to body weight, to that of an adult. However, because neonatal alveolar ventilation is twice that of an adult, the ratio of alveolar ventilation to FRC in the neonate is twice that of the adult. The high ratio of minute ventilation to FRC causes a much more rapid wash-out or wash-in of oxygen and anesthetic drugs in response to changes in inspired concentrations.

The active mechanisms utilized by the newborn to protect lung volume are exquisitely sensitive to the effects of general anesthesia. Therefore, the neonatal FRC may decrease significantly during anesthesia, particularly during periodic breathing and apnea. The combination of increased oxygen consumption and a reduced FRC means that apnea and hypoventilation are associated with marked and rapid arterial oxygen desaturation.

Although the peripheral chemoreceptors are active from 28 weeks of gestation, their function is immature until several days after birth. Therefore, the neonate and preterm infant exhibit an altered response to hypoxia and

TABLE 60-1.
ACTIVE MECHANISMS USED BY NEONATES TO MAINTAIN LUNG VOLUME*

Rapid respiratory rate—early termination of expiration
Intercostal muscle activity in expiration—stabilizes compliant chest wall
Expiration against partially closed glottis—retards expiratory flow

*Significantly attenuated by general anesthesia.

hypercarbia. When challenged with hypoxic inspired gas mixtures, both the term and preterm infant have an initial 1- or 2-minute period of hyperventilation followed by sustained hypoventilation. As postnatal age increases, the hyperventilatory response becomes sustained. However, this protective response develops more slowly in the preterm infant and the ventilatory response to hypercarbia is impaired. The impaired neonatal ventilatory responses to hypoxia and hypercarbia are contributing factors to the development of life-threatening apnea and hypoventilation in the postoperative period.

Although airway resistance is relatively low in infants, in absolute terms, the airways are very narrow. Relatively minor quantities of secretions or trivial inflammatory disease can produce serious respiratory embarrassment in small infants.

Neonatal Thermoregulation

The neonate tends to become hypothermic during general anesthesia much more rapidly than the adult. Accelerated heat loss in the neonate is related to its relatively large surface area, thinner layer of insulating subcutaneous fat, and a limited capability for thermogenesis. The neonate primarily relies on nonshivering or chemical thermogenesis in brown adipose tissue for heat production. Thermogenesis in brown fat is mediated by the sympathetic nervous system and is stimulated by norepinephrine, resulting in triglyceride hydrolysis. The thermoregulatory range is the ambient temperature range within which an unclothed subject can maintain normal body temperature. The lower limit of the thermoregulatory range (critical temperature) is 1°C for an adult, but is as high as 23°C and 28°C for the full-term infant and premature infant respectively. Therefore, the thermoregulatory range of the neonate is much narrower than that of the adult. During anesthesia and surgery, heat loss in the pediatric patient is further enhanced by decrease in the thermoregulatory threshold, low ambient temperatures of the operating suite (20°C to 22°C), preparation of skin with cold solutions, infusion of cold solutions, anesthesia-induced vasodilatation, and use of dry anesthetic gases in high flow, nonrebreathing systems. Intraoperative hypothermia will markedly delay emergence. Furthermore, with the return of the thermostatic reflexes, oxygen consumption increases by three- to fourfold as the metabolic rate is increased in an attempt to generate heat. This additional demand on an immature cardiorespiratory system that is already compromised due to the residual effects of anesthesia and surgery may precipitate cardiorespiratory failure. However, the loss of heat during anesthesia and surgery can be prevented by a number of simple measures, such as raising operating room temperature to 28°C to 30°C, radiant heat lamps, wrapping the extremities with insulating material, using nonvolatile warmed solutions for skin preparation, and administration of warmed intravenous fluids and blood products. Inhaled gases should be heated and humidified. Forced air warming devices are also effective in maintaining perioperative normothermia.

Neonatal Fluid, Electrolyte, and Renal Physiology

The neonate is characterized by an increased total body water, increased extracellular fluid volume, increased water turnover rate, and reduced glomerular filtration rate. The neonatal renal tubules have a decreased ability to absorb sodium, bicarbonate, glucose, amino acids, and phosphates. The neonates are obligate sodium losers and require sodium supplementation. All of these factors contribute to the potential for overhydration, dehydration, metabolic acidosis, and hyponatremia, necessitating meticulous attention to intraoperative fluid therapy. Although third-space translocation of fluids is relatively similar in neonates and adults, neonatal insensible losses vary greatly. Fever, radiant warmers, phototherapy, increased ambient temperature, and decreased humidity all increase insensible loss.

Neonates have decreased glycogen stores and are prone to hypoglycemia after relatively brief periods of starvation. The preterm infant is at even greater risk for hypoglycemia. Glucose is therefore an essential element of the intraoperative fluid plan. The term neonate requires 3 to 5 mg/kg/minute and preterm neonates 5 to 6 mg/kg/minute of glucose to maintain serum glucose between 35 and 125 mg/dL.

Neonatal Neurophysiology

The neural connections required for the transmission and perception of pain are functional by the 24th week of gestation. Although myelination is incomplete, and nerve conduction velocity may be diminished, the shorter conduction distances found in the neonate facilitate rapid transmission of nociceptive impulses to the brain (Benatar and Benatar, 2001). Furthermore, even in adults, most nociceptive impulses are transmitted by unmyelinated C-fibers and by thinly myelinated Aδ fibers. Painful stimuli produce withdrawal, autonomic stimulation, and neuroendocrine stress responses. The concept of plasticity of the nervous system has important implications for the management of pain in newborns. The failure to provide analgesia for neonatal pain causes up-regulation of the nociceptive pathways in the dorsal horn of the spinal cord. Thus, future painful insults result in exaggerated pain perception. Indeed, in human newborns, the failure to provide adequate anesthesia or analgesia for circumcision is associated with long-term changes, including an increased response to immunization at a later date. The adequate treatment of pain in the neonatal period is challenging because of the fear of respiratory depression associated with opioid administration. Fortunately, several nonpharmacologic behavioral interventions have antinociceptive effects in infants (Kaufman et al., 2002). Analgesia may be induced by the administration of sucrose and by suckling. These effects are mediated via descending endogenous opioid mechanisms originating in the brainstem and may be reversed by the administration of naloxone.

The germinal matrix has a rich blood supply, thin vessel walls, and scant vascular supporting tissue, causing the vessels of this region to be susceptible to rupture. With increasing gestational age the germinal matrix involutes and is absent in the full term infant. Intraventricular hemorrhage originates predominantly in the germinal matrix and occasionally in the choroid plexus. Periventricular-intraventricular hemorrhage occurs in 40% to 50% of premature infants and is a major cause of neonatal morbidity and mortality. The factors in the pathogenesis of intraventricular hemorrhage include abrupt changes in cerebral hemodynamics, changes in intracranial pressure, disturbances in osmotic equilibrium, and coagulopathy. Preterm infants are also at risk for retinopathy of prematurity (ROP) in which abnormal growth of retinal vessels can lead to scarring and blindness. Though the degree of prematurity is the primary etiologic factor in the development of ROP, hyperoxia, hypocarbia, vitamin E deficiency, and acidemia have also been implicated as contributing factors. The brain is comparatively large at birth compared to the adult. Although myelination is incomplete at birth, it is typically complete before the third year of age.

THE PHYSIOLOGY OF THE ELDERLY

Aging and the Cardiovascular System

Increasing age is associated with increasing cardiac morbidity. Aging is associated with an increasing prevalence of cardiovascular disease and decreasing cardiovascular functional reserve (Lakatta and Levy, 2003). Heart failure is the most frequent cause of hospitalization in patients older than 65 years of age. However, it is important to separate the cardiovascular effects of aging from those of common coexisting disease processes such as atherosclerosis, hypertension, and diabetes mellitus. The decline in cardiac function that occurs with aging in the healthy individual appears to be related in part to decreasing functional demand. Indeed, when exercise and conditioning are maintained into the later decades, the decline in cardiovascular function is markedly attenuated. It has been suggested that cardiovascular function is directly related to skeletal muscle mass. Aging has discrete effects upon the heart, large vessels, endothelial function, conduction system, and the cardiovascular autonomic response.

Heart

The heart increases in size during aging as a result of concentric ventricular hypertrophy. This occurs in response to the increase in left ventricular afterload resulting from a reduction in arterial distensibility. Hypertrophy of cardiac myocytes is typical, and accounts for an approximately 30% increase in left ventricular wall thickness. However, the number of myocytes is decreased. Despite these changes, resting systolic function tends to be well preserved in healthy individuals. However, increases in cardiac output in response to severe exertion are attenuated by approximately 20% to 30% in the elderly, principally because the heart rate response to severe exercise is diminished. There is an age-related increase in cardiac connective tissue that, when combined with ventricular hypertrophy, increases wall stiffness and reduces diastolic compliance. Ventricular filling in the elderly is especially dependant upon active diastolic relaxation. In this process, calcium is removed from troponin C-binding sites, triggering the dissociation of actin and myosin, thus facilitating isometric relaxation. Active diastolic relaxation utilizes approximately 15% of the energy consumed during the cardiac cycle. This process is significantly impaired in the elderly and exacerbates the adverse effects of ventricular hypertrophy on diastolic filling. Thus, the elderly heart is markedly dependent upon the atrial "kick" for adequate ventricular preload. It is estimated that atrial contraction contributes approximately 30% of ventricular filling in the elderly versus 10% in younger individuals. Because of the importance of atrial contraction, and because filling is delayed by reduced ventricular compliance, ventricular filling is typically not complete until very late in diastole. Tachycardia and shortened diastolic intervals are associated with marked decreases in ventricular preload in the elderly. Loss of the atrial "kick," such as during atrial fibrillation, is particularly poorly tolerated. Perioperative events that reduce venous return, such as hypovolemia, positive pressure ventilation, and increased venous capacitance, may be accompanied by significant decreases in cardiac output. Conversely, excessive perioperative increases in blood volume or decreases in contractility can precipitate congestive cardiac failure. Diastolic dysfunction is now recognized as a major contributor to cardiovascular disease in the elderly population and is exacerbated by several coexisting diseases (Phillip et al., 2003; Aurigemma and Gaasch, 2004) (Table 60-2). It is difficult to distinguish systolic dysfunc-

TABLE 60-2.
DISEASES COMMONLY ENCOUNTERED IN THE ELDERLY THAT ARE ASSOCIATED WITH DIASTOLIC DYSFUNCTION

Systemic hypertension
Coronary artery disease
Cardiomyopathy
Aortic stenosis
Atrial fibrillation
Diabetes
Chronic renal disease

tion from diastolic dysfunction during routine clinical evaluation. Furthermore, routine preoperative echocardiographic indices of function such as left ventricular ejection fraction will fail to identify diastolic dysfunction. However, diastolic filling can be evaluated by comparing Doppler echocardiographic measurements of mitral valve inflow velocities during the early and late (atrial contraction) phases of diastole. Dyspnea in the elderly may indicate congestive cardiac failure and/or pulmonary disease. B-type natriuretic peptide is released in response to ventricular myocyte stretch. Plasma B-type natriuretic peptide measurements may help differentiate between cardiac and respiratory origins of dyspnea (Mueller et al., 2004).

Large Vessels

Structural changes in the large vessels are an important element of the aging process and contribute significantly to the age-related changes in the heart described above (Ferrari et al., 2003). The large vessels are elongated, tortuous, and dilated in the elderly. Their intima and media are thickened, causing these vessels to be less distensible. The normal cushioning function of the large vessels is impaired; causing accelerated and enhanced pulse wave propagation. In the elderly, the pulse wave is reflected back from the peripheral circulation and augments systolic pressure. In young adults, the reflected pulse wave generally has a lower amplitude and its return from the peripheral circulation is delayed such that diastolic rather than systolic pressure is augmented. As a result, diastolic pressure tends to be lower in the elderly than in younger individuals. Thus, in the elderly, both systolic pressure and pulse pressure are increased and left ventricular afterload is elevated. All of the aforementioned age-related vascular structural changes are accelerated in the presence of hypertension or atherosclerosis.

Endothelial Function

The endothelium is an important regulator of vasomotor response, coagulation, fibrinolysis, immunomodulation, and vascular growth and proliferation. Endothelial dysfunction is an important element in the early pathogenesis of atherosclerosis, diabetes mellitus, and systemic hypertension (Matz and Andrianstitohaina, 2003). Aging is associated with altered endothelial structure and function, even in the absence of disease. Reactive oxygen species, such as superoxide anions, have been implicated in age-related endothelial dysfunction. Endothelial dysfunction is accelerated by smoking, diabetes, hypertension, and hyperlipidemia. In the elderly, endothelial nitric oxide release is decreased in all vascular beds, including the coronary circulation. Furthermore, the vasodilator response to nitric oxide of the adjacent vascular smooth muscle is also reduced. Vasodilator responses to beta-2 agonists and vasoconstrictor responses to alpha-adrenergic stimulation are similarly attenuated in the elderly. Thus, age-related endothelial dysfunction can be characterized as a decrease in the ability of the endothelium to dilate blood vessels in response to physiologic and pharmacologic stimuli.

Conduction System

There are several important age-related structural and functional changes in the cardiac conduction system (Lakatta and Levy, 2003). The sinoatrial node undergoes a progressive change over time such that the proportion of pacemaker cells decreases from 50% in late childhood to less than 10% at 75 years. The sinoatrial node, atrioventricular node, and conduction bundles also become infiltrated with fibrous and fatty tissue. These changes are responsible for the increased incidence of first- and second-degree heart block, sick sinus syndrome, and atrial fibrillation in the elderly. The development of atrial fibrillation is also facilitated by left atrial enlargement, which typically accompanies aging in otherwise healthy individuals. Otherwise, healthy elderly men also experience an age-related increase in the prevalence, frequency, and complexity, of ventricular ectopy.

Autonomic and Integrated Cardiovascular Responses

Aging is associated with increased norepinephrine entry into the circulation and deficient catecholamine reuptake at nerve endings. Therefore, elevated circulating concentrations of norepinephrine are usual, generating chronically increased adrenergic receptor occupancy. However, the cardiovascular response to increased adrenergic stimulation is attenuated by down-regulation of postreceptor signaling, decreased receptor density, and reduced contractile response of the myocardium. The response to exogenously administered beta agonists, such as isoproterenol, is similarly attenuated. Receptor down-regulation is responsible for the age-related decline in maximum heart rate during exercise. Indeed, receptor down-regulation in the elderly makes their cardiovascular function similar to that of a younger individual who has received beta-adrenergic antagonists.

Orthostatic hypotension is common in the elderly and is associated with syncope, falls, and cognitive decline. Impaired baroreceptor reflexes and attenuated peripheral vasoconstriction are partially responsible. Hypovolemia and salt depletion also contribute and are the result of diuretic administration or increased atrial natriuretic peptide release. Orthostatic hypotension is more common in hypertensive patients. Baroreceptor responses to elevated arterial pressure are attenuated in the elderly. However, it is difficult to separate the effects of aging per se from those of age-related chronic increases in systolic pressure. Straining against a closed glottis (Valsalva maneuver) typically produces a decrease in venous return and cardiac output. The normal baroreceptor response to this maneuver includes an increase in heart rate and peripheral vascular tone and restoration of blood pressure. However, this response is markedly attenuated in the elderly. Age-related impairment of baroreceptor responses make hypotension more likely after the initiation of positive pressure ventilation, particularly in the presence of hypovolemia. Similarly, neuroaxial local anesthetic-induced sympathetic blockade is more likely to be accompanied by hypotension in the presence of an impaired baroreceptor response.

Anesthetic and Ischemic Preconditioning in the Aging Heart

It is now recognized that, under certain circumstances, exposure to volatile anesthetics (anesthetic preconditioning) or several brief periods of ischemia (ischemic preconditioning) may enhance tolerance to subsequent ischemia, enhance cardiac function, and reduce infarction size (Zaugg et al., 2004). Because the incidence of atherosclerosis and coronary artery disease is age-related, the elderly would seem be most likely to benefit from a preconditioning strategy. However, anesthetic preconditioning may be markedly attenuated in the elderly. Furthermore, potent volatile drugs may induce significant cardiovascular depression in this age group. Therefore, the utility of preconditioning strategies in this age group is uncertain.

Aging and the Respiratory System

The respiratory system undergoes a multifactorial decline in functional reserve with aging (Tables 60-3 and 60-4) (Chan and Welsh, 1998). Under normal circumstances, this decrease in respiratory function is not associated with significant limitation of daily activity. However, decreased respiratory reserve may be unmasked by illness, surgery, anesthesia, and other perioperative events. Common respiratory diseases and the effects of smoking and environmental pollution frequently exacerbate the decline in respiratory function with aging.

Respiratory System Mechanics and Architecture

The chest wall becomes less compliant with aging, presumably related to changes in the thoracic skeleton and a decline in costovertebral joint mobility. These changes produce a restrictive functional impairment. The noncompliant thoracic cage makes intercostal muscle activity less efficient. Therefore, the diaphragm and abdominal muscles assume a greater role in tidal breathing. However, diaphragmatic function declines with age, predisposing the elderly to respiratory fatigue when required to significantly increase minute ventilation. Although the diaphragm does not appear to undergo significant atrophy or change in muscle fiber type with aging, it does occupy a flatter position and therefore has a less favorable mechanical advantage.

Aging is associated with a loss of lung elasticity that is responsible for a decrease in lung recoil, thus making the lung more distensible. Changes in surfactant function may also contribute to age-related changes in lung compliance. The net result of these changes in the elastic properties of the lung and chest wall is an increase in intrapleural pressure that significantly impacts upon respiratory function. Intrapleural pressure is a critical determinant of small airway caliber. Increased intrapleural pressures increase the tendency for small airway collapse to occur, thus causing gas trapping and/or expiratory airflow limitation.

TABLE 60-3.
INTRINSIC AND EXTRINSIC EVENTS THAT INFLUENCE THE RESPIRATORY SYSTEM DURING AGING

Intrinsic to the Aging Process	Environmental, Behavioral, and Disease Related
Decreased bronchiolar caliber	Industrial and environmental pollution
Decreased alveolar surface area	Smoking
Increased lung collagen content	General deconditioning
Decreased lung elastin content	Co-existing disease
Kyphoscoliosis	
Increased thoracic cage rigidity	
Decreased diaphragmatic strength	

TABLE 60-4.
FUNCTIONAL CONSEQUENCES OF THE INTRINSIC AND EXTRINSIC EVENTS THAT INFLUENCE THE RESPIRATORY SYSTEM DURING AGING

Decrease in lung elastic recoil
Increase in lung compliance
Decrease in oxygen diffusing capacity
Premature airway closure causing V/Q mismatch and increased alveolar-to-arterial oxygen gradient
Small airway closure and gas trapping
Decreased expiratory flow rates

Lung Volumes and Capacities

Vital Capacity

Vital capacity (VC) is the volume generated when a maximal inspiration is followed by a maximal expiration. There is a progressive loss of VC with aging that results from increased chest wall stiffness, decreased lung elastic recoil, and decreased respiratory muscle strength.

Residual Volume

The residual volume is the volume remaining in the lungs after a maximal expiration. In young individuals, the residual volume is determined primarily by ability of the expiratory muscles to overcome the elastic recoil properties of the lung and chest wall. However, in the elderly, dynamic airway closure also limits expiration. Therefore, aging is associated with a progressive increase in residual volume of up to 10% per decade.

Total Lung Capacity

Total lung capacity is the sum of the residual volume and the vital capacity. Thus, the combined effect of the decline in vital capacity and increase in residual volume is that the total lung capacity remains relatively constant with aging.

Functional Residual Capacity

The functional residual capacity (FRC) is the volume remaining in the lungs at the end of a normal expiration. The FRC is the volume at which the elastic recoil forces of the lung and chest wall are at equilibrium. The opposing recoil forces of the lung and chest wall generate the subatmospheric intrapleural pressure. Aging is associated with a progressive increase in FRC that occurs as a result of the decreased elastic recoil force of the lungs. However, the increase in FRC is less than would be predicted from the change in lung elastic recoil alone. This is because the increased stiffness of the chest wall counteracts the increase in lung volume.

Closing Capacity

Airway closure may occur in small airways (<1 mm) whose caliber is determined by their transmural pressure. Airway closure typically occurs in dependant areas of the lung where the surrounding intrapleural pressure is likely to be greater. In young adults airway closure occurs only at low lung volumes (approximately 10% of vital capacity). Thus, airway closure is unlikely during normal tidal breathing. However, as intrapleural pressure increases with age, airway closure occurs at progressively greater lung volumes. Indeed, in the elderly, airway closure occurs at approximately 40% of the VC reflecting lung volumes that exceed FRC. Although the FRC increases by up to 3% per decade, closing capacity increases at a greater rate. Thus, gas exchange impairment due to shunting in regions of airway closure is typical in the elderly during normal tidal breathing. The supine position is associated with a decrease in FRC when compared to the standing position. In this regard the supine position makes airway closure during normal tidal breathing more likely. Indeed, airway closure may occur during tidal breathing as early as the mid-forties in the supine position.

Expiratory Flow

There is a progressive decline in forced exhaled volume in 1 second (FEV_1) and forced vital capacity (FVC) with age that is independent of smoking or environmental exposure. Age-related loss of lung elastic recoil predisposes to dynamic airway collapse during forced expiratory maneuvers. Expiratory muscle strength also declines with age.

Diffusing Capacity and Alveolar-to-Arterial Oxygen Gradient

Gas-exchange efficiency declines with aging as a result of increasing intrapulmonary shunting and decreasing lung-diffusing capacity. The result is a linear decline in resting supine Pao_2 between early adulthood and 65 years of age (about 0.5 mm Hg/year). Small airway closure causes ventilation to perfusion (V/Q) mismatch and shunting. Cardiac output is often decreased in the elderly to the extent that mixed venous oxygen tension is decreased. Thus, even modest amounts of shunting may produce a significant decrease in Pao_2 because of the contribution of desaturated venous blood. The diameter of the alveolar ducts is increased and their respective alveoli are wider and shallower. These architectural changes significantly reduce alveolar surface area. As a result, diffusing capacity for carbon monoxide may decline by up to 50% between early adulthood and 80 years of age.

Upper Airway Protective Reflexes

Cough effectiveness is reduced in the elderly because of diminished reflex sensitivity and impaired muscle function. Cough reflex attenuation is associated with an increased incidence of aspiration pneumonia. The mechanisms of cough reflex impairment include desensitization of airway epithelial cough receptors. Smoking causes airway sensory nerve neuropeptide depletion and nicotine inhibits C-fiber transmission in the lower respiratory tract (Watando et al., 2004). Coexisting medical conditions that are associated with cough reflex suppression include stroke, laryngectomy, and Parkinson disease. Cough reflex sensitivity may be improved by angiotensin-converting enzyme inhibitor administration.

Control of Breathing, Chemoreceptors, and Integrated Responses

The cardiorespiratory responses to hypoxia and hypercarbia are mediated via central and peripheral chemoreceptors. The increases in heart rate and minute ventilation in response to elevations in $Paco_2$ or decreases in Pao_2 are markedly attenuated in the elderly. The attenuated ventilatory response is multifactorial and reflects decreased peripheral chemoreceptor sensitivity, reduced respiratory muscle activity, decreased respiratory mechanical efficiency, and general respiratory deconditioning. The ventilatory responses to hypercarbia and hypoxia are very important protective mechanisms. However, these responses are further attenuated by the administration of opioids and sedative/hypnotic drugs. Thus, the elderly are at particular risk from life-threatening respiratory depression in the perioperative period.

Exercise Capacity

In healthy young individuals the intensity and duration of strenuous exertion is limited by cardiovascular and musculoskeletal function rather than by the respiratory system.

However, exercise in the elderly may be limited by both decreased cardiovascular and respiratory reserve. Respiratory function during exercise is limited as a result of airflow limitation, respiratory muscle strength decline, and chest wall rigidity. The age-related increase in FRC places the inspiratory muscles at a mechanical disadvantage and increases the work of breathing.

Sleep Disordered Breathing

The incidence of sleep disordered breathing increases with age, especially in men. It is estimated that approximately one-third of elderly men have clinically significant obstructive sleep apnea. The prevalence of snoring is highest in the seventh decade and is associated with an increased risk of stroke. Morbidity associated with sleep apnea includes systemic and pulmonary hypertension, dysrhythmias, myocardial infarction, stroke, sudden death, and automobile accidents.

Thermoregulation in the Elderly

There is ample evidence that hyperthermia and hypothermia in the elderly are poorly tolerated and that extreme cold and heat stress are associated with increased mortality compared to younger individuals (Kenney and Munce, 2003). However, it is not clear whether the greater susceptibility to thermal stress is related to aging per se, or to underlying socioeconomic conditions, general fitness, activity levels, and the effects of coexisting disease.

Resting Core Temperature

Aging is associated with a greater variability in core temperature. Indeed, it is estimated that up to 10% of people >65 years of age have early morning core temperatures of <35.5°C (Table 60-5). However, when the effects of coexisting disease, socioeconomic circumstances, and medication are eliminated, there is no evidence of declining body temperature with advancing age in healthy individuals under thermoneutral conditions. Circadian temperature variations are not significantly different in the healthy elderly compared to younger individuals.

TABLE 60-5.
FACTORS ASSOCIATED WITH REDUCED RESTING CORE TEMPERATURES IN THE ELDERLY

Neurologic disease
Diabetes
Low body weight
Lack of self-sufficiency
Consumption of less than two meals per day
Smoking
Alcohol consumption

TABLE 60-6.
FACTORS RESPONSIBLE FOR ATTENUATED THERMAL STRESS RESPONSES IN THE ELDERLY

Heat Stress Response	Cold Stress Response
Reduced sweat gland output	Loss of muscle mass
Reduced ability to increase cutaneous blood flow	Reduced ability for cutaneous vasoconstriction
Reduced ability to increase cardiac output	
Less redistribution of cardiac output from core to peripheral circulations	

Response to Cold Stress

The usual physiologic response to cold stress is to decrease heat loss by peripheral vasoconstriction, and to increase heat production via shivering and nonshivering thermogenesis. Aging is associated with attenuated vasoconstrictor responses to cold (Table 60-6). The inability to efficiently conserve heat in the elderly is exacerbated by the age-related decrease in skeletal muscle mass. Loss of skeletal muscle mass is responsible for the age-related decline in basal heat production. It is estimated that resting heat production declines by 20% between the ages of 30 and 70 years. There is a significant gender-related difference in cold stress response in the elderly. Mortality during cold weather is higher in men compared to age-matched women. It is likely that the higher percentage of body fat and lower surface area-to-mass ratio in females is responsible for this difference. The attenuated cold-stress responses of the elderly are further diminished by general and regional anesthesia. Perioperative hypothermia is very likely in the elderly patient unless active measures are taken to maintain normothermia.

Response to Heat Stress

Heat stress is less common than cold stress in the perioperative period. However, the response to heat stress may be markedly attenuated in the elderly and places a significant burden on the cardiovascular system (see Table 60-6). The normal heat stress response includes sweat gland activation and peripheral vasodilatation. Sweat gland activation during heat stress is under sympathetic cholinergic control and may be induced experimentally by cholinergic analogues such as methylcholine (MCh). Aging is associated with progressive declines in MCh-stimulated sweat gland output. Furthermore, the core temperature threshold at which sweating is triggered is elevated in the elderly. The heat stress-induced increase in cutaneous blood flow is attenuated with aging. It is likely that structural changes in the cutaneous circulation are partly responsible for this effect. Aging is associated with loss of the vessels of the microcirculation in dermal papillary and superficial vascular plexuses. The integrated cardiovascular response to heat stress is significantly attenuated. The normal heat stress response is associated with distribution of blood away from the splanchnic and renal circulations, increased cutaneous flow, and increased cardiac output. In the elderly, the heat stress-induced increase in cardiac output is limited by the inability to increase stroke volume to a significant degree. Although heart rate response to thermal stress is relatively well preserved, the obligatory increase in cardiac output requires that the elderly utilize a greater proportion of their heart rate reserve (Kenney and Munce, 2003). Because heat stress response requires almost maximal utilization of the cardiac reserve, additional cardiovascular stresses during heat stress are likely to be poorly tolerated. For example, the vasoconstrictor response to orthostatic hypotension is markedly attenuated in the elderly during heat stress. Thus, it is likely that perioperative insults such as hypovolemia, myocardial depression, positive pressure ventilation, and decreases in heart rate, will be associated with significant declines in cardiac output in the heat stressed elderly patient.

Gastrointestinal Function in the Elderly

Liver

Although aging is associated with a decrease in liver mass and hepatic blood flow, hepatocellular function appears to be relatively well preserved. However, protein synthetic function may be diminished in some elderly individuals, particularly those with poor nutritional intake. Reduced serum albumin concentrations will affect drug binding. On the other hand, the concentration of another important drug-binding protein, alpha-1-acid glycoprotein, is typically increased in the elderly. Hepatic synthesis of plasma cholinesterase may be diminished, particularly in men. Although hepatic enzyme function may be qualitatively normal in the elderly, the reduction in hepatic mass and blood flow is responsible for a significant decrease in first-pass metabolism of several drugs that are important in the aging population (Mangoni and Jackson, 2004). Thus, the oral bioavailability of propanolol and labetalol are increased in the elderly. Conversely, several ACE inhibitors, including enalapril, are prodrugs that require activation by the liver before they exert their pharmacologic effect. Therefore, the bioavailability of these drugs may be decreased in the elderly.

Gastroesophageal Physiology

Gastric emptying of solid material appears to be relatively normal in the healthy elderly population. However, gastric emptying of liquids may be delayed compared to younger individuals (Thompson, 2001). Emptying of both liquids and solids is commonly delayed in the presence of coexisting disease. Gastroesophageal reflux disease (GERD) is more frequent in the elderly (Table 60-7). The typical symptoms of GERD seen in the younger population, (heartburn and regurgitation) are less frequent in the elderly. Dysphagia, vomiting, respiratory symptoms, weight loss, and anemia are more common presenting symptoms in the elderly. Several medications that are commonly prescribed in the elderly population predispose to GERD by decreasing lower esophageal sphincter tone (Table 60-8).

TABLE 60-7.
FACTORS THAT PREDISPOSE TO THE INCREASED INCIDENCE OF GASTROESOPHAGEAL REFLUX DISEASE IN THE ELDERLY

Increased prevalence of sliding hiatal hernia
Shortened intraabdominal segment of the lower esophageal sphincter
Impaired clearance of refluxed acid
Use of medications that reduce lower esophageal sphincter pressure
Decreased esophageal peristalsis pressure

Renal Function in the Elderly

Aging is accompanied by a decrease in the cortical nephron population and a reduction in renal mass. Renal blood flow and glomerular filtration rate (GFR) both decline with age (Mangoni and Jackson, 2004). The average male GFR is 125 mL/minute. This value decreases by approximately 1 mL/minute/yr after the age of 40 as a result of the decline in nephron population and hyalinization of cortical afferent arterioles. The medullary nephron population is relatively preserved and age-related vascular changes in the medulla are minimal. Despite the significant decline in GFR with aging, the serum creatinine concentration does not increase because there is also an age-related decrease in skeletal muscle mass. Although renal function is diminished in the elderly, it is sufficient to maintain homeostasis under normal physiologic conditions. However, the renal response to common perioperative stresses may be insufficient to maintain homeostasis (Mangoni and Jackson,

TABLE 60-8.
MEDICATIONS THAT ARE COMMONLY ADMINISTERED IN THE ELDERLY THAT REDUCE LOWER ESOPHAGEAL SPHINCTER TONE AND PREDISPOSE TO GASTROESOPHAGEAL REFLUX

Anticholinergics
Antidepressants
Nitrates
Calcium channel blockers
Theophylline

2004). Although the elderly individual is able to maintain acid–base balance under every day physiologic conditions, the response to increased acid loads is attenuated due to impaired renal tubular ammonium secretion.

The renal response to volume depletion is similarly attenuated. Urine concentrating ability is critically dependent upon the presence of a hypertonic renal medulla. However, medullary perfusion is relatively increased in the elderly, resulting in a washout of solute and a reduction in osmolality in that region. Thus, the collecting tubules are not exposed to the usual concentration gradient necessary to produce concentrated urine (Guyton and Hall, 2000). Reduced numbers of cortical nephrons also contribute to impaired salt conservation. This suboptimal renal response to dehydration is compounded by age-related deficiencies in thirst mechanisms. Water deprivation is associated with a reduced thirst response in elderly subjects, despite significant increases in plasma osmolality (Phillips et al., 1984).

The response to water loading is similarly attenuated in the elderly. This is particularly relevant because the perioperative neuroendocrine stress response is associated with arginine vasopressin (antidiuretic hormone) release and water retention. When combined with iatrogenic hypotonic fluid administration, these factors make the elderly patient particularly susceptible to perioperative free water excess and hyponatremia.

Skeletal Muscle Mass and Aging

Aging is associated with a significant decline in neuromuscular performance. Loss of neuromuscular function causes functional disability and loss of independence (Doherty, 2003). By the seventh and eighth decades maximal voluntary contractile strength is reduced by 20% to 40%. Neuromuscular decline results predominantly from loss of skeletal muscle mass, which declines by approximately 40% between the ages of 20 and 60 years (sarcopenia). However, strength losses with aging may be attenuated by continued physical activity, particularly resistance training.

TABLE 60-9.
FACTORS THAT ARE THOUGHT TO BE RESPONSIBLE FOR THE SIGNIFICANT DECREASE IN LEAN MUSCLE MASS THAT OCCURS WITH AGING

Decreased motor neuron innervation
Decreased physical activity
Endocrine shift towards catabolism (reduced insulin-like-growth factor-1 secretion)
Decreased androgen (testosterone and estrogen) secretion
Decreased total caloric intake
Decreased protein consumption and protein synthesis
Inflammatory mediators and cytokines (Interleukins 1 and 6, tumor necrosis factor)

TABLE 60-10.
PERIOPERATIVE FUNCTIONAL CONSEQUENCES OF THE LOSS OF SKELETAL MUSCLE MASS THAT TYPICALLY ACCOMPANIES AGING

Impaired postoperative mobilization and ambulation
Reduced cough effectiveness
Reduced shivering thermogenesis
Altered drug disposition
Reduced neuromuscular functional reserve
Prolonged recovery and hospitalization

The decline in muscle function is multifactorial (Table 60-9). Diminished skeletal muscle mass has significant implications for the elderly patient in the perioperative period (Table 60-10).

Neurophysiology of Aging

The elderly demonstrate increased sensitivity to benzodiazepines, opioids, and volatile anesthetic drugs. The minimum effective concentration (MAC) of potent volatile anesthetic drugs is decreased by approximately 25% at 80 years of age when compared to MAC values obtained at 40 years of age (Gold, 1993). The addition of nitrous oxide is more effective in reducing the requirements for potent inhaled anesthetic drugs in the elderly.

Postoperative delirium is very common in the elderly population and often delays return to full cognitive function. Delirium is equally common after both regional and general anesthesia (Jolles, 1995). The pathophysiology of acute postoperative delirium in the elderly is undetermined. However, disturbance of the circadian sleep-awake cycle may be an important factor as suggested by the successful use of melatonin to treat delirium (Hanania, 2002). Postoperative delirium may also predispose to long-term postoperative cognitive impairment in a significant proportion of elderly patients undergoing major procedures. Aging is associated with changes in the neuroendocrine response to stress, particularly in the hypothalamic-pituitary-adrenal (HPA) axis. HPA activation during stress is associated with glucocorticoid hypersecretion in the elderly. This hyperacute neuroendocrine response to perioperative stress may cause dendritic atrophy in hippocampal neurons, thus contributing to memory and learning impairment and contributing to postoperative cognitive decline. Furthermore, hippocampal injury results in impaired feedback inhibition of the HPA, thus predisposing to further corticosteroid release. This positive feedback phenomenon is called the glucocorticoid cascade hypothesis (Sapolski, 1985).

REFERENCES

Aurigemma GP, Gaasch WH. Diastolic heart failure. *N Engl J Med* 2004;351:1097–1105.

Benatar D, Benatar M. A pain in the fetus: toward ending confusion about fetal pain. *Bioethics* 2001;15:57–76.
Chan ED, Welsch CH. Geriatric respiratory medicine. *Chest* 1998;114: 1704–1733.
Doherty TJ. Invited review: aging and sarcopenia. *J Appl Physiol* 2003; 95:1717–1727.
Ferrari AU, Radaelli A, Centola M. Aging and the cardiovascular system. *J Appl Physiol* 2003;95:2591–2597.
Gold MI, Abello D, Herrington C. Minimum alveolar concentration of desflurane in patients older than 65yr. *Anesthesiology* 1993;79: 710–714.
Guyton AC, Hall JE. *Textbook of medical physiology,* 10th ed. Philadelphia: Saunders 2000.
Hanania M, Kitain E. Melatonin for the treatment and prevention of postoperative delirium. *Anesth Analg.* 2002;94:338–339.
Hillier SC, Krishna G, Brasoveanu E. Neonatal anesthesia. *Semin Ped Surg* 2004;13:142–151.
Jolles J, Verhey FR, Riedel WJ, et al. Cognitive impairment in elderly people; predisposing factors and implications for experimental drug studies. *Drugs and Aging* 1995;7:459–479.
Kaufman GE, Cimo S, Miller LW, et al. An evaluation of the effects of sucrose on neonatal pain with 2 commonly used circumcision methods. *Am J Obstet Gynecol* 2002;186:564–568.
Kenny WL, Munce TA. Aging and human temperature regulation. *J Appl Physiol* 2003;95:2598–2603.
Lakatta EG, Levy D. Arterial and cardiac aging: major shareholders in cardiovascular disease enterprises. Part II: The aging heart in health: Links to disease. *Circulation* 2003;107:346–354.
Mangoni AA, Jackson SHD. Age-related changes in pharmacokinetics and pharmacodynamics: Basic principles and applications. *Br J Clin Pharm* 2004;57:6–14.
Matz RL, Andriantsitohaina R. Age-related endothelial dysfunction. *Drugs and Aging.* 2003;20:527–550.
Mueller CM, Scholer A, Laule-Kilian K, et al. Use of B-type natriuretic peptide in the evaluation and management of acute dyspnea. *N Engl J Med* 2004;350:647–54.
Phillip BK, Pastor D, Bellows W, et al. The prevalence of preoperative diastolic filling abnormalities in geriatric surgical patients. *Anesth Analg* 2003;97:1214–1221.
Phillips PA, Rolls BJ, Ledingham JG, et al. Reduced thirst after water deprivation in healthy elderly men. *N Engl J Med* 1984;311:753–759.
Sapolski RM, Krey LC, McEwen BS. Prolonged glucocorticoid exposure reduces hippocampal neuron number: Implications for aging. *J Neurosci* 1985;5:1222–1227.
Thompson ABR. Gastro-esophageal reflux in the elderly. Role of drug therapy in management. *Drugs and Aging* 2001;18:409–414.
Watando A, Ebihara S, Ebihara T, et al. Daily oral care and cough reflex sensitivity in elderly nursing home patients. *Chest* 2004;126: 1066–1070.
Zaugg M, Schaub MC, Foex P. Myocardial injury and its prevention in the perioperative setting. *Br J Anaesth* 2004;93:21–33.

Drug Index

Note: Page numbers followed by *f* indicate figures; page numbers followed by *t* indicate tables.

Subject Index

Note: Page numbers followed by *f* indicate figures; page numbers followed by *t* indicate tables.

C

Q

R